Pediatric Dosage Handbook

including

Neonatal Dosing, Drug Administration, & Extemporaneous Preparations

8ᵗʰ Edition *2001-2002*

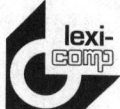

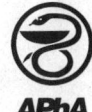

Pediatric Dosage Handbook

including

Neonatal Dosing, Drug Administration, & Extemporaneous Preparations

8th Edition ▌▌ *2001-2002*

Carol K. Taketomo, PharmD
Pharmacy Manager
Children's Hospital of Los Angeles
Los Angeles, California

Jane Hurlburt Hodding, PharmD
Director, Pharmacy Services
Miller Children's Hospital
Long Beach, California

Donna M. Kraus, PharmD, FAPhA
Associate Professor of Pharmacy Practice
Departments of Pharmacy Practice and Pediatrics
Pediatric Clinical Pharmacist
University of Illinois at Chicago
Chicago, Illinois

LEXI-COMP INC
Hudson (Cleveland)

AMERICAN
PHARMACEUTICAL
ASSOCIATION APhA

NOTICE

This data is intended to serve the user as a handy reference and not as a complete drug information resource. It does not include information on every therapeutic agent available. The publication covers 670 commonly used drugs and is specifically designed to present important aspects of drug data in a more concise format than is typically found in medical literature or product material supplied by manufacturers.

The nature of drug information is that it is constantly evolving because of ongoing research and clinical experience and is often subject to interpretation. While great care has been taken to ensure the accuracy of the information presented, the reader is advised that the authors, editors, reviewers, contributors, and publishers cannot be responsible for the continued currency of the information or for any errors, omissions, or the application of this information, or for any consequences arising therefrom. Therefore, the author(s) and/or the publisher shall have no liability to any person or entity with regard to claims, loss, or damage caused, or alleged to be caused, directly or indirectly, by the use of information contained herein. Because of the dynamic nature of drug information, readers are advised that decisions regarding drug therapy must be based on the independent judgment of the clinician, changing information about a drug (eg, as reflected in the literature and manufacturer's most current product information), and changing medical practices. Therefore, this data is designed to be used in conjunction with other necessary information and is not designed to be solely relied upon by any user. The user of this data hereby and forever releases the authors of this data for any and all liability of any kind that might arise out of the use of this data. The editors are not responsible for any inaccuracy of quotation or for any false or misleading implication that may arise due to the text or formulas as used or due to the quotation of revisions no longer official.

The authors, editors, and contributors have written this book in their private capacities. No official support or endorsement by any federal or state agency or pharmaceutical company is intended or inferred.

The publishers have made every effort to trace the copyright holders for borrowed material. If they have inadvertently overlooked any, they will be pleased to make the necessary arrangements at the first opportunity.

If you have any suggestions or questions regarding any information presented in this data, please contact our drug information pharmacist at

1-877-837-LEXI (5394)

This manual was produced using the FormuLex™ Program —
A complete publishing service of Lexi-Comp Inc.

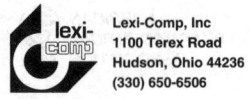

lexi-comp

Lexi-Comp, Inc
1100 Terex Road
Hudson, Ohio 44236
(330) 650-6506

ISBN 1-930598-75-0 (Domestic Edition)

ISBN 1-930598-76-9 (International Edition)

TABLE OF CONTENTS

PREFACE

This eighth edition of the *Pediatric Dosage Handbook* is designed to be a practical and convenient guide to the dosing and usage of medications in children. The pediatric population is a dynamic group, with major changes in pharmacokinetics and pharmacodynamics taking place throughout infancy and childhood. Therefore, the need for the evaluation and establishment of medication dosing regimens in children of different ages is great.

Special considerations must be taken into account when dosing medications in pediatric patients. Unfortunately, due to a lack of appropriate studies, most medications commonly used in children do not have FDA approved labeling for use in pediatric patients. Only 30% of drugs used in children in a 1988 survey carried FDA approval in their labeling. Seventy-five percent of medications listed in the *1990 Physicians Desk Reference* carry some type of precaution or disclaimer statement for use in children.[1]

The FDA Modernization Act of 1997, the 1998 Pediatric Final Rule, and the Children's Health Act of 2000 will help to increase pediatric drugs studies. The FDA Modernization Act of 1997 was signed into law on November 21, 1997 (Section 111, Public Law 105-115, 105th Congress). This bill **encourages** pharmaceutical companies to conduct pediatric drug studies by allowing 6 months of market exclusivity to certain designated drugs. A list of drugs, for which additional pediatric information may produce pediatric healthcare benefits, was required by this law to be developed by the U.S. Department of Health and Human Services (HHS), with input from the American Academy of Pediatrics, the Pediatric Pharmacology Research Unit Network,[2] and the U.S. Pharmacopoeia. To date, the FDA has received 237 proposals from pharmaceutical companies to conduct pediatric drug studies under this Act and has issued 194 written requests for studies. If these pediatric studies are completed as the FDA has specified, then these medications will qualify for the 6 month patent extension or additional market exclusivity. Thirty-one products have already had their marketing patents extended by this law and pediatric labeling changes have occurred for 18 of these products[3]. Unfortunately, the pediatric section of the FDA Modernization Act will sunset January 1, 2002 and will require renewal by Congress to continue. The FDA submitted a required report on the Pediatric Exclusivity Provision to Congress in January 2001[4]. This report describes the effectiveness, short comings, and economic impact of the Pediatric Exclusivity Provision. It also gives suggestions for modifications and ways to address gaps in the statute.

The 1998 Pediatric Final Rule is an FDA regulation, titled "Regulations Requiring Manufacturers to Assess the Safety and Effectiveness of New Drugs and Biological Products in Pediatric Patients; Final Rule,"[5]. This important regulation **requires** that manufacturers conduct pediatric studies for certain new and marketed drugs and biological products. This requirement is mandatory, and its scope includes new drugs (ie, new chemical entities, new dosage forms, new indications, new routes of administration, and new dosing regimens) and certain marketed drugs (ie, where the drug product offers meaningful therapeutic benefit or has substantial use in pediatric patients, AND the absence of pediatric labeling poses a risk). This FDA regulation became effective April 1, 1999, but studies mandated under this rule were not required to be submitted to the FDA before December 2, 2000.

The Children's Health Act of 2000 was signed into law on October 17, 2000. This important law establishes a Pediatric Research Initiative (headed by the Director of the NIH) and provides funds to increase support for pediatric clinical research. These two important laws and FDA regulation, plus other FDA regulations, such as the FDA labeling changes[6] that required expanded information in the Pediatric Use section of the package insert for all prescription drugs, will certainly help to increase and disseminate pediatric drug information.

Currently, however, most commonly used pharmacy references do not include information regarding pediatric dosing, drug administration, or special pediatric concerns. It is, therefore, not surprising that in order to obtain pediatric dosing information, oftentimes the pediatric clinician is faced with extensive literature searches to arrive at a logical dose. This handbook was developed with the intent

PREFACE *(Continued)*

to serve as a compilation of recommended pediatric doses found in the literature and to provide relevant clinical information regarding the use of drugs in children.

This new edition incorporates additions and revisions in a format which we hope the user will find beneficial. As with each edition, drug monographs have been updated and revised. Nineteen new medications have been added. Seven monographs have been deleted: 3 medications (phenylpropanolamine; brompheniramine and phenylpropanolamine; and guaifenesin, phenylpropanolamine and phenylephrine) were withdrawn from the US market; 2 medications (methicillin and sultilains) are no longer available; and 2 monographs (iron dextran complex and ferric gluconate) were combined with iron sucrose into a new monograph [Iron supplements, (parenteral)]. This brings the total number of drug monographs to 670. New monographs added to this edition include: Abacavir, lamivudine, and zidovudine; acarbose; albendazole; alteplase; brompheniramine and pseudoephedrine; cefdinir; cidofovir; ciprofloxacin and hydrocortisone; dihydroergotamine; glipizide; glyburide; iron supplements (parenteral); levofloxacin; lopinavir and ritonavir; metformin; oseltamivir; oxycodone; rosiglitazone; and sertraline.

The information and format of the Brand Names, Available Salts, and Dosage Forms fields have been significantly revised. Brand Names has been separated into two fields: U.S. Brand Names and Canadian Brand Names. Dosage form descriptors (eg oral, injection) have been removed from the Brand Names field and brand names have been inserted into the Dosage Forms field where appropriate. The Available Salts field has been deleted for most monographs and this information can now also be found in the Dosage Forms field. Cytochrome P-450 enzyme information (which is found on the first line of the Drug Interactions field) has been added to additional monographs, bringing the total number of monographs with cytochrome P-450 information to 152. In addition, 8 new extemporaneous preparations have been added to this edition, including 4 new extemporaneous preparations for drugs that did not previously have one. This brings the total number of drug monographs with extemporaneous preparations to 66 and the total number of "recipes" to 88.

Appendix material has been updated to include the 2001 Childhood Immunization Schedule. Information from the new "Guidelines 2000 for Cardiopulmonary Resuscitation and Emergency Cardiovascular Care" has been added, including the new Neonatal, PALS, and ACLS algorithms. In addition, the following tables were also updated or revised: CPR Pediatric Drug Dosages, OTC Cough and Cold Preparations, Cytochrome P-450 Enzymes and Drug Metabolism, Adult and Adolescent HIV, and Contraindications and Precautions to Immunizations.

We hope this edition continues to be a valuable and practical source of clinical drug information for the pediatric healthcare professional. We welcome comments to further improve future editions.

Footnotes

1. Food and Drug Letter, Washington Business Information, Inc. November 23, 1990.

2. "NIH Funds Network of Centers for Pediatric Drug Research," *Am J Hosp Pharm*, 1994, 51:2546.

3. Center for Drug Evaluation and Research, U.S. Food and Drug Administration," Approved Active Moieties to Which FDA has Granted Exclusivity for Pediatric Studies Under Section 505A of the Federal Food, Drug, and Cosmetic Act," June 14, 2001, http://www.fda.gov/cder/pediatric/exgrant.htm

4. Department of Health and Human Services, U.S. Food and Drug Administration, "The Pediatric Exclusivity Provision, January 2001: Status Report to Congress," http://www.fda.gov/cder/pediatric/reportcong01.pdf.

5. Department of Health and Human Services, Food and Drug Administration, 21CFR Parts 201, 312, 314, and 601, Regulations Requiring Manufacturers to Assess the Safety and Effectiveness of New Drugs and Biological Products in Pediatric Patients; Final Rule,' *Fed Regist* 1998, 63(231):66631-72.

6. "Pediatric Use Drug Labeling NDA Supplements Due by December 1996 - FDA Final Rule; Agency Establishing Pediatric Subcommittee to Track Implementation," *F-D-C Reports - The Pink Sheet*, Wallace Werble Jr, Publisher, December 19, 1994.

ACKNOWLEDGMENTS

The *Pediatric Dosage Handbook* exists in its present form as the result of the concerted efforts of the following individuals: Robert D. Kerscher, publisher and president of Lexi-Comp Inc; Lynn D. Coppinger, managing editor; Barbara F. Kerscher, production manager; Mark F Bonfiglio, BS, PharmD, RPh, director of pharmacotherapy resources; Elizabeth Tomsik, BS, PharmD, pharmacotherapy specialist; Joni L. Stahura, BS, PharmD, pharmacotherapy specialist; Matthew Fuller, PharmD, clinical pharmacy specialist, psychiatry (VA Medical Center, Brecksville, OH); Leonard L. Lance, RPh, BSPharm, pharmacist; David C. Marcus, director of information systems; Stacy S. Robinson, project manager; and Julian I. Graubart, American Pharmaceutical Association (APhA), Director of Books and Electronic Products.

Special acknowledgment goes to all Lexi-Comp staff for their contributions to this handbook.

Special thanks goes to Chris Lomax, PharmD, director of pharmacy, Children's Hospital, Los Angeles, who played a significant role in bringing APhA and Lexi-Comp together.

Some of the material contained in the book was a result of pediatric pharmacy contributors throughout the United States and Canada. Lexi-Comp has assisted many pediatric medical institutions to develop hospital-specific formulary manuals that contain clinical drug information as well as dosing. Working with these pediatric clinical pharmacists, pediatric hospital pharmacy and therapeutics committees, and hospital drug information centers, Lexi-Comp has developed an evolutionary drug database that reflects the practice of pediatric pharmacy in these major pediatric institutions.

The authors wish to thank their families, friends, and colleagues who supported them in their efforts to complete this handbook.

In addition, Dr Taketomo would like to thank Robert Taketomo, PharmD, MBA and Chris Lomax, PharmD for their professional guidance and continued support, and the pharmacy staff at Childrens Hospital, Los Angeles for their assistance.

Dr Kraus would like to especially thank Keith A. Rodvold, PharmD, for his ongoing professional and personal support.

Dr Hodding would like to thank Glenn Hodding, PharmD, Carl Kildoo, PharmD, and the pediatric pharmacists at Miller Children's Hospital for their continued professional and personal support.

EDITORIAL ADVISORY PANEL

Andrew J. Donnelly, PharmD, MBA
Clinical Pharmacist
Operating Room/Anesthesia
Assistant Director of Pharmacy
Rush-Presbyterian-St Luke's Medical Center
Chicago, Illinois

Matthew A. Fuller, PharmD, MBA
Clinical Pharmacy Specialist
Psychiatry
Cleveland Department of Veterans Affairs Medical Center
Brecksville, Ohio

Mark Geraci, PharmD, BCOP
Clinical Assistant Professor
Department of Pharmacy Practice
University of Illinois
Chicago, Illinois

Morton P. Goldman, PharmD
Assistant Director
Pharmacotherapy Services
Cleveland Clinic Foundation
Cleveland, Ohio

Harold J. Grady, PhD
Director of Clinical Chemistry
Truman Medical Center
Kansas City, Missouri

Larry D. Gray, PhD
TriHealth Clinical Microbiology Laboratory
Bethesda Oak Hospital
Cincinnati, Ohio

Martin D. Higbee, PharmD, CGP
Associate Professor
Department of Pharmacy Practice and Science
The University of Arizona
Tucson, Arizona

Rebecca T. Horvat, PhD
Assistant Professor of Pathology and Laboratory Medicine
University of Kansas Medical Center
Kansas City, Kansas

Carlos M. Isada, MD
Department of Infectious Disease
Cleveland Clinic Foundation
Cleveland, Ohio

David S. Jacobs, MD
President, Pathologists Chartered
Overland Park, Kansas

Bernard L. Kasten, Jr, MD, FCAP
Vice-President/Chief Medical Officer
Quest Diagnostics Inc
Teteroboro, New Jersey

EDITORIAL ADVISORY PANEL *(Continued)*

Bradley G. Phillips, PharmD, BCPS
Associate Professor
University of Iowa College of Pharmacy
Clinical Pharmacist
Veterans Affairs Medical Center
Iowa City, Iowa

Martha Sajatovic, MD
Assistant Professor of Psychiatry
Case Western Reserve University
Cleveland, Ohio

Todd P. Semla, PharmD
Associate Director of the Psychopharmacology Clinical and Research Center
Department of Psychiatry and Behavioral Sciences
Evanston Northwestern Healthcare
Evanston, Illinois
*Clinical Assistant Professor of Pharmacy Practice in Medicine,
Section of Geriatric Medicine*
University of Illinois at Chicago
Chicago, Illinois

Dominic A. Solimando, Jr, MA
Oncology Pharmacist
Director of Oncology Drug Information
cancer**education**.com
Arlington, VA

Virend K. Somers, MD, DPhil
Consultant in Hypertension and in Cardiovascular Disease
Mayo Clinic
Professor
Mayo Medical School
Rochester, MN

Lowell L. Tilzer, MD
Associate Medical Director
Community Blood Center of Greater Kansas City
Kansas City, Missouri

Beatrice B. Turkoski, RN, PhD
Professor, Advanced Pharmacology and Applied Therapeutics
Kent State University School of Nursing
Kent, Ohio

Richard L. Wynn, PhD
Professor and Chairman of Pharmacology
Baltimore College of Dental Surgery
Dental School
University of Maryland at Baltimore
Baltimore, Maryland

ABOUT THE AUTHORS

Carol K. Taketomo, PharmD

Dr Taketomo received her doctorate from the University of Southern California School of Pharmacy. Subsequently, she completed a clinical pharmacy residency at the University of California Medical Center in San Diego. With over 24 years of clinical experience at one of the largest pediatric teaching hospitals in the nation, she is an acknowledged expert in the practical aspects of pediatric drug distribution and clinical pharmacy practice. She currently holds the appointment of Adjunct Assistant Professor of Pharmacy Practice at the University of Southern California School of Pharmacy.

In her current capacity as Pharmacy Manager at Children's Hospital of Los Angeles, Dr Taketomo plays an active role in the education and training of the medical, pharmacy, and nursing staff. She coordinates the Pharmacy Department's quality assurance and drug use evaluation programs; maintains the hospital's strict formulary program; and is the editor of the house staff manual. Her particular interests are strategies to influence physician prescribing patterns and methods to decrease medication errors in the pediatric setting. She has been the author of numerous publications, and is an active presenter at professional meetings.

Dr Taketomo is a member of the American Pharmaceutical Association (APhA), American Society of Health-System Pharmacists (ASHP), California Society of Hospital Pharmacists (CSHP), and Southern California Pediatric Pharmacy Group.

Jane Hurlburt Hodding, PharmD

Dr Hodding earned a doctorate and completed her pharmacy residency at the University of California School of Pharmacy in San Francisco. She has held teaching positions as Assistant Clinical Professor of Pharmacy at UCSF as well as Assistant Clinical Professor of Pharmacy Practice at the University of Southern California in Los Angeles. Currently, Dr Hodding is the Director, Pharmacy Services at Miller Children's Hospital in Long Beach, California.

Throughout her 24 years of pediatric pharmacy practice, Dr Hodding has actively pursued methods to improve neonatal intensive care, pediatric intensive care, pediatric hematology/oncology, and parenteral nutrition. She has published numerous articles covering neonatal medication administration and aminoglycoside and theophylline clearance in premature infants.

Dr Hodding is a member of the American Pharmaceutical Association (APhA), American Society of Health-System Pharmacists (ASHP), California Society of Hospital Pharmacists (CSHP), Children's Oncology Group, and Southern California Pediatric Pharmacy Group. She is frequently an invited speaker on the topics of Monitoring Drug Therapy in the NICU, Fluid and Electrolyte Therapy in Children, Drug Therapy Considerations in Children, and Parenteral Nutrition in the Premature Infant.

Donna M. Kraus, PharmD

Dr Kraus received her Bachelor of Science in Pharmacy from the University of Illinois at Chicago (UIC). She worked for several years as a hospital pediatric/obstetric satellite pharmacist before earning her doctorate degree at the UIC. Dr Kraus then completed a postdoctoral pediatric specialty residency at the University of Texas Health Science Center in San Antonio. She has served as a pediatric intensive care clinical pharmacist for 15 years and currently is an ambulatory care pediatric clinical pharmacist, specializing in pediatric HIV pharmacotherapy and patient/parent medication adherence. Dr Kraus has also served as a clinical pharmacist consultant to a pediatric long-term care facility for over 16 years. She currently holds the appointment of Associate Professor of Pharmacy Practice in both the Departments of Pharmacy Practice and Pediatrics at the University of Illinois in Chicago.

In her 24 years of active pharmacy experience, Dr Kraus has dealt with pediatric pharmacy issues and pharmacotherapy problems. She is an active educator and has been a guest lecturer in China, Thailand, and Hong Kong. Dr Kraus has played a leading role in the advanced training of postgraduate pharmacists and has been the Director of the UIC (ASHP accredited) Pediatric Residency and Fellowship Program for 14 years. Dr Kraus' research areas include pediatric drug dosing and developmental pharmacokinetics and pharmacodynamics. She has published a number of articles on various issues of pediatric pharmacy and pharmacotherapy.

Dr Kraus has been an active member of numerous professional associations including the American Pharmaceutical Association (APhA), American Society of Health-System Pharmacists (ASHP), Illinois Pharmacists Association (IPhA), American College of Clinical Pharmacy (ACCP), Illinois College of Clinical Pharmacy (ICCP), and the Pediatric Pharmacy Advocacy Group (PPAG). She served as Chairperson of the ASHP Commission on Therapeutics, and was an APhA, Academy of Pharmaceutical Research and Science, Member-at-Large. Dr. Kraus also served as an Editorial Board member of the *American Journal of Health-System Pharmacy* and the *Journal of Pediatric Pharmacy Practice*. Currently, she serves as an Editorial Board member of *The Journal of Pediatric Pharmacology and Therapeutics*. Dr. Kraus was recently awarded Fellow status by the American Pharmaceutical Association and is the APhA designated author for this handbook.

DESCRIPTION OF SECTIONS AND FIELDS USED IN THIS HANDBOOK

The *Pediatric Dosage Handbook, 8th Edition* is organized into a drug information section, an appendix, and a therapeutic category & key word index.

Drug information is presented in a consistent format and provides the following:

Generic Name	U.S. adopted name
Pronunciation Guide	Phonetic listing of generic name
Related Information	Cross-reference to other pertinent drug information found in the Appendix
U.S. Brand Names	Common trade names used in the U.S
Canadian Brand Names	Common trade names used in Canada
Available Salts	Lists the various salt forms of the drug for selected monographs. For the majority of drugs, this information can be found in the dosage forms field.
Synonyms	Other names or accepted abbreviations for the generic drug
Therapeutic Category	Unique systematic classification of medications
Generic Available	Indicated by a "Yes" or "No" as to whether a generic form of the drug is available
Use	Information pertaining to appropriate indications or use of the drug
Restrictions	Drug Enforcement Agency (DEA) classification for federally scheduled controlled substances
Pregnancy Risk Factor	Five categories established by the FDA to indicate the potential of a systemically absorbed drug for causing birth defects
Contraindications	Information pertaining to inappropriate use of the drug, or disease states and patient populations in which the drug should not be used
Warnings	Hazardous conditions related to use of the drug
Precautions	Disease states or patient populations in which the drug should be cautiously used
Adverse Reactions	Side effects are grouped by body system and include a listing of the more common and/or serious side effects. Due to space limitations, every reported side effect is not listed.
Drug Interactions	For select drugs that have demonstrated involvement with cytochrome P-450 enzymes, the initial line of this field identifies the drug as a substrate, inducer, or inhibitor of specific isoenzymes (eg, CYP1A2). A summary of this information can also be found in a tabular format within the appendix. The remainder of the field presents a description of common or significant interactions between the drug listed in the monograph and other drugs or drug classes that are commonly used in pediatric patients. Due to space limitations, the reader is advised to read the drug interaction field of both drugs involved in the interaction.
Food Interactions	Possible interactions between the drug listed in the monograph and certain foods and/or nutritional substances
Stability	Storage, refrigeration, and compatibility information
Mechanism of Action	How the drug works in the body to elicit a response

Pharmacodynamics	Dose-response relationships including onset of action, time of peak action, and duration of action
Pharmacokinetics	Drug movement through the body over time. Pharmacokinetics deals with absorption, distribution, protein binding, metabolism, bioavailability, half-life, time to peak concentration, elimination, and clearance of drugs. Pharmacokinetic parameters help predict drug concentration and dosage requirements.
Usual Dosage	The amount of the drug to be typically given or taken during therapy
	Please note that doses for neonates are often listed by postnatal age (PNA) (eg, PNA ≤7 days) and/or by body weight (eg, 1200-2000 g)
	When both milligram and milligram per kilogram doses are listed, the milligram per kilogram dosing method is preferred. If using a milligram dosing guideline according to age, special care and lower doses should be used in children who have a low weight for their age. When ranges of doses are listed, initiate therapy at the lower end of the range and titrate the dose accordingly. References are listed at the end of drug monographs to support doses listed when little dosing information exists.
	For select drugs, the dosing adjustment in renal impairment or dosing interval in renal impairment is given according to creatinine clearance (Cl_{cr}). Since most studies that recommend dosing guidelines in renal dysfunction are conducted in adult patients, Cl_{cr} is usually expressed in units of mL/minute. However, in order to extrapolate the adult information to the pediatric population, one must assume that the adults studied were of standard surface area (ie, 1.73 m^2). Therefore, although the value of Cl_{cr} listed for dosing adjustment in renal impairment or dosing interval in renal impairment may be expressed in mL/minute, it is assumed to be equal to the same value in mL/minute/1.73 m^2.
	To calculate the dose in a pediatric patient with renal dysfunction, first calculate the normal dose (ie, the dose for a patient without renal dysfunction), then use the guidelines to adjust the dose. For example, the normal piperacillin dose for a 20 kg child is 200-300 mg/kg/day divided every 4-6 hours. If one selected 300 mg/kg/day divided every 6 hours, the dose would be 1.5 g every 6 hours in normal renal function. If Cl_{cr} was 20-40 mL/minute/1.73 m^2, the dose would be 1.5 g every 8 hours and if Cl_{cr} was <20 mL/minute/1.73 m^2, the dose would be 1.5 g every 12 hours.
Administration	Information regarding the recommended final concentrations and rates for administration of parenteral drugs are listed when appropriate, along with pertinent oral, ophthalmic, and topical administration information.
Monitoring Parameters	Laboratory tests and patient physical parameters that should be monitored for safety and efficacy of drug therapy are listed when appropriate.
Reference Range	Therapeutic and toxic serum concentrations are listed when appropriate
Test Interactions	Listing of assay interferences when relevant; (S) = Serum; (U) = Urine

DESCRIPTION OF SECTIONS AND FIELDS USED IN THIS HANDBOOK *(Continued)*

Patient Information	Advice, warnings, precautions, and other information of which the patient should be informed
Nursing Implications	Comments regarding nursing care of the patient are offered when appropriate
Additional Information	Other data and facts about the drug are offered when appropriate
Dosage Forms	Information with regard to form, strength, and availability of the drug
Extemporaneous Preparations	Directions for preparing liquid formulations from solid drug products. May include stability information and references (listed when appropriate).
References	Bibliographic information referring to specific pediatric literature findings, especially doses

Appendix

The appendix offers a compilation of tables, guidelines, and conversion information which can often be helpful when considering patient care. This section is broken down into various sections for ease of use.

Therapeutic Category & Key Word Index

This index provides a useful listing by an easy-to-use therapeutic classification system. Also listed are controlled substances, preservative free, sugar free, and alcohol free medications.

DEFINITION OF AGE GROUP TERMINOLOGY

Information in this handbook is listed according to specific age or by age group. The following are definitions of age groups and age-related terminologies. These definitions should be used unless otherwise specified in the monograph.

Gestational age (GA)	The time from conception until birth. More specifically, gestational age is defined as the number of weeks from the first day of the mother's last menstrual period (LMP) until the birth of the baby. Gestational age at birth is assessed by the date of the LMP and by physical exam (Dubowitz score).
Postnatal age (PNA)	Chronological age since birth
Postconceptional age (PCA)	Age since conception. Postconceptional age is calculated as gestational age plus postnatal age (PCA = GA + PNA).
Neonate	A full-term newborn 0-4 weeks postnatal age. This term may also be applied to a premature neonate whose postconceptional age (PCA) is 42-46 weeks.
Premature neonate	Neonate born at <38 weeks gestational age
Full-term neonate	Neonate born at 38-42 weeks (average ~40 weeks) gestational age
Infant	1 month to 1 year of age
Child/Children	1-12 years of age
Adolescent	13-18 years of age
Adult	>18 years of age

FDA PREGNANCY CATEGORIES

Throughout this book there is a field labeled Pregnancy Risk Factor and the letter A, B, C, D, or X immediately following which signifies a category. The FDA has established these five categories to indicate the potential of a systemically absorbed drug for causing birth defects. The key differentiation among the categories rests upon the reliability of documentation and the risk:benefit ratio. Pregnancy Category X is particularly notable in that if any data exists that may implicate a drug as a teratogen and the risk:benefit ratio is clearly negative, the drug is contraindicated during pregnancy.

These categories are summarized as follows:

A   Controlled studies in pregnant women fail to demonstrate a risk to the fetus in the first trimester with no evidence of risk in later trimesters. The possibility of fetal harm appears remote.

B   Either animal-reproduction studies have not demonstrated a fetal risk but there are no controlled studies in pregnant women, or animal-reproduction studies have shown an adverse effect (other than a decrease in fertility) that was not confirmed in controlled studies in women in the first trimester and there is no evidence of a risk in later trimesters.

C   Either studies in animals have revealed adverse effects on the fetus (teratogenic or embryocidal effects or other) and there are no controlled studies in women, or studies in women and animals are not available. Drugs should be given only if the potential benefits justify the potential risk to the fetus.

D   There is positive evidence of human fetal risk, but the benefits from use in pregnant women may be acceptable despite the risk (eg, if the drug is needed in a life-threatening situation or for a serious disease for which safer drugs cannot be used or are ineffective).

X   Studies in animals or human beings have demonstrated fetal abnormalities or there is evidence of fetal risk based on human experience, or both, and the risk of the use of the drug in pregnant women clearly outweighs any possible benefit. The drug is contraindicated in women who are or may become pregnant.

SYMBOLS & ABBREVIATIONS USED IN THIS HANDBOOK*

°C	degrees Celsius (Centigrade)
<	less than
>	greater than
≤	less than or equal to
≥	greater than or equal to
μg	microgram
μmol	micromole
AAP	American Academy of Pediatrics
AAPC	antibiotic associated pseudomembranous colitis
ABG	arterial blood gas
ABMT	autologous bone marrow transplant
ACE	angiotensin-converting enzyme
ACLS	advanced cardiac life support
ADH	antidiuretic hormone
AED	antiepileptic drug
AHCPR	Agency for Health Care Policy and Research
AIDS	acquired immunodeficiency syndrome
ALL	acute lymphoblastic leukemia
ALT	alanine aminotransferase (formerly called SGPT)
AML	acute myeloblastic leukemia
ANA	antinuclear antibodies
ANC	absolute neutrophil count
ANLL	acute nonlymphoblastic leukemia
APTT	activated partial thromboplastin time
ARDS	adult respiratory distress syndrome
ASA (class I-IV)	American Society of Anesthesiology physical status classification of surgical patients according to their baseline health
	ASA I: Normal healthy patients
	ASA II: Patients having controlled disease states (eg, controlled hypertension)
	ASA III: Patients having a disease which compromises their organ function (eg, decompensated CHF, end stage renal failure)
	ASA IV: Patients who are extremely critically ill
AST	aspartate aminotransferase (formerly called SGOT)
ATP	adenosine triphosphate
AUC	area under the curve (area under the serum concentration-time curve)
A-V	atrial-ventricular
BMT	bone marrow transplant
BPD	bronchopulmonary disease
BUN	blood urea nitrogen
CADD	computer ambulatory drug delivery
cAMP	cyclic adenosine monophosphate
CBC	complete blood count
CDC	center for Disease Control and Prevention
CF	cystic fibrosis
CHF	congestive heart failure
CI	cardiac index
Cl_{cr}	creatinine clearance

SYMBOLS & ABBREVIATIONS USED IN THIS HANDBOOK* *(Continued)*

CLL	chronic lymphocytic leukemia
CML	chronic myelogenous leukemia
CMV	cytomegalovirus
CNS	central nervous system
COPD	chronic obstructive pulmonary disease
CRF	chronic renal failure
CSF	cerebrospinal fluid
CT	computed tomography
CVA	cerebral vascular accident
CVP	central venous pressure
CYP	cytochrome
d	day
D_5/LR	dextrose 5% in lactated Ringer's
D_5/NS	dextrose 5% in sodium chloride 0.9%
D_5W	dextrose 5% in water
$D_5/^1/_4$ NS	dextrose 5% in sodium chloride 0.2%
$D_5/^1/_2$ NS	dextrose 5% in sodium chloride 0.45%
D_{10}W	dextrose 10% in water
DIC	disseminated intravascular coagulation
DL_{co}	pulmonary diffusion capacity for carbon monoxide
DNA	deoxyribonucleic acid
DVT	deep vein thrombosis
ECHO	echocardiogram
ECMO	extracorporeal membrane oxygenation
EEG	electroencephalogram
EKG	electrocardiogram
ESR	erythrocyte sedimentation rate
ESRD	end stage renal disease
E.T.	endotracheal
FDA	Food and Drug Administration (United States)
FEV_1	forced expiratory volume exhaled after 1 second
FSH	follicle-stimulating hormone
FVC	forced vital capacity
g	gram
G-6-PD	glucose-6-phosphate dehydrogenase
GA	gestational age
GABA	gamma-aminobutyric acid
GE	gastroesophageal
GERD	gastroesophageal reflux disease
GI	gastrointestinal
GVHD	graft versus host disease
GU	genitourinary
h	hour
Hct	hematocrit
Hgb	hemoglobin
HIV	human immunodeficiency virus
HPLC	high performance liquid chromatography
HSV	herpes simplex virus
ICP	intracranial pressure
IDDM	insulin-dependent diabetes mellitus

IgG	immune globulin G
I.M.	intramuscular
INR	international normalized ratio
ILCOR	International Liaison Committee on Resuscitation
I.O.	intraosseous
I & O	input and output
IOP	intraocular pressure
I.T.	intrathecal
I.V.	intravenous
IVH	intraventricular hemorrhage
IVP	intravenous push
JRA	juvenile rheumatoid arthritis
kg	kilogram
L	liter
LDH	lactate dehydrogenase
LE	lupus erythematosus
LH	luteinizing hormone
LP	lumbar puncture
LR	lactated Ringer's
M	molar
MAC	*Mycobacterium avium* complex
MAO	monoamine oxidase
MAP	mean arterial pressure
mcg	microgram
mg	milligram
MI	myocardial infarction
min	minute
mL	milliliter
mM	millimole
mo	month
MOPP	mustargen (mechlorethamine), Oncovin® (vincristine), procarbazine, and prednisone
mOsm	milliosmoles
MRI	magnetic resonance image
MRSA	methicillin-resistant *Staphylococcus aureus*
NCI	National Cancer Institute
ND	nasoduodenal
ng	nanogram
NG	nasogastric
NIDDM	noninsulin-dependent diabetes mellitus
NMDA	n-methyl-d-aspartate
nmol	nanomole
NPO	nothing per os (nothing by mouth)
NS	normal saline (0.9% sodium chloride)
½NS	0.45% sodium chloride
NSAID	nonsteroidal anti-inflammatory drug
NYHA	New York Heart Association
O.R.	operating room
OTC	over-the-counter (nonprescription)
PABA	para-aminobenzoic acid
PALS	pediatric advanced life support
PCA	postconceptional age
PCP	*Pneumocystis carinii* pneumonia

SYMBOLS & ABBREVIATIONS USED IN THIS HANDBOOK* *(Continued)*

PCWP	pulmonary capillary wedge pressure
PDA	patent ductus arteriosus
PICU	Pediatric Intensive Care Unit
PIP	peak inspiratory pressure
PNA	postnatal age
prn	as needed
PSVT	paroxysmal supraventricular tachycardia
PT	prothrombin time
PTH	parathyroid hormone
PTT	partial thromboplastin time
PUD	peptic ulcer disease
PVC	premature ventricular contraction
PVR	peripheral vascular resistance
qsad	add an amount sufficient to equal
RAP	right arterial pressure
RDA	recommended daily allowance
RIA	radioimmunoassay
RNA	ribonucleic acid
RSV	respiratory syncytial virus
S-A	sino-atrial
S.C.	subcutaneous
S_{cr}	serum creatinine
SIADH	syndrome of inappropriate antidiuretic hormone
S.L.	sublingual
SLE	systemic lupus erythematosus
STD	sexually-transmitted disease
SVR	systemic vascular resistance
SVT	supraventricular tachycardia
SWI	sterile water for injection
T_3	triiodothyronine
T_4	thyroxine
TCA	tricyclic antidepressant
TIA	transient ischemic attack
TIBC	total iron binding capacity
TNF	tissue necrosis factor
TPN	total parenteral nutrition
TSH	thyroid stimulating hormone
TT	thrombin time
UA	urine analysis
UTI	urinary tract infection
V_d	volume of distribution
V_{dss}	volume of distribution at steady-state
VF	ventricular fibrillation
VMA	vanillylmandelic acid
VT	ventricular tachycardia
VZV	varicella zoster virus
w/v	weight for volume
w/w	weight for weight
y	year

*Other than drug synonyms

SAFE WRITING

Health professionals and their support personnel frequently produce handwritten copies of information they see in print; therefore, such information is subjected to even greater possibilities for error or misinterpretation on the part of others. Thus, particular care must be given to how drug names and strengths are expressed when creating written health-care documents.

The following are a few examples of safe writing rules suggested by the Institute for Safe Medication Practices, Inc.*

1. There should be a space between a number and its units as it is easier to read. There should be no periods after the abbreviations mg or mL.

Correct	Incorrect
10 mg	10mg
100 mg	100mg

2. Never place a decimal and a zero after a whole number (2 mg is correct and 2.0 mg is **incorrect**). If the decimal point is not seen because it falls on a line or because individuals are working from copies where the decimal point is not seen, this causes a tenfold overdose.

3. Just the opposite is true for numbers less than one. Always place a zero before a naked decimal (0.5 mL is correct, .5 mL is **incorrect**).

4. Never abbreviate the word unit. The handwritten U or u, looks like a 0 (zero), and may cause a tenfold overdose error to be made.

5. IU is not a safe abbreviation for international units. The handwritten IU looks like IV. Write out international units or use int. units.

6. Q.D. is not a safe abbreviation for once daily, as when the Q is followed by a sloppy dot, it looks like QID which means four times daily.

7. O.D. is not a safe abbreviation for once daily, as it is properly interpreted as meaning "right eye" and has caused liquid medications such as saturated solution of potassium iodide and Lugol's solution to be administered incorrectly. There is no safe abbreviation for once daily. It must be written out in full.

8. Do not use chemical names such as 6-mercaptopurine or 6-thioguanine, as sixfold overdoses have been given when these were not recognized as chemical names. The proper names of these drugs are mercaptopurine or thioguanine.

9. Do not abbreviate drug names (5FC, 6MP, 5-ASA, MTX, HCTZ, CPZ, PBZ, etc) as they are misinterpreted and cause error.

10. Do not use the apothecary system or symbols.

11. Do not abbreviate microgram as µg; instead use mcg as there is less likelihood of misinterpretation.

12. When writing an outpatient prescription, write a complete prescription. A complete prescription can prevent the prescriber, the pharmacist, and/or the patient from making a mistake and can eliminate the need for further clarification. The legible prescriptions should contain:

   a. patient's full name

   b. for pediatric or geriatric patients: their age (or weight where applicable)

   c. drug name, dosage form and strength; if a drug is new or rarely prescribed, print this information

   d. number or amount to be dispensed

   e. complete instructions for the patient, including the purpose of the medication

   f. when there are recognized contraindications for a prescribed drug, indicate to the pharmacist that you are aware of this fact (ie, when prescribing a potassium salt for a patient receiving an ACE inhibitor, write "K serum leveling being monitored")

---

*From "Safe Writing" by Davis NM, PharmD and Cohen MR, MS, Lecturers and Consultants for Safe Medication Practices, 1143 Wright Drive, Huntington Valley, PA 19006. Phone: (215) 947-7566.

SELECTED REFERENCES

Dorr RT and Von Hoff DD, *Cancer Chemotherapy Handbook*, 2nd ed, Norwalk, CT: Appleton & Lange, 1994.

Drug Interaction Facts, St Louis, MO: J.B. Lippincott Co (Facts and Comparisons Division), 2001.

Facts and Comparisons, St Louis, MO: J.B. Lippincott Co (Facts and Comparisons Division), 2001.

Feigin RD and Cherry JD, *Textbook of Pediatric Infectious Diseases,* 4th ed, Philadelphia, PA: WB Saunders Company, 1998.

Hale T, *Medications and Mother's Milk*, 8th ed, Amarillo, TX: Pharmasoft Medical Publishing, 1999.

Handbook on Extemporaneous Formulations, Bethesda, MD: American Society of Health-System Pharmacists, 1987.

Handbook of Nonprescription Drugs, 12th ed, Washington, DC: American Pharmaceutical Association, 1998.

Jacobs DS, DeMott WR, Grady HJ, et al, *Laboratory Test Handbook with Key Word Index*, 4th ed, Hudson, OH: Lexi-Comp Inc, 1996.

Jenson HB and Baltimore RS, *Pediatric Infectious Diseases - Principles and Practice*, Norwalk, CT: Appleton & Lange, 1995.

Lacy CF, Armstrong LL, Goldman MP, et al, *Drug Information Handbook*, 9th ed, Hudson, OH: Lexi-Comp, Inc, 2001.

Mandell GL, Bennett JE, and Dolin R, *Principles and Practice of Infectious Diseases*, 4th ed, New York, NY: Churchill Livingstone, 1995.

McEvoy GK and Litvak K, *AHFS Drug Information*, 43rd ed, Bethesda, MD: American Society of Health-System Pharmacists, 2001.

Nahata MC and Hipple TF, *Pediatric Drug Formulations*, 4th ed, Cincinnati, OH: Harvey Whitney Books Company, 2000.

Nelson JD and Bradley JS, *Nelson's Pocket Book of Pediatric Antimicrobial Therapy*, 14th ed, Philadelphia, PA: Lippincott Williams & Wilkins, 2000.

PDR® Generics™, 2nd ed, Montvale, New Jersey: Medical Economics Co, 1996.

Phelps SJ and Hak EB, *Guidelines for Administration of Intravenous Medications to Pediatric Patients*, 5th ed, Bethesda, MD: American Society of Health-System Pharmacists, 1996.

Physician's Desk Reference, 55th ed, Montvale, NJ: Medical Economics Co, 2001.

Pickering LK, ed, *2000 Red Book, Report of the Committee on Infectious Diseases*, 25th ed, Elk Grove Village, IL: American Academy of Pediatrics, 2000.

Piscitelli SC and Rodvold KA, eds, *Drug Interactions in Infectious Diseases*, Totowa, NJ: Humana Press Inc, 2001.

Pizzo PA and Poplack DG, *Principles and Practice of Pediatric Oncology*, 3rd ed, Philadelphia, PA: Lippincott Raven Publishers, 1996.

Pronsky ZM, *Powers and Moore's Food Medication Interactions*, 11th ed, Pottstown, PA: Food Medication Interactions, 2000.

Radde IC and MacLead SM, *Pediatric Pharmacology and Therapeutics*, St. Louis, MO: Mosby, 1993.

Rogers MC and Helfaer MA, *Handbook of Pediatric Intensive Care*, 2nd ed, Baltimore, MD: Williams & Wilkins, 1995.

Rogers MC and Nichols DG, *Textbook of Pediatric Intensive Care*, 3rd ed, Baltimore, MD: Williams & Wilkins, 1996.

Rudolph AM, *Rudolph's Pediatrics*, 20th ed, Norwalk, CT: Appleton & Lange, 1996.

Toro-Figueroa LO, Levin DL, and Morriss FC, *Essentials of Pediatric Intensive Care Manual*, St Louis, MO: Quality Medical Pub, Inc, 1992.

Trissel L, *Handbook of Injectable Drugs*, 11th ed, Bethesda, MD: American Society of Health-System Pharmacists, 2000.

Trissel LA, *Trissel's Stability of Compounded Formulations*, Washington, DC: American Pharmaceutical Association, 1996.

United States Pharmacopeia Dispensing Information (USP DI), 21st ed, Englewood, CO: Micromedex, Inc, 2001.

Yaffe SJ and Aranda JV, *Pediatric Pharmacology: Therapeutic Principles in Practice,* Philadelphia, PA: WB Saunders Company, 1992.

ALPHABETICAL LISTING OF DRUGS

♦ **A-ase** *see* Asparaginase *on page 107*

Abacavir (uh BACK ah veer)

Related Information
Adult and Adolescent HIV *on page 1166*
Pediatric HIV *on page 1162*

U.S. Brand Names Ziagen®

Therapeutic Category Antiretroviral Agent; HIV Agents (Anti-HIV Agents); Nucleoside Reverse Transcriptase Inhibitor (NRTI)

Generic Available No

Use Treatment of HIV-1 infection in combination with other antiretroviral agents. (**Note:** HIV regimens consisting of **three** antiretroviral agents are strongly recommended)

Pregnancy Risk Factor C

Contraindications Hypersensitivity to abacavir or any component; **do not rechallenge** patients who have experienced hypersensitivity reactions to abacavir, potentially fatal hypersensitivity reactions may occur (see Warnings)

Warnings Fatal hypersensitivity reactions may occur; discontinue therapy immediately in patients who show signs or symptoms of hypersensitivity reaction such as fever, fatigue, skin rash, respiratory symptoms (cough, dyspnea, pharyngitis), and GI symptoms (nausea, vomiting, diarrhea, or abdominal pain). Carefully consider the diagnosis of hypersensitivity reaction in patients who present with acute onset respiratory symptoms, even if other diagnoses, such as bronchitis, flu-like illness, pharyngitis, or pneumonia, are possible. Skin rash may be maculopapular or urticarial, but hypersensitivity reaction may occur without a rash; other symptoms may include edema, lethargy, malaise, arthralgia, myolysis, myalgia, paresthesia, shortness of breath, mouth ulcerations, conjunctivitis, headache, and lymphadenopathy. Laboratory abnormalities include increase in liver function tests, creatine phosphokinase, creatinine, and lymphopenia.

Do not restart abacavir after a hypersensitivity reaction occurs; more severe symptoms can recur within hours and may include: Anaphylaxis, renal failure, hepatic failure, life-threatening hypotension and death. Fatal hypersensitivity reactions have occurred following the reintroduction of abacavir in patients whose therapy was interrupted for other reasons. These patients had no identified history or had unrecognized symptoms of abacavir hypersensitivity. Reactions occurred within hours. In some cases, signs of a hypersensitivity reaction may have been previously present, but attributed to other medical conditions (acute onset respiratory diseases, gastroenteritis, reactions to other medications). If abacavir (or Trizivir™) is to be restarted following an interruption in therapy, the patient must first be evaluated for previously unsuspected symptoms of hypersensitivity. **Do not restart** abacavir (or Trizivir™) if hypersensitivity is suspected or cannot be ruled out. Hypersensitivity reactions occur in ~5% of adult and pediatric patients; most hypersensitivity reactions occur within the first 6 weeks of therapy, but can occur at any time; call the Abacavir Hypersensitivity Reaction Registry at 1-800-270-0425 to facilitate reporting and collection of information on patients experiencing abacavir hypersensitivity reactions

Cases of lactic acidosis, severe hepatomegaly with steatosis and death have been reported; prolonged nucleoside use, obesity, and prior liver disease may be risk factors; use with extreme caution in patients with other risk factors for liver disease; discontinue abacavir in patients who develop laboratory or clinical evidence of lactic acidosis or pronounced hepatotoxicity

Precautions Always use abacavir in combination with other antiretroviral agents; do not add abacavir as a single agent to antiretroviral regimens that are failing; resistance to abacavir develops relatively slowly, but cross resistance between abacavir and other nucleoside reverse transcriptase inhibitors (NRTIs) may occur; limited response may be seen in patients with HIV isolates containing multiple mutations conferring resistance to NRTIs or in patients with a prolonged prior NRTI exposure

Adverse Reactions
Central nervous system: Insomnia, fever, headache, malaise, fatigue
Dermatologic: Rash
Endocrine & metabolic: Mild elevations of blood glucose, hypertriglyceridemia, lactic acidosis
Gastrointestinal: Nausea, vomiting, diarrhea, anorexia
Hepatic: Hepatomegaly with steatosis
Neuromuscular & skeletal: Asthenia
Respiratory: Cough
Miscellaneous: Hypersensitivity reaction (see Warnings)

Drug Interactions Use with ethanol increases abacavir AUC by 41% and prolongs half-life by 26%

Food Interactions Food does not significantly affect AUC

Stability Store tablets and oral solution at room temperature; oral solution may be refrigerated; do not freeze

Mechanism of Action A carbocyclic analogue that is converted within cells to the active metabolite carbovir triphosphate; carbovir triphosphate serves as an alternative substrate to deoxyguanosine-5'-triphosphate (dGTP), a natural substrate for cellular DNA polymerase and reverse transcriptase; carbovir triphosphate inhibits HIV viral reverse transcriptase by competing with natural dGTP and by becoming incorporated into viral DNA causing chain termination

Pharmacokinetics

Absorption: Rapid and extensive

Distribution: Apparent V_d: Adults: 0.86 ± 0.15 L/kg

CSF to plasma AUC ratio: 27% to 33%

Protein binding: 50%

Metabolism: In the liver by alcohol dehydrogenase and glucuronyl transferase to inactive carboxylate and glucuronide metabolites; not significantly metabolized by cytochrome P-450 enzymes

Bioavailability: Tablet: 83%; solution and tablet provide comparable AUCs

Half-life:

Children 3 months to 13 years: 1-1.5 hours (range)

Adults: 1.54 ± 0.63 hours

Time to peak concentration: Children 3 months to 13 years: Within 1.5 hours

Clearance (apparent): Single dose 8 mg/kg:

Children 3 months to 13 years: 17.84 mL/minute/kg

Adults: 10.14 mL/minute/kg

Elimination: ~83% of dose excreted in the urine as unchanged drug (1.2%) and metabolites (30% as 5'-carboxylic acid metabolite, 36% as the glucuronide, and 15% as other metabolites); 16% eliminated in feces

Usual Dosage Oral (use in combination with other antiretroviral agents):

Neonates: Not approved for use

Infants 1-3 months: Not approved for use; doses of 8 mg/kg twice daily are being studied

Infants ≥3 months, Children, and Adolescents: 8 mg/kg twice daily (maximum: 300 mg twice daily)

Adults: 300 mg twice daily

Administration Oral: May be administered without regard to food

Monitoring Parameters Signs and symptoms of hypersensitivity reaction; serum glucose and triglycerides, viral load, CD4 counts

Patient Information Abacavir is not a cure for HIV. Stop taking abacavir and notify physician immediately if skin rash or 2 or more of the following sets of symptoms occur: Fever, GI symptoms (nausea, vomiting, diarrhea or abdominal pain), flu-like symptoms (severe tiredness, achiness, or generally ill feeling), or respiratory symptoms (sore throat, shortness of breath, cough). If you experience an allergic (hypersensitivity) reaction to abacavir, **never** take abacavir (or Trizivir™) again. Take abacavir everyday as prescribed; do not change dose or discontinue without physician's advice. If abacavir is stopped for any reason, notify physician before restarting therapy. If a dose is missed, take it as soon as possible, then return to normal dosing schedule; if a dose is skipped, do **not** double the next dose

Nursing Implications Inform patients of the possibility of a fatal hypersensitivity reaction and the signs and symptoms (see Warnings)

Additional Information The patient Medication Guide, which includes written manufacturer information, should be dispensed to the patient with each new prescription and refill; the Warning Card describing the hypersensitivity reaction should be given to the patient to carry with them; oral solution contains methylparaben and propylparaben (preservatives) and propylene glycol

Dosage Forms Available as abacavir sulfate; mg strength refers to abacavir

Oral solution: 20 mg/mL [strawberry-banana flavor] (240 mL)

Tablet: 300 mg

References

Collura JM and Kraus DM, "New Pediatric Antiretroviral Agents," *J Pediatr Health Care*, 2000, 14(4):183-90.

Foster RH and Faulds D, "Abacavir," *Drugs*, 1998, 55(5):729-36.

Hughes W, McDowell JA, Shenep J, et al, "Safety and Single-Dose Pharmacokinetics of Abacavir (1592U89) in Human Immunodeficiency Virus Type 1-Infected Children," *Antimicrob Agents Chemother*, 1999, 43(3):609-15.

Kline MW, Blanchard S, Fletcher CV, et al, "A Phase I Study of Abacavir (1592U89) Alone and in Combination With Other Antiretroviral Agents in Infants and Children With Human Immunodeficiency Virus Infection," *Pediatrics*, 1999, 103(4):e47; http://www.pediatrics.org/cgi/content/full/103/4/e47.

Panel on Clinical Practices for Treatment of HIV Infection, "Guidelines for the Use of Antiretroviral Agents in HIV-Infected Adults and Adolescents," April 23, 2001, http://www.hivatis.org.

(Continued)

Abacavir *(Continued)*

Working Group on Antiretroviral Therapy and Medical Management of HIV-Infected Children, "Guidelines for the Use of Antiretroviral Agents in Pediatric HIV Infection," January 7, 2000, http://www.hivatis.org.

♦ **Abacavir, 3TC, and AZT** *see* Abacavir, Lamivudine, and Zidovudine *on page 26*

♦ **Abacavir, 3TC, and ZDV** *see* Abacavir, Lamivudine, and Zidovudine *on page 26*

♦ **Abacavir, Lamivudine, and Azidothymidine** *see* Abacavir, Lamivudine, and Zidovudine *on page 26*

Abacavir, Lamivudine, and Zidovudine

(uh BACK ah veer, la MI vyoo deen, & zye DOE vyoo deen)

U.S. Brand Names Trizivir™

Synonyms Abacavir, 3TC, and AZT; Abacavir, 3TC, and ZDV; Abacavir, Lamivudine, and Azidothymidine; Abacavir, Zidovudine, and Lamivudine; ABC, 3TC, and AZT; ABC, 3TC, and ZDV; Azidothymidine, Abacavir, and Lamivudine; Azidothymidine, Lamivudine and Abacavir; AZT, Abacavir, and 3TC; AZT, Abacavir, and Lamivudine; AZT, ABC, and 3TC; Compound S, Abacavir, and 3TC; Compound S, Abacavir, and Lamivudine; Compound S, ABC, and 3TC; Lamivudine, Abacavir, and Zidovudine; Lamivudine, Zidovudine, and Abacavir; 3TC, Abacavir, and AZT; 3TC, Abacavir, and ZDV; 3TC, Abacavir, and Zidovudine; 3TC, ABC, and AZT; 3TC, ABC, and ZDV; ZDV, Abacavir, and 3TC; ZDV, Abacavir, and Lamivudine; ZDV, ABC, and 3TC; Zidovudine, Abacavir, and Lamivudine

Therapeutic Category Antiretroviral Agent; HIV Agents (Anti-HIV Agents); Nucleoside Analog Reverse Transcriptase Inhibitor (NRTI)

Generic Available No

Use Treatment of HIV-1 infection (either alone or in combination with other antiretroviral agents) **(Note:** HIV regimens consisting of **three** antiretroviral agents are strongly recommended; data on the use of this triple NRTI combination regimen in patients with baseline viral loads >100,000 copies/mL is limited)

Pregnancy Risk Factor C

Contraindications Hypersensitivity to abacavir, lamivudine, zidovudine, or any component. **Do not rechallenge** patients who have experienced hypersensitivity reactions to abacavir, potentially fatal hypersensitivity reactions may occur (see Warnings)

Warnings Fatal hypersensitivity reactions may occur; discontinue therapy immediately in patients who show signs or symptoms of hypersensitivity reaction such as fever, fatigue, skin rash, respiratory symptoms (cough, dyspnea, pharyngitis) and GI symptoms (nausea, vomiting, diarrhea, or abdominal pain). Carefully consider the diagnosis of hypersensitivity reaction in patients who present with acute onset respiratory symptoms, even if other diagnoses, such as bronchitis, flu-like illness, pharyngitis, or pneumonia, are possible. Skin rash may be maculopapular or urticarial, but hypersensitivity reaction may occur without a rash; other symptoms may include edema, lethargy, malaise, arthralgia, myolysis, myalgia, paresthesia, shortness of breath, mouth ulcerations, conjunctivitis, headache, and lymphadenopathy. Laboratory abnormalities include increase in liver function tests, creatine phosphokinase, creatinine, and lymphopenia.

Do not restart abacavir or Trizivir™ after a hypersensitivity reaction occurs; more severe symptoms can recur within hours and may include: Anaphylaxis, renal failure, hepatic failure, life-threatening hypotension, and death. Fatal hypersensitivity reactions have occurred following the reintroduction of abacavir in patients whose therapy was interrupted for other reasons. These patients had no identified history or had unrecognized symptoms of abacavir hypersensitivity. Reactions occurred within hours. In some cases, signs of a hypersensitivity reaction may have been previously present, but attributed to other medical conditions (acute onset respiratory diseases, gastroenteritis, reactions to other medications). If abacavir or Trizivir™ is to be restarted following an interruption in therapy, the patient must first be evaluated for previously unsuspected symptoms of hypersensitivity. **Do not restart** abacavir or Trizivir™ if hypersensitivity is suspected or cannot be ruled out. Hypersensitivity reactions occur in ~5% of adult and pediatric patients; most hypersensitivity reactions occur within the first 6 weeks of therapy, but can occur at any time; call the Abacavir Hypersensitivity Reaction Registry at 1-800-270-0425 to facilitate reporting and collection of information on patients experiencing abacavir hypersensitivity reactions.

Cases of lactic acidosis, severe hepatomegaly with steatosis, and death have been reported in patients receiving nucleoside analogues; prolonged nucleoside use, obesity, and prior liver disease may be risk factors; use with extreme caution in patients with other risk factors for liver disease; discontinue Trizivir™ in patients who develop laboratory or clinical evidence of lactic acidosis or pronounced hepatotoxicity.

The major clinical toxicity of lamivudine in pediatric patients is pancreatitis; discontinue therapy if clinical signs, symptoms, or laboratory abnormalities suggestive of pancreatitis occur. Zidovudine is associated with hematologic toxicity including granulocytopenia and severe anemia requiring transfusions; use with caution in patients with ANC <1000 cells/mm^3 or hemoglobin <9.5 g/dL; discontinue treatment in children with an ANC <500 cells/mm^3 until marrow recovery is observed; use of erythropoietin, or filgrastim may be necessary in some patients; prolonged use of zidovudine may cause myositis and myopathy; zidovudine has been shown to be carcinogenic in rats and mice.

Trizivir™ contains abacavir, lamivudine, and zidovudine as a fixed-dose combination; do not use in patients weighing <40 kg or in patients who require dosage adjustment (eg, patients with Cl$_{cr}$ ≤50 mL/minute); concomitant use of Trizivir™ with abacavir, lamivudine, or zidovudine is not recommended.

Precautions Resistance to abacavir develops relatively slowly, but cross resistance between abacavir and other nucleoside reverse transcriptase inhibitors (NRTIs) may occur; limited response may be seen in patients with HIV isolates containing multiple mutations conferring resistance to NRTIs or in patients with a prolonged prior NRTI exposure. HIV-infected patients who are coinfected with hepatitis B may experience clinical symptoms or laboratory evidence of hepatitis when lamivudine is discontinued.

Adverse Reactions See Abacavir *on page 24*, Lamivudine *on page 572*, and Zidovudine *on page 1022*

Drug Interactions See Abacavir *on page 24*, Lamivudine *on page 572*, and Zidovudine *on page 1022*

Food Interactions Food decreases the rate, but not the extent of absorption (see Yuen, 2001).

Stability Store at room temperature 25°C (77°F)

Mechanism of Action See Abacavir *on page 24*, Lamivudine *on page 572*, and Zidovudine *on page 1022*

Pharmacokinetics One Trizivir™ tablet is bioequivalent, in the extent (AUC) and rate of absorption (peak concentration and time to peak concentration), to one abacavir 300 mg tablet, one lamivudine 150 mg tablet, plus one zidovudine 300 mg tablet; See Abacavir *on page 24*, Lamivudine *on page 572*, and Zidovudine *on page 1022*

Usual Dosage Oral:

Children: Not intended for pediatric use; product is a fixed-dose combination

Adolescents and Adults:

<40 kg: Not recommended; product is a fixed-dose combination

≥40 kg: 1 tablet twice daily

Dosing adjustment in renal impairment: Cl$_{cr}$ ≤50 mL/minute: Not recommended (use individual antiretroviral agents to reduce dosage)

Administration May be administered without regard to meals

Monitoring Parameters Signs and symptoms of abacavir hypersensitivity reaction, lactic acidosis, pronounced hepatotoxicity, anemia, bone marrow suppression, and pancreatitis; serum glucose and triglycerides, viral load, CD4 counts, CBC with differential, hemoglobin, MCV, reticulocyte count, liver enzymes, serum amylase, bilirubin, renal and hepatic function tests

Patient Information Trizivir™ is not a cure for HIV. Trizivir™ contains abacavir (also called Ziagen®). Abacavir may cause a potentially fatal allergic (hypersensitivity) reaction. Stop taking Trizivir™ and notify physician immediately if skin rash or 2 more of the following sets of symptoms occur: Fever, GI symptoms (nausea, vomiting, diarrhea, or abdominal pain), flu-like symptoms (severe tiredness, achiness, or generally ill feeling), or respiratory symptoms (sore throat, shortness of breath, cough). If you experience an allergic (hypersensitivity) reaction to Trizivir™ (or abacavir or Ziagen®), **never** take Trizivir™, abacavir or Ziagen® again. Take Trizivir™ every day as prescribed; do not change dose or discontinue without physician's advice. If Trizivir™ is stopped for any reason, notify physician before restarting therapy. If a dose is missed, take it as soon as possible, then return to normal dosing schedule; if a dose is skipped, do **not** double the next dose. Avoid alcohol. Notify physician if persistent severe abdominal pain, nausea, or vomiting occurs.

Nursing Implications Inform patients of the possibility of a fatal abacavir hypersensitivity reaction and the signs and symptoms (see Warnings and Patient Information)

Additional Information The Patient Medication Guide, which includes written manufacturer information, should be dispensed to the patient with each new

(Continued)

Abacavir, Lamivudine, and Zidovudine *(Continued)*

prescription and refill; a Warning Card describing the hypersensitivity reaction should be given to the patient to carry with them

Dosage Forms Tablet: Abacavir 300 mg [as abacavir sulfate], lamivudine 150 mg, and zidovudine 300 mg

References

Panel on Clinical Practices for Treatment of HIV Infection, "Guidelines for the Use of Antiretroviral Agents in HIV-Infected Adults and Adolescents," April 23, 2001, http://www.hivatis.org.

Saez-Llorens X, Nelson RP, Emmanuel P, et al, "A Randomized, Double-Blind Study of Triple Nucleoside Therapy of Abacavir, Lamivudine, and Zidovudine Versus Lamivudine and Zidovudine in Previously Treated Human Immunodeficiency Virus Type 1-Infected Children," *Pediatrics*, 2001, 107(1), URL: http://www.pediatrics.org/cgi/content/full/107/1/e4.

Yuen GJ, Lou Y, Thompson NF, et al, "Abacavir/Lamivudine/Zidovudine as a Combined Formulation Tablet: Bioequivalence Compared With Each Component Administered Concurrently and the Effect of Food on Absorption," *J Clin Pharmacol*, 2001, 41(3):277-88.

♦ **Abacavir, Zidovudine, and Lamivudine** *see* Abacavir, Lamivudine, and Zidovudine *on page 26*

♦ **Abbokinase®** *see* Urokinase *on page 995*

♦ **ABC, 3TC, and AZT** *see* Abacavir, Lamivudine, and Zidovudine *on page 26*

♦ **ABC, 3TC, and ZDV** *see* Abacavir, Lamivudine, and Zidovudine *on page 26*

♦ **Abelcet®** *see* Amphotericin B Lipid Complex *on page 86*

♦ **Abenol (Can)** *see* Acetaminophen *on page 29*

♦ **ABLC** *see* Amphotericin B Lipid Complex *on page 86*

♦ **Absorbine Jr.® Antifungal [OTC]** *see* Tolnaftate *on page 969*

♦ **ABT-378/Ritonavir** *see* Lopinavir and Ritonavir *on page 604*

♦ **A-Caine® Rectal [OTC]** *see* Hemorrhoidal Preparations *on page 490*

Acarbose *(AY car bose)*

U.S. Brand Names Precose®

Canadian Brand Names Prandase

Therapeutic Category Antidiabetic Agent, Oral; Antidiabetic Agent, Alpha-glucosidase Inhibitor

Generic Available No

Use Management of type II diabetes mellitus (noninsulin-dependent, NIDDM) when hyperglycemia cannot be managed by diet alone; may be used concomitantly with metformin, a sulfonylurea, or insulin to improve glycemic control

Pregnancy Risk Factor B

Contraindications Hypersensitivity to acarbose or any component; diabetic ketoacidosis; cirrhosis; patients with inflammatory bowel disease, colonic ulceration, partial intestinal obstruction, or patients predisposed to intestinal obstruction; patients who have chronic intestinal diseases associated with marked disorders of digestion or absorption; patients who have conditions that may deteriorate as a result of increased gas formation in the intestine

Warnings Dose-related elevations in serum transaminases occurred in 15% of acarbose-treated patients in long-term studies; these elevations were asymptomatic, reversible, more common in females, and not associated with other evidence of liver dysfunction; acarbose serum levels are proportionately higher in patients with renal dysfunction (S_{cr} >2 mg/dL); until long term clinical studies are completed, use in renally-compromised patients is not recommended

Precautions Hypoglycemia may occur when used in combination with sulfonylureas or insulin; oral glucose (absorption is not affected by acarbose) should be used instead of sucrose (table sugar) for the treatment of mild to moderate hypoglycemia

Adverse Reactions

Central nervous system: Headache, vertigo, drowsiness

Dermatologic: Urticaria, erythema

Endocrine & metabolic: Hypoglycemia

Gastrointestinal: Abdominal pain, diarrhea, flatulence

Hepatic: Elevated LFTs

Neuromuscular & skeletal: Weakness

Drug Interactions Drugs that produce hyperglycemia (eg, diuretics, corticosteroids, phenothiazines, thyroid products, estrogens, oral contraceptives, phenytoin, nicotinic acid, sympathomimetics, calcium channel blocking drugs, rifampin, and isoniazid) may lead to a loss of glycemic control; intestinal adsorbents; digestive enzyme preparations

Mechanism of Action Competitive inhibitor of pancreatic α-glucosidases, resulting in delayed hydrolysis of ingested complex carbohydrates and disaccharides and absorption of glucose; dose-dependent reduction in postprandial serum insulin and glucose peaks; inhibits the metabolism of sucrose to glucose and fructose

Pharmacodynamics Average decrease in fasting blood sugar: 20-30 mg/dL
Pharmacokinetics
   Absorption: <2% absorbed as active drug
   Metabolism: Metabolized exclusively within the GI tract, principally by intestinal
      bacteria and by digestive enzymes; 13 metabolites have been identified
   Bioavailability: Low systemic bioavailability of parent compound
   Elimination: Fraction absorbed as intact drug is almost completely excreted in urine
Usual Dosage Oral:
   Adolescents and Adults: Dosage must be individualized on the basis of effective-
      ness and tolerance; do not exceed the maximum recommended dose (use slow
      titration to prevent or minimize GI effects):
      Initial: 25 mg once or twice daily; increase in 25 mg/day increments in 2-4 week
         intervals to maximum dose
      Maximum dose:
         Patients ≤60 kg: 50 mg 3 times/day
         Patients >60 kg: 100 mg 3 times/day
   Dosing adjustment in renal impairment: See Warnings
Administration Oral: Administer with first bite of each main meal
Monitoring Parameters Fasting blood glucose; hemoglobin A_{1c}; LFTs every 3
months for the first year of therapy and periodically thereafter
Reference Range Target range:
   Blood glucose: Fasting and preprandial: 80-120 mg/dL; bedtime: 100-140 mg/dL
   Glycosylated hemoglobin (hemoglobin A_{1c}): <7%
Dosage Forms Tablet: 25 mg, 50 mg, 100 mg
References
   DeFronzo RA, "Pharmacologic Therapy for Type 2 Diabetes Mellitus," *Ann Intern Med*, 1999, 131(4):281-
   303.

♦ **Accolate**® *see* Zafirlukast *on page 1019*
♦ **Accutane**® *see* Isotretinoin *on page 557*
♦ **Acephen**® [OTC] *see* Acetaminophen *on page 29*
♦ **Acet (Can)** *see* Acetaminophen *on page 29*
♦ **Aceta**® [OTC] *see* Acetaminophen *on page 29*

Acetaminophen (a seet a MIN oh fen)

Related Information
   Acetaminophen Toxicity Nomogram *on page 1237*
   Carbohydrate and Alcohol Content of Liquid Medications for Use in Patients
      Receiving Ketogenic Diets *on page 1258*
   OTC Cough & Cold Preparations, Pediatric *on page 1072*
   Overdose and Toxicology *on page 1222*
U.S. Brand Names Acephen® [OTC]; Aceta® [OTC]; Apacet® [OTC]; Aspirin Free
Anacin® [OTC]; Feverall™ [OTC]; Genapap® [OTC]; Genebs® [OTC]; Halenol®
[OTC]; Mapap® [OTC]; Meda-Cap® [OTC]; Meda® Tab [OTC]; Redutemp® [OTC];
Ridenol® [OTC]; Silapap® [OTC]; Tapanol® [OTC]; Tempra® [OTC]; Tylenol® [OTC]
Canadian Brand Names Abenol; Acet; Alisiphene Forte; Artritol; Atasol; Cephanol;
Childrens Feverhalt; Novo-Gesic; Pain Aid Free; Panadol; Pediatrix; Robigesic;
Tantaphen
Synonyms APAP; N-Acetyl-P-Aminophenol; Paracetamol
Therapeutic Category Analgesic, Non-narcotic; Antipyretic
Generic Available Yes
Use Treatment of mild to moderate pain and fever; does not have antirheumatic or
systemic anti-inflammatory effects
Pregnancy Risk Factor B
Contraindications Hypersensitivity to acetaminophen or any component
Warnings May cause severe hepatic toxicity with overdose
Precautions Some products (eg, Children's Tylenol® chewable tablets) contain
aspartame; aspartame is metabolized to phenylalanine and must be avoided or
used with caution in patients with phenylketonuria

G-6-PD deficiency: Although several case reports of acetaminophen-associated
hemolytic anemia have been reported in patients with G-6-PD deficiency, a direct
cause and effect relationship has not been well established (concurrent illnesses
such as fever or infection may precipitate hemolytic anemia in patients with G-6-PD
deficiency); therefore, acetaminophen is generally thought to be safe when given in
therapeutic doses to patients with G-6-PD deficiency.
Adverse Reactions
   Dermatologic: Rash
   Hematologic: Blood dyscrasias (neutropenia, pancytopenia, leukopenia)
   (Continued)

Acetaminophen *(Continued)*

Hepatic: Hepatic necrosis with overdose

Renal: Renal injury with chronic use

Miscellaneous: Hypersensitivity reactions (rare)

Drug Interactions Cytochrome P-450 isoenzyme CYP1A2 substrate (minor), CYP2E1 and CYP3A3/4 isoenzyme substrate

Enzyme inducers (barbiturates, carbamazepine, phenytoin), carmustine (with high dose acetaminophen), alcohol (especially chronic use) can increase hepatotoxicity; rifampin may decrease acetaminophen's therapeutic effect; anticholinergic agents (scopolamine) may effect GI absorption; acetaminophen may increase the clearance of lamotrigine; acetaminophen may increase zidovudine concentration and toxicity

Food Interactions Rate of absorption may be decreased when given with food high in carbohydrates

Mechanism of Action Inhibits the synthesis of prostaglandins in the central nervous system and peripherally blocks pain impulse generation; produces antipyresis from inhibition of hypothalamic heat-regulating center

Pharmacokinetics

Protein binding: 20% to 50%

Metabolism: At normal therapeutic dosages the parent compound is metabolized in the liver to sulfate and glucuronide metabolites, while a small amount is metabolized by microsomal mixed function oxidases to a highly reactive intermediate (N-acetyl-imidoquinone) which is conjugated with glutathione and inactivated; at toxic doses (as little as 4 g in a single day) glutathione can become depleted, and conjugation becomes insufficient to meet the metabolic demand causing an increase in N-acetyl-imidoquinone concentration, which is thought to cause hepatic cell necrosis.

Half-life:

Neonates: 2-5 hours

Adults: 1-3 hours

Time to peak serum concentration: 10-60 minutes after normal oral doses, but may be delayed in acute overdoses

Usual Dosage Oral, rectal:

Neonates: 10-15 mg/kg/dose every 6-8 hours as needed

Infants and Children: 10-15 mg/kg/dose every 4-6 hours as needed; do **not** exceed 5 doses in 24 hours; alternatively, the following doses may be used. See table.

Acetaminophen Dosing

Age	Dosage (mg)	Age	Dosage (mg)
0-3 mo	40	4-5 y	240
4-11 mo	80	6-8 y	320
1-2 y	120	9-10 y	400
2-3 y	160	11 y	480

Children ≥12 years and Adults: 325-650 mg every 4-6 hours or 1000 mg 3-4 times/ day; do **not** exceed 4 g/day

Administration Oral: Administer with food to decrease GI upset; shake suspension well before use; do not crush or chew extended release products

Reference Range Acute ingestions: Toxic concentration with probable hepatotoxicity: >200 µg/mL at 4 hours or 50 µg/mL at 12 hours after ingestion of overdose

Patient Information Avoid alcohol; do not take longer than 10 days without physician's advice

Additional Information Some elixir preparations contain sodium benzoate; drops contain saccharin

Acetaminophen (15 mg/kg/dose given orally every 6 hours for 24 hours) did **not** relieve the intraoperative or the immediate postoperative pain associated with neonatal circumcision; some benefit was seen 6 hours after circumcision (see Howard, 1994).

There is currently no scientific evidence to support alternating acetaminophen with ibuprofen in the treatment of fever (see Mayoral, 2000).

Dosage Forms Most commonly available concentrations for nonsolid dosage forms are **bolded** when more than one concentration is available

Caplet: 500 mg

Caplet, extended: 650 mg

Capsule: 500 mg

Drops: See Solution, oral drops; suspension, oral drops

Elixir: 120 mg/5 mL (120 mL); **160 mg/5 mL** (5 mL, 10 mL, 20 mL, 120 mL, 240 mL, 500 mL, 3780 mL)

Gelcap: 500 mg

Liquid, oral: **160 mg/5 mL** (5 mL, 60 mL, 120 mL, 240 mL, 480 mL, 3870 mL); 500 mg/15 mL (240 mL)

Solution, oral drops: 100 mg/mL [droppers are marked at 0.4 mL (40 mg) and at 0.8 mL (80 mg)] (15 mL, 30 mL)

Suppository, rectal: 80 mg, 120 mg, 325 mg, 650 mg

Suspension, oral: 160 mg/5 mL (120 mL)

Suspension, oral drops: 100 mg/mL [droppers are marked at 0.4 mL (40 mg) and at 0.8 mL (80 mg)] (15 mL, 30 mL)

Syrup, oral: 160 mg/5 mL (120 mL)

Tablet: 160 mg, 325 mg, 500 mg

Tablet, chewable: 80 mg, 160 mg

References

Howard CR, Howard FM, and Weitzman ML, "Acetaminophen Analgesia in Neonatal Circumcision: The Effect on Pain," *Pediatrics*, 1994, 93(4):641-646.

Mayoral CE, Marino RV, Rosenfeld W, et al, "Alternating Antipyretics: Is This An Alternative?" *Pediatrics*, 2000, 105(5):1009-12.

Acetaminophen and Codeine (a seet a MIN oh fen & KOE deen)

Related Information

Carbohydrate and Alcohol Content of Liquid Medications for Use in Patients Receiving Ketogenic Diets *on page 1258*

Overdose and Toxicology *on page 1222*

U.S. Brand Names Capital® and Codeine; Phenaphen® With Codeine; Tylenol® With Codeine

Canadian Brand Names Acet Codeine; Empracet; Empracet 30, 60; Emtec-30; Lenoltec No 4; Rounox + Codeine; Triatec-30; Tylenol No. 3 with Codeine without Caffeine; Tylenol with Codeine; Tylenol with Codeine No 4

Synonyms Codeine and Acetaminophen

Therapeutic Category Analgesic, Narcotic

Generic Available Yes

Use Relief of mild to moderate pain

Restrictions C-III; C-V

Pregnancy Risk Factor C

Contraindications Hypersensitivity to acetaminophen, codeine phosphate, or any component

Warnings Tablets contain metabisulfite which may cause allergic reactions

Precautions Use with caution in patients with hypersensitivity reactions to other phenanthrene derivative opioid agonists (morphine, hydrocodone, hydromorphone, levorphanol, oxycodone, oxymorphone) or respiratory disease/compromise.

G-6-PD deficiency: Although several case reports of acetaminophen-associated hemolytic anemia have been reported in patients with G-6-PD deficiency, a direct cause and effect relationship has not been well established (concurrent illnesses such as fever or infection may precipitate hemolytic anemia in patients with G-6-PD deficiency); therefore, acetaminophen is generally thought to be safe when given in therapeutic doses to patients with G-6-PD deficiency.

Adverse Reactions

Acetaminophen:

Dermatologic: Rash

Hematologic: Blood dyscrasias (neutropenia, pancytopenia, leukopenia)

Hepatic: Hepatic necrosis with overdose

Renal: Renal injury with chronic use

Miscellaneous: Hypersensitivity reactions (rare)

Codeine:

Cardiovascular: Palpitations, hypotension, bradycardia, peripheral vasodilation

Central nervous system: CNS depression, dizziness, drowsiness, sedation, increased intracranial pressure

Dermatologic: Pruritus

Endocrine & metabolic: Antidiuretic hormone release

Gastrointestinal: Nausea, vomiting, constipation, biliary tract spasm

Genitourinary: Urinary retention

Ocular: Miosis

Respiratory: Respiratory depression

Miscellaneous: Histamine release, physical and psychological dependence with prolonged use

(Continued)

Acetaminophen and Codeine *(Continued)*

Drug Interactions See Acetaminophen *on page 29* and Codeine *on page 262*

Food Interactions Rate of absorption of acetaminophen may be decreased when given with food high in carbohydrates

Mechanism of Action See individual monographs for Acetaminophen *on page 29* and Codeine *on page 262*

Pharmacokinetics See individual monographs for Acetaminophen *on page 29* and Codeine *on page 262*

Usual Dosage Oral (doses should be titrated to appropriate analgesic effect):
  Children: Analgesic: 0.5-1 mg codeine/kg/dose every 4-6 hours
    3-6 years: 5 mL 3-4 times/day as needed
    7-12 years: 10 mL 3-4 times/day as needed
    >12 years: 15 mL every 4 hours as needed
  Adults: 1-2 tablets every 4 hours; maximum dose: 12 tablets/24 hours

Administration Oral: Administer with food to decrease GI upset; shake suspension well before use

Patient Information Codeine may be habit-forming; avoid abrupt discontinuation after prolonged use; may cause drowsiness and impair ability to perform activities requiring mental alertness or coordination; avoid alcohol

Nursing Implications Observe patient for excessive sedation, respiratory depression

Additional Information Tylenol® With Codeine elixir contains sodium benzoate and saccharin

Dosage Forms
  Capsule:
    #3: Acetaminophen 325 mg and codeine phosphate 30 mg (C-III)
    #4: Acetaminophen 325 mg and codeine phosphate 60 mg (C-III)
  Elixir, oral: Acetaminophen 120 mg and codeine phosphate 12 mg per 5 mL [with alcohol 7%] (C-V) (5 mL, 10 mL, 15 mL, 60 mL, 100 mL, 120 mL, 480 mL, 3840 mL)
  Suspension, oral: Acetaminophen 120 mg and codeine phosphate 12 mg per 5 mL [alcohol free] (C-V) (480 mL)
  Tablet: Acetaminophen 500 mg and codeine phosphate 30 mg (C-III); acetaminophen 650 mg and codeine phosphate 30 mg (C-III)
  Tablet:
    #2: Acetaminophen 300 mg and codeine phosphate 15 mg (C-III)
    #3: Acetaminophen 300 mg and codeine phosphate 30 mg (C-III)
    #4: Acetaminophen 300 mg and codeine phosphate 60 mg (C-III)

♦ **Acetaminophen and Hydrocodone** *see* Hydrocodone and Acetaminophen *on page 505*

♦ **Acetaminophen and Oxycodone** *see* Oxycodone and Acetaminophen *on page 747*

♦ **Acetaminophen and Propoxyphene** *see* Propoxyphene and Acetaminophen *on page 846*

♦ **Acetaminophen Toxicity Nomogram** *see page 1237*

♦ **Acetazolam (Can)** *see* Acetazolamide *on page 32*

Acetazolamide *(a set a ZOLE a mide)*

Related Information
  Antiepileptic Drugs *on page 1208*

U.S. Brand Names Diamox®; Diamox Sequels®

Canadian Brand Names Acetazolam; Apo-Acetazolamide; Novo-Zolamide

Therapeutic Category Anticonvulsant, Miscellaneous; Carbonic Anhydrase Inhibitor; Diuretic, Carbonic Anhydrase Inhibitor

Generic Available Yes

Use Reduce elevated intraocular pressure in glaucoma; diuretic; adjunct to the treatment of refractory seizures; prevent acute altitude sickness; treatment of centrencephalic epilepsies

Pregnancy Risk Factor C

Contraindications Hypersensitivity to acetazolamide, any component, or other sulfonamides; patients with hepatic disease or insufficiency; decreased serum sodium and/or potassium; adrenocortical insufficiency; hyperchloremic acidosis; or severe renal disease

Warnings Tolerance to antiepileptic effects may require dosage adjustment

Precautions Use with caution in patients with respiratory acidosis, COPD, diabetes mellitus, and gout

Adverse Reactions

Cardiovascular: Cyanosis

Central nervous system: Drowsiness, fatigue, vertigo, fever, seizures, dizziness, depression, malaise

Dermatologic: Rash, erythema multiforme, photosensitivity, Stevens-Johnson syndrome

Endocrine & metabolic: Hypokalemia, hyperchloremic metabolic acidosis, hyperglycemia

Gastrointestinal: GI irritation, anorexia, nausea, vomiting, xerostomia, melena, dysgeusia, metallic taste, black stools

Genitourinary: Dysuria, polyuria

Hematologic: Bone marrow suppression, thrombocytopenia, hemolytic anemia, pancytopenia, agranulocytosis

Hepatic: Hepatic insufficiency

Neuromuscular & skeletal: Paresthesia, muscle weakness

Ocular: Myopia

Renal: Renal calculi, phosphaturia, renal colic

Respiratory: Hyperpnea

Drug Interactions Increases lithium excretion; may decrease the rate of excretion of other drugs such as procainamide, flecainide, quinidine, and tricyclic antidepressants; may increase the excretion of salicylates and phenobarbital; may inactivate methenamine in the urine; may increase cyclosporine levels; may increase the risk of developing osteomalacia in patients receiving phenytoin or phenobarbital; topiramate may increase risk of nephrolithiasis and paresthesia; salicylates increase acetazolamide serum levels resulting in CNS toxicity; ammonium chloride increases plasma concentration of nonionized acetazolamide; increased toxicity with propofol (cardiorespiratory instability)

Food Interactions Avoid natural licorice (causes sodium and water retention and increases potassium loss)

Stability After reconstitution, acetazolamide injection is stable for 12 hours at room temperature and for 1 week when refrigerated; physically incompatible with parenteral multivitamins

Mechanism of Action Competitive, reversible inhibition of the enzyme carbonic anhydrase resulting in increased renal excretion of sodium, potassium, bicarbonate, and water and decreased formation of aqueous humor; also inhibits carbonic anhydrase in CNS to retard abnormal and excessive discharge from CNS neurons

Pharmacodynamics

Onset of action:

Capsule, extended release: 2 hours

Tablet: 1-1.5 hours

I.V.: 2 minutes

Peak effect:

Capsule, extended release: 3-6 hours

Tablet: 1-4 hours

I.V.: 15 minutes

Duration:

Capsule, extended release: 18-24 hours

Tablet: 8-12 hours

I.V.: 4-5 hours

Pharmacokinetics

Absorption: Appears to be dose dependent; erratic with daily doses >10 mg/kg

Distribution: Into erythrocytes, kidneys, and breast milk (breast milk to plasma ratio of 0.25 has been reported); crosses the blood-brain barrier and the placenta;

Protein binding: 95%

Half-life: 2.4-5.8 hours

Time to peak level: Tablet: 2-4 hours

Dialysis: 20% to 50% removed by hemodialysis

Elimination: 70% to 100% of an I.V. or tablet dose and 47% of an extended release capsule excreted unchanged in urine within 24 hours

Usual Dosage

Neonates and Infants: Hydrocephalus: To slow the progression of hydrocephalus in neonates and infants who may not be good candidates for surgery, acetazolamide I.V. or oral doses of 5 mg/kg/dose every 6 hours increased by 25 mg/kg/day to a maximum of 100 mg/kg/day, if tolerated, have been used. Furosemide was used in combination with acetazolamide.

Children:

Glaucoma:

Oral: 8-30 mg/kg/day or 300-900 mg/m^2/day divided every 8 hours

I.V.: 20-40 mg/kg/day divided every 6 hours, not to exceed 1 g/day

(Continued)

Acetazolamide *(Continued)*

Edema: Oral, I.V.: 5 mg/kg/dose or 150 mg/m²/dose once daily

Epilepsy: Oral: 4-16 mg/kg/day in 1-4 divided doses, not to exceed 30 mg/kg/day or 1 g/day; **extended release capsule is not recommended for treatment of epilepsy**

Adults:

Glaucoma:

Chronic simple (open-angle): Oral: 250 mg 1-4 times/day or 500 mg sustained release capsule twice daily

Secondary, acute (closed-angle): I.V.: 250-500 mg, may repeat in 2-4 hours to a maximum of 1 g/day

Edema: Oral, I.V.: 250-375 mg/day

Epilepsy: Oral: 4-16 mg/kg/day in 1-4 divided doses, not to exceed 30 mg/kg/day or 1 g/day; **extended release capsule is not recommended for treatment of epilepsy**

Altitude sickness: Oral: 250 mg every 8-12 hours or 500 mg extended release capsules every 12-24 hours; therapy should begin 24-48 hours before and continued during ascent and for at least 48 hours after arrival at the high altitude

Urine alkalinization: Oral: 5 mg/kg/dose repeated 2-3 times over 24 hours

Dosing interval in renal impairment: Children and Adults:

Cl_{cr} 10-50 mL/minute: Administer every 12 hours

Cl_{cr} <10 mL/minute: Avoid use

Administration

Oral: Administer with food to decrease GI upset; tablet may be crushed and suspended in cherry or chocolate syrup to disguise the bitter taste of the drug (See Extemporaneous Preparations)

Parenteral:

I.V.: Reconstitute with at least 5 mL sterile water to provide a solution containing not more than 100 mg/mL; maximum concentration: 100 mg/mL; maximum rate of I.V. infusion: 500 mg/minute

I.M.: Not generally recommended as the drug's alkaline pH makes it very painful

Monitoring Parameters Serum electrolytes, periodic hematologic determinations

Test Interactions May cause false-positive results for urinary protein with Albustix®, Labstix®, Albutest®, Bumintest®

Patient Information Do not crush or chew long-acting capsule

Additional Information Sodium content of 500 mg injection: 2.049 mEq

Extended release capsules are indicated only for use for the adjunctive treatment of open-angle or secondary glaucoma and the prevention of high altitude sickness; avoid using extended release capsules for anticonvulsant or diuretic therapy

Dosage Forms

Capsule, sustained release: 500 mg

Powder for injection, as sodium: 500 mg

Tablet: 125 mg, 250 mg

Extemporaneous Preparations

A 25 mg/mL suspension may be made by crushing twelve 250 mg tablets and mixing with 120 mL of a 1:1 mixture of Ora-Sweet® and Ora-Plus® or a 1:1 mixture of Ora-Sweet® SF and Ora-Plus®. The resulting suspension is stable for 60 days refrigerated (Allen, 1996).

A 25 mg/mL suspension may be made by crushing one hundred 250 mg tablets; add 100 mL flavor/purified water; add a mixture of 10 g Veegum (already mixed with 200 mL purified water), 300 mL 1% methylcellulose and 300 mL syrup; qsad to 1000 mL with flavor/purified water and 10 mL paraben concentrate (methylparaben 120 mg, propylparaben 12 mg, propylene glycol qsad to 100 mL); stable 79 days refrigerated (Alexander, 1991).

Allen LV and Erickson MA, "Stability of Acetazolamide, Allopurinol, Azathioprine, Clonazepam, and Flucytosine in Extemporaneously Compounded Oral Liquids," *Am J Health Sys Pharm*, 1996, 53:1944-9.

Alexander KS, Haribhakti RP, and Parker GA, "Stability of Acetazolamide in Suspension Compounded From Tablets," *Am J Hosp Pharm*, 1991, 48(6):1241-4.

References

Libenson MH, Kaye EM, Rosman NP, et al, "Acetazolamide and Furosemide for Posthemorrhagic Hydrocephalus of the Newborn," *Pediatr Neurol*, 1999, 20(3):185-91.

Reiss WG and Oles KS, "Acetazolamide in the Treatment of Seizures," *Ann Pharmacother*, 1996, 30(5):514-9.

Shinnar S, Gammon K, Bergman EW Jr, et al, "Management of Hydrocephalus in Infancy: Use of Acetazolamide and Furosemide to Avoid Cerebrospinal Fluid Shunts," *J Pediatr*, 1985, 107(1):31-7.

♦ **Acet Codeine (Can)** *see* Acetaminophen and Codeine *on page 31*

♦ **Acetoxyl (Can)** *see* Benzoyl Peroxide *on page 136*
♦ **Acetoxymethylprogesterone** *see* Medroxyprogesterone *on page 624*

Acetylcholine (a se teel KOE leen)

U.S. Brand Names Miochol-E®
Therapeutic Category Cholinergic Agent, Ophthalmic; Ophthalmic Agent, Miotic
Generic Available No
Use Produces complete miosis in cataract surgery, keratoplasty, iridectomy and other anterior segment surgery where rapid miosis is required
Pregnancy Risk Factor C
Contraindications Hypersensitivity to acetylcholine chloride or any component; acute iritis and acute inflammatory disease of the anterior chamber
Warnings Open under aseptic conditions only
Precautions Systemic effects rarely occur, but can cause problems for patients with acute CHF, bronchial asthma, peptic ulcer, hyperthyroidism, GI spasm, and urinary tract obstruction
Adverse Reactions
  Cardiovascular: Transient bradycardia and hypotension
  Central nervous system: Headache
  Ocular: Iris atrophy, temporary lens opacities (attributed to osmotic effect of 5% mannitol present in preparation)
  Respiratory: Dyspnea
  Miscellaneous: Diaphoresis
Drug Interactions Flurbiprofen decreases effectiveness; sodium nitrate antagonizes acetylcholine's effects
Stability Prepare solution immediately before use; do not use solution which is not clear and colorless
Mechanism of Action Causes contraction of the sphincter muscles of the iris, resulting in miosis and contraction of the ciliary muscle, leading to accommodation
Pharmacodynamics
  Onset of action: Miosis occurs promptly
  Duration: ~10-20 minutes
Usual Dosage Adults: 0.5-2 mL of 1% injection (5-20 mg)
Administration Ophthalmic: Instill into anterior chamber before or after securing one or more sutures; instillation should be gentle and parallel to the iris face and tangential to the pupil border; in cataract surgery, acetylcholine should be used only after delivery of the lens
Dosage Forms Powder, intraocular, as chloride: 1% 1:100 [10 mg/mL] (2 mL)

Acetylcysteine (a se teel SIS teen)

U.S. Brand Names Mucomyst®; Mucosil™
Canadian Brand Names Parvolex
Synonyms Mercapturic Acid; NAC; *N*-Acetylcysteine; *N*-Acetyl-L-Cysteine
Therapeutic Category Antidote, Acetaminophen; Mucolytic Agent
Generic Available Yes
Use Adjunctive therapy in patients with abnormal or viscid mucous secretions in bronchopulmonary diseases, pulmonary complications of surgery, and cystic fibrosis; diagnostic bronchial studies; antidote for acute acetaminophen toxicity; enema to treat bowel obstruction due to meconium ileus or its equivalent
Pregnancy Risk Factor B
Contraindications Hypersensitivity to acetylcysteine or any component
Warnings Since increased bronchial secretions may develop after inhalation, percussion, postural drainage and suctioning should follow
Precautions If bronchospasm occurs, administer a bronchodilator; discontinue acetylcysteine if bronchospasm progresses
Adverse Reactions
  Cardiovascular: Tachycardia, hypotension, hypertension (after large oral doses)
  Central nervous system: Drowsiness, chills
  Dermatologic: Generalized urticaria, rash
  Gastrointestinal: Stomatitis, nausea, vomiting, hemoptysis
  Hepatic: Mild elevations in liver function tests have occurred after oral therapy
  Respiratory: Bronchospasm, rhinorrhea
  Miscellaneous: Unpleasant odor during administration
Drug Interactions May potentiate the effects of nitrates; adsorbed by activated charcoal
(Continued)

35

Acetylcysteine *(Continued)*

Stability Store opened vials in the refrigerator; use within 96 hours; contact with rubber, copper, iron, and cork may inactivate the drug; the light purple color of solution does **not** affect its activity

Mechanism of Action Exerts mucolytic action through its free sulfhydryl group which opens up the disulfide bonds in the mucoproteins thus lowering the viscosity. The exact mechanism of action in acetaminophen toxicity is unknown. It may act by maintaining or restoring glutathione levels or by acting as an alternative substrate for conjugation with the toxic metabolite.

Pharmacodynamics

Onset of action: Upon inhalation, mucus liquefaction occurs maximally within 5-10 minutes

Duration of mucus liquefaction: More than 1 hour

Pharmacokinetics

Protein binding: ~50%

Half-life:

Reduced acetylcysteine: 2 hours

Total acetylcysteine: 5.5 hours

Time to peak serum concentration: 1-2 hours

Usual Dosage

Acetaminophen poisoning: Children and Adults: Oral: 140 mg/kg; followed by 17 doses of 70 mg/kg every 4 hours; repeat dose if emesis occurs within 1 hour of administration; therapy should continue until all doses are administered even though the acetaminophen plasma level has dropped below the toxic range

Inhalation:

Infants: 1-2 mL of 20% solution or 2-4 mL of 10% solution until nebulized, given 3-4 times/day

Children: 3-5 mL of 20% solution or 6-10 mL of 10% solution until nebulized, given 3-4 times/day

Adolescents: 5-10 mL of 10% to 20% solution until nebulized, given 3-4 times/day

Note: Patients should receive an aerosolized bronchodilator 10-15 minutes prior to acetylcysteine

Intratracheal: Children and Adults: 1-2 mL of 10% to 20% solution every 1-4 hours as needed

Meconium ileus equivalent: Children and Adults (varying regimens have been reported): Oral, Rectal Irrigation: 5-30 mL of 10% to 20% solution 3-6 times/day for at least 24 hours and symptom improvement

Administration

Oral: For treatment of acetaminophen overdosage, administer as a 5% solution; dilute the 20% solution 1:3 with a cola, orange juice, or other soft drink; use within 1 hour of preparation

Oral inhalation: May be administered either undiluted (both 10% and 20%) or diluted in NS

Monitoring Parameters When used in acetaminophen overdose, determine acetaminophen level as soon as possible, but no sooner than 4 hours after ingestion (to ensure peak levels have been obtained) (see Acetaminophen Serum Level Nomogram *on page 1237* in the appendix); liver function tests

Patient Information Clear airway by coughing deeply before aerosol treatment

Nursing Implications Assess patient for nausea, vomiting, and skin rash following oral administration for treatment of acetaminophen poisoning; intermittent aerosol treatments are commonly given when patient arises, before meals, and just before retiring at bedtime

Additional Information I.V. route is investigational in the U.S.; contact a poison control center for more information

Dosage Forms Solution, as sodium: 10% [100 mg/mL] (4 mL, 10 mL, 30 mL); 20% [200 mg/mL] (4 mL, 10 mL, 30 mL, 100 mL)

References

Hanly JG and Fitzgerald MX, "Meconium Ileus Equivalent in Older Patients With Cystic Fibrosis," *Br Med J (Clin Res Ed)*, 1983, 286(6375):1411-3.

Walson PD and Groth JF Jr, "Acetaminophen Hepatotoxicity After Prolonged Ingestion," *Pediatrics*, 1993, 91(5):1021-2.

- ◆ **Acetylsalicylic Acid** *see* Aspirin *on page 109*
- ◆ **Aciclovir** *see* Acyclovir *on page 37*
- ◆ **Acid Control (Can)** *see* Famotidine *on page 417*
- ◆ **Acid Halt (Can)** *see* Famotidine *on page 417*
- ◆ **Acid Mantle® [OTC]** *see* Aluminum Acetate *on page 62*
- ◆ **Acilac (Can)** *see* Lactulose *on page 571*

- ◆ **Acnex (Can)** see Salicylic Acid on page 886
- ◆ **ACT** see Dactinomycin on page 294
- ◆ **ACT**® **[OTC]** see Fluoride on page 441
- ◆ **Act-D** see Dactinomycin on page 294
- ◆ **ACTH** see Corticotropin on page 267
- ◆ **Acti-B₁₂ (Can)** see Hydroxocobalamin on page 512
- ◆ **Actidose-Aqua**® **[OTC]** see Charcoal on page 213
- ◆ **Actidose**® **With Sorbitol [OTC]** see Charcoal on page 213
- ◆ **Actifed**® **Cold and Allergy [OTC]** see Triprolidine and Pseudoephedrine on page 989
- ◆ **Actigall**™ see Ursodiol on page 996
- ◆ **Actinomycin D** see Dactinomycin on page 294
- ◆ **Action (Can)** see Ascorbic Acid on page 106
- ◆ **Actiq**® see Fentanyl on page 422
- ◆ **Activase**® see Alteplase on page 58
- ◆ **Activated Carbon** see Charcoal on page 213
- ◆ **Activated Charcoal** see Charcoal on page 213
- ◆ **Activated Dimethicone** see Simethicone on page 902
- ◆ **Activated Ergosterol** see Ergocalciferol on page 392
- ◆ **Activated Methylpolysiloxane** see Simethicone on page 902
- ◆ **Acular**® see Ketorolac on page 565
- ◆ **Acular**® **P.F.** see Ketorolac on page 565
- ◆ **ACV** see Acyclovir on page 37
- ◆ **Acycloguanosine** see Acyclovir on page 37

Acyclovir (ay SYE kloe veer)

Related Information
  Carbohydrate and Alcohol Content of Liquid Medications for Use in Patients Receiving Ketogenic Diets on page 1258

U.S. Brand Names Zovirax®

Canadian Brand Names Apo-Acyclovir; Avirax; Nu-Acyclovir

Synonyms Aciclovir; ACV; Acycloguanosine

Therapeutic Category Antiviral Agent, Oral; Antiviral Agent, Parenteral; Antiviral Agent, Topical

Generic Available Yes; Capsule

Use Treatment of initial and prophylaxis of recurrent mucosal and cutaneous herpes simplex (HSV 1 and HSV 2) infections; herpes simplex encephalitis; herpes zoster infections; varicella-zoster infections in healthy, nonpregnant persons >13 years of age, children >12 months of age who have a chronic skin or lung disorder or are receiving long-term aspirin therapy, and immunocompromised patients

Pregnancy Risk Factor C

Contraindications Hypersensitivity to acyclovir, valacyclovir, or any component

Warnings HSV and VZV with reduced susceptibility to acyclovir have been isolated from immunocompromised patients, especially with advanced HIV infection; renal failure, in some cases resulting in death, has occurred with acyclovir

Precautions Use with caution in patients with renal disease, dehydration, underlying neurologic disease, and in patients with hypoxia, hepatic, or electrolyte abnormalities; dosage should be reduced in patients with renal impairment

Adverse Reactions
  Central nervous system: Headache, lethargy, delirium, coma, dizziness, seizures, pain, insomnia, fever, hallucinations
  Dermatologic: Skin rash, pruritus, alopecia, erythema multiforme, urticaria, photosensitivity, Stevens-Johnson syndrome
  Gastrointestinal: Nausea, vomiting, diarrhea
  Hematologic: Bone marrow suppression, thrombotic thrombocytopenic purpura/hemolytic uremic syndrome
  Hepatic: Elevated liver enzymes, hepatitis, jaundice
  Local: Phlebitis at injection site, local pain and stinging with topical use
  Neuromuscular & skeletal: Tremulousness, myalgia, paresthesia
  Renal: Nephrotoxicity, hematuria, elevated BUN and serum creatinine
  Respiratory: Sore throat
  Miscellaneous: Diaphoresis, anaphylaxis

Drug Interactions Zidovudine (neurotoxicity); probenecid decreases renal clearance of acyclovir

Food Interactions Food does not appear to affect absorption

  (Continued)

Acyclovir *(Continued)*

Stability Incompatible with blood products and protein-containing solutions; reconstituted 50 mg/mL solution should be used within 12 hours; do not refrigerate reconstituted solutions as they may precipitate

Mechanism of Action Inhibits DNA synthesis and viral replication by competing with deoxyguanosine triphosphate for viral DNA polymerase and by incorporation into viral DNA

Pharmacokinetics

Absorption: Oral: 15% to 30%

Distribution: Widely distributed throughout the body including brain, kidney, lungs, liver, spleen, muscle, uterus, vagina, and the CSF; CSF acyclovir concentration is 50% of serum concentration; crosses the placenta; excreted into breast milk; V_d:

Neonates to 3 months of age: 28.8 L/1.73 m^2

Children 1-2 years: 31.6 L/1.73 m^2

Children 2-7 years: 42 L/1.73 m^2

Protein binding: <30%

Half-life, terminal phase:

Neonates: 4 hours

Children 1-12 years: 2-3 hours

Adults: 2-3.5 hours (with normal renal function)

Time to peak serum concentration: Oral: Within 1.5-2 hours

Elimination: Primary route is the kidney with 30% to 90% of a dose excreted unchanged in the urine; requires dosage adjustment with renal impairment; hemodialysis removes ~60% of a dose while removal by peritoneal dialysis is to a much lesser extent; supplemental dose recommended after hemodialysis

Usual Dosage

Children and Adults: Oral:

Genital herpes simplex virus (HSV), first infection: 1000 mg/day in 5 divided doses **or** 1200 mg/day in 3 divided doses for 7-10 days; maximum dose in children: 80 mg/kg/day in 3-5 divided doses

Genital HSV infection recurrence: 1000 mg/day in 5 divided doses **or** 1200 mg/day in 3 divided doses or 1600 mg/day in 2 divided doses for 5 days; maximum dose in children: 80 mg/kg/day in 2-5 divided doses

Recurrent genital HSV: Chronic suppressive therapy for frequent recurrences: 800-1000 mg/day in 2-5 divided doses; maximum dose in children: 80 mg/kg/day in 2-5 divided doses

HSV in immunocompromised host: 1000 mg/day in 3-5 divided doses for 7-14 days; maximum dose in children: 80 mg/kg/day in 3-5 divided doses

Prophylaxis of HSV in immunocompromised HSV-seropositive patient: 600-1000 mg/day in 3-5 divided doses during risk period; maximum dose in children: 80 mg/kg/day in 3-5 divided doses

Zoster in immunocompetent host: 4000 mg/day in 5 divided doses for 5-7 days; maximum dose in children: 80 mg/kg/day in 5 divided doses

Herpes zoster in immunocompromised patients:

Children: 250-600 mg/m^2/dose 4-5 times/day

Adults: 800 mg every 4 hours (5 times/day) for 7-10 days; prophylaxis: 400 mg 5 times/day

Varicella zoster (chickenpox) in immunocompetent host: 80 mg/kg/day in 4 divided doses for 5 days; maximum daily dose: 3200 mg/day; start treatment within the first 24 hours of rash onset

Prophylaxis of CMV infection in immunocompromised host: 800-3200 mg/day in 1-4 divided doses during risk period; maximum dose in children: 80 mg/kg/day in 3-4 divided doses

Premature neonates: HSV infection: I.V.: 20 mg/kg/day divided every 12 hours for 14-21 days

Neonates: HSV infection: I.V.: 1500 mg/m^2/day divided every 8 hours **or** 30 mg/kg/day divided every 8 hours for 14-21 days. Doses as high as 45-60 mg/kg/day divided every 8 hours have been used in term infants with normal renal function.

Children and Adults: I.V. (dosage for obese patients should be based on ideal body weight):

HSV infection: 750 mg/m^2/day divided every 8 hours **or** 15 mg/kg/day divided every 8 hours for 5-7 days

HSV in immunocompromised host:

Children <1 year: 15-30 mg/kg/day divided every 8 hours for 7-14 days

Children ≥1 year: 750-1500 mg/m^2/day divided every 8 hours or 15-30 mg/kg/day divided every 8 hours for 7-14 days

Prophylaxis of HSV in immunocompromised HSV-seropositive patients: 750 mg/ m^2/day divided every 8 hours during risk period

HSV encephalitis: 1500 mg/m^2/day divided every 8 hours **or** 30 mg/kg/day divided every 8 hours for 14-21 days

Varicella or zoster in immunocompromised host or zoster in immunocompetent host:

Children <1 year (some experts also recommend this dose for children ≥1 year): 30 mg/kg/day divided every 8 hours for 7-10 days

Children ≥1 year: 1500 mg/m^2/day divided every 8 hours or 30 mg/kg/day divided every 8 hours for 7-10 days

Prophylaxis of CMV infection in immunocompromised host: 1500 mg/m^2 /day divided every 8 hours during risk period

Prophylaxis of bone marrow transplant recipients:

Autologous patients who are HSV-seropositive: 250 mg/m^2/dose every 8 hours

Autologous patients who are CMV seropositive: 500 mg/m^2/dose every 8 hours; for clinically symptomatic CMV infection, consider replacing acyclovir with ganciclovir

Children and Adults: Topical: Apply ½" ribbon of ointment for a 4" square surface area every 3 hours (6 times/day) for 7 days

Dosing interval in renal impairment: Children ≥6 months and Adults:

Oral:

Usual Dose	Creatinine Clearance	Adjusted Dose
200 mg 5 times/day	Cl$_{cr}$ <10 mL/minute	Administer 200 mg q12h
800 mg 5 times/day	Cl$_{cr}$ 10-25 mL/minute	Administer 800 mg q8h
800 mg 5 times/day	Cl$_{cr}$ <10 mL/minute	Administer 800 mg q12h

I.V.:

Cl$_{cr}$ 25-50 mL/minute: Administer normal dose every 12 hours

Cl$_{cr}$ 10-25 mL/minute: Administer normal dose every 24 hours

Cl$_{cr}$ <10 mL/minute: 50% decrease in dose, administer every 24 hours

Administration

Oral: May administer with food; shake suspension well before use

Parenteral: Reconstitute vial for injection with paraben-free sterile water; administer by slow I.V. infusion over at least 1 hour at a final concentration not to exceed 7 mg/mL since rapid infusions can cause nephrotoxicity with crystalluria and renal tubular damage; in patients who require fluid restriction, a concentration of up to 10 mg/mL has been infused; concentration >10 mg/mL increases the risk of phlebitis

Monitoring Parameters Urinalysis, BUN, serum creatinine, I & O; liver enzymes, CBC

Nursing Implications Maintain adequate hydration and urine output the first 2 hours after I.V. infusion to decrease the risk of nephrotoxicity; check infusion site for phlebitis

Additional Information Sodium content of 1 g: 4.2 mEq

Dosage Forms

Capsule: 200 mg

Injection: 500 mg (10 mL); 1000 mg (20 mL)

Ointment, topical: 5% (3 g, 15 g)

Suspension, oral: 200 mg/5 mL [banana flavor] (473 mL)

Tablet: 400 mg, 800 mg

References

American Academy of Pediatrics Committee on Infectious Diseases, "The Use of Oral Acyclovir in Otherwise Healthy Children With Varicella," *Pediatrics*, 1993, 91(3):674-6.

Dunkle LM, Arvin AM, Whitley RJ, et al, "A Controlled Trial of Acyclovir for Chickenpox in Normal Children," *N Engl J Med*, 1991, 325(22):1539-44.

Englund JA, Fletcher CV, and Balfour HH Jr, "Acyclovir Therapy in Neonates," *J Pediatr*, 1991, 119(1 Pt 1):129-35.

Meyers JD, Reed EC, Shepp DH, et al, "Acyclovir for Prevention of Cytomegalovirus Infection and Disease After Allogenic Marrow Transplantation," *N Engl J Med*, 1988, 318(2):70-5.

Novelli VM, Marshall WC, Yeo J, et al, "High-Dose Oral Acyclovir for Children at Risk of Disseminated Herpes Virus Infections," *J Infect Dis*, 1985, 151(2):372.

♦ **Adalat® CC** *see* Nifedipine *on page 714*

♦ **Adalat PA (Can)** *see* Nifedipine *on page 714*

♦ **Adamantanamine** *see* Amantadine *on page 62*

♦ **Adderall®** *see* Dextroamphetamine and Amphetamine *on page 314*

♦ **Adek®** *see page 1069*

♦ **Adenine Arabinoside** *see* Vidarabine *on page 1009*

♦ **Adenocard®** *see* Adenosine *on page 40*

Adenosine (a DEN oh seen)

Related Information

Adult ACLS Algorithm, Narrow-Complex Supraventricular Tachycardia *on page 1046*
Adult ACLS Algorithm, Tachycardia Overview *on page 1045*
CPR Pediatric Drug Dosages *on page 1031*
Pediatric ALS Algorithm, Tachycardia - Rapid Rhythm and Adequate Perfusion *on page 1037*
Pediatric ALS Algorithm, Tachycardia - Rapid Rhythm and Evidence of Poor Perfusion *on page 1038*

U.S. Brand Names Adenocard®

Synonyms 9-Beta-D-ribofuranosyladenine

Therapeutic Category Antiarrhythmic Agent, Miscellaneous

Generic Available No

Use Treatment of paroxysmal supraventricular tachycardia (PSVT); used in adult ACLS algorithms for narrow-complex tachycardias, stable narrow-complex supraventricular tachycardias, and wide-complex tachycardias that are supraventricular in origin; used in PALS algorithms for probable supraventricular tachycardia; investigationally used as a continuous infusion for the treatment of primary pulmonary hypertension in adults and persistent pulmonary hypertension of the newborn (see Konduri, 1996)

Pregnancy Risk Factor C

Contraindications Hypersensitivity to adenosine or any component; second and third degree A-V block or sick sinus syndrome unless pacemaker placed

Warnings Heart block, including transient or prolonged asystole may occur as well as other arrhythmias; episodes of asystole or other arrhythmias may be fatal; if arrhythmia is not due to re-entry pathway through A-V node or sinus node (ie, atrial fibrillation, flutter, or tachycardia or ventricular tachycardia), adenosine will not terminate the arrhythmia but can produce transient ventriculoatrial or A-V block; possible mutagenic effects

Precautions Bronchoconstriction may occur in patients with bronchospasm or bronchoconstriction); use with caution in patients with underlying dysfunction of sinus or A-V node, obstructive lung disease, and those taking digoxin or verapamil; initial adenosine dose should be significantly decreased in patients receiving dipyridamole

Adverse Reactions

Cardiovascular: Flushing, arrhythmias, palpitations, chest pain, bradycardia, heart block, minimal hemodynamic disturbances, hypotension (<1%)
Central nervous system: Irritability, headaches, lightheadedness, dizziness
Gastrointestinal: Nausea, metallic taste
Respiratory: Dyspnea, hyperventilation, bronchoconstriction in asthmatics

Drug Interactions Dipyridamole potentiates effects of adenosine (dose of adenosine should be significantly reduced); methylxanthines (aminophylline, theophylline, caffeine) antagonize adenosine's effects so that larger doses of adenosine or an alternative agent may be required; carbamazepine may increase heart block; digoxin and verapamil may cause ventricular fibrillation (rare cases reported)

Stability Do **not** refrigerate, precipitation may occur; contains no preservatives, discard unused portion

Mechanism of Action Slows conduction time through the A-V node, interrupting the re-entry pathways through the A-V node, restoring normal sinus rhythm

Pharmacodynamics

Onset of action: Rapid
Duration: Very brief

Pharmacokinetics

Metabolism: Removed from systemic circulation primarily by vascular endothelial cells and erythrocytes (by cellular uptake); rapidly metabolized intracellularly; phosphorylated by adenosine kinase to adenosine monophosphate (AMP) which is then incorporated into high-energy pool; intracellular adenosine is also deaminated by adenosine deaminase to inosine; inosine can be metabolized to hypoxanthine, then xanthine and finally to uric acid.
Half-life: <10 seconds

Usual Dosage Note: Adequate controlled studies in pediatric patients have not been conducted.

Manufacturer's recommendations: Rapid I.V.:
Neonates, Infants, Children, and Adolescents weighing <50 kg: Initial dose: 0.05-0.1 mg/kg; if not effective within 1-2 minutes, increase dose by 0.05-0.1 mg/kg increments every 1-2 minutes to a maximum single dose of 0.3 mg/kg or until termination of PSVT

Children and Adolescents weighing ≥50 kg and Adults: 6 mg, if not effective within 1-2 minutes, 12 mg may be given; may repeat 12 mg bolus if needed

Alternative pediatric dosing:

Neonates: Rapid I.V.: Initial dose: 0.05 mg/kg; if not effective within 2 minutes, increase dose by 0.05 mg/kg increments every 2 minutes to a maximum dose of 0.25 mg/kg or until termination of PSVT

Infants and Children: **PALS dose for treatment of SVT**: Rapid I.V.; I.O.: Initial: 0.1 mg/kg (maximum: 6 mg); if not effective, give 0.2 mg/kg (maximum: 12 mg)

Administration Parenteral: For rapid bolus I.V. use, administer over 1-2 seconds at peripheral I.V. site closest to patient's heart; follow each bolus with NS flush (infants and children: 5-10 mL; adults: 20 mL); if given peripherally in adults, elevate the extremity for 10-20 seconds after the NS flush. To administer doses <600 mcg (0.2 mL of commercial product), a dilution with NS (final concentration: 300 mcg/mL) may be made. **Note:** Preliminary results in adults suggest adenosine may be administered via a **central line** at lower doses (eg, Adults: Initial dose: 3 mg); FDA approved labeling for pediatric patients weighing <50 kg states that doses listed may be administered either peripherally or centrally (further studies are needed)

Monitoring Parameters Continuous EKG, heart rate, blood pressure, respirations

Nursing Implications Be alert for dyspnea, shortness of breath, and possible exacerbation of asthma

Additional Information Not effective in atrial flutter, atrial fibrillation, or ventricular tachycardia; short action an advantage as adverse effects are usually rapidly self-limiting; effects may be prolonged in patients with denervated transplanted hearts. Individualize treatment of prolonged adverse effects: Give I.V. fluids for hypotension, aminophylline/theophylline may antagonize effects.

Adenosine is also available as Adenoscan®, which is used in adults as an adjunct to thallium-201 myocardial perfusion scintigraphy; see package insert for further information for this use.

Dosage Forms Injection, preservative free: 3 mg/mL (2 mL, 4 mL)

References

Eubanks AP and Artman M, "Administration of Adenosine to a Newborn of 26 Weeks' Gestation," *Pediatr Cardiol*, 1994, 15(3):157-8.

"Guidelines 2000 for Cardiopulmonary Resuscitation and Emergency Cardiovascular Care, Part 6: Advanced Cardiovascular Life Support, The American Heart Association in Collaboration With the International Liaison Committee on Resuscitation," *Circulation*, 2000, 102(8 Suppl):I86-171.

"Guidelines 2000 for Cardiopulmonary Resuscitation and Emergency Cardiovascular Care, Part 10: Pediatric Advanced Life Support, The American Heart Association in Collaboration With the International Liaison Committee on Resuscitation," *Circulation*, 2000, 102(8 Suppl): I291-342.

Konduri GG, Garcia DC, Kazzi NJ, et al, "Adenosine Infusion Improves Oxygenation in Term Infants With Respiratory Failure," *Pediatrics*, 1996, 97(3):295-300.

McIntosh-Yellin NL, Drew BJ, and Scheinman MM, "Safety and Efficacy of Central Intravenous Bolus Administration of Adenosine for Termination of Supraventricular Tachycardia," *J Am Coll Cardiol*, 1993, 22(3):741-5.

Till J, Shinebourne EA, Rigby ML, et al, "Efficacy and Safety in the Treatment of Supraventricular Tachycardia in Infants and Children," *Br Heart J*, 1989, 62(3):204-11.

Zeigler V, "Adenosine in the Pediatric Population: Nursing Implications," *Pediatr Nurs*, 1991, 17(6):600-2.

♦ **Advanced Formula Oxy® Sensitive Gel [OTC]** *see* Benzoyl Peroxide *on page 136*

♦ **Advil® [OTC]** *see* Ibuprofen *on page 520*

♦ **Advil® Migraine [OTC]** *see* Ibuprofen *on page 520*

♦ **AeroBid®** *see* Flunisolide *on page 438*

♦ **AeroBid®-M** *see* Flunisolide *on page 438*

♦ **Aerolate III®** *see* Theophylline *on page 943*

♦ **Aerolate® JR** *see* Theophylline *on page 943*

♦ **Aerolate® SR** *see* Theophylline *on page 943*

♦ **Aerosporin® Injection** *see* Polymyxin B *on page 812*

♦ **Afrin® [OTC]** *see* Oxymetazoline *on page 749*

♦ **Afrin® Extra Moisturizing [OTC]** *see* Oxymetazoline *on page 749*

♦ **Afrin® Saline Mist [OTC]** *see* Sodium Chloride *on page 906*

♦ **Afrin® Sinus [OTC]** *see* Oxymetazoline *on page 749*

♦ **Afrin® with Menthol [OTC]** *see* Oxymetazoline *on page 749*

♦ **Aftate® [OTC]** *see* Tolnaftate *on page 969*

♦ **Afterburn (Can)** *see* Lidocaine *on page 590*

♦ **Agenerase™** *see* Amprenavir *on page 91*

♦ **Agoral® Plain [OTC]** *see* Mineral Oil *on page 675*

♦ **AHF** *see* Antihemophilic Factor (Human) *on page 98*

♦ **AHG** *see* Antihemophilic Factor (Human) *on page 98*

♦ **A-hydroCort®** *see* Hydrocortisone *on page 506*

♦ **Airet®** *see* Albuterol *on page 45*

♦ **Airomir (Can)** *see* Albuterol *on page 45*

♦ **AKBeta®** *see* Levobunolol *on page 584*

♦ **Ak-Chlor (Can)** *see* Chloramphenicol *on page 218*

♦ **AK-Con®** *see* Naphazoline *on page 698*

♦ **AK-Dex®** *see* Dexamethasone *on page 307*

♦ **AK-Dilate®** *see* Phenylephrine *on page 789*

♦ **AK-Mycin®** *see* Erythromycin *on page 394*

♦ **AK-NaCl® [OTC]** *see* Sodium Chloride *on page 906*

♦ **AK-Nefrin®** *see* Phenylephrine *on page 789*

♦ **Akne-Mycin®** *see* Erythromycin *on page 394*

♦ **AK-Pentolate®** *see* Cyclopentolate *on page 279*

♦ **AK-Poly-Bac® Ophthalmic** *see* Bacitracin and Polymyxin B *on page 129*

♦ **AK-Pred®** *see* Prednisolone *on page 821*

♦ **AK-Spore H.C.® Otic** *see* Neomycin, (Bacitracin) Polymyxin B, and Hydrocortisone *on page 705*

♦ **AK-Spore® Ointment** *see* Neomycin, Polymyxin B, and Bacitracin *on page 707*

♦ **AK-Sulf®** *see* Sulfacetamide *on page 922*

♦ **Ak-Tate (Can)** *see* Prednisolone *on page 821*

♦ **AK-T-Caine™** *see* Tetracaine *on page 940*

♦ **AKTob®** *see* Tobramycin *on page 963*

♦ **AK-Tracin®** *see* Bacitracin *on page 127*

♦ **AK-Trol®** *see* Dexamethasone, Neomycin, and Polymyxin B *on page 309*

♦ **Ala-Cort®** *see* Hydrocortisone *on page 506*

♦ **Ala-Scalp®** *see* Hydrocortisone *on page 506*

♦ **Albalon® Liquifilm®** *see* Naphazoline *on page 698*

Albendazole (al BEN da zole)

Therapeutic Category Anthelmintic

Generic Available No

Use Treatment of parenchymal neurocysticercosis due to active lesions caused by larval forms of *Taenia solium*; treatment of cystic hydatid disease of the liver, lung, and peritoneum caused by the larval form of *Echinococcus granulosus*; active against *Ascaris lumbricoides* (roundworm), *Ancylostoma duodenale* and *Necator americanus* (hookworm), *Enterobius vermicularis* (pinworm), *Clonorchis sinensis* (Chinese liver fluke), *Trichuris trichiura* (whipworm), and *Capillaria philippinensis*

Pregnancy Risk Factor C

Contraindications Hypersensitivity to albendazole, any component, or the benzimidazole class of compounds

Warnings Fatalities due to granulocytopenia or pancytopenia associated with the use of albendazole have been reported; women of childbearing age should only begin treatment after a negative pregnancy test and should be cautioned against becoming pregnant during and for at least one month after treatment cessation with albendazole since it may cause harm to fetus.

Precautions Use with caution in patients with hepatic impairment or decreased total leukocyte count; discontinue albendazole if significant elevation of liver function tests occur; may restart therapy when LFT decreases to pretreatment values; corticosteroids should be administered 1-2 days before initiating albendazole therapy in patients with neurocysticercosis to minimize inflammatory reactions and should be followed by concurrent steroid and anticonvulsant therapy for the first week of therapy to prevent cerebral hypertension. Albendazole may induce further retinal damage in patients having retinal lesions with neurocysticercosis.

Adverse Reactions
Central nervous system: Headache, dizziness, vertigo, increased intracranial pressure, meningeal signs, fever, seizures
Dermatologic: Rash, urticaria, alopecia
Gastrointestinal: Abdominal pain, nausea, vomiting
Hematologic: Leukopenia, pancytopenia, thrombocytopenia, granulocytopenia, agranulocytosis
Hepatic: Elevated liver function tests
Renal: Acute renal failure
Miscellaneous: Hypersensitivity reactions, migration of *Ascaris* through mouth and nose

Drug Interactions Cytochrome P-450 isoenzyme CYP1A2 inducer; isoenzyme CYP1A2 substrate (minor) and CYP3A4 substrate (major)
Dexamethasone, cimetidine, and praziquantel increase albendazole sulfoxide (active metabolite) concentration

Food Interactions Bioavailability is increased when taken with a fatty meal

Stability Store at room temperature

Mechanism of Action Binds to β-tubulin in parasite cells inhibiting tubulin polymerization which results in the loss of cytoplasmic microtubules and inhibition of glucose uptake

Pharmacokinetics
Absorption: Poorly absorbed from the GI tract
Distribution: Widely distributed throughout the body including urine, bile, liver, cyst wall, cyst fluid, and CSF
Protein binding: 70%
Metabolism: Extensive first-pass metabolism; hepatic metabolism to albendazole sulfoxide, an active metabolite
Half-life: Albendazole sulfoxide: 8-12 hours
Time to peak serum concentrations: 2-5 hours for the metabolite
Elimination: Biliary

Usual Dosage Children and Adults: Oral:
Neurocysticercosis: (patients should receive appropriate corticosteroid and anticonvulsant therapy as required):
<60kg: 15 mg/kg/day in 2 divided doses (maximum: 800 mg/day) for 8-30 days
≥60kg: 400 mg twice daily for 8-30 days
Hydatid disease:
<60kg: 15 mg/kg/day in 2 divided doses (maximum: 800 mg/day) for 1-6 months
≥60kg: 400 mg twice daily for 1-6 months
Ancylostoma caninum, ascariasis (roundworm), hookworm, trichuriasis (whipworm): 400 mg as a single dose
Capillariasis: 400 mg once daily for 10 days
Clonorchis sinensis (Chinese liver fluke): 10 mg/kg/day once daily for 7 days
Cutaneous larva migrans: 400 mg once daily for 3 days
Enterobius vermicularis (pinworm): 400 mg as a single dose; repeat in 2 weeks
Filariasis (*Mansonella perstans*): 400 mg twice daily for 10 days
Trichinosis (*Trichinella spiralis*): 400 mg twice daily for 8-14 days
Visceral larva migrans: 400 mg twice daily for 5 days

Administration Oral: Administer with food

Monitoring Parameters Monitor liver function tests, CBC at start of each cycle and every 2 weeks during therapy

Dosage Forms Tablet: 200 mg

References
Baranwal AK, Singhi PD, Khandelwal N, et al, "Albendazole Therapy in Children With Focal Seizures and Single Small Enhancing Computerized Tomographic Lesions: A Randomized, Placebo-Controlled, Double Blind Trial," *Pediatr Infect Dis J*, 1998, 17(8):696-700.
Jung H, Sanchez M, Gonzalez-Astiazaran A, et al, "Clinical Pharmacokinetics of Albendazole in Children With Neurocysticercosis," *Am J Ther*, 1997, 4(1):23-6.
Paul I, Gnanamani G, and Nallam NR, "Intestinal Helminth Infections Among School Children in Visakhapatnam," *Indian J Pediatr*, 1999, 66(5):669-73.
(Continued)

Albendazole *(Continued)*

Pengsaa K, Sirivichayakul C, Pojjaroen-anant C, et al, "Albendazole Treatment for *Giardia intestinalis* Infections in School Children," *Southeast Asian J Trop Med Public Health*, 1999, 30(1):78-83.

- ◆ **Albert Docusate (Can)** *see* Docusate *on page 350*
- ◆ **Albert Glyburide (Can)** *see* Glyburide *on page 476*
- ◆ **Albert Oxybutynin (Can)** *see* Oxybutynin *on page 744*
- ◆ **Albert Pentoxifylline (Can)** *see* Pentoxifylline *on page 781*

Albumin *(al BYOO min)*

U.S. Brand Names Albuminar®; Albutein®; Buminate®; Plasbumin®

Synonyms Albumin Human; Normal Human Serum Albumin; Normal Serum Albumin (Human); Salt Poor Albumin

Therapeutic Category Blood Product Derivative; Plasma Volume Expander

Generic Available Yes

Use Treatment of hypovolemia; plasma volume expansion and maintenance of cardiac output in the treatment of certain types of shock or impending shock; hypoproteinemia resulting in generalized edema or decreased intravascular volume (eg, hypoproteinemia associated with acute nephrotic syndrome, premature neonates)

> **Note:** PALS and Neonatal Resuscitation 2000 Guidelines recommend isotonic crystalloid solutions (eg, NS or LR) as initial volume expansion; albumin is used less frequently due to limited supply, potential risk of infections, and an association with an increase in mortality (identified by meta-analyses); few studies in these analyses included children, so no firm conclusions in pediatric patients can be made

Pregnancy Risk Factor C

Contraindications Patients with severe anemia or cardiac failure; hypersensitivity to albumin or any component

Warnings Avoid 25% concentration in preterm neonates due to risk of IVH

Precautions Rapid infusion of albumin solutions may cause vascular overload. Do not administer albumin to burn patients for the first 24 hours after the burn (capillary exudation of albumin will occur); use with caution in patients with hepatic or renal failure (added protein load) and in patients who require sodium restriction; monitor for signs of hypervolemia

> Due to the occasional shortage of 5% human albumin, 5% solutions may at times be prepared by diluting 25% human albumin with NS or with D_5W (if sodium load is a concern); however, **do not use sterile water** to dilute albumin solutions, as this may result in hypotonic-associated hemolysis which can be fatal

Adverse Reactions

Cardiovascular: Precipitation of CHF or pulmonary edema, hypertension, tachycardia, hypervolemia, hypotension due to hypersensitivity reaction

Central nervous system: Fever, chills

Dermatologic: Rash

Gastrointestinal: Nausea, vomiting

Stability Use within 4 hours after opening vial, do not use if turbid or contains a deposit; do not use sterile water to dilute albumin (see Precautions)

Mechanism of Action Provides increase in intravascular oncotic pressure and causes mobilization of fluids from interstitial into intravascular space

Pharmacodynamics Duration of volume expansion: ~24 hours

Pharmacokinetics Half-life: 21 days

Usual Dosage 5% should be used in hypovolemic or intravascularly depleted patients; 25% should be used in patients with fluid or sodium restrictions (eg, patients with hypoproteinemia and generalized edema). Dose depends on condition of patient. I.V.:

Hypoproteinemia: Neonates, Infants, Children: 0.5-1 g/kg/dose; may repeat every 1-2 days; see Administration

Hypovolemia:

Neonates: Usual dose: 0.5 g/kg/dose (10 mL/kg/dose of 5% albumin); range: 0.25-0.5 g/kg/dose (5-10 mL/kg/dose of 5% albumin)

Infants and Children: 0.5-1 g/kg/dose (10-20 mL/kg/dose of 5% albumin); may repeat as needed; maximum dose: 6 g/kg/day (120 mL/kg/day of 5% albumin); see Administration

Adults: 25 g; no more than 250 g should be administered within 48 hours

Administration Parenteral: I.V.:

Albuminar®: May administer via the administration set provided (in-line 60 micron filter) or via any administration set; use of filter is optional; size of filter may vary according to institutional policy. Method of filter sterilization used by manufacturer includes 0.2 micron filter; however, aggregates may form under storage, shipping, and handling. Administration via very small filter will not damage product, but will slow flow rate.

Buminate®: Administer via the administration set provided (in-line 15 micron filter) or via any filtered administration set; use ≥5 micron filter to ensure adequate flow rate

Plasbumin®: May administer with or without an I.V. filter; filter as small as 0.22 microns may be used

Too rapid infusion may result in vascular overload

Hypoproteinemia: Infuse over 2-4 hours; for neonates, dose may be added to hyperalimentation fluid and infused over 24 hours

Hypovolemia: Rate of infusion depends on severity of hypovolemia and patient's symptoms; usually infuse dose over 30-60 minutes (faster infusion rates may be clinically necessary)

Maximum rates of I.V. infusion after initial volume replacement:
5%: 2-4 mL/minute
25%: 1 mL/minute

To prepare 5% albumin from 25%, see Precautions.

Monitoring Parameters Observe for signs of hypervolemia, pulmonary edema, and cardiac failure

Nursing Implications Albumin administration must be completed within 6 hours after entering container, provided that administration is begun within 4 hours of entering the container

Additional Information In certain conditions (eg, hypoproteinemia with generalized edema, nephrotic syndrome), doses of albumin may be followed with I.V. furosemide: 0.5-1 mg/kg/dose. Both 5% and 25% albumin contain 130-160 mEq of sodium/L; osmolarity: 5% albumin = 300 mOsm/L; 25% albumin = 1500 mOsm/L

Dosage Forms Injection, as human: 5% [50 mg/mL] (50 mL, 250 mL, 500 mL, 1000 mL); 25% [250 mg/mL] (10 mL, 20 mL, 50 mL, 100 mL)

References

"Guidelines 2000 for Cardiopulmonary Resuscitation and Emergency Cardiovascular Care, Part 10: Pediatric Advanced Life Support, The American Heart Association in Collaboration With the International Liaison Committee on Resuscitation," *Circulation*, 2000, 102(8 Suppl):I306.

"Guidelines 2000 for Cardiopulmonary Resuscitation and Emergency Cardiovascular Care, Part 11: Neonatal Resuscitation, The American Heart Association in Collaboration With the International Liaison Committee on Resuscitation," *Circulation*, 2000, 102(8 Suppl):I352.

♦ **Albuminar®** *see* Albumin *on page 44*
♦ **Albumin Human** *see* Albumin *on page 44*
♦ **Albutein®** *see* Albumin *on page 44*

Albuterol (al BYOO ter ole)

Related Information

Asthma Guidelines *on page 1210*
Carbohydrate and Alcohol Content of Liquid Medications for Use in Patients Receiving Ketogenic Diets *on page 1258*

U.S. Brand Names Airet®; Proventil®; Proventil® HFA; Ventolin®; Ventolin® Rotocaps®; Volmax®

Canadian Brand Names Airomir; Apo-Salvent; Asmavent; Gen-Salbutamol; Novo-Salmol; Nu-Salbutamol; PMS-Salbutamol; Rhoxal-Salbutamol; Sabulin; Ventodisk

Synonyms Salbutamol

Therapeutic Category Adrenergic Agonist Agent; Antiasthmatic; Beta$_2$-Adrenergic Agonist Agent; Bronchodilator; Sympathomimetic

Generic Available Yes

Use Prevention and relief of bronchospasm in patients with reversible airway obstruction due to asthma or COPD; prevention of exercise-induced bronchospasm

Pregnancy Risk Factor C

Contraindications Hypersensitivity to albuterol, any component, or adrenergic amine

Precautions Use with caution in patients with hyperthyroidism, diabetes mellitus; cardiovascular disorders including coronary insufficiency or hypertension; excessive or prolonged use can lead to tolerance

Adverse Reactions

Cardiovascular: Tachycardia, palpitations, hypertension, chest pain

Central nervous system: Nervousness, CNS stimulation, hyperactivity and insomnia occur more frequently in younger children than adults; dizziness, lightheadedness, drowsiness, headache

Dermatologic: Angioedema, urticaria

Endocrine & metabolic: Hypokalemia

(Continued)

Albuterol (Continued)

Gastrointestinal: GI upset, xerostomia, heartburn, vomiting, nausea, unusual taste, hoarseness (inhalation only)

Genitourinary: Dysuria

Neuromuscular & skeletal: Tremor, weakness, muscle cramping

Respiratory: Irritation of oropharynx, coughing, paradoxical bronchospasm (oral inhalation only)

Miscellaneous: Diaphoresis (increased)

Drug Interactions Action of albuterol is antagonized by beta-adrenergic blocking agents such as propranolol; cardiovascular effects are potentiated in patients also receiving MAO inhibitors or tricyclic antidepressants; concomitant administration of sympathomimetics may result in enhanced cardiovascular effects

Food Interactions Caffeinated beverages may increase side effects of albuterol

Stability Liquid, tablets, Rotocaps®, and oral inhalation solutions are stable at room temperature; Nebules® should be refrigerated, but may be kept at room temperature for 2 weeks; compatible with cromolyn and ipratropium nebulizer solutions

Mechanism of Action Relaxes bronchial smooth muscle by action on beta$_2$-receptors with little effect on heart rate

Pharmacodynamics

Nebulization/oral inhalation:
  Peak bronchodilation: Within 0.5-2 hours nebulization
  Duration: 2-5 hours
Oral:
  Peak bronchodilatation: 2-3 hours
  Duration: 4-6 hours
Extended release tablets: Duration: Up to 12 hours

Pharmacokinetics

Metabolism: By the liver to an inactive sulfate
Half-life:
  Oral: 2.7-5 hours
  Inhalation: 3.8 hours
Elimination: 30% appears in urine as unchanged drug

Usual Dosage

Oral:
  Children 2-6 years: 0.1-0.2 mg/kg/dose 3 times/day; maximum dose not to exceed 4 mg 3 times/day
  Children 6-12 years: 2 mg/dose 3-4 times/day; Repetabs®: 4 mg 2 times/day (maximum daily dosage: 24 mg)
  Children >12 years to Adults: 2-4 mg/dose 3-4 times/day; Repetabs®: 4-8 mg 2 times/day (maximum daily dosage: 32 mg)
Inhalation: MDI: 90 mcg/spray:
  Children <12 years: 1-2 inhalations 4 times/day
  Children ≥12 years to Adults: 1-2 inhalations every 4-6 hours; maximum 12 inhalations/day
Exercise-induced bronchospasm: Children ≥12 years to Adults: 2 inhalations 30 minutes before exercising
Inhalation: Children and Adults: Nebulization: See dosage table; administer every 4-6 hours

Albuterol Nebulization Dosage

Age	Dose (by weight)	0.5% Solution (mL/kg)	0.083% Solution (mL/kg)
Children <12 y	0.15-0.25 mg/kg (maximum: 5 mg)*	0.01-0.05 (maximum: 1 mL)*	0.06-0.3 (maximum 6 mL)*
Children 12 y - Adults	2.5 mg	0.5 mL	3 mL

*Doses >2.5 mg have been associated with a higher frequency of adverse systemic effects.

Intensive care patients may require more frequent administration; continuous nebulized albuterol at 0.3 mg/kg/hour has been used safely in the treatment of severe status asthmaticus in children; continuous nebulized doses of 3 mg/kg/hour ± 2.2 mg/kg/hour (Katz, 1993) in children whose mean age was 20.7 months resulted in no cardiotoxicity; the optimal dosage for continuous nebulization remains to be determined

Oral inhalation (Rotahaler®): Children >4 years and Adults: 200-400 mcg every 4-6 hours

Administration

Inhalation: Nebulization: Using 0.5% solution, dilute dosage in 1-2 mL NS (0.083% solution does not require further dilution); adjust nebulizer flow to deliver dosage over 5-15 minutes

Oral: Administer with food; do not crush or chew extended release tablets (Repetabs® or Volmax®)

Oral inhalation: Prime the inhaler (before first use or if it has not been used for more than 2 weeks) by releasing 4 test sprays into the air away from the face; shake well before use; use spacer for children <8 years of age

Monitoring Parameters Serum potassium, heart rate, pulmonary function tests, respiratory rate; arterial or capillary blood gases (if patient's condition warrants)

Patient Information Do not exceed recommended dosage; rinse mouth with water following each inhalation to help with dry throat and mouth; if more than one inhalation is necessary, wait at least 1 full minute between inhalations; notify physician if palpitations, tachycardia, chest pain, muscle tremors, dizziness, headache, flushing, or if breathing difficulty persists; limit caffeinated beverages

Dosage Forms

Aerosol, as sulfate (Proventil® HFA): 90 mcg/dose [chlorofluorocarbon free] (3.7 g, 6.7 g, 17 g)

Aerosol, oral: 90 mcg/spray [200 inhalations] (17 g)

Capsule, microfine, for inhalation, as sulfate (Rotacaps®): 200 mcg [to be used with Rotahaler® inhalation device]

Solution, inhalation, as sulfate: 0.083% [0.83 mg/mL] (3 mL); 0.5% [5 mg/mL] (20 mL)

Syrup, as sulfate: 2 mg/5 mL [alcohol and sugar free, strawberry flavor] (60 mL, 120 mL, 480 mL)

Tablet, as sulfate: 2 mg, 4 mg

Tablet, extended release, as sulfate:
Proventil®, Repetabs®: 4 mg
Volmax®: 4 mg, 8 mg

References

Katz RW, Kelly HW, Crowley MR, et al, "Safety of Continuous Nebulized Albuterol for Bronchospasm in Infants and Children," *Pediatrics*, 1993, 92(5):666-69.

O'Callaghan C, Milner AD, and Swarbrick A, "Nebulized Salbutamol Does Have a Protective Effect on Airways in Children Under One Year Old," *Arch Dis Child*, 1988, 63(5):479-83.

Papo MC, Frank J, and Thompson AE, "A Prospective, Randomized Study of Continuous Versus Intermittent Nebulized Albuterol for Severe Status Asthmaticus in Children," *Crit Care Med*, 1993, 21(10):1479-86.

Rachelefsky GS and Siegel SC, "Asthma in Infants and Children - Treatment of Childhood Asthma: Part II," *J Allergy Clin Immunol*, 1985, 76(3):409-25.

Schuh S, Parkin P, Rajan A, et al, "High- Versus Low-Dose, Frequently Administered, Nebulized Albuterol in Children With Severe, Acute Asthma," *Pediatrics*, 1989, 83(4):513-8.

Schuh S, Reider MJ, Canny G, et al, "Nebulized Albuterol in Acute Childhood Asthma: Comparison of Two Doses," *Pediatrics*, 1990, 86(4):509-13.

♦ **Alcaine®** *see* Proparacaine *on page 841*

♦ **Alcohol** *see* Ethyl Alcohol *on page 409*

♦ **Alcomicin (Can)** *see* Gentamicin *on page 469*

♦ **Aldactazide®** *see* Hydrochlorothiazide and Spironolactone *on page 504*

♦ **Aldactone®** *see* Spironolactone *on page 911*

Aldesleukin (al des LOO kin)

U.S. Brand Names Proleukin®

Synonyms Epidermal Thymocyte Activating Factor; ETAF; IL-2; Interleukin-2; Lymphocyte Mitogenic Factor; NSC-373364; T-Cell Growth Factor; TCGF; Thymocyte Stimulating Factor

Therapeutic Category Antineoplastic Agent, Miscellaneous; Biological Response Modulator

Generic Available No

Use Treatment of metastatic renal cell carcinoma and metastatic melanoma; for investigational use in tumors known to have a response to immunotherapy such as colorectal cancer and non-Hodgkin's lymphoma (alone or in combination with lymphokine-activated killer cells); investigational treatment of Kaposi's sarcoma in combination with zidovudine and acute myelogenous leukemia (AML)

Pregnancy Risk Factor C

Contraindications Hypersensitivity to aldesleukin or any component; abnormal thallium stress test or pulmonary function tests; organ allografts (due to increased risk of rejection); **retreatment** in patients who have experienced sustained ventricular tachycardia (≥5 beats), cardiac rhythm disturbances not controlled or unresponsive to management, recurrent chest pain with EKG changes (consistent with angina or myocardial infarction), intubation required >72 hours, pericardial tamponade; renal
(Continued)

Aldesleukin *(Continued)*

dysfunction requiring dialysis >72 hours, coma or toxic psychosis lasting >48 hours, repetitive or difficult to control seizures, bowel ischemia/perforation, and GI bleeding requiring surgery

Warnings High-dose aldesleukin therapy is associated with capillary leak syndrome (CLS) resulting in hypotension and reduced organ perfusion (occurring within 2-12 hours after start of treatment) which may be severe and fatal; CLS may be associated with cardiac arrhythmias, angina, MI, respiratory insufficiency requiring intubation, GI bleeding or infarction, renal insufficiency, edema, and mental status changes; therapy should be restricted to patients with normal cardiac and pulmonary functions as defined by thallium stress and formal pulmonary function testing; hold aldesleukin administration in patients developing moderate to severe lethargy or somnolence as continued administration may result in coma; may exacerbate disease symptoms in patients with clinically unrecognized or untreated CNS metastases; thoroughly evaluate and treat all patients with CNS metastases prior to therapy

Precautions Use with extreme caution in patients with normal thallium stress tests and pulmonary functions tests who have a history of prior cardiac or pulmonary disease; intensive aldesleukin treatment is associated with impaired neutrophil function (reduced chemotaxis) and with an increased risk of disseminated infection (particularly with *Staphylococcus aureus*) including sepsis and bacterial endocarditis; patients with indwelling central lines are particularly at increased risk of infection; treat pre-existing bacterial infections prior to initiation of aldesleukin therapy; standard supportive care during high-dose aldesleukin treatment includes acetaminophen to relieve fever and chills and an H_2 antagonist to reduce the risk of GI ulceration and/or bleeding; aldesleukin may exacerbate autoimmune disease; closely monitor for thyroid abnormalities or other potentially autoimmune phenomena; use with caution in patients with known seizure disorders

Adverse Reactions Many adverse effects of aldesleukin are dosage and schedule dependent; greater toxicity occurs with high dose, bolus administration and the least toxicity with low dose, subcutaneous administration

Cardiovascular: Hypotension (dose-limiting, possibly fatal), sinus tachycardia, arrhythmias, edema, angina, MI, CHF, capillary leak syndrome

Central nervous system: Confusion, drowsiness, transient memory loss, dizziness, cognitive changes, fatigue, chills, malaise, somnolence, disorientation, headaches, insomnia, paranoid delusion, seizures, coma, fever, pain

Dermatologic: Macular erythematous rash, pruritus, erythema, exfoliative dermatitis, dry skin, alopecia, petechiae, purpura, vitiligo

Endocrine & metabolic: Hypomagnesemia, hypocalcemia, hypokalemia, hypophosphatemia, hyponatremia, hypoglycemia, hyperglycemia, hypermagnesemia, hypercalcemia, hyperkalemia, hyperphosphatemia, hypernatremia, thyroid dysfunction

Gastrointestinal: Nausea, vomiting, diarrhea, stomatitis, GI bleeding, anorexia, weight gain, pancreatitis

Hematologic: Anemia, thrombocytopenia, leukopenia, eosinophilia

Hepatic: Transient elevations of bilirubin and liver enzymes, jaundice, ascites, decreased clotting factors

Neuromuscular & skeletal: Weakness, rigors, arthralgia, myalgia

Renal: Oliguria, proteinuria, transient increase in BUN, hematuria

Respiratory: Congestion, dyspnea, pleural effusion, pulmonary edema

Miscellaneous: Allergic reactions

Drug Interactions Corticosteroids may decrease efficacy; increased CNS depression when administered concomitantly with other sedating agents; increased toxicity when administered concomitantly with other potentially nephrotoxic, myelotoxic, cardiotoxic, or hepatotoxic agents; increased hypotensive effects with antihypertensives or beta-blocking agents; acute reactions including fever, chills, nausea, vomiting, pruritus, rash, diarrhea, hypotension, edema, and oliguria with iodinated contrast media (may occur within 4 weeks to several months after aldesleukin administration); hypersensitivity reactions have been reported when combined with dacarbazine, cis-platinum, tamoxifen, and interferon-alfa; exacerbation of autoimmune and inflammatory disorders and myocardial injury when used in combination with interferon-alfa

Stability Store in refrigerator; do not freeze; reconstituted solution is stable 48 hours in refrigerator or at room temperature; since aldesleukin contains no preservatives, refrigerated storage of the reconstituted solution is preferred; compatible **only** with D_5W; incompatible with sodium chloride solutions; do not mix with other medications

Mechanism of Action Aldesleukin, a human recombinant interleukin-2 product, promotes proliferation, differentiation, and recruitment of T and B cells, natural killer cells, and thymocytes; also causes cytolytic activity in some lymphocytes and subsequent interactions between lymphokine-activated killer cells and tumor-infiltrating lymphocytes; causes multiple immunological effects including activation of cellular immunity with lymphocytosis, eosinophilia, and thrombocytopenia; production of cytokines (including tumor necrosis factor, interleukin-1), and inhibition of tumor growth

Final Dilution Concentration (mcg/mL)	Final Dilution Concentration (10^6 international units/mL)	Stability
<30	<0.49	Albumin must be added to bag **prior to addition** of aldesleukin at a final concentration of 0.1% (1 mg/mL) albumin; stable at room temperature for 6 days*
≥30 to ≤70	≥0.49 to ≤1.1	Stable at room temperature for 6 days*
71-99	1.2-1.6	Unstable; avoid use
100-500	1.7-8.2	Unstable at room temperature; avoid use; stable at ≥32°C (89°F) for 6 days*†

*These solutions do not contain a preservative; use for more than 24 hours may not be advisable.
†Continuous infusion via CADD pump or similar infusion device raises aldesleukin to this temperature.

Pharmacokinetics

Absorption: Oral: Not absorbed

Distribution: Primarily into plasma, lymphocytes, lungs, liver, kidney, and spleen
V_d: Adults: 4-7 L

Metabolism: Metabolized to amino acids in the cells lining the proximal convoluted tubules of the kidney

Bioavailability: I.M.: 30% to 37%

Half-life:
Children:
Distribution: 14 ± 6 minutes
Elimination: 51 ± 11 minutes
Adults:
Distribution: 6-27 minutes
Elimination: 85 minutes

Time to peak concentration: S.C.: 2-3 hours

Clearance: Adults: 7.2-16.1 L/hour

Usual Dosage A wide variety of dosages have been or are currently under investigation (refer to individual protocols):

AML: Children: (Investigational use only, Sievers, 1998): Continuous I.V. infusion: 9 million international units (9 x 10^6 international units) daily for 4 days; repeat 4 days later with 1.6 million international units (1.6 x 10^6 international units) daily for 10 days

Metastatic renal cell carcinoma and metastatic melanoma: Adults:
I.V.:
Initial: Treatment consists of two 5-day treatment cycles separated by a rest period: 600,000 international units/kg (0.037 mg/kg) every 8 hours for a total of 14 doses; followed by a rest period of 9 days, then repeat the 14-dose regimen; these two cycles constitute one course of therapy

Retreatment: Each treatment course should be separated by a rest period of at least 7 weeks from the date of completion; patients should be evaluated for response approximately 4 weeks after completion of a course of therapy and again immediately prior to the scheduled start of the next treatment course

S.C.: (Investigational): 11 million international units (11 x 10^6 international units) daily for 4 days per week for 4 consecutive weeks; repeat every 6 weeks, or alternatively, 18 million international units (18 x 10^6 international units) daily for 5 days followed by a 2-day rest period, then 9 million international units (9 x 10^6 international units) for 2 days, followed by 18 million international units (18 x 10^6 international units) daily for 3 days

Dosage modification for toxicity: In high-dose therapy, see manufacturer's guidelines (or refer to specific protocol for recommendations) for holding and restarting therapy; hold or interrupt a dose, **do not dose reduce**

(Continued)

Aldesleukin *(Continued)*

Administration Parenteral:

I.V.: Reconstitute with 1.2 mL SWI (swirl, do not shake); resulting concentration is 1.1 mg/mL [18 million (18 x 10^6) international units/mL]; further dilute dosage in D$_5$W to a final concentration between 30-70 mcg/mL (0.49-1.1 million international units/mL) and infuse over 15 minutes; for continuous infusions, dilute in D$_5$W maintaining the same final concentration; final dilutions <30 mcg/mL or >70 mcg/mL have shown increased variability in drug stability and bioactivity; addition of albumin has been used to improve stability if final dilution concentrations <30 mcg/mL are necessary; when continuous infusion is via devices which expose aldesleukin to temperatures higher than room temperature (≥32°C/89.6°F) (eg, CADD pump or similar infusion device), drug stability is also altered; see Stability for more detailed information; do not use in-line filter when administering

S.C.: Reconstituted solution may be administered subcutaneously without further dilution (**Note**: Subcutaneous administration is a non-FDA approved route)

Monitoring Parameters Baseline chest x-ray, pulmonary function tests and thallium stress study; CBC with differential, platelet counts, electrolytes, BUN, serum creatinine, hepatic enzymes, vital signs, weight, pulse oximetry, arterial blood gases (if pulmonary symptoms), fluid intake and output

Nursing Implications See Warnings and Precautions

Additional Information

1 Cetus Unit = 6 international units

1 Roche Unit (Teceleukin) = 3 international units

1.1 mg = 18 x 10^6 international units or 3 x 10^6 Cetus units

Dosage Forms Powder for injection, lyophilized: 22 x 10^6 international units (1.3 mg) [18 x 10^6 international units/mL] [1.1 mg/mL]

References

Sievers EL, Lange BJ, Sondel PM, et al, "Feasibility, Toxicity, and Biologic Response of Interleukin-2 After Consolidation Chemotherapy for Acute Myelogenous Leukemia: A Report From the Children's Cancer Group," *J Clin Oncol*, 1998, 16(3):914-9.

Whittington R and Faulds D, "Interleukin-2: A Review of Its Pharmacological Properties and Therapeutic Use in Patients With Cancer," *Drugs*, 1993, 46(3):446-514.

♦ **Aldomet**® *see* Methyldopa *on page 651*

♦ **Aleve**® **[OTC]** *see* Naproxen *on page 699*

♦ **Alfenta**® **Injection** *see* Alfentanil *on page 50*

Alfentanil *(al FEN ta nil)*

Related Information

Narcotic Analgesics Comparison *on page 1070*

Overdose and Toxicology *on page 1222*

U.S. Brand Names Alfenta® Injection

Therapeutic Category Analgesic, Narcotic; General Anesthetic

Generic Available Yes

Use Analgesia; analgesia adjunct; anesthetic agent

Restrictions C-II

Pregnancy Risk Factor C (D if used for prolonged periods or high doses at term)

Contraindications Hypersensitivity to alfentanil hydrochloride or any component; increased intracranial pressure; severe respiratory depression

Warnings Rapid I.V. infusion may result in skeletal muscle and chest wall rigidity → impaired ventilation → respiratory distress/arrest; inject slowly over 3-5 minutes; nondepolarizing skeletal muscle relaxant may be required

Precautions Use with caution in patients with bradycardia

Adverse Reactions

Cardiovascular: Bradycardia, peripheral vasodilation, hypotension

Central nervous system: Drowsiness, dizziness, sedation, CNS depression, increased intracranial pressure

Dermatologic: Pruritus

Endocrine & metabolic: Antidiuretic hormone release

Gastrointestinal: Nausea, vomiting, constipation, biliary tract spasm

Genitourinary: Urinary tract spasm

Neuromuscular & skeletal: Skeletal muscle and chest wall rigidity especially following rapid I.V. administration

Ocular: Miosis

Respiratory: Respiratory depression, apnea, respiratory arrest

Miscellaneous: Histamine release, physical and psychological dependence with prolonged use

Drug Interactions Cytochrome P-450 isoenzyme CYP3A3/4 substrate

CNS depressants, phenothiazines, tricyclic antidepressants may potentiate the adverse effects of opiate agonists; erythromycin may significantly decrease alfentanil clearance; chronic beta-blocker therapy may potentiate alfentanil-induced bradycardia; propofol may increase serum concentrations of alfentanil

Mechanism of Action Binds with stereospecific receptors at many sites within the CNS, increases pain threshold, alters pain reception, inhibits ascending pain pathways

Pharmacodynamics

Onset: Within 5 minutes

Duration: <15-20 minutes

Pharmacokinetics

Distribution: V_d beta:

Newborns, premature: 1 L/kg

Children: 0.163-0.48 L/kg

Adults: 0.46 L/kg

Protein binding:

Neonates: 67%

Adults: 88% to 92%

Bound to alpha$_1$-acid glycoprotein

Metabolism: Hepatic

Half-life, elimination:

Newborns, premature: 320-525 minutes

Children: 40-60 minutes

Adults: 83-97 minutes

Usual Dosage Doses should be titrated to appropriate effects; wide range of doses is dependent upon desired degree of analgesia/anesthesia

Neonates, Infants, and Children <12 years: Dose not established; A high percent of newborn infants receiving alfentanil (prior to procedures) at doses of 9-15 mcg/kg (mean dose: 11.7 mcg/kg) developed chest wall rigidity; 9 out of 20 newborns (45%) developed mild or moderate rigidity that did not affect ventilation, while 4 out of 20 (20%) had severe rigidity interfering with respiration for ~5-10 minutes; use of a skeletal muscle relaxant to prevent chest wall rigidity is recommended; however, smaller alfentanil doses may be required in newborns. Further studies are needed to determine appropriate doses of alfentanil in pediatric patients.

Adults: Use lean body weight for patients who weigh >20% over ideal body weight; see table.

Alfentanil: Adult Dosing

Indication	Approximate Duration of Anesthesia (min)	Induction Period (Initial Dose) (mcg/kg)	Maintenance Period (Increments/ Infusion)	Total Dose (mcg/kg)	Effects
Incremental injection	≤30	8-20	3-5 mcg/kg or 0.5-1 mcg/kg/min	8-40	Spontaneously breathing or assisted ventilation when required.
	30-60	20-50	5-15 mcg/kg	Up to 75	Assisted or controlled ventilation required. Attenuation of response to laryngoscopy and intubation.
Continuous infusion	>45	50-75	0.5-3 mcg/kg/min; average infusion rate: 1-1.5 mcg/kg/min	Dependent on duration of procedure	Assisted or controlled ventilation required. Some attenuation of response to intubation and incision, with intraoperative stability.
Anesthetic induction	>45	130-245	0.5-1.5 mcg/kg/min or general anesthetic	Dependent on duration of procedure	Assisted or controlled ventilation required. Administer slowly (over 3 minutes). Concentration of inhalation agents reduced by 30% to 50% for initial hour.

Administration Parenteral: I.V.: Inject slowly over 3-5 minutes or by I.V. continuous infusion

Monitoring Parameters Respiratory rate, blood pressure, heart rate, neurological status (for degree of analgesia/anesthesia)

(Continued)

Alfentanil *(Continued)*

Nursing Implications Alfentanil may produce more hypotension compared to fentanyl, therefore, be sure to administer slowly and ensure patient has adequate hydration

Dosage Forms Injection, preservative free, as hydrochloride: 500 mcg/mL (2 mL, 5 mL, 10 mL, 20 mL)

References

Davis PJ, Killian A, Stiller RL, et al, "Pharmacokinetics of Alfentanil in Newborn Premature Infants and Older Children," *Dev Pharmacol Ther*, 1989, 13(1):21-7.

Marlow N, Weindling AM, Van Peer A, et al, "Alfentanil Pharmacokinetics in Preterm Infants," *Arch Dis Child*, 1990, 65(4 Spec No):349-51.

Meistelman C, Saint-Maurice C, Lepaul M, et al, "A Comparison of Alfentanil Pharmacokinetics in Children and Adults," *Anesthesiology*, 1987, 66(1):13-6.

Pokela ML, Ryhanen PT, Koivisto ME, et al, "Alfentanil-Induced Rigidity in Newborn Infants," *Anesth Analg*, 1992, 75(2):252-7.

Alglucerase *(al GLOO ser ase)*

U.S. Brand Names Ceredase®

Synonyms Glucocerebrosidase

Therapeutic Category Enzyme, Glucocerebrosidase; Gaucher's Disease, Treatment Agent

Generic Available No

Use Long-term enzyme replacement in patients with confirmed Type I Gaucher's disease who exhibit one or more of the following conditions: Moderate to severe anemia; thrombocytopenia and bleeding tendencies; bone disease; hepatomegaly or splenomegaly

Pregnancy Risk Factor C

Contraindications Hypersensitivity to alglucerase or any component

Precautions Alglucerase is prepared from pooled human placental tissue that may contain the causative agents of some viral diseases; the risk of contamination from slowly active or latent viruses is believed to be remote due to steps taken in the manufacturing process; observe for signs of early virilization in males <10 years of age

Adverse Reactions

Central nervous system: Fever, chills, fatigue

Gastrointestinal: Abdominal discomfort, nausea, vomiting, diarrhea, oral ulcerations

Local: Discomfort, burning, and edema at the site of injection

Neuromuscular: Weakness, backache

Miscellaneous: Hypersensitivity reactions

Drug Interactions No information available at this time

Stability When diluted to 100-200 mL with NS, resultant solution is stable up to 18 hours when stored at 2°C to 8°C

Mechanism of Action Glucocerebrosidase is an enzyme prepared from human placental tissue. Gaucher's disease is an inherited metabolic disorder caused by the defective activity of beta-glucosidase and the resultant accumulation of glucosyl ceramide laden macrophages in the liver, bone, and spleen. Alglucerase acts by replacing the missing enzyme associated with Gaucher's disease.

Pharmacodynamics

Onset of significant improvement in symptoms:

Hepatosplenomegaly and hematologic abnormalities: Occurs within 6 months

Improvement in bone mineralization: Noted at 80-104 weeks of therapy

Pharmacokinetics

Distribution: V_d: 0.05-0.28 L/kg

Half-life, elimination: ~4-10 minutes

Usual Dosage Children and Adults: I.V. infusion: Dosage varies with the severity of disease; the recommended dosage ranges from 1.15 units/kg 3 times/week to 60 units/kg administered as frequently as once weekly or as infrequently as every 4 weeks; a common low-dose high-frequency protocol is 30 units/kg/month divided into 3 infusions weekly; after a response is firmly established, the dosage may be progressively lowered at periods of 3-6 months

Administration Parenteral: Dilute to a final volume of 100-200 mL NS and infuse I.V. over 1-2 hours; an in-line filter should be used; do not shake solution as it denatures the enzyme

Monitoring Parameters CBC, platelets, liver function tests

Dosage Forms Injection: 10 units/mL (5 mL); 80 units/mL (5 mL)

References

Barton NW, Brady RO, Dambrosia JM, et al, "Replacement Therapy for Inherited Enzyme Deficiency - Macrophage-Targeted Glucocerebrosidase for Gaucher's Disease," *N Engl J Med*, 1991, 324(21):1464-70.

♦ **Alisiphene Forte (Can)** *see* Acetaminophen *on page 29*
♦ **Alka-Mints® [OTC]** *see* Calcium Supplements *on page 167*
♦ **Alka-Seltzer® Gas Relief [OTC]** *see* Simethicone *on page 902*
♦ **Alkeran®** *see* Melphalan *on page 626*
♦ **Aller-Aide (Can)** *see* Diphenhydramine *on page 342*
♦ **Aller-Chlor® Oral [OTC]** *see* Chlorpheniramine *on page 225*
♦ **Allerdryl (Can)** *see* Diphenhydramine *on page 342*
♦ **Allerfrin® [OTC]** *see* Triprolidine and Pseudoephedrine *on page 989*
♦ **Allergen® Ear Drops** *see* Antipyrine and Benzocaine *on page 99*
♦ **Allergy Elixir (Can)** *see* Diphenhydramine *on page 342*
♦ **Allergy Formula (Can)** *see* Diphenhydramine *on page 342*
♦ **Allergy Tablets (Can)** *see* Diphenhydramine *on page 342*
♦ **AllerMax® [OTC]** *see* Diphenhydramine *on page 342*
♦ **Allernix (Can)** *see* Diphenhydramine *on page 342*
♦ **Allerphed® [OTC]** *see* Triprolidine and Pseudoephedrine *on page 989*
♦ **Alloprin (Can)** *see* Allopurinol *on page 53*

Allopurinol (al oh PURE i nole)

Related Information
Tumor Lysis Syndrome, Management *on page 1158*

U.S. Brand Names Aloprim™; Zyloprim®

Canadian Brand Names Alloprin; Apo-Allopurinol; Novo-Purol

Therapeutic Category Antigout Agent; Uric Acid Lowering Agent

Generic Available Yes (oral forms only)

Use Prevention of attacks of gouty arthritis and nephropathy; also used in treatment of secondary hyperuricemia which may occur during treatment of tumors or leukemia; prevention of recurrent calcium oxalate calculi

Pregnancy Risk Factor C

Contraindications Hypersensitivity to allopurinol or any component

Warnings Do not treat asymptomatic hyperuricemia; monitor liver function and complete blood counts before initiating therapy and periodically

Precautions Reduce dosage in renal impairment; discontinue drug at the first sign of rash; risk of skin rash may be increased in patients receiving amoxicillin or ampicillin; risk of hypersensitivity may be increased in patients receiving thiazides and possibly ACE inhibitors

Adverse Reactions
Cardiovascular: (reported with I.V. administration) Hypotension, flushing, hypertension, bradycardia, heart failure
Central nervous system: Drowsiness, fever, headache, chills, somnolence, agitation
Dermatologic: Pruritic maculopapular rash, exfoliative dermatitis, erythema multiforme, alopecia
Gastrointestinal: GI irritation, dyspepsia, nausea, vomiting, diarrhea, abdominal pain, gastritis
Genitourinary: Hematuria
Hematologic: Leukocytosis, leukopenia, thrombocytopenia, eosinophilia, bone marrow suppression
Hepatic: Hepatitis, elevated liver enzymes, hepatomegaly, hyperbilirubinemia, jaundice
Local: Local injection site reaction
Neuromuscular & skeletal: Peripheral neuropathy, paresthesia, neuritis, arthralgia, myoclonus
Ocular: Cataracts, optic neuritis
Renal: Renal impairment
Respiratory: Epistaxis; (reported with I.V. administration) apnea, hyperpnea, ARDS
Vascular: Necrotizing angiitis, vasculitis

Drug Interactions Inhibits metabolism of azathioprine and mercaptopurine; use with ampicillin or amoxicillin may increase the incidence of skin rash; may increase myelosuppressive effects of cyclophosphamide; large doses may decrease theophylline clearance; increased risk of hypersensitivity reactions when coadministered with ACE inhibitors and thiazide diuretics; decreased allopurinol effectiveness when coadministered with uricosuric agents; increases kidney stone formation when taken with large doses of vitamin C; aluminum hydroxide antacids decrease allopurinol's absorption; increases chlorpropamide levels; may increase risk of osteomalacia in patients receiving phenytoin or phenobarbital; prolongs the half-life of oral anticoagulants; may increase cyclosporine serum levels

(Continued)

Allopurinol *(Continued)*

Stability Reconstituted parenteral solution should be stored at room temperature; do not refrigerate; use within 10 hours of preparation; physically **incompatible** when mixed with or infused through the same line with the following: Amikacin, amphotericin B, carmustine, cefotaxime, chlorpromazine, cimetidine, clindamycin, cytarabine, dacarbazine, daunorubicin, diphenhydramine, doxorubicin, doxycycline, droperidol, floxuridine, gentamicin, haloperidol, hydroxyzine, idarubicin, imipenem-cilastatin, mechlorethamine, meperidine, metoclopramide, methylprednisolone sodium succinate, minocycline, nalbuphine, netilmicin, ondansetron, prochlorperazine, promethazine, sodium bicarbonate, streptozocin, tobramycin, vinorelbine

Mechanism of Action Decreases the production of uric acid by inhibiting the action of xanthine oxidase, an enzyme that converts hypoxanthine to xanthine and xanthine to uric acid

Pharmacodynamics Decrease in serum uric acid occurs in 1-2 days with a nadir achieved in 1-3 weeks

Pharmacokinetics

Absorption: Oral: ~80% from the GI tract

Distribution: Into breast milk; breast milk to plasma ratio: 0.9-1.4

Protein binding: <1%

Metabolism: ~75% of drug metabolized to active metabolites, chiefly oxypurinol

Half-life:

Parent: 1-3 hours

Oxypurinol metabolite: 18-30 hours in patients with normal renal function

Time to peak serum concentration: Within 2-6 hours

Allopurinol and oxypurinol are dialyzable

Usual Dosage

Prevention of acute uric acid nephropathy in myeloproliferative neoplastic disorders (beginning 1-2 days before chemotherapy): Daily doses >300 mg should be administered in divided doses:

Children ≤10 years:

I.V.: 200 mg/m^2/day in 1-3 divided doses; maximum dose: 600 mg/day

Oral: 10 mg/kg/day in 2-3 divided doses or 200-300 mg/m^2/day in 2-4 divided doses; maximum dose: 800 mg/day

Alternative:

<6 years: 150 mg/day in 3 divided doses

6-10 years: 300 mg/day in 2-3 divided doses

Children >10 years and Adults:

I.V.: 200-400 mg/m^2/day in 1-3 divided doses; maximum: 600 mg/day

Oral: 600-800 mg/day in 2-3 divided doses

Gout: Children >10 years and Adults: Oral:

Mild: 200-300 mg/day

Severe: 400-600 mg/day

Recurrent calcium oxalate stones: Children >10 years and Adults: Oral: 200-300 mg daily in divided or single daily dosage

Dosing adjustment in renal impairment:

Cl$_{cr}$ >50 mL/minute: No dosage change

Cl$_{cr}$ 10-50 mL/minute: Reduce dosage to 50% of recommended

Cl$_{cr}$ <10 mL/minute: Reduce dosage to 30% of recommended

Administration

Oral: Administer after meals with plenty of fluid

Parenteral: Reconstitute 500 mg vial with 25 mL sterile water; prior to administration, further dilute with D$_5$W or NS to a maximum concentration of 6 mg/mL; rate of infusion is dependent upon the volume of infusate (in research studies, 100-300 mg doses were infused over 30 minutes)

Monitoring Parameters CBC, liver function tests, renal function, serum uric acid; 24-hour urinary urate (when treating calcium oxalate stones)

Reference Range

Uric acid: Male: 3.0-7.0 mg/dL; Female: 2.0-6.0 mg/dL

Urinary urate excretion: Male: <800 mg/day; Female: <750 mg/day

Patient Information Report any skin rash, painful urination, blood in urine, irritation of the eyes, or swelling of lips or mouth; avoid alcohol; drink plenty of fluids; may produce drowsiness; use with caution when performing hazardous activities which require mental alertness or physical coordination

Dosage Forms

Injection, as sodium: 500 mg

Tablet: 100 mg, 300 mg

Extemporaneous Preparations

A 20 mg/mL suspension may be made by crushing eight 300 mg tablets and mixing with 120 mL of either a 1:1 mixture of Ora-Sweet® and Ora-Plus® or a 1:1 mixture of Ora-Sweet® SF and Ora-Plus®. The resulting suspension is stable for 60 days refrigerated (Allen, 1996).

A 20 mg/mL suspension may be made by crushing one 100 mg tablet; wet crushed tablet with small amount of 1% methylcellulose then add syrup NF to a final volume of 5 mL; stable 56 days refrigerated (Dressman, 1983).

Allen LV and Erickson MA, "Stability of Acetazolamide, Allopurinol, Azathioprine, Clonazepam, and Flucytosine in Extemporaneously Compounded Oral Liquids," *Am J Health Sys Pharm,* 1996, 53:1944-9.

Dressman JB and Poust RI, "Stability of Allopurinol and of Five Antineoplastics in Suspension," *Am J Hosp Pharm,* 1983, 40(4):616-8.

References

Bennett WM, Aronoff GR, Golper TA, et al, *Drug Prescribing in Renal Failure,* Philadelphia, PA: American College of Physicians, 1987.

Krakoff IH and Murphy ML, "Hyperuricemia in Neoplastic Disease in Children: Prevention With Allopurinol, A Xanthine Oxidase Inhibitor" *Pediatrics,* 1968, 41(1):52-6.

♦ **Almora® [OTC]** *see* Magnesium Supplements *on page 614*

♦ **Alocril™** *see* Nedocromil *on page 701*

♦ **Aloprim™** *see* Allopurinol *on page 53*

♦ **Alora®** *see* Estradiol *on page 400*

♦ **Alphanate®** *see* Antihemophilic Factor (Human) *on page 98*

♦ **Alphatrex®** *see* Betamethasone *on page 140*

Alprazolam (al PRAY zoe lam)

Related Information

Carbohydrate and Alcohol Content of Liquid Medications for Use in Patients Receiving Ketogenic Diets *on page 1258*
Overdose and Toxicology *on page 1222*
Serotonin Syndrome *on page 1247*

U.S. Brand Names Alprazolam Intensol®; Xanax®

Canadian Brand Names Alti-Alprazolam; Apo-Alpraz; Gen-Alprazolam; Novo-Alprazol; Nu-Alpraz

Therapeutic Category Antianxiety Agent; Benzodiazepine

Generic Available Yes

Use Treatment of generalized anxiety disorder (GAD); symptoms of anxiety (short-term treatment); anxiety associated with depression; management of panic attacks

Restrictions C-IV

Pregnancy Risk Factor D

Contraindications Hypersensitivity to alprazolam, any component, or other benzodiazepines; severe uncontrolled pain, narrow-angle glaucoma, severe respiratory depression, pre-existing CNS depression; not to be used in pregnancy or lactation or in patients taking certain medications (see Drug Interactions)

Warnings Withdrawal symptoms including seizures have occurred 18 hours to 3 days after abrupt discontinuation; when discontinuing therapy, decrease daily dose by no more than 0.5 mg every 3 days; reduce dose in patients with significant hepatic disease

Precautions Safety and effectiveness have not been established in children <18 years of age

Adverse Reactions

Central nervous system: Drowsiness, dizziness, confusion, sedation, headache, ataxia
Gastrointestinal: Xerostomia, constipation, diarrhea, nausea, vomiting
Ocular: Blurred vision
Miscellaneous: Physical and psychological dependence with prolonged use

Drug Interactions Cytochrome P-450 isoenzyme CYP3A3/4 substrate

Enzyme inducers may increase metabolism of alprazolam; CNS depressants including alcohol may enhance CNS effects; cimetidine, fluvoxamine, fluoxetine, propoxyphene, and oral contraceptives may decrease the metabolism of alprazolam; delavirdine, ritonavir, ketoconazole, or itraconazole may decrease the metabolism of alprazolam and significantly increase alprazolam levels; concurrent use of delavirdine, ritonavir, ketoconazole, or itraconazole with alprazolam is not recommended

Mechanism of Action Depresses all levels of the CNS, including the limbic and reticular formation, by binding to the benzodiazepine site on the gamma-aminobutyric acid (GABA) receptor complex and modulating GABA, which is a major inhibitory neurotransmitter in the brain

(Continued)

Alprazolam (Continued)

Pharmacokinetics
Absorption: Oral: Rapidly and well absorbed

Distribution: 0.9-1.2 L/kg; distributes into breast milk

Protein binding: 80%

Metabolism: Extensive in the liver; major metabolites: alpha-hydroxy-alprazolam (about half as active as alprazolam) and a benzophenone metabolite (inactive)

Half-life: Adults: 6.3-26.9 hours; mean: 11.2 hours

Time to peak serum concentration: Within 1-2 hours

Elimination: Excretion of metabolites and parent compound in urine

Usual Dosage Oral:
Children <18 years: Dose not established; investigationally in children 7-16 years of age (n=13), initial doses of 0.005 mg/kg or 0.125 mg/dose were given 3 times/day for situational anxiety and increments of 0.125-0.25 mg/dose were used to increase doses to maximum of 0.02 mg/kg/dose or 0.06 mg/kg/day; a range of 0.375-3 mg/day was needed (see Pfefferbaum, 1987). **Note:** A more recent study in 17 children (8-17 years of age) with overanxious disorder or avoidant disorders used initial daily doses of 0.25 mg for children <40 kg and 0.5 mg for those >40 kg. The dose was titrated at 2-day intervals to a maximum of 0.04 mg/kg/day. Required doses ranged from 0.5-3.5 mg/day with a mean of 1.6 mg/day. Based on clinical global ratings, alprazolam appeared to be better than placebo, however, this difference was **not** statistically significant (see Simeon, 1992); further studies are needed.

Adults: 0.25-0.5 mg 2-3 times/day, titrate dose upward; maximum dose: 4 mg/day (antianxiety); 10 mg/day (antipanic)

Administration Oral: Administer with food to decrease GI upset

Monitoring Parameters CNS status, respiratory rate

Patient Information May cause drowsiness and impair ability to perform activities requiring mental alertness or coordination; may be habit-forming; avoid abrupt discontinuation after prolonged use; avoid alcohol; limit caffeine

Nursing Implications Assist with ambulation during beginning of therapy; allow patient to rise slowly to avoid fainting

Dosage Forms
Solution, oral: 1 mg/mL (30 mL)

Tablet: 0.25 mg, 0.5 mg, 1 mg, 2 mg

References
Bernstein GA, Garfinkel BD, and Borchardt CM, "Comparative Studies of Pharmacotherapy for School Refusal," *J Am Acad Child Adolesc Psychiatry*, 1990, 29(5):773-81.

Pfefferbaum B, Overall JE, Boren HA, et al, "Alprazolam in the Treatment of Anticipatory and Acute Situational Anxiety in Children With Cancer," *J Am Acad Child Adolesc Psychiatry*, 1987, 26(4):532-5.

Simeon JG and Ferguson HB, "Alprazolam Effects in Children With Anxiety Disorders," *Can J Psychiatry*, 1987, 32(7):570-4.

Simeon JG, Ferguson HB, Knott V, et al, "Clinical, Cognitive, and Neurophysiological Effects of Alprazolam in Children and Adolescents With Overanxious and Avoidant Disorders," *J Am Acad Child Adolesc Psychiatry*, 1992, 31(1):29-33.

♦ **Alprazolam Intensol**® *see Alprazolam on page 55*

Alprostadil (al PROS ta dill)

U.S. Brand Names Caverject® Injection; Edex® Injection; Muse® Pellet; Prostin VR Pediatric® Injection

Synonyms PGE$_1$; Prostaglandin E$_1$

Therapeutic Category Prostaglandin

Generic Available Yes: Injection (500 mcg/mL)

Use Temporary maintenance of patency of ductus arteriosus in neonates with ductal-dependent congenital heart disease until surgery can be performed. These defects include cyanotic (eg, pulmonary atresia, pulmonary stenosis, tricuspid atresia, Fallot's tetralogy, transposition of the great vessels) and acyanotic (eg, interruption of aortic arch, coarctation of aorta, hypoplastic left ventricle) heart disease.

Investigationally used for the treatment of pulmonary hypertension in infants and children with congenital heart defects with left-to-right shunts

Adult males: Diagnosis and treatment of erectile dysfunction

Pregnancy Risk Factor X

Contraindications Respiratory distress syndrome or persistent fetal circulation

Warnings Apnea occurs in 10% to 12% of neonates with congenital heart defects (especially in those weighing <2 kg at birth) and usually appears during the first hour of drug infusion

Precautions Use cautiously in neonates with bleeding tendencies; if hypotension or pyrexia occurs, the infusion rate should be reduced until symptoms subside; severe hypotension, apnea, or bradycardia requires drug discontinuation with cautious reinstitution at a lower dose

Adverse Reactions

Cardiovascular: Systemic hypotension, flushing, bradycardia, rhythm disturbances, tachycardia

Central nervous system: Seizure-like activity, fever

Endocrine & metabolic: Hypocalcemia, hypoglycemia; cortical proliferation of long bones (cortical hyperostosis) has been seen with long-term infusions (incidence and severity are related to duration of therapy and cumulative dose)

Gastrointestinal: Diarrhea, gastric-outlet obstruction secondary to antral hyperplasia (occurrence related to duration of therapy and cumulative dose)

Hematologic: Inhibition of platelet aggregation

Respiratory: Respiratory depression, apnea

Stability Compatible in D_5W, $D_{10}W$, and saline solutions; refrigerate ampuls at 2°C to 8°C

Mechanism of Action Causes vasodilation by means of direct effect on vascular and ductus arteriosus smooth muscle

Pharmacodynamics

Maximum effect:

Acyanotic congenital heart disease: Usual: 1.5-3 hours; range: 15 minutes to 11 hours

Cyanotic congenital heart disease: Usual: ~30 minutes

Duration: Ductus arteriosus will begin to close within 1-2 hours after drug is stopped

Pharmacokinetics

Metabolism: ~70% to 80% metabolized by oxidation during a single pass through the lungs; metabolite (13,14 dihydro-PGE_1) is active and has been identified in neonates

Half-life: 5-10 minutes; since the half-life is so short, the drug must be administered by continuous infusion

Elimination: Metabolites excreted in urine

Usual Dosage Neonates and Infants: 0.05-0.1 mcg/kg/minute; with therapeutic response, rate is reduced to lowest effective dosage; with unsatisfactory response, rate is increased gradually; maintenance: 0.01-0.4 mcg/kg/minute

PGE_1 is usually given at an infusion rate of 0.1 mcg/kg/minute; but it is often possible to reduce the dosage to $1/2$ or even $1/10$ without losing the therapeutic effect. The mixing schedule is shown in the table.

Add 1 Ampul (500 mcg) to:	Concentration (mcg/mL)	Infusion Rate to Deliver 0.1 mcg/kg/min		
		mL/kg/min	mL/kg/h	mL/kg/24 h
250 mL	2	0.05	3	72
100 mL	5	0.02	1.2	28.8
50 mL	10	0.01	0.6	14.4
25 mL	20	0.005	0.3	7.2

Administration Parenteral: I.V. continuous infusion into a large vein or alternatively through an umbilical artery catheter placed at the ductal opening; maximum concentration listed (per package insert) for I.V. infusion: 20 mcg/mL; has also been administered via continuous infusion into the right pulmonary artery for investigational treatment of pulmonary hypertension in infants and children with congenital heart defects with left-to-right shunts; rate of infusion (mL/hour) = dose (mcg/kg/minute) x weight (kg) x 60 minutes/hour divided by the concentration (mcg/mL)

Monitoring Parameters Arterial pressure, respiratory rate, heart rate, temperature, pO_2; monitor for gastric obstruction in patients receiving PGE_1 for longer than 120 hours; x-rays may be needed to assess cortical hyperostosis in patients receiving prolonged PGE_1 therapy

Nursing Implications Prepare fresh solution every 24 hours; flushing of arm or face may indicate misplacement of intra-arterial catheter and infusion of drug into subclavian or carotid artery; reposition catheter

Additional Information Therapeutic response is indicated by an increase in systemic blood pressure and pH in those with restricted systemic blood flow and acidosis, or by an increase in oxygenation (pO_2) in those with restricted pulmonary blood flow. Most cases of bone changes occurred 4-6 weeks after starting alprostadil, but it has occurred as early as 9 days; cortical hyperostosis usually resolves over 6-12 months after stopping PGE_1 therapy

Dosage Forms

Injection:

Caverject®, powder for injection: 5 mcg, 10 mcg, 20 mcg, 40 mcg

(Continued)

Alprostadil *(Continued)*

  Caverject®: 10 mcg/mL (1 mL); 20 mcg/mL (1 mL, 2 mL)

  Edex®, powder for injection: 10 mcg, 20 mcg, 40 mcg

  Prostin VR Pediatric®: 500 mcg/mL (1 mL)

  Pellet, urethral: 125 mcg, 250 mcg, 500 mcg, 1000 mcg

References
Kaufman MB and El-Chaar GM, "Bone and Tissue Changes Following Prostaglandin Therapy in Neonates," *Ann Pharmacother*, 1996, 30(3):269-74, 277.

Peled N, Dagan O, Babyn P, et al, "Gastric-Outlet Obstruction Induced by Prostaglandin Therapy in Neonates," *N Engl J Med*, 1992, 327(8):505-10.

Weesner KM, "Hemodynamic Effects of Prostaglandin E₁ in Patients With Congenital Heart Disease and Pulmonary Hypertension," *Cathet Cardiovasc Diagn*, 1991, 24(1):10-5.

Woo K, Emery J, and Peabody J, "Cortical Hyperostosis: A Complication of Prolonged Prostaglandin Infusion in Infants Awaiting Cardiac Transplantation," *Pediatrics*, 1994, 93(3):417-20.

Alteplase *(AL te plase)*

U.S. Brand Names Activase®

Canadian Brand Names Lysatec-rt-PA

Synonyms Alteplase, Recombinant; Tissue Plasminogen Activator, Recombinant; t-PA

Therapeutic Category Thrombolytic Agent

Generic Available No

Use Thrombolytic agent used in treatment of acute MI, acute ischemic stroke, acute massive pulmonary embolism, and occluded arteriovenous cannulas

Pregnancy Risk Factor C

Contraindications Hypersensitivity to alteplase or any component

  Contraindications for use in the treatment of acute MI or pulmonary embolism: Active internal bleeding; known bleeding diathesis; history of CVA; intracranial neoplasm, arteriovenous malformation, or aneurysm; recent intracranial or intraspinal surgery or trauma; severe uncontrolled hypertension

  Contraindications for use in the treatment of acute ischemic stroke: Active internal bleeding; known bleeding diathesis (including but not limited to: Current use of oral anticoagulants or an INR >1.7 or PT >15 seconds, use of heparin within 48 hours before the onset of stroke and an elevated aPTT at presentation, platelet count <100,000/mm³); evidence of intracranial hemorrhage on pretreatment evaluation; history of intracranial hemorrhage; suspicion of subarachnoid hemorrhage; recent (within 3 months) intracranial or intraspinal surgery, serious head trauma, or previous stroke; intracranial neoplasm, arteriovenous malformation, or aneurysm; seizure at the onset of stroke; uncontrolled hypertension at time of treatment (eg, adults with blood pressures of >185 mm Hg systolic or >110 mm Hg diastolic)

Warnings May cause bleeding (internal, superficial, or surface bleeding); concurrent use of heparin anticoagulation may increase bleeding; monitor all potential bleeding sites. Avoid I.M. injections and nonessential handling of patient; carefully perform venipunctures and only when necessary. If an arterial puncture is required, use vessel in an upper extremity that can be manually compressed. Stop alteplase (and heparin) if serious bleeding occurs (effects of heparin can be reversed by protamine). Do not exceed recommended doses; do not use doses of 150 mg to treat acute MI as this dose has been associated with an increase in intracranial hemorrhage.

  Risks from alteplase may be increased in the following conditions (risks versus benefits should be weighed carefully before use): Recent major surgery (eg, organ biopsy, previous puncture of noncompressible vessels, coronary artery bypass graft, obstetrical delivery), recent trauma, recent GI or GU bleeding, current use of oral anticoagulants, cerebrovascular disease, diabetic hemorrhagic retinopathy or other hemorrhagic ophthalmic conditions, hypertension (eg, adults with systolic BP ≥175 mm Hg and/or diastolic BP ≥110 mm Hg), patients with an increased risk of left heart thrombus (eg, mitral stenosis with atrial fibrillation), acute pericarditis, subacute bacterial endocarditis, hemostatic defects including ones caused by severe renal or hepatic dysfunction, significant hepatic dysfunction, pregnancy, septic thrombophlebitis or occluded AV cannula at seriously infected site, advanced age (eg, >75 years old), any other condition in which bleeding would be a significant risk or would be especially difficult to manage due to its location.

  Cholesterol embolism may occur (rare). Risk of stroke in acute MI patients who are at low risk for death from cardiac causes and who present with high blood pressure, may be greater than the survival benefit from thrombolytic therapy. Reperfusion arrhythmias may occur following coronary thrombolysis. In patients with pulmonary embolism, alteplase has not been proven to adequately treat underlying DVT; possible re-embolization from DVT may occur.

Acute ischemic stroke: Risks of alteplase therapy may be increased in patients with major early signs of infarct on CT and in those with severe neurological deficit at presentation (risks versus benefits should be weighed carefully); treatment of patients >3 hours after onset of symptoms and those with rapidly improving symptoms or minor neurological deficit is not recommended.

Precautions Use with caution if drug is readministered; discontinue immediately if anaphylactoid reaction occurs. For treatment of acute ischemic stroke, frequent monitoring and control of blood pressure during and after alteplase administration is recommended. For systemic use, pretreatment lab studies should include platelet count, PT/PTT, fibrinogen, fibrin degradation products, plasminogen, antithrombin III, protein S, protein C.

Adverse Reactions
Cardiovascular: Hypotension; reperfusion arrhythmias (following coronary thrombolysis)

Central nervous system: Fever, intracranial hemorrhage

Dermatologic: Bruising (1%), rash, urticaria (rare)

Gastrointestinal: GI bleeding (5%), nausea, vomiting

Genitourinary: GU bleeding (4%)

Hematologic: Surface bleeding, internal bleeding, cerebral hemorrhage

Local: Bleeding at catheter puncture site; bruising and inflammation with extravasation

Respiratory: Epistaxis (<1%), laryngeal edema (rare)

Miscellaneous: Anaphylactoid reaction (rare)

Drug Interactions Anticoagulants (warfarin, heparin) and drugs that affect platelet function (aspirin, NSAIDs, dipyridamole) may increase the risk of bleeding. Aspirin and heparin have been given concurrently with and after alteplase infusions in patients with acute MI or pulmonary embolism (careful monitoring for bleeding is recommended). However, the concurrent use of aspirin or heparin with alteplase within the first 24 hours after the onset of symptoms of stroke was prohibited in the major stroke trial; therefore, safety of the use of these agents with alteplase in patients with acute ischemic stroke is unknown. Antifibrinolytic agents (aminocaproic acid) may decrease effectiveness.

Stability Store lyophilized product at room temperature [not to exceed 86°F (30°C)] or under refrigeration; protect from excessive light exposure during extended storage. Reconstitute vials with supplied diluent (SWI); do not reconstitute with bacteriostatic water for injection; use large bore needle and syringe to reconstitute 50 mg vial and accompanying transfer device to reconstitute 100 mg vial (100 mg vial does not contain vacuum); swirl gently, do not shake; final concentration after reconstitution: 1 mg/mL; reconstituted solution must be used within 8 hours (manufacturer's recommendations).

Solutions of 0.5 mg/mL, 1 mg/mL, and 2 mg/mL in sterile water retained ≥94% of fibrinolytic activity at 48 hours when stored at 2°C in plastic syringes; these solutions retained ≥90% of fibrinolytic activity when stored in plastic syringes at -25°C or -70°C for 7 or 14 days, thawed at room temperature and then stored at 2°C for 48 hours (see Davis, 2000). Solutions of 1 mg/mL in sterile water were stable for 22 weeks in plastic syringes when stored at -30°C and for ~1 month in glass vials when stored at -20°C; bioactivity remained unchanged for 6 months in propylene containers when stored at -20°C and for 2 weeks in glass vials when stored at -70°C (see review by Generali, 2001).

Prepare bolus dose using one of the following methods: 1) Remove bolus dose from reconstituted vial using syringe and needle; for 50 mg vial: do not prime syringe with air, insert needle into vial stopper; for 100 mg vial, insert needle away from puncture mark created by transfer device; 2) Remove bolus dose from a port on the infusion line after priming; 3) Program an infusion pump to deliver the bolus at the beginning of the infusion. Administer the remaining dose as follows: From 50 mg vial: Use polyvinyl chloride I.V. bag or glass vial and infusion set; from 100 mg vial: Use same puncture site made by transfer device to insert spike end of infusion set and infuse from vial.

The 1 mg/mL solution may be diluted further (immediately before use) with an equal volume of NS or D_5W to yield a final concentration of 0.5 mg/mL; swirl gently, do not shake to dilute; diluted solutions are stable for 8 hours; do not add other medications to alteplase solutions. Alteplase is incompatible with bacteriostatic water, dobutamine, dopamine, heparin, and nitroglycerin infusions; physically compatible with lidocaine, metoprolol, and propranolol when administered via Y site.

Mechanism of Action A naturally-occurring serine protease (enzyme) that initiates local fibrinolysis by binding to fibrin in a thrombus (clot) and directly activating entrapped plasminogen to plasmin; plasmin degrades fibrin, fibrinogen, and other procoagulant proteins into soluble fragments

(Continued)

Alteplase *(Continued)*

Pharmacokinetics
Distribution: Initial: Approximates plasma volume
Metabolism: In the liver
Half-life: <5 minutes
Clearance: Plasma: Adults: 380-570 mL/minute

Usual Dosage I.V.:
Neonates, Infants, and Children:
Occluded I.V. catheters: *Chest*, 2001 dosing recommendations:
Central venous catheter: **Dose listed is per lumen; for multilumen catheters, treat one lumen at a time:** [**Note:** Some institutions use lower doses (eg, 0.25 mg/0.5 mL) in neonates and infants <3 months]
Patients ≤10 kg: 0.5 mg diluted in NS to a volume equal to the internal volume of the lumen; instill in each lumen over 1-2 minutes; leave in lumen for 1-2 hours, then **aspirate out of catheter, do not infuse into patient;** flush catheter with NS
Patients >10 kg: 1 mg in 1 mL of NS; use a volume equal to the internal volume of the lumen; maximum: 2 mg in 2 mL per lumen; instill in each lumen over 1-2 minutes; leave in lumen for 1-2 hours; then **aspirate out of catheter, do not infuse into patient;** flush catheter with NS
S.C. port:
Patients ≤10 kg: 0.5 mg diluted with NS to 3 mL
Patients >10 kg: 2 mg diluted with NS to 3 mL
Systemic thromboses: I.V. (**Note:** Dose must be titrated to effect): *Chest*, 2001 recommendations: 0.1-0.6 mg/kg/hour for 6 hours (some patients may require longer or shorter duration of therapy). **Note:** The optimal dose for various thrombotic conditions is not established in pediatric patients; most published papers consist of case reports; few prospective pediatric studies have been conducted; several studies have used the following doses (see Levy, 1991 and Weiner, 1998). **Note:** Bleeding complications were associated with doses in the higher range.
Initial: 0.1 mg/kg/hour for 6 hours; monitor patient closely for bleeding, monitor fibrinogen levels; if no response after 6 hours, increase infusion by 0.1 mg/kg/hour at 6-hour intervals to a maximum of 0.5 mg/kg/hour; maintain fibrinogen >100 mg/dL (**Note:** Some centers maintain fibrinogen >150 mg/dL in newborns); duration of therapy is based on clinical response
Low-dose (local) infusion for occluded catheters: **Note:** No pediatric studies have compared local to systemic thrombolytic therapy; therefore, there is no evidence to suggest that local infusions are superior. The pediatric patients' small vessel size may increase the chance of local damage to blood vessels and formation of a new thrombus; however, local infusion may be appropriate for catheter related thromboses if the catheter is already in place (See *Chest*, 2001). Various "low-dose" regimens have been used; the following dosing recommendations are based on Doyle, 1992 and Anderson, 1991:
Initial: 0.01 mg/kg/hour for 6 hours; if no response after 6 hours, increase infusion by 0.01 mg/kg/hour at 6-hour intervals to a maximum of 0.05 mg/kg/hour; monitor patient closely; systemic fibrinolysis (decreased plasma fibrinogen levels) or bleeding has been reported in some neonates and infants receiving 0.05 mg/kg/hour; duration of therapy is based on clinical response
Adults:
Acute MI:
Accelerated infusion:
Patients >67 kg: Total dose: 100 mg given in 3 divided doses as follows: Infuse 15 mg I.V. bolus over 1-2 minutes, then infuse 50 mg over the next 30 minutes, then 35 mg over the next 60 minutes. Maximum total dose: 100 mg
Patients ≤67 kg: Infuse 15 mg I.V. bolus over 1-2 minutes, then infuse 0.75 mg/kg (maximum: 50 mg) over the next 30 minutes, then 0.5 mg/kg (maximum 35 mg) over the next 60 minutes. Maximum total dose: 100 mg
3-hour infusion:
Patients ≥65 kg: Total dose: 100 mg given as follows: Infuse 60 mg over the first hour with 6-10 mg given as an I.V. bolus, then infuse 20 mg/hour for 2 hours
Patients <65 kg: Total dose: 1.25 mg/kg given over 3 hours as described above
Acute ischemic stroke: (**Note:** Alteplase therapy should only be started within 3 hours after the onset of symptoms of stroke and after exclusion of intracranial hemorrhage by CT scan or other sensitive diagnostic imaging method): Total

dose: 0.9 mg/kg (maximum: 90 mg) given over 1 hour as follows: Infuse 10% of total dose (0.09 mg/kg) I.V. bolus over 1 minute, then infuse the rest of the total dose (0.81 mg/kg) over 60 minutes

Pulmonary embolism: 100 mg infused over 2 hours

Occluded central venous catheter: Standard dose: 2 mg (1 mg/mL); instill in each lumen; leave in lumen for 2 hours, then **aspirate out of catheter, do not infuse into patient**; flush catheter with NS; **Note:** A recent study using escalating doses of 0.5 mg, 1 mg, and 2 mg (60 minute dwell time) found that 86.2% of catheters were cleared with the 0.5 mg dose (see Davis, 2000).

Administration Parenteral: I.V.: May administer at a final concentration of 1 mg/mL or may dilute and administer as 0.5 mg/mL (see Stability); for treatment of acute MI: Administer dose as soon as possible after symptom onset; for treatment of acute ischemic stroke: Administer dose within 3 hours of onset of symptoms

Monitoring Parameters Blood pressure; CBC, reticulocyte, platelet count; fibrinogen level, plasminogen, fibrin/fibrinogen degradation products, D-dimer, PT, PTT, antithrombin III, protein C; urinalysis, signs of bleeding

Nursing Implications Extravasation may cause bruising or inflammation; monitor infusion site for patency of I.V.; if extravasation occurs, discontinue infusion at site of extravasation and apply local treatment; avoid I.M. injections; assess patient for bleeding

Additional Information Advantages of alteplase include: Low immunogenicity, short half-life, direct activation of plasminogen, and a strong and specific affinity for fibrin. Failure of thrombolytic agents in newborns/neonates may occur due to the low plasminogen concentrations (~50% to 70% of adult levels); supplementing plasminogen (via administration of fresh frozen plasma) may possibly help. Osmolality of 1 mg/mL solution is ~215 mOsm/kg.

Dosage Forms Powder for injection, lyophilized (recombinant): 50 mg [29 million units] (50 mL); 100 mg [58 million units] (100 mL)

References

Anderson BJ, Keeley SR, and Johnson ND, "Caval Thrombolysis in Neonates Using Low Doses of Recombinant Human Tissue-Type Plasminogen Activator," *Anaesth Intensive Care*, 1991, 19(1):22-7.

Andrew M, Brooker L, Leaker M, et al, "Fibrin Clot Lysis by Thrombolytic Agents is Impaired in Newborns Due to a Low Plasminogen Concentration," *Thromb Haemost*, 1992, 68(3):325-30.

Davis SN, Vermeulen L, Banton J, et al, "Activity and Dosage of Alteplase Dilution for Clearing Occlusions of Venous-Access Devices," *Am J Health Syst Pharm*, 2000, 57(11):1039-45.

Doyle E, Britto J, Freeman J, et al, "Thrombolysis With Low Dose Tissue Plasminogen Activator," *Arch Dis Child*, 1992, 67(12):1483-4.

Farnoux C, Camard O, Pinquier D, et al, "Recombinant Tissue-Type Plasminogen Activator Therapy of Thrombosis in 16 Neonates," *J Pediatr*, 1998, 133(1):137-40.

Generali J and Cada DJ, "Alteplase (t-PA) Bolus: Occluded Catheters," *Hospital Pharmacy*, 2001, 36(1):93-103.

Kothari SS, Varma S, and Wasir S, "Thrombolytic Therapy in Infants and Children," *Am Heart J*, 1994, 127(3):651-7.

Levy M, Benson LN, Burrows PE, et al, "Tissue Plasminogen Activator for the Treatment of Thromboembolism in Infants and Children," *J Pediatr*, 1991, 118(3):467-72.

Monagle P, Michelson AD, Bovill E, et al, "Antithrombotic Therapy in Children," *Chest*, 2001, 119(1 Suppl):344S-370S.

Nowak-Gottl U, Auberger K, Halimeh S, et al, "Thrombolysis in Newborns and Infants," *Thromb Haemost*, 1999, 82 (Suppl 1):112-6.

Weiner GM, Castle VP, DiPietro MA, et al, "Successful Treatment of Neonatal Arterial Thromboses With Recombinant Tissue Plasminogen Activator," *J Pediatr*, 1998, 133(1):133-6.

♦ **Alti-Nortriptyline (Can)** *see* Nortriptyline *on page 724*
♦ **Alti-Piroxicam (Can)** *see* Piroxicam *on page 806*
♦ **Alti-Prazosin (Can)** *see* Prazosin *on page 820*
♦ **Alti-Ranitidine (Can)** *see* Ranitidine *on page 865*
♦ **Alti-Sulfasalazine (Can)** *see* Sulfasalazine *on page 926*
♦ **Alti-Trazodone (Can)** *see* Trazodone *on page 977*
♦ **Alti-Valproic (Can)** *see* Valproic Acid and Derivatives *on page 998*
♦ **Alti-Verapamil (Can)** *see* Verapamil *on page 1007*

Aluminum Acetate (a LOO mi num AS e tate)

U.S. Brand Names Acid Mantle® [OTC]; Bluboro® [OTC]; Boropak®; Domeboro® [OTC]; Pedi-Boro® [OTC]
Synonyms Burow's Solution
Therapeutic Category Topical Skin Product
Generic Available Yes
Use Astringent wet dressing for relief of inflammatory conditions of the skin and to reduce weeping that may occur in dermatitis
Pregnancy Risk Factor C
Contraindications Use with topical collagenase
Precautions Do not use plastic or other impervious material to prevent evaporation
Adverse Reactions Local: Irritation
Usual Dosage Children and Adults: Topical: Soak the affected area in the solution 2-4 times/day for 15-30 minutes or apply wet dressing soaked in the solution 2-4 times/day for 30-minute treatment periods; rewet dressing with solution every few minutes to keep it moist
Administration Topical: Keep away from eyes, external use only; one tablet dissolved in a pint of water makes a modified Burow's solution equivalent to a 1:40 dilution, 2 tablets: 1:20 dilution, 4 tablets: 1:10 dilution; one powder packet dissolved in a pint of water makes a modified Burow's solution equivalent to a 1:40 dilution
Dosage Forms
Powder, to make topical solution: 1 packet/pint of water = 1:40 solution
Tablet: 1 tablet/pint = 1:40 dilution

♦ **Aluminum Carbonate** *see* Antacid Preparations *on page 95*
♦ **Aluminum Carbonate Gel** *see* Antacid Preparations *on page 95*
♦ **Aluminum Hydroxide** *see* Antacid Preparations *on page 95*
♦ **Aluminum Hydroxide and Magnesium Hydroxide** *see* Antacid Preparations *on page 95*
♦ **Aluminum Hydroxide and Magnesium Trisilicate** *see* Antacid Preparations *on page 95*
♦ **Aluminum Hydroxide Gel** *see* Antacid Preparations *on page 95*
♦ **Aluminum Hydroxide, Magnesium Hydroxide, and Simethicone** *see* Antacid Preparations *on page 95*
♦ **Aluminum Sucrose Sulfate, Basic** *see* Sucralfate *on page 919*
♦ **Alupent®** *see* Metaproterenol *on page 637*

Amantadine (a MAN ta deen)

U.S. Brand Names Symadine®; Symmetrel®
Canadian Brand Names Endantadine; Gen-Amantadine; PMS-Amantadine
Synonyms Adamantanamine
Therapeutic Category Anti-Parkinson's Agent; Antiviral Agent, Oral
Generic Available Yes
Use Prophylaxis and treatment of influenza A viral infection; symptomatic and adjunct treatment of parkinsonism
Pregnancy Risk Factor C
Contraindications Hypersensitivity to amantadine hydrochloride or any component
Precautions Use with caution in patients with liver disease, epilepsy, history of recurrent eczematoid dermatitis, uncontrolled psychosis, and in patients receiving CNS stimulant drugs; may increase seizure activity or EEG disturbances in patients with pre-existing seizure disorders; modify dosage in patients with renal impairment and in patients with active seizure disorders
Adverse Reactions
Cardiovascular: Orthostatic hypotension, edema
Central nervous system: Dizziness, confusion, headache, insomnia, difficulty in concentrating, anxiety, restlessness, irritability, hallucinations, seizures
Dermatologic: Livedo reticularis
Gastrointestinal: Nausea, vomiting, xerostomia

Genitourinary: Urinary retention

Drug Interactions Additive anticholinergic effects in patients receiving drugs with anticholinergic activity; additive CNS stimulant effect with CNS stimulants

Mechanism of Action As an antiviral, blocks the uncoating of influenza A virus preventing penetration of virus into host and inhibits M_2 protein in the assembly of progeny virions; antiparkinsonian activity may be due to its blocking the reuptake of dopamine into presynaptic neurons and causing direct stimulation of postsynaptic receptors

Pharmacokinetics

Absorption: Well absorbed from the GI tract

Half-life, patients with normal renal function: 10-28 hours

Time to peak serum concentration: 1-4 hours

Elimination: 80% to 90% excreted unchanged in the urine by glomerular filtration and tubular secretion

Dialysis: 0% to 5% removed by hemodialysis; no supplemental dose needed after hemodialysis or peritoneal dialysis

Usual Dosage Oral:

Children: Influenza A prophylaxis and treatment:

1-9 years: 5 mg/kg/day in 1-2 divided doses; maximum dose: 150 mg/day

≥10-12 years: 5 mg/kg/day in 1-2 divided doses; maximum dose: 200 mg/day

Note: After first influenza A virus vaccine dose, amantadine prophylaxis may be administered for up to 6 weeks, or until 2 weeks after the second dose of vaccine; administer a 10-day course of therapy following exposure; for symptomatic treatment, administer within 24-48 hours of symptom onset with usual duration of therapy between 2-5 days or for 24-48 hours after patient becomes asymptomatic

Alternative dosage for influenza A prophylaxis: Children >20 kg and Adults: 100 mg/day in 1-2 divided doses

Adults:

Parkinson's disease: 100 mg twice daily

Influenza A viral infection: 200 mg/day in 1-2 divided doses

Prophylaxis: Minimum 10-day course of therapy following exposure, or continue for 2-3 weeks after influenza A virus vaccine is given

Dosing interval in renal impairment: Adults:

Cl_{cr} 30-50 mL/minute: Administer 100 mg/day

Cl_{cr} 15-29 mL/minute: Administer 100 mg every other day

Cl_{cr} <15 mL/minute: Administer 200 mg every 7 days

Monitoring Parameters Renal function; monitor for signs of neurotoxicity

Patient Information Causes drowsiness and may impair ability to perform activities requiring mental alertness or coordination; do not abruptly discontinue therapy, may precipitate a parkinsonian crisis; avoid alcohol

Nursing Implications If insomnia occurs, the last daily dose should be taken several hours before retiring

Dosage Forms

Capsule, as hydrochloride: 100 mg

Syrup, as hydrochloride: 50 mg/5 mL (480 mL)

References

Strong DK, Eisenstat DD, Bryson SM, et al, "Amantadine Neurotoxicity in a Pediatric Patient With Renal Insufficiency," *DICP*, 1991, 25(11):1175-7.

♦ **Ambi 10**® **[OTC]**   *see* Benzoyl Peroxide *on page 136*

♦ **AmBisome**®   *see* Amphotericin B Liposome *on page 87*

♦ **AMCA**   *see* Tranexamic Acid *on page 975*

♦ **Amcort**®   *see* Triamcinolone *on page 979*

♦ **Americaine**® **[OTC]**   *see* Benzocaine *on page 135*

♦ **A-methaPred**®   *see* Methylprednisolone *on page 655*

♦ **Amethocaine**   *see* Tetracaine *on page 940*

♦ **Amethopterin**   *see* Methotrexate *on page 648*

♦ **Ametop (Can)**   *see* Tetracaine *on page 940*

♦ **Amicar**®   *see* Aminocaproic Acid *on page 68*

Amifostine (am i FOS teen)

U.S. Brand Names Ethyol®

Therapeutic Category Antidote, Cisplatin; Cytoprotective Agent

Use Cytoprotective agent which scavenges free radicals and binds to reactive drug derivatives due to radiation therapy, cisplatin, carboplatin, cyclophosphamide, ifosfamide, carmustine, melphalan, and mechlorethamine to selectively protect normal

(Continued)

Amifostine *(Continued)*

tissues against toxicity due to these agents; reduction of moderate to severe xerostomia from radiation treatment of the head and neck where the radiation port includes a substantial portion of the parotid glands

Pregnancy Risk Factor C

Contraindications Hypersensitivity to amifostine, aminothiol compounds, or any component; patients who are hypotensive or dehydrated

Warnings Due to limited experience and the possibility of amifostine interference with antineoplastic efficacy, amifostine should not be administered to patients in settings where chemotherapy can produce a significant survival benefit or cure, except in the context of a clinical study. Monitor serum calcium levels in patients at risk of hypocalcemia (eg, those patients receiving multiple doses of amifostine, patients with nephrotic syndrome).

Precautions Use with caution in patients with pre-existing cardiovascular or cerebrovascular conditions such as ischemic heart disease, arrhythmias, CHF, history of stroke or transient ischemic attacks; may cause hypotension; use special caution in situations where concomitant antihypertensive therapy cannot be interrupted 24 hours prior to starting amifostine or in patients in whom the adverse effects of nausea/vomiting may be more likely to have serious consequences

Adverse Reactions

Cardiovascular: Transient hypotension (62%; incidence is higher in patients with head and neck cancer, esophageal cancer, non-small cell lung cancer, prior neck irradiation, or hypercalcemia), flushing, warm sensation

Central nervous system: Chills, fever, dizziness, somnolence, hiccups, anxiety, malaise

Dermatologic: Rash

Endocrine & metabolic: Hypocalcemia, hypomagnesemia

Gastrointestinal: Nausea, vomiting, metallic taste in mouth

Genitourinary: Urinary retention (reversible)

Respiratory: Sneezing

Drug Interactions Antihypertensive agents may potentiate the hypotensive effects of amifostine

Stability When 500 mg amifostine is reconstituted with 9.7 mL of NS, the resultant solution is stable for 5 hours at room temperature or up to 24 hours if refrigerated; amifostine solutions diluted to 5-40 mg/mL in NS are chemically stable for 5 hours at room temperature or 24 hours if refrigerated; decreased stability in low pH conditions; incompatible with acyclovir, amphotericin B, chlorpromazine, cisplatin, ganciclovir, hydroxyzine, prochlorperazine

Mechanism of Action Amifostine is a prodrug that is converted by the alkaline membrane-bound enzyme alkaline phosphatase to the active free sulfhydryl compound WR-1065, which is further oxidized to a symmetrical disulfide (WR-33278) or to mixed disulfides. The active drug scavenges free radicals, donates hydrogen ions to free radicals, and binds to active derivatives of antineoplastic agents, thus preventing the alkylation of nucleic acid. Selective protection of normal tissue is demonstrated by:

1) decreased alkaline phosphatase activity in tumor cells,

2) decreased vascularity of tumors, and

3) lower pH in tumor tissues due to the predominance of anaerobic metabolism (WR-1065 requires a pH in the range of 6.6-8.2 for uptake into tissues)

Pharmacokinetics

Distribution: V_d: Adults: 6.4 L; unmetabolized prodrug is largely confined to the intravascular compartment; active metabolite is distributed into normal tissues with high concentrations in bone marrow, GI mucosa, skin, liver, and salivary glands

Protein binding: 4%

Metabolism: Amifostine (phosphorylated prodrug) is hydrolyzed by alkaline phosphatase to an active free sulfhydryl compound (WR-1065)

Half-life: 8 minutes (amifostine)

Elimination: Metabolites excreted in urine

Usual Dosage I.V. (refer to individual protocols):

Children: Limited data available on use in pediatric patients; dosing based on a prior clinical phase I trial and single case reports: 740 mg/m^2 once daily administered 30 minutes prior to chemotherapy; doses as high as 1650 mg/m^2 administered 30 minutes prior to melphalan have been used in phase II trials; repeat amifostine doses may be required when using a cytotoxic agent with a long half-life or long infusion time

Adults: 910 mg/m^2 once daily administered 30 minutes prior to chemotherapy; reduce dose to 740 mg/m^2 in patients who have a higher incidence of hypotension

Reduction of moderate to severe xerostomia from radiation of the head and neck: 200 mg/m² once daily starting 15-30 minutes prior to standard fraction radiation therapy

Administration Parenteral: I.V.: Reconstituted amifostine dose must be further diluted with NS to a final volume of 50 mL (adults) or a final concentration of 5-40 mg/mL (children). Administer amifostine doses >740 mg/m² as an I.V. intermittent infusion over 15 minutes since the 15-minute infusion is better tolerated than a more prolonged infusion. Administer 200 mg/m² dose as a 3-minute infusion. Amifostine should be interrupted if the blood pressure decreases significantly from baseline or if the patient develops symptoms related to decreased cerebral or cardiovascular perfusion. Patients experiencing decreased blood pressure should receive a rapid infusion of NS and be kept supine or placed in the Trendelenburg position. Amifostine can be restarted if the blood pressure returns to the baseline level.

Monitoring Parameters Baseline blood pressure followed by a blood pressure reading every 3-5 minutes during the 15-minute infusion; monitor electrolytes, urinalysis, serum calcium, serum magnesium; monitor I & O

Nursing Implications Pretreat patient with antiemetics; patients should be well hydrated prior to amifostine infusion; patients taking antihypertensive medications should discontinue therapy 24 hours before administration of amifostine; begin chemotherapy or radiation therapy 15 minutes after completion of amifostine

Dosage Forms Injection: 500 mg vial

References
Adamson PC, Balis FM, Belasco JE, et al, "A Phase I Trial of Amifostine (WR-2721) and Melphalan in Children With Refractory Cancer," *Cancer Res*, 1995, 55(18): 4069-72.

Bukowski R, "Cytoprotection in the Treatment of Pediatric Cancer: Review of Current Strategies in Adults and Their Application to Children," *Med Pediatr Oncol*, 1999, 32(2):124-34.

Schuchter LM, "Guidelines for the Administration of Amifostine," *Semin Oncol*, 1996, 23(4 Suppl 8):40-3.

Shaw LM, Bonner H, and Lieberman R, "Pharmacokinetic Profile of Amifostine," *Semin Oncol*, 1996, 23(4 Suppl 8):18-22.

Amikacin (am i KAY sin)

Related Information
Blood Level Sampling Time Guidelines *on page 1220*
Overdose and Toxicology *on page 1222*

U.S. Brand Names Amikin®

Therapeutic Category Antibiotic, Aminoglycoside

Generic Available Yes

Use Treatment of documented gram-negative enteric infection resistant to gentamicin and tobramycin; documented infection of mycobacterial organisms susceptible to amikacin

Pregnancy Risk Factor D

Contraindications Hypersensitivity to amikacin sulfate or any component; cross-sensitivity may exist with other aminoglycosides

Warnings Aminoglycosides are associated with significant nephrotoxicity or ototoxicity; the ototoxicity is directly proportional to the amount of drug given and the duration of treatment. Tinnitus or vertigo are indications of vestibular injury and impending bilateral irreversible deafness. Risk of nephrotoxicity increases when used concurrently with other potentially nephrotoxic drugs; renal damage is usually reversible. Aminoglycosides can cause fetal harm when administered to a pregnant woman, and have been associated with several reports of total irreversible bilateral congenital deafness in pediatric patients exposed *in utero*.

Precautions Use with caution in neonates (due to renal immaturity that results in a prolonged half-life); patients with pre-existing renal impairment, auditory or vestibular impairment, hypocalcemia, myasthenia gravis, and in conditions which depress neuromuscular transmission; dose and/or frequency of administration must be modified in patients with renal impairment

Adverse Reactions
Central nervous system: Fever, headache, dizziness, drowsiness, ataxia, vertigo
Dermatologic: Rash
Gastrointestinal: Nausea, vomiting
Hematologic: Eosinophilia, anemia, leukopenia
Neuromuscular & skeletal: Neuromuscular blockade, tremor, paresthesia, weakness, gait instability
Otic: Ototoxicity
Renal: Nephrotoxicity

Drug Interactions Extended-spectrum penicillins (decrease serum amikacin concentration in patients with renal failure); loop diuretics may potentiate the ototoxicity of the aminoglycosides; amphotericin, vancomycin, acyclovir, cisplatin, or (Continued)

Amikacin *(Continued)*

cephalosporins may increase nephrotoxicity; may potentiate the effects of neuro-muscular blocking agents and general anesthetics; indomethacin may increase serum amikacin concentrations

Mechanism of Action Inhibits protein synthesis in susceptible bacteria by binding to ribosomal subunits

Pharmacokinetics

Distribution: Primarily into extracellular fluid (highly hydrophilic); 12% of serum concentration penetrates into bronchial secretions; poor penetration into the blood-brain barrier even when meninges are inflamed; V_d is increased in neonates and patients with edema, ascites, fluid overload; V_d is decreased in patients with dehydration; crosses the placenta

Half-life:

Infants:

Low birth weight, 1-3 days of age: 7 hours

Full-term >7 days: 4-5 hours

Children: 1.6-2.5 hours

Adolescents: 1.5 ± 1 hour

Adults: 2-3 hours

Anuria: 28-86 hours; half-life and clearance are dependent on renal function

Time to peak serum concentration:

I.M.: Within 45-120 minutes

I.V.: Within 30 minutes following a 30-minute infusion

Elimination: 94% to 98% is excreted unchanged in the urine via glomerular filtration within 24 hours

Dialyzable (50% to 100%); supplemental dose recommended after hemodialysis or peritoneal dialysis

Usual Dosage I.M., I.V. (dosage should be based on an estimate of ideal body weight except in neonates; neonatal dosage should be based on actual weight unless the patient has hydrocephalus or hydrops fetalis):

Neonates:

0-4 weeks, <1200 g: 7.5 mg/kg/dose every 18-24 hours

Postnatal age ≤7 days:

1200-2000 g: 7.5 mg/kg/dose every 12 hours

>2000 g: 7.5-10 mg/kg/dose every 12 hours

Postnatal age >7 days:

1200-2000 g: 7.5-10 mg/kg/dose every 8-12 hours

>2000 g: 10 mg/kg/dose every 8 hours

Infants and Children: 15-22.5 mg/kg/day divided every 8 hours; some consultants recommend initial doses of 30 mg/kg/day divided every 8 hours in patients who may require larger doses; see Note

Treatment for nontuberculous mycobacterial infection: 15-30 mg/kg/day divided every 12-24 hours as part of a multiple drug regimen; maximum dose: 1.5 g/day

Adults: 15 mg/kg/day divided every 8-12 hours; maximum: 1.5 g/day

Treatment of *M. avium* complex infection: 7.5-15 mg/kg/day divided every 12-24 hours as part of a multiple drug regimen

Dosing interval in renal impairment: Loading dose: 5-7.5 mg/kg; subsequent dosages and frequency of administration are best determined by measurement of serum levels and assessment of renal insufficiency

Note: Some patients may require larger or more frequent doses if serum levels document the need (ie, cystic fibrosis or febrile granulocytopenic patients)

Administration Parenteral: Administer by intermittent I.V. infusion over 30 minutes at a final concentration not to exceed 5 mg amikacin/mL

Monitoring Parameters Urinalysis, urine output, BUN, serum creatinine, peak and trough serum amikacin concentrations; be alert to ototoxicity

Not all infants and children who receive aminoglycosides require monitoring of serum aminoglycoside concentrations. Indications for use of aminoglycoside serum concentration monitoring include:

• treatment course >5 days

• patients with decreased or changing renal function

• patients with poor therapeutic response

• infants <3 months of age

• atypical body constituency (obesity, expanded extracellular fluid volume)

• clinical need for higher doses or shorter intervals (eg, cystic fibrosis, burns, endocarditis, meningitis, critically ill patients, relatively resistant organisms)

• patients on hemodialysis or chronic ambulatory peritoneal dialysis

• signs of nephrotoxicity or ototoxicity

• concomitant use of other nephrotoxic agents

Reference Range
Peak: 20-30 µg/mL
Trough: <10 µg/mL

Patient Information Report loss of hearing, ringing or roaring in the ears, or feeling of fullness in head

Nursing Implications Aminoglycoside levels measured from blood taken from Silastic® central catheters can sometimes give falsely elevated readings; peak serum levels should be drawn 30 minutes after the end of a 30-minute infusion; trough levels are drawn within 30 minutes before the next dose; provide optimal patient hydration

Dosage Forms Injection, as sulfate: 50 mg/mL (2 mL); 250 mg/mL (2 mL, 4 mL)

References

Kenyon CF, Knoppert DC, Lee SK, et al, "Amikacin Pharmacokinetics and Suggested Dosage Modifications for the Preterm Infant," *Antimicrob Agents Chemother*, 1990, 34(2):265-8.

Public Health Service Task Force on Prophylaxis and Therapy for *Mycobacterium avium* Complex, "Recommendations on Prophylaxis and Therapy for Disseminated *Mycobacterium avium* Complex Disease in Patients Infected With the Human Immunodeficiency Virus," *N Engl J Med*, 1993, 329(12):898-904.

Starke JR and Correa AG, "Management of Mycobacterial Infection and Disease in Children," *Pediatr Infect Dis J*, 1995, 14(6):455-69.

Vogelstein B, Kowarski A, and Lietman PS, "The Pharmacokinetics of Amikacin in Children," *J Pediatr*, 1977, 91(2):333-9.

♦ **Amikin®** *see* Amikacin *on page 65*

Amiloride (a MIL oh ride)

U.S. Brand Names Midamor®

Therapeutic Category Antihypertensive Agent; Diuretic, Potassium Sparing

Generic Available Yes

Use Management of edema associated with CHF, hepatic cirrhosis, and hyperaldosteronism; hypertension; primary hyperaldosteronism; hypokalemia induced by kaliuretic diuretics

Pregnancy Risk Factor B

Contraindications Hypersensitivity to amiloride or any component; hyperkalemia; anuria

Warnings Due to potential severe hyperkalemia, amiloride should be discontinued in diabetic patients for at least 3 days prior to glucose tolerance testing; discontinue if serum potassium >5.5 mEq/L

Precautions Use with caution in patients with dehydration, electrolyte imbalance, metabolic or respiratory acidosis, diabetes (particularly those with nephropathy), hyponatremia, impaired renal function, or hepatic dysfunction; patients receiving potassium or other potassium-sparing diuretics

Adverse Reactions

Cardiovascular: Angina, orthostatic hypotension, arrhythmia, palpitations

Central nervous system: Headache, dizziness, encephalopathy, vertigo, nervousness, mental confusion, insomnia, depression, somnolence

Dermatologic: Skin rash, pruritus, alopecia

Endocrine & metabolic: Hyperkalemia, hyperchloremic metabolic acidosis, dehydration, hyponatremia, gynecomastia

Gastrointestinal: Nausea, anorexia, diarrhea, vomiting, abdominal pain, appetite changes, constipation, GI bleeding, xerostomia, heartburn, flatulence, dyspepsia

Genitourinary: Impotence, dysuria, urinary frequency, bladder spasms

Hematologic: Aplastic anemia, neutropenia

Hepatic: Abnormal liver function

Neuromuscular & skeletal: Weakness, muscle cramps, joint and back pain, paresthesia, tremors

Ophthalmic: Visual disturbances, increased intraocular pressure

Otic: Tinnitus

Renal: Polyuria

Respiratory: Cough, dyspnea, nasal congestion, shortness of breath

Drug Interactions Potassium, other potassium-sparing diuretics, and ACE inhibitors (eg, captopril) may additively increase the serum potassium; may decrease digoxin clearance and attenuate its inotropic effect; decreases lithium clearance; decreased diuresis and antihypertensive effects with concomitant NSAID use

Food Interactions Avoid natural licorice (causes sodium and water retention and increases potassium loss) and salt substitutes; food decreases absorption to ~30%

Mechanism of Action Acts directly on the distal renal tubule to inhibit sodium-potassium ion exchange; decreases sodium reabsorption in the distal tubule by inhibiting cellular sodium transport mechanisms such as the conductive sodium

(Continued)

Amiloride *(Continued)*

influx pathway and possibly the sodium-hydrogen ion exchange system; also inhibits hydrogen ion secretion; its diuretic activity is **independent** of aldosterone.

Pharmacodynamics
Onset of action: 2 hours
Peak effect: 6-10 hours
Duration: 24 hours

Pharmacokinetics
Absorption: 50%
Distribution: Adults: V_d: 350-380 L
Metabolism: No active metabolites
Half-life: Adults:
  Normal renal function: 6-9 hours
  End stage renal disease: 21-144 hours
Elimination: Unchanged drug, equally in urine and feces

Usual Dosage Oral:
Children 6-20 kg: 0.625 mg/kg/day once daily; maximum dose: 10 mg/day
Children >20 kg and Adults: 5-10 mg/day; maximum dose: 20 mg/day
  Dosing adjustment in renal impairment:
  Cl_{cr} 10-50 mL/minute: Administer at 50% of normal dose
  Cl_{cr} <10 mL/minute: Avoid use

Administration Oral: Administer with food or milk

Monitoring Parameters Serum potassium, sodium, creatinine, BUN, blood pressure, fluid balance

Test Interactions May falsely elevate serum digoxin levels done by radioimmunoassay

Patient Information Report to your physician any muscle cramps, weakness, nausea, or dizziness; may cause drowsiness and impair ability to perform hazardous tasks which require mental alertness or physical coordination

Additional Information Studies utilizing aerosolized amiloride (5 mmol/L in 0.3% saline) in adult cystic fibrosis patients (Tomkiewicz, 1993) have suggested that inhaled amiloride is capable of improving the rheologic properties of the abnormally thickened mucus by increasing mucus sodium content

Dosage Forms Tablet, as hydrochloride: 5 mg

Extemporaneous Preparations A 1 mg/mL oral liquid may be prepared from crushed tablets added to a small quantity of sterile water to which glycerin (final concentration of 40% w/v) is added; sterile water is then added in sufficient quantity to make the desired volume; stable 21 days when refrigerated

Fawcett JP, Woods DJ, Ferry DG, et al, "Stability of Amiloride Hydrochloride Oral Liquids Prepared From Tablets and Powder," *Aust J Hosp Pharm*, 1995, 25:10-23.

References
Tomkiewicz RP, App, EM, Zayas JG, et al, "Amiloride Inhalation Therapy in Cystic Fibrosis. Influence on Ion Content, Hydration, and Rheology of Sputum," *Am Rev Resp Dis*, 1993, 148:1002-7.

♦ **2-Amino-6-mercaptopurine** *see* Thioguanine *on page 950*
♦ **Aminobenzylpenicillin** *see* Ampicillin *on page 88*

Aminocaproic Acid *(a mee noe ka PROE ik AS id)*

Related Information
Carbohydrate and Alcohol Content of Liquid Medications for Use in Patients Receiving Ketogenic Diets *on page 1258*

U.S. Brand Names Amicar®

Therapeutic Category Hemostatic Agent

Generic Available Yes: Injection

Use Treatment of excessive bleeding resulting from systemic hyperfibrinolysis, urinary fibrinolysis, or traumatic ocular hyphema

Pregnancy Risk Factor C

Contraindications Disseminated intravascular coagulation; evidence of an intravascular clotting process; use of factor IX concentrate or anti-inhibitor coagulant concentrate; injectable product contains benzyl alcohol, avoid use in newborns

Warnings Aminocaproic acid may accumulate in patients with decreased renal function; intrarenal obstruction may occur secondary to glomerular capillary thrombosis or clots in the renal pelvis and ureters; do not use in hematuria of upper urinary tract origin unless benefits outweigh potential risks; inhibition of fibrinolysis may promote clotting or thrombosis

Precautions Use with caution in patients with cardiac, renal or hepatic disease; use with caution in patients at risk for veno-occlusive disease of the liver

Adverse Reactions

Cardiovascular: Hypotension, bradycardia and arrhythmias (following rapid I.V. administration)

Central nervous system: Dizziness, headache, malaise, seizures, confusion

Dermatologic: Rash

Endocrine & metabolic: Hyperkalemia

Gastrointestinal: GI irritation, nausea, cramps, diarrhea

Hematologic: Decreased platelet function, agranulocytosis, leukopenia

Neuromuscular & skeletal: Myopathy, acute rhabdomyolysis, weakness

Ocular: Glaucoma, watery eyes

Otic: Tinnitus, deafness

Renal: Renal failure

Respiratory: Nasal congestion, dyspnea, pulmonary embolism

Drug Interactions Increased risk of thrombosis with oral contraceptives, estrogens, and factor IX

Mechanism of Action Competitively inhibits activation of plasminogen thereby reducing fibrinolysin, without inhibiting lysis of clot

Pharmacodynamics Onset of action: Inhibition of fibrinolysis: Within 1-72 hours (onset shortened substantially if loading dose is used)

Pharmacokinetics

Distribution: Widely distributes through intravascular and extravascular compartments

Metabolism: Hepatic metabolism is minimal

Bioavailability: Oral: 100%

Half-life: 1-2 hours

Elimination: 40% to 60% excreted as unchanged drug in the urine within 12 hours

Usual Dosage

Children:

Oral, I.V.: Loading dose: 100-200 mg/kg; maintenance: 100 mg/kg/dose every 6 hours; maximum daily dose: 30 g

or as an alternative: I.V. loading dose: 100 mg/kg or 3 g/m^2 followed by a continuous infusion of 33.3 mg/kg/hour or 1 g/m^2/hour; total dosage should not exceed 18 g/m^2/day

Traumatic hyphema: Oral, I.V.: 100 mg/kg/dose every 4 hours (maximum dose: 5 g/dose; maximum daily dose: 30 g/day)

Adults:

Oral: For the treatment of acute bleeding syndromes due to elevated fibrinolytic activity, give 5 g during first hour, followed by 1-1.25 g/hour for about 8 hours or until bleeding stops; daily dose should not exceed 30 g

I.V.: Give 4-5 g during first hour followed by continuous infusion at the rate of 1-1.25 g/hour, continue for 8 hours or until bleeding stops

Dosing adjustment in renal impairment: Oliguria or ESRD: Reduce dose to 25% of normal

Administration

Oral: May administer without regard to food

Parenteral: Maximum concentration for I.V. administration: 20 mg/mL; administer single doses over at least 1 hour

Monitoring Parameters Fibrinogen, fibrin split products, serum creatinine kinase (long-term therapy); serum potassium (may be elevated by aminocaproic acid, especially if the patient has impaired renal function)

Reference Range Therapeutic concentration: >130 µg/mL (concentration necessary for inhibition of fibrinolysis)

Nursing Implications Rapid I.V. injection (IVP) should be avoided since hypotension, bradycardia, and arrhythmias may result

Dosage Forms

Injection: 250 mg/mL (20 mL)

Syrup: 250 mg/mL [raspberry flavor] (480 mL)

Tablet: 500 mg

References

McGetrick JJ, Jampol LM, Goldberg MP, et al, "Aminocaproic Acid Decreases Secondary Hemorrhage After Traumatic Hyphema," *Arch Ophthalmol*, 1983, 101(7):1031-3.

♦ **Aminohydroxypropylidene Diphosphonate** *see* Pamidronate *on page 753*

♦ **Aminophyllin**™ *see* Aminophylline *on page 69*

Aminophylline (am in OFF i lin)

Related Information

Asthma Guidelines *on page 1210*

Overdose and Toxicology *on page 1222*

(Continued)

Aminophylline *(Continued)*

Theophylline *on page 943*

U.S. Brand Names Aminophyllin™

Canadian Brand Names Phyllocontin

Synonyms Theophylline Ethylenediamine

Therapeutic Category Antiasthmatic; Bronchodilator; Respiratory Stimulant; Theophylline Derivative

Generic Available Yes

Use Bronchodilator in reversible airway obstruction due to asthma or COPD; increase diaphragmatic contractility; neonatal idiopathic apnea of prematurity

Pregnancy Risk Factor C

Contraindications Uncontrolled arrhythmias

Warnings Some commercial products may contain sulfites which may produce hypersensitivity reactions in sensitive individuals

Adverse Reactions See Theophylline *on page 943*

Drug Interactions Cytochrome P-450 isoenzyme CYP1A2, CYP2E1 (minor), and CYP3A3/4 substrate

Clinical Factors Reported to Affect Theophylline Clearance

Decreased Theophylline Level	Increased Theophylline Level
Smoking (cigarettes, marijuana)	Acute pulmonary edema
High protein/low carbohydrate diet	Cessation of smoking (after chronic use)
Charcoal broiled beef	Cor pulmonale
	Congestive heart failure
	Hypothyroidism
	Fever (≥102° for 24 hours or more, or lesser temperature elevations for longer periods)
	Hepatic cirrhosis/acute hepatitis
	Renal failure in infants <3 mo of age
	Sepsis with multisystem organ failure
	Shock
	Viral illness

Medications Affecting Theophylline Clearance Resulting in Either Increased or Decreased Serum Levels

Decreased Theophylline Level	Increased Theophylline Level
Aminoglutethimide	Alcohol
Carbamazepine	Allopurinol (>600 mg/day)
Isoproterenol (I.V.)	Beta-blockers
Isoniazid*	Calcium channel blockers
Ketoconazole	Cimetidine
Loop diuretics*	Ciprofloxacin
Nevirapine	Clarithromycin
Phenobarbital	Corticosteroids
Phenytoin	Disulfiram
Rifampin	Ephedrine
Ritonavir	Erythromycin
Sulfinpyrazone	Esmolol
Sympathomimetics	Influenza virus vaccine
	Interferon, human recombinant alpha 2-a and 2-b
	Isoniazid*
	Loop diuretics*
	Methotrexate
	Mexiletine
	Oral contraceptives
	Propafenone
	Propranolol
	Tacrine
	Thiabendazole
	Thyroid hormones
	Troleandomycin (TAO®)
	Verapamil
	Zileuton

*Both increased and decreased theophylline levels have been reported.

Decreases adenosine, benzodiazepines, and pancuronium effects; decreases zafirlukast serum levels; increases lithium clearance; increases CNS side effects with ephedrine; increases risk of cardiac arrhythmias with halothane; for medications which change aminophylline (theophylline) clearance, see tables.

Food Interactions Food does not appreciably affect absorption; avoid extremes of dietary protein and carbohydrate intake; limit charcoal-broiled foods and caffeinated beverages

Mechanism of Action See Theophylline *on page 943*

Pharmacokinetics Aminophylline is the ethylenediamine salt of theophylline, pharmacokinetic parameters are those of **theophylline**; fraction available: 80% (eg, 100 mg aminophylline = 80 mg theophylline); see Theophylline *on page 943*

Usual Dosage All dosages based upon **aminophylline**
Neonates:
Apnea of prematurity: Oral, I.V.:
Loading dose: 5 mg/kg
Maintenance: Initial: 5 mg/kg/day every 12 hours; increased dosages may be indicated as liver metabolism matures (usually >30 days of life); monitor serum levels to determine appropriate dosages
Theophylline levels should be initially drawn after 3 days of therapy; repeat levels are indicated 3 days after each increase in dosage or weekly if on a stabilized dosage
Infants, Children, and Adults: Treatment of acute bronchospasm: I.V.: Loading dose (in patients not currently receiving aminophylline or theophylline): 6 mg/kg (based on aminophylline) given I.V. over 20-30 minutes

Approximate I.V. maintenance dosages are based upon **continuous infusions**; intermittent dosing (often used in children <6 months of age) may be determined by multiplying the hourly infusion rate by 24 hours and dividing by the desired number of doses/day (usually in 3-4 doses/day)
6 weeks to 6 months: 0.5 mg/kg/hour
6 months to 1 year: 0.6-0.7 mg/kg/hour
1-9 years: 1-1.2 mg/kg/hour
9-12 years and young adult smokers: 0.9 mg/kg/hour
12-16 years: 0.7 mg/kg/hour
Adults (healthy, nonsmoking): 0.7 mg/kg/hour
Older patients and patients with cor pulmonale, patients with CHF or liver failure: 0.25 mg/kg/hour
Oral dose: See Theophylline *on page 943*, (consider mg theophylline available when using aminophylline products)
Dosage should be adjusted according to serum level measurements during the first 12- to 24-hour period. Avoid using suppositories due to erratic, unreliable absorption. See table.

Guidelines for Drawing Theophylline Serum Levels

Dosage Form	Time to Draw Level*
I.V. bolus	30 min after end of 30-min infusion
I.V. continuous infusion	12-24 h after initiation of infusion
P.O. liquid, fast-release formulation	Peak: 1 h postdose after at least 1 day of therapy Trough: Just before a dose after at least 1 day of therapy

*The time to achieve steady-state serum levels is prolonged in patients with longer half-lives (eg, premature neonates, infants, and adults with cardiac or liver failure (see theophylline half-life table). In these patients, serum theophylline levels should be drawn after 48-72 hours of therapy; serum levels may need to be done prior to steady-state to assess the patient's current progress or evaluate potential toxicity.

Administration
Oral: May be administered without regard to meals
Parenteral: Dilute with I.V. fluid to a concentration of 1 mg/mL and infuse over 20-30 minutes; maximum concentration: 25 mg/mL; maximum rate of infusion: 0.36 mg/kg/minute, and no greater than 25 mg/minute
Monitoring Parameters Serum theophylline levels, heart rate, respiratory rate, number and severity of apnea spells (when used for apnea of prematurity); arterial or capillary blood gases (if applicable); pulmonary function tests
(Continued)

Aminophylline *(Continued)*

Reference Range Therapeutic: For asthma 10-20 µg/mL; for neonatal apnea 6-13 µg/mL (serum levels are reduced for neonatal apnea due to decreased binding of theophylline to fetal albumin resulting in a greater amount of free "active" theophylline)

Dosage Forms Theophylline (anhydrous) equivalent listed in brackets

Injection, I.V. (Aminophyllin™): 25 mg/mL [19.7 mg/mL] (10 mL, 20 mL)

Liquid, oral: 105 mg/5 mL [90 mg/5 mL] (10 mL, 240 mL, 500 mL)

Suppository, rectal: 250 mg [197.5 mg], 500 mg [395 mg]

Tablet (Aminophyllin™): 100 mg [79 mg], 200 mg [158 mg]

♦ **5-Aminosalicylic Acid** *see* Mesalamine *on page 634*

Amiodarone (a MEE oh da rone)

Related Information

Adult ACLS Algorithm, Narrow-Complex Supraventricular Tachycardia *on page 1046*

Adult ACLS Algorithm, Stable Ventricular Tachycardia *on page 1047*

Adult ACLS Algorithm, V. Fib and Pulseless VT *on page 1041*

CPR Pediatric Drug Dosages *on page 1031*

Pediatric ALS Algorithm, Pulseless Arrest *on page 1036*

Pediatric ALS Algorithm, Tachycardia - Rapid Rhythm and Adequate Perfusion *on page 1037*

Pediatric ALS Algorithm, Tachycardia - Rapid Rhythm and Evidence of Poor Perfusion *on page 1038*

U.S. Brand Names Cordarone®; Pacerone®

Canadian Brand Names Alti-Amiodarone; Gen-Amiodarone; Novo-Amiodarone

Therapeutic Category Antiarrhythmic Agent, Class III

Generic Available Yes

Use

Oral: Management of life-threatening ventricular arrhythmias [eg, recurrent ventricular fibrillation (VF) or recurrent hemodynamically unstable ventricular tachycardia (VT)] unresponsive to other therapy

I.V.: Initiation of management and prophylaxis of frequently recurrent VF and hemodynamically unstable VT unresponsive to other therapy; VF and VT in patients requiring amiodarone who are not able to take oral therapy

Note: Also has been used to treat supraventricular arrhythmias unresponsive to other therapy. A benzyl alcohol-free injectable product is available from the manufacturer via orphan drug status or compassionate use for acute treatment and prophylaxis of life-threatening ventricular tachycardia or ventricular fibrillation (see Dosage Forms)

Pregnancy Risk Factor D

Contraindications Hypersensitivity to amiodarone or any component; severe sinus node dysfunction; marked sinus bradycardia, second and third degree A-V block; cardiogenic shock; bradycardia-induced syncope, except if pacemaker is placed

Warnings Not considered first-line antiarrhythmic due to high incidence of toxicity; 75% of patients experience adverse effects with large doses. Discontinuation is required in 5% to 20% of patients. Pulmonary and hepatic toxicities may be fatal (see Adverse Reactions); reserve for use in life-threatening arrhythmias refractory to other therapy. Optic neuropathy and/or optic neuritis resulting in visual impairment may occur at any time and can progress to permanent blindness; prompt ophthalmic exam is recommended if visual impairment occurs; re-evaluate amiodarone therapy if optic neuropathy or neuritis occurs. Hypotension with I.V. product occurs in about 16% of patients and may be associated with infusion rate. Bradycardia and AV block may occur; temporary pacemaker should be available when I.V. product is used in patients with known predisposition to bradycardia or AV block. Patients should be hospitalized for initiation of therapy and loading dose administration.

Precautions Amiodarone HCl contains 37% iodine by weight; avoid use during pregnancy and while breast-feeding (fetal/neonatal goiters, hypothyroidism, and possible cerebral damage may occur); use with caution and monitor closely in patients with thyroid disease. May worsen or precipitate arrhythmias; when possible, hypokalemia and hypomagnesemia should be corrected prior to I.V. amiodarone use due to increased risk for torsade de pointes. Use with caution in neonates as injectable product (Cordarone®) contains benzyl alcohol and polysorbate (Tween®) 80; benzyl alcohol may displace bilirubin from protein binding sites and at larger doses can cause a potentially fatal gasping syndrome in neonates. Serious drug interactions may occur (see Drug Interactions).

Safety and efficacy of amiodarone have not been established in pediatric patients. The I.V. product (Cordarone®) has been shown to leach out plasticizers [eg, DEHP or di-(2-ethylhexyl)phthalate] from I.V. tubing, including polyvinyl chloride tubing. In immature animals, exposure to DEHP may adversely affect the development of the male reproductive tract. In order to decrease the potential exposure of infants to plasticizers, consider the use of bolus dosing in 1 mg/kg oliquots as described by Perry, 1996; see Usual Dosage. See also http://www.fda.gov/medwatch/safety/2001/safety01.htm#cordar.

Adverse Reactions

Cardiovascular: Proarrhythmia (including torsade de pointes), atropine-resistant bradycardia, heart block, sinus arrest, myocardial depression, CHF, paroxysmal ventricular tachycardia, cardiogenic shock, hypotension (**Note:** In adults, I.V. daily doses >2100 mg are associated with a greater risk of hypotension.)

Central nervous system (20% to 40% incidence): Lack of coordination, fatigue, malaise, abnormal gait, dizziness, headache, insomnia, nightmares, ataxia, behavioral changes, fever

Dermatologic: Discoloration of skin (slate blue), photosensitivity, rash, angioedema

Endocrine & metabolic: Hypothyroidism (or less commonly hyperthyroidism, see Additional Information), hyperglycemia, increased triglycerides

Gastrointestinal: Nausea, vomiting, anorexia, constipation

Genitourinary: Sterile epididymitis

Hematologic: Coagulation abnormalities, thrombocytopenia

Hepatic: Elevated liver enzymes, severe hepatic toxicity (potentially fatal), increased bilirubin, increased serum ammonia

Local: Phlebitis (with I.V. formulation; concentration dependent)

Neuromuscular & skeletal: Paresthesia, tremor, peripheral neuropathy (rare)

Ocular: Corneal microdeposits, halos or blurred vision (10% incidence), photophobia, optic neuropathy, optic neuritis, visual impairment, permanent blindness (**Note:** Asymptomatic corneal microdeposits alone do not require dose reduction or discontinuation)

Respiratory (potentially fatal): Interstitial pneumonitis, hypersensitivity pneumonitis, pulmonary fibrosis (may present with cough, fever, dyspnea, malaise, chest x-ray changes); adult respiratory distress syndrome following surgery

Drug Interactions
Cytochrome P-450 isoenzyme CYP3A3/4 substrate; isoenzyme CYP2C9, CYP2D6, and CYP3A3/4 inhibitor

Amiodarone inhibits P-450 enzymes and may increase plasma concentrations of digoxin, cyclosporine, flecainide, lidocaine, methotrexate, theophylline, procainamide, quinidine, warfarin, and phenytoin resulting in toxicities. **Note:** Dosage reduction of these agents and follow-up serum concentration monitoring are recommended (eg, a 50% dosage reduction in digoxin, 30% dosage reduction in flecainide, and a 30% to 50% dosage reduction in warfarin have been recommended). Combined use with beta-blockers, digitalis glycosides, or calcium channel blockers may result in bradycardia, sinus arrest; use with class I antiarrhythmics may cause ventricular arrhythmias; amiodarone and general anesthetics may result in bradycardia, hypotension, heart block; use with fentanyl may cause bradycardia, hypotension, decreased cardiac output; amiodarone may inhibit the metabolism of dextromethorphan; phenytoin and cholestyramine may decrease and cimetidine may increase amiodarone serum levels. Concurrent use of amiodarone with ritonavir or nelfinavir is not recommended.

Food Interactions
Food increases rate and extent of oral absorption (high fat meal increased AUC by a mean of 2.3 times)

Stability

Storage: Tablets and I.V. product should be kept at room temperature and protected from light during storage; injection should also be protected from excessive heat; there is no need to protect diluted solutions from light during I.V. administration

Compatibility: Injection is compatible in D_5W at concentrations of 1-6 mg/mL for 24 hours in glass or polyolefin bottles and for 2 hours in polyvinyl chloride bags; although amiodarone adsorbs to polyvinyl chloride tubing, all clinical studies used polyvinyl chloride tubing and the recommended doses take adsorption into account, therefore, polyvinyl chloride tubing is recommended; amiodarone I.V. in D_5W is **not** compatible with aminophylline, cefamandole, cefazolin, mezlocillin, heparin, or sodium bicarbonate when administered together at the Y-site (a precipitate will occur)

Mechanism of Action
A class III antiarrhythmic agent which inhibits adrenergic stimulation, prolongs the action potential and refractory period in myocardial tissue; decreases A-V conduction and sinus node function; possesses vasodilatory and negative inotropic effects

(Continued)

Amiodarone *(Continued)*

Pharmacodynamics

Onset of effect: Oral: 2-3 days to 1-3 weeks after starting therapy; I.V.: (electrophysiologic effects) within hours; antiarrhythmic effects: 2-3 days to 1-3 weeks; mean onset of effect may be shorter in children vs adults and in patients receiving I.V. loading doses

Maximum effect: Oral: 1 week to 5 months

Duration of effects after discontinuation of oral therapy: Variable, 2 weeks to months: Children: less than a few weeks; adults: several months

Pharmacokinetics

Absorption: Oral: Slow and incomplete

Distribution: Amiodarone and its active metabolite cross the placenta; both distribute to breast milk in concentrations higher than maternal plasma concentrations

I.V.: Rapid redistribution with a decrease to 10% of peak values within 30-45 minutes after completion of infusion

V_{dss}: I.V. single dose in adults: Mean range: 40-84 L/kg

V_d: Oral dose in adults: 66 L/kg: range: 18-148 L/kg

Protein binding: >96%

Metabolism: In the liver and possibly the GI tract via cytochrome P-450 enzymes; the major metabolite N-desethylamiodarone is active

Bioavailability: Oral: ~50% (range: 35% to 65%)

Half-life:

Amiodarone:

Single dose in adults: Mean: 58 days (range 15-142 days)

Oral chronic therapy in adults: Mean range: 40-55 days (range: 26-107 days)

I.V. single dose in adults: Mean range: 20-47 days

Half-life is shortened in children vs adults

N-desethylamiodarone (active metabolite):

Single dose in adults: Mean: 36 days (range 14-75 days)

Oral chronic therapy in adults: Mean: 61 days

Elimination: Via biliary excretion; possible enterohepatic recirculation; <1% excreted unchanged in urine

Dialysis: Nondialyzable (parent and metabolite)

Usual Dosage

Infants and Children:

Oral: **Note:** Calculate dose using body surface area for children <1 year of age: Loading dose: 10-15 mg/kg/day or 600-800 mg/1.73 m²/day in 1-2 divided doses/day for 4-14 days or until adequate control of arrhythmia or prominent adverse effects occur; dosage should then be reduced to 5 mg/kg/day or 200-400 mg/1.73 m²/day given once daily for several weeks; if arrhythmia does not recur, reduce to lowest effective dosage possible; usual daily minimal dose: 2.5 mg/kg; maintenance doses may be given for 5 of 7 days/week.

Note: A more aggressive dosing regimen was used in neonates and infants (n=50; mean age: 1 ±1.5 months) <9 months of age, treated for various types of SVT; 90% of patients at discharge and 100% of patients within 3 months of discharge were free of tachycardia; however, patients who received a higher loading dose (20 mg/kg/day in 2 divided doses) were more likely to have a prolongation of the corrected QT interval (see Etheridge, 2001); further studies are needed.

I.V., I.O.:

PALS dose for treatment of pulseless VF or VT: 5 mg/kg rapid I.V. bolus or I.O.

PALS dose for treatment of perfusing tachycardias: Loading dose: 5 mg/kg I.V. over 20-60 minutes or I.O.; may repeat up to maximum dose: 15 mg/kg/day. **Note:** Routine use with drugs that prolong the QT interval is **not** recommended; monitor for hypotension.

I.V.: Limited data is available. Four retrospective studies (Figa, 1994; Raja, 1994; Soult, 1995; Celiker, 1998) used I.V. loading doses of 5 mg/kg. Loading doses were administered over 1 hour in three of these studies to treat various life-threatening tachyarrhythmias including junctional ectopic tachycardia after cardiac surgery (in conjunction with atrial pacing). Soult 1995 used I.V. amiodarone for short-term treatment of paroxysmal supraventricular tachycardia (PSVT) and administered the loading dose via slow I.V. bolus over 5 minutes. For continuous infusion, Figa 1994 and Celiker 1998, used initial maintenance doses of 5 mcg/kg/minute (7.2 mg/kg/day) which was increased incrementally until the desired effect was seen or a maximum dose of 15 mcg/kg/minute (21.6 mg/kg/day) was reached. The mean effective dose in the study by Figa 1994 (n=30) was 9.5 mcg/kg/minute (13.7 mg/kg/day) and in Celiker 1998 (n=12) was 10 ±4.7 mcg/kg/minute (range: 5-15 mg/kg/minute).

A multicenter study (Perry, 1996; n=40; mean age 5.4 years with 24 of 40 children <2 years of age) used an I.V. loading dose of 5 mg/kg that was divided into five 1 mg/kg aliquots, with each aliquot given over 5-10 minutes. Additional 1-5 mg/kg doses could be administered 30 minutes later in a similar fashion if needed. The mean loading dose was 6.3 mg/kg. A maintenance dose (continuous infusion of 10-15 mg/kg/day) was administered to 21 of the 40 patients. Further studies are needed.

Adults:

ACLS dose for cardiac arrest due to pulseless VT or VF: I.V.: Initial: 300 mg diluted in 20-30 mL D_5W or NS given rapid I.V. push; supplemental bolus doses of 150 mg rapid I.V. infusion may be given for recurring VF or pulseless VT; maximum total dose: 2.2 g/24 hours

Ventricular arrhythmias:

Oral: Loading dose: 800-1600 mg/day divided in 1-2 doses/day for 1-3 weeks, then 600-800 mg/day in 1-2 doses/day for 1 month; maintenance: 400 mg/day; lower doses are recommended for supraventricular arrhythmias.

I.V.: Loading dose: ~1000 mg delivered over 24 hours as follows: 150 mg given over 10 minutes (at a rate of 15 mg/minute) followed by 360 mg given over 6 hours (at a rate of 1 mg/minute); follow with maintenance dose: 540 mg given over the next 18 hours (at a rate of 0.5 mg/minute); after the first 24 hours the maintenance dose is continued at 0.5 mg/minute; additional supplemental bolus doses of 150 mg infused over 10 minutes may be given for breakthrough VF or hemodynamically unstable VT; maintenance dose infusion may be increased to control arrhythmia; maximum daily dose: 2 g

Atrial fibrillation (see Goldschlager, 2000):

Oral: Loading dose: 600-800 mg/day divided in 2 doses/day for 2-4 weeks, then 400 mg/day; at 3-6 months, dose may be reduced further to 100-300 mg/day based on clinical efficacy and adverse effects; usual maintenance: 200 mg/day; **Note:** some patients may require higher maintenance doses or increased maintenance doses for short periods of time for breakthrough arrhythmias; some patients can be maintained with 200 mg/day given for 5 of 7 days/week

Transition from I.V. to oral therapy: Optimal initial daily dose depends on I.V. dose administered and oral bioavailability; use the following as a guide for an initial daily dose, assuming patient received 0.5 mg/minute for the listed duration of I.V. infusion:

<1 week infusion: 800-1600 mg/day
1-3 week infusion: 600-800 mg/day
>3 week infusion: 400 mg/day

Dosing adjustment in renal impairment: No adjustment necessary

Administration

Oral: Administer at same time in relation to meals

I.V.: Injection must be diluted before I.V. use. Adults: Usual dilutions: First loading infusion: 150 mg in 100 mL D_5W (1.5 mg/mL) for infusion over 10 minutes; then 900 mg in 500 mL D_5W (1.8 mg/mL) to deliver rest of dose; administer via central venous catheter, if possible; increased phlebitis may occur with peripheral infusions >3 mg/mL in D_5W, but concentrations ≤2.5 mg/mL may be less irritating; the use of a central venous catheter with concentrations >2 mg/mL for infusions >1 hour is recommended; maximum concentration for infusion: 6 mg/mL; use glass or polyolefin bottles for infusions >2 hours; the use of polyvinyl chloride tubing is recommended (see Stability); must be infused via volumetric infusion device; drop size of I.V. solution may be reduced and underdosage may occur if drop counter infusion sets are used; use in-line filter during administration; adults: Do not exceed 30 mg/minute initial infusion rate; infants and children: See Usual Dosage I.V.

Monitoring Parameters Heart rate and rhythm, blood pressure, EKG, chest x-ray, pulmonary function tests, thyroid function tests (see Additional Information), serum glucose, triglycerides, liver enzymes, ophthalmologic exams including fundoscopy and slit-lamp examinations, physical signs and symptoms of thyroid dysfunction (lethargy, edema of hands and feet, weight gain or loss), and pulmonary toxicity (dyspnea, cough)

Reference Range Therapeutic: Chronic oral dosing: 1-2.5 mg/L (SI: 2-4 μmol/L) (parent); desethyl metabolite (active) is present in equal concentration to parent drug; serum levels may not be of great value for predicting toxicity and efficacy; toxicity may occur even at therapeutic concentrations

Patient Information Avoid exposure to sunlight; use sunscreen and sunglasses; may discolor skin to a slate blue color; notify physician if persistent dry cough, shortness of breath, or decreased vision occurs

(Continued)

Amiodarone *(Continued)*

Nursing Implications Ambulation of patient may be impaired due to adverse effects; due to possible infusion rate-related hypotension, the I.V. infusion rate should be carefully monitored

Additional Information Intoxication with amiodarone necessitates EKG monitoring; bradycardia may be atropine resistant, I.V. isoproterenol or cardiac pacemaker may be required; hypotension, cardiogenic shock, heart block, QT prolongation and hepatotoxicity may also be seen; patients should be monitored for several days following overdose due to long half-life

I.V. product is used for acute treatment; the duration of I.V. treatment is usually 48-96 hours, however, in adults, infusions may be used cautiously for 2-3 weeks; there is limited experience with administering infusions for >3 weeks

Use of amiodarone 300 mg I.V. in adults with cardiac arrest (out-of-hospital) due to refractory ventricular arrhythmias improved the rate of survival to hospital admission (see Kudenchuk, 1999).

Thyroid function tests: Amiodarone partially inhibits the peripheral conversion of thyroxine (T_4) to triiodothyronine (T_3); serum T_4 and reverse triiodothyronine (RT_3) concentrations may be increased and serum T_3 may be decreased; most patients remain clinically euthyroid, however, clinical hypothyroidism or hyperthyroidism may occur

Dosage Forms

Injection, as hydrochloride:

Cordarone®: 50 mg/mL [contains benzyl alcohol and polysorbate (Tween®) 80] (3 mL)

Amio-Aqueous®: 15 mg/mL [benzyl alcohol free and polysorbate free; contains an aqueous acetate buffer; available via orphan drug status or compassionate use from the manufacturer Academic Pharmaceuticals, Inc (847) 735-1170] (10 mL)

Tablet, scored, as hydrochloride:

Cordarone®: 200 mg

Pacerone®: 200 mg, 400 mg

Extemporaneous Preparations

A 5 mg/mL oral suspension can be made from tablets; two stability studies using different vehicles exist; a 5 mg/mL oral suspension made with simple syrup NF containing methylcellulose 1% (50:50, v/v) was stable for 42 days at room temperature (25°C) and 91 days under refrigeration (4°C) in both glass and plastic prescription bottles (Nahata, 1997); label "shake well" and "protect from light"

Five 200 mg tablets were crushed in a mortar, the vehicle (either a 1:1 mixture of Ora-Sweet® and Ora-Plus® or a 1:1 mixture of Ora-Sweet® SF and Ora-Plus®) was adjusted to a pH between 6-7 using a sodium bicarbonate solution (5 g/100 mL of distilled water). A small amount of the vehicle was added to the mortar to make a uniform paste; geometric amounts of the vehicle were added while mixing to **almost** the desired volume; suspension was transferred to a graduate and qsad to 200 mL while mixing. Suspensions prepared in both vehicles were stable for 42 days at room temperature (25°C) and 91 days under refrigeration (4°C) in plastic prescription bottles (Nahata 1999); label "shake well" and "protect from light"

Neither of these 2 studies determined microbial growth; extended storage under refrigeration is recommended

Nahata MC, "Stability of Amiodarone in an Oral Suspension Stored Under Refrigeration and at Room Temperature," *Ann Pharmacother*, 1997, 31(7-8):851-2.

Nahata MC, Morosco RS, and Hipple TF, "Stability of Amiodarone in Extemporaneous Oral Suspensions Prepared From Commercially Available Vehicles," *J Ped Pharmacy Practice*, 1999, 4(4):186-9.

References

Celiker A, Ceviz N, and Ozme S, "Effectiveness and Safety of Intravenous Amiodarone in Drug-Resistant Tachyarrhythmias of Children," *Acta Paediatr Jpn*, 1998, 40(6):567-72.

Coumel P and Fidelle J, "Amiodarone in the Treatment of Cardiac Arrhythmias in Children: One Hundred Thirty-Five Cases," *Am Heart J*, 1980, 100(6 Pt 2):1063-9.

Drago F, Mazza A, Guccione P, et al, "Amiodarone Used Alone or in Combination With Propranolol: A Very Effective Therapy for Tachyarrhythmias in Infants and Children," *Pediatr Cardiol*, 1998, 19(6):445-9.

Etheridge SP, Craig JE, and Compton SJ, "Amiodarone is Safe and Highly Effective Therapy for Supraventricular Tachycardia in Infants," *Am Heart J*, 2001, 141(1):105-10.

Figa FH, Gow RM, Hamilton RM, et al, "Clinical Efficacy and Safety of Intravenous Amiodarone in Infants and Children," *Am J Cardiol*, 1994, 74(6):573-7.

Garson A Jr, Gillette PC, McVey P, et al, "Amiodarone Treatment of Critical Arrhythmias in Children and Young Adults," *J Am Coll Cardiol*, 1984, 4(4):749-55.

Goldschlager N, Epstein AE, Naccarelli G, et al, "Practical Guidelines for Clinicians Who Treat Patients With Amiodarone," *Arch Intern Med*, 2000, 160(12):1741-8.

"Guidelines 2000 for Cardiopulmonary Resuscitation and Emergency Cardiovascular Care, Part 6: Advanced Cardiovascular Life Support, The American Heart Association in Collaboration With the International Liasion Committee on Resuscitation," *Circulation*, 2000, 102(8 Suppl):I86-171.

"Guidelines 2000 for Cardiopulmonary Resuscitation and Emergency Cardiovascular Care, Part 10: Pediatric Advanced Life Support, The American Heart Association in Collaboration With the International Liaison Committee on Resuscitation," *Circulation*, 2000, 102(8 Suppl): I291-342.

Kudenchuk PJ, Cobb LA, Copass MK, et al, "Amiodarone for Resuscitation After Out-of-Hospital Cardiac Arrest Due to Ventricular Fibrillation," *N Engl J Med*, 1999, 341(12):871-8.

Paul T and Guccione P, "New Antiarrhythmic Drugs in Pediatric Use: Amiodarone," *Pediatr Cardiol*, 1994, 15(3):132-8.

Perry JC, Fenrich AL, Hulse JE, et al, "Pediatric Use of Intravenous Amiodarone: Efficacy and Safety in Critically III Patients From a Multicenter Protocol," *J Am Coll Cardiol*, 1996, 27(5):1246-50.

Raja P, Hawker RE, Chaikitpinyo A, et al, "Amiodarone Management of Junctional Ectopic Tachycardia After Cardiac Surgery in Children," *Br Heart J*, 1994, 72(3):261-5.

Shahar E, Barzilay Z, Frand M, et al, "Amiodarone in Control of Sustained Tachyarrhythmias in Children With Wolff-Parkinson-White Syndrome," *Pediatrics*, 1983, 72(6):813-6.

Shuler CO, Case CL, and Gillette PC, "Efficacy and Safety of Amiodarone in Infants," *Am Heart J*, 1993, 125(5 Pt 1):1430-2.

Soult JA, Munoz M, Lopez JD, et al, "Efficacy and Safety of Intravenous Amiodarone for Short-Term Treatment of Paroxysmal Supraventricular Tachycardia in Children," *Pediatr Cardiol*, 1995, 16(1):16-9.

♦ **Amitone®** [OTC]   *see* Calcium Supplements *on page 167*

Amitriptyline (a mee TRIP ti leen)

Related Information
Comparison of Adverse Effects of Antidepressants *on page 1066*
Comparison of Usual Adult Dosage and Mechanism of Action of Antidepressants *on page 1065*
Drugs and Breast-Feeding *on page 1243*
Overdose and Toxicology *on page 1222*
Serotonin Syndrome *on page 1247*

U.S. Brand Names Elavil®
Canadian Brand Names Apo-Amitriptyline; Levate; Novo-Triptyn
Therapeutic Category Antidepressant, Tricyclic; Antimigraine Agent
Generic Available Yes
Use Treatment of various forms of depression, often in conjunction with psychotherapy; analgesic for certain chronic and neuropathic pain; migraine prophylaxis
Pregnancy Risk Factor C
Contraindications Hypersensitivity to amitriptyline (cross-sensitivity with other tricyclics may occur) or any component; narrow-angle glaucoma; use of MAO inhibitors within 14 days (potentially fatal reactions may occur, see Drug Interactions); concurrent use of cisapride; use during acute recovery phase after MI
Warnings Do not discontinue abruptly in patients receiving high doses chronically
Precautions Use with caution in patients with cardiac conduction disturbances, cardiovascular disease, seizure disorders, narrow-angle glaucoma, history of urinary retention or bowel obstruction, hepatic or renal dysfunction, hyperthyroidism or those receiving thyroid hormone replacement; degree of sedation, anticholinergic effects, and risk of orthostatic hypotension are very high relative to other antidepressants
Adverse Reactions Anticholinergic effects may be pronounced; moderate to marked sedation can occur (tolerance to these effects usually occurs)

Cardiovascular: Postural hypotension, arrhythmias, tachycardia, sudden death
Central nervous system: Sedation, fatigue, anxiety, confusion, insomnia, impaired cognitive function, seizures; extrapyramidal symptoms are possible
Dermatologic: Photosensitivity, urticaria, rash
Endocrine & metabolic: Rarely SIADH
Gastrointestinal: Xerostomia, constipation, decrease of lower esophageal sphincter tone, GE reflux, increased appetite, weight gain
Genitourinary: Urinary retention, discoloration of urine (blue-green)
Hematologic: Rarely agranulocytosis, leukopenia, eosinophilia
Hepatic: Increased liver enzymes, cholestatic jaundice
Neuromuscular & skeletal: Tremor, weakness
Ocular: Blurred vision, increased intraocular pressure
Miscellaneous: Allergic reactions

Drug Interactions Cytochrome P-450 isoenzyme CYP1A2, CYP2C9, CYP2C19, CYP2D6 and CYP3A3/4 substrate
Amitriptyline may decrease the effects of clonidine and guanethidine; with clonidine, hypertensive crisis may occur following discontinuation of clonidine; amitriptyline may increase the effects of CNS depressants (including alcohol), adrenergic agents (epinephrine, isoproterenol), anticholinergic agents and warfarin. With MAO inhibitors, hyperpyrexia, tachycardia, hypertension, confusion, seizures, and death have been reported. The herbal medicine St John's wort (*Hypericum*
(Continued)

Amitriptyline *(Continued)*

perforatum) may increase serious side effects; its use is **not** recommended. Cimetidine, fluoxetine, and methylphenidate may decrease the metabolism and phenobarbital, carbamazepine, and rifampin may increase the metabolism of amitriptyline; amitriptyline may potentiate the cardiac effects of cisapride (do not administer concurrently)

Food Interactions Riboflavin dietary requirements may be increased; increased dietary fiber may decrease drug effect

Stability Protect injection and Elavil® 10 mg tablets from light; store injection at <40°C (preferably 15°C to 30°C)

Mechanism of Action Increases the synaptic concentration of serotonin and/or norepinephrine in the central nervous system by inhibition of their reuptake by the presynaptic neuronal membrane

Pharmacodynamics Onset of action: Therapeutic antidepressant effects begin in 7-21 days; maximum effects may not occur for ≥2 weeks and as long as 4-6 weeks

Pharmacokinetics

Absorption: Oral: Rapid, well absorbed

Distribution: Crosses placenta; enters breast milk

Protein binding: >90%

Metabolism: In the liver to nortriptyline (active), hydroxy derivatives and conjugated derivatives

Half-life, adults: 9-25 hours (15-hour average)

Time to peak serum concentration: Within 4 hours

Elimination: Renal excretion of 18% as unchanged drug; small amounts eliminated in feces by bile

Nondialyzable

Usual Dosage

Chronic pain management: Children: Oral: Initial: 0.1 mg/kg at bedtime, may advance as tolerated over 2-3 weeks to 0.5-2 mg/kg at bedtime

Depressive disorders: Oral:

Children: Investigationally initial doses of 1 mg/kg/day given in 3 divided doses with increases to 1.5 mg/kg/day have been reported in a small number of children (n=9) 9-12 years of age; clinically, doses up to 3 mg/kg/day (5 mg/kg/day if monitored closely) have been proposed

Adolescents: Initial: 25-50 mg/day; may give in divided doses; increase gradually to 100 mg/day in divided doses; maximum dose: 200 mg/day

Migraine prophylaxis: Children: Limited studies exist; one small study (n=24; mean age: 8 years; range: 6-12 years) used increasing doses over 5 days to reach a final dose of 1.5 mg/kg/day; effectiveness was seen in 19 of 24 patients, but 5 children dropped out of the trial due to adverse effects (see Sorge, 1982). A recent large open-label trial in 192 children (mean age 12 ±3 years) with >3 headaches/month (61% with migraine, 8% with migraine with aura, and 10% with tension-type headaches) used an initial dose of 0.25 mg/kg/day given before bedtime; doses were increased every 2 weeks by 0.25 mg/kg/day to a final dose of 1 mg/kg/day; patients also used appropriate abortive medications and lifestyle adjustments; at initial re-evaluation (mean: 67 days after initiation of therapy), the mean number of headaches per month significantly decreased from 17.1 to 9.2; the mean duration of headaches decreased from 11.5 to 6.3 hours; continued improvement was observed at follow-up visits; minimal adverse effects were reported. **Note:** Mean final dose was 0.99 ±0.23 mg/kg; range: 0.16-1.7 mg/kg/day; EKGs were obtained on children receiving >1 mg/kg/day or in those describing a cardiac side effect (see Hershey, 2000). Further studies are needed.

Adults:

Oral: 30-100 mg/day single dose at bedtime or in divided doses; dose may be gradually increased up to 300 mg/day; once symptoms are controlled, decrease gradually to lowest effective dose

I.M.: 20-30 mg 4 times/day

Administration

Oral: May administer with food to decrease GI upset

Parenteral: Administer by I.M. route only; do not administer I.V.

Monitoring Parameters Heart rate, blood pressure, mental status, weight

Reference Range Note: Plasma levels do not always correlate with clinical effectiveness

Therapeutic:

Amitriptyline plus nortriptyline (active metabolite): 100-250 ng/mL (SI: 360-900 nmol/L)

Nortriptyline 50-150 ng/mL (SI: 190-570 nmol/L)

Toxic: >500 ng/mL (SI: >1800 nmol/L)

Patient Information Avoid alcohol and the herbal medicine St John's wort; limit caffeine intake; may cause drowsiness and impair ability to perform activities requiring mental alertness or coordination; may cause dry mouth; do not discontinue abruptly; may discolor urine to a blue-green color

Additional Information Due to promotion of weight gain with amitriptyline, other antidepressants (ie, imipramine or desipramine) may be preferred in heavy or obese children and adolescents

Dosage Forms

Injection, as hydrochloride: 10 mg/mL (10 mL)

Tablet, as hydrochloride: 10 mg, 25 mg, 50 mg, 75 mg, 100 mg, 150 mg

References

Elser JM and Woody RC, "Migraine Headache in the Infant and Young Child," *Headache*, 1990, 30(6):366-8.

Hershey AD, Powers SW, Bentti AL, et al, "Effectiveness of Amitriptyline in the Prophylactic Management of Childhood Headaches," *Headache*, 2000, 40(7):539-49.

Kashani JH, Shekim WO, and Reid JC, "Amitriptyline in Children With Major Depressive Disorder: A Double-Blind Crossover Pilot Study," *J Am Acad Child Psychiatry*, 1984, 23(3):348-51.

Levy HB, Harper CR, and Weinberg WA, "A Practical Approach to Children Failing in School," *Pediatr Clin North Am*, 1992, 39(4):895-928.

Sorge F, Barone P, Steardo L, et al, "Amitriptyline as a Prophylactic for Migraine in Children," *Acta Neurol (Napoli)*, 1982, 4(5):362-7.

♦ **Ammens® Medicated Deodorant [OTC]** *see* Zinc Oxide *on page 1026*

♦ **Ammonapse** *see* Sodium Phenylbutyrate *on page 907*

Ammonium Chloride (a MOE nee um KLOR ide)

Synonyms NH_4Cl

Therapeutic Category Metabolic Alkalosis Agent; Urinary Acidifying Agent

Generic Available Yes

Use Diuretic or systemic and urinary acidifying agent; treatment of hypochloremic states

Pregnancy Risk Factor C

Contraindications Severe hepatic and renal dysfunction; patients with primary respiratory acidosis

Adverse Reactions

Cardiovascular: Bradycardia

Central nervous system: Mental confusion, coma, headache

Dermatologic: Rash

Endocrine & metabolic: Metabolic acidosis secondary to hyperchloremia

Gastrointestinal: GI irritation

Local: Pain at site of injection

Respiratory: Hyperventilation

Drug Interactions Chlorpropamide's effects may be enhanced due to decreased urinary excretion; may decrease flecainide levels due to increased urinary excretion; systemic acidosis may occur when used with spironolactone

Mechanism of Action Its dissociation to ammonium and chloride ions increases acidity by increasing free hydrogen ion concentration which combines with bicarbonate ion to form CO_2 and water; the net result is the replacement of bicarbonate ions by chloride ions

Pharmacokinetics

Metabolism: In the liver

Elimination: In urine

Usual Dosage

The following equations represent different methods of chloride or alkalosis correction utilizing either the serum HCO_3^-, the serum Cl^- or the base excess: Children and Adults: I.V.:

Correction of refractory hypochloremic metabolic alkalosis: mEq NH_4Cl = 0.5 L/kg x wt in kg x [serum HCO_3^- - 24] mEq/L; give $1/2$ to $2/3$ of the calculated dose, then re-evaluate

Correction of hypochloremia: mEq NH_4Cl = 0.2 L/kg x wt in kg x [103 - serum Cl^-] mEq/L, give $1/2$ to $2/3$ of calculated dose, then re-evaluate

Correction of alkalosis via base excess method: mEq NH_4Cl = 0.3 L/kg x wt in kg x base excess (mEq/L), give $1/2$ to $2/3$ of calculated dose, then re-evaluate

Children: I.V.: 75 mg/kg/day in 4 divided doses for urinary acidification; maximum daily dose: 6 g

Adults: I.V.: 1.5 g/dose every 6 hours

Administration

Parenteral: Dilute to 0.2 mEq/mL and infuse I.V. over 3 hours; maximum concentration: 0.4 mEq/mL; maximum rate of infusion: 1 mEq/kg/hour

Monitoring Parameters Serum electrolytes, serum ammonia

(Continued)

Ammonium Chloride *(Continued)*

Nursing Implications Rapid I.V. injection may increase the likelihood of ammonia toxicity

Dosage Forms Injection: 26.75% [267.5 mg/mL, 5 mEq/mL] (20 mL)

♦ **Ammonium Molybdate** *see* Trace Metals *on page 972*

Amoxicillin (a moks i SIL in)

Related Information

Carbohydrate and Alcohol Content of Liquid Medications for Use in Patients Receiving Ketogenic Diets *on page 1258*

Endocarditis Prophylaxis *on page 1160*

U.S. Brand Names Amoxil®; Biomox®; Polymox®; Trimox®; Wymox®

Canadian Brand Names Apo-Amoxi; Gen-Amoxicillin; Lin-Amox; Novamoxin; Nu-Amoxi; Pro-Amox

Synonyms Amoxycillin; *p*-Hydroxyampicillin

Therapeutic Category Antibiotic, Penicillin

Generic Available Yes

Use Treatment of otitis media, sinusitis, and infections involving the respiratory tract, skin, and urinary tract due to susceptible *H. influenzae*, *N. gonorrhoeae*, *E. coli*, *P. mirabilis*, *E. faecalis*, streptococci, and nonpenicillinase-producing staphylococci; treatment of Lyme disease in children <8 years of age; prophylaxis of bacterial endocarditis

Pregnancy Risk Factor B

Contraindications Hypersensitivity to amoxicillin, penicillin, or any component

Warnings Epstein-Barr virus infection, acute lymphocytic leukemia or cytomegalovirus infection increases risk for amoxicillin-induced maculopapular rash

Precautions In patients with renal dysfunction, doses and/or frequency of administration should be modified in response to the degree of renal impairment; use with caution in patients with history of cephalosporin allergy

Adverse Reactions

Central nervous system: Fever

Dermatologic: Rash, exfoliative dermatitis, Stevens-Johnson syndrome, urticaria

Gastrointestinal: Diarrhea, nausea, vomiting, pseudomembranous colitis

Hematologic: Anemia, neutropenia, eosinophilia, thrombocytopenia, prolongation of bleeding time

Miscellaneous: Superinfection, hypersensitivity reactions, serum sickness, vasculitis, anaphylaxis

Drug Interactions Probenecid (increases serum amoxicillin concentration); allopurinol may increase frequency for amoxicillin rash; decreases oral contraceptive efficacy

Food Interactions Food does not interfere with absorption

Stability Suspensions are stable for 14 days at room temperature or if refrigerated; refrigeration is preferred

Mechanism of Action Interferes with bacterial cell wall synthesis during active multiplication by binding to one or more of the penicillin-binding proteins, causing cell wall death and resultant bactericidal activity against susceptible bacteria

Pharmacokinetics

Absorption: Oral: Rapid and nearly complete

Distribution: Into liver, lungs, prostate, muscle, middle ear effusions, maxillary sinus secretions, bile, and into ascitic and synovial fluids; excreted into breast milk

Protein binding: 17% to 20%, lower in neonates

Half-life:

Neonates, full-term: 3.7 hours

Infants and children: 1-2 hours

Adults with normal renal function: 0.7-1.4 hours

Patients with Cl_{cr} <10 mL/minute: 7-21 hours

Metabolism: Partial

Time to peak serum concentration:

Capsule: Within 2 hours

Suspension: Neonates: 3-4.5 hours; children: 1 hour

Elimination: Renal excretion (80% unchanged drug)

Moderately dialyzable (20% to 50%); ~30% removed by 3-hour hemodialysis; supplemental dose is recommended after hemodialysis

Usual Dosage Oral:

Neonates and Infants: ≤3 months: 20-30 mg/kg/day in divided doses every 12 hours

Infants >3 months and Children: 25-50 mg/kg/day in divided doses every 8 hours or 25-50 mg/kg/day in divided doses every 12 hours

Acute otitis media due to highly resistant strains of *S. pneumoniae*: 80-90 mg/kg/day divided every 12 hours

Uncomplicated gonorrhea:

<2 years, probenecid is contraindicated in this age group

≥2 years: 50 mg/kg plus probenecid 25 mg/kg as a single dose

Endocarditis prophylaxis: 50 mg/kg 1 hour before procedure, not to exceed adult dose

Adults: 250-500 mg every 8 hours or 500-875 mg tablets twice daily; maximum dose: 2-3 g/day

Uncomplicated gonorrhea: 3 g plus probenecid 1 g as a single dose

Endocarditis prophylaxis: 2 g 1 hour before procedure

Dosing interval in renal impairment:

Cl_{cr} 10-30 mL/minute: Administer every 12 hours

Cl_{cr} <10 mL/minute: Administer every 24 hours

Administration Oral: May be administered on an empty or full stomach; may be mixed with formula, milk, or juice; shake suspension well before use

Monitoring Parameters With prolonged therapy, monitor renal, hepatic, and hematologic function periodically; monitor for diarrhea

Additional Information Appearance of a rash should be carefully evaluated to differentiate a nonallergic amoxicillin rash from a hypersensitivity reaction. Amoxicillin rash occurs in 5% to 10% of children receiving amoxicillin and is a generalized dull, red, maculopapular rash, generally appearing 3-14 days after the start of therapy. It normally begins on the trunk and spreads over most of the body. It may be most intense at pressure areas, elbows, and knees. Incidence of amoxicillin rash is higher in patients with viral infections, cytomegalovirus infections, infectious mononucleosis, lymphocytic leukemia, or patients with hyperuricemia who are receiving allopurinol.

Dosage Forms

Capsule, as trihydrate: 250 mg, 500 mg

Powder for oral suspension, as trihydrate: 125 mg/5 mL (80 mL, 100 mL, 150 mL, 200 mL); 200 mg/5 mL (5 mL, 50 mL, 75 mL, 100 mL); 250 mg/5 mL (80 mL, 100 mL, 150 mL, 200 mL); 400 mg/5 mL (5 mL, 50 mL, 75 mL, 100 mL)

Powder for oral suspension, drops, as trihydrate: 50 mg/mL (15 mL, 30 mL)

Tablet, chewable, as trihydrate: 125 mg, 200 mg, 250 mg, 400 mg

Tablet, film coated, as trihydrate: 500 mg, 875 mg

References

Boguniewicz M and Leung DY, "Hypersensitivity Reactions to Antibiotics Commonly Used in Children," *Pediatr Infect Dis J*, 1995, 14(3):221-31.

Canafax, DM, Yuan Z, Chonmaitree T, et al, "Amoxicillin Middle Ear Fluid Penetration and Pharmacokinetics in Children with Acute Otitis Media," *Pediatr Infect Dis J*, 1998, 17(2):149-56.

Dajani AS, Taubert KA, Wilson WW, et al, "Prevention of Bacterial Endocarditis. Recommendations by the American Heart Association," *JAMA*, 1997, 277(22):1794-1801.

Amoxicillin and Clavulanic Acid

(a moks i SIL in & klav yoo LAN ic AS id)

Related Information

Carbohydrate and Alcohol Content of Liquid Medications for Use in Patients Receiving Ketogenic Diets *on page 1258*

U.S. Brand Names Augmentin®

Canadian Brand Names Clavulin

Synonyms Clavulanic Acid and Amoxicillin

Therapeutic Category Antibiotic, Beta-lactam and Beta-lactamase Combination; Antibiotic, Penicillin

Generic Available No

Use Infections caused by susceptible organisms involving the lower respiratory tract, otitis media, sinusitis, skin and skin structure, and urinary tract; spectrum same as amoxicillin in addition to beta-lactamase producing *M. catarrhalis*, *H. influenzae*, *N. gonorrhoeae*, and *S. aureus* (not MRSA)

Pregnancy Risk Factor B

Contraindications Hypersensitivity to amoxicillin, clavulanic acid, penicillins, or any component; concomitant use of disulfiram; history of amoxicillin/clavulanic acid-associated cholestatic jaundice or hepatic dysfunction

Warnings Epstein-Barr virus infection, acute lymphocytic leukemia or cytomegalovirus infection increase the risk for amoxicillin-induced maculopapular rash

Precautions Use with caution in patients with history of cephalosporin hypersensitivity; in patients with renal dysfunction, doses and/or frequency of administration should be modified in response to the degree of renal impairment; avoid using the "BID" formulation in patients with phenylketonuria since it contains phenylalanine

(Continued)

Amoxicillin and Clavulanic Acid *(Continued)*

Adverse Reactions
Central nervous system: Headache

Dermatologic: Rash, urticaria, exfoliative dermatitis, Stevens-Johnson syndrome

Gastrointestinal: Nausea, vomiting, pseudomembranous colitis; incidence of diarrhea (9%) is higher than with amoxicillin alone

Genitourinary: Vaginal candidiasis

Hepatic: Elevated AST, ALT, alkaline phosphatase, and bilirubin

Miscellaneous: Superinfection, hypersensitivity reactions, serum sickness, vasculitis, anaphylaxis

Drug Interactions Probenecid (increases serum amoxicillin concentration), allopurinol, disulfiram

Stability Reconstituted oral suspension should be refrigerated; discard unused suspension after 10 days

Mechanism of Action Clavulanic acid binds and inhibits beta-lactamases that inactivate amoxicillin resulting in amoxicillin having an expanded spectrum of activity; amoxicillin interferes with bacterial cell wall synthesis by binding to one or more of the penicillin-binding proteins and causing cell wall death

Pharmacokinetics
Absorption: Both amoxicillin and clavulanate are well absorbed

Distribution: Both widely distributed into lungs, pleural, peritoneal, synovial, and ascitic fluid as well as bone, gynecologic tissue, and middle ear fluid; crosses the placenta; excreted in breast milk

Metabolism: Clavulanic acid: Metabolized in the liver

Half-life of both agents in adults with normal renal function: ~1 hour; amoxicillin pharmacokinetics are not affected by clavulanic acid

Time to peak serum concentration: Within 2 hours

Elimination: Amoxicillin: Excreted primarily unchanged in the urine

Dialysis: ~30% of amoxicillin removed by 3-hour hemodialysis; supplemental dose recommended after hemodialysis

Usual Dosage Oral (dosing based on amoxicillin component):

Neonates and Infants <3 months: 30 mg/kg/day divided every 12 hours using the 125 mg/5 mL suspension

Children <40 kg: 20-40 mg (amoxicillin component)/kg/day in divided doses every 8 hours **or** 25-45 mg (amoxicillin component)/kg/day divided every 12 hours using either 200 mg/5 mL or 400 mg/5 mL suspension, or 200 mg, 400 mg chewable tablet formulation

Multidrug-resistant pneumococcal otitis media: 80-90 mg/kg/day divided every 12 hours (use a 7:1 "BID" formulation)

Adults:

Less severe infection: 250 mg every 8 hours or 500 mg every 12 hours

More severe infections and respiratory tract infections: 500 mg every 8 hours or 875 mg every 12 hours

Dosing interval in renal impairment:

Cl_{cr} 10-30 mL/minute: Administer 250-500 mg every 12 hours; do not administer the 875 mg tablet

Cl_{cr} <10 mL/minute: Administer 250-500 mg every 24 hours

Administration Oral: Administer at the start of a meal to decrease the frequency or severity of GI side effects; may mix with milk, formula, or juice; shake suspension well before use

Monitoring Parameters With prolonged therapy, monitor renal, hepatic, and hematologic function periodically

Test Interactions May interfere with urinary glucose determinations using Clinitest®

Patient Information Adverse GI effects may occur less frequently if taken with food

Additional Information Potassium content: 0.16 mEq of potassium per 31.25 mg of clavulanic acid; since both the 250 mg and 500 mg tablets contain the same amount of clavulanic acid, two 250 mg tablets are not equivalent to one 500 mg tablet; the "q12h" chewable tablet and oral suspension (200 mg, 400 mg) formulations contain phenylalanine

Appearance of a rash should be carefully evaluated to differentiate a nonallergic amoxicillin rash from a hypersensitivity reaction. Amoxicillin rash occurs in 5% to 10% of children receiving amoxicillin and is a generalized dull, red, maculopapular rash, generally appearing 3-14 days after the start of therapy. It normally begins on the trunk and spreads over most of the body. It may be most intense at pressure areas, elbows, and knees. Incidence of amoxicillin rash is higher in patients with viral infections, *Salmonella* infections, lymphocytic leukemia, or patients with hyperuricemia who are receiving allopurinol.

Dosage Forms
Suspension, oral:
  125: Amoxicillin, as trihydrate, 125 mg and clavulanic potassium 31.25 mg per 5 mL [banana flavor] (75 mL, 150 mL)
  200: Amoxicillin, as trihydrate, 200 mg and clavulanic potassium 28.5 mg per 5 mL [banana flavor] (50 mL, 75 mL, 100 mL) **["BID" formulation]**
  250: Amoxicillin, as trihydrate, 250 mg and clavulanic potassium 62.5 mg per 5 mL [banana flavor] (75 mL, 150 mL)
  400: Amoxicillin, as trihydrate, 400 mg and clavulanic potassium 57 mg per 5 mL [banana flavor] (50 mL, 75 mL, 100 mL) **["BID" formulation]**
Tablet:
  250: Amoxicillin, as trihydrate, 250 mg and clavulanic potassium 125 mg
  500: Amoxicillin, as trihydrate, 500 mg and clavulanic potassium 125 mg
  875: Amoxicillin, as trihydrate, 875 mg and clavulanic potassium 125 mg: **["BID" formulation]**
Tablet, chewable:
  125: Amoxicillin, as trihydrate, 125 mg and clavulanic potassium 31.25 mg
  200: Amoxicillin, as trihydrate, 200 mg and clavulanic potassium 28.5 mg: **["BID" formulation]**
  250: Amoxicillin, as trihydrate, 250 mg and clavulanic potassium 62.5 mg
  400: Amoxicillin, as trihydrate, 400 mg and clavulanic potassium 57 mg: **["BID" formulation]**

References
Gan VN, Kusmiesz H, Shelton S, et al, "Comparative Evaluation of Loracarbef and Amoxicillin-Clavulanate for Acute Otitis Media," *Antimicrob Agents Chemother*, 1991, 35(5):967-71.

Hoberman A, Paradise JL, Burch DJ, et al, "Equivalent Efficiency and Reduced Occurrence of Diarrhea From a New Formulation of Amoxicillin/Clavulanate Potassium (Augmentin®) for Treatment of Acute Otitis Media in Children," *Pediatr Infect Dis J*, 1997, 16(5):463-70.

Reed MD, "Clinical Pharmacokinetics of Amoxicillin and Clavulanate," *Pediatr Infect Dis J*, 1996, 15(10):949-54.

Thoene DE and Johnson CE, "Pharmacotherapy of Otitis Media," *Pharmacotherapy*, 1991, 11(3):212-21.

Todd PA and Benfield P, "Amoxicillin/Clavulanic Acid. An Update of Its Antibacterial Activity, Pharmacokinetic Properties and Therapeutic Use," *Drugs*, 1990, 39(2):264-307.

♦ **Amoxil®** *see* Amoxicillin *on page 80*

♦ **Amoxycillin** *see* Amoxicillin *on page 80*

♦ **Amphetamine and Dextroamphetamine** *see* Dextroamphetamine and Amphetamine *on page 314*

♦ **Amphojel® [OTC]** *see* Antacid Preparations *on page 95*

Amphotericin B (Conventional)
(am foe TER i sin bee con VEN sha nal)

U.S. Brand Names Fungizone®

Therapeutic Category Antifungal Agent, Systemic; Antifungal Agent, Topical

Generic Available Yes

Use Treatment of severe systemic infections and meningitis caused by susceptible fungi such as *Candida* species, *Histoplasma capsulatum*, *Cryptococcus neoformans*, *Aspergillus* species, *Mucor* species, *Blastomyces dermatitidis*, *Torulopsis glabrata*, *Sporothrix schenckii*, *Paracoccidioides brasiliensis*, and *Coccidioides immitis*; fungal peritonitis; irrigant for bladder fungal infections; treatment of amebic meningoencephalitis caused by *Naegleria fouleri*; topically for cutaneous and mucocutaneous candidal infections

Pregnancy Risk Factor B

Contraindications Hypersensitivity to amphotericin or any component

Warnings I.V. amphotericin is used primarily for the treatment of patients with progressive and potentially fatal fungal infections; not to be used for common clinically inapparent forms of fungal disease; anaphylaxis has been reported with amphotericin B-containing drugs; facilities for cardiopulmonary resuscitation should be available during administration due to the possibility of anaphylactic reaction

Precautions Due to the nephrotoxic potential of amphotericin, other nephrotoxic drugs should be avoided

Adverse Reactions
Cardiovascular: Hypotension, hypertension, cardiac arrhythmias, flushing
Central nervous system: Fever, chills, and headache are the most common adverse effects reported with amphotericin B infusion; delirium, seizures, malaise
Endocrine & metabolic: Hypokalemia, hypomagnesemia
Gastrointestinal: Anorexia, nausea, vomiting, steatorrhea, weight loss
Hematologic: Anemia, leukopenia, thrombocytopenia
Hepatic: Acute hepatic failure, jaundice
Local: Phlebitis
(Continued)

Amphotericin B (Conventional) *(Continued)*

Renal: Renal tubular acidosis, renal failure (oliguria, azotemia, elevated serum creatinine)

Respiratory: Wheezing, hypoxemia

Miscellaneous: Anaphylactoid reaction

Adverse effects due to intrathecal amphotericin:

Central nervous system: Headache, pain along lumbar nerves, arachnoiditis

Gastrointestinal: Nausea, vomiting

Genitourinary: Urinary retention

Neuromuscular & skeletal: Paresthesia, leg and back pain, foot drop

Ocular: Vision changes

Drug Interactions Nephrotoxic drugs may cause additive toxic effects; corticosteroids may increase potassium depletion caused by amphotericin; may predispose patients receiving cardiac glycosides or skeletal muscle relaxants to toxicity secondary to hypokalemia; imidazole derivatives (eg, miconazole, fluconazole, ketoconazole) may antagonize the effect and induce fungal resistance to amphotericin; may increase toxicity of flucytosine by increasing cellular uptake and/or impairing its renal excretion; may potentiate renal toxicity, bronchospasm, and hypotension of antineoplastic agents

Stability Reconstitute only with sterile water without preservatives, not bacteriostatic water; benzyl alcohol, sodium chloride, or other electrolyte solutions may cause precipitation; can be diluted in D_5W, $D_{10}W$, up to $D_{20}W$; for I.V. infusion, an in-line filter (>1 micron mean pore diameter) may be used; irrigating solutions should be diluted in sterile water; short-term exposure (<24 hours) to light during I.V. infusion does **not** appreciably affect potency

Mechanism of Action Binds to ergosterol altering cell membrane permeability in susceptible fungi and causing leakage of cell components with subsequent cell death

Pharmacokinetics

Absorption: Poor oral absorption

Distribution: Minimal amounts enter the aqueous humor, bile, amniotic fluid, pericardial fluid, pleural fluid, and synovial fluid; poor CSF penetration

Protein binding: 90%

Half-life: Increased in small neonates and young infants

Initial: 15-48 hours

Terminal phase: 15 days

Elimination: 2% to 4% of dose eliminated in urine unchanged; ~40% eliminated over 7-day period and may be detected in urine for up to 8 weeks after discontinued use

Dialysis: Poorly dialyzed

Usual Dosage Medication errors, including deaths, have resulted from confusion between lipid-based forms of amphotericin (Abelcet®, Amphotec®, AmBisome®) and conventional amphotericin B for injection; conventional amphotericin B for injection doses should not exceed 1.5 mg/kg/day

Neonates, Infants, and Children:

I.V.: Test dose: 0.1 mg/kg/dose to a maximum of 1 mg; infuse over 20-60 minutes; an alternative method to the 0.1 mg/kg test dose is to initiate therapy with 0.25 mg/kg amphotericin administered over 6 hours; frequent observation of the patient and assessment of vital signs during the first several hours of the infusion is recommended

Initial therapeutic dose: If the 0.1 mg/kg test dose is tolerated without the occurrence of serious adverse effects, a therapeutic dose of 0.4 mg/kg can be given the same day as the test dose

The daily dose can then be gradually increased, usually in 0.25 mg/kg increments on each subsequent day until the desired daily dose is reached; in critically ill patients, more rapid dosage acceleration (up to 0.5 mg/kg increments on each subsequent day) may be warranted

Maintenance dose: 0.25-1 mg/kg/day given once daily; infuse over 2-6 hours; rapidly progressing disease may require short-term use of doses to 1.5 mg/kg/day; once therapy has been established, amphotericin B can be administered on an every-other-day basis at 1-1.5 mg/kg/dose

Intrathecal, intraventricular, or intracisternal (preferably into the lateral ventricles through a cisternal Ommaya reservoir): 25-100 mcg every 48-72 hours; increase to 500 mcg as tolerated

Adults:

I.V.: Test dose: 1 mg infused over 20-30 minutes

Initial therapeutic dose (if the test dose is tolerated): 0.25 mg/kg

The daily dose can then be gradually increased, usually in 0.25 mg/kg increments on each subsequent day until the desired daily dose is reached

Maintenance dose: 0.25-1 mg/kg/day once daily, infuse over 2-6 hours; or 1-1.5 mg/kg/dose every other day; do not exceed 1.5 mg/kg/day

Intrathecal, intraventricular, or intracisternal (preferably into the lateral ventricles through a cisternal Ommaya reservoir): 25-100 mcg every 48-72 hours; increase to 500 mcg as tolerated

Children and Adults:

Bladder irrigation: 5-15 mg amphotericin/100 mL of sterile water irrigation solution at 100-300 mL/day. Fluid is instilled into the bladder; the catheter is clamped for 60-120 minutes and the bladder drained. Perform irrigation 3-4 times/day for 2-5 days.

Dialysate: 1-4 mg/L of peritoneal dialysis fluid either with or without low-dose I.V. amphotericin B therapy

Topical: Apply to affected areas 2-4 times/day

Note: Amphotericin B has been administered intranasally to reduce the frequency of invasive aspergillosis in neutropenic patients; 7 mg amphotericin B in 7 mL sterile water was placed in a De Vilbiss atomizer and the aerosolized solution was instilled intranasally to each nostril 4 times/day delivering an average of 5 mg amphotericin/day

Dosing adjustment in renal impairment: Dosage adjustments are not necessary with pre-existing renal impairment; if decreased renal function is due to amphotericin, the daily dose can be decreased by 50% or the dose can be given every other day. Therapy may be held until serum creatinine concentrations begin to decline.

Administration Parenteral: Amphotericin is administered by I.V. infusion over 2-3 hours (range: 1-6 hours) at a final concentration not to exceed 0.1 mg/mL through a peripheral venous catheter; in patients unable to tolerate a large fluid volume, amphotericin B at a final concentration not to exceed 0.5 mg/mL in D_5W or $D_{10}W$ may be administered through a central venous catheter

Monitoring Parameters BUN and serum creatinine levels should be determined every other day while therapy is increased and at least weekly thereafter; serum potassium and magnesium should be monitored closely; monitor electrolytes, liver function, hematocrit, CBC regularly; monitor I & O; monitor for signs of hypokalemia (muscle weakness, cramping, drowsiness, EKG changes, etc); blood pressure, temperature, pulse, respiration

Patient Information Amphotericin cream may slightly discolor skin and stain clothing; personal hygiene is very important to help reduce the spread and recurrence of lesions; avoid covering topical applications with occlusive bandages; most skin lesions require 1-3 weeks of therapy

Nursing Implications Cardiovascular collapse has been reported after rapid amphotericin injection; may premedicate patients who experience mild adverse reactions with acetaminophen and diphenhydramine 30 minutes prior to the amphotericin infusion. Meperidine and ibuprofen may help to reduce fevers and chills. Hydrocortisone can be added to the infusion solution to reduce febrile and other systemic reactions.

Additional Information Amphotericin B-induced nephrotoxicity may be minimized by sodium loading with 10-15 mL/kg of NS infused prior to each amphotericin B dose or pentoxifylline, and avoiding use of other nephrotoxic agents

Dosage Forms

Cream: 3% (20 g)

Lotion: 3% (30 mL)

Ointment, topical: 3% (20 g)

Powder for injection, lyophilized: 50 mg

References

The Ad Hoc Advisory Panel on Peritonitis Management. "Continuous Ambulatory Peritoneal Dialysis (CAPD) Peritonitis Treatment Recommendations: 1989 Update," *Perit Dial Int*, 1989, 9(4):247-56.

Benson JM and Nahata MC, "Pharmacokinetics of Amphotericin B in Children," *Antimicrob Agents Chemother*, 1989, 33(11):1989-93.

Bianco JA, Almgren J, Kern DL, et al, "Evidence That Oral Pentoxifylline Reverses Acute Renal Dysfunction in Bone Marrow Transplant Recipients Receiving Amphotericin B and Cyclosporine," *Transplantation*, 1991, 51(4):925-7.

Branch RA, "Prevention of Amphotericin B-Induced Renal Impairment. A Review on the Use of Sodium Supplementation," *Arch Intern Med*, 1988, 148(11):2389-94.

Jeffery GM, Beard ME, Ikram RB, et al, "Intranasal Amphotericin B Reduces the Frequency of Invasive Aspergillosis in Neutropenic Patients," *Am J Med*, 1991, 90(6):685-92.

Kintzel PE and Smith GH, "Practical Guidelines for Preparing and Administering Amphotericin B," *Am J Hosp Pharm*, 1992, 49(5):1156-64.

Koren G, Lau A, Klein J, et al, "Pharmacokinetics and Adverse Effects of Amphotericin B in Infants and Children," *J Pediatr*, 1988, 113(3):559-63.

Amphotericin B Lipid Complex
(am foe TER i sin bee LIP id KOM pleks)

U.S. Brand Names Abelcet®

Synonyms ABLC

Therapeutic Category Antifungal Agent, Systemic

Generic Available No

Use Treatment of aspergillosis or invasive fungal infections in patients who are refractory to or intolerant of conventional amphotericin B therapy (refractory to or intolerant is defined as renal dysfunction with a serum creatinine ≥1.5 mg/dL that develops during therapy, or disease progression after a total dose of conventional amphotericin B of at least 10 mg/kg). This indication is primarily based on results of emergency studies for the treatment of aspergillosis; may be useful in the treatment of hepatosplenic candidiasis and cryptococcal meningitis.

Pregnancy Risk Factor B

Contraindications Hypersensitivity to amphotericin B, dimyristoylphosphatidylcholine (DMPC) and dimirystoylphosphatidylglycerol (DMPG) which are two phospholipids in the formulation, or any component

Warnings Anaphylaxis has been reported with amphotericin B-containing drugs; facilities for cardiopulmonary resuscitation should be available during administration due to the possibility of anaphylactic reaction

Precautions Due to the nephrotoxic potential of amphotericin B, other nephrotoxic drugs should be avoided

Adverse Reactions
Cardiovascular: Hypotension, cardiac arrest, arrhythmias, flushing
Central nervous system: Headache; transient chills and fever and during infusion of the drug are the most common effects reported with ABLC
Dermatologic: Rash, pruritus
Endocrine & metabolic: Hypokalemia, bilirubinemia, hypomagnesemia
Gastrointestinal: Diarrhea, abdominal pain
Hematologic: Thrombocytopenia, leukopenia, anemia
Renal: Renal tubular acidosis, elevated serum creatinine (occurs to a lesser degree than with conventional amphotericin B), azotemia, oliguria
Respiratory: Dyspnea, respiratory failure
Miscellaneous: Anaphylactoid and other allergic reactions

Drug Interactions Nephrotoxic drugs may cause additive nephrotoxic effects; corticosteroids may increase potassium depletion caused by amphotericin; may predispose patients receiving cardiac glycosides or skeletal muscle relaxants to toxicity secondary to hypokalemia; may increase myelotoxicity and nephrotoxicity of zidovudine; imidazole derivatives (eg, miconazole, fluconazole, ketoconazole) may antagonize the effect and induce fungal resistance to amphotericin; may increase toxicity of flucytosine by increasing cellular uptake and/or impairing its renal excretion; may potentiate renal toxicity, bronchospasm, and hypotension of antineoplastic agents

Stability Prior to admixture, refrigerate vial and protect from light; diluted ABLC infusion solution is stable up to 15 hours refrigerated and an additional 6 hours at room temperature. Do not freeze. Do not dilute with saline solutions or mix with other drugs or electrolytes.

Mechanism of Action Binds to ergosterol altering cell membrane permeability in susceptible fungi and causing leakage of cell components with subsequent cell death

Pharmacokinetics Exhibits nonlinear kinetics; volume of distribution and clearance from blood increases with increasing dose
Distribution: High tissue concentration found in the liver, spleen, and lung
Half-life, terminal: 173 hours
Elimination: 0.9% of dose excreted in urine over 24 hours; effects of hepatic and renal impairment on drug disposition are unknown
Dialysis: ABLC is not hemodialyzable

Usual Dosage Children and Adults: I.V.: 2.5-5 mg/kg given as a once daily infusion
Dosing adjustment in renal failure: Renal toxicity is dose dependent; there are no firm guidelines for dose adjustment based on lab test results (serum creatinine levels).

Administration Parenteral: I.V.: Prior to administration, assure serum potassium is >3.2 mEq/L; do not use an in-line filter less than 5 microns; administer at a rate of 2.5 mg/kg/hour (over 2 hours) at a final concentration of 1 mg/mL in D$_5$W. A maximum concentration of 2 mg/mL may be used in fluid-restricted patients

Monitoring Parameters BUN, serum creatinine, liver function tests, serum electrolytes, CBC; vital signs, I & O; monitor for signs of hypokalemia (muscle weakness, cramping, drowsiness, EKG changes, etc)

Nursing Implications If infusion time exceeds 2 hours, mix the contents by gently rotating the infusion bag every 2 hours.

Additional Information Management of side effects is similar to conventional amphotericin B. [See Amphotericin B (Conventional) *on page 83* for suggested management guidelines of side effects.]

Dosage Forms Injection: 100 mg of Abelcet® in 20 mL of suspension (single use only)

References

De Marie S, "Clinical Use of Liposomal and Lipid-Complexed Amphotericin B," *J Antimicrob Chemother*, 1994, 33(5):907-16.

Kline S, Larsen TA, Fieber L, et al, "Limited Toxicity of Prolonged Therapy With High Doses of Amphotericin B Lipid Complex," *Clin Infect Dis*, 1995, 21(5):1154-8.

Amphotericin B Liposome (am foe TER i sin bee LYE po som)

U.S. Brand Names AmBisome®

Synonyms L-AmB

Therapeutic Category Antifungal Agent, Systemic

Use Treatment of aspergillosis, candidiasis, or cryptococcosis in patients who are refractory to or intolerant of conventional amphotericin B therapy (refractory to or intolerant is defined as renal dysfunction with a serum creatinine ≥1.5 mg/dL that develops during therapy, or disease progression after a total dose of conventional amphotericin B of at least 10 mg/kg); empiric therapy for presumed fungal infection in febrile, neutropenic bone marrow transplant patients or febrile, neutropenic acute nonlymphocytic leukemia patients after an unsuccessful trial of antibiotics; treatment of suspected or proven fungal infections in patients with renal impairment

Pregnancy Risk Factor B

Contraindications Hypersensitivity to amphotericin B or any component

Warnings Anaphylaxis has been reported with amphotericin B-containing drugs; facilities for cardiopulmonary resuscitation should be available during administration due to the possibility of anaphylactic reaction

Precautions Due to the nephrotoxic potential of amphotericin B, other nephrotoxic drugs should be avoided

Adverse Reactions

Cardiovascular: Hypotension, arrhythmias, chest pain, cardiac arrest, vasodilatation

Central nervous system: Headache, transient chills or rigors (18%), fever (17%), anxiety, insomnia, dizziness, hallucinations

Dermatologic: Pruritus, rash, diaphoresis

Endocrine & metabolic: Hypokalemia, bilirubinemia, hypomagnesemia, hyperglycemia, hypocalcemia

Gastrointestinal: Diarrhea, nausea, vomiting

Hematologic: Anemia, thrombocytopenia

Hepatic: Elevated ALT, AST, and alkaline phosphatase

Renal: Renal tubular acidosis, elevated serum creatinine and BUN (19%; occurs to a lesser degree than with conventional amphotericin B), oliguria, hematuria

Respiratory: Dyspnea, respiratory failure, cough

Miscellaneous: Anaphylactoid and other allergic reactions

Drug Interactions Nephrotoxic drugs may cause additive nephrotoxic effects; corticosteroids may increase potassium depletion caused by amphotericin; may predispose patients receiving cardiac glycosides or skeletal muscle relaxants to toxicity secondary to hypokalemia; may result in acute pulmonary toxicity in patients simultaneously receiving leukocyte transfusions; ketoconazole, fluconazole may induce fungal resistance to amphotericin B; may increase toxicity of flucytosine by increasing cellular uptake and/or impairing its renal excretion; may potentiate renal toxicity, bronchospasm and hypotension of antineoplastic agents

Stability Store unopened vials under refrigeration; reconstituted drug is stable for 24 hours under refrigeration. Do not dilute with saline solutions or mix with other drugs or electrolytes since this may cause precipitation of AmBisome®. AmBisome® is stable when further diluted to a concentration of 0.5-2.2 mg/mL in D_5W, $D_{10}W$, and $D_{20}W$ for 72 hours at room temperature or when further diluted in D_5W for 14 days if refrigerated

Pharmacokinetics Exhibits nonlinear kinetics (greater than proportional increase in serum concentration with an increase in dose)

Distribution: V_d: 0.1-0.16 L/kg

Half-life (terminal): 100-153 hours

Usual Dosage Children and Adults: I.V.: 3-5 mg/kg/day given as a once daily infusion; doses as high as 6 mg/kg/day have been used in patients with documented *Aspergillus* infection

Administration Parenteral: I.V.: Do not use in-line filter less than 1 micron to administer AmBisome®. Flush line with D_5W prior to infusion; infusion of diluted

(Continued)

Amphotericin B Liposome (Continued)

AmBisome® should start within 6 hours of preparation; infuse over 2 hours; infusion time may be reduced to 1 hour in patients who tolerate the treatment; AmBisome® may be diluted with D_5W, $D_{10}W$, or $D_{20}W$ to a final concentration in 1-2 mg/mL; lower concentrations (0.2-0.5 mg/mL) may be administered to infants and small children to provide sufficient volume for infusion

Monitoring Parameters BUN, serum creatinine, liver function tests, serum electrolytes, CBC, vital signs, I & O; monitor for signs of hypokalemia (muscle weakness, cramping, drowsiness, EKG changes)

Nursing Implications Management of side effects is similar to conventional amphotericin B. [See Amphotericin B (Conventional) *on page 83* for suggested management guidelines of side effects.]

Dosage Forms Injection: 50 mg

References

Emminger W, Graninger W, Emminger-Schmidmeir W, et al, "Tolerance of High Doses of Amphotericin B by Infusion of a Liposomal Formulation in Children With Cancer," *Ann Hematol*, 1994, 68:27-31.

Ringden O, Andstrom E, Remberger M, et al, "Safety of Liposomal Amphotericin B (AmBisome®) In 187 Transplant Recipients Treated With Cyclosporin," *Bone Marrow Transplant*, 1994, 14 Suppl 5:S10-4.

Walsh TJ, Finberg RW, Arndt C, et al, "Liposomal Amphotericin B for Empirical Therapy in Patients With Persistent Fever and Neutropenia," *N Engl J Med*, 1999, 340:764-71.

Ampicillin (am pi SIL in)

Related Information

Carbohydrate and Alcohol Content of Liquid Medications for Use in Patients Receiving Ketogenic Diets *on page 1258*

Endocarditis Prophylaxis *on page 1160*

U.S. Brand Names Marcillin®; Omnipen®; Omnipen®-N; Polycillin®; Polycillin-N®; Principen®; Totacillin®; Totacillin®-N

Canadian Brand Names Ampicin; Apo-Ampi; Jaa Amp; Novo-Ampicillin; Nu-Ampi; Pro-Ampi

Synonyms Aminobenzylpenicillin

Therapeutic Category Antibiotic, Penicillin

Generic Available Yes

Use Treatment of susceptible bacterial infections caused by streptococci, pneumococci, enterococci, nonpenicillinase-producing staphylococci, *Listeria*, meningococci; some strains of *H. influenzae*, *P. mirabilis*, *Salmonella*, *Shigella*, *E. coli*, *Enterobacter*, and *Klebsiella*; initial empiric treatment of neonates with suspected bacterial sepsis or meningitis used in combination with an aminoglycoside or cefotaxime; endocarditis prophylaxis

Pregnancy Risk Factor B

Contraindications Hypersensitivity to ampicillin (penicillins) or any component

Warnings Epstein-Barr virus infection, acute lymphocytic leukemia or cytomegalovirus infection increases risk for ampicillin-induced maculopapular rash

Precautions Dosage adjustment may be necessary in patients with renal impairment (Cl_{cr} <10-15 mL/minute); use with caution in patients allergic to cephalosporins

Adverse Reactions

Central nervous system: Seizures, headache, dizziness, drug fever

Dermatologic: Rash, urticaria, exfoliative dermatitis, Stevens-Johnson syndrome

Gastrointestinal: Diarrhea (20%), nausea, vomiting, glossitis, pseudomembranous enterocolitis, oral candidiasis

Hematologic: Eosinophilia, hemolytic anemia, thrombocytopenia, neutropenia, prolongation of bleeding time

Renal: Interstitial nephritis

Miscellaneous: Anaphylaxis, hypersensitivity reactions, serum sickness, vasculitis, superinfection

Drug Interactions Estrogen-containing oral contraceptives (decreases contraceptive effectiveness), aminoglycosides, probenecid (increases ampicillin serum levels), chloroquine (decreases bioavailability of ampicillin), allopurinol (possible increased frequency of ampicillin rash)

Food Interactions Food decreases rate and extent of absorption

Stability Oral suspension is stable for 14 days under refrigeration; reconstituted solutions for I.M. or direct I.V. should be used within 1 hour; solutions for I.V. infusion will be inactivated by dextrose at room temperature; if dextrose-containing solutions are to be used as a diluent, the resultant solution will only be stable for 2 hours vs 8 hours in solutions containing NS

Mechanism of Action Interferes with bacterial cell wall synthesis by binding to one or more penicillin-binding proteins during active multiplication; inhibits the final transpeptidation step of peptidoglycan synthesis causing cell wall death and resultant bactericidal activity against susceptible bacteria

Pharmacokinetics

Absorption: Oral: 50%

Distribution: Into bile; penetration into CSF occurs with inflamed meninges only; low excretion into breast milk

Protein binding:

Neonates: 10%

Adults: 15% to 18%

Half-life:

Neonates:

2-7 days: 4 hours

8-14 days: 2.8 hours

15-30 days: 1.7 hours

Children and Adults: 1-1.8 hours

Anuric patients: 8-20 hours

Time to peak serum concentration: Oral: Within 1-2 hours

Elimination: ~90% of drug excreted unchanged in urine within 24 hours; excreted in bile

Dialysis: ~40% is removed by hemodialysis

Usual Dosage

Children: Oral: 50-100 mg/kg/day divided every 6 hours; maximum dose: 2-3 g/day

Adults: Oral: 250-500 mg every 6 hours

Neonates: I.M., I.V.:

Postnatal age ≤7 days:

≤2000 g: 50 mg/kg/day divided every 12 hours; meningitis: 100 mg/kg/day divided every 12 hours

>2000 g: 75 mg/kg/day divided every 8 hours; meningitis: 150 mg/kg/day divided every 8 hours

Group B streptococcal meningitis: 200 mg/kg/day divided every 8 hours

Postnatal age >7 days:

<1200 g: 50 mg/kg/day divided every 12 hours; meningitis: 100 mg/kg/day divided every 12 hours

1200-2000 g: 75 mg/kg/day divided every 8 hours; meningitis: 150 mg/kg/day divided every 8 hours

>2000 g: 100 mg/kg/day divided every 6 hours; meningitis: 200 mg/kg/day divided every 6 hours

Group B streptococcal meningitis: 300 mg/kg/day divided every 6 hours

Infants and Children: I.M., I.V.: 100-200 mg/kg/day divided every 6 hours; meningitis: 200-400 mg/kg/day divided every 6 hours; maximum dose: 12 g/day

Endocarditis prophylaxis:

50 mg/kg within 30 minutes before procedure (dental, oral, respiratory tract, or esophageal procedures)

50 mg/kg plus gentamicin 1.5 mg/kg within 30 minutes of starting the procedure; 25 mg/kg 6 hours later (for high-risk patients undergoing genitourinary and GI tract procedures)

Adults: I.M., I.V.: 500 mg to 3 g every 6 hours; maximum dose: 14 g/day

Endocarditis prophylaxis:

2 g within 30 minutes before procedure (dental, oral, respiratory tract, or esophageal procedures)

2 g plus gentamicin 1.5 mg/kg (maximum dose: 120 mg) within 30 minutes of starting the procedure; 1 g 6 hours later (for high-risk patients undergoing genitourinary and GI tract procedures)

Adults: I.M., I.V.: 500 mg to 3 g every 4-6 hours

Dosing interval in renal impairment: Adults:

Cl_{cr} 10-30 mL/minute: Administer every 6-12 hours

Cl_{cr} <10 mL/minute: Administer every 12 hours

Administration

Oral: Administer with water 1-2 hours prior to food on an empty stomach; shake suspension well before using

Parenteral: Ampicillin may be administered IVP over 3-5 minutes at a rate not to exceed 100 mg/minute or I.V. intermittent infusion over 15-30 minutes; final concentration for I.V. administration should not exceed 100 mg/mL (IVP) or 30 mg/mL (I.V. intermittent infusion)

Monitoring Parameters With prolonged therapy monitor renal, hepatic, and hematologic function periodically; observe for change in bowel frequency

(Continued)

Ampicillin *(Continued)*

Test Interactions False-positive urinary glucose (Benedict's solution, Clinitest®); + Coombs' [direct]

Nursing Implications Ampicillin and gentamicin should not be mixed in the same I.V. tubing or administered concurrently

Additional Information Appearance of a rash should be carefully evaluated to differentiate a nonallergic ampicillin rash from a hypersensitivity reaction. Ampicillin rash occurs in 5% to 10% of children receiving ampicillin and is a generalized dull red, maculopapular rash, generally appearing 3-14 days after the start of therapy. It normally begins on the trunk and spreads over most of the body. It may be most intense at pressure areas, elbows, and knees. Incidence of ampicillin rash is higher in patients with viral infections, infectious mononucleosis, lymphocytic leukemia, or patients with hyperuricemia who are receiving allopurinol.

Sodium content of suspension (250 mg/5 mL, 5 mL): 10 mg (0.4 mEq)
Sodium content of 1 g: 66.7 mg (3 mEq)

Dosage Forms

Capsule, as anhydrous: 250 mg, 500 mg
Capsule, as trihydrate: 250 mg, 500 mg
Powder for injection, as sodium: 125 mg, 250 mg, 500 mg, 1 g, 2 g, 10 g
Powder for oral suspension, as trihydrate: 125 mg/5 mL (5 mL unit dose, 80 mL, 100 mL, 150 mL, 200 mL); 250 mg/5 mL (5 mL unit dose, 80 mL, 100 mL, 150 mL, 200 mL); 500 mg/5 mL (5 mL unit dose, 100 mL)
Powder for oral suspension, drops, as trihydrate: 100 mg/mL (20 mL)

References

Boguniewicz M and Leung DY, "Hypersensitivity Reactions to Antibiotics Commonly Used in Children," *Pediatr Infect Dis J*, 1995, 14(3):221-31.

Brown RD, Campoli-Richards DM, "Antimicrobial Therapy in Neonates, Infants, and Children," *Clin Pharmacokinet*, 1989, 17(Suppl 1):105-15.

Ampicillin and Sulbactam *(am pi SIL in & SUL bak tam)*

U.S. Brand Names Unasyn®

Synonyms Sulbactam and Ampicillin

Therapeutic Category Antibiotic, Beta-lactam and Beta-lactamase Combination; Antibiotic, Penicillin

Generic Available No

Use Treatment of susceptible bacterial infections involved with skin and skin structure, intra-abdominal infections, gynecological infections; spectrum is that of ampicillin plus organisms producing beta-lactamases such as *S. aureus*, *H. influenzae*, *E. coli*, *Klebsiella*, *Acinetobacter*, *Enterobacter*, and anaerobes

Pregnancy Risk Factor B

Contraindications Hypersensitivity to ampicillin, sulbactam, any component, or penicillins

Warnings Epstein-Barr virus infection, acute lymphocytic leukemia or cytomegalovirus infection increases risk for ampicillin-induced maculopapular rash; not FDA approved for children <12 years of age

Precautions Modify dosage in patients with renal impairment; use with caution in patients allergic to cephalosporins

Adverse Reactions

Cardiovascular: Chest pain
Central nervous system: Fatigue, malaise, headache, chills, dizziness
Dermatologic: Rash (2%), itching, urticaria, exfoliative dermatitis, Stevens-Johnson syndrome
Gastrointestinal: Diarrhea (3%), nausea, vomiting, candidiasis, flatulence, pseudomembranous colitis, hairy tongue
Genitourinary: Dysuria, hematuria
Hematologic: Decreased WBC, neutrophils, platelets, hemoglobin, and hematocrit
Hepatic: Increased liver enzymes
Local: Pain at injection site (I.M.: 16%, I.V.: 3%), thrombophlebitis (3%)
Renal: Elevated BUN, elevated serum creatinine
Miscellaneous: Hypersensitivity reactions, anaphylaxis, serum sickness, vasculitis, superinfection

Drug Interactions Probenecid (decreased elimination of ampicillin and sulbactam); allopurinol (possible increased frequency of ampicillin rash); efficacy of oral contraceptives may be reduced

Stability Ampicillin/sulbactam infusion solution is stable for 8 hours in NS at room temperature; incompatible when mixed with aminoglycosides

Mechanism of Action Sulbactam has very little antibacterial activity by itself. The addition of sulbactam, a beta-lactamase inhibitor, to ampicillin extends the spectrum of ampicillin to include beta-lactamase producing organisms; ampicillin acts by inhibiting bacterial cell wall synthesis during the stage of active multiplication

Pharmacokinetics

Distribution: Into bile, blister and tissue fluids; poor penetration into CSF with uninflamed meninges; higher concentrations attained with inflamed meninges

Protein binding:

Ampicillin: 28%

Sulbactam: 38%

Half-life: Ampicillin and sulbactam are similar: 1-1.8 hours and 1-1.3 hours, respectively in patients with normal renal function

Elimination: ~75% to 85% of both drugs are excreted unchanged in urine within 8 hours following administration

Usual Dosage Unasyn® (ampicillin/sulbactam) is a combination product; each 3 g vial contains 2 g of ampicillin and 1 g of sulbactam. Dosage recommendations are based on the **ampicillin** component.

I.M., I.V.:

Infants ≥1 month: 100-150 mg/kg/day divided every 6 hours

Meningitis: 200-300 mg/kg/day divided every 6 hours

Children: 100-200 mg ampicillin/kg/day divided every 6 hours

Meningitis: 200-400 mg/kg/day divided every 6 hours; maximum dose: 8 g ampicillin/day

Adults: 1-2 g ampicillin every 6-8 hours; maximum dose: 12 g ampicillin/day

Dosing interval in renal impairment:

Cl_{cr} 15-29 mL/minute: Administer every 12 hours

Cl_{cr} 5-14 mL/minute: Administer every 24 hours

Administration Parenteral: May be administered by slow I.V. injection over 10-15 minutes at a final concentration for administration not to exceed 45 mg Unasyn® (30 mg ampicillin and 15 mg sulbactam)/mL

Monitoring Parameters With prolonged therapy monitor hematologic, renal, and hepatic function; observe for change in bowel frequency

Test Interactions False-positive urinary glucose levels (Benedict's solution, Clinitest®)

Additional Information Sodium content of 1.5 g (1 g ampicillin plus 0.5 g sulbactam): 5 mEq

Dosage Forms Powder for injection: 1.5 g [ampicillin sodium 1 g and sulbactam sodium 0.5 g]; 3 g [ampicillin sodium 2 g and sulbactam sodium 1 g]

References

Dajani AS, "Sulbactam/Ampicillin in Pediatric Infections," *Drugs*, 1988, 35(Suppl 7):35-8.

Goldfarb J, Aronoff SC, Jaffé A, et al, "Sultamicillin in the Treatment of Superficial Skin and Soft Tissue Infections in Children," *Antimicrob Agents Chemother*, 1987, 31(4):663-4.

Kulhanjian J, Dunphy MG, Hamstra S, et al, "Randomized Comparative Study of Ampicillin/Sulbactam vs Ceftriaxone for Treatment of Soft Tissue and Skeletal Infections in Children," *Pediatr Infect Dis J*, 1989, 8(9):605-10.

Syriopoulou V, Bitsi M, Theodoridis C, et al, "Clinical Efficacy of Sulbactam/Ampicillin in Pediatric Infections Caused by Ampicillin-Resistant or Penicillin-Resistant Organisms," *Rev Infect Dis*, 1986, 8(Suppl 5):S630-3.

♦ **Ampicin (Can)** *see Ampicillin on page 88*

Amprenavir (am PRE na veer)

Related Information

Adult and Adolescent HIV *on page 1166*

Pediatric HIV *on page 1162*

U.S. Brand Names Agenerase™

Therapeutic Category Antiretroviral Agent; HIV Agents (Anti-HIV Agents); Protease Inhibitor

Generic Available No

Use Treatment of HIV infection in combination with other antiretroviral agents (Note: HIV regimens consisting of **three** antiretroviral agents are strongly recommended)

Pregnancy Risk Factor C

Contraindications Hypersensitivity to amprenavir or any component; concurrent therapy with astemizole, bepridil, cisapride, dihydroergotamine, ergotamine, midazolam, or triazolam; due to the high amount of propylene glycol, amprenavir oral **solution** is contraindicated in infants and children <4 years, pregnancy, renal or hepatic failure, and in patients receiving disulfiram or metronidazole

Warnings Amprenavir is a potent CYP3A isoenzyme inhibitor that interacts with numerous drugs. Due to potential serious and/or life-threatening drug interactions, some drugs are contraindicated (see Contraindications and Drug interactions) and the following drugs require concentration monitoring if coadministered with (Continued)

Amprenavir *(Continued)*

amprenavir: amiodarone, systemic lidocaine, tricyclic antidepressants, and quinidine. Concurrent use with rifampin or certain cholesterol-lowering agents (lovastatin, simvastatin) is not recommended.

Amprenavir oral solution contains a high amount of propylene glycol and should only be used when the capsules or other protease inhibitors are not options; women and certain ethnic groups (Native Americans, Eskimos, Asians) may have a decreased capacity to metabolize propylene glycol and therefore, may be at a higher risk for adverse effects of propylene glycol; when using the oral solution, monitor patients for propylene glycol adverse effects (see Monitoring Parameters); change patient to capsule formulation as soon as patient is able to take capsules.

Severe and life-threatening skin reactions (eg, Stevens-Johnson syndrome) may occur; discontinue amprenavir in patients who develop severe or life-threatening rashes or in patients with moderate rashes and systemic symptoms. Spontaneous bleeding episodes have been reported in patients with hemophilia type A and B receiving protease inhibitors. New onset diabetes mellitus, exacerbations of diabetes, and hyperglycemia have been reported in HIV-infected patients receiving protease inhibitors. Acute hemolytic anemia has been reported.

Precautions Use with caution in patients with diabetes mellitus, sulfonamide allergy, hepatic impairment, or hemophilia. Capsules and oral solution contain high amounts of vitamin E; additional supplements of vitamin E should be avoided.

Adverse Reactions

Central nervous system: Depression or mood disorders (4% to 15%), headache, fatigue

Dermatologic: Rash (28% incidence; usually mild to moderate, maculopapular, some pruritic; median onset: 10 days, range: 7-73 days), Stevens-Johnson syndrome (1% of patients, 4% of patients who develop a rash)

Endocrine & metabolic: Hyperglycemia (37% to 41%), hypertriglyceridemia (36% to 47%), hypercholesterolemia (4% to 9%), new onset diabetes, exacerbation of diabetes mellitus; central redistribution of body fat: central obesity, buffalo hump, facial atrophy, and breast enlargement

Gastrointestinal: Nausea (38% to 73%), vomiting (20% to 29%), diarrhea (33% to 56%), taste disorders (1% to 10%)

Hematologic: Acute hemolytic anemia (rare, one case reported), spontaneous bleeding in hemophiliacs

Neuromuscular & skeletal: Paresthesia (perioral or peripheral)

Drug Interactions Cytochrome P-450 isoenzyme CYP3A4 substrate and inhibitor

Amprenavir may inhibit the metabolism of the following drugs and cause serious or life-threatening adverse effects: Astemizole, bepridil, cisapride, dihydroergotamine, ergotamine, midazolam, and triazolam (concurrent therapy with these drugs and amprenavir is contraindicated); amprenavir may increase the toxic effects of amiodarone, lidocaine, quinidine, warfarin, and tricyclic antidepressants (serum concentration monitoring of these drugs is necessary); amprenavir significantly increases the AUC of rifabutin by 193% (rifabutin dose should be decreased by at least $\frac{1}{2}$ the recommended dose when used in combination with amprenavir); amprenavir may increase the AUC of ketoconazole and zidovudine and decrease the AUC of indinavir and saquinavir; amprenavir may increase serum concentrations or toxicity of diltiazem, nifedipine, alprazolam, clorazepate, diazepam, flurazepam, itraconazole, dapsone, erythromycin, loratadine, sildenafil, carbamazepine, pimozide, and cholesterol-lowering agents (concurrent use of lovastatin or simvastatin is not recommended)

Rifampin significantly reduces amprenavir plasma concentrations (AUC decreased 82%) and should **not** be used concurrently; the herbal medicine, St John's wort (*Hypericum perforatum*), may significantly decrease concentrations of amprenavir and is **not** recommended for concurrent use; efavirenz decreases amprenavir concentrations by 39%; saquinavir decreases amprenavir AUC by 32%; phenobarbital, phenytoin, or carbamazepine may decrease amprenavir concentrations; abacavir, clarithromycin, indinavir, ketoconazole, or zidovudine may increase the AUC of amprenavir; nelfinavir may increase the trough concentrations of amprenavir; cimetidine or ritonavir may increase amprenavir concentrations

Amprenavir may decrease the efficacy of hormonal contraceptives (reliable barrier method should be used); antacids or didanosine should be given at least 1 hour before or after amprenavir; vitamin E supplements should be avoided (amprenavir products contain high amounts of vitamin E); alcohol may interact with the high amount of propylene glycol in the oral solution and should be avoided

Food Interactions A high fat meal may decrease mean AUC by 14%

Stability Store at room temperature

Mechanism of Action A protease inhibitor which acts on an enzyme (protease) late in the HIV replication process after the virus has entered into the cell's nucleus; amprenavir binds to the protease activity site and inhibits the activity of the enzyme, thus preventing cleavage of viral polyprotein precursors (gag-pol protein precursors) into individual functional proteins found in infectious HIV; this results in the formation of immature, noninfectious viral particles

Pharmacokinetics

Distribution: V_d (apparent): Adults: 430 L

Protein binding: 90%; high affinity binding protein: alpha$_1$ acid glycoprotein

Metabolism: In the liver via cytochrome P-450 CYP3A4 isoenzyme system; glucuronide conjugation of oxidized metabolites also occurs

Bioavailability: Absolute bioavailability not established; oral solution is 14% less bioavailable than capsules (do not interchange on a mg per mg basis)

Half-life: Adults: 7.1-10.6 hours

Time to peak serum concentration (single dose): 1-2 hours

Elimination: Minimal excretion of unchanged drug in urine (<3%) and feces; 75% of dose excreted as metabolites via biliary tract into feces and 14% excreted as metabolites in urine

Usual Dosage Oral (use in combination with other antiretroviral agents): **Note:** Due to differences in bioavailability, capsules and solution are **not** interchangeable on a mg per mg basis:

Neonates, Infants, and Children <4 years:

Solution: Contraindicated due to potential toxicity from propylene glycol

Capsules: Not approved for use

Children 4-12 years and Adolescents 13-16 years with a body weight <50 kg:

Solution: 22.5 mg/kg twice daily or 17 mg/kg 3 times/day; maximum: 2800 mg/day

Capsules: 20 mg/kg twice daily or 15 mg/kg 3 times/day; maximum: 2400 mg/day

Adolescents 13-16 years with a body weight >50 kg and Adults:

Capsules: 1200 mg twice daily

Dosing adjustment in hepatic impairment: Adults: Oral: Capsules:

Child-Pugh score 5-8: 450 mg twice daily

Child-Pugh score 9-12: 300 mg twice daily

Administration May be administered without regard to meals; avoid administration with high fat meals; do not administer concurrently with antacids

Monitoring Parameters Signs and symptoms of rash or adverse effects; serum glucose, triglycerides, cholesterol, CBC with differential, CD4 cell count, viral load; patients treated with amprenavir oral solution need to be monitored for adverse effects of propylene glycol, such as hyperosmolality, lactic acidosis, seizures, stupor, tachycardia, renal toxicity, and hemolysis

Patient Information Inform your physician if you have a sulfa allergy; amprenavir is not a cure for HIV; notify physician immediately if rash develops; report the use of other medications, nonprescription medications, and herbal or natural products to your physician and pharmacist; take amprenavir everyday as prescribed; do not change dose or discontinue without physician's advice; if a dose is missed, take it as soon as possible, then return to normal dosing schedule; if a dose is skipped, do not double the next dose; avoid alcohol if taking amprenavir oral solution

Additional Information To increase amprenavir solubility, propylene glycol has been added to the oral solution. **Note:** The recommended pediatric dose of the oral solution delivers 1650 mg/kg/day of propylene glycol; the acceptable amount of propylene glycol (when used as an excipient) is not known; treatment of overdose of the oral solution should include monitoring and management of propylene glycol adverse effects including acid-base abnormalities (see Monitoring Parameters); hemodialysis for removal of propylene glycol may be needed.

To increase amprenavir bioavailability, d-alpha tocopherol polyethylene glycol 1000 succinate (a form of vitamin E) has been added in significant concentrations to the product formulations; vitamin E content: 150 mg capsule: 109 international units; oral solution: 46 international units/mL. **Note:** The recommended pediatric dose of the oral solution delivers 138 international units/kg/day of vitamin E; this significantly exceeds the pediatric RDA of 10 international units.

Dosage Forms

Capsules: 50 mg, 150 mg

Solution, oral: 15 mg/mL [grape bubblegum peppermint flavor] (240 mL)

References

Adkins JC and Faulds D, "Amprenavir," *Drugs*, 1998, 55(6):837-42.

Collura JM and Kraus DM, "New Pediatric Antiretroviral Agents," *J Pediatr Health Care*, 2000, 14(4):183-90.

Panel on Clinical Practices for Treatment of HIV Infection, "Guidelines for the Use of Antiretroviral Agents in HIV-Infected Adults and Adolescents," April 23, 2001, http://www.hivatis.org.

(Continued)

Amprenavir *(Continued)*

Piscitelli SC, Burstein AH, Chaitt D, et al, "Indinavir Concentrations and St. John's Wort," *Lancet*, 2000, 355(9203):547-8.

Sadler BM, Hanson CD, Chittick GE, et al, "Safety and Pharmacokinetics of Amprenavir (141W94), a Human Immunodeficiency Virus (HIV) Type 1 Protease Inhibitor, Following Oral Administration of Single Doses to HIV-Infected Adults," *Antimicrob Agents Chemother*, 1999, 43(7):1686-92.

Working Group on Antiretroviral Therapy and Medical Management of HIV-Infected Children, "Guidelines for the Use of Antiretroviral Agents in Pediatric HIV Infection," January 7, 2000, http://www.hivatis.org.

♦ **Amrinone** *see* Inamrinone *on page 532*

Amyl Nitrite (AM il NYE trite)

Synonyms Isoamyl Nitrite

Therapeutic Category Antidote, Cyanide; Vasodilator, Coronary

Generic Available Yes

Use Coronary vasodilator in angina pectoris; an adjunct in treatment of cyanide poisoning

Pregnancy Risk Factor C

Contraindications Severe anemia; hypersensitivity to nitrates or any component; recent head trauma or cerebral hemorrhage; hyperthyroidism; recent MI

Precautions Use with caution in patients with increased intracranial pressure, glaucoma, low systolic blood pressure

Adverse Reactions
Cardiovascular: Postural hypotension; cutaneous flushing of head, neck, and clavicular area; tachycardia; palpitations; vasodilation; syncope
Central nervous system: Headache, dizziness, restlessness
Dermatologic: Skin rash (contact dermatitis)
Gastrointestinal: Nausea, vomiting
Hematologic: Hemolytic anemia
Ocular: Increased intraocular pressure

Drug Interactions Alcohol; medications that cause hypotension may increase the postural hypotensive effects of amyl nitrite

Stability Store in cool place, protect from light; flammable, avoid exposure to heat or flame

Mechanism of Action Vasodilator (vascular smooth muscle relaxant) which decreases afterload and improves myocardial blood supply via coronary artery vasodilation; antidote for cyanide poisoning: promotes formation of methemoglobin which combines with cyanide molecule to form cyanmethemoglobin (nontoxic)

Pharmacodynamics
Onset of action: Within 30 seconds
Duration: 3-5 minutes

Pharmacokinetics
Absorption: Inhalation: Readily absorbed through respiratory tract
Metabolism: In the liver to form inorganic nitrates (less potent)
Half-life:
    Amyl nitrite: <1 hour
    Methemoglobin: 1 hour
Elimination: Renal; ~33%

Usual Dosage Nasal inhalation:
Children and Adults: Cyanide poisoning: Inhale the vapor from a 0.3 mL crushed ampul every minute for 15-30 seconds until I.V. sodium nitrite infusion is available
Adults: Angina: 1-6 inhalations from 1 crushed ampul; may repeat in 3-5 minutes

Administration Give by nasal inhalation; crush ampul in woven covering between finger and hold under patient's nostrils

Monitoring Parameters Blood pressure; with treatment for cyanide poisoning: methemoglobin levels, arterial blood gas

Patient Information Remain seated or lying down during administration because of possible hypotension and dizziness; do not get up suddenly after use; avoid alcohol; if angina pain is not relieved after 2 doses, seek immediate medical attention

Additional Information Amyl nitrite has been used to treat penile erections after urological surgery (eg, circumcisions in adults) and has been used to change the intensity of heart murmurs to aid in their diagnosis

Dosage Forms Inhalant: 0.3 mL crushable glass perles (ampuls)

♦ **Anaprox®** *see* Naproxen *on page 699*
♦ **Anaprox® DS** *see* Naproxen *on page 699*
♦ **Anaspaz®** *see* Hyoscyamine *on page 517*
♦ **Anbesol® [OTC]** *see* Benzocaine *on page 135*
♦ **Anbesol® Maximum Strength [OTC]** *see* Benzocaine *on page 135*

+ **Ancef®**   *see* Cefazolin *on page 189*
+ **Ancobon®**   *see* Flucytosine *on page 432*
+ **Andriol (Can)**   *see* Testosterone *on page 938*
+ **Androderm®**   *see* Testosterone *on page 938*
+ **AndroGel®**   *see* Testosterone *on page 938*
+ **Anebesol Baby (Can)**   *see* Benzocaine *on page 135*
+ **Anectine®**   *see* Succinylcholine *on page 918*
+ **Anestacon®**   *see* Lidocaine *on page 590*
+ **Aneurine**   *see* Thiamine *on page 948*
+ **Anexate (Can)**   *see* Flumazenil *on page 436*
+ **Anexsia®**   *see* Hydrocodone and Acetaminophen *on page 505*
+ **Anhydrous Glucose**   *see* Dextrose *on page 317*
+ **Ansaid®**   *see* Flurbiprofen *on page 450*
+ **Ansamycin**   *see* Rifabutin *on page 875*

Antacid Preparations (ant AS id prep a RAE shuns)

Related Information
Calcium Supplements *on page 167*
Carbohydrate and Alcohol Content of Liquid Medications for Use in Patients Receiving Ketogenic Diets *on page 1258*
Magnesium Supplements *on page 614*
Sodium Bicarbonate *on page 904*

U.S. Brand Names Amphojel® [OTC]; Basaljel® [OTC]; Gaviscon® [OTC]; Maalox® [OTC]; Maalox® Plus Extra Strength [OTC]; Mylanta® [OTC]; Mylanta®-II [OTC]; Riopan® [OTC]; Tums® [OTC]

Available Salts Aluminum Carbonate; Aluminum Carbonate Gel; Aluminum Hydroxide; Aluminum Hydroxide and Magnesium Hydroxide; Aluminum Hydroxide and Magnesium Trisilicate; Aluminum Hydroxide Gel; Aluminum Hydroxide, Magnesium Hydroxide, and Simethicone; Hydroxide and Magnesium Carbonate

Therapeutic Category Antacid; Gastrointestinal Agent, Gastric or Duodenal Ulcer Treatment

Generic Available Yes

Use Adjunct for the relief of peptic ulcer pain and to promote healing of peptic ulcers; relief of stomach upset associated with hyperacidity; prevention of stress ulcer bleeding; treatment of duodenal ulcer and gastroesophageal reflux disease. Aluminum hydroxide is also used to reduce phosphate absorption in hyperphosphatemia; calcium carbonate is used to treat calcium deficiency and to bind phosphate; magnesium oxide is used to treat hypomagnesemia

Warnings Use aluminum-containing antacids with caution in patients with decreased bowel motility and dehydration, in patients with gastric outlet obstruction, in patients with renal failure, and in patients who have an upper GI hemorrhage; use magnesium-containing products with caution in patients with renal impairment; use sodium-containing antacids with caution in patients on low-sodium diets, and in patients with CHF, edema, renal failure, or hepatic failure

Adverse Reactions
Aluminum-containing antacids:
Central nervous system: Dementia, encephalopathy, malaise, seizures, confusion, coma
Endocrine & metabolic: Hypophosphatemia, hyperaluminemia, osteoporosis
Gastrointestinal: Constipation, anorexia
Genitourinary: Urinary calculi
Neuromuscular & skeletal: Muscle weakness, osteomalacia
Calcium-containing antacids:
Endocrine & metabolic: Milk-alkali syndrome (hypercalcemia, metabolic alkalosis), hypophosphatemia
Gastrointestinal: Constipation, flatulence
Magnesium-containing antacids:
Endocrine & metabolic: Hypermagnesemia, fluid and electrolyte imbalance
Gastrointestinal: Laxative effects, diarrhea
Sodium-containing antacids:
Cardiovascular: Fluid retention
Endocrine & metabolic: Metabolic alkalosis, sodium overload
Gastrointestinal: Flatulence

Drug Interactions Aluminum-, calcium-, or magnesium-containing antacids (decrease tetracycline and quinolone absorption); antacids decrease absorption of iron, digoxin, phenytoin, indomethacin; chlorpromazine, increased absorption of buffered or enteric-coated aspirin; aluminum hydroxide (decreased absorption of *(Continued)*

Antacid Preparations (Continued)

isoniazid); sucralfate antacids (may impair binding of sucralfate to ulcerated mucosa)

Stability Avoid freezing aluminum hydroxide and magnesium hydroxide

Mechanism of Action Neutralizes gastric acidity increasing gastric pH; inhibits proteolytic activity of pepsin when gastric pH is increased >4

Pharmacodynamics

Duration of action: Dependent on gastric emptying time

Fasting state: 20-60 minutes

1 hour after meals: May be up to 3 hours

Antacid Preparations

Generic/Therapeutic Groupings Brand Names	Al(OH)₃*	Mg(OH)₂*	CaCO₃*	Other Content	Sodium† (mEq)	ANC‡ (mEq)	How Supplied
Aluminum carbonate gel (basic)	400			Simethicone, saccharin, sorbitol	0.13	12	Suspension
Basaljel®	500				0.12	12	Capsule
	500				0.12	13	Tablet
Aluminum hydroxide gel	600			Saccharin, sorbitol	<0.13	16	Suspension
Amphojel®	320			Saccharin, sorbitol	<0.1	10	Suspension
	300				0.08	9	Tablet
	600				0.13	16	Tablet
Aluminum/magnesium hydroxide	225	200		Saccharin, sorbitol	0.06	13.3	Suspension
Maalox®	200	200		Saccharin, sorbitol	0.03	9.7	Tablet/chewable
Maalox® Antacid/Anti-Gas Extra Strength	500	450		Simethicone 40 mg, saccharin, sorbitol (sugar-free)	0.05	29	Suspension
	350	350		Simethicone 30 mg, saccharin, sorbitol (sugar-free)			Tablet
Mylanta®	200	200		Simethicone 20 mg	0.03	12.7	Suspension
	200	200		Simethicone 20 mg	0.03	11.5	Tablet
Mylanta® Maximum Strength	400	400		Simethicone 40 mg	0.05	25.4	Suspension
	400	400		Simethicone 40 mg	0.06	23	Tablet
Riopan®				Magaldrate 540 mg	0.013	15	Suspension
				Magaldrate 480 mg	≤0.004	13.5	Tablet

Usual Dosage Oral: Aluminum/magnesium hydroxide combination (for extra strength or concentrated suspension, use half the volume of the stated dose):

Peptic ulcer disease:

Infants: 1-2 mL/kg/dose 1-3 hours after meals and at bedtime

Children: 5-15 mL/dose every 3-6 hours or 1-3 hours after meals and at bedtime

Adults: 15-45 mL every 3-6 hours or 1-3 hours after meals and at bedtime

Prophylaxis against GI bleeding:

Neonates: 1 mL/kg every 4 hours as needed

Infants: 2-5 mL/dose every 1-2 hours, titrate to gastric pH >3.5

Children: 5-15 mL/dose every 1-2 hours, titrate to gastric pH >3.5

Adults: 30-60 mL every 1-2 hours, titrate to gastric pH >3.5

Hyperphosphatemia:

Children: Use Al(OH)$_3$ or aluminum carbonate gel product only: 50-150 mg/kg/day (as aluminum hydroxide gel) divided every 4-6 hours; titrate to normal serum phosphorus level

Adults: 30-40 mL of Al(OH)$_3$ 3-4 times/day between meals and at bedtime

Antacid Preparations (continued)

Generic/Therapeutic Groupings Brand Names	Al(OH)$_3$*	Mg(OH)$_2$*	CaCO$_3$*	Other Content	Sodium† (mEq)	ANC‡ (mEq)	How Supplied
Aluminum hydroxide/magnesium carbonate	31.7				0.57		Tablet
Gaviscon®				Magnesium carbonate 119.3 mg, sodium alginate, EDTA, saccharin, sorbitol, parabens		4	Suspension
Aluminum hydroxide/magnesium trisilicate	80						
Gaviscon®				Magnesium trisilicate 20 mg, alginic acid, sodium bicarbonate	0.8	0.5	Tablet/chewable
Calcium carbonate tablets							
Tums®			500		≤0.087	10	Tablet/chewable
Tums E-X® Extra Strength			750		≤0.087		Tablet/chewable
Tums® Ultra			1000	Sodium ≤4 mg			Tablet/chewable
Calcium carbonate suspension			1250		<0.217		Suspension
Mylanta® Children's Upset Stomach Relief			400		0.0065	11	Suspension
Titralac Plus®			500	Simethicone 20 mg	0.0065	11	Suspension
			420	Simethicone 21 mg	≤0.001	7.5	Tablet

*Liquids in mg per 5 mL; capsules and tablets in mg.

†mEq of sodium per tablet, capsule, or 5 mL of liquid (23 mg = 1 mEq sodium).

‡ANC = Acid neutralizing capacity per tablet, capsule, or 5 mL of liquid.

Administration Oral: Thoroughly chew tablets before swallowing; shake suspensions well before use

Monitoring Parameters GI complaints, stool frequency; serum phosphate concentrations in patients on hemodialysis receiving chronic aluminum-containing antacid therapy; serum calcium in patients receiving large doses of calcium carbonate; serum electrolytes in patients with renal impairment receiving magnesium-containing antacids

(Continued)

Antacid Preparations *(Continued)*

Patient Information Antacids may impair or increase absorption of many drugs, do not take oral medications within 1-2 hours of an antacid dose unless specifically instructed to do so

Dosage Forms See tables on previous pages.

References

Nord KS, "Peptic Ulcer Disease in the Pediatric Population," *Pediatr Clin North Am*, 1988, 35(1):117-140.

♦ **Anti-Acne Control Formula (Can)** *see* Salicylic Acid *on page 886*

♦ **Anti-Acne Spot Treatment (Can)** *see* Salicylic Acid *on page 886*

♦ **Antibiotic Ointment (Can)** *see* Bacitracin and Polymyxin B *on page 129*

♦ **AntibiOtic® Otic** *see* Neomycin, (Bacitracin) Polymyxin B, and Hydrocortisone *on page 705*

♦ **Antibiotique Onguent (Can)** *see* Bacitracin and Polymyxin B *on page 129*

♦ **Anti-Diarrheal (Can)** *see* Loperamide *on page 603*

♦ **Antidigoxin Fab Fragments** *see* Digoxin Immune Fab *on page 333*

♦ **Antidiuretic Hormone** *see* Vasopressin *on page 1003*

♦ **Antiepileptic Drugs** *see page 1208*

Antihemophilic Factor (Human)

(an tee hee moe FIL ik FAK tor HYU man)

U.S. Brand Names Alphanate®; Hemofil® M; Humate-P®; Koate®-DVI; Monarc® M; Monoclate-P®

Synonyms AHF; AHG; Factor VIII

Therapeutic Category Antihemophilic Agent; Blood Product Derivative

Generic Available Yes

Use Management of hemophilia A in patients whom a deficiency in factor VIII has been demonstrated

Pregnancy Risk Factor C

Contraindications Hypersensitivity to mouse protein [Monoclate-P®; Hemofil® M (Method M, Monoclonal Purified); Antihemophilic Factor, Human (Method M, Monoclonal Purified) contain trace amounts of mouse protein]

Precautions Human antihemophilic factor is prepared from pooled plasma and even with heat treated or other viral attenuated processes, the risk of viral transmission (ie, viral hepatitis, HIV) is not totally eradicated. The use of recombinant antihemophilic factor products (such as Bioclate®, Helixate®, Kogenate®, or Recombinate™) substantially decreases the risk of viral transmission because these products are biosynthetically prepared. Progressive anemia and hemolysis may occur in individuals with blood groups A, B, and AB who receive large or frequent doses of human antihemophilic factor due to trace amounts of blood group A and B isohemagglutinins.

Adverse Reactions

Cardiovascular: Flushing, tachycardia

Central nervous system: Headache

Gastrointestinal: Nausea, vomiting

Neuromuscular & skeletal: Paresthesia

Miscellaneous: Allergic vasomotor reactions, tightness in neck or chest, development of inhibitor antibodies (3% to 52%); inhibitor antibodies are IgG immunoglobulins that neutralize the activity of factor VIII; an increase of inhibitor antibody concentration is seen at 2-7 days, with peak concentrations at 1-3 weeks after therapy. Children <5 years of age are at greatest risk; higher doses of AHF may be needed if antibody is present; if antibody concentration is >10 Bethesda units/mL, patients may not respond to larger doses and alternative treatment modalities may be needed.

Stability Dried concentrate should be refrigerated, but may be stored at room temperature for up to 6 months depending upon specific product; if refrigerated, the dried concentrate and diluent should be warmed to room temperature before reconstitution; gently agitate or rotate vial after adding diluent, do not shake vigorously; do **not** refrigerate after reconstitution, precipitation may occur; administer within 3 hours after reconstitution; Method M, monoclonal purified products should be administered within 1 hour after reconstitution

Mechanism of Action Factor VIII is a protein in normal plasma which is necessary for clot formation and maintenance of hemostasis; it activates factor X in conjunction with activated factor IX; activated factor X converts prothrombin to thrombin, which converts fibrinogen to fibrin and with factor XIII forms a stable clot

Pharmacodynamics Maximal effect: 1-2 hours

Pharmacokinetics
    Distribution: Does not readily cross the placenta
    Half-life: 4-24 hours; mean = 12 hours (biphasic)
Usual Dosage Children and Adults: I.V. (individualize dosage based on coagulation studies performed prior to and during treatment at regular intervals):

    Hospitalized patients: 20-50 units/kg/dose; may be higher for special circumstances. Dose can be given every 12-24 hours and more frequently in special circumstances.
    Hemophilia A with high titer of inhibitor antibody: 50-75 units/kg/hour has been given Formula to approximate percentage increase in plasma antihemophilic factor: Units required = body weight (kg) x 0.5 x desired increase factor VIII (% of normal)
Administration Parenteral: I.V. administration only; administer through a separate line, do not mix with drugs or other I.V. fluids; maximum rate of administration is product dependent: Monoclate-P® 2 mL/minute; Humate-P® 4 mL/minute; administration of other AHF products should not exceed 10 mL/minute; use filter needle to draw product into syringe
Monitoring Parameters Heart rate before and during I.V. administration; plasma antihemophilic factor levels prior to and during treatment; inhibitor antibody concentration
Reference Range Plasma antihemophilic factor level: Desired: ~30% of normal for effective hemostasis in patients with hemorrhage; ~5% to 10% of normal for hemarthrosis; ~30% to 50% of normal to prevent hemorrhage for minor surgical procedures; ~80% to 100% of normal for major surgical procedures (give dose 1 hour prior to O.R.); ~30% to 60% of normal may be required for at least 10-14 days postoperatively
Nursing Implications Reduce rate of administration or temporarily discontinue if patient becomes tachycardiac
Additional Information Products using a heat treatment process for viral attenuation include Humate-P® and Monoclate-P®; a solvent/detergent viral inactivation process is used in making Alphanate®
Dosage Forms Injection, human (approximate factor VIII activity per vial): 200 units, 250 units, 500 units, 750 units, 1000 units, 1250 units, 1500 units [exact potency labeled on each vial]

◆ **Antiminth® [OTC]** *see* Pyrantel Pamoate *on page 855*
◆ **Anti-Nauseant (Can)** *see* Dimenhydrinate *on page 339*
◆ **Antiphogistine Rub A-535 Capsaicin (Can)** *see* Capsaicin *on page 172*

Antipyrine and Benzocaine (an tee PYE reen & BEN zoe kane)
U.S. Brand Names Allergen® Ear Drops; Auralgan®; Auroto®; Oto®; Otocalm® Ear
Synonyms Benzocaine and Antipyrine
Therapeutic Category Otic Agent, Analgesic; Otic Agent, Cerumenolytic
Generic Available Yes
Use Temporary relief of pain and reduction of inflammation associated with acute congestive and serous otitis media, swimmer's ear, otitis externa; facilitates ear wax removal
Contraindications Hypersensitivity to antipyrine, benzocaine, or any component; perforated tympanic membrane
Warnings Use of otic anesthetics may mask symptoms of a fulminating middle ear infection (acute otitis media); not intended for prolonged use
Adverse Reactions
    Hematologic: Methemoglobinemia
    Local: Burning, stinging, tenderness, edema
    Miscellaneous: Hypersensitivity reactions
Usual Dosage Infants, Children, and Adults: Otic: Fill ear canal; moisten cotton pledget, place in external ear, repeat every 1-2 hours until pain and congestion is relieved; for ear wax removal instill drops 3-4 times/day for 2-3 days
Dosage Forms Solution, otic: Antipyrine 5.4% and benzocaine 1.4% (10 mL, 15 mL)
References
    Rodriguez LF, Smolik LM, and Zbehlik AJ, "Benzocaine-Induced Methemoglobinemia: Report of a Severe Reaction and Review of the Literature," *Ann Pharmacother*, 1994, 28(5):643-9.

◆ **Antithymocyte Globulin (equine)** *see* Lymphocyte Immune Globulin *on page 612*

Antivenin (*Crotalidae*) Polyvalent
(an tee VEN in (kroe TAL ih die) pol i VAY lent)
Synonyms Crotaline Antivenin, Polyvalent; North and South American Antisnakebite Serum; Snake (Pit Vipers) Antivenin
(Continued)

Antivenin (*Crotalidae*) Polyvalent *(Continued)*

Therapeutic Category Antivenin

Generic Available No

Use Neutralization of venoms of North and South American crotalids: rattlesnake, copperhead, cottonmouth, tropical moccasins, fer-de-lance, bushmaster

Pregnancy Risk Factor C

Contraindications Not effective against the venoms of coral snakes

Warnings Desensitization may need to be performed on patients with positive skin test reaction or history of sensitivity to equine serum

Precautions Patients with a negative skin test may still react when antivenin is administered; skin test should not be performed unless antivenin is to be used

Adverse Reactions

Cardiovascular: Flushing, cyanosis, shock, edema of the face

Central nervous system: Apprehension

Dermatologic: Urticaria

Gastrointestinal: Vomiting

Neuromuscular & skeletal: Muscle weakness, peripheral neuritis

Respiratory: Dyspnea, cough

Miscellaneous: Anaphylaxis, serum sickness (dose-related; occurs in 83% of patients receiving more than 8 vials)

Stability Avoid storage temperatures >37°C; reconstituted solutions should be used within 48 hours

Usual Dosage The initial dose of antivenin should be administered as soon as possible to be most effective (within 4 hours after the bite). Intradermal sensitivity test should be performed prior to administering antivenin; see Additional Information.

Children and Adults: I.V.:

Minimal envenomation: 20-40 mL

Moderate envenomation: 50-90 mL

Severe envenomation: 100-150 mL

See table.

Dosage Based on Severity of Clinical Picture

Clinical Severity		# of Vials
Minimal	Symptoms confined to bite area; absent of insignificant systemic symptoms	0
Mild	Edema progressing slowly; bite site reveals small amount of ecchymosis; only systemic sign is metallic taste	5
Moderate	Tissue damage beyond immediate bite area; moderate laboratory changes; perioral fasciculation; paresthesias	10
Severe	Tissue damage to entire extremity; major systemic symptoms; significant laboratory abnormalities	>15

Gold BS and Barish RA, "Venomous Snakebites: Current Concepts in Diagnosis, Treatment, and Management," *Emerg Med Clin North Am*, 1992, 10(2):249-67.

Additional doses of antivenin are based on clinical response to the initial dose. If swelling continues to progress, symptoms increase in severity, hypotension occurs, or decrease in hematocrit appears, an additional 10-50 mL should be administered.

Administration Parenteral: Antivenin may be administered I.M. into a large muscle mass for minimal envenomation. I.V. administration of antivenin is preferred for moderate to severe envenomation or in the presence of shock; for I.V. infusion, prepare a 1:1 to 1:10 dilution of reconstituted antivenin in NS or D_5W; infuse the initial 5-10 mL dilution over 3-5 minutes while carefully observing the patient for signs and symptoms of sensitivity reactions. If no reaction occurs, continue infusion at a safe I.V. fluid delivery rate.

Monitoring Parameters Vital signs, hematocrit

Nursing Implications **Do not inject into a finger or toe**; immediate sensitivity reactions usually occur within 30 minutes after administration; if an immediate reaction occurs, temporarily discontinue antivenin, administer epinephrine and/or an antihistamine; then reinstate infusion at a slower rate after control of the reaction; serum-sickness reaction may occur 5-24 days after a dose

Additional Information Intradermal skin test: 0.02-0.03 mL of a 1:10 dilution of antivenin in NS. If the patient has a history of equine serum sensitivity, administer a 1:100 or greater dilution skin test. Test site is read after 5-30 minutes.

Dosage Forms Injection: Lyophilized serum, diluent (10 mL); one vacuum vial to yield 10 mL of serum

- **Antivert®** *see* Meclizine *on page 622*
- **Antizol®** *see* Fomepizole *on page 455*
- **Anucort™ HC** *see* Hydrocortisone *on page 506*
- **Anumed [OTC]** *see* Hemorrhoidal Preparations *on page 490*
- **Anusol® [OTC]** *see* Hemorrhoidal Preparations *on page 490*
- **Anusol-HC®** *see* Hydrocortisone *on page 506*
- **Anusol® HC-1 [OTC]** *see* Hydrocortisone *on page 506*
- **Anzemet®** *see* Dolasetron *on page 352*
- **Apacet® [OTC]** *see* Acetaminophen *on page 29*
- **APAP** *see* Acetaminophen *on page 29*
- **APD** *see* Pamidronate *on page 753*
- **A.P.L.®** *see* Chorionic Gonadotropin *on page 232*
- **Apo-Acetazolamide (Can)** *see* Acetazolamide *on page 32*
- **Apo-Acyclovir (Can)** *see* Acyclovir *on page 37*
- **Apo-Allopurinol (Can)** *see* Allopurinol *on page 53*
- **Apo-Alpraz (Can)** *see* Alprazolam *on page 55*
- **Apo-Amitriptyline (Can)** *see* Amitriptyline *on page 77*
- **Apo-Amoxi (Can)** *see* Amoxicillin *on page 80*
- **Apo-Ampi (Can)** *see* Ampicillin *on page 88*
- **Apo-ASA (Can)** *see* Aspirin *on page 109*
- **Apo-Atenol (Can)** *see* Atenolol *on page 111*
- **Apo-Baclofen (Can)** *see* Baclofen *on page 129*
- **Apo-Beclomethasone (Can)** *see* Beclomethasone *on page 131*
- **Apo-Benztropine (Can)** *see* Benztropine *on page 137*
- **Apo-Bisacodyl (Can)** *see* Bisacodyl *on page 143*
- **Apo-Buspirone (Can)** *see* Buspirone *on page 159*
- **Apo-C (Can)** *see* Ascorbic Acid *on page 106*
- **Apo-Capto (Can)** *see* Captopril *on page 173*
- **Apo-Carbamazepine (Can)** *see* Carbamazepine *on page 175*
- **Apo-Cefaclor (Can)** *see* Cefaclor *on page 186*
- **Apo-Cefadroxil (Can)** *see* Cefadroxil Monohydrate *on page 188*
- **Apo-Cephalex (Can)** *see* Cephalexin *on page 207*
- **Apo-Cetirizine (Can)** *see* Cetirizine *on page 212*
- **Apo-Chlorpromazine (Can)** *see* Chlorpromazine *on page 226*
- **Apo-Cimetidine (Can)** *see* Cimetidine *on page 234*
- **Apo-Clonazepam (Can)** *see* Clonazepam *on page 254*
- **Apo-Clonidine (Can)** *see* Clonidine *on page 255*
- **Apo-Clorazepate (Can)** *see* Clorazepate *on page 257*
- **Apo-Cloxi (Can)** *see* Cloxacillin *on page 260*
- **Apo-Cromolyn (Can)** *see* Cromolyn *on page 273*
- **Apo-Desipramine (Can)** *see* Desipramine *on page 303*
- **Apo-Diazepam (Can)** *see* Diazepam *on page 320*
- **Apo-Diclo (Can)** *see* Diclofenac *on page 324*
- **Apo-Diltiaz (Can)** *see* Diltiazem *on page 337*
- **Apo-Dimenhydrinate (Can)** *see* Dimenhydrinate *on page 339*
- **Apo-Dipyridamole FC (Can)** *see* Dipyridamole *on page 346*
- **Apo-Dipyridamole SC (Can)** *see* Dipyridamole *on page 346*
- **Apo-Divalproex (Can)** *see* Valproic Acid and Derivatives *on page 998*
- **Apo-Doxepin (Can)** *see* Doxepin *on page 358*
- **Apo-Doxy (Can)** *see* Doxycycline *on page 362*
- **Apo-Enalapril (Can)** *see* Enalapril/Enalaprilat *on page 377*
- **Apo-Erythro Base (Can)** *see* Erythromycin *on page 394*
- **Apo-Erythro E-C (Can)** *see* Erythromycin *on page 394*
- **Apo-Erythro ES (Can)** *see* Erythromycin *on page 394*
- **Apo-Erythro S (Can)** *see* Erythromycin *on page 394*
- **Apo-Famotidine (Can)** *see* Famotidine *on page 417*

+ **Apo-Fluconazole (Can)** *see* Fluconazole *on page 430*
+ **Apo-Flunisolide (Can)** *see* Flunisolide *on page 438*
+ **Apo-Fluoxetine (Can)** *see* Fluoxetine *on page 445*
+ **Apo-Flurazepam (Can)** *see* Flurazepam *on page 449*
+ **Apo-Flurbiprofen (Can)** *see* Flurbiprofen *on page 450*
+ **Apo-Folic (Can)** *see* Folic Acid *on page 454*
+ **Apo-Furosemide (Can)** *see* Furosemide *on page 462*
+ **Apo-Gain (Can)** *see* Minoxidil *on page 676*
+ **Apo-Glyburide (Can)** *see* Glyburide *on page 476*
+ **Apo-Haloperidol (Can)** *see* Haloperidol *on page 488*
+ **Apo-Hydralazine (Can)** *see* Hydralazine *on page 501*
+ **Apo-Hydro (Can)** *see* Hydrochlorothiazide *on page 503*
+ **Apo-Hydroxyzine (Can)** *see* Hydroxyzine *on page 516*
+ **Apo-Ibuprofen (Can)** *see* Ibuprofen *on page 520*
+ **Apo-Imipramine (Can)** *see* Imipramine *on page 528*
+ **Apo-Indomethacin (Can)** *see* Indomethacin *on page 536*
+ **Apo-Ipravent (Can)** *see* Ipratropium *on page 547*
+ **Apo-Ketoconazole (Can)** *see* Ketoconazole *on page 564*
+ **Apo-Ketorolac (Can)** *see* Ketorolac *on page 565*
+ **Apo-Lisinopril (Can)** *see* Lisinopril *on page 598*
+ **Apo-Loperamide (Can)** *see* Loperamide *on page 603*
+ **Apo-Lorazepam (Can)** *see* Lorazepam *on page 609*
+ **Apo-Metformin (Can)** *see* Metformin *on page 639*
+ **Apo-Methyldopa (Can)** *see* Methyldopa *on page 651*
+ **Apo-Metoclop (Can)** *see* Metoclopramide *on page 657*
+ **Apo-Metoprolol (Type L) (Can)** *see* Metoprolol *on page 660*
+ **Apo-Metronidazole (Can)** *see* Metronidazole *on page 662*
+ **Apo-Nadol (Can)** *see* Nadolol *on page 691*
+ **Apo-Napro-Na (Can)** *see* Naproxen *on page 699*
+ **Apo-Naproxen (Can)** *see* Naproxen *on page 699*
+ **Apo-Nifed (Can)** *see* Nifedipine *on page 714*
+ **Apo-Nitrofurantoin (Can)** *see* Nitrofurantoin *on page 716*
+ **Apo-Nizatidine (Can)** *see* Nizatidine *on page 720*
+ **Apo-Nortriptyline (Can)** *see* Nortriptyline *on page 724*
+ **Apo-Oxybutynin (Can)** *see* Oxybutynin *on page 744*
+ **Apo-Pentoxifylline SR (Can)** *see* Pentoxifylline *on page 781*
+ **Apo-Pen-VK (Can)** *see* Penicillin V Potassium *on page 774*
+ **Apo-Piroxicam (Can)** *see* Piroxicam *on page 806*
+ **Apo-Prazo (Can)** *see* Prazosin *on page 820*
+ **Apo-Prednisone (Can)** *see* Prednisone *on page 824*
+ **Apo-Primidone (Can)** *see* Primidone *on page 827*
+ **Apo-Procainamide (Can)** *see* Procainamide *on page 829*
+ **Apo-Propranolol (Can)** *see* Propranolol *on page 847*
+ **Apo-Quinidine (Can)** *see* Quinidine *on page 860*
+ **Apo-Ranitidine (Can)** *see* Ranitidine *on page 865*
+ **Apo-Salvent (Can)** *see* Albuterol *on page 45*
+ **Apo-Sertraline (Can)** *see* Sertraline *on page 898*
+ **Apo-Spirozide (Can)** *see* Hydrochlorothiazide and Spironolactone *on page 504*
+ **Apo-Sucralfate (Can)** *see* Sucralfate *on page 919*
+ **Apo-Sulfamethoxazole (Can)** *see* Sulfamethoxazole *on page 925*
+ **Apo-Sulfasalazine (Can)** *see* Sulfasalazine *on page 926*
+ **Apo-Sulfatrim (Can)** *see* Co-Trimoxazole *on page 270*
+ **Apo-Sulin (Can)** *see* Sulindac *on page 930*
+ **Apo-Tetra (Can)** *see* Tetracycline *on page 941*
+ **Apo-Theo LA (Can)** *see* Theophylline *on page 943*
+ **Apo-Thioridazine (Can)** *see* Thioridazine *on page 953*
+ **Apo-Timol (Can)** *see* Timolol *on page 962*
+ **Apo-Timop (Can)** *see* Timolol *on page 962*
+ **Apo-Trazodone (Can)** *see* Trazodone *on page 977*
+ **Apo-Triazo (Can)** *see* Triazolam *on page 982*
+ **Apo-Trihex (Can)** *see* Trihexyphenidyl *on page 984*

- ♦ **Apo-Valproic (Can)** *see* Valproic Acid and Derivatives *on page 998*
- ♦ **Apo-Verap (Can)** *see* Verapamil *on page 1007*
- ♦ **Apo-Zidovudine (Can)** *see* Zidovudine *on page 1022*
- ♦ **APPG** *see* Penicillin G Procaine *on page 773*
- ♦ **Apresoline®** *see* Hydralazine *on page 501*
- ♦ **Aprodine® [OTC]** *see* Triprolidine and Pseudoephedrine *on page 989*

Aprotinin (a proe TYE nin)

U.S. Brand Names Trasylol®

Therapeutic Category Hemostatic Agent

Use Prophylactic use to reduce perioperative blood loss and the need for blood transfusion in patients undergoing cardiopulmonary bypass in the course of coronary artery bypass graft surgery (CABG); in selected repeat cases of primary CABG surgery where the risk of bleeding is especially high or where transfusion is unavailable or unacceptable

Pregnancy Risk Factor B

Contraindications Hypersensitivity to aprotinin or any component

Warnings Patients with a previous exposure to aprotinin (particularly when re-exposure is within 6 months) are at an increased risk for hypersensitivity reactions including anaphylactic or anaphylactoid reactions; pretreatment with an antihistamine and H_2-blocker before administration of the loading dose is recommended in these patients; delay the addition of aprotinin into the pump prime solution until the loading dose has safely been administered.

Precautions All patients treated with aprotinin should first receive a test dose at least 10 minutes before the loading dose to assess the potential for allergic reactions

Adverse Reactions

Cardiovascular: Atrial fibrillation, MI, heart failure, atrial flutter, ventricular tachycardia, cerebral embolism, cerebrovascular events, chest pain, hypotension, pericardial effusion, pulmonary hypertension

Central nervous system: Fever, mental confusion, seizures, agitation, dizziness, anxiety

Endocrine & metabolic: Hyperglycemia, hypokalemia, acidosis

Gastrointestinal: Nausea, vomiting, constipation, diarrhea, GI hemorrhage

Hematologic: Hemolysis, anemia, thrombosis

Hepatic: Liver damage, jaundice

Local: Phlebitis

Neuromuscular & skeletal: Arthralgia

Renal: Decreased renal function

Respiratory: Dyspnea, bronchoconstriction, pulmonary edema, apnea, increased cough

Miscellaneous: Anaphylaxis (see Warnings)

Drug Interactions Decreases effects of fibrinolytic agents such as streptokinase or anistreplase; decreases effects of captopril; prolonged activated clotting time when used with heparin

Stability Store between 2°C to 25°C (36°F to 77°F); do not freeze; do not mix with other medications; incompatible with corticosteroids, heparin, amino acids, and fat emulsion

Mechanism of Action Aprotinin, a serine protease inhibitor, modulates the systemic inflammatory response associated with cardiopulmonary bypass surgery; inhibits plasmin, kallikrein, and platelet activation producing antifibrinolytic effects; is a weak inhibitor of plasma pseudocholinesterase; inhibits the contact phase activation of coagulation and preserves adhesive platelet glycoproteins making them resistant to damage from increased circulating plasmin or mechanical injury occurring during bypass

Pharmacokinetics

Metabolism: Aprotinin is slowly degraded by lysosomal enzymes

Half-life, elimination: 150 minutes; terminal elimination: 10 hours

Elimination: <10% excreted unchanged in the urine

Usual Dosage I.V.: Test dose: All patients should receive a test dose at least 10 minutes prior to the loading dose to assess the potential for allergic reactions

Infants and Children: No conclusive dosage regimen has been established; variable dosage recommendations in the literature. Test dose: (dosage not well documented in studies) 0.1 mg/kg (maximum: 1.4 mg) has been used. Two of the more common recommendations follow (see References for other recommendations):

Body surface area: ≤1.16 m²:

240 mg/m² loading dose

240 mg/m² into pump prime volume

56 mg/m²/hour continuous infusion during surgery

(Continued)

Aprotinin *(Continued)*

Body surface area: >1.16 m²:
280 mg/m² loading dose
280 mg/m² into pump prime volume
70 mg/m²/hour continuous infusion during surgery
Alternative (based upon body weight only):
30,000 units/kg (4.2 mg/kg) loading dose
30,000 units/kg (4.2 mg/kg) into pump prime volume
30,000 units/kg/hour (4.2 mg/kg/hour) continuous infusion

Adults: Test dose: 1 mL (1.4 mg)
Regimen A (standard dose):
2 million units (280 mg) loading dose
2 million units (280 mg) into pump prime volume
500,000 units/hour (70 mg/hour) continuous infusion during surgery
Regimen B (low dose):
1 million units (140 mg) loading dose
1 million units (140 mg) into pump prime volume
250,000 units/hour (35 mg/hour) continuous infusion during surgery

Administration Parenteral: For I.V. use only; all I.V. doses should be administered through a central line; infuse test dose over at least 10 minutes; infuse loading dose over 20-30 minutes with patient in the supine position

Monitoring Parameters Bleeding times, prothrombin time, activated clotting time, platelet count, red blood cell counts, hematocrit, hemoglobin, and fibrinogen degradation products

Test Interactions Aprotinin prolongs whole blood clotting time of heparinized blood as determined by the Hemochrom® method or similar surface activation methods; patients may require additional heparin even in the presence of activated clotting time levels that appear to represent adequate anticoagulation

Dosage Forms Injection: 1.4 mg/mL [10,000 units/mL] (100 mL, 200 mL)

References

Boldt J, "Endothelial-Related Coagulation in Pediatric Surgery," *Ann Thorac Surg*, 1998, 65(6 Suppl):S56-9.

Carrel TP, Schwanda M, Vogt P, et al, "Aprotinin in Pediatric Cardiac Operations: A Benefit in Complex Malformations and With High-Dose Regimen Only," *Ann Thorac Surg*, 1998, 66(1):153-8.

Miller BE, Tosone SR, Tam VK, et al, "Hematologic and Economic Impact of Aprotinin in Reoperative Pediatric Cardiac Operations," *Ann Thorac Surg*, 1998, 66(2):535-41.

Penkoske P, Entwistle LM, Marchak BE, et al, "Aprotinin in Children Undergoing Repair of Congenital Heart Defects," *Ann Thorac Surg*, 1995, 60(6 Suppl):S529-32.

Spray TL, "Use of Aprotinin in Pediatric Organ Transplantation," *Ann Thorac Surg*, 1998, 65(6 Suppl):S71-3.

♦ **Aquachloral® Supprettes®** *see* Chloral Hydrate *on page 215*
♦ **Aquacort (Can)** *see* Hydrocortisone *on page 506*
♦ **AquaMEPHYTON®** *see* Phytonadione *on page 798*
♦ **Aquasol A®** [OTC] *see* Vitamin A *on page 1013*
♦ **Aquasol E® Oral [OTC]** *see* Vitamin E *on page 1014*
♦ **Aquatab® DM** *see* Guaifenesin and Dextromethorphan *on page 487*
♦ **AquaTar® [OTC]** *see* Coal Tar *on page 260*
♦ **Aquavit-E®** *see* Vitamin E *on page 1014*
♦ **Aqueous Procaine Penicillin G** *see* Penicillin G Procaine *on page 773*
♦ **Aqueous Testosterone** *see* Testosterone *on page 938*
♦ **Ara-A** *see* Vidarabine *on page 1009*
♦ **Arabinofuranosyladenine** *see* Vidarabine *on page 1009*
♦ **Arabinosylcytosine** *see* Cytarabine *on page 290*
♦ **Ara-C** *see* Cytarabine *on page 290*
♦ **Aralen®** *see* Chloroquine *on page 222*
♦ **Aralen Phosphate (Can)** *see* Chloroquine *on page 222*
♦ **Aramine®** *see* Metaraminol *on page 638*
♦ **Aredia™** *see* Pamidronate *on page 753*
♦ **Arfonad® Injection** *see* Trimethaphan Camsylate *on page 985*

Arginine *(AR ji neen)*

U.S. Brand Names R-Gene®
Therapeutic Category Diagnostic Agent, Growth Hormone Function; Metabolic Alkalosis Agent; Urea Cycle Disorder (UCD) Treatment Agent
Generic Available No

Use Pituitary function test (growth hormone); management of severe, uncompensated, metabolic alkalosis (pH ≥7.55) **after** optimizing therapy with sodium, potassium, or ammonium chloride supplements; treatment agent for urea cycle disorders

Contraindications Hypersensitivity to arginine or any component; renal or hepatic failure

Precautions Arginine hydrochloride is metabolized to nitrogen-containing products for excretion; the temporary effect of a high nitrogen load on the kidneys should be evaluated; accumulation of excess arginine may result in an overproduction of nitric oxide, leading to vasodilation and hypotension

Adverse Reactions

Cardiovascular: Flushing (after rapid I.V. administration), hypotension

Central nervous system: Headache (after rapid I.V. administration)

Endocrine & metabolic: Hyperglycemia, hyperkalemia, metabolic acidosis secondary to hyperchloremia

Gastrointestinal: Nausea, vomiting, abdominal pain, bloating

Local: Venous irritation, severe tissue necrosis with extravasation

Miscellaneous: Increased serum gastrin concentration

Drug Interactions Estrogen-progesterone combinations, spironolactone (potentially fatal hyperkalemia has been reported in patients with hepatic disease)

Mechanism of Action Stimulates pituitary release of growth hormone and prolactin and pancreatic release of glucagon and insulin; patients with impaired pituitary function have lower or no increase in plasma concentrations of growth hormone after administration of arginine. Arginine hydrochloride has been used for severe metabolic alkalosis due to its high chloride content. Arginine becomes an essential amino acid in ASL deficiency due to a decrease in the conversion of argininosuccinate to arginine; in other urea cycle disorders, arginine is used not only to increase its serum concentration but also to prevent the breakdown of endogenous protein.

Pharmacokinetics

Absorption: Oral: Well absorbed

Time to peak serum concentration: Within 2 hours

Usual Dosage I.V.:

Growth hormone reserve test:

Children: 500 mg/kg over 30 minutes

Adults: 300 mL over 30 minutes

Treatment of urea cycle disorders: Neonates, Infants, Children, and Adults:

Argininosuccinic acid lyase (ASL) or argininosuccinic acid synthetase (ASS) disorders or pending definitive diagnosis: 600 mg/kg as a loading dose followed by 600 mg/kg/day as a continuous infusion

Carbamyl phosphate synthetase (CPS) or ornithine transcarbamylase (OTC) disorder: 200 mg/kg as a loading dose followed by 200 mg/kg/day as a continuous infusion

Intermittent hyperammonemic crisis in patients with urea cycle disorders: Neonates, Infants, Children, and Adults:

ASL or ASS: 0.6 g/kg or 12 g/m^2 loading dose followed by 0.6 g/kg/day or 12 g/m^2/day continuous infusion

CPS or OTC: 0.2 g/kg or 4 g/m^2 loading dose followed by 0.2 g/kg/day or 4 g/m^2/day continuous infusion

Metabolic alkalosis: Infants, Children, and Adults: Arginine hydrochloride dose (g) = weight (kg) x 0.1 x [HCO$_3^-$ - 24] where HCO$_3^-$ = the patient's serum bicarbonate concentration in mEq/L; give $^1/_2$ to $^2/_3$ of calculated dose and re-evaluate

Note: Arginine hydrochloride is a fourth-line treatment for uncompensated metabolic alkalosis after sodium chloride, potassium chloride, and ammonium chloride supplementation has been optimized

To correct hypochloremia: Infants, Children, and Adults: Arginine hydrochloride dose (mEq) = 0.2 x weight (kg) x [103 - Cl$^-$] where Cl$^-$ = the patient's serum chloride concentration in mEq/L; give $^1/_2$ to $^2/_3$ of calculated dose and re-evaluate

Note: Arginine hydrochloride should never be used as initial therapy for chloride supplementation but as an alternative in the patient who is unresponsive to sodium chloride or potassium chloride supplementation.

Administration Parenteral: May be infused without further dilution; maximum rate of I.V. infusion: 1 g/kg/hour (4.75 mEq/kg/hour) (maximum dose: 60 g/hour = 285 mEq over 1 hour); administration through a central line is recommended; infuse loading doses for urea cycle disorders over 90 minutes

Monitoring Parameters Acid-base status (arterial or capillary blood gases), serum electrolytes, BUN, glucose, plasma growth hormone concentrations (when evaluating growth hormone reserve), plasma ammonia and amino acids (when treating urea cycle disorders)

(Continued)

Arginine *(Continued)*

Reference Range If intact pituitary function, human growth hormone levels should rise after arginine administration to 10-30 ng/mL (control range: 0-6 ng/mL)

Nursing Implications I.V. infiltration of arginine hydrochloride may cause necrosis and phlebitis; prolongation of the infusion may diminish the stimulus to the pituitary gland and nullify the test

Additional Information When treating urea cycle disorders, sodium bicarbonate use may be necessary to neutralize the acidifying effects of arginine HCl.

Dosage Forms Injection, as hydrochloride: 10% [0.475 mEq chloride/mL] (500 mL)

References

Batshaw ML, MacArthur RB, and Tuchman M, "Alternative Pathway Therapy for Urea Cycle Disorders: Twenty Years Later," *J Pediatr*, 2001, 138(1 Suppl):S46-54.

Bushinsky DA and Gennari FJ, "Life-Threatening Hyperkalemia Induced by Arginine," *Ann Intern Med*, 1978, 89(5 Pt 1):632-4.

Summar M, "Current Strategies for the Management of Neonatal Urea Cycle Disorders," *J Pediatr*, 2001, 138(1 Suppl):S30-9.

- ◆ **8-Arginine Vasopressin** *see* Vasopressin *on page 1003*
- ◆ **Aristocort®** *see* Triamcinolone *on page 979*
- ◆ **Aristocort® A** *see* Triamcinolone *on page 979*
- ◆ **Aristocort® Forte** *see* Triamcinolone *on page 979*
- ◆ **Aristospan®** *see* Triamcinolone *on page 979*
- ◆ **Artane®** *see* Trihexyphenidyl *on page 984*
- ◆ **Arthrotec (Can)** *see* Diclofenac *on page 324*
- ◆ **Artritol (Can)** *see* Acetaminophen *on page 29*
- ◆ **ASA** *see* Aspirin *on page 109*
- ◆ **5-ASA** *see* Mesalamine *on page 634*
- ◆ **Asacol®** *see* Mesalamine *on page 634*
- ◆ **Asaphen (Can)** *see* Aspirin *on page 109*
- ◆ **Ascorbex (Can)** *see* Ascorbic Acid *on page 106*

Ascorbic Acid *(a SKOR bik AS id)*

U.S. Brand Names Cecon® [OTC]; Cevi-Bid® [OTC]; Dull-C® [OTC]; Vita-C® [OTC]

Canadian Brand Names Action; Apo-C; Ascorbex; Balanced C Complex; C-1000; C-3000; C Forte; Kamu Jay; Nutrol C; Orti C; Revitalose-C-1000; Super C; Vita-C

Synonyms Vitamin C

Therapeutic Category Nutritional Supplement; Urinary Acidifying Agent; Vitamin, Water Soluble

Generic Available Yes

Use Prevention and treatment of scurvy; urinary acidification; dietary supplementation; prevention and reduction in the severity of colds

Pregnancy Risk Factor A (C if used in doses above RDA recommendation)

Contraindications Large doses during pregnancy

Warnings Some products contain tartrazine or sulfites which may cause allergic reactions in susceptible individuals

Adverse Reactions

Cardiovascular: Flushing

Central nervous system: Faintness, dizziness, headache, fatigue

Gastrointestinal: Nausea, vomiting, heartburn, diarrhea

Renal: Hyperoxaluria

Drug Interactions Aspirin, iron, oral contraceptives (increases estrogen levels), decreased warfarin effect

Stability Injectable form should be stored under refrigeration (2°C to 8°C); protect oral dosage forms from light; ascorbic acid solution is rapidly oxidized

Mechanism of Action Necessary for collagen formation and tissue repair in the body; involved in some oxidation-reduction reactions as well as many other metabolic reactions

Pharmacodynamics Reversal of scurvy symptoms: 2 days to 3 weeks

Pharmacokinetics

Absorption: Oral: Readily absorbed; absorption is an active process and is thought to be dose-dependent

Distribution: Widely distributed

Protein binding: 25%

Metabolism: In the liver by oxidation and sulfation

Elimination: In urine; there is an individual specific renal threshold for ascorbic acid; when blood levels are high, ascorbic acid is excreted in urine, whereas when the levels are subthreshold very little if any ascorbic acid is excreted into urine

Usual Dosage Oral, I.M., I.V., S.C.:

Recommended adequate intake (AI):

0-6 months: 40 mg

6-12 months: 50 mg

Recommended daily allowance (RDA):

1-3 years: 15 mg

4-8 years: 25 mg

9-13 years: 45 mg

14-18 years: Males: 75 mg, females: 65 mg

19 years to Adults: Males: 90 mg, females: 75 mg

Children:

Scurvy: 100-300 mg/day in divided doses

Urinary acidification: 500 mg every 6-8 hours

Dietary supplement (variable): 35-100 mg/day

Adults:

Scurvy: 100-250 mg 1-2 times/day

Urinary acidification: 4-12 g/day in 3-4 divided doses

Dietary supplement (variable): 50-200 mg/day

Prevention and treatment of cold: 1-3 g/day

Children and Adults: To increase iron excretion during deferoxamine administration: 100-200 mg/day during deferoxamine therapy

Administration

Oral: May be administered without regard to meals

Parenteral: Use only in circumstances when the oral route is not possible; I.M. preferred parenteral route due to improved utilization; for I.V. use dilute in equal volume D_5W or NS, and infuse over at least 10 minutes

Reference Range

Normal levels: 10-20 µg/mL

Scurvy: <1-1.5 µg/mL

Test Interactions False-positive urinary glucose with cupric sulfate reagent, false-negative urinary glucose with glucose oxidase method, false-negative amine-dependent stool occult blood test

Additional Information Sodium content of 1 g: ~5 mEq

Dosage Forms

Capsule: 500 mg, 1000 mg

Capsule, timed release: 500 mg

Crystals: 4 g/teaspoonful (100 g, 500 g)

Injection: 250 mg/mL (2 mL, 30 mL); 500 mg/mL (2 mL, 50 mL)

Powder: 4 g/teaspoonful (100 g, 500 g)

Solution, oral: 100 mg/mL (50 mL)

Tablet: 100 mg, 250 mg, 500 mg, 1000 mg

Tablet:

Chewable: 100 mg, 500 mg

Timed release: 500 mg, 1000 mg

References

"Dietary Reference Intakes for Vitamin C, Vitamin E, Selenium, and Carotenoids. A Report of the Panel on Dietary Antioxidants and Related Compounds Food and Nutrition Board, Institute of Medicine," National Academy of Sciences, Washington, DC: National Academy Press, 2000.

♦ **Ascriptin® [OTC]** see Aspirin on page 109

♦ **Asmavent (Can)** see Albuterol on page 45

♦ **ASN-ase** see Asparaginase on page 107

Asparaginase (a SPIR a ji nase)

Related Information

Emetogenic Potential of Single Chemotherapeutic Agents on page 1129

U.S. Brand Names Elspar®

Canadian Brand Names Kidrolase

Synonyms A-ase; ASN-ase; Colaspase

Therapeutic Category Antineoplastic Agent, Miscellaneous

Generic Available No

Use In combination therapy for the treatment of acute lymphocytic leukemia, lymphoma

Pregnancy Risk Factor C

Contraindications Pancreatitis; hypersensitivity to *E. coli*, asparaginase, or any component (if a reaction to Elspar® occurs, obtain investigational *Erwinia* preparation from McKesson BioServices at (301) 762-0069 or pegaspargase from Gentiva Health Services at (888) 276-2217 is another alternative - use with caution)

(Continued)

Asparaginase *(Continued)*

Warnings The FDA currently recommends that procedures for proper handling and disposal of antineoplastic agents be considered; be prepared to treat anaphylaxis at each administration

Precautions Use with caution in patients with impaired renal function; discontinue asparaginase at the first sign of renal failure or pancreatitis

Adverse Reactions

Cardiovascular: Hypotension

Central nervous system: Fever, drowsiness, seizures, chills, malaise, coma, headache, stroke, confusion, dizziness, hallucinations

Dermatologic: Rash, pruritus, urticaria

Endocrine & metabolic: Hyperglycemia, transient diabetes mellitus, hyperammonemia, hyperuricemia, hypoalbuminemia; decreased thyroxine and thyroxine-binding globulin concentration

Gastrointestinal: Vomiting, pancreatitis, nausea, anorexia, abdominal cramps

Hematologic: Leukopenia, coagulation abnormalities (prolonged thrombin, PT, and partial prothrombin times), reduced fibrinogen

Hepatic: Hepatotoxicity (elevated liver enzymes, hyperbilirubinemia)

Renal: Azotemia

Respiratory: Coughing, laryngeal edema, bronchospasm

Miscellaneous: Hypersensitivity reactions (incidence in children is 20% with *E. coli* asparaginase and <5% with *Erwinia* asparaginase); anaphylaxis

Drug Interactions Methotrexate (decreased antineoplastic effect if given prior to methotrexate); vincristine (increases toxicity if given concomitantly); prednisone (increases hyperglycemic effect)

Stability Refrigerate; no loss in potency was noted after storage for 1 week at room temperature, however, the manufacturer recommends that reconstituted solutions should be discarded after 8 hours since there is no preservative; discard immediately if solution becomes cloudy; use of a 0.2 micron filter may result in some loss of potency

Mechanism of Action Inhibits protein synthesis by deaminating asparagine and depriving tumor cells of this essential amino acid

Pharmacokinetics

Absorption: Not absorbed from GI tract, therefore requires parenteral administration

Distribution: Asparaginase not detected in CSF but CSF asparagine is depleted

Half-life:

E. coli L-asparaginase: 24-36 hours

Patients who have had a hypersensitivity reaction to asparaginase have a decreased half-life

Erwinia L-asparaginase: Significantly shorter than for the *E. coli*-derived product; mean half-life *Erwinia* L-asparaginase: 10-15 hours

Elimination: Clearance is unaffected by age, renal function, or hepatic function

Usual Dosage Children and Adults: Refer to individual protocols

Perform intradermal sensitivity testing with 2 units of asparaginase before the initial dose and when a week or more has elapsed between doses:

I.M. (preferred): 6000-10,000 units/m^2/dose 3 times/week for 3 weeks for combination therapy; high-dose I.M. regimen of 25,000 units/m^2/dose once weekly for 9 doses has also been used

I.V.: 1000 units/kg/day for 10 days for combination therapy or 200 units/kg/day for 28 days if combination therapy is inappropriate

Administration

I.M.: Maximum 2 mL volume is recommended for I.M. injections; if the volume to be administered is >2 mL, use multiple injection sites

I.V.: Must be infused over a minimum of 30 minutes

Monitoring Parameters Vital signs during administration, CBC, urinalysis, amylase, liver enzymes, bilirubin, prothrombin time, renal function tests, urine glucose, blood glucose

Patient Information Notify physician if fever, sore throat, painful/burning urination, bruising, bleeding, or shortness of breath occurs

Nursing Implications I.M. route is associated with a more delayed, less severe anaphylactoid reaction compared to the I.V. route; patients should be observed for one hour following an I.M. injection for signs of severe hypersensitivity; appropriate agents for maintenance of an adequate airway and treatment of a hypersensitivity reaction (antihistamine, epinephrine, oxygen, I.V. corticosteroids) should be readily available

Dosage Forms Injection: 10,000 units/vial

References
Asselin BL, Whitin JC, Coppola DJ, et al, "Comparative Pharmacokinetic Studies of Three Asparaginase Preparations," *J Clin Oncol*, 1993, 11(9):1780-6.

Clavell LA, Gelber RD, Cohen HJ, et al, "Four-Agent Induction and Intensive Asparaginase Therapy for Treatment of Childhood Acute Lymphoblastic Leukemia," *N Engl J Med*, 1986, 315(11):657-63.

Nesbit M, Chard R, Evans A, et al, "Evaluation of Intramuscular Versus Intravenous Administration of L-Asparaginase in Childhood Leukemia," *Am J Pediatr Hematol Oncol*, 1979, 1(1):9-13.

Ortega JA, Nesbit ME Jr, and Donaldson MH, "L-Asparaginase, Vincristine, and Prednisone for Induction of First Remission in Acute Lymphocytic Leukemia," *Cancer Res*, 1977, 37(2):535-40.

♦ **A-Spas® S/L** *see* Hyoscyamine *on page 517*

♦ **Aspergum® [OTC]** *see* Aspirin *on page 109*

Aspirin (AS pir in)
Related Information
Drugs and Breast-Feeding *on page 1243*
Overdose and Toxicology *on page 1222*
U.S. Brand Names Ascriptin® [OTC]; Aspergum® [OTC]; Bayer® Aspirin [OTC]; Bufferin® [OTC]; Easprin®; Ecotrin® [OTC]; Empirin® [OTC]; Halfprin® [OTC]; Measurin® [OTC]; ZORprin®

Canadian Brand Names Apo-ASA; ASA; Asaphen; Entrophen; MSD Enteric Coated ASA; Novasen

Synonyms Acetylsalicylic Acid; ASA

Therapeutic Category Analgesic, Non-narcotic; Anti-inflammatory Agent; Anti-platelet Agent; Antipyretic; Nonsteroidal Anti-inflammatory Drug (NSAID), Oral; Salicylate

Generic Available Yes

Use Treatment of mild to moderate pain, inflammation and fever; adjunctive treatment of Kawasaki disease; prevention of vascular mortality during suspected acute MI; prevention of recurrent MI; prevention of MI in patients with angina; prevention of recurrent stroke and mortality following TIA or stroke

Pregnancy Risk Factor C (D if full-dose aspirin in 3rd trimester)

Contraindications Bleeding disorders; hypersensitivity to salicylates, any component, or other NSAIDs; hepatic failure

Warnings Do not use aspirin in children <16 years of age for chickenpox or flu symptoms due to the association with Reye's syndrome

Precautions Use with caution in patients with impaired renal function, erosive gastritis, peptic ulcer, gout, platelet and bleeding disorders

Adverse Reactions
Dermatologic: Rash, urticaria
Gastrointestinal: Nausea, vomiting, GI distress, GI bleeding, ulcers
Hematologic: Inhibition of platelet aggregation
Hepatic: Hepatotoxicity
Respiratory: Bronchospasm

Drug Interactions Aspirin may increase methotrexate serum levels and may displace valproic acid from binding sites which can result in toxicity; aspirin may increase free (unbound) buspirone concentrations; use of warfarin, heparin, low molecular weight heparins, urokinase, streptokinase, alteplase, and platelet inhibitors (eg, dipyridamole) with aspirin may cause an increase in bleeding; use of NSAIDs with aspirin may cause an increase in GI adverse effects and a possible decrease in serum concentration of NSAIDs; aspirin may antagonize effects of probenecid; aspirin, especially high doses, may decrease the antihypertensive effects of ACE inhibitors; buffered preparations may decrease the oral absorption of tetracycline or ketoconazole, therefore, administer 3-4 hours apart

Food Interactions Aspirin may increase the renal excretion of vitamin C and may decrease serum folate levels; some suggest increasing the dietary intake of foods that are high in vitamin C and folic acid

Stability Keep suppositories in refrigerator, do not freeze; hydrolysis of aspirin occurs upon exposure to water or moist air, resulting in salicylate and acetate; acetate possesses a vinegar-like odor; do not use if a strong odor is present

Mechanism of Action Inhibits prostaglandin synthesis, acts on the hypothalamus heat-regulating center to reduce fever, blocks prostaglandin synthetase action which prevents formation of the platelet-aggregating substance thromboxane A_2

Pharmacokinetics
Absorption: From the stomach and small intestine
Distribution: Readily distributes into most body fluids and tissues; hydrolyzed to salicylate (active) by esterases in the GI mucosa, red blood cells, synovial fluid and blood
Metabolism: Primarily by hepatic microsomal enzymes
(Continued)

Aspirin *(Continued)*

Half-life: 15-20 minutes; metabolic pathways are saturable such that salicylate half-life is dose-dependent ranging from 3 hours at lower doses (300-600 mg), 5-6 hours (after 1 g) and 10 hours with higher doses

Time to peak serum concentration: Salicylate: ~1-2 hours; may be delayed with controlled or timed-release preparations

Elimination: Renal as salicylate and conjugated metabolites

Dialyzable: 50% to 100%

Usual Dosage

Children:

Analgesic and antipyretic: Oral, rectal: 10-15 mg/kg/dose every 4-6 hours; maximum dose: 4 g/day

Anti-inflammatory: Oral: Initial: 60-90 mg/kg/day in divided doses; usual maintenance: 80-100 mg/kg/day divided every 6-8 hours; monitor serum concentrations

Antiplatelet effects: Adequate pediatric studies have not been performed; pediatric dosage is derived from adult studies and clinical experience and is not well established; suggested doses have ranged from 3-5 mg/kg/day to 5-10 mg/kg/day given as a single daily dose. Doses are rounded to a convenient amount (eg, $\frac{1}{2}$ of 80 mg tablet).

Mechanical prosthetic heart valves: 6-20 mg/kg/day given as a single daily dose (used in combination with an oral anticoagulant in children who have systemic embolism despite adequate oral anticoagulation therapy (INR 2.5-3.5) and used in combination with low-dose anticoagulation (INR 2-3) and dipyridamole when full-dose oral anticoagulation is contraindicated)

Blalock-Taussig shunts: 3-5 mg/kg/day given as a single daily dose

Kawasaki disease: Oral: 80-100 mg/kg/day divided every 6 hours; monitor serum concentrations; after fever resolves: 3-5 mg/kg/day once daily; in patients without coronary artery abnormalities, give lower dose for at least 6-8 weeks or until ESR and platelet count are normal; in patients with coronary artery abnormalities, low-dose aspirin should be continued indefinitely

Adults:

Analgesic and antipyretic: Oral, rectal: 325-1000 mg every 4-6 hours up to 4 g/day

Anti-inflammatory: Oral: Initial: 2.4-3.6 g/day in divided doses; usual maintenance: 3.6-5.4 g/day; monitor serum concentrations

Suspected acute MI: Oral: Initial: 160-162.5 mg as soon as MI is suspected; then 160-162.5 mg once daily for 30 days post MI; then consider further aspirin treatment

MI prophylaxis: Oral: 75-325 mg once daily (continue indefinitely)

Prevention of stroke following ischemic stroke or TIA: Oral: 50-325 mg once daily (continue indefinitely)

Administration Oral: Administer with water, food, or milk to decrease GI upset. Do not crush controlled release, timed release, or enteric coated tablets; these preparations should be swallowed whole

Monitoring Parameters Serum salicylate concentration with chronic use

Reference Range

Therapeutic levels:

Anti-inflammatory effect: 150-300 μg/mL

Serum Salicylate: Clinical Correlations

Serum Salicylate Concentration (μg/mL)	Desired Effects	Adverse Effects/Intoxication
~100	Antiplatelet Antipyresis Analgesia	GI intolerance and bleeding, hypersensitivity, hemostatic defects
150-300	Anti-inflammatory	Mild salicylism
250-400	Treatment of rheumatic fever	Nausea/vomiting, hyperventilation, salicylism, flushing, sweating, thirst, headache, diarrhea, and tachycardia
>400-500		Respiratory alkalosis, hemorrhage, excitement, confusion, asterixis, pulmonary edema, convulsions, tetany, metabolic acidosis, fever, coma, cardiovascular collapse, renal and respiratory failure

Analgesic and antipyretic effect: 30-50 µg/mL

Timing of serum samples: Peak levels usually occur 2 hours after normal doses but may occur 6-24 hours after acute toxic ingestion.

Salicylate serum concentrations correlate with the pharmacological actions and adverse effects observed. See table on previous page.

Test Interactions False-negative results for glucose oxidase urinary glucose tests (Clinistix®); false-positives using the cupric sulfate method (Clinitest®); interferes with Gerhardt test, VMA determination; 5-HIAA, xylose tolerance test and T_3 and T_4

Patient Information Watch for bleeding gums or signs of GI bleeding, (bright red blood in emesis or stool, coffee ground-like emesis, black tarry stools); notify physician if ringing in the ears, persistent GI pain, or GI bleeding occurs

Additional Information Bayer® Aspirin has received 5 new FDA indications (see http://www.wonderdrug.com/practitioners3.html)

Dosage Forms

Chewing gum (Aspergum®): 227 mg

Suppository, rectal: 60 mg, 120 mg, 125 mg, 200 mg, 300 mg, 325 mg, 600 mg, 650 mg

Tablet: 325 mg, 500 mg

Tablet, buffered:

Bufferin®: 325 mg (with calcium carbonate, magnesium carbonate, and magnesium hydroxide)

Ascriptin®: 325 mg (with aluminum hydroxide, calcium carbonate, and magnesium hydroxide)

Ascriptin® Extra Strength: 500 mg (with aluminum hydroxide, calcium carbonate, and magnesium hydroxide)

Tablet, chewable: 81 mg

Tablet, controlled release (ZORprin®): 800 mg

Tablet, delayed release (Bayer® Low Adult Strength): 81 mg

Tablet, enteric coated: 80 mg, 165 mg, 325 mg, 500 mg, 650 mg, 975 mg

Tablet, extended release (Bayer® 8-Hour): 650 mg

References

Hathaway WE, "Use of Antiplatelet Agents in Pediatric Hypercoagulable States," *Am J Dis Child*, 1984, 138(3):301-4.

Monagle P, Michelson AD, Bovill E, et al, "Antithrombotic Therapy in Children," *Chest*, 2001, 119(1 Suppl):344S-370S.

Pickering LK, ed, *2000 Red Book, Report of the Committee on Infectious Diseases*, 25th ed, Elk Grove Village IL: American Academy of Pediatrics, 2000, 360-3.

♦ **Aspirin and Oxycodone** *see* Oxycodone and Aspirin *on page 748*

♦ **Aspirin Free Anacin® [OTC]** *see* Acetaminophen *on page 29*

♦ **Astelin® Nasal Spray** *see* Azelastine *on page 123*

♦ **Asthma Guidelines** *see page 1210*

♦ **AsthmaHaler® Mist [OTC]** *see* Epinephrine *on page 385*

♦ **Astramorph/PF™** *see* Morphine Sulfate *on page 683*

♦ **Atarax®** *see* Hydroxyzine *on page 516*

♦ **Atasol (Can)** *see* Acetaminophen *on page 29*

Atenolol (a TEN oh lole)

Related Information

Overdose and Toxicology *on page 1222*

U.S. Brand Names Tenormin®

Canadian Brand Names Apo-Atenol; Gen-Atenolol; Novo-Atenol; Nu-Atenol; PMS-Atenolol; Rhoxal-Atenolol; Tenolin

Therapeutic Category Antianginal Agent; Antihypertensive Agent; Beta-Adrenergic Blocker

Generic Available Yes

Use Treatment of hypertension, alone or in combination with other agents; management of angina pectoris; antiarrhythmic; post-MI patients; acute alcohol withdrawal

Pregnancy Risk Factor D

Contraindications Hypersensitivity to atenolol or any component; Pulmonary edema, cardiogenic shock, bradycardia, heart block, or uncompensated CHF

Warnings Abrupt withdrawal of the drug should be avoided; drug should be discontinued over 1-2 weeks

Precautions Use with caution and modify dosage in patients with renal impairment; use with caution in patients with CHF, bronchospastic disease, diabetes mellitus, and hyperthyroidism. Patients who have a history of anaphylactic hypersensitivity reactions to various substances may be more reactive while receiving beta-blockers; these patients may not be responsive to the normal doses of epinephrine used to treat hypersensitivity reactions.

(Continued)

Atenolol *(Continued)*

Adverse Reactions

Cardiovascular: Bradycardia, hypotension, second or third degree A-V block, CHF, chest pain, edema, Raynaud's phenomenon

Central nervous system: Dizziness, fatigue, lethargy, headache, nightmares, insomnia, confusion, mental impairment

Gastrointestinal: Constipation, nausea, diarrhea

Respiratory: Wheezing and dyspnea have occurred with higher doses (eg, >100 mg/day in adults)

Drug Interactions

Catecholamine-depleting drugs, such as reserpine, may have additive effects (hypotension, bradycardia); hypotensive agents, diuretics, cardiac glycosides, amiodarone, calcium channel blockers, agents that slow AV conduction, and myocardial depressant general anesthetics may have additive effects with beta-blockers; abrupt withdrawal of clonidine while receiving beta-blockers may result in an exaggerated hypertensive crisis; NSAIDs may decrease the antihypertensive effects of beta-blockers; atenolol (especially at higher doses) may reverse the therapeutic effects of theophylline

Mechanism of Action

Competitively blocks response to beta-adrenergic stimulation; selectively blocks $beta_1$-receptors with little or no effect on $beta_2$-receptors except at high doses; does not possess membrane stabilizing or intrinsic sympathomimetic (partial agonist) activities

Pharmacokinetics

Absorption: Incomplete from the GI tract; ~50% absorbed

Distribution: Does not cross the blood-brain barrier; low lipophilicity

Protein binding: Low (6% to 16%)

Half-life, beta:

Neonates: Mean: 16 hours, up to 35 hours

Children 5-16 years of age: Mean: 4.6 hours; range: 3.5-7 hours; children >10 years of age may have longer half-life (>5 hours) compared to children 5-10 years of age (<5 hours)

Adults: 6-7 hours

Prolonged half-life with renal dysfunction

Time to peak serum concentration: Oral: Within 2-4 hours

Elimination: 40% as unchanged drug in urine, 50% in feces

Dialysis: Moderately dialyzable (20% to 50%)

Usual Dosage

Oral:

Children: Initial: 0.8-1 mg/kg/dose given daily; range: 0.8-1.5 mg/kg/day; maximum dose: 2 mg/kg/day

Adults:

Initial: 25-50 mg/dose given daily; usual dose: 50-100 mg/dose given daily

Maximum dose: Hypertension: 100 mg given daily; angina: 200 mg given daily

See table for oral dosing interval in renal impairment.

Creatinine Clearance	Maximum Oral Dose	Frequency of Administration
15-35 mL/min	50 mg or 1 mg/kg/dose	Daily
<15 mL/min	50 mg or 1 mg/kg/dose	Every other day

I.V.: Adults: For early treatment of MI: 5 mg slow I.V. over 5 minutes; may repeat in 10 minutes; if both doses are tolerated, may start oral atenolol 50 mg every 12 hours for 6-9 days post MI

Administration

Oral: May be administered without regard to food

Parenteral: Administer by slow I.V. injection at a rate not to exceed 1 mg/minute; the injection can be administered undiluted or diluted with a compatible I.V. solution

Monitoring Parameters

Blood pressure, heart rate, EKG, fluid intake and output, daily weight, respiratory rate

Patient Information

Abrupt withdrawal of the drug should be avoided

Additional Information

In diabetic patients, atenolol may potentiate hypoglycemia and mask signs and symptoms of hypoglycemia; limited data suggests that atenolol may have a shorter half-life and faster clearance in patients with Marfan syndrome. Higher doses (2 mg/kg/day divided every 12 hours) have been used in patients with Marfan syndrome (6-22 years of age) to decrease aortic root growth rate and prevent aortic dissection or rupture; further studies are needed.

Dosage Forms

Injection: 0.5 mg/mL (10 mL)

Tablet: 25 mg, 50 mg, 100 mg

Extemporaneous Preparations A 2 mg/mL atenolol oral liquid compounded from tablets and a commercially available oral diluent was found to be stable for up to 40 days when stored at 5°C or 25°C

Garner SS, Wiest DB, and Reynolds ER, "Stability of Atenolol in an Extemporaneously Compounded Oral Liquid," *Am J Hosp Pharm*, 1994, 51(4):508-11.

References

Buck ML, Wiest D, Gillette PC, et al, "Pharmacokinetics and Pharmacodynamics of Atenolol in Children," *Clin Pharmacol Ther*, 1989, 46(6):629-33.

Case CL, Trippel DL, and Gillette PC, "New Antiarrhythmic Agents in Pediatrics," *Pediatr Clin North Am*, 1989, 36(5):1293-320.

Trippel DL and Gillette PC, "Atenolol in Children With Supraventricular Tachycardia," *Am J Cardiol*, 1989, 64(3):233-6.

Trippel DL and Gillette PC, "Atenolol in Children With Ventricular Arrhythmias," *Am Heart J*, 1990, 119(6):1312-6.

♦ **ATG** *see* Lymphocyte Immune Globulin *on page 612*

♦ **Atgam®** *see* Lymphocyte Immune Globulin *on page 612*

♦ **Ativan®** *see* Lorazepam *on page 609*

Atovaquone (a TOE va kwone)

U.S. Brand Names Mepron®

Synonyms Hydroxy-1,4-naphthoquinone

Therapeutic Category Antiprotozoal

Generic Available No

Use Second-line treatment of mild to moderate *Pneumocystis carinii* pneumonia (PCP) in patients intolerant of trimethoprim/sulfamethoxazole (TMP/SMX); mild to moderate PCP is defined as an alveolar-arterial oxygen diffusion gradient ≤45 mm Hg and PaO_2 ≥60 mm Hg on room air; patients intolerant of TMP/SMX are defined as having a significant rash (ie, Stevens-Johnson-like syndrome), neutropenia, or hemolysis; prevention of PCP in patients who are intolerant to TMP/SMX; treatment of babesiosis

Pregnancy Risk Factor C

Contraindications Hypersensitivity to atovaquone or any component

Warnings Clinical experience with atovaquone has been limited to patients with mild to moderate PCP; treatment of more severe episodes of PCP has not been systematically studied

Precautions For patients who have difficulty taking atovaquone with food or who have chronic diarrhea, stomach or intestinal problems which may result in drug malabsorption, parenteral therapy with other agents should be considered since a low serum atovaquone concentration could lead to treatment failure

Adverse Reactions

Central nervous system: Fever, headache, insomnia, dizziness, pain

Dermatologic: Maculopapular rash, erythema multiforme, pruritus

Endocrine & metabolic: Hyponatremia

Gastrointestinal: Nausea, vomiting, diarrhea, abdominal pain, constipation, anorexia, elevated amylase

Hematologic: Rare: Neutropenia, anemia

Hepatic: Elevated hepatic enzymes, cholestasis

Respiratory: Cough, sinusitis

Miscellaneous: Diaphoresis

Drug Interactions Rifampin may decrease plasma atovaquone concentration; since atovaquone is highly protein bound, it may compete for protein binding sites with other highly protein-bound agents like warfarin (however, there have been no drug-drug interactions of this type reported to date)

Food Interactions Administration with food increases bioavailability of atovaquone 1.4 fold over that achieved in a fasting state

Stability Store at room temperature; do not freeze

Mechanism of Action The mechanism of action against *Pneumocystis carinii* has not been fully elucidated; in *Plasmodium* species, atovaquone selectively inhibits the mitochondrial electron-transport system at the cytochrome bc_1 complex resulting in depletion of dihydroorotate dehydrogenase and ultimately resulting in the inhibition of nucleic acid and adenosine triphosphate synthesis

Pharmacokinetics

Absorption: Oral:

Infants and Children <2 years of age: Decreased absorption

Adults: Oral suspension: Absorption is enhanced twofold with food; decreased absorption with single doses exceeding 750 mg

Distribution: V_{dss}: 0.6 L/kg; CSF concentration is <1% of the plasma concentration

Protein binding: >99%

(Continued)

Atovaquone (Continued)

Bioavailability: Suspension (administered with food): 47%

Half-life, elimination:

Children (4 months to 12 years): 60 hours (range: 31-163 hours)

Adults: 2.9 days

Adults with AIDS: 2.2 days

Time to peak serum concentration: Dual peak serum concentrations at 1 to 8 hours and at 24 to 96 hours after dose due to enterohepatic cycling

Elimination: ~94% is recovered as unchanged drug in feces; 0.6% excreted in urine

Usual Dosage Oral:

Children:

Treatment: Dose of 40 mg/kg/day divided twice daily (maximum dose: 1500 mg/day) may be necessary to attain comparable plasma concentrations associated with the successful treatment of PCP as seen in adults.

Prophylaxis of *Pneumocystis carinii* pneumonia:

1-3 months of age and >24 months of age: 30 mg/kg/day once daily (maximum dose: 1500 mg/day)

4-24 months of age: 45 mg/kg/day once daily (maximum dose: 1500 mg/day)

Babesiosis: 40 mg/kg/day divided twice daily (maximum dose: 1500 mg/day) with azithromycin 12 mg/kg/day once daily for 7-10 days

Adolescents 13-16 years and Adults:

Treatment: 750 mg/dose twice daily for 21 days

Prophylaxis of *Pneumocystis carinii* pneumonia: 1500 mg once daily

Babesiosis: 750 mg/dose twice daily for 7-10 days with azithromycin 1000 mg once daily for 3 days then 500 mg once daily for 7 days

Administration Oral: Administer with food or a high-fat meal; shake suspension well before using

Monitoring Parameters CBC with differential, liver enzymes, serum chemistries, serum amylase

Additional Information The suspension contains the inactive ingredients benzyl alcohol and poloxamer 188

Dosage Forms Suspension, oral: 750 mg/5 mL [citrus flavor] (210 mL)

References

Centers for Disease Control and Prevention, "1999 USPHS/IDSA Guidelines for the Prevention of Opportunistic Infections in Persons Infected With Human Immunodeficiency Virus," *MMWR Morb Mortal Wkly Rep*, 1999, 48(RR-10):1-59.

Haile LG and Flaherty JF, "Atovaquone: A Review," *Ann Pharmacother*, 1993, 27(12):1488-94.

Hughes W, Dorenbaum A, Yogev R, et al, "Phase I Safety and Pharmacokinetics Study of Micronized Atovaquone Human Immunodeficiency Virus-Infected Infants and Children. Pediatric AIDS Clinical Trials Group," *Antimicrob Agents Chemother*, 1998, 42(6):1315-8.

Hughes W, Leoung G, Kramer F, et al, "Comparison of Atovaquone (566C80) With Trimethoprim-Sulfamethoxazole to Treat *Pneumocystis carinii* Pneumonia in Patients With AIDS," *N Engl J Med*, 1993, 328(21):1521-7.

Atracurium (a tra KYOO ree um)

U.S. Brand Names Tracrium®

Therapeutic Category Neuromuscular Blocker Agent, Nondepolarizing; Skeletal Muscle Relaxant, Paralytic

Generic Available No

Use Eases endotracheal intubation as an adjunct to general anesthesia and relaxes skeletal muscle during surgery or mechanical ventilation

Pregnancy Risk Factor C

Contraindications Hypersensitivity to atracurium besylate or any component

Clinical Conditions Affecting Neuromuscular Blockade

Potentiation	Antagonism
Electrolyte abnormalities	Alkalosis
Severe hyponatremia	Hypercalcemia
Severe hypocalcemia	Demyelinating lesions
Severe hypokalemia	Peripheral neuropathies
Hypermagnesemia	Diabetes mellitus
Neuromuscular diseases	
Acidosis	
Acute intermittent porphyria	
Renal failure	
Hepatic failure	

ATRACURIUM

Warnings Reduce initial dosage and inject slowly (over 1-2 minutes) in patients in whom substantial histamine release would be potentially hazardous (eg, patients with clinically important cardiovascular disease); maintenance of an adequate airway and respiratory support is critical; avoid use of preservative-containing formulation in neonates; certain clinical conditions may result in potentiation or antagonism of neuromuscular blockade, see table on previous page.

Increased sensitivity in patients with myasthenia gravis, Eaton-Lambert syndrome; resistance to neuromuscular blockade in burn patients (>30% of body) for period of 5-70 days postinjury; resistance in patients with muscle trauma, denervation, immobilization, infection, chronic treatment with atracurium. When used in conjunction with anesthetics, bradycardia may be more common with atracurium than with other neuromuscular blocking agents; it has no clinically significant effects on heart rate to counteract the bradycardia produced by anesthetics.

Precautions Due to potential histamine release, use with caution in patients in whom histamine release may be hazardous (eg, cardiovascular disease, asthma); patients with severe electrolyte disorders; patients with myasthenia gravis

Adverse Reactions
Cardiovascular: Effects are minimal and transient
Dermatologic: Erythema, itching, urticaria
Respiratory: Wheezing, bronchial secretions (increased)

Drug Interactions See table.

Potential Drug Interactions

Potentiation	Antagonism
Inhalation anesthetics	Calcium
Desflurane, sevoflurane, enflurane and isoflurane > halothane > nitrous oxide	Carbamazepine
	Phenytoin
	Steroids (chronic administration)
Antibiotics	Theophylline
Aminoglycosides, polymyxins, clindamycin, vancomycin	Anticholinesterases*
Magnesium	Neostigmine, pyridostigmine, edrophonium, echothiophate ophthalmic solution
Antiarrhythmics	Caffeine
Quinidine, procainamide, bretylium, and possibly lidocaine	Azathioprine
Diuretics	
Furosemide, mannitol, thiazides	
Amphotericin B (secondary to hypokalemia)	
Local anesthetics	
Dantrolene (directly depresses skeletal muscle)	
Beta blockers	
Calcium channel blockers	
Ketamine	
Lithium	
Succinylcholine (when administered prior to nondepolarizing neuromuscular-blocking agent)	
Cyclosporine	

*Can prolong the effects of acetylcholine

Stability Refrigerate; stable at room temperature for 14 days; unstable in alkaline solutions; compatible with D_5W, D_5NS, and NS; do not dilute in LR

Mechanism of Action Blocks neural transmission at the myoneural junction by binding with cholinergic receptor sites

Pharmacodynamics
Onset of action: I.V.: 1-4 minutes
Peak effect: Within 3-5 minutes
Duration: Recovery begins in 20-35 minutes when anesthesia is balanced

Pharmacokinetics
Distribution: V_d:
Infants: 0.21 L/kg
Children: 0.13 L/kg
(Continued)

115

Atracurium (Continued)

Adults: 0.1 L/kg

Metabolism: Some metabolites are active; undergoes rapid nonenzymatic degradation (Hofmann elimination) in the bloodstream; additional metabolism occurs via ester hydrolysis

Half-life: Elimination:

Infants: 20 minutes

Children: 17 minutes

Adults: 16 minutes

Elimination: Clearance:

Infants: 7.9 mL/kg/minute

Children: 6.8 mL/kg/minute

Adults: 5.3 mL/kg/minute

Usual Dosage I.V.:

Neonates, Infants, and Children ≤2 years:

0.3-0.4 mg/kg initially followed by maintenance doses of 0.3-0.4 mg/kg as needed to maintain neuromuscular blockade

or

Continuous infusion: 0.6-1.2 mg/kg/hour or 10-20 mcg/kg/minute

Children >2 years to Adults:

0.4-0.5 mg/kg then 0.08-0.1 mg/kg 20-45 minutes after initial dose to maintain neuromuscular block

or

Continuous infusion: 0.4-0.8 mg/kg/hour or 6.7-13 mcg/kg/minute (range: 2-15 mcg/kg/minute)

Dosage adjustment in hepatic or renal impairment: Not necessary

Dosage adjustment with enflurane or isoflurane: Reduce dosage by 33%

Dosage adjustment with induced hypothermia (cardio-bypass surgery): Reduce dosage by 50%

Administration Parenteral: May be administered without further dilution by rapid I.V. injection; for continuous infusions, dilute to a maximum concentration of 0.5 mg/mL (more concentrated solutions have reduced stability, ie, <24 hours at room temperature); not for I.M. injection due to tissue irritation

Monitoring Parameters Muscle twitch response to peripheral nerve stimulation, heart rate, blood pressure

Additional Information Neuromuscular blockade may be reversed with neostigmine; atropine or glycopyrrolate should be available to treat excessive cholinergic effects from neostigmine

Dosage Forms

Injection, as besylate: 10 mg/mL (5 mL, 10 mL)

Injection, preservative free, as besylate: 10 mg/mL (5 mL)

References

Martin LD, Bratton SL, and O'Rourke PP, "Clinical Uses and Controversies of Neuromuscular Blocking Agents in Infants and Children," *Crit Care Med*, 1999, 27(7):1358-68.

♦ **Atrial Fibrillation / Atrial Flutter** *see page 1049*

Atropine (A troe peen)

Related Information

Adult ACLS Algorithm, Asystole *on page 1043*

Adult ACLS Algorithm, Bradycardia *on page 1044*

Adult ACLS Algorithm, Pulseless Electrical Activity *on page 1042*

Asthma Guidelines *on page 1210*

Compatibility of Medications Mixed in a Syringe *on page 1238*

CPR Pediatric Drug Dosages *on page 1031*

Overdose and Toxicology *on page 1222*

Pediatric ALS Algorithm, Bradycardia *on page 1035*

U.S. Brand Names Atropine-Care®; Atropisol®; Isopto® Atropine; Ocu-Trpoine®; Sal-Tropine™

Therapeutic Category Antiasthmatic; Anticholinergic Agent; Anticholinergic Agent, Ophthalmic; Antidote, Organophosphate Poisoning; Antispasmodic Agent, Gastrointestinal; Bronchodilator; Ophthalmic Agent, Mydriatic

Generic Available Yes

Use Preoperative medication to inhibit salivation and secretions; treatment of sinus bradycardia; treatment of asystole and pulseless electrical activity (adults); management of peptic ulcer; reversal of the muscarinic effects of cholinergic agents such as neostigmine and pyridostigmine; treatment of exercise-induced bronchospasm; antidote for organophosphate pesticide poisoning; used to produce mydriasis and cycloplegia for examination of the retina and optic disk and accurate measurement of refractive errors; treatment of uveitis

Pregnancy Risk Factor C

Contraindications Hypersensitivity to atropine sulfate or any component; narrow-angle glaucoma; tachycardia; thyrotoxicosis; obstructive disease of the GI tract; obstructive uropathy

Precautions Use with caution in children with spastic paralysis or brain damage; children are at increased risk for rapid rise in body temperature due to suppression of sweat gland activity; paradoxical hyperexcitability may occur in children given large doses; infants with Down's syndrome have both increased sensitivity to cardiac effects and mydriasis

Adverse Reactions
Cardiovascular: Tachycardia, palpitations
Central nervous system: Fatigue, delirium, headache, restlessness, ataxia
Dermatologic: Dry hot skin
Gastrointestinal: Impaired GI motility
Neuromuscular & skeletal: Tremor
Ocular: Blurred vision

Drug Interactions Additive effects when administered with other anticholinergic agents; may alter response to beta-adrenergic blockers

Mechanism of Action Blocks the action of acetylcholine at parasympathetic sites in smooth muscle, secretory glands, and the CNS; increases cardiac output, dries secretions, antagonizes histamine and serotonin

Pharmacodynamics
Inhibition of salivation:
Onset:
Oral: 30-60 minutes
I.M.: 30 minutes
Peak effect:
Oral: 2 hours
I.M.: 1-1.6 hours
Duration: Oral, I.M.: Up to 4 hours
Increased heart rate:
Onset:
Oral: 30 minutes to 2 hours
I.M.: 5-40 minutes
Peak effect:
Oral: 1-2 hours
I.M.: 20 minutes to 1 hour
I.V.: 2-4 minutes
Bronchodilation: Oral Inhalation:
Onset: 15 minutes
Peak effect: 15 minutes to 1.5 hours

Pharmacokinetics
Absorption: Well absorbed from all dosage forms
Distribution: Widely distributes throughout the body; crosses the placenta; trace amounts appear in breast milk; crosses the blood-brain barrier
Protein binding: 20%
Metabolism: In the liver
Half-life: Adults: 2-3 hours
Elimination: Both metabolites and unchanged drug (30% to 50%) are excreted into urine

Usual Dosage Note: Doses <0.1 mg have been associated with paradoxical bradycardia

Neonates, Infants and Children:
Preanesthetic: Oral, I.M., I.V., S.C.:
<5 kg: 0.02 mg/kg/dose 30-60 minutes preop then every 4-6 hours as needed; use of a minimum dosage of 0.1 mg in neonates <5 kg will result in dosages >0.02 mg/kg; there is no documented minimum dosage in this age group
>5 kg: 0.01-0.02 mg/kg/dose to a maximum 0.4 mg/dose 30-60 minutes preop; minimum dose: 0.1 mg
Bradycardia: I.V., intratracheal, I.O.: 0.02 mg/kg, minimum dose 0.1 mg, maximum single dose: 0.5 mg in children and 1 mg in adolescents; may repeat in 5 minutes; maximum total dose of 1 mg in children or 2 mg in adolescents.
(**Note:** For intratracheal administration, must be diluted; see Administration.)
(Continued)

Atropine *(Continued)*

When treating bradycardia in neonates, reserve use for those patients unresponsive to improved oxygenation and epinephrine.

Children:

Bronchospasm: Inhalation: 0.03-0.05 mg/kg/dose 3-4 times/day; maximum: 2.5 mg/dose

Refraction: Ophthalmic:

Infants <1 year: Instill 1 drop of 0.25% solution 3 times/day for 3 days before the procedure

Children: 1-5 years: Instill 1 drop of 0.5% solution 3 times/day for 3 days before the procedure

Children >5 years or Children with dark irides: Instill 1 drop of 1% solution 3 times/day for 3 days before the procedure

Uveitis: Ophthalmic: Instill 1 drop of 0.5% solution 1-3 times daily

Adults (doses <0.5 mg have been associated with paradoxical bradycardia):

Asystole and slow pulseless electrical activity: I.V.: 1 mg; may repeat every 3-5 minutes as needed to a total dose of 0.04 mg/kg

Preanesthetic: Oral, I.M., I.V., S.C.: 0.4-0.6 mg 30-60 minutes preop

Bradycardia: I.V.: 0.5-1 mg every 5 minutes, not to exceed a total of 2 mg or 0.04 mg/kg

Bronchospasm: Inhalation: 0.025-0.05 mg/kg/dose every 4-6 hours as needed; maximum: 2.5 mg/dose

Refraction: Ophthalmic: Instill 1-2 drops of 1% solution before the procedure

Uveitis: Ophthalmic: Instill 1-2 drops of 1% solution up to 4 times/day

Administration

Intratracheal: Dilute with NS to a total volume of 3-5 mL followed by several positive-pressure ventilations

Parenteral: Administer undiluted by rapid I.V. injection; slow injection may result in paradoxical bradycardia

Oral: Administer without regard to food

Ophthalmic: Due to the discontinuance of 0.5% ophthalmic solutions commercially, 0.5% and 0.25% solutions may be prepared by dilution of 1% atropine ophthalmic solution with artificial tears; a 1:1 dilution for 0.5% and a 1:4 dilution for 0.25%; instill solution into conjunctival sac of affected eye(s); avoid contact of bottle tip with eye or skin

Monitoring Parameters Heart rate

Dosage Forms

Injection, as sulfate: 0.1 mg/mL (5 mL, 10 mL); 0.3 mg/mL (1 mL, 30 mL); 0.4 mg/mL (1 mL, 20 mL, 30 mL); 0.5 mg/mL (1 mL, 5 mL, 30 mL); 0.8 mg/mL (0.5 mL, 1 mL); 1 mg/mL (1 mL, 10 mL)

Ointment, ophthalmic, as sulfate: 1% (3.5 g)

Solution, ophthalmic, as sulfate: 1% (1 mL, 2 mL, 5 mL, 15 mL); 2% (2 mL)

Tablet, as sulfate (Sal-Tropine™): 0.4 mg

References

"Guidelines 2000 for Cardiopulmonary Resuscitation and Emergency Cardiovascular Care. Part 10: Pediatric Advanced Life Support. The American Heart Association in Collaboration With the International Liaison Committee on Resuscitation," *Circulation*, 2000, 102(8 Suppl):I291-342.

♦ **Atropine and Diphenoxylate** *see* Diphenoxylate and Atropine *on page 343*

♦ **Atropine-Care®** *see* Atropine *on page 116*

♦ **Atropine, Hyoscyamine, Scopolamine, and Phenobarbital** *see* Hyoscyamine, Atropine, Scopolamine, and Phenobarbital *on page 519*

♦ **Atropisol®** *see* Atropine *on page 116*

♦ **Atrovent®** *see* Ipratropium *on page 547*

♦ **A/T/S®** *see* Erythromycin *on page 394*

Attapulgite *(at a PULL gite)*

U.S. Brand Names Children's Kaopectate® [OTC]; Diasorb® [OTC]; Kaopectate® Advanced Formula [OTC]; Kaopectate® Maximum Strength; K-Pek® [OTC]

Canadian Brand Names Fowlers

Therapeutic Category Antidiarrheal

Generic Available Yes

Use Treatment of uncomplicated diarrhea

Pregnancy Risk Factor B

Contraindications Hypersensitivity to attapulgite or any component

Warnings Not to be used for self-medication for diarrhea >48 hours or in the presence of high fever in infants and children <3 years of age; do not use for diarrhea associated with pseudomembranous enterocolitis or in diarrhea caused by toxigenic bacteria

Adverse Reactions

Gastrointestinal: Constipation

Respiratory: Pneumoconiosis (from inhalation of the powder chronically as it contains large amounts of silica)

Drug Interactions May inhibit GI absorption of promazine, digoxin, clindamycin, tetracycline, and penicillamine

Mechanism of Action Controls diarrhea because of its absorbent action

Usual Dosage Adequate controlled clinical studies documenting the efficacy of attapulgite are lacking; its usage and dosage has been primarily empiric; the following are manufacturer's recommended dosages

Oral: Give after each bowel movement

Children:

3-6 years: 300-750 mg/dose; maximum dose: 7 doses/day or 2250 mg/day

6-12 years: 600-1500 mg/dose; maximum dose: 7 doses/day or 4500 mg/day

Children >12 years and Adults: 1200-3000 mg/dose; maximum dose: 8 doses/day or 9000 mg/day

Administration May be administered without regard to meals; shake liquid preparation well before use

Patient Information Do not exceed maximum number of doses per day; drink plenty of fluids; contact your physician if diarrhea persists more than 48 hours or if fever develops in children <3 years of age

Dosage Forms

Liquid: Oral concentrate: 600 mg activated attapulgite/15 mL (120 mL, 180 mL, 240 mL); 750 mg activated attapulgite/15 mL (120 mL, 360 mL)

Tablet: 750 mg

Tablet, chewable: 600 mg

♦ **Augmentin**® *see* Amoxicillin and Clavulanic Acid *on page 81*

♦ **Auralgan**® *see* Antipyrine and Benzocaine *on page 99*

Auranofin (au RANE oh fin)

U.S. Brand Names Ridaura®

Therapeutic Category Gold Compound

Generic Available No

Use Management of active stage of classic or definite rheumatoid or psoriatic arthritis in patients who do not respond to or tolerate other agents; adjunctive or alternative therapy for pemphigus

Pregnancy Risk Factor C

Contraindications Renal disease; hypersensitivity to auranofin or any component; history of blood dyscrasias; CHF; exfoliative dermatitis; necrotizing enterocolitis; urticaria, eczema, SLE, bone marrow aplasia, pulmonary fibrosis; history of severe toxicity resulting from previous exposure to other heavy metals; patients who have recently received radiation therapy

Warnings Explain the possibility of adverse reactions before initiating therapy; signs of gold toxicity include decrease in hemoglobin, leukocytes, granulocytes and platelets, proteinuria, hematuria, pruritus, stomatitis or persistent diarrhea; advise patients to report any symptoms of toxicity; therapy should be discontinued if platelet count falls to <100,000/mm³

Adverse Reactions

Central nervous system: Confusion, hallucinations, seizures

Dermatologic: Dermatitis, pruritus, alopecia, chrysiasis, rash, angioedema

Gastrointestinal: Diarrhea, loose stools, stomatitis, abdominal cramping, metallic taste, glossitis, ulcerative enterocolitis, GI hemorrhage, gingivitis, dysphagia

Hematologic: Thrombocytopenia, aplastic anemia, eosinophilia, leukopenia

Hepatic: Elevated liver enzymes, jaundice, hepatitis

Neuromuscular & skeletal: Peripheral neuropathy

Ocular: Conjunctivitis, iritis, corneal ulcers

Renal: Proteinuria, hematuria, nephrotic syndrome

Respiratory: Interstitial pneumonitis, fibrosis, gold bronchitis

Drug Interactions Possible increase of phenytoin serum levels (1 case reported); penicillamine, antimalarials, hydroxychloroquine, cytotoxic drugs, or immunosuppressive agents

Mechanism of Action Unknown, acts principally via immunomodulating effects and by decreasing lysosomal enzyme release; may alter cellular mechanisms by inhibiting sulfhydryl systems

(Continued)

Auranofin *(Continued)*

Pharmacodynamics Onset of action: Therapeutic response may not be seen for 3-4 months after start of therapy

Pharmacokinetics
Absorption: Oral: Only about 20% to 25% of gold in a dose is absorbed
Protein binding: 60%
Half-life: 21-31 days (half-life dependent upon single or multiple dosing)
Time to peak blood concentrations: Within 2 hours
Elimination: 60% of absorbed gold is eliminated in urine while the remainder is eliminated in feces

Usual Dosage Oral:
Children: Initial: 0.1 mg/kg/day in 1-2 divided doses; usual maintenance: 0.15 mg/kg/day in 1-2 divided doses; maximum dose: 0.2 mg/kg/day in 1-2 divided doses
Adults: 6 mg/day in 1-2 divided doses; after 3 months may be increased to 9 mg/day in 3 divided doses; if still no response after 3 months at 9 mg/day, discontinue drug

Dosing adjustment in renal impairment:
Cl_{cr} 50-80 mL/minute: Reduce dose to 50%
Cl_{cr} <50 mL/minute: Avoid use

Monitoring Parameters CBC with differential, platelet count, urinalysis, baseline renal and liver function tests

Reference Range Gold: Normal: 0-0.1 μg/mL (SI: 0-0.0064 μmol/L); Therapeutic: 1-3 μg/mL (SI: 0.06-0.18 μmol/L); Urine <0.1 μg/24 hours

Test Interactions May enhance the response to a tuberculin skin test

Patient Information Minimize exposure to sunlight; notify your physician of pruritus, sore mouth, indigestion, metallic taste; observe careful oral hygiene

Additional Information Metallic taste may indicate stomatitis

Dosage Forms Capsule: 3 mg [gold 29%]

♦ **Auro**® **[OTC]** *see* Carbamide Peroxide *on page 178*
♦ **Aurolate**® *see* Gold Sodium Thiomalate *on page 481*

Aurothioglucose *(aur oh thye oh GLOO kose)*

U.S. Brand Names Solganal®

Therapeutic Category Gold Compound

Generic Available No

Use Management of active stage of classic or definite rheumatoid or psoriatic arthritis in patients that do not respond to or tolerate other agents

Pregnancy Risk Factor C

Contraindications Renal disease; hypersensitivity to aurothioglucose or any component; history of blood dyscrasias; CHF; exfoliative dermatitis; necrotizing enterocolitis; urticaria, eczema, SLE, bone marrow aplasia, pulmonary fibrosis; history of severe toxicity resulting from previous exposure to other heavy metals; patients who have recently received radiation therapy

Warnings Explain the possibility of adverse reactions before initiating therapy; signs of gold toxicity include: decrease in hemoglobin, leukocytes, granulocytes and platelets; proteinuria, hematuria, pruritus, stomatitis, persistent diarrhea, rash, or metallic taste; advise patients to report any symptoms of toxicity; therapy should be discontinued if platelet count <100,000/mm³, WBC <4000/mm³, or granulocytes <1500/mm³

Adverse Reactions
Central nervous system: Confusion, hallucinations, seizures, encephalitis, EEG abnormalities, fever
Dermatologic: Alopecia, urticaria, mild to severe dermatitis, pruritus, chrysiasis, exfoliative dermatitis
Gastrointestinal: Diarrhea, stomatitis, glossitis, metallic taste, gingivitis, ulcerative enterocolitis
Genitourinary: Vaginitis
Hematologic: Eosinophilia, leukopenia, thrombocytopenia, aplastic anemia
Hepatic: Hepatitis, jaundice, elevated liver enzymes
Neuromuscular & skeletal: Peripheral neuropathy
Ocular: Conjunctivitis, corneal ulcers, iritis
Renal: Hematuria, proteinuria, nephrotic syndrome, glomerulitis
Respiratory: Interstitial pneumonitis, fibrosis, gold bronchitis, pharyngitis, pulmonary fibrosis
Miscellaneous: Anaphylactic shock, allergic reaction

Drug Interactions Increased toxicity with penicillamine, antimalarials, hydroxychloroquine, cytotoxic agents, and immunosuppressants

Mechanism of Action Unknown, may decrease prostaglandin synthesis or may alter cellular mechanisms by inhibiting sulfhydryl systems; may decrease lysosomal enzyme release

Pharmacokinetics
Absorption: I.M.: Erratic and slow
Distribution: Crosses the placenta; appears in breast milk
Protein binding: 95% to 99%
Metabolism: Unknown
Half-life: 3-27 days (single dose); 14-40 days (third dose); up to 168 days (11th dose)
Time to peak serum concentration: Within 4-6 hours
Elimination: Majority ultimately excreted in urine (70%) and the remainder in feces (30%)

Usual Dosage I.M. (doses should initially be given at weekly intervals):
Children: Initial: 0.25 mg/kg/dose first week; increase by 0.25 mg/kg/dose increments with each weekly dose; maintenance: 0.75-1 mg/kg/dose weekly not to exceed 25 mg/dose to a total of 20 doses, then every 2-4 weeks
Adults: 10 mg first week; 25 mg second and third week; then 50 mg/week until 800 mg to 1 g cumulative dose has been given; if improvement occurs without adverse reactions, give 25-50 mg every 2-3 weeks, then every 3-4 weeks

Administration Parenteral: Deep I.M. injection into the upper outer quadrant of the gluteal region; vial should be thoroughly shaken before withdrawing a dose. Do not administer I.V.

Monitoring Parameters CBC with differential, platelet count, urinalysis, baseline renal and liver function tests

Reference Range Gold: Normal: 0-0.1 μg/mL (SI: 0-0.0064 μmol/L); Therapeutic: 1-3 μg/mL (SI: 0.06-0.18 μmol/L); Urine <0.1 μg/24 hours

Patient Information Minimize exposure to sunlight; notify physician of pruritus, sore mouth, indigestion, metallic taste; observe careful oral hygiene

Dosage Forms Injection, suspension: 50 mg/mL [gold 50%] (10 mL)

Azathioprine (ay za THYE oh preen)

U.S. Brand Names Imuran®
Canadian Brand Names Alti-Azathioprine; Gen-Azathioprine
Therapeutic Category Antineoplastic Agent, Adjuvant; Immunosuppressant Agent
Generic Available Yes
Use Adjunct with other agents in prevention of transplant rejection; used as an immunosuppressant in a variety of autoimmune diseases such as SLE, severe rheumatoid arthritis unresponsive to other agents, and nephrotic syndrome
Pregnancy Risk Factor D
Contraindications Hypersensitivity to azathioprine or any component; pregnancy and lactation
Warnings Chronic immunosuppression increases the risk of neoplasia, particularly lymphoma and skin cancers; mutagenic potential in both men and women; may cause irreversible bone marrow suppression
Precautions Use with caution in patients with liver disease, renal impairment, and those with cadaveric kidneys; modify dosage in patients with renal impairment; reduce dosage to 25% to 33% of usual dosage in patients receiving allopurinol and azathioprine concurrently; discontinue azathioprine therapy in patients with hepatic veno-occlusive disease
Adverse Reactions
Central nervous system: Fever, chills
(Continued)

Azathioprine *(Continued)*

Dermatologic: Alopecia, erythematous or maculopapular rash

Gastrointestinal: Nausea, vomiting, anorexia, diarrhea, aphthous stomatitis, pancreatitis

Hematologic: Bone marrow depression (leukopenia, thrombocytopenia, anemia)

Hepatic: Hepatotoxicity, jaundice, hepatic veno-occlusive disease

Neuromuscular & skeletal: Arthralgias

Ocular: Retinopathy

Miscellaneous: Rare hypersensitivity reactions which include myalgias, rigors, dyspnea, hypotension, serum sickness, rash

Drug Interactions Allopurinol inhibits the metabolic pathway of azathioprine by inhibiting xanthine oxidase and blocking the conversion of mercaptopurine to inactive products which increases azathioprine's effects; nondepolarizing neuromuscular blockers (decreased blockade); captopril or enalapril in combination with azathioprine has resulted in severe anemia

Stability Reconstituted 10 mg/mL injection is stable for 24 hours at room temperature; stable in neutral or acid solutions, but is hydrolyzed to mercaptopurine in alkaline solutions

Mechanism of Action Antagonizes purine metabolism and may inhibit synthesis of DNA, RNA, and proteins; may also interfere with cellular metabolism and inhibit mitosis

Pharmacokinetics

Distribution: Crosses the placenta

Protein binding: ~30%

Metabolism: Extensive by hepatic xanthine oxidase to 6-mercaptopurine (active)

Bioavailability: ~50%

Half-life:

Parent: 12 minutes

6-mercaptopurine: 0.7-3 hours; with anuria: 50 hours

Elimination: Small amount eliminated as unchanged drug; metabolites eliminated eventually in the urine

Dialysis: Slightly dialyzable (5% to 20%)

Usual Dosage Children and Adults:

Transplantation: Oral, I.V.: Initial: 2-5 mg/kg/dose once daily; maintenance: 1-3 mg/kg/dose once daily

Lupus nephritis: Oral: 2-3 mg/kg/dose once daily

Rheumatoid arthritis: Oral: 1 mg/kg/dose once daily for 6-8 weeks; increase by 0.5 mg/kg every 4 weeks until response or up to 2.5 mg/kg/day

Dosing interval in renal impairment:

Cl_{cr} 10-50 mL/minute: Administer every 36 hours or administer 75% of dose once daily

Cl_{cr} <10 mL/minute: Administer every 48 hours or administer 50% of dose once daily

Administration

Oral: Administer with food to decrease GI upset

Parenteral: Administer IVP over 5 minutes at a concentration not to exceed 10 mg/mL; or may be further diluted with NS or D_5W and administered by intermittent infusion over 15-60 minutes

Monitoring Parameters CBC, platelet counts, creatinine, total bilirubin, alkaline phosphatase, liver function tests

Patient Information Response in rheumatoid arthritis may not occur for up to 2-3 months; inform physician of persistent sore throat, unusual bleeding or bruising, or fatigue

Dosage Forms

Lyophilized powder for injection, as sodium: 100 mg

Tablet: 50 mg

Extemporaneous Preparations A 50 mg/mL suspension compounded from one-hundred twenty 50 mg tablets comminuted to a fine powder in a mortar with 40 mL of a 1:1 mixture of Ora-Sweet® and Ora-Plus® added and mixed to a fine paste, and then adding the 1:1 mixture of Ora-Sweet® and Ora-Plus® to a total volume of 120 mL, was stable for 60 days at 5°C and 25°C when protected from light. Label "shake well before using" and "protect from light."

Allen LV Jr and Erickson MA, "Stability of Acetazolamide, Allopurinol, Azathioprine, Clonazepam, and Flucytosine in Extemporaneously Compounded Oral Liquids," *Am J Health Syst Pharm*, 1996, 53(16):1944-9.

References

American College of Rheumatology Ad Hoc Committee on Clinical Guidelines, "Guidelines for Monitoring Drug Therapy in Rheumatoid Arthritis," *Arthritis Rheum*, 1996, 39(5):723-31.

Baum D, Bernstein D, Starnes VA, et al, "Pediatric Heart Transplantation at Stanford: Results of a 15-Year Experience," *Pediatrics*, 1991, 88(2):203-14.

Leichter HE, Sheth KJ, Gerlach MJ, et al, "Outcome of Renal Transplantation in Children Aged 1-5 and 6-18 Years," *Child Nephrol Urol*, 1992, 12(1):1-5.

Azelastine (a ZEL as teen)

U.S. Brand Names Astelin® Nasal Spray; Optivar™

Therapeutic Category Antiallergic, Ophthalmic; Antihistamine, Nasal

Generic Available No

Use

Nasal: Treatment of the symptoms of seasonal allergic rhinitis (SAR), perennial allergic rhinitis (PAR)

Ophthalmic: Treatment of itching of the eye associated with allergic conjunctivitis

Pregnancy Risk Factor C

Contraindications Hypersensitivity to azelastine or any component

Warnings Ophthalmic solution not for use in contact lens-related irritation; preservative in ophthalmic solution may be absorbed by soft contact lenses; wait at least 10 minutes after instillation before inserting soft contact lenses

Precautions Use with caution in asthmatics; patients with hepatic or renal dysfunction may require lower doses

Adverse Reactions

Cardiovascular: Flushing, hypertension, tachycardia

Central nervous system: Drowsiness, headache, somnolence, fatigue, vertigo, depression, nervousness, hypoesthesia

Dermatologic: Contact dermatitis, eczema, hair and follicle infection, furunculosis

Endocrine & metabolic: Weight gain

Gastrointestinal: Nausea, xerostomia, bitter taste, glossitis, ulcerative stomatitis, aphthous stomatitis, constipation, abdominal pain

Genitourinary: Urinary frequency, hematuria

Neuromuscular & skeletal: Myalgia, hyperkinesia

Ocular: Conjunctivitis, watery eyes, eye pain, transient eye burning/stinging (ophthalmic use)

Respiratory: Nasal burning, paroxysmal sneezing, rhinitis, epistaxis, bronchospasm, coughing, throat burning, laryngitis (nasal use)

Drug Interactions May cause additive sedation when concomitantly administered with other CNS depressant medications

Stability Stable 3 months after opening

Mechanism of Action Competes with histamine for H_1-receptor sites on effector cells in the blood vessels and respiratory tract; reduces hyper-reactivity of the airways; increases the motility of bronchial epithelial cilia, improving mucociliary transport

Pharmacodynamics

Onset of action: 30 minutes to 1 hour

Peak effect: 3 hours

Duration of action: 12 hours

Pharmacokinetics

Protein binding: 88%

Metabolism: Metabolized by cytochrome P-450 enzyme system; active metabolite desmethylazelastine

Bioavailability: After intranasal administration: 40%

Half-life, elimination: 22 hours

Time to peak serum concentration: 2-3 hours

Usual Dosage

Intranasal:

Children 5-12 years: 1 spray each nostril twice daily

Children ≥12 years and Adults: 2 sprays each nostril twice daily

Ophthalmic: Children ≥3 years and Adults: Instill 1 drop into each affected eye twice daily

Administration

Intranasal: Before use, the child-resistant screw cap on the bottle should be replaced with the pump unit and the delivery system should be primed with 4 sprays or until a fine mist appears; when 3 or more days have elapsed since the last use, the pump should be reprimed with 2 sprays or until a fine mist appears

Ophthalmic: Apply finger pressure to lacrimal sac during and for 1-2 minutes after instillation to decrease risk of systemic effects; avoid contact of bottle tip with skin or eye

Patient Information May cause drowsiness and impair ability to perform hazardous activities requiring mental alertness or physical coordination

(Continued)

Azelastine *(Continued)*

Dosage Forms

Solution, nasal: 1 mg/mL (137 mcg/spray) (17 mL)

Solution, ophthalmic (Optivar™): 0.05% (6 mL)

References

McNeely W and Wiseman LR, "Intranasal Azelastine. A Review of Its Efficacy in the Management of Allergic Rhinitis," *Drugs*, 1988, 56(1):91-114.

♦ **Azidothymidine** *see Zidovudine on page 1022*

♦ **Azidothymidine, Abacavir, and Lamivudine** *see Abacavir, Lamivudine, and Zidovudine on page 26*

♦ **Azidothymidine, Lamivudine and Abacavir** *see Abacavir, Lamivudine, and Zidovudine on page 26*

Azithromycin *(az ith roe MYE sin)*

Related Information

Carbohydrate and Alcohol Content of Liquid Medications for Use in Patients Receiving Ketogenic Diets *on page 1258*

Endocarditis Prophylaxis *on page 1160*

U.S. Brand Names Zithromax™

Therapeutic Category Antibiotic, Macrolide

Generic Available No

Use Treatment of mild to moderate upper and lower respiratory tract infections, infections of the skin and skin structure, acute otitis media, and urethritis and cervicitis due to susceptible strains of *C. trachomatis*, *N. gonorrhoeae*, *M. catarrhalis*, *H. influenzae*, *S. aureus*, *S. pneumoniae*, *Mycoplasma pneumoniae*, *M. avium* complex, *C. psittaci*, and *C. pneumoniae*; treatment of babesiosis; endocarditis prophylaxis

Pregnancy Risk Factor B

Contraindications Hypersensitivity to azithromycin, erythromycin, any component, or macrolide antibiotics

Warnings Oral azithromycin should not be used to treat pneumonia that is considered inappropriate for outpatient oral therapy; may mask or delay symptoms of incubating gonorrhea or syphilis so appropriate culture and susceptibility tests should be performed prior to initiating azithromycin; pseudomembranous colitis has been reported with use of macrolide antibiotics; patients who experience allergic reactions to azithromycin may require prolonged periods of observation and symptomatic treatment possibly due to the drug's long tissue half-life

Precautions Use with caution in patients with impaired hepatic function

Adverse Reactions

Cardiovascular: Palpitations, chest pain

Central nervous system: Headache, dizziness, agitation, nervousness, insomnia

Dermatologic: Rash, pruritus, angioedema, photosensitivity, Stevens-Johnson syndrome, toxic epidermal necrolysis

Gastrointestinal: Diarrhea (6%), nausea (2%), abdominal pain (2.5%), vomiting, anorexia

Genitourinary: Vaginitis

Hepatic: Elevated hepatic enzymes, cholestatic jaundice

Local: Pain at injection site, inflammation

Otic: Ototoxicity

Renal: Nephritis

Miscellaneous: Anaphylaxis

Drug Interactions Cytochrome P-450 isoenzyme CYP3A3/4 inhibitor (mild)

Aluminum- and magnesium-containing antacids decrease azithromycin peak serum levels by 24%; monitor patients receiving azithromycin and drugs known to interact with erythromycin (ie, theophylline, cisapride, anticoagulants) since there are still very few studies examining drug-drug interactions with azithromycin; azithromycin may increase levels of tacrolimus, phenytoin, ergot alkaloids, alfentanil, astemizole, terfenadine, bromocriptine, carbamazepine, cyclosporine, digoxin, disopyramide, and triazolam; avoid use with pimozide due to risk of cardiotoxicity

Food Interactions Food decreases bioavailability of the **capsule and suspension formulation** by up to 50%; presence of food does not affect bioavailability of the **tablet formulation or the 1 g suspension regimen**

Stability

Oral suspension: After reconstitution, multiple dose oral suspension may be stored for 10 days at room temperature or in the refrigerator.

Injection: After reconstituting 500 mg vial at a concentration of 100 mg/mL, solution is stable for 24 hours at room temperature. If solution is further diluted with a compatible diluent to a 1-2 mg/mL concentration, this solution is stable for 24 hours at room temperature or 7 days if refrigerated.

Mechanism of Action Inhibits bacterial RNA-dependent protein synthesis by binding to the 50S ribosomal subunit which results in the blockage of transpeptidation

Pharmacokinetics

Absorption: Oral: Rapid from the GI tract

Distribution: Extensive tissue distribution into skin, lungs, bone, prostate, cervix; CSF concentrations are low

Protein binding: 7% to 50% (concentration-dependent and dependent on alpha$_1$-acid glycoprotein levels)

Metabolism: In the liver to inactive metabolites

Bioavailability: Capsule, tablet, oral suspension: 34% to 52%

Half-life, terminal: 68 hours

Time to peak serum concentration: Oral: 2-3 hours

Elimination: 50% of dose is excreted unchanged in bile; 6% of dose is excreted unchanged in urine

Usual Dosage

Oral:

Children ≥6 months: Otitis media and respiratory tract infections: 10 mg/kg on day 1 (maximum dose: 500 mg/day) followed by 5 mg/kg/day once daily on days 2-5 (maximum dose: 250 mg/day)

Children ≥2 years: Pharyngitis, tonsillitis: 12 mg/kg/day once daily for 5 days (maximum dose: 500 mg/day)

Children:

Chancroid: Single 20 mg/kg dose (maximum dose: 1 g)

Uncomplicated chlamydial urethritis or cervicitis: Single 10 mg/kg dose (maximum dose: 1 g)

Primary prevention of disseminated MAC: 5 mg/kg/day once daily (maximum: 250 mg/day) or 20 mg/kg (maximum dose: 1200 mg) once weekly given alone or in combination with rifabutin

Treatment and secondary prevention of disseminated MAC: 5 mg/kg/day once daily (maximum: 250 mg/day) in combination with ethambutol, with or without rifabutin

Babesiosis: 12 mg/kg/day once daily for 7-10 days with oral atovaquone 40 mg/kg/day divided twice daily

Endocarditis prophylaxis: 15 mg/kg/dose 1 hour before procedure

Adolescents ≥16 years and Adults:

Respiratory tract, skin and soft tissue infections: 500 mg on day 1 followed by 250 mg/day once daily on days 2-5

Chancroid or nongonococcal urethritis and cervicitis due to *C. trachomatis*: Single 1 g dose

Urethritis and cervicitis due to *N. gonorrhoeae*: Single 2 g dose

Prevention of disseminated MAC: 1200 mg once weekly alone or in combination with rifabutin

Treatment and secondary prevention of disseminated MAC: 500 mg once daily in combination with ethambutol, with or without rifabutin

I.V.: Adults: 500 mg once daily for 2 days followed by a switch to oral azithromycin therapy

Administration

Oral: Administer capsule or oral suspension on an empty stomach at least 1 hour prior to a meal or 2 hours after a meal; shake suspension well before use; tablet or the 1 g suspension regimen formulation may be administered with or without food; do not administer with antacids that contain aluminum or magnesium; azithromycin 1 g oral suspension for a single dose regimen should be prepared by mixing contents of 1 packet with approximately 60 mL of water. Have the patient drink the entire contents immediately; add an additional 60 mL of water, mix, and drink (1 g suspension regimen can be taken with or without food).

Parenteral: Administer infusion at a final concentration of 1 mg/mL over 3 hours; for a 2 mg/mL concentration, infuse over 1 hour; do not infuse over a period of less than 60 minutes

Monitoring Parameters Liver function tests, WBC with differential; monitor patients receiving azithromycin and drugs known to interact with erythromycin (ie, theophylline, digoxin, anticoagulants, triazolam) since there are still very few studies examining drug-drug interactions with azithromycin

Patient Information Report any symptoms of chest pain, heart palpitations, and yellowing of skin or eyes

(Continued)

Azithromycin (Continued)

Dosage Forms
Capsule, as dihydrate: 250 mg
Powder for injection: 500 mg vial
Suspension: 100 mg/5 mL (15 mL); 200 mg/5 mL (15 mL, 22.5 mL, 30 mL); 1 g (single-dose packet)
Tablet, as dihydrate: 250 mg, 600 mg

References
Drew RH and Gallis HA, "Azithromycin-Spectrum of Activity, Pharmacokinetics, and Clinical Applications, " *Pharmacotherapy*, 1992, 12(3):161-73.

Foulds G, Shepard RM, and Johnson RB, "The Pharmacokinetics of Azithromycin in Human Serum and Tissues," *J Antimicrob Chemother*, 1990, 25(Suppl A):73-82.

Hammerschlag MR, Golden NH, Oh MK, et al, "Single Dose of Azithromycin for the Treatment of Genital Chlamydial Infections in Adolescents," *J Pediatr*, 1993, 122(6):961-5.

Nahata MC, Koranyi KI, Gadgil SD, et al, "Pharmacokinetics of Azithromycin After Oral Administration of Multiple Doses of Suspension," *Antimicrob Agents Chemother*, 1993, 37(2):314-16.

Starke JR and Correa AG, "Management of Mycobacterial Infection and Disease in Children," *Pediatr Infect Dis J*, 1995, 14(6):455-69.

"1999 USPHS/IDSA Guidelines for the Prevention of Opportunistic Infections in Persons Infected With Human Immunodeficiency Virus. USPHS/IDSA Prevention of Opportunistic Working Group," *MMWR Morb Mortal Wkly Rep*, 1999, 48(RR-10):1-61.

♦ **Azmacort®** see Triamcinolone on page 979
♦ **Azo-Standard® [OTC]** see Phenazopyridine on page 784
♦ **AZT** see Zidovudine on page 1022
♦ **AZT, Abacavir, and 3TC** see Abacavir, Lamivudine, and Zidovudine on page 26
♦ **AZT, Abacavir, and Lamivudine** see Abacavir, Lamivudine, and Zidovudine on page 26
♦ **AZT, ABC, and 3TC** see Abacavir, Lamivudine, and Zidovudine on page 26
♦ **AZT and 3TC** see Lamivudine and Zidovudine on page 574
♦ **Azthreonam** see Aztreonam on page 126

Aztreonam (AZ tree oh nam)

U.S. Brand Names Azactam®
Synonyms Azthreonam
Therapeutic Category Antibiotic, Miscellaneous
Generic Available No

Use Treatment of patients with documented multidrug resistant aerobic gram-negative infection in which beta-lactam therapy is contraindicated; used for UTI, lower respiratory tract infections, septicemia, skin/skin structure infections, intra-abdominal infections and gynecological infections caused by susceptible *Enterobacteriaceae*, *E. coli*, *K. pneumoniae*, *P. mirabilis*, *H. influenzae*, and *P. aeruginosa*

Pregnancy Risk Factor B

Contraindications Hypersensitivity to aztreonam or any component

Warnings Check for hypersensitivity to other beta-lactams (hypersensitivity reactions to aztreonam have occurred rarely in patients with a history of penicillin or cephalosporin hypersensitivity); prolonged use may result in superinfection

Precautions Use with caution and reduce dose in patients with renal impairment

Adverse Reactions
Cardiovascular: Hypotension, transient EKG changes
Central nervous system: Seizures, confusion
Dermatologic: Rash
Gastrointestinal: Diarrhea, nausea, vomiting, abdominal pain, pseudomembranous colitis
Hematologic: Eosinophilia, leukopenia, neutropenia, thrombocytopenia
Hepatic: Elevated liver enzymes
Local: Pain at injection site, thrombophlebitis, swelling at injection site
Renal: Elevated BUN and serum creatinine

Drug Interactions Avoid antibiotics that induce beta-lactamase production (cefoxitin, imipenem)

Stability Reconstituted solution is stable 48 hours at room temperature and 7 days when refrigerated; incompatible when mixed with nafcillin, metronidazole

Mechanism of Action Binds to penicillin-binding protein 3 which produces filamentation of the bacterium inhibiting bacterial cell wall synthesis and causing cell wall destruction

Pharmacokinetics
Absorption: I.M.: Well absorbed
Distribution: Widely distributed into body tissues, cerebrospinal fluid, bronchial secretions, peritoneal fluid, bone, and breast milk

V_d:
   Neonates: 0.26-0.36 L/kg
   Children: 0.2-0.29 L/kg
   Adults: 0.2 L/kg
Protein binding: 56%
Half-life:
   Neonates:
      <7 days, ≤2.5 kg: 5.5-9.9 hours
      <7 days, >2.5 kg: 2.6 hours
      1 week to 1 month: 2.4 hours
   Children 2 months to 12 years: 1.7 hours
   Children with cystic fibrosis: 1.3 hours
   Adults: 1.3-2.2 hours (half-life prolonged in renal failure)
Time to peak serum concentration: Within 60 minutes after an I.M. dose
Elimination: 60% to 70% excreted unchanged in the urine and partially excreted in feces
Dialysis: Moderately dialyzable
   Hemodialysis: 27% to 58% in 4 hours
   Peritoneal dialysis: 10% with a 6-hour dwell time
Usual Dosage I.M., I.V.:
Neonates:
   Postnatal age ≤7 days:
      ≤2000 g: 60 mg/kg/day divided every 12 hours
      >2000 g: 90 mg/kg/day divided every 8 hours
   Postnatal age >7 days:
      <1200 g: 60 mg/kg/day divided every 12 hours
      1200-2000 g: 90 mg/kg/day divided every 8 hours
      >2000 g: 120 mg/kg/day divided every 6 hours
Children >1 month: 90-120 mg/kg/day divided every 6-8 hours
   Cystic fibrosis: 50 mg/kg/dose every 6-8 hours (ie, up to 200 mg/kg/day); maximum dose: 8 g/day
Adults:
   Urinary tract infection: 500 mg to 1 g every 8-12 hours
   Moderately severe systemic infections: 1 g I.V. or I.M. or 2 g I.V. every 8-12 hours
   Severe systemic or life-threatening infections (especially if caused by *Pseudomonas aeruginosa*): I.V.: 2 g every 6-8 hours; maximum dose: 8 g/day
Dosing adjustment in renal impairment:
   Cl_{cr} 10-30 mL/minute: Reduce dose by 50%; give at the usual interval
   Cl_{cr} <10 mL/minute: Reduce dose by 75%; give at the usual interval
Administration Parenteral: Administer by IVP over 3-5 minutes at a maximum concentration of 66 mg/mL or by intermittent infusion over 20-60 minutes at a final concentration not to exceed 20 mg/mL
Monitoring Parameters Periodic liver function test
Test Interactions Urine glucose (Clinitest®)
Dosage Forms Powder for injection: 500 mg (15 mL, 100 mL); 1 g (15 mL, 100 mL); 2 g (15 mL, 100 mL)
References
Bosso JA and Black PG, "The Use of Aztreonam in Pediatric Patients: A Review," *Pharmacotherapy*, 1991, 11(1):20-5.
Stutman HR, Chartrand SA, Tolentino T, et al, "Aztreonam Therapy for Serious Gram-Negative Infections in Children," *Am J Dis Child*, 1986, 140(11):1147-51.

♦ **Azulfidine®** *see* Sulfasalazine *on page 926*
♦ **Azulfidine® EN-tabs®** *see* Sulfasalazine *on page 926*
♦ **Babee® Teething [OTC]** *see* Benzocaine *on page 135*
♦ **Baby Orajel (Can)** *see* Benzocaine *on page 135*
♦ **Babys Own Ointment (Can)** *see* Zinc Oxide *on page 1026*
♦ **Bacid® [OTC]** *see Lactobacillus acidophilus* and *Lactobacillus bulgaricus* on page 571
♦ **Baciguent® [OTC]** *see* Bacitracin *on page 127*
♦ **Baci-IM®** *see* Bacitracin *on page 127*
♦ **Bacimyxin (Can)** *see* Bacitracin and Polymyxin B *on page 129*
♦ **Bacitin (Can)** *see* Bacitracin *on page 127*

Bacitracin (bas i TRAY sin)
U.S. Brand Names AK-Tracin®; Baciguent® [OTC]; Baci-IM®
Canadian Brand Names Bacitin
Therapeutic Category Antibiotic, Ophthalmic; Antibiotic, Topical; Antibiotic, Miscellaneous
(Continued)

Bacitracin *(Continued)*

Generic Available Yes

Use Treatment of pneumonia and empyema caused by susceptible staphylococci; prevention or treatment of superficial skin infections or infections of the eye caused by susceptible organisms; due to its toxicity, use of bacitracin systemically or as an irrigant should be limited to situations where less toxic alternatives would not be effective; treatment of antibiotic-associated colitis

Pregnancy Risk Factor C

Contraindications Hypersensitivity to bacitracin or any component; I.M. use is contraindicated in patients with renal impairment

Warnings I.M. use may cause renal failure due to tubular and glomerular necrosis; do **not** administer intravenously because severe thrombophlebitis occurs; bacitracin may be absorbed from denuded areas and irrigation sites

Precautions Prolonged use may result in overgrowth of nonsusceptible organisms

Adverse Reactions
  Cardiovascular: Hypotension, tightness of chest
  Central nervous system: Pain
  Dermatologic: Rash, itching
  Gastrointestinal: Anorexia, nausea, vomiting, diarrhea, rectal itching and burning
  Hematologic: Blood dyscrasias
  Renal: With I.M. use: Renal tubular and glomerular necrosis, azotemia, renal failure
  Miscellaneous: Diaphoresis, edema of lips and face

Drug Interactions Nephrotoxic drugs (increase toxicity), neuromuscular blocking agents and anesthetics (increase neuromuscular blockade)

Stability Sterile powder should be stored in the refrigerator; once reconstituted, bacitracin is stable for 1 week under refrigeration (2°C to 8°C); incompatible with diluents containing parabens

Mechanism of Action Inhibits bacterial cell wall synthesis by preventing transfer of mucopeptides into the growing cell wall

Pharmacokinetics
  Absorption: Poor from mucous membranes and intact skin; rapid following I.M. administration
  Protein binding: Minimally bound to plasma proteins
  Time to peak serum concentration: I.M.: Within 1-2 hours
  Elimination: Slow elimination into the urine with 10% to 40% of a dose excreted within 24 hours

Usual Dosage
  I.M. (not recommended):
    Infants:
      ≤2.5 kg: 900 units/kg/day in 2-3 divided doses
      >2.5 kg: 1000 units/kg/day in 2-3 divided doses
    Children: 800-1200 units/kg/day divided every 8 hours
    Adults: 10,000-25,000 units/dose every 6 hours; not to exceed 100,000 units/day
  Children and Adults:
    Topical: Apply 1-5 times/day
    Ophthalmic ointment: Instill ¼" to ½" ribbon directly into conjunctival sac(s) every 3-4 hours; reduce frequency of administration as the infection is brought under control to 1-3 times/day
    Irrigation, solution: 50-100 units/mL in NS, LR, or sterile water for irrigation; soak sponges in solution for topical compresses 1-5 times/day or as needed during surgical procedures
  Antibiotic-associated colitis: Adults: Oral: 25,000 units every 6 hours for 7-10 days

Administration
  Ophthalmic: Do not use topical ointment in the eyes; avoid contact of tube tip with skin or eye
  Parenteral: For I.M. administration, pH of urine should be kept above 6 by using sodium bicarbonate; bacitracin sterile powder should be dissolved in NS injection containing 2% procaine hydrochloride; administer I.M. injection into the upper outer quadrant of the buttocks; alternate injection sites

Monitoring Parameters I.M.: Urinalysis, renal function tests

Patient Information Ophthalmic ointment may cause blurred vision; topical bacitracin should not be used for longer than 1 week unless directed by a physician

Dosage Forms
  Injection: 50,000 units
  Ointment:
    Ophthalmic: 500 units/g (3.5 g, 3.75 g)
    Topical: 500 units/g (1 g, 15 g, 30 g, 120 g, 454 g)

References
Kelly CP, Pothoulakis C, and LaMont JT, "*Clostridium difficile* Colitis," *N Engl J Med*, 1994, 330(4):257-62.

Bacitracin and Polymyxin B (bas i TRAY sin & pol i MIKS in bee)

U.S. Brand Names AK-Poly-Bac® Ophthalmic; Betadine® First Aid Antibiotics + Moisturizer [OTC]; Polysporin® Ophthalmic; Polysporin® Topical

Canadian Brand Names Antibiotic Ointment; Antibiotique Onguent; Bacimyxin; Band-Aid Antibiotic; Bioderm; Lid-Pack; Optimyxin; Polycidin; Polyderm; Polytopic Ointment; Polytracin

Synonyms Polymyxin B and Bacitracin

Therapeutic Category Antibiotic, Ophthalmic; Antibiotic, Topical

Generic Available Yes

Use Treatment of superficial infections involving the conjunctiva and/or cornea caused by susceptible organisms; prevent infection in minor cuts, scrapes and burns

Pregnancy Risk Factor C

Contraindications Hypersensitivity to polymyxin, bacitracin, or any component

Precautions Prolonged use may result in overgrowth of nonsusceptible organisms

Adverse Reactions
Local: Rash, itching, burning, edema
Ocular: Conjunctival erythema
Miscellaneous: Anaphylactoid reactions

Pharmacokinetics Absorption: Insignificant from intact skin or mucous membrane

Usual Dosage Children and Adults:
Ophthalmic: Instill ¼" to ½" directly into conjunctival sac(s) every 3-4 hours depending on severity of the infection
Topical: Apply a small amount of ointment or dusting of powder to the affected area 1-3 times/day

Administration Ophthalmic: Do not use topical ointment in the eyes; avoid contact of tube tip with skin or eye

Patient Information Do not use longer than 1 week unless directed by physician; ophthalmic ointment may cause blurred vision

Dosage Forms
Ointment:
Ophthalmic: Bacitracin 500 units and polymyxin B sulfate 10,000 units per g (3.5 g)
Topical: Bacitracin 500 units and polymyxin B sulfate 10,000 units per g in white petrolatum (15 g, 30 g)
Powder, topical: Polymyxin B sulfate 10,000 units and bacitracin 500 units per g (10 g)

♦ **Bacitracin, Neomycin, and Polymyxin B** *see* Neomycin, Polymyxin B, and Bacitracin *on page 707*

♦ **Bacitracin, Neomycin, Polymyxin B, and Hydrocortisone** *see* Neomycin, (Bacitracin) Polymyxin B, and Hydrocortisone *on page 705*

Baclofen (BAK loe fen)

U.S. Brand Names Lioresal®

Canadian Brand Names Apo-Baclofen; Gen-Baclofen; Liotec; Novo-Baclofen; Nu-Baclo; PMS-Baclofen

Therapeutic Category Skeletal Muscle Relaxant, Nonparalytic

Generic Available Yes: Tablets only

Use Treatment of cerebral spasticity, reversible spasticity associated with multiple sclerosis or spinal cord lesions; intrathecal use for the management of spasticity in patients who are unresponsive to oral baclofen or experience intolerable CNS side effects; treatment of trigeminal neuralgia; adjunctive treatment of tardive dyskinesia

Pregnancy Risk Factor C

Contraindications Hypersensitivity to baclofen or any component

Warnings Should not be used when spasticity is used to maintain posture or balance; abrupt withdrawal of baclofen has been reported to precipitate hallucinations and/or seizures; due to the life-threatening complications of intrathecal use, physicians must be adequately trained in its use; physostigmine should be available to reverse life-threatening central nervous side effects (eg, respiratory depression); injection for intrathecal use is not recommended or intended for I.V., I.M., S.C. or epidural administration

Precautions Use with caution in patients with seizure disorder, impaired renal function, peptic ulcer disease, stroke, ovarian cysts, psychotic disorders, autonomic dysreflexia (intrathecal therapy)
(Continued)

Baclofen *(Continued)*

Adverse Reactions

Cardiovascular: Hypotension, cardiovascular collapse (with intrathecal therapy), chest pain, palpitations

Central nervous system: Drowsiness, fatigue, vertigo, dizziness, psychiatric disturbances, insomnia, slurred speech, headache, hypotonia, ataxia, life-threatening CNS depression (with intrathecal use)

Dermatologic: Rash, pruritus

Gastrointestinal: Nausea, constipation, anorexia, dysgeusia, diarrhea, abdominal pain, xerostomia

Genitourinary: Impotence, urinary frequency, nocturia

Renal: Hematuria

Respiratory: Respiratory failure (with intrathecal administration), dyspnea

Miscellaneous: Diaphoresis

Drug Interactions
Increased CNS depression when administered with other CNS depressants (eg, opiates, alcohol, benzodiazepines), tricyclic antidepressants; MAO inhibitors; baclofen may decrease lithium's effect

Mechanism of Action
Inhibits the transmission of both monosynaptic and polysynaptic reflexes at the spinal cord level, possibly by hyperpolarization of primary afferent fiber terminals, with resultant relief of muscle spasticity

Pharmacodynamics

Oral: Muscle relaxation effects require 3-4 days and maximal clinical effects are not seen for 5-10 days

Intrathecal:

Bolus:

Onset of effect: 30 minutes to 1 hour

Peak effect: 4 hours

Duration: 4-8 hours

Continuous intrathecal infusion:

Onset of action: 6-8 hours

Maximum activity: 24-48 hours

Pharmacokinetics

Oral:

Absorption: Rapid; absorption from the GI tract is thought to be dose dependent

Protein binding: 30%

Metabolism: Minimal in the liver (15%)

Half-life: 2.5-4 hours

Time to peak serum concentration: Oral: Within 2-3 hours

Elimination: 85% of dose excreted in urine and feces as unchanged drug

Intrathecal:

Half-life, CSF elimination: 1.5 hours

Clearance, CSF: 30 mL/hour

Usual Dosage

Oral:

Children:

2-7 years: Initial: 10-15 mg/day divided every 8 hours; titrate dose every 3 days in increments of 5-15 mg/day to a maximum of 40 mg/day

≥8 years: Titrate dosage as above to a maximum of 60 mg/day

Adults: 5 mg 3 times/day, may increase 5 mg/dose every 3 days to a maximum of 80 mg/day

Intrathecal: Children and Adults:

Screening dosage: 50 mcg for 1 dose and observe for 4-8 hours; very small children may receive 25 mcg; if ineffective, a repeat dosage increased by 50% (eg, 75 mcg) may be repeated in 24 hours: if still suboptimal, a third dose increased by 33% (eg, 100 mcg) may be repeated in 24 hours; patients who do not respond to 100 mcg intrathecally should not be considered for continuous chronic administration via an implantable pump

Maintenance dose: Continuous infusion: Initial: Depending upon the screening dosage and its duration:

If the screening dose duration >8 hours: Daily dose = effective screening dose

If the screening dose duration <8 hours: Daily dose = **twice** effective screening dose

Continuous infusion dose mcg/hour = daily dose divided by 24 hours

Note: Further adjustments in infusion rate may be done every 24 hours as needed; for spinal cord-related spasticity, increase in 10% to 30% increments/ 24 hours; for spasticity of cerebral origin, increase in 5% to 10% increments/ 24 hours

Average daily dose:
Children ≤12 years: 100-300 mcg/day (4.2-12.5 mcg/hour); doses as high as 1000 mcg/day have been used
Children >12 years and Adults: 300-800 mcg/day (12.5-33 mcg/hour); doses as high as 2000 mcg/day have been used

Administration
Oral: Administer with food or milk
Parenteral: Intrathecal: Test dosage: Use dilute concentration (50 mcg/mL) and inject over at least 1 minute; for maintenance infusions, concentrations of 500-2000 mcg/mL may be used

Monitoring Parameters Muscle rigidity, spasticity (decrease in number and severity of spasms), modified Ashworth score

Patient Information Avoid alcohol and other CNS depressants; causes drowsiness and impairs ability to perform hazardous activities requiring mental alertness or physical coordination

Dosage Forms
Injection, intrathecal, preservative free: 0.05 mg/mL (1 mL); 0.5 mg/mL (20 mL); 2 mg/mL (5 mL)
Tablet: 10 mg, 20 mg

Extemporaneous Preparations Make a 10 mg/mL oral suspension by crushing one hundred twenty 10 mg tablets; gradually add 60 mL Ora-Sweet® or Ora-Plus® and mix until a uniform paste, then add more vehicle to make a total volume of 120 mL; refrigerate; shake well; stable 60 days
Allen LV Jr and Erickson MA 3rd, "Stability of Baclofen, Captopril, Diltiazem Hydrochloride, Dipyridamole, and Flecainide Acetate in Extemporaneously Compounded Oral Liquids," *Am J Health Syst Pharm*, 1996, 53(18):2179-84.

♦ **Bacticort® Otic** *see* Neomycin, (Bacitracin) Polymyxin B, and Hydrocortisone *on page 705*
♦ **Bactocill®** *see* Oxacillin *on page 740*
♦ **Bactopen (Can)** *see* Cloxacillin *on page 260*
♦ **Bactrim™** *see* Co-Trimoxazole *on page 270*
♦ **Bactrim™ DS** *see* Co-Trimoxazole *on page 270*
♦ **Bactroban®** *see* Mupirocin *on page 687*
♦ **Baking Soda** *see* Sodium Bicarbonate *on page 904*
♦ **Balanced C Complex (Can)** *see* Ascorbic Acid *on page 106*
♦ **BAL in Oil®** *see* Dimercaprol *on page 340*
♦ **Balmex® [OTC]** *see* Zinc Oxide *on page 1026*
♦ **Balminil Decongestant (Can)** *see* Pseudoephedrine *on page 852*
♦ **Balminil DM (Can)** *see* Dextromethorphan *on page 316*
♦ **Balminil DM E (Can)** *see* Guaifenesin and Dextromethorphan *on page 487*
♦ **Balminil Expectorant (Can)** *see* Guaifenesin *on page 485*
♦ **Balnetar (Can)** *see* Coal Tar *on page 260*
♦ **Bancap HC®** *see* Hydrocodone and Acetaminophen *on page 505*
♦ **Band-Aid Antibiotic (Can)** *see* Bacitracin and Polymyxin B *on page 129*
♦ **Banophen® [OTC]** *see* Diphenhydramine *on page 342*
♦ **Barbilixir (Can)** *see* Phenobarbital *on page 785*
♦ **Baridium® [OTC]** *see* Phenazopyridine *on page 784*
♦ **Barriere-HC (Can)** *see* Hydrocortisone *on page 506*
♦ **Basaljel® [OTC]** *see* Antacid Preparations *on page 95*
♦ **Baxedin (Can)** *see* Chlorhexidine Gluconate *on page 220*
♦ **Bayer® Aspirin [OTC]** *see* Aspirin *on page 109*
♦ **BCNU** *see* Carmustine *on page 182*
♦ **B Complex** *see page 1069*
♦ **B-D Glucose® [OTC]** *see* Dextrose *on page 317*
♦ **Bebulin® VH** *see* Factor IX Complex (Human) *on page 414*

Beclomethasone (be kloe METH a sone)
Related Information
Asthma Guidelines *on page 1210*
Estimated Comparative Daily Dosages for Inhaled Corticosteroids *on page 1216*
U.S. Brand Names Beclovent®; Beconase®; Beconase® AQ; QVAR™ 40 mcg; QVAR™ 80 mcg; Vancenase®; Vancenase® AQ; Vancenase® AQ 84 mcg; Vanceril®; Vanceril® 84 mcg Double Strength
Canadian Brand Names Alti-Beclomethasone; Apo-Beclomethasone; Gen-Beclo AQ; Nu-Beclomethasone; Propaderm; Rivenase AQ
(Continued)

Beclomethasone (Continued)

Therapeutic Category Adrenal Corticosteroid; Antiasthmatic; Anti-inflammatory Agent; Corticosteroid, Inhalant (Oral); Corticosteroid, Intranasal; Glucocorticoid

Generic Available No

Use

Oral inhalation: Long-term (chronic) control of persistent bronchial asthma; **NOT** indicated for the relief of acute bronchospasm. Also used to help reduce or discontinue oral corticosteroid therapy for asthma.

Intranasal: Management of seasonal or perennial rhinitis and nasal polyposis

Pregnancy Risk Factor C

Contraindications Hypersensitivity to beclomethasone or any component; primary treatment of status asthmaticus or other acute episodes of bronchial asthma where intensive treatment is needed

Warnings Fatalities have occurred due to adrenal insufficiency in asthmatic patients during and after switching from systemic corticosteroids to aerosol steroids; several months may be required for full recovery of the adrenal glands; patients receiving higher doses of systemic corticosteroids (eg, adults receiving ≥20 mg of prednisone per day) may be at greater risk; during this period of adrenal suppression, aerosol steroids do **not** provide the systemic corticosteroid needed to treat patients requiring stress doses (ie, patients with major stress such as trauma, surgery, or infections). When used at high doses hypothalamic - pituitary - adrenal (HPA) suppression may occur; use with inhaled or systemic corticosteroids (even alternate-day dosing) may increase risk of HPA suppression; withdrawal and discontinuation of corticosteroids should be done carefully. Switching from systemic corticosteroids to inhalation may unmask allergic conditions (such as eczema, conjunctivitis, and rhinitis) that were previously suppressed by systemic steroids. Immunosuppression may occur

Precautions Avoid using higher than recommended dosages; suppression of HPA function, suppression of linear growth, or hypercorticism (Cushing's syndrome) may occur; use with extreme caution in patients with respiratory tuberculosis, untreated systemic infections, or ocular herpes simplex; rare cases of increased IOP, glaucoma, or cataracts may occur

Adverse Reactions

Central nervous system: Headache

Endocrine & metabolic: Potential adrenal suppression, dysmenorrhea

Gastrointestinal: Xerostomia, sore throat, pharyngitis

Local: Growth of *Candida* in the mouth, throat, or nares

Neuromuscular & skeletal: Growth velocity suppression (reported in asthmatic children receiving oral inhalation 2 puffs 4 times/day)

Respiratory: Cough, sneezing, hoarseness, irritation and burning of the nasal mucosa, nasal ulceration, epistaxis, rhinorrhea, nasal congestion

Drug Interactions Cytochrome P-450 isoenzyme CYP3A substrate

Interactions similar to other corticosteroids may potentially occur

Stability Do not store near heat or open flame; store QVAR™ so inhaler rests on concave end of canister (with plastic actuator on top); use Vanceril® within 6 months after removal from moisture protective package

Mechanism of Action Controls the rate of protein synthesis, depresses the migration of polymorphonuclear leukocytes and fibroblasts, reverses capillary permeability, and stabilizes lysosomal membranes at the cellular level to prevent or control inflammation

Pharmacodynamics

Onset:

Oral inhalation: Within 1-2 days in some patients; usually within 1-2 weeks

Nasal inhalation: Within a few days up to 2 weeks

Maximum effects: Oral inhalation: 3-4 weeks

Pharmacokinetics

Absorption: Inhalation: Readily absorbed; quickly hydrolyzed by pulmonary esterases prior to absorption; oral: 90%

Distribution: 10% to 25% of inhaled dose reaches respiratory tract (50% with QVAR™); secreted into breast milk

Protein binding: 87%

Metabolism: In the liver via cytochrome P-450 isoenzyme CYP3A to 3 major metabolites: Beclomethasone-17-monopropionate (17-BMP), beclomethasone-21-monopropionate (21-BMP), and beclomethasone (BOH); most active metabolite is 17-BMP

Half-life: Biphasic: Initial 3 hours; terminal: 15 hours

Elimination: Primary route of excretion is via feces; 12% to 15% of oral dose excreted in urine as metabolites

Usual Dosage

Aqueous inhalation, nasal:

Vancenase® AQ, Beconase® AQ: Children ≥6 years and Adults: 1-2 inhalations each nostril twice daily

Vancenase® AQ 84 mcg: Children ≥6 years and Adults: 1-2 inhalations in each nostril once daily

Intranasal (Vancenase®, Beconase®):

Children 6-12 years: 1 inhalation in each nostril 3 times/day

Children ≥12 years and Adults: 1 inhalation in each nostril 2-4 times/day or 2 inhalations each nostril twice daily; usual maximum maintenance: 1 inhalation in each nostril 3 times/day

Oral inhalation (doses should be titrated to the lowest effective dose once asthma is controlled):

Beclovent®, Vanceril®:

Children 6-12 years: 1-2 inhalations 3-4 times/day (alternatively: 2-4 inhalations twice daily); maximum dose: 10 inhalations/day

Children ≥12 years and Adults: 2 inhalations 3-4 times/day (alternatively: 4 inhalations twice daily); maximum dose: 20 inhalations/day; patients with severe asthma: Initial: 12-16 inhalations/day (divided 3-4 times/day); dose should be adjusted downward according to patient's response

Vanceril® 84 mcg Double Strength:

Children 6-12 years: 2 inhalations twice daily; maximum dose: 5 inhalations/day

Children ≥12 years and Adults: 2 inhalations twice daily; maximum dose: 10 inhalations/day; patients with severe asthma: Initial: 6-8 inhalations/day (divided twice daily); dose should be adjusted downward according to patient's response

QVAR™: Children ≥12 years and Adults:

No previous inhaled corticosteroids: Initial: 40-80 mcg twice daily; maximum dose: 320 mcg twice daily

Previous inhaled corticosteroid use: Initial: 40-160 mcg twice daily; maximum dose: 320 mcg twice daily

Note: Therapeutic ratio between QVAR™ and other beclomethasone inhalers has not been established; when switching to QVAR™, monitor patients for efficacy and adverse effects

NIH Guidelines (NIH, 1997) [give in divided doses]:

Children:

"Low" dose: 84-336 mcg/day (42 mcg/puff: 2-8 puffs/day or 84 mcg/puff: 1-4 puffs/day)

"Medium" dose: 336-672 mcg/day (42 mcg/puff: 8-16 puffs/day or 84 mcg/puff: 4-8 puffs/day)

"High" dose: >672 mcg/day (42 mcg/puff: >16 puffs/day or 84 mcg/puff >8 puffs/day)

Adults:

"Low" dose: 168-504 mcg/day (42 mcg/puff: 4-12 puffs/day or 84 mcg/puff: 2-6 puffs/day)

"Medium" dose: 504-840 mcg/day (42 mcg/puff: 12-20 puffs/day or 84 mcg/puff: 6-10 puffs/day)

"High" dose: >840 mcg/day (42 mcg/puff: >20 puffs/day or 84 mcg/puff: >10 puffs/day)

Administration

Oral inhalation: Use a spacer device for children <8 years of age

Nasal and oral inhalation (all products except QVAR™): Shake container well before use

Monitoring Parameters Check mucous membranes for signs of fungal infection; monitor growth in pediatric patients

Patient Information Notify physician if condition being treated persists or worsens; do not decrease dose or discontinue without physician approval; avoid spraying in eyes; avoid exposure to chicken pox or measles; if exposed, seek medical advice without delay; discard canister when labeled number of metered doses (sprays) have been used. QVAR™ may taste differently and have a different feeling during inhalation compared to other inhalers containing chlorofluorocarbons (CFCs).

Oral inhalant: Rinse mouth after inhalation to decrease chance of oral candidiasis; report sore mouth or mouth lesions to physician

Additional Information

Oral inhalation: If bronchospasm with wheezing occurs after use, a fast-acting bronchodilator may be used.

QVAR™: Does not contain chlorofluorocarbons (CFCs), uses hydrofluoroalkane (HFA) as the propellant; is a solution formulation (other beclomethasone

(Continued)

133

Beclomethasone *(Continued)*

inhalers are suspension aerosols); uses smaller-size particles which results in a higher percent of drug delivered to the respiratory tract and lower recommended doses than other products

Aqueous beclomethasone nasal spray (2 sprays in each nostril twice daily for 4 weeks, followed by 1 spray in each nostril twice daily) may be useful in reducing adenoidal hypertrophy and nasal airway obstruction in children 5-11 years of age (Demain, 1995)

Dosage Forms

Inhalation, as dipropionate:

Nasal:

Beconase®, Vancenase®: 42 mcg/inhalation [80 metered doses] (6.7 g); [200 metered doses] (16.8 g)

Vancenase® Pockethaler: 42 mcg/inhalation [200 metered doses] (7 g)

Oral:

Beclovent®, Vanceril®: 42 mcg/inhalation [80 metered doses] (6.7 g); [200 metered doses] (16.8 g)

QVAR™ 40 mcg: 40 mcg/inhalation [100 metered doses] (7.3 g)

QVAR™ 80 mcg: 80 mcg/inhalation [100 metered doses] (7.3 g)

Vanceril® 84 mcg Double Strength: 84 mcg/inhalation [40 metered doses] (5.4 g); [120 metered doses] (12.2 g)

Spray, aqueous, nasal, as dipropionate

Beconase® AQ, Vancenase® AQ: 42 mcg/inhalation [200 metered doses] (25 g)

Vancenase® AQ 84 mcg: 84 mcg/inhalation [120 metered doses] (19 g)

References

Demain JG and Goetz DW, "Pediatric Adenoidal Hypertrophy and Nasal Airway Obstruction: Reduction With Aqueous Nasal Beclomethasone," *Pediatrics*, 1995, 95(3):355-64.

Expert Panel Report 2, "Guidelines for the Diagnosis and Management of Asthma," *Clinical Practice Guidelines*, National Institutes of Health, National Heart, Lung, and Blood Institute, NIH Publication No. 94-4051, April, 1997.

Kobayashi RH, Tinkelman DG, Reese ME, et al, "Beclomethasone Dipropionate Aqueous Nasal Spray for Seasonal Allergic Rhinitis in Children," *Ann Allergy*, 1989, 62(3):205-8.

Tinkelman DG, Reed CE, Nelson HS, et al, "Aerosol Beclomethasone Dipropionate Compared With Theophylline as Primary Treatment of Chronic, Mild to Moderately Severe Asthma in Children," *Pediatrics*, 1993, 92(1):64-77.

Wyatt R, Waschek J, Weinberger M, et al, "Effects of Inhaled Beclomethasone Dipropionate and Alternate-Day Prednisone on Pituitary-Adrenal Function in Children With Chronic Asthma," *N Engl J Med*, 1978, 299(25):1387-92.

- **Beclovent®** *see* Beclomethasone *on page 131*
- **Beconase®** *see* Beclomethasone *on page 131*
- **Beconase® AQ** *see* Beclomethasone *on page 131*
- **Bedoz (Can)** *see* Cyanocobalamin *on page 277*
- **Beepen-VK®** *see* Penicillin V Potassium *on page 774*
- **Benadryl® [OTC]** *see* Diphenhydramine *on page 342*
- **Benadryl® Allergy [OTC]** *see* Diphenhydramine *on page 342*
- **Benadryl® Injection** *see* Diphenhydramine *on page 342*
- **Ben-Aqua® [OTC]** *see* Benzoyl Peroxide *on page 136*
- **Benoxyl®** *see* Benzoyl Peroxide *on page 136*
- **Bentyl®** *see* Dicyclomine *on page 326*
- **Bentylol (Can)** *see* Dicyclomine *on page 326*
- **Benuryl (Can)** *see* Probenecid *on page 828*
- **Benylin® Adult [OTC]** *see* Dextromethorphan *on page 316*
- **Benylin DM (Can)** *see* Dextromethorphan *on page 316*
- **Benylin DM-E (Can)** *see* Guaifenesin and Dextromethorphan *on page 487*
- **Benylin-E (Can)** *see* Guaifenesin *on page 485*
- **Benylin® Expectorant [OTC]** *see* Guaifenesin and Dextromethorphan *on page 487*
- **Benylin® Pediatric [OTC]** *see* Dextromethorphan *on page 316*
- **Benzac AC® Gel** *see* Benzoyl Peroxide *on page 136*
- **Benzac AC® Wash** *see* Benzoyl Peroxide *on page 136*
- **Benzac W® Gel** *see* Benzoyl Peroxide *on page 136*
- **Benzac W® Wash** *see* Benzoyl Peroxide *on page 136*
- **5-Benzagel®** *see* Benzoyl Peroxide *on page 136*
- **10-Benzagel®** *see* Benzoyl Peroxide *on page 136*
- **Benzashave® Cream** *see* Benzoyl Peroxide *on page 136*
- **Benzathine Benzylpenicillin** *see* Penicillin G Benzathine *on page 770*

- **Benzathine Penicillin G** *see* Penicillin G Benzathine *on page 770*
- **Benzazoline** *see* Tolazoline *on page 967*
- **Benzene Hexachloride** *see* Lindane *on page 595*
- **Benzhexol** *see* Trihexyphenidyl *on page 984*

Benzocaine (BEN zoe kane)

U.S. Brand Names Americaine® [OTC]; Anbesol® [OTC]; Anbesol® Maximum Strength [OTC]; Babee® Teething [OTC]; Benzodent® [OTC]; Chiggerex® [OTC]; Chiggertox® [OTC]; Cylex® [OTC]; Dermoplast® [OTC]; Detane® [OTC]; Foille® [OTC]; Foille® Medicated First Aid [OTC]; HDA Toothache® [OTC]; Hurricaine®; Lanacane® [OTC]; Mycinettes® [OTC]; Numzit Teething® [OTC]; Orabase®-B [OTC]; Orajel® Maximum Strength [OTC]; Orajel® Mouth-Aid [OTC]; Orasept® [OTC]; Orasol® [OTC]; Solarcaine® [OTC]; Zilactin®-B Medicated [OTC]

Canadian Brand Names Anebesol Baby; Baby Orajel; Outgro; Sirop Dentition; Zilactin Baby

Synonyms Ethyl Aminobenzoate

Therapeutic Category Analgesic, Topical; Local Anesthetic, Oral; Local Anesthetic, Topical

Generic Available Yes

Use Temporary relief of pain associated with pruritic dermatosis, pruritus, minor burns, toothache, minor sore throat pain, canker sores, hemorrhoids, rectal fissures; anesthetic lubricant for passage of catheters and endoscopic tubes

Pregnancy Risk Factor C

Contraindications Hypersensitivity to benzocaine, other ester-type local anesthetics, or any component; secondary bacterial infection of area; perforated tympanic membrane (otic formulations only)

Adverse Reactions
  Cardiovascular: Edema
  Dermatologic: Angioedema, urticaria
  Genitourinary: Urethritis
  Hematologic: Methemoglobinemia in infants
  Local: Contact dermatitis, burning, stinging, tenderness

Mechanism of Action Blocks both the initiation and conduction of nerve impulses from sensory nerves by decreasing the neuronal membrane's permeability to sodium ions, which results in inhibition of depolarization with resultant blockade of conduction

Pharmacokinetics
  Absorption: Poor after topical administration to intact skin, but well absorbed from mucous membranes and traumatized skin
  Metabolism: Hydrolyzed in plasma and to a lesser extent in the liver by cholinesterase
  Elimination: Excretion of the metabolites in urine

Usual Dosage Children and Adults:
  Mucous membranes: Dosage varies depending on area to be anesthetized and vascularity of tissues
  Oral mouth/throat preparations: Do not administer for >2 days or in children <2 years of age, unless directed by a physician; refer to specific package labeling
  Otic: 4-5 drops into ear canal; may repeat every 1-2 hours as needed
  Topical: Apply to affected area as needed

Administration
  Mucous membranes: Apply to mucous membrane; do not eat for 1 hour after application to oral mucosa
  Otic: After instilling into external ear canal, insert cotton pledget into ear canal
  Topical: Apply evenly; do not apply to deep or puncture wounds or to serious burns

Patient Information Do not eat for 1 hour after application to oral mucosa; do not chew gum while mouth or throat is anesthetized due to potential biting trauma; do not overuse; do not apply to infected areas or to large areas of broken skin

Dosage Forms
  Topical for mucus membranes:
    Gel (Americaine® Anesthetic Lubricant, Hurricane®): 20% [Americaine® contains 0.1% benzethonium chloride; Hurricane® contains 60% alcohol] (2.5 g, 7 g, 30 g)
  Topical for skin disorders:
    Cream: 5% (30 g, 454 g)
    Liquid (Chiggertox®): 2% (30 mL)
    Ointment:
      Chiggerex®: 2% (52 g)
(Continued)

Benzocaine *(Continued)*

Foille® Medicated First Aid: 5% [with 0.1% chloroxylenol, benzyl alcohol; corn oil base] (3.5 g, 28 g)

Spray:

Foille®: 5% [with 0.63% chloroxylenol] (97.5 mL)

Americaine®, Hurricane®, Solarcaine®: 20% [Hurricane® is cherry flavor; Solarcaine® contains 0.13% triclosan, alcohol] (60 mL, 90 mL, 120 mL)

Mouth and throat preparations:

Gel:

Anbesol®: 6.3% (7.5 g)

HDA Toothache®: 6.5% [with benzyl alcohol] (15 mL)

Anbesol® Baby, Detane®, Numz-It®, Orajel® Baby: 7.5% (7.5 g, 10 g, 15 g)

Orajel® Denture, Orajel® Baby Nighttime, Zilactin®-B: 10% (6 g, 7.5 g, 10 g)

Anbesol® Maximum Strength, Orajel® Maximum Strength: 20% (7.5 g, 10.5 g)

Liquid:

Anbesol®, Orasol®: 6.3% [Anbesol® contains 0.5% phenol, povidone iodine, 70% alcohol, camphor, menthol] (9 mL, 15mL)

Orajel® Maximum Strength, Orajel® Mouth-Aid: 20% [Anbesol® Maximum Strength contains 50% alcohol; Orajel® Mouth-Aid contains 0.1% cetylpyridinium chloride, 70% alcohol, tartrazine, saccharin] (9 mL, 14 mL)

Lotion (Babee® Teething): 2.5% (15 mL)

Lozenges:

Trocaine®: 10 mg

Cylex®, Mycinettes®: 15 mg [Cylex contains 5 mg cetylpyrudinium chloride]

Ointment (Benzodent®): 20% (30 g)

Paste (Orabase® with benzocaine): 20% (5 g)

♦ **Benzocaine and Antipyrine** *see Antipyrine and Benzocaine on page 99*

♦ **Benzodent® [OTC]** *see Benzocaine on page 135*

Benzoyl Peroxide (BEN zoe il peer OKS ide)

U.S. Brand Names Advanced Formula Oxy® Sensitive Gel [OTC]; Ambi 10® [OTC]; Ben-Aqua® [OTC]; Benoxyl®; Benzac AC® Gel; Benzac AC® Wash; Benzac W® Gel; Benzac W® Wash; 5-Benzagel®; 10-Benzagel®; Benzashave® Cream; BlemErase® Lotion [OTC]; Brevoxyl® Gel; Clear By Design® Gel [OTC]; Clearsil® Maximum Strength [OTC]; Del Aqua-5® Gel; Del Aqua-10® Gel; Desquam-E® Gel; Desquam-X® Gel; Desquam-X® Wash; Dryox® Gel [OTC]; Dryox® Wash [OTC]; Exact® Cream [OTC]; Fostex® 10% BPO Gel [OTC]; Fostex® 10% Wash [OTC]; Fostex® Bar [OTC]; Loroxide® [OTC]; Neutrogena® Acne Mask [OTC]; Oxy-5® Advanced Formula for Sensitive Skin [OTC]; Oxy-5® Tinted [OTC]; Oxy-10® Advanced Formula for Sensitive Skin [OTC]; Oxy 10® Wash [OTC]; PanOxyl®-AQ; PanOxyl® Bar [OTC]; Perfectoderm® Gel [OTC]; Peroxin A5®; Peroxin A10®; Persa-Gel®; Theroxide® Wash [OTC]; Vanoxide® [OTC]

Canadian Brand Names Acetoxyl; Benoxyl; Clearasil B.P. Plus; Clear & Clean Persa; Dermacne; Dermoxyl; Neutrogena Acne Mask; Neutrogena On-The-Spot Acne Lotion; Oxyderm; Solugel

Therapeutic Category Acne Products; Topical Skin Product

Generic Available Yes

Use Adjunctive treatment of mild to moderate acne vulgaris

Pregnancy Risk Factor C

Contraindications Hypersensitivity to benzoyl peroxide, benzoic acid, or any component

Warnings Discontinue if burning, swelling, or undue dryness occurs

Precautions For external use only; may bleach colored fabrics; avoid contact with eyes, eyelids, lips, mucous membranes, and highly inflamed or denuded skin

Adverse Reactions

Dermatologic: Contact dermatitis

Local: Irritation, stinging, dryness, peeling, erythema

Mechanism of Action Releases free-radical oxygen which oxidizes bacterial proteins in the sebaceous follicles decreasing the number of anaerobic bacteria and irritating free fatty acids; exerts a keratolytic activity and a comedolytic effect

Pharmacokinetics

Absorption: ~5% through the skin

Metabolism: Major metabolite is benzoic acid

Elimination: In the urine as benzoate

Usual Dosage Children and Adults: Topical: Apply sparingly 1-3 times/day; initially apply for 15 minutes; length of exposure, strength, and frequency of application are increased as tolerated

Administration Topical: Shake lotion before using; cleanse skin before applying; for external use only; avoid contact with eyes and mucous membranes

Additional Information Granulation may indicate effectiveness; gels are more penetrating than creams and last longer than creams or lotions

Dosage Forms
Bar: 5% (113 g); 10% (106 g, 113 g)
Cream: 5% (18 g, 113.4 g); 10% (18 g, 28 g, 113.4 g)
Gel: 2.5% (30 g, 42.5 g, 45 g, 57 g, 60 g, 90 g, 113 g); 5% (42.5 g, 45 g, 60 g, 80 g, 90 g, 113.4 g); 10% (30 g, 42.5 g, 45 g, 56.7 g, 60 g, 90 g, 113.4 g, 120 g); 20% (30 g, 60 g)
Liquid: 5% (120 mL, 150 mL, 240 mL); 10% (120 mL, 150 mL, 240 mL)
Lotion: 5% (25 mL, 30 mL); 5.5% (25 mL); 10% (12 mL, 29 mL, 30 mL, 60 mL)
Mask: 5% (30 mL, 60 mL, 60 g)

References
Winston MH and Shalita AR, "Acne Vulgaris: Pathogenesis and Treatment," *Pediatr Clin North Am,* 1991, 38(4):889-903.

Benztropine (BENZ troe peen)

Related Information
Overdose and Toxicology *on page 1222*
U.S. Brand Names Cogentin®
Canadian Brand Names Apo-Benztropine; PMS-Benztropine
Therapeutic Category Anticholinergic Agent; Antidote, Drug-induced Dystonic Reactions; Anti-Parkinson's Agent
Generic Available Yes: Tablet
Use Adjunctive treatment of parkinsonism; also used in treatment of drug-induced extrapyramidal effects (except tardive dyskinesia) and acute dystonic reactions
Pregnancy Risk Factor C
Contraindications Hypersensitivity to benztropine mesylate or any component; children <3 years of age; patients with narrow-angle glaucoma, pyloric or duodenal obstruction, stenosing peptic ulcers; bladder neck obstructions; achalasia; myasthenia gravis
Precautions Use with caution in hot weather or during exercise; may cause anhydrosis and hyperthermia; increased risk of hyperthermia in alcoholics, patients with CNS disease, and with prolonged outdoor exposure
Adverse Reactions
Cardiovascular: Tachycardia, orthostatic hypotension, ventricular fibrillation, palpitations
Central nervous system: Drowsiness, nervousness, hallucinations, coma
Dermatologic: Dry skin, photosensitivity
Endocrine & metabolic: Decreased flow of breast milk
Gastrointestinal: Nausea, vomiting, xerostomia, constipation, dry throat, dysphagia
Neuromuscular & skeletal: Weakness
Ocular: Blurred vision, mydriasis, increased intraocular pain
Respiratory: Dry nose
Miscellaneous: Diaphoresis (decreased)
Drug Interactions As an anticholinergic, benztropine may potentiate the CNS depressant effects of CNS depressants; may inhibit the therapeutic response to neuroleptics; central and/or peripheral anticholinergic syndrome can occur when administered with amantadine, rimantadine, narcotic analgesics, phenothiazides, TCAs, quinidine, and antihistamines
Mechanism of Action Thought to partially block striatal cholinergic receptors to help balance cholinergic and dopaminergic activity
Pharmacodynamics
Onset of action:
Oral: Within 1 hour
Parenteral: Within 15 minutes
Duration of action: 6-48 hours
Usual Dosage
Drug-induced extrapyramidal reaction: Oral, I.M., I.V.:
Children >3 years: 0.02-0.05 mg/kg/dose 1-2 times/day; use in children <3 years should be reserved for life-threatening emergencies
Adults: 1-4 mg/dose 1-2 times/day
Acute dystonia: Adults: I.M., I.V.: 1-2 mg as a single dose
Parkinsonism: Oral: 0.5-6 mg/day in 1-2 divided doses; begin with 0.5 mg/day; increase in 0.5 mg increments at 5- to 6-day intervals to achieve the desired effect
Administration
Oral: Administer with food to decrease GI upset
(Continued)

Benztropine *(Continued)*

Parenteral: I.V. route should be reserved for situations when oral or I.M. are not appropriate

Patient Information Causes drowsiness and may impair ability to perform hazardous tasks requiring mental alertness

Dosage Forms

Injection, as mesylate: 1 mg/mL (2 mL)

Tablet, as mesylate: 0.5 mg, 1 mg, 2 mg

♦ **Benzylpenicillin Benzathine** *see* Penicillin G Benzathine *on page 770*

Benzylpenicilloyl-polylysine (BEN zil pen i SIL oyl pol i LIE seen)

U.S. Brand Names Pre-Pen®

Synonyms Penicilloyl-polylysine; PPL

Therapeutic Category Diagnostic Agent, Penicillin Allergy Skin Test

Generic Available No

Use Adjunct in assessing the risk of administering penicillin (penicillin or benzylpenicillin) in patients with a history of clinical penicillin hypersensitivity

Pregnancy Risk Factor C

Contraindications Patients known to be extremely hypersensitive to penicillin

Warnings PPL test alone has a sensitivity rate of 76% and does not identify those patients who react to a minor antigenic determinant; does not appear to reliably predict the occurrence of late reactions and patients at risk for anaphylaxis can be missed; PPL test alone is estimated to miss 3% to 6% of penicillin-allergic patients who are at risk for serious or fatal reactions

Adverse Reactions

Dermatologic: Erythema, urticaria

Local: Pruritus, wheal, edema

Miscellaneous: Systemic allergic reactions occur rarely

Drug Interactions Antihistamines, tricyclic antidepressants, and sympathomimetic agents may affect skin response

Stability Store in refrigerator; discard if left at room temperature for longer than 1 day

Mechanism of Action Elicits IgE antibodies which produce type I accelerated urticarial reactions to penicillins

Usual Dosage Children and Adults:

Scratch test: Use scratch technique with a 20-gauge needle to make 3-5 mm non-bleeding scratch on epidermis, apply a small drop of solution to scratch, rub in gently with applicator or toothpick. A positive reaction consists of a pale wheal surrounding the scratch site which develops within 10 minutes and ranges from 5-15 mm or more in diameter.

Intradermal test: Use intradermal test with a tuberculin syringe with a 26- to 30-gauge short bevel needle; a dose of 0.01-0.02 mL is injected intradermally. A control of NS should be injected at least 1½" from the PPL test site. Most skin responses to the intradermal test will develop within 5-15 minutes.

Interpretation:

(-) Negative: No reaction

(+/-) Equivocal: Wheal only slightly larger than original bleb with or without erythematous flare and larger than control site

(+) Positive: Itching and marked increase in size of original bleb

Control site should not exhibit any reaction

Administration Parenteral: PPL is administered by a scratch technique or by intradermal injection. For initial testing, PPL should always be applied via the scratch technique. Do not administer intradermally to patients who have positive reactions to a scratch test.

Nursing Implications Always use scratch test for initial testing

Additional Information Hydroxyzine and diphenhydramine should be discontinued for at least 4 days and astemizole for 6-8 weeks before skin testing

Dosage Forms Injection, for intradermal use or scratch test: 0.25 mL

References

Boguniewicz M and Leung DYM, "Hypersensitivity Reactions to Antibiotics Commonly Used in Children," *Pediatr Infect Dis J*, 1995, 14(3):221-31.

Beractant (ber AKT ant)

U.S. Brand Names Survanta®

Synonyms Bovine Lung Surfactant; Natural Lung Surfactant

Therapeutic Category Lung Surfactant

Generic Available No

Use Prevention and treatment of respiratory distress syndrome (RDS) in premature infants

Prophylactic therapy: Infants with body weight <1250 g who are at risk for developing or with evidence of surfactant deficiency

Rescue therapy: Treatment of infants with RDS confirmed by x-ray and requiring mechanical ventilation

Warnings Rapidly affects oxygenation and lung compliance and should be restricted to a highly supervised use in a clinical setting with immediate availability of clinicians experienced with intubation and ventilatory management of premature infants. If transient episodes of bradycardia and decreased oxygen saturation occur, discontinue the dosing procedure and initiate measures to alleviate the condition; produces rapid improvements in lung oxygenation and compliance that may require immediate reductions in ventilator settings and FiO_2.

Precautions Use of beractant in infants <600 g birth weight or >1750 g birth weight has not been evaluated

Adverse Reactions During the dosing procedure:

Cardiovascular: Transient bradycardia, vasoconstriction, hypotension, hypertension, pallor

Respiratory: Oxygen desaturation, endotracheal tube blockage, hypocarbia, hypercarbia, apnea, pulmonary air leaks, pulmonary interstitial emphysema, pulmonary hemorrhage

Miscellaneous: Increased probability of post-treatment nosocomial sepsis

Stability Refrigerate; protect from light; prior to administration warm by standing at room temperature for 20 minutes or hold in hand for 8 minutes; artificial warming methods should **not** be used; unused, unopened vials warmed to room temperature may be returned to the refrigerator within 8 hours of warming only once

Mechanism of Action Replaces deficient or ineffective endogenous lung surfactant in neonates with respiratory distress syndrome (RDS) or in neonates at risk of developing RDS. Surfactant prevents the alveoli from collapsing during expiration by lowering surface tension between air and alveolar surfaces.

Usual Dosage Intratracheal: Neonates:

Prophylactic treatment: Give 4 mL/kg as soon as possible; as many as 4 doses may be administered during the first 48 hours of life, no more frequently than 6 hours apart. The need for additional doses is determined by evidence of continuing respiratory distress or if the infant is still intubated and requiring at least 30% inspired oxygen to maintain a PaO_2 ≤80 torr.

Rescue treatment: Give 4 mL/kg as soon as the diagnosis of RDS is made; may repeat if needed, no more frequently than every 6 hours to a maximum of 4 doses

Administration Intratracheal: For intratracheal administration only. Do not shake; if settling occurs during storage, gently swirl. Suction infant prior to administration; inspect solution to verify complete mixing of the suspension. Administer intratracheally by instillation through a 5-French end-hole catheter inserted into the infant's endotracheal tube. Administer the dose in four 1 mL/kg aliquots. Each quarter-dose is instilled over 2-3 seconds; each quarter-dose is administered with the infant in a different position; slightly downward inclination with head turned to the right, then repeat with head turned to the left; then slightly upward inclination with head turned to the right, then repeat with head turned to the left.

Monitoring Parameters Continuous heart rate and transcutaneous O_2 saturation should be monitored during administration; frequent ABG sampling is necessary to prevent postdosing hyperoxia and hypocarbia.

Dosage Forms Suspension: 25 mg/mL (4 mL, 8 mL)

♦ **Betacort (Can)** see Betamethasone on page 140
♦ **Betaderm (Can)** see Betamethasone on page 140
♦ **Betadine® First Aid Antibiotics + Moisturizer [OTC]** see Bacitracin and Polymyxin B on page 129
♦ **9-Beta-D-ribofuranosyladenine** see Adenosine on page 40
♦ **Betagan® Liquifilm®** see Levobunolol on page 584

Betaine Anhydrous (BAY tayne an HY drus)

U.S. Brand Names Cystadane®

Therapeutic Category Homocystinuria, Treatment Agent

Generic Available No

Use Treatment of homocystinuria

Pregnancy Risk Factor C

Contraindications Hypersensitivity to betaine or any component

Adverse Reactions Gastrointestinal: Nausea, vomiting, diarrhea, GI distress

(Continued)

Betaine Anhydrous *(Continued)*

Mechanism of Action Betaine reduces homocysteine blood concentrations by acting as a methyl group donor in the remethylation of homocysteine to methionine

Usual Dosage Oral:

Children <3 years: 100 mg/kg/day divided into 2 doses; increase at weekly intervals in 100 mg/kg/day increments

Children ≥3 years and Adults: 3 g twice daily; doses up to 20 g/day have been needed to control homocysteine plasma concentrations in some patients

Administration Oral: Shake bottle lightly before opening; measure prescribed amount with provided measuring scoop and dissolve in 4-6 ounces of water, juice, milk, or formula; administer immediately; do not use if powder does not completely dissolve or gives a colored solution

Monitoring Parameters Plasma homocysteine concentration (should be low or undetectable)

Additional Information Orphan drug; may only be obtained by contacting Chronimed Inc at 1-800-900-4267; vitamin B_6, vitamin B_{12}, and folate have been helpful in the management of homocystinuria and are often used in conjunction

Dosage Forms Powder: 1 g/scoop (1 scoop = 1.7 mL) (180 g)

♦ **Betaject (Can)** *see Betamethasone on page 140*
♦ **Betaloc (Can)** *see Metoprolol on page 660*
♦ **Betaloc Durules (Can)** *see Metoprolol on page 660*

Betamethasone (bay ta METH a sone)

Related Information

Corticosteroids Comparison, Topical *on page 1068*

U.S. Brand Names Alphatrex®; Betatrex®; Beta-Val®; Celestone®; Celestone® Phosphate; Celestone® Soluspan®; Diprolene®; Diprolene® AF; Diprosone®; Luxiq™; Maxivate®

Canadian Brand Names Betacort; Betaderm; Betaject; Betnesol; Betnovate; Celestoderm; Diprolene Glycol; Ectosone; Prevex B; Rivasone; Rolene; Rosone; Taro-Sone; Topilene; Topisone

Synonyms Flubenisolone

Therapeutic Category Adrenal Corticosteroid; Anti-inflammatory Agent; Corticosteroid, Systemic; Corticosteroid, Topical; Glucocorticoid

Generic Available Yes

Use Anti-inflammatory; immunosuppressant agent; corticosteroid replacement therapy

Topical: Inflammatory dermatoses such as psoriasis, seborrheic or atopic dermatitis, neurodermatitis, inflammatory phase of xerosis, late phase of allergic dermatitis or irritant dermatitis; Foam: Inflammatory and pruritic symptoms of scalp dermatoses responsive to corticosteroids

Pregnancy Risk Factor C

Contraindications Systemic fungal infections; hypersensitivity to betamethasone or any component

Precautions Use with caution in patients with hypothyroidism, cirrhosis, ulcerative colitis; use topical products sparingly in children, systemic effects may be seen

Adverse Reactions

Cardiovascular: Edema, hypertension

Central nervous system: Convulsions, vertigo, confusion, headache

Dermatologic: Thin fragile skin, hyperpigmentation or hypopigmentation, acne, impaired wound healing

Endocrine & metabolic: Cushingoid state, sodium retention, potential pituitary-adrenal axis suppression, potential growth suppression, glucose intolerance, hypokalemia

Gastrointestinal: Peptic ulcer, nausea, vomiting

Local: Burning, itching, stinging, sterile abscess

Neuromuscular & skeletal: Muscle weakness, osteoporosis, fractures

Ocular: Cataracts, glaucoma

Drug Interactions Cytochrome P-450 isoenzyme CYP3A substrate

Barbiturates, phenytoin and rifampin will decrease corticosteroid effects; salicylates; NSAIDs; diuretics (potassium depleting); caffeine and alcohol may increase risk for GI ulcer; with systemic use: Live virus vaccines (increase risk of viral infection), vaccines may have decreased effects

Food Interactions Systemic use of corticosteroids may require a diet with increased potassium, vitamins A, B_6, C, D, folate, calcium, zinc, and phosphorus and decreased sodium

Stability Foam canister is flammable; store at controlled room temperature; avoid fire, flame, heat; do not store at >120°F (49°C)

Mechanism of Action Controls the rate of protein synthesis, depresses the migration of polymorphonuclear leukocytes and fibroblasts, reverses capillary permeability, and causes lysosomal stabilization at the cellular level to prevent or control inflammation

Pharmacokinetics
Protein binding: 64%
Metabolism: Hepatic
Elimination: <5% of dose excreted renally as unchanged drug; small amounts eliminated via biliary tract

Usual Dosage Base dosage on severity of disease and patient response
Children: Use lowest dose listed as initial dose for adrenocortical insufficiency (physiologic replacement)
I.M.: 0.0175-0.125 mg base/kg/day divided every 6-12 hours **or** 0.5-7.5 mg base/m^2/day divided every 6-12 hours
Oral: 0.0175-0.25 mg/kg/day divided every 6-8 hours **or** 0.5-7.5 mg/m^2/day divided every 6-8 hours
Adolescents and Adults:
I.M.: 0.6-9 mg/day divided every 12-24 hours
Oral: 2.4-4.8 mg/day in 2-4 doses; range: 0.6-7.2 mg/day
Children and Adults: Topical: Apply thin film 1-3 times/day
Adolescents ≥16 years and Adults: Topical, foam: Apply twice daily (in morning and at night)

Administration
Oral: Administer with food to decrease GI effects
Parenteral: Do not administer injectable suspension I.V.; shake injectable suspension before use
Topical: Apply sparingly, rub in gently until it disappears; do not apply to face or inguinal areas; not for use on broken skin or in areas of infection
Foam: Invert can, dispense small amount of foam onto saucer or other cool surface; foam will melt upon contact with warm skin (do not dispense directly into hands); use fingers to apply small amounts of foam to affected scalp area; rub in gently until it disappears; avoid fire, flame, or smoking during use; contents of can are flammable and under pressure

Test Interactions Skin tests

Patient Information Topical use: Avoid contact with eyes; do not use occlusive dressings unless directed by physician

Additional Information Medium to high potency topical corticosteroid; long-acting corticosteroid with minimal or no sodium-retaining potential

Dosage Forms
Base (Celestone®):
Syrup: 0.6 mg/5 mL (120 mL)
Tablet: 0.6 mg
Dipropionate (Alphatrex®, Diprosone®, Maxivate®):
Cream: 0.05% (15 g, 45 g)
Lotion: 0.05% (20 mL, 30 mL, 60 mL)
Ointment, topical: 0.05% (15 g, 45 g)
Dipropionate, augmented (Diprolene®, Diprolene® AF):
Cream, emollient base: 0.05% (15 g, 45 g)
Gel, topical: 0.05% (15 g, 45 g)
Lotion: 0.05% (30 mL, 60 mL)
Ointment, topical: 0.05% (15 g, 45 g)
Valerate (Betatrex®, Beta-Val®):
Cream: 0.1% (15 g, 45 g)
Foam (Luxiq™): 0.12% (100 g)
Lotion: 0.1% (60 mL)
Ointment, topical: 0.1% (15 g, 45 g)
Sodium phosphate (Celestone® Phosphate):
Injection: Equivalent to 3 mg/mL betamethasone base (5 mL)
Sodium phosphate and acetate (Celestone® Soluspan®):
Injection, suspension: 6 mg/mL [3 mg betamethasone as betamethasone sodium phosphate and 3 mg betamethasone acetate per mL] (5 mL)

♦ **Betapen®-VK** *see* Penicillin V Potassium *on page 774*
♦ **Betasept® [OTC]** *see* Chlorhexidine Gluconate *on page 220*
♦ **Beta-Tim (Can)** *see* Timolol *on page 962*
♦ **Betatrex®** *see* Betamethasone *on page 140*
♦ **Beta-Val®** *see* Betamethasone *on page 140*

♦ **Betaxin (Can)** see Thiamine *on page 948*

Bethanechol (be THAN e kole)

U.S. Brand Names Urecholine®

Canadian Brand Names Duvoid; Myotonachol; PMS-Bethanechol Chloride

Therapeutic Category Cholinergic Agent

Generic Available Yes: Tablet

Use Treatment of nonobstructive urinary retention and retention due to neurogenic bladder; gastroesophageal reflux

Pregnancy Risk Factor C

Contraindications Hypersensitivity to bethanechol chloride or any component; do not use in patients with mechanical obstruction of the GI or GU tract; do not use in patients with hyperthyroidism, peptic ulcer, bronchial asthma, or cardiac disease; contraindicated for I.M. or I.V. use due to severe cholinergic activity

Adverse Reactions

Cardiovascular: Hypotension, cardiac arrest, flushed skin (vasomotor response)

Central nervous system: Headache

Gastrointestinal: Abdominal cramps, diarrhea, nausea, vomiting, salivation

Genitourinary: Urinary frequency

Hepatic: Elevated liver enzymes, increased bilirubin

Ocular: Miosis, lacrimation

Respiratory: Bronchial constriction

Miscellaneous: Diaphoresis

Drug Interactions Ganglionic blockers may cause a critical fall in blood pressure; additive effects with other cholinergic agents, epinephrine, and other sympathomimetics; quinidine and procainamide may antagonize cholinergic effects

Mechanism of Action Stimulates cholinergic receptors in the smooth muscle of the urinary bladder and GI tract resulting in increased peristalsis, increased GI and pancreatic secretions, bladder muscle contraction, and increased ureteral peristaltic waves

Pharmacodynamics

Onset of action:

Oral 30-90 minutes

S.C.: 5-15 minutes

Duration:

Oral: Up to 6 hours

S.C.: 2 hours

Pharmacokinetics

Absorption: Oral: Variable

Metabolic fate and excretion have not been determined

Usual Dosage

Children:

Oral:

Abdominal distention or urinary retention: 0.6 mg/kg/day divided 3-4 times/day

Gastroesophageal reflux: 0.1-0.2 mg/kg/dose or 3 mg/m^2/dose given 30 minutes to 1 hour before each meal to a maximum of 4 times/day

S.C.: 0.12-0.2 mg/kg/day divided 3-4 times/day

Adults:

Oral: 10-50 mg 2-4 times/day

S.C.: 2.5-5 mg 3-4 times/day, up to 7.5-10 mg every 4 hours for neurogenic bladder

Administration

Oral: Administer on an empty stomach to reduce nausea and vomiting

Parenteral: For S.C. injection only; do not administer I.M. or I.V.

Patient Information Dizziness, lightheadedness, or fainting may occur especially when getting up from a lying position

Dosage Forms

Injection, as chloride: 5 mg/mL (1 mL)

Tablet, as chloride: 5 mg, 10 mg, 25 mg, 50 mg

Extemporaneous Preparations

An oral solution of bethanechol 1 mg/mL diluted in sterile water for irrigation is stable for at least 30 days refrigerated (Schlatter, 1997).

A 5 mg/mL suspension may be made by crushing twelve 50 mg tablets; add to a total volume of 120 mL of a 1:1 mixture of Ora-Plus®:Ora-Sweet® or Ora-Plus®:Ora-Sweet® SF; stable 60 days refrigerated; label "shake well" and protect from light (Allen, 1998).

Allen LV Jr and Erickson MA, "Stability of Bethanechol Chloride, Pyrazinamide, Quinidine Sulfate, Rifampin, and Tetracycline Hydrochloride in Extemporaneously Compounded Oral Liquids," *Am J Health Syst Pharm*, 1998, 55(17):1804-9.

Schlatter JL and Saulnier J, "Bethanechol Chloride Oral Solutions: Stability and Use in Infants," *Ann Pharmacother*, 31:294-296, 1997.

♦ **Betimol**® *see* Timolol *on page 962*
♦ **Betnesol (Can)** *see* Betamethasone *on page 140*
♦ **Betnovate (Can)** *see* Betamethasone *on page 140*
♦ **Biaxin**® *see* Clarithromycin *on page 247*
♦ **Biaxin**® **XL** *see* Clarithromycin *on page 247*
♦ **Bicillin**® **L-A** *see* Penicillin G Benzathine *on page 770*
♦ **Bicitra**® *see* Citrate and Citric Acid *on page 244*
♦ **BiCNU**®, **Gliadel**® *see* Carmustine *on page 182*
♦ **Biltricide**® *see* Praziquantel *on page 819*
♦ **Biobase (Can)** *see* Ethyl Alcohol *on page 409*
♦ **Biocef**® *see* Cephalexin *on page 207*
♦ **Bioderm (Can)** *see* Bacitracin and Polymyxin B *on page 129*
♦ **Biomox**® *see* Amoxicillin *on page 80*
♦ **Bio-Tab**® *see* Doxycycline *on page 362*

Biotin (BYE oh tin)

U.S. Brand Names Biotin® Forte [OTC]; d-Biotin [OTC]; Meribin [OTC]
Therapeutic Category Biotinidase Deficiency, Treatment Agent; Nutritional Supplement; Vitamin, Water Soluble
Generic Available Yes
Use Treatment of primary biotinidase deficiency; nutritional biotin deficiency; component of the vitamin B complex
Contraindications Hypersensitivity to biotin or any component
Food Interactions Large amounts of raw egg whites prevent biotin absorption
Mechanism of Action A member of the B-complex group of vitamins; biotin is required for various metabolic functions such as gluconeogenesis, lipogenesis, fatty acid biosynthesis, propionate metabolism, and the catabolism of branched-chain amino acids; there are 9 known biotin-dependent enzymes; the enzyme biotinidase regenerates biotin in the body and is also required for the release of dietary protein-bound biotin.

Biotinidase deficiency is an autosomal recessively inherited metabolic disorder characterized by deficient activity of the enzyme in serum. Children with the disorder usually exhibit seizures, hypotonia, ataxia, skin rash, alopecia, metabolic ketoacidosis, and organic aciduria.

Usual Dosage Oral:
RDA: Infants, Children, and Adults: There is no official RDA, however 100-200 mcg/day is considered adequate
Biotinidase deficiency: Neonates, Infants, Children, and Adults: 5-10 mg once daily
Biotin deficiency: Children and Adults: 5-20 mg once daily
Administration Oral: May be administered without regard to meals
Reference Range Serum biotinidase activity
Dosage Forms
Capsule: 5 mg
Tablet: 300 mcg, 2.5 mg, 3 mg, 5 mg, 10 mg
References

McVoy JR, Levy HL, Lawler M, et al, "Partial Biotinidase Deficiency: Clinical and Biochemical Features," 1990, *J Pediatr*, 116(1):78-83.
Salbert BA, Pellock JM, and Wolf B, "Characterization of Seizures Associated With Biotinidase Deficiency," *Neurology*, 1993, 43(7):1351-5.
Wastell HJ, Bartlett K, Dale G, et al, "Biotinidase Deficiency: A Survey of 10 Cases," *Arch Dis Child*, 1988, 63(10):1244-9.

♦ **Biotin**® **Forte [OTC]** *see* Biotin *on page 143*
♦ **Biquin (Can)** *see* Quinidine *on page 860*
♦ **Bisac-Evac**® **[OTC]** *see* Bisacodyl *on page 143*

Bisacodyl (bis a KOE dil)

U.S. Brand Names Bisac-Evac® [OTC]; Bisacodyl Uniserts®; Bisco-Lax® [OTC]; Carter's Little Pills® [OTC]; Clysodrast®; Dacodyl® [OTC]; Deficol® [OTC]; Dulcolax® [OTC]; Fleet® Laxative [OTC]
Canadian Brand Names Apo-Bisacodyl; Bisacolax; Feen-A-Mint; Soflax EX
(Continued)

Bisacodyl *(Continued)*

Therapeutic Category Laxative, Stimulant

Generic Available Yes

Use Treatment of constipation; colonic evacuation prior to procedures or examination

Pregnancy Risk Factor C

Contraindications Hypersensitivity to bisacodyl or any component; do not use in patients with abdominal pain, appendicitis, obstruction, nausea or vomiting; not to be used during pregnancy or lactation

Warnings Safety of bisacodyl tannex usage in children <10 years of age has not been established

Precautions Bisacodyl tannex powder for preparation as a rectal solution should be used with caution in patients with ulceration of the colon

Adverse Reactions

Endocrine & metabolic: Electrolyte and fluid imbalance (metabolic acidosis or alkalosis, hypocalcemia)

Gastrointestinal: Abdominal cramps, nausea, vomiting, diarrhea, rectal burning, proctitis (rare)

Food Interactions Administration within 1 hour of ingesting antacids, alkaline material, milk, or dairy products will cause premature dissolution of the enteric coating and resultant gastric irritation

Stability Store enteric-coated tablets and rectal suppositories at <30°C. Reconstituted bisacodyl tannex solution should be used immediately after preparation.

Mechanism of Action Stimulates peristalsis by directly irritating the smooth muscle of the intestine, possibly the colonic intramural plexus; alters water and electrolyte secretion producing net intestinal fluid accumulation and laxation

Pharmacodynamics Onset of action:

Oral: Within 6-10 hours

Rectal: 15-60 minutes

Pharmacokinetics

Absorption: Oral, rectal: <5% absorbed systemically

Metabolism: In the liver

Elimination: Conjugated metabolites excreted in breast milk, bile, and urine

Usual Dosage

Bisacodyl (Dulcolax®) tablet: Oral:

Children 3-12 years: 5-10 mg or 0.3 mg/kg/day as a single dose

Children ≥12 years and Adults: 5-15 mg/day as a single dose

Bisacodyl (Dulcolax®) suppository: Rectal:

Children:

<2 years: 5 mg/day as a single dose

2-11 years: 5-10 mg/day as a single dose

Children ≥12 years and Adults: 10 mg/day as a single dose

Administration Oral: Administer on an empty stomach with water; patient should swallow tablet whole; do not break or chew enteric-coated tablet; do not administer within 1 hour of ingesting antacids, alkaline material, milk, or dairy products

Patient Information Should not be used regularly for more than 1 week

Additional Information In a randomized prospective study of 70 patients, bisacodyl tablets were given orally once daily in the morning for 2 days before colonoscopy to 19 patients (dose for children <5 years: 5 mg; 5-12 years: 10 mg; >12 years: 15 mg) with a Fleet® enema given on the morning of the procedure without any dietary restriction. Results showed that bisacodyl without dietary restriction provided unsatisfactory colon cleansing.

Dosage Forms

Enema: 10 mg/30 mL

Powder: 1.5 mg with tannic acid 2.5 g per packet (25s, 50s)

Suppository, rectal: 5 mg, 10 mg

Tablet, enteric coated: 5 mg

References

BaKer SS, Liptak GS, Colletti RB, et al, "Constipation in Infants and Children: Evaluation and Treatment," 2000, www.naspgn.org/constipation.

Dahshan A, Lin CH, Peters J, et al, "A Randomized, Prospective Study to Evaluate the Efficacy and Acceptance of Three Bowel Preparations for Colonoscopy in Children," *Am J Gastroenterol*, 1999, 94(12):3497-501.

♦ **Bisacodyl Uniserts®** *see* Bisacodyl *on page 143*

♦ **Bisacolax (Can)** *see* Bisacodyl *on page 143*

♦ **Bisco-Lax® [OTC]** *see* Bisacodyl *on page 143*

♦ **Bismatrol® [OTC]** *see* Bismuth *on page 145*

Bismuth (BIZ muth)

U.S. Brand Names Bismatrol® [OTC]; Pepto-Bismol® [OTC]

Synonyms BSS

Therapeutic Category Antidiarrheal; Gastrointestinal Agent, Gastric or Duodenal Ulcer Treatment

Generic Available Yes

Use Symptomatic treatment of mild, nonspecific diarrhea including traveler's diarrhea; chronic infantile diarrhea; adjunctive treatment of *Helicobacter pylori*-associated antral gastritis

Pregnancy Risk Factor C (D in 3rd trimester)

Contraindications Do not use subsalicylate in patients with influenza or chickenpox because of risk of Reye's syndrome; do not use in patients with hypersensitivity to salicylates; history of severe GI bleeding or coagulopathy

Warnings Subsalicylate should be used with caution if patient is taking aspirin, due to additive toxicity; use with caution in children <3 years of age and those with viral illness; be aware of salicylate content when prescribing for use in children

Precautions May interfere with radiologic examinations of GI tract as bismuth is radiopaque

Adverse Reactions
Central nervous system: Anxiety, confusion, slurred speech, headache, mental depression

Gastrointestinal: Impaction (infants and debilitated patients), grayish-black stools, darkened tongue

Neuromuscular & skeletal: Muscle spasms, weakness

Otic: Tinnitus, loss of hearing

Drug Interactions Decreases absorption of tetracycline; increases toxicity of aspirin (due to absorption of salicylate), warfarin, hypoglycemics

Mechanism of Action Adsorbs extra water in large intestine, as well as toxins; forms a protective coat on the intestinal mucosa; appears to have antisecretory (salicylate moiety) and antimicrobial effects (bismuth moiety) against bacterial and viral pathogens

Pharmacokinetics
Absorption: Bismuth is minimally absorbed (<1%) across the GI tract while salicylate salt is readily absorbed (80%)

Distribution: Salicylate: V_d: 170 mL/kg

Protein binding, plasma: Bismuth and salicylate: >90%

Metabolism: Bismuth salts undergo chemical dissociation after oral administration; salicylate is extensively metabolized in the liver

Half-life:
Bismuth: Terminal: 21-72 days
Salicylate: Terminal: 2-5 hours

Elimination:
Bismuth: Renal, biliary
Salicylate: Only 10% excreted unchanged in urine

Usual Dosage Oral (bismuth subsalicylate liquid dosages expressed in mL of 262 mg/15 mL concentration):
Nonspecific diarrhea: Bismuth subsalicylate: 100 mg/kg/day divided into 5 equal doses for 5 days (maximum: 4.19 g/day) **or**
Children: Up to 8 doses/24 hours:
3-6 years: $^1/_3$ tablet or 5 mL every 30 minutes to 1 hour as needed
6-9 years: $^2/_3$ tablet or 10 mL every 30 minutes to 1 hour as needed
9-12 years: 1 tablet or 15 mL every 30 minutes to 1 hour as needed
Adults: 2 tablets or 30 mL every 30 minutes to 1 hour as needed up to 8 doses/24 hours

Chronic infantile diarrhea: Bismuth subsalicylate:
2-24 months: 2.5 mL every 4 hours
24-48 months: 5 mL every 4 hours
48-70 months: 10 mL every 4 hours

Prevention of traveler's diarrhea: Adults:
Bismuth subgallate: 1-2 tablets 3 times/day with meals
Bismuth subsalicylate: 2.1 g/day or 2 tablets 4 times/day before meals and at bedtime

Helicobacter pylori-associated antral gastritis: Bismuth subsalicylate: Dosage in children is not well established, the following dosages have been used [in conjunction with ampicillin and metronidazole or (in adults) tetracycline and metronidazole]:
Children ≤10 years: 15 mL (262 mg) 4 times/day for 6 weeks
Children >10 years and Adults: 30 mL of 262 mg/15 mL solution or two 262 mg tablets 4 times/day for 6 weeks
(Continued)

Bismuth *(Continued)*

Dosing adjustment in renal impairment: Avoid use in patients with renal failure

Administration Oral: Shake liquid well before using; chew tablets or allow to dissolve in mouth before swallowing

Test Interactions Bismuth absorbs x-rays and may interfere with diagnostic procedures of GI tract

Patient Information May darken stools; if diarrhea persists for more than 2 days, consult a physician; may turn tongue black

Additional Information Bismuth subsalicylate: 262 mg = 130 mg nonaspirin salicylate; 525 mg = 236 mg nonaspirin salicylate

Dosage Forms
Liquid, as subsalicylate: 262 mg/15 mL (120 mL, 240 mL, 360 mL, 480 mL); 525 mg/ 15 mL (maximum strength) (120 mL, 240 mL, 360 mL)
Tablet, chewable, as subsalicylate: 262 mg

References
Drumm B, Sherman P, Karmali M, et al, "Treatment of *Campylobacter pylori*-associated Antral Gastritis in Children With Bismuth Subsalicylate and Ampicillin," *J Pediatr,* 1988, 113(5):908-12.
Soriano-Brucher HE, Avendano P, O'Ryan M, et al, "Use of Bismuth Subsalicylate in Acute Diarrhea in Children," *Rev Infect Dis,* 1990, 12(Suppl 1):S51-5.
Walsh JH and Peterson WL, "The Treatment of *Helicobacter pylori* Infection in the Management of Peptic Ulcer Disease," *N Engl J Med,* 1995, 333(15):984-91.

♦ **Bistropamide** *see* Tropicamide *on page 991*

Bitolterol *(bye TOLE ter ole)*

Related Information
Asthma Guidelines *on page 1210*

U.S. Brand Names Tornalate®

Therapeutic Category Adrenergic Agonist Agent; Antiasthmatic; Beta$_2$-Adrenergic Agonist Agent; Bronchodilator; Sympathomimetic

Use Prevention and treatment of bronchial asthma and bronchospasm

Pregnancy Risk Factor C

Contraindications Hypersensitivity to bitolterol or any component

Warnings Excessive use may result in cardiac arrest and death

Precautions Use with caution in patients with unstable vasomotor symptoms, diabetes, hyperthyroidism, prostatic hypertrophy or a history of seizures, cardiovascular disorders such as coronary artery disease, arrhythmias, and hypertension; do not use concurrently with other sympathomimetic bronchodilators

Adverse Reactions
Cardiovascular: Flushing of face, hypertension, pounding heartbeat, chest pain, arrhythmias, tachycardia
Central nervous system: Dizziness, lightheadedness, nervousness, insomnia
Gastrointestinal: Xerostomia, nausea, unpleasant taste, mouth and throat irritation
Neuromuscular & skeletal: Tremors, hyperkinesia, paresthesia
Respiratory: Bronchial irritation, coughing, paradoxical bronchospasm

Drug Interactions Bitolterol decreases the effects of beta-adrenergic blockers (eg, propranolol); inhaled ipratropium may increase duration of bronchodilation; nifedipine may increase FEV-1; increased toxicity with MAO inhibitors, tricyclic antidepressants, sympathomimetic agents, inhaled anesthetics (eg, enflurane)

Stability Solution for nebulization should not be mixed with cromolyn sodium or acetylcysteine; stability when mixed with other nebulized drugs has not been established

Mechanism of Action Bitolterol, a prodrug, undergoes hydrolysis in the lungs to the active agent, colterol. Colterol selectively stimulates beta$_2$-adrenergic receptors in the lungs producing bronchial smooth muscle relaxation. Colterol possesses minor beta$_1$ activity.

Pharmacodynamics
Onset of effect: After oral inhalation: 3-5 minutes
Maximum effect: 0.5-2 hours
Duration of action: 4-8 hours

Pharmacokinetics Since blood levels of colterol (active drug) are too low to be measured by currently available assay methods, the pharmacokinetics of this agent following inhalation are not known.

Usual Dosage Children >12 years and Adults:
Bronchospasm: Oral inhalation: 2 inhalations at an interval of at least 1-3 minutes, followed by a third inhalation if needed
Prevention of bronchospasm: Oral inhalation: 2 inhalations every 8 hours; maximum daily dosage: 3 inhalations every 6 hours or 2 inhalations every 4 hours

Intermittent nebulization: 1 mg (0.5 mL) [range: 0.5-1.5 mg (0.25-0.75 mL)] every 8 hours; treatments may be increased to four times daily, however, the interval between treatments should **not** be less than 4 hours; a dosage of 2 mg (1 mL) may be used in severely obstructed patients; maximum daily dosage: 8 mg (4 mL)

Continuous flow nebulization: 2.5 mg (1.25 mL) 3 times/day [range: 1.5-3.5 mg (0.75-1.75 mL)]; maximum daily dosage 14 mg (7 mL); treatments should be at least 4 hours apart

Administration

Oral inhalation: Shake canister well before use; administer pressurized inhalation during the second half of inspiration, as the airways are open and the aerosol distribution is more extensive. If more than one inhalation per dose is necessary, wait at least 1 full minute between inhalations - second inhalation is best delivered after 10 minutes. Administer every 8 hours rather than 3 times/day, to promote less variation in peak and trough serum levels

Nebulization: Dilute with NS to a total volume of 2-4 mL prior to use; after adding to nebulizer reservoir, swirl contents gently; the patient should breathe deeply until the nebulizer chamber is empty (approximately 5-15 minutes)

Monitoring Parameters Assess lung sounds, heart rate, respiratory rate, peak flow; arterial or capillary blood gases (if patient's condition warrants)

Patient Information Do not exceed recommended dosage, excessive use may lead to adverse effects or loss of effectiveness. May cause nervousness, restlessness, and insomnia; if these effects continue after dosage reduction, notify physician. Also notify physician if palpitations, tachycardia, chest pain, muscle tremors, dizziness, headache, flushing, or if breathing difficulty persists.

Dosage Forms

Aerosol, oral, as mesylate: 0.8% [370 mcg/metered spray, 300 inhalations] (15 mL)

Solution, inhalation, as mesylate: 0.2% (10 mL, 30 mL, 60 mL)

♦ **Black Draught® [OTC]** *see* Senna *on page 896*

♦ **BlemErase® Lotion [OTC]** *see* Benzoyl Peroxide *on page 136*

♦ **Blemish Control (Can)** *see* Salicylic Acid *on page 886*

♦ **Blenoxane®** *see* Bleomycin *on page 147*

Bleomycin (blee oh MYE sin)

Related Information

Emetogenic Potential of Single Chemotherapeutic Agents *on page 1129*

U.S. Brand Names Blenoxane®

Synonyms BLM

Therapeutic Category Antineoplastic Agent, Antibiotic

Generic Available Yes

Use Palliative treatment of squamous cell carcinoma, testicular carcinoma, and germ cell tumors; Hodgkin's lymphoma, non-Hodgkin's lymphoma, renal carcinoma, and soft tissue sarcoma; sclerosing agent to control malignant effusions

Pregnancy Risk Factor D

Contraindications Hypersensitivity to bleomycin sulfate or any component

Warnings The FDA currently recommends that procedures for proper handling and disposal of antineoplastic agents be considered. Occurrence of pulmonary fibrosis is higher in elderly patients and in those receiving a total cumulative dose >400 units; pulmonary toxicity has occurred at a total dosage <200 units or 250 units/m^2 in younger patients; pulmonary irradiation and use of supplemental oxygen increase the chance for developing toxic pulmonary reactions in patients previously treated with bleomycin; a severe idiosyncratic reaction consisting of hypotension, mental confusion, fever, chills, and wheezing is possible.

Precautions Use with caution in patients with renal or pulmonary impairment; dosage modification is recommended in patients with renal impairment; dosage modification may be necessary in patients with a 20% decrease from baseline in FEV_1, FVC, or DL_{co}; administer test dose to lymphoma patients prior to starting therapy

Adverse Reactions

Cardiovascular: Cerebrovascular accident, hypotension, Raynaud's phenomenon

Central nervous system: Fever, chills, malaise

Dermatologic: Hyperpigmentation, hyperkeratosis of hands and nails, rash, alopecia, desquamation

Gastrointestinal: Stomatitis, vomiting, anorexia, mild nausea

Hematologic: Thrombocytopenia, leukopenia

Local: Phlebitis

(Continued)

Bleomycin *(Continued)*

Respiratory: Interstitial pneumonitis (10%), pulmonary fibrosis (cumulative lifetime dose should not exceed 400 units or 250 units/m^2 in younger patients), dyspnea, tachypnea, nonproductive cough, rales

Miscellaneous: Anaphylactoid reactions

Drug Interactions Phenytoin (decreases phenytoin concentrations), cisplatin (decreases bleomycin clearance), bleomycin may decrease digoxin absorption; concurrent use with amphotericin B products may increase nephrotoxicity and risk for hypotension and bronchospasm

Stability Refrigerate; intact vials are stable 28 days at room temperature; reconstituted solution is stable for 24 hours at room temperature; incompatible with amino acid solutions, ascorbic acid, cefazolin, furosemide, diazepam, hydrocortisone, mitomycin, nafcillin, penicillin G, aminophylline, copper; dilution in dextrose solutions may result in a 10% loss of activity within 24 hours

Mechanism of Action Inhibits synthesis of DNA; binds to DNA leading to single- and double-strand breaks by a Fe^{++}-O$_2$-catalyzed free radical reaction

Pharmacokinetics

Distribution: Into skin, lungs, kidneys, peritoneum, and lymphatics

Protein binding: <10%

Half-life: Dependent upon renal function

Children: 2.1-3.5 hours

Adults, with normal renal function: 2-3 hours

Time to peak serum concentration: I.M.: Within 30-60 minutes

Elimination: 60% to 70% of a dose excreted in the urine as active drug

Dialysis: Not removed by hemodialysis

Usual Dosage Refer to individual protocol

Children and Adults:

I.M., I.V., S.C.:

Test dose for lymphoma patients: 1-2 units of bleomycin for the first 2 doses; monitor vital signs every 15 minutes; wait a minimum of 1 hour before administering remainder of dose

Treatment: 10-20 units/m^2 (0.25-0.5 units/kg) 1-2 times/week in combination regimens or once every 2-4 weeks

Germ cell tumors: 15 units/m^2/dose once weekly for 3 weeks per regimen

Hodgkin's disease: 10 units/m^2/dose on days 1 and 15 of cycle

I.V. continuous infusion: 15-20 units/m^2/day over 24 hours for 3-5 days

Adults: Intracavitary injection for pleural effusion: 15-60 units (dose generally does not exceed 1 unit/kg); drug is diluted with 50-100 mL of NS and is instilled into the pleural cavity via a thoracostomy tube

Dosing adjustment in renal impairment:

Cl$_{cr}$ 25-50 mL/minute: Reduce dose by 25%

Cl$_{cr}$ <25 mL/minute: Reduce dose by 50% to 75%

Administration Parenteral:

I.V.: Administer I.V. slowly over at least 10 minutes (no greater than 1 unit/minute) at a concentration not to exceed 3 units/mL; bleomycin for I.V. continuous infusion can be further diluted in NS (preferred) or D$_5$W; administration by continuous infusion may produce less severe pulmonary toxicity.

I.M., S.C.: 15 units/mL concentration may be used for I.M., S.C. administration

Monitoring Parameters Pulmonary function tests (total lung volume, FVC, DL$_{co}$), renal function tests, chest x-ray; vital signs and temperature initially; CBC with differential and platelet count

Patient Information Report any coughing, shortness of breath, or wheezing to physician

Nursing Implications Fever and chills can occur 2-6 hours following parenteral administration; pretreatment with acetaminophen, antihistamine, and hydrocortisone may decrease the severity of fever and chills

Dosage Forms Powder for injection, as sulfate: 15 units (1 unit = 1 mg)

References

Alberts DS, Chen HS, Liu R, et al, "Bleomycin Pharmacokinetics in Man. I. Intravenous Administration," *Cancer Chemother Pharmacol*, 1978, 1(3):177-81.

Berg SL, Grisell DL, Delaney TF, et al, "Principles of Treatment of Pediatric Solid Tumors," *Pediatr Clin North Am*, 1991, 38(2):249-67.

♦ **Bleph®-10** *see* Sulfacetamide *on page 922*

♦ **BLM** *see* Bleomycin *on page 147*

♦ **Blocadren®** *see* Timolol *on page 962*

♦ **Blood Level Sampling Time Guidelines** *see page 1220*

♦ **Bluboro® [OTC]** *see* Aluminum Acetate *on page 62*

♦ **Bonamine (Can)** *see* Meclizine *on page 622*
♦ **Bonine**® **[OTC]** *see* Meclizine *on page 622*
♦ **Boropak**® *see* Aluminum Acetate *on page 62*
♦ **Botox**® *see* Botulinum Toxin Type A *on page 149*

Botulinum Toxin Type A (BOT yoo lin num TOKS in type aye)

U.S. Brand Names Botox®

Synonyms *Clostridium botulinum* Toxin Type A; Oculinum®

Therapeutic Category Muscle Contracture, Treatment; Ophthalmic Agent, Toxin

Generic Available No

Use Treatment of strabismus and blepharospasm associated with dystonia (including benign essential blepharospasm or VII nerve disorders); treatment of dynamic muscle contracture in pediatric cerebral palsy patients (orphan drug); treatment of cervical dystonia

Pregnancy Risk Factor C

Contraindications Hypersensitivity to botulinum A toxin or any component

Warnings The European formulation of botulinum A toxin (Dysport®) is not equivalent in potency to Botox®; the Dysport®:Botox® equivalency ratio is ~3:1 or 4:1, respectively; patients treated for cervical dystonia may experience dysphagia which rarely may result in dyspnea, aspiration, and pneumonia

Precautions Presence of antibodies to botulinum toxin type A may reduce the effectiveness of therapy; to minimize the development of antibodies, keep the dose of botulinum toxin type A as low as possible; reduced blinking from botulinum toxin type A injection of the orbicularis muscle can lead to corneal exposure, persistent epithelial defect, and corneal ulceration, especially in patients with VII nerve disorders; carefully test corneal sensation in eyes previously operated upon, avoid injection into the lower lid area to avoid ectropion, and vigorously treat any epithelial defect (this may require protective drops, ointment, therapeutic soft contact lenses, or closure of the eye by patching); retrobulbar hemorrhages sufficient to compromise retinal circulation have occurred from needle penetrations into the orbit; have appropriate instruments to decompress the orbit accessible; ocular (globe) penetrations by needles have also occurred (an ophthalmoscope to diagnose this condition should be available); use with caution in patients with peripheral motor neuropathic diseases or neuromuscular junction disorders; use cautiously if there is inflammation present at the proposed injection site or when excessive weakness or atrophy is present in the target muscles

Adverse Reactions
Cardiovascular: Arrhythmia, MI (rare)
Central nervous system: Fever
Dermatologic: Rash, keratitis, pruritus, erythema multiforme, psoriasiform eruption
Gastrointestinal: Dysphagia (particularly after treatment of cervical dystonia), dyspepsia, dry mouth
Local: Pain, bruising at injection site
Neuromuscular & skeletal: Weakness, temporary loss of function
Ocular: Dry eyes, lagophthalmos, ptosis, photophobia, vertical deviation, tearing, diplopia, eyelid edema, spatial disorientation, blepharospasm, ectropion, entropion, retrobulbar hemorrhage

Drug Interactions Effects of botulinum toxin may be potentiated by aminoglycoside antibiotics, or any other drug that interferes with neuromuscular transmission

Stability Store lyophilized product in freezer at or below -5°C (23°F); administer within 4 hours after the vial is removed from the freezer and reconstituted; store reconstituted solution in refrigerator (2°C to 8°C/36°F to 46°F)

Mechanism of Action Botulinum A toxin is a neurotoxin produced by *Clostridium botulinum*, a spore-forming anaerobic bacillus; it blocks neuromuscular conduction by binding to receptor sites on motor nerve terminals, entering the nerve terminals and inhibiting the release of acetylcholine. When injected intramuscularly at therapeutic doses, it produces a localized chemical denervation muscle paralysis. When the muscle is chemically denervated, it atrophies and may develop extrajunctional acetylcholine receptors. There is evidence that the nerve can sprout and reinnervate the muscle, with the weakness being reversible. Following several weeks of paralysis, alignment of the eye is measurably changed, despite return of innervation to the injected muscle.

Pharmacodynamics
Strabismus:
Onset of action: 1-2 days after injection
Duration of paralysis: 2-6 weeks
Blepharospasm:
Onset of action: 3 days after injection
(Continued)

Botulinum Toxin Type A *(Continued)*

Peak effect: 1-2 weeks
Duration of paralysis: 3 months
Spasticity associated with cerebral palsy
Onset of action: Several days
Duration of paralysis: 3-8 months

Usual Dosage I.M.

Strabismus:

Children 2 months to 12 years:

Horizontal or vertical deviations <20 prism diopters: 1.25 units into any one muscle

Horizontal or vertical deviations 20-25 prism diopters: 1-2.5 units into any one muscle

Persistent VI nerve palsy of ≥1 month duration: 1-1.25 units into the medial rectus muscle

Children ≥12 years and Adults:

Horizontal or vertical deviations <20 prism diopters: 1.25-2.5 units into any one muscle

Horizontal or vertical deviations 20-50 prism diopters: 2.5-5 units into any one muscle

Persistent VI nerve palsy of ≥1 month duration: 1.25-2.5 units into the medial rectus muscle

Note: Re-examine patient 7-14 days after each injection to assess effects; dosage may be increased up to twofold of the previously administered dose; do not exceed 25 units as a single injection for any one muscle

Blepharospasm: Adults: Initial: 1.25-2.5 units injected into the medial and lateral pretarsal orbicularis oculi of the upper lid and into the lateral pretarsal orbicularis oculi of the lower lid; dose may be increased up to 2.5-5 units at repeat treatment sessions; do not exceed 5 units per injection or cumulative dose of 200 units in a 30-day period

Spasticity associated with cerebral palsy: Children >18 months to Adolescents: Small muscle: 1-2 units/kg; large muscle: 3-6 units/kg; maximum dose per injection site: 50 units; maximum dose for any one visit: 12 units/kg, up to 400 units; no more than 400 units should be administered during a 3-month period

Cervical dystonia: Adults: Initial and sequential doses should be individualized related to the patient's head and neck position, localization of pain, muscle hypertrophy, and patient response; mean dosage used in research trials: 236 units (range: 198-300 units) divided among affected muscles; limit total dose into sternocleidomastoid muscles to ≤100 units

Administration Parenteral: For I.M. administration only by individuals understanding the relevant neuromuscular and orbital anatomy and any alterations to the anatomy due to prior surgical procedures and standard electromyographic techniques; reconstitute vial with preservative-free NS to obtain an optimal injection volume of 0.1 mL; suggested volumes and concentrations: 1 mL (10 units/0.1 mL); 2 mL (5 units/0.1 mL), 4 mL (2.5 units/0.1 mL) or 8 mL (1.25 units/0.1 mL); gently swirl as botulinum toxin type A is denatured by violent agitation

Patient Information Patients with blepharospasm may have been extremely sedentary for a long time; sedentary patients should be cautioned to resume activity slowly and carefully following injection

Dosage Forms Powder for injection, lyophilized: 100 units *Clostridium botulinum* toxin type A

References

Scott AB, Magoon EH, McNeer KW, et al, "Botulinum Treatment of Childhood Strabismus," *Ophthalmology*, 1990, 97(11):1434-8.

Russman BS, Tilton A, and Gormley ME Jr, "Cerebral Palsy: A Rational Approach to a Treatment Protocol, and the Role of Botulinum Toxin in Treatment," *Muscle Nerve Suppl*, 1997, 6:S181-S193.

Bretylium *(bre TIL ee um)*

Therapeutic Category Antiarrhythmic Agent, Class III
Generic Available Yes

Use Ventricular tachycardia or ventricular fibrillation; other serious ventricular arrhythmias resistant to lidocaine

Note: Bretylium has been removed from the 2000 Adult ACLS and PALS Guidelines due to the limited supply, high incidence of adverse effects (eg, hypotension), and availability of safer agents; studies of its use in children are lacking and effectiveness in treatment of VT has not been demonstrated

Pregnancy Risk Factor C

Contraindications Digitalis intoxication-induced arrhythmias

Precautions Hypotension; patients with fixed cardiac output (severe pulmonary hypertension or aortic stenosis) may experience severe hypotension due to decrease in peripheral resistance without ability to increase cardiac output; reduce dose in renal failure patients

Adverse Reactions
Cardiovascular: Hypotension (incidence 50% to 75%), transient initial hypertension, increase in PVCs, bradycardia, flushing, syncope
Central nervous system: Vertigo, confusion, anxiety, lethargy, hyperthermia
Dermatologic: Rash
Gastrointestinal: Nausea and vomiting with rapid I.V. administration; rarely diarrhea, abdominal pain
Local: Muscle atrophy and necrosis with repeated I.M. injections at same site
Ocular: Conjunctivitis
Renal: Renal impairment
Respiratory: Nasal congestion
Miscellaneous: Hiccups, diaphoresis

Drug Interactions Other antiarrhythmic agents may potentiate or antagonize cardiac effects, toxic effects may be additive; the pressor effects of catecholamines may be enhanced by bretylium; may potentiate digitalis toxicity; methylphenidate may antagonize effects of bretylium

Mechanism of Action Class III antiarrhythmic; after an initial release of norepinephrine at the peripheral adrenergic nerve terminals, bretylium inhibits further release by postganglionic nerve endings in response to sympathetic nerve stimulation

Pharmacodynamics
Onset of antiarrhythmic effects:
I.M.: Up to 2 hours
I.V.: Within 6-20 minutes
Maximum effect: Within 6-9 hours

Pharmacokinetics
Protein binding: 1% to 6%
Half-life, adults: 7-11 hours; increases with decreased renal function
Elimination: Unchanged in urine

Usual Dosage Note: Bretylium has been removed from the 2000 Adult ACLS and PALS Guidelines (see note in Use section); if used patients should undergo defibrillation/cardioversion before and after bretylium doses as necessary

Children: (**Note:** Dose not well established; the following dose has been recommended):
I.M.: 2-5 mg/kg as a single dose
I.V.: 5 mg/kg/dose, may repeat every 10-20 minutes as needed to a total dose of 30 mg/kg
1992 PALS guidelines for treatment of ventricular fibrillation **(see note in Use section):** Initial: 5 mg/kg, then attempt electrical defibrillation; repeat with 10 mg/kg and then reattempt electrical defibrillation if ventricular fibrillation persists; may repeat as needed to a total dose of 30 mg/kg
Maintenance dose: I.M., I.V.: 5 mg/kg every 6-8 hours
Adults **(see note in Use section):**
Immediately life-threatening ventricular arrhythmias, ventricular fibrillation, unstable ventricular tachycardia:
Initial dose: I.V.: 5 mg/kg (undiluted) over 1 minute; if arrhythmia persists, give 10 mg/kg (undiluted) over 1 minute and repeat as necessary (usually at 15- to 30-minute intervals) up to a total dose of 30-35 mg/kg
Maintenance dose (for continuous suppression):
I.V. (diluted): 5-10 mg/kg every 6 hours
I.V. continuous infusion (diluted): 1-2 mg/minute (little experience with doses >40 mg/kg/day)
Other ventricular arrhythmias:
Initial dose: I.M., I.V.: 5-10 mg/kg, may repeat every 1-2 hours if arrhythmia persists; give I.V. dose (diluted) over 8-10 minutes
Maintenance dose:
I.M.: 5-10 mg/kg every 6-8 hours
(Continued)

Bretylium *(Continued)*

       I.V. (diluted): 5-10 mg/kg every 6 hours
       I.V. continuous infusion (diluted): 1-2 mg/minute (little experience with doses >40 mg/kg/day)

Dosing interval in renal impairment:
  Cl$_{cr}$ 10-50 mL/minute: Administer 25% to 50% of normal dose
  Cl$_{cr}$ <10 mL/minute: Administer 25% of normal dose or use alternative agent

Administration Parenteral:
  I.M.: Not recommended for ventricular fibrillation; no more than 5 mL should be injected I.M. per site (adults); rotate injection sites
  I.V.:
    Life-threatening situations: May administer undiluted I.V. push over <30 seconds
    Nonlife-threatening situations: Dilute to 10 mg/mL and administer slow I.V. push over at least 8 minutes

Monitoring Parameters EKG, heart rate, rhythm, blood pressure

Nursing Implications Avoid extravasation

Additional Information Change patient to oral antiarrhythmic agent as soon as possible (when indicated) for maintenance therapy

Dosage Forms
Injection, as tosylate: 50 mg/mL (10 mL)
Injection, as tosylate, premixed in D$_5$W: 2 mg/mL (250 mL); 4 mg/mL (250 mL)

References

Emergency Cardiac Care Committee and Subcommittees, American Heart Association, "Guidelines for Cardiopulmonary Resuscitation and Emergency Cardiac Care, III: Adult Advanced Cardiac Life Support," and "VI: Pediatric Advanced Life Support," *JAMA*, 1992, 268(16):2199-241 and 2262-75.

"Guidelines 2000 for Cardiopulmonary Resuscitation and Emergency Cardiovascular Care, Part 6: Advanced Cardiovascular Life Support, The American Heart Association in Collaboration With the International Liaison Committee on Resuscitation," *Circulation*, 2000, 102(8 Suppl):I86-171.

"Guidelines 2000 for Cardiopulmonary Resuscitation and Emergency Cardiovascular Care, Part 10: Pediatric Advanced Life Support, The American Heart Association in Collaboration With the International Liaison Committee on Resuscitation," *Circulation*, 2000, 102(8 Suppl): I291-342.

♦ **Brevibloc®** *see* Esmolol *on page 399*
♦ **Brevital® Sodium** *see* Methohexital *on page 646*
♦ **Brevoxyl® Gel** *see* Benzoyl Peroxide *on page 136*
♦ **Brexidol (Can)** *see* Piroxicam *on page 806*
♦ **Bricanyl (Can)** *see* Terbutaline *on page 937*
♦ **Brietal (Can)** *see* Methohexital *on page 646*
♦ **Brioschi (Can)** *see* Sodium Bicarbonate *on page 904*

Brompheniramine *(brome fen IR a meen)*

Related Information
OTC Cough & Cold Preparations, Pediatric *on page 1072*
Overdose and Toxicology *on page 1222*

Synonyms Parabromdylamine

Therapeutic Category Antihistamine

Generic Available Yes

Use Perennial and seasonal allergic rhinitis and other allergic symptoms including urticaria

Pregnancy Risk Factor C

Contraindications Hypersensitivity to brompheniramine or any component; narrow-angle glaucoma, bladder neck obstruction, symptomatic prostatic hypertrophy, stenosing peptic ulcer, and pyloroduodenal obstruction

Precautions Use with caution in patients with asthma, heart disease, hypertension, and thyroid disease

Adverse Reactions
Cardiovascular: Palpitations
Central nervous system: Paradoxical excitability, drowsiness, dizziness, headache, fever, nervousness, depression
Dermatologic: Rash, photosensitivity, angioedema
Gastrointestinal: Nausea, anorexia, xerostomia, appetite increase, weight gain, diarrhea, abdominal pain
Hepatic: Hepatitis
Neuromuscular & skeletal: Myalgia, paresthesia
Respiratory: Bronchospasm, epistaxis, thickening of bronchial secretions

Drug Interactions May cause additive sedation with other CNS depressants; may cause additive anticholinergic effects with other anticholinergic agents; MAO inhibitors

Stability Solutions may crystallize if stored below 0°C, crystals will dissolve when warmed

Mechanism of Action Competes with histamine for H_1-receptor sites on effector cells in the GI tract, blood vessels, and respiratory tract

Pharmacodynamics
Peak effect: Maximal clinical effects seen within 3-9 hours
Duration: Varies with formulation

Pharmacokinetics
Metabolism: Extensive by the liver
Half-life: 12-34 hours
Time to peak serum concentration: Oral: Within 2-5 hours
Elimination: In urine as inactive metabolites

Usual Dosage
Oral:
Children:
<6 years: 0.125 mg/kg/dose given every 6 hours; maximum dose: 6-8 mg/day
6-12 years: 2-4 mg every 6-8 hours; maximum dose: 12-16 mg/day
Adults: 4-8 mg every 4-6 hours or 8 mg of sustained release form every 8-12 hours or 12 mg of sustained release form every 12 hours; maximum dose: 24 mg/day
I.M., I.V., S.C.:
Children <12 years: 0.5 mg/kg/day or 15 mg/m^2/day divided every 6-8 hours
Children ≥12 years and Adults: 10 mg (range: 5-20 mg) every 6-12 hours; maximum dose: 40 mg/day

Administration
Oral: Administer with food or milk; sustained release tablets should be swallowed whole; do not crush or chew
Parenteral: I.V.: Dilute in 1-10 mL D_5W or NS and infuse over several minutes; the patient should be in a recumbent position during the infusion

Patient Information Causes drowsiness and may impair ability to perform hazardous activities requiring mental alertness or physical coordination

Dosage Forms
Elixir, as maleate: 2 mg/5 mL (120 mL, 480 mL, 4000 mL)
Injection, as maleate: 10 mg/mL (10 mL)
Tablet, as maleate: 4 mg
Tablet, sustained release, as maleate: 12 mg

Brompheniramine and Pseudoephedrine
(brome fen IR a meen & soo doe e FED rin)

Related Information
OTC Cough & Cold Preparations, Pediatric on page 1072

U.S. Brand Names Children's Dimetapp® Elixir Cold & Allergy

Canadian Brand Names Dimedrine

Synonyms Pseudoephedrine and Brompheniramine

Therapeutic Category Antihistamine/Decongestant Combination

Generic Available Yes

Use Temporary relief of nasal congestion, running nose, sneezing, and itchy, watery eyes; also promotes nasal or sinus drainage

Pregnancy Risk Factor C

Contraindications Hypersensitivity to brompheniramine, pseudoephedrine, or any component; MAO inhibitor therapy, severe hypertension, severe coronary artery disease

Precautions Use with caution in patients with mild-moderate hypertension, heart disease, arrhythmias, diabetes mellitus, thyroid disease, asthma, glaucoma, and prostatic hypertrophy

Adverse Reactions See individual monographs for Brompheniramine on page 152 and Pseudoephedrine on page 852.

Drug Interactions See individual monographs for Brompheniramine on page 152 and Pseudoephedrine on page 852.

Pharmacodynamics See individual monographs

Pharmacokinetics See individual monographs

Usual Dosage Oral:
Manufacturer's recommendations:
Children 6-12 years: 10 mL (pseudoephedrine 30 mg) every 4 hours
Children >12 years and Adults: 20 mL (pseudoephedrine 60 mg) every 4 hours
Alternative pediatric dosing: May dose according to the pseudoephedrine component:
Infants and Children <2 years: 4 mg/kg/day in divided doses every 6 hours
(Continued)

Brompheniramine and Pseudoephedrine *(Continued)*

Children 2-5 years: 15 mg every 6 hours; maximum dose: 60 mg/24 hours
Children 6-12 years: 30 mg every 6 hours; maximum dose: 120 mg/24 hours
Children >12 years and Adults: 30-60 mg every 6 hours; maximum dose: 240 mg/24 hours

Administration Oral: Administer with food

Test Interactions False-positive test for amphetamines by EMIT assay

Patient Information Causes drowsiness and may impair ability to perform hazardous activities requiring mental alertness or physical coordination

Dosage Forms Elixir: Brompheniramine maleate 1 mg and pseudoephedrine hydrochloride 15 mg per 5 mL [grape flavor]

♦ **Broncho-Grippol-DM (Can)** *see* Dextromethorphan *on page 316*
♦ **Broncho® Saline [OTC]** *see* Sodium Chloride *on page 906*
♦ **Brontex®** *see* Guaifenesin and Codeine *on page 486*
♦ **BSS** *see* Bismuth *on page 145*
♦ **Buckley's DM (Can)** *see* Dextromethorphan *on page 316*

Budesonide *(byoo DES oh nide)*

Related Information

Asthma Guidelines *on page 1210*
Estimated Comparative Daily Dosages for Inhaled Corticosteroids *on page 1216*

U.S. Brand Names Pulmicort® Respules™; Pulmicort® Turbuhaler®; Rhinocort®; Rhinocort® Aqua™

Canadian Brand Names Entocort; Gen-Budesonide

Therapeutic Category Adrenal Corticosteroid; Antiasthmatic; Anti-inflammatory Agent; Corticosteroid, Inhalant (Oral); Corticosteroid, Intranasal; Glucocorticoid

Generic Available No

Use

Intranasal:
Children and Adults: Management of seasonal or perennial allergic rhinitis
Adults: Nonallergic perennial rhinitis

Nebulization: Children 12 months to 8 years: Maintenance therapy and prophylaxis of bronchial asthma; **not** indicated for the relief of acute bronchospasm

Oral inhalation: Long-term (chronic) control of persistent bronchial asthma; **NOT** indicated for the relief of acute bronchospasm; also indicated in bronchial asthma patients requiring oral corticosteroids (inhalation may decrease or eliminate need for oral steroids over time)

Pregnancy Risk Factor C

Contraindications Hypersensitivity to budesonide or any component; primary treatment of status asthmaticus or other acute episodes of bronchial asthma where intensive treatment is needed

Warnings Fatalities have occurred due to adrenal insufficiency in asthmatic patients during and after switching from systemic corticosteroids to aerosol steroids; several months may be required for full recovery of the adrenal glands; patients receiving ≥20 mg of prednisone per day may be at higher risk; during this period of adrenal suppression, aerosol steroids do **not** provide the systemic corticosteroid needed to treat patients requiring stress doses (ie, patients with major stress such as trauma, surgery, or infections); when used at high doses, hypothalamic-pituitary-adrenal (HPA) suppression may occur; use with inhaled or systemic corticosteroids (even alternate-day dosing) may increase risk of HPA suppression; withdrawal and discontinuation of corticosteroids should be done carefully; immunosuppression may occur

Precautions Avoid using higher than recommended dosages; suppression of HPA function, suppression of linear growth, or hypercorticism (Cushing's syndrome) may occur; use with extreme caution in patients with respiratory tuberculosis, untreated systemic infections, or ocular herpes simplex; rare cases of increased IOP, glaucoma, or cataracts may occur

Adverse Reactions

Cardiovascular: Facial edema
Central nervous system: Nervousness, migraine, insomnia
Dermatologic: Rash, pruritus, contact dermatitis
Endocrine & metabolic: Potential adrenal suppression
Gastrointestinal: Xerostomia, dysgeusia, GI irritation, nausea, weight gain, abdominal pain, vomiting, diarrhea
Local: Nasal irritation, burning, or ulceration; pharyngitis; growth of *Candida* in the mouth, throat, or nares

Neuromuscular & skeletal: Potential growth suppression, fracture, myalgia, arthralgia

Ocular: Conjunctivitis

Otic: Otitis media

Respiratory: Cough, epistaxis, wheezing, decreased sense of smell, hoarseness, respiratory infection, rhinitis, sinusitis

Drug Interactions Cytochrome P-450 isoenzyme CYP3A substrate

Ketoconazole, cimetidine may increase budesonide serum concentrations; interactions similar to other corticosteroids may potentially occur

Stability

Intranasal inhaler: Use within 6 months after opening; avoid storage in high humidity; do not store or use by heat or open flame

Nebulization: Store Respules™ upright at room temperature (68°F to 77°F); do not refrigerate or freeze; do not mix with other medications; after foil packet has been opened, Respules™ are stable for 2 weeks when protected from light; return unused Respules™ to foil packet to protect from light; use opened Respules™ promptly

Oral inhaler: Keep clean and dry; store at room temperature 68°F to 77°F

Mechanism of Action Controls the rate of protein synthesis, depresses the migration of polymorphonuclear leukocytes and fibroblasts, reverses capillary permeability, and stabilizes lysosomal membranes at the cellular level to prevent or control inflammation

Pharmacodynamics Clinical effects are due to direct local effect, rather than systemic absorption

Onset of action: Within 24 hours; nebulization (control of asthma symptoms): Within 2-8 days

Maximum effect:

Intranasal: Inhaler: 3-7 days; spray: 2 weeks

Nebulization: 4-6 weeks

Oral inhalation: 1-2 weeks or more

Duration after discontinuation: Intranasal: Several days

Pharmacokinetics

Absorption:

Intranasal:

Inhaler: 20% of dose delivered reaches systemic circulation

Spray: 34% of dose delivered reaches systemic circulation

Oral inhalation: 39% of the metered dose is systemically available

Distribution: V_d:

Children 4-6 years: 3 L/kg

Adults: ~200 L or 2-3 L/kg

Protein binding: 85% to 90%

Metabolism: Extensively metabolized by the liver via cytochrome P-450 CYP3A isoenzyme to 2 major metabolites: 16α-hydroxyprednisolone and 6β-hydroxybudesonide; both are <1% as active as parent

Bioavailability:

Nebulization: Children 4-6 years: 6%; **Note:** AUC of single 1 mg dose was comparable to a single 2 mg dose in healthy adults

Oral: ~10% (large first pass effect)

Half-life:

Children: 4-6 years: 2.3 hours (after nebulization)

Children 10-14 years: 1.5 hours

Adults: 2-3 hours

Elimination: 60% to 66% of dose renally excreted as metabolites; 0% unchanged drug found in urine

Clearance: Children 4-6 years: 0.5 L/minute (~50% greater than healthy adults after weight adjustment)

Usual Dosage

Intranasal: Children ≥6 years and Adults:

Rhinocort®: Initial: 8 sprays (4 sprays/nostril) per day (256 mcg/day), given as either 2 sprays in each nostril in the morning and evening or as 4 sprays in each nostril in the morning; after symptoms decrease (usually by 3-7 days), reduce dose slowly every 2-4 weeks to the smallest effective dose

Rhinocort® Aqua™ (32 mcg/spray): Initial: 2 sprays (1 spray/nostril) once daily (64 mcg/day); dose may be increased if needed

Maximum dose:

Children <12 years: 4 sprays (2 sprays/nostril) once daily (128 mcg/day)

Children ≥12 years and Adults: 8 sprays (4 sprays/nostril) once daily (256 mcg/day)

(Continued)

Budesonide *(Continued)*

Nebulization: Children 12 months to 8 years: Pulmicort® Respules™: Doses should be titrated to the lowest effective dose once asthma is controlled:

Previously treated with bronchodilators alone: Initial: 0.25 mg twice daily or 0.5 mg once daily; maximum dose: 0.5 mg/day

Previously treated with inhaled corticosteroids: Initial: 0.25 mg twice daily or 0.5 mg once daily; maximum dose: 1 mg/day

Previously treated with oral corticosteroids: Initial: 0.5 mg twice daily or 1 mg once daily; maximum dose: 1 mg/day

Symptomatic children not responding to nonsteroidal medications: Initial: 0.25 mg once daily may be considered

Oral inhalation: **Note:** Doses should be titrated to the lowest effective dose once asthma is controlled; Manufacturer's recommendations:

Children ≥6 years:

Previously treated with bronchodilators alone or with inhaled corticosteroids: Initial: 200 mcg (1 puff) twice daily; maximum dose: 400 mcg (2 puffs) twice daily

Treated with oral corticosteroids: Initial: 400 mcg (2 puffs) twice daily (maximum dose)

Adults:

Previously treated with bronchodilators alone: Initial: 200-400 mcg (1-2 puffs) twice daily; maximum dose: 400 mcg (2 puffs) twice daily

Treated with inhaled corticosteroids: Initial: 200-400 mcg (1-2 puffs) twice daily; maximum dose: 800 mcg (4 puffs) twice daily

Treated with oral corticosteroids: Initial: 400-800 mcg (2-4 puffs) twice daily; maximum dose: 800 mcg (4 puffs) twice daily

NIH Guidelines (NIH, 1997) [give in divided doses twice daily]:

Children:

"Low" dose: 100-200 mcg/day

"Medium" dose: 200-400 mcg/day (1-2 inhalations/day)

"High" dose: >400 mcg/day (>2 inhalation/day)

Adults:

"Low" dose: 200-400 mcg/day (1-2 inhalations/day)

"Medium" dose: 400-600 mcg/day (2-3 inhalations/day)

"High" dose: >600 mcg/day (>3 inhalation/day)

Administration

Intranasal inhaler and intranasal spray: Clear nasal passage by blowing nose prior to use

Intranasal inhaler: Shake well before each use

Intranasal spray: Shake gently before use

Nebulization: Shake gently with a circular motion before use. Administer only with a compressed air driven jet nebulizer; do not use an ultrasonic nebulizer; use adequate flow rates and administer via appropriate size face mask or mouthpiece; avoid exposure of nebulized medication to eyes

Oral inhaler: Do **not** shake inhaler; do not use inhaler with a spacer

Monitoring Parameters Check mucous membranes for signs of fungal infection; monitor growth in pediatric patients

Patient Information Notify physician if condition being treated persists or worsens; do not decrease dose or discontinue without physician approval; avoid exposure to chicken pox or measles; if exposed, seek medical advice without delay

Nebulization: Rinse mouth after treatment and wash face after using face mask to decrease chance of oral candidiasis and steroid effects on skin

Oral inhaler: Rinse mouth after inhalation to decrease chance of oral candidiasis; report sore mouth or mouth lesions to physician. A red mark will appear on the indicator window of the Pulmicort Turbuhaler® when 20 doses are left.

Additional Information If bronchospasm with wheezing occurs after use of oral inhaler, a fast-acting bronchodilator may be used. Pulmicort Turbuhaler® delivers budesonide as a fine powder. Children and adolescents (n=18; 6-15 years) receiving budesonide nebulizations of 1 and 2 mg twice daily showed a significant reduction in urinary cortisol excretion; this reduction was not seen when patients were dosed at 1 mg/day (maximum recommended dose). Long-term effects of chronic use of budesonide nebulization on immunological or developmental processes of upper airways, mouth, and lung are unknown.

Dosage Forms

Oral inhaler (Pulmicort Turbuhaler®): 200 mcg per metered dose [200 doses]

Nasal inhaler (Rhinocort®): 50 mcg released per actuation to deliver ~32 mcg to patient via nasal adapter [200 metered doses] (7 g)

Nasal spray (Rhinocort® Aqua™): 32 mcg per spray [60 metered sprays]
Suspension, for inhalation (Pulmicort® Respules™): 0.25 mg/2 mL (30 doses); 0.5 mg/2 mL (30 doses)

References

Expert Panel Report 2, "Guidelines for the Diagnosis and Management of Asthma," *Clinical Practice Guidelines*, National Institutes of Health, National Heart, Lung, and Blood Institute, NIH Publication No. 94-4051, April, 1997.

Szefler SJ, "A Review of Budesonide Inhalation Suspension in the Treatment of Pediatric Asthma," *Pharmacotherapy*, 2001, 21(2):195-206.

♦ **Bufferin® [OTC]** *see* Aspirin *on page 109*

Bumetanide (byoo MET a nide)

U.S. Brand Names Bumex®
Canadian Brand Names Burinex
Therapeutic Category Antihypertensive Agent; Diuretic, Loop
Generic Available Yes
Use Management of edema secondary to CHF or hepatic or renal disease including nephrotic syndrome; may also be used alone or in combination with antihypertensives in the treatment of hypertension
Pregnancy Risk Factor C
Contraindications Hypersensitivity to bumetanide or any component; in anuria or increasing azotemia
Warnings Loop diuretics are potent diuretics; excess amounts can lead to profound diuresis with fluid and electrolyte loss; close medical supervision and dose evaluation is required; *in vitro* studies using pooled sera from critically ill neonates have shown bumetanide to be a potent displacer of bilirubin; avoid use in neonates at risk for kernicterus; increased risk of ototoxicity with rapid I.V. administration, renal impairment, excessive doses, and concurrent use of other ototoxins
Precautions Use with caution in patients with cirrhosis; allergy to sulfonamides may result in cross hypersensitivity to bumetanide
Adverse Reactions
  Cardiovascular: Hypotension, chest pain
  Central nervous system: Dizziness, headache, encephalopathy, vertigo
  Dermatologic: Rash, pruritus
  Endocrine & metabolic: Hyperglycemia, hypokalemia, hypochloremia, hyponatremia
  Gastrointestinal: Cramps, nausea, vomiting, diarrhea, abdominal pain
  Hepatic: Elevated liver enzymes
  Neuromuscular & skeletal: Weakness, muscle cramps, arthritic pain
  Otic: Ototoxicity (with rapid I.V. administration)
  Renal: Decreased uric acid excretion, elevated serum creatinine
Drug Interactions Decreased blood pressure when used with other antihypertensive agents and ACE inhibitors (may need to decrease dose of one or both agents); indomethacin and probenecid may decrease bumetanide's effect; decreased lithium excretion; ototoxic drugs (aminoglycoside antibiotics, cisplatin); cholestyramine may decrease absorption
Stability Light sensitive, may discolor when exposed to light
Mechanism of Action Inhibits reabsorption of sodium and chloride in the ascending loop of Henle and proximal renal tubule, interfering with the chloride-binding cotransport system, thus causing increased excretion of water, sodium, chloride, magnesium, calcium, and phosphate
Pharmacodynamics
  Onset of clinical effects:
    Oral, I.M.: Within 30-60 minutes
    I.V.: Within a few minutes
  Peak effects:
    Oral, I.M.: 1-2 hours
    I.V.: 15-30 minutes
  Duration:
    Oral: 4-6 hours
    I.V.: 2-3 hours
Pharmacokinetics
  Protein binding: 95%
    Newborns: 97%
  Metabolism: Partial metabolism occurs in the liver
  Bioavailability: 72% to 96%
  Half-life:
    Infants <2 months: 2.5 hours
    Infants 2-6 months: 1.5 hours
    Adults: 1-1.5 hours
(Continued)

Bumetanide *(Continued)*

Time to peak serum concentration: 0.5-2 hours
Elimination: Unchanged drug excreted in urine (50%)

Usual Dosage

Oral, I.M., I.V.:

Neonates (see Warnings): 0.01-0.05 mg/kg/dose every 24-48 hours

Infants and Children: 0.015-0.1 mg/kg/dose every 6-24 hours (maximum dose: 10 mg/day)

Adults:

Edema:

Oral: 0.5-2 mg/dose (maximum dose: 10 mg/day) 1-2 times/day

I.M., I.V.: 0.5-1 mg/dose; may repeat in 2-3 hours for up to 2 doses if needed (maximum dose: 10 mg/day)

Continuous I.V. infusion: 0.9-1 mg/hour

Hypertension: Oral: 0.5 mg daily (range: 1-4 mg/day, maximum dose: 5 mg/day); for larger doses, divide into 2-3 doses daily

Administration

Oral: Administer with food to decrease GI irritation

Parenteral: Administer without additional dilution by direct I.V. injection over 1-2 minutes; for continuous infusion, dilute in D_5W, NS, or LR; stability and maximum dilution in I.V. fluid has not been determined

Monitoring Parameters Blood pressure, serum electrolytes, renal function, urine output

Additional Information Patients with impaired hepatic function must be monitored carefully, often requiring reduced doses; larger doses may be necessary in patients with impaired renal function to obtain the same therapeutic response

Dosage Forms

Injection: 0.25 mg/mL (2 mL, 4 mL, 10 mL)

Tablet: 0.5 mg, 1 mg, 2 mg

References

Wells TG, "The Pharmacology and Therapeutics of Diuretics in the Pediatric Patient," *Pediatr Clin North Am*, 1990, 37(2):463-504.

♦ **Bumex**® *see* Bumetanide *on page 157*

♦ **Buminate**® *see* Albumin *on page 44*

♦ **Buphenyl**® *see* Sodium Phenylbutyrate *on page 907*

Bupivacaine *(byoo PIV a kane)*

U.S. Brand Names Marcaine®; Sensorcaine®; Sensorcaine-MPF®

Therapeutic Category Local Anesthetic, Injectable

Generic Available Yes

Use Local anesthetic (injectable) for peripheral nerve block, infiltration, sympathetic block, caudal or epidural block, retrobulbar block

Pregnancy Risk Factor C

Contraindications Hypersensitivity to bupivacaine hydrochloride, PABA, parabens, or any component; not recommended for I.V. regional anesthesia (Bier block)

Warnings Convulsions due to systemic toxicity leading to cardiac arrest have been reported, presumably following unintentional I.V. injection; some commercially available formulations contain sodium metabisulfite, which may cause allergic-type reactions; **do not use solutions containing preservatives for caudal or epidural block**

Precautions Use with caution in patients with liver disease

Adverse Reactions

Cardiovascular: Cardiac arrest, hypotension, bradycardia, palpitations

Central nervous system: Headache, restlessness, anxiety, dizziness, seizures

Dermatologic: Pruritus, angioneurotic edema

Gastrointestinal: Nausea, vomiting

Neuromuscular & skeletal: Weakness

Ocular: Blurred vision

Otic: Tinnitus

Respiratory: Apnea, sneezing

Mechanism of Action Blocks both the initiation and conduction of nerve impulses by decreasing the neuronal membrane's permeability to sodium ions, which results in inhibition of depolarization with resultant blockade of conduction

Pharmacodynamics

Onset of anesthetic action: Dependent on route administered, but generally occurs within 4-10 minutes

Duration: 1.5-8.5 hours (depending upon route of administration)

Pharmacokinetics
  Protein binding: 84% to 95%
  Metabolism: In the liver
  Half-life (age-dependent):
    Neonates: 8.1 hours
    Adults: 1.5-5.5 hours
  Elimination: Small amounts (~6%) excreted in urine unchanged
Usual Dosage Dose varies with procedure, depth of anesthesia, vascularity of tissues, duration of anesthesia and condition of patient

  Caudal block (with or without epinephrine):
    Children: 1-3.7 mg/kg
    Adults: 15-30 mL of 0.25% or 0.5%
  Epidural block (other than caudal block):
    Children: 1.25 mg/kg/dose
    Adults: 10-20 mL of 0.25%, 0.5%, or 0.75%
  Peripheral nerve block: 5 mL dose of 0.25% or 0.5% (12.5-25 mg); maximum dose: 400 mg/day
  Sympathetic nerve block: 20-50 mL of 0.25% (no epinephrine) solution
Administration Solutions containing preservatives should not be used for epidural or caudal blocks
Additional Information Metabisulfites (in epinephrine-containing injection)
Dosage Forms
  Injection, as hydrochloride:
    Preservative free: 0.25% [2.5 mg/mL] (10 mL, 30 mL); 0.5% [5 mg/mL] (10 mL, 30 mL); 0.75% [7.5 mg/mL] (10 mL, 30 mL)
    With preservative: 0.25% [2.5 mg/mL] (50 mL); 0.5% [5 mg/mL] (50 mL)
  Injection, as hydrochloride with epinephrine [1:200,000] injection:
    Preservative free: 0.25% [2.5 mg/mL] (10 mL, 30 mL); 0.5% [5 mg/mL] (3 mL, 5 mL, 10 mL, 30 mL); 0.75% [7.5 mg/mL] (10 mL, 30 mL)
    With preservative: 0.25% [2.5 mg/mL] (50 mL); 0.5% [5 mg/mL] (50 mL)
  Injection (spinal), as hydrochloride in dextrose [8.25%]: Preservative free: 0.75% [7.5 mg/mL] (2 mL)

♦ **Burinex (Can)** *see* Bumetanide *on page 157*
♦ **Burow's Solution** *see* Aluminum Acetate *on page 62*
♦ **Buscopan (Can)** *see* Scopolamine *on page 892*
♦ **BuSpar®** *see* Buspirone *on page 159*
♦ **Buspirex (Can)** *see* Buspirone *on page 159*

Buspirone (byoo SPYE rone)

Related Information
  Serotonin Syndrome *on page 1247*
U.S. Brand Names BuSpar®
Canadian Brand Names Apo-Buspirone; Buspirex; Bustab; Lin-Buspirone; Novo-Buspirone; Nu-Buspirone; PMS-Buspirone
Therapeutic Category Antianxiety Agent
Generic Available No
Use Management of anxiety
Pregnancy Risk Factor B
Contraindications Hypersensitivity to buspirone or any component
Warnings Do not use concurrently with MAO inhibitors or within 10 days of MAO inhibitors as significant increases in blood pressure may occur
Precautions Use with caution in patients with hepatic or renal dysfunction; use in severe hepatic or renal impairment is not recommended; buspirone does not prevent or treat withdrawal from benzodiazepines or sedative/hypnotic drugs
Adverse Reactions
  Cardiovascular: Chest pain, tachycardia
  Central nervous system: Dizziness, lightheadedness, headache, fatigue, restlessness, confusion, insomnia, nightmares, sedation (about $\frac{1}{3}$ of that with benzodiazepines), disorientation, excitement, fever, drowsiness (more common with ≥20 mg/day), akathisia; possible psychotic deterioration has been reported (two pediatric cases, see Soni, 1992)
  Dermatologic: Rash, urticaria
  Gastrointestinal: Nausea, vomiting, diarrhea, flatulence, xerostomia
  Hematologic: Rare: Leukopenia, eosinophilia, thrombocytopenia
  Neuromuscular & skeletal: Muscle weakness, numbness
  Ocular: Blurred vision
  Otic: Tinnitus
  (Continued)

Buspirone *(Continued)*

Drug Interactions Cytochrome P-450 isoenzyme CYP3A4 substrate

Use with MAO inhibitors may cause significant increases in blood pressure; alcohol or other CNS depressants may increase CNS adverse effects; buspirone may increase haloperidol levels; buspirone may displace digoxin from serum proteins; fluoxetine; use with warfarin may increase PT; erythromycin, itraconazole, and nefazodone increase buspirone plasma concentrations (the dose of buspirone should be reduced); when used with diazepam, buspirone may increase nordiazepam serum concentrations; aspirin may increase and flurazepam may decrease free (unbound) buspirone concentrations

Food Interactions Food may delay oral absorption, decrease the first-pass metabolism effect and increase oral bioavailability; grapefruit juice may greatly increase buspirone concentrations

Stability Protect from light; store at room temperature

Mechanism of Action Decreases the spontaneous firing of serotonin-containing neurons in the CNS by selectively binding to and acting as agonist at presynaptic CNS serotonin 5-HT$_1$A receptors; possesses partial agonist activity (mixed agonist/antagonist) at postsynaptic 5-HT$_2$A receptors; does not bind to benzodiazepine-GABA receptors; binds to dopamine$_2$ receptors; may have other effects on other neurotransmitter systems; buspirone is "anxiolytic-select" and does not possess the anticonvulsant, muscle relaxant, or sedative effects of the benzodiazepines; little potential for abuse, tolerance, or withdrawal reactions

Pharmacodynamics

Onset of effect: Within 2 weeks

Time to maximum effect: 3-4 weeks, up to 4-6 weeks

Pharmacokinetics

Absorption: Rapid and complete, but bioavailability is limited by extensive first-pass effect; only 1.5% to 13% (mean 4%) of the oral dose reaches the systemic circulation unchanged

Protein binding: 86%

Metabolism: In the liver by oxidation (by cytochrome P-450 isoenzyme CYP3A4) to several metabolites including 1-pyrimidinyl piperazine (about $^1\!/_4$ as active as buspirone)

Half-life: Adults: Mean: 2-3 hours; increased with renal or liver dysfunction

Elimination: 29% to 63% excreted in urine (primarily as metabolites)

Usual Dosage Oral:

Children and Adolescents: Anxiety disorders: Limited information is available from pediatric case studies and open-labeled trials; dose is not well established; one pilot study of 15 children, 6-14 years of age (mean 10 years), with mixed anxiety disorders, used initial doses of 5 mg daily; doses were individualized with increases in increments of 5 mg/day every week as needed to a maximum dose of 20 mg/day divided into 2 doses; the mean dose required = 18.6 mg/day; some authors (Carrey, 1996 and Kutcher, 1992), based on their clinical experience, recommend higher doses

Adults: Initial: 7.5 mg twice daily; increase in increments of 5 mg/day every 2-3 days as needed to a maximum of 60 mg/day; usual dose: 20-30 mg/day in 2 or 3 divided doses

Dosing adjustment in renal impairment:

Mild to moderate renal dysfunction: Dose reductions not required

Patients with anuria: Reduce dose by 25% to 50%; further studies are needed

Administration Oral: May be administered without regard to food; may administer with food to decrease GI upset; use caution if administered with grapefruit juice; avoid large amounts of grapefruit juice (see Food Interactions)

Monitoring Parameters Mental status, signs and symptoms of anxiety, liver and renal function

Patient Information Avoid alcohol; may cause drowsiness and impair the ability to perform tasks which require mental alertness or physical coordination

Additional Information Not appropriate for "as needed" (prn) use or for brief, situational anxiety; buspirone is equipotent to diazepam on a milligram to milligram basis in the treatment of anxiety; however, unlike diazepam, the onset of buspirone is delayed (see Pharmacodynamics)

Dosage Forms Tablet, as hydrochloride: 5 mg, 10 mg, 15 mg, 30 mg

References

Carrey NJ, Wiggins DM, and Milin RP, "Pharmacological Treatment of Psychiatric Disorders in Children and Adolescents," *Drugs*, 1996, 51(5):750-9.

Hanna GL, Feibusch EL, and Albright KJ, "Buspirone Treatment of Anxiety, Associated With Pharyngeal Dysphagia in a Four-Year Old," *J Child Adolesc Psychopharmacol*, 1997, 7(2):137-43.

Kivisto KT, Lamberg TS, and Kantola T, "Plasma Buspirone Concentrations Are Greatly Increased by Erythromycin and Itraconazole," *Clin Pharmacol Ther*, 1997, 62(3):348-54.

Kutcher SP, Reiter S, Gardner DM, et al, "The Pharmacotherapy of Anxiety Disorders in Children and Adolescents," *Psychiatr Clin North Am*, 1992, 15(1):41-67.

Simeon JG, Knott VJ, DuBois C, et al, "Buspirone Therapy of Mixed Anxiety Disorders in Childhood and Adolescence: A Pilot Study," *J Child Adolesc Psychopharmacol*, 1994, 4(3):159-70.

Soni P and Weintraub AL, "Buspirone-Associated Mental Status Changes," *J Am Acad Child Adolesc Psychiatry*, 1992, 31(6):1098-9.

♦ **Bustab (Can)** *see* Buspirone *on page 159*

Busulfan (byoo SUL fan)

Related Information
Emetogenic Potential of Single Chemotherapeutic Agents *on page 1129*

U.S. Brand Names Busulfex®; Myleran®

Therapeutic Category Antineoplastic Agent, Alkylating Agent

Generic Available No

Use Chronic myelogenous leukemia (CML); component of marrow-ablative conditioning regimen prior to bone marrow transplantation (BMT) for refractory leukemias, lymphomas, and pediatric solid tumors

Pregnancy Risk Factor D

Contraindications Hypersensitivity to busulfan or any component; failure to respond to previous courses; should not be used in pregnancy or lactation

Warnings The FDA currently recommends that procedures for proper handling and disposal of antineoplastic agents be considered; discontinue busulfan if lung toxicity develops; busulfan is potentially carcinogenic; malignant tumors and acute leukemias have been reported in patients who received busulfan; busulfan is associated with ovarian failure including failure to achieve puberty in females

Precautions May induce severe bone marrow hypoplasia; reduce dosage in patients with bone marrow suppression; use with extreme caution in patients who have recently received other myelosuppressive drugs or radiation therapy; use with caution in patients with a history of seizure disorder, head trauma, or when receiving other epileptogenic drugs

Adverse Reactions

Central nervous system: Dizziness, seizures

Dermatologic: Hyperpigmentation, alopecia, rash, urticaria

Endocrine & metabolic: Addisonian-like syndrome (hyperpigmentation, wasting, hypotension), hyperuricemia, gynecomastia, testicular atrophy, amenorrhea, sterility

Gastrointestinal: Nausea, vomiting, mucositis, diarrhea

Genitourinary: Hemorrhagic cystitis

Hematologic: Myelosuppression with nadirs of 14-21 days for leukopenia and thrombocytopenia; anemia, aplastic anemia

Hepatic: Hepatic impairment, hepatic veno-occlusive disease, hyperbilirubinemia

Ocular: Blurred vision, subcapsular cataracts, corneal thinning

Respiratory: Pulmonary fibrosis

Drug Interactions Cytochrome P-450 isoenzyme CYP3A3/4 substrate

Thioguanine (may increase hepatotoxicity); itraconazole (may decrease busulfan clearance by 25% and increase busulfan toxicity); phenytoin lowers busulfan plasma AUC by 15%; acetaminophen may decrease busulfan clearance

Food Interactions No clear or firm data on the effect of food on busulfan bioavailability

Stability Store intact ampuls in the refrigerator; diluted busulfan solution is stable for up to 8 hours at room temperature; infusion must be completed within that 8 hour time frame. If diluted in NS, the solution is stable for 12 hours if refrigerated, but the infusion must be completed within that 12-hour time frame.

Mechanism of Action Interferes with the normal function of DNA by alkylation of intracellular nucleophiles and cross-linking the strands of DNA

Pharmacokinetics

Absorption: Oral: 70% absorbed

Distribution: Crosses into CSF, saliva, placenta, and liver

Protein binding: 32% to 55%

Metabolism: Extensive in the liver

Half-life:

Children: 2.5 hours

Adults: 2.3-2.6 hours

Time to peak plasma concentration: Oral: Within 1-2 hours

Elimination: 10% to 50% excreted in urine as metabolites, 1% excreted unchanged in urine within 24 hours; total plasma clearance rate is 2-4 times higher in children than in adults

Usual Dosage Refer to individual protocols; dose should be based on ideal body weight

(Continued)

Busulfan *(Continued)*

Children: Oral:
Remission induction of CML: 0.06-0.12 mg/kg once daily **or** 1.8-4.6 mg/m²/day once daily; titrate dose to maintain a leukocyte count >40,000/mm³; discontinue busulfan if counts fall to ≤20,000/mm³
BMT marrow-ablative conditioning regimen: 1 mg/kg/dose every 6 hours for 16 doses
Children ≤6 years of age in the hematopoietic stem cell transplant program may receive 40 mg/m²/dose every 6 hours for 16 doses

Adults:
Oral:
Remission induction of CML: 4-8 mg/day or 0.06 mg/kg/day
Maintenance dose: Controversial; range is from 1-4 mg/day to 2 mg/week; reduce dose in proportion to the decrease in leukocyte count or discontinue busulfan when the leukocyte count falls to ≤20,000/mm³
I.V.: High-dose BMT conditioning regimen: 0.8 mg/kg/dose every 6 hours for 16 doses ending on day 3 before transplantation

Administration

Oral: May be administered without regard to meals
Parenteral: Dilute busulfan injection with either NS or D₅W to a final concentration of ≥0.5 mg/mL (diluent volume should be 10 times the volume of busulfan injection); infuse over 2 hours through a central venous catheter; flush line before and after each infusion with D₅W or NS

Monitoring Parameters CBC with differential and platelet count, hemoglobin, liver function tests, bilirubin, alkaline phosphatase; monitor busulfan plasma concentration

Patient Information Report any difficulty in breathing, cough, fever, sore throat, bleeding or bruising to physician

Additional Information One method used to prevent seizures during high-dose busulfan (16 mg/kg over 4 days) is to initiate a standard loading dose of phenytoin (15 mg/kg) 1 day prior to starting busulfan therapy followed by a maintenance dose adjusted to maintain a therapeutic phenytoin concentration until 24 hours after the final busulfan dose

Dosage Forms

Injection: 6 mg/mL (10 mL ampul)
Tablet, scored: 2 mg

References

Bolinger AM, Zangwill AB, Slattery JT, et al, "An Evaluation of Engraftment, Toxicity and Busulfan Concentration in Children Receiving Bone Marrow Transplantation for Leukemia or Genetic Disease," *Bone Marrow Transplant*, 2000, 25(9):925-30.
Heard BE and Cooke RA, "Busulphan Lung," *Thorax*, 1968, 23(2):187-93.
Ozkaynak MF, Weinberg K, Kohn D, et al, "Hepatic Veno-Occlusive Disease Post-Bone Marrow Transplantation in Children Conditioned With Busulfan and Cyclophosphamide: Incidence, Risk Factors, and Clinical Outcome," *Bone Marrow Transplant*, 1991, 7(6):467-74.
Regazzi MB, Locatelli F, Buggia I, et al, "Disposition of High Dose Busulfan in Pediatric Patients Undergoing Bone Marrow Transplantation," *Clin Pharmacol Ther*, 1993, 54(1):45-52.
Vassal G, Gouyette A, Hartmann O, et al, "Pharmacokinetics of High-Dose Busulfan in Children," *Cancer Chemother Pharmacol*, 1989, 24(6):386-90.

- ♦ **Busulfex®** *see* Busulfan *on page 161*
- ♦ **BW-430C** *see* Lamotrigine *on page 575*
- ♦ **C-1000 (Can)** *see* Ascorbic Acid *on page 106*
- ♦ **C-3000 (Can)** *see* Ascorbic Acid *on page 106*
- ♦ **Caelyx (Can)** *see* Doxorubicin *on page 360*
- ♦ **Cafcit®** *see* Caffeine (Citrated) *on page 162*
- ♦ **Cafergot®** *see* Ergotamine *on page 393*

Caffeine (Citrated) (KAF een, SIT rated)

Related Information
Overdose and Toxicology *on page 1222*
U.S. Brand Names Cafcit®
Therapeutic Category Central Nervous System Stimulant, Nonamphetamine; Respiratory Stimulant
Generic Available No
Use Treatment of idiopathic apnea of prematurity
Pregnancy Risk Factor C
Contraindications Hypersensitivity to caffeine or any component
Warnings Do not interchange the caffeine citrate salt formulation with the caffeine sodium benzoate formulation; the sodium benzoate salt has been reported to

produce kernicterus (by displacement of bilirubin) and neonatal "gasping syndrome"; its use (sodium benzoate) should be avoided in neonates; during a Cafcit® double-blind, placebo-controlled study, 6 of 85 patients developed necrotizing enterocolitis (NEC); 5 of these 6 patients had received caffeine citrate; although no causal relationship has been established, neonates who receive caffeine citrate should be closely monitored for the development of NEC.

Precautions Use with caution in patients with a history of peptic ulcer, impaired renal or hepatic function, seizure disorders, or cardiovascular disease; avoid in patients with symptomatic cardiac arrhythmias

Adverse Reactions

Cardiovascular: Cardiac arrhythmias, tachycardia, extrasystoles

Central nervous system: Insomnia, restlessness, agitation, irritability, hyperactivity, jitteriness, headache

Endocrine & metabolic: Hypoglycemia, hyperglycemia

Gastrointestinal: Nausea, vomiting, gastric irritation, necrotizing enterocolitis, GI hemorrhage

Genitourinary: Increased urine output

Neuromuscular & skeletal: Muscle tremors or twitches

Drug Interactions Cytochrome P-450 isoenzyme CYP1A2, CYP2E1, and CYP3A3/4 substrate

Enhances the positive cardiac inotropic and chronotropic effects of beta-adrenergic agonists; cimetidine and phenylpropanolamine may impair caffeine metabolism; decreases hemodynamic effect of adenosine; fluconazole, mexiletine and cimetidine increase caffeine serum levels

Stability Injection and oral solution contain no preservatives; injection is chemically stable for at least 24 hours at room temperature when diluted to 10 mg/mL (as caffeine citrate) with D_5W, $D_{50}W$, Intralipid® 20%, and Aminosyn® 8.5%; also compatible with dopamine (600 mcg/mL), calcium gluconate 10%, heparin (1 unit/mL), and fentanyl (10 mcg/mL) at room temperature for 24 hours

Mechanism of Action Increases levels of 3-5-AMP by inhibiting phosphodiesterase; CNS stimulant which increases medullary respiratory center sensitivity to carbon dioxide, stimulates central inspiratory drive, and improves skeletal muscle contraction (diaphragmatic contractility); prevention of apnea may occur by competitive inhibition of adenosine

Pharmacokinetics

Distribution: V_d:

Neonates: 0.8-0.9 L/kg

Children >9 months to Adults: 0.6 L/kg

Protein binding: 17%

Metabolism: Interconversion between caffeine and theophylline has been reported in preterm neonates (caffeine levels are ~25% of measured theophylline after theophylline administration and ~3% to 8% of caffeine would be expected to be converted to theophylline)

Half-life:

Neonates: 72-96 hours (range: 40-230 hours)

Adults: 5 hours

Time to peak serum concentration: Oral: Within 30 minutes to 2 hours

Elimination:

Neonates ≤1 month: 86% excreted unchanged in urine

Infants >1 month and Adults: Extensively liver metabolized to a series of partially demethylated xanthines and methyluric acids

Clearance:

Neonates: 8.9 mL/hour/kg (range: 2.5-17)

Adults: 94 mL/hour/kg

Usual Dosage Apnea of prematurity: Neonates: Oral, I.V.:

Loading dose: 10-20 mg/kg as caffeine citrate (5-10 mg/kg as caffeine base). If theophylline has been administered to the patient within the previous 3 days, a full or modified loading dose (50% to 75% of a loading dose) may be given (caffeine is a significant metabolite of theophylline in the newborn; see Pharmacokinetics).

Maintenance dose: 5 mg/kg/day as caffeine citrate (2.5 mg/kg/day as caffeine base) once daily starting 24 hours after the loading dose. Maintenance dose is adjusted based on patient's response (efficacy and adverse effects), and serum caffeine concentrations.

Administration

Oral: May be administered without regard to feedings or meals; may administer injectable formulation orally

Parenteral: Infuse loading dose over at least 30 minutes; maintenance dose may be infused over at least 10 minutes; may administer without dilution or diluted with D_5W to 10 mg/mL (caffeine citrate)

(Continued)

Caffeine (Citrated) *(Continued)*

Monitoring Parameters Heart rate, number and severity of apnea spells, serum caffeine levels

Reference Range

Therapeutic: Apnea of prematurity: 8-20 µg/mL

Potentially toxic: >20 µg/mL

Toxic: >50 µg/mL

Dosage Forms

Injection: 20 mg/mL as caffeine citrate [equivalent to 10 mg/mL caffeine base] (3 mL)

Solution, oral: 20 mg/mL as caffeine citrate [equivalent to 10 mg/mL caffeine base] (3 mL)

Extemporaneous Preparations An oral solution of 20 mg/mL caffeine citrate, prepared from 10 g caffeine (anhydrous) combined with 10 g citric acid USP and 1000 mL SWI is stable for 3 months refrigerated (Nahata, 1987).

An oral solution 20 mg/mL caffeine citrate may be made by dissolving 5 g anhydrous caffeine and 5 g citric acid USP in 250 mL SWI. Stir solution until completely clear; add 2:1 simple syrup:cherry syrup mixture to a final volume of 500 mL; stable refrigerated 90 days (Eisenberg, 1984).

Eisenberg MG and Kang N, "Stability of Citrated Caffeine Solutions for Injectable and Enteral Use," *Am J Hosp Pharm*, 1984, 41(11):2405-6.

Nahata MC and Roberts DL, "Formulation of Caffeine Injection for I.V. Administration," *Am J Hosp Pharm*, 1987, 44(6):1308, 1312.

References

Erenberg A, Leff RD, Haack DG, et al, "Caffeine Citrate for the Treatment of Apnea of Prematurity: A Double-Blind, Placebo-Controlled Study," *Pharmacotherapy*, 2000, 20(6):644-52.

Kriter KE and Blanchard J, "Management of Apnea in Infants," *Clin Pharm*, 1989, 8(8):577-87.

Calamine Lotion *(KAL a myne loe shun)*

Therapeutic Category Topical Skin Product

Generic Available Yes

Use Employed primarily as an astringent, protectant, and soothing agent for conditions such as poison ivy, poison oak, poison sumac, sunburn, insect bites, or minor skin irritations

Precautions For external use only

Adverse Reactions

Dermatologic: Rash

Local: Irritation

Usual Dosage Topical: Apply 1-4 times/day as needed; reapply after bathing

Administration Topical: Shake well before using; avoid contact with the eyes; do not use on open wounds or burns

Additional Information Active ingredients: Calamine, zinc oxide

Dosage Forms Lotion, topical:

Calamine, USP: Calamine 8%, zinc oxide 8%, glycerin 2% and bentonite magma in calcium hydroxide solution (120 mL, 240 mL, 480 mL)

Calamine, USP, phenolated: Calamine 8%, zinc oxide 8%, glycerin 2%, bentonite magma, and phenol 1% in calcium hydroxide solution (120 mL, 240 mL)

♦ **Calan**® *see* Verapamil *on page 1007*

♦ **Calan**® **SR** *see* Verapamil *on page 1007*

♦ **Calax (Can)** *see* Docusate *on page 350*

♦ **Calci-Chew**™ **[OTC]** *see* Calcium Supplements *on page 167*

♦ **Calciferol**™ *see* Ergocalciferol *on page 392*

♦ **Calcijex**™ *see* Calcitriol *on page 166*

♦ **Calcimar (Can)** *see* Calcitonin *on page 164*

♦ **Calci-Mix**™ **[OTC]** *see* Calcium Supplements *on page 167*

Calcitonin *(kal si TOE nin)*

U.S. Brand Names Miacalcin®

Canadian Brand Names Calcimar; Caltine

Therapeutic Category Antidote, Hypercalcemia

Generic Available No

Use Calcitonin (salmon): Treatment of Paget's disease of bone and as adjunctive therapy for hypercalcemia; also used in postmenopausal osteoporosis and osteogenesis imperfecta

Pregnancy Risk Factor C

Contraindications Hypersensitivity to salmon protein or gelatin diluent

Precautions A skin test should be performed prior to initiating therapy; the skin test is 0.1 mL of 10 unit/mL calcitonin injection in NS (must be prepared) injected intradermally; observe injection site for 15 minutes for wheal or significant erythema

Adverse Reactions
Cardiovascular: Flushing of the face, edema
Central nervous system: Dizziness, headache, chills
Dermatologic: Rash
Gastrointestinal: Nausea, vomiting, diarrhea, anorexia, metallic taste
Local: Inflammatory reactions at the injection site
Neuromuscular & skeletal: Weakness, tingling of palms and soles, back and joint pain
Renal: Diuresis
Respiratory: Shortness of breath, nasal congestion, epistaxis, nasal sores, and sore bridge of nose (nasal spray)

Stability
Salmon calcitonin: Injection: Store under refrigeration; stable for up to 2 weeks at room temperature
Salmon calcitonin: Nasal spray: Store unopened bottle under refrigeration; once the pump has been activated, store at room temperature; stable at room temperature for 30 days

Mechanism of Action Salmon calcitonin directly inhibits osteoclastic bone resorption; promotes the renal excretion of calcium, phosphate, sodium, magnesium and potassium by decreasing tubular reabsorption; increases the jejunal secretion of water, sodium, potassium, and chloride

Pharmacodynamics
Hypercalcemia:
Onset of action:
I.M., S.C.: 15 minutes
I.V.: Immediate
Peak effect: I.M., S.C.: 4 hours
Duration of effect:
I.M., S.C.: 8-24 hours
I.V.: 30 minutes to 12 hours

Pharmacokinetics
Absorption: Intranasal: Rapidly but highly variable and lower than I.M. administration
Metabolism: Rapidly in the kidneys, blood, and peripheral tissues
Half-life, elimination: Intranasal: 43 minutes
Time to peak serum concentration: Intranasal: 31-39 minutes
Elimination: As inactive metabolites in urine
Clearance: Salmon calcitonin: 3.1 mL/kg/minute

Usual Dosage Dosage for children not established; Adults:
Paget's disease:
I.M., S.C.: Initial: 100 units/day; maintenance dose: 50 units/day or 50-100 units every 1-3 days
Intranasal: 200-400 units (1-2 sprays) per day
Hypercalcemia: Initial: I.M., S.C.: 4 units/kg every 12 hours; may increase up to 8 units/kg every 12 hours to a maximum of every 6 hours
Osteogenesis imperfecta: I.M., S.C.: 2 units/kg 3 times/week
Postmenopausal osteoporosis:
I.M., S.C.: 100 units/day
Intranasal: 200 units (1 spray) per day

Administration
Intranasal: Alternate spray into each nostril daily
Parenteral: Do not exceed 2 mL volume per injection site; may be administered S.C. or I.M.

Monitoring Parameters Serum electrolytes and calcium; alkaline phosphatase and 24-hour urine collection for hydroxyproline excretion (Paget's disease); serum calcium

Reference Range Therapeutic: <19 pg/mL (SI: 19 ng/L) basal, depending on the assay

Patient Information Nasal spray: Notify physician if you develop significant nasal irritation; alternate nostrils; in treatment of postmenopausal osteoporosis, maintain adequate vitamin D intake and supplemental calcium

Dosage Forms
Injection: **Salmon** (Miacalcin®): 200 units/mL (2 mL)
Spray, nasal: **Salmon** (Miacalcin®): 200 units/activation (0.09 mL/dose) (2 mL glass bottle with pump)

♦ **Cal-Citrate®** [OTC] *see* Calcium Supplements *on page 167*

Calcitriol (kal si TRYE ole)

U.S. Brand Names Calcijex™; Rocaltrol®

Synonyms 1,25 dihydroxycholecalciferol

Therapeutic Category Rickets, Treatment Agent; Vitamin D Analog; Vitamin, Fat Soluble

Generic Available No

Use Management of hypocalcemia associated with hypoparathyroidism, pseudohypothyroidism, and in patients on chronic renal dialysis; rickets

Pregnancy Risk Factor C

Contraindications Hypercalcemia; vitamin D toxicity; abnormal sensitivity to the effects of vitamin D

Adverse Reactions
Cardiovascular: Increased blood pressure, cardiac arrhythmias
Central nervous system: Somnolence, headache, hyperthermia
Dermatologic: Pruritus
Endocrine & metabolic: Hypercholesterolemia, hypercalcemia, polydipsia
Gastrointestinal: Nausea, vomiting, constipation, anorexia, xerostomia, pancreatitis, metallic taste, weight loss
Genitourinary: Nocturia
Hepatic: Elevated liver enzymes
Neuromuscular & skeletal: Myalgia, bone pain, weakness
Ocular: Calcific conjunctivitis, photophobia
Renal: Polyuria, uremia, albuminuria
Respiratory: Rhinorrhea

Drug Interactions May antagonize the effects of calcium channel blockers by increasing serum calcium level; may be associated with digoxin toxicity by increasing calcium levels; may result in an additive increase in calcium levels due to decreased calcium excretion by thiazide diuretics; magnesium-containing antacids (potential development of hypermagnesemia); cholestyramine, colestipol, orlistat, and excessive use of mineral oil decrease absorption

Stability Protect from light and heat

Mechanism of Action Promotes absorption of calcium in the intestines and retention via the kidneys thereby increasing calcium levels in the serum; decreases excessive serum phosphatase levels, parathyroid hormone levels, and decreases bone resorption

Pharmacodynamics Oral:
Onset of effect: 2 hours
Peak effect: 10 hours
Duration: 3-5 days

Pharmacokinetics
Metabolism: Primarily to 1,24,25-trihydroxycholecalciferol and 1,24,25-trihydroxy ergocalciferol
Half-life: 4-6 hours
Elimination: Principally in bile and feces

Usual Dosage Individualize dosage to maintain calcium levels of 9-10 mg/dL
Management of hypocalcemia in patients with chronic renal failure:
Hemodialysis patients:
I.V.:
Children: 0.01-0.05 mcg/kg 3 times/week
Adults: 0.5 mcg (0.01 mcg/kg) 3 times/week; may increase dosage by 0.25-0.5 mcg increments at 2- to 4-week intervals until an optimal response is achieved; range: 0.5-3 mcg (0.01-0.05 mcg/kg)
Oral:
Children: 0.25-2 mcg/day
Adults: 0.25 mcg; may increase in 0.25 mcg increments at 4- to 8-week intervals; range: 0.5-1 mcg/day
Nonhemodialysis patients: Moderate to severe renal failure (Cl$_{cr}$ 15-55 mL/minute; corrected for surface area in children): Oral:
Children <3 years: 0.01-0.015 mcg/kg once daily
Children ≥3 years and Adults: 0.25 mcg/day (maximum dose: 0.5 mcg/day)
Hypoparathyroidism/pseudohypoparathyroidism: Oral (evaluate dosage at 2- to 4-week intervals):
Children:
<1 year: 0.04-0.08 mcg/kg once daily
1-5 years: 0.25-0.75 mcg once daily
Children >6 years and Adults: 0.5-2 mcg once daily
Vitamin D-dependent rickets: Children and Adults: Oral: 1 mcg once daily

Vitamin D-resistant rickets (familial hypophosphatemia): Children and Adults: Oral: Initial: 0.015-0.02 mcg/kg once daily; maintenance: 0.03-0.06 mcg/kg once daily; maximum dose: 2 mcg once daily

Hypocalcemia in premature infants: Oral: 1 mcg once daily for 5 days

Hypocalcemic tetany in premature infants: I.V.: 0.05 mcg/kg once daily for 5-12 days

Administration

Oral: When administering small doses from the liquid-filled capsules, consider the following concentration for Rocaltrol®:

0.25 mcg capsule = 0.25 mcg per 0.17 mL

0.5 mcg capsule = 0.5 mcg per 0.17 mL

Parenteral: May be administered undiluted as a bolus dose I.V. through the catheter at the end of hemodialysis

Monitoring Parameters Serum calcium and phosphorus levels at least twice weekly at the onset of therapy and after each dosage adjustment; weekly for 12 weeks, then monthly after stabilization of dosage; magnesium, 24-hour urinary calcium

Dosage Forms

Capsule (Rocaltrol®): 0.25 mcg, 0.5 mcg

Injection (Calcijex™): 1 mcg/mL (1 mL); 2 mcg/mL (1 mL)

Solution, oral (Rocaltrol®): 1 mcg/mL (15 mL)

- ◆ **Calcium Acetate** *see* Calcium Supplements *on page 167*
- ◆ **Calcium Carbonate** *see* Calcium Supplements *on page 167*
- ◆ **Calcium Chloride** *see* Calcium Supplements *on page 167*
- ◆ **Calcium Citrate** *see* Calcium Supplements *on page 167*
- ◆ **Calcium Disodium Edathamil** *see* Edetate Calcium Disodium *on page 371*
- ◆ **Calcium Disodium Edetate** *see* Edetate Calcium Disodium *on page 371*
- ◆ **Calcium Disodium Versenate®** *see* Edetate Calcium Disodium *on page 371*
- ◆ **Calcium Edetate** *see* Edetate Calcium Disodium *on page 371*
- ◆ **Calcium EDTA** *see* Edetate Calcium Disodium *on page 371*
- ◆ **Calcium Glubionate** *see* Calcium Supplements *on page 167*
- ◆ **Calcium Gluconate** *see* Calcium Supplements *on page 167*
- ◆ **Calcium Lactate** *see* Calcium Supplements *on page 167*
- ◆ **Calcium Phosphate, Tribasic** *see* Calcium Supplements *on page 167*

Calcium Supplements (KAL see um SUP la ments)

Related Information

Antacid Preparations *on page 95*

Carbohydrate and Alcohol Content of Liquid Medications for Use in Patients Receiving Ketogenic Diets *on page 1258*

CPR Pediatric Drug Dosages *on page 1031*

Extravasation Treatment *on page 1085*

U.S. Brand Names Alka-Mints® [OTC]; Amitone® [OTC]; Calci-Chew™ [OTC]; Calci-Mix™ [OTC]; Cal-Citrate® [OTC]; Cal-lac® [OTC]; Caltrate® 600 [OTC]; Chooz® [OTC]; Citracal® [OTC]; Citracal® Liquitab [OTC]; Florical® [OTC]; Mallamint® [OTC]; Mylanta® Calci Tabs Extra Strength [OTC]; Mylanta® Calci Tabs Ultra [OTC]; Mylanta® Children's [OTC]; Neo-Calglucon® [OTC]; Nephro-Calci® [OTC]; Os-Cal® 500 [OTC]; Oysco®; Oyst-Cal 500 [OTC]; Oystercal® 500; PhosLo® Posture® [OTC]; Rolaids® [OTC]; Titralac® [OTC]; Tums® [OTC]; Tums® E-X [OTC]; Tums® Ultra® [OTC]

Available Salts Calcium Acetate; Calcium Carbonate; Calcium Chloride; Calcium Citrate; Calcium Glubionate; Calcium Gluconate; Calcium Lactate; Calcium Phosphate, Tribasic

Therapeutic Category Antacid; Antidote, Hydrofluoric Acid; Calcium Salt; Electrolyte Supplement, Oral; Electrolyte Supplement, Parenteral

Generic Available Yes

Use Treatment and prevention of calcium depletion; relief of acid indigestion, heartburn; emergency treatment of hypocalcemic tetany; treatment of hypermagnesemia, cardiac disturbances of hyperkalemia, hypocalcemia, or calcium channel blocking agent toxicity; topical treatment of hydrofluoric acid burns

Pregnancy Risk Factor C

Contraindications Hypercalcemia, renal calculi, ventricular fibrillation

Precautions Use cautiously in patients with sarcoidosis, respiratory failure, acidosis, renal or cardiac disease; avoid too rapid I.V. administration; avoid extravasation; use with caution in digitalized patients; Quick Dissolve Maalox® Maximum Strength tablets contain aspartame, avoid or use with caution in phenylketonuria

(Continued)

Calcium Supplements *(Continued)*

Adverse Reactions

Cardiovascular: Vasodilation, hypotension, bradycardia, cardiac arrhythmias, ventricular fibrillation, syncope

Central nervous system: Headache, mental confusion, dizziness, lethargy, coma

Dermatologic: Erythema

Endocrine & metabolic: Hypercalcemia, milk-alkali syndrome, hypophosphatemia, hypercalciuria, hypomagnesemia

Gastrointestinal: Constipation, nausea, vomiting, xerostomia, elevated serum amylase

Local: Tissue necrosis (I.V. administration)

Neuromuscular & skeletal: Muscle weakness

Drug Interactions May potentiate digoxin toxicity; may antagonize the effects of calcium channel blockers (eg, verapamil); when administered orally, calcium decreases the absorption of tetracycline, atenolol, iron, quinolone antibiotics, alendronate, sodium fluoride, and zinc; high doses of calcium with thiazide diuretics may result in milk-alkali syndrome and hypercalcemia; decreases potassium-binding ability of polystyrene sulfonate

Food Interactions Do not give orally with bran, foods high in oxalates, or whole grain cereals which may decrease calcium absorption

Stability Incompatible with bicarbonates, phosphates, and sulfates

Mechanism of Action Moderates nerve and muscle performance via action potential excitation threshold regulation; neutralizes acidity of stomach (carbonate salt)

Usual Dosage Note: Multiple salt forms of calcium exist; close attention must be paid to the salt form when ordering and administering calcium; incorrect selection or substitution of one salt for another without proper dosage adjustment may result in serious over- or underdosing.

Oral: **Note:** For comparison information of calcium salts, see table.

Elemental Calcium Content of Calcium Salts

Calcium Salt	Elemental Calcium (mg/1 g of salt form)	mEq calcium per gram	Approximate Equivalent Doses (mg of calcium salt)
Calcium acetate	250	12.7	354
Calcium carbonate	400	20	225
Calcium chloride	270	13.5	330
Calcium citrate	211	10.6	425
Calcium glubionate	64	3.2	1400
Calcium gluconate	90	4.5	1000
Calcium lactate	130	6.5	700
Calcium phosphate, tribasic	390	19.3	233

Recommended daily allowance (RDA): Dosage is in terms of elemental calcium:

<6 months: 400 mg/day

6-12 months: 600 mg/day

1-10 years: 800 mg/day

11-24 years: 1200 mg/day

Adults >24 years: 800 mg/day

Adequate intake (1997 National Academy of Science Recommendations): **Dosage is in terms of elemental calcium:**

0-6 months: 210 mg/day

7-12 months: 270 mg/day

1-3 years: 500 mg/day

4-8 years: 800 mg/day

9-18 years: 1300 mg/day

19-50 years: 1000 mg/day

>50 years: 1200 mg/day

Hypocalcemia (dose depends on clinical condition and serum calcium level): **Oral:** Dose expressed in mg of **elemental calcium:**

Neonates: 50-150 mg/kg/day in 4-6 divided doses; not to exceed 1 g/day

Children: 45-65 mg/kg/day in 4 divided doses

Adults: 1-2 g or more per day in 3-4 divided doses

Dose expressed in mg of **calcium gluconate:**
Neonates: 500-1500 mg/kg/day in 4-6 divided doses
Infants and Children: 500-725 mg/kg/day in 3-4 divided doses
Adults: 10-20 g daily in 3-4 divided doses
Dose expressed in mg of **calcium glubionate:**
Neonates: 1200 mg/kg/day in 4-6 divided doses
Infants and Children: 600-2000 mg/kg/day in 4 divided doses up to a maximum of 9 g/day
Adults: 6-18 g/day in divided doses
Dose expressed in mg of **calcium lactate:**
Neonates and Infants: 400-500 mg/kg/day divided every 4-6 hours
Children: 500 mg/kg/day divided every 6-8 hours; maximum daily dose 9 g
Adults: 1.5-3 g divided every 8 hours
Hypocalcemia: I.V.:
Dosage expressed in mg of **calcium chloride:**
Manufacturer's recommendations: Children: 2.7-5 mg/kg/dose every 4-6 hours
Alternative pediatric dosing: Neonates, Infants, and Children: 10-20 mg/kg/dose, repeat every 4-6 hours if needed
Adults: 500 mg to 1 g/dose every 6 hours
Dose expressed in mg of **calcium gluconate:**
Neonates: 200-800 mg/kg/day as a continuous infusion or in 4 divided doses
Infants and Children: 200-500 mg/kg/day as a continuous infusion or in 4 divided doses
Adults: 2-15 g/day as a continuous infusion or in divided doses
Cardiac arrest in the presence of hyperkalemia or hypocalcemia, magnesium toxicity, or calcium antagonist toxicity: I.V., I.O.:
Dosage expressed in mg of **calcium chloride:**
Neonates, Infants, and Children: 20 mg/kg; may repeat in 10 minutes if necessary
Adults: 2-4 mg/kg; may repeat in 10 minutes if necessary
Dosage expressed in mg of **calcium gluconate:**
Neonates, Infants, and Children: 60-100 mg/kg/dose (maximum 3 g/dose)
Adults: 500-800 mg (maximum 3 g/dose)
Hypocalcemia secondary to citrated blood infusion: I.V.: Give 0.45 mEq **elemental** calcium for each 100 mL citrated blood infused
Tetany: I.V.:
Dose expressed in mg of **calcium chloride:**
Neonates, Infants, and Children: 10 mg/kg over 5-10 minutes; may repeat after 6 hours or follow with an infusion with a maximum dose of 200 mg/kg/day
Adults: 1 g over 10-30 minutes; may repeat after 6 hours
Dose expressed in mg of **calcium gluconate:**
Neonates: 100-200 mg/kg/dose; may follow with 500 mg/kg/day in 3-4 divided doses or as a continuous infusion
Infants and Children: 100-200 mg/kg/dose over 5-10 minutes; may repeat after 6 hours or follow with an infusion of 500 mg/kg/day
Adults: 1-3 g may be administered until therapeutic response occurs
Antacid (calcium carbonate): See Antacid Preparations *on page 95*
Hydrofluoric acid (HF) burns (HF concentration <20%): Topical: Various topical calcium preparations have been used anecdotally for treatment of dermal exposure to HF solutions; both calcium gluconate and carbonate at concentrations ranging from 2.5% to 33% have been used: Massage calcium gluconate gel or slurry into exposed area for 15 minutes; topical calcium preparations must be compounded (see Extemporaneous Preparations)
Administration
Oral: Administer with plenty of fluids with or following meals
Parenteral:
I.V.: For direct I.V. injection infuse at a maximum rate of 50-100 mg/minute of calcium salt (gluconate, chloride, or gluceptate)
I.V. infusion: Dilution and infusion rates are dependent upon the salt form; dilute with I.V. fluid to a final concentration not to exceed maximums listed below; infuse over 1 hour without exceeding maximum rates of infusion listed below
Salt form (Maximum dilution; Maximum rate of infusion)
Calcium **chloride:** 20 mg/mL; 45-90 mg/kg over 1 hour; 0.6-1.2 mEq/kg over 1 hour
Calcium **gluconate:** 50 mg/mL; 120-240 mg/kg over 1 hour ; 0.6-1.2 mEq/kg over 1 hour
Do not inject calcium salts I.M. or administer S.C. since severe necrosis and sloughing may occur; extravasation of calcium can result in severe necrosis and
(Continued)

Calcium Supplements *(Continued)*

tissue sloughing. Do not use scalp vein or small hand or foot veins for I.V. administration. Not for endotracheal administration.

Monitoring Parameters Serum calcium (ionized calcium preferred if available, see Additional Information), phosphate, magnesium, heart rate, EKG

Reference Range

Calcium: Newborns: 7.0-12.0 mg/dL; 0-2 years: 8.8-11.2 mg/dL; 2 years to adults: 9.0-11.0 mg/dL

Calcium, ionized, whole blood: 4.4-5.4 mg/dL

Additional Information Due to a poor correlation between the serum ionized calcium (free) and total serum calcium, particularly in states of low albumin or acid/base imbalances, direct measurement of ionized calcium is recommended. If ionized calcium is unavailable, in low albumin states, the corrected **total** serum calcium may be estimated by this equation (assuming a normal albumin of 4 g/dL); corrected total calcium = total serum calcium + 0.8 (4 - measured serum albumin)

Dosage Forms Elemental calcium listed in brackets

Calcium acetate:

Capsule (PhosLo®): 333.5 mg [84.5 mg], 667 mg [169 mg]

Gelcap (PhosLo®): 667 mg [169 mg]

Calcium carbonate:

Capsule: 1500 mg [600 mg]

Florical®: 364 mg [145.6 mg] with sodium fluoride 8.3 mg

Suspension, oral: 1250 mg/5 mL [500 mg]

Children's Mylanta®: 400 mg/5 mL

Tablet: 650 mg [260 mg], 1500 mg [600 mg]

Os-Cal® 500, Oyst-Cal 500, Oystercal® 500: 1250 mg [500 mg]

Caltrate® 600, Nephro-Calci®: 1500 mg [600 mg]

Tablet, chewable:

Alka-Mints®: 850 mg [340 mg]

Calci-Chew™, Os-Cal® 500, Oysco® 500: 1250 mg [500 mg]

Children's Mylanta®: 400 mg [160 mg]

Chooz®, Tums®: 500 mg [200 mg]

Mallamint®: 420 mg [168 mg]

Rolaids®: 550 mg [220 mg] [with 110 mg magnesium hydroxide (45 mg elemental magnesium)]

Mylanta® Calci Tabs Extra Strength, Tums® E-X: 750 mg [300 mg]

Mylanta® Calci Tabs Ultra, Tums® Ultra®: 1000 mg [400 mg]

Calcium chloride:

Injection: 10% 100 mg/mL [27.2 mg/mL] (10 mL) (1.4 mEq calcium/mL)

Calcium citrate:

Tablet (Cal-Citrate®): 250 mg [53 mg]; (Citracal®): 950 mg [200 mg]

Tablet, effervescent (Citracal® Liquitab): 2376 mg [500 mg] (also contains 12 mg phenylalanine; citrus flavor)

Calcium glubionate: Syrup: 1.8 g/5 mL [115 mg/5mL] (480 mL) (1.2 mEq calcium/mL)

Calcium gluconate:

Injection: 10% 100 mg/mL [9 mg/mL] (10 mL, 50 mL, 100 mL, 200 mL) (0.45 mEq/mL)

Tablet: 500 mg [45 mg], 650 mg [58.5 mg], 975 mg [87.75 mg], 1 g [90 mg]

Calcium lactate:

Capsule (Cal-lac®): 500 mg [96 mg]

Tablet: 325 mg [42.25 mg], 650 mg [84.5 mg]

Calcium phosphate, tribasic: Tablet, sugar free (Posture®): 1565.2 mg [600 mg]

Extemporaneous Preparations

Calcium gluconate gel: Crush 3.5 g calcium gluconate tablets into a fine powder; add to 5 oz tube of water-soluble surgical lubricant (eg, K-Y® Jelly) or add 3.5 g calcium gluconate injection to 5 oz of water-soluble surgical lubricant (calcium carbonate may be substituted; do not use calcium chloride due to potential for irritation)

Calcium carbonate slurry: 32.5% slurry can be prepared by triturating ten 650 mg tablets into a fine powder and adding 20 mL of water-soluble lubricant gel (eg, K-Y® Jelly)

References

Baker SS, Cochran WJ, Flores CA, et al, "American Academy of Pediatrics. Committee on Nutrition: Calcium Requirements of Infants, Children, and Adolescents," *Pediatrics*, 1999, 104(5):1152-7.

"Dietary Reference Intakes for Calcium, Phosphorus, Magnesium, Vitamin D, and Fluoride. Standing Committee on the Scientific Evaluation of Dietary Reference Intakes, Food and Nutrition Board, Institute of Medicine," National Academy of Sciences, Washington, DC: National Academy Press, 1997.

"Guidelines 2000 for Cardiopulmonary Resuscitation and Emergency Cardiovascular Care. Part 10: Pediatric Advanced Life Support. The American Heart Association in Collaboration With the International Liaison Committee on Resuscitation," *Circulation*, 2000, 102(8 Suppl):I291-342.

NIH Consensus Conference, "Optimal Calcium Intake," *JAMA*, 1994, 272(24):1942-8.

♦ **CaldeCORT® [OTC]** *see* Hydrocortisone *on page 506*

♦ **Caldesene® Topical [OTC]** *see* Undecylenic Acid and Derivatives *on page 994*

Calfactant (cal FAC tant)

U.S. Brand Names Infasurf®

Synonyms Bovine Lung Surfactant

Therapeutic Category Lung Surfactant

Generic Available No

Use Prevention and treatment of respiratory distress syndrome (RDS) in premature infants

Prophylactic therapy: Infants <29 weeks at significant risk for RDS

Treatment: Infants ≤72 hours of age with RDS (confirmed by clinical and radiologic findings and requiring endotracheal intubation)

Warnings Rapidly affects oxygenation and lung compliance and should be restricted to a highly supervised use in a clinical setting with immediate availability of clinicians experienced with intubation and ventilatory management of premature infants; if transient episodes of bradycardia and decreased oxygen saturation occur, discontinue the dosing procedure and initiate measures to alleviate the condition; produces rapid improvement in lung oxygenation and compliance that may require immediate reductions in ventilator settings and FiO_2; for intratracheal administration only

Precautions Transient episodes of reflux of calfactant into the endotracheal tube, cyanosis, bradycardia, or airway obstruction have occurred during dosing procedures; such episodes may require stopping administration and taking appropriate measures to alleviate the condition before resuming therapy

Adverse Reactions Most adverse reactions occur during the dosing procedure

Cardiovascular: Bradycardia, cyanosis

Respiratory: Airway obstruction, pneumothorax, pulmonary hemorrhage, apnea

Stability Refrigerate; protect from light; unopened, unused warmed vials of calfactant may be returned to refrigerator within 24 hours for future use; repeated warming to room temperature should be avoided

Mechanism of Action Replaces deficient or ineffective endogenous lung surfactant in neonates with RDS or in neonates at risk of developing RDS; surfactant prevents the alveoli from collapsing during expiration by lowering surface tension between air and alveolar surfaces

Usual Dosage Intratracheal: Neonates: 3 mL/kg every 12 hours up to a total of 3 doses; repeat doses have been administered as early as 6 hours after the previous dose for a total of up to four doses (if the infant was still intubated and required at least 30% inspired oxygen to maintain a PaO_2 ≤80 torr)

Administration Intratracheal: Gently swirl to redisperse suspension; do not shake; administer dosage divided into two aliquots of 1.5 mL/kg each into the endotracheal tube; after each instillation, reposition the infant with either the right or left side dependent; administration is made while ventilation is continued over 20-30 breaths for each aliquot, with small bursts timed only during the inspiratory cycles; a pause followed by evaluation of the respiratory status and repositioning should separate the two aliquots; calfactant dosage has also been divided into four equal aliquots and administered with repositioning in four different positions (prone, supine, right and left lateral)

Monitoring Parameters Continuous heart rate and transcutaneous O_2 saturation should be monitored during administration; frequent ABG sampling is necessary to prevent postdosing hyperoxia and hypocarbia

Dosage Forms Suspension, intratracheal: 35 mg/mL (6 mL)

References

Hudak ML, Martin DJ, Egan EA, et al, "A Multicenter Randomized Masked Comparison Trail of Synthetic Surfactant Versus Calf Lung Surfactant Extract in the Prevention of Neonatal Respiratory Distress Syndrome," *Pediatrics*, 1997, 100(1):39-50.

Bloom BT, Kattwinkel J, Hall RT, et al, "Comparison of Infasurf® (Calf Lung Surfactant Extract) to Survanta® (Beractant) in the Treatment and Prevention of Respiratory Distress Syndrome," *Pediatrics*, 1997, 100(1):31-8.

♦ **Cal-lac® [OTC]** *see* Calcium Supplements *on page 167*

♦ **Calmex (Can)** *see* Diphenhydramine *on page 342*

♦ **Calmol 4®** *see* Hemorrhoidal Preparations *on page 490*

♦ **Calm-X® [OTC]** *see* Dimenhydrinate *on page 339*

♦ **Calmylin-1 (Can)** *see* Dextromethorphan *on page 316*

♦ **Calmylin Expectorant (Can)** *see* Guaifenesin *on page 485*

- ◆ **Caltine (Can)** *see* Calcitonin *on page 164*
- ◆ **Caltrate® 600 [OTC]** *see* Calcium Supplements *on page 167*
- ◆ **Camphorated Tincture of Opium** *see* Paregoric *on page 761*
- ◆ **Candistatin (Can)** *see* Nystatin *on page 729*
- ◆ **Canesten (Can)** *see* Clotrimazole *on page 259*
- ◆ **Cankaid® [OTC]** *see* Carbamide Peroxide *on page 178*
- ◆ **Capex®** *see* Fluocinolone *on page 439*
- ◆ **Capital® and Codeine** *see* Acetaminophen and Codeine *on page 31*
- ◆ **Capoten®** *see* Captopril *on page 173*

Capsaicin (kap SAY sin)

U.S. Brand Names Capsin® [OTC]; Rid-a-Pain-HP® [OTC]; Zostrix® [OTC]; Zostrix®-HP [OTC]

Canadian Brand Names Antiphogistine Rub A-535 Capsaicin

Therapeutic Category Analgesic, Topical; Topical Skin Product

Generic Available No

Use FDA approved for the topical treatment of pain associated with postherpetic neuralgia, rheumatoid arthritis, osteoarthritis, diabetic neuropathy, and postsurgical pain.

Unlabeled use: Treatment of pain associated with psoriasis, chronic neuralgias unresponsive to other forms of therapy, and intractable pruritus

Contraindications Hypersensitivity to capsaicin or any component

Warnings Avoid contact with eyes, mucous membrane, or with damaged or irritated skin

Precautions Since warm water or excessive sweating may intensify the localized burning sensation after capsaicin application, the affected area should not be tightly bandaged or exposed to direct sunlight or a heat lamp

Adverse Reactions

Dermatologic: Erythema

Local: Itching, burning, or stinging sensation

Respiratory: Cough

Mechanism of Action Induces release of substance P, the principal chemomediator of pain impulses from the periphery to the CNS, from peripheral sensory neurons. After repeated application, capsaicin depletes the neuron of substance P and prevents reaccumulation.

Pharmacodynamics

Onset of action: Pain relief is usually seen within 14-28 days of regular topical application; maximal response may require 4-6 weeks of continuous therapy

Duration: Several hours

Usual Dosage Children ≥2 years and Adults: Topical: Apply to affected area at least 3-4 times/day; application frequency less than 3-4 times/day prevents the total depletion, inhibition of synthesis, and transport of substance P resulting in decreased clinical efficacy and increased local discomfort

Administration Topical: Should not be applied to wounds or damaged skin; avoid eye and mucous membrane exposure

Patient Information For external use only. Avoid washing treated areas for 30 minutes after application

Nursing Implications Wash hands with soap and water after applying to avoid spreading cream to eyes or other sensitive areas of the body

Additional Information In patients with severe and persistent local discomfort, pretreatment with topical lidocaine 5% ointment or concurrent oral analgesics for the first 2 weeks of therapy have been effective in alleviating the initial burning sensation and enabling continuation of topical capsaicin

Dosage Forms

Cream:

Zostrix®: 0.025% (45 g, 90 g)

Rid-a-Pain-HP®, Zostrix®-HP: 0.075% (30 g, 45 g, 60 g)

Gel: 0.025% (60 g); 0.075% (30 g)

Lotion (Capsin®): 0.025% (59 mL); 0.075% (59 mL)

References

Bernstein JE, Korman NJ, Bickers DR, et al, "Topical Capsaicin Treatment of Chronic Postherpetic Neuralgia," *J Am Acad Dermatol*, 1989, 21(2 Pt 1):265-70.

- ◆ **Capsin® [OTC]** *see* Capsaicin *on page 172*

Captopril (KAP toe pril)

U.S. Brand Names Capoten®

Canadian Brand Names Alti-Captopril; Apo-Capto; Captril; Gen-Captopril; Novo-Captopril; Nu-Capto; PMS-Captopril

Therapeutic Category Angiotensin-Converting Enzyme (ACE) Inhibitor; Antihypertensive Agent

Generic Available Yes

Use Management of hypertension; treatment of CHF; in post-MI patients, improves survival in clinically stable patients with left-ventricular dysfunction

Pregnancy Risk Factor C (1st trimester); D (may cause injury and death to the developing fetus when used during the second and third trimester of pregnancy)

Contraindications Hypersensitivity to captopril, any component, or other ACE inhibitors

Warnings Serious adverse effects including angioedema, anaphylactoid reactions, neutropenia, agranulocytosis, proteinuria, hypotension, and hepatic failure may occur (see Adverse Reactions); risk of neutropenia is increased 15 fold to 1 per 500 in patients with renal dysfunction, and increased to 3.7% in patients with both collagen vascular disease and renal dysfunction

Precautions Use with caution and modify dosage in patients with renal impairment, especially those with severe renal artery stenosis; elevated BUN and serum creatinine may occur in these patients after decrease in blood pressure with captopril; dosage reduction of captopril or discontinuation of concurrent diuretic may be needed; control of blood pressure while maintaining adequate renal perfusion may not be possible in some of these patients. Use with caution in patients with collagen vascular disease.

Adverse Reactions

Cardiovascular: Hypotension, tachycardia

Central nervous system: Headache, dizziness, fatigue, insomnia, fever

Dermatologic: Rash, angioedema. **Note:** The relative risk of angioedema with ACE inhibitors is higher within the first 30 days of use (compared to >1 year of use), for Black Americans (compared to Whites), for lisinopril or enalapril (compared to captopril), and for patients previously hospitalized within 30 days (Brown, 1996).

Endocrine & metabolic: Hyperkalemia

Gastrointestinal: Ageusia

Hematologic: Neutropenia, agranulocytosis, eosinophilia

Hepatic: Cholestatic jaundice, fulminant hepatic necrosis (rare, but potentially fatal)

Respiratory: Cough, dyspnea; **Note:** An isolated dry cough lasting >3 weeks was reported in 7 of 42 pediatric patients (17%) receiving ACE inhibitors (see von Vigier, 2000)

Renal: Elevated BUN and serum creatinine, proteinuria, oliguria

Drug Interactions Cytochrome P-450 isoenzyme CYP2D6 substrate

Captopril plus potassium supplements or potassium-sparing diuretics may cause an additive hyperkalemic effect; captopril plus indomethacin or NSAIDs may result in a reduced antihypertensive response to captopril

Food Interactions Absorption of captopril may be reduced by food; long-term use of captopril may result in a zinc deficiency which can result in a decrease in taste perception; zinc supplements may be used; limit salt substitutes or potassium-rich diet; avoid natural licorice (causes sodium and water retention and increases potassium loss)

Stability Unstable in aqueous solutions

Mechanism of Action Competitive inhibitor of angiotensin-converting enzyme (ACE); prevents conversion of angiotensin I to angiotensin II, a potent vasoconstrictor; results in lower levels of angiotensin II which causes an increase in plasma renin activity and a reduction in aldosterone secretion

Pharmacodynamics

Onset of action: Decrease in blood pressure within 15 minutes

Maximum effect: 60-90 minutes; may require several weeks of therapy before full hypotensive effect is seen

Duration: Dose-related

Pharmacokinetics

Absorption: 60% to 75%

Distribution: 7 L/kg

Protein binding: 25% to 30%

Metabolism: 50% metabolized

Half-life:

Infants with CHF: 3.3 hours; range: 1.2-12.4 hours

Children: 1.5 hours; range: 0.98-2.3 hours

Normal adults (dependent upon renal and cardiac function): 1.9 hours

(Continued)

Captopril (Continued)

Adults with CHF: 2.1 hours
Anuria: 20-40 hours

Time to peak serum concentration: Within 1-2 hours
Elimination: 95% excreted in urine in 24 hours

Usual Dosage Note: Dosage must be titrated according to patient's response; use lowest effective dose; lower doses (~½ of those listed) should be used in patients who are sodium and water depleted due to diuretic therapy; Oral:

Newborns and premature Neonates: Initial: 0.01 mg/kg/dose every 8-12 hours; titrate dose

Neonates: Initial: 0.05-0.1 mg/kg/dose every 8-24 hours; titrate dose up to 0.5 mg/kg/dose given every 6-24 hours

Infants: Initial: 0.15-0.3 mg/kg/dose; titrate dose upward to maximum of 6 mg/kg/day in 1-4 divided doses; usual required dose: 2.5-6 mg/kg/day

Children: Initial: 0.3-0.5 mg/kg/dose; titrate upward to maximum of 6 mg/kg/day in 2-4 divided doses

Older Children: Initial: 6.25-12.5 mg/dose every 12-24 hours; titrate upward to maximum of 6 mg/kg/day in 2-4 divided doses

Adolescents and Adults: Initial: 12.5-25 mg/dose given every 8-12 hours; increase by 25 mg/dose to maximum of 450 mg/day

Dosing adjustment in renal impairment:
Cl_{cr} 10-50 mL/minute: Administer 75% of dose
Cl_{cr} <10 mL/minute: Administer 50% of dose

Administration Oral: Administer on an empty stomach 1 hour before meals or 2 hours after meals

Monitoring Parameters Blood pressure, BUN, serum creatinine, renal function, urine dipstick for protein, WBC with differential, serum potassium

Patient Information Limit alcohol; notify physician if swelling of face, lips, tongue, difficulty in breathing, or persistent cough occurs; do not use salt substitute (potassium-containing) without physician advice

Nursing Implications Discontinue if angioedema occurs; monitor blood pressure for hypotension within 1-3 hours after first dose or after a new higher dose

Additional Information Severe hypotension may occur in patients who are sodium and/or volume depleted

Dosage Forms Tablet: 12.5 mg, 25 mg, 50 mg, 100 mg

Extemporaneous Preparations

Captopril has limited stability in aqueous preparations. The addition of an antioxidant [sodium ascorbate (using an injectable product) or ascorbic acid (using tablets)] has been shown to increase the stability of captopril in solution; captopril (1 mg/mL) in syrup with methylcellulose is stable for 7 days stored either at 4°C or 22°C. Captopril (1 mg/mL) in distilled water (no additives) is stable for 14 days if stored at 4°C and 7 days if stored at 22°C; captopril (1 mg/mL) with sodium ascorbate (5 mg/mL) in distilled water is stable for 56 days at 4°C and 14 days at 22°C (Nahata MC, et al, *Am J Hosp Pharm*, 1994, 51(1):95-6); captopril (1 mg/mL) with ascorbic acid (5 mg/mL) in distilled water is stable for 56 days at 4°C and 28 days at 22°C (Nahata MC, et al, *Am J Hosp Pharm*, 1994, 51(13):1707-8); captopril (1 mg/mL) in an undiluted syrup containing preservatives is stable for 30 days at 5°C in amber glass containers (Lye, 1997).

Captopril (0.75 mg/mL) in cherry syrup is stable for only 2 days in amber clear plastic containers stored at room temperature or under refrigeration; captopril (0.75 mg/mL) in either a 1:1 mixture of Ora-Sweet® and Ora-Plus® or a 1:1 mixture of Ora-Sweet® SF and Ora-Plus® is stable for 10 days or less depending on the storage temperature (see Allen, 1996).

Powder papers can also be made; powder papers are stable for 12 weeks when stored at room temperature (Taketomo, 1990).

Allen LV and Erickson MA, "Stability of Baclofen, Captopril, Diltiazem Hydrochloride, Dipyridamole, and Flecainide Acetate in Extemporaneously Compounded Oral Liquids," *Am J Health Sys Pharm*, 1996, 53(18):2179-84.

Lye MY, Yow KL, Lim LY, et al, "Effects of Ingredients on Stability of Captopril in Extemporaneously Prepared Oral Liquids," *Am J Health Syst Pharm*, 1997, 54(21):2483-7.

Nahata MC, Morosco RS, and Hipple TF, "Stability of Captopril in Liquid Containing Ascorbic Acid or Sodium Ascorbate," *Am J Hosp Pharm*, 1994, 51(13):1707-8.

Nahata MC, Morosco RS, and Hipple TF, "Stability of Captopril in Three Liquid Dosage Forms," *Am J Hosp Pharm*, 1994, 51(1):95-6.

Taketomo CK, Chu SA, Cheng MH, et al, "Stability of Captopril in Powder Papers Under Three Storage Conditions," *Am J Hosp Pharm*, 1990, 47(8):1799-801.

References

Brown NJ, Ray WA, Snowden M, et al, "Black Americans Have an Increased Rate of Angiotensin-Converting Enzyme Inhibitor-Associated Angioedema," *Clin Pharmacol Ther*, 1996, 60(1):8-13.

Friedman WF and George BL, "New Concepts and Drugs in the Treatment of Congestive Heart Failure," *Pediatr Clin North Am*, 1984, 31(6):1197-227.

Levy M, Koren G, Klein J, et al, "Captopril Pharmacokinetics, Blood Pressure Response and Plasma Renin Activity in Normotensive Children With Renal Scarring," *Dev Pharmacol Ther*, 1991, 16(4):185-93.

Mirkin BL and Newman TJ, "Efficacy and Safety of Captopril in the Treatment of Severe Childhood Hypertension: Report of the International Collaborative Study Group," *Pediatrics*, 1985, 75(6):1091-100.

Pereira CM, Tam YK, Collins-Nakai RL, "The Pharmacokinetics of Captopril in Infants With Congestive Heart Failure," *Ther Drug Monit*, 1991, 13(3):209-14.

von Vigier RO, Mozzettini S, Truttmann AC, et al, "Cough is Common in Children Prescribed Converting Enzyme Inhibitors," *Nephron*, 2000, 84(1):98.

♦ **Captril (Can)** *see* Captopril *on page 173*
♦ **Carafate®** *see* Sucralfate *on page 919*

Carbamazepine (kar ba MAZ e peen)

Related Information

Antiepileptic Drugs *on page 1208*
Blood Level Sampling Time Guidelines *on page 1220*
Carbohydrate and Alcohol Content of Liquid Medications for Use in Patients Receiving Ketogenic Diets *on page 1258*
Overdose and Toxicology *on page 1222*
Serotonin Syndrome *on page 1247*

U.S. Brand Names Carbatrol®; Epitol®; Tegretol®; Tegretol®-XR

Canadian Brand Names Apo-Carbamazepine; Gen-Carbamazepine; Mazepine; Novo-Carbamaz; Nu-Carbamazepine; PMS-Carbamazepine; Taro-Carbamazepine

Synonyms CBZ

Therapeutic Category Anticonvulsant, Miscellaneous

Generic Available Yes: Tablet

Use Prophylaxis of generalized tonic-clonic, partial (especially complex partial), and mixed partial or generalized seizure disorder; to relieve pain in trigeminal neuralgia or diabetic neuropathy; treatment of bipolar disorders

Pregnancy Risk Factor D

Contraindications Patients with a history of bone marrow suppression; hypersensitivity to carbamazepine or any component; cross-sensitivity with tricyclic antidepressants may occur; concomitant therapy with MAO inhibitors

Warnings Potentially fatal blood cell abnormalities have been reported following treatment; early detection of hematologic change is important; advise patients of early signs and symptoms which are: fever, sore throat, mouth ulcers, infections, easy bruising, petechial or purpuric hemorrhage

Substitution of Tegretol® with generic carbamazepine has resulted in decreased carbamazepine levels and increased seizure activity, as well as increased carbamazepine levels and toxicity. Monitoring of carbamazepine serum concentrations is mandatory when patients are switched from any product to another.

Precautions MAO inhibitors should be discontinued for a minimum of 14 days before carbamazepine is begun; administer with caution to patients with history of cardiac disease, hepatic disease, renal failure, or history of hypersensitivity reactions to other anticonvulsants (eg, phenobarbital, phenytoin); hepatic failure (rare) and multiorgan hypersensitivity reactions may occur (see Adverse Reactions); consider discontinuation of carbamazepine if any evidence of hypersensitivity occurs; higher peak concentrations occur with the suspension, so treatment is initiated with lower amounts per dose and increased slowly to avoid adverse effects

Adverse Reactions

Cardiovascular: Edema, CHF, syncope, dysrhythmias, heart block
Central nervous system: Sedation, dizziness, drowsiness, fatigue, slurred speech, ataxia, confusion
Dermatologic: Rash, Stevens-Johnson syndrome
Endocrine & metabolic: SIADH, hyponatremia
Gastrointestinal: Nausea, diarrhea, vomiting, abdominal cramps, pancreatitis
Genitourinary: Urinary retention
Hematologic: Neutropenia (can be transient), aplastic anemia, agranulocytosis, thrombocytopenia
Hepatic: Elevated liver enzymes, jaundice, hepatitis; hepatic failure (very rare)
Ocular: Nystagmus, diplopia, blurred vision
(Continued)

Carbamazepine *(Continued)*

Miscellaneous: Multi-organ hypersensitivity reactions (rare): Reactions may include vasculitis, lymphadenopathy, fever, rash, lymphoma-like symptoms, arthralgia, eosinophilia, leukopenia, elevated liver function tests, hepato-splenomegaly

Drug Interactions Cytochrome P-450 isoenzyme CYP2C8 and CYP3A3/4 substrate; isoenzyme CYP1A2, CYP2C, and CYP3A3/4 inducer

Clarithromycin, erythromycin, isoniazid, danazol, fluoxetine, ketoconazole, itraconazole, propoxyphene, verapamil, diltiazem, and cimetidine may inhibit hepatic metabolism of carbamazepine with resultant increase of carbamazepine serum concentrations and toxicity; carbamazepine may induce the metabolism of warfarin, cyclosporine, doxycycline, oral or subdermal contraceptives (consider alternative or back-up methods of contraception), phenytoin, theophylline, ritonavir, saquinavir, delavirdine, benzodiazepines, ethosuximide, valproic acid, lamotrigine, tigabine, topiramate, midazolam, corticosteroids, teniposide, etoposide, doxorubicin, vincristine, methotrexate, and thyroid hormones; use with lithium may increase neurotic side effects; ritonavir and cefixime may affect the metabolism of carbamazepine; administration of Tegretol® suspension in combination with liquid chlorpromazine or thioridazine results in an orange rubbery precipitate

Food Interactions Extended release capsules (Carbatrol®): A high fat meal may increase the rate of absorption, reduce time to peak concentration (from 24 hours to 14 hours), and increase peak concentrations, but does not effect extent of absorption (AUC)

Stability Store tablets in dry place, protect from moisture

Mechanism of Action May depress activity in the nucleus ventralis of the thalamus or decrease synaptic transmission or decrease summation of temporal stimulation leading to neural discharge, by limiting influx of sodium ions across cell membrane; other unknown mechanisms; stimulates the release of ADH and potentiates its action in promoting reabsorption of water; chemically related to tricyclic antidepressants; in addition to anticonvulsant effects, carbamazepine has anticholinergic, antineuralgic, antidiuretic, muscle relaxant and antiarrhythmic properties

Pharmacokinetics

Absorption: Slowly from the GI tract

Distribution: V_d:

Neonates: 1.5 L/kg

Children: 1.9 L/kg

Adults: 0.59-2 L/kg

Protein binding: 75% to 90%, bound to alpha$_1$-acid glycoprotein and nonspecific binding sites on albumin; protein binding may be decreased in newborns

Metabolism: Induces liver enzymes to increase metabolism and shorten half-life over time; metabolized in the liver by cytochrome P-450 3A4 to active epoxide metabolite; ratio of serum epoxide to carbamazepine concentrations may be higher in patients receiving polytherapy (vs monotherapy) and in infants (vs older children); boys may have faster carbamazepine clearances and may, therefore, require higher mg/kg/day doses of carbamazepine compared to girls of similar age and weight

Bioavailability, oral: 75% to 85%; relative bioavailability of extended release tablet to suspension: 89%

Half-life:

Initial: 25-65 hours

Multiple dosing:

Children: 8-14 hours

Adults: 12-17 hours

Time to peak serum concentration: Unpredictable, within 4-8 hours

Chronic administration:

Suspension: 1.5 hours

Tablet: 4-5 hours

Extended release tablet: 3-12 hours

Elimination: 1% to 3% excreted unchanged in urine

Usual Dosage Dosage must be adjusted according to patient's response and serum concentrations. Administer tablets (chewable or conventional) in 2-3 divided doses daily and suspension in 4 divided doses daily. (See Additional Information for investigational oral loading dose information.) Oral:

Children:

<6 years: Initial: 10-20 mg/kg/day divided twice or 3 times daily as tablets or 4 times/day as suspension; increase dose every week until optimal response and therapeutic levels are achieved; maintenance dose: Divide into 3-4 doses daily (tablets or suspension); maximum recommended dose: 35 mg/kg/day

6-12 years: Initial: 100 mg twice daily (tablets or extended release tablets) or 50 mg of suspension 4 times/day (200 mg/day); increase by up to 100 mg/day at weekly intervals using a twice daily regimen of extended release tablets or 3-4 times daily regimen of other formulations until optimal response and therapeutic levels are achieved; usual maintenance: 400-800 mg/day; maximum recommended dose: 1000 mg/day

Note: Children <12 years who receive ≥400 mg/day of carbamazepine may be converted to extended release capsules (Carbatrol®) using the same total daily dosage divided twice daily

Children >12 years and Adults: Initial: 200 mg twice daily (tablets, extended release tablets, or extended release capsules) or 100 mg of suspension 4 times/day (400 mg daily); increase by up to 200 mg/day at weekly intervals using a twice daily regimen of extended release tablets or capsules, or a 3-4 times/day regimen of other formulations until optimal response and therapeutic levels are achieved; usual dose: 800-1200 mg/day

Maximum recommended doses:

Children 12-15 years: 1000 mg/day

Children >15 years: 1200 mg/day

Adults: 1600 mg/day; however, some patients have required up to 1.6-2.4 g/day

Dosing adjustment in renal impairment: Cl_{cr} <10 mL/minute: Administer 75% of recommended dose; monitor serum levels

Administration

Oral: Administer with food to decrease GI upset; extended release capsules (Carbatrol®) may be taken without regard to meals; suspension dosage should be administered on a 3-4 times/day schedule vs tablet (conventional or chewable) which can be administered 2-4 times/day; extended release (XR) tablets should be dosed twice daily; do not crush or chew XR tablets; examine XR tablets for cracks or chips; do not use damaged XR tablets or XR tablets without a release portal; chewable tablet should be chewed well and swallowed. Swallow extended release capsules whole or open and sprinkle contents on small amount of soft food (eg, 1 teaspoonful of applesauce); swallow sprinkle/food mixture immediately; do not chew; do not store for later use; drink fluids after dose to make sure mixture is completely swallowed

Suspension: Tegretol® should not be administered with diluents or other liquid medicines due to the possibility of a component interaction (see Drug Interactions); shake suspension well before use

Monitoring Parameters CBC with platelet count, liver function tests, serum drug concentration; observe patient for excessive sedation especially when instituting or increasing therapy

Reference Range Therapeutic: 4-12 µg/mL (SI: 17-51 µmol/L). Patients who require higher levels [8-12 µg/mL (SI: 34-51 µmol/L)] should be carefully monitored. Side effects (especially CNS) occur commonly at higher levels. If other anticonvulsants (enzyme inducers) are given, therapeutic range is 4-8 µg/mL (SI: 17-34 µmol/L) due to increase in unmeasured active epoxide metabolite.

Patient Information Avoid alcohol; may cause drowsiness and impair ability to perform activities requiring mental alertness or physical coordination; report fever, sore throat, infection, mouth ulcers, easy bruising, bleeding, loss of appetite, nausea, vomiting, or yellow skin or eyes to physician; the tablet coating of Tegretol®-XR tablet is not absorbed and may appear in the stool

Additional Information Carbamazepine is not effective in absence, myoclonic, akinetic, or febrile seizures; exacerbation of certain seizure types have been seen after initiation of carbamazepine therapy in children with mixed seizure disorders

Investigationally, loading doses of the suspension (10 mg/kg for children <12 years of age and 8 mg/kg for children >12 years) were given (via NG or ND tubes followed by 5-10 mL of water to flush through tube) to PICU patients with frequent seizures/status; 5 of 6 patients attained mean plasma concentrations of 4.3 mcg/mL and 7.3 mcg/mL at 1 and 2 hours postload; concurrent enteral feeding or ileus may delay absorption of loading dose (Miles, 1990)

A recent study (Relling, 2000) demonstrated that enzyme-inducing antiepileptic drugs (AEDs) (carbamazepine, phenobarbital, and phenytoin) increased systemic clearance of antileukemic drugs (teniposide and methotrexate) and were associated with a worse event-free survival, CNS relapse, and hematologic relapse, (ie, lower efficacy), in B-lineage ALL children receiving chemotherapy; the authors recommend using nonenzyme-inducing AEDs in patients receiving chemotherapy for ALL.

Dosage Forms

Capsule, extended release (Carbatrol®): 200 mg, 300 mg

Suspension, oral (Tegretol®): 100 mg/5 mL [citrus-vanilla flavor] (450 mL)

Tablet (Epitol®, Tegretol®): 200 mg

(Continued)

Carbamazepine *(Continued)*

Tablet, chewable (Tegretol®): 100 mg
Tablet, extended release (Tegretol® XR): 100 mg, 200 mg, 400 mg

References

Gilman JT, "Carbamazepine Dosing for Pediatric Seizure Disorders: The Highs and Lows," *DICP*, 1991, 25(10):1109-12.

Korinthenberg R, Haug C, and Hannak D, "The Metabolization of Carbamazepine to CBZ-10,11 Epoxide in Children From the Newborn Age to Adolescence," *Neuropediatrics*, 1994, 25(4):214-6.

Liu H and Delgado MR, "Influence of Sex, Age, Weight, and Carbamazepine Dose on Serum Concentrations, Concentration Ratios, and Level/Dose Ratios of Carbamazepine and Its Metabolites," *Ther Drug Monit*, 1994, 16(5):469-76.

Miles MV, Lawless ST, Tennison MB, et al, "Rapid Loading of Critically Ill Patients With Carbamazepine Suspension," *Pediatrics*, 1990, 86(2):263-6.

Relling MV, Pui CH, Sandlund JT, et al, "Adverse Effect of Anticonvulsants on Efficacy of Chemotherapy for Acute Lymphoblastic Leukaemia," *Lancet*, 2000, 356(9226):285-90.

Carbamide Peroxide (KAR ba mide per OKS ide)

U.S. Brand Names Auro® [OTC]; Cankaid® [OTC]; Debrox® [OTC]; E•R•O [OTC]; Gly-Oxide® [OTC]; Mollifene® Ear Wax Removing Formula [OTC]; Murine® Ear [OTC]; Orajel® Perioseptic [OTC]; Proxigel® [OTC]

Synonyms Urea Peroxide

Therapeutic Category Otic Agent, Cerumenolytic

Generic Available Yes

Use

Oral: Relief of minor inflammation of gums, oral mucosal surfaces and lips including canker sores and dental irritation; adjunct in oral hygiene

Otic: Emulsify and disperse ear wax

Pregnancy Risk Factor C

Contraindications Otic preparation should not be used in patients with a perforated tympanic membrane or following otic surgery; ear drainage, ear pain, or rash in the ear; dizziness; oral preparation should not be used for self medication in children <3 years of age; hypersensitivity to carbamide peroxide or any component

Warnings With prolonged use of oral carbamide peroxide, there is a potential for overgrowth of opportunistic organisms, damage to periodontal tissues, delayed wound healing

Adverse Reactions

Central nervous system: Dizziness

Dermatologic: Rash

Local: Irritation, tenderness, pain, redness

Stability Protect from heat and direct light

Mechanism of Action Carbamide peroxide releases hydrogen peroxide which serves as a source of nascent oxygen upon contact with catalase; deodorant action is probably due to inhibition of odor-causing bacteria; softens impacted cerumen due to its foaming action

Pharmacodynamics Onset of effect: Otic: Slight disintegration of hard ear wax in 24 hours

Usual Dosage

Oral: Children and Adults:

Gel: Massage on affected area 4 times/day for up to 7 days

Solution: Apply several drops undiluted to affected area of the mouth 4 times/day and at bedtime for up to 7 days, expectorate after 2-3 minutes; as an adjunct to oral hygiene after brushing, swish 10 drops for 2-3 minutes, then expectorate

Otic: Solution:

Children <12 years: Individualize the dose according to patient size; 3 drops (range: 1-5 drops) twice daily for up to 4 days

Children ≥12 years and Adults: Instill 5-10 drops twice daily for up to 4 days

Administration

Oral: Apply undiluted solution with an applicator or cotton swab to the affected area after meals and at bedtime; or place drops on the tongue, mix with saliva, swish in the mouth for several minutes, then expectorate

Otic: Instill drops into the external ear canal; keep drops in ear for several minutes by keeping head tilted or placing cotton in ear

Patient Information Contact physician if dizziness or otic redness, rash, irritation, tenderness, pain, drainage or discharge develop; do not use in the eye

Nursing Implications Drops foam on contact with ear wax

Dosage Forms

Gel, oral (Proxigel®): 10% (36 g)

Solution: Oral:
   Cankaid®, Gly-Oxide®: 10% in anhydrous glycerol (15 mL, 60 mL)
   Orajel® Perioseptic: 15% in anhydrous glycerin (13.3 mL)
Solution: Otic (Auro®, Debrox®, E•R•O, Mollifene® Ear Wax Removing Formula, Murine® Ear): 6.5% in glycerin (15 mL, 30 mL)

♦ **Carbatrol®** see Carbamazepine on page 175

Carbenicillin (kar ben i SIL in)

U.S. Brand Names Geocillin®
Synonyms Carindacillin
Therapeutic Category Antibiotic, Penicillin (Antipseudomonal)
Generic Available No
Use Treatment of urinary tract infections, asymptomatic bacteriuria, or prostatitis caused by susceptible strains of *Pseudomonas aeruginosa*, *E. coli*, indole-positive *Proteus*, and *Enterobacter*
Pregnancy Risk Factor B
Contraindications Hypersensitivity to carbenicillin, any component, or penicillins
Warnings Oral carbenicillin should be limited to treatment of urinary tract infections
Precautions Use with caution in patients with history of cephalosporin hypersensitivity; do not use in patients with severe renal impairment (Cl_{cr} <10 mL/minute) since drug concentration in urine is reduced and inadequate for treatment of UTIs
Adverse Reactions
   Dermatologic: Rash, urticaria, pruritus
   Gastrointestinal: Nausea, vomiting, diarrhea, abdominal cramps, furry tongue
   Genitourinary: Vaginitis
   Hematologic: Eosinophilia, hemolytic anemia, neutropenia, leukopenia, thrombocytopenia
   Hepatic: Elevated liver enzymes, hepatotoxicity
Drug Interactions Probenecid, lithium
Mechanism of Action Interferes with bacterial cell wall synthesis during active multiplication
Pharmacokinetics
   Absorption: Oral: 30% to 40%; in patients with normal renal function, serum concentrations of carbenicillin following oral absorption are inadequate for the treatment of systemic infections
   Protein binding: 50%
   Half-life:
      Neonates:
         <7 days, ≤2.5 kg: 4 hours
         <7 days, >2.5 kg: 2.7 hours
      Children: 0.8-1.8 hours
      Adults: 1-1.5 hours; prolonged to 10-20 hours with renal insufficiency
   Time to peak serum concentration: Within 30-120 minutes
   Elimination: Carbenicillin and its metabolites are excreted in the urine; ~80% to 99% of the dose is excreted unchanged in the urine
   Dialysis: Moderately dialyzable (20% to 50%)
Usual Dosage Oral:
   Children: 30-50 mg/kg/day divided every 6 hours; maximum dose: 2-3 g/day
   Adults:
      Urinary tract infections: 1-2 tablets every 6 hours
      Prostatitis: 2 tablets every 6 hours
Administration Oral: Administer with water
Monitoring Parameters Renal, hepatic, and hematologic function tests
Test Interactions False-positive urine or serum proteins; false-positive urine glucose (Clinitest®)
Patient Information Tablets have a bitter taste
Additional Information Sodium content of 382 mg tablet: 23 mg (1 mEq)
Dosage Forms Tablet, film coated, as indanyl sodium ester: 382 mg [base]

Carbinoxamine and Pseudoephedrine
(kar bi NOKS a meen & soo doe e FED rin)

U.S. Brand Names Carbiset®; Cardec-S®; Palgic® D; Palgic® DS; Rondec®; Rondec-TR®
Synonyms Pseudoephedrine and Carbinoxamine
Therapeutic Category Antihistamine/Decongestant Combination
Generic Available Yes
(Continued)

179

Carbinoxamine and Pseudoephedrine *(Continued)*

Use Temporary relief of nasal congestion, running nose, sneezing, itching of nose or throat, and itchy, watery eyes due to the common cold, hay fever, or other respiratory allergies

Pregnancy Risk Factor C

Contraindications Hypersensitivity to carbinoxamine, pseudoephedrine, or any component; severe hypertension or coronary artery disease, MAO inhibitor therapy, GI or GU obstruction, narrow-angle glaucoma

Precautions Use with caution in patients with mild to moderate hypertension, heart disease, diabetes, asthma, thyroid disease, or prostatic hypertrophy

Adverse Reactions

Cardiovascular: Hypertension, tachycardia, arrhythmias edema, palpitations

Central nervous system: Sedation, CNS stimulation, headache, seizures, drowsiness, fatigue, nervousness, depression

Dermatologic: Angioedema, photosensitivity, rash

Gastrointestinal: Nausea, vomiting, xerostomia, anorexia, diarrhea, heart burn

Genitourinary: Dysuria

Hepatic: Hepatitis

Neuromuscular & skeletal: Weakness, myalgia, paresthesia

Ocular: Diplopia

Respiratory: Bronchospasm, epistaxis

Renal: Polyuria

Drug Interactions May produce severe hypertensive episodes when used with MAO inhibitors; may inhibit hypotensive effects of beta-adrenergic blocking agents; additive effects with other sympathomimetics, sedatives, alcohol, barbiturates, and other CNS depressants

Mechanism of Action Carbinoxamine competes with histamine for H_1-receptor sites on effector cells in the GI tract, blood vessels, and respiratory tract; pseudoephedrine directly stimulates alpha-adrenergic receptors of respiratory mucosa causing vasoconstriction; directly stimulates beta-adrenergic receptors causing bronchial relaxation, increased heart rate and contractility

Usual Dosage Oral:

Children: May dose according to pseudoephedrine component: 4 mg/kg/day **or** the carbinoxamine component: 0.2-0.4 mg/kg/day

Alternative dosing (manufacturer's recommendation):

Drops:

1-3 months: 1/4 dropperful (0.25 mL) 4 times/day

3-6 months: 1/2 dropperful (0.5 mL) 4 times/day

6-9 months: 3/4 dropperful (0.75 mL) 4 times/day

9-18 months: 1 dropperful (1 mL) 4 times/day

Syrup or tablet:

18 months to 6 years: 2.5 mL 4 times/day

6 years to Adults: 5 mL or 1 tablet 4 times/day

Extended release tablet: Children >12 years and Adults: 1 tablet 2 times/day

Administration Oral: Do not crush or chew extended release tablets

Patient Information May cause drowsiness or impair ability to perform activities requiring mental alertness or physical coordination; may cause blurred vision; may also cause CNS excitation and difficulty sleeping

Dosage Forms

Drops (Rondec®): Carbinoxamine maleate 2 mg and pseudoephedrine hydrochloride 25 mg per mL (30 mL with dropper)

Syrup:

Palgic® DS: Carbinoxamine maleate 2 mg and pseudoephedrine hydrochloride 15 mg per 5 mL (480 mL)

Cardec® S: Carbinoxamine maleate 4 mg and pseudoephedrine hydrochloride 60 mg per 5 mL (120 mL, 480 mL)

Tablet:

Film-coated (Carbiset®, Rondec®): Carbinoxamine maleate 4 mg and pseudoephedrine hydrochloride 60 mg

Sustained release:

Palgic® D: Carbinoxamine maleate 8 mg and pseudoephedrine hydrochloride 90 mg

Rondec-TR®: Carbinoxamine maleate 8 mg and pseudoephedrine hydrochloride 120 mg

- **Carbiset®** *see* Carbinoxamine and Pseudoephedrine *on page 179*
- **Carbohydrate and Alcohol Content of Liquid Medications for Use in Patients Receiving Ketogenic Diets** *see page 1258*

Carboplatin (KAR boe pla tin)

Related Information
Emetogenic Potential of Single Chemotherapeutic Agents *on page 1129*

U.S. Brand Names Paraplatin®

Synonyms CBDCA

Therapeutic Category Antineoplastic Agent, Alkylating Agent

Generic Available No

Use Treatment of ovarian carcinoma; used in the treatment of small cell lung cancer, squamous cell carcinoma of the esophagus; solid tumors of the bladder, cervix and testes; pediatric brain tumor, neuroblastoma, bony and soft tissue sarcomas, germ cell tumors, and high-dose therapy with stem cell/bone marrow transplants

Pregnancy Risk Factor D

Contraindications Hypersensitivity to carboplatin, cisplatin, any component, other platinum-containing compounds, or mannitol; severe bone marrow suppression or excessive bleeding

Warnings The FDA currently recommends that procedures for proper handling and disposal of antineoplastic agents be considered. When carboplatin is dosed using AUC as the endpoint, note that the calculated dose is the dose administered, not the dose based on body surface area

Precautions Bone marrow suppression, which may be severe, and vomiting are dose-related; high doses have also resulted in severe abnormalities of liver function; reduce dosage in patients with bone marrow suppression and impaired renal function (creatinine clearance values <60 mL/minute)

Adverse Reactions
Cardiovascular: Hypotension
Central nervous system: Pain
Dermatologic: Urticaria, rash, alopecia, pruritus, erythema
Endocrine & metabolic: Electrolyte abnormalities such as hypocalcemia, hypokalemia, hypomagnesemia
Gastrointestinal: Nausea, vomiting, diarrhea, anorexia, hemorrhagic colitis, mucositis, constipation
Hematologic: Neutropenia, leukopenia, thrombocytopenia (platelet count reaches a nadir between 14-21 days), anemia
Hepatic: Abnormal liver function tests
Neuromuscular & skeletal: Peripheral neuropathy, weakness
Otic: Tinnitus, hearing loss at high tones
Renal: Nephrotoxicity, elevated BUN and serum creatinine, hematuria
Respiratory: Bronchospasm, interstitial pneumonia
Miscellaneous: Anaphylactic-like reactions

Drug Interactions Aminoglycosides (increased ototoxicity and nephrotoxicity); nephrotoxic drugs (increased renal toxicity); decreases phenytoin serum levels

Stability Store unopened vials at room temperature; protect from light; after reconstitution, solutions are stable for 8 hours; 2 mg/mL solutions diluted in D_5W for infusion are stable for 24 hours; 7 mg/mL solutions diluted in NS for infusion are stable for 24 hours; aluminum reacts with carboplatin resulting in a precipitate and loss of potency

Mechanism of Action Platination of DNA results in possible cross-linking and interference with the function of DNA

Pharmacokinetics
Distribution: V_d: 16 L/kg
Protein binding: 0%; however, platinum is 30% protein bound
Half-life: Patients with Cl_{cr} >60 mL/minute: 2.5-5.9 hours
Elimination: ~60% to 80% is excreted renally

Usual Dosage I.V. (refer to individual protocols):
Infants and Children <3 years or ≤12 kg: Various protocols calculate dosage on the basis of body weight rather than body surface area
Children:
Dosing based on target AUC (modified Calvert formula for use in children): Total dose (mg) = [Target AUC (mg/mL/minute)] x [GFR (mL/minute) + (0.36 x body weight in kilograms)]; **Note:** GFR is measured by the plasma clearance of ^{51}Cr-EDTA
Note: The dose of carboplatin calculated is TOTAL mg DOSE not mg/m²
Target AUC will vary depending upon: Number of agents in the regimen and treatment status (ie, previously untreated or treated)
Solid tumor: 300-600 mg/m² once every 4 weeks
Brain tumor: 175 mg/m² once weekly for 4 weeks with a 2-week recovery period between courses; dose is then adjusted on platelet count and neutrophil count values; courses should not be repeated until the platelet count is ≥100,000/mm³ and the neutrophil count is ≥2000/mm³

(Continued)

Carboplatin *(Continued)*

Bone marrow transplant preparative regimen: 500 mg/m^2/day for 3 days

Note: Retinoblastoma: Subconjunctival injection of carboplatin for intraocular retinoblastoma has been administered using 1-2 mL of a 10 mg/mL solution per
dose to affected eye(s)

Adults:

Single agent: 360 mg/m^2 once every 4 weeks; dose is then adjusted on platelet
count and neutrophil count values; courses should not be repeated until the
platelet count is ≥100,000/mm^3 and the neutrophil count is ≥2000/mm^3

Calvert formula: See table

Single Agent Carboplatin/No Prior Chemotherapy	Total dose (mg): 6-8 (GFR + 25)
Single Agent Carboplatin/Prior Chemotherapy	Total dose (mg): 4-6 (GFR + 25)
Combination Chemotherapy/No Prior Chemotherapy	Total dose (mg): 4.5-6 (GFR + 25)
Combination Chemotherapy/Prior Chemotherapy	Use a target AUC value <5 for the initial cycle

Dosing adjustment in renal impairment: Adults: Calvert formula:

Total dose (mg) = [Target AUC (mg/mL/minute)] x [GFR (mL/minute) + 25]

Note: The dose of carboplatin calculated is TOTAL mg DOSE not mg/m^2; AUC will
vary depending upon: Number of agents in the regimen and treatment status
(ie, previously untreated or treated)

Administration Parenteral: Administer by I.V. intermittent infusion over 15 minutes
to 1 hour, or by continuous infusion (continuous infusion regimens may be less toxic
than the bolus route); reconstituted carboplatin 10 mg/mL should be further diluted
to a final concentration of 0.5-2 mg/mL with D$_5$W or NS for administration

Monitoring Parameters CBC with differential and platelet count, serum electrolytes,
urinalysis, creatinine clearance, liver function tests

Nursing Implications Needle or intravenous administration sets containing
aluminum parts should not be used in the administration or preparation of carboplatin (aluminum can interact with carboplatin resulting in precipitate formation and
loss of potency)

Dosage Forms Powder for injection, lyophilized: 50 mg, 150 mg, 450 mg

References

Abramson DH, Frank CM, and Dunkel IJ, "A Phase I/II Study of Subconjunctival Carboplatin for Intraocular Retinoblastoma," *Ophthalmology*, 1999, 106(10):1947-50.

Lovett D, Kelsen D, Eisenberger M, et al, "A Phase II Trial of Carboplatin and Vinblastine in the Treatment
of Advanced Squamous Cell Carcinoma of the Esophagus," *Cancer*, 1991, 67(2):354-6.

Newell DR, Pearson AD, Balmanno K, et al, "Carboplatin Pharmacokinetics in Children: The Development
of a Pediatric Dosing Formula. The United Kingdom Children's Cancer Study Group," *J Clin Oncol*,
1993, 11(12):2314-23.

Oguri S, Sakakibara T, Mase H, et al, "Clinical Pharmacokinetics of Carboplatin," *J Clin Pharmacol*, 1988,
28(3):208-15.

Reece PA, Stafford I, Abbott RI, et al, "Two- Versus 24-Hour Infusion of Cisplatin: Pharmacokinetic
Considerations," *J Clin Oncol*, 1989, 7(2):270-5.

Zeltzer PM, Epport K, Nelson MD Jr, et al, "Prolonged Response to Carboplatin in an Infant With Brain
Stem Glioma," *Cancer*, 1991, 67(1):43-7.

♦ **Cardec-S**® *see* Carbinoxamine and Pseudoephedrine *on page 179*

♦ **Cardizem**® *see* Diltiazem *on page 337*

♦ **Cardizem**® **CD** *see* Diltiazem *on page 337*

♦ **Cardizem**® **SR** *see* Diltiazem *on page 337*

♦ **Carindacillin** *see* Carbenicillin *on page 179*

Carmustine *(kar MUS teen)*

Related Information

Emetogenic Potential of Single Chemotherapeutic Agents *on page 1129*

U.S. Brand Names BiCNU®, Gliadel®

Synonyms BCNU

Therapeutic Category Antineoplastic Agent, Alkylating Agent (Nitrosourea)

Generic Available No

Use Treatment of brain tumors, multiple myeloma, Hodgkin's disease, and non-
Hodgkin's lymphomas; some activity in malignant melanoma, lung and colon cancer

Pregnancy Risk Factor D

Contraindications Hypersensitivity to carmustine or any component

Warnings The FDA currently recommends that procedures for proper handling and
disposal of antineoplastic agents be considered. Bone marrow suppression, notably

thrombocytopenia and leukopenia, may lead to bleeding and overwhelming infection in an already compromised patient; myelosuppressive effects will last for at least 6 weeks after a dose, do not give courses more frequently than every 6 weeks because the toxicity is cumulative; pulmonary toxicity is more common in patients receiving a cumulative dose >1400 mg/m^2, patients with recent mediastinal irradiation, and in patients with a past history of lung disease; acute leukemia has been reported in patients receiving long-term carmustine.

Precautions Administer with caution to patients with depressed platelet, leukocyte or erythrocyte counts and in patients with renal or hepatic impairment; dosage reduction is recommended in patients with compromised bone marrow function (decreased leukocyte and platelet counts)

Adverse Reactions

Cardiovascular: Flushing; high dose (≥300 mg/m^2) can produce hypotension, tachycardia, and confusion

Central nervous system: Ataxia, dizziness

Dermatologic: Dermatitis, hyperpigmentation, alopecia

Gastrointestinal: Nausea, vomiting, diarrhea, esophagitis, anorexia, mucositis, metallic taste

Hematologic: Myelosuppression (leukopenia, thrombocytopenia) with nadir at 28 days, anemia

Hepatic: Hepatotoxicity, elevated liver enzymes and serum bilirubin, jaundice, veno-occlusive disease with high doses

Local: Pain and thrombophlebitis at injection site, burning sensation

Ocular: Retinitis, optic neuritis

Renal: Renal failure, azotemia

Respiratory: Pulmonary fibrosis, cough, dyspnea, tachypnea

Drug Interactions Cimetidine (potentiates myelosuppressive effects); may potentiate hepatotoxicity with high doses of acetaminophen; may decrease serum digoxin and phenytoin levels; metronidazole (disulfiram reaction)

Stability Store in refrigerator, protect from light and heat; discard vial if oily film is found on the bottom of the vial; reconstituted solution is stable for 8 hours at room temperature, 24 hours when refrigerated, or 48 hours when refrigerated after further dilution in D$_5$W or NS in a glass bottle to a concentration of 0.2 mg/mL; incompatible with sodium bicarbonate; adsorption of carmustine to plastics and polyvinyl chloride-based infusion containers has been documented

Mechanism of Action Inhibits key enzymatic reactions involved with DNA synthesis; carbamoylation of amine groups on proteins; interferes with the normal function of DNA by alkylation and forms DNA-protein cross-links

Pharmacokinetics

Distribution: Readily crosses the blood-brain barrier since it is highly lipid soluble; CSF:plasma ratio >90%; distributes into breast milk

Protein binding: 75%

Metabolism: Denitrosation through action of microsomal enzymes; some enterohepatic circulation occurs

Half-life, terminal: 20-70 minutes (active metabolites may persist for days)

Elimination: ~60% to 70% excreted as metabolites in the urine and 6% to 10% excreted as CO$_2$ by the lungs

Usual Dosage I.V. infusion (refer to individual protocols):

Children: 200-250 mg/m^2 every 4-6 weeks as a single dose; next dose is to be determined based on clinical and hematologic response to the previous dose (a repeat course should not be given until platelets are >100,000/mm^3 and leukocytes are >4000/mm^3)

BMT-conditioning agent: 300-600 mg/m^2 over at least 2 hours or may be divided into 2 doses administered 12 hours apart

Adults: 150-200 mg/m^2 every 6 weeks as a single dose or divided into 75-100 mg/m^2/dose on 2 successive days; next dose is to be determined based on clinical and hematologic response to the previous dose (a repeat course should not be given until platelets are >100,000/mm^3 and leukocytes are >4000/mm^3)

Administration Parenteral: Further dilute the 3.3 mg of carmustine per mL solution with NS or D$_5$W in a glass or polyolefin container to a final concentration of 0.2-1 mg/mL and administer by I.V. infusion over 1-2 hours to prevent vein irritation; carmustine has also been administered over 15-45 minutes diluted in 100-250 mL D$_5$W with monitoring for vein irritation; burning sensation and pain at I.V. site can be decreased with reduction of infusion rate and further dilution of solution or placing ice pack on I.V. site; flush line before and after carmustine administration to ensure vein patency

Monitoring Parameters CBC with differential and platelet count; pulmonary function, liver function, and renal function tests

(Continued)

Carmustine *(Continued)*

Patient Information Report occurrence of fever, sore throat, unusual bleeding or bruising to physician; may discolor skin brown

Nursing Implications Must administer in glass containers; do not mix or administer with solutions containing sodium bicarbonate; accidental skin contact may cause transient burning and brown discoloration of the skin

Additional Information Myelosuppressive effects:
WBC: Moderate (nadir: 5-6 weeks)
Platelets: Severe (nadir: 4-5 weeks)

Dosage Forms
Powder for injection (BiCNU®): 100 mg/vial packaged with 3 mL of absolute alcohol for use as a sterile diluent
Wafer (Gliadel®): 7.7 mg

References
Aronin PA, Mahaley MS Jr, Rudnick SA, et al, "Prediction of BCNU Pulmonary Toxicity in Patients With Malignant Gliomas," *N Engl J Med*, 1980, 303(4):183-8.
Colvin M, Hartner J and Summerfield M, "Stability of Carmustine in the Presence of Sodium Bicarbonate," *Am J Hosp Pharm*, 1980, 37(5):677-8.
O'Driscoll BR, Hasleton PS, Taylor PM, et al, "Active Lung Fibrosis Up to 17 Years After Chemotherapy With Carmustine (BCNU) in Childhood," *N Engl J Med*, 1990, 323(6):378-82.

♦ **Carnation (Can)** *see* Salicylic Acid *on page 886*

Carnitine *(KAR ni teen)*

Related Information
Carbohydrate and Alcohol Content of Liquid Medications for Use in Patients Receiving Ketogenic Diets *on page 1258*

U.S. Brand Names Carnitor®; Vitacarn®

Synonyms L-carnitine; Levocarnitine

Therapeutic Category Nutritional Supplement

Generic Available Yes

Use Treatment of primary or secondary carnitine deficiency; prevention and treatment of carnitinic deficiency (injection) in patients undergoing dialysis for end stage renal disease (ESRD)

Pregnancy Risk Factor B

Precautions Use with caution in patients with seizure disorders; both new onset seizure activity and increased frequency of seizures have been reported

Adverse Reactions
Central nervous system: Myasthenia (in uremic patients on D,L-carnitine not L-carnitine), dizziness, fever, depression, seizures
Gastrointestinal: Nausea, vomiting, abdominal cramps, diarrhea, gastritis
Neuromuscular & skeletal: Weakness, paresthesia
Miscellaneous: Body odor (dose-related), allergic reactions

Drug Interactions Valproic acid, sodium benzoate; D,L-carnitine sold in health food stores as vitamin B_T, competitively inhibits L-carnitine

Stability Protect from light

Mechanism of Action Endogenous substance required in energy metabolism; facilitates long chain fatty acid entry into the mitochondria; modulates intracellular coenzyme A homeostasis; carnitine deficiency exists when there is insufficient carnitine to buffer toxic acyl-Co A compounds; secondary carnitine deficiency may be a consequence of inborn errors of metabolism

Pharmacokinetics
Metabolism: Major metabolites: Trimethylamine-N-oxide and acylcarnitine
Half-life, terminal: Adults: 17.4 hours
Bioavailability: 16%
Time to peak serum concentration: Oral: 3.3 hours
Elimination: Renal excretion of free and conjugated metabolites (acylcarnitine)

Usual Dosage
Primary carnitine deficiency:
Oral:
Children: 50-100 mg/kg/day divided 2-3 times/day, maximum 3 g/day; dosage must be individualized based upon patient response; higher dosages have been used
Adults: 330-990 mg/dose 2-3 times/day
I.V.: Children and Adults: 50 mg/kg as a loading dose, followed (in severe cases) by 50 mg/kg/day infusion; maintenance: 50 mg/kg/day divided every 4-6 hours, increase as needed to a maximum of 300 mg/kg/day
ESRD patients on hemodialysis: Adults: I.V.: Predialysis carnitine levels below normal (30-60 µmol): 10-20 mg/kg after each dialysis session; maintenance doses

as low as 5 mg/kg may be used after 3-4 weeks of therapy depending upon response (carnitine level)

Supplement to parenteral nutrition: I.V.: Neonates: 10-20 mg/kg/day in parenteral nutrition solution

Administration
Oral: Dilute in beverages or liquid food; administer with meals; consume slowly
Parenteral: May be administered by direct I.V. infusion over 2-3 minutes or as a continuous infusion

Monitoring Parameters Serum triglycerides, fatty acids, and carnitine levels

Reference Range Plasma free carnitine level: >20 μmol/L; plasma total carnitine level 30-60 μmol/L; to evaluate for carnitine deficiency determine the plasma acylcarnitine/free carnitine ratio (A/F ratio)
A/F ratio = [plasma total carnitine - free carnitine] divided by free carnitine
Normal plasma A/F ratio = 0.25; in carnitine deficiency A/F ratio >0.4

Additional Information Routine prophylactic use of carnitine in children receiving valproic acid to avoid carnitine deficiency and hepatotoxicity is probably not indicated

Dosage Forms
Capsule: 250 mg
Injection: 200 mg/mL (2.5 mL, 5 mL)
Liquid: 100 mg/mL [cherry flavor] (10 mL)
Tablet: 330 mg

References
Bonner CM, De Brie KL, Hug G, et al, "Effects of Parenteral L-Carnitine Supplementation on Fat Metabolism and Nutrition in Premature Neonates," *J Pediatr*, 1995, 126(2):287-92.
Borum PR, "Carnitine in Neonatal Nutrition," *J Child Neurol*, 1995, 10(Suppl 2):S25-31.
Helms RA, Mauer EC, and Hay WW Jr, "Effect of Intravenous L-Carnitine on Growth Parameters and Fat Metabolism During Parenteral Nutrition in Neonates," *JPEN J Parenter Enteral Nutr*, 1990, 14(5):448-53.

♦ **Carnitor**® *see* Carnitine *on page 184*
♦ **Carter's Little Pills**® **[OTC]** *see* Bisacodyl *on page 143*
♦ **Cartia XT**™ *see* Diltiazem *on page 337*
♦ **Casanthranol and Docusate** *see* Docusate and Casanthranol *on page 351*

Cascara Sagrada (kas KAR a sah GRAH dah)

Canadian Brand Names Le 500 D
Therapeutic Category Laxative, Stimulant
Generic Available Yes
Use Temporary relief of constipation; sometimes used with milk of magnesia ("black and white" mixture)
Pregnancy Risk Factor C
Contraindications Nausea, vomiting, abdominal pain, fecal impaction, intestinal obstruction, GI bleeding, appendicitis, CHF
Warnings Long-term use may result in laxative dependence
Adverse Reactions
Cardiovascular: Faintness
Endocrine & metabolic: Electrolyte and fluid imbalance
Gastrointestinal: Abdominal cramps, nausea, diarrhea, benign pigmentation of the colonic mucosa (with prolonged use)
Genitourinary: Discoloration of urine (reddish, pink, or brown)
Stability Protect from light and heat
Mechanism of Action Direct chemical irritation of the intestinal mucosa resulting in an increased rate of colonic motility and change in fluid and electrolyte secretion
Pharmacodynamics Onset of action: 6-10 hours
Pharmacokinetics
Absorption: Oral: Small amount from small intestine
Metabolism: In the liver
Usual Dosage Oral (**aromatic** fluid extract):
Infants: 1.25 mL/day as a single dose (range: 0.5-2 mL) as needed
Children 2-11 years: 2.5 mL/day as a single dose (range: 1-3 mL) as needed
Children ≥12 years and Adults: 5 mL/day (range: 2-6 mL) as needed at bedtime
Administration Oral: Administer on an empty stomach; drink plenty of fluids
Patient Information Should not be used regularly for more than 1 week; may discolor urine reddish, pink, or brown
Additional Information Cascara sagrada fluid extract is 5 times more potent than cascara sagrada aromatic fluid extract
Dosage Forms
Liquid, aromatic fluid extract: 120 mL, 473 mL
Tablet: 325 mg

Castor Oil (KAS tor oyl)

U.S. Brand Names Emulsoil® [OTC]; Neoloid® [OTC]; Purge® [OTC]
Synonyms Oleum Ricini
Therapeutic Category Laxative, Stimulant
Generic Available Yes
Use Preparation for rectal or bowel examination or surgery; rarely used to relieve constipation; also applied to skin as emollient and protectant
Pregnancy Risk Factor X
Contraindications Hypersensitivity to castor oil; nausea, vomiting, abdominal pain, fecal impaction, GI bleeding, appendicitis, CHF, menstruation, dehydration
Warnings Long-term use may result in laxative dependence
Adverse Reactions
Central nervous system: Dizziness
Endocrine & metabolic: Electrolyte disturbance, dehydration
Gastrointestinal: Abdominal cramps, nausea, diarrhea
Stability Protect from heat (emulsion should be protected from freezing)
Mechanism of Action Acts primarily in the small intestine; hydrolyzed to ricinoleic acid which reduces net absorption of fluid and electrolytes and stimulates peristalsis
Pharmacodynamics Onset of action: Oral: Within 2-6 hours
Usual Dosage Oral:
Castor oil:
Infants <2 years: 1-5 mL or 15 mL/m^2/dose as a single dose
Children 2-11 years: 5-15 mL as a single dose
Children ≥12 years and Adults: 15-60 mL as a single dose
Emulsified castor oil:
Infants: 2.5-7.5 mL/dose
Children:
<2 years: 5-15 mL/dose
2-11 years: 7.5-30 mL/dose
Children ≥12 years and Adults: 30-60 mL/dose
Administration Oral: Do not administer at bedtime because of rapid onset of action; chill or administer with juice or carbonated beverage to improve palatability; administer on an empty stomach
Monitoring Parameters I & O, serum electrolytes, stool frequency
Dosage Forms
Emulsion, oral:
Emulsoil®: 95% (63 mL)
Neoloid®: 36.4% [mint flavor] (118 mL)
Liquid, oral:
100% (60 mL, 120 mL, 480 mL)
Purge®: 95% [lemon flavor] (30 mL, 60 mL)

Cefaclor (SEF a klor)

Related Information
Carbohydrate and Alcohol Content of Liquid Medications for Use in Patients Receiving Ketogenic Diets on page 1258
U.S. Brand Names Ceclor®; Ceclor® CD
Canadian Brand Names Apo-Cefaclor; Novo-Cefaclor; Nu-Cefaclor; PMS-Cefaclor

Therapeutic Category Antibiotic, Cephalosporin (Second Generation)

Generic Available Yes

Use Infections caused by susceptible organisms including *Staph aureus*, *S. pneumoniae*, and *H. influenzae*; treatment of otitis media, sinusitis, and infections involving the respiratory tract, skin and skin structure, bone and joint, and urinary tract

Pregnancy Risk Factor B

Contraindications Hypersensitivity to cefaclor, any component, or cephalosporins

Warnings Prolonged use may result in superinfection; do not use in patients with immediate-type hypersensitivity reactions to penicillin

Precautions Use with caution in patients with impaired renal function, history of colitis, or history of penicillin hypersensitivity; modify dosage in patients with severe renal impairment

Adverse Reactions

Dermatologic: Rash, urticaria, pruritus

Gastrointestinal: Nausea, vomiting, diarrhea

Hematologic: Eosinophilia, neutropenia

Hepatic: Elevated liver enzymes, cholestatic jaundice

Miscellaneous: Serum sickness-like reaction (estimated incidence ranges from 0.024% to 0.2% per drug course); majority of reactions have occurred in children <5 years of age with symptoms of rash and arthralgia, often occurring during the second or third exposure

Drug Interactions Probenecid (increased cefaclor concentration); magnesium- or aluminum-containing antacids administered with cefaclor extended-release tablet (decreased cefaclor absorption)

Food Interactions

Capsules and suspension: Food or milk delays and decreases peak concentration

Extended release tablets: Food increases extent of absorption and peak concentrations

Stability Refrigerate suspension after reconstitution; discard after 14 days

Mechanism of Action Inhibits bacterial cell wall synthesis by binding to one or more of the penicillin-binding proteins and interfering with the final transpeptidation step of peptidoglycan synthesis resulting in cell wall death

Pharmacokinetics

Absorption: Oral: Well absorbed; acid stable

Distribution: Distributes into tissues and fluids including bone, pleural and synovial fluid; crosses the placenta; appears in breast milk

Protein binding: 25%

Half-life: 30-60 minutes (prolonged with renal impairment)

Time to peak serum concentration:

Capsule: 60 minutes

Suspension: 45 minutes

Tablet, extended release: 1.5-2.7 hours

Elimination: Most of dose (80%) excreted unchanged in urine

Dialysis: Moderately dialyzable (20% to 50%)

Usual Dosage Oral:

Children >1 month: 20-40 mg/kg/day divided every 8-12 hours; maximum dose: 2 g/day (twice daily option is for treatment of otitis media or pharyngitis)

Adults: 250-500 mg every 8 hours or daily dose can be given in 2 divided doses (twice daily option is for treatment of otitis media or pharyngitis)

Acute bronchitis: 500 mg extended release tablet every 12 hours for 7 days

Pharyngitis and/or tonsillitis: 375 mg extended release tablet every 12 hours for 10 days

Uncomplicated skin and skin structure infection: 375 mg extended release tablet every 12 hours for 7-10 days

Dosing adjustment in renal impairment: Cl_{cr} <10 mL//minute: Administer 50% of dose

Administration Oral:

Capsule, suspension: Administer 1 hour before or 2 hours after a meal; shake suspension well before use

Extended release tablet: Administer with food; do not crush, cut, or chew tablet

Monitoring Parameters With prolonged therapy, monitor CBC and stool frequency periodically

Test Interactions Positive Coombs' [direct], false-positive urine glucose (Clinitest®), false ↑ of serum or urine creatinine

Dosage Forms

Capsule: 250 mg, 500 mg

(Continued)

Powder for oral suspension: 125 mg/5 mL [strawberry flavor] (75 mL, 150 mL); 187 mg/5 mL [strawberry flavor] (50 mL, 100 mL); 250 mg/5 mL [strawberry flavor] (75 mL, 150 mL); 375 mg/5 mL [strawberry flavor] (50 mL, 100 mL)

Tablet, extended release (Ceclor® CD): 375 mg, 500 mg

References
Boguniewicz M and Leung DYM, "Hypersensitivity Reactions to Antibiotics Commonly Used in Children," *Pediatr Infect Dis J*, 1995, 14(3):221-31.

Hyslop DL, "Cefaclor Safety Profile: A Ten Year Review," *Clin Ther*, 1988, 11(Suppl A):83-94.

Levine LR, "Quantitative Comparison of Adverse Reactions to Cefaclor vs Amoxicillin in a Surveillance Study," *Pediatr Infect Dis*, 1985, 4(4):358-61.

Cefadroxil Monohydrate (sef a DROKS il mon o HYE drate)

Related Information
Carbohydrate and Alcohol Content of Liquid Medications for Use in Patients Receiving Ketogenic Diets *on page 1258*

U.S. Brand Names Duricef®

Canadian Brand Names Apo-Cefadroxil; Novo-Cefadroxil

Therapeutic Category Antibiotic, Cephalosporin (First Generation)

Generic Available Yes

Use Treatment of susceptible bacterial infections including group A beta-hemolytic streptococcal pharyngitis or tonsillitis; skin and soft tissue infections caused by streptococci or staphylococci; urinary tract infections caused by *Klebsiella*, *E. coli*, and *Proteus mirabilis*

Pregnancy Risk Factor B

Contraindications Hypersensitivity to cefadroxil, any component, or cephalosporins

Warnings Prolonged use may result in superinfection; do not use in patients with immediate-type hypersensitivity reaction to penicillin

Precautions Use with caution in patients who are hypersensitive to penicillin; modify dosage in patients with renal impairment

Adverse Reactions
Dermatologic: Rash
Gastrointestinal: Nausea, vomiting, diarrhea, pseudomembranous colitis
Genitourinary: Vaginitis
Hematologic: Transient neutropenia

Drug Interactions Probenecid may decrease renal tubular secretion and increase cefadroxil serum concentrations

Food Interactions Concomitant administration with food, infant formula, or cow's milk does **not** significantly affect absorption

Stability Refrigerate suspension after reconstitution; discard after 14 days

Mechanism of Action Interferes with bacterial cell wall synthesis during active replication, causing cell wall death and resultant bactericidal activity against susceptible bacteria

Pharmacokinetics
Absorption: Oral: Rapid; well absorbed from GI tract
Distribution: V_d: 0.31 L/kg; crosses the placenta; appears in breast milk
Protein binding: 20%
Half-life: 1-2 hours; 20-24 hours in renal failure
Time to peak serum concentration: Within 70-90 minutes
Elimination: >90% of dose excreted unchanged in urine within 24 hours

Usual Dosage Oral:
Infants and Children: 30 mg/kg/day divided twice daily up to a maximum of 2 g/day
Adolescents and Adults: 1-2 g/day in 1-2 divided doses; maximum dose for adults: 4 g/day

Dosing interval in renal impairment:
Cl_{cr} 10-25 mL/minute: Administer every 24 hours
Cl_{cr} <10 mL/minute: Administer every 36 hours

Administration Oral: May be administered without regard to food; administration with food may decrease nausea or vomiting; shake suspension well before use

Monitoring Parameters Stool frequency, resolution of infection

Test Interactions Positive Coombs' [direct], false-positive with urinary glucose tests using cupric sulfate (Clinitest®, Benedict's solution)

Patient Information Report persistent diarrhea; entire course of medication (eg, 10-14 days) should be taken to ensure eradication of organism

Dosage Forms
Capsule: 500 mg
Powder for oral suspension: 125 mg/5 mL (50 mL, 100 mL); 250 mg/5 mL (50 mL, 100 mL); 500 mg/5 mL (50 mL, 75 mL, 100 mL)
Tablet: 1 g

Cefazolin (sef A zoe lin)

Related Information
Endocarditis Prophylaxis *on page 1160*
U.S. Brand Names Ancef®; Kefzol®

Therapeutic Category Antibiotic, Cephalosporin (First Generation)

Generic Available Yes

Use Treatment of respiratory tract, skin and skin structure, urinary tract, biliary tract, bone and joint infections and septicemia due to susceptible gram-positive cocci (except enterococcus); some gram-negative bacilli including *E. coli*, *Proteus*, and *Klebsiella* may be susceptible; perioperative prophylaxis; bacterial endocarditis prophylaxis for dental and upper respiratory procedures

Pregnancy Risk Factor B

Contraindications Hypersensitivity to cefazolin sodium, any component, or cephalosporins

Warnings Prolonged use may result in superinfection; do not use in patients with immediate-type hypersensitivity reactions to penicillin

Precautions Use with caution in patients with a history of colitis or in patients with a history of hypersensitivity to penicillins; modify dosage in patients with renal impairment

Adverse Reactions
Central nervous system: Fever, CNS irritation, seizures
Dermatologic: Rash, urticaria
Hematologic: Leukopenia, thrombocytopenia
Hepatic: Transient elevation of liver enzymes
Local: Thrombophlebitis

Drug Interactions Probenecid may decrease renal tubular secretion and increase cefazolin serum concentrations; nephrotoxic agents

Stability Reconstituted solution is stable for 24 hours at room temperature or 96 hours when refrigerated; thawed solutions of the commercially available frozen cefazolin injections are stable for 48 hours at room temperature or 10 days when refrigerated

Mechanism of Action Inhibits bacterial cell wall synthesis by binding to one or more of the penicillin-binding proteins and interfering with the final transpeptidation step of peptidoglycan synthesis resulting in cell wall death

Pharmacokinetics
Distribution: Crosses the placenta; small amounts appear in breast milk; CSF penetration is poor; penetrates bone and synovial fluid well; distributes into bile
Protein binding: 74% to 86%
Metabolism: Hepatic is minimal
Half-life:
Neonates: 3-5 hours
Adults: 90-150 minutes (prolonged with renal impairment)
Time to peak serum concentration:
I.M.: Within 0.5-2 hours
I.V.: Within 5 minutes
Elimination: 80% to 100% excreted unchanged in urine
Dialysis: Moderately dialyzable (20% to 50%)

Usual Dosage I.M., I.V.:
Neonates:
Postnatal age ≤7 days: 40 mg/kg/day divided every 12 hours
Postnatal age >7 days:
≤2000 g: 40 mg/kg/day divided every 12 hours
>2000 g: 60 mg/kg/day divided every 8 hours
Infants and Children: 50-100 mg/kg/day divided every 8 hours; maximum dose: 6 g/day
Bacterial endocarditis prophylaxis for dental and upper respiratory procedures in penicillin allergic patients (see Precautions): 25 mg/kg 30 minutes before procedure; maximum dose: 1 g
Adults: 0.5-2 g every 6-8 hours; maximum dose: 12 g/day
Bacterial endocarditis prophylaxis for dental and upper respiratory procedures in penicillin allergic patients (see Precautions): 1 g 30 minutes before procedure
Perioperative prophylaxis: 1 g 30-60 minutes prior to surgery; 0.5-1 g every 8 hours for 24 hours postoperatively depending on the procedure
Dosing interval in renal impairment:
Cl$_{cr}$ 10-30 mL/minute: Administer every 12 hours
Cl$_{cr}$ <10 mL/minute: Administer every 24 hours
(Continued)

Cefazolin *(Continued)*

Administration Parenteral: Cefazolin may be administered IVP over 3-5 minutes at a maximum concentration of 100 mg/mL or I.V. intermittent infusion over 10-60 minutes at a final concentration for I.V. administration of 20 mg/mL. In fluid-restricted patients, a concentration of 138 mg/mL has been administered IVP.

Monitoring Parameters Renal function periodically when used in combination with other nephrotoxic drugs, hepatic function tests, and CBC

Test Interactions False-positive urine glucose using Clinitest®, positive Coombs' [direct], false $\uparrow$ serum or urine creatinine

Additional Information Sodium content of 1 g: 2 mEq

Dosage Forms

Infusion, premixed, as sodium, in D_5W (frozen) (Ancef®): 500 mg (50 mL); 1 g (50 mL)

Powder for injection, as sodium (Ancef®, Kefzol®, Zolicef®): 500 mg, 1 g, 10 g, 20 g

References

Dajani AS, Taubert KA, Wilson WW, et al, "Prevention of Bacterial Endocarditis. Recommendations by the American Heart Association," *JAMA*, 1997, 277(22):1794-801.

Pickering LK, O'Connor DM, Anderson D, et al, "Clinical and Pharmacologic Evaluation of Cefazolin in Children," *J Infect Dis* 1973, 128(Suppl):S407-1.

Robinson DC, Cookson TL, and Grisafe JA, "Concentration Guidelines for Parenteral Antibiotics in Fluid-Restricted Patients," *Drug Intell Clin Pharm*, 1987, 21(12):985-9.

Cefdinir *(SEF di ner)*

U.S. Brand Names Omnicef®

Therapeutic Category Antibiotic, Cephalosporin (Third Generation)

Generic Available No

Use Infections caused by susceptible organisms including *S. pneumoniae* (penicillin-susceptible strains only; inadequate activity against resistant pneumococcus), *H. influenzae* (including beta-lactamase-producing strains), *M. catarrhalis* (including beta-lactamase-producing strains), *S. aureus*, and *S. pyogenes*; treatment of infections involving the respiratory tract, skin and skin structure, and otitis media

Pregnancy Risk Factor B

Contraindications Hypersensitivity to cefdinir, any component, or cephalosporins

Warnings Pseudomembranous colitis has been reported with cefdinir; prolonged use may result in superinfection; serum sickness-like reactions have been reported with signs and symptoms occurring after a few days of therapy and resolving a few days after drug discontinuation.

Precautions Use with caution in patients with impaired renal function, history of colitis, or in penicillin-sensitive patients; modify dosage in patients with severe renal impairment

Adverse Reactions

Central nervous system: Headache, hyperactivity, insomnia, somnolence, seizures

Dermatologic: Rash, pruritus, diaper rash, Stevens-Johnson syndrome

Gastrointestinal: Diarrhea, nausea, vomiting, abdominal pain, pseudomembranous colitis, dyspepsia

Genitourinary: Vaginitis, microhematuria

Hematologic: Leukopenia, neutropenia, hemolytic anemia, eosinophilia, thrombocytopenia

Hepatic: Elevated AST, ALT, alkaline phosphatase; cholestatic jaundice, prolonged PT

Renal: Elevated BUN/serum creatinine

Miscellaneous: Serum sickness-like reactions, anaphylaxis

Drug Interactions Probenecid increases cefdinir serum levels; aluminum- or magnesium-containing antacids decrease cefdinir absorption by 40%; iron decreases cefdinir absorption by 80%

Food Interactions Total absorption is not affected by food.

Stability Store at room temperature; reconstituted suspension stable for 10 days at room temperature

Mechanism of Action Inhibits bacterial cell wall synthesis by binding to one or more of the penicillin-binding proteins resulting in disruption of cell wall synthesis and cell lysis

Pharmacokinetics

Absorption: High-fat meal decreases extent of absorption by 10%

Distribution: Penetrates into blister fluid, middle ear fluid, tonsils, sinus, and lung tissues

V_d:

Children 6 months to 12 years: 0.67 L/kg

Adults: 0.35 L/kg

Protein binding: 60% to 70%

Bioavailability:

Capsules: 16% to 21%

Suspension: 25%

Half-life, elimination: 1.7 (±0.6) hours with normal renal function

Time to peak serum concentrations: 2-4 hours

Elimination: 11.6% to 18.4% of a dose is excreted unchanged in urine

Hemodialysis: ~63% is removed by hemodialysis

Usual Dosage Oral:

Infants and Children (≥6 months to 12 years):

Otitis media or pharyngitis/tonsillitis: 14 mg/kg/day divided every 12 hours for 5-10 days or 14 mg/kg/day once daily for 10 days; maximum: 600 mg/day

Skin and skin structure infection: 14 mg/kg/day divided twice daily for 10 days; maximum: 600 mg/day

Acute maxillary sinusitis: 14 mg/kg/day divided every 12 hours for 10 days or 14 mg/kg/day once daily for 10 days; maximum: 600 mg/day

Children >12 years and Adults:

Acute exacerbations of chronic bronchitis or pharyngitis/tonsillitis: 600 mg once daily for 10 days or 300 mg every 12 hours for 5-10 days

Skin and skin structure infection or community-acquired pneumonia: 300 mg every 12 hours for 10 days

Acute maxillary sinusitis: 600 mg once daily for 10 days or 300 mg every 12 hours for 10 days

Dosing adjustment in renal impairment: Cl_{cr} <30 mL/minute:

Children ≥6 months to 12 years: 7 mg/kg/dose once daily

Adults: 300 mg once daily

Patients receiving hemodialysis: 300 mg or 7 mg/kg/dose starting at the conclusion of each hemodialysis session with subsequent doses every other day

Administration Oral: May administer with or without food; administer with food if stomach upset occurs; administer cefdinir at least 2 hours before or after antacids or iron supplements; shake suspension before use

Monitoring Parameters Evaluate renal function before and during therapy; with prolonged therapy, monitor coagulation tests, CBC, and liver function test periodically

Test Interactions Positive Coombs' [direct]; may produce false-positive reaction to urine glucose with Clinitest®; may produce false-positive reaction for ketones in the urine with tests using nitroprusside

Patient Information Report persistent diarrhea to physician; may discolor stools red if taken with iron

Additional Information Oral suspension contains 2.86 g of sucrose per teaspoon.

Dosage Forms

Capsule: 300 mg

Suspension, oral: 125 mg/5 mL (60 mL, 100 mL)

References

Klein JO and McCracken GH Jr, "Summary: Role of a New Oral Cephalosporin, Cefdinir, for Therapy of Infections of Infants and Children," *Pediatr Infect Dis J*, 2000, 19(12 Suppl):S181-3.

Cefepime (SEF e pim)

U.S. Brand Names Maxipime®

Therapeutic Category Antibiotic, Cephalosporin (Fourth Generation)

Use Treatment of lower respiratory tract infections, cellulitis, other skin and soft tissue infections, and urinary tract infections; empiric monotherapy in febrile neutropenia; considered a fourth generation cephalosporin because it is active against aerobic gram-negative bacteria, including *Pseudomonas aeruginosa*, active against some gram-negative bacteria that are resistant to third-generation cephalosporins, and more active than third-generation cephalosporins against gram-positive bacteria such as *Staphylococcus aureus*

Pregnancy Risk Factor B

Contraindications Hypersensitivity to cefepime, any component, or cephalosporins

Warnings Modify dosage in patients with severe renal impairment; prolonged use may result in superinfection; use with caution in patients with penicillin hypersensitivity; do not use in patients with immediate-type hypersensitivity reactions to penicillin

Adverse Reactions

Central nervous system: Headache, lightheadedness, fever, encephalopathy

Dermatologic: Maculopapular rash, pruritus, urticaria

Gastrointestinal: Dyspepsia, diarrhea, nausea, vomiting, pseudomembranous colitis

(Continued)

Cefepime *(Continued)*

Hematologic: Neutropenia after extended therapy, transient leukopenia and thrombocytopenia, agranulocytosis

Hepatic: Transient elevations in LFTs

Local: Phlebitis

Ocular: Blurred vision

Renal: Elevated BUN, elevated serum creatinine

Miscellaneous: Anaphylaxis including anaphylactic shock

Drug Interactions Probenecid decreases the clearance of cefepime; aminoglycosides increase nephrotoxic potential

Stability Store vial at room temperature and protect from light; incompatible with metronidazole, vancomycin, aminoglycosides, and aminophylline

Mechanism of Action Inhibits bacterial cell wall synthesis by binding to one or more of the penicillin-binding proteins; inhibits the final transpeptidation step of peptidoglycan synthesis in bacterial cell walls

Pharmacokinetics

Distribution: V_d:

Children (2 months to 6 years): 0.32-0.35 L/kg

Adults: 14-20 L; penetrates into inflammatory fluid at concentrations ~80% of serum levels and into bronchial mucosa at levels ~60% of plasma levels; excreted in breast milk at very low concentrations

Protein binding: 16% to 19%

Metabolism: Very little

Half-life:

Children 2 months to 6 years: 1.77-1.96 hours

Adults: 2 hours

Elimination: At least 85% eliminated as unchanged drug in urine

Dialysis: 45% to 68% removed by hemodialysis

Usual Dosage I.M., I.V.:

Children 2 months to 16 years, ≤40 kg in weight: 50 mg/kg/dose every 12 hours

Febrile neutropenic patients: 50 mg/kg/dose every 8 hours

Cefepime has been studied in 12 cystic fibrosis patients (ages 4-41 years) with bronchopulmonary infection at a dose of 50 mg/kg/dose every 8 hours (maximum dose: 2 g/dose every 8 hours); cefepime was as effective as cefotaxime in 90 children <15 years of age who were randomized to receive cefepime 50 mg/kg/dose every 8 hours (n=43) or cefotaxime 50 mg/kg/dose every 6 hours (n=47) for the treatment of bacterial meningitis

Adults: 1-2 g every 12 hours; high doses or more frequent administration may be required in pseudomonal infections

UTIs: 500 mg every 12 hours

Empiric monotherapy in febrile neutropenia: 2 g every 8 hours

Dosing Adjustment in Renal Impairment, Adults

Cl_{cr} (mL/min)	Infection		
	Mild to Moderate	Moderate to Severe	Severe
30-60	0.5-1 g I.M./I.V. every 24 hours	1-2 g I.V. every 24 hours	2 g I.V. every 24 hours
11-29	0.5 g I.M./I.V. every 24 hours	0.5-1 g I.V. every 24 hours	1 g I.V. every 24 hours
≤10	0.25 g I.M./I.V. every 24 hours	0.25-0.5 g I.V. every 24 hours	0.5 g I.V. every 24 hours

Administration Parenteral: Cefepime may be administered by I.V. intermittent infusion over 20-30 minutes; final concentration for I.V. administration should not exceed 40 mg/mL in D_5W, NS, $D_{10}W$, D_5/NS, or D_5/LR; in clinical trials, cefepime was administered by direct I.V. injection over 3-5 minutes at a final concentration of 100 mg/mL for mild to moderate infections

Monitoring Parameters With prolonged therapy, monitor renal and hepatic function periodically; number and type of stools/day for diarrhea; CBC with differential

Test Interactions Positive Coombs' [direct]; may falsely elevate creatinine values when Jaffé reaction is used; may cause false-positive results in urine glucose tests when using Clinitest®; false-positive urinary proteins and steroids

Patient Information Report side effects such as diarrhea, dyspepsia, headache, blurred vision, and lightheadedness to your physician

Nursing Implications Do not admix with aminoglycosides

Dosage Forms Powder for injection, as hydrochloride: 500 mg, 1 g, 2 g

References

Arguedas AG, Stutman HR, Zaleska M, et al, "Cefepime. Pharmacokinetics and Clinical Response in Patients With Cystic Fibrosis," *Am J Dis Child*, 1992, 146(7):797-802.

Blumer JL, Reed MD, Lemon E, et al, "Pharmacokinetics (PK) of Cefepime in Pediatric Patients Administered Single and Multiple 50 mg/kg Doses Every 8 Hours by the Intravenous (I.V.) or Intramuscular (I.M.) Route," 34th Interscience Conference on Antimicrobial Agents and Chemotherapy, 1994, Orlando, Fl. Abs. A69.

Saez-Llorens X, Castano E, Garcia R, et al, "Prospective Randomized Comparison of Cefepime and Cefotaxime for Treatment of Bacterial Meningitis in Infants and Children", *Antimicrob Agents Chemother*, 1995, 39(4):937-40.

Wynd MA and Paladino JA, "Cefepime: A Fourth-Generation Parenteral Cephalosporin," *Ann Pharmacother*, 1996, 30(12):1414-24.

Cefixime (sef IKS eem)

U.S. Brand Names Suprax®

Therapeutic Category Antibiotic, Cephalosporin (Third Generation)

Generic Available No

Use Treatment of urinary tract infections, otitis media, respiratory infections due to susceptible organisms including *S. pneumoniae* and *pyogenes*, *H. influenzae*, *M. catarrhalis*, and many *Enterobacteriaceae*; documented poor compliance with other oral antimicrobials; outpatient therapy of serious soft tissue or skeletal infections due to susceptible organisms; single-dose oral treatment of uncomplicated cervical/urethral gonorrhea due to *N. gonorrhoeae*; treatment of shigellosis in areas with a high rate of resistance to TMP-SMX

Pregnancy Risk Factor B

Contraindications Hypersensitivity to cefixime, any component, or cephalosporins

Warnings Prolonged use may result in superinfection; do not use in patients with immediate-type hypersensitivity reactions to penicillin

Precautions Use with caution in patients hypersensitive to penicillin, patients with impaired renal function, and patients with a history of colitis; modify dosage in patients with renal impairment

Adverse Reactions

Central nervous system: Headache, fever, dizziness, fatigue

Dermatologic: Skin rash, urticaria, pruritus

Gastrointestinal: Nausea, diarrhea (up to 15% of children), abdominal pain, pseudomembranous colitis

Genitourinary: Vaginitis

Hematologic: Eosinophilia, thrombocytopenia, leukopenia

Hepatic: Transient elevation of liver enzymes

Renal: Transient elevation of BUN and serum creatinine

Drug Interactions Probenecid (increases cefixime concentration); cefixime may increase carbamazepine serum concentrations

Food Interactions Food delays the time to reach peak concentrations

Stability After reconstitution, suspension may be stored for 14 days at room temperature

Mechanism of Action Inhibits bacterial cell wall synthesis by binding to one or more of the penicillin-binding proteins; inhibits the final transpeptidation step of peptidoglycan synthesis resulting in cell wall death

Pharmacokinetics

Absorption: Oral: 40% to 50%

Distribution: Into bile, sputum, middle ear fluid; crosses the placenta

Protein binding: 65%

Half-life:

Normal renal function: 3-4 hours

Renal failure: Up to 11.5 hours

Time to peak serum concentration: Within 2-6 hours; peak serum concentrations are 15% to 50% higher for the oral suspension versus tablets

Elimination: 50% of absorbed dose excreted as active drug in urine and 10% in bile

Dialysis: 10% removed by hemodialysis

Usual Dosage Oral:

Infants and Children: 8 mg/kg/day divided every 12-24 hours; maximum dose: 400 mg/day

Treatment of acute UTI: 16 mg/kg/day divided every 12 hours on day 1, then 8 mg/kg/day every 24 hours for 13 days

Prophylaxis after sexual victimization: 8 mg/kg in a single dose (maximum dose: 400 mg) **plus** azithromycin 20 mg/kg in a single dose (maximum dose: 1 g); also begin or complete hepatitis B virus immunization and consider prophylaxis for trichomoniasis and bacterial vaginosis

Adolescents and Adults: 400 mg/day divided every 12-24 hours

(Continued)

Cefixime *(Continued)*

Uncomplicated cervical/urethral gonorrhea due to *N. gonorrhoeae*: 400 mg as a single dose plus azithromycin 1 g orally in a single dose **or** doxycycline 100 mg orally twice daily for 7 days

Prophylaxis after sexual victimization: 400 mg in a single dose **plus** azithromycin 1 g orally in a single dose **or** doxycycline 100 mg orally twice daily for 7 days **plus** metronidazole 2 g orally in a single dose **plus** hepatitis B virus immunization if not fully immunized plus consider prophylaxis for HIV depending on circumstances

Dosing adjustment in renal impairment:
Cl_{cr} 21-60 mL/minute: Administer 75% of the standard dose
Cl_{cr} <20 mL/minute: Administer 50% of the standard dose

Administration Oral: May be administered with or without food; administer with food to decrease GI distress; shake suspension well before use

Monitoring Parameters With prolonged therapy, monitor renal and hepatic function periodically; number and type of stools/day for diarrhea

Test Interactions False-positive reaction for urine glucose using Clinitest®; false-positive urine ketones using tests with nitroprusside

Patient Information Report problems with diarrhea

Additional Information Otitis media should be treated with the suspension since it results in higher peak blood levels than the tablet

Dosage Forms

Powder for oral suspension: 100 mg/5 mL [strawberry flavor] (50 mL, 75 mL, 100 mL)

Tablet, film coated: 200 mg, 400 mg

References

Ashkenazi S, Amir J, Waisman Y, et al, "A Randomized, Double-Blind Study Comparing Cefixime and Trimethoprim-Sulfamethoxazole in the Treatment of Childhood Shigellosis," *J Pediatr*, 1993, 123(5):817-21.

"1998 Guidelines for the Treatment of Sexually Transmitted Diseases. Centers for Disease Control and Prevention," *MMWR Morb Mortal Wkly Rep*, 1998, 47(RR-1):1-111.

Hoberman A, Wald ER, Hickey RW, et al, "Oral Versus Initial Intravenous Therapy for Urinary Tract Infections in Young Febrile Children," *Pediatrics*, 1999, 104(1 Pt 1):79-86.

Johnson CE, Carlin SA, Super DM, et al, "Cefixime Compared With Amoxicillin for Treatment of Acute Otitis Media," *J Pediatr*, 1991, 119(1):117-22.

♦ **Cefizox®** *see* Ceftizoxime *on page 202*

♦ **Cefobid®** *see* Cefoperazone *on page 194*

Cefoperazone *(sef oh PER a zone)*

U.S. Brand Names Cefobid®

Therapeutic Category Antibiotic, Cephalosporin (Third Generation)

Generic Available No

Use Treatment of susceptible bacterial infections, mainly respiratory tract, skin and skin structure, urinary tract and sepsis; as a third generation cephalosporin, cefoperazone has activity against gram-negative bacilli (eg, *E. coli*, *Klebsiella*, and *Haemophilus*) but variable activity against *Streptococcus* and *Staphylococcus* species; it has activity against *Pseudomonas aeruginosa*, but less than ceftazidime

Pregnancy Risk Factor B

Contraindications Hypersensitivity to cefoperazone, any component, or cephalosporins

Warnings Modify dosage in patients who have both severe renal impairment and hepatic dysfunction; prolonged use may result in superinfection; do not use in patients with immediate-type hypersensitivity reactions to penicillin

Precautions Use with caution in patients who are hypersensitive to penicillins

Adverse Reactions

Dermatologic: Rash

Gastrointestinal: Nausea, vomiting, diarrhea, pseudomembranous colitis

Hematologic: Bleeding, bruising, positive Coombs' test

Local: Pain and induration at I.M. injection site, phlebitis

Drug Interactions Disulfiram-like reaction may occur if taken with alcohol; concomitant use of anticoagulants or other agents that affect blood clotting may increase the risk of severe hemorrhage

Food Interactions Cefoperazone may decrease vitamin K synthesis by suppressing GI flora; vitamin K deficiency may occur and result in an increased risk of hemorrhage; patients at risk include those with malabsorption states (eg, cystic fibrosis) or poor nutritional status; monitor prothrombin time and administer vitamin K as needed

Stability Reconstituted solution and I.V. infusion in NS or D$_5$W are stable for 24 hours at room temperature, 5 days when refrigerated or 3 weeks when frozen; after freezing, thawed solution is stable for 48 hours at room temperature or 10 days when refrigerated; do not refreeze, do not mix with aminoglycosides

Mechanism of Action Interferes with bacterial cell wall synthesis during active replication, causing cell wall death and resultant bactericidal activity against susceptible bacteria

Pharmacokinetics
Half-life:
Neonates (low birth weight): 6-10 hours
Adults: 2 hours; half-life increases with hepatic disease or biliary obstruction
Time to peak serum concentration:
I.M.: Within 1-2 hours
I.V.: Within 15-20 minutes (serum levels 2-3 times the serum levels following I.M. administration)
Elimination: Excreted primarily in the bile (70% to 75%); 20% to 30% recovered unchanged in urine within 12 hours

Usual Dosage I.M., I.V.:
Neonates: 50 mg/kg/dose every 12 hours
Infants and Children: 100-150 mg/kg/day divided every 8-12 hours; up to 12 g/day
Adults: 2-4 g/day in divided doses every 12 hours; maximum dose: 12 g/day divided every 6-12 hours; 16 g/day has been given via continuous infusion to severely immunocompromised patients
Maximum dose with impaired hepatic function and/or biliary obstruction: 4 g/day
Maximum dose with combined hepatic and renal dysfunction: 1-2 g/day

Administration Parenteral:
I.M.: For concentrations ≥250 mg/mL, may dilute using SWI and 2% lidocaine to make final concentration of 0.5% lidocaine (see package insert)
Intermittent I.V.: Administer over 15-30 minutes at a maximum concentration of 50 mg/mL
I.V. continuous infusion: Infuse at a concentration of 2-25 mg/mL

Monitoring Parameters Prothrombin time; number and type of stools/day for diarrhea; resolution of infection

Test Interactions False-positive with urinary glucose tests using cupric sulfate (Clinitest®, Benedict's solution)

Patient Information Avoid alcohol

Nursing Implications Monitor for coagulation abnormalities and diarrhea

Additional Information Sodium content of 1 g cefoperazone sodium: 1.5 mEq (34 mg); chemical structure contains the N-methylthiotetrazole side chain which may be responsible for the increased risk of bleeding and the disulfiram-like reaction with alcohol

Dosage Forms
Injection, as sodium, premixed (frozen): 1 g (50 mL); 2 g (50 mL)
Powder for injection, as sodium: 1 g, 2 g, 10 g

♦ **Cefotan**® *see Cefotetan on page 197*

Cefotaxime (sef oh TAKS eem)

U.S. Brand Names Claforan®
Therapeutic Category Antibiotic, Cephalosporin (Third Generation)
Generic Available No
Use Treatment of susceptible lower respiratory tract, skin and skin structure, bone and joint, intra-abdominal and genitourinary tract infections; treatment of a documented or suspected meningitis due to susceptible organisms such as *H. influenzae* and *N. meningitidis*; indicated for *Neisseria gonorrhoeae* infections (including uncomplicated cervical and urethral gonorrhea and gonorrhea pelvic inflammatory disease); nonpseudomonal gram-negative rod infection in a patient at risk of developing aminoglycoside-induced nephrotoxicity and/or ototoxicity; infection due to an organism whose susceptibilities clearly favor cefotaxime over cefuroxime or an aminoglycoside

Pregnancy Risk Factor B
Contraindications Hypersensitivity to cefotaxime, any component, or cephalosporins
Warnings Prolonged use may result in superinfection; do not use in patients with immediate-type hypersensitivity reactions to penicillin
Precautions Use with caution in patients with history of penicillin hypersensitivity, impaired renal function, or history of colitis; modify dosage in patients with Cl$_{cr}$ <20 mL/minute
(Continued)

Cefotaxime *(Continued)*

Adverse Reactions

Central nervous system: Fever, headache

Dermatologic: Rash, pruritus

Gastrointestinal: Antibiotic-associated pseudomembranous colitis, diarrhea, nausea, vomiting

Hematologic: Transient neutropenia, thrombocytopenia, eosinophilia, leukopenia

Hepatic: Transient elevation of liver enzymes

Local: Phlebitis, pain at injection site

Renal: Transient elevation of BUN and serum creatinine

Drug Interactions Probenecid (increases cefotaxime concentration)

Stability Reconstituted solution is stable for 24 hours at room temperature and 10 days when refrigerated

Mechanism of Action Inhibits bacterial cell wall synthesis by binding to one or more of the penicillin-binding proteins; inhibits the final transpeptidation step of peptidoglycan synthesis resulting in cell wall death

Pharmacokinetics

Distribution: Into bronchial secretions, middle ear effusions, bone, bile; penetration into CSF when meninges are inflamed; crosses the placenta; appears in breast milk

Protein binding: 31% to 50%

Metabolism: Partially metabolized in the liver to active metabolite, desacetylcefotaxime

Half-life:

Cefotaxime:

Neonates, premature: <1 week: 5-6 hours

Neonates, full-term: <1 week: 2-3.4 hours; 1-4 weeks: 2 hours

Children: 1.5 hours

Adults: 1-1.5 hours (prolonged with renal and/or hepatic impairment)

Desacetylcefotaxime: Adults: 1.5-1.9 hours (prolonged with renal impairment)

Time to peak serum concentration: I.M.: Within 30 minutes

Elimination: 40% to 60% of a dose excreted as unchanged drug and 24% excreted as desacetylcefotaxime in the urine

Dialysis: Moderately dialyzable (20% to 50%)

Usual Dosage I.M., I.V.:

Neonates: 0-4 weeks: <1200 g: 100 mg/kg/day divided every 12 hours

Postnatal age ≤7 days:

1200-2000 g: 100 mg/kg/day divided every 12 hours

>2000 g: 100-150 mg/kg/day divided every 8-12 hours

Postnatal age >7 days:

1200-2000 g: 150 mg/kg/day divided every 8 hours

>2000 g: 150-200 mg/kg/day divided every 6-8 hours

Infants and Children 1 month to 12 years:

<50 kg: 100-200 mg/kg/day divided every 6-8 hours

Meningitis: 200 mg/kg/day divided every 6 hours; 225-300 mg/kg/day divided every 6-8 hours has been used to treat invasive pneumococcal meningitis

≥50 kg: Moderate to severe infection: 1-2 g every 6-8 hours; life-threatening infection: 2 g/dose every 4 hours; maximum dose: 12 g/day

Children >12 years and Adults: 1-2 g every 6-8 hours (up to 12 g/day)

Dosing adjustment in renal impairment: Cl$_{cr}$ <20 mL/minute: Reduce dose by 50%

Administration Parenteral: Cefotaxime may be administered IVP over 3-5 minutes at a maximum concentration of 100 mg/mL or I.V. intermittent infusion over 15-30 minutes at a final concentration of 20-60 mg/mL; in fluid-restricted patients, a concentration of 150 mg/mL may be administered IVP

Monitoring Parameters With prolonged therapy, monitor renal, hepatic, and hematologic function periodically; number and type of stools/day for diarrhea

Test Interactions Positive Coombs' [direct]

Additional Information Sodium content of 1 g: 2.2 mEq

Dosage Forms

Infusion, as sodium, premixed, in D$_5$W (frozen): 1 g (50 mL); 2 g (50 mL)

Powder for injection, as sodium: 500 mg, 1 g, 2 g, 10 g

References

Spritzer R, Kamp HJ, Dzoljic G, et al, "Five Years of Cefotaxime Use in a Neonatal Intensive Care Unit," *Pediatr Infect Dis J*, 1990, 9(2):92-6.

Cefotetan (SEF oh tee tan)

U.S. Brand Names Cefotan®

Therapeutic Category Antibiotic, Cephalosporin (Second Generation)

Generic Available No

Use Treatment of susceptible lower respiratory tract, skin and skin structure, bone and joint, genitourinary tract, sepsis, gynecologic, and intra-abdominal infections; active against anaerobes including *Bacteroides* species of gastrointestinal tract, gram-negative enteric bacilli including *E. coli*, *Klebsiella*, and *Proteus*; active against many strains of *N. gonorrhoeae*; perioperative prophylaxis

Pregnancy Risk Factor B

Contraindications Hypersensitivity to cefotetan, any component, or cephalosporins

Warnings Prolonged use may result in superinfection; do not use in patients with immediate-type hypersensitivity reactions to penicillin

Precautions Use with caution and modify dosage in patients with renal impairment; use with caution in patients with history of colitis or penicillin hypersensitivity

Adverse Reactions

Central nervous system: Seizures, fever

Dermatologic: Rash, pruritus, urticaria

Gastrointestinal: Diarrhea, nausea, vomiting, pseudomembranous colitis

Hematologic: Neutropenia, leukopenia, thrombocytopenia, hemolytic anemia, bleeding, prolongation of PT

Hepatic: Elevated serum AST, ALT, alkaline phosphatase, LDH

Local: Phlebitis, pain at the injection site, edema

Renal: Elevated BUN, elevated serum creatinine

Drug Interactions Alcohol (disulfiram-like reaction), anticoagulants (may increase the risk of hemorrhage)

Stability Reconstituted solution is stable for 24 hours at room temperature and 96 hours when refrigerated; thawed solutions of the commercially available frozen cefotetan injections are stable for 48 hours at room temperature or 21 days when refrigerated; do not refreeze; incompatible with aminoglycosides, heparin, and tetracycline

Mechanism of Action Inhibits bacterial cell wall synthesis by binding to one or more of the penicillin-binding proteins; inhibits the final transpeptidation step of peptidoglycan synthesis resulting in cell wall death

Pharmacokinetics

Absorption: I.M.: Completely absorbed

Distribution: Distributes into tissues and fluids including gallbladder, kidney, skin, tonsils, uterus, sputum, prostatic and peritoneal fluids; poor penetration into CSF; cross the placenta; small amounts appear in breast milk

Protein binding: 76% to 91%

Half-life: 3.5 hours, prolonged in patients with impaired renal function (up to 10 hours)

Time to peak serum concentration: I.M.: Within 1.5-3 hours

Elimination: 49% to 81% excreted as unchanged drug in urine, 20% of dose is excreted in bile

Dialysis: <10% removed by hemodialysis

Usual Dosage I.M., I.V.: Safety and efficacy in children have not been established

Children: 40-80 mg/kg/day divided every 12 hours; up to 6 g/day

Adolescents and Adults: 2-4 g/day divided every 12 hours; maximum dose: 6 g/day

Urinary tract infections: 1-2 g/day divided every 12-24 hours

Perioperative prophylaxis: I.V.: 1-2 g 30-60 minutes prior to procedure

Pelvic inflammatory disease: I.V.: 2 g every 12 hours continued for 24-48 hours after significant clinical improvement is demonstrated **plus** doxycycline 100 mg I.V. or orally every 12 hours for 14 days

Dosing interval in renal impairment:

Cl_{cr} 10-30 mL/minute: Administer every 24 hours

Cl_{cr} <10 mL/minute: Administer every 48 hours

Administration Parenteral:

IVP: Administer over 3-5 minutes at a maximum concentration of 100 mg/mL

I.V. intermittent: Infuse over 20-60 minutes at a concentration of 10-40 mg/mL

Monitoring Parameters Prothrombin time, renal function tests; number and type of stools/day for diarrhea

Test Interactions Positive Coombs' [direct], false-positive urine glucose (Clinitest®), falsely elevated serum or urinary creatinine (Jaffé reaction)

Patient Information Avoid alcohol

(Continued)

Cefotetan (Continued)

Additional Information Sodium content of 1 g: 3.5 mEq; chemical structure contains a methyltetrazolethiol side chain which may be responsible for the disulfiram-like reaction with alcohol and increased risk of bleeding

Dosage Forms

Infusion, as disodium, premixed (frozen): 1 g (50 mL); 2 g (50 mL)

Powder for injection, as disodium: 1 g, 2 g, 10 g

References

Martin C, Thomachot L, and Albanese J, "Clinical Pharmacokinetics of Cefotetan," *Clin Pharmacokinet*, 1994, 26(4):248-58.

Cefoxitin (se FOKS i tin)

U.S. Brand Names Mefoxin®

Therapeutic Category Antibiotic, Cephalosporin (Second Generation)

Generic Available No

Use Treatment of susceptible lower respiratory tract, skin and skin structure, bone and joint, genitourinary tract, sepsis, gynecologic, and intra-abdominal infections; active against anaerobes including *Bacteroides* species of the gastrointestinal tract, gram-negative enteric bacilli including *E. coli*, *Klebsiella*, and *Proteus*; active against many strains of *N. gonorrhoeae*; perioperative prophylaxis

Pregnancy Risk Factor B

Contraindications Hypersensitivity to cefoxitin, any component, or cephalosporins

Warnings Prolonged use may result in superinfection; high doses in children have been associated with an increased incidence of eosinophilia and elevation of serum AST; safety and efficacy in infants <3 months have not been established; do not use in patients with immediate-type hypersensitivity reactions to penicillin

Precautions Use with caution and modify dosage in patients with renal impairment; use with caution in patients with history of colitis or penicillin hypersensitivity

Adverse Reactions

Central nervous system: Fever, headache

Dermatologic: Rash, pruritus, exfoliative dermatitis

Gastrointestinal: Pseudomembranous colitis, diarrhea, nausea, vomiting

Hematologic: Transient leukopenia, thrombocytopenia, neutropenia, anemia, eosinophilia

Hepatic: Transient elevation of liver enzymes, AST, ALT, and alkaline phosphatase

Local: Thrombophlebitis, pain at injection site

Renal: Transient elevation of BUN and serum creatinine

Drug Interactions Probenecid (increases serum concentration of cefoxitin)

Stability Reconstituted solution is stable for 24 hours at room temperature and for 1 week under refrigeration; thawed solutions of the commercially available frozen cefoxitin injections are stable for 24 hours at room temperature or 5 days when refrigerated

Mechanism of Action Inhibits bacterial cell wall synthesis by binding to one or more of the penicillin-binding proteins; inhibits the final transpeptidation step of peptidoglycan synthesis resulting in cell wall death

Pharmacokinetics

Distribution: Distributes into tissues and fluids including ascitic, pleural, bile, and synovial fluids; poor penetration into CSF even with inflamed meninges; crosses the placenta; small amounts appear in breast milk

Protein binding: 65% to 79%

Half-life:

Infants (10-53 days of age): 1.4 hours

Adults: 45-60 minutes, increases significantly with renal insufficiency

Time to peak serum concentration: I.M.: Within 20-30 minutes

Elimination: Rapidly excreted as unchanged drug (85%) in the urine

Dialysis: Moderately dialyzable (20% to 50%)

Usual Dosage I.M., I.V.:

Neonates: 90-100 mg/kg/day divided every 8 hours

Infants ≥3 months and Children:

Mild-moderate infection: 80-100 mg/kg/day divided every 6-8 hours

Severe infection: 100-160 mg/kg/day divided every 4-6 hours; maximum dose: 12 g/day

Perioperative prophylaxis: 30-40 mg/kg 30-60 minutes prior to surgery followed by 30-40 mg/kg/dose every 6 hours for no more than 24 hours after surgery depending on the procedure

Adolescents and Adults: 1-2 g every 6-8 hours (I.M. injection is painful); maximum dose: 12 g/day

Pelvic inflammatory disease: I.V.: 2 g every 6 hours continued for 24-48 hours after significant clinical improvement is demonstrated **plus** doxycycline 100 mg I.V. or orally every 12 hours for 14 days

Perioperative prophylaxis: 1-2 g 30-60 minutes prior to surgery followed by 1-2 g every 6-8 hours for no more than 24 hours after surgery depending on the procedure

Dosing interval in renal impairment:
Cl_{cr} 30-50 mL/minute: Administer every 8-12 hours
Cl_{cr} 10-30 mL/minute: Administer every 12-24 hours
Cl_{cr} <10 mL/minute: Administer every 24-48 hours

Administration Parenteral:
IVP: Administer over 3-5 minutes at a maximum concentration of 200 mg/mL
I.V. intermittent infusion: Administer over 10-60 minutes at a final concentration not to exceed 40 mg/mL

Monitoring Parameters Renal function periodically when used in combination with other nephrotoxic drugs; liver function and hematologic function tests; number and type of stools/day for diarrhea

Test Interactions Positive Coombs' [direct]; false-positive urine glucose (Clinitest®), false ↑ in serum or urine creatinine

Additional Information Sodium content of 1 g: 2.3 mEq

Dosage Forms
Infusion, as sodium, premixed, in D_5W (frozen): 1 g (50 mL); 2 g (50 mL)
Powder for injection, as sodium: 1 g, 2 g, 10 g

References
Feldman WE, Moffitt S, and Sprow N, "Clinical and Pharmacokinetic Evaluation of Parenteral Cefoxitin in Infants and Children," *Antimicrob Agents Chemother*, 1980, 17(4):669-74.
Regazzi MB, Chirico G, Cristiani D, et al, "Cefoxitin in Newborn Infants. A Clinical and Pharmacokinetic Study," *Eur J Clin Pharmacol*, 1983, 25(4):507-9.

Cefpodoxime (sef pode OKS eem)

Related Information
Carbohydrate and Alcohol Content of Liquid Medications for Use in Patients Receiving Ketogenic Diets *on page 1258*

U.S. Brand Names Vantin®

Therapeutic Category Antibiotic, Cephalosporin (Third Generation)

Generic Available No

Use Treatment of susceptible acute, community-acquired pneumonia caused by *S. pneumoniae* or nonbeta-lactamase producing *H. influenzae*; alternative regimen for acute uncomplicated gonorrhea caused by *N. gonorrhoeae*; uncomplicated skin and skin structure infections caused by *S. aureus* or *S. pyogenes*; acute otitis media caused by *S. pneumoniae*, *H. influenzae*, or *M. catarrhalis*; pharyngitis or tonsillitis; and uncomplicated urinary tract infections caused by *E. coli*, *Klebsiella*, and *Proteus*

Pregnancy Risk Factor B

Contraindications Hypersensitivity to cefpodoxime, any component, or cephalosporins

Warnings Prolonged use may result in superinfection; do not use in patients with immediate-type hypersensitivity reactions to penicillin

Precautions Use with caution in patients with history of penicillin hypersensitivity, impaired renal function, and patients with a history of colitis; modify dosage in patients with renal impairment

Adverse Reactions
Central nervous system: Headache
Dermatologic: Rash
Gastrointestinal: Nausea (3.8%), vomiting, abdominal pain, diarrhea (7.1%), pseudomembranous colitis
Genitourinary: Vaginal fungal infections (3.3%)
Hematologic: Eosinophilia, leukocytosis, thrombocytosis, decrease in hemoglobin or hematocrit, leukopenia, prolonged PT and PTT
Hepatic: Transient elevation in AST, ALT, bilirubin
Renal: Elevated BUN, elevated serum creatinine

Drug Interactions Antacids and H_2-receptor antagonists (reduce absorption and serum concentration of cefpodoxime); probenecid (inhibits renal excretion of cefpodoxime)

Food Interactions Food increases oral bioavailability

Stability After reconstitution, suspension may be stored in refrigerator for 14 days

Mechanism of Action Inhibits bacterial cell wall synthesis by binding to one or more of the penicillin-binding proteins; inhibits the final transpeptidation step of peptidoglycan synthesis resulting in cell wall death
(Continued)

Cefpodoxime *(Continued)*

Pharmacokinetics

Absorption: Enhanced in the presence of food or low gastric pH

Distribution: Good tissue penetration, including lung and tonsils; penetrates into pleural fluid

Protein binding: 18% to 23%

Metabolism: Following oral administration, cefpodoxime proxetil is de-esterified in the GI tract to the active metabolite, cefpodoxime

Bioavailability: Oral: 50%

Half-life: 2.2 hours (prolonged with renal impairment)

Time to peak serum concentration: Within 2-3 hours

Elimination: Primarily by the kidney with 80% of absorbed dose excreted unchanged in urine in 24 hours

Usual Dosage Oral:

Children >6 months to 12 years: 10 mg/kg/day divided every 12 hours; maximum dose: 800 mg/day

Children ≥13 years and Adults: 100-400 mg/dose every 12 hours

Uncomplicated gonorrhea: 200 mg as a single dose

Dosing adjustment in renal impairment: Cl_{cr} <30 mL/minute: Administer every 24 hours; patients on hemodialysis, administer dose 3 times/week

Dosing adjustment in hepatic impairment: Not necessary in patient with cirrhosis

Administration Oral:

Tablet: Administer with food

Suspension: May administer with or without food; shake suspension well before use

Monitoring Parameters Observe patient for diarrhea; with prolonged therapy, monitor renal function periodically

Test Interactions Positive Coombs' [direct]

Dosage Forms

Granules for oral suspension, as proxetil: 50 mg/5 mL [lemon creme flavor] (100 mL); 100 mg/5 mL [lemon creme flavor] (100 mL)

Tablet, film coated, as proxetil: 100 mg, 200 mg

References

Borin MT, "A Review of the Pharmacokinetics of Cefpodoxime Proxetil," *Drugs*, 1991, 42(Suppl 3):13-21.

Fujii R, "Clinical Trials of Cefpodoxime Proxetil Suspension in Pediatrics," *Drugs*, 1991, 42(Suppl 3):57-60.

Mendelman PM, Del-Beccaro MA, McLinn SE, et al, "Cefpodoxime Proxetil Compared With Amoxicillin-Clavulanate for the Treatment of Otitis Media," *J Pediatr*, 1992, 121(3):459-65.

Cefprozil *(sef PROE zil)*

Related Information

Carbohydrate and Alcohol Content of Liquid Medications for Use in Patients Receiving Ketogenic Diets *on page 1258*

U.S. Brand Names Cefzil®

Therapeutic Category Antibiotic, Cephalosporin (Second Generation)

Generic Available No

Use Infections caused by susceptible organisms including *S. pneumoniae, H. influenzae, M. catarrhalis, S. aureus, S. pyogenes*; treatment of infections involving the respiratory tract, skin and skin structure, and otitis media

Pregnancy Risk Factor B

Contraindications Hypersensitivity to cefprozil, any component, or cephalosporins

Warnings Prolonged use may result in superinfection; do not use in patients with immediate-type hypersensitivity reactions to penicillin

Precautions Use with caution in patients with impaired renal function, history of colitis, or in penicillin-sensitive patients; modify dosage in patients with severe renal impairment

Adverse Reactions

Central nervous system: Headache, hyperactivity, insomnia, confusion, dizziness

Dermatologic: Rash, pruritus, diaper rash

Gastrointestinal: Diarrhea, nausea, vomiting, abdominal pain

Genitourinary: Vaginitis

Hematologic: Decrease in leukocyte and platelet count, eosinophilia

Hepatic: Elevated AST, ALT, and alkaline phosphatase; cholestatic jaundice; prolonged PT

Renal: Elevated BUN and serum creatinine

Miscellaneous: Serum sickness-like reactions

Drug Interactions Probenecid increases cefprozil serum levels

Food Interactions Total absorption is not affected by food

Stability Refrigerate suspension after reconstitution; discard after 14 days

Mechanism of Action Inhibits bacterial cell wall synthesis by binding to one or more of the penicillin-binding proteins resulting in disruption of cell wall synthesis and cell lysis

Pharmacokinetics
Absorption: Oral: Well absorbed (95%)
Distribution: Low excretion into breast milk
Protein binding: 35% to 45%
Bioavailability: 94%
Half-life, elimination: 1.3 hours (normal renal function)
Time to peak serum concentration: 1.5 hours (fasting state)
Elimination: 61% excreted unchanged in urine
Dialysis: ~55% is removed by hemodialysis

Usual Dosage Oral:
Infants and Children (>6 months to 12 years):
Otitis media: 30 mg/kg/day divided every 12 hours; maximum dose: 1 g/day
Pharyngitis/tonsillitis: 2-12 years: 15 mg/kg/day divided every 12 hours; maximum dose: 1 g/day
Children >12 years and Adults: 250-500 mg every 12 hours or 500 mg every 24 hours
Dosing adjustment in renal impairment: Cl_{cr} <30 mL/minute: Reduce dose by 50%

Administration Oral: May administer with or without food; administer with food if stomach upset occurs; chilling improves flavor of suspension (do not freeze); shake suspension well before use

Monitoring Parameters Evaluate renal function before and during therapy; with prolonged therapy, monitor coagulation tests, CBC, and liver function tests periodically

Test Interactions Positive Coombs' [direct]; may produce false-positive reaction for urine glucose with Clinitest®

Patient Information Report persistent diarrhea to physician

Additional Information Suspension also contains aspartame, FD&C red No. 3, glycine, sodium benzoate, carboxymethylcellulose, sucrose, and phenylalanine

Dosage Forms
Powder for oral suspension, as anhydrous: 125 mg/5 mL [bubblegum flavor] (50 mL, 75 mL, 100 mL); 250 mg/5 mL [bubblegum flavor] (50 mL, 75 mL, 100 mL)
Tablet, as anhydrous: 250 mg, 500 mg

References
Arguedas AG, Zaleska M, Stutman HR, et al, "Comparative Trial of Cefprozil vs Amoxicillin Clavulanate Potassium in the Treatment of Children With Acute Otitis Media With Effusion," *Pediatr Infect Dis J,* 1991, 10(5):375-80.
Barriere SL, "Review of *In Vitro* Activity, Pharmacokinetic Characteristics, Safety, and Clinical Efficacy of Cefprozil, a New Oral Cephalosporin," *Ann Pharmacother,* 1993, 27(9):1082-9.
Lowery N, Kearns GL, Young RA, et al, "Serum Sickness-Like Reactions Associated With Cefprozil Therapy," *J Pediatr,* 1994, 125(2):325-8.

Ceftazidime (SEF tay zi deem)

U.S. Brand Names Ceptaz™; Fortaz®; Tazicef®; Tazidime®
Therapeutic Category Antibiotic, Cephalosporin (Third Generation)
Generic Available No
Use Treatment of infections of the respiratory tract, urinary tract, skin and skin structure, intra-abdominal, osteomyelitis, sepsis, and meningitis caused by susceptible gram-negative aerobic organisms such as Enterobacteriaceae and *Pseudomonas*; pseudomonal infection in patient at risk of developing aminoglycoside-induced nephrotoxicity and/or ototoxicity; empiric therapy for febrile, granulocytopenic patients
Pregnancy Risk Factor B
Contraindications Hypersensitivity to ceftazidime, any component, or cephalosporins
Warnings Prolonged use may result in superinfection; do not use in patients with immediate-type hypersensitivity reactions to penicillin
Precautions Use with caution and modify dosage in patients with impaired renal function; use with caution in patients with history of colitis or patients with penicillin hypersensitivity
Adverse Reactions
Central nervous system: Fever, headache, dizziness
Dermatologic: Rash, pruritus
Gastrointestinal: Pseudomembranous colitis, diarrhea, nausea, vomiting, candidiasis
(Continued)

201

Ceftazidime *(Continued)*

Hematologic: Transient leukopenia, thrombocytopenia, eosinophilia, thrombocytosis, hemolytic anemia

Hepatic: Transient elevation of liver enzymes

Local: Phlebitis, pain at injection site

Renal: Transient elevation of BUN and serum creatinine

Drug Interactions Probenecid decreases renal clearance of ceftazidime; aminoglycosides may increase risk of nephrotoxicity

Stability Reconstituted solution is stable for 24 hours at room temperature and 10 days when refrigerated; incompatible with sodium bicarbonate; potentially incompatible with aminoglycosides

Mechanism of Action Bactericidal antibiotic with a mechanism similar to that of penicillins by binding to one or more of the penicillin-binding proteins; inhibits mucopeptide synthesis in the bacterial cell wall

Pharmacokinetics

Distribution: Widely distributed throughout the body including bone, bile, skin, CSF (diffuses into CSF at higher concentrations when the meninges are inflamed), endometrium, heart, pleural and lymphatic fluids; distributes into breast milk

Protein binding: 17%

Half-life:

Neonates <23 days: 2.2-4.7 hours

Adults: 1-2 hours (prolonged with renal impairment)

Time to peak serum concentration: I.M.: Within 60 minutes

Elimination: By glomerular filtration with 80% to 90% of the dose excreted as unchanged drug in urine within 24 hours

Dialysis: Dialyzable (50% to 100%)

Usual Dosage I.M., I.V.:

Neonates: 0-4 weeks: <1200 g: 100 mg/kg/day divided every 12 hours

Postnatal age ≤7 days:

1200-2000 g: 100 mg/kg/day divided every 12 hours

>2000 g: 100-150 mg/kg/day divided every 8-12 hours

Postnatal age >7 days: ≥1200 g: 150 mg/kg/day divided every 8 hours

Infants and Children 1 month to 12 years: 100-150 mg/kg/day divided every 8 hours; maximum dose: 6 g/day

Meningitis: 150 mg/kg/day divided every 8 hours; maximum dose: 6 g/day

Adults: 1-2 g every 8-12 hours

Urinary tract infections: 250-500 mg every 12 hours

Dosing interval in renal impairment:

Cl_{cr} 30-50 mL/minute: Administer every 12 hours

Cl_{cr} 10-30 mL/minute: Administer every 24 hours

Cl_{cr} <10 mL/minute: Administer every 24-48 hours

Administration Parenteral: Any carbon dioxide bubbles that may be present in the withdrawn solution should be expelled prior to injection

IVP: Administer over 3-5 minutes at a maximum concentration of 180 mg/mL

I.V. intermittent infusion: Administer over 15-30 minutes at a final concentration ≤40 mg/mL

Monitoring Parameters Renal function periodically when used in combination with aminoglycosides; with prolonged therapy also monitor hepatic and hematologic function periodically; number and type of stools/day for diarrhea

Test Interactions Positive Coombs' [direct], false-positive urine glucose (Clinitest®)

Additional Information Sodium content of 1 g: 2.3 mEq

Dosage Forms

Infusion, premixed (frozen), as sodium (Fortaz®): 1 g (50 mL); 2 g (50 mL)

Powder for injection: 500 mg, 1 g, 2 g, 6 g, 10 g

References

McCracken GH Jr, Threlkeld N, and Thomas ML, "Pharmacokinetics of Ceftazidime in Newborn Infants," *Antimicrob Agents Chemother,* 1984, 26(4):583-4.

Robinson DG, Cookson TL, and Frisafe JA, "Concentration Guidelines for Parenteral Antibiotics in Fluid-Restricted Patients," *Drug Intell Clin Pharm,* 1987, 21(12):985-9.

♦ **Ceftin®** *see Cefuroxime on page 205*

Ceftizoxime (sef ti ZOKS eem)

U.S. Brand Names Cefizox®

Therapeutic Category Antibiotic, Cephalosporin (Third Generation)

Generic Available No

Use Treatment of susceptible bacterial infections, mainly respiratory tract, skin and skin structure, bone and joint, urinary tract and sepsis; as a third generation cephalosporin, ceftizoxime has activity against gram-negative enteric bacilli (eg, *E. coli,*

Klebsiella), and cocci (eg, *Neisseria*), and variable activity against gram-positive cocci (*Staphylococcus* and *Streptococcus*); ceftizoxime has some anaerobic coverage but is less active against *B. fragilis* than cefoxitin; also indicated for *Neisseria gonorrhoeae* infections (including uncomplicated cervical and urethral gonorrhea and gonorrhea pelvic inflammatory disease), and *Haemophilus influenzae* meningitis

Pregnancy Risk Factor B

Contraindications Hypersensitivity to ceftizoxime, any component, or cephalosporins

Warnings Prolonged use may result in superinfection; do not use in patients with immediate-type hypersensitivity reaction to penicillin

Precautions Use with caution in patients who are hypersensitive to penicillins; use with caution and modify dosage in patients with renal impairment

Adverse Reactions
  Central nervous system: Fever
  Dermatologic: Rash, pruritus
  Gastrointestinal: Diarrhea, occasionally nausea and vomiting
  Genitourinary: Vaginitis (rare)
  Hematologic: Positive Coombs' test, eosinophilia, thrombocytosis (transient); rarely: anemia, leukopenia, neutropenia, thrombocytopenia
  Hepatic: Elevated bilirubin; transient elevation of AST, ALT, alkaline phosphatase
  Local: Pain, burning at injection site
  Neuromuscular & skeletal: Numbness
  Renal: Transient elevations of BUN and serum creatinine

Drug Interactions Probenecid may decrease renal tubular secretion and increase ceftizoxime serum concentrations

Stability Reconstituted solution is stable for 24 hours at room temperature and 96 hours when refrigerated; for I.V. infusion in NS or D_5W solution is stable for 24 hours at room temperature, 96 hours when refrigerated or 12 weeks when frozen; after freezing, thawed solution is stable for 24 hours at room temperature or 10 days when refrigerated; do not refreeze; do not mix with aminoglycosides

Mechanism of Action Interferes with bacterial cell wall synthesis during active replication, causing cell wall death and resultant bactericidal activity against susceptible bacteria

Pharmacokinetics
  Distribution: V_d: 0.35-0.5 L/kg; penetrates CSF
  Protein binding: 30%
  Half-life: 1.6 hours, increases to 25 hours when Cl_{cr} falls to <10 mL/minute
  Time to peak serum concentration: I.M.: Within 0.5-1 hour
  Elimination: Excreted unchanged in urine
  Dialysis: Moderately dialyzable (20% to 50%)

Usual Dosage I.M., I.V.:
  Children ≥6 months: 150-200 mg/kg/day divided every 6-8 hours; maximum dose: 12 g/24 hours
  Adults: 1-2 g every 8-12 hours
    Life-threatening infections: Up to 2 g every 4 hours or 4 g every 8 hours
    Uncomplicated gonorrhea: I.M.: 1 g (single dose)
  Dosing interval in renal impairment:
    Cl_{cr} 50-80 mL/minute: Administer every 8-12 hours
    Cl_{cr} 10-50 mL/minute: Administer every 36-48 hours
    Cl_{cr} <10 mL/minute: Administer every 48-72 hours

Administration Parenteral:
  I.V. intermittent infusion: Administer over 30 minutes; usual dilution: 1 g/50 mL, doses >1 g are usually diluted to 100 mL
  I.V. direct (bolus) injection: Administer slowly over 3-5 minutes at a concentration of 95 mg/mL

Test Interactions May falsely elevate creatine values when Jaffé reaction is used; may cause false-positive urinary glucose tests using cupric sulfate (Clinitest®, Benedict's solution)

Additional Information Sodium content of 1 g ceftizoxime: 60 mg (2.6 mEq); ceftizoxime does not cover *Chlamydia trachomatis* infections and must, therefore, be used with appropriate antichlamydial agents when treating pelvic inflammatory disease if *C. trachomatis* is suspected

Dosage Forms
  Injection, as sodium, in D_5W (frozen): 1 g (50 mL); 2 g (50 mL)
  Powder for injection, as sodium: 500 mg, 1 g, 2 g, 10 g

Ceftriaxone (sef trye AKS one)

U.S. Brand Names Rocephin®

Therapeutic Category Antibiotic, Cephalosporin (Third Generation)

Generic Available No

Use Treatment of sepsis, meningitis, infections of the lower respiratory tract, skin and skin structure, bone and joint, intra-abdominal and urinary tract due to susceptible organisms; as a third generation cephalosporin, ceftriaxone has activity against gram-negative aerobic bacteria (ie, *H. influenzae*, Enterobacteriaceae, *Neisseria*), and variable activity against gram-positive cocci; documented or suspected infection due to susceptible organisms in home care patients and patients without I.V. line access; treatment of documented or suspected gonococcal infection or chancroid; emergency room management of patients at high risk for bacteremia, periorbital or buccal cellulitis, salmonellosis or shigellosis and pneumonia of unestablished etiology (<5 years of age); treatment of resistant acute otitis media; in children with acute otitis media who are unable to take oral antibiotics

Pregnancy Risk Factor B

Contraindications Hypersensitivity to ceftriaxone sodium, any component, or cephalosporins; do not use in hyperbilirubinemic neonates, particularly those who are premature since ceftriaxone is reported to displace bilirubin from albumin binding sites increasing the risk for kernicterus

Warnings Prolonged use may result in superinfection with yeasts, enterococci, *B. fragilis*, or *P. aeruginosa*; do not use in patients with immediate-type hypersensitivity reactions to penicillin

Precautions Use with caution in patients with gallbladder, biliary tract, liver, or pancreatic disease; or in patients with history of colitis or penicillin hypersensitivity

Adverse Reactions
Central nervous system: Fever, chills, headache, dizziness
Dermatologic: Rash, pruritus
Gastrointestinal: Diarrhea, nausea, vomiting, sludging in the gallbladder, cholelithiasis, pseudomembranous colitis
Genitourinary: Vaginitis, casts in urine
Hematologic: Eosinophilia, leukopenia, anemia, thrombocytopenia, thrombocytosis, bleeding, neutropenia
Hepatic: Transient elevation in liver enzymes, jaundice, elevation in serum bilirubin
Local: Pain at injection site
Renal: Elevated BUN and serum creatinine

Drug Interactions High-dose probenecid (decreases elimination half-life of ceftriaxone); aminoglycosides may increase risk of nephrotoxicity

Stability Reconstituted solution (100 mg/mL) is stable for 3 days at room temperature and 10 days when refrigerated; reconstituted solution (250 mg/mL) is stable for 24 hours at room temperature and 3 days when refrigerated

Mechanism of Action Inhibits bacterial cell wall synthesis by binding to one or more of the penicillin-binding proteins; inhibits the final transpeptidation step of peptidoglycan synthesis resulting in cell wall death

Pharmacokinetics
Distribution: Widely distributed throughout the body including gallbladder, lungs, bone, bile, CSF (diffuses into the CSF at higher concentrations when the meninges are inflamed); crosses the placenta
Protein binding: 85% to 95%
Half-life:
Neonates:
1-4 days: 16 hours
9-30 days: 9 hours
Adults: 5-9 hours (with normal renal and hepatic function)
Time to peak serum concentration: I.M.: Within 1-2 hours
Elimination: Unchanged in the urine (33% to 65%) by glomerular filtration and in feces via bile
Dialysis: Not dialyzable (0% to 5%)

Usual Dosage I.M., I.V.:
Neonates:
Postnatal age ≤7 days: 50 mg/kg/day given every 24 hours
Postnatal age >7 days:
≤2000 g: 50 mg/kg/day given every 24 hours
>2000 g: 50-75 mg/kg/day given every 24 hours
Gonococcal prophylaxis: 25-50 mg/kg as a single dose (dose not to exceed 125 mg)
Gonococcal infection: 25-50 mg/kg/day (maximum dose: 125 mg) given every 24 hours for 7 days, up to 10-14 days if meningitis is documented

Note: Use cefotaxime in place of ceftriaxone in hyperbilirubinemic neonates

Infants and Children: 50-75 mg/kg/day divided every 12-24 hours

Meningitis: 80-100 mg/kg/day divided every 12-24 hours; loading dose of 75 mg/kg may be administered at the start of therapy; maximum dose: 4 g/day

Chemoprophylaxis for high-risk contacts of patients with invasive meningococcal disease:

≤12 years: I.M.: 125 mg in a single dose

>12 years: I.M.: 250 mg in a single dose

Uncomplicated gonococcal infections, sexual assault, and STD prophylaxis: I.M.: 125 mg in a single dose

Complicated gonococcal infections: I.M., I.V.:

<45 kg:

Peritonitis, arthritis, or bacteremia: 50 mg/kg/day once daily for 7 days; maximum dose: 1 g/day

Conjunctivitis: 50 mg/kg (maximum dose: 1 g) in a single dose

Meningitis or endocarditis: 50 mg/kg/day divided every 12 hours for 10-14 days (meningitis), for 28 days (endocarditis); maximum dose: 2 g/day

>45 kg:

Disseminated gonococcal infections: 1 g/day once daily for 7 days

Meningitis: 1-2 g/dose every 12 hours for 10-14 days

Endocarditis: 1-2 g/dose every 12 hours for 28 days

Conjunctivitis: I.M.: 1 g in a single dose

Chancroid: I.M.: 50 mg/kg as a single dose (maximum dose: 250 mg)

Acute epididymitis: I.M.: 250 mg in a single dose

Acute otitis media: 50 mg/kg once daily for 3 days (maximum dose: 1 g/day)

Adults: 1-2 g every 12-24 hours depending on the type and severity of the infection; maximum dose: 4 g/day

Dosing interval in renal impairment: No change necessary with dose ≤2 g/day

Administration Parenteral:

IVP: Administer over 2-4 minutes at a maximum concentration of 40 mg/mL

I.V. intermittent infusion: Administer over 10-30 minutes; final concentration for I.V. administration should not exceed 40 mg/mL

I.M. injection: May be diluted with sterile water or 1% lidocaine to a final concentration of 250 mg/mL or may be concentrated by using the manufacturer's recommended diluent volume of 1% lidocaine with a resultant concentration of 350 mg/mL; administer I.M. injections deep into a large muscle mass

Monitoring Parameters CBC with differential, PT, renal and hepatic function tests periodically; number and type of stools/day for diarrhea

Test Interactions False-positive urine glucose with Clinitest®

Additional Information Sodium content of 1 g: 3.6 mEq

Dosage Forms

Infusion, as sodium, premixed (frozen): 1 g in $D_{3.8}W$ (50 mL); 2 g in $D_{2.4}W$ (50 mL)

Powder for injection, as sodium: 250 mg, 500 mg, 1 g, 2 g, 10 g

References

Bradley JS, Compogiannis LS, Murray WE, et al, "Pharmacokinetics and Safety of Intramuscular Injection of Concentrated Ceftriaxone in Children," *Clin Pharm*, 1992, 11(11):961-4.

Centers for Disease Control and Prevention, "1998 Guidelines for Treatment of Sexually Transmitted Diseases," *MMWR Morb Mortal Wkly Rep*, 1998, 47(RR-1):1-111.

Committee on Adolescence, American Academy of Pediatrics, "Sexual Assault and the Adolescent," *Pediatrics*, 1994, 94(5):761-5.

Dowell SF, Butler JC, Giebink GS, et al, "Acute Otitis Media: Management and Surveillance in an era of Pneumococcal Resistance--A Report From the Drug-Resistant *Streptococcus pneumoniae* Therapeutic Working Group," *Pediatr Infect Dis J*, 1999, 18(1):1-9.

Richards DM, Heel RC, Brogden RN, et al, "Ceftriaxone: A Review of Its Antibacterial Activity, Pharmacological Properties and Therapeutic Use," *Drugs*, 1984, 27(6):469-527.

Cefuroxime (se fyoor OKS eem)

Related Information

Carbohydrate and Alcohol Content of Liquid Medications for Use in Patients Receiving Ketogenic Diets *on page 1258*

U.S. Brand Names Ceftin®; Kefurox®; Zinacef®

Therapeutic Category Antibiotic, Cephalosporin (Second Generation)

Generic Available Yes

Use A second generation cephalosporin useful in infections caused by susceptible staphylococci, group B streptococci, pneumococci, *H. influenzae* (type A and B), *E. coli*, *Enterobacter*, and *Klebsiella*; treatment of susceptible infections of the upper and lower respiratory tract, otitis media, acute bacterial maxillary sinusitis, urinary tract, skin and soft tissue, bone and joint, and sepsis

Pregnancy Risk Factor B

(Continued)

Cefuroxime *(Continued)*

Contraindications Hypersensitivity to cefuroxime, any component, or cephalosporins

Warnings Prolonged use may result in superinfection; safety and efficacy in infants <3 months of age have not been established; do not use in patients with immediate-type hypersensitivity reactions to penicillin

Precautions Use with caution and modify dosage in patients with renal impairment; use with caution in patients with history of colitis or history of penicillin hypersensitivity

Adverse Reactions

Central nervous system: Fever, headache, dizziness, vertigo, seizures

Dermatologic: Rash, pruritus, erythema multiforme, diaper rash

Gastrointestinal: Nausea, vomiting, diarrhea, stomach cramps, GI bleeding, antibiotic-associated colitis, stomatitis

Genitourinary: Vaginitis

Hematologic: Transient neutropenia and leukopenia, decreased hemoglobin and hematocrit, eosinophilia

Hepatic: Transient elevation in liver enzymes

Local: Pain at injection site, thrombophlebitis

Renal: Elevated BUN and serum creatinine

Drug Interactions Probenecid (increases serum cefuroxime concentration); aminoglycosides may increase risk of nephrotoxicity

Food Interactions Food and milk increase bioavailability and peak levels

Stability Reconstituted injectable solution (100 mg/mL) or injectable suspension (200-220 mg/mL) is stable for 24 hours at room temperature or 48 hours when refrigerated; reconstituted oral suspension can be stored in the refrigerator or at room temperature; discard after 10 days

Mechanism of Action Inhibits bacterial cell wall synthesis by binding to one or more of the penicillin-binding proteins; inhibits the final transpeptidation step of peptidoglycan synthesis resulting in cell wall death

Pharmacokinetics

Absorption: Oral: Increased when given with or shortly after food or infant formula

Distribution: Into bronchial secretions, synovial and pericardial fluid, kidneys, heart, liver, bone and bile; penetrates into CSF with inflamed meninges; crosses the placenta; excreted into breast milk

Protein binding: 33% to 50%

Bioavailability: Oral cefuroxime axetil tablets: 37% to 52%; cefuroxime axetil suspension is less bioavailable than the tablet (91% of the AUC for tablets)

Half-life:

Neonates:

≤3 days: 5.1-5.8 hours

6-14 days: 2-4.2 hours

3-4 weeks: 1-1.5 hours

Adults: 1-2 hours (prolonged in renal impairment)

Time to peak serum concentration:

Oral: 2-3 hours

I.M.: Within 15-60 minutes

Elimination: Primarily 66% to 100% as unchanged drug in urine by both glomerular filtration and tubular secretion

Dialysis: Dialyzable

Usual Dosage

I.M., I.V.:

Neonates: 20-100 mg/kg/day divided every 12 hours

Children: 75-150 mg/kg/day divided every 8 hours; maximum dose: 6 g/day

Meningitis: Not recommended (doses of 200-240 mg/kg/day divided every 6-8 hours have been used); maximum dose: 9 g/day

Adults: 750 mg to 1.5 g/dose every 8 hours

Oral: **Cefuroxime axetil film-coated tablets and oral suspension are not bioequivalent and are not substitutable on a mg/mg basis**

Children:

Pharyngitis, tonsillitis:

Suspension: 20 mg/kg/day (maximum dose: 500 mg/day) in 2 divided doses

Tablet: 125 mg every 12 hours

Acute otitis media, acute bacterial maxillary sinusitis, impetigo:

Suspension: 30 mg/kg/day (maximum dose: 1 g/day) in 2 divided doses

Tablet: 250 mg every 12 hours

Adults: 250-500 mg twice daily; uncomplicated urinary tract infection: 125-250 mg every 12 hours

Dosing interval in renal impairment:
Cl_{cr} 10-20 mL/minute: Administer every 12 hours
Cl_{cr} <10 mL/minute: Administer every 24 hours

Administration
Oral: Cefuroxime axetil suspension must be administered with food; shake suspension well before use; tablets may be administered with or without food; administer with food to decrease GI upset; avoid crushing the tablet due to its bitter taste
Parenteral:
IVP: Administer over 3-5 minutes at a maximum concentration of 100 mg/mL
I.V. intermittent infusion: Administer over 15-30 minutes at a final concentration for administration ≤30 mg/mL; in fluid restricted patients, a concentration of 137 mg/mL may be administered
I.M.: I.M. injection is less painful when administered as an injectable suspension rather than a solution, and is less painful when administered into the buttock rather than the thigh

Monitoring Parameters With prolonged therapy, monitor renal, hepatic, and hematologic function periodically; number and type of stools/day for diarrhea

Test Interactions Positive Coombs' [direct]; false-positive urine glucose with Clinitest®

Additional Information Sodium content of 1 g: 2.4 mEq

Dosage Forms
Infusion, premixed (frozen), as sodium (Zinacef®): 750 mg (50 mL); 1.5 g (50 mL)
Powder for injection, as sodium (Kefurox®, Zinacef®): 750 mg, 1.5 g, 7.5 g
Powder for oral suspension, as axetil (Ceftin®): 125 mg/5 mL [tutti-frutti flavor] (50 mL, 100 mL, 200 mL); 250 mg/5 mL [tutti-frutti flavor] (50 mL, 100 mL)
Tablet, as axetil (Ceftin®): 125 mg, 250 mg, 500 mg

References
de Louvois J, Mulhall A, and Hurley R, "Cefuroxime in the Treatment of Neonates," *Arch Dis Child*, 1982, 57(1):59-62.
Gooch WM 3rd, Blair E, Puopolo A, et al, "Effectiveness of Five Days of Therapy With Cefuroxime Axetil Suspension for Treatment of Acute Otitis Media," *Pediatr Infect Dis J*, 1996, 15(2):157-64.
Nelson JD, "Cefuroxime: A Cephalosporin With Unique Applicability to Pediatric Practice," *Pediatr Infect Dis*, 1983, 2(5):394-6.
Thoene DE and Johnson CE, "Pharmacotherapy of Otitis Media," *Pharmacotherapy*, 1991, 11(3):212-21.

♦ **Cefzil®** *see Cefprozil on page 200*
♦ **Celestoderm (Can)** *see Betamethasone on page 140*
♦ **Celestone®** *see Betamethasone on page 140*
♦ **Celestone® Phosphate** *see Betamethasone on page 140*
♦ **Celestone® Soluspan®** *see Betamethasone on page 140*
♦ **CellCept®** *see Mycophenolate on page 689*
♦ **Celontin®** *see Methsuximide on page 650*
♦ **Cenafed® [OTC]** *see Pseudoephedrine on page 852*
♦ **Cena-K®** *see Potassium Supplements on page 816*
♦ **Cepacol Viractin® [OTC]** *see Tetracaine on page 940*

Cephalexin (sef a LEKS in)

Related Information
Carbohydrate and Alcohol Content of Liquid Medications for Use in Patients Receiving Ketogenic Diets *on page 1258*
Endocarditis Prophylaxis *on page 1160*

U.S. Brand Names Biocef®; Keflex®; Keftab®

Canadian Brand Names Apo-Cephalex; Ceporex; Novo-Lexin; Nu-Cephalex; PMS-Cephalexin

Therapeutic Category Antibiotic, Cephalosporin (First Generation)

Generic Available Yes

Use Treatment of susceptible bacterial infections, including those caused by group A beta-hemolytic *Streptococcus*, *Staphylococcus*, *Klebsiella pneumoniae*, *E. coli*, and *Proteus mirabilis*; not active against enterococci; used to treat susceptible infections of the respiratory tract, skin and skin structure, bone, genitourinary tract, and otitis media

Pregnancy Risk Factor B

Contraindications Hypersensitivity to cephalexin, any component, or cephalosporins

Warnings Prolonged use may result in gastrointestinal or genitourinary superinfection; do not use in patients with immediate-type hypersensitivity reactions to penicillin

(Continued)

Cephalexin *(Continued)*

Precautions Use with caution and modify dosage in patients with renal impairment; use with caution in patients with history of colitis or history of penicillin hypersensitivity

Adverse Reactions
Central nervous system: Dizziness, headache, fatigue, fever
Dermatologic: Rash
Gastrointestinal: Nausea, vomiting, pseudomembranous colitis, diarrhea, cramps
Hematologic: Transient neutropenia, anemia, eosinophilia
Hepatic: Transient elevation in liver enzymes

Drug Interactions Probenecid increases serum concentration of cephalexin

Food Interactions Food may delay absorption

Stability Refrigerate suspension after reconstitution; discard after 14 days

Mechanism of Action Inhibits bacterial cell wall synthesis by binding to one or more of the penicillin-binding proteins; inhibits the final transpeptidation step of peptidoglycan synthesis resulting in cell wall death

Pharmacokinetics
Absorption: Delayed in young children and may be decreased up to 50% in neonates
Distribution: Into tissues and fluids including bone, pleural and synovial fluid; crosses the placenta; appears in breast milk
Protein binding: 6% to 15%
Half-life:
Neonates: 5 hours
Children 3-12 months: 2.5 hours
Adults: 0.5-1.2 hours (prolonged with renal impairment)
Time to peak serum concentration: Oral: Within 60 minutes
Elimination: 80% to 100% of dose excreted as unchanged drug in urine within 8 hours
Dialysis: Moderately dialyzable (20% to 50%)

Usual Dosage Oral:
Children: 25-100 mg/kg/day divided every 6-8 hours; maximum dose: 4 g/day
Adults: 250-500 mg every 6 hours; maximum dose: 4 g/day
Dosing interval in renal impairment:
Cl_{cr} 10-40 mL/minute: Administer every 8-12 hours
Cl_{cr} <10 mL/minute: Administer every 12-24 hours

Administration Oral: Administer on an empty stomach (ie, 1 hour prior to, or 2 hours after meals); administer with food if GI upset occurs; shake suspension well before use

Monitoring Parameters With prolonged therapy, monitor renal, hepatic, and hematologic function periodically; number and type of stools/day for diarrhea

Test Interactions False-positive urine glucose with Clinitest®; positive Coombs' [direct]; false ↑ serum or urine creatinine

Dosage Forms
Capsule, as monohydrate: 250 mg, 500 mg
Powder for oral suspension, as monohydrate: 125 mg/5 mL (100 mL, 200 mL); 250 mg/5 mL (100 mL, 200 mL)
Tablet, as monohydrate: 250 mg, 500 mg, 1 g
Tablet, as hydrochloride (Keftab®): 500 mg

Cephalothin *(sef A loe thin)*

Canadian Brand Names Ceporacin

Therapeutic Category Antibiotic, Cephalosporin (First Generation)

Generic Available Yes

Use Treatment of respiratory tract, skin and skin structure, urinary tract, bone and joint infections, endocarditis, and septicemia due to susceptible gram-positive cocci (except enterococcus); some gram-negative bacilli including *E. coli*, *Proteus*, and *Klebsiella* may be susceptible; perioperative prophylaxis

Pregnancy Risk Factor B

Contraindications Hypersensitivity to cephalothin, any component, or cephalosporins

Warnings Prolonged use may result in superinfection; do not use in patients with immediate-type hypersensitivity reactions to penicillin

Precautions Use with caution in patients with a history of colitis or in patients with a history of hypersensitivity to penicillins; modify dosage in patients with renal impairment

Adverse Reactions
Central nervous system: Dizziness, headache, fever
Dermatologic: Rash, urticaria, pruritus
Gastrointestinal: Nausea, vomiting, diarrhea, dyspepsia, pseudomembranous colitis
Hematological: Hemolytic anemia, granulocytopenia, eosinophilia, thrombocytopenia, prolonged PT, bleeding
Hepatic: Transient elevation in AST and alkaline phosphatase
Local: Severe phlebitis (especially with doses >6 g/day for longer than 3 days), thrombophlebitis, pain and induration at injection site
Renal: Elevated BUN and serum creatinine, nephrotoxicity

Drug Interactions Probenecid decreases renal clearance of cephalothin; aminoglycosides may increase risk of nephrotoxicity

Stability Reconstituted solution is stable for 12-24 hours at room temperature and 96 hours when refrigerated; thawed solution of the commercially available frozen cephalothin injection is stable for 12 hours at room temperature or 7 days when refrigerated

Mechanism of Action Inhibits bacterial cell wall synthesis by binding to one or more of the penicillin-binding proteins and interfering with the final transpeptidation step of peptidoglycan synthesis

Pharmacokinetics
Distribution: Widely distributed throughout the body but with poor penetration into CSF and bile; crosses the placenta
Protein binding: 65% to 80%
Metabolism: 10% to 40% metabolized in the liver and kidneys to desacetylcephalothin (active metabolite)
Half-life:
Neonates <7 days: 90-120 minutes
Adults with normal renal function: 30-60 minutes (cephalothin) and 12 minutes (desacetylcephalothin)
Time to peak serum concentration: I.M.: Within 30 minutes
Elimination: 50% to 75% of a dose is excreted in the urine as unchanged drug

Usual Dosage
Neonates: I.V.:
Postnatal age ≤7 days:
≤2000 g: 40 mg/kg/day divided every 12 hours
>2000 g: 60 mg/kg/day divided every 8 hours
Postnatal age >7 days:
<1200 g: 40 mg/kg/day divided every 12 hours
1200-2000 g: 60 mg/kg/day divided every 8 hours
>2000 g: 80 mg/kg/day divided every 6 hours
Children: I.M., I.V.: 80-150 mg/kg/day divided every 4-6 hours; maximum dose: 12 g/day
Perioperative prophylaxis: I.V.: 20-30 mg/kg 30-60 minutes prior to surgery and 20-30 mg/kg every 6 hours for no more than 24 hours after surgery depending on the procedure
Adults: I.M., I.V.: 500 mg to 2 g every 4-6 hours; maximum dose: 12 g/day
Perioperative prophylaxis: I.V.: 1-2 g 30-60 minutes prior to surgery and 1-2 g every 6 hours for no more than 24 hours after surgery depending on the procedure

Dosing interval in renal impairment:
Cl_{cr} 10-50 mL/minute: Administer every 6-8 hours
Cl_{cr} <10 mL/minute: Administer every 12 hours

Administration Parenteral:
IVP: Administer over 3-5 minutes at a maximum concentration of 100 mg/mL
I.V. intermittent infusion: Administer over 30-60 minutes at a final concentration for I.V. administration ≤100 mg/mL

Monitoring Parameters Periodic renal function tests when used in combination with other nephrotoxic drugs, hepatic function tests, and CBC; number and type of stools/day for diarrhea

Test Interactions False-positive urine glucose, using Clinitest®, positive Coombs' [direct], false ↑ serum or urine creatinine

Nursing Implications Monitor patient for vein irritation

Additional Information Sodium content of 1 g: 2.8 mEq

Dosage Forms
Infusion, as sodium, in $D_{1.1}W$ (frozen): 2 g (50 mL)
Infusion, as sodium, in $D_{3.5}W$ (frozen): 1 g (50 mL)

References
Pickering LK, O'Connor DM, Anderson D, et al, "Comparative Evaluation of Cefazolin and Cephalothin in Children," *J Pediatr*, 1974, 85(6):842-7.

♦ **Cephanol (Can)** *see* Acetaminophen *on page 29*

Cephapirin (sef a PYE rin)

Therapeutic Category Antibiotic, Cephalosporin (First Generation)

Generic Available No

Use Treatment of respiratory tract, skin and skin structure, urinary tract, bone and joint infections, endocarditis and septicemia due to susceptible gram-positive cocci (except enterococcus); some gram-negative bacilli including *E. coli*, *Proteus*, and *Klebsiella*, may be susceptible; perioperative prophylaxis

Pregnancy Risk Factor B

Contraindications Hypersensitivity to cephapirin sodium, any component, or cephalosporins

Warnings Prolonged use may result in superinfection; safety and efficacy in infants <3 months of age have not been established; do not use in patients with immediate-type hypersensitivity reactions to penicillin

Precautions Use with caution in patients with a history of colitis or in patients with a history of hypersensitivity to penicillins; modify dosage in patients with renal impairment

Adverse Reactions

Central nervous system: Fever

Dermatologic: Rash, urticaria

Gastrointestinal: Diarrhea, pseudomembranous colitis

Hematologic: Neutropenia, eosinophilia, leukopenia, thrombocytopenia

Hepatic: Elevated AST, ALT, alkaline phosphatase, and bilirubin; jaundice

Local: Thrombophlebitis, pain on injection

Renal: Nephrotoxicity, acute interstitial nephritis, elevated BUN, elevated serum creatinine

Drug Interactions Probenecid decreases renal clearance of cephapirin; aminoglycosides may increase risk of nephrotoxicity

Stability Reconstituted solution is stable for 12 hours at room temperature and 10 days when refrigerated; after freezing, thawed solution is stable for 12 hours at room temperature or 10 days when refrigerated

Mechanism of Action Inhibits bacterial cell wall synthesis by binding to one or more of the penicillin-binding proteins and interfering with the final transpeptidation step of peptidoglycan synthesis

Pharmacokinetics

Distribution: Widely distributed to tissues and fluids including heart, bone, pericardial, pleural and synovial fluid; crosses the placenta; only small amounts distribute into CSF and breast milk

Protein binding: 44% to 50%

Metabolism: Partially metabolized in the liver, kidneys, and plasma to desacetylcephapirin (active metabolite)

Half-life: 21-48 minutes (adults with normal renal function); desacetylcephapirin: 26 minutes

Time to peak serum concentration: I.M.: Within 30 minutes

Elimination: 30% to 70% excreted as unchanged drug in urine

Dialysis: 23% of a dose is removed by hemodialysis

Usual Dosage I.M., I.V.:

Infants >3 months of age and Children: 40-80 mg/kg/day divided every 6 hours; maximum dose: 12 g/day

Adults: 500 mg to 1 g every 6 hours up to 12 g/day

Perioperative prophylaxis: 1-2 g 30-60 minutes prior to surgery and 1-2 g every 6 hours for no more than 24 hours after surgery depending on the procedure

Dosing interval in renal impairment:

Cl$_{cr}$ 10-50 mL/minute: Administer every 6-8 hours

Cl$_{cr}$ <10 mL/minute: Administer every 12 hours

Administration Parenteral:

IVP: Administer over 3-5 minutes at a maximum concentration of 100 mg/mL

I.V. intermittent infusion: Administer over 30 minutes; maximum cephapirin concentration that can be administered to fluid-restricted patients is 200 mg/mL

Monitoring Parameters Periodic renal function tests, CBC; number and type of stools/day for diarrhea

Test Interactions False-positive urine glucose using Clinitest®; positive Coombs' [direct]; false ↑ serum or urine creatinine

Nursing Implications Monitor patient for vein irritation

Additional Information Sodium content of 1 g: 2.4 mEq

Dosage Forms Powder for injection, as sodium: 1 g

References
Khan AJ and Pryles CV, "Clinical and Pharmacological Evaluation of Cephapirin Sodium (BL-P-1322) in Infants and Children (Cephapirin in Pediatric Patients)," *Curr Ther Res Clin Exp*, 1973, 15(4):198-204.

Cephradine (SEF ra deen)
Related Information
Carbohydrate and Alcohol Content of Liquid Medications for Use in Patients Receiving Ketogenic Diets *on page 1258*

U.S. Brand Names Velosef®

Therapeutic Category Antibiotic, Cephalosporin (First Generation)

Generic Available Yes

Use Treatment of susceptible bacterial infections, including skin and skin structure infections caused by *Streptococcus* or *Staphylococcus*; urinary tract infections caused by *Klebsiella*, *E. coli*, and *Proteus mirabilis*; respiratory tract infections caused by group A beta-hemolytic streptococci and *Streptococcus pneumoniae*; otitis media caused by group A beta-hemolytic streptococci, *Streptococcus pneumoniae*, or *H. influenzae*

Pregnancy Risk Factor B

Contraindications Hypersensitivity to cephradine, any component, or cephalosporins

Warnings Prolonged use may result in superinfection; do not use in patients with immediate-type hypersensitivity reaction to penicillin

Precautions Use with caution in patients with a history of penicillin hypersensitivity; reduce dose in patients with renal impairment

Adverse Reactions
Dermatologic: Rash
Gastrointestinal: Diarrhea, nausea, vomiting, pseudomembranous colitis
Genitourinary: Vaginitis
Hematologic: Transient neutropenia
Hepatic: Elevated hepatic enzymes, elevated bilirubin
Neuromuscular & skeletal: Arthralgia
Renal: Elevated BUN and serum creatinine

Drug Interactions Probenecid may decrease renal tubular secretion and increase cephradine serum concentrations

Food Interactions Food will decrease the rate, but not the extent of oral absorption

Stability Oral suspension: Stable for 7 days at room temperature, or 14 days at 2°C to 8°C after reconstitution

Mechanism of Action Interferes with bacterial cell wall synthesis during active replication, causing cell wall death and resultant bactericidal activity against susceptible bacteria

Pharmacokinetics
Absorption: Well absorbed from GI tract
Distribution: V_d: 0.25 L/kg; crosses the placenta; appears in breast milk
Protein binding: 6% to 20%
Half-life: Adults: 0.7-2 hours; Children: 1 hour; half-life increases with renal dysfunction
Time to peak serum concentration: Oral: Within 1-2 hours
Elimination: Excreted unchanged in the urine (80% to 90%) via glomerular filtration and tubular secretion

Usual Dosage Oral:
Infants ≥9 months and children:
Usual: 25-50 mg/kg/day in divided doses every 6-12 hours
Otitis media: 75-100 mg/kg/day in divided doses every 6-12 hours
Maximum dose: 4 g/day
Adults: Oral: 250-500 mg every 6-12 hours
Dosing adjustment in renal impairment:
Cl_{cr} 10-50 mL/minute: Administer 50% of dose given at normal interval
Cl_{cr} <10 mL/minute: Administer 25% of dose given at normal interval
or
Cl_{cr} 25-50 mL/minute: Administer normal dose every 12 hours
Cl_{cr} 10-25 mL/minute: Administer normal dose every 24 hours
Cl_{cr} <10 mL/minute: Administer normal dose every 36 hours

Administration Oral: May be administered without regard to food; shake suspension well before use

Test Interactions False-positive Coombs' test; may falsely elevate creatinine values when Jaffé reaction is used; may cause false-positive results in urine glucose tests using cupric sulfate (Benedict's solution, Clinitest®)
(Continued)

Cephradine *(Continued)*

Patient Information Report persistent diarrhea; entire course of medication (eg, 10-14 days) should be taken to ensure eradication of organism

Additional Information Efficacy not established for twice daily dosing in infants <9 months of age; parenteral product no longer available in the United States

Dosage Forms

Capsule: 250 mg, 500 mg

Powder for oral suspension: 125 mg/5 mL (100 mL, 200 mL); 250 mg/5 mL (100 mL, 200 mL)

References

Donowitz GR and Mandell GL, "Drug Therapy. Beta-Lactam Antibiotics (1)," *N Engl J Med*, 1988, 318(7):419-26.

Donowitz GR and Mandell GL, "Drug Therapy. Beta-Lactam Antibiotics (2)," *N Engl J Med*, 1988, 318(8):490-500.

Gustaferro CA and Steckelberg JM, "Cephalosporin Antimicrobial Agents and Related Compounds," *Mayo Clin Proc*, 1991, 66(10):1064-73.

Smith GH, "Oral Cephalosporins in Perspective," *DICP*, 1990, 24(1):45-51.

♦ **Cephulac®** *see* Lactulose *on page 571*

♦ **Ceporacin (Can)** *see* Cephalothin *on page 208*

♦ **Ceporex (Can)** *see* Cephalexin *on page 207*

♦ **Ceptaz™** *see* Ceftazidime *on page 201*

♦ **Cerebyx®** *see* Fosphenytoin *on page 458*

♦ **Ceredase®** *see* Alglucerase *on page 52*

♦ **Cerezyme®** *see* Imiglucerase *on page 525*

♦ **Certified Nasal (Can)** *see* Sodium Chloride *on page 906*

♦ **Cerubidine®** *see* Daunorubicin *on page 298*

♦ **Cerumenex® Otic** *see* Triethanolamine Polypeptide Oleate-Condensate *on page 983*

♦ **C.E.S.** *see* Estrogens (Conjugated) *on page 402*

♦ **Cetacort®** *see* Hydrocortisone *on page 506*

♦ **Cetamide®** *see* Sulfacetamide *on page 922*

♦ **Ceta-Plus®** *see* Hydrocodone and Acetaminophen *on page 505*

Cetirizine *(se TI ra zeen)*

U.S. Brand Names Zyrtec®

Canadian Brand Names Apo-Cetirizine; Reactine

Synonyms P-071; UCB-P071

Therapeutic Category Antihistamine

Generic Available No

Use Perennial and seasonal allergic rhinitis; chronic idiopathic urticaria

Pregnancy Risk Factor B

Contraindications Hypersensitivity to cetirizine, hydroxyzine, or any component

Warnings Doses >10 mg/day may cause significant drowsiness

Precautions Use with caution in patients with hepatic or renal dysfunction

Adverse Reactions

Central nervous system: Headache, drowsiness, somnolence, fatigue, dizziness, depression, confusion, vertigo, ataxia

Gastrointestinal: Diarrhea, flatulence, constipation, xerostomia, dyspepsia, abdominal pain, pharyngitis

Neuromuscular & skeletal: Paresthesias, hyperkinesia, hypertonia, tremor, leg cramps

Respiratory: Cough, epistaxis, bronchospasm

Drug Interactions Increased cetirizine toxicity: CNS depressants, anticholinergics; theophylline may decrease cetirizine clearance with potential increased toxicity

Stability Store at room temperature; protect syrup from light

Mechanism of Action Cetirizine, a metabolite of hydroxyzine, competes with histamine for H_1-receptor sites on effector cells in the GI tract, blood vessels, and respiratory tract

Pharmacodynamics

Onset of effect: 20-60 minutes

Duration of effect: 24 hours

Pharmacokinetics

Absorption: Well absorbed from the GI tract

Distribution: V_d:

Children: 0.7 L/kg

Adults: 0.5-0.8 L/kg

Protein binding: 93%

Metabolism: Exact fate is unknown, limited hepatic metabolism

Half-life:

Children: 6.2 hours

Adults: 7.4-9 hours

Adults with mild-moderate renal failure: 19-21 hours

Time to peak serum concentration: 1 hour

Elimination: 60% to 70% excreted unchanged in urine

Usual Dosage Oral:

Children <2 years: Limited data: 0.25 mg/kg/day as a single dose

Children 2-5 years: 2.5 mg/day; may be increased to a maximum of 5 mg/day given either as a single dose or divided into 2 doses

Children ≥6 years to Adults: 5-10 mg/day as a single dose or divided into 2 doses

Dosing interval in renal or hepatic impairment: Adults with Cl_{cr} ≤31 mL/minute, dialysis patients with Cl_{cr} <7 mL/minute, or hepatic impairment: Administer 5 mg/day

Administration Oral: Administer with or without food

Patient Information Causes drowsiness and may impair ability to perform hazardous tasks requiring mental alertness

Dosage Forms

Syrup, as hydrochloride: 5 mg/5 mL [banana-grape flavor] (120 mL, 480 mL)

Tablet, film-coated, as hydrochloride: 5 mg, 10 mg

♦ **Cevi-Bid® [OTC]** *see* Ascorbic Acid *on page 106*

♦ **C Forte (Can)** *see* Ascorbic Acid *on page 106*

♦ **CG** *see* Chorionic Gonadotropin *on page 232*

♦ **Charac (Can)** *see* Charcoal *on page 213*

♦ **CharcoAid® [OTC]** *see* Charcoal *on page 213*

♦ **CharcoAid G® [OTC]** *see* Charcoal *on page 213*

Charcoal (CHAR kole)

U.S. Brand Names Actidose-Aqua® [OTC]; Actidose® With Sorbitol [OTC]; CharcoAid® [OTC]; CharcoAid G® [OTC]; Charcoal Plus® DS [OTC]; Charcocaps® [OTC]; Kerr Insta-Char® [OTC]; Liqui-Char® [OTC]

Canadian Brand Names Charac; Charcodote

Synonyms Activated Carbon; Activated Charcoal; Adsorbent Charcoal; Liquid Antidote; Medicinal Carbon; Medicinal Charcoal

Therapeutic Category Antidiarrheal; Antidote, Adsorbent; Antiflatulent

Generic Available Yes

Use Emergency treatment in poisoning by drugs and chemicals (see Additional Information); repetitive doses for gastrointestinal dialysis in drug overdose to enhance the elimination of certain drugs (eg, theophylline, phenobarbital, carbamazepine, dapsone, quinine) and in uremia to adsorb various waste products

Pregnancy Risk Factor C

Contraindications Patients with an unprotected airway (eg, depressed CNS state without endotracheal intubation); patients at increased risk and severity of aspiration (eg, ingestion of hydrocarbon with a high potential for aspiration); patients at risk of GI perforation or hemorrhage due to medical conditions, recent surgery, or other pathology; **Note:** Ingestion of a corrosive (caustic) substance is **not** a contraindication if charcoal is used for co-ingested systemic toxin. Charcoal is not effective for cyanide, mineral acids, caustic alkalis, organic solvents, iron, ethanol, methanol or lithium poisonings; do not use charcoal with sorbitol in patients with fructose intolerance; charcoal with sorbitol is not recommended in children <1 year of age

Warnings If charcoal in sorbitol is administered, doses should be limited to prevent excessive fluid and electrolyte losses

Precautions When using ipecac with charcoal, induce vomiting with ipecac before administering activated charcoal since charcoal adsorbs ipecac syrup; charcoal may cause vomiting which is hazardous in petroleum distillate and caustic ingestions; charcoal (especially in multiple doses) may adsorb maintenance medications and place the patient at risk for exacerbation of concomitant disorders

Adverse Reactions

Gastrointestinal: Vomiting (**Note:** Use of charcoal with sorbitol may increase rate of emesis), constipation, intestinal obstruction, black stools; diarrhea if product contains sorbitol

Ocular: Corneal abrasions if spilled into eyes

Miscellaneous: Aspiration may cause tracheal obstruction in infants, but usually not a major problem in adults; aspiration pneumonitis, bronchiolitis obliterans, and
(Continued)

Charcoal *(Continued)*

ARDS have been reported following aspiration of charcoal; however, these problems may be due to the aspiration of gastric contents and not charcoal per se

Food Interactions Milk, ice cream, sherbet, or marmalade may reduce charcoal's effectiveness; chocolate or fruit syrup do not appear to reduce efficacy

Stability Adsorbs gases from air; store in closed container

Mechanism of Action Adsorbs toxic substances or irritants, thus inhibiting GI absorption; for select drugs, increases drug clearance by interfering with enterohepatic recycling or causing dialysis across intestinal membrane; adsorbs intestinal gas; the addition of sorbitol results in hyperosmotic laxative action causing catharsis

Pharmacodynamics In studies using adult human volunteers: Mean **reduction** in drug absorption following a single dose of activated charcoal:

All size doses of activated charcoal:
Given within 30 minutes after ingestion: 69.1% reduction
Given at 60 minutes after ingestion: 34.4% reduction
50 g activated charcoal:
Given within 30 minutes after ingestion: 88.6% reduction
Given at 60 minutes after ingestion: 37.3% reduction

Pharmacokinetics
Absorption: Not absorbed from the GI tract
Metabolism: Not metabolized
Elimination: Excreted as charcoal in feces

Usual Dosage Oral:
Acute poisoning:
Single dose: Charcoal with sorbitol (**Note:** The use of repeated oral charcoal with sorbitol doses is not recommended):
Infants <1 year: Not recommended
Children 1-12 years: 1-2 g/kg or 25-50 g or approximately 5-10 times the weight of the ingested poison on a gram-to-gram basis; 1 g adsorbs 100-1000 mg of poison; in young children sorbitol should be repeated **no more** than 1-2 times/day
Adolescents and Adults: 30-100 g
Single dose: Charcoal in water (a cathartic such as sorbitol should be added in appropriate doses):
Infants <1 year: 1 g/kg
Children 1-12 years: 1-2 g/kg or 25-50 g
Adolescents and Adults: 30-100 g or 1-2 g/kg
Multiple dose: Charcoal in water (doses are repeated until clinical observations of toxicity subside and serum drug concentrations have returned to a subtherapeutic range or until the development of absent bowel sounds or ileus; use only one dose of cathartic daily):
Infants <1 year: 1 g/kg every 4-6 hours
Children 1-12 years: 1-2 g/kg or 15-30 g every 2-6 hours
Adolescents and Adults: 25-60 g or 1-2 g/kg every 2-6 hours
Gastric dialysis: Adults: 20-50 g every 6 hours for 1-2 days

Administration Oral: Administer as soon as possible after ingestion, preferably within 1 hour for greatest effect; shake well before use; do not mix with milk, ice cream, sherbet, or marmalade; may be mixed with chocolate or fruit syrup to increase palatability; instruct patient to drink slowly, rapid administration may increase frequency of vomiting; if patient has persistent vomiting, multiple doses may be administered as a continuous enteral infusion

Monitoring Parameters Fluid status, sorbitol intake, number of stools, electrolytes if increase in stools or diarrhea occurs

Patient Information Charcoal causes the stools to turn black

Nursing Implications Charcoal slurries that are too concentrated may clog airways, if aspirated

Additional Information 5-6 tablespoonfuls is approximately equal to 30 g of activated charcoal; minimum dilution of 240 mL water per 20-30 g activated charcoal should be mixed as an aqueous slurry; multiple dose activated charcoal has been shown to be effective in increasing the elimination of certain drugs (carbamazepine, theophylline, phenobarbital) even after these drugs have been absorbed

The Position Statement of The American Academy of Clinical Toxicology and The European Association of Poisons Centres and Clinical Toxicologists does not advocate **routine** use of single dose activated charcoal in the treatment of poisoned patients; scientific literature supports the use of activated charcoal within 1 hour of toxin ingestion, when it will be more likely to produce benefit. Therefore, this publication states that activated charcoal may be considered up to 1 hour following ingestion of a potentially toxic amount of poison; the use of activated charcoal may be considered greater than 1 hour following ingestion, but there are no studies to support or exclude its use; furthermore, based on current literature, the routine administration of a cathartic with activated charcoal is not recommended; when cathartics are used, only a single dose should be administered so as to decrease adverse effects.

Dosage Forms

Capsule (Charcocaps®): 260 mg

Granules, activated (CharcoAid® G): 15 g (120 mL)

Liquid, activated:

Actidose-Aqua®: 12.5 g (60 mL); 25 g (120 mL); 50 g (240 mL)

Liqui-Char®: 12.5 g (60 mL); 15 g (75 mL); 25 g (120 mL); 30 g (120 mL); 50 g (240 mL)

Kerr Insta-Char®: 25 g (120 mL); 50 g (240 mL)

Liquid, activated, with sorbitol (Actidose® With Sorbitol, Kerr Insta-Char®): 25 g (120 mL); 50 g (240 mL)

Powder for suspension, activated: 15 g, 30 g, 40 g, 120 g, 240 g

Tablets (Charcol Plus® DS): 250 mg

References

Burns MM, "Activated Charcoal as the Sole Intervention for Treatment After Childhood Poisoning," *Curr Opin Pediatr*, 2000, 12(2):166-71.

Farley TA, "Severe Hypernatremic Dehydration After Use of an Activated Charcoal-Sorbitol Suspension," *J Pediatr*, 1986, 109(4):719-22.

"Position Statement and Practice Guidelines on the Use of Multi-dose Activated Charcoal in the Treatment of Acute Poisoning. American Academy of Clinical Toxicology; European Association of Poisons Centres and Clinical Toxicologists," *J Toxicol Clin Toxicol*, 1999, 37(6):731-51.

"Position Statement: Cathartics. American Academy of Clinical Toxicology; European Association of Poisons Centres and Clinical Toxicologists," *J Toxicol Clin Toxicol*, 1997, 35(7):743-52.

"Position Statement: Single-Dose Activated Charcoal. American Academy of Clinical Toxicology; European Association of Poisons Centres and Clinical Toxicologists," *J Toxicol Clin Toxicol*, 1997, 35(7):721-41.

Shannon M, "Ingestion of Toxic Substances by Children," *N Engl J Med*, 2000, 342(3):186-91.

- ♦ **Charcoal Plus® DS [OTC]** *see* Charcoal *on page 213*
- ♦ **Charcocaps® [OTC]** *see* Charcoal *on page 213*
- ♦ **Charcodote (Can)** *see* Charcoal *on page 213*
- ♦ **Chemet®** *see* Succimer *on page 917*
- ♦ **Cheracol D® [OTC]** *see* Guaifenesin and Dextromethorphan *on page 487*
- ♦ **Cheracol® With Codeine** *see* Guaifenesin and Codeine *on page 486*
- ♦ **Chiggerex® [OTC]** *see* Benzocaine *on page 135*
- ♦ **Chiggertox® [OTC]** *see* Benzocaine *on page 135*
- ♦ **Children's Advil® [OTC]** *see* Ibuprofen *on page 520*
- ♦ **Children's Advil® Suspension** *see* Ibuprofen *on page 520*
- ♦ **Children's Dimetapp® Elixir Cold & Allergy** *see* Brompheniramine and Pseudoephedrine *on page 153*
- ♦ **Childrens Feverhalt (Can)** *see* Acetaminophen *on page 29*
- ♦ **Children's Kaopectate® [OTC]** *see* Attapulgite *on page 118*
- ♦ **Childrens Motion Sickness Liquid (Can)** *see* Dimenhydrinate *on page 339*
- ♦ **Children's Motrin® [OTC]** *see* Ibuprofen *on page 520*
- ♦ **Children's Nasalcrom® [OTC]** *see* Cromolyn *on page 273*
- ♦ **Children's Silfedrine® [OTC]** *see* Pseudoephedrine *on page 852*
- ♦ **Chloral** *see* Chloral Hydrate *on page 215*

Chloral Hydrate (KLOR al HYE drate)

Related Information

Carbohydrate and Alcohol Content of Liquid Medications for Use in Patients Receiving Ketogenic Diets *on page 1258*

Preprocedure Sedatives in Children *on page 1201*

U.S. Brand Names Aquachloral® Supprettes®

Canadian Brand Names Novo-Chlorhydrate; PMS-Chloral Hydrate

Synonyms Chloral; Hydrated Chloral; Trichloroacetaldehyde Monohydrate

Therapeutic Category Hypnotic; Sedative

Generic Available Yes

Use Short-term sedative and hypnotic (<2 weeks), sedative/hypnotic prior to nonpainful therapeutic or diagnostic procedures (eg, EEG, CT scan, MRI, ophthalmic exam, dental procedure)

Restrictions C-IV

(Continued)

Chloral Hydrate *(Continued)*

Pregnancy Risk Factor C

Contraindications Hypersensitivity to chloral hydrate or any component; hepatic or renal impairment; gastritis or ulcers; severe cardiac disease

Warnings Trichloroethanol (TCE), an active metabolite of chloral hydrate, is a carcinogen in mice; there is no data in humans

Precautions Use with caution in neonates, drug and metabolites may accumulate with repeated use; prolonged use in neonates is associated with direct hyperbilirubinemia (active metabolite [TCE] competes with bilirubin for glucuronide conjugation in the liver); use with caution in patients with porphyria. Tolerance to hypnotic effect develops, therefore, not recommended for use >2 weeks; taper dosage to avoid withdrawal with prolonged use. Avoid use in patients with moderate to severe renal failure (Cl_{cr} <50 mL/minute).

Adverse Reactions

Central nervous system: Disorientation, sedation, excitement (paradoxical), dizziness, fever, headache, ataxia

Dermatologic: Rash, urticaria

Gastrointestinal: Gastric irritation, nausea, vomiting, diarrhea, flatulence

Hematologic: Leukopenia, eosinophilia

Respiratory: Respiratory depression when combined with other sedatives or narcotics

Miscellaneous: Physical and psychological dependence with prolonged use

Drug Interactions May potentiate effects of warfarin, central nervous system depressants, alcohol; vasodilation reaction (flushing, tachycardia, etc) may occur with concurrent use of alcohol; concomitant use of furosemide (I.V.) may result in flushing, sweating, and blood pressure changes; chloral hydrate may increase the conversion of cyclophosphamide and ifosfamide to active metabolites and may increase toxicity

Stability Sensitive to light; exposure to air causes volatilization; store in light-resistant, airtight container

Mechanism of Action Central nervous system depressant effects are primarily due to its active metabolite trichloroethanol, mechanism unknown; in neonates, chloral hydrate itself may play a role in the immediate sedative effects

Pharmacodynamics

Onset of action: 10-20 minutes

Peak effects: Within 30-60 minutes

Duration: 4-8 hours

Pharmacokinetics

Absorption: Oral, rectal: Well absorbed

Distribution: Crosses the placenta; negligible amounts appear in breast milk

Protein binding: Trichloroethanol: 35% to 40%; trichloroacetic acid: ~94% (may compete with bilirubin for albumin binding sites)

Metabolism: Rapidly metabolized by alcohol dehydrogenase to trichloroethanol (active metabolite); trichloroethanol undergoes glucuronidation in the liver; variable amounts of chloral hydrate and trichloroethanol are metabolized in liver and kidney to trichloroacetic acid (inactive)

Half-life:

Chloral hydrate: Infants: 1 hour

Trichloroethanol (active metabolite):

Neonates: Range: 8.5-66 hours

Half-life decreases with increasing postconceptional age (PCA):

Preterm infants (PCA 31-37 weeks): Mean half-life: 40 hours

Term infants (PCA 38-42 weeks): Mean half-life: 28 hours

Older children (PCA 57-708 weeks): Mean half-life: 10 hours

Adults: 8-11 hours

Trichloroacetic acid: Adults: 67.2 hours

Elimination: Metabolites excreted in urine; small amounts excreted in feces via bile

Dialysis: Dialyzable (50% to 100%)

Usual Dosage Oral, rectal:

Neonates: 25 mg/kg/dose for sedation prior to a procedure; **Note:** Repeat doses should be used with great caution, as drug and metabolites accumulate with repeated use; toxicity has been reported after 3 days in a preterm neonate and after 7 days in a term neonate receiving chloral hydrate 40-50 mg/kg every 6 hours

Infants and Children:

Sedation, anxiety: 25-50 mg/kg/day divided every 6-8 hours, maximum dose: 500 mg/dose

Prior to EEG: 25-50 mg/kg/dose 30-60 minutes prior to EEG; may repeat in 30 minutes to a total maximum of 100 mg/kg or 1 g total for infants and 2 g total for children

Hypnotic: 50 mg/kg; maximum dose: 2 g/dose/day

Sedation, nonpainful procedure: 50-75 mg/kg/dose 30-60 minutes prior to procedure; may repeat 30 minutes after initial dose if needed, to a total maximum dose of 120 mg/kg or 1 g total for infants and 2 g total for children

Adults:

Sedation, anxiety: 250 mg 3 times/day

Hypnotic: 500-1000 mg at bedtime or 30 minutes prior to procedure, not to exceed 2 g/24 hours

Dosing adjustment in renal impairment:

Cl_{cr} ≥50 mL/minute: No dosage adjustment needed

Cl_{cr} <50 mL/minute: Avoid use

Administration Oral: Minimize unpleasant taste and gastric irritation by administering with water, infant formula, fruit juice, or ginger ale; do not crush capsule, contains drug in liquid form with unpleasant taste

Monitoring Parameters Level of sedation; vital signs and O_2 saturation with doses used for sedation prior to procedure

Test Interactions False-positive urine glucose using Clinitest® method; may interfere with fluorometric urine catecholamine and urinary 17-hydroxycorticosteroid tests

Patient Information May cause drowsiness and impair ability to perform hazardous duties requiring mental alertness; avoid alcohol and other CNS depressants

Nursing Implications May cause irritation of skin and mucous membranes

Additional Information Not an analgesic; osmolality of 500 mg/5 mL syrup is approximately 3500 mOsm/kg

Dosage Forms

Capsule: 500 mg

Suppository, rectal (Aquachloral® Supprettes®): 324 mg, 648 mg

Syrup: 500 mg/5 mL (5 mL, 480 mL)

References

American Academy of Pediatrics, Committee on Drugs and Committee on Environmental Health, "Use of Chloral Hydrate for Sedation in Children," *Pediatrics*, 1993, 92(3):471-3.

Buck ML, "Chloral Hydrate Use During Infancy," *Neonatal Pharmacology Quarterly*, 1992, 1(1):31-7.

Mayers DJ, Hindmarsh KW, Gorecki DK, et al, "Sedative/Hypnotic Effects of Chloral Hydrate in the Neonate: Trichloroethanol or Parent Drug?" *Dev Pharmacol Ther*, 1992, 19(2-3):141-6.

Mayers DJ, Hindmarsh KW, Sankaran K, et al, "Chloral Hydrate Disposition Following Single-Dose Administration to Critically Ill Neonates and Children," *Dev Pharmacol Ther*, 1991, 16(2):71-7.

Steinberg AD, "Should Chloral Hydrate be Banned?" *Pediatrics*, 1993, 92(3)442-6.

Chlorambucil (klor AM byoo sil)

Related Information

Emetogenic Potential of Single Chemotherapeutic Agents *on page 1129*

U.S. Brand Names Leukeran®

Therapeutic Category Antineoplastic Agent, Alkylating Agent (Nitrogen Mustard)

Generic Available No

Use Treatment of chronic lymphocytic leukemia (CLL), Hodgkin's and non-Hodgkin's lymphoma; breast and ovarian carcinoma, testicular carcinoma, choriocarcinoma; Waldenström's macroglobulinemia, and nephrotic syndrome unresponsive to conventional therapy

Pregnancy Risk Factor D

Contraindications Hypersensitivity to chlorambucil or any component, or previous resistance

Warnings The FDA currently recommends that procedures for proper handling and disposal of antineoplastic agents be considered. Chlorambucil can severely suppress bone marrow function; affects human fertility; carcinogenic in humans and probably mutagenic and teratogenic as well; chromosomal damage has been documented; secondary AML may be associated with chronic therapy.

Precautions Use with caution in patients with seizure disorder and bone marrow suppression; reduce initial dosage if patient has received radiation therapy, myelosuppressive drugs or has a depressed baseline leukocyte or platelet count within the previous 4 weeks

Adverse Reactions

Central nervous system: Seizures, fever, agitation, irritability, hyperactivity, confusion, ataxia

Dermatologic: Rash, pruritus, erythema multiforme, toxic epidermal necrolysis

Endocrine & metabolic: Hyperuricemia, menstrual cramps, amenorrhea

Gastrointestinal: Nausea, vomiting, abdominal pain, stomatitis, diarrhea

(Continued)

Chlorambucil *(Continued)*

Genitourinary: Oligospermia

Hematologic: Leukopenia, thrombocytopenia, anemia, lymphocytopenia, neutropenia

Hepatic: Hepatotoxicity, jaundice

Neuromuscular & skeletal: Tremor, muscular twitching, weakness

Respiratory: Pulmonary fibrosis

Drug Interactions Phenobarbital (possible increased chlorambucil toxicity)

Food Interactions Avoid acidic foods, hot foods, and spices; increased bioavailability when administered with food

Mechanism of Action Interferes with DNA replication and RNA transcription by alkylation and cross-linking the strands of DNA; immunosuppressive activity due to suppression of lymphocytes

Pharmacokinetics

Absorption: Oral: 70% to 80% from GI tract

Distribution: To liver, ascitic fluid, fat; extensively bound to plasma and tissue proteins; crosses the placenta

Protein binding: ~99%

Metabolism: In the liver to an active metabolite, phenylacetic acid mustard

Bioavailability: 56% to 100% (increased when taken with food)

Half-life: Chlorambucil: 1.5 hours; phenylacetic acid mustard: 2.5 hours

Elimination: 60% excreted in urine within 24 hours principally as metabolites; <1% excreted as unchanged drug in urine

Dialysis: Probably not dialyzable

Usual Dosage Oral (refer to individual protocols):

Children:

General short courses: 0.1-0.2 mg/kg/day or 4.5 mg/m²/day once daily for 3-6 weeks for remission induction (usual: 4-10 mg/day); maintenance therapy: 0.03-0.1 mg/kg/day (usual: 2-4 mg/day)

Nephrotic syndrome: 0.1-0.2 mg/kg/day every day for 5-12 weeks with low dose prednisone

CLL:

Biweekly regimen: Initial: 0.4 mg/kg/dose every 2 weeks; increase dose by 0.1 mg/kg every 2 weeks until a response occurs and/or myelosuppression occurs

Monthly regimen: Initial: 0.4 mg/kg every 4 weeks, increase dose by 0.2 mg/kg every 4 weeks until a response occurs and/or myelosuppression occurs

Malignant lymphomas:

Non-Hodgkin's lymphoma: 0.1 mg/kg/day

Hodgkin's: 0.2 mg/kg/day

Adults: 0.1-0.2 mg/kg/day or 3-6 mg/m²/day once daily for 3-6 weeks, then adjust dose on basis of blood counts

Administration Oral: Administer with food

Monitoring Parameters Liver function tests, CBC, leukocyte and platelet counts, serum uric acid

Patient Information Notify physician if fever, sore throat, or bleeding occurs

Additional Information Myelosuppressive effects:

WBC: Moderate

Platelets: Moderate

Onset (days): 7

Nadir (days): 14-21

Dosage Forms Tablet, sugar coated: 2 mg

Extemporaneous Preparations A 2 mg/mL suspension was stable for 7 days when refrigerated and compounded as follows: Pulverize sixty 2 mg tablets; levigate with a small amount of glycerin; add 20 mL Cologel® and levigate until a uniform mixture is obtained; add a 2:1 simple syrup/cherry syrup mixture to make a total volume of 60 mL; label "refrigerate" and "shake well before use"

Dressman JB and Poust RI, "Stability of Allopurinol and of Five Antineoplastics in Suspension," *Am J Hosp Pharm*, 1983, 40(4):616-8.

References

Baluarte HJ, Hiner L, and Gruskin AB, "Chlorambucil Dosage in Frequently Relapsing Nephrotic Syndrome: A Controlled Clinical Trial," *J Pediatr*, 1978, 92(2):295-8.

Chloramphenicol *(klor am FEN i kole)*

Related Information

Blood Level Sampling Time Guidelines *on page 1220*

Drugs and Breast-Feeding *on page 1243*

U.S. Brand Names Chloromycetin®; Chloroptic®; Chloroptic® S.O.P

Canadian Brand Names Ak-Chlor; Diochloram; Novo-Chlorocap; Pentamycetin

Therapeutic Category Antibacterial, Otic; Antibiotic, Ophthalmic; Antibiotic, Otic; Antibiotic, Miscellaneous

Generic Available Yes

Use Treatment of serious infections due to organisms resistant to other less toxic antibiotics or when its penetrability into the site of infection is clinically superior to other antibiotics to which the organism is sensitive; useful in infections caused by *Bacteroides, H. influenzae, Neisseria meningitidis, S. pneumoniae, Salmonella*, and *Rickettsia*

Pregnancy Risk Factor C

Contraindications Hypersensitivity to chloramphenicol or any component

Warnings Serious and fatal blood dyscrasias have occurred after both short-term and prolonged therapy; should not be used when less potentially toxic agents are effective; prolonged use may result in superinfection; breast-feeding is not recommended

Precautions Use with caution in patients with G-6-PD deficiency, impaired renal or hepatic function and in neonates; monitor serum concentrations and CBC in all patients; reduce dose in patients with hepatic and renal impairment

Adverse Reactions
Cardiovascular: Cardiotoxicity (left ventricular dysfunction), gray baby syndrome (see Additional Information)
Central nervous system: Nightmares, headache
Dermatologic: Rash
Gastrointestinal: Diarrhea, stomatitis, enterocolitis, vomiting, nausea
Hematologic: Bone marrow suppression, aplastic anemia, neutropenia, thrombocytopenia, hemolysis in patients with G-6-PD deficiency, anemia (see Additional Information)
Hepatic: Hepatitis-pancytopenia syndrome
Neuromuscular & skeletal: Peripheral neuropathy
Ocular: Optic neuritis
Miscellaneous: Anaphylaxis

Drug Interactions Cytochrome P-450 isoenzyme CYP2C9 inhibitor
Chloramphenicol inhibits the metabolism of chlorpropamide, phenytoin, oral anticoagulants; phenobarbital and rifampin may decrease concentration of chloramphenicol; phenytoin may increase chloramphenicol concentration

Food Interactions May decrease intestinal absorption of vitamin B_{12}; may have increased dietary need for riboflavin, pyridoxine, and vitamin B_{12}

Stability Store ophthalmic solution in the refrigerator; reconstituted parenteral solution (100 mg/mL) is stable for 30 days at room temperature

Mechanism of Action Reversibly binds to 50S ribosomal subunits of susceptible organisms preventing amino acids from being transferred to growing peptide chains thus inhibiting protein synthesis

Pharmacokinetics
Distribution: Readily crosses the placenta; appears in breast milk; distributes to most tissues and body fluids; good CSF and brain penetration
CSF concentration with uninflamed meninges: 21% to 50% of plasma concentration
CSF concentration with inflamed meninges: 45% to 89% of plasma concentration
Protein binding: 60%
Metabolism: Extensive in the liver (90%) to inactive metabolites, principally by glucuronidation; chloramphenicol sodium succinate must be hydrolyzed by esterases to active base.
Half-life:
Neonates:
1-2 days: 24 hours
10-16 days: 10 hours
Adults: 1.6-3.3 hours (prolonged with hepatic insufficiency)
Elimination: 5% to 15% excreted as unchanged drug in urine and 4% excreted in bile; in neonates, 6% to 80% of the dose may be excreted unchanged in urine
Dialysis: Slightly dialyzable (5% to 20%)

Usual Dosage
Neonates: Initial loading dose: I.V. (I.M. administration is not recommended): 20 mg/kg (the first maintenance dose should be given 12 hours after the loading dose)
Maintenance dose: Postnatal age:
≤7 days: 25 mg/kg/day once every 24 hours
>7 days, ≤2000 g: 25 mg/kg/day once every 24 hours
>7 days, >2000 g: 50 mg/kg/day divided every 12 hours
(Continued)

Chloramphenicol *(Continued)*

Meningitis: I.V.: Infants and Children: Maintenance dose: 75-100 mg/kg/day divided every 6 hours

Other infections: I.V.:

Infants and Children: 50-75 mg/kg/day divided every 6 hours; maximum daily dose: 4 g/day

Adults: 50 mg/kg/day in divided doses every 6 hours; maximum daily dose: 4 g/day

Dosing adjustment in renal and/or hepatic impairment: Dose reduction should be based upon serum chloramphenicol concentrations

Children and Adults:

Ophthalmic: Apply 1-2 drops or small amount of ointment every 3-6 hours; increase interval between applications after 48 hours

Otic: Place 2-3 drops into the affected ear 3 times/day

Topical: Gently rub into the affected area 3-4 times/day

Administration

Ophthalmic: Solution: Avoid contact of tube or bottle tip with skin or eye; reconstitute powder with sterile water to make a final concentration of 0.5%, 0.25%, or 0.16% chloramphenicol; apply finger pressure to lacrimal sac during and for 1-2 minutes after instillation to decrease risk of absorption and systemic effects

Otic: Apply topically to external ear

Parenteral:

IVP: Administer over 5 minutes at a maximum concentration of 100 mg/mL

I.V. intermittent infusion: Administer over 15-30 minutes at a final concentration for administration ≤20 mg/mL

Monitoring Parameters CBC with reticulocyte and platelet counts, serum iron level, iron-binding capacity, periodic liver and renal function tests, serum drug concentration

Reference Range

Meningitis:

Peak: 15-25 µg/mL

Trough: 5-15 µg/mL

Other infections:

Peak: 10-20 µg/mL

Trough: 5-10 µg/mL

Nursing Implications Draw peak levels 90 minutes after the end of a 30-minute infusion; trough levels should be drawn just prior to the next dose

Additional Information Sodium content of 1 g injection: 2.25 mEq

Three major toxicities associated with chloramphenicol include:

Aplastic anemia, an idiosyncratic reaction which can occur with any route of administration; usually occurs 3 weeks to 12 months after initial exposure to chloramphenicol; incidence: 1 in 40,000 cases

Bone marrow suppression is thought to be dose-related with serum concentrations >25 mcg/mL and reversible once chloramphenicol is discontinued; anemia and neutropenia may occur during the first week of therapy

Gray baby syndrome is characterized by circulatory collapse, hypothermia, cyanosis, acidosis, abdominal distention, myocardial depression, coma, and death; reaction appears to be associated with serum levels ≥50 mcg/mL; may result from drug accumulation in patients with impaired hepatic or renal function; may occur after 3-4 days of therapy or within hours of initiating therapy

Dosage Forms

Ointment, ophthalmic (Chloromycetin®, Chloroptic® S.O.P.): 1% [10 mg/g] (3.5 g)

Powder for injection, as sodium succinate (Chloromycetin®): 1 g

Solution:

Ophthalmic (Chloroptic®): 0.5% [5 mg/mL] (2.5 mL, 7.5 mL, 15 mL)

Otic (Chloromycetin®): 0.5% (15 mL)

References

Nahata MC and Powell DA, "Bioavailability and Clearance of Chloramphenicol After Intravenous Chloramphenicol Succinate," *Clin Pharmacol Ther*, 1981, 30(3):368-72.

Chlorhexidine Gluconate *(klor HEKS i deen GLOO koe nate)*

U.S. Brand Names Betasept® [OTC]; Dyna-Hex® [OTC]; Hibiclens® [OTC]; Peridex®; PerioGard®; Stat Touch 2® [OTC]

Canadian Brand Names Baxedin; Chlorhexseptic; Hibidil; Hibitane; Oro-Clense; Spectro Gram

Therapeutic Category Antibacterial, Topical; Antibiotic, Oral Rinse

Generic Available Yes

Use Skin cleanser for surgical scrub; cleanser for skin wounds; germicidal hand rinse; antibacterial dental rinse to reduce plaque formation and control gingivitis; prophylactic dental rinse to prevent oral infections in immunocompromised patients, particularly bone marrow transplant patients receiving cytotoxic therapy; and short-term substitute for toothbrushing in situations where the patient is unable to tolerate mechanical stimulation of the gums

Pregnancy Risk Factor B

Contraindications Hypersensitivity to chlorhexidine gluconate or any component; do not use as a preoperative skin preparation of the face or head (except Hibiclens® liquid) as serious, permanent eye injury has occurred when chlorhexidine gluconate enters and remains in the eye during surgery.

Warnings For topical use only; there have been several case reports of anaphylaxis following disinfection with chlorhexidine; a case of bradycardic episodes after breast-feeding in a 2 day old infant whose mother used chlorhexidine gluconate topically on her breasts to prevent mastitis has been reported

Precautions Staining of oral surfaces, teeth, restorations, and dorsum of tongue may occur and may be visible as soon as 1 week after therapy begins; staining is more pronounced when there is a heavy accumulation of unremoved plaque and when teeth fillings have rough surfaces; stain does not have clinically adverse effect, but because removal may not be possible, patients with frontal restoration should be advised of the potential permanency of the stain; avoid contact with meninges; corneal injury has been associated with direct eye contact (see Contraindications); deafness has been associated with direct instillation into the middle ear through a perforated eardrum

Adverse Reactions

Dermatologic: Skin irritation, photosensitivity (rare)

Gastrointestinal: Tongue irritation, minor irritation and superficial desquamation of oral mucosa (particularly among children), increased tartar on teeth, staining of oral surfaces (mucosa, teeth, and dorsum of tongue; see Warnings), dysgeusia, transient parotiditis; toothache (chip)

Ophthalmic: Corneal damage (see Precautions)

Otic: Deafness (see Precautions)

Respiratory: Nasal congestion, shortness of breath

Miscellaneous: Edema of face, anaphylactoid reactions

Drug Interactions When combined with nystatin, *in vitro*, the minimum inhibitory concentrations (MIC) of susceptible organisms, were increased to both agents.

Stability Store away from heat and direct light; do not freeze

Mechanism of Action The bactericidal effect of chlorhexidine is a result of the binding of this cationic molecule to negatively charged bacterial cell walls and extramicrobial complexes. At low concentrations, this causes an alteration of bacterial cell osmotic equilibrium and leakage of potassium and phosphorous resulting in a bacteriostatic effect. At high concentrations of chlorhexidine, the cytoplasmic contents of the bacterial cell precipitate and result in cell death. Chlorhexidine is active against gram-positive and gram-negative organisms, facultative anaerobes, anaerobes, and yeast.

Pharmacokinetics

Absorption: ~30% of chlorhexidine is retained in the oral cavity following rinsing and is slowly released into the oral fluids; chlorhexidine is poorly absorbed from the GI tract and is not absorbed topically through intact skin

Serum concentrations: Detectable levels are not present in the plasma 12 hours after administration

Elimination: Primarily through the feces (~90%); <1% excreted in the urine

Usual Dosage

Oral rinse (Peridex® or PerioGard®) (see Administration: Oral):

Children and Adults: 15 mL twice daily

Immunocompromised patient: 10-15 mL, 2-3 times/day

Cleanser: Children and Adults: Apply 5 mL per scrub or hand wash; apply 25 mL per body wash or hair wash

Administration

Oral rinse: Precede use of solution by flossing and brushing teeth, completely rinse toothpaste from mouth; swish undiluted oral rinse around in mouth for 30 seconds, then expectorate; caution patient not to swallow the medicine; avoid eating for 2-3 hours after treatment.

Topical:

Surgical scrub: Scrub 3 minutes and rinse thoroughly, wash for an additional 3 minutes

Hand wash: Wash for 15 seconds and rinse

Hand rinse: Rub vigorously for 15 seconds

(Continued)

Chlorhexidine Gluconate *(Continued)*

Body wash: Wet body and/or hair, apply, rinse thoroughly, repeat.

Monitoring Parameters Improvement in gingival inflammation and bleeding; development of teeth or denture discoloration; dental prophylaxis to remove stains at regular intervals of no greater than 6 months.

Test Interactions If chlorhexidine is used as a disinfectant before midstream urine collection, a false-positive urine protein may result (when using dipstick method based upon a pH indicator color change).

Patient Information

Oral rinse: Use after tooth brushing; do not swallow, do not rinse after use; may cause reduced taste perception which is reversible; may cause discoloration of teeth which may be removed with professional dental cleaning; notify dentist or physician if difficulty breathing or flushing or swelling of face occurs

Topical administration is for external use only; if accidentally enters eyes or ears, rinse out promptly and thoroughly with water

Dosage Forms

Liquid, topical (Stat Touch 2®): 2% (946 mL, 3800 mL)

Liquid, topical, with isopropyl alcohol 4%:

Skin cleanser:

Dyna-Hex® 2: 2% (120 mL, 240 mL, 480 mL, 960 mL, 4000 mL)

Dyna-Hex®, Hibiclens®: 4% (120 mL, 480 mL, 960 mL, 4000 mL)

Sponge/brush (Hibiclens®): 4% (22 mL)

Rinse:

Oral (Peridex®, PerioGard®): 0.12% with alcohol 11.6% (480 mL)

References

Quinn MW and Bini RM, "Bradycardia Associated With Chlorhexidine Spray," *Arch Dis Child*, 1989, 64(6):892-3.

Yong D, Parker FC, and Foran SM, "Severe Allergic Reactions and Intra-Urethral Chlorhexidine Gluconate," *Med J Aust*, 1995, 162(5):257-8.

♦ **Chlorhexseptic (Can)** *see* Chlorhexidine Gluconate *on page 220*

♦ **2-Chlorodeoxyadenosine** *see* Cladribine *on page 245*

♦ **Chloromycetin®** *see* Chloramphenicol *on page 218*

♦ **Chloroptic®** *see* Chloramphenicol *on page 218*

♦ **Chloroptic® S.O.P** *see* Chloramphenicol *on page 218*

Chloroquine *(KLOR oh kwin)*

U.S. Brand Names Aralen®

Canadian Brand Names Aralen Phosphate

Therapeutic Category Amebicide; Antimalarial Agent

Generic Available Yes

Use Suppression or chemoprophylaxis of malaria in chloroquine-sensitive areas; treatment of uncomplicated or mild-moderate malaria due to susceptible *Plasmodium* species, except chloroquine-resistant *Plasmodium falciparum*; extraintestinal amebiasis; rheumatoid arthritis; discoid lupus erythematosus, scleroderma, pemphigus

Pregnancy Risk Factor C

Contraindications Retinal or visual field changes; patients with psoriasis; hypersensitivity to chloroquine or any component

Precautions Use with caution in patients with liver disease, G-6-PD deficiency, or in conjunction with hepatotoxic drugs

Adverse Reactions

Cardiovascular: Hypotension, EKG changes

Central nervous system: Fatigue, personality changes, headache, confusion, agitation, psychotic episodes, seizures

Dermatologic: Pruritus, hair bleaching, skin eruptions, exfoliative dermatitis

Gastrointestinal: Anorexia, nausea, vomiting, diarrhea, stomatitis, weight loss

Hematologic: Blood dyscrasias (neutropenia, aplastic anemia, thrombocytopenia)

Neuromuscular & skeletal: Peripheral neuropathy, neuromyopathy, myalgia

Ocular: Retinopathy, blurred vision, corneal opacity, photophobia

Otic: Tinnitus, deafness

Drug Interactions Intradermally administered rabies vaccine; cimetidine increases levels of chloroquine; urinary acidifiers increase the elimination of chloroquine

Stability Protect from light

Mechanism of Action Binds to and inhibits DNA and RNA polymerase; interferes with metabolism and hemoglobin utilization by parasites; inhibits prostaglandin effects

Pharmacokinetics

Absorption: Oral: Rapid

Distribution: Widely distributed in body tissues including eyes, heart, kidneys, liver, and lungs where retention is prolonged; crosses the placenta; appears in breast milk

Protein binding: 50% to 65%

Metabolism: Partial hepatic

Half-life: 3-5 days

Time to peak serum concentration: Oral: Within 1-2 hours

Elimination: ~70% of dose excreted unchanged in urine; acidification of the urine increases elimination of drug; small amounts of drug may be present in urine months following discontinuation of therapy

Dialysis: Minimally removed by hemodialysis

Usual Dosage (Dosage expressed in terms of base):

Oral:

Suppression or prophylaxis of malaria:

Children: Administer 5 mg base/kg/week on the same day each week (not to exceed 300 mg base/dose); begin 1-2 weeks prior to exposure; continue for 4 weeks after leaving endemic area; if suppressive therapy is not begun prior to exposure, double the initial loading dose to 10 mg base/kg and give in 2 divided doses 6 hours apart, followed by the usual dosage regimen

Adults: 300 mg/week (base) on the same day each week; begin 1-2 weeks prior to exposure; continue for 4 weeks after leaving endemic area; if suppressive therapy is not begun prior to exposure, double the initial loading dose to 600 mg base and give in 2 divided doses 6 hours apart, followed by the usual dosage regimen

Acute attack:

Children: 10 mg base/kg (maximum dose: 600 mg) stat, then 5 mg base/kg (maximum dose: 300 mg base) 6 hours later and then 5 mg base/kg/day (maximum daily dose: 300 mg base) once daily for 2 days

Adults: 600 mg base/dose one time, then 300 mg base/dose 6 hours later, and then 300 mg base/dose once daily for 2 days

Extraintestinal amebiasis:

Children: 10 mg base/kg once daily for 2-3 weeks (up to 300 mg base/day)

Adults: 600 mg base/day for 2 days followed by 300 mg base/day for at least 2-3 weeks

Rheumatoid arthritis: Adults: 150 mg base once daily

I.M.:

Severe malaria when oral therapy is not feasible:

Children: 5 mg base/kg (maximum dose: 200 mg base); dose may be repeated in 6 hours; maximum dose: 10 mg base/kg in a 24-hour period

Adults: 200 mg base every 6 hours

Administration

Oral: Administer with meals to decrease GI upset; chloroquine phosphate tablets have also been mixed with chocolate syrup or enclosed in gelatin capsules to mask the bitter taste

Parenteral: Cautious administration of frequent small doses by I.M. or S.C. injection in children with severe malaria may reduce risk of severe adverse effects (eg, 2.5 mg base/kg every 4 hours not to exceed 10 mg base/kg in a 24-hour period)

Monitoring Parameters Periodic CBC, examination for muscular weakness and ophthalmologic examination in patients receiving prolonged therapy

Patient Information Report any visual disturbances, muscular weakness, or difficulty in hearing or ringing in the ears; tablets are bitter tasting

Dosage Forms

Injection, as hydrochloride: 50 mg/mL **[40 mg base/mL]** (5 mL)

Tablet, as phosphate: 250 mg [150 mg base]; 500 mg [300 mg base]

Extemporaneous Preparations A 15 mg chloroquine base/mL suspension is made by pulverizing three Aralen® 500 mg phosphate = 300 mg base/tablet, levigating with 15 mL of a 1:1 vehicle of Ora-Sweet® and Ora-Plus®, and adding vehicle by geometric proportion, levigating until a uniform mixture is obtained; qsad to 100 mL with vehicle, stable for up to 60 days when stored at 5°C or 25°C and protected from light. Label "shake well before using" and "protect from light."

Allen LV Jr and Erickson MA, "Stability of Alprazolam, Chloroquine Phosphate, Cisapride, Enalapril Maleate, and Hydralazine Hydrochloride in Extemporaneously Compounded Oral Liquids," *Am J Health Syst Pharm*, 1998, 55(18):1915-20.

References

Wyler DJ, "Malaria Chemoprophylaxis for the Traveler," *N Engl J Med*, 1993, 329(1):31-7.

Chlorothiazide (klor oh THYE a zide)

Related Information
Carbohydrate and Alcohol Content of Liquid Medications for Use in Patients Receiving Ketogenic Diets *on page 1258*

U.S. Brand Names Diuril®

Therapeutic Category Antihypertensive Agent; Diuretic, Thiazide

Generic Available Yes: Tablet

Use Management of mild to moderate hypertension; edema associated with CHF, pregnancy, or nephrotic syndrome

Pregnancy Risk Factor C

Contraindications Hypersensitivity to chlorothiazide or any component; cross-sensitivity with other thiazides or sulfonamides; do not use in anuric patients

Warnings The injection must not be administered subcutaneously or I.M.

Precautions Use with caution in patients with severe renal disease, impaired hepatic function, moderate-high cholesterol concentrations, and in patients with high triglycerides

Adverse Reactions
Cardiovascular: Hypotension, arrhythmia, weak pulse
Central nervous system: Dizziness, vertigo, headache, fever
Dermatologic: Rash, photosensitivity
Endocrine & metabolic: Hypokalemia, hypochloremic alkalosis, hyperglycemia, hyperlipidemia, hyperuricemia
Gastrointestinal: Anorexia, nausea, vomiting, cramping, diarrhea, pancreatitis, constipation
Hematologic: Rarely blood dyscrasias, thrombocytopenia
Hepatic: Intrahepatic cholestasis
Neuromuscular & skeletal: Muscle weakness, paresthesia
Ophthalmic: Blurred vision
Renal: Prerenal azotemia, hematuria

Drug Interactions NSAIDs with chlorothiazide may result in decreased antihypertensive effect; additive potassium losses with steroids, loop diuretics and amphotericin B; decreases lithium clearance; increases hypersensitivity reactions to allopurinol; increases hyperglycemia with diazoxide; decreased absorption of chlorothiazide when administered with cholestyramine; milk-alkali syndrome with high calcium dosages

Food Interactions Avoid natural licorice (causes sodium and water retention and increases potassium loss); may need to decrease sodium and calcium, may need to increase potassium, zinc, magnesium, and riboflavin in diet

Stability Reconstituted injection is stable for 24 hours at room temperature

Mechanism of Action Inhibits sodium reabsorption in the distal tubules causing increased excretion of sodium, chloride, potassium, bicarbonate, magnesium, phosphate, calcium (transiently) and water

Pharmacodynamics
Diuresis: Onset of effect: Oral: Within 2 hours
Duration:
  Oral: ~6-12 hours
  I.V.: 2 hours

Pharmacokinetics
Absorption: Oral: Poor (~10% to 20%); dose dependent
Distribution: Breast milk to plasma ratio: 0.05
Half-life: Adults: 45-120 minutes
Time to peak serum concentration: Within 4 hours
Elimination: Excreted unchanged in urine

Usual Dosage I.V. dosage in infants and children has not been well established. The following I.V. dosages in infants and children have been extrapolated from oral absorption data (~10% to 20%) and have been used successfully. Equivalent I.V./oral doses have been used safely in adult patients.

Neonates and Infants <6 months:
  Oral: 20-40 mg/kg/day in 2 divided doses; maximum: 375 mg/day
  I.V.: 2-8 mg/kg/day in 2 divided doses
Infants >6 months and Children:
  Oral: 20 mg/kg/day in 2 divided doses; maximum: 1 g/day
  I.V.: 4 mg/kg/day divided in 1-2 doses
Adults:
  Oral: 500 mg to 2 g/day divided in 1-2 doses
  I.V.: 100-500 mg/day divided in 1-2 doses

Administration
Oral: Administer with food; shake suspension well before use
Parenteral: Dilute 500 mg vial with 18 mL sterile water (resulting in 27.8 mg/mL concentration); administer by direct I.V. infusion over 3-5 minutes or infusion over 30 minutes in dextrose or NS; avoid extravasation of parenteral solution since it is extremely irritating to tissues

Monitoring Parameters Serum electrolytes (sodium, potassium, chloride, and bicarbonate), glucose, uric acid, triglycerides

Dosage Forms
Powder for injection, lyophilized, as sodium: 500 mg
Suspension, oral: 250 mg/5 mL (237 mL)
Tablet: 250 mg, 500 mg

Chlorpheniramine (klor fen IR a meen)

Related Information
OTC Cough & Cold Preparations, Pediatric *on page 1072*
Overdose and Toxicology *on page 1222*

U.S. Brand Names Aller-Chlor® Oral [OTC]; Chlor-Trimeton® [OTC]; Polaramine®

Canadian Brand Names Chlor-Tripolon; Novo-Pheniram

Therapeutic Category Antihistamine

Generic Available Yes

Use Perennial and seasonal allergic rhinitis and other allergic symptoms including urticaria

Pregnancy Risk Factor B

Contraindications Hypersensitivity to chlorpheniramine maleate or any component; narrow-angle glaucoma, bladder neck obstruction, symptomatic prostatic hypertrophy, stenosing peptic ulcer, pyloroduodenal obstruction

Precautions Use with caution in patients with asthma; young children may be more susceptible to side effects and CNS stimulation

Adverse Reactions
Cardiovascular: Palpitations
Central nervous system: Drowsiness, vertigo, headache, excitability (children may be at increased risk for developing CNS stimulation), nervousness, fatigue, dizziness, depression
Dermatologic: Dermatitis, photosensitivity, angioedema
Gastrointestinal: Nausea, xerostomia, diarrhea, abdominal pain, appetite increase, weight gain
Genitourinary: Urinary retention
Neuromuscular & skeletal: Weakness, arthralgia, paresthesia
Ocular: Diplopia, blurred vision
Renal: Polyuria
Respiratory: Thickening of bronchial secretions, pharyngitis, epistaxis

Drug Interactions Cytochrome P-450 isoenzyme CYP2D6 substrate
May cause additive sedation when concomitantly administered with other CNS depressant medications

Mechanism of Action Competes with histamine for H_1-receptor sites on effector cells in the GI tract, blood vessels, and respiratory tract

Pharmacodynamics
Onset: Oral: 6 hours
Duration: Oral: 24 hours

Pharmacokinetics (Data from chlorpheniramine maleate)
Distribution: V_d:
Children: 3.8 L/kg
Adults: 2.5-3.2 L/kg
Protein binding: 69% to 72%
Metabolism: Substantial metabolism in GI mucosa and on first pass through liver
Bioavailability: Chlorpheniramine:
Solution: 35% to 60%
Tablet: 25% to 45%
Half-life:
Children: Average: 9.6-13.1 hours (range: 5.2-23.1 hours)
Adults: 12-43 hours
Time to peak serum concentration: Oral (solution and conventional tablets): 2-6 hours
Elimination: 35% excreted in 48 hours
(Continued)

Chlorpheniramine *(Continued)*

Usual Dosage

Chlorpheniramine maleate: Oral:
Children <12 years: Oral: 0.35 mg/kg/day in divided doses every 4-6 hours or as an alternative

2-5 years: 1 mg every 4-6 hours

6-11 years: 2 mg every 4-6 hours, not to exceed 12 mg/day or timed release 8 mg every 12 hours

Children ≥12 years and Adults: 4 mg every 4-6 hours, not to exceed 24 mg/day or timed release 8-12 mg every 12 hours

Chlorpheniramine maleate: I.M., I.V., S.C.:
Children <12 years: 0.0875 mg/kg or 2.5 mg/m^2 4 times/day

Children ≥12 years and Adults: 5-20 mg as a single dose; not to exceed 40 mg/day

Dexchlorpheniramine maleate: Oral:
Children 2-5 years: 0.5 mg every 4-6 hours, not to exceed 3 mg/day

Children 6-11 years: 1 mg every 4-6 hours, not to exceed 6 mg/day **or** as timed release tablets: 4 mg once daily at bedtime

Children ≥12 years and Adults: 2 mg every 4-6 hours **or** as timed release tablets: 4-6 mg at bedtime or every 8-10 hours; not to exceed 12 mg/day

Administration
Oral: Administer with food to decrease GI distress; do not crush or chew timed release tablets

Parenteral: May be given I.M., I.V., or S.C.; do not administer intradermally

Patient Information
Causes drowsiness and may impair ability to perform hazardous activities requiring mental alertness or physical coordination

Dosage Forms
Capsule, timed release, as chlorpheniramine maleate: 8 mg, 12 mg

Injection: as chlorpheniramine maleate: 10 mg/mL (30 mL)

Solution, as dexchlorpheniramine maleate (Polaramine®): 2 mg/5 mL (480 mL)

Syrup, as chlorpheniramine maleate (Aller-Chlor®, Chlor-Trimeton®): 2 mg/5 mL (120 mL, 473 mL)

Tablet, as chlorpheniramine maleate (Aller-Chlor®, Chlor-Trimeton®): 4 mg

Tablet, as dexchlorpheniramine maleate (Polaramine®): 2 mg

Tablet, timed release, as chlorpheniramine maleate (Aller-Chlor®, Chlor-Trimeton®): 8 mg, 12 mg

Tablet, timed release, as dexchlorpheniramine maleate (Polaramine®): 4 mg, 6 mg

♦ **Chlorpromanyl (Can)** *see* Chlorpromazine *on page 226*

Chlorpromazine *(klor PROE ma zeen)*

Related Information
Carbohydrate and Alcohol Content of Liquid Medications for Use in Patients Receiving Ketogenic Diets *on page 1258*

Compatibility of Medications Mixed in a Syringe *on page 1238*

Drugs and Breast-Feeding *on page 1243*

Overdose and Toxicology *on page 1222*

Prochlorperazine *on page 834*

U.S. Brand Names
Thorazine®

Canadian Brand Names
Apo-Chlorpromazine; Chlorpromanyl; Largactil; Novo-Chlorpromazine

Therapeutic Category
Antiemetic; Antipsychotic Agent; Phenothiazine Derivative

Generic Available
Yes

Use
Treatment of nausea and vomiting, psychoses, Tourette's syndrome, mania, intractable hiccups (adults), behavioral problems (children)

Pregnancy Risk Factor
C

Contraindications
Hypersensitivity to chlorpromazine hydrochloride or any component; cross-sensitivity with other phenothiazines may exist; avoid use in patients with narrow-angle glaucoma, bone marrow suppression, severe liver or cardiac disease

Warnings
Significant hypotension may occur, especially when the drug is administered parenterally; extended release capsules and injection contain benzyl alcohol; injection also contains sulfites which may cause allergic reaction

Precautions
Use with caution in patients with cardiovascular, renal, or hepatic disease; seizures; significant medical disorders or children with acute illnesses

Adverse Reactions
Cardiovascular: Hypotension (especially with I.V. use), orthostatic hypotension, tachycardia, arrhythmias

Central nervous system: Sedation, drowsiness, restlessness, anxiety, extrapyramidal reactions, pseudoparkinsonian signs and symptoms, tardive dyskinesia, neuroleptic malignant syndrome, seizures, altered central temperature regulation

Dermatologic: Hyperpigmentation, pruritus, rash, photosensitivity; oral solution or injection may cause contact dermatitis (avoid contact with skin)

Endocrine & metabolic: Amenorrhea, galactorrhea, gynecomastia

Gastrointestinal: Xerostomia, constipation, GI upset, weight gain

Genitourinary: Impotence, urinary retention

Hematologic: Agranulocytosis, leukopenia (usually in patients with large doses for prolonged periods), thrombocytopenia, hemolytic anemia, eosinophilia

Hepatic: Cholestatic jaundice (rare)

Local: Thrombophlebitis

Ocular: Retinal pigmentation, blurred vision

Miscellaneous: Anaphylactoid reactions

Drug Interactions Cytochrome P-450 isoenzyme CYP1A2, CYP2D6, and CYP3A3/4 substrate; isoenzyme CYP2D6 inhibitor

Additive effects with other CNS depressants; epinephrine may cause hypotension in patients receiving chlorpromazine due to phenothiazine-induced alpha-adrenergic blockade and unopposed epinephrine beta$_2$ action; chlorpromazine may increase valproic acid serum concentrations; absorption may be decreased if administered concomitantly with aluminum- or magnesium-containing antacids; liquid preparations of chlorpromazine will form an orange rubbery precipitate if mixed with or administered simultaneously with carbamazepine suspension; may interact with metyrapone and reduce test effectiveness; may interact with tranexamic acid

Food Interactions Increases riboflavin elimination and may induce depletion; some may recommend increasing riboflavin in diet; may also decrease absorption of vitamin B$_{12}$; undiluted oral concentrate may precipitate when mixed with tube feeding; brown precipitate may occur when chlorpromazine is mixed with caffeine-containing liquids

Stability Protect oral dosage forms from light; discard solution if markedly discolored; diluted injection (1 mg/mL) with NS stored in 5 mL vials remains stable for 30 days

Mechanism of Action Blocks postsynaptic mesolimbic dopaminergic receptors in the brain; exhibits a strong alpha-adrenergic blocking effect and depresses the release of hypothalamic and hypophyseal hormones

Pharmacodynamics

Onset of action:
Oral tablet: 30-60 minutes
Rectal suppository: >60 minutes
Antipsychotic effects: Gradual, may take up to several weeks

Time to peak antipsychotic effects: 6 weeks to 6 months

Duration of action:
Oral tablets: 4-6 hours
Rectal suppository: 3-4 hours

Pharmacokinetics

Absorption: Oral: Rapid and virtually complete; large first-pass effect due to metabolism during absorption in the GI mucosa

Distribution: Widely distributed into most body tissues and fluids; crosses blood-brain barrier and placenta; appears in breast milk; V$_d$: 8-160 L/kg (adults)

Protein binding: 90% to 99%

Metabolism: Extensively in the liver by demethylation (followed by glucuronide conjugation) and amine oxidation

Bioavailability: Oral: ~32%

Half-life, biphasic:
Initial: 2 hours
Terminal: 30 hours

Elimination: <1% excreted in urine as unchanged drug within 24 hours

Dialysis: Not dialyzable (0% to 5%)

Usual Dosage

Neonates: Neonatal abstinence syndrome (withdrawal from maternal narcotic use): I.M. and Oral: Initial: I.M.: 0.5-0.7 mg/kg/dose given every 6 hours; change to oral after ~4 days, decrease dose gradually over 2-3 weeks. **Note:** Chlorpromazine is rarely used for neonatal abstinence syndrome due to adverse effects such as hypothermia and eosinophilia. Other agents (eg, phenobarbital or a 25-fold dilution of tincture of opium) are preferred.

Children >6 months:
Psychosis:
Oral: 0.5-1 mg/kg/dose every 4-6 hours; older children may require 200 mg/day or higher
I.M., I.V.: 0.5-1 mg/kg/dose every 6-8 hours

(Continued)

Chlorpromazine *(Continued)*

Maximum recommended doses:
Children <5 years (<22.7 kg): 40 mg/day
Children 5-12 years (22.7-45.5 kg): 75 mg/day
Nausea and vomiting:
Oral: 0.5-1 mg/kg/dose every 4-6 hours as needed
I.M., I.V.: 0.5-1 mg/kg/dose every 6-8 hours; maximum dose: Same as psychosis
Rectal: 1 mg/kg/dose every 6-8 hours as needed
Adults:
Psychosis:
Oral: Range: 30-800 mg/day in 1-4 divided doses, initiate at lower doses and titrate as needed; usual dose is 200 mg/day; some patients may require 1-2 g/day
I.M., I.V.: 25 mg initially, may repeat (25-50 mg) in 1-4 hours, gradually increase to a maximum of 400 mg/dose every 4-6 hours until patient controlled; usual dose 300-800 mg/day
Nausea and vomiting:
Oral: 10-25 mg every 4-6 hours
I.M., I.V.: 25-50 mg every 4-6 hours
Rectal: 50-100 mg every 6-8 hours

Administration
Oral: Administer with water, food, or milk to decrease GI upset; swallow sustained release capsule whole; do not chew; dilute oral concentrate solution in water, tomato or fruit juice, milk, simple syrup, orange syrup, or carbonated beverages just before administration; do not mix undiluted oral concentrate with tube feeding (see Food Interactions); do not administer chlorpromazine liquid preparations simultaneously with carbamazepine suspension (see Drug Interactions)
Parenteral: Do not administer S.C. (tissue damage and irritation may occur); for direct I.V. injection: Dilute with NS to a maximum concentration of 1 mg/mL, administer slow I.V. at a rate not to exceed 1 mg/minute in adults and 0.5 mg/minute in children

Monitoring Parameters Periodic eye exam with prolonged therapy; blood pressure with parenteral administration; CBC with differential

Reference Range Relationship of plasma concentration to clinical response is not well established
Therapeutic: 50-300 ng/mL (SI: 157-942 nmol/L)
Toxic: >750 ng/mL (SI: >2355 nmol/L)

Test Interactions False-positives for phenylketonuria, amylase, uroporphyrins, urobilinogen; possible false-negative pregnancy urinary test

Patient Information May cause drowsiness and impair ability to perform activities requiring mental alertness or physical coordination; may cause dry mouth, photosensitivity; avoid excessive sunlight; use sunscreen; avoid alcohol

Nursing Implications Avoid contact of oral solution or injection with skin (may cause contact dermatitis)

Additional Information Although chlorpromazine has been used in combination with meperidine and promethazine as a premedication ("lytic cocktail"), this combination may have a higher rate of adverse effects compared to alternative sedatives/analgesics; see References. Use decreased doses in elderly or debilitated patients; dystonic reactions may be more common in patients with hypocalcemia; extrapyramidal reactions may be more common in pediatric patients, especially those with dehydration or acute illnesses (viral or CNS infections); avoid rectal administration in immunocompromised patients.

Dosage Forms
Capsule, as hydrochloride, sustained action: 30 mg, 75 mg, 150 mg
Concentrate, oral, as hydrochloride: 30 mg/mL (120 mL); 100 mg/mL (240 mL)
Injection, as hydrochloride: 25 mg/mL (1 mL, 2 mL, 10 mL)
Suppository, rectal, as base: 25 mg, 100 mg
Syrup, as hydrochloride: 10 mg/5 mL [orange-custard flavor] (120 mL)
Tablet, as hydrochloride: 10 mg, 25 mg, 50 mg, 100 mg, 200 mg

References
American Academy of Pediatrics Committee on Drugs, "Reappraisal of Lytic Cocktail/Demerol®, Phenergan®, and Thorazine® (DPT) for the Sedation of Children," *Pediatrics*, 1995, 95(4):598-602.

♦ **Chlor-Trimeton® [OTC]** *see* Chlorpheniramine *on page 225*
♦ **Chlor-Tripolon (Can)** *see* Chlorpheniramine *on page 225*

Chlorzoxazone (klor ZOKS a zone)

U.S. Brand Names Parafon Forte™ DSC; Remular® S

Therapeutic Category Skeletal Muscle Relaxant, Nonparalytic

Generic Available Yes

Use Symptomatic treatment of muscle spasm and pain associated with acute musculoskeletal conditions

Pregnancy Risk Factor C

Contraindications Hypersensitivity to chlorzoxazone or any component; impaired liver function

Warnings Serious (including fatal) hepatocellular toxicity has been reported rarely

Adverse Reactions

Cardiovascular: Tachycardia, tightness in chest, flushing of face, syncope

Central nervous system: Drowsiness, dizziness, lightheadedness, headache, paradoxical stimulation, ataxia

Dermatologic: Rash, urticaria, petechiae, angioneurotic edema, erythema multiforme

Gastrointestinal: Nausea, vomiting, diarrhea, GI bleeding (rare), stomach cramps

Genitourinary: Discoloration of urine (orange or purple-red)

Hematologic: Anemia, granulocytopenia, eosinophilia

Hepatic: Hepatitis

Neuromuscular & skeletal: Paresthesia, trembling

Ocular: Burning of eyes

Respiratory: Shortness of breath

Miscellaneous: Hiccups

Drug Interactions Cytochrome P-450 isoenzyme CYP2E1 substrate

May cause additive sedation when concomitantly administered with other CNS depressant medications

Food Interactions Watercress may decrease chlorzoxazone clearance

Mechanism of Action Acts on the spinal cord and subcortical levels by depressing polysynaptic reflexes

Pharmacodynamics

Onset of effects: Within 60 minutes

Duration: 3-4 hours

Pharmacokinetics

Absorption: Oral: Readily

Metabolism: Extensive in the liver by glucuronidation

Half-life: ~60 minutes

Elimination: In urine as conjugates

Usual Dosage Oral:

Children: 20 mg/kg/day or 600 mg/m^2/day in 3-4 divided doses

Adults: 250-750 mg 3-4 times/day

Administration Oral: Administer with food

Monitoring Parameters Periodic liver function tests

Patient Information May color urine orange or purple-red; causes drowsiness and may impair ability to perform hazardous activities requiring mental alertness; notify physician if experiencing fever, rash, anorexia, right upper quadrant pain, dark urine, or jaundice

Dosage Forms

Caplet (Parafon Forte™ DSC): 500 mg

Tablet (Remular®): 250 mg, 500 mg

♦ **Cholac**® see Lactulose on page 571

Cholestyramine Resin (koe LES tir a meen REZ in)

U.S. Brand Names LoCHOLEST®; LoCHOLEST® Light; Prevalite®; Questran®; Questran® Light

Canadian Brand Names Novo-Cholamine; PMS-Cholestyramine

Therapeutic Category Antilipemic Agent

Generic Available Yes

Use Adjunct in the management of primary hypercholesterolemia; pruritus associated with elevated levels of bile acids; diarrhea associated with excess fecal bile acids; pseudomembraneous colitis

Pregnancy Risk Factor C

Contraindications Hypersensitivity to cholestyramine or any component; avoid using in complete biliary obstruction or biliary atresia

(Continued)

Cholestyramine Resin *(Continued)*

Precautions Use with caution in patients with constipation or recent abdominal surgery (see Additional Information); Prevalite®, LoCHOLEST® Light, and Questran® Light contain aspartame; aspartame is metabolized to phenylalanine and must be avoided or used with caution in patients with phenylketonuria

Adverse Reactions
Dermatologic: Rash
Endocrine & metabolic: Hyperchloremic acidosis
Gastrointestinal: Constipation, nausea, vomiting, abdominal distention and pain, malabsorption of fat-soluble vitamins
Genitourinary: Increased urinary calcium excretion
Local: Irritation of perianal area, skin, or tongue

Drug Interactions May decrease oral absorption of digitalis glycosides, warfarin, thyroid hormones, thiazide diuretics, propranolol, phenobarbital, amiodarone, methotrexate, NSAIDs, and other drugs by binding to the drug in the intestine

Food Interactions Cholestyramine (especially high doses or long-term therapy) may decrease the absorption of fat-soluble vitamins (vitamins A, D, E, and K), folic acid, calcium, iron, zinc, and magnesium; deficiencies may occur including hypoprothrombinemia and increased bleeding from vitamin K deficiency; supplementation of vitamins A, D, E, and K, folic acid, and iron may be required with high-dose, long-term therapy

Mechanism of Action Forms a nonabsorbable complex with bile acids in the intestine, releasing chloride ions in the process; inhibits enterohepatic reuptake of intestinal bile salts and thereby increases the fecal loss of bile salt-bound low density lipoprotein cholesterol

Pharmacodynamics
Peak effect on serum cholesterol levels: Within 4 weeks

Pharmacokinetics
Absorption: Not absorbed from the GI tract
Elimination: Forms an insoluble complex with bile acids which is excreted in feces

Usual Dosage Oral (dosages are expressed in terms of anhydrous resin):
Children: 240 mg/kg/day in 3 divided doses; need to titrate dose depending on indication
Hypercholesterolemia (**Note:** Doses >8 g/day may not provide additional significant cholesterol-lowering effects, but may increase adverse effects): Some centers use the following doses (see Sprecher, 1996):
Children ≤10 years: Initial: 2 g/day; titrate dose based on efficacy and tolerance; range: 1-4 g/day
Children >10 years and Adolescents: Initial: 2 g/day; titrate dose based on efficacy and tolerance, up to 8 g/day
Adults: 3-4 g 3-4 times/day to a maximum of 16-32 g/day in 2-4 divided doses

Administration Oral: Administer before meals; do not administer the powder in its dry form; just prior to administration, mix with 2-6 ounces of water, noncarbonated liquid, or applesauce; to minimize binding of concomitant medications, administer other drugs including vitamins or mineral supplements at least 1 hour before or at least 4-6 hours after cholestyramine

Monitoring Parameters Serum cholesterol, serum triglycerides; with prolonged use, prothrombin time, liver enzymes, CBC, electrolytes; number of stools/day

Nursing Implications Maintain adequate oral fluid intake to avoid constipation; with high-dose, long-term therapy, use of daily multivitamin with iron and folic acid is recommended

Additional Information Overdose may result in GI obstruction; intestinal obstruction has been reported in patients with recent abdominal surgery (see Tonstad, 1996)

Dosage Forms
Powder (LoCHOLEST®, Questran®): 4 g of resin/9 g of powder (9 g, 378 g)
Powder, for oral suspension, with aspartame:
LoCHOLEST® Light: 4 g of resin/5.7 g of powder (5.7 g, 231 g)
Prevalite®: 4 g of resin/5.5 g of powder (5.5 g)
Questran® Light: 4 g of resin/5 g of powder (5 g, 210 g)

References
McCrindle BW, O'Neill MB, Cullen-Dean G, et al, "Acceptability and Compliance With Two Forms of Cholestyramine in the Treatment of Hypercholesterolemia in Children: A Randomized, Crossover Trial," *J Pediatr*, 1997, 130(2):266-73.
Sprecher DL and Daniels SR, "Rational Approach to Pharmacologic Reduction of Cholesterol Levels in Children," *J Pediatr*, 1996, 129(1):4-7.
Tonstad S, Knudtzon J, Sivertsen M, et al, "Efficacy and Safety of Cholestyramine Therapy in Peripubertal and Prepubertal Children With Familial Hypercholesterolemia," *J Pediatr*, 1996, 129(1):42-9.

Choline Magnesium Trisalicylate
(KOE leen mag NEE zhum trye sa LIS i late)

Related Information
Overdose and Toxicology *on page 1222*

U.S. Brand Names Tricosal®; Trilisate®

Therapeutic Category Analgesic, Non-narcotic; Anti-inflammatory Agent; Antipyretic; Nonsteroidal Anti-inflammatory Drug (NSAID), Oral; Salicylate

Generic Available Yes

Use Management of osteoarthritis, rheumatoid arthritis, and other arthritides; treatment of acute painful shoulder, mild to moderate pain, and fever

Pregnancy Risk Factor C (D in 3rd trimester)

Contraindications Hypersensitivity to salicylates, any component, or other nonacetylated salicylates

Warnings Avoid use in patients with suspected varicella or influenza (salicylates have been associated with Reye's syndrome in children <16 years of age when used to treat symptoms of chickenpox or the flu)

Precautions Use with extreme caution in patients with impaired renal function, erosive gastritis or peptic ulcer

Adverse Reactions
Dermatologic: Rash, pruritus, urticaria
Gastrointestinal: Nausea, vomiting, GI distress, ulceration
Hepatic: Hepatotoxicity
Otic: Tinnitus
Respiratory: Pulmonary edema

Drug Interactions Antacids may decrease salicylate concentration; salicylates may increase hypoprothrombinemic effect of warfarin

Mechanism of Action Inhibits prostaglandin synthesis; acts on the hypothalamus heat-regulating center to reduce fever; blocks the generation of pain impulses

Pharmacokinetics
Absorption: From stomach and small intestine
Distribution: Readily distributes into most body fluids and tissues; crosses the placenta; appears in breast milk
Protein binding: 90% to 95%
Metabolism: Hepatic microsomal enzyme system
Half-life: Dose-dependent, ranging from 2-3 hours at low doses to 30 hours at high doses
Time to peak serum concentration:
Solution: 20-35 minutes
Tablet: Within ~2 hours
Elimination: 10% excreted as unchanged drug

Usual Dosage Oral (based on **total salicylate content**):
Children: 30-60 mg/kg/day given in 3-4 divided doses
Adults: 500 mg to 1.5 g 1-3 times/day

Administration Oral: Administer with food or milk to decrease GI upset; liquid may be mixed with fruit juice just before drinking; do not administer with antacids

Monitoring Parameters Serum salicylate levels; serum magnesium with high doses or in patients with decreased renal function

Reference Range
Salicylate blood levels for anti-inflammatory effect: 150-300 µg/mL
Analgesia and antipyretic effect: 30-50 µg/mL

Test Interactions False-negative results for Clinistix® urine test; false-positive results with Clinitest®

Choline Magnesium Trisalicylate

Brand Name	Dosage Form	Labeled Strength (Total Salicylate)	Choline Salicylate	Magnesium Salicylate
Trilisate® [cherry cordial flavor]	Liquid	500 mg/5 mL	293 mg/5 mL	362 mg/5 mL
Trilisate®, Tricosal®	Tablet	500 mg	293 mg	362 mg
Trilisate®, Tricosal®	Tablet	750 mg	440 mg	544 mg
Trilisate®, Tricosal®	Tablet	1000 mg	587 mg	725 mg

(Continued)

Choline Magnesium Trisalicylate *(Continued)*

Patient Information Avoid alcohol; notify physician if ringing in ears or persistent GI pain occurs

Additional Information Salicylate salts do not inhibit platelet aggregation and, therefore, should not be substituted for aspirin in the prophylaxis of thrombosis (ie, for aspirin's antiplatelet effects)

Dosage Forms See table on previous page.

References

Berde C, Ablin A, Glazer J, et al, "American Academy of Pediatrics Report of the Subcommittee on Disease-Related Pain in Childhood Cancer," *Pediatrics*, 1990, 86(5 Pt 2):818-25.

◆ **Chooz®** [OTC] *see* Calcium Supplements *on page 167*
◆ **Chorex®** *see* Chorionic Gonadotropin *on page 232*

Chorionic Gonadotropin (kor ee ON ik goe NAD oh troe pin)

U.S. Brand Names A.P.L.®; Chorex®; Novarel™; Pregnyl®; Profasi®

Synonyms CG; hCG

Therapeutic Category Gonadotropin; Ovulation Stimulator

Generic Available Yes

Use Treatment of hypogonadotropic hypogonadism, prepubertal cryptorchidism; induce ovulation

Pregnancy Risk Factor X

Contraindications Hypersensitivity to chorionic gonadotropin or any component; precocious puberty, prostatic carcinoma or similar neoplasms

Warnings hCG is **not** effective in the treatment of obesity; Pregnyl® contains benzyl alcohol; avoid use in neonates

Precautions Use with caution in patients with asthma, seizure disorders, migraine, cardiac or renal disease; may induce precocious puberty

Adverse Reactions

Cardiovascular: Edema

Central nervous system: Irritability, restlessness, depression, fatigue, headache, aggressive behavior

Endocrine & metabolic: Gynecomastia, precocious puberty

Local: Pain at the injection site

Neuromuscular & skeletal: Premature closure of epiphyses

Stability Following reconstitution with provided diluent, stable for 30-90 days (depending upon preparation) when stored at 2°C to 15°C

Mechanism of Action Stimulates production of gonadal steroid hormones by causing production of androgen by the testis; as a substitute for luteinizing hormone (LH) to stimulate ovulation

Pharmacokinetics

Half-life, biphasic:

Initial: 11 hours

Terminal: 23 hours

Elimination: Excreted unchanged in urine within 3-4 days

Usual Dosage Children: I.M. (many regimens have been described):

Prepubertal cryptorchidism:

1000-2000 units/m² /dose 3 times/week for 3 weeks or 4000 units 3 times/week for 3 weeks

or

5000 units every second day for 4 injections

or

500 units 3 times/week for 4-6 weeks

Hypogonadotropic hypogonadism:

500-1000 units 3 times/week for 3 weeks, followed by the same dose twice weekly for 3 weeks

or

1000-2000 units 3 times/week

or

4000 units 3 times/week for 6-9 months; reduce dosage to 2000 units 3 times/week for additional 3 months

Induction of ovulation: 5000-10,000 units the day following the last dose of menotropins

Administration Parenteral: Administer I.M. only

Reference Range Depends on application and methodology; <3 milli international units/mL (SI: <3 units/L) usually normal (nonpregnant)

Dosage Forms Powder for injection: 500 units/mL (10 mL); 1000 units/mL (10 mL); 2000 units/mL (10 mL)

+ **Chromium Chloride** *see* Trace Metals *on page 972*
+ **Chronovera (Can)** *see* Verapamil *on page 1007*
+ **Chronulac®** *see* Lactulose *on page 571*

Cidofovir (si DOF o veer)

Synonyms HPMPC

Therapeutic Category Antiviral Agent, Parenteral

Generic Available No

Use Treatment of cytomegalovirus (CMV) retinitis in patients with acquired immuno-deficiency syndrome; antiviral agent with activity against ganciclovir-resistant CMV, foscarnet-resistant CMV, acyclovir-resistant HSV or VZV, and adenovirus

Pregnancy Risk Factor C

Contraindications Hypersensitivity to cidofovir or any component; history of clinically severe hypersensitivity to probenecid or other sulfa-containing medications; patients with a serum creatinine >1.5 mg/dL, creatinine clearance ≤55 mL/minute, urine protein ≥100 mg/dL (≥2 plus proteinuria); patients who are receiving other nephrotoxic agents; direct intraocular injection

Warnings Safety and efficacy have not been established in children; due to risk of long-term carcinogenicity and reproductive toxicity, administration of cidofovir to children warrants extreme caution. Prepare admixture in a Class II laminar flow hood, administer, and dispose according to guidelines issued for cytotoxic drugs. Acute renal failure resulting in dialysis and/or contributing to death has been reported to occur after as few as one or two cidofovir doses; neutropenia and ocular hypotony have been reported in association with cidofovir treatment.

Precautions Modify dose in patients with changing renal function due to dose-dependent nephrotoxicity. Cidofovir administration must be accompanied by oral probenecid and normal saline I.V. prehydration to reduce possible nephrotoxicity.

Adverse Reactions

Cardiovascular: Hypotension, pallor, syncope, tachycardia, cardiomyopathy, edema, hypertension

Central nervous system: Headache, agitation, dizziness, fever, chills, amnesia, confusion, seizures, insomnia, personality/mood disorder, hallucinations, anxiety, somnolence, malaise

Dermatologic: Alopecia, rash, acne, skin discoloration, pruritus, urticaria

Endocrine & metabolic: Metabolic acidosis, hyperglycemia, hyperlipidemia, hypocalcemia, hypokalemia, dehydration, hypomagnesemia, hyponatremia, hypophosphatemia

Gastrointestinal: Nausea, vomiting, diarrhea, anorexia, abdominal pain, constipation, dyspepsia, gastritis, abnormal taste, stomatitis, colitis, cholangitis, pancreatitis, dysphagia

Genitourinary: Glycosuria, urinary incontinence, hematuria, proteinuria

Hematologic: Neutropenia (not dose-related; occurs in up to 24% of AIDS patients), thrombocytopenia, anemia

Hepatic: Hepatomegaly, elevated SGOT and SGPT

Neuromuscular & skeletal: Weakness, paresthesia, skeletal pain, peripheral neuropathy

Ocular: Amblyopia, conjunctivitis, iritis, uveitis, decreased intraocular pressure, ocular hypotony, retinal detachment

Renal: Tubular damage (dose-dependent), elevated BUN and serum creatinine, Fanconi-like syndrome

Respiratory: Asthma, bronchitis, coughing, dyspnea, pharyngitis, pneumonia, rhinitis, sinusitis

Miscellaneous: Diaphoresis, allergic reactions

Drug Interactions Aminoglycosides, amphotericin B, foscarnet, vancomycin, I.V. pentamidine and NSAIDs increase nephrotoxicity (cidofovir is contraindicated in patients who are receiving other nephrotoxic drugs); probenecid may decrease zidovudine clearance (temporarily discontinue zidovudine or decrease its dose by 50% on the days of cidofovir administration only); probenecid reduces the risk of cidofovir-induced nephrotoxicity by decreasing its concentration in proximal tubular cells; ganciclovir ocular implant (increased toxicity)

Stability Store vial at room temperature; cidofovir admixture is stable for 24 hours under refrigeration.

Mechanism of Action Cidofovir is converted to cidofovir diphosphate which is the active intracellular metabolite; suppresses CMV replication by selective inhibition of viral DNA polymerase; incorporation of cidofovir into the growing viral DNA chain results in reduction in the rate of viral DNA synthesis

Pharmacokinetics

Distribution: V_d: 0.54 L/kg; does not cross significantly into the CSF

(Continued)

Cidofovir (Continued)

Protein binding: <6%

Metabolism: Cidofovir is phosphorylated intracellularly to the active metabolite cidofovir diphosphate

Half-life: ~2.6 hours (cidofovir); 17 hours (cidofovir diphosphate)

Elimination: Renal tubular secretion and glomerular filtration

Renal clearance without probenecid: 130-170 mL/minute/1.73 m^2

Renal clearance with probenecid: 70-125 mL/minute/1.73 m^2

Usual Dosage I.V.: Administration of cidofovir must be accompanied by concomitant oral probenecid and intravenous saline hydration

Children: **Note:** Limited information regarding cidofovir use in pediatric patients is currently available in the literature; some centers have used doses of 1 mg/kg/dose 3 times/week for the treatment of adenovirus infection after bone marrow transplantation. Oral probenecid 1.25 g/m^2/dose is administered 3 hours prior to and 1 hour and 8 hours after completion of each 1-hour cidofovir infusion. NS bolus equal to 3 times the maintenance fluid is administered for 1 hour before cidofovir infusion and 1 hour after, then decrease to 2 times the maintenance fluid for the subsequent 2 hours.

Adults: Cytomegalovirus (CMV) retinitis: Administer 2 g probenecid orally 3 hours prior to each cidofovir dose and 1 g at 2 and 8 hours after completion of the cidofovir infusion (total probenecid dose: 4 g); infuse one liter NS over 1-2 hours prior to the cidofovir infusion; may administer second liter of NS over 1-3 hours with or immediately after the cidofovir infusion if tolerated

Induction: 5 mg/kg/dose once weekly for 2 consecutive weeks

Maintenance: 5 mg/kg/dose once every other week

Dosing adjustment in renal impairment: If the serum creatinine increases by 0.3-0.4 mg/dL above baseline, reduce the cidofovir dose to 3 mg/kg; discontinue cidofovir therapy for increases ≥0.5 mg/dL above baseline or development of ≥3+ proteinuria.

Administration Do **not** administer by direct intraocular injection due to risk of iritis, ocular hypotony, and permanent visual impairment.

Parenteral: Administer by I.V. infusion over 1 hour. Dilute in 100 mL NS or D$_5$W or to a final concentration not to exceed 8 mg/mL.

Monitoring Parameters Monitor renal function (BUN, serum creatinine), urinalysis (urine glucose and protein), CBC with differential (neutrophil count), electrolytes (calcium, magnesium, phosphorus, uric acid), liver function tests (SGOT/SGPT), intraocular pressure and visual acuity

Patient Information Cidofovir is not a cure for CMV retinitis; regular follow-up ophthalmologic exams and careful monitoring of renal function are necessary; report any rash immediately to your physician; use contraception during and for 3 months following treatment

Nursing Implications Administration of probenecid with a meal may decrease associated nausea; acetaminophen and antihistamines may ameliorate hypersensitivity reactions. Handle and dispose of cidofovir according to guidelines issued for cytotoxic drugs. Maintain adequate patient hydration.

Dosage Forms Injection, as dihydrate: 75 mg/mL (5 mL single-use vial)

References

Izadifar-legrand F, Berrebi D, Faye A, et al, "Early Diagnosis of Adenovirus Infection and Treatment With Cidofovir After Bone Marrow Transplantation in Children," Blood, 1999, 94:341a.

Lalezari JP, Holland GN, Kramer F, et al, "Randomized, Controlled Study of the Safety and Efficacy of Intravenous Cidofovir for the Treatment of Relapsing Cytomegalovirus Retinitis in Patients With AIDS," J Acquir Immune Defic Syndr Hum Retrovirol, 1998, 17(4):339-44.

Ribaud P, Scieux C, Freymuth F, et al, "Successful Treatment of Adenovirus Disease With Intravenous Cidofovir in an Unrelated Stem-Cell Transplant Recipient," Clinical Infectious Diseases, 1999, 28(3):690-1.

♦ **Cilastatin and Imipenem** see Imipenem and Cilastatin on page 526

♦ **Ciloxan**™ see Ciprofloxacin on page 236

Cimetidine (sye MET i deen)

Related Information

Carbohydrate and Alcohol Content of Liquid Medications for Use in Patients Receiving Ketogenic Diets on page 1258

U.S. Brand Names Tagamet®; Tagamet-HB® [OTC]

Canadian Brand Names Apo-Cimetidine; Gen-Cimetidine; Novo-Cimetine; Nu-Cimet; Peptol; PMS-Cimetidine

Therapeutic Category Gastrointestinal Agent, Gastric or Duodenal Ulcer Treatment; Histamine H$_2$ Antagonist

Generic Available Yes

Use Short-term treatment of active duodenal ulcers and benign gastric ulcers; long-term prophylaxis of duodenal ulcer; gastric hypersecretory states; gastroesophageal reflux (GERD); prevention of upper GI bleeding in critically ill patients; over-the-counter (OTC) formulation for relief of acid indigestion, heartburn, or sour stomach

Pregnancy Risk Factor B

Contraindications Hypersensitivity to cimetidine or any component

Warnings Rapid I.V. administration may cause hypotension or cardiac arrhythmias

Precautions Modify dosage in patients with renal and/or hepatic impairment; multiple drug interactions exist requiring dose modifications of other medications or cimetidine (see Drug Interactions)

Adverse Reactions

Cardiovascular: Bradycardia, hypotension, cardiac arrhythmias (after rapid I.V. administration), tachycardia

Central nervous system: Dizziness, mental confusion, agitation, headache, psychosis, drowsiness, fever

Dermatologic: Rash

Endocrine & metabolic: Gynecomastia

Gastrointestinal: Mild diarrhea, nausea, vomiting

Hematologic: Neutropenia, agranulocytosis, thrombocytopenia

Hepatic: Elevated AST and ALT

Neuromuscular & skeletal: Myalgia

Renal: Elevated serum creatinine

Drug Interactions Cytochrome P-450 isoenzyme CYP1A2, CYP2C9, CYP2C19, CYP2D6, CYP3A3/4, and CYP2C18 inhibitor; isoenzyme CYP3A3/4 substrate

Cimetidine reduces the hepatic metabolism of drugs metabolized by the cytochrome P-450 pathway which may result in decreased elimination of lidocaine, diazepam, theophylline, phenytoin, gabapentin, metronidazole, triamterene, procainamide, quinidine, propranolol, carbamazepine, chloroquine, lomustine, warfarin, flecainide, and tricyclic antidepressants; antacids, metoclopramide, and anticholinergics may reduce the absorption of cimetidine; cimetidine may decrease the absorption of iron, melphalan, indomethacin, ketoconazole, tetracyclines, delavirdine, and possibly fluconazole; cimetidine may decrease digoxin serum levels; may increase diltiazem, flecainide, praziquantel, tacrolimus, cyclosporin, nevirapine, mexiletine, and pentoxifylline serum levels; cimetidine decreases the renal clearance of zalcitabine and zidovudine; potentiates myelosuppressive effects of carmustine; may increase didanosine absorption

Food Interactions Limit xanthine-containing foods and beverages

Stability Protect from light; store at room temperature; do not refrigerate the injection since precipitation may occur (can be redissolved by warming without degradation); stable in parenteral nutrition solutions for up to 7 days when protected from light

Mechanism of Action Competitive inhibition of histamine at H_2-receptors of the gastric parietal cells resulting in reduced gastric acid secretion

Pharmacokinetics

Distribution: Crosses the placenta; breast milk to plasma ratio: 4.6-11.76

Protein binding: 13% to 25%

Bioavailability: 60% to 70%

Half-life:

Neonates: 3.6 hours

Children: 1.4 hours

Adults with normal renal function: 2 hours

Time to peak serum concentration: Oral: Within 1-2 hours

Elimination: Principally as unchanged drug by the kidney; some excretion in bile and feces

Usual Dosage

Neonates: Oral, I.M., I.V.: 5-10 mg/kg/day in divided doses every 8-12 hours

Infants: Oral, I.M., I.V.: 10-20 mg/kg/day divided every 6-12 hours

Children: Oral, I.M., I.V.: 20-40 mg/kg/day in divided doses every 6 hours

Adults:

Short-term treatment of active ulcers:

Oral: 300 mg 4 times/day or 800 mg at bedtime or 400 mg twice daily for up to 8 weeks

I.M., I.V.: 300 mg every 6 hours or 150 mg single dose followed by 37.5 mg/hour by continuous infusion; adjust dosage to maintain an intragastric pH ≥5 or acid secretory rate of <10 mEq/hour; (average dose 160 mg/hour; range: 40-600 mg/hour)

Duodenal ulcer prophylaxis: Oral: 400-800 mg at bedtime

Gastric hypersecretory conditions: Oral, I.M., I.V.: 300-600 mg every 6 hours; dosage not to exceed 2.4 g/day

(Continued)

Cimetidine *(Continued)*

GERD: Oral: 800 mg twice daily or 400 mg 4 times/day for 12 weeks

Acid indigestion, heartburn, sour stomach relief (OTC use): Oral: 100 mg right before or up to 30 minutes before a meal; no more than 2 tablets per day

Prevention of upper GI bleeding: Continuous I.V. infusion of 50 mg/hour

Dosing interval in renal impairment using 5-10 mg/kg/dose in children or 300 mg in adults (titrate dose to gastric pH and Cl_{cr}):

Cl_{cr} >40 mL/minute: Administer every 6 hours

Cl_{cr} 20-40 mL/minute: Administer every 8 hours or reduce dose by 25%

Cl_{cr} <20 mL/minute: Administer every 12 hours or reduce dose by 50%

Hemodialysis: Administer after dialysis and every 12 hours during the interdialysis period

Dosing adjustment in hepatic impairment: Reduce dosage in severe liver disease

Administration

Oral: Administer with food; do not administer with antacids

Parenteral: Can be administered as a slow I.V. push over 15 minutes (minimum 5 minutes; rapid administration has been associated with hypotension and cardiac arrhythmias) at a concentration not to exceed 15 mg/mL; or preferably as an I.V. intermittent or I.V. continuous infusion. Intermittent infusions are administered over 15-30 minutes at a final concentration not to exceed 6 mg/mL; for patients with an active bleed, preferred method of administration is continuous infusion; may be administered intramuscularly

Monitoring Parameters Blood pressure and heart rate with I.V. push administration; CBC; gastric pH

Patient Information Avoid excessive amount of coffee and aspirin; when self medicating, if symptoms of heartburn, acid indigestion, or sour stomach persist after 2 weeks of continuous use of the drug, consult a clinician; notify your physician if taking other medications (multiple drug interactions exist)

Dosage Forms

Infusion, as hydrochloride, in NS: 300 mg (50 mL)

Injection, as hydrochloride: 150 mg/mL (2 mL, 8 mL)

Liquid, oral, as hydrochloride: 300 mg/5 mL with alcohol 2.8% [mint-peach flavor] (5 mL, 240 mL, 480 mL)

Tagamet-HB®: 200 mg/20 mL [cool mint flavor] (355 mL)

Tablet: 200 mg, 300 mg, 400 mg, 800 mg

References

Lambert J, Mobassaleh M, and Grand RJ, "Efficacy of Cimetidine for Gastric Acid Suppression in Pediatric Patients," *J Pediatr*, 1992, 120(3):474-8.

Lloyd CW, Martin WJ, Taylor BD, et al, "Pharmacokinetics and Pharmacodynamics of Cimetidine and Metabolites in Critically Ill Children," *J Pediatr*, 1985, 107(2):295-300.

Lloyd CW, Martin WJ, and Taylor BD, "The Pharmacokinetics of Cimetidine and Metabolites in a Neonate," *Drug Intell Clin Pharm*, 1985, 19(3):203-5.

Somogyi A and Gugler R, "Clinical Pharmacokinetics of Cimetidine," *Clin Pharmacokinet*, 1983, 8(6):463-95.

♦ **Cipro®** *see* Ciprofloxacin *on page 236*

Ciprofloxacin *(sip roe FLOKS a sin)*

U.S. Brand Names Ciloxan™; Cipro®

Therapeutic Category Antibiotic, Ophthalmic; Antibiotic, Quinolone

Generic Available No

Use Treatment of documented or suspected pseudomonal infection of the respiratory or urinary tract, skin and soft tissue, bone and joint, eye and ear; documented multidrug-resistant, aerobic gram-negative bacilli, some gram-positive staphylococci, and *Mycobacterium tuberculosis*; documented infectious diarrhea due to *Campylobacter jejuni*, *Shigella*, or *Salmonella*; osteomyelitis caused by susceptible organisms in which parenteral therapy is not feasible; pulmonary exacerbation of cystic fibrosis; used ophthalmically for treatment of corneal ulcers and conjunctivitis due to susceptible organisms

Pregnancy Risk Factor C

Contraindications Hypersensitivity to ciprofloxacin, any component, or other quinolones; not recommended for use in pregnant women or during breast-feeding

Warnings Not recommended in children <18 years of age; ciprofloxacin has caused arthropathy with erosions of the cartilage in weight bearing joints of immature animals; green discoloration of teeth in newborns has been reported; Achilles tendonitis and tendon rupture have been reported with fluoroquinolones; prolonged use may result in superinfection; CNS stimulation may occur resulting in tremors, restlessness, confusion, and very rarely hallucinations or convulsive seizures

Precautions Use with caution in patients with seizure disorders or renal impairment; modify dosage in patients with renal impairment

Adverse Reactions

Central nervous system: Headache, restlessness, dizziness, confusion, seizures, insomnia, hallucinations

Dermatologic: Rash, photosensitivity, pruritus, urticaria

Gastrointestinal: Nausea, diarrhea, vomiting, GI bleeding, abdominal pain, pseudo-membranous colitis

Genitourinary: Crystalluria

Hematologic: Anemia, eosinophilia, neutropenia

Hepatic: Elevated liver enzymes

Local: With I.V.: Phlebitis, burning, pain, erythema, and swelling (occurs more frequently with infusion time <30 minutes)

Neuromuscular & skeletal: Arthralgia, joint and back pain, tremor, joint stiffness, arthritis, tendonitis

Renal: Elevated BUN and serum creatinine, acute renal failure, interstitial nephritis

Miscellaneous: Anaphylaxis

Drug Interactions Cytochrome P-450 isoenzyme CYP1A2 inhibitor

Magnesium-, aluminum- or calcium-containing antacids and sucralfate decrease ciprofloxacin absorption by up to 90% if given at the same time; antacids in didanosine formulation chelate ciprofloxacin and decrease its absorption (administer ciprofloxacin 2 hours before or 6 hours after didanosine); probenecid decreases renal clearance of ciprofloxacin and can increase ciprofloxacin concentrations; ciprofloxacin decreases theophylline, warfarin, and cyclosporine clearance; NSAID (increase CNS stimulation)

Food Interactions Dairy foods (milk, yogurt) and mineral supplements decrease ciprofloxacin concentrations; ciprofloxacin increases caffeine concentrations; use caution with xanthine-containing foods and beverages

Stability Premixed bags: Out of overwrap stability: 14 days at room temperature; reconstituted oral suspension: Stable for 14 days when stored at room temperature or refrigerated; store tablets at room temperature; protect from intense light

Mechanism of Action Inhibits DNA-gyrase in susceptible organisms; inhibits relaxation of supercoiled DNA and promotes breakage of double-stranded DNA

Pharmacokinetics

Absorption: Oral: Well absorbed

Distribution: Widely distributed into body tissues and fluids with high concentration in bile, urine, sputum, stool, lungs, liver, skin, muscle, and bone; low concentration in CSF; crosses the placenta; appears in breast milk

Protein binding: 16% to 43%

Metabolism: Partially in the liver to active metabolites

Bioavailability: Oral: 50% to 85%; younger CF patients have a lower bioavailability of 68% versus CF patients >13 years of age with bioavailability of 95%

Half-life:

Infants: 2.73 hours

Children:

1-5 years: 1.28 hours

6-12 years: 2.5-2.6 hours

Adults with normal renal function: 3-5 hours

Time to peak serum concentration: Oral: Within 0.5-2 hours

Elimination: 30% to 50% excreted as unchanged drug in urine; 20% to 40% excreted in feces primarily from biliary excretion

Clearance: After I.V.:

CF child: 0.84 L/hour/kg

Adult: 0.5-0.6 L/hour/kg

Dialysis: Only small amounts of ciprofloxacin are removed by dialysis (<10%)

Usual Dosage

Neonates: I.V. ciprofloxacin has been used in 23 neonates at doses ranging from 7-40 mg/kg/day divided every 12 hours (Schaad, 1995)

Children:

Oral: 20-30 mg/kg/day in 2 divided doses; maximum dose: 1.5 g/day

I.V.: 20-30 mg/kg/day divided every 12 hours; maximum dose: 800 mg/day

Cystic fibrosis:

Oral: 40 mg/kg/day divided every 12 hours; maximum dose: 2 g/day

I.V.: 30 mg/kg/day divided every 8-12 hours; maximum dose: 1.2 g/day

Adults:

Oral: 250-750 mg every 12 hours, depending on severity of infection and susceptibility

Chemoprophylaxis regimen for high-risk contacts of invasive meningococcal disease: 500 mg as a single dose

(Continued)

Ciprofloxacin *(Continued)*

Uncomplicated gonorrhea: 500 mg as a single dose

Chancroid: 500 mg twice daily for 3 days

I.V.: 200-400 mg every 12 hours depending on severity of infection

Ophthalmic: Instill 1-2 drops into the affected eye(s) every 2 hours while awake for 2 days, then 1-2 drops every 4 hours while awake for the next 5 days **or** instill $\frac{1}{2}$" ointment ribbon 3 times/day for 2 days, then twice daily for the next 5 days

Treatment of corneal ulcers: Instill 2 drops every 15 minutes for the first 6 hours, then 2 drops every 30 minutes for the remainder of the first day; on the second day, 2 drops every hour; then 2 drops every 4 hours thereafter

Dosing interval in renal impairment: Cl_{cr} <30 mL/minute: Administer every 18-24 hours

Administration

Oral: Administer tablets 2 hours after a meal; may administer with food to minimize GI upset; oral suspension may be administered with or without food; to prepare oral suspension, pour the microcapsules (small bottle) completely into the large bottle of diluent - DO NOT ADD WATER TO THE SUSPENSION. Shake suspension vigorously before use. Avoid antacid use. Drink plenty of fluids to maintain proper hydration and urine output

Parenteral: Administer by slow I.V. infusion over 60 minutes to reduce the risk of venous irritation (burning, pain, erythema, and swelling); final concentration for administration should not exceed 2 mg/mL

Ophthalmic:

Ointment: Instill ointment in the lower conjunctival sac

Solution: Apply finger pressure to lacrimal sac during and for 1-2 minutes after instillation to decrease risk of absorption and systemic effects

Monitoring Parameters Monitor renal, hepatic, and hematopoietic function periodically; number and type of stools/day for diarrhea. Patients receiving concurrent ciprofloxacin and theophylline should have serum levels of theophylline monitored; monitor INR in patients receiving warfarin; patients receiving concurrent ciprofloxacin and cyclosporine should have cyclosporine levels monitored

Reference Range Avoid peak serum concentrations >5 µg/mL

Patient Information Do not chew microcapsules of the oral suspension; avoid caffeine; may cause dizziness or lightheadedness and impair ability to perform activities which require mental alertness; avoid excessive exposure to sunlight; notify physician if tendon pain or swelling occurs; remove contact lenses prior to administration of ophthalmic solution and ointment

Nursing Implications Do not administer antacids with or within 4 hours of a ciprofloxacin dose; ensure adequate patient hydration

Dosage Forms

Infusion, as lactate, in D_5W: 400 mg (200 mL)

Infusion, as lactate, in D_5W: 200 mg (100 mL)

Injection, as lactate: 10 mg/mL (20 mL, 40 mL, 120 mL)

Ointment, ophthalmic, as hydrochloride (Ciloxan™): 0.3% (3.5 g)

Solution, ophthalmic, as hydrochloride (Ciloxan™): 3.5 mg/mL (2.5 mL, 5 mL, 10 mL)

Suspension, oral, as base: 5% (50 mg/mL) [strawberry flavor] (100 mL); 10% (100 mg/mL) [strawberry flavor] (100 mL)

Tablet, as hydrochloride: 100 mg, 250 mg, 500 mg, 750 mg

References

Campoli-Richards DM, Monk JP, Price A, et al, "Ciprofloxacin: A Review of Its Antibacterial Activity, Pharmacokinetic Properties and Therapeutic Use," *Drugs*, 1988, 35(4):373-447.

Rodriguez WJ, and Wiedermann BL, "The Role of Newer Oral Cephalosporins, Fluoroquinolones, and Macrolides in the Treatment of Pediatric Infections," *Adv Pediatr Infect Dis*, 1994, 9:125-59.

Rubio TT, Miles MV, Lettieri JT, et al, "Pharmacokinetic Disposition of Sequential Intravenous/Oral Ciprofloxacin in Pediatric Cystic Fibrosis Patients with Acute Pulmonary Exacerbation," *Pediatr Infect Dis J*, 1997, 16:112-7

Schaad UB, abdus Salam M, Aujard Y, et al, "Use of Fluoroquinolones in Pediatrics: Consensus Report of an International Society of Chemotherapy Commission," *Pediatr Infect Dis J*, 1995, 14(1):1-9.

Ciprofloxacin and Hydrocortisone

(sip roe FLOKS a sin & hye droe KOR ti sone)

Related Information

Ciprofloxacin *on page 236*

Hydrocortisone *on page 506*

U.S. Brand Names Cipro® HC Otic

Therapeutic Category Antibiotic/Corticosteroid, Otic

Generic Available No

Use Treatment of acute bacterial otitis externa due to susceptible strains of *S. aureus*, *P. aeruginosa*, or *Proteus mirabilis*

Contraindications Hypersensitivity to ciprofloxacin, hydrocortisone, any component, or other quinolones; patients with perforated tympanic membrane; patients with viral infections of the external ear canal

Adverse Reactions
Central nervous system: Headache
Dermatologic: Pruritus, fungal dermatitis, rash, urticaria, alopecia
Neuromuscular & skeletal: Paresthesia, hypoesthesia
Respiratory: Cough

Usual Dosage Children ≥1 year and Adults: Otic: Instill 3 drops into the affected ear(s) twice daily for 7 days

Administration Otic: Warm suspension by holding bottle in hand prior to instillation; shake well before use; patient should lie with affected ear upward and maintain position for 30-60 seconds after suspension is instilled into the ear canal

Dosage Forms Suspension, otic: Ciprofloxacin hydrochloride 0.2% and hydrocortisone 1% (10 mL)

♦ **Cipro® HC Otic** *see* Ciprofloxacin and Hydrocortisone *on page 238*

Cisapride *U.S. - Available Via Limited-Access Protocol Only* (SIS a pride)

Related Information
Carbohydrate and Alcohol Content of Liquid Medications for Use in Patients Receiving Ketogenic Diets *on page 1258*

U.S. Brand Names Propulsid®

Therapeutic Category Gastrointestinal Agent, Prokinetic

Generic Available No

Use Treatment of nocturnal symptoms of gastroesophageal reflux disease (GERD), also demonstrated effectiveness for gastroparesis, refractory constipation, and nonulcer dyspepsia in patients failing other therapies (see Warnings)

Pregnancy Risk Factor C

Contraindications Hypersensitivity to cisapride or any component; GI hemorrhage, mechanical obstruction, GI perforation, or other situations when GI motility stimulation is dangerous; patients with CHF, renal failure, multisystem organ failure, and COPD; patients at risk for developing or who have hypokalemia, hypocalcemia, or hypomagnesemia (eg, severe dehydration, vomiting, diarrhea, malnutrition, or receiving chronic diuretic therapy); patients with a known family history of congenital long-QT syndrome; prolonged QT intervals (QT_c >450), ventricular arrhythmias, ischemic heart disease, sinus node dysfunction, clinically significant bradycardia, and second or third degree AV block; patients receiving medications known to prolong the QT interval such as quinidine, procainamide, sotalol, amitriptyline (and other tricyclic antidepressants), maprotiline, phenothiazines, sertindole, astemizole, bepridil, or sparfloxacin, (see Warnings and Drug Interactions); serious cardiac arrhythmias including ventricular tachycardia, ventricular fibrillation, torsade de pointes, and QT prolongations have been reported in patients taking medications which inhibit cytochrome P-450 3A4; some of these events have been fatal; do not coadminister with ketoconazole, itraconazole, fluconazole, miconazole, erythromycin, clarithromycin, nefazodone, delavirdine, indinavir, nelfinavir, ritonavir, saquinavir, or troleandomycin; do not coadminister with grapefruit juice

Warnings Serious cardiac arrhythmias including ventricular tachycardia, ventricular fibrillation, torsade de pointes, and QT prolongation have been reported in patients receiving cisapride; more than 270 cases have been reported including 70 fatalities; 85% of these cases occurred in patients with known risk factors (see Contraindications); for this reason, cisapride is available only for use in patients with severely debilitating conditions who meet specific criteria for a limited-access program directly through Janssen Pharmaceutical Company; for more information contact Janssen at 1-800-Janssen

Precautions Use with caution in neonates, particularly if premature due to a potential increased risk of serious cardiac arrhythmias; decreased cisapride clearance found in neonates may result in increased serum levels; a 12-lead EKG (measuring QT intervals) should be done in all patients before beginning therapy

Adverse Reactions
Cardiovascular: Sinus tachycardia, QT interval prolongation, serious cardiac arrhythmias (see Warnings and Contraindications)
Central nervous system: Headache, insomnia, anxiety, nervousness, confusion
Dermatologic: Rash, pruritus, photosensitivity
Endocrine & metabolic: Hypoglycemia with acidosis, hyperglycemia
Gastrointestinal: Diarrhea, abdominal pain, nausea, flatulence, dyspepsia, constipation, xerostomia
(Continued)

Cisapride *U.S. - Available Via Limited-Access Protocol Only* (Continued)

Genitourinary: Vaginitis (rare), urinary frequency

Hematologic: Thrombocytopenia, leukopenia, aplastic anemia, pancytopenia, hemolytic anemia, methemoglobinemia

Hepatic: Hepatitis, elevated liver enzymes

Neuromuscular & skeletal: Arthralgia, tremor

Respiratory: Rhinitis, sinusitis, cough, apnea

Miscellaneous: Positive ANA

Drug Interactions Cytochrome P-450 isoenzyme CYP3A3/4 substrate

Decreased absorption of digoxin; decreased effect with atropine

Increased effect/toxicity of warfarin, diazepam (increased levels); increased bioavailability of cisapride with cimetidine and ranitidine use

Concomitant administration with ketoconazole has resulted in markedly elevated cisapride plasma concentrations and prolonged QT intervals on the EKG. These prolonged intervals have rarely been associated with serious ventricular arrhythmias and torsade de pointes; some of these adverse reactions have been fatal. Since the interaction is due to a decrease in cytochrome P-450 metabolism induced by ketoconazole, it is expected that similar reactions would occur with itraconazole, miconazole, fluconazole, troleandomycin, delavirdine, indinavir, erythromycin, clarithromycin, nefazodone, nelfinavir, amprenavir, ritonavir, and saquinavir; see Contraindications and Food Interactions

Food Interactions Do not use with grapefruit juice which increases cisapride bioavailability

Mechanism of Action A GI prokinetic agent which enhances the release of acetylcholine at the myenteric plexus. *In vitro* studies have shown cisapride to have serotonin-4 receptor agonistic properties; it has no dopamine receptor blocking activity and, therefore, no extrapyramidal side effects or central antiemetic activity. It increases lower esophageal sphincter pressure, increases the amplitude of peristalsis, accelerates gastric emptying, improves antroduodenal coordination, increases colonic motility, and enhances cecal and ascending colonic emptying.

Pharmacodynamics Onset of effect: 0.5-1 hour

Pharmacokinetics

Distribution: Breast milk to plasma ratio: 0.045

Protein binding: 98%

Metabolism: Extensive in liver via cytochrome P-450 isoenzyme CYP 3A3/4 to norcisapride, which is eliminated in urine and feces

Bioavailability: 40% to 50%

Half-life: 7-10 hours

Elimination: <10% of dose excreted into feces and urine

Usual Dosage Oral:

Neonates: 0.15-0.2 mg/kg/dose 3-4 times/day; maximum dose: 0.8 mg/kg/day

Infants and Children: 0.15-0.3 mg/kg/dose 3-4 times/day; maximum dose: 10 mg/dose

Adults: Initial: 10 mg 4 times/day at least 15 minutes before meals and at bedtime; in some patients the dosage will need to be increased to 20 mg to obtain a satisfactory result

Dosage adjustment in liver dysfunction: Reduce daily dosage by 50%

Administration Oral: Administer 15 minutes before meals or feeding

Monitoring Parameters EKG (prior to beginning therapy), serum electrolytes in patients on diuretic therapy (prior to beginning therapy and periodically thereafter); see Contraindications

Dosage Forms

Suspension: 1 mg/mL [cherry cream flavor] (450 mL)

Tablet: 10 mg, 20 mg

References

Cucchiara S, Staiano A, Boccieri A, et al, "Effects of Cisapride on Parameters of Oesophageal Motility and on the Prolonged Intraoesophageal pH Test in Infants With Gastro-Oesophageal Reflux Disease," *Gut*, 1990, 31(1):21-5.

Hill SL, Evangelista KJ, Pizzi AM, et al, "Proarrhythmia Associated With Cisapride in Children," *Pediatrics*, 1998, 101(6):1053-6.

Khongphatthanayothin A, Lane J, Thomas D, et al, "Effects of Cisapride on QT Interval in Children," *J Pediatr*, 1998, 133(1):51-6.

Lander A, "The Risks and Benefits of Cisapride in Premature Neonates, Infants and Children," *Arch Dis Child*, 1998, 79:469-71.

Lewin MB, Bryant RM, Fenrich AL, et al, "Cisapride-Induced QT Interval," *J Pediatr*, 1996, 128(2):279-81.

Tolia V, "Long-Term Use of Cisapride in Premature Neonates of <34 Weeks Gestational Age," *J Pediatr Gastroenterol Nutr*, 1990, 11:420-2.

Van Eygen M and Van Ravensteyn H, "Effect of Cisapride on Excessive Regurgitation in Infants," *Clin Ther*, 1989, 11(5):669-77.

Cisatracurium (sis a tra KYOO ree um)

U.S. Brand Names Nimbex®

Therapeutic Category Neuromuscular Blocker Agent, Nondepolarizing; Skeletal Muscle Relaxant, Paralytic

Generic Available No

Use Eases endotracheal intubation as an adjunct to general anesthesia and relaxes skeletal muscle during surgery or mechanical ventilation

Pregnancy Risk Factor B

Contraindications Hypersensitivity to cisatracurium or any component

Warnings Maintenance of an adequate airway and respiratory support is critical; 10 mL multiple use vials contain benzyl alcohol as a preservative; avoid use in neonates; due to its intermediate onset of action, it is not recommended for rapid sequence intubation; certain clinical conditions may result in potentiation or antagonism of neuromuscular blockade, see table on next page.

Increased sensitivity in patients with myasthenia gravis, Eaton-Lambert syndrome, resistance to neuromuscular blockade in burn patients (>30% of body) for period of 5-70 days postinjury; resistance to neuromuscular blockade in patients with muscle trauma, denervation, immobilization, infection

Precautions Certain clinical conditions may result in potentiation or antagonism of neuromuscular blockade, see table on next page.

Adverse Reactions

Cardiovascular: Rarely mild histamine release, cardiovascular effects are minimal and transient

Dermatologic: Rash

Respiratory: Bronchospasm

Miscellaneous: Hypersensitivity reactions including anaphylaxis

Drug Interactions See table below.

Stability Protect from light; refrigerate; once removed from refrigerator, stable 21 days even if re-refrigerated; unstable in alkaline solutions; **compatible** with D_5W, D_5NS, and NS; do not dilute in LR; **incompatible** for Y-site administration with propofol or ketorolac; **compatible** for Y-site administration with sufentanil, alfentanil, fentanyl, midazolam, and droperidol.

Potential Drug Interactions

Potentiation	Antagonism
Inhalation anesthetics	Calcium
Desflurane, sevoflurane, enflurane and	Carbamazepine
isoflurane > halothane > nitrous	Phenytoin
oxide	Steroids (chronic administration)
Antibiotics	Theophylline
Aminoglycosides, polymyxins,	Anticholinesterases*
clindamycin, vancomycin	Neostigmine, pyridostigmine,
Magnesium	edrophonium, echothiophate
Antiarrhythmics	ophthalmic solution
Quinidine, procainamide, bretylium, and	Caffeine
possibly lidocaine	Azathioprine
Diuretics	
Furosemide, mannitol, thiazides	
Amphotericin B (secondary to hypokalemia)	
Local anesthetics	
Dantrolene (directly depresses skeletal muscle)	
Beta blockers	
Calcium channel blockers	
Ketamine	
Lithium	
Succinylcholine (when administered prior to nondepolarizing neuromuscular-blocking agent)	
Cyclosporine	

*Can prolong the effects of acetylcholine

(Continued)

Cisatracurium *(Continued)*

Clinical Conditions Affecting Neuromuscular Blockade

Potentiation	Antagonism
Electrolyte abnormalities	Alkalosis
Severe hyponatremia	Hypercalcemia
Severe hypocalcemia	Demyelinating lesions
Severe hypokalemia	Peripheral neuropathies
Hypermagnesemia	Diabetes mellitus
Neuromuscular diseases	
Acidosis	
Acute intermittent porphyria	
Renal failure	
Hepatic failure	

Mechanism of Action Blocks neural transmission at the myoneural junction by binding with cholinergic receptor sites

Pharmacodynamics
  Onset of action: I.V.: Within 2-3 minutes
  Peak effect: Within 3-5 minutes
  Clinical duration: Dose dependent, 35-45 minutes after a single 0.1 mg/kg dose; recovery begins in 20-35 minutes when anesthesia is balanced; recovery is attained in 90% of patients in 25-93 minutes

Pharmacokinetics
  Distribution: V_d: Adults: 0.16 L/kg
  Metabolism: Some metabolites are active; 80% of drug clearance is via a rapid nonenzymatic degradation (Hofmann elimination) in the bloodstream; additional metabolism occurs via ester hydrolysis
  Half-life: 22-31 minutes
  Elimination: <10% of dose excreted as unchanged drug in urine
  Clearance: Adults: 5.1 mL/kg/minute

Usual Dosage I.V.:
  Children 2-12 years: Initial: 0.1 mg/kg followed by maintenance dose of 0.03 mg/kg as needed to maintain neuromuscular blockade
  Children >12 years to Adults: Initial: 0.15-0.2 mg/kg followed by maintenance dose of 0.03 mg/kg 40-65 minutes later or as needed to maintain neuromuscular blockade
  Continuous infusion: Children ≥2 years to Adults: 1-3 mcg/kg/minute (range 0.5-10 mcg/kg/minute) or 0.06-0.18 mg/kg/hour

Administration Parenteral: May be administered without further dilution by rapid I.V. injection over 5-10 seconds; for continuous infusions, dilute to a concentration of 0.1-0.4 mg/mL in D_5W or NS; not for I.M. injection due to tissue irritation

Monitoring Parameters Muscle twitch response to peripheral nerve stimulation, heart rate, blood pressure

Additional Information Neuromuscular blocking potency is 3 times that of atracurium; maximum block is up to 2 minutes longer than for equipotent doses of atracurium; laudanosine, a metabolite without neuromuscular blocking activity has been associated with hypotension and seizure activity in animal studies.

Dosage Forms Injection, as besylate: 2 mg/mL (5 mL, 10 mL); 10 mg/mL (20 mL)

References
Martin LD, Bratton SL, and O'Rourke PP, "Clinical Uses and Controversies of Neuromuscular Blocking Agents in Infants and Children," *Crit Care Med*, 1999, 27(7):1358-68.

Cisplatin *(SIS pla tin)*

Related Information
Emetogenic Potential of Single Chemotherapeutic Agents *on page 1129*
Extravasation Treatment *on page 1085*

U.S. Brand Names Platinol®-AQ

Synonyms CDDP

Therapeutic Category Antineoplastic Agent, Alkylating Agent

Generic Available No

Use Treatment of testicular, ovarian, and breast cancer; advanced bladder cancer, osteosarcoma, Hodgkin's and non-Hodgkin's lymphoma, head or neck cancer, cervical cancer, lung cancer, brain tumors, neuroblastoma; used alone or in combination with other agents

Pregnancy Risk Factor D

Contraindications Hypersensitivity to cisplatin, platinum-containing agents, or any component; pre-existing renal impairment, hearing impairment, and myelosuppression; pregnancy

Warnings The FDA currently recommends that procedures for proper handling and disposal of antineoplastic agents be considered. Cumulative renal toxicity may be severe; dose-related toxicities include myelosuppression, nausea and vomiting; ototoxicity, especially pronounced in children, is manifested by tinnitus or loss of high frequency hearing and occasionally, deafness

Precautions All patients should receive adequate hydration prior to and for 24 hours after cisplatin administration with a sodium chloride-containing intravenous solution to promote chloruresis, with or without mannitol and/or furosemide, to ensure good urine output and decrease the chance of nephrotoxicity; reduce dosage in renal impairment and in infants <6 months of age due to their decreased renal function and renal tubular secretion; serum magnesium, as well as electrolytes, should be monitored before and within 48 hours after cisplatin therapy. Patients who are magnesium-depleted should receive replacement therapy before the start of cisplatin.

Adverse Reactions

Cardiovascular: Bradycardia, arrhythmias, Raynaud's phenomenon

Central nervous system: Seizures, encephalopathy

Dermatologic: Mild alopecia

Endocrine & metabolic: Hypomagnesemia, hypocalcemia, hypokalemia, hypophosphatemia, hyperuricemia

Gastrointestinal: Nausea and vomiting occur in 76% to 100% of patients and is dose-related

Hematologic: Myelosuppression

Hepatic: Elevated liver enzymes

Local: Phlebitis

Neuromuscular & skeletal: Peripheral neuropathy (related to cumulative doses >200 mg/m^2)

Ocular: Papilledema, optic neuritis

Otic: Ototoxicity (especially pronounced in children; hearing loss in the high-frequency range is related to a cumulative dose of cisplatin >400 mg/m^2)

Renal: Nephrotoxicity (damage to the proximal tubules), azotemia, elevated BUN and serum creatinine

Miscellaneous: Anaphylactoid reactions

Drug Interactions Aminoglycosides, amphotericin B, and other nephrotoxic drugs (increase risk of nephrotoxicity); loop diuretics, aminoglycosides (potentiate ototoxicity); synergistic antineoplastic activity with cytarabine, 5-fluorouracil, etoposide; reduces renal elimination of methotrexate

Stability Reconstituted powder for injection is stable for 20 hours at room temperature; do not refrigerate reconstituted solution since precipitation may occur; protect from light; incompatible with sodium bicarbonate; do not infuse in solutions containing <0.2% sodium chloride; stable when combined with mannitol (12.5-50 g mannitol/L)

Mechanism of Action Platination of DNA leads to reactive intermediates that bind to DNA and form intrastrand and interstrand DNA cross-links

Pharmacokinetics

Distribution: I.V.: Rapid tissue distribution; CSF unbound platinum concentration: 40% of the plasma concentration

Protein binding: >90%; only the free (unbound) platinum and parent drug are cytotoxic

Metabolism: Undergoes nonenzymatic metabolism

Half-life, terminal: Children:

Free drug: 1.3 hours

Total platinum: 44 hours

Elimination: ~50% of dose excreted in urine within 5 days in an inactive form

Dialysis: Minimally removed by hemodialysis

Usual Dosage Children and Adults: I.V. (refer to individual protocols): **TO PREVENT POSSIBLE OVERDOSE, VERIFY ANY CISPLATIN DOSE EXCEEDING 120 mg/ m^2 PER COURSE**:

Intermittent dosing schedule: 37-75 mg/m^2 once every 2-3 weeks or 50-100 mg/m^2 over 4-6 hours, once every 21-28 days

Daily dosing schedule: 15-20 mg/m^2/day for 5 days every 3-4 weeks

Osteogenic sarcoma or neuroblastoma: 60-100 mg/m^2 on day 1 every 3-4 weeks

Recurrent brain tumors: 60 mg/m^2 once daily for 2 consecutive days every 3-4 weeks

(Continued)

Cisplatin *(Continued)*

Bone marrow/blood cell transplantation: Continuous infusion: High dose: 55 mg/m^2/day for 72 hours; total dose = 165 mg/m^2

Dosing adjustment in renal impairment:

Cl$_{cr}$ 10-50 mL/minute: Administer 75% of dose

Cl$_{cr}$ <10 mL/minute: Administer 50% of dose

Administration Parenteral: I.V.: Administer according to protocol; rate of administration has varied from a 15- to 20-minute infusion, 1 mg/minute infusion, 6- to 8-hour infusion or 24-hour infusion; rapid I.V. injection may be associated with increased nephrotoxicity or ototoxicity compared to a slower I.V. infusion

Monitoring Parameters Renal function tests (serum creatinine, BUN, Cl$_{cr}$), electrolytes (particularly magnesium, calcium, potassium), hearing test, neurologic exam (with high dose), liver function tests periodically, CBC with differential and platelet count, urine output, urinalysis

Nursing Implications Needles, syringes, catheters, or I.V. administration sets that contain aluminum parts should not be used for administration of drug; methods to prevent nephrotoxicity include prehydration, diuresis with mannitol, and administration of hypertonic sodium chloride solutions to promote chloruresis. Adequate hydration and urinary output should be maintained for 24 hours after administration.

Additional Information Myelosuppressive effects:

WBC: Mild

Platelets: Mild

Onset (days): 10

Nadir (days): 18-23

Recovery (days): 21-40

Dosage Forms Injection, aqueous: 1 mg/mL (50 mL, 100 mL)

References

Costello MA, Dominick C, and Clerico A, "A Pilot Study of 5-Day Continuous Infusion of High-Dose Cisplatin and Pulsed Etoposide in Childhood Solid Tumors," *Am J Pediatr Hematol Oncol*, 1988, 10:103-8.

Reece PA, Stafford I, Abbott RL, et al, "Two-Versus 24-Hour Infusion of Cisplatin: Pharmacokinetic Considerations," *J Clin Oncol*, 1989, 7(2):270-5.

♦ **13-*cis*-Retinoic Acid** *see* Isotretinoin *on page 557*

♦ **Citracal® [OTC]** *see* Calcium Supplements *on page 167*

♦ **Citracal® Liquitab [OTC]** *see* Calcium Supplements *on page 167*

Citrate and Citric Acid *(SIT rate & SIT rik AS id)*

Related Information

Carbohydrate and Alcohol Content of Liquid Medications for Use in Patients Receiving Ketogenic Diets *on page 1258*

U.S. Brand Names Bicitra®; Cytra-3®; Cytra-K®; Oracit®; Polycitra®; Polycitra K®; Polycitra-LC®; Urocit®-K

Synonyms Citrate/Citric Acid; Citric Acid and Citrate; Shohl's Solution, Modified

Therapeutic Category Alkalinizing Agent, Oral

Generic Available No

Use Treatment of metabolic acidosis; alkalinizing agent in conditions where long-term maintenance of an alkaline urine is desirable

Potassium citrate: Prevention of uric acid nephrolithiasis, prevention of calcium renal stones in patients with hypocitraturia; urinary alkalizer when sodium citrate is contraindicated

Pregnancy Risk Factor C

Contraindications Patients receiving sodium-restricted diet (sodium salts); severe renal impairment with oliguria, azotemia, or anuria; untreated Addison's disease, acute dehydration, heat cramps, severe myocardial damage, hyperkalemia (potassium salts); Urocit®-K (wax matrix tablet) is contraindicated in patients with delayed gastric emptying, intestinal obstruction, or stricture, patients receiving anticholinergic medications and in patients with peptic ulcer disease

Warnings Conversion to bicarbonate may be impaired in patients with hepatic failure, in shock, or who are severely ill

Precautions Use sodium salts with caution in patients with CHF, hypertension, pulmonary edema; may predispose patient to urolithiasis

Adverse Reactions

Central nervous system: Tetany

Endocrine & metabolic: Metabolic alkalosis, hypernatremia (if sodium salt used), hypocalcemia, hyperkalemia (if potassium salt used)

Gastrointestinal: Diarrhea, nausea, vomiting, stenotic or ulcerative lesions (wax matrix tablets)

Drug Interactions

Decreased effect/levels of chlorpropamide, lithium, methenamine, methotrexate, salicylates, and tetracycline due to urinary alkalinization

Increased toxicity/levels of amphetamines, flecainide, ephedrine, pseudoephedrine, quinidine, and quinine due to urinary alkalinization

Potassium-sparing diuretics, salt substitutes, captopril, and enalapril may result in increased serum potassium (potassium-containing salt forms only)

Mechanism of Action Citrate salts are oxidized in the body to form bicarbonate

Usual Dosage Oral (dilute in water or juice):

Infants and Children: 2-3 mEq/kg/day in divided doses 3-4 times/day **or** 5-15 mL with water after meals and at bedtime

Adults:

Solution: 15-30 mL with water after meals and at bedtime

Wax matrix tablet (Urocit®-K): 30-60 mEq/day in divided doses 3-4 times/day

Administration Oral: Dilute with water or juice and administer after meals; do not crush or chew wax matrix tablets (Urocit®-K)

Monitoring Parameters Serum sodium, bicarbonate, potassium, urine pH

Dosage Forms

Solution, oral:

Bicitra® (alcohol free): Sodium citrate 500 mg and citric acid 334 mg per 5 mL **(1 mEq sodium and 1 mEq bicarbonate equivalent per mL)** (15 mL unit dose, 30 mL unit dose, 480 mL)

Cytra-3® (sugar free): Potassium citrate 550 mg, sodium citrate 500 mg and citric acid 334 mg per 5 mL **(1 mEq potassium and 1 mEq sodium per mL, equivalent to 2 mEq bicarbonate)** (480 mL)

Oracit®: Sodium citrate 490 mg and citric acid 640 mg per 5 mL **(1 mEq sodium and 1 mEq bicarbonate equivalent per mL)** (15 mL unit dose, 30 mL unit dose, 480 mL, 4000 mL)

Polycitra® (alcohol free): Sodium citrate 500 mg and citric acid 334 mg with potassium citrate 550 mg per 5 mL **(1 mEq potassium, 1 mEq sodium, 2 mEq bicarbonate equivalent per mL)** (480 mL)

Polycitra-LC® (alcohol free and sugar free): Potassium citrate monohydrate 550 mg, sodium citrate dihydrate 500 mg, citric acid monohydrate 334 mg per 5 mL **(1 mEq potassium, 1 mEq sodium, 2 mEq bicarbonate equivalent per mL)** (480 mL)

Cytra-K®, Polycitra K® (alcohol free): Crystals and solution: Potassium citrate monohydrate 1100 mg, citric acid monohydrate 334 mg per 5 mL **(2 mEq potassium and 2 mEq bicarbonate equivalent per mL)** (473 mL)

Tablet, extended release (Urocit®-K): Potassium citrate monohydrate: 5 mEq, 10 mEq

Cladribine (KLA dri been)

U.S. Brand Names Leustatin™

Synonyms 2-CdA; 2-Chlorodeoxyadenosine

Therapeutic Category Antineoplastic Agent, Antimetabolite (Purine)

Use Treatment of hairy cell leukemia, chronic myeloid leukemia, and chronic lymphocytic leukemia; cladribine has activity in the treatment of Langerhans cell histiocytosis (LCH), non-Hodgkin's lymphomas, T-cell lymphomas, relapsed acute lymphocytic leukemia and relapsed acute myeloid leukemia

Pregnancy Risk Factor D

Contraindications Hypersensitivity to cladribine or any component

Warnings The FDA currently recommends that procedures for proper handling and disposal of antineoplastic agents be considered. Serious neurological toxicity has been reported in patients who received cladribine by continuous infusion at high doses (0.4-0.8 mg/kg/day or >16 mg/m^2/day); neurologic toxicity appears to be dose-related. Severe neurologic toxicity has been reported rarely with standard dosing regimens. Acute nephrotoxicity has been observed with cladribine doses of 0.4-0.8 mg/kg/day, especially in patients concurrently receiving other nephrotoxic agents.

(Continued)

Cladribine *(Continued)*

Precautions Dose-limiting toxicity is myelosuppression; use with caution in patients with pre-existing hematologic or immunologic abnormalities; prophylactic administration of allopurinol should be considered in patients receiving cladribine due to the potential for hyperuricemia secondary to tumor lysis; appropriate antibiotic therapy should be administered promptly in patients exhibiting signs and symptoms of neutropenia and infection.

Adverse Reactions

Cardiovascular: Edema, tachycardia

Central nervous system: Fever (69%), fatigue (45%), headache, dizziness, insomnia, malaise, irreversible neurologic toxicity (paraparesis/quadriparesis) at high doses (0.4-0.8 mg/kg/day or >16 mg/m^2/day)

Dermatologic: Pruritus, erythema, rash

Gastrointestinal: Constipation, abdominal pain, nausea, vomiting, decreased appetite, diarrhea

Hematologic: Myelosuppression (prolonged pancytopenia), aplastic anemia, hemolytic anemia

Hepatic: Reversible, mild elevations of bilirubin and transaminase levels

Local: Injection site reactions, pain

Neuromuscular & skeletal: Myalgia, trunk pain

Renal: Acute nephrotoxicity reported at high doses (rare)

Respiratory: Abnormal breath sounds, cough, shortness of breath

Stability Refrigerate unopened vials (2°C to 8°C/36°F to 46°F); protect from light. Solutions should be administered immediately after the initial dilution or stored in the refrigerator (2°C to 8°C) for ≤8 hours. **The use of D$_5$W as a diluent is not recommended due to increased degradation of cladribine;** should not be mixed with other intravenous drugs or additives or infused simultaneously via a common intravenous line. Diluted solution of cladribine in NS is stable for 24 hours at room temperature under normal room light in polyvinyl chloride infusion containers.

Mechanism of Action A purine nucleoside analogue; prodrug which enters the cells through a transport system and is activated via phosphorylation by deoxycytidine kinase to a 5'-triphosphate derivative. This active form incorporates into DNA resulting in inhibition of DNA synthesis and early chain termination. The induction of strand breaks results in a drop in the cofactor nicotinamide adenine dinucleotide and disruption of cell metabolism. ATP is depleted to deprive cells of an important source of energy. Cladribine kills both resting as well as dividing cells.

Pharmacokinetics

Distribution: V$_d$:

Children: 305 L/m^2

Adults: 0.5-9 L/kg (53-160 L/m^2)

CSF: Plasma concentration ratio: 18.2%

Protein binding: 20%

Bioavailability: S.C.: 100%

Half-life: 19.7 hours ± 3.4 hours; (range: 14.3-25.8 hours)

Elimination: 21% to 44% renally excreted

Usual Dosage I.V.: (refer to individual protocols):

Children:

Hairy cell leukemia: 0.09 mg/kg/day continuous infusion for 7 days

AML:

<3 years: 0.3 mg/kg/day over 2 hours daily for 5 days

≥3 years: 9 mg/m^2/day over 2 hours daily for 5 days

Langerhans cell histiocytosis: 5-10 mg/m^2/day over 2 hours daily for 5 days; do not administer if platelet count <100,000

Adults: 0.09-0.1 mg/kg/day continuous infusion for 7 consecutive days

Administration Parenteral: I.V.: **Single daily infusion:** May administer diluted in NS as an intermittent infusion or continuous infusion; administer through a 0.22 micron in-line filter

Monitoring Parameters CBC with differential and platelet count; creatinine clearance before initial dose; periodic renal and hepatic function tests

Nursing Implications Cladribine I.V. solution for administration should be inspected visually for particulates. A precipitate may occur at low temperatures and may be resolubilized at room temperature or by shaking the solution vigorously.

Dosage Forms Injection, preservative free: 1 mg/mL (10 mL)

References

Kearns CM, Biakley RL, Santane VM, et al, "Pharmacokinetics of Cladribine (2-Chlorodeoxyadenosine) in Children with Acute Leukemia," *Cancer Research*, 1994, 54:1235-39.

Larson RA, et al, "Dose Escalation Trial of Cladribine Using 5 Daily I.V. Infusions in Patients with Advanced Hematologic Malignancies," *J Clin Oncol*, 1996, 14(1):188-95.

Liliemark J, "The Clinical Pharmacokinetics of Cladribine," *Clin Pharmacokinet*, 1997, 32:120-131.

Stine KC, Saylors RL, Williams LL, et al, "2-Chlorodeoxyadenosine (2-CDA) for the Treatment of Refractory or Recurrent Langerhans Cell Histiocytosis (LCH) in Pediatric Patients," *Med Pediatr Oncol*, 1997, 29:288-92.

♦ **Claforan**® *see* Cefotaxime *on page 195*

Clarithromycin (kla RITH roe mye sin)

Related Information
Carbohydrate and Alcohol Content of Liquid Medications for Use in Patients Receiving Ketogenic Diets *on page 1258*
Endocarditis Prophylaxis *on page 1160*

U.S. Brand Names Biaxin®; Biaxin® XL

Therapeutic Category Antibiotic, Macrolide

Generic Available No

Use Treatment of upper and lower respiratory tract infections, acute otitis media, and infections of the skin and skin structure due to susceptible strains of *S. aureus*, *S. pyogenes*, *S. pneumoniae*, *H. influenzae*, *M. catarrhalis*, *Mycoplasma pneumoniae*, *C. trachomatis*, and *Legionella* sp; prophylaxis and treatment of *Mycobacterium avium* complex (MAC) disease in patients with advanced HIV infection; treatment of *Helicobacter pylori* infection; prophylaxis of bacterial endocarditis in penicillin-allergic patients

Pregnancy Risk Factor C

Contraindications Hypersensitivity to clarithromycin, any component, erythromycin, or any macrolide antibiotics; concomitant administration of terfenadine, astemizole, or cisapride with clarithromycin may result in QT interval prolongation, ventricular tachycardia, ventricular fibrillation, hypotension, palpitations, cardiac arrest, and death

Warnings Safety and efficacy of clarithromycin have not been established in children <6 months of age; pseudomembranous colitis has been reported with use of clarithromycin

Precautions Use with caution in patients with hepatic or renal impairment; reduce dosage or prolong dosing interval in patients with severe renal impairment with or without coexisting hepatic impairment

Adverse Reactions
Central nervous system: Headache, hallucinations
Dermatologic: Pruritus, rash, Stevens-Johnson syndrome
Gastrointestinal: Diarrhea, nausea, vomiting, abdominal pain, dysgeusia, stomatitis; incidence of adverse GI effects (diarrhea, nausea, vomiting, dyspepsia, abdominal pain) is lower (13%) compared to erythromycin treated patients (32%)
Hematologic: Increased prothrombin time, decreased WBC
Hepatic: Elevated liver enzymes, hyperbilirubinemia
Otic: Hearing loss
Renal: Elevated BUN and serum creatinine

Drug Interactions Cytochrome P-450 isoenzyme CYP3A3/4 substrate; CYP1A2 and CYP3A3/4 isoenzyme inhibitor
Clarithromycin has been shown to increase serum **theophylline** levels by as much as 20%; **carbamazepine** levels have been shown to increase after a single dose of clarithromycin; hepatic metabolism of terfenadine, astemizole, and cisapride are reduced by clarithromycin (see Contraindications); increases serum level of digoxin, cyclosporine, tacrolimus, ergot alkaloids, omeprazole, lovastatin, simvastatin, and triazolam; potentiates the effects of warfarin; fluconazole and ritonavir increase serum level of clarithromycin; efavirenz decreases clarithromycin levels while increasing the levels of its metabolite

Food Interactions Food may delay the rate but not the extent of oral absorption

Stability Reconstituted oral suspension should **not** be refrigerated because it might gel; microencapsulated particles of clarithromycin in suspension is stable for 14 days when stored at room temperature

Mechanism of Action Inhibits bacterial RNA-dependent protein synthesis by binding to the 50S ribosomal subunit; the 14-hydroxy metabolite of clarithromycin is twice as active as the parent compound

Pharmacokinetics
Absorption: Rapid from the GI tract; food delays onset of absorption and formation of active metabolite, but does not affect the extent of tablet absorption; in pediatric patients, coadministration of the suspension with food did not significantly alter the extent of clarithromycin absorption or formation of the 14-OH metabolite
Distribution: Widely distributed throughout the body with tissue concentrations higher than serum concentrations
Protein binding: 65% to 70%
(Continued)

Clarithromycin *(Continued)*

Metabolism: In the liver to active and inactive metabolites; undergoes extensive first-pass metabolism

Bioavailability: 50% to 68%

Half-life: Dose-dependent, prolonged with renal dysfunction

Clarithromycin:
- 250 mg dose: 3-4 hours
- 500 mg dose: 5-7 hours

14-hydroxy metabolite:
- 250 mg dose: 5-6 hours
- 500 mg dose: 7 hours

Time to peak serum concentration: 1-4 hours

Elimination: After a 250 mg dose, 20% is excreted unchanged in urine, 10% to 15% is excreted as active metabolite 14-OH clarithromycin, and 4% is excreted in feces

Usual Dosage Oral:

Infants and Children:

Acute otitis media: 15 mg/kg/day divided every 12 hours for 10 days

Respiratory, skin and skin structure infections: 15 mg/kg/day divided every 12 hours for 7-14 days

Prophylaxis for bacterial endocarditis: 15 mg/kg 1 hour before procedure

Prophylaxis for first episode of MAC with the following CD4+ T-lymphocyte counts (see below): 15 mg/kg/day divided every 12 hours; maximum dose: 1 g/day

Children <12 months: <750 cells/μL
- 1-2 years: <500 cells/μL
- 2-6 years: <75 cells/μL
- ≥6 years: <50 cells/μL

Prophylaxis for recurrence of MAC: 15 mg/kg/day divided every 12 hours; maximum dose: 1 g/day (use in combination with ethambutol and with or without rifabutin)

Adolescents and Adults: 250 mg every 12 hours for 7-14 days for all indications except sinusitis and chronic bronchitis due to *H. influenzae*; for these indications, 500 mg every 12 hours for 7-14 days

Prophylaxis for bacterial endocarditis: 500 mg 1 hour before procedure

Prophylaxis for first episode of MAC in patients with CD4+ T-lymphocyte count <50 cells/μL: 500 mg twice daily

Prophylaxis for recurrence of MAC: 500 mg twice daily in combination with ethambutol and with or without rifabutin

Helicobacter pylori (combination therapy with omeprazole or with bismuth subsalicylate, tetracycline, and an H₂-receptor antagonist): 250 mg twice daily up to 500 mg 3 times/day

Dosing adjustment in renal impairment: Cl$_{cr}$ <30 mL/minute: Decrease dose by 50% and administer once or twice daily

Administration Oral: May administer with or without meals; may administer with milk; shake suspension well before use

Monitoring Parameters Monitor serum concentration of other drugs in patients receiving clarithromycin and drugs known to interact with erythromycin (ie, theophylline, digoxin, anticoagulants, triazolam) since there are still very few studies examining drug-drug interactions with clarithromycin; liver function tests; hearing (in patients receiving long-term treatment with clarithromycin); observe for changes in bowel frequency

Dosage Forms

Granules for suspension, oral: 125 mg/5 mL (50 mL, 100 mL); 250 mg/5 mL (50 mL, 100 mL)

Tablet, film coated: 250 mg, 500 mg

Tablet, extended release: 500 mg

References

Aspin MM, Hoberman A, McCarty J, et al, "Comparative Study of the Safety and Efficacy of Clarithromycin and Amoxicillin-Clavulanate in the Treatment of Acute Otitis Media in Children," *J Pediatr*, 1994, 125(1):136-41.

Guay DR and Craft JC, "Overview of the Pharmacology of Clarithromycin Suspension in Children and a Comparison With That in Adults," *Pediatr Infect Dis J*, 1993, 12(12 Suppl 3):S106-11.

Husson RN, Ross LA, Sandelli S, et al, "Orally Administered Clarithromycin for the Treatment of Systemic *Mycobacterium avium* Complex Infection in Children With Acquired Immunodeficiency Syndrome," *J Pediatr*, 1994, 124(5 Pt 1):807-14.

Neu HC, "The Development of Macrolides: Clarithromycin in Perspective," *J Antimicrob Chemother*, 1991, 27(Suppl A):1-9.

"1999 USPHS/IDSA Guidelines for the Prevention of Opportunistic Infections in Persons Infected With Human Immunodeficiency Virus. USPHS/IDSA Prevention of Opportunistic Infections Working Group," *MMWR Morb Mortal Wkly Rep*, 1999, 48(RR-10):1-66.

♦ **Claritin**® *see* Loratadine *on page 608*

♦ **Claritin® RediTab®** *see* Loratadine *on page 608*
♦ **Clavulanate Potassium and Ticarcillin** *see* Ticarcillin and Clavulanate Potassium *on page 960*
♦ **Clavulanic Acid and Amoxicillin** *see* Amoxicillin and Clavulanic Acid *on page 81*
♦ **Clavulin (Can)** *see* Amoxicillin and Clavulanic Acid *on page 81*
♦ **Clean & Clear Deep Cleaning Astringent (Can)** *see* Salicylic Acid *on page 886*
♦ **Clean & Clear Invisible Blemish (Can)** *see* Salicylic Acid *on page 886*
♦ **Clearasil B.P. Plus (Can)** *see* Benzoyl Peroxide *on page 136*
♦ **Clearasil Cleanser (Can)** *see* Salicylic Acid *on page 886*
♦ **Clearasil Clearstick (Can)** *see* Salicylic Acid *on page 886*
♦ **Clearasil Pads (Can)** *see* Salicylic Acid *on page 886*
♦ **Clear By Design® Gel [OTC]** *see* Benzoyl Peroxide *on page 136*
♦ **Clear & Clean Persa (Can)** *see* Benzoyl Peroxide *on page 136*
♦ **Clear Eyes® [OTC]** *see* Naphazoline *on page 698*
♦ **Clear Eyes® ACR [OTC]** *see* Naphazoline *on page 698*
♦ **Clear Pore Treatment (Can)** *see* Salicylic Acid *on page 886*
♦ **Clearsil® Maximum Strength [OTC]** *see* Benzoyl Peroxide *on page 136*
♦ **Clearskin Medicated Wash (Can)** *see* Salicylic Acid *on page 886*
♦ **Clearskin Overnight Acne Treatment (Can)** *see* Salicylic Acid *on page 886*

Clemastine (KLEM as teen)
Related Information
Carbohydrate and Alcohol Content of Liquid Medications for Use in Patients Receiving Ketogenic Diets *on page 1258*
Drugs and Breast-Feeding *on page 1243*
U.S. Brand Names Tavist®; Tavist®-1 [OTC]
Synonyms Meclastine; Mecloprodin
Therapeutic Category Antihistamine
Generic Available Yes
Use Perennial and seasonal allergic rhinitis and other allergic symptoms including urticaria
Pregnancy Risk Factor C
Contraindications Narrow-angle glaucoma; hypersensitivity to clemastine or any component; patients receiving MAO inhibitors
Precautions Use with caution in patients with stenosing peptic ulcer, GI or GU obstruction, asthma, or prostatic hypertrophy
Adverse Reactions
Cardiovascular: Bradycardia, edema, palpitations
Central nervous system: Drowsiness, fatigue, headache, dizziness, vertigo, ataxia, CNS stimulation (more common in children)
Dermatologic: Rash, angioedema, photosensitivity
Gastrointestinal: Nausea, vomiting, xerostomia, gastritis, appetite increase, weight gain, diarrhea, abdominal pain
Hepatic: Hepatitis
Neuromuscular & skeletal: Arthralgia, myalgia, paresthesia
Respiratory: Shortness of breath, pharyngitis, bronchospasm, epistaxis
Drug Interactions Increased toxicity (CNS depression or excessive anticholinergic activity): CNS depressants, MAO inhibitors, tricyclic antidepressants, phenothiazines
Mechanism of Action Competes with histamine for H_1-receptor sites on effector cells in the GI tract, blood vessels, and respiratory tract
Pharmacodynamics
Onset of effect: 2 hours after administration
Peak effect: 5-7 hours
Duration of action: 10-12 hours
Pharmacokinetics
Absorption: Oral: Well absorbed
Distribution: Breast milk to plasma ratio: 0.25-0.5
Metabolism: In the liver
Time to peak serum concentration: 2-4 hours
Elimination: Majority of an oral dose eliminated in the urine
Usual Dosage Oral:
Infants and Children <6 years: 0.05 mg/kg/day as **clemastine base** or 0.335-0.67 mg/day clemastine fumarate (0.25-0.5 mg base/day) divided into two or three doses; maximum daily dosage: 1.34 mg (1 mg base)
(Continued)

Clemastine (Continued)

Children 6-12 years: 0.67-1.34 mg clemastine fumarate (0.5-1 mg base) twice daily; do not exceed 4.02 mg/day (3 mg/day base)

Children ≥12 years and Adults: 1.34 mg clemastine fumarate (1 mg base) twice daily to 2.68 mg (2 mg base) 3 times/day; do not exceed 8.04 mg/day (6 mg base)

Administration Oral: Administer with food

Monitoring Parameters Look for a reduction of rhinitis, urticaria, eczema, pruritus, or other allergic symptoms

Patient Information Avoid alcohol; may cause drowsiness and impair ability to perform hazardous activities requiring mental alertness or physical coordination

Dosage Forms

Syrup, as fumarate: 0.67 mg/5 mL (0.5 mg base/5 mL) with alcohol 5.5% (120 mL)

Tablet, as fumarate: 1.34 mg (1 mg base), 2.68 mg (2 mg base)

- ◆ **Cleocin®** *see* Clindamycin *on page 250*
- ◆ **Cleocin T®** *see* Clindamycin *on page 250*
- ◆ **Climara®** *see* Estradiol *on page 400*
- ◆ **Clinacort®** *see* Triamcinolone *on page 979*
- ◆ **Clinda-Derm®** *see* Clindamycin *on page 250*

Clindamycin (klin da MYE sin)

Related Information

Carbohydrate and Alcohol Content of Liquid Medications for Use in Patients Receiving Ketogenic Diets *on page 1258*

Endocarditis Prophylaxis *on page 1160*

U.S. Brand Names Cleocin®; Cleocin T®; Clinda-Derm®; Clindets®

Canadian Brand Names Dalacin C; Dalacin T; Dalacin Vaginal

Therapeutic Category Acne Products; Antibiotic, Anaerobic; Antibiotic, Miscellaneous

Generic Available Yes

Use Useful agent against most aerobic gram-positive staphylococci and streptococci (except enterococci); useful against *Fusobacterium*, *Bacteroides* sp and *Actinomyces* for treatment of respiratory tract infections, skin and soft tissue infections, sepsis, intra-abdominal infections, and infections of the female pelvis and genital tract; bacterial endocarditis prophylaxis for dental and upper respiratory procedures in penicillin-allergic patients; treatment of babesiosis; used topically in treatment of severe acne; used intravaginally for treatment of bacterial vaginosis

Pregnancy Risk Factor B

Contraindications Hypersensitivity to clindamycin or any component; previous pseudomembranous colitis, hepatic impairment

Warnings Can cause severe and possibly fatal colitis characterized by severe persistent diarrhea, severe abdominal cramps and possibly, the passage of blood and mucus; discontinue drug if significant diarrhea occurs

Precautions Use with caution and modify dosage in patients with severe renal and/or hepatic impairment

Adverse Reactions

Cardiovascular: Hypotension, cardiac arrest (with rapid I.V. administration); arrhythmia due to QT_c prolongation

Dermatologic: Urticaria, rash, Stevens-Johnson syndrome

Gastrointestinal: Diarrhea, nausea, vomiting, pseudomembranous colitis, esophagitis

Hematologic: Eosinophilia, granulocytopenia, thrombocytopenia

Hepatic: Elevated liver enzymes

Local: Sterile abscess at I.M. injection site; thrombophlebitis, erythema, pain, swelling

Renal: Rare: Renal dysfunction

Drug Interactions Cytochrome P-450 isoenzyme CYP3A3/4 substrate

Clindamycin may increase the neuromuscular blocking action of tubocurarine, pancuronium

Stability Do **not** refrigerate the reconstituted oral solution because it will thicken; oral solution stable for 2 weeks at room temperature following reconstitution; I.V. clindamycin is incompatible with aminophylline, tobramycin

Mechanism of Action Reversibly binds to 50S ribosomal subunits preventing peptide bond formation thus inhibiting bacterial protein synthesis; bacteriostatic or bactericidal depending on drug concentration, infection site, and organism

Pharmacokinetics

Absorption:

Oral: 90% of clindamycin hydrochloride is rapidly absorbed; clindamycin palmitate must be hydrolyzed in the GI tract before it is active

Topical: ~10% absorbed systemically

Distribution: No significant levels are seen in CSF, even with inflamed meninges; crosses the placenta; distributes into breast milk, saliva, ascites fluid, pleural fluid, bone, and bile

Protein binding: 94%

Bioavailability: Oral: ~90%

Half-life:

Neonates:

Premature: 8.7 hours

Full-term: 3.6 hours

Infants 1 month to 1 year: 3 hours

Children and Adults with normal renal function: 2-3 hours

Time to peak serum concentration:

Oral: Within 60 minutes

I.M.: Within 1-3 hours

Elimination: Most of the drug is eliminated by hepatic metabolism; 10% of an oral dose excreted in urine and 3.6% excreted in feces as active drug and metabolites

Dialysis: Not dialyzable (0% to 5%)

Usual Dosage

Neonates: I.M., I.V.:

Postnatal age ≤7 days:

≤2000 g: 10 mg/kg/day divided every 12 hours

>2000 g: 15 mg/kg/day divided every 8 hours

Postnatal age >7 days:

<1200 g: 10 mg/kg/day divided every 12 hours

1200-2000 g: 15 mg/kg/day divided every 8 hours

>2000 g: 20-30 mg/kg/day divided every 6-8 hours

Infants and Children:

Oral: 10-30 mg/kg/day divided every 6-8 hours; maximum dose: 1.8 g/day

I.M., I.V.: 25-40 mg/kg/day divided every 6-8 hours; maximum dose: 4.8 g/day

Bacterial endocarditis prophylaxis for dental and upper respiratory procedures in penicillin allergic patients:

Oral: 20 mg/kg 1 hour before procedure **or** I.V.: 20 mg/kg 30 minutes before procedure; maximum dose: 600 mg

Babesiosis: Oral: 20-40 mg/kg/day divided every 8 hours for 7 days plus quinine

Children and Adults: Topical: Apply twice daily

Adolescents and Adults:

Oral: 150-450 mg/dose every 6-8 hours; maximum dose: 1.8 g/day

I.M., I.V.: 1.2-1.8 g/day in 2-4 divided doses; maximum dose: 4.8 g/day

Vaginal: One full applicator (100 mg) inserted intravaginally once daily before bedtime for seven consecutive days

Bacterial endocarditis prophylaxis for dental and upper respiratory procedures in penicillin allergic patients:

Oral: 600 mg 1 hour before procedure **or** I.V.: 600 mg 30 minutes before procedure

Pelvic inflammatory disease: 900 mg I.V. every 8 hours for 24-48 hours after significant clinical improvement, followed by 600 mg orally 3 times/day to complete a 14-day course

Babesiosis:

I.V.: 1.2 g twice daily plus quinine

or

Oral: 600 mg 3 times/day for 7 days plus quinine

Dosing interval in renal/hepatic impairment: Reduce dosage in patients with severe renal or hepatic impairment

Administration

Intravaginal: Do not use for topical therapy, instillation in the eye, or oral administration

Oral: Capsule should be taken with a full glass of water to avoid esophageal irritation; shake oral solution well before use; may administer with or without meals

Parenteral: Administer by I.V. intermittent infusion over at least 10-60 minutes, at a rate **not** to exceed 30 mg/minute; hypotension and cardiopulmonary arrest have been reported following rapid I.V. administration; final concentration for administration should not exceed 18 mg/mL

Topical: Do not use intravaginally, instill in the eye, or administer orally

(Continued)

Clindamycin (Continued)

Monitoring Parameters Observe for changes in bowel frequency; during prolonged therapy monitor CBC, liver and renal function tests periodically

Patient Information Report any severe diarrhea immediately; clindamycin vaginal cream (oil-based) may weaken latex condoms for up to 72 hours after completing therapy

Dosage Forms

Capsule, as hydrochloride (Cleocin®): 75 mg, 150 mg, 300 mg

Cream, vaginal, as phosphate (Cleocin®): 2% (40 g)

Gel, topical, as phosphate (Cleocin T®): 1% (30 g)

Granules for oral solution, as palmitate (Cleocin® Pediatric): 75 mg/5 mL (100 mL)

Infusion, as phosphate, in D_5W: 300 mg (50 mL); 600 mg (50 mL); 900 mg (50 mL)

Injection, as phosphate: 150 mg/mL (2 mL, 4 mL, 6 mL, 60 mL)

Lotion, as phosphate (Cleocin T®): 1% (60 mL)

Solution, topical, as phosphate (Cleocin T®, Clindaderm®): 1% (30 mL, 60 mL)

Suppositories, vaginal, as phosphate (Cleocin®): 100 mg (3)

Swabs, topical (Clindets®): 1% (60s)

References

Dajani AS, Taubert KA, Wilson W, et al, "Prevention of Bacterial Endocarditis. Recommendations by the American Heart Association," *JAMA*, 1997, 277(22):1794-801.

♦ **Clindets**® see Clindamycin on page 250

♦ **Clinoril**® see Sulindac on page 930

Clioquinol (klye oh KWIN ole)

U.S. Brand Names Vioform® [OTC]

Synonyms Iodochlorhydroxyquin

Therapeutic Category Antifungal Agent, Topical

Generic Available Yes: Cream

Use Used topically in the treatment of tinea pedis, tinea cruris, and skin infections caused by dermatophytic fungi (ringworm)

Contraindications Not effective in the treatment of scalp or nail fungal infections; children <2 years of age; hypersensitivity to clioquinol, hydroxyquinoline, quinoline derivatives, iodides, or any component

Warnings Topical application poses a potential risk of toxicity to infants and children; known to cause serious and irreversible optic atrophy, optic neuritis, and peripheral neuropathy with muscular weakness, sensory loss, and blindness

Precautions Routine use is not recommended; may irritate sensitized skin; use with caution in patients with iodine intolerance

Adverse Reactions

Dermatologic: Skin irritation, rash, discoloration of skin

Neuromuscular & skeletal: Peripheral neuropathy

Ocular: Optic atrophy

Stability Store in tight, light-resistant container; avoid freezing

Mechanism of Action Chelates bacterial surface and trace metals needed for bacterial growth

Pharmacokinetics

Absorption: With an occlusive dressing up to 40% of a dose can be absorbed systemically during a 12-hour period; drug absorption is enhanced when applied under diapers

Metabolism: Undergoes conjugation in the liver

Half-life: 11-14 hours

Elimination: Excreted renally as the glucuronide and sulfate metabolites and free clioquinol

Usual Dosage Children ≥2 years and Adults: Topical: Apply 2-4 times/day; do not use for >7 days

Administration Topical: Do not apply to the eyes; apply after cleansing the affected area with soap and water and drying thoroughly

Test Interactions Thyroid function tests (decreases ^{131}I uptake); false-positive ferric chloride test for phenylketonuria

Patient Information Can stain skin and fabrics; for external use only; avoid contact with eyes and mucous membranes

Dosage Forms

Cream: 3% (30 g)

Ointment, topical: 3% (30 g)

References

American Academy of Pediatrics Committee on Drugs, "Clioquinol (Iodochlorhydroxyquin, Vioform®) and Iodoquinol (Diiodohydroxyquin): Blindness and Neuropathy," *Pediatrics*, 1990, 86(5):797-8.

Clofazimine (kloe FA zi meen)

U.S. Brand Names Lamprene®

Therapeutic Category Antibiotic, Miscellaneous; Leprostatic Agent

Generic Available No

Use Treatment of dapsone-resistant lepromatous leprosy (*Mycobacterium leprae*); multibacillary dapsone-sensitive leprosy; erythema nodosum leprosum; **Note:** Clofazimine has been associated with an adverse outcome in the treatment of MAC disease and should not be used

Pregnancy Risk Factor C

Contraindications Hypersensitivity to clofazimine or any component

Precautions Well tolerated when administered in dosages ≤100 mg/day; dosages >100 mg/day should be used for as short a duration as possible; use with caution in patients with GI problems; patients with abdominal pain, colic, nausea, vomiting, or diarrhea during clofazimine therapy may require a dosage adjustment or discontinuation of therapy

Adverse Reactions

Central nervous system: Dizziness, drowsiness, fatigue, headache, fever

Dermatologic: Discoloration of the skin and conjunctiva (pink to brownish-black), dry skin, rash, pruritus, acneiform eruptions, erythema multiforme, phototoxicity

Endocrine & metabolic: Hyperglycemia

Gastrointestinal: Constipation, abdominal pain, diarrhea, nausea, anorexia, vomiting, bowel obstruction, GI bleeding, dysgeusia

Hepatic: Hepatitis, jaundice

Ocular: Irritation of the eyes

Neuromuscular & skeletal: Peripheral neuropathy

Drug Interactions Isoniazid increases clofazimine plasma and urinary concentration and decreases clofazimine skin concentration

Food Interactions Food increases the extent of absorption

Stability Protect from moisture

Mechanism of Action Binds preferentially to mycobacterial DNA at the guanine base to inhibit mycobacterial growth; also has some anti-inflammatory activity through an unknown mechanism

Pharmacokinetics

Absorption: Oral: 45% to 70% slowly absorbed

Distribution: Remains in tissues for prolonged periods and distributes into fatty tissues of the reticuloendothelial system, mesenteric lymph nodes, adrenal glands, liver, bile, spleen, small intestine, lungs, muscles, bone, skin, breast milk; does not appear to penetrate into the CSF

Metabolism: In the liver to three metabolites

Half-life:
Terminal: 8 days
Tissue: 70 days

Elimination: Principally in feces; only negligible amounts excreted unchanged in the urine; small amounts excreted in sputum, saliva, and sweat

Usual Dosage Oral:

Children: Leprosy: 1 mg/kg/day every 24 hours in combination with dapsone and rifampin

Adults:

Dapsone-resistant leprosy: 50-100 mg once daily in combination with one or more antileprosy drugs for 2 years; then alone 50-100 mg/day

Dapsone-sensitive multibacillary leprosy: 50-100 mg once daily in combination with two or more antileprosy drugs for at least 2 years and continue until negative skin smears are obtained, then institute single-drug therapy with appropriate agent

Erythema nodosum leprosum: 100-200 mg/day for up to 3 months or longer then taper dose to 100 mg/day when possible

Administration Oral: Administer with meals or milk to maximize absorption

Monitoring Parameters GI complaints, periodic liver function tests

Patient Information May discolor skin, conjunctiva, tears, sweat, urine, feces, and nasal secretions to a pink to brownish-black color; skin discoloration reversal may take several months after discontinuation of clofazimine

Nursing Implications Clofazimine-induced dry skin may be relieved by applying petrolatum or an emollient lotion containing 25% urea to the affected areas

Dosage Forms Capsule: 50 mg, 100 mg

References

Chesney PJ, "New Concepts for Antimicrobial Use in Opportunistic Infections," *Semin Pediatr Infect Dis*, 1991, 2(1):67-73.

(Continued)

Clofazimine *(Continued)*

Garrelts JC, "Clofazimine: A Review of Its Use in Leprosy and *Mycobacterium avium* Complex Infection," *DICP*, 1991, 25(5):525-31.

"1999 USPHS/IDSA Guidelines for the Prevention of Opportunistic Infections in Persons Infected With Human Immunodeficiency Virus. USPHS/IDSA Prevention of Opportunistic Infections Working Group," *MMWR Morb Mortal Wkly Rep*, 1999, 48(RR-10):1-66.

♦ **Clonapam (Can)** *see* Clonazepam *on page 254*

Clonazepam (kloe NA ze pam)

Related Information
Antiepileptic Drugs *on page 1208*
Overdose and Toxicology *on page 1222*

U.S. Brand Names Klonopin™

Canadian Brand Names Alti-Clonazepam; Apo-Clonazepam; Clonapam; Novo-Clonazepam; Nu-Clonazepam; PMS-Clonazepam; Rho-Clonazepam; Rivotril

Therapeutic Category Anticonvulsant, Benzodiazepine; Benzodiazepine

Generic Available Yes

Use Treatment of absence (petit mal), petit mal variant (Lennox-Gastaut), infantile spasms, akinetic, and myoclonic seizures

Restrictions C-IV

Pregnancy Risk Factor D

Contraindications Hypersensitivity to clonazepam, any component, or other benzodiazepines; severe liver disease, acute narrow-angle glaucoma

Precautions Use with caution in patients with chronic respiratory disease or impaired renal function; abrupt discontinuance may precipitate withdrawal symptoms, status epilepticus or seizures

Adverse Reactions
Cardiovascular: Hypotension
Central nervous system: Drowsiness, changes in behavior or personality, vertigo, confusion, memory impairment, decreased concentration, headache, ataxia, choreiform movements, hypotonia
Dermatologic: Rash
Gastrointestinal: Nausea, xerostomia, vomiting, diarrhea, constipation, anorexia, hypersalivation
Hematologic: Thrombocytopenia, anemia, leukopenia, eosinophilia
Neuromuscular & skeletal: Tremor
Ocular: Nystagmus, blurred vision
Respiratory: Bronchial hypersecretion, respiratory depression
Miscellaneous: Physical and psychological dependence

Drug Interactions Cytochrome P-450 isoenzyme CYP3A3/4 substrate
CNS depressants or alcohol increase sedation; phenytoin, carbamazepine, rifampin, or barbiturates increase clonazepam clearance; drugs that inhibit cytochrome P-450 isoenzyme CYP3A3/4 may increase levels and effects of clonazepam; monitor for altered benzodiazepine response

Mechanism of Action Suppresses the spike-and-wave discharge in absence seizures by depressing nerve transmission in the motor cortex; depresses all levels of the CNS, including the limbic and reticular formation, by binding to the benzodiazepine site on the gamma-aminobutyric acid (GABA) receptor complex and modulating GABA, which is a major inhibitory neurotransmitter in the brain

Pharmacodynamics
Onset of effect: 20-60 minutes
Duration:
Infants and young children: Up to 6-8 hours
Adults: Up to 12 hours

Pharmacokinetics
Absorption: Oral: Well absorbed
Distribution: V_d: Adults: 1.5-4.4 L/kg
Protein binding: 85%
Metabolism: Extensively metabolized in the liver; undergoes nitroreduction to 7-aminoclonazepam, followed by acetylation to 7-acetamidoclonazepam; nitroreduction and acetylation are via cytochrome P-450 enzyme system; metabolites undergo glucuronide and sulfate conjugation
Half-life:
Children: 22-33 hours
Adults: 19-50 hours
Elimination: Metabolites excreted as glucuronide or sulfate conjugates; less than 2% excreted unchanged in urine

Usual Dosage Oral:
Infants and Children <10 years or 30 kg:
Initial daily dose: 0.01-0.03 mg/kg/day (maximum dose: 0.05 mg/kg/day) given in 2-3 divided doses; increase by no more than 0.5 mg every third day until seizures are controlled or adverse effects seen
Maintenance dose: 0.1-0.2 mg/kg/day divided 3 times/day; not to exceed 0.2 mg/kg/day
Children ≥10 years (>30 kg) and Adults:
Initial daily dose not to exceed 1.5 mg given in 3 divided doses; may increase by 0.5-1 mg every third day until seizures are controlled or adverse effects seen
Maintenance dose: 0.05-0.2 mg/kg/day; do not exceed 20 mg/day

Administration Oral: May administer with food or water to decrease GI distress

Reference Range Relationship between serum concentration and seizure control is not well established; measurement at random times postdose may contribute to this problem; predose concentrations are recommended
Proposed therapeutic levels: 20-80 ng/mL
Potentially toxic concentration: >80 ng/mL

Patient Information Avoid alcohol; limit caffeine; may cause drowsiness and impair ability to perform hazardous activities requiring mental alertness or physical coordination

Additional Information Ethosuximide or valproic acid may be preferred for treatment of absence (petit mal) seizures; clonazepam-induced behavioral disturbances may be more frequent in mentally handicapped patients; when discontinuing therapy in children, the clonazepam dose may be safely reduced by ≤0.04 mg/kg/week and discontinued when the daily dose is ≤0.04 mg/kg/day

Dosage Forms Tablet: 0.5 mg, 1 mg, 2 mg

Extemporaneous Preparations A 0.1 mg/mL oral liquid can be made using 3 different vehicles (cherry syrup; a 1:1 mixture of Ora-Sweet® and Ora-Plus®; or a 1:1 mixture of Ora-Sweet® SF and Ora-Plus®); crush six 2 mg tablets into a fine powder in a mortar; add 10 mL of the vehicle and mix to make a uniform paste; mix while adding the vehicle in geometric portions to **almost** 120 mL; transfer to a calibrated bottle and qsad with vehicle to 120 mL; preparation is stable for 60 days when stored in amber prescription bottles in the dark at room temperature (25°C) or under refrigeration (5°C); label "shake well" and "protect from light"
Allen LV and Erickson MA, "Stability of Acetazolamide, Allopurinol, Azathioprine, Clonazepam, and Flucytosine in Extemporaneously Compounded Oral Liquids," *Am J Health Syst Pharm*, 1996, 53(16):1944-9.

References
Sugai K, "Seizures With Clonazepam: Discontinuation and Suggestions for Safe Discontinuation Rates in Children," *Epilepsia*, 1993, 34(6):1089-97.
Walson PD and Edge JH, "Clonazepam Disposition in Pediatric Patients," *Ther Drug Monit*, 1996, 18(1):1-5.

Clonidine (KLOE ni deen)

U.S. Brand Names Catapres®; Catapres-TTS®; Duraclon™
Canadian Brand Names Apo-Clonidine; Dixarit; Novo-Clonidine; Nu-Clonidine
Therapeutic Category Adrenergic Agonist Agent; Alpha-Adrenergic Agonist; Analgesic, Non-narcotic (Epidural); Antihypertensive Agent
Generic Available Yes: Tablet
Use Management of hypertension; aid in the diagnosis of pheochromocytoma and growth hormone deficiency; used for heroin withdrawal and smoking cessation therapy in adults; alternate agent for the treatment of attention-deficit/hyperactivity disorder (ADHD); epidural form is used in combination with opiates for relief of severe pain in cancer patients whose pain was not relieved by opiates alone
Pregnancy Risk Factor C
Contraindications Hypersensitivity to clonidine hydrochloride or any component; epidural injection is contraindicated in patients receiving anticoagulation therapy and in patients with a bleeding diathesis or an infection at the injection site. Administration of epidural clonidine above the C_4 dermatome is contraindicated.
Warnings Do not abruptly discontinue as rapid increase in blood pressure and symptoms of sympathetic overactivity (such as increased heart rate, tremors, agitation, anxiety, insomnia, sweating, palpitations) may occur; if need to discontinue, taper dose gradually over more than 1 week. EKG abnormalities and 4 cases of sudden cardiac death have been reported in children receiving clonidine with methylphenidate; reduce dose of methylphenidate by 40% when used concurrently with clonidine; consider EKG monitoring. Epidural clonidine is not recommended for perioperative, obstetrical, or postpartum pain [due to the risk of hemodynamic instability (hypotension, bradycardia)], in patients with severe cardiovascular disease, or those who are hemodynamically unstable.
(Continued)

Clonidine *(Continued)*

Precautions Dosage modification is required in patients with renal impairment; use with caution in cerebrovascular disease, coronary insufficiency, renal impairment, sinus node dysfunction; monitor patients for signs of depression (especially those with a history of affective disorders)

Adverse Reactions

Cardiovascular: Raynaud's phenomenon, hypotension, bradycardia, palpitations, tachycardia, CHF, rebound hypertension if discontinued abruptly

Central nervous system: Drowsiness, sedation, headache, dizziness, fatigue, insomnia, anxiety, depression

Dermatologic: Rash, local skin reactions with patch

Endocrine & metabolic: Sodium and water retention, parotid pain

Gastrointestinal: Constipation, anorexia, xerostomia

Respiratory: Respiratory depression and ventilatory abnormalities with high epidural doses

Drug Interactions Use with methylphenidate may potentially increase EKG effects (see Warnings); tricyclic antidepressants antagonize hypotensive effects of clonidine; beta-blockers may potentiate bradycardia in patients receiving clonidine and may increase the rebound hypertension seen with clonidine withdrawal; discontinue beta-blocker several days before clonidine is tapered off; CNS depressants and alcohol may increase sedative effects; use with opiates may increase hypotension; epidural clonidine may prolong the effects of epidural local anesthetics

Food Interactions Avoid natural licorice (causes sodium and water retention and increases potassium loss)

Stability Epidural injection: Discard unused portion of vial (preservative free); do not use with preservative

Mechanism of Action Stimulates alpha$_2$-adrenoreceptors in the brain stem, thus activating an inhibitory neuron, resulting in reduced sympathetic outflow, producing a decrease in vasomotor tone and heart rate

Epidural use: Prevents pain signal transmission to the brain and produces analgesia at presynaptic and postjunctional alpha$_2$-adrenoreceptors in the spinal cord

Pharmacodynamics Antihypertensive effects: Oral:

Onset of effects: 30-60 minutes

Peak effects: Within 2-4 hours

Duration: 6-10 hours

Pharmacokinetics

Distribution: V_d: Adults: 2.1 L/kg

Protein binding: 20% to 40%

Metabolism: Hepatic to inactive metabolites

Bioavailability, oral: 75% to 95%

Half-life, serum:

Neonates: 44-72 hours

Children: 8-12 hours

Adults:

Normal renal function: 6-20 hours

Renal impairment: 18-41 hours

Half-life, CSF: Adults: 1.3 ± 0.5 hours

Elimination: 65% excreted in urine (32% unchanged) and 22% excreted in feces via enterohepatic recirculation

Dialysis: Not dialyzable (0% to 5%)

Usual Dosage

Children:

Hypertension: Oral: Initial: 5-10 mcg/kg/day in divided doses every 8-12 hours; increase gradually, if needed, to 5-25 mcg/kg/day in divided doses every 6 hours; maximum dose: 0.9 mg/day

ADHD: Oral: Initial: 0.05 mg/day, increase every 3-7 days by 0.05 mg/day to 3-5 mcg/kg/day given in divided doses 3-4 times/day; usual maximum dose: 0.3-0.4 mg/day. **Note:** Some centers use doses as high as 8 mcg/kg/day or 0.5 mg/day (see Hunt, 1990).

Clonidine tolerance test (test of growth hormone release from the pituitary): Oral: 0.15 mg/m^2 or 4 mcg/kg as a single dose

Analgesia: Epidural (continuous infusion): Reserved for cancer patients with severe intractable pain, unresponsive to other analgesics or epidural or spinal opiates: Initial: 0.5 mcg/kg/hour; adjust with caution, based on clinical effect; do not exceed adult doses

Transdermal: Children may be switched to the transdermal delivery system after oral therapy is titrated to an optimal and stable dose; a transdermal dose approximately equivalent to the total oral daily dose may be used (see Hunt, 1990; see Administration)

Adults:

Hypertension:

Oral: Initial dose: 0.1 mg twice daily, usual maintenance dose: 0.2-1.2 mg/day in 2-4 divided doses; maximum recommended dose: 2.4 mg/day

Transdermal: Applied once weekly as transdermal delivery system; initial therapy with 0.1 mg/24 hours applied once every 7 days; adjust dosage based on response; hypotensive action may not begin until 2-3 days after initial application

Analgesia: Epidural (continuous infusion): Initial: 30 mcg/hour; titrate to clinical effect; usual maximum dose: 40 mcg/hour

Administration

Epidural: Dilute the 500 mcg/mL product with preservative free NS to a final concentration of 100 mcg/mL prior to use; visually inspect for particulate matter and discoloration prior to administration (whenever permitted by container and solution)

Oral: May be administered without regard to meals

Transdermal: Patches should be applied at bedtime to a clean, hairless area of the upper arm or chest; rotate patch sites weekly in adults; in children, the patch may need to be changed more frequently (eg, every 3-5 days); **Note:** Transdermal patch is a membrane-controlled system; do **not** cut the patch to deliver partial doses; rate of drug delivery, reservoir contents, and adhesion may be affected if cut; if partial dose is needed, surface area of patch can be blocked proportionally using adhesive bandage (see Lee, 1997)

Monitoring Parameters Blood pressure, heart rate; consider EKG monitoring in patients with history of heart disease or concurrent use of medications affecting conduction

Patient Information Avoid alcohol; may cause drowsiness and impair ability to perform hazardous duties requiring mental alertness; do not stop drug abruptly

Nursing Implications Counsel patient/parent about compliance and danger of withdrawal reaction if doses are missed or drug is discontinued

Additional Information Epidural clonidine may be more effective in the treatment of neuropathic pain compared to somatic or visceral pain; clonidine-induced symptomatic bradycardia may be treated with atropine

Dosage Forms

Injection, epidural, preservative free, as hydrochloride (Duraclon™): 100 mcg/mL (10 mL); 500 mcg/mL (10 mL)

Patch, transdermal (Catapress-TTS®): 1, 2, and 3 (0.1 mg, 0.2 mg, 0.3 mg/day to 7-day duration)

Tablet, as hydrochloride (Catapres®): 0.1 mg, 0.2 mg, 0.3 mg

Extemporaneous Preparations A 0.1 mg/mL oral suspension compounded from tablets is stable for 28 days when stored in amber glass bottles and refrigerated (4°C); thirty 0.2 mg tablets are crushed in a glass mortar and ground to a fine powder; 2 mL Purified Water USP is slowly added, and triturated to make a fine paste; Simple Syrup, NF is slowly added in 15 mL increments and triturated; qsad 60 mL; shake well before use

Levinson ML and Johnson CE, "Stability of an Extemporaneously Compounded Clonidine Hydrochloride Oral Liquid," *Am J Hosp Pharm*, 1992, 49(1):122-5.

References

Chafin CC, Hovinga CA,and Phelps SJ, "Clonidine in the Treatment of Attention Deficit Hyperactivity Disorder," *Journal of Pediatric Pharmacy Practice*, 1999, 4(6):308-15.

Hart-Santora D and Hart LL, "Clonidine in Attention Deficit Hyperactivity Disorder," *Ann Pharmacother*, 1992, 26(1):37-9.

Hunt RD, Capper L, and O'Connell P, "Clonidine in Child and Adolescent Psychiatry," *J Child Adol Psychpharm*, 1990, 1(1):87-102.

Hunt RD, Minderaa RB, and Cohen DJ, "The Therapeutic Effect of Clonidine in Attention Deficit Disorder With Hyperactivity: A Comparison With Placebo and Methylphenidate," *Psychopharmacol Bull*, 1986, 22(1):229-35.

Lee NA and Anderson PO, "Giving Partial Doses of Transdermal Patches," *Am J Health Syst Pharm*, 1997, 54(15):1759-60.

Rocchini AP, "Childhood Hypertension: Etiology, Diagnosis, and Treatment," *Pediatr Clin North Am*, 1984, 31(6):1259-73.

Sinaiko AR, "Pharmacologic Management of Childhood Hypertension," *Pediatr Clin North Am*, 1993, 40(1):195-212.

Clorazepate (klor AZ e pate)

Related Information

Antiepileptic Drugs *on page 1208*
Overdose and Toxicology *on page 1222*

U.S. Brand Names Gen-XENE®; Tranxene®; Tranxene® SD

(Continued)

Clorazepate *(Continued)*

Canadian Brand Names Apo-Clorazepate; Novo-Clopate

Therapeutic Category Anticonvulsant, Benzodiazepine; Benzodiazepine; Sedative

Generic Available Yes

Use Treatment of generalized anxiety and panic disorders; management of alcohol withdrawal; adjunct anticonvulsant in management of partial seizures

Restrictions C-IV

Pregnancy Risk Factor D

Contraindications Hypersensitivity to clorazepate dipotassium or any component; cross-sensitivity with other benzodiazepines may exist; avoid using in patients with pre-existing CNS depression, severe uncontrolled pain, or narrow-angle glaucoma

Warnings Abrupt discontinuation may cause withdrawal symptoms or seizures

Precautions Use with caution in patients with hepatic or renal disease

Adverse Reactions

Cardiovascular: Hypotension

Central nervous system: Drowsiness, dizziness, confusion, amnesia, headache, depression, ataxia

Dermatologic: Rash

Gastrointestinal: Nausea, xerostomia

Hematologic: Reduced hematocrit (with long-term use)

Ocular: Blurred vision

Miscellaneous: Physical and psychological dependence with long-term use; long-term use may also be associated with renal or hepatic injury

Drug Interactions Cytochrome P-450 isoenzyme CYP3A3/4 substrate

Cimetidine or other hepatic enzyme inhibitors may decrease hepatic clearance, monitor for altered benzodiazepine response; concurrent use of clorazepate with ritonavir is not recommended

Stability Unstable in water

Mechanism of Action Depresses all levels of the CNS, including the limbic and reticular formation, by binding to the benzodiazepine site on the gamma-aminobutyric acid (GABA) receptor complex and modulating GABA, which is a major inhibitory neurotransmitter in the brain

Pharmacokinetics

Absorption: Rapidly decarboxylated to desmethyldiazepam (active) in acidic stomach prior to absorption

Distribution: Crosses the placenta

Metabolism: In the liver to oxazepam (active)

Half-life, adults:

Desmethyldiazepam: 48-96 hours

Oxazepam: 6-8 hours

Time to peak serum concentration: Oral: Within 1 hour

Elimination: Primarily in urine

Usual Dosage Oral:

Anticonvulsant:

Children 9-12 years: Initial: 3.75-7.5 mg/dose twice daily; increase dose by 3.75 mg at weekly intervals, not to exceed 60 mg/day in 2-3 divided doses

Children >12 years and Adults: Initial: Up to 7.5 mg/dose 2-3 times/day; increase dose by 7.5 mg at weekly intervals; usual dose: 0.5-1 mg/kg/day; not to exceed 90 mg/day (up to 3 mg/kg/day has been used)

Anxiety: Adults: 7.5-15 mg 2-4 times/day, or given as single dose of 15-22.5 mg at bedtime

Alcohol withdrawal: Adults: Initial: 30 mg, then 15 mg 2-4 times/day on first day; maximum daily dose: 90 mg; gradually decrease dose over subsequent days

Administration Oral: May administer with food or water to decrease GI upset

Monitoring Parameters Excessive CNS depression, respiratory rate, and cardiovascular stress

Reference Range Therapeutic: 0.12-1 µg/mL (SI: 0.36-3.01 µmol/L)

Patient Information Avoid alcohol; may cause drowsiness and impair ability to perform hazardous duties requiring mental alertness

Dosage Forms

Tablet, as dipotassium (Gen-XENE®, Tranxene®): 3.75 mg, 7.5 mg, 15 mg

Tablet, as dipotassium, extended release (Tranxene® SD): 11.25 mg, 22.5 mg

♦ *Clostridium botulinum* **Toxin Type A** *see Botulinum Toxin Type A on page 149*

♦ **Clotrimaderm (Can)** *see Clotrimazole on page 259*

Clotrimazole (kloe TRIM a zole)

U.S. Brand Names Gyne-Lotrimin® Vaginal [OTC]; Lotrimin AF® Topical [OTC]; Lotrimin® Topical; Mycelex®-G Topical; Mycelex®-G Vaginal [OTC]; Mycelex® Troche

Canadian Brand Names Canesten; Clotrimaderm; Neo-Zol

Therapeutic Category Antifungal Agent, Oral Nonabsorbed; Antifungal Agent, Topical; Antifungal Agent, Vaginal

Generic Available Yes

Use Treatment of susceptible fungal infections, including oropharyngeal candidiasis, dermatophytoses, superficial mycoses, cutaneous candidiasis, as well as vulvovaginal candidiasis; limited data suggests that the use of clotrimazole troches may be effective for prophylaxis against oropharyngeal candidiasis in neutropenic patients

Pregnancy Risk Factor B (topical); C (troches)

Contraindications Hypersensitivity to clotrimazole or any component

Warnings Clotrimazole troches should not be used for treatment of systemic fungal infection

Precautions Safety and effectiveness of clotrimazole lozenges (troches) in children <3 years of age have not been established

Adverse Reactions

Dermatologic: Erythema, pruritus, urticaria, skin fissures, blistering

Gastrointestinal: Nausea and vomiting may occur in patients on clotrimazole troches; lower abdominal cramps may occur in patients receiving clotrimazole vaginal tablets

Hepatic: Abnormal liver function tests (causal relationship between troches and elevated LFTs not clearly established)

Local: Mild burning, irritation, stinging of skin or vaginal area

Mechanism of Action Binds to phospholipids in the fungal cell membrane altering cell wall permeability resulting in loss of essential intracellular elements

Pharmacokinetics

Absorption: Negligible through intact skin when administered topically; 3% to 10% of an intravaginal dose is absorbed

Distribution: Following oral/topical administration, clotrimazole is present in saliva for up to 3 hours following 30 minutes of dissolution time in the mouth

Usual Dosage

Children >3 years and Adults:

Topical/Oral: 10 mg troche dissolved slowly 5 times/day

Topical: Apply twice daily

Children >12 years and Adults: Vaginal: 100 mg/day at bedtime for 7 days or 200 mg/day at bedtime for 3 days or 500 mg single dose; or 5 g (= 1 applicatorful) of 1% vaginal cream daily at bedtime for 7-14 days

Administration

Oral: Dissolve lozenge (troche) in mouth over 15-30 minutes

Topical: Apply sparingly and rub gently into the cleansed, affected area and surrounding skin; do not apply to the eye

Vaginal: Wash hands before using. Insert full applicator into vagina gently and expel cream, or insert tablet into vagina. Wash applicator with soap and water following use. Remain lying down for 30 minutes following administration.

Monitoring Parameters Periodic liver function tests during oral therapy with clotrimazole lozenges

Patient Information Vaginal cream and tablet are oil-based and may weaken latex condoms and diaphragms; avoid intercourse during therapy. Do not use tampons until therapy is complete.

Dosage Forms

Cream:

Topical (Lotrimin®, Lotrimin® AF, Mycelex®, Mycelex® OTC): 1% (15 g, 30 g, 45 g, 90 g)

Vaginal (Gyne-Lotrimin®, Mycelex®-G): 1% (45 g, 90 g)

Lotion (Lotrimin®): 1% (30 mL)

Solution, topical (Lotrimin®, Lotrimin® AF, Mycelex®, Mycelex® OTC): 1% (10 mL, 30 mL)

Tablet, vaginal (Gyne-Lotrimin®, Mycelex®-G): 100 mg (7s); 500 mg (1s)

Troche (Mycelex®): 10 mg

Twin pack (Mycelex®): Tablet 500 mg (1's) and vaginal cream 1% (7 g)

Cloxacillin (kloks a SIL in)

Related Information
Carbohydrate and Alcohol Content of Liquid Medications for Use in Patients Receiving Ketogenic Diets *on page 1258*

U.S. Brand Names Cloxapen®; Tegopen®

Canadian Brand Names Apo-Cloxi; Bactopen; Novo-Cloxin; Nu-Cloxi; Orbenin

Therapeutic Category Antibiotic, Penicillin (Antistaphylococcal)

Generic Available Yes

Use Treatment of susceptible bacterial infections of the respiratory tract, skin and skin structure, bone and joint caused by penicillinase-producing staphylococci

Pregnancy Risk Factor B

Contraindications Hypersensitivity to cloxacillin, any component, or penicillins

Precautions Use with caution in patients with a history of cephalosporin hypersensitivity

Adverse Reactions
Central nervous system: Fever

Dermatologic: Rash

Gastrointestinal: Nausea, vomiting, diarrhea

Hematologic: Eosinophilia, leukopenia, neutropenia, thrombocytopenia, agranulocytosis

Hepatic: Hepatotoxicity

Renal: Hematuria, elevated BUN and serum creatinine

Miscellaneous: Serum sickness-like reactions

Drug Interactions Probenecid (increases serum cloxacillin concentration)

Food Interactions Food decreases extent of absorption

Stability Refrigerate oral solution after reconstitution; discard after 14 days; stable for 3 days at room temperature

Mechanism of Action Inhibits bacterial cell wall synthesis by binding to one or more of the penicillin-binding proteins; inhibits the final transpeptidation step of peptidoglycan synthesis resulting in cell wall death

Pharmacokinetics
Absorption: Oral: ~50%

Distribution: Into pleural and synovial fluid, bone, liver, and kidneys; poor penetration into CSF; crosses the placenta; appears in breast milk

Protein binding: 90% to 98%

Metabolism: Significant in the liver to active and inactive metabolites

Half-life: 30-90 minutes (prolonged with renal impairment and in neonates)

Time to peak serum concentration: Oral: Within 0.5-2 hours

Elimination: In the urine and through the bile

Dialysis: Not dialyzable (0% to 5%)

Usual Dosage Oral:
Children >1 month: 50-100 mg/kg/day in divided doses every 6 hours; up to a maximum of 4 g/day

Adults: 250-500 mg every 6 hours

Administration Oral: Administer 1 hour before or 2 hours after meals; shake suspension well before use

Monitoring Parameters CBC with differential, urinalysis, BUN, serum creatinine, and liver enzymes

Test Interactions False-positive urine and serum proteins

Additional Information
Sodium content of 250 mg capsule: 0.6 mEq

Sodium content of 5 mL of 125 mg/5 mL solution, oral: 0.48 mEq

Dosage Forms
Capsule, as sodium: 250 mg, 500 mg

Powder for oral suspension, as sodium: 125 mg/5 mL (100 mL, 200 mL)

♦ **Cloxapen®** *see Cloxacillin on page 260*

♦ **Clysodrast®** *see Bisacodyl on page 143*

Coal Tar (KOLE tar)

U.S. Brand Names AquaTar® [OTC]; Denorex® [OTC]; DHS® Tar [OTC]; Duplex® T [OTC]; Estar® [OTC]; Fototar® [OTC]; Neutrogena® T/Derm; Pentrax® [OTC]; Polytar® [OTC]; psoriGel® [OTC]; T/Gel® [OTC]; Zetar® [OTC]

Canadian Brand Names Balnetar; Doak-Oil; Mazon Medicated Soap; Spectro Tar; Tar Distillate; Targel; Tersa-Tar

Synonyms LCD

Therapeutic Category Antipsoriatic Agent, Topical; Antiseborrheic Agent, Topical

Generic Available Yes

Use Topically for controlling dandruff, seborrheic dermatitis, or psoriasis

Contraindications Hypersensitivity to coal tar or any ingredient in the formulation

Warnings Due to a potential carcinogenic risk, do not use around the rectum or in the genital area or groin

Precautions Do not apply to acutely inflamed skin; avoid exposure to sunlight for at least 24 hours

Adverse Reactions Dermatologic: Dermatitis, folliculitis, irritation, acneiform eruption, photosensitization

Drug Interactions Tetracyclines, phenothiazines, tretinoin, and sulfonamides also have phototoxic potential

Mechanism of Action Reduces the number and size of epidermal cells produced

Usual Dosage Children and Adults: Topical:
  Bath: 60-90 mL of a 5% to 20% solution or 15-25 mL of 30% lotion is added to bath water; soak 5-20 minutes, then pat dry; use once daily to once every 3 days
  Shampoo: Apply twice weekly for the first 2 weeks then once weekly or more often if needed
  Skin: Apply to the affected area 1-4 times/day; decrease frequency to 2-3 times/week once condition has been controlled
    Atopic dermatitis: 2% to 5% coal tar cream may be applied once daily or every other day to reduce inflammation
  Scalp psoriasis: Tar oil bath or coal tar solution may be painted sparingly to the lesions 3-12 hours before each shampoo
  Psoriasis of the body, arms, legs: Apply at bedtime; if thick scales are present, use product with salicylic acid and apply several times during the day

Administration Topical:
  Bath: Add appropriate amount of coal tar to lukewarm bath water and mix thoroughly
  Shampoo: Rub shampoo onto wet hair and scalp, rinse thoroughly; repeat; leave on 5 minutes; rinse thoroughly

Patient Information Avoid contact with eyes, genital, or rectal area; coal tar preparations frequently stain the skin and hair; avoid exposure to direct sunlight; shake suspension well before use

Dosage Forms
  Cream: 1% to 5%
  Gel: Coal tar 5%
  Lotion: 2.5% to 30%
  Lotion: Coal tar 2% to 5%
  Shampoo: Coal tar extract 2% with salicylic acid 2% (60 mL)
  Shampoo, topical: Coal tar: 0.5% to 5%
  Solution:
    Coal tar: 2.5%, 5%, 20%
    Coal tar extract: 5%
  Suspension, coal tar: 30% to 33.3%

References
Greaves MW, Weinstein GD, "Treatment of Psoriasis," *N Engl J Med*, 1995, 332(9):581-8.
Hanifin JM, "Atopic Dermatitis in Infants and Children," *Pediatr Clin North Am*, 1991, 38(4):763-89.

Cocaine (koe KANE)

Related Information
  Drugs and Breast-Feeding *on page 1243*
  Laboratory Detection of Drugs in Urine *on page 1234*

Therapeutic Category Analgesic, Topical; Local Anesthetic, Topical

Generic Available Yes

Use Topical anesthesia for mucous membranes

Restrictions C-II

Pregnancy Risk Factor C (X if nonmedical use)

Contraindications Systemic use; hypersensitivity to cocaine or any component

Precautions Use with caution in patients with hypertension, severe cardiovascular disease, thyrotoxicosis, and in infants; use with caution in patients with severely traumatized mucosa in the region of intended application

Adverse Reactions
  Cardiovascular: Hypertension, tachycardia, cardiac arrhythmias
  Central nervous system: Restlessness, nervousness, euphoria, excitement, hallucinations, seizures
  Gastrointestinal: Vomiting
  Neuromuscular & skeletal: Tremor
  Ocular: Topical: Sloughing of the corneal epithelium, ulceration of the cornea
  Respiratory: Tachypnea
  (Continued)

Cocaine (Continued)

Drug Interactions Cytochrome P-450 isoenzyme CYP3A3/4 substrate
MAO inhibitors, inhalational anesthetics, levodopa, methyldopa, sympathomimetics and ethanol may increase risk of cardiac arrhythmias; CNS stimulants; beta-adrenergic blocking agents; cholinesterase inhibitors

Stability Store in well closed, light-resistant containers

Mechanism of Action Blocks both the initiation and conduction of nerve impulses by decreasing the neuronal membrane's permeability to sodium ions. This results in inhibition of depolarization with resultant blockade of conduction; interferes with the uptake of norepinephrine by adrenergic nerve terminals producing vasoconstriction.

Pharmacodynamics Following topical administration to mucosa:
Onset of action: Within 1 minute
Peak action: Within 5 minutes
Duration: ≥30 minutes, depending upon route and dosage administered

Pharmacokinetics
Absorption: Well absorbed through mucous membranes; absorption is limited by drug-induced vasoconstriction and enhanced by inflammation
Distribution: V_d: ~2 L/kg; appears in breast milk (see Additional Information)
Metabolism: In the liver; major metabolites are ecgonine methyl ester and benzoyl ecgonine
Half-life: 75 minutes
Elimination: Primarily in urine as metabolites and unchanged drug (<10%); cocaine metabolites may appear in the urine of neonates for up to 5 days after birth due to maternal cocaine use shortly before birth

Usual Dosage Topical application (ear, nose, throat, bronchoscopy): Concentrations of 1% to 4% are used; use lowest effective dose; do not exceed 1 mg/kg; patient tolerance, anesthetic technique, vascularity of tissue, and area to be anesthetized will determine dose needed. Solutions >4% are not recommended due to increased risk and severity of systemic toxicities.

Administration Topical: Use only on mucous membranes of the oral, laryngeal, and nasal cavities; do not use on extensive areas of broken skin; do not apply commercially available products to the eye (an extemporaneously prepared ophthalmic product must be made)

Monitoring Parameters Heart rate, blood pressure, respiratory rate, temperature

Additional Information Repeated ophthalmic applications to the eye may cause cornea to become clouded or pitted, therefore, NS should be used to irrigate and protect cornea during surgery; not for injection; cocaine intoxication of infants who are receiving breast milk from their mothers abusing cocaine has been reported

Dosage Forms
Powder, as hydrochloride: 5 g, 25 g
Solution, topical, as hydrochloride: 4% [40 mg/mL] (4 mL, 10 mL); 10% [100 mg/mL] (4 mL, 10 mL)

References

Chasnoff IJ, Lewis DE, and Squires L, "Cocaine Intoxication in Breast-Fed Infants," *Pediatrics*, 1987, 80(6):836-8.

Greenglass EJ, "The Adverse Effects of Cocaine on the Developing Human," Yaffe SJ and Arana JV, eds, *Pediatric Pharmacology: Therapeutic Principles in Practice*, 2nd ed, Philadelphia, PA: WB Saunders Co, 1992, 598-604.

Codeine (KOE deen)

Related Information
Compatibility of Medications Mixed in a Syringe *on page 1238*
Laboratory Detection of Drugs in Urine *on page 1234*
Narcotic Analgesics Comparison *on page 1070*
Overdose and Toxicology *on page 1222*

Canadian Brand Names Codeine Contin; Linctus Codeine Blac

Synonyms Methylmorphine

Therapeutic Category Analgesic, Narcotic; Antitussive; Cough Preparation

Generic Available Yes

Use Treatment of mild to moderate pain; antitussive in lower doses

Restrictions C-II

Pregnancy Risk Factor C (D if used for prolonged periods or in high doses at term)

Contraindications Hypersensitivity to codeine or any component

Warnings Some preparations contain sulfites which may cause allergic reactions

Precautions Use with caution in patients with hypersensitivity reactions to other phenanthrene derivative opioid agonists (morphine, hydrocodone, hydromorphone, levorphanol, oxycodone, oxymorphone); respiratory diseases including: asthma, emphysema, COPD or severe liver or renal insufficiency

Adverse Reactions

Cardiovascular: Palpitations, bradycardia, peripheral vasodilation, hypotension due to vasodilation from histamine release

Central nervous system: CNS depression, increased intracranial pressure, dizziness, drowsiness, sedation

Dermatologic: Pruritus from histamine release

Endocrine & metabolic: Antidiuretic hormone release

Gastrointestinal: Nausea, vomiting, constipation, biliary tract spasm

Genitourinary: Urinary tract spasm

Ocular: Miosis

Respiratory: Respiratory depression

Miscellaneous: Physical and psychological dependence, histamine release

Drug Interactions
Cytochrome P-450 isoenzyme CYP2D6 and CYP3A3/4 substrate; isoenzyme CYP2D6 inhibitor

CNS depressants, phenothiazines, tricyclic antidepressants may potentiate the adverse effects of codeine

Mechanism of Action
Binds to opiate receptors in the CNS, causing inhibition of ascending pain pathways, altering the perception of and response to pain; causes cough suppression by direct central action in the medulla; produces generalized CNS depression

Pharmacodynamics

Onset:
Oral: 30-60 minutes
I.M.: 10-30 minutes

Peak action:
Oral: 60-90 minutes
I.M.: 30-60 minutes

Duration: 4-6 hours

Pharmacokinetics

Absorption: Oral: Adequate

Distribution: Crosses the placenta; appears in breast milk

Protein binding: 7%

Metabolism: Hepatic to morphine (active); undergoes hydroxylation and O-demethylation via cytochrome P-450 isoenzyme CYP2D6 and demethylation via CYP3A3/4

Bioavailability: 60% to 70%

Half-life: 2.5-3.5 hours

Elimination: 3% to 16% in urine as unchanged drug, norcodeine, and free and conjugated morphine

Usual Dosage
Doses should be titrated to appropriate analgesic effect; when changing routes of administration, note that oral dose is $2/3$ as effective as parenteral dose

Analgesic: Oral, I.M., S.C.:
Children: 0.5-1 mg/kg/dose every 4-6 hours as needed; maximum dose: 60 mg/dose
Adults: Usual: 30 mg/dose; range: 15-60 mg every 4-6 hours as needed

Antitussive: Oral (for nonproductive cough):
Infants and Children <2 years: Not recommended
Children ≥2 years: 1-1.5 mg/kg/day in divided doses every 4-6 hours as needed: Alternatively dose according to age:
2-5 years: 2.5-5 mg every 4-6 hours as needed; maximum dose: 30 mg/day
6-12 years: 5-10 mg every 4-6 hours as needed; maximum dose: 60 mg/day
Children >12 years and Adults: 10-20 mg/dose every 4-6 hours as needed; maximum dose: 120 mg/day

Dosing adjustment in renal impairment:
Cl_{cr} 10-50 mL/minute: Administer 75% of dose
Cl_{cr} <10 mL/minute: Administer 50% of dose

Administration

Oral: Administer with food or water to decrease nausea and GI upset

Parenteral: I.M., S.C.: Not intended for I.V. use due to large histamine release and cardiovascular effects

Monitoring Parameters
Respiratory rate, heart rate, blood pressure, pain relief

Patient Information
Increase fluid and fiber intake to avoid constipation; avoid alcohol; may cause drowsiness and impair ability to perform hazardous duties requiring mental alertness; may be habit-forming with long term use

Nursing Implications
Observe patient for excessive sedation and respiratory depression; implement safety measures; may need to assist with ambulation

(Continued)

Codeine (Continued)

Additional Information Not recommended for use for cough control in patients with a productive cough; equianalgesic doses: 120 mg codeine phosphate I.M. approximately equals morphine 10 mg I.M.

Dosage Forms
Injection, as phosphate: 15 mg/mL (2 mL); 30 mg/mL (2 mL); 60 mg/mL (1 mL)
Solution, oral, as phosphate: 15 mg/5 mL [strawberry flavor] (5 mL, 500 mL)
Tablet, as sulfate: 15 mg, 30 mg, 60 mg
Tablet, as phosphate: 30 mg, 60 mg

♦ **Codeine and Acetaminophen** *see* Acetaminophen and Codeine *on page 31*
♦ **Codeine and Glycerol Guaiacolate** *see* Guaifenesin and Codeine *on page 486*
♦ **Codeine and Guaifenesin** *see* Guaifenesin and Codeine *on page 486*
♦ **Codeine and Promethazine** *see* Promethazine and Codeine *on page 838*
♦ **Codeine Contin (Can)** *see* Codeine *on page 262*
♦ **Codeine, Promethazine, and Phenylephrine** *see* Promethazine, Phenylephrine, and Codeine *on page 840*
♦ **Cogentin®** *see* Benztropine *on page 137*
♦ **Co-Gesic®** *see* Hydrocodone and Acetaminophen *on page 505*
♦ **Colace® [OTC]** *see* Docusate *on page 350*
♦ **Colaspase** *see* Asparaginase *on page 107*

Colchicine (KOL chi seen)

Therapeutic Category Antigout Agent; Anti-inflammatory Agent
Generic Available Yes
Use Treatment of acute gouty arthritis attacks and prevention of recurrences of such attacks; management of familial Mediterranean fever
Pregnancy Risk Factor D
Contraindications Hypersensitivity to colchicine or any component; severe renal, GI disease, or cardiac disorders
Warnings Patients who become pregnant while receiving colchicine therapy may be at greater risk of producing trisomic offspring
Precautions Modify dosage in patients with renal impairment
Adverse Reactions
Dermatologic: Rash, alopecia
Endocrine & metabolic: Azoospermia, hypothyroidism
Gastrointestinal: Nausea, vomiting, diarrhea, abdominal pain, steatorrhea, paralytic ileus
Hematologic: Agranulocytosis, aplastic anemia
Hepatic: Elevated liver enzymes
Local: Irritation if extravasation occurs
Neuromuscular & skeletal: Myopathy, peripheral neuropathy
Renal: Hematuria, renal damage
Drug Interactions Colchicine may decrease absorption of Vitamin B_{12}
Food Interactions May need low purine diet during acute gouty attack
Stability I.V. colchicine is incompatible with dextrose or I.V. solutions with preservatives; protect from light
Mechanism of Action Decreases leukocyte motility, phagocytosis in joints and lactic acid production, thereby reducing the deposition of urate crystals that perpetuates the inflammatory response; inhibits secretion of serum amyloid A protein
Pharmacodynamics Onset of effect:
Oral: Relief of pain and inflammation occurs after 24-48 hours
I.V.: 6-12 hours
Pharmacokinetics
Distribution: Concentrates in leukocytes, kidney, spleen, and liver; does not distribute in heart, skeletal muscle, and brain
Metabolism: Partially deacetylated in the liver
Half-life, terminal: 9.3-10.6 hours
Time to peak serum concentration: Oral: Within 30-120 minutes then declines for 2 hours before increasing again due to enterohepatic recycling
Elimination: Primarily in the feces via bile; 10% to 20% excreted in urine
Dialysis: Not dialyzable (0% to 5%)
Usual Dosage
Prophylaxis of familial Mediterranean fever: Oral:
Children:
≤5 years: 0.5 mg/day
>5 years: 1-1.5 mg/day in 2-3 divided doses

Adults: 1-2 mg/day in 2-3 divided doses

Gouty arthritis: Acute attacks: Adults:

Oral: Initial: 0.5-1.2 mg, then 0.5-0.6 mg every 1-2 hours or 1-1.2 mg every 2 hours until relief or GI side effects occur to a maximum total dose of 8 mg

I.V.: Initial: 1-3 mg, then 0.5 mg every 6 hours until response, not to exceed 4 mg/day; if pain recurs, it may be necessary to administer a daily dose of 1-2 mg for several days, however, do not give more colchicine by any route for at least 7 days after a full course of I.V. therapy (4 mg); transfer to oral colchicine in a dose similar to that being given I.V.

Prophylaxis of recurrent attacks: Oral: 0.5-0.6 mg every day or every other day

Dosing adjustment in renal impairment: Cl_{cr} <10 mL/minute: Decrease dose by 50%

Administration

Oral: Administer with water and maintain adequate fluid intake

Parenteral: Administer I.V. over 2-5 minutes into tubing of free-flowing I.V. with compatible fluid

Monitoring Parameters CBC and renal function test

Test Interactions May cause false-positive results in urine tests for erythrocytes or hemoglobin

Patient Information If taking for acute gouty attacks, discontinue if pain is relieved or if nausea, vomiting or diarrhea occur; avoid alcohol

Nursing Implications Severe local irritation can occur if inadvertently administered S.C. or I.M.; extravasation can cause tissue irritation

Dosage Forms

Injection: 0.5 mg/mL (2 mL)

Tablet: 0.5 mg, 0.6 mg

References

Levy M, Spino M, and Read SE, "Colchicine: A State-of-the-Art Review," *Pharmacotherapy*, 1991, 11(3):196-211.

Majeed HA, Carroll JE, Khuffash FA, et al, "Long-term Colchicine Prophylaxis in Children With Familial Mediterranean Fever (Recurrent Hereditary Polyserositis)," *J Pediatr*, 1990, 116(6):997-9.

♦ **Cold-Eeze®** [OTC] *see* Zinc Supplements *on page 1026*

Colfosceril (kole FOS er il)

U.S. Brand Names Exosurf® Neonatal

Synonyms Dipalmitoylphosphatidylcholine; DPPC; Synthetic Lung Surfactant

Therapeutic Category Lung Surfactant

Generic Available No

Use Neonatal respiratory distress syndrome (RDS):

Prophylactic therapy: Infants at risk for developing RDS with body weight <1350 g; infants with evidence of pulmonary immaturity with body weight >1350 g

Rescue therapy: Treatment of infants with RDS based on respiratory distress not attributable to any other causes and chest radiographic findings consistent with RDS

Warnings This drug may rapidly affect oxygenation and lung compliance. If chest expansion improves substantially the ventilator peak inspiratory pressure setting should be reduced immediately. Hyperoxia and hypocarbia (hypocarbia can decrease blood flow to the brain) may occur requiring appropriate ventilator adjustments.

Adverse Reactions Respiratory: Pulmonary hemorrhage, apnea, mucous plugging, decrease in transcutaneous O_2 >20%

Stability Reconstituted suspension is stable 12 hours after reconstitution; **do not refrigerate**

Mechanism of Action Replaces deficient or ineffective endogenous lung surfactant in neonates with RDS or in neonates at risk of developing RDS; reduces surface tension and stabilizes the alveoli from collapsing

Pharmacokinetics Absorption: Following intratracheal administration, colfosceril is absorbed from the alveolus; catabolized and reutilized for further synthesis and secretion in lung tissue

Usual Dosage Intratracheal: Neonates:

Prophylactic treatment: Give 5 mL/kg as soon as possible; the second and third doses should be administered at 12 and 24 hours later to those infants remaining on ventilators

Rescue treatment: Give 5 mL/kg as soon as the diagnosis of RDS is made. The second 5 mL/kg dose should be administered 12 hours later

Administration Reconstitute with 8 mL preservative SWI; each mL contains 13.5 mg colfosceril; if the suspension appears to separate, gently swirl vial to resuspend contents; do not use if persistent large flakes or particulates appear

(Continued)

Colfosceril *(Continued)*

Intratracheal: For intratracheal administration only. Suction infant prior to administration; inspect solution to verify complete mixing of the suspension. Administer via sideport on the special endotracheal tube adapter without interrupting mechanical ventilation. Administer the dose in two 2.5 mL/kg aliquots. Each half-dose is instilled slowly over 1-2 minutes in small bursts with each inspiration. After the first 2.5 mL/kg dose turn the infants head and torso 45° right for 30 seconds, then return to the midline position and administer the second dose as above. Following the second dose, turn the infant's head and torso 45° to the left for 30 seconds and return the infant to the midline position.

Monitoring Parameters Continuous EKG and transcutaneous O_2 saturation should be monitored during administration; frequent ABG sampling is necessary to prevent postdosing hyperoxia and hypocarbia.

Dosage Forms Suspension, intratracheal, as palmitate: 108 mg (10 mL)

♦ **Colocort**™ *see* Hydrocortisone *on page 506*
♦ **Colonic Lavage Solution** *see* Polyethylene Glycol-Electrolyte Solution *on page 811*
♦ **CoLyte®** *see* Polyethylene Glycol-Electrolyte Solution *on page 811*
♦ **CoLyte®-Flavored** *see* Polyethylene Glycol-Electrolyte Solution *on page 811*
♦ **Combantrin (Can)** *see* Pyrantel Pamoate *on page 855*
♦ **Combivir®** *see* Lamivudine and Zidovudine *on page 574*
♦ **Comparison of Adverse Effects of Antidepressants** *see page 1066*
♦ **Comparison of Usual Adult Dosage and Mechanism of Action of Antidepressants** *see page 1065*
♦ **Compatibility of Medications Mixed in a Syringe** *see page 1238*
♦ **Compazine®** *see* Prochlorperazine *on page 834*
♦ **Compound F** *see* Hydrocortisone *on page 506*
♦ **Compound S** *see* Zidovudine *on page 1022*
♦ **Compound S, Abacavir, and 3TC** *see* Abacavir, Lamivudine, and Zidovudine *on page 26*
♦ **Compound S, Abacavir, and Lamivudine** *see* Abacavir, Lamivudine, and Zidovudine *on page 26*
♦ **Compound S, ABC, and 3TC** *see* Abacavir, Lamivudine, and Zidovudine *on page 26*
♦ **Compound W® [OTC]** *see* Salicylic Acid *on page 886*
♦ **Compound W® One Step Wart Remover [OTC]** *see* Salicylic Acid *on page 886*
♦ **Compoz® Nighttime Sleep Aid [OTC]** *see* Diphenhydramine *on page 342*
♦ **Concerta**™ *see* Methylphenidate *on page 653*
♦ **Congest (Can)** *see* Estrogens (Conjugated) *on page 402*
♦ **Congest Aid (Can)** *see* Pseudoephedrine *on page 852*
♦ **Congest-Eze (Can)** *see* Pseudoephedrine *on page 852*
♦ **Conjugated Estrogens** *see* Estrogens (Conjugated) *on page 402*
♦ **Constilac®** *see* Lactulose *on page 571*
♦ **Constulose®** *see* Lactulose *on page 571*
♦ **Contac Cold Nondrowsy (Can)** *see* Pseudoephedrine *on page 852*
♦ **Copper Sulfate** *see* Trace Metals *on page 972*
♦ **Cordarone®** *see* Amiodarone *on page 72*
♦ **Corgard®** *see* Nadolol *on page 691*
♦ **Correctol Stool Softener (Can)** *see* Docusate *on page 350*
♦ **Cortacet (Can)** *see* Hydrocortisone *on page 506*
♦ **CortaGel® Extra Strength [OTC]** *see* Hydrocortisone *on page 506*
♦ **Cortaid® Intensive Therapy [OTC]** *see* Hydrocortisone *on page 506*
♦ **Cortaid® Maximum Strength [OTC]** *see* Hydrocortisone *on page 506*
♦ **Cortamed (Can)** *see* Hydrocortisone *on page 506*
♦ **Cortastat®** *see* Dexamethasone *on page 307*
♦ **Cortastat® LA** *see* Dexamethasone *on page 307*
♦ **Cortate (Can)** *see* Hydrocortisone *on page 506*
♦ **Cortatrigen® Otic** *see* Neomycin, (Bacitracin) Polymyxin B, and Hydrocortisone *on page 705*
♦ **Cortef®** *see* Hydrocortisone *on page 506*
♦ **Cortenema®** *see* Hydrocortisone *on page 506*
♦ **Corticosteroids Comparison, Systemic** *see page 1067*

♦ **Corticosteroids Comparison, Topical** *see page 1068*

Corticotropin (kor ti koe TROE pin)

Related Information
  Antiepileptic Drugs *on page 1208*

U.S. Brand Names H.P. Acthar® Gel

Synonyms ACTH; Adrenocorticotropic Hormone; Corticotropin, Repository

Therapeutic Category Adrenal Corticosteroid; Diagnostic Agent, Adrenocortical Insufficiency; Infantile Spasms, Treatment

Generic Available Yes

Use Infantile spasms; diagnostic aid in adrenocortical insufficiency; acute exacerbations of multiple sclerosis; severe muscle weakness in myasthenia gravis

Pregnancy Risk Factor C

Contraindications Scleroderma, osteoporosis, systemic fungal infections, ocular herpes simplex, peptic ulcer, hypertension, CHF; hypersensitivity to corticotropin, porcine proteins, or any component

Warnings May mask signs of infection; do not administer live vaccines; long-term therapy in children may retard bone growth; acute adrenal insufficiency may occur with abrupt withdrawal after chronic use or with stress

Precautions Use with caution in patients with hypothyroidism, cirrhosis, thromboembolic disorders, seizure disorders or renal insufficiency

Adverse Reactions
  Cardiovascular: Hypertension
  Central nervous system: Seizures, mood swings, headache, pseudotumor cerebri
  Dermatologic: Skin atrophy, bruising, hyperpigmentation, acne, hirsutism
  Endocrine & metabolic: Amenorrhea, sodium and water retention, Cushing's syndrome, hyperglycemia, bone growth suppression, hypokalemia
  Gastrointestinal: Abdominal distention, ulcerative esophagitis, pancreatitis
  Neuromuscular & skeletal: Muscle wasting
  Miscellaneous: Hypersensitivity reactions, including anaphylaxis

Drug Interactions NSAIDs (increase risk of ulcers, increase clearance of NSAIDs), loop diuretics, thiazide diuretics, amphotericin B (increases potassium wasting), antidiabetic agents (may require increased doses due to hyperglycemic activity of adrenal glucocorticoids), live virus vaccines (increase risk of viral infection), vaccines may have decreased effect

Food Interactions May increase renal loss of potassium, calcium, zinc, and vitamin C; may need to increase dietary intake or give supplements

Stability Store repository injection (gel) in the refrigerator; warm gel before administration

Mechanism of Action Stimulates the adrenal cortex to secrete adrenal steroids (including hydrocortisone, cortisone), androgenic substances, and a small amount of aldosterone. Exact mechanism of action for treatment of infantile spasms is unknown, but may be an independent antiepileptic effect (unrelated to stimulation of release of adrenocorticosteroids). One theory is that ACTH suppresses corticotropin-releasing hormone (CRH). CRH is an excitatory neuropeptide that has a greater potency in infants. Infants with infantile spasms may have increased CRH activity. ACTH may decrease CRH release and, therefore, decrease infantile spasms.

Pharmacodynamics
  Peak effect on cortisol levels: I.M., S.C. (gel): 3-12 hours
  Duration: Repository (gel): 10-25 hours, up to 3 days

Pharmacokinetics
  Absorption: I.M. (repository): Over 8-16 hours
  Half-life: 15 minutes
  Elimination: In urine

Usual Dosage
  Children: I.M.: Gel (repository) formulation:
    Anti-inflammatory/immunosuppressant: 0.8 units/kg/day or 25 units/m²/day divided every 12-24 hours
    Infantile spasms: Various regimens have been used. Some neurologists recommend low-dose ACTH (5-40 units/day) for short periods (1-6 weeks), while others recommend larger doses of ACTH (40-160 units/day) for long periods of treatment (3-12 months)
      A prospective, single-blind study (Hrachovy, 1994) found no major difference in effectiveness between high-dose long-duration versus low-dose short-duration ACTH therapy. Hypertension, however, occurred more frequently in the

(Continued)

Corticotropin *(Continued)*

high-dose group. Further studies comparing long-term outcomes are needed. Low-dose regimen used in this study:

Initial: 20 units/day for 2 weeks, if patient responds, taper and discontinue over a 1-week period; if patient does not respond, increase dose to 30 units/day for 4 weeks then taper and discontinue over a 1-week period

Usual dose: 20-40 units/day or 5-8 units/kg/day in 1-2 divided doses; range: 5-160 units/day

Adults: I.M.: Gel (repository) formulation:

Acute exacerbation of multiple sclerosis: 80-120 units/day in divided doses for 2-3 weeks

Diagnostic purposes: 25 units

Anti-inflammatory/immunosuppressant: 40-80 units every 24-72 hours

Administration Parenteral: Gel should be administered I.M. only

Monitoring Parameters Electrolytes, glucose, blood pressure, height, and weight; for infantile spasms, monitor seizure frequency, type, and duration

Test Interactions Skin tests

Patient Information Do not abruptly discontinue the medication; tell your physician you are using this drug if you are going to have skin tests, immunizations, surgery, emergency treatment, or if you have a serious infection or injury

Additional Information Cosyntropin is preferred over corticotropin for diagnostic test of adrenocortical insufficiency (cosyntropin is less allergenic and test is shorter in duration); oral prednisone (2 mg/kg/day) was as effective as I.M. ACTH gel (20 units/day) in controlling infantile spasms; corticotropin zinc hydroxide (Cortrophin® Zinc) and corticotropin aqueous (Acthar®) have been discontinued by the manufacturer

Dosage Forms Injection, repository (H.P. Acthar® Gel): 80 units/mL (5 mL)

References
Haines ST and Casto DT, "Treatment of Infantile Spasms," *Ann Pharmacother*, 1994, 28(6):779-91.
Hrachovy RA and Frost JD Jr, "Infantile Spasms," *Pediatr Clin North Am*, 1989, 36(2):311-29.
Hrachovy RA, Frost JD Jr, and Glaze DG, "High-Dose, Long-Duration Versus Low-Dose, Short-Duration Corticotropin Therapy for Infantile Spasms," *J Pediatr*, 1994, 124(5 Pt 1):803-6.
Hrachovy RA, Frost JD Jr, Kellaway P, et al, "Double-Blind Study of ACTH vs Prednisone Therapy in Infantile Spasms," *J Pediatr*, 1983, 103(4):641-5.

♦ **Corticotropin, Repository** *see Corticotropin on page 267*
♦ **Cortifoam®** *see Hydrocortisone on page 506*
♦ **Cortimyxin (Can)** *see Neomycin, (Bacitracin) Polymyxin B, and Hydrocortisone on page 705*
♦ **Cortisol** *see Hydrocortisone on page 506*

Cortisone *(KOR ti sone)*

Related Information
Corticosteroids Comparison, Systemic *on page 1067*

Canadian Brand Names Cortone

Therapeutic Category Adrenal Corticosteroid; Anti-inflammatory Agent; Corticosteroid, Systemic; Glucocorticoid

Generic Available Yes

Use Management of adrenocortical insufficiency

Pregnancy Risk Factor D

Contraindications Serious infections, except septic shock or tuberculous meningitis; hypersensitivity to corticosteroids; systemic fungal or viral infections

Warnings May retard bone growth; acute adrenal insufficiency may occur with abrupt withdrawal after long-term therapy or with stress

Precautions Use with caution in patients with hypothyroidism, cirrhosis, hypertension, CHF, ulcerative colitis, thromboembolic disorders, osteoporosis, peptic ulcer, diabetes mellitus, seizure disorders; avoid using higher than recommended dosages; supression of hypothalamic - pituitary - adrenal function, suppression of linear growth, or hypercorticism (Cushing's syndrome) may occur

Adverse Reactions
Cardiovascular: Edema, hypertension
Central nervous system: Vertigo, seizures, headache, psychoses, pseudotumor cerebri
Dermatologic: Acne, skin atrophy
Endocrine & metabolic: Cushing's syndrome, pituitary-adrenal axis suppression, growth suppression, glucose intolerance, hypokalemia, alkalosis, weight gain
Gastrointestinal: Peptic ulcer, nausea, vomiting
Neuromuscular & skeletal: Muscle weakness, osteoporosis, fractures
Ocular: Cataracts, glaucoma

Drug Interactions Cytochrome P-450 isoenzyme CYP3A3/4 substrate
Barbiturates, phenytoin, rifampin, salicylates, estrogens, NSAID, diuretics (potassium depleting), anticholinesterase agents, warfarin; caffeine and alcohol may increase risk for GI ulcer; live virus vaccines (increase risk of viral infection); vaccines may have decreased effects

Food Interactions Systemic use of corticosteroids may require a diet with increased potassium, vitamins A, B_6, C, D, folate, calcium, zinc, phosphorus, and decreased sodium

Mechanism of Action Controls the rate of protein synthesis, depresses the migration of polymorphonuclear leukocytes and fibroblasts, reverses capillary permeability, and stabilizes lysosomal membranes at the cellular level to prevent or control inflammation

Pharmacodynamics
Peak effect: Oral: Within 2 hours
Duration: 30-36 hours

Pharmacokinetics
Distribution: Crosses the placenta; appears in breast milk; distributes to muscles, liver, skin, intestines, and kidneys
Metabolism: In the liver to inactive metabolites
Half-life: 30 minutes
Elimination: In bile and urine

Usual Dosage Depends upon the condition being treated and the response of the patient. Supplemental doses may be warranted during times of stress in the course of withdrawing therapy. Oral:

Children:
Anti-inflammatory or immunosuppressive: 2.5-10 mg/kg/day or 20-300 mg/m^2/day in divided doses every 6-8 hours
Physiologic replacement: 0.5-0.75 mg/kg/day or 20-25 mg/m^2/day in divided doses every 8 hours
Adults: 20-300 mg/day divided every 12-24 hours

Administration Oral: Administer with meals, food, or milk to decrease GI effects

Monitoring Parameters Long-term use: Electrolytes, glucose, blood pressure, height, weight

Test Interactions Skin tests

Patient Information Do not discontinue or reduce dose without physician's approval; limit caffeine; avoid alcohol

Nursing Implications Taper dose gradually with long-term use

Additional Information Insoluble in water

Dosage Forms Tablet, as acetate: 5 mg, 10 mg, 25 mg

♦ **Cortisone® 10 Quick Shot** see Hydrocortisone on page 506
♦ **Cortisporin® Ophthalmic Suspension** see Neomycin, (Bacitracin) Polymyxin B, and Hydrocortisone on page 705
♦ **Cortisporin® Otic** see Neomycin, (Bacitracin) Polymyxin B, and Hydrocortisone on page 705
♦ **Cortisporin® Topical Cream** see Neomycin, (Bacitracin) Polymyxin B, and Hydrocortisone on page 705
♦ **Cortizone®-5 [OTC]** see Hydrocortisone on page 506
♦ **Cortizone®-10 [OTC]** see Hydrocortisone on page 506
♦ **Cortizone® for Kids [OTC]** see Hydrocortisone on page 506
♦ **Cortoderm (Can)** see Hydrocortisone on page 506
♦ **Cortone (Can)** see Cortisone on page 268
♦ **Cortrosyn®** see Cosyntropin on page 269
♦ **Cosmegen®** see Dactinomycin on page 294

Cosyntropin (koe sin TROE pin)

U.S. Brand Names Cortrosyn®
Canadian Brand Names Synacthen Depot
Synonyms Synacthen; Tetracosactide
Therapeutic Category Adrenal Corticosteroid; Diagnostic Agent, Adrenocortical Insufficiency
Generic Available No
Use Diagnostic test to differentiate primary adrenal from secondary (pituitary) adrenocortical insufficiency
Pregnancy Risk Factor C
Contraindications Hypersensitivity to cosyntropin or any component

(Continued)

Cosyntropin *(Continued)*

Precautions Use with caution in patients with pre-existing allergic disease or a history of allergic reactions to corticotropin

Adverse Reactions

Dermatologic: Pruritus, flushing

Endocrine & metabolic: Decreased carbohydrate tolerance; increased requirements for insulin or oral hypoglycemic agents in diabetics; activation of latent diabetes mellitus

Miscellaneous: Hypersensitivity reactions, including anaphylaxis

Drug Interactions Cortisone, hydrocortisone, estrogens, spironolactone

Stability Reconstituted solution is stable for 24 hours at room temperature and 21 days when refrigerated; when diluted in NS or D_5W, I.V. infusion is stable for 12 hours at room temperature

Mechanism of Action Stimulates the adrenal cortex to secrete adrenal steroids (including hydrocortisone, cortisone), androgenic substances, and a small amount of aldosterone

Pharmacodynamics I.M., I.V.:

Onset of action: Plasma cortisol levels rise in healthy individuals in 5 minutes

Peak levels: Within 45-60 minutes

Pharmacokinetics Metabolism: Unknown

Usual Dosage Diagnostic test doses:

Adrenocortical insufficiency: I.M., I.V.:

Preterm neonates: Dose not well defined; Korte 1996 used physiologic doses of cosyntropin (0.1 mcg/kg) to test adrenal function in VLBW infants [mean weight 900 g; mean gestational age 27 weeks (range: 23-32 weeks)]; only 36% of infants responded; increasing the dose to 0.2 mcg/kg resulted in 67% of the infants responding, but sensitivity of the test was decreased. Cole 1999 used cosyntropin doses of 3.5 mcg/kg to test adrenal function in 44 preterm infants [mean birthweight 823 g; mean gestational age 26.2 weeks; mean postmenstrual age 30.1 weeks] during inhaled beclomethasone therapy.

Neonates: 0.015 mg/kg/dose

Children <2 years: 0.125 mg

Children >2 years and Adults: 0.25 mg

When greater cortisol stimulation is needed, an I.V. infusion may be used:

Children >2 years and Adults: 0.25 mg administered over 4-8 hours (usually 6 hours)

Congenital adrenal hyperplasia evaluation: 1 mg/m^2/dose up to a maximum of 1 mg

Administration Parenteral: Administer I.V. push doses over 2 minutes; for I.V. infusion, may dilute with D_5W or NS

Reference Range Plasma cortisol concentrations should be measured immediately before and exactly 30 minutes after the dose; dose should be given in the early morning; normal morning baseline cortisol >5 µg/dL (SI: >138 nmol/L); normal response 30 minutes after cosyntropin injection: an increase in serum cortisol concentration of ≥7 µg/dL (SI: ≥193 nmol/L) or peak response >18 µg/dL (SI: >497 nmol/L).

Nursing Implications Patient should not receive corticosteroids or spironolactone the day prior to and the day of the test

Additional Information Each 0.25 mg of cosyntropin is equivalent to 25 units of corticotropin.

Dosage Forms Powder for injection: 0.25 mg

References

Cole CH, Shah B, Abbasi S, et al, "Adrenal Function in Premature Infants During Inhaled Beclomethasone Therapy," *J Pediatr*, 1999, 135(1):65-70.

Korte C, Styne D, Merritt TA, et al, "Adrenocortical Function in the Very Low Birth Weight Infant: Improved Testing Sensitivity and Association With Neonatal Outcome," *J Pediatr*, 1996, 128(2):257-63.

- ◆ **Cotazym®** *see* Pancrelipase *on page 755*
- ◆ **Cotazym-S®** *see* Pancrelipase *on page 755*
- ◆ **Cotrim®** *see* Co-Trimoxazole *on page 270*
- ◆ **Cotrim® DS** *see* Co-Trimoxazole *on page 270*

Co-Trimoxazole *(koe trye MOKS a zole)*

Related Information

Carbohydrate and Alcohol Content of Liquid Medications for Use in Patients Receiving Ketogenic Diets *on page 1258*

U.S. Brand Names Bactrim™; Bactrim™ DS; Cotrim®; Cotrim® DS; Septra®; Septra® DS; Sulfamethoprim®; Sulfatrim®; Sulfatrim® DS; Uroplus® DS; Uroplus® SS

Canadian Brand Names Apo-Sulfatrim; Novo-Trimel; Nu-Cotrimox; Protrin; Trisulfa; Trisulfa-S

Synonyms SMX-TMP; Sulfamethoxazole and Trimethoprim; TMP-SMX; Trimethoprim and Sulfamethoxazole

Therapeutic Category Antibiotic, Sulfonamide Derivative

Generic Available Yes

Use Treatment of urinary tract infections caused by susceptible *E. coli*, *Klebsiella*, *Enterobacter*, *Proteus mirabilis*, *Proteus* (indole positive); acute otitis media due to amoxicillin-resistant *H. influenzae*, *S. pneumoniae*, and *M. catarrhalis*; acute exacerbations of chronic bronchitis; prophylaxis and treatment of *Pneumocystis carinii* pneumonitis (PCP); treatment of susceptible shigellosis, typhoid fever, *Nocardia asteroides* infection, and *Xanthomonas maltophilia* infection; the I.V. preparation is used for treatment of *Pneumocystis carinii* pneumonitis, *Shigella*, and severe urinary tract infections

Pregnancy Risk Factor C

Contraindications Hypersensitivity to any sulfa drug, trimethoprim, or any component; porphyria; megaloblastic anemia due to folate deficiency; infants <2 months of age (for exception, see Additional Information)

Warnings Fatalities associated with sulfonamides, although rare, have occurred due to severe reactions including Stevens-Johnson syndrome, toxic epidermal necrolysis, hepatic necrosis, agranulocytosis, aplastic anemia, and other blood dyscrasias; discontinue use at first sign of rash or any sign of adverse reaction; injectable formulation contains benzyl alcohol, propylene glycol, and sodium metabisulfite; metabisulfites may cause allergic type reactions in susceptible patients

Precautions Use with caution in patients with G-6-PD deficiency, impaired renal or hepatic function; adjust dosage in patients with renal impairment

Adverse Reactions

Cardiovascular: Allergic myocarditis, hypotension

Central nervous system: Confusion, depression, hallucinations, seizures, fever, ataxia, kernicterus in neonates, aseptic meningitis, headache, insomnia

Dermatologic: Rash (more common in patients taking large dosages or in patients with AIDS), erythema multiforme, epidermal necrolysis, Stevens-Johnson syndrome, pruritus, urticaria

Endocrine & metabolic: Hyperkalemia

Gastrointestinal: Nausea, vomiting, glossitis, stomatitis, diarrhea, pseudomembranous colitis, pancreatitis, splenomegaly, anorexia

Hematologic: Thrombocytopenia, megaloblastic anemia, granulocytopenia, aplastic anemia, hemolysis (with G-6-PD deficiency)

Hepatic: Hepatitis, cholestatic jaundice

Local: Local irritation, pain, phlebitis

Neuromuscular & skeletal: Arthralgia, myalgia, rhabdomyolysis

Renal: Interstitial nephritis, renal tubular acidosis

Respiratory: Shortness of breath, cough, pulmonary infiltrates

Miscellaneous: Serum sickness, angioedema

Drug Interactions Cytochrome P-450 isoenzyme CYP2C9 inhibitor

Co-trimoxazole decreases the clearance of warfarin; methotrexate (displaced from protein binding sites); increases the effect of sulfonylureas, phenytoin, digoxin, and thiopental; decreases serum cyclosporine concentrations

Stability Do not refrigerate concentrate for injection; for I.V. administration, a 1:25 dilution is stable for 48 hours in D_5W or NS; 1:20 dilution is stable for 24 hours in D_5W or 14 hours in NS; 1:15 dilution is stable for 4 hours in D_5W or 2 hours in NS; 1:10 dilution is stable for 1 hour in D_5W or NS; do not mix with other drugs or solutions

Mechanism of Action Sulfamethoxazole interferes with bacterial folic acid synthesis and growth via inhibition of dihydrofolic acid formation from para-aminobenzoic acid; trimethoprim inhibits dihydrofolic acid reduction to tetrahydrofolate resulting in sequential inhibition of enzymes of the folic acid pathway

Pharmacokinetics

Absorption: Oral: Almost completely (90% to 100%)

Distribution: Crosses the placenta; distributes into breast milk, joint fluid, sputum, middle ear fluid, bile, and CSF

Protein binding:

TMP: 45%

SMX: 68%

Metabolism:

TMP: Metabolized to oxide and hydroxylated metabolites

SMX: N-acetylated and glucuronidated

(Continued)

Co-Trimoxazole *(Continued)*

Half-life:
TMP: 6-11 hours, prolonged in renal failure
SMX: 9-12 hours, prolonged in renal failure
Time to peak serum concentration: Oral: Within 1-4 hours
Elimination: Both excreted in urine as metabolites and unchanged drug

Usual Dosage Oral, I.V. **(dosage recommendations are based on the trimethoprim (TMP) component):**

Children >2 months and Adults:
Mild-moderate infections: 6-12 mg TMP/kg/day in divided doses every 12 hours
Serious infection/*Pneumocystis*: 15-20 mg TMP/kg/day in divided doses every 6-8 hours
Prophylaxis of *Pneumocystis* (see Note in Additional Information): 150 mg TMP/m^2/day in divided doses every 12 hours 3 days/week on consecutive days; acceptable alternative dosage schedules include 150 mg TMP/m^2/day as a single daily dose 3 times/week on consecutive days or 150 mg TMP/m^2/day in divided doses every 12 hours administered 7 days/week, or 150 mg TMP/m^2/day in divided doses every 12 hours administered 3 times/week on alternate days; dose should not exceed 320 mg trimethoprim and 1600 mg sulfamethoxazole/day
Urinary tract infection prophylaxis: 2 mg TMP/kg/dose daily or 5 mg TMP/kg/dose twice weekly

Adults:
Urinary tract infection/chronic bronchitis: 1 double strength tablet every 12 hours for 10-14 days
Prophylaxis of *Pneumocystis*: One double-strength tablet daily or an acceptable alternative is 1 single-strength tablet daily

Dosing adjustment in renal impairment (frequency may need to be adjusted):
Cl_{cr} 15-30 mL/minute: Reduce dose by 50%
Cl_{cr} <15 mL/minute: Not recommended

Administration
Oral: May administer with water on an empty stomach; shake suspension well before use
Parenteral: Infuse I.V. co-trimoxazole over 60-90 minutes; must be further diluted 1:25 (5 mL drug to 125 mL diluent, ie, D_5W); in patients who require fluid restriction, a 1:15 dilution (5 mL drug to 75 mL diluent, ie, D_5W) or a 1:10 dilution (5 mL drug to 50 mL diluent, ie, D_5W) may be administered; see Stability

Monitoring Parameters CBC, renal function test, liver function test, urinalysis; observe for change in bowel frequency

Patient Information Maintain adequate fluid intake

Additional Information Note: Guidelines for prophylaxis of *Pneumocystis carinii* pneumonia: Initiate PCP prophylaxis in the following patients: Children born to HIV-infected mothers should be given prophylaxis with TMP/SMZ beginning at 4-6 weeks of age and continue through the first year of life or until HIV infection has been reasonably excluded; children 1-5 years of age with CD4+ count <500 or CD4+ percentage <15%; children 6-12 years of age with CD4+ count <200 or CD4+ percentage <15%; adolescents and adults with CD4+ count <200 or oropharyngeal candidiasis. Folinic acid should be given if bone marrow suppression occurs.

Dosage Forms The 5:1 ratio (SMX to TMP) remains constant in all dosage forms:
Injection: Sulfamethoxazole 80 mg and trimethoprim 16 mg per mL (5 mL, 10 mL, 20 mL, 30 mL, 50 mL)
Suspension, oral: Sulfamethoxazole 200 mg and trimethoprim 40 mg per 5 mL (20 mL, 100 mL, 150 mL, 200 mL, 480 mL)
Tablet: Sulfamethoxazole 400 mg and trimethoprim 80 mg
Tablet, double strength: Sulfamethoxazole 800 mg and trimethoprim 160 mg

References
Jarosinki PF, Kennedy PE, and Gallelli JF, "Stability of Concentrated Trimethoprim-Sulfamethoxazole Admixtures," *AJHP*, 1989, 46(4):732-7.

Hughes WT, "*Pneumocystis carinii* Pneumonia: New Approaches to Diagnosis, Treatment, and Prevention," *Pediatr Infect Dis J*, 1991, 10(5):391-9.

"1999 USPHS/IDSA Guidelines for the Prevention of Opportunistic Infections in Persons Infected With Human Immunodeficiency Virus. USPHS/IDSA Prevention of Opportunistic Infections Working Group," *MMWR Morb Mortal Wkly Rep*, 1999, 48(RR-10):1-66.

♦ **Cough Syrup DM (Can)** *see* Dextromethorphan *on page 316*
♦ **Cough Syrup DM-E (Can)** *see* Guaifenesin and Dextromethorphan *on page 487*
♦ **Cough Syrup DM Expectorant (Can)** *see* Guaifenesin and Dextromethorphan *on page 487*
♦ **Cough Syrup Expectorant (Can)** *see* Guaifenesin *on page 485*

- **Cough Syrup with Guaifenesin & Dextromethorphan (Can)** *see* Guaifenesin and Dextromethorphan *on page 487*
- **Coumadin**® *see* Warfarin *on page 1016*
- **Covera-HS**® *see* Verapamil *on page 1007*
- **CPI**® **[OTC]** *see* Hemorrhoidal Preparations *on page 490*
- **CPM** *see* Cyclophosphamide *on page 281*
- **CPR Pediatric Drug Dosages** *see page 1031*
- **Creon**® **5** *see* Pancrelipase *on page 755*
- **Creon**® **10** *see* Pancrelipase *on page 755*
- **Creon**® **20** *see* Pancrelipase *on page 755*
- **Creo-Terpin**® **[OTC]** *see* Dextromethorphan *on page 316*
- **Critic-Aid Skin Care**® **[OTC]** *see* Zinc Oxide *on page 1026*
- **Crixivan**® *see* Indinavir *on page 534*
- **Crolom**® *see* Cromolyn *on page 273*
- **Cromoglycic Acid** *see* Cromolyn *on page 273*

Cromolyn (KROE moe lin)

Related Information
Asthma Guidelines *on page 1210*

U.S. Brand Names Children's Nasalcrom® [OTC]; Crolom®; Gastrocrom®; Intal®; Nasalcrom® [OTC]; Opticrom®

Canadian Brand Names Apo-Cromolyn; Nalcom; Novo-Cromolyn; PMS-Sodium Cromoglycate; Solu-Crom

Synonyms Cromoglycic Acid; Disodium Cromoglycate; DSCG

Therapeutic Category Antiasthmatic; Inhalation, Miscellaneous

Generic Available Yes

Use
Oral inhalation and nebulization: Prophylactic agent used for long-term (chronic) control of persistent asthma; **NOT** indicated for the relief of acute bronchospasm; also used for the prevention of allergen- or exercise-induced bronchospasm
Intranasal: Management of seasonal or perennial allergic rhinitis
Ophthalmologic: Vernal conjunctivitis, vernal keratoconjunctivitis, and vernal keratitis
Systemic: Mastocytosis, food allergy, and treatment of inflammatory bowel disease

Pregnancy Risk Factor B

Contraindications Hypersensitivity to cromolyn or any component; primary treatment of status asthmaticus

Warnings Cromolyn is a prophylactic drug with no benefit for acute situations; rare but severe anaphylactic reactions can occur; discontinue if eosinophilic pneumonia occurs

Precautions Use with caution and decrease dose in patients with renal and hepatic impairment; use inhalation aerosol with caution in patients with coronary artery disease or history of cardiac arrhythmias (due to propellants); use with caution when tapering the dose or withdrawing the drug since symptoms may reoccur; patients should not wear contact lenses during treatment with ophthalmic solution

Adverse Reactions
Central nervous system: Dizziness, headache
Dermatologic: Rash, urticaria, angioedema
Gastrointestinal: Nausea, vomiting, diarrhea, xerostomia, unpleasant taste (inhalation aerosol)
Local: Nasal burning
Neuromuscular & skeletal: Arthralgia
Ocular (topical): Ocular stinging, lacrimation
Respiratory: Coughing, wheezing, sneezing, nasal congestion, throat irritation, eosinophilic pneumonia, pulmonary infiltrates, hoarseness

Stability Protect from direct light and heat; nebulization solution is compatible with beta agonists, anticholinergic solutions, acetylcysteine and NS; incompatible with alkaline solutions, calcium and magnesium salts; store oral concentrate ampuls in foil pouch until ready for use

Mechanism of Action Prevents the mast cell release of histamine, leukotrienes and slow-reacting substance of anaphylaxis by inhibiting degranulation after contact with antigens

Pharmacodynamics Not effective for immediate relief of symptoms in acute asthmatic attacks; must be used at regular intervals for 2-4 weeks to be effective
(Continued)

273

Cromolyn *(Continued)*

Pharmacokinetics

Absorption:

Oral: 0.5% to 2%

Inhalation: ~8% of dose reaches the lungs upon inhalation of the powder and is well absorbed

Half-life: 80-90 minutes

Time to peak serum concentration: Within 15 minutes after inhalation

Elimination: Equally excreted unchanged in urine and feces (via bile); small amounts after inhalation are exhaled

Usual Dosage

Inhalation:

For chronic control of asthma, taper frequency to the lowest effective dose (ie, 4 times/day to 3 times/day to twice daily):

Nebulization solution: Children >2 years and Adults: Initial: 20 mg 4 times/day; usual dose: 20 mg 3-4 times/day

Metered spray:

Children 5-12 years: Initial: 2 inhalations 4 times/day; usual dose: 1-2 inhalations 3-4 times/day

Children ≥12 years and Adults: Initial: 2 inhalations 4 times/day; usual dose: 2-4 inhalations 3-4 times/day

Prevention of allergen- or exercise-induced bronchospasm: Administer 10-15 minutes prior to exercise or allergen exposure but no longer than 1 hour before:

Nebulization solution: Children >2 years and Adults: Single dose of 20 mg

Metered spray: Children >5 years and Adults: Single dose of 2 inhalations

Intranasal: Children ≥6 years and Adults: 1 spray in each nostril 3-6 times/day

Ophthalmic: Children >4 years and Adults: Instill 1-2 drops 4-6 times/day

Oral:

Systemic mastocytosis:

Neonates and Preterm Infants: Not recommended

Infants and Children <2 years: 20 mg/kg/day in 4 divided doses; may increase in patients 6 months to 2 years of age if benefits not seen after 2-3 weeks; do not exceed 30 mg/kg/day

Children 2-12 years: 100 mg 4 times/day; not to exceed 40 mg/kg/day

Children >12 years and Adults: 200 mg 4 times/day

Food allergy and inflammatory bowel disease:

Children <2 years: Not recommended

Children 2-12 years: Initial dose: 100 mg 4 times/day; may double the dose if effect is not satisfactory within 2-3 weeks; not to exceed 40 mg/kg/day

Children >12 years and Adults: Initial dose: 200 mg 4 times/day; may double the dose if effect is not satisfactory within 2-3 weeks; up to 400 mg 4 times/day

Once desired effect is achieved, dose may be tapered to lowest effective dose

Administration

Oral concentrate: Open ampul and squeeze contents into glass of water; stir well; administer at least 30 minutes before meals and at bedtime; do not mix with juice, milk, or food

Oral inhalation: Shake canister gently before use; do not immerse canister in water

Nasal inhalation: Clear nasal passages by blowing nose prior to use

Monitoring Parameters Asthma: Periodic pulmonary function tests; signs and symptoms of disease state when tapering dose

Additional Information Reserve systemic use in children <2 years of age for severe disease; avoid systemic use in premature infants; inhalation aerosol contains fluorocarbon propellants

Dosage Forms

Inhalation, as sodium, oral (Intal®): 800 mcg/spray [112 metered inhalations (56 doses)] (8.1 g); [200 metered inhalation (100 doses)] (14.2 g)

Oral concentrate, as sodium, (Gastrocrom®): 100 mg/5 mL ampul

Solution, as sodium, for nebulization (Intal®): 10 mg/mL (2 mL)

Solution, as sodium, nasal (Children's Nasalcrom®, Nasalcrom® [OTC]): 40 mg/mL [5.2 mg/inhalation] (13 mL, 26 mL)

Solution, as sodium, ophthalmic (Crolom®, Opticrom®): 4% (10 mL)

References

Expert Panel Report 2, "Guidelines for the Diagnosis and Management of Asthma," *Clinical Practice Guidelines*, National Institutes of Health, National Heart, Lung, and Blood Institute, NIH Publication No. 94-4051, April, 1997.

♦ **Crotaline Antivenin, Polyvalent** *see* Antivenin *(Crotalidae)* Polyvalent *on page 99*

Crotamiton (kroe TAM i tonn)

U.S. Brand Names Eurax®
Therapeutic Category Scabicidal Agent
Generic Available No
Use Treatment of scabies (*Sarcoptes scabiei*) in infants and children
Pregnancy Risk Factor C
Contraindications Hypersensitivity to crotamiton or any component; patients who manifest a primary irritation response to topical medications
Precautions Avoid contact with face, eyes, mucous membranes, and urethral meatus; do not apply to acutely inflamed or raw skin
Adverse Reactions
Dermatologic: Pruritus, contact dermatitis
Local: Irritation
Mechanism of Action Mechanism for scabicidal activity is unknown
Usual Dosage Scabicide: Topical: Infants, Children, and Adults: Apply over entire body below the head; apply once daily for 2 days followed by a cleansing bath 48 hours after the last application; treatment may be repeated after 7-10 days if mites appear
Administration Topical: Wash thoroughly and scrub away loose scales, then towel dry; apply a thin layer and gently massage drug onto skin of the entire body from the neck to the toes (with special attention to skin folds, creases, and interdigital spaces); since scabies can affect the head, scalp, and neck in infants and young children, apply to head, neck, and body of this age group; do not apply to the face, eyes, mouth, mucous membranes, or urethral meatus; shake lotion well before use
Patient Information For topical use only; all contaminated clothing and bed linen should be washed to avoid reinfestation
Additional Information Treatment may be repeated after 7-10 days if live mites are still present
Dosage Forms
Cream: 10% (60 g)
Lotion: 10% (60 mL, 480 mL)
References
Eichenfield LF, Honig PJ, "Blistering Disorders in Childhood," *Pediatr Clin North Am*, 1991, 38(4):959-76.
Hogan DJ, Schachner L, Tanglertsampan C, "Diagnosis and Treatment of Childhood Scabies and Pediculosis," *Pediatr Clin North Am*, 1991, 38(4):941-57.

Cyanide Antidote Kit (SYE a nide AN tee dote kit)

Therapeutic Category Antidote, Cyanide
Generic Available Yes
Use Treatment agents for cyanide poisoning
Pregnancy Risk Factor Sodium thiosulfate and sodium nitrite: C; amyl nitrite: C
Contraindications Hypersensitivity to amyl nitrite, sodium nitrite, sodium thiosulfate, or any component
Warnings Excessive methemoglobin results when sodium nitrite dosage is exceeded; use only enough sodium nitrite to achieve a satisfactory clinical response; avoid methemoglobin levels >30%; patients with malignancy and G6PD deficiency have increased sensitivity to the methemoglobin-generating activities of sodium nitrite
Precautions When cyanide poisoning is related to smoke inhalation, if possible, the patient should be at pressure in a hyperbaric chamber before the kit is administered; the methemoglobin initially produced by sodium nitrite injection may otherwise exacerbate concomitant carbon monoxide poisoning that has already severely diminished oxygen-carrying capacity in red cells
(Continued)

Cyanide Antidote Kit *(Continued)*

Adverse Reactions Reactions listed are those of sodium nitrite; see individual monographs for Amyl Nitrite *on page 94* and Sodium Thiosulfate *on page 909*:
Cardiovascular: Tachycardia, syncope, cyanosis, hypotension (associated with rapid infusion), flushing
Central nervous system: Dizziness, headache
Gastrointestinal: Nausea, vomiting
Miscellaneous: Methemoglobin formation

Drug Interactions Sodium nitrite antagonizes acetylcholine, epinephrine, and histamine effects; sodium nitrite potentiates hypotensive effects and/or anticholinergic effects of tricyclic antidepressants, antihistamines, and meperidine and related CNS depressants; also see Amyl Nitrite *on page 94*

Stability Sodium nitrite is stable at room temperature; do not mix with other medications; see individual monographs Amyl Nitrite *on page 94* and Sodium Thiosulfate *on page 909*

Mechanism of Action Amyl nitrite and sodium nitrite promote the formation of methemoglobin which binds with cyanide to form cyanomethemoglobin (nontoxic); sodium thiosulfate, by providing an extra sulfur group to the enzyme rhodanese, increases the rate of detoxification of cyanide

Usual Dosage Administer in sequential order:
Amyl nitrite: Infants, Children, and Adults: Inhale vapors from 1 ampul continuously for 15-30 seconds, followed by a rest for 15 seconds (this interrupted schedule is important because continuous use of amyl nitrite may prevent adequate oxygenation); reapply until sodium nitrite can be administered
Sodium nitrite: I.V.:
Infants and Children ≤25 kg: See table

Variation of Sodium Nitrite and Sodium Thiosulfate Dose With Hemoglobin Concentration*

Hemoglobin (g/dL)	Initial Dose Sodium Nitrite (mg/kg)	Initial Dose Sodium Nitrite 3% (mL/kg)	Initial Dose Sodium Thiosulfate 25% (mL/kg)
7	5.8	0.19	0.95
8	6.6	0.22	1.10
9	7.5	0.25	1.25
10	8.3	0.27	1.35
11	9.1	0.30	1.50
12	10.0	0.33	1.65
13	10.8	0.36	1.80
14	11.6	0.39	1.95

*Adapted from Berlin DM Jr, "The Treatment of Cyanide Poisoning in Children," *Pediatrics*, 1970, 46:793.

Follow immediately with sodium thiosulfate
Children >25 kg, Adolescents, and Adults: 300 mg; follow immediately with sodium thiosulfate
Sodium thiosulfate: I.V.:
Infants and Children ≤25 kg: See table
Children >25 kg, Adolescents, and Adults: 12.5 g
Patients should be watched for at least 24-48 hours; if signs of poisoning reappear, injection of both sodium nitrite and sodium thiosulfate should be repeated, but each in $^{1}/_{2}$ of the original dose; even if the patient is asymptomatic, repeat $^{1}/_{2}$ doses of both sodium nitrite and sodium thiosulfate may be given for prophylactic purposes 2 hours after the first injection

Administration
Inhalation: **Amyl nitrite:** Crush ampul in cloth and hold under patient's nares for 15-30 seconds; remove for 15 seconds; repeat
Parenteral: I.V.:
Sodium nitrite: Administer undiluted at a rate of 2.5-5 mL/minute
Sodium thiosulfate: Administer undiluted over at least 10 minutes; rapid administration may cause hypotension

Monitoring Parameters Blood cyanide levels, methemoglobin levels, arterial blood gases, oxygen saturation, vital signs

Reference Range Symptoms associated with blood cyanide levels:
Flushing and tachycardia: 0.5-1 µg/mL
Obtundation: 1-2.5 µg/mL
Coma and respiratory depression: >2.5 µg/mL
Death: >3 µg/mL

Dosage Forms Kit:
Injection: Sodium nitrite 300 mg/10 mL (2 ampuls); sodium thiosulfate 12.5 g/50 mL (2 ampuls)
Inhalant: Amyl nitrite 0.3 mL (12 crushable ampuls)

Cyanocobalamin (sye an oh koe BAL a min)

U.S. Brand Names LA-12®; Nascobal®
Canadian Brand Names Bedoz; Rubion
Synonyms Vitamin B_{12}
Therapeutic Category Nutritional Supplement; Vitamin, Water Soluble
Generic Available Yes
Use Pernicious anemia; vitamin B_{12} deficiency; increased B_{12} requirements due to pregnancy, thyrotoxicosis, hemorrhage, malignancy, liver or kidney disease; nutritional supplement
Pregnancy Risk Factor A (C if dose exceeds RDA recommendation)
Contraindications Hypersensitivity to cyanocobalamin, any component, or cobalt; patients with hereditary optic nerve atrophy
Warnings Vitamin B_{12} deficiency for >3 months results in irreversible degenerative CNS lesions; vegetarian diets may result in vitamin B_{12} deficiency
Precautions Serum potassium concentrations should be monitored early as severe hypokalemia has occurred after the conversion of megaloblastic anemia to normal erythropoiesis
Adverse Reactions
Cardiovascular: Peripheral vascular thrombosis
Dermatologic: Itching, urticaria, exanthema
Endocrine & metabolic: Hypokalemia
Gastrointestinal: Diarrhea
Miscellaneous: Allergic reactions
Drug Interactions Cytochrome P-450 isoenzyme CYP2D6 and CYP3A3/4 substrate
Decreased absorption of cyanocobalamin from GI tract: aminoglycoside antibiotics, colchicine, extended release potassium products, aminosalicylic acid, phenytoin, and phenobarbital; antagonism of hematopoietic response to cyanocobalamin: chloramphenicol; chemical degradation of cyanocobalamin: large doses of ascorbic acid
Stability Clear pink to red solutions are stable at room temperature; protect from light; **incompatible** with chlorpromazine, phytonadione, prochlorperazine, warfarin, ascorbic acid, dextrose, heavy metals, oxidizing or reducing agents
Mechanism of Action Coenzyme for various metabolic functions, including fat and carbohydrate metabolism and protein synthesis, used in cell replication and hematopoiesis
Pharmacodynamics Onset:
Megaloblastic anemia: I.M.:
Conversion of megaloblastic to normoblastic erythroid hyperplasia within bone marrow: 8 hours
Increased reticulocytes: 2-5 days
Complicated vitamin B_{12} deficiency: I.M., S.C.: Resolution of:
Psychiatric sequelae: 24 hours
Thrombocytopenia: 10 days
Granulocytopenia: 2 weeks
Pharmacokinetics
Absorption: Oral: Drug is absorbed from the terminal ileum in the presence of calcium; for absorption to occur, gastric "intrinsic factor" must be present to transfer the compound across the intestinal mucosa
Distribution: Principally stored in the liver, also stored in the kidneys and adrenals
Protein binding: Bound to transcobalamin II
Metabolism: Converted in the tissues to active coenzymes methylcobalamin and deoxyadenosylcobalamin
Bioavailability: Oral: Pernicious anemia: 1.2%
Time to peak serum concentration:
I.M., S.C.: 30 minutes to 2 hours
Intranasal: 1.6 hours
Elimination: 50% to 98% unchanged in the urine
Usual Dosage
I.M. or deep S.C. (oral use is recommended only as a nutritional supplement or as maintenance of vitamin B_{12} deficiency):
Recommended daily allowance (RDA):
Children: 0.3-2 mcg
(Continued)

Cyanocobalamin *(Continued)*

Adults: 2 mcg
Adults, pregnancy: 2.2 mcg
Adults, lactation: 2.6 mcg
Adults, vegetarians: 6 mcg
Pernicious anemia, congenital (if evidence of neurologic involvement): 1000 mcg/day for at least 2 weeks; maintenance: 50 mcg/month
Children: 30-50 mcg/day for 2 or more weeks (to a total dose of 1000 mcg), then follow with 100 mcg monthly as maintenance dosage
Adults: 100 mcg/day for 6-7 days; if improvement, give same dose on alternate days for 7 doses; then every 3-4 days for 2-3 weeks; once hematologic values have returned to normal, maintenance dosage: 100 mcg/month

Vitamin B_{12} deficiency:
Children (dosage in children not well established): I.M., S.C.: 0.2 mcg/kg for 2 days followed by 1000 mcg/day for 2-7 days followed by 100 mcg/week for a month; for malabsorptive causes of B_{12} deficiency, monthly maintenance doses of 100 mcg have been recommended or as an alternative 100 mcg/day for 10-15 days (total dose of 1-1.5 mg), then once or twice weekly for several months; may taper to 60 mcg every month
Adults:
Uncomplicated: Initial: (I.M. or deep S.C. are the preferred routes)
Oral: 25-1000 mcg/day until remission is complete
I.M. or deep S.C.: 100 mcg/day for 5-10 days, followed by 100-200 mcg monthly until remission is complete **or** as an alternative: 100 mcg/day for 7 days, followed by 100 mcg every other day for 2 weeks, followed by 100 mcg every 3-4 days until remission is complete
Complicated (severe anemia, CHF, thrombocytopenia with bleeding, severe neurologic damage or granulocytopenia with infection): Initial: I.M. or deep S.C.: 1000 mcg with I.M. or I.V. folic acid 15 mg as single doses, followed by 1000 mcg/day plus oral folic acid 5 mg/day for 1 week; **Note:** Oral cyanocobalamin therapy is **not** indicated for treatment of complicated deficiency
Maintenance: Oral, I.M., deep S.C.: 100-200 mcg monthly
Note: Low initial B_{12} doses combined with potassium supplementation (as needed) may prevent a hypokalemia seen in patients with severe deficiency
Dosage adjustment in renal impairment: Increased dosage may be required in vitamin B_{12}-deficient patients

Administration
Oral: Not generally recommended for treatment of severe vitamin B_{12} deficiency due to poor oral absorption (lack of intrinsic factor); oral administration may be used in less severe deficiencies and maintenance therapy; may be administered without regard to food
Parenteral: I.M. or deep S.C.: Avoid I.V. administration due to a more rapid system elimination with resulting decreased utilization

Monitoring Parameters Serum potassium, erythrocyte and reticulocyte count, hemoglobin, hematocrit, serum B_{12} level

Reference Range Serum vitamin B_{12} levels: Normal: 200-900 pg/mL; vitamin B_{12} deficiency: <200 pg/mL; megaloblastic anemia: <100 pg/mL

Dosage Forms
Gel, nasal (Nascobal®): 500 mcg/0.1 mL (2.3 mL)
Injection (LA-12®): 1000 mcg/mL (10 mL, 30 mL)
Lozenge: 100 mcg, 250 mcg, 500 mcg
Tablet [OTC]: 50 mcg, 100 mcg, 250 mcg, 500 mcg, 1000 mcg, 5000 mcg

References
Rasmussen SA, Fernhoff PM, and Scanlon KS, "Vitamin B_{12} Deficiency in Children and Adolescents," *J Pediatr*, 2001, 138(1):10-7.

Cyclobenzaprine *(sye kloe BEN za preen)*

U.S. Brand Names Flexeril®
Canadian Brand Names Flexitec; Gen-Cyclobenzaprine; Novo-Cycloprine; Nu-Cyclobenzaprine
Therapeutic Category Skeletal Muscle Relaxant, Nonparalytic
Generic Available Yes
Use Treatment of muscle spasm associated with acute painful musculoskeletal conditions; supportive therapy in tetanus
Pregnancy Risk Factor B
Contraindications Hypersensitivity to cyclobenzaprine or any component; hyperthyroidism, CHF, arrhythmias, heart block; do not use concomitantly or within 14 days of MAO inhibitors

Warnings Abrupt withdrawal after prolonged administration may result in nausea, headache, and malaise; not effective in the treatment of spasticity due to cerebral or spinal cord disease

Precautions Use with caution in patients with urinary retention, angle-closure glaucoma

Adverse Reactions

Cardiovascular: Tachycardia, hypotension, arrhythmias, edema of face/lips, syncope

Central nervous system: Drowsiness, headache, dizziness, fatigue, nervousness, confusion

Dermatologic: Rash

Gastrointestinal: Dyspepsia, nausea, constipation, xerostomia, vomiting, diarrhea, paralytic ileus, dysgeusia, stomach cramps

Genitourinary: Urinary frequency or retention

Hepatic: Hepatitis, cholestasis, jaundice

Neuromuscular & skeletal: Weakness, muscle twitching

Ocular: Blurred vision

Otic: Tinnitus

Drug Interactions Cytochrome P-450 isoenzyme CYP1A2, CYP2D6, CYP3A3/4 substrate

MAO inhibitors; additive effects with sedatives, alcohol, anticholinergic agents, and other CNS depressants

Mechanism of Action Centrally-acting skeletal muscle relaxant pharmacologically related to tricyclic antidepressants; reduces tonic somatic motor activity influencing both alpha and gamma motor neurons

Pharmacodynamics

Onset of action: Within 1 hour

Duration: 12-24 hours

Pharmacokinetics

Absorption: Oral: Complete

Metabolism: Hepatic

Half-life: 1-3 days

Time to peak serum concentration: Within 3-8 hours

Elimination: Primarily renal as inactive metabolites and in the feces (via bile) as unchanged drug; may undergo enterohepatic recycling

Usual Dosage Oral:

Children: Dosage has not been established

Adults: 10 mg 3 times/day (range: 20-40 mg/day in 2-4 divided doses); maximum dose: 60 mg/day; usage for more than 2-3 weeks is not recommended

Administration Oral: May be administered without regard to meals

Patient Information Avoid alcohol; causes drowsiness and may impair ability to perform hazardous tasks involving mental alertness or physical coordination

Dosage Forms Tablet, as hydrochloride: 10 mg

♦ **Cyclogyl**® see Cyclopentolate on page 279

♦ **Cyclomydril**® see Cyclopentolate and Phenylephrine on page 280

Cyclopentolate (sye kloe PEN toe late)

U.S. Brand Names AK-Pentolate®; Cyclogyl®; Ocu-Pentolate®

Canadian Brand Names Diopentolate; Minims-Cyclopentolate

Therapeutic Category Anticholinergic Agent, Ophthalmic; Ophthalmic Agent, Mydriatic

Generic Available Yes

Use Diagnostic procedures requiring mydriasis and cycloplegia

Pregnancy Risk Factor C

Contraindications Narrow-angle glaucoma; hypersensitivity to cyclopentolate or any component

Warnings Use of cyclopentolate has been associated with psychotic reactions and behavioral disturbances in pediatric patients; increased susceptibility to these effects has been reported in young infants, young children, and in children with spastic paralysis or brain damage, particularly with concentrations >1%; observe neonates and infants closely for at least 30 minutes after administration; may cause transient elevation of intraocular pressure

Adverse Reactions Central nervous system and cardiovascular reactions most commonly seen in children after receiving 2% solution:

Cardiovascular: Tachycardia, hypertension

(Continued)

Cyclopentolate *(Continued)*

Central nervous system: Psychotic and behavioral disturbances manifested by ataxia, restlessness, hallucinations, psychosis, hyperactivity, seizures, incoherent speech

Local: Burning sensation

Ocular: Increase in intraocular pressure, loss of visual accommodation

Miscellaneous: Allergic reactions

Mechanism of Action Prevents the muscle of the ciliary body and the sphincter muscle of the iris from responding to cholinergic stimulation, causing mydriasis and cycloplegia

Pharmacodynamics

Peak effects:

Cycloplegia: 15-60 minutes

Mydriasis: Within 15-60 minutes, with recovery taking up to 24 hours

Usual Dosage Ophthalmic:

Neonates and Infants: See Cyclopentolate and Phenylephrine *on page 280* (preferred agent for use in neonates and infants due to lower cyclopentolate concentration and reduced risk for systemic reactions)

Children: 1 drop of 0.5% or 1% in eye followed by 1 drop of 0.5% or 1% in 5 minutes, if necessary, approximately 40-50 minutes before procedure

Adults: 1 drop of 1% followed by another drop in 5 minutes; approximately 40-50 minutes prior to the procedure, may use 2% solution in heavily pigmented iris

Administration Ophthalmic: Instill drops into conjunctival sac of affected eye(s); avoid contact of bottle tip with skin or eye; to avoid excessive systemic absorption, finger pressure should be applied on the lacrimal sac during and for 1-2 minutes following application

Patient Information May cause blurred vision and increased sensitivity to light

Additional Information Pilocarpine ophthalmic drops applied after the examination may reduce recovery time to 3-6 hours

Dosage Forms Solution, ophthalmic, as hydrochloride: 0.5% (15 mL); 1% (2 mL, 5 mL, 15 mL); 2% (2 mL, 5 mL)

Cyclopentolate and Phenylephrine

(sye kloe PEN toe late & fen il EF rin)

U.S. Brand Names Cyclomydril®

Synonyms Phenylephrine and Cyclopentolate

Therapeutic Category Adrenergic Agonist Agent, Ophthalmic; Anticholinergic Agent, Ophthalmic; Ophthalmic Agent, Mydriatic

Generic Available No

Use Diagnostic procedures requiring mydriasis and cycloplegia; preferred agent for use in neonates and infants

Pregnancy Risk Factor C

Contraindications Narrow-angle glaucoma or untreated anatomically narrow angles; hypersensitivity to cyclopentolate, phenylephrine, or any component

Warnings Use of cyclopentolate has been associated with psychotic reactions and behavioral disturbances in pediatric patients; increased susceptibility to these effects has been reported in young infants, young children, and in children with spastic paralysis or brain damage, particularly with concentrations >1%; observe neonates and infants closely for at least 30 minutes after administration; may cause transient elevation of intraocular pressure

Precautions Use with caution in patient's with Down's syndrome, cardiovascular disease, hypertension, and hyperthyroidism; feeding intolerance may follow ophthalmic use of this product in neonates and infants; withhold feedings for 4 hours after examination

Adverse Reactions

Cardiovascular: Tachycardia, hypertension

Central nervous system: Psychotic and behavioral disturbances manifested by ataxia, restlessness, hallucinations, psychosis, hyperactivity, seizures, incoherent speech, hyperpyrexia

Gastrointestinal: Feeding intolerance, decreased gastric motility

Genitourinary: Urinary retention

Local: Burning sensation

Ocular: Increased intraocular pressure, loss of visual accommodation, transient stinging, browache, photophobia, lacrimation, superficial punctate keratitis

Miscellaneous: Allergic reactions

Drug Interactions May interfere with the ocular antihypertensive action of carbachol, pilocarpine, or ophthalmic cholinesterase inhibitors

Stability Store at room temperature

Mechanism of Action See individual monographs for Cyclopentolate *on page 279* and Phenylephrine *on page 789*

Pharmacodynamics Onset of action and duration of effect are partially dependent upon eye pigment; dark eyes have a prolonged onset of action and shorter duration than blue eyes

Onset: 15-60 minutes

Duration: 4-12 hours

Usual Dosage Ophthalmic:

Neonates, Infants, Children, and Adults: Instill 1 drop into the eye every 5-10 minutes, for up to 3 doses, approximately 40-50 minutes before the examination

Administration Ophthalmic: Instill drops into conjunctival sac of affected eye(s); avoid contact of bottle tip with skin or eye; to avoid excessive systemic absorption, finger pressure should be applied on the lacrimal sac during and for 1-2 minutes following application

Patient Information May cause blurred vision and increased sensitivity to light

Nursing Implications Do not repeat dosage within at least 4 hours, but preferably 24 hours, after initial treatment to prevent drug accumulation and potential systemic toxicity; see Warnings

Additional Information Cyclomydril® is the preferred agent for use in neonates and infants because lower concentrations of both cyclopentolate and phenylephrine provide optimal dilation while minimizing the systemic side effects noted with a higher concentration of each agent used alone

Dosage Forms Solution, ophthalmic: Cyclopentolate hydrochloride 0.2% and phenylephrine hydrochloride 1% (2 mL, 5 mL)

Cyclophosphamide (sye kloe FOS fa mide)

Related Information

Drugs and Breast-Feeding *on page 1243*

Emetogenic Potential of Single Chemotherapeutic Agents *on page 1129*

U.S. Brand Names Cytoxan®; Neosar®

Canadian Brand Names Procytox

Synonyms CPM; CTX; CYT

Therapeutic Category Antineoplastic Agent, Alkylating Agent (Nitrogen Mustard)

Generic Available No

Use Treatment of Hodgkin's disease, malignant lymphomas, multiple myeloma, leukemias, sarcomas, mycosis fungoides, neuroblastoma, ovarian carcinoma, breast carcinoma, a variety of other tumors; conditioning regimen for bone marrow transplantation; nephrotic syndrome, lupus erythematosus, severe rheumatoid arthritis, and rheumatoid vasculitis

Pregnancy Risk Factor D

Contraindications Hypersensitivity to cyclophosphamide or any component

Warnings The FDA currently recommends that procedures for proper handling and disposal of antineoplastic agents be considered; cyclophosphamide is potentially carcinogenic and mutagenic; it may impair fertility or cause sterility and birth defects

Precautions Use with caution in patients with bone marrow suppression and impaired renal or hepatic function; modify dosage in patients with renal impairment or compromised bone marrow function. Patients with compromised bone marrow function may require a 33% to 50% reduction in initial dose.

Adverse Reactions

Cardiovascular: Cardiotoxicity with high-dose therapy, pericardial effusion, CHF

Dermatologic: Alopecia, rash

Endocrine & metabolic: Hypokalemia, amenorrhea, SIADH, hyperuricemia, hyperkalemia, hyponatremia, oligospermia, sterility (interferes with oogenesis and spermatogenesis) which may be irreversible

Gastrointestinal: Nausea, vomiting, dysgeusia, anorexia, diarrhea, mucositis

Genitourinary: Hemorrhagic cystitis (5% to 10%)

Hematologic: Leukopenia nadir at 8-15 days, hemolytic anemia, thrombocytopenia, hypothrombinemia

Hepatic: Dose-related hepatotoxicity, jaundice

Renal: Nephrotoxicity

Respiratory: Interstitial pulmonary fibrosis, nasal stuffiness

Drug Interactions Cytochrome P-450 isoenzyme CYP2B6, CYP2D6, and CYP3A3/4 substrate

Allopurinol (increases myelotoxicity of cyclophosphamide); phenobarbital, phenytoin, and chloral hydrate may increase conversion of cyclophosphamide to active

(Continued)

Cyclophosphamide *(Continued)*

metabolites; chloramphenicol, phenothiazines, imipramine may inhibit the metabolism of cyclophosphamide (increased bone marrow suppression); cyclophosphamide may prolong the neuromuscular blocking activity of succinylcholine

Stability Reconstituted I.V. solution is stable for 24 hours at room temperature or 6 days if refrigerated

Mechanism of Action Interferes with the normal function of DNA by alkylation and cross-linking the strands of DNA, and by possible protein modification

Pharmacokinetics

Absorption: 75% to 95% with low doses

Distribution: Crosses the placenta; appears in breast milk; distributes throughout the body including the brain and CSF, but not in concentrations high enough to treat meningeal leukemia

Protein binding: 20%; metabolite: 60%

Metabolism: Inactive prodrug must undergo hydroxylation to form active alkylating mustards; further oxidation leads to formation of inactive metabolites

Half-life: Range 3-12 hours

Children: 4 hours

Adults: 6-8 hours

Time to peak serum concentration: Oral: Within 1 hour

Elimination: In urine as unchanged drug (<20%) and as metabolites (85% to 90%)

Dialysis: Moderately dialyzable (20% to 50%)

Usual Dosage Refer to individual protocols

Children and Adults with no hematologic problems:

Induction:

Oral, I.V.: Children: 2-8 mg/kg or 60-250 mg/m^2/day

I.V.: 40-50 mg/kg (1.5-1.8 g/m^2) in divided doses over 2-5 days

Maintenance:

Oral: Children: 2-5 mg/kg or 50-150 mg/m^2 twice weekly

Oral: Adults: 1-5 mg/kg/day

I.V.: 10-15 mg/kg (350-550 mg/m^2) every 7-10 days or 3-5 mg/kg (110-185 mg/m^2) twice weekly

Children:

SLE: I.V.: 500-750 mg/m^2 every month; maximum dose: 1 g/m^2

JRA/vasculitis: I.V.: 10 mg/kg every 2 weeks

BMT conditioning regimen: I.V.: 50 mg/kg/day once daily for 3-4 days

Nephrotic syndrome: Oral: 2-3 mg/kg/day every day for up to 12 weeks when corticosteroids are unsuccessful

Dosing adjustment in renal impairment:

Cl_{cr} >10 mL/minute: Administer 100% of normal dose

Cl_{cr} ≤10 mL/minute: Administer 75% of normal dose

Administration

Oral: Administer with food only if GI distress occurs

Parenteral: May administer IVP, I.V. intermittent, or continuous infusion at a final maximum concentration for administration of 20-25 mg/mL; usually administered as a single bolus dose or in fractionated doses over 2-3 days. Most protocols use a 30-60 minute infusion time; doses >1800 mg/m^2 need to be infused over a longer period (ie, 4- or 6-hour infusions)

Monitoring Parameters CBC with differential and platelet count, ESR, BUN, urinalysis, serum electrolytes, serum creatinine, urine specific gravity, urine output

Test Interactions Positive Coombs' [direct]

Patient Information Maintain high fluid intake and urine output. Report any difficulty or pain with urination, unusual bleeding or bruising, persistent fever or sore throat, blood in urine or stool, skin rash, or yellowing of skin or eyes. You may be more susceptible to infection; avoid crowds and unnecessary exposure to infection.

Nursing Implications Encourage adequate hydration and frequent voiding to help prevent hemorrhagic cystitis; before initiating cyclophosphamide therapy, verify that urine specific gravity is <1.010 and that urine output is >100 mL/m^2/hour (or 3 mL/kg/hour)

Additional Information Aggressive hydration using fluid containing at least 0.45% sodium chloride at 125 mL/m^2/hour, frequent emptying of the bladder, and concurrent administration of mesna are used to reduce the potential of hemorrhagic cystitis (use mesna with cyclophosphamide doses >1 g/m^2/day; doses ≤1 g/m^2/day may not require use of mesna)

Myelosuppressive effects:

WBC: Moderate

Platelets: Moderate

Onset (days): 7
Nadir (days): 8-14
Recovery (days): 21

Dosage Forms
Powder for injection: 100 mg, 200 mg, 500 mg, 1 g, 2 g
Tablet: 25 mg, 50 mg

Extemporaneous Preparations To make a 2 mg/mL oral elixir, reconstitute a 200 mg vial with aromatic elixir, withdraw the solution, and add sufficient aromatic elixir to make a final volume of 100 mL in a graduate; store in amber glass; stable for 14 days in the refrigerator

Brook D, Davis RE, and Bequette RJ, "Chemical Stability of Cyclophosphamide in Aromatic Elixir USP," *Am J Hosp Pharm*, 1973, 30:618-20.

References
Bostrom BC, Weisdorf DJ, Kim TH, et al, "Bone Marrow Transplantation for Advanced Acute Leukemia: A Pilot Study of High-Energy Total Body Irradiation, Cyclophosphamide and Continuous Infusion Etoposide," *Bone Marrow Transplant*, 1990, 5(2):83-9.

McCune WJ, Golbus J, Zeldes W, et al, "Clinical and Immunologic Effects of Monthly Administration of Intravenous Cyclophosphamide in Severe Systemic Lupus Erythematosus," *N Engl J Med*, 1988, 318(22):1423-31.

Cycloserine (sye kloe SER een)

U.S. Brand Names Seromycin® Pulvules®
Therapeutic Category Antibiotic, Miscellaneous; Antitubercular Agent
Generic Available No
Use Adjunctive treatment in pulmonary or extrapulmonary tuberculosis; treatment of acute urinary tract infections caused by *E. coli* or *Enterobacter* species when less toxic conventional therapy has failed or is contraindicated
Pregnancy Risk Factor C
Contraindications Hypersensitivity to cycloserine or any component; epilepsy, depression, severe anxiety or psychosis, severe renal insufficiency, chronic alcoholism
Precautions Dosage must be adjusted in patients with renal impairment
Adverse Reactions
Cardiovascular: Cardiac arrhythmias, CHF
Central nervous system: Drowsiness, headache, dizziness, vertigo, seizures, confusion, psychosis, paresis, coma, anxiety, nervousness, depression, personality changes
Dermatologic: Rash, photosensitivity
Endocrine & metabolic: Vitamin B_{12} deficiency, folate deficiency
Hepatic: Elevated liver enzymes
Neuromuscular & skeletal: Tremor, dysarthria
Drug Interactions Cycloserine inhibits metabolism of phenytoin; alcohol may increase risk of seizures; ethionamide, isoniazid (additive neurotoxicity with cycloserine)
Food Interactions May increase vitamin B_{12} and folic acid dietary requirements
Mechanism of Action Inhibits bacterial cell wall synthesis by competing with amino acid (D-alanine) for incorporation into the bacterial cell wall
Pharmacokinetics
Absorption: ~70% to 90% from the GI tract
Distribution: Crosses the placenta; appears in breast milk, bile, sputum, synovial fluid and CSF
Protein binding: Not plasma protein bound
Half-life: Patients with normal renal function: 10 hours
Time to peak serum concentration: Within 3-4 hours
Elimination: 60% to 70% of an oral dose excreted unchanged in urine by glomerular filtration within 72 hours, small amounts excreted in feces, remainder is metabolized
Usual Dosage Oral:
Tuberculosis:
Children: 10-20 mg/kg/day divided every 12 hours up to 1000 mg/day
Adults: Initial: 250 mg every 12 hours for 14 days, then give 500 mg to 1 g/day in 2 divided doses
Urinary tract infection: Adults: 250 mg every 12 hours for 14 days
Dosing adjustment in renal impairment:
Cl_{cr} 10-50 mL/minute: Administer every 24 hours
Cl_{cr} <10 mL/minute: Administer every 36-48 hours
Administration Oral: May administer without regard to meals
Monitoring Parameters Periodic renal, hepatic, hematological tests, and plasma cycloserine concentrations
(Continued)

Cycloserine *(Continued)*

Reference Range Adjust dosage to maintain blood cycloserine concentrations <30 µg/mL

Patient Information May cause drowsiness and impair ability to perform tasks requiring mental alertness or physical coordination; avoid alcohol

Nursing Implications Some of the neurotoxic effects may be relieved or prevented by the concomitant administration of pyridoxine; sedatives may be effective in reducing anxiety or tremor

Dosage Forms Capsule: 250 mg

Cyclosporine *(SYE kloe spor een)*

Related Information

Blood Level Sampling Time Guidelines *on page 1220*

Carbohydrate and Alcohol Content of Liquid Medications for Use in Patients Receiving Ketogenic Diets *on page 1258*

Drugs and Breast-Feeding *on page 1243*

U.S. Brand Names Neoral®; Sandimmune®; SangCya™

Synonyms CsA; CyA; Cyclosporine A

Therapeutic Category Immunosuppressant Agent

Generic Available No

Use Immunosuppressant used with corticosteroids to prevent graft vs host disease in patients with kidney, liver, lung, heart, and bone marrow transplants; treatment of nephrotic syndrome in patients with documented focal glomerulosclerosis when corticosteroids and cyclophosphamide are unsuccessful; severe psoriasis; severe autoimmune disease that is resistant to corticosteroids and other therapy

Pregnancy Risk Factor C

Contraindications Hypersensitivity to cyclosporine or any component (ie, polyoxyl 35 castor oil is an ingredient of the parenteral formulation and polyoxyl 40 hydrogenated castor oil is an ingredient of the cyclosporine capsules and solution for microemulsion)

Warnings Immunosuppression with cyclosporine may result in an increased susceptibility to infection and an increased risk of malignancy (lymphomas, lymphoproliferative disorders and squamous cell carcinoma); closely monitor and be prepared to treat anaphylaxis in patients receiving I.V. cyclosporine; serious nephrotoxicity, hypertension, and/or seizures may occur in children receiving cyclosporine; **adjust dosage to avoid toxicity or possible organ rejection via cyclosporine blood or plasma concentration monitoring.**

Precautions Close monitoring and dosage adjustment is required in patients with renal and hepatic impairment

Adverse Reactions

Cardiovascular: Hypertension, flushing, edema

Central nervous system: Seizures, headache, confusion, fever

Dermatologic: Hirsutism, gingival hyperplasia, acne

Endocrine & metabolic: Hyperkalemia, hypomagnesemia, hyperuricemia, hyperchloremic metabolic acidosis, gynecomastia, hyperlipidemia (in patients receiving I.V. cyclosporine)

Gastrointestinal: Abdominal discomfort, diarrhea, nausea, vomiting, anorexia, pancreatitis, hiccups, peptic ulcer

Hematologic: Leukopenia, anemia, thrombocytopenia

Hepatic: Hepatotoxicity (elevated liver enzymes, hyperbilirubinemia)

Neuromuscular & skeletal: Myositis, tremor, paresthesia, leg cramps

Renal: Nephrotoxicity (elevated BUN and serum creatinine)

Respiratory: Sinusitis

Miscellaneous: Lymphoproliferative disorder, increased susceptibility to infection, sensitivity to temperature extremes, anaphylaxis in patients receiving I.V. cyclosporine (reaction includes flushing of the face, respiratory distress with dyspnea and wheezing, hypotension, tachycardia)

Drug Interactions Cytochrome P-450 isoenzyme CYP3A3/4 substrate

Ketoconazole, itraconazole, clarithromycin, fluconazole, azithromycin, clarithromycin, allopurinol, erythromycin, tacrolimus, diltiazem, verapamil, and methylprednisolone increase cyclosporine concentration by inhibiting hepatic metabolism; acyclovir, amphotericin B, aminoglycosides, diclofenac, co-trimoxazole, melphalan, and vancomycin may increase nephrotoxicity of cyclosporine; erythromycin and metoclopramide increase cyclosporine absorption; phenytoin and octreotide decrease cyclosporine bioavailability; phenytoin, phenobarbital, carbamazepine, primidone, ticlopidine, rifabutin, rifampin, trimethoprim, and nafcillin decrease cyclosporine concentration by increasing hepatic metabolism of cyclosporine; potassium-sparing diuretics increase risk of hyperkalemia; lovastatin, simvastatin, and cimetidine may increase cyclosporine concentration; the herbal medicine St John's wort (*Hypericum perforatum*) may significantly decrease concentrations of cyclosporine

Food Interactions High-fat meal increases volume of distribution of cyclosporine; grapefruit and grapefruit juice may affect cyclosporine metabolism resulting in increased cyclosporine concentrations

Stability Do **not** store oral solution or oral solution for emulsion in the refrigerator; store oral solutions in original container only and use contents within 2 months after opening; I.V. cyclosporine prepared in NS is stable 6 hours in a polyvinyl chloride container or 12 hours in a glass container; I.V. cyclosporine diluted in D_5W to a final concentration of 2 mg/mL is stable for 24 hours in glass or polyvinyl chloride containers; I.V. cyclosporine may bind to the plastic tubing in I.V. administration sets and to polyvinyl chloride bags. Polyoxyethylated castor oil (Cremophor El®) surfactant in cyclosporine injection may leach phthalate from polyvinyl chloride containers such as bags and tubing.

Mechanism of Action Inhibition of production and release of interleukin II and inhibits interleukin II-induced activation of resting T lymphocytes

Pharmacokinetics

Absorption: Oral:
Solution or soft gelatin capsule (Sandimmune®): Erratically and incompletely absorbed; dependent on the presence of food, bile acids, and GI motility; larger oral doses of cyclosporine are needed in pediatric patients vs adults due to a shorter bowel length resulting in limited intestinal absorption

Solution in a microemulsion or soft gelatin capsule in a microemulsion are bioequivalent (Neoral®): Erratically and incompletely absorbed; increased absorption, up to 30% when compared to Sandimmune®; absorption is less dependent on food intake, bile, or GI motility when compared to Sandimmune®

Distribution: Widely distributed in tissues and body fluids including the liver, pancreas, and lungs; crosses the placenta; excreted into breast milk
V_{dss}: 4-6 L/kg in renal, liver, and marrow transplant recipients (slightly lower values in cardiac transplant patients; children <10 years of age have higher values)

Protein binding: 90% to 98% of dose binds to blood lipoproteins

Metabolism: Undergoes extensive first-pass metabolism following oral administration; extensively metabolized by the cytochrome P-450 system in the liver

Bioavailability:
Solution or soft gelatin capsule (Sandimmune®): Dependent on patient population and transplant type (<10% in adult liver transplant patients and as high as 89% in renal patients)
Children: 28% (range: 17% to 42%); with gut dysfunction commonly seen in BMT recipients, oral bioavailability is further reduced
Solution or soft gelatin capsule in a microemulsion (Neoral®):
Children: 43% (range: 30% to 68%)
Adults: 23% greater than with Sandimmune® in renal transplant patients, 50% greater in liver transplant patients

Half-life:
Solution or soft gelatin capsule (Sandimmune®): Biphasic
Alpha phase: 1.4 hours
Terminal phase: 6-24 hours, prolonged in patients with hepatic dysfunction
Solution or soft gelatin capsule in a microemulsion (Neoral®): 8.4 hours; lower in pediatric patients vs adults due to a higher metabolism rate

Time to peak serum concentration:
Oral solution or capsule (Sandimmune®): 2-6 hours; some patients have a second peak at 5-6 hours
Oral solution or capsule in a microemulsion (Neoral®): 1.5-2 hours (in renal transplant patients)

Elimination: Primarily biliary with 6% of the dose excreted in urine as unchanged drug (0.1%) and metabolites; clearance is more rapid in pediatric patients than in adults

Usual Dosage Children and Adults (oral dosage is ~3 times the I.V. dosage):
I.V.:
Initial: 5-6 mg/kg/dose administered 4-12 hours prior to organ transplantation
Maintenance: 2-10 mg/kg/day in divided doses every 8-24 hours; patients should be switched to oral cyclosporine as soon as possible; cyclosporine doses should be adjusted to maintain whole blood HPLC trough concentrations in the reference range
Oral: Solution or soft gelatin capsule:
Initial: 14-18 mg/kg/dose administered 4-12 hours prior to organ transplantation
(Continued)

Cyclosporine *(Continued)*

Maintenance, postoperative: 5-15 mg/kg/day divided every 12-24 hours; maintenance dose is usually tapered to 3-10 mg/kg/day

Focal segmental glomerulosclerosis: Initial: 3 mg/kg/day divided every 12 hours

Oral: Solution or soft gelatin capsule in a microemulsion (Neoral®): Based on the organ transplant population:

Initial: Same as the initial dose for solution or soft gelatin capsule
  or
Renal: 9 mg/kg/day (range: 6-12 mg/kg/day)
Liver: 8 mg/kg/day (range: 4-12 mg/kg/day)
Heart: 7 mg/kg/day (range: 4-10 mg/kg/day)

Note: A 1:1 ratio conversion from Sandimmune® to Neoral® has been recommended initially; however, lower doses of Neoral® may be required after conversion to prevent overdose. Total daily doses should be adjusted based on the cyclosporine trough blood concentration and clinical assessment of organ rejection. Cyclosporine blood trough levels should be determined prior to conversion. After conversion to Neoral®, cyclosporine trough levels should be monitored every 4-7 days. **Neoral®, SangCya™, and Sandimmune® are not bioequivalent and cannot be used interchangeably. (SangCya™ oral solution was voluntarily withdrawn form the market.)**

Conditions for dosage adjustments, see table.

Cyclosporine

Condition	Cyclosporine Dosing Adjustment
Switch from I.V. to oral therapy	Threefold increase in dose
T-tube clamping	Decrease dose; increase availability of bile facilitates absorption of cyclosporine
Pediatric patients	May require higher weight-based dose compared to adults
Hepatic dysfunction	Decrease I.V. dose; increase oral dose
Renal dysfunction	Monitor drug levels; may need to decrease dose
Dialysis	Not removed
Inhibitors of hepatic metabolism	Decrease dose
Inducers of hepatic metabolism	Monitor drug level; may need to increase dose

Administration

Oral: Administer consistently at the same time twice daily; use oral syringe, glass dropper, or glass container (not plastic or styrofoam cup); to improve palatability, oral solution may be mixed with milk, chocolate milk, orange juice, or apple juice that is at room temperature; dilution of Neoral® with milk can be unpalatable; stir well and drink at once; do not allow to stand before drinking; rinse with more diluent to ensure that the total dose is taken; after use, dry outside of glass dropper, do not rinse with water or other cleaning agents

Parenteral: May administer by I.V. intermittent infusion or continuous infusion; for intermittent infusion, administer over 2-6 hours at a final concentration not to exceed 2.5 mg/mL

Monitoring Parameters Blood/serum drug concentration (trough), renal and hepatic function tests, serum electrolytes, lipid profile, blood pressure, heart rate

Reference Range Reference ranges are method dependent and specimen dependent; use the same analytical method consistently; trough levels should be obtained immediately prior to next dose

Therapeutic: Not well defined, dependent on organ transplanted, time after transplant, organ function, and cyclosporine toxicity. Empiric therapeutic concentration ranges for trough cyclosporine concentrations:
Kidney: 100-200 ng/mL (serum, RIA)
BMT: 100-250 ng/mL (serum, RIA)
Heart: 100-200 ng/mL (serum, RIA)
Liver: 100-400 ng/mL (blood, HPLC)
Method dependent (optimum cyclosporine trough concentrations):
Serum, RIA: 150-300 ng/mL; 50-150 ng/mL (late post-transplant period)
Whole blood, RIA: 250-800 ng/mL; 150-450 ng/mL (late post-transplant period)
Whole blood, HPLC: 100-500 ng/mL

Test Interactions Cyclosporine adsorbs to silicone; specific whole blood assay for cyclosporine may be falsely elevated if sample is drawn from the same central venous line through which dose was administered (even if flush has been administered and/or dose was given hours before); cyclosporine metabolites cross-react with radioimmunoassay and fluorescence polarization immunoassay

Patient Information Take dose at the same time each day; do not allow diluted oral solution to stand before drinking; do not change brands of cyclosporine unless directed by your physician

Nursing Implications Adequate airway, supportive measures, and agents for treating anaphylaxis should be present when I.V. cyclosporine is administered

Additional Information Diltiazem has been used to prevent cyclosporine nephrotoxicity, reduce the frequency of delayed graft function when administered before and after surgery, and used to treat the mild hypertension that occurs in most patients after transplantation; diltiazem increases cyclosporine blood concentration by delaying its clearance resulting in decreased dosage requirements for cyclosporine

Dosage Forms
Capsule (in a microemulsion): Neoral®: 25 mg, 100 mg
Capsule, soft gelatin: Sandimmune®: 25 mg, 50 mg, 100 mg
Injection: 50 mg/mL (5 mL)
Solution (in a microemulsion): Neoral®: 100 mg/mL

References
Burckart GJ, Canafax DM, and Yee GC, "Cyclosporine Monitoring," *Drug Intell Clin Pharm*, 1986, 20(9):649-52.

Holt DW, Mueller EA, Kovarik JM, et al, "Sandimmune® Neoral® Pharmacokinetics: Impact of the New Oral Formulation," *Transplant Proc*, 1995, 27(1):1434-7.

Lin CY and Lee SF, "Comparison of Pharmacokinetics Between CsA Capsules and Sandimmune® in Pediatric Patients," *Transplant Proc*, 1994, 26(5):2973-4.

Niese D, "A Double-Blind Randomized Study of Sandimmune® Neoral® vs Sandimmune® in New Renal Transplant Recipients: Results After 12 Months," *Transplant Proc*, 1995, 27(2):1849-56.

Taesch S, Niese D, and Mueller EA, "Sandimmune® Neoral®, A New Oral Formulation of Cyclosporine With Improved Pharmacokinetic Characteristics: Safety and Tolerability in Renal Transplant Patients," *Transplant Proc*, 1994, 26(6):3147-9.

Wandstrat TL, Schroeder TJ, and Myre SA, "Cyclosporine Pharmacokinetics in Pediatric Transplant Recipients," *Ther Drug Monit*, 1989, 11(5):493-6.

Yee GC, "Recent Advances in Cyclosporine Pharmacokinetics," *Pharmacotherapy*, 1991, 11(5):130S-134S.

♦ **Cyclosporine A** *see* Cyclosporine *on page 284*
♦ **Cyklokapron®** *see* Tranexamic Acid *on page 975*
♦ **Cylert®** *see* Pemoline *on page 767*
♦ **Cylex® [OTC]** *see* Benzocaine *on page 135*

Cyproheptadine (si proe HEP ta deen)

Related Information
Overdose and Toxicology *on page 1222*

U.S. Brand Names Periactin®

Canadian Brand Names PMS-Cyproheptadine

Therapeutic Category Antihistamine

Generic Available Yes

Use Perennial and seasonal allergic rhinitis and other allergic symptoms including urticaria; appetite stimulant (useful in the management of anorexia nervosa); prophylactic treatment of cluster and migraine headaches; spasticity associated with spinal cord damage associated with spasticity

Pregnancy Risk Factor B

Contraindications Hypersensitivity to cyproheptadine or any component; narrow-angle glaucoma, bladder neck obstruction, acute asthmatic attack, stenosing peptic ulcer, GI tract obstruction, those on MAO inhibitors

Adverse Reactions
Cardiovascular: Tachycardia, palpitations, edema
Central nervous system: Sedation, CNS stimulation, seizures, fatigue, headache, nervousness, depression
Dermatologic: Photosensitivity, rash, angioedema
Gastrointestinal: Appetite stimulation, xerostomia, nausea, diarrhea, abdominal pain
Hematologic: Hemolytic anemia, leukopenia, thrombocytopenia
Hepatic: Hepatitis
Neuromuscular & skeletal: Myalgia, paresthesia, arthralgia
Respiratory: Bronchospasm, epistaxis, pharyngitis
Miscellaneous: Allergic reactions

Drug Interactions MAO inhibitors; enhances sedative effects of other CNS depressants; enhances anticholinergic effects of other anticholinergic agents
(Continued)

Cyproheptadine *(Continued)*

Mechanism of Action A potent antihistamine and serotonin antagonist, competes with histamine for H_1-receptor sites on effector cells in the GI tract, blood vessels, and respiratory tract

Pharmacokinetics
Absorption: Well absorbed
Metabolism: Extensively by conjugation
Elimination: >50% excreted in urine (primarily as metabolites); approximately 25% excreted in feces

Usual Dosage Oral:
Allergic conditions:
Children: 0.25 mg/kg/day or 8 mg/m^2/day in 2-3 divided doses **or**
2-6 years: 2 mg every 8-12 hours (not to exceed 12 mg/day)
7-14 years: 4 mg every 8-12 hours (not to exceed 16 mg/day)
Adults: 4-20 mg/day divided every 8 hours (not to exceed 0.5 mg/kg/day)
Appetite stimulation (anorexia nervosa): Children >13 years and Adults: 2 mg 4 times/day; may be increased gradually over a 3-week period to 8 mg 4 times/day
Cluster headaches: Adults: 4 mg 4 times/day
Migraine headaches:
Children: 4 mg 2-3 times/day
Adults: 4-8 mg 3 times/day
Spasticity associated with spinal cord damage: Children ≥12 years and Adults: 4 mg at bedtime; increase by a 4 mg dose every 3-4 days; average daily dose: 16 mg in divided doses; not to exceed 36 mg/day
Dosage adjustment in hepatic impairment: Reduce dosage in patients with significant hepatic dysfunction

Administration Oral: Administer with food or milk

Test Interactions Diagnostic antigen skin tests; ↑ amylase (S); ↓ fasting glucose (S)

Patient Information Causes drowsiness and may impair ability to perform hazardous duties requiring mental alertness or physical coordination

Dosage Forms
Syrup, as hydrochloride: 2 mg/5 mL with alcohol 5% (120 mL, 473 mL, 4000 mL)
Tablet, as hydrochloride: 4 mg

References
Gracies JM, Nance P, Elovic E, et al, "Traditional Pharmacological Treatments for Spasticity. Part II: General and Regional Treatments," *Muscle Nerve Suppl*, 1997, 6:S92-120.

♦ **Cystadane**® *see Betaine Anhydrous on page 139*
♦ **Cystagon**® *see Cysteamine on page 288*

Cysteamine *(sis TEE a meen)*

U.S. Brand Names Cystagon®

Therapeutic Category Cystinosis, Treatment Agent

Use Management of nephropathic cystinosis

Pregnancy Risk Factor C

Contraindications Hypersensitivity to cysteamine, penicillamine, or any component

Warnings Leukocyte cystine levels should be monitored during oral cysteamine therapy; cysteamine should be given in the lowest doses possible to achieve adequate leukocyte cystine depletion; toxicity can be reduced by initiating therapy with a slowly increasing dose schedule (See Usual Dosage)

Precautions Use with caution in patients with a history of blood dyscrasias, gastric or duodenal ulcer, or neurologic disorder

Adverse Reactions
Cardiovascular: Hypertension
Central nervous system: Somnolence, encephalopathy, headache, seizures, ataxia, confusion, dizziness, jitteriness, nervousness, impaired cognition, emotional changes, hallucinations, nightmares, fever, lethargy
Dermatologic: Urticaria, rash
Endocrine & metabolic: Dehydration
Gastrointestinal: Bad breath, abdominal pain, dyspepsia, constipation, gastroenteritis, duodenitis, duodenal ulceration, vomiting, anorexia, diarrhea
Hematologic: Anemia, leukopenia
Hepatic: Abnormal liver enzymes
Neuromuscular & skeletal: Tremor, hyperkinesia
Otic: Decreased hearing

Mechanism of Action Reacts with cystine in the lysosome to convert it to cysteine and to a cysteine-cysteamine mixed disulfide, both of which can then exit the lysosome in patients with cystinosis, an inherited defect of lysosomal transport

Pharmacokinetics
Absorption: Rapid
Protein binding: 10% to 18%
Half-life: 1 hour

Usual Dosage Oral:
Children <12 years: Initial: 10 mg/kg/day divided into 4 doses; increase by 10 mg/kg/day every 3 weeks to a maximum of 90 mg/kg/day (average effective dose: 50-60 mg/kg/day) **or** 0.16-0.32 g/m^2/day divided into 4 doses; increasing every 3 weeks to a maximum of 1.3 g/m^2/day
Children ≥12 years and Adults (>110 lb): 2 g/day in 4 divided doses; dosage may be increased gradually to 1.95 g/m^2/day

Administration Oral: Contents of capsule may be sprinkled over food

Monitoring Parameters Blood counts and liver enzymes during therapy; monitor leukocyte cystine measurements to determine adequate dosage and compliance (measure 5-6 hours after administration)

Reference Range Leukocyte cystine: <1 nmol of half-cystine/mg protein

Patient Information May cause drowsiness or impair ability to perform activities which require mental alertness or physical coordination

Dosage Forms Capsule, as bitartrate: 50 mg, 150 mg

Cysteine (SIS teen)

Therapeutic Category Nutritional Supplement

Generic Available Yes

Use Supplement to crystalline amino acid solutions, in particular the specialized pediatric formulas (eg, Aminosyn® PF, TrophAmine®) to meet the intravenous amino acid nutritional requirements of infants receiving parenteral nutrition (PN)

Contraindications Hypersensitivity to cysteine or any component; patients with hepatic coma or metabolic disorders involving impaired nitrogen utilization

Warnings Metabolic acidosis has occurred in infants related to the "hydrochloride" component of cysteine; each 1 mmol cysteine (175 mg) delivers 1 mEq chloride and 1 mEq hydrogen ion; to balance the extra hydrochloride ions and prevent acidosis addition to the PN solution of a 1 mEq acetate electrolyte salt for each mmole (175 mg) of cysteine may be needed; each 40 mg cysteine (equal to every 1 g amino acid when used in the recommended ratio) adds 0.228 mEq chloride and hydrogen

Precautions Use with caution in patients with renal dysfunction and hepatic insufficiency

Adverse Reactions
Central nervous system: Fever
Endocrine & metabolic: Metabolic acidosis (see Warnings)
Gastrointestinal: Nausea
Renal: Elevated BUN, azotemia

Stability Avoid excessive heat, do not freeze; when combined with parenteral amino acid solutions, cysteine is relatively unstable; it is intended to be added immediately prior to administration to the patient; infusion of the admixture should begin within 1 hour of mixing or refrigerated until use; stable 24 hours in PN solution; opened vials must be used within 4 hours of entry

Mechanism of Action Cysteine is a sulfur-containing amino acid synthesized from methionine via the transsulfuration pathway. It is a precursor of the tripeptide glutathione and also of taurine. Newborn infants have a relative deficiency of the enzyme necessary to affect this conversion. Cysteine may be considered an essential amino acid in infants.

Usual Dosage I.V.: Neonates and Infants: Added as a fixed ratio to crystalline amino acid solution: 40 mg cysteine per g of amino acids; dosage will vary with the daily amino acid dosage (eg, 0.5-2.5 g/kg/day amino acids would result in 20-100 mg/kg/day cysteine); individual doses of cysteine of 0.8-1 mmol/kg/day have also been added directly to the daily PN solution; the duration of treatment relates to the need for PN; patients on chronic PN therapy have received cysteine until 6 months of age and in some cases until 2 years of age

Administration Parenteral: Use only after dilution into PN solution; dilute with amino acid solution in a ratio of 40 mg cysteine to 1 g amino acid: eg, 500 mg cysteine is added to 12.5 g (250 mL) of 5% amino acid solution

Monitoring Parameters BUN, ammonia, electrolytes, pH, acid-base balance, serum creatinine, liver function tests, growth curve

Additional Information Addition of cysteine to PN solutions enhances the solubility of calcium and phosphate by lowering the overall pH of the solution

Dosage Forms Injection, as hydrochloride: 50 mg/mL [~0.285 mmol/mL] (10 mL)

♦ **Cystospaz®** see Hyoscyamine on page 517

♦ **Cystospaz-M**® *see* Hyoscyamine *on page 517*

♦ **CYT** *see* Cyclophosphamide *on page 281*

Cytarabine (sye TARE a been)

Related Information
    Emetogenic Potential of Single Chemotherapeutic Agents *on page 1129*
U.S. Brand Names Cytosar-U®; Tarabine® PFS
Synonyms Arabinosylcytosine; Ara-C; Cytosine Arabinosine
Therapeutic Category Antineoplastic Agent, Antimetabolite
Generic Available Yes
Use Used in combination regimens for the treatment of leukemias, meningeal leukemia, Hodgkin's lymphoma, and non-Hodgkin's lymphoma
Pregnancy Risk Factor D
Contraindications Hypersensitivity to cytarabine or any component
Warnings The FDA currently recommends that procedures for proper handling and disposal of antineoplastic agents be considered. Must monitor for drug toxicity; drug toxicity includes bone marrow suppression with leukopenia, thrombocytopenia, and anemia along with nausea, vomiting, diarrhea, abdominal pain, oral ulceration, and hepatic dysfunction; irreversible cerebellar toxicity may occur with a cumulative dose ≥ 30 g/m^2; cytarabine is potentially mutagenic and carcinogenic.
Precautions Marked bone marrow suppression necessitates dosage reduction or a reduction in the number of days of administration; with severe hepatic dysfunction, dosage may need to be reduced
Adverse Reactions
    Cardiovascular: Cardiomegaly, chest pain, pericarditis
    Central nervous system: Headache, malaise, confusion, seizures, fever, irritability, cerebral and cerebellar dysfunction (somnolence, personality changes, coma, ataxia)
    Dermatologic: Alopecia, rash
    Endocrine & metabolic: Hyperuricemia
    Gastrointestinal: Nausea, vomiting, oral and anal inflammation with ulceration, anorexia, diarrhea, GI hemorrhage, mucositis
    Hematologic: Myelosuppression (leukopenia, thrombocytopenia, anemia)
    Hepatic: Hepatic dysfunction, jaundice, elevated serum bilirubin and liver enzymes
    Local: Thrombophlebitis
    Neuromuscular & skeletal: Myalgia, bone pain, peripheral neuropathy, weakness, gait disturbances
    Ocular: Conjunctivitis, hemorrhagic conjunctivitis, corneal toxicity, photophobia, blurred vision
    Respiratory: Syndrome of sudden respiratory distress progressing to pulmonary edema and diffuse interstitial pneumonitis have been reported with high-dose regimens
    Miscellaneous: Ara-C syndrome (fever, myalgia, bone pain, rash, conjunctivitis, malaise occurring 6-12 hours after administration); headache and vomiting with I.T. administration; anaphylactoid reaction
Drug Interactions Decreases digoxin oral tablet absorption
Stability Reconstituted solutions containing 20-100 mg/mL cytarabine are stable for 48 hours at room temperature; I.T. Ara-C is compatible with methotrexate and hydrocortisone mixed in the same syringe; physically incompatible with fluorouracil, heparin
Mechanism of Action Converted intracellularly to the active metabolite cytarabine triphosphate; inhibits DNA polymerase via competing with deoxycytidine triphosphate resulting in inhibition of DNA synthesis; incorporated into DNA chain resulting in termination of chain elongation; cell cycle-specific for the S-phase of cell division
Pharmacokinetics
    Distribution: Penetrates the CSF in limited amounts, crosses the placenta
    Protein binding: 13%
    Metabolism: Deactivated by cytidine deaminase primarily in the liver, but also in kidneys, GI mucosa, and granulocytes
    Half-life, terminal: 1-3 hours
    Elimination: ~80% of dose excreted in urine as metabolites within 24 hours; 10% excreted in urine as unchanged drug
Usual Dosage Children and Adults (refer to individual protocols):
    Induction remission:
        I.V.: 200 mg/m^2/day for 5 days at 2-week intervals as a single agent; in combination chemotherapy, 100-200 mg/m^2/day for 5- to 10-day therapy course every 2-4 weeks, or every day until remission, given as an I.V. continuous drip or in 2 divided doses/day

I.T.: 5-75 mg/m² every 2-7 days until CNS findings normalize

Maintenance remission:

I.V.: 70-200 mg/m²/day for 2-5 days at monthly intervals

I.M., S.C.: 1-1.5 mg/kg single dose for maintenance at 1- to 4-week intervals

I.T.: 5-75 mg/m² every 2-7 days until CNS findings normalize **or**

<1 year: 20 mg

1-2 years: 30 mg

2-3 years: 50 mg

>3 years: 70 mg

High-dose regimen: Refractory leukemias or refractory non-Hodgkin's lymphoma:

I.V. infusion: 3 g/m²/dose every 12 hours for up to 12 doses

Administration Parenteral: May administer S.C., I.M., IVP, I.V. infusion, or I.T. at a concentration not to exceed 100 mg/mL

High-dose regimens or for use in neonates: Diluents containing benzyl alcohol should not be used to reconstitute the drug; high-dose regimens (dose >1 g/m²) are usually administered by I.V. infusion over 2 hours or longer, or as an I.V. continuous infusion

IVP: May administer over 15 minutes; rapid administration is associated with greater neurotoxicity

I.T. administration: Reconstitute with preservative free NS, Elliotts B solution, or preservative free LR solution; use preservative free injection formulation for I.T. use; filter through a 0.22 micron filter; the volume to be given I.T. is in the range of 3-10 mL and should correspond to an equivalent volume of CSF removed; antiemetic therapy should be administered prior to intrathecal doses of cytarabine

S.C. administration: Rotate injection sites to thigh, abdomen, and flank regions; avoid repeated administration to a single site

Monitoring Parameters Liver function tests, CBC with differential and platelet count, serum creatinine, BUN, serum uric acid; signs of neurotoxicity

Patient Information Notify physician of any fever, sore throat, bleeding, or bruising

Nursing Implications Administer corticosteroid eye drops for prophylaxis of conjunctivitis around-the-clock prior to, during, and for 2-7 days after high-dose Ara-C; pyridoxine has been administered on days of high-dose Ara-C therapy for prophylaxis of CNS toxicity.

Additional Information Myelosuppressive effects:

WBC: Severe

Platelets: Severe

Onset (days): 4-7

Nadir (days): 14-18

Recovery (days): 21-28

Dosage Forms

Injection, preservative free, as hydrochloride (Tarabine® PFS): 20 mg/mL (5 mL, 50 mL)

Powder for injection, as hydrochloride (Cytosar-U®): 100 mg, 500 mg, 1 g, 2 g

References

Baker WJ, Royer GL, and Weiss RB, "Cytarabine and Neurologic Toxicity," *J Clinical Oncology,* 1991, 9(4):679-93.

Grossman L, Baker MA, Sutton DM, et al, "Central Nervous System Toxicity of High-Dose Cytosine Arabinoside," *Med Pediatr Oncol,* 1983, 11(4):246-50.

♦ **D₇₀W** *see* Dextrose *on page 317*

Dacarbazine (da KAR ba zeen)

Related Information
  Emetogenic Potential of Single Chemotherapeutic Agents *on page 1129*
U.S. Brand Names DTIC-Dome®
Canadian Brand Names DTIC
Synonyms DIC; Imidazole Carboxamide
Therapeutic Category Antineoplastic Agent, Miscellaneous
Generic Available Yes
Use Treatment of malignant melanoma, Hodgkin's disease, soft-tissue sarcomas (fibrosarcomas, rhabdomyosarcoma), islet cell carcinoma, medullary carcinoma of the thyroid, and neuroblastoma
Pregnancy Risk Factor C
Contraindications Hypersensitivity to dacarbazine or any component
Warnings The FDA currently recommends that procedures for proper handling and disposal of antineoplastic agents be considered. Hematopoietic depression is common; hepatic necrosis is also possible; dacarbazine has been reported to cause sterility and is mutagenic and teratogenic in rats
Precautions Use with caution in patients with bone marrow suppression, renal and/ or hepatic impairment; dosage reduction may be necessary in patients with renal or hepatic insufficiency; avoid extravasation of the drug
Adverse Reactions
  Cardiovascular: Facial flushing, hypotension
  Central nervous system: Malaise, headache, fever, seizure
  Dermatologic: Alopecia, rash, photosensitivity
  Gastrointestinal: Anorexia, nausea, vomiting, metallic taste
  Hematologic: Myelosuppression (nadir: 2-4 weeks): Leukopenia, thrombocytopenia
  Hepatic: Hepatotoxicity, hepatic vein thrombosis, hepatocellular necrosis
  Local: Pain and burning at infusion site, thrombophlebitis
  Neuromuscular & skeletal: Myalgia, paresthesia
  Ocular: Blurred vision
  Respiratory: Sinus congestion
  Miscellaneous: Flu-like syndrome, anaphylactic reactions
Drug Interactions Phenytoin, phenobarbital may induce dacarbazine metabolism
Stability Store in refrigerator; intact vials are stable for 4 weeks at room temperature; protect dacarbazine solutions from light; reconstituted dacarbazine solution 10 mg/ mL is stable for 72 hours when refrigerated or 8 hours at room temperature; drug decomposition has occurred if the solution turns pink; dacarbazine is incompatible with hydrocortisone sodium succinate
Mechanism of Action Alkylating agent which forms methyldiazonium ions that attack nucleophilic groups in DNA; inhibits DNA, RNA, and protein synthesis by cross-linking DNA strands
Pharmacokinetics
  Distribution: Distributes to the liver; very little distribution into CSF with CSF concentrations ~14% of plasma concentrations
    V_{dss}: Adults: 17 L/m²
  Protein binding: Minimal, 5%
  Metabolism: N-demethylated in the liver by microsomal enzymes; metabolites may also have an antineoplastic effect
  Half-life, biphasic: Initial: 20-40 minutes; terminal: 5 hours (in patients with normal renal/hepatic function)
  Elimination: ~30% to 50% of dose excreted in urine by tubular secretion, 15% to 25% is excreted in urine as unchanged drug
Usual Dosage I.V. (refer to individual protocols):
  Children:
    Pediatric solid tumors: 200-470 mg/m²/day over 5 days every 21-28 days
    Pediatric neuroblastoma: 800-900 mg/m² as a single dose on day 1 of therapy every 3-4 weeks in combination therapy
    Hodgkin's disease: 375 mg/m² on days 1 and 15 of treatment course, repeat every 28 days
  Adults:
    Malignant melanoma: 2-4.5 mg/kg/day for 10 days, repeat in 4 weeks or may use 250 mg/m²/day for 5 days, repeat in 3 weeks
    Hodgkin's disease: 150 mg/m²/day for 5 days, repeat every 4 weeks **or** 375 mg/ m² on day 1, repeat in 15 days of each 28-day cycle in combination with other agents

Administration Parenteral: Reconstitute vial for IVP doses with at least 2 mL of D_5W or NS; administer dose diluted in 5-10 mL D_5W or NS by slow IVP over 2-3 minutes or by I.V. infusion over 15-120 minutes at a concentration not to exceed 10 mg/mL

Monitoring Parameters CBC with differential, erythrocytes and platelet count; liver function tests

Patient Information Avoid exposure to sunlight; restrict intake of food for 4-6 hours prior to dacarbazine dose to decrease vomiting; flu-like symptoms (ie, malaise, fever, myalgia) may occur 1 week after infusion

Nursing Implications Avoid extravasation; use a D_5W or NS flush before and after a dacarbazine infusion; local pain, burning sensation, and irritation at the injection site may be relieved by local application of hot packs, slowing the I.V. rate and further dilution in I.V. fluid

Dosage Forms Injection: 100 mg (10 mL, 20 mL); 200 mg (20 mL, 30 mL); 500 mg (50 mL)

References

Berg SL, Grisell DL, DeLaney TF, et al, "Principles of Treatment of Pediatric Solid Tumors," *Pediatr Clin North Am*, 1991, 38(2):249-67.

Finklestein JZ, Albo V, Ertel I, et al, "5-(3,3-Dimethyl-l-triazeno) imidazole-4-carboxamide (NSC-45388) in the Treatment of Solid Tumors in Children," *Cancer Chemother Rep*, 1975, 59(2 Pt 1):351-7.

Mutz ID and Urban CE, "Dimethyl-triazeno-imidazole-carboxamide (DTIC) in Combination Chemotherapy for Childhood Neuroblastoma," *Wien Klin Wochenschr*, 1978, 90(24):867-70.

Daclizumab (da CLI zoo mab)

U.S. Brand Names Zenapax®

Synonyms HAT Antibody; Humanized Anti-CD25 mo Ab; Humanized Anti-interleukin-2 Receptor mo Ab; Humanized Anti-Tac mo Ab

Therapeutic Category Immunosuppressant Agent

Use In combination with an immunosuppressive regimen, including cyclosporine and corticosteroids, for prophylaxis of acute organ rejection in patients receiving renal transplants; daclizumab has also been studied in pediatric bone marrow patients; steroid-refractory graft-versus-host disease

Pregnancy Risk Factor C

Contraindications Hypersensitivity to daclizumab or any component

Warnings Should only be used by physicians experienced in immunosuppressive therapy or management of transplant patients; adequate laboratory and supportive medical resources must be readily available in the facility for patient management; may result in an increased susceptibility to infection or an increased risk for developing lymphoproliferative disorders

Adverse Reactions

Cardiovascular: Edema, hypertension (48% in pediatric patients), hypotension, tachycardia, thrombosis

Central nervous system: Headache, dizziness, insomnia, depression, anxiety, fever, chills

Dermatologic: Impaired wound healing, acne, pruritus, rash, hirsutism

Endocrine & metabolic: Dehydration (frequency may be higher for pediatric patients than for adults), diabetes mellitus

Genitourinary: Oliguria, dysuria

Gastrointestinal: Constipation, nausea, diarrhea (36%), vomiting (32%), abdominal pain, abdominal distention

Neuromuscular & skeletal: Tremors, back pain, arthralgia, myalgia

Ocular: Blurred vision

Renal: Renal tubular necrosis, hematuria

Respiratory: Atelectasis, congestion, hypoxia, pharyngitis, pleural effusion

Miscellaneous: Diaphoresis

Stability Refrigerate; do not shake or freeze; protect from direct light; diluted daclizumab solution is stable for 24 hours if refrigerated or for 4 hours at room temperature; discard solution if colored or if particulate matter is present

Mechanism of Action A humanized IgG1 monoclonal antibody produced by recombinant DNA technology that binds specifically to the alpha subunit (p55 alpha, CD25, or Tac subunit) of the human high affinity interleukin-2 receptor (IL-2R) on the surface of activated lymphocytes inhibiting IL-2 binding; inhibits IL-2 mediated activation of lymphocytes which is involved in allograft rejection

Pharmacokinetics Daclizumab serum levels appeared to be somewhat lower in pediatric renal transplant patients than in adult transplant patients administered the same 1 mg/kg dosing regimen

Distribution: V_d: Adults: ~6 L

Half-life: Adults: 20 days

(Continued)

Daclizumab *(Continued)*

Usual Dosage I.V. (refer to individual protocols): Children and Adults:

Initial dose: 1 mg/kg given no more than 24 hours before transplantation, followed by 1 mg/kg/dose administered every 14 days for a total of 5 doses; maximum dose: 100 mg

Steroid-refractory graft-versus-host disease: 0.5-1.5 g/kg as a single dose administered for transient response (repeat doses have been given 11-48 days following the initial dose)

Dosing interval in renal impairment: No dosage adjustment necessary

Administration Parenteral: Daclizumab dose should be diluted in 50 mL NS solution. In fluid-restricted patients, a final concentration of 1 mg/mL can be administered over 15 minutes. When mixing the solution, gently invert the bag to avoid foaming; do not shake. Daclizumab solution should be administered within 4 hours of preparation if stored at room temperature; infuse over a 15-minute period via a peripheral or central vein

Monitoring Parameters CBC with differential, vital signs, immunologic monitoring of T cells, renal function tests, serum glucose

Reference Range Serum trough levels: 5-10 µg/mL

Dosage Forms Injection: 5 mg/mL (5 mL)

References

Vincenti F, Kirkman R, Light S, et al, "Interleukin-2-Receptor Blockade With Daclizumab to Prevent Acute Rejection in Renal Transplantation. Daclizumab Triple Therapy Study Group," *N Engl J Med*, 1998, 338(3):161-5.

♦ **Dacodyl**® **[OTC]** *see* Bisacodyl *on page 143*

Dactinomycin *(dak ti noe MYE sin)*

Related Information

Emetogenic Potential of Single Chemotherapeutic Agents *on page 1129*

U.S. Brand Names Cosmegen®

Synonyms ACT; Act-D; Actinomycin D

Therapeutic Category Antineoplastic Agent, Antibiotic

Generic Available No

Use Management (either alone or in combination with other treatment modalities) of Wilms' tumor, rhabdomyosarcoma, neuroblastoma, retinoblastoma, Ewing's sarcoma, trophoblastic neoplasms, testicular tumors and uterine sarcomas

Pregnancy Risk Factor C

Contraindications Hypersensitivity to dactinomycin or any component; patients with chickenpox or herpes zoster; avoid in infants <6 months of age since the incidence of adverse effects is increased in infants

Warnings The FDA currently recommends that procedures for proper handling and disposal of antineoplastic agents be considered. Dactinomycin is extremely irritating to tissues. If extravasation occurs during I.V. use, severe damage to soft tissue may occur leading to pain, swelling, ulceration, and necrosis.

Precautions Use with caution in patients with hepatobiliary dysfunction or in patients who have received radiation therapy; reduce dosage in patients receiving concurrent radiation therapy and in patients with hepatobiliary dysfunction; avoid administering live virus vaccinations after dactinomycin

Adverse Reactions

Central nervous system: Fatigue, fever

Dermatologic: Alopecia, erythema, hyperpigmentation of skin, desquamation, acne, maculopapular rash

Endocrine & metabolic: Hypocalcemia, hyperuricemia

Gastrointestinal: Anorexia, vomiting, diarrhea, stomatitis, proctitis, nausea

Hematologic: Myelosuppression (nadir: 2-3 weeks), leukopenia, thrombocytopenia, anemia

Hepatic: Hepatitis, hepatic veno-occlusive disease, elevated liver enzymes

Local: Soft tissue damage with extravasation

Miscellaneous: Anaphylactoid reaction, immunosuppression

Drug Interactions Dactinomycin potentiates the effects of radiation therapy; enflurane, halothane (increased hepatotoxicity); decreased effectiveness of vaccines given following dactinomycin

Stability Binds to cellulose filters, therefore, avoid in-line filtration; adsorbs to glass and plastic so dactinomycin should not be given by continuous or intermittent infusion; use of a diluent containing preservatives for reconstitution may result in a precipitate; any unused portion of the reconstituted 0.5 mg/mL solution should be discarded after 24 hours

Mechanism of Action Binds to the guanine portion of DNA intercalating between guanine and cytosine base pairs blocking replication and transcription of the DNA template; causes topoisomerase-mediated single-strand breaks in DNA

Pharmacokinetics

Distribution: Concentrates in nucleated cells and bone marrow; crosses the placenta; poor penetration into CSF (CSF:plasma ratio is <10%); distributes into submaxillary gland, liver, and kidney

Half-life: 3.5 hours (using radioimmunoassay)

Time to peak serum concentration: I.V.: Within 2-5 minutes

Elimination: ~10% of dose excreted as unchanged drug in urine; 15% recovered in feces; 50% appears in bile

Usual Dosage Dosage should be based on body surface area in obese or edematous patients

Children >6 months and Adults: I.V. (refer to individual protocols): 15 mcg/kg/day or 400-600 mcg/m²/day (maximum dose: 500 mcg/day) for 5 days, may repeat every 3-6 weeks; or 2.5 mg/m² given in divided doses over 1 week; or 0.75-2 mg/m² as a single dose given at intervals of 3-6 weeks has been used

Administration Parenteral: I.V.: For I.V. administration only; since drug is extremely irritating to tissues, **do not give I.M. or S.C.**; avoid extravasation; use a D_5W or NS flush before and after a dactinomycin dose to ensure venous patency; administer by slow IVP over a few minutes at a concentration not to exceed 500 mcg/mL into the side-port of a freely flowing I.V. infusion; if extravasation occurs, apply cold compresses to the site

Monitoring Parameters CBC with differential and platelet count, liver function tests and renal function tests

Patient Information Notify physician if fever, sore throat, bleeding, or bruising occurs

Dosage Forms Powder for injection, lyophilized: 0.5 mg

References

Berg SL, Grisell DL, DeLaney TF, et al, "Principles of Treatment of Pediatric Solid Tumors," *Pediatr Clin North Am*, 1991, 38(2):249-67.

Berkowitz RS and Goldstein DP, "Gestational Trophoblastic Disease," *Cancer*, 1995, 76(10 Suppl):2079-85.

Carli M, Pastore G, Perilongo G, et al, "Tumor Response and Toxicity After Single High-Dose Versus Standard Five-Day Divided Dose Dactinomycin in Childhood Rhabdomyosarcoma," *J Clin Oncol*, 1988, 6(4):654-8.

Dantrolene (DAN troe leen)

U.S. Brand Names Dantrium®

Therapeutic Category Antidote, Malignant Hyperthermia; Hyperthermia, Treatment; Skeletal Muscle Relaxant, Nonparalytic

Generic Available No

Use Treatment of spasticity associated with upper motor neuron disorders such as spinal cord injury, stroke, cerebral palsy, or multiple sclerosis; also used as treatment of malignant hyperthermia

Pregnancy Risk Factor C

Contraindications Active hepatic disease; should not be administered where spasticity is used to maintain posture or balance

Warnings May cause hepatotoxicity; overt hepatitis has been most frequently observed between the third and twelfth month of therapy; hepatic injury appears to be greater in females and in patients >35 years of age

Precautions Use with caution in patients with impaired cardiac or pulmonary function or history of previous liver disease

Adverse Reactions

Cardiovascular/respiratory: Pleural effusion with pericarditis, tachycardia

Central nervous system: Seizures, drowsiness, dizziness, lightheadedness, confusion, headache, fatigue, speech disturbances, mental depression, chills, fever

Dermatologic: Rash, photosensitization, acne-like rash, pruritus, urticaria, abnormal hair growth

Gastrointestinal: Diarrhea, nausea, vomiting, severe constipation, GI bleeding, abdominal cramps, dysphagia

(Continued)

Dantrolene *(Continued)*

Genitourinary: Urinary retention or frequency, urinary incontinence

Hepatic: Hepatitis

Local: Phlebitis

Neuromuscular & skeletal: Muscle weakness, myalgia, backache

Ocular: Visual disturbances, excessive tearing

Renal: Hematuria

Drug Interactions Use with verapamil may result in hyperkalemia and myocardial depression; estrogen increases incidence of hepatotoxicity when used concomitantly; additive CNS depressive effects with other CNS depressants; increased toxicity with MAO inhibitors, phenothiazines, clindamycin, warfarin, clofibrate, and tolbutamide

Stability Protect from light; use reconstituted injection within 6 hours; incompatible with dextrose, NS, or bacteriostatic water for injection; precipitates when placed in glass containers for infusion

Mechanism of Action Acts directly on skeletal muscle by interfering with release of calcium ion from the sarcoplasmic reticulum; prevents or reduces the increase in myoplasmic calcium ion concentration that activates the acute catabolic processes associated with malignant hyperthermia

Pharmacokinetics

Absorption: Oral: 35%

Metabolism: Extensive

Half-life:

Children: 7.3 hours

Adults: 8.7 hours

Elimination: 25% excreted in urine as metabolites and unchanged drug; 45% to 50% excreted in feces via bile

Usual Dosage

Spasticity: Oral:

Children: Initial: 0.5 mg/kg/dose twice daily, increase frequency to 3-4 times/day at 4- to 7-day intervals, then increase dose by 0.5 mg/kg to a maximum of 3 mg/kg/dose 2-4 times/day up to 400 mg/day

Adults: 25 mg/day to start, increase frequency to 2-4 times/day, then increase dose by 25 mg every 4-7 days to a maximum of 100 mg 2-4 times/day or 400 mg/day

Hyperthermia: Children and Adults:

Preoperative prophylaxis:

Oral: 4-8 mg/kg/day in 4 divided doses given 1-2 days prior to surgery for those patients at risk; to prevent recurrence, administer last dosage 3-4 hours before scheduled surgery

I.V.: 2.5 mg/kg 1¼ hours before surgery and infused over 1 hour; additional doses may be needed during surgery especially for prolonged surgery

Crisis: I.V.: 1 mg/kg; may repeat as needed to a maximum cumulative dose of 10 mg/kg; if physiologic and metabolic abnormalities reappear, repeat regimen

Postcrisis follow-up: Oral: 4-8 mg/kg/day in 4 divided doses for 1-3 days; I.V. dantrolene may be used when oral therapy is not practical; individualize dosage beginning with 1 mg/kg or more as the clinical situation dictates

Administration

Oral: Contents of capsule may be mixed with juice or liquid

Parenteral: Reconstitute by adding 60 mL sterile water (**not bacteriostatic water for injection**), resultant concentration 0.333 mg/mL; administer by rapid I.V. injection; for infusion, do **not** further dilute with NS or dextrose; place solution in plastic container for continuous infusion

Monitoring Parameters Baseline and periodic liver function tests; temperature (hyperthermia use)

Patient Information Avoid unnecessary exposure to sunlight; avoid alcohol; causes drowsiness and may impair ability to perform hazardous functions requiring mental alertness or physical coordination

Nursing Implications Avoid extravasation since dantrolene is a tissue irritant

Dosage Forms

Capsule, as sodium: 25 mg, 50 mg, 100 mg

Powder for injection, as sodium: 20 mg

Extemporaneous Preparations A 5 mg/mL suspension may be made by adding five 100 mg capsules to a citric acid solution (150 mg citric acid powder in 10 mL water) and then adding syrup to a total volume of 100 mL; shake well; stable 2 days in refrigerator

Nahata MC and Hipple TF, *Pediatric Drug Formulations*, 4th ed, Cincinnati, OH: Harvey Whitney Books Co, 2000.

Dapsone (DAP sone)

U.S. Brand Names Avlosulfon®

Synonyms Diaminodiphenylsulfone

Therapeutic Category Antibiotic, Sulfone; Leprostatic Agent

Generic Available Yes

Use Treatment of leprosy due to susceptible strains of *M. leprae*; treatment of dermatitis herpetiformis; prophylaxis against *Pneumocystis carinii* pneumonia (PCP) in patients who cannot tolerate co-trimoxazole or aerosolized pentamidine; prophylaxis against toxoplasmic encephalitis in patients who cannot tolerate co-trimoxazole

Pregnancy Risk Factor C

Contraindications Hypersensitivity to dapsone or any component; patients with severe anemia

Precautions Use with caution in patients with G-6-PD deficiency, methemoglobin reductase deficiency or hemoglobin M; in patients receiving drugs capable of inducing hemolysis; hypersensitivity to other sulfonamides

Adverse Reactions

Cardiovascular: Tachycardia

Central nervous system: Psychotic episodes, hallucinations, insomnia, vertigo, irritability, headache, fever, uncoordinated speech

Dermatologic: Exfoliative dermatitis, erythema multiforme, toxic epidermal necrolysis, urticaria, morbilliform reactions, erythema nodosum, photosensitivity

Endocrine & metabolic: Hyperkalemia, hypoalbuminemia

Gastrointestinal: Nausea, vomiting, abdominal pain, anorexia

Hematologic: Hemolytic anemia, methemoglobinemia, leukopenia, agranulocytosis, aplastic anemia, neutropenia

Hepatic: Hepatitis, cholestatic jaundice; elevated alkaline phosphatase, AST, bilirubin, and LDH

Neuromuscular & skeletal: Muscle weakness, peripheral neuropathy

Ocular: Blurred vision

Otic: Tinnitus

Renal: Acute tubular necrosis, nephrotic syndrome, albuminuria

Miscellaneous: Lupus erythematosus, mononucleosis-like syndrome

Drug Interactions Cytochrome P-450 isoenzyme CYP2C9, CYP2E1, and CYP3A3/4 substrate

Didanosine (decreases dapsone absorption); rifampin (decreases dapsone concentrations); trimethoprim (increases dapsone concentration); pyrimethamine, nitrofurantoin, primaquine (increase risk of hematologic side effects)

Food Interactions Do not administer with antacids, alkaline foods, or alkaline drugs (may decrease dapsone absorption)

Stability Protect from light

Mechanism of Action Dapsone is a sulfone antimicrobial. The mechanism of action of the sulfones is similar to that of the sulfonamides. Sulfonamides are competitive antagonists of para-aminobenzoic acid (PABA) and inhibit folic acid synthesis in susceptible organisms.

Pharmacokinetics

Absorption: Oral: 86% to 100%

Distribution: Distributes into skin, muscle, kidneys, liver, sweat, sputum, tears, and bile; distributes into breast milk

Protein binding: 50% to 90%

Metabolism: Acetylated and hydroxylated in the liver

Half-life:

Children: 15.1 hours

Adults: 13-83 hours (mean: 20-30 hours)

Time to peak serum concentration: Within 2-8 hours

Elimination: 5% to 20% of dose excreted in urine as unchanged drug; 70% to 85% excreted in urine as metabolites; small amount excreted in feces

Usual Dosage Oral:

Children ≥1 month of age:

Prophylaxis for first episode of opportunistic disease due to *Toxoplasma gondii:* 2 mg/kg or 15 mg/m^2 (maximum dose: 25 mg) once daily in combination with pyrimethamine 1 mg/kg once daily and leucovorin 5 mg every 3 days

Primary and secondary PCP prophylaxis (see "Note" in Additional Information): 2 mg/kg/day once daily (maximum dose: 100 mg/day), or 4 mg/kg/dose once weekly (maximum dose: 200 mg)

Children:

Leprosy: 1-2 mg/kg/day given once daily in combination therapy; maximum dose: 100 mg/day

(Continued)

297

Dapsone *(Continued)*

Adults:

Leprosy: 50-100 mg once daily; combination therapy with one or more antileprosy drugs is recommended to avoid dapsone resistance

Dermatitis herpetiformis: Initial: 50 mg once daily; maintenance dosage range: 25-400 mg/day

PCP treatment: 100 mg once daily in combination with trimethoprim

Primary and secondary PCP prophylaxis: 50 mg twice daily; or dapsone 50 mg once daily plus pyrimethamine 50 mg orally every week plus leucovorin 25 mg orally every week; or dapsone 200 mg orally plus pyrimethamine 75 mg orally plus leucovorin 25 mg orally every week

Toxoplasma gondii prophylaxis: 50 mg once daily plus pyrimethamine 50 mg orally every week, plus leucovorin 25 mg orally every week

Administration Oral: Administer with water

Monitoring Parameters CBC with differential, platelet count, hemoglobin, hematocrit, liver function tests, and urinalysis

Patient Information May cause photosensitivity; notify physician if fever, sore throat, pallor, fatigue, rash, purpura, or jaundice occurs

Additional Information Note: Guidelines for prophylaxis of *Pneumocystis carinii* pneumonia: Initiate PCP prophylaxis in the following patients: In all HIV-exposed children at 4-6 weeks of age and continue through the first year of life or until HIV infection has been reasonably excluded; children 1-5 years of age with CD4+ count <500 or CD4+ percentage <15%; children 6-12 years of age with CD4+ count <200 or CD4+ percentage <15%; adolescents and adults with CD4+ count <200 or oropharyngeal candidiasis. Folinic acid (leucovorin) should be given if bone marrow suppression occurs.

Dosage Forms Tablet: 25 mg, 100 mg

Extemporaneous Preparations One report indicated that dapsone may not be well absorbed when administered to children as suspensions made from pulverized tablets

Mirochnick M, Clarke D, Brenn A, et al, "Low Serum Dapsone Concentrations in Children Receiving an Extemporaneously Prepared Oral Formulation," [Abstract Th B 365], APS-SPR, Baltimore, MD: 1992.

Jacobus Pharmaceutical Company (609) 921-7447 makes a 2 mg/mL proprietary liquid formulation available under an IND for the prophylaxis of *Pneumocystis carinii* pneumonia

References

"1999 USPHS/IDSA Guidelines for the Prevention of Opportunistic Infections in Persons Infected With Human Immunodeficiency Virus. USPHS/IDSA Prevention of Opportunistic Infections Working Group," *MMWR Morb Mortal Wkly Rep*, 1999, 48(RR-10): 1-66.

Barnett ED, Pelton SI, Mirochnick M, et al, "Dapsone for Prevention of *Pneumocystis* Pneumonia in Children With Acquired Immunodeficiency Syndrome," *Pediatr Infect Dis J*, 1994, 13(1):72-4.

Mirochnick M, Michaels M, Clarke D, et al, "Pharmacokinetics of Dapsone in Children," *J Pediatr*, 1993, 122(5 Pt 1):806-9.

Stavola JJ and Noel GJ, "Efficacy and Safety of Dapsone Prophylaxis Against *Pneumocystis carinii* Pneumonia in Human Immunodeficiency Virus-Infected Children," *Pediatr Infect Dis J*, 1993, 12(8):644-7.

♦ **Daraprim**® *see* Pyrimethamine *on page 859*

♦ **Darvocet-N**® **50** *see* Propoxyphene and Acetaminophen *on page 846*

♦ **Darvocet-N**® **100** *see* Propoxyphene and Acetaminophen *on page 846*

♦ **Darvon**® *see* Propoxyphene *on page 845*

♦ **Darvon-N**® *see* Propoxyphene *on page 845*

♦ **Daunomycin** *see* Daunorubicin *on page 298*

Daunorubicin *(daw noe ROO bi sin)*

Related Information

Extravasation Treatment *on page 1085*

U.S. Brand Names Cerubidine®

Synonyms Daunomycin; DNR; Rubidomycin

Therapeutic Category Antineoplastic Agent, Anthracycline; Antineoplastic Agent, Antibiotic

Generic Available No

Use In combination with other agents in the treatment of leukemias (ALL, AML)

Pregnancy Risk Factor D

Contraindications Hypersensitivity to daunorubicin or any component; CHF, left ventricular ejection fraction <30% to 40%, or arrhythmias; pre-existing bone marrow suppression

Warnings The FDA currently recommends that procedures for proper handling and disposal of antineoplastic agents be considered; I.V. use only; severe local tissue necrosis will result if extravasation occurs; irreversible myocardial toxicity may occur as total dosage approaches 550 mg/m^2 in adults, 400 mg/m^2 in patients receiving chest radiation, 300 mg/m^2 in children ≥2 years of age, or 10 mg/kg in children <2 years; this may occur during therapy or several months after therapy; total cumulative dose should take into account previous or concomitant treatment with cardiotoxic agents or irradiation of chest; infants and children may be more susceptible to anthracycline-induced cardiotoxicity than adults; severe myelosuppression is possible when used in therapeutic doses

Precautions Reduce dosage in patients with hepatic, biliary, or renal impairment

Adverse Reactions
   Cardiovascular: Cardiotoxicity, CHF (dose-related, may occur 7-8 years after treatment), arrhythmias, EKG abnormalities
   Central nervous system: Fever, chills
   Dermatologic: Alopecia, hyperpigmentation of skin and nail beds, urticaria, pruritus
   Endocrine & metabolic: Hyperuricemia, infertility, sterility
   Gastrointestinal: Stomatitis, esophagitis, nausea, vomiting, diarrhea
   Genitourinary: Discoloration of urine (red-orange)
   Hematologic: Myelosuppression (thrombocytopenia, leukopenia)
   Hepatic: Elevated serum bilirubin, AST, and alkaline phosphatase
   Local: Severe tissue necrosis with extravasation

Stability Protect from light; reconstituted solution is stable for 48 hours when refrigerated and 24 hours at room temperature; a color change from red to blue/purple indicates decomposition of the drug; unstable in solutions with a pH >8; incompatible with heparin, sodium bicarbonate, 5-FU, and dexamethasone

Mechanism of Action Inhibition of DNA and RNA synthesis by intercalating between DNA base pairs, uncoiling of the helix, and by steric obstruction; not cell cycle-specific for the S-phase of cell division; may cause free radical damage to DNA

Pharmacokinetics
   Distribution: Widely distributed in tissues such as spleen, heart, kidneys, liver, and lungs; does not cross the blood-brain barrier; crosses the placenta
   Metabolism: To daunorubicinol (active)
   Half-life, terminal: 14-18.5 hours
      Daunorubicinol, active metabolite: 26.7 hours
   Elimination: 40% of dose excreted in bile; ~14% to 23% excreted in urine as metabolite and unchanged drug

Usual Dosage I.V. (refer to individual protocols):
   Children <2 years or <0.5 m^2: Dosage should be calculated on the basis of body weight rather than body surface area: 1 mg/kg or per protocol with frequency dependent on regimen employed
   Children:
      ALL combination therapy: Remission induction: 25-45 mg/m^2 on days 1 and 8 of cycle, or 30-45 mg/m^2/day for 3 days every 3-4 weeks, or 25 mg/m^2 every week for 4 weeks
      AML combination therapy: Induction: I.V. continuous infusion: 30-60 mg/m^2/day on days 1-3 of cycle, or 20 mg/m^2/day for 4 days every 14 days
   Adults: 30-60 mg/m^2/day for 3-5 days, repeat dose in 3-4 weeks; total cumulative dose should not exceed 400-600 mg/m^2
      AML: Single agent induction: 60 mg/m^2/day for 3 days; repeat every 3-4 weeks
      AML: Combination therapy induction: 45 mg/m^2/day for 3 days of the first course of induction therapy; subsequent courses: Every day for 2 days
      ALL: Combination therapy: Remission induction: 45 mg/m^2 on days 1, 2, and 3 of induction course
   Dosing adjustment in hepatic or renal impairment: Reduce dose by 25% in patients with serum bilirubin of 1.2-3 mg/dL; reduce dose by 50% in patients with serum bilirubin and/or creatinine >3 mg/dL

Administration Parenteral: Drug is very irritating, do not inject I.M. or S.C.; administer IVP diluting the reconstituted dose in 10-15 mL NS and administering over 2-3 minutes into the tubing of a rapidly infusing I.V. solution of D$_5$W or NS; daunorubicin has also been diluted in 100 mL of D$_5$W or NS and infused over 30-45 minutes or as a continuous 24-hour infusion

Monitoring Parameters CBC with differential and platelet count, liver function test, EKG, ventricular ejection fraction, renal function test; patency of I.V. line

Patient Information Transient red-orange discoloration of urine can occur for up to 48 hours after a dose; notify physician if fever, sore throat, bleeding, or bruising occurs
(Continued)

Daunorubicin *(Continued)*

Nursing Implications Leukemic patients should receive prophylactic allopurinol to prevent acute urate nephropathy; avoid extravasation; if extravasation occurs, apply a cold compress immediately for 30-60 minutes, then alternate off/on every 15 minutes for 1 day; apply 1.5 mL of dimethylsulfoxide 99% (w/v) solution to the site every 6 hours for 14 days; allow to air-dry; do not cover

Additional Information Myelosuppressive effects:

WBC: Severe
Platelets: Severe
Onset (days): 7
Nadir (days): 10-14
Recovery (days): 21-28

Dosage Forms

Injection, as hydrochloride: 5 mg/mL (4 mL)
Powder for injection, lyophilized, as hydrochloride: 20 mg

References

Crom WR, Glynn-Barnhart AM, Rodman JH, et al, "Pharmacokinetics of Anticancer Drugs in Children," *Clin Pharmacokinet*, 1987, 12(3):168-213.

♦ **d-Biotin [OTC]** *see Biotin on page 143*
♦ **DC 240® Softgel® [OTC]** *see Docusate on page 350*
♦ **DDAVP®** *see Desmopressin on page 305*
♦ **ddC** *see Zalcitabine on page 1020*
♦ **DDI** *see Didanosine on page 327*
♦ **1-Deamino-8-D-Arginine Vasopressin** *see Desmopressin on page 305*
♦ **Debrox® [OTC]** *see Carbamide Peroxide on page 178*
♦ **Decadron®** *see Dexamethasone on page 307*
♦ **Decadron® Phosphate** *see Dexamethasone on page 307*
♦ **Declomycin®** *see Demeclocycline on page 302*
♦ **Decofed® Syrup [OTC]** *see Pseudoephedrine on page 852*
♦ **Decongestant Nasal Mist (Can)** *see Oxymetazoline on page 749*
♦ **Decongestant Tablets (Can)** *see Pseudoephedrine on page 852*

Deferoxamine *(de fer OKS a meen)*

U.S. Brand Names Desferal®

Therapeutic Category Antidote, Aluminum Toxicity; Antidote, Iron Toxicity; Chelating Agent, Parenteral

Generic Available No

Use Acute iron intoxication; chronic iron overload secondary to multiple transfusions; diagnostic test for iron overload; used investigationally in the treatment of aluminum accumulation in renal failure

Pregnancy Risk Factor C

Contraindications Patients with severe renal disease, anuria, or primary hemochromatosis

Warnings Cataracts, decreased visual acuity, impaired peripheral and color vision, impaired night vision, and retinal pigmentary abnormalities have been reported after usage for prolonged periods at high dosages or in patients with low ferritin levels; periodic eye exams are recommended while on chronic therapy; neurotoxicity-related auditory abnormalities have been reported including high frequency sensorineural hearing loss; periodic auditory exams are recommended

Precautions Use with caution in patients with pyelonephritis; may increase susceptibility to *Yersinia enterocolitica* infections; flushing of the skin, urticaria, hypotension, and shock have been reported after rapid I.V. administration

Adverse Reactions

Cardiovascular: Flushing, hypotension with rapid I.V. injection, tachycardia, shock, edema
Central nervous system: Fever
Dermatologic: Erythema, urticaria, pruritus, rash, cutaneous wheal formation
Endocrine & Metabolic: Growth impairment
Gastrointestinal: Abdominal discomfort, diarrhea
Genitourinary: Discoloration of urine (reddish color)
Local: Pain, induration at injection site
Neuromuscular & skeletal: Leg cramps
Ocular: Blurred vision; cataracts; impaired peripheral, color, and night vision; retinal pigmentary abnormalities
Otic: Hearing loss, tinnitus

Miscellaneous: Anaphylaxis, possible increased risk of infections particularly with *Y. enterocolitica*

Stability Protect from light; reconstituted solutions are stable for 7 days at room temperature

Mechanism of Action Complexes with trivalent ions (ferric ions) to form ferrioxamine, which is removed by the kidneys

Pharmacokinetics

Absorption: Oral: <15%

Metabolism: By plasma enzymes to ferrioxamine

Half-life:

Deferoxamine: 6.1 hours

Ferrioxamine: 5.8 hours

Elimination: Renal excretion of the metabolite iron chelate and unchanged drug

Usual Dosage

Children:

Acute iron intoxication:

I.M.: 50 mg/kg/dose every 6 hours; maximum dose: 6 g/day

I.V.: 15 mg/kg/hour; maximum dose: 6 g/day

Alternative dosing I.M. or I.V.: 20 mg/kg or 600 mg/m^2 initially followed by 10 mg/kg or 300 mg/m^2 at 4-hour intervals for 2 doses; subsequent doses of 10 mg/kg or 300 mg/m^2 every 4-12 hours may be repeated depending upon the clinical response; maximum dose: 6 g/day

Chronic iron overload:

I.V.: 15 mg/kg/hour; maximum dose: 12 g/day

S.C. infusion via a portable, controlled infusion device: 20-50 mg/kg/day over 8-12 hours; maximum dose: 2 g/day

Adults:

Acute iron intoxication:

I.M.: 1 g stat, then 0.5 g every 4 hours for two doses, additional doses of 0.5 g every 4-12 hours up to 6 g/day may be needed depending upon the clinical response

I.V.: 15 mg/kg/hour; maximum dose: 6 g/day

Chronic iron overload:

I.M.: 0.5-1 g/day

I.V.: 15 mg/kg/hour; maximum dose: 12 g/day

S.C. infusion via a portable, controlled infusion device: 1-2 g/day over 8-24 hours

Aluminum-induced bone disease: 20-40 mg/kg every hemodialysis treatment, frequency dependent on clinical status of the patient

Administration Parenteral: Add 2 mL sterile water to 500 mg vial; for I.M. or S.C. administration, no further dilution is required; for I.V. infusion, dilute in dextrose, NS, LR: 10 mg/mL (maximum concentration: 250 mg/mL); maximum rate of infusion: 15 mg/kg/hour; local reactions at the site of subcutaneous infusion may be minimized by diluting the deferoxamine in 5-10 mL sterile water and adding 1 mg hydrocortisone to each mL of deferoxamine solution

Monitoring Parameters Serum ferritin, iron, total iron binding capacity; ophthalmologic exam and audiometry with chronic use

Reference Range Effective plasma concentration: 3-15 mcg/mL

Patient Information Report any hearing loss, night blindness, decreased visual acuity, impaired peripheral vision, or loss of color vision; may cause the urine to turn a reddish color

Nursing Implications Local injection site reactions may be minimized by daily rotation of subcutaneous injection sites and by applying topical corticosteroids; painful lumps formed under the skin may indicate that the rate of S.C. administration exceeds the rate of absorption from the injection site or the needle is inserted too close to the dermis

Additional Information Has been used investigationally as a single 40 mg/kg I.V. dose over 2 hours, to promote mobilization of aluminum from tissue stores as an aid in the diagnosis of aluminum-associated osteodystrophy

Dosage Forms Powder for injection, as mesylate: 500 mg

References

Bentur Y, McGuigan M, and Koren G, "Deferoxamine (Desferrioxamine): New Toxicities for an Old Drug," *Drug Saf*, 1991, 6(1):37-46.

Cohen AR, Mizanin J, and Schwartz E, "Rapid Removal of Excessive Iron With Daily, High-Dose Intravenous Chelation Therapy," *J Pediatr*, 1989, 115(1):151-5.

Freedman MH, Olivieri N, Benson L, et al, "Clinical Studies on Iron Chelation in Patients With Thalassemia Major," *Haematologica*, 1990, 75(Suppl 5):74-83.

Giardina PJ, Grady RW, Ehlers KH, et al, "Current Therapy of Cooley's Anemia: A Decade of Experience With Subcutaneous Desferrioxamine," *Ann N Y Acad Sci*, 1990, 612:275-85.

Kirking MH, "Treatment of Chronic Iron Overload," *Clin Pharm*, 1991, 10(10):775-83.

(Continued)

Deferoxamine *(Continued)*

Pippard MJ, "Iron Metabolism and Iron Chelation in the Thalassemia Disorders," *Haematologica*, 1990, 75(Suppl 5):66-71.

♦ **Deficol® [OTC]** *see* Bisacodyl *on page 143*
♦ **Dehydral (Can)** *see* Methenamine *on page 643*
♦ **Dehydrated Alcohol Injection** *see* Ethyl Alcohol *on page 409*
♦ **Delacort®** *see* Hydrocortisone *on page 506*
♦ **Del Aqua-5® Gel** *see* Benzoyl Peroxide *on page 136*
♦ **Del Aqua-10® Gel** *see* Benzoyl Peroxide *on page 136*
♦ **Delatestryl®** *see* Testosterone *on page 938*
♦ **Delestrogen®** *see* Estradiol *on page 400*
♦ **Delsym® [OTC]** *see* Dextromethorphan *on page 316*
♦ **Deltacortisone** *see* Prednisone *on page 824*
♦ **Deltadehydrocortisone** *see* Prednisone *on page 824*
♦ **Deltahydrocortisone** *see* Prednisolone *on page 821*
♦ **Deltasone®** *see* Prednisone *on page 824*
♦ **Demadex®** *see* Torsemide *on page 971*

Demeclocycline *(dem e kloe SYE kleen)*

U.S. Brand Names Declomycin®
Synonyms Demethylchlortetracycline
Therapeutic Category Antibiotic, Tetracycline Derivative
Generic Available No
Use Treatment of susceptible bacterial infections (acne, gonorrhea, pertussis, chronic bronchitis, and urinary tract infections) caused by both gram-negative and gram-positive organisms; treatment of chronic syndrome of inappropriate antidiuretic hormone (SIADH) secretion
Pregnancy Risk Factor D
Contraindications Hypersensitivity to demeclocycline, tetracyclines, or any component
Warnings Photosensitivity reactions occur frequently with this drug, avoid prolonged exposure to sunlight; do not use tanning equipment. Do not administer to children ≤8 years of age; use of tetracyclines during tooth development may cause permanent discoloration of the teeth and enamel hypoplasia; do not administer to pregnant women; use of tetracyclines in pregnant women may result in retardation of bone growth and skeletal development of the fetus; prolonged use may result in superinfection. Use of outdated tetracyclines have caused a Fanconi-like syndrome.
Precautions Modify dosage in patients with impaired renal function
Adverse Reactions
Central nervous system: Increased intracranial pressure, bulging fontanels in infants
Dermatologic: Rash, pruritus, photosensitivity, exfoliative dermatitis, discoloration of nails, Stevens-Johnson syndrome
Endocrine & metabolic: Diabetes insipidus syndrome
Gastrointestinal: Nausea, vomiting, diarrhea, anorexia, pancreatitis
Hematologic: Leukopenia, neutropenia, thrombocytopenia
Hepatic: Hepatotoxicity
Neuromuscular & skeletal: Paresthesia
Renal: Azotemia
Miscellaneous: Superinfections
Drug Interactions Antacids, calcium, magnesium, zinc, and iron preparations may decrease absorption of demeclocycline
Food Interactions Food, milk, milk formulas, and dairy products decrease absorption of demeclocycline
Mechanism of Action Inhibits protein synthesis by binding with the 30S ribosomal subunits and preventing the binding of transfer RNA to those ribosomes of susceptible bacteria; may also cause alterations in the cytoplasmic membrane
Pharmacodynamics Onset of action for diuresis in SIADH: Within 5 days
Pharmacokinetics
Absorption: ~60% to 80% of dose absorbed from the GI tract; food and dairy products reduce absorption by 50% or more
Distribution: Excreted into breast milk
Protein binding: 90% to 95%
Metabolism: Small amounts metabolized in the liver to inactive metabolites; enterohepatically recycled
Half-life: 10-17 hours (prolonged with reduced renal function)
Time to peak serum concentration: Oral: Within 3-6 hours

Elimination: Excreted as unchanged drug (42% to 50%) in urine
Usual Dosage Oral:
   Children >8 years: 8-12 mg/kg/day divided every 6-12 hours
   Adults: 150 mg 4 times/day or 300 mg twice daily
      Uncomplicated gonorrhea: 600 mg stat, 300 mg every 12 hours for 4 days (3 g total)
      SIADH: 900-1200 mg/day or 13-15 mg/kg/day divided every 6-8 hours initially, then decrease to 600-900 mg/day
Dosing adjustment in renal impairment: Not recommended for use
Administration Oral: Administer 1 hour before or 2 hours after food or milk with plenty of fluids; do not administer with food, milk, dairy products, antacids, zinc, or iron supplements
Monitoring Parameters CBC, renal and hepatic function tests
Test Interactions May interfere with tests for urinary glucose (false-negative urine glucose using Clinistix®, Tes-Tape®)
Patient Information Avoid prolonged exposure to sunlight or sunlamps; sunscreens provide only limited protection against photosensitivity reactions; may discolor fingernails; avoid taking dosages at bedtime
Dosage Forms
   Capsule, as hydrochloride: 150 mg
   Tablet, as hydrochloride: 150 mg, 300 mg
References
Abdi EA and Bishop S, "The Syndrome of Inappropriate Antidiuretic Hormone Secretion With Carcinoma of the Tongue," *Med Pediatr Oncol*, 1988, 16(3):210-5.
Troyer AD, "Demeclocycline. Treatment for Syndrome of Inappropriate Antidiuretic Hormone Secretion," *JAMA*, 1977, 237(25):2723-6.

♦ **Demerol®** *see* Meperidine *on page 628*
♦ **4-Demethoxydaunorubicin** *see* Idarubicin *on page 523*
♦ **Demethylchlortetracycline** *see* Demeclocycline *on page 302*
♦ **Denorex® [OTC]** *see* Coal Tar *on page 260*
♦ **Deodorized Opium Tincture** *see* Opium Tincture *on page 737*
♦ **2'-Deoxy-3'-Thiacytidine** *see* Lamivudine *on page 572*
♦ **Depacon™** *see* Valproic Acid and Derivatives *on page 998*
♦ **Depakene®** *see* Valproic Acid and Derivatives *on page 998*
♦ **Depakote®** *see* Valproic Acid and Derivatives *on page 998*
♦ **Depakote®-ER** *see* Valproic Acid and Derivatives *on page 998*
♦ **Depen®** *see* Penicillamine *on page 769*
♦ **Depo®-Estradiol** *see* Estradiol *on page 400*
♦ **Depogen®** *see* Estradiol *on page 400*
♦ **Depo-Medrol®** *see* Methylprednisolone *on page 655*
♦ **Deponit®** *see* Nitroglycerin *on page 717*
♦ **Depopred®** *see* Methylprednisolone *on page 655*
♦ **Depo-Provera®** *see* Medroxyprogesterone *on page 624*
♦ **Depo®-Testosterone** *see* Testosterone *on page 938*
♦ **Deproic (Can)** *see* Valproic Acid and Derivatives *on page 998*
♦ **Dermacne (Can)** *see* Benzoyl Peroxide *on page 136*
♦ **Dermarest Dricort® [OTC]** *see* Hydrocortisone *on page 506*
♦ **Derma-Smoothe/FS®** *see* Fluocinolone *on page 439*
♦ **Dermazin (Can)** *see* Silver Sulfadiazine *on page 901*
♦ **Dermoplast® [OTC]** *see* Benzocaine *on page 135*
♦ **Dermoxyl (Can)** *see* Benzoyl Peroxide *on page 136*
♦ **Dermtex® HC [OTC]** *see* Hydrocortisone *on page 506*
♦ **Desenex (Can)** *see* Undecylenic Acid and Derivatives *on page 994*
♦ **Desferal®** *see* Deferoxamine *on page 300*

Desipramine (des IP ra meen)
Related Information
   Comparison of Adverse Effects of Antidepressants *on page 1066*
   Comparison of Usual Adult Dosage and Mechanism of Action of Antidepressants *on page 1065*
   Drugs and Breast-Feeding *on page 1243*
   Overdose and Toxicology *on page 1222*
U.S. Brand Names Norpramin®
Canadian Brand Names Alti-Desipramine; Apo-Desipramine; Novo-Desipramine; Nu-Desipramine; PMS-Desipramine
(Continued)

Desipramine *(Continued)*

Therapeutic Category Antidepressant, Tricyclic

Generic Available Yes: Tablet

Use Treatment of various forms of depression, often in conjunction with psychotherapy; analgesic in chronic pain, peripheral neuropathies

Pregnancy Risk Factor C

Contraindications Hypersensitivity to desipramine (cross-sensitivity with other tricyclic antidepressants may occur) or any component; use of MAO inhibitors within 14 days (potentially fatal reactions may occur, see Drug Interactions); narrow-angle glaucoma

Warnings Do not discontinue abruptly in patients receiving long-term high-dose therapy

Precautions Use with caution in patients with cardiovascular disease, conduction disturbances, urinary retention, seizure disorders, hyperthyroidism or those receiving thyroid replacement

Adverse Reactions Less sedation and anticholinergic adverse effects than amitriptyline or imipramine

> Cardiovascular: Arrhythmias, hypotension; asymptomatic EKG changes and minor increases in diastolic blood pressure and heart rate have been noted in children receiving >3.5 mg/kg/day; **Note:** 4 cases of sudden death have been reported in children 5-14 years of age; an association between desipramine and sudden death was not shown to be significant in one retrospective study; further studies are needed
>
> Central nervous system: Sedation, confusion, dizziness
>
> Dermatologic: Photosensitivity
>
> Endocrine & metabolic: SIADH
>
> Gastrointestinal: Constipation, nausea, vomiting, xerostomia, weight gain
>
> Genitourinary: Urinary retention, discoloration of urine (blue-green)
>
> Hematologic: Blood dyscrasias
>
> Hepatic: Hepatitis
>
> Ocular: Blurred vision, increases intraocular pressure
>
> Otic: Tinnitus
>
> Miscellaneous: Hypersensitivity reactions

Drug Interactions Cytochrome P-450 isoenzyme CYP1A2 and CYP2D6 substrate; isoenzyme CYP2D6 inhibitor

> May decrease effects of guanethidine and clonidine; may increase effects of CNS depressants, alcohol, adrenergic agents, anticholinergic agents; with MAO inhibitors, fever, tachycardia, hypertension, seizures, and death may occur; cimetidine may decrease desipramine clearance and increase plasma concentrations; the herbal medicine St John's wort (*Hypericum perforatum*) may increase serious side effects, its use is **not** recommended; interactions similar to other tricyclics may occur

Food Interactions May increase riboflavin dietary requirements

Mechanism of Action Increases the synaptic concentration of serotonin and/or norepinephrine in the central nervous system by inhibition of their reuptake by the presynaptic neuronal membrane

Pharmacodynamics

> Onset of antidepressant effects: Occasionally seen in 2-5 days
>
> Maximum antidepressant effects: After more than 2 weeks

Pharmacokinetics

> Absorption: Well absorbed from the GI tract
>
> Distribution: V_d: Adults: 21 L/kg; distributes into breast milk (concentrations approximately equal to maternal plasma)
>
> Protein binding: 90%
>
> Metabolism: In the liver
>
> Half-life, adults: 12-57 hours
>
> Elimination: 70% in urine

Usual Dosage Oral:

> Children 6-12 years: 1-3 mg/kg/day in divided doses; monitor carefully with doses >3 mg/kg/day; maximum dose: 5 mg/kg/day
>
> Adolescents: Initial: 25-50 mg/day; gradually increase to 100 mg/day in single or divided doses; maximum dose: 150 mg/day
>
> Adults: Initial: 75 mg/day in divided doses; increase gradually to 150-200 mg/day in divided or single dose; maximum dose: 300 mg/day

Administration Oral: Administer with food to decrease GI upset

Monitoring Parameters Blood pressure, heart rate, EKG, mental status, weight

> Long-term use: CBC with differential, liver enzymes, serum concentrations

Reference Range
Therapeutic: 150-300 ng/mL (SI: 560-1125 nmol/L)
Possible toxicity: >300 ng/mL (SI: >1070 nmol/L)
Toxic: >1000 ng/mL (SI: >3750 nmol/L)

Patient Information May cause drowsiness and impair ability to perform activities requiring mental alertness or physical coordination; may cause dry mouth; avoid alcohol and the herbal medicine, St John's wort; limit caffeine; may discolor urine to blue-green color; do not discontinue medication abruptly; may increase appetite; avoid unnecessary exposure to sunlight

Additional Information Place in therapy (treatment of depression): Desipramine is considered by some clinicians to be the first or second drug of choice for depressed children with excessive daytime sleepiness

Dosage Forms Tablet, as hydrochloride (Norpramin®): 10 mg, 25 mg, 50 mg, 75 mg, 100 mg, 150 mg

References
Biederman J, Thisted RA, Greenhill LL, et al, "Estimation of the Association Between Desipramine and the Risk for Sudden Death in 5-14 Year-Old Children," *J Clin Psychiatry*, 1995, 56(3):87-93.
Levy HB, Harper CR, and Weinberg WA, "A Practical Approach to Children Failing in School," *Pediatr Clin North Am*, 1992, 39(4):895-928.

♦ **Desitin® [OTC]** *see* Zinc Oxide *on page 1026*
♦ **Desitin® Creamy [OTC]** *see* Zinc Oxide *on page 1026*

Desmopressin (des moe PRES in)

U.S. Brand Names DDAVP®; Stimate®
Canadian Brand Names Octostim
Synonyms 1-Deamino-8-D-Arginine Vasopressin
Therapeutic Category Antihemophilic Agent; Hemostatic Agent; Vasopressin Analog, Synthetic
Generic Available Yes (injection)
Use Treatment of diabetes insipidus, control of bleeding in hemophilia A (with factor VIII levels >5%), mild to moderate type I von Willebrand disease, and thrombocytopenia; primary nocturnal enuresis
Pregnancy Risk Factor B
Contraindications Hypersensitivity to desmopressin or any component; avoid using in patients with severe type I, type IIB or platelet-type (pseudo) von Willebrand disease, hemophilia A with factor VIII levels ≤5% or hemophilia B
Warnings Avoid intranasal use in patients with nasal mucosa changes (scarring, edema, discharge, obstruction, or severe atopic rhinitis)
Precautions Use with caution in patients with predisposition to thrombus formation, conditions associated with fluid and electrolyte imbalance (eg, cystic fibrosis), and in patients with coronary artery disease and/or hypertensive cardiovascular disease
Adverse Reactions
Cardiovascular: Facial flushing, increase in blood pressure, chest pain, palpitations, tachycardia
Central nervous system: Headache, somnolence, dizziness, insomnia, agitation
Endocrine & metabolic: Hyponatremia, water intoxication
Gastrointestinal: Nausea, abdominal cramps, dyspepsia, vomiting
Genitourinary: Vulval pain, balanitis
Local: Pain at the injection site
Ocular: Itchy or light-sensitive eyes
Respiratory: Rhinitis, upper respiratory infections, epistaxis, nasal congestion
Drug Interactions Decreased antidiuretic response with lithium, large doses of epinephrine, demeclocycline, and heparin; increased antidiuretic response with carbamazepine, chlorpropamide, fludrocortisone, and clofibrate
Stability Refrigerate injection, nasal solution and Stimate® nasal spray; nasal solution and Stimate® nasal spray are stable for 3 weeks when stored at room temperature if unopened; injection is stable for 2 weeks at room temperature; DDAVP® nasal spray is stable at room temperature
Mechanism of Action Enhances reabsorption of water in the kidneys by increasing cellular permeability of the collecting ducts; possibly causes smooth muscle constriction with resultant vasoconstriction; dose-dependent increase in plasma factor VIII and plasminogen activator
Pharmacodynamics
Oral administration:
Onset of ADH effects: 1 hour
Peak effect: 2-7 hours
Duration: 6-8 hours
(Continued)

Desmopressin *(Continued)*

Intranasal administration:
Onset of ADH effects: Within 1 hour
Peak effect: Within 1.5 hours
Duration: 5-21 hours

I.V. infusion:
Onset of increased factor VIII activity: Within 15-30 minutes
Peak effect: 90 minutes to 3 hours

Pharmacokinetics

Absorption:
Oral tablets: 5% to 15%
Nasal solution: 10% to 20%
Nasal spray (1.5 mg/mL concentration): 3.3% to 4.1%
Metabolism: Unknown
Half-life:
Oral: 1.5-2.5 hours
I.V.:
Initial: 7.8 minutes
Terminal: 75.5 minutes (range: 0.4-4 hours)
Intranasal: 3.3-3.5 hours

Usual Dosage

Diabetes insipidus:
Oral:
Children ≤12 years: Initial: 0.05 mg 2 times daily; titrate to desired response (range: 0.1-0.8 mg daily)
Children >12 years and Adults: 0.05 mg 2 times daily; titrate to desired response (range: 0.1-1.2 mg divided 2-3 times/day)
Intranasal:
Children 3 months to ≤12 years: Initial (using 100 mcg/mL nasal solution): 5 mcg/day (0.05 mL) divided 1-2 times/day; range: 5-30 mcg/day (0.05-0.3 mL/day); adjust morning and evening doses separately for an adequate diurnal rhythm of water turnover
Children >12 years and Adults: Initial (using 100 mcg/mL nasal solution): 5-40 mcg (0.05-0.4 mL) divided 1-3 times/day; adjust morning and evening doses separately for an adequate diurnal rhythm of water turnover. **Note:** The nasal spray pump can only deliver doses of 10 mcg (0.1 mL) or multiples of 10 mcg (0.1 mL), if doses other than this are needed, the rhinal tube delivery system is preferred
I.V., S.C.: Children >12 years and Adults: 2-4 mcg/day in 2 divided doses or $^1/_{10}$ of the maintenance intranasal dose

Hemophilia:
I.V.: Children ≥3 months and Adults: 0.3 mcg/kg beginning 30 minutes before procedure; may repeat dose if needed
Intranasal: Children >12 years and Adults: Using high concentration Stimate® nasal spray:
≤50 kg: 150 mcg (1 spray)
>50 kg: 300 mcg (1 spray each nostril)
Repeat use is determined by the patient's clinical condition and laboratory work; if using preoperatively, administer 2 hours before surgery

Nocturnal enuresis:
Intranasal: Children ≥6 years: (Using 100 mcg/mL nasal solution): Initial: 20 mcg (0.2 mL) at bedtime; range: 10-40 mcg; it is recommended that $^1/_2$ of the dose be given in each nostril
Oral: Children >12 years: 0.2-0.4 mg once before bedtime

Administration

Intranasal: Using rhinal tube delivery system, draw solution into flexible, calibrated rhinal tube; insert one end into nostril; blow on the other end to deposit the solution deep into the nasal cavity. The Stimate® spray pump must be primed prior to first use; to prime pump, press down 4 times. Avoid spray use in children <6 years of age due to difficulty in titrating dosage; discard any solution remaining after 25 or 50 doses (2.5 or 5 mL vials, respectively) because the amount delivered may be substantially less than prescribed

Parenteral: I.V.: Dilute to a maximum concentration of 0.5 mcg/mL in NS and infuse over 15-30 minutes; if desmopressin I.V. is given preoperatively, administer 30 minutes prior to surgery

Monitoring Parameters I.V. infusion: Blood pressure and pulse should be monitored

Diabetes insipidus: Fluid intake, urine volume, specific gravity, plasma and urine osmolality, serum electrolytes

Hemophilia: Factor VIII antigen levels, APTT, Factor VIII activity level

Patient Information Avoid overhydration; blow nose before using nasal solution or spray; notify physician if headache, shortness of breath, heartburn, nausea, abdominal cramps, or vulval pain occur

Dosage Forms

Injection, as acetate (DDAVP®): 4 mcg/mL (1 mL, 10 mL)

Solution, nasal, as acetate, (DDAVP®): 100 mcg/mL [with rhinal tube] (2.5 mL)

Spray, nasal, as acetate:

DDAVP®: 10 mcg/spray (5 mL)

Stimate®: 1.5 mg/mL (2.5 mL)

Tablet, as acetate (DDAVP®): 0.1 mg, 0.2 mg

References

Stenberg A and Läckgren G, "Desmopressin Tablets in the Treatment of Severe Nocturnal Enuresis in Adolescents," *Pediatrics*, 1994, 94(6 Pt 1):841-46.

♦ **Desquam-E® Gel** *see* Benzoyl Peroxide *on page 136*

♦ **Desquam-X® Gel** *see* Benzoyl Peroxide *on page 136*

♦ **Desquam-X® Wash** *see* Benzoyl Peroxide *on page 136*

♦ **Desyrel®** *see* Trazodone *on page 977*

♦ **Detane® [OTC]** *see* Benzocaine *on page 135*

♦ **Dex4 Glucose [OTC]** *see* Dextrose *on page 317*

♦ **Dexacidin®** *see* Dexamethasone, Neomycin, and Polymyxin B *on page 309*

Dexamethasone (deks a METH a sone)

Related Information

Carbohydrate and Alcohol Content of Liquid Medications for Use in Patients Receiving Ketogenic Diets *on page 1258*

Corticosteroids Comparison, Systemic *on page 1067*

U.S. Brand Names AK-Dex®; Cortastat®; Cortastat® LA; Dalalone D.P.®; Decadron®; Decadron® Phosphate; Dexamethasone Intensol®; Dexasone®; Dexasone® L.A.; Dexone® LA; Maxidex®; Solurex®; Solurex L.A.®

Canadian Brand Names Alti-Dexamethasone; Dexasone; Diodex; Hexadrol Phosphate; PMS-Dexamethasone

Therapeutic Category Adrenal Corticosteroid; Antiasthmatic; Antiemetic; Anti-inflammatory Agent; Anti-inflammatory Agent, Ophthalmic; Corticosteroid, Ophthalmic; Corticosteroid, Systemic; Glucocorticoid

Generic Available Yes

Use Treatment of chronic inflammation, allergic, hematologic, neoplastic, and autoimmune diseases; may be used in management of cerebral edema, septic shock, and as a diagnostic agent; adjunctive antiemetic agent in the treatment of chemotherapy-induced emesis

Pregnancy Risk Factor C

Contraindications Active untreated infections; viral, fungal, or tuberculous diseases of the eye; hypersensitivity to dexamethasone or any component

Warnings Hypothalamic - pituitary - adrenal (HPA) suppression may occur; withdrawal and discontinuation of corticosteroids should be done carefully; acute adrenal insufficiency may occur with abrupt withdrawal after long term therapy or with stress; immunosuppression may occur

Precautions Suppression of HPA function, suppression of linear growth, or hypercorticism (Cushing's syndrome) may occur; use with extreme caution in patients with respiratory tuberculosis, untreated systemic infections, or ocular herpes simplex; use with caution in patients with hyperthyroidism, cirrhosis, ulcerative colitis, hypertension, osteoporosis, thromboembolic tendencies, CHF, convulsive disorders, myasthenia gravis, thrombophlebitis, peptic ulcer, diabetes; prolonged use may result in cataracts or glaucoma

Adverse Reactions

Cardiovascular: Edema, hypertension

Central nervous system: Headache, vertigo, seizures, psychosis, pseudotumor cerebri, insomnia, nervousness

Dermatologic: Acne, skin atrophy

Endocrine & metabolic: Pituitary-adrenal axis suppression, growth suppression, glucose intolerance, hypokalemia, alkalosis, Cushing's syndrome

Gastrointestinal: Peptic ulcer, nausea, vomiting

Neuromuscular & skeletal: Muscle weakness, osteoporosis, fractures

Ocular: Cataracts, glaucoma

Miscellaneous: Immunosuppression

(Continued)

Dexamethasone *(Continued)*

Drug Interactions Cytochrome P-450 isoenzyme CYP3A3/4 substrate; isoenzyme CYP3A3/4 inducer; isoenzyme CYP3A3/4 inhibitor

Barbiturates, phenytoin, rifampin, ritonavir, saquinavir, salicylates, NSAIDs, toxoids; alcohol and caffeine may increase adverse GI effects; live virus vaccines (increase risk of viral infection); vaccines may have decreased effects

Food Interactions Systemic use of corticosteroids may require a diet with increased potassium, vitamins A, B_6, C, D, folate, calcium, zinc, and phosphorus and decreased sodium

Stability Dilution of dexamethasone sodium phosphate injection with D_5W or NS is stable for at least 24 hours

Mechanism of Action Decreases inflammation by suppression of migration of polymorphonuclear leukocytes and reversal of increased capillary permeability; suppresses normal immune response

Pharmacodynamics Duration: Metabolic effects can last for 72 hours

Pharmacokinetics

Metabolism: In the liver

Half-life: Terminal:

Extremely low birth weight infants with BPD: 9.3 hours

Children 3 months to 16 years: 4.3 hours

Healthy adults: 3 hours

Time to peak serum concentration:

Oral: Within 1-2 hours

I.M.: Within 8 hours

Elimination: In urine and bile

Usual Dosage

Neonates:

Airway edema or extubation: I.V.: Usual: 0.25 mg/kg/dose given ~4 hours prior to scheduled extubation and then every 8 hours for 3 doses total; range: 0.25-1 mg/kg/dose for 1-3 doses; maximum dose: 1 mg/kg/day. **Note:** A longer duration of therapy may be needed with more severe cases.

Bronchopulmonary dysplasia (to facilitate ventilator weaning): Oral, I.V.: Numerous dosing schedules have been proposed; range: 0.5-0.6 mg/kg/day given in divided doses every 12 hours for 3-7 days, then taper over 1-6 weeks

Children:

Airway edema or extubation: Oral, I.M., I.V.: 0.5-2 mg/kg/day in divided doses every 6 hours; begin 24 hours prior to extubation and continue for 4-6 doses after extubation

Antiemetic (chemotherapy induced): I.V.: Initial: 10 mg/m^2/dose (maximum dose: 20 mg) then 5 mg/m^2/dose every 6 hours

Anti-inflammatory: Oral, I.M., I.V.: 0.08-0.3 mg/kg/day or 2.5-10 mg/m^2/day in divided doses every 6-12 hours

Bacterial meningitis: Infants and Children >2 months: I.V.: 0.6 mg/kg/day divided every 6 hours for the first 4 days of antibiotic treatment; start dexamethasone at the time of the first dose of antibiotic

Cerebral edema: Oral, I.M., I.V.: Loading dose: 1-2 mg/kg/dose as a single dose; maintenance: 1-1.5 mg/kg/day (maximum dose: 16 mg/day) in divided doses every 4-6 hours

Physiologic replacement: Oral, I.M., I.V.: 0.03-0.15 mg/kg/day or 0.6-0.75 mg/m^2/day in divided doses every 6-12 hours

Children and Adults: Ophthalmic:

Ointment: Apply thin coating to conjunctival sac 3-4 times/day, gradually taper dose to discontinue

Suspension: Instill 2 drops every hour during the day and every other hour during the night; gradually reduce dose to every 3-4 hours, then to 3-4 times/day

Adults:

Acute nonlymphoblastic leukemia (ANLL) protocol: I.V.: 2 mg/m^2/dose every 8 hours for 12 doses

Anti-inflammatory: Oral, I.M., I.V.: 0.75-9 mg/day in divided doses every 6-12 hours

Cerebral edema: I.V.: Initial: 10 mg then 4 mg I.M./I.V. every 6 hours

Diagnosis for Cushing's syndrome: Oral: 1 mg at 11 PM, draw blood at 8 AM

Administration

Ophthalmic: Avoid contact of container tip with skin or eye

Solution: Apply finger pressure to lacrimal sac during and for 1-2 minutes after instillation to decrease risk of absorption and systemic effects

Oral: May administer with food or milk to decrease GI adverse effects

Parenteral: **Acetate injection is not for I.V. use**; I.V. (as sodium phosphate): Administer undiluted solution (4 mg/mL) I.V. push over 1-4 minutes if dose is <10 mg; high-dose therapy must be diluted in D₅W or NS and administered by I.V. intermittent infusion over 15-30 minutes

Monitoring Parameters Hemoglobin, occult blood loss, blood pressure, serum potassium and glucose

Reference Range Dexamethasone suppression test: 8 AM cortisol less than 6 µg/100 mL in adults given dexamethasone 1 mg at 11 PM the previous night

Test Interactions Skin tests

Patient Information Avoid alcohol; limit caffeine; do not decrease dose or discontinue drug without physician's approval; inform physician you are taking corticosteroid prior to any surgery or with any injury

Additional Information Due to long duration of effect, not suitable for every other day dosing

Dosage Forms
Dexamethasone **acetate**:
Injection:
Cortastat® LA, Dexasone® L.A., Dexone® LA, Solurex L.A.®: 8 mg/mL (5 mL)
Dalalone D.P.®: 16 mg/mL (1 mL, 5 mL)
Dexamethasone **base**:
Elixir: 0.5 mg/5 mL (5 mL, 100 mL, 120 mL, 240 mL)
Solution, oral: 0.5 mg/5 mL (5 mL, 500 mL)
Solution, oral concentrate (Dexamethasone Intensol®): 0.5 mg/0.5 mL (30 mL)
Suspension, ophthalmic (Maxidex®): 0.1% (5 mL, 15 mL)
Tablet (Decadron®): 0.25 mg, 0.5 mg, 0.75 mg, 1 mg, 1.5 mg, 2 mg, 4 mg, 6 mg
Therapeutic pack: Six 1.5 mg tablets and eight 0.75 mg tablets
Dexamethasone **sodium phosphate**:
Injection:
Cortastat®, Decadron® Phosphate, Dexasone®, Solurex®: 4 mg/mL (1 mL, 5 mL, 10 mL, 25 mL, 30 mL); 10 mg/mL (10 mL)
Decadron® Phosphate: 24 mg/mL (5 mL)
Ointment, ophthalmic: 0.05% (3.5 g)
Solution, ophthalmic (AK-Dex®, Decadron® Phosphate): 0.1% (5 mL)

References
American Academy of Pediatrics Committee on Infectious Diseases, "Dexamethasone Therapy for Bacterial Meningitis in Infants and Children," *Pediatrics*, 1990, 86(1):130-3.
Bahal N and Nahata MC, "The Role of Corticosteroids in Infants and Children With Bacterial Meningitis," *DICP*, 1991, 25(5):542-5.
Couser RJ, Ferrara TB, Falde B, et al, "Effectiveness of Dexamethasone in Preventing Extubation Failure in Preterm Infants at Increased Risk for Airway Edema," *J Pediatr*, 1992, 121(4):591-6.
Durand M, Sardesai S, and McEvoy C, "Effects of Early Dexamethasone Therapy on Pulmonary Mechanics and Chronic Lung Disease in Very Low Birth Weight Infants: A Randomized, Controlled Trial," *Pediatrics*, 1995, 95(4):584-90.
Ng PC, "The Effectiveness and Side Effects of Dexamethasone in Preterm Infants With Bronchopulmonary Dysplasia," *Arch Dis Child*, 1993, 68(3 Spec No):330-6.

♦ **Dexamethasone Intensol®** see Dexamethasone on page 307

Dexamethasone, Neomycin, and Polymyxin B

(deks a METH a sone, nee oh MYE sin, & pol i MIKS in bee)

U.S. Brand Names AK-Trol®; Dexacidin®; Dexasporin®; Infectrol®; Maxitrol®; Ocu-Trol®

Canadian Brand Names Dioptrol

Synonyms Neomycin, Dexamethasone, and Polymyxin B Polymyxin B, Dexamethasone, and Neomycin

Therapeutic Category Antibiotic, Ophthalmic; Corticosteroid, Ophthalmic

Generic Available Yes

Use Steroid-responsive inflammatory ocular conditions in which a corticosteroid is indicated and where bacterial infection or a risk of bacterial infection exists

Pregnancy Risk Factor C

Contraindications Hypersensitivity to dexamethasone, polymyxin, neomycin, or any component; viral diseases of the cornea and conjunctiva; mycobacterial infection of the eye; fungal disease of ocular structures; dendritic keratitis; use after uncomplicated removal of a corneal foreign body

Warnings Prolonged use may result in glaucoma, defects in visual acuity, posterior subcapsular cataract formation, and secondary ocular infections

Adverse Reactions
Dermatologic: Contact dermatitis, cutaneous sensitization (sensitivity to topical neomycin has been reported to occur in 5% to 15% of patients)
Local: Pain, stinging
(Continued)

Dexamethasone, Neomycin, and Polymyxin B *(Continued)*

Ocular: Development of glaucoma, cataract, increased intraocular pressure, optic nerve damage, visual defects, blurred vision

Miscellaneous: Delayed wound healing, secondary infections

Usual Dosage Children and Adults: Ophthalmic:

Ointment: Apply a small amount (~1/2") in the affected eye 3-4 times/day or apply at bedtime as an adjunct with drops

Suspension: Instill 1-2 drops into affected eye(s) every 4-6 hours; in severe disease, drops may be used hourly and tapered to discontinuation

Administration Ophthalmic: Shake suspension well before using; instill drop into affected eye; avoid contacting bottle tip with skin or eye; apply finger pressure to lacrimal sac during and for 1-2 minutes after instillation to decrease risk of absorption and systemic effects

Monitoring Parameters Intraocular pressure with use >10 days

Patient Information May cause temporary blurring of vision or stinging following administration

Dosage Forms

Ointment, ophthalmic: Dexamethasone 0.1%, neomycin sulfate 3.5 mg, and polymyxin B sulfate 10,000 units per g (3.5 g)

Suspension, ophthalmic: Dexamethasone 0.1%, neomycin sulfate 3.5 mg, and polymyxin B sulfate 10,000 units per mL (5 mL)

Dexrazoxane (deks ray ZOKS ane)

U.S. Brand Names Zinecard®

Therapeutic Category Antineoplastic Agent; Chelating Agent; Chemoprotectant Agent

Use Reduction of anthracycline-induced (doxorubicin, daunorubicin) cardiotoxicity. Not generally recommended for use with the initiation of anthracycline therapy. Most dexrazoxane studies have been done in women with metastatic breast cancer who had received a cumulative doxorubicin dose of 300 mg/m^2.

Pregnancy Risk Factor C

Contraindications Hypersensitivity to dexrazoxane or any component; should only be used with chemotherapy regimens containing an anthracycline

Warnings Due to limited experience, the possibility of dexrazoxane interference with antineoplastic efficacy may exist; dose-limiting toxicity is myelosuppression; dexrazoxane may add to the myelosuppression caused by chemotherapeutic agents; dexrazoxane should be handled, prepared, and disposed as an antineoplastic agent

Precautions Do not give doxorubicin prior to dexrazoxane administration. Doxorubicin should be given within 30 minutes after the beginning of a dexrazoxane infusion.

Adverse Reactions

Central nervous system: Low grade fever

Dermatologic: Alopecia (possibly dose-related)

Endocrine/metabolic: Elevated serum iron and serum triglyceride levels, decreased serum zinc and calcium levels

Gastrointestinal: Mild nausea and vomiting, diarrhea, elevated serum amylase levels

Hepatic: Transient elevation of serum transaminase level

Hematologic: **Dose-limiting, additive myelosuppression** (leukopenia and thrombocytopenia at high doses >1000 mg/m^2)

Local: Pain at injection site (13%)

Drug Interactions Dexrazoxane can have either a synergistic or inhibitory activity with different anthracylines

Stability Reconstituted solution is stable for 6 hours at room temperature or under refrigeration. Dexrazoxane degrades rapidly at pH >7.

Mechanism of Action Dexrazoxane is a piperazine EDTA derivative that rapidly penetrates the myocardial cell membrane. It binds intracellular iron and prevents generation of oxygen free radicals by anthracyclines. Dexrazoxane is hydrolyzed intracellularly to an open-ring chelating agent which is responsible for chelating heavy metals and preventing formation of superhydroxide free radicals believed to be responsible for anthracycline-induced cardiomyopathy. Dexrazoxane may also have antitumor activity and have synergistic activity with certain cytotoxic agents.

Pharmacokinetics Minimal data in the pediatric population

Distribution: V_d:
  Children: 0.67 L/kg
  Adults: 1.3 L/kg
Protein binding: Insignificant
Half-life: Biphasic
  Distribution half-life: 8-21 minutes
  Terminal half-life: 2-3 hours
Elimination: 40% to 60% of dose excreted renally within 24 hours; removed by peritoneal or hemodialysis

Usual Dosage I.V. (refer to individual protocols):

Children: 10:1 dose ratio with doxorubicin (example: 250 mg/m^2 dexrazoxane: 25 mg/m^2 doxorubicin) is currently recommended; 20:1 ratio with doxorubicin has been studied, but due to higher incidence of adverse reactions is no longer recommended

Adults: 10:1 ratio with doxorubicin (example: 500 mg/m^2 dexrazoxane: 50 mg/m^2 doxorubicin); administer 30 minutes before doxorubicin

Administration Parenteral: Reconstitute with 0.167 Molar sodium lactate injection to a concentration of 10 mg/mL. Administer slow I.V. push or further dilute in NS or D$_5$W to a final concentration of 1.3-5 mg/mL and give as a rapid I.V. infusion over 15-30 minutes

Monitoring Parameters Complete blood count; cardiac function tests; serum iron, calcium, and zinc levels; liver function tests

Nursing Implications To ensure optimal chemoprotectant effect, do not allow chemotherapy to be delayed following completion of dexrazoxane

Dosage Forms Injection: 250 mg

References

Sehested M, et al, "Dexrazoxane for Protection Against Cardiotoxic Effects of Anthracyclines," *J Clin Oncol*, 1996, 14:2884.

Swain SM, et al, "Cardioprotection With Dexrazoxane for Doxorubicin-Containing Therapy in Advanced Breast Cancer," *J Clin Oncol*, 1997, 15:1318-32.

Swain SM, et al, "Delayed Administration of Dexrazoxane Provides Cardioprotection for Patients With Advanced Breast Cancer Treated With Doxorubicin-Containing Therapy," *J Clin Oncol*, 1997, 15:1333-40.

Wexler LH, et al, "Randomized Trial of the Cardioprotective Agent ICRF-187 in Pediatric Sarcoma Patients Treated With Doxorubicin," *J Clin Oncol*, 1996, 14:362-72.

Dextran (DEKS tran)

U.S. Brand Names Gentran®; LMD®; Macrodex®; Rheomacrodex®

Synonyms Dextran 40; Dextran 70; Dextran, High Molecular Weight; Dextran, Low Molecular Weight

Therapeutic Category Plasma Volume Expander

Generic Available Yes

Use Fluid replacement and blood volume expander used in the treatment of hypovolemia, shock, or near shock states

Pregnancy Risk Factor C

Contraindications Hypersensitivity to dextrans or any component; renal failure, severe thrombocytopenia

Warnings Use with caution in patients with CHF, pulmonary edema, renal insufficiency, thrombocytopenia, or active hemorrhage; watch for anaphylactoid reactions, have epinephrine and diphenhydramine at bedside

Precautions Use with caution in patients with extreme dehydration, renal failure may occur

Adverse Reactions

Cardiovascular: Mild hypotension
Central nervous system: Fever
Dermatologic: Urticaria
Gastrointestinal: Nausea, vomiting
Hematologic: Prolongation of bleeding time with higher doses (may interfere with platelet function)
Neuromuscular & skeletal: Arthralgia
Respiratory: Wheezing, pulmonary edema with high doses, tightness of chest, nasal congestion
Miscellaneous: Anaphylaxis

Stability Store at room temperature; discard partially used containers

(Continued)

Dextran (Continued)

Mechanism of Action Produces plasma volume expansion due to high colloidal osmotic effect (similar to albumin); draws interstitial fluid into the intravascular space; dextran 40 may also increase blood flow in microcirculation

Pharmacodynamics

Maximum effect on plasma volume:

Dextran 40: Within several minutes

Dextran 70 and dextran 75: ~1 hour

Pharmacokinetics

Metabolism: Molecules with molecular weight ≥50,000 are metabolized to glucose

Elimination:

Molecules with molecular weight ≤15,000: Rapidly eliminated in the kidney

Dextran 40: ~70% excreted in urine (unchanged) within 24 hours

Dextran 70 & 75: ~50% excreted in urine within 24 hours

Usual Dosage I.V. (dose and infusion rate are dependent upon the patient's fluid status and must be individualized):

Volume expansion/shock:

Children: Total dose should not be >20 mL/kg during first 24 hours and not >10 mL/kg/day thereafter; do not treat for >5 days

Adults: 500-1000 mL at rate of 20-40 mL/minute

Maximum daily dose: First 24 hours: 20 mL/kg and 10 mL/kg/day thereafter; therapy should not continue beyond 5 days

Administration Parenteral: I.V. infusion only; usual maximum infusion rate (adults): 4 mL/minute; maximum infusion rate in emergency situations (adults): 20-40 mL/minute

Monitoring Parameters Vital signs, signs of allergic/anaphylactoid reaction especially when starting infusions; signs of circulatory overload (ie, heart rate, blood pressure, central venous pressure, hematocrit), urine output; urine specific gravity

Nursing Implications Be prepared to treat anaphylaxis with epinephrine, antihistamines, supportive therapy, and alternative agents to dextran to maintain circulation; do not administer if cloudy or if solution contains dextran flakes; discontinue dextran if urine specific gravity is low, if oliguria or anuria occur, or if there is a rapid acute rise in central venous pressure or other signs of circulatory overload

Additional Information Dextran in sodium chloride 0.9% contains sodium chloride 154 mEq/L

Dosage Forms Injection:

High molecular weight:

Gentran®: 6% dextran 75 in sodium chloride 0.9% (500 mL)

Gentran®, Macrodex®: 6% dextran 70 in sodium chloride 0.9% (500 mL)

Low molecular weight: Gentran®, LMD®, Rheomacrodex®:

10% dextran 40 in dextrose 5% (500 mL)

10% dextran 40 in sodium chloride 0.9% (500 mL)

♦ **Dextran 40** see Dextran on page 311

♦ **Dextran 70** see Dextran on page 311

♦ **Dextran, High Molecular Weight** see Dextran on page 311

♦ **Dextran, Low Molecular Weight** see Dextran on page 311

Dextroamphetamine (deks troe am FET a meen)

Related Information

Drugs and Breast-Feeding on page 1243

Laboratory Detection of Drugs in Urine on page 1234

U.S. Brand Names Dexedrine®; Dextrostat®

Therapeutic Category Amphetamine; Anorexiant; Central Nervous System Stimulant, Amphetamine

Generic Available Yes

Use Adjunct in treatment of attention-deficit/hyperactivity disorder (ADHD) in children, narcolepsy, exogenous obesity

Restrictions C-II

Pregnancy Risk Factor C

Contraindications Hypersensitivity to dextroamphetamine or any component; advanced arteriosclerosis, hypertension, hyperthyroidism, glaucoma; concurrent use or use within 14 days of MAO inhibitors (hypertensive crisis may occur)

Warnings High potential for abuse; use in weight reduction programs only when alternative therapy has been ineffective; prolonged administration may lead to drug dependence; use in psychotic children may exacerbate symptoms of thought disorder and behavior disturbance; may potentially be associated with growth inhibition (monitor growth); tablets and capsules contain tartrazine

Precautions Use with caution in patients with psychopathic personalities

Adverse Reactions

Cardiovascular: Hypertension, tachycardia, palpitations, cardiac arrhythmias

Central nervous system: Insomnia, headache, nervousness, dizziness, irritability, depression

Endocrine & metabolic: Growth suppression, weight loss

Gastrointestinal: Anorexia, nausea, vomiting, diarrhea, abdominal cramps, metallic taste, xerostomia

Neuromuscular & skeletal: Movement disorders, tremor

Ocular: Mydriasis

Miscellaneous: Physical and psychologic dependence with long-term use

Drug Interactions Amphetamines may decrease hypotensive effects of antihypertensives and sedative effect of antihistamines; may increase effects of tricyclic antidepressants or sympathomimetics; may delay oral absorption of ethosuximide, phenobarbital, and phenytoin; may precipitate hypertensive crisis in patients receiving MAO inhibitors (avoid use within 14 days); the herb medicine St John's wort (*Hypericum perforatum*) may increase serious side effects, its use is **not** recommended; amphetamine may precipitate arrhythmias in patients receiving general anesthetics. With propoxyphene overdose, CNS stimulation from amphetamines is potentiated (fatal convulsions may occur); tricyclic antidepressants may enhance the effects of amphetamines (avoid use or monitor for cardiovascular effects); chlorpromazine and haloperidol may inhibit the CNS stimulant effects of amphetamines. Antacids may increase the oral absorption of amphetamines; urinary alkalinizers or large doses of antacids may decrease urinary excretion of amphetamines and increase their half-life and duration of action (dosage decrease may be needed). Acids or acidifiers may decrease the oral absorption of amphetamines; urinary acidifiers may increase urinary excretion of amphetamines and decrease their half-life and duration of action (dosage adjustment may be needed).

Food Interactions Acidic foods, juices, or vitamin C may decrease GI absorption

Mechanism of Action Blocks reuptake of dopamine and norepinephrine from the synapse, thus increases the amounts of circulating dopamine and norepinephrine in cerebral cortex to reticular activating system; inhibits the action of monoamine oxidase and causes catecholamines to be released; peripherally increases blood pressure and acts as a respiratory stimulant and weak bronchodilator

Pharmacodynamics Onset of action: Oral: 60-90 minutes

Pharmacokinetics

Metabolism: In the liver

Half-life, adults: 34 hours (pH dependent)

Time to peak serum concentration: Oral: Within 3 hours

Elimination: In urine as unchanged drug and inactive metabolites; urinary excretion is pH dependent and is increased with acid urine (low pH)

Usual Dosage Oral: **Note:** Use lowest effective individualized dose; administer first dose as soon as awake

ADHD: Children:

<3 years: Not recommended

3-5 years: Initial: 2.5 mg/day given every morning; increase by 2.5 mg/day at weekly intervals until optimal response is obtained, usual range is 0.1-0.5 mg/kg/dose every morning with maximum of 40 mg/day given in 1-3 divided doses per day

≥6 years: 5 mg once or twice daily; increase in increments of 5 mg/day at weekly intervals until optimal response is reached, usual range is 0.1-0.5 mg/kg/dose every morning (5-20 mg/day) with maximum of 40 mg/day given in 1-3 divided doses per day

Narcolepsy:

Children 6-12 years: Initial: 5 mg/day, may increase at 5 mg increments at weekly intervals until optimal response is obtained; maximum dose: 60 mg/day

Children >12 and Adults: Initial: 10 mg/day, may increase at 10 mg increments at weekly intervals until optimal response is obtained; maximum dose: 60 mg/day

Exogenous obesity: Children >12 years and Adults: 5-30 mg/day in divided doses of 5-10 mg given 30-60 minutes before meals

Administration Oral: Sustained release preparations should be used for once daily dosing; do not crush or chew sustained release preparations; to avoid insomnia, last daily dose should be administered no less than 6 hours before retiring

Monitoring Parameters CNS activity, blood pressure, height, weight

(Continued)

313

Dextroamphetamine (Continued)

Patient Information May impair ability to perform potentially hazardous activities; may be habit-forming; do not discontinue abruptly; limit caffeine; avoid alcohol and the herbal medicine, St. John's wort

Additional Information Treatment for ADHD should include "drug holiday" or periodic discontinuation in order to assess the patient's requirements, decrease tolerance, and limit suppression of linear growth and weight

Dosage Forms

Capsule, sustained release, as sulfate (Dexedrine® Spansule® capsules contain tartrazine): 5 mg, 10 mg, 15 mg

Tablet, as sulfate:

Dexedrine®: 5 mg [with tartrazine]

Dextrostat®: 5 mg, 10 mg [with tartrazine]

Dextroamphetamine and Amphetamine

(deks troe am FET a meen & am FET a meen)

Related Information

Dextroamphetamine *on page 312*

Drugs and Breast-Feeding *on page 1243*

Laboratory Detection of Drugs in Urine *on page 1234*

U.S. Brand Names Adderall®

Synonyms Amphetamine and Dextroamphetamine

Therapeutic Category Amphetamine; Anorexiant; Central Nervous System Stimulant, Amphetamine

Generic Available No

Use Attention-deficit/hyperactivity disorder (ADHD); narcolepsy

Restrictions C-II

Pregnancy Risk Factor C

Contraindications Hypersensitivity or idiosyncrasy to dextroamphetamine, amphetamine, sympathomimetic amines, or any component; advanced arteriosclerosis, moderate to severe hypertension, symptomatic cardiovascular disease, hyperthyroidism, glaucoma, agitated states, history of drug abuse; concurrent use or use within 14 days of MAO inhibitors (hypertensive crisis may occur)

Warnings High potential for abuse; prolonged administration may lead to drug dependence; use in psychotic children may exacerbate symptoms of thought disorder and behavior disturbance; may potentially be associated with growth inhibition (monitor growth)

Precautions Use with caution in patients with mild hypertension; prescribe or dispense least amount feasible to minimize chance of overdose

Adverse Reactions

Cardiovascular system: Hypertension: tachycardia, palpitations; cardiomyopathy (chronic use)

Central nervous system: Insomnia, headache, nervousness, overstimulation, dizziness, euphoria, dysphoria, dyskinesia, exacerbation of phonic and motor tics; psychotic episodes (rare at recommended doses)

Dermatologic: Rash, urticaria

Endocrine and metabolic: Growth suppression, weight loss

Gastrointestinal: Anorexia, diarrhea, constipation, xerostomia, unpleasant taste

Neuromuscular and skeletal: Tremor

Miscellaneous: Physical and psychological dependence with long-term use

Drug Interactions Amphetamines may decrease hypotensive effects of antihypertensives and sedative effect of antihistamines; may increase effects of tricyclic antidepressants or sympathomimetics; may delay oral absorption of ethosuximide, phenobarbital, and phenytoin; may precipitate hypertensive crisis in patients receiving MAO inhibitors (avoid use within 14 days); the herbal medicine St John's wort (*Hypericum perforatum*) may increase serious side effects, its use is **not** recommended; amphetamines may precipitate arrhythmias in patients receiving general anesthetics. With propoxyphene overdose, CNS stimulation from amphetamines is potentiated (fatal convulsions may occur); tricyclic antidepressants may enhance the effects of amphetamines (avoid use or monitor for cardiovascular effects); chlorpromazine and haloperidol may inhibit the CNS stimulant effects of amphetamines. Antacids may increase the oral absorption of amphetamines; urinary alkalinizers or large doses of antacids may decrease urinary excretion of amphetamines and increase their half-life and duration of action (dosage decrease may be needed). Acids or acidifiers may decrease the oral absorption of amphetamines; urinary acidifiers may increase urinary excretion of amphetamines and decrease their half-life and duration of action (dosage adjustment may be needed).

Food Interactions Acidic foods, juices, or vitamin C may decrease oral absorption

Stability Store tablets at controlled room temperature; dispense in tight, light-resistant container

Mechanism of Action Blocks reuptake of dopamine and norepinephrine from the synapse, thus increases the amounts of circulating dopamine and norepinephrine in cerebral cortex to reticular activating system; inhibits the action of monoamine oxidase and causes catecholamines to be released; peripherally increases blood pressure and acts as a respiratory stimulant and weak bronchodilator

Pharmacodynamics Oral:
  Onset: 30-60 minutes
  Duration: 4-6 hours

Pharmacokinetics
  Absorption: Oral: Well-absorbed
  Distribution: V_d: Adults: 3.5-4.6 L/kg; concentrates in breast milk (avoid breast-feeding); distributes into CNS, mean CSF concentrations are 80% of plasma
  Metabolism: In the liver by cytochrome P-450 mono-oxygenase and glucuronidation
  Elimination: 70% of a single dose is eliminated within 24 hours; excreted as unchanged amphetamine (30%), benzoic acid, hydroxy-amphetamine, hippuric acid, norephedrine and p-hydroxynorephedrine

Usual Dosage Oral: **Note:** Use lowest effective individualized dose; administer first dose as soon as awake; use intervals of 4-6 hours between additional doses
  ADHD:
    Children: <3 years: Not recommended
    Children: 3-5 years: Initial 2.5 mg/day given every morning; increase daily dose by 2.5 mg at weekly intervals until optimal response is obtained; maximum dose: 40 mg/day given in 1-3 divided doses per day
    Children: ≥6 years: Initial: 5 mg once or twice daily; increase daily dose by 5 mg at weekly intervals until optimal response is obtained; usual maximum dose: 40 mg/day given in 1-3 divided doses per day
  Narcolepsy:
    Children: 6-12 years: Initial: 5 mg/day; increase daily dose by 5 mg at weekly intervals until optimal response is obtained; maximum dose: 60 mg/day given in 1-3 divided doses per day
    Children >12 years and Adults: Initial: 10 mg/day; increase daily dose by 10 mg at weekly intervals until optimal response is obtained; maximum dose: 60 mg/day given in 1-3 divided doses per day

Administration Oral: To avoid insomnia, last daily dose should be administered no less than 6 hours before retiring

Monitoring Parameters CNS activity, blood pressure, height, weight

Patient Information May impair ability to perform potentially hazardous activities; may be habit forming; do not discontinue abruptly; limit caffeine; avoid alcohol and the herbal medicine, St John's wort

Additional Information Treatment of ADHD should include "drug holidays" or periodic discontinuation of medication in order to assess the patient's requirments, decrease tolerance, and limit suppression of linear growth and weight; the combination of equal parts of d, l-amphetamine aspartate, d, l-amphetamine sulfate, dextroamphetamine saccharate and dextroamphetamine sulfate results in a 75:25 ratio of the dextro- and levo isomers of amphetamine.

The duration of action of Adderall® is longer than methylphenidate; behavioral effects of a single morning dose of Adderall® may last throughout the school day; a single morning dose of Adderall® has been shown in several studies to be as effective as twice daily dosing of methylphenidate for the treatment of ADHD (see Pelham et al, Pediatrics, 1999, 104(6):1300-11; Manos 1999, Pliszka 2000).

A recent randomized, double-blind, placebo-controlled crossover trial of Adderall® in children with ADHD demonstrated efficacy rates of 82% based on parent response, 77% based on teacher response, and 59% based on concurrence between parent and teacher response; reported side effects included decreased appetite, stomach aches, insomnia, and headaches; decreased appetite and insomnia were more problematic on the high dose (0.3 mg/kg/dose twice daily) versus the low dose (0.15 mg/kg/dose twice daily); headaches occurred more frequently on the high dose, suggesting a dose-dependency (Ahmann, 2001).

Dosage Forms Tablet:
  5 mg (amphetamine aspartate 1.25 mg, amphetamine sulfate 1.25 mg, dextroamphetamine saccharate 1.25 mg, dextroamphetamine sulfate 1.25 mg) [total amphetamine base equivalence: 3.13 mg]
  7.5 mg (amphetamine aspartate 1.875 mg, amphetamine sulfate 1.875 mg, dextroamphetamine saccharate 1.875 mg, dextroamphetamine sulfate 1.875 mg) [total amphetamine base equivalence: 4.7 mg]
  (Continued)

Dextroamphetamine and Amphetamine *(Continued)*

10 mg (amphetamine aspartate 2.5 mg, amphetamine sulfate 2.5 mg, dextroamphetamine saccharate 2.5 mg, dextroamphetamine sulfate 2.5 mg) [total amphetamine base equivalence: 6.3 mg]

12.5 mg (amphetamine aspartate 3.125 mg, amphetamine sulfate 3.125 mg, dextroamphetamine saccharate 3.125 mg, dextroamphetamine sulfate 3.125 mg) [total amphetamine base equivalence: 7.8 mg]

15 mg (amphetamine aspartate 3.75 mg, amphetamine sulfate 3.75 mg, dextroamphetamine saccharate 3.75 mg, dextroamphetamine sulfate 3.75 mg) [total amphetamine base equivalence: 9.4 mg]

20 mg (amphetamine aspartate 5 mg, amphetamine sulfate 5 mg, dextroamphetamine saccharate 5 mg, dextroamphetamine sulfate 5 mg) [total amphetamine base equivalence: 12.6 mg]

30 mg (amphetamine aspartate 7.5 mg, amphetamine sulfate 7.5 mg, dextroamphetamine saccharate 7.5 mg, dextroamphetamine sulfate 7.5 mg) [total amphetamine base equivalence: 18.8 mg]

References

Ahmann PA, Theye FW, Berg R, et al, "Placebo-Controlled Evaluation of Amphetamine Mixture - Dextroamphetamine Salts and Amphetamine Salts (Adderall): Efficacy Rate and Side Effects," *Pediatrics*, 2001, 107(1), http://www.pediatrics.org/cgi/content/full/107/1/e10.

Manos MJ, Short EJ, and Findling RL, "Differential Effectiveness of Methylphenidate and Adderall® in School-Age Youths With Attention-Deficit/Hyperactivity Disorder," *J Am Acad Child Adolesc Psychiatry*, 1999, 38(7):813-9.

Pelham WE, Aronoff HR, Midlam JK, et al, "A Comparison of Ritalin® and Adderall®: Efficacy and Time-Course in Children With Attention-Deficit/Hyperactivity Disorder," *Pediatrics*, 1999, 103(4):e43. URL: http://www.pediatrics.org/cgi/content/full/103/4/e43

Pelham WE, Gnagy EM, Chronis AM, et al, "A Comparison of Morning-Only and Morning/Late Afternoon Adderall® to Morning-Only, Twice-Daily, and Three Times-Daily Methylphenidate in Children With Attention-Deficit/Hyperactivity Disorder," *Pediatrics*, 1999, 104(6):1300-11.

Pliszka SR, Browne RG, Olvera RL, et al, "A Double-Blind, Placebo-Controlled Study of Adderall® and Methylphenidate in the Treatment of Attention-Deficit/Hyperactivity Disorder," *J Am Acad Child Adolesc Psychiatry*, 2000, 39(5):619-26.

Swanson JM, Wigal S, Greenhill LL, et al, "Analog Classroom Assessment of Adderall® in Children With ADHD," *J Am Acad Child Adolesc Psychiatry*, 1998, 37(5):519-26.

Dextromethorphan *(deks troe meth OR fan)*

U.S. Brand Names Benylin® Adult [OTC]; Benylin® Pediatric [OTC]; Creo-Terpin® [OTC]; Delsym® [OTC]; Hold® DM [OTC]; Pertussin® CS [OTC]; Pertussin® DM [OTC]; Robitussin® Cough Calmers [OTC]; Robitussin® Pediatric [OTC]; Scot-Tussin® Diabetes Cough Formula [OTC]; Silphen DM® [OTC]; St. Joseph® Cough Suppressant [OTC]; Sucrets® 4-Hour Cough [OTC]; Vicks Formula 44® Cough Relief [OTC]

Canadian Brand Names Balminil DM; Benylin DM; Broncho-Grippol-DM; Buckley's DM; Calmylin-1; Cough Syrup DM; DM Cough Syrup; DM Sans Sucre; Formula 44; Koffex DM; Novahistex DM; Novahistine DM; Pharmilin-DM; Pharminil DM; Robitussin Children's; Sedatuss DM; Sucrets Cough Control; Syrup DM; Tussin DM Antitussive

Synonyms DM

Therapeutic Category Antitussive; Cough Preparation

Generic Available Yes

Use Symptomatic relief of coughs caused by minor viral upper respiratory tract infections or inhaled irritants

Pregnancy Risk Factor C

Contraindications Hypersensitivity to dextromethorphan or any component; concomitant use or use within 14 days of MAO inhibitors

Warnings Do not use for persistent or chronic cough, or for cough accompanied by excessive secretions

Precautions Anecdotal reports of abuse of dextromethorphan-containing cough/cold products have increased, especially among teenagers

Adverse Reactions

Central nervous system: Drowsiness, dizziness

Gastrointestinal: Nausea

Drug Interactions Cytochrome P-450 isoenzyme CYP2D6, CYP2E1, and CYP3A3/4 substrate

MAO inhibitors (increased risk of serotonin syndrome); haloperidol and fluoxetine decrease dextromethorphan metabolism; dextromethorphan decreases fluoxetine metabolism

Mechanism of Action Non-narcotic chemical relative of morphine; controls cough by depressing the medullary cough center

Pharmacodynamics
Onset of antitussive action: Within 15-30 minutes
Duration: Up to 6 hours

Pharmacokinetics
Metabolism: In the liver
Half-Life: 1.4-3.9 hours
Time to peak serum concentration: 2-2.5 hours
Elimination: Principally in urine

Usual Dosage Dosage in children <2 years of age is not well established; the following dosage recommendations in children <2 years are consistent with the dosages received when using combination products containing dextromethorphan.
Oral:
Children:
1-3 months: 0.5-1 mg every 6-8 hours
3-6 months: 1-2 mg every 6-8 hours
7 months to 1 year: 2-4 mg every 6-8 hours
≥2-6 years : 2.5-7.5 mg every 4-8 hours; extended release formulation: 15 mg twice daily (maximum: 30 mg/24 hours)
7-12 years: 5-10 mg every 4 hours or 15 mg every 6-8 hours; extended release formulation: 30 mg twice daily (maximum: 60 mg/24 hours)
Children >12 years and Adults: 10-30 mg every 4-8 hours or extended release formulation: 60 mg twice daily (maximum: 120 mg/24 hours)

Administration Oral: May administer without regard to meals

Monitoring Parameters Cough, mental status

Test Interactions Can give a false-positive on phencyclidine qualitative immunoassay screen

Patient Information If cough lasts more than 1 week or is accompanied by fever or headache, notify physician

Additional Information Dextromethorphan 15-30 mg equals 8-15 mg codeine as an antitussive

Dosage Forms
Liquid, as hydrobromide:
Creo-Terpin®: 10 mg/15 mL [with tartrazine, 25% alcohol] (120 mL)
Vicks Formula 44® Cough Relief: 10 mg/5 mL (120 mL)
Pertussin® CS: 3.5 mg/5 mL [wild berry flavor, alcohol free] (120 mL)
Benylin® Pediatric, Robitussin® Pediatric, St. Joseph® Cough Suppressant: 7.5 mg/5 mL (60 mL, 120 mL)
Benylin® Adult: 15 mg/5 mL (120 mL)
Liquid, sustained release, as polistirex, as hydrobromide (Delsym®): 30 mg/5 mL [orange flavor] (89 mL)
Lozenges, as hydrobromide
Hold® DM, Robitussin® Cough Calmers: 5 mg
Sucrets® 4-Hour Cough: 15 mg
Syrup, as hydrobromide:
Silphen DM®, Scot-Tussin® Diabetes Cough Formula: 10 mg/5 mL (120 mL)
Pertussin® DM: 15 mg/15 mL (120 mL)

♦ **Dextromethorphan and Glycerol Guaiacolate** *see* Guaifenesin and Dextromethorphan *on page 487*
♦ **Dextromethorphan and Guaifenesin** *see* Guaifenesin and Dextromethorphan *on page 487*
♦ **Dextropropoxyphene** *see* Propoxyphene *on page 845*

Dextrose (DEKS trose)
Related Information
Fluid and Electrolyte Requirements in Children *on page 1102*
Parenteral Nutrition (PN) *on page 1106*
U.S. Brand Names B-D Glucose® [OTC]; Dex4 Glucose [OTC]; Glutose® [OTC]; Insta-Glucose® [OTC]; Insulin Reaction [OTC]
Canadian Brand Names Glucodex
Synonyms Anhydrous Glucose; D_5W; $D_{10}W$; $D_{25}W$; $D_{30}W$; $D_{40}W$; $D_{50}W$; $D_{60}W$; $D_{70}W$; Dextrose Monohydrate; Glucose; Glucose Monohydrate; Glycosum
Therapeutic Category Antidote, Insulin; Antidote, Oral Hypoglycemic; Fluid Replacement, Enteral; Fluid Replacement, Parenteral; Hyperglycemic Agent; Hyperkalemia, Adjunctive Treatment Agent; Intravenous Nutritional Therapy
Generic Available Yes
Use
5% and 10% solutions: Peripheral infusion to provide calories and fluid replacement
10% solution: Treatment of hypoglycemia in premature neonates
(Continued)

Dextrose (Continued)

25% (hypertonic) solution: Treatment of acute symptomatic episodes of hypoglycemia in infants and children to restore depressed blood glucose levels; adjunctive treatment of hyperkalemia when combined with insulin

50% (hypertonic) solution: Treatment of insulin-induced hypoglycemia (hyperinsulinemia or insulin shock) and adjunctive treatment of hyperkalemia in adolescents and adults

≥10% solutions: Infusion after admixture with amino acids for nutritional support

Pregnancy Risk Factor C

Contraindications Diabetic coma with hyperglycemia; hypertonic solutions in patients with intracranial or intraspinal hemorrhage; patients with delirium tremens and dehydration; patients with anuria, hepatic coma, or glucose-galactose malabsorption syndrome

Warnings Hypertonic solutions (>10%) may cause thrombosis if infused via peripheral veins; administer hypertonic solutions via a central venous catheter; rapid administration of hypertonic solutions may produce significant hyperglycemia, glycosuria, and shifts in electrolytes; this may result in dehydration, hyperosmolar syndrome, coma, and death especially in patients with chronic uremia or carbohydrate intolerance; hyperglycemia and glycosuria may be functions of the rate of administration of dextrose; to minimize these effects, reduce the rate of infusion; addition of insulin may be necessary; administration of potassium free I.V. dextrose solutions may result in significant hypokalemia, particularly if highly concentrated solutions are used; add potassium to dextrose solutions for patients with adequate renal function; abrupt withdrawal of dextrose solution may be associated with rebound hypoglycemia; an unexpected rise in blood glucose level in an otherwise stable patient may be an early symptom of infection; glucose is not absorbed from the buccal cavity; it must be swallowed to be effective; do not use oral forms in unconscious patients

Precautions Use with caution in premature infants, especially very low birth weight infants, as rapid changes is osmolality may produce profound effects on the brain, including intraventricular hemorrhage; small incremental changes in infusion rates are necessary in these patients; use with caution also in patients with diabetes mellitus

Adverse Reactions Note: Most adverse effects are associated with excessive dosage or rate of infusion

Cardiovascular: Venous thrombosis, phlebitis, hypovolemia, hypervolemia, dehydration, edema

Central nervous system: Fever, mental confusion, unconsciousness, hyperosmolar syndrome

Endocrine & metabolic: Hyperglycemia, hypokalemia, acidosis, hypophosphatemia, hypomagnesemia

Local: Pain, vein irritation, tissue necrosis

Genitourinary: Polyuria, glycosuria, ketonuria

Gastrointestinal: Polydipsia, nausea

Respiratory: Tachypnea, pulmonary edema

Drug Interactions Corticosteroids

Stability Stable at room temperature; protect from freezing and extreme heat; store oral dextrose in airtight containers

Mechanism of Action Dextrose, a monosaccharide, is a source of calories and fluid for patients unable to obtain an adequate oral intake; may decrease body protein and nitrogen losses; promotes glycogen deposition in the liver; for the treatment of hyperkalemia, when combined with insulin, dextrose stimulates the uptake of potassium by cells, especially in muscle tissue

Pharmacodynamics

Onset: Treatment of hypoglycemia: Oral: 10 minutes

Peak effect: Treatment of hyperkalemia: I.V.: 30 minutes

Pharmacokinetics

Absorption: Rapidly from the small intestine by an active mechanism

Metabolism: Metabolized to carbon dioxide and water

Time to peak concentration: Oral: 40 minutes

Usual Dosage

Hypoglycemia: Doses may be repeated in severe cases

I.V.:

Premature neonates: 0.1-0.2 g/kg/dose (1-2 mL/kg/dose of 10% solution); followed by continuous infusion at a rate of 4-6 mg/kg/minute

Infants ≤6 months: 0.25-0.5 g/kg/dose (1-2 mL/kg/dose of 25% solution); maximum: 25 g/dose

Infants >6 months and Children: 0.5-1 g/kg/dose (2-4 mL/kg/dose of 25% solution); maximum: 25 g/dose

Adolescents and Adults: 10-25 g (40-100 mL of 25% solution or 20-50 mL of 50% solution)

Oral:

Children >2 years and Adults: 10-20 g as single dose; repeat in 10 minutes if necessary

Treatment of Hyperkalemia: I.V. (in combination with insulin):

Infants and Children: 0.5-1 g/kg (using 25% or 50% solution) combined with regular insulin 1 unit for every 4-5 g dextrose given; infuse over 2 hours (infusions as short as 30 minutes have been recommended); repeat as needed

Adolescents and Adults: 0.1 mL/kg (using 50% solution) combined with regular insulin 1 unit for every 4-5 g dextrose given (repeat as needed) **or** as an alternative 10 units regular insulin added to 250 mL $D_{10}W$ and infuse over 30-60 minutes

Fluid therapy: See Fluid and Electrolyte Requirements in Children *on page 1102*

Nutrition: See Parenteral Nutrition (PN) *on page 1106*

Administration

Oral: Must be swallowed to be absorbed (see Warnings)

Parenteral: Not for S.C. or I.M. administration; dilute concentrated dextrose solutions for peripheral venous administration to a maximum concentration of 12.5%; in emergency situations, 25% dextrose has been used peripherally; for direct I.V. infusion, infuse at a maximum rate of 200 mg/kg over 1 minute; continuous infusion rates vary with tolerance (see Parenteral Nutrition (PN) *on page 1106*) and range from 4.5-15 mg/kg/minute; hyperinsulinemic neonates may require up to 15-25 mg/kg/minute infusion rates

Monitoring Parameters Blood and urine sugar, serum electrolytes, I & O, caloric intake

Reference Range Normal blood sugar:

Neonates: 110-270 mg/dL

0-2 years: 60-105 mg/dL

Children >2 years and Adults: 70-110 mg/dL

Additional Information Each g of I.V. dextrose contains 3.4 kcal; glucose monohydrate 1 g is equal to 1 g anhydrous dextrose

Dosage Forms

Gel, as 40% dextrose: (Glutose®, Insta-Glucose®, Insulin Reaction): 25 g, 30.8 g, 80 g

Infusion, as 5% dextrose: 10 mL, 25 mL, 50 mL, 150 mL, 250 mL, 500 mL, 1000 mL

Infusion, as 10% dextrose: 3 mL, 250 mL, 500 mL, 1000 mL

Infusion, as 20% dextrose: 500 mL, 1000 mL

Infusion, as 25% dextrose: 10 mL

Infusion, as 30% dextrose: 500 mL, 1000 mL

Infusion, as 40% dextrose: 500 mL, 1000 mL

Infusion, as 50% dextrose: 50 mL, 500 mL, 1000 mL, 2000 mL

Infusion, as 60% dextrose: 500 mL, 1000 mL

Infusion, as 70% dextrose: 70 mL, 500 mL, 1000 mL, 2000 mL

Tablet, chewable (B-D Glucose®): 5 g

- ◆ **Dextrose Monohydrate** *see* Dextrose *on page 317*
- ◆ **Dextrostat®** *see* Dextroamphetamine *on page 312*
- ◆ **Dey-Drop® Ophthalmic Solution** *see* Silver Nitrate *on page 900*
- ◆ **DHAD** *see* Mitoxantrone *on page 679*
- ◆ **DHE** *see* Dihydroergotamine *on page 334*
- ◆ **D.H.E. 45® Injection** *see* Dihydroergotamine *on page 334*
- ◆ **DHPG** *see* Ganciclovir *on page 466*
- ◆ **DHS Sal®** *see* Salicylic Acid *on page 886*
- ◆ **DHS® Tar [OTC]** *see* Coal Tar *on page 260*
- ◆ **DHT™** *see* Dihydrotachysterol *on page 336*
- ◆ **Diaβeta®** *see* Glyburide *on page 476*
- ◆ **Diabetic Tussin DM® [OTC]** *see* Guaifenesin and Dextromethorphan *on page 487*
- ◆ **Diabetic Tussin EX® [OTC]** *see* Guaifenesin *on page 485*
- ◆ **Diahalt (Can)** *see* Loperamide *on page 603*
- ◆ **Dialose® [OTC]** *see* Docusate *on page 350*
- ◆ **Dialose® Plus Capsule [OTC]** *see* Docusate and Casanthranol *on page 351*
- ◆ **Diaminodiphenylsulfone** *see* Dapsone *on page 297*
- ◆ **Diamox®** *see* Acetazolamide *on page 32*

+ **Diamox Sequels**® *see* Acetazolamide *on page 32*
+ **Diaper Rash (Can)** *see* Zinc Oxide *on page 1026*
+ **Diarr-Eze (Can)** *see* Loperamide *on page 603*
+ **Diarrhea Relief (Can)** *see* Loperamide *on page 603*
+ **Diasorb**® [OTC] *see* Attapulgite *on page 118*
+ **Diastat**® **Rectal Delivery System** *see* Diazepam *on page 320*
+ **Diazemuls (Can)** *see* Diazepam *on page 320*

Diazepam (dye AZ e pam)

Related Information

Adult ACLS Algorithm, Synchronized Cardioversion *on page 1048*
Carbohydrate and Alcohol Content of Liquid Medications for Use in Patients Receiving Ketogenic Diets *on page 1258*
Drugs and Breast-Feeding *on page 1243*
Laboratory Detection of Drugs in Urine *on page 1234*
Overdose and Toxicology *on page 1222*
Preprocedure Sedatives in Children *on page 1201*

U.S. Brand Names Diastat® Rectal Delivery System; Diazepam Intensol®; Valium®

Canadian Brand Names Apo-Diazepam; Diazemuls; E Pam; Novo-Dipam; PMS-Diazepam; Vivol

Therapeutic Category Antianxiety Agent; Anticonvulsant, Benzodiazepine; Benzodiazepine; Hypnotic; Sedative

Generic Available

Yes: Injection, tablets, solution
No: Extended release capsules, rectal gel

Use Management of general anxiety disorders, panic disorders; to provide preoperative sedation, light anesthesia, and amnesia; treatment of status epilepticus, alcohol withdrawal symptoms; used as a skeletal muscle relaxant; rectal gel is indicated for intermittent episodes of markedly increased seizure activity in epilepsy patients on stable regimens of anticonvulsants

Restrictions C-IV

Pregnancy Risk Factor D

Contraindications Hypersensitivity to diazepam or any component; possible cross-sensitivity with other benzodiazepines; do not use in a comatose patient, in those with pre-existing CNS depression, respiratory depression, narrow-angle glaucoma, or severe uncontrolled pain

Warnings Rapid I.V. push may cause sudden respiratory depression, apnea, or hypotension

Precautions Use with caution in patients receiving other CNS depressants, patients with low albumin, renal or hepatic dysfunction, and in young infants and the elderly; use with extreme caution in neonates; injection and rectal gel contain sodium benzoate and benzoic acid which may displace bilirubin from protein binding sites and at larger doses can cause the gasping syndrome; neonates have decreased metabolism of diazepam and desmethyldiazepam (active metabolite), both can accumulate with repeated use and cause increased toxicity

Adverse Reactions

Cardiovascular: Cardiac arrest, hypotension, bradycardia, cardiovascular collapse
Central nervous system: Drowsiness, somnolence, confusion, dizziness, fatigue, amnesia, slurred speech, ataxia, impaired coordination, paradoxical excitement or rage (rare)
Dermatologic: Rash, dermatitis
Local: Phlebitis, pain with injection
Ocular: Blurred vision, diplopia
Respiratory: Decrease in respiratory rate, apnea, laryngospasm
Miscellaneous: Physical and psychological dependence with prolonged use

Drug Interactions Cytochrome P-450 isoenzyme CYP1A2, CYP2C8, CYP2C19 (minor), and CYP3A3/4 (minor) substrate; desmethyldiazepam is a CYP2C19 isoenzyme substrate

CNS depressants (alcohol, barbiturates, opioids) may enhance sedation and respiratory depression of diazepam; enzyme inducers may increase the hepatic metabolism of diazepam; cimetidine and erythromycin may decrease the metabolism of diazepam; valproic acid may displace diazepam from binding sites which may result in an increase in sedative effects; concurrent use of diazepam with ritonavir is not recommended

Stability Injection: Do not mix with other medications; protect from light

Mechanism of Action Depresses all levels of the CNS, including the limbic and reticular formation by binding to the benzodiazepine site on the gamma-aminobutyric acid (GABA) receptor complex and modulating GABA, which is a major inhibitory neurotransmitter in the brain

Pharmacodynamics Status epilepticus:

Onset of action:

I.V.: 1-3 minutes

Rectal: 2-10 minutes

Duration: 15-30 minutes

Pharmacokinetics

Absorption:

Oral: 85% to 100%

I.M.: Poor

Rectal (gel): Well absorbed

Distribution: Widely distributed; crosses blood-brain barrier and placenta; distributes into breast milk

Protein binding:

Neonates: 84% to 86%

Adults: 98%

Metabolism: In the liver to desmethyldiazepam (active metabolite) and N-methyloxazepam (active metabolite); these are metabolized to oxazepam (active) which undergoes glucuronide conjugation before being excreted

Bioavailability: Rectal (gel): 90%

Half-life:

Diazepam:

Infants 1 month to 2 years: 40-50 hours

Children 2-12 years: 15-21 hours

Children 12-16 years: 18-20 hours

Adults: 20-50 hours

Increased half-life in neonates (50-95 hours), elderly, and those with severe hepatic disorders

Desmethyldiazepam (active metabolite): 50-100 hours and can be prolonged in neonates

Time to peak serum concentration: Rectal (gel): 1.5 hours

Elimination: In urine, primarily as conjugated oxazepam (75%), desmethyldiazepam, and N-methyloxazepam

Usual Dosage

Children:

Conscious sedation for procedures: Oral: 0.2-0.3 mg/kg (maximum dose: 10 mg) 45-60 minutes prior to procedure

Febrile seizure prophylaxis: Oral: 1 mg/kg/day divided every 8 hours; initiate therapy at first sign of fever and continue for 24 hours after fever is gone

Sedation or muscle relaxation or anxiety:

Oral: 0.12-0.8 mg/kg/day in divided doses every 6-8 hours

I.M., I.V.: 0.04-0.3 mg/kg/dose every 2-4 hours to a maximum of 0.6 mg/kg within an 8-hour period if needed

Status epilepticus: I.V.:

Neonates: (Not recommended as a first-line agent; injection contains sodium benzoate and benzoic acid; see Precautions) 0.1-0.3 mg/kg/dose given over 3-5 minutes, every 15-30 minutes to a maximum total dose of 2 mg

Infants >30 days and Children <5 years: 0.05-0.3 mg/kg/dose given over 3-5 minutes, every 15-30 minutes to a maximum total dose of 5 mg **or** 0.2-0.5 mg/dose every 2-5 minutes to a maximum total dose of 5 mg; repeat in 2-4 hours as needed

Children ≥5 years: 0.05-0.3 mg/kg/dose given over 3-5 minutes, every 15-30 minutes to a maximum total dose of 10 mg **or** 1 mg/dose every 2-5 minutes to a maximum of 10 mg; repeat in 2-4 hours as needed

Muscle spasm associated with tetanus: I.V., I.M.:

Infants >30 days: 1-2 mg/dose every 3-4 hours as needed

Children ≥5 years: 5-10 mg/dose every 3-4 hours as needed

Anticonvulsant: Acute treatment:

Rectal gel formulation:

Infants <6 months: Not recommended

Children <2 years: Safety and efficacy have not been studied

Children 2-5 years: 0.5 mg/kg

Children 6-11 years: 0.3 mg/kg

Children ≥12 years and Adults: 0.2 mg/kg

(Continued)

Diazepam *(Continued)*

Note: Round dose to 2.5, 5, 10, 15, and 20 mg/dose; dose may be repeated in 4-12 hours if needed; do not use more than 5 times per month or more than once every 5 days

Rectal: Undiluted 5 mg/mL parenteral formulation (filter if using ampul): 0.5 mg/kg/dose then 0.25 mg/kg/dose in 10 minutes if needed

Adolescents: Conscious sedation for procedures:
Oral: 10 mg
I.V.: 5 mg; may repeat with 2.5 mg if needed

Adults:
Anxiety:
Oral: 2-10 mg 2-4 times/day
I.M., I.V.: 2-10 mg, may repeat in 3-4 hours if needed
Skeletal muscle relaxation:
Oral: 2-10 mg 2-4 times/day
I.M., I.V.: 5-10 mg, may repeat in 2-4 hours
Status epilepticus: I.V.: 5-10 mg every 10-15 minutes up to 30 mg in an 8-hour period; may repeat in 2-4 hours
Preoperative medication: I.M.: 10 mg before surgery

Administration

Oral: Administer with food or water; oral concentrate solution (5 mg/mL) should be diluted or mixed with water, juice, soda, applesauce, or pudding before use

Parenteral: I.V.: Infants and children: Do not exceed 1-2 mg/minute I.V. push; adult maximum infusion rate: 5 mg/minute; rapid injection may cause respiratory depression or hypotension

Rectal: Diastat®: Place patient on their side; remove protective cap and seal pin from syringe; lubricate rectal tip with lubricating jelly (provided in twin pack); turn patient on side facing you; bend upper leg forward and separate buttocks to expose rectum; insert syringe tip gently into rectum until rim fits snug against rectal opening; administer dose while slowly counting to 3 while gently pushing on plunger; slowly count to 3 again before removing syringe; hold buttocks together while slowing counting to 3 to prevent leakage; keep patient on their side, facing towards you and continue to observe patient; discard syringe and all used materials safely away from children; do not reuse

Monitoring Parameters Heart rate, respiratory rate, blood pressure

Reference Range Effective therapeutic range not well established
Proposed therapeutic:
Diazepam: 0.2-1.5 µg/mL (SI: 0.7-5.3 µmol/L)
N-desmethyldiazepam (nordiazepam): 0.1-0.5 µg/mL (SI: 0.35-1.8 µmol/L)

Test Interactions False-negative urinary glucose determinations with Clinistix® or Diastix®

Patient Information Avoid alcohol; limit caffeine; may cause drowsiness and impair ability to perform activities that require mental alertness or physical coordination; avoid abrupt discontinuation after prolonged use

Nursing Implications Avoid extravasation; infuse I.V. into secure line using larger veins

Additional Information Diazepam does not have any analgesic effects; diarrhea in a 9 month old infant receiving high-dose oral diazepam was attributed to the diazepam oral solution that contained polyethylene glycol and propylene glycol (both are osmotically active); diarrhea resolved when crushed tablets were substituted for the oral solution (see Marshall, 1995); rectal gel contains sodium benzoate, benzyl alcohol (1.5%), benzoic acid, and ethyl alcohol (10%)

Dosage Forms

Gel, rectal delivery system (Diastat®):
Pediatric rectal tip (4.4 cm): 5 mg/mL (2.5 mg, 5 mg) [twin packs]
Universal rectal tip [for pediatric and adult use] (4.4 cm): 5 mg/mL (10 mg) [twin pack]
Adult rectal tip (6 cm): 5 mg/mL (15 mg, 20 mg) [twin packs]
Injection: 5 mg/mL (1 mL, 2 mL, 10 mL)
Solution, oral: 5 mg/5 mL [wintergreen-spice flavor] (5 mL, 10 mL, 500 mL)
Solution, oral concentrate (Diazepam Intensol®): 5 mg/mL (30 mL)
Tablet: 2 mg, 5 mg, 10 mg

References

Dreifuss FE, Rosman NP, Cloyd JC, et al, "A Comparison of Rectal Diazepam Gel and Placebo for Acute Repetitive Seizures," *N Engl J Med*, 1998, 338(26):1869-75.

Marshall JD, Farrar HC, and Kearns GL, "Diarrhea Associated With Enteral Benzodiazepine Solutions," *J Pediatr*, 1995, 126(4):657-9.

Rosman NP, Colton T, Labazzo J, et al, "A Controlled Trial of Diazepam Administered During Febrile Illnesses to Prevent Recurrence of Febrile Seizures," *N Engl J Med*, 1993, 329(2):79-84.

Zeltzer LK, Altman A, Cohen D, et al, "Report of the Subcommittee on the Management of Pain Associated With Procedures in Children With Cancer," *Pediatrics*, 1990, 86(5 Pt 2):826-31.

♦ **Diazepam Intensol®** *see* Diazepam *on page 320*

Diazoxide (dye az OKS ide)

U.S. Brand Names Hyperstat®; Proglycem®

Therapeutic Category Antihypertensive Agent; Antihypoglycemic Agent; Vasodilator

Generic Available Yes: Injection

Use
  I.V.: Emergency lowering of blood pressure
  Oral: Hypoglycemia related to hyperinsulinism secondary to: Islet cell adenoma, carcinoma, or hyperplasia; adenomatosis; nesidioblastosis (persistent hyperinsulinemic hypoglycemia of infancy); leucine sensitivity, or extrapancreatic malignancy

Pregnancy Risk Factor C

Contraindications Hypersensitivity to diazoxide, any component, thiazides, or other sulfonamide derivatives; aortic coarctation, arteriovenous shunts, dissecting aortic aneurysm

Precautions Diabetes mellitus, renal or liver disease, coronary artery disease, or cerebral vascular insufficiency

Adverse Reactions
  Cardiovascular: Hypotension, tachycardia, flushing
  Central nervous system: Dizziness, seizure, headache
  Dermatologic: Rash, hirsutism
  Endocrine & metabolic: Hyperglycemia, ketoacidosis, hyperuricemia, sodium and water retention, edema (more common in young infants and adults)
  Gastrointestinal: Nausea, vomiting, anorexia, constipation
  Hematologic: Leukopenia, thrombocytopenia
  Local: Pain, burning, cellulitis/phlebitis upon extravasation
  Neuromuscular & skeletal: Weakness
  Miscellaneous: Extrapyramidal symptoms and development of abnormal facies with chronic oral use

Drug Interactions Diuretics and hypotensive agents may potentiate diazoxide adverse effects; diazoxide may increase phenytoin metabolism or free fraction; diazoxide may decrease warfarin protein binding

Stability Protect from light, heat, and freezing; avoid using darkened solutions

Mechanism of Action Inhibits insulin release from the pancreas; produces direct smooth muscle relaxation of the peripheral arterioles which results in decrease in blood pressure and reflex increase in heart rate and cardiac output

Pharmacodynamics
  Hyperglycemic effects (oral):
    Onset of action: Within 1 hour
    Duration (normal renal function): 8 hours
  Hypotensive effects (I.V.):
    Peak: Within 5 minutes
    Duration: Usually 3-12 hours

Pharmacokinetics
  Protein binding: 90%
  Half-life:
    Children: 9-24 hours
    Adults: 20-36 hours
  Elimination: 50% excreted unchanged in urine

Usual Dosage
  Hyperinsulinemic hypoglycemia: Oral (**Note**: Use lower dose listed as initial dose):
    Newborns and Infants: 8-15 mg/kg/day in divided doses every 8-12 hours
    Children and Adults: 3-8 mg/kg/day in divided doses every 8-12 hours
  Hypertension: I.V.: Children and Adults: 1-3 mg/kg (maximum dose: 150 mg in a single injection); repeat dose in 5-15 minutes until blood pressure adequately reduced; repeat administration every 4-24 hours; monitor blood pressure closely

Administration
  Oral: Administer on an empty stomach 1 hour before or 1 hour after meals; shake suspension well before use
  Parenteral: Do not administer I.M. or S.C.; administer I.V. (undiluted) by rapid I.V. injection over a period of 30 seconds or less

Monitoring Parameters Blood pressure, blood glucose

Additional Information Patients may require a diuretic with repeated doses
(Continued)

Diazoxide *(Continued)*

Dosage Forms
Injection (Hyperstat®): 15 mg/mL (20 mL)
Suspension, oral (Proglycem®): 50 mg/mL [chocolate-mint flavor] (30 mL)

♦ **Dibenzyline®** *see* Phenoxybenzamine *on page 787*

Dibucaine *(DYE byoo kane)*

U.S. Brand Names Nupercainal® [OTC]
Therapeutic Category Analgesic, Topical; Local Anesthetic, Topical
Generic Available Yes
Use Fast, temporary relief of pain and itching due to hemorrhoids, minor burns, other minor skin conditions
Pregnancy Risk Factor C
Contraindications Hypersensitivity to amide-type anesthetics
Warnings Products may contain sulfites; avoid use in sensitive individuals
Adverse Reactions
Cardiovascular: Edema
Dermatologic: Urticaria, cutaneous lesions, contact dermatitis
Local: Burning, tenderness, irritation, inflammation
Mechanism of Action Blocks both the initiation and conduction of nerve impulses by decreasing the neuronal membrane's permeability to sodium ions, which results in inhibition of depolarization with resultant blockade of conduction
Pharmacodynamics
Onset of action: Within 15 minutes
Duration: 2-4 hours
Pharmacokinetics Absorption: Poor through intact skin, but well absorbed through mucous membranes and excoriated skin
Usual Dosage Children and Adults:
Rectal: Hemorrhoids: Administer each morning, evening, and after each bowel movement
Topical: Apply gently to the affected areas; no more than 30 g for adults or 7.5 g for children should be used in any 24-hour period
Administration
Rectal: Insert ointment into rectum using a rectal applicator
Topical: Apply gently to affected areas; do not use near the eyes or over denuded surfaces or blistered areas
Dosage Forms
Cream: 0.5% (45 g)
Ointment, topical: 1% (30 g, 60 g)

♦ **DIC** *see* Dacarbazine *on page 292*
♦ **Dichysterol** *see* Dihydrotachysterol *on page 336*

Diclofenac *(dye KLOE fen ak)*

U.S. Brand Names Cataflam®; Voltaren®; Voltaren®-XR
Canadian Brand Names Apo-Diclo; Arthrotec; Diclotec; Novo-Difenac; Novo-Difenac-SR; Nu-Diclo; PMS-Diclofenac; Riva-Diclofenac; Voltaren Ophtha; Voltaren Rapide
Therapeutic Category Analgesic, Non-narcotic; Anti-inflammatory Agent; Nonsteroidal Anti-inflammatory Drug (NSAID), Ophthalmic; Nonsteroidal Anti-inflammatory Drug (NSAID), Oral
Generic Available Yes
Use
Oral: Acute treatment of mild to moderate pain; acute and chronic treatment of rheumatoid arthritis, ankylosing spondylitis, and osteoarthritis; used for juvenile rheumatoid arthritis, gout, dysmenorrhea
Ophthalmic solution: Postoperative inflammation after cataract extraction; temporary relief of pain and photophobia in patients undergoing corneal refractive surgery
Pregnancy Risk Factor Oral: B (D in 3rd trimester); Ophthalmic: C
Contraindications Hypersensitivity to diclofenac, any component, aspirin, or NSAIDs; porphyria
Precautions Use with caution in patients with CHF, hypertension, decreased renal or hepatic function, history of GI disease, or those receiving anticoagulants; patients should not wear soft contact lenses while using ophthalmic solution
Adverse Reactions
Central nervous system: Dizziness, headache
Dermatologic: Rash, pruritus

Endocrine & metabolic: Fluid retention

Gastrointestinal: Abdominal pain, indigestion, peptic ulcer, GI bleeding, GI perforation, constipation, diarrhea

Hematologic: Agranulocytosis, aplastic anemia (rare), inhibition of platelet aggregation

Hepatic: Elevated ALT or AST, possible hepatitis

Ocular: With ophthalmic use, itching, tearing (allergic reaction); irritation, redness, burning; ocular irritation with use of hydrogel soft contact lenses

Otic: Tinnitus

Renal: Renal impairment, nephrotic-like syndrome

Drug Interactions Cytochrome P-450 isoenzyme CYP2C8 and CYP2C9 substrate; CYP2C9 isoenzyme inhibitor

Diclofenac may increase serum concentrations of digoxin, methotrexate and lithium; may increase nephrotoxicity of cyclosporine; may decrease diuretic and antihypertensive effects of thiazides and furosemide; may decrease antihypertensive effects of ACE inhibitors and angiotensin II antagonists; diclofenac plus potassium-sparing diuretics may increase serum potassium; concomitant insulin or oral hypoglycemic agents may increase or decrease serum glucose; aspirin may decrease serum concentration of diclofenac (combination not recommended); gastric irritants (eg, aspirin, other NSAIDs, potassium supplements) may increase risk of GI irritation

Food Interactions Delayed oral absorption has been reported with food for single doses but not with chronic multiple-dose administration

Stability Ophthalmic solution: Store at room temperature; protect from light

Mechanism of Action Inhibits prostaglandin synthesis by decreasing the activity of the enzyme, cyclo-oxygenase, which results in decreased formation of prostaglandin precursors

Usual Dosage Note: Cataflam® tablets are immediate release and is the formulation which should be used when prompt onset of pain relief is desired; Voltaren®-XR should not be used for acute pain relief due to its extended release

Oral:

Children: 2-3 mg/kg/day divided 2-4 times/day

Adults:

Rheumatoid arthritis:

Cataflam® or Voltaren®: 100-200 mg/day in 2-4 divided doses; maximum dose: 225 mg/day

Voltaren®-XR: 100 mg/day; dose may be increased to 100 mg twice daily; maximum dose: 200 mg/day

Osteoarthritis:

Cataflam® or Voltaren®: 100-150 mg/day in 2-3 divided doses

Voltaren®-XR: 100 mg/day

Ankylosing spondylitis: Voltaren®: 100-125 mg/day in 4-5 divided doses

Analgesia and primary dysmenorrhea: Cataflam®: 50 mg given 3 times/day; some patients may have better relief with an initial dose of 100 mg

Ophthalmic:

Cataract surgery: Instill 1 drop into affected eye 4 times/day beginning 24 hours after cataract surgery and continuing for 2 weeks

Corneal refractive surgery: Instill 1-2 drops into operative eye within the hour prior to surgery, within 15 minutes after surgery, and continuing 4 times/day for up to 3 days

Administration

Ophthalmic: Avoid contact of bottle tip with skin or eye; apply finger pressure to lacrimal sac during and for 1-2 minutes after instillation to decrease risk of absorption and systemic effects

Oral: Administer with milk or food to decrease GI upset; do not chew or crush delayed release or extended release tablets, swallow whole

Monitoring Parameters CBC, liver enzymes; monitor urine output, BUN, serum creatinine in patients receiving diuretics

Patient Information Avoid alcohol; report any signs of blood in stool; do not use hydrogel soft contact lenses during ophthalmic diclofenac therapy

Additional Information Vomiting, drowsiness, and acute renal failure have been reported with overdoses

Dosage Forms

Solution, ophthalmic, as sodium (Voltaren®): 0.1% (2.5 mL, 5 mL)

Tablet, delayed release, as sodium (Voltaren®): 25 mg, 50 mg, 75 mg

Tablet, extended release, as sodium (Voltaren®-XR): 100 mg

Tablet, as potassium (Cataflam®): 50 mg

(Continued)

Diclofenac *(Continued)*

References

Brogden RN, Heel RC, Pakes GE, et al, "Diclofenac Sodium: A Review of Its Pharmacological Properties and Therapeutic Use in Rheumatic Diseases and Pain of Varying Origin," *Drugs*, 1980, 20(1):24-48.
Haapasaari J, Wuolijoki E, and Ylijoki H, "Treatment of Juvenile Rheumatoid Arthritis With Diclofenac Sodium" *Scand J Rheumatol*, 1983, 12(4):325-30.

♦ **Diclotec (Can)** *see* Diclofenac *on page 324*

Dicloxacillin (dye kloks a SIL in)

U.S. Brand Names Dycill®; Dynapen®; Pathocil®

Therapeutic Category Antibiotic, Penicillin (Antistaphylococcal)

Generic Available Yes

Use Treatment of skin and soft tissue infections, pneumonia and follow-up therapy of osteomyelitis caused by susceptible penicillinase-producing staphylococci

Pregnancy Risk Factor B

Contraindications Hypersensitivity to dicloxacillin, penicillin, or any component

Warnings Elimination is prolonged in neonates

Adverse Reactions

Central nervous system: Fever

Dermatologic: Rash

Gastrointestinal: Nausea, vomiting, diarrhea, *C. difficile* colitis

Hematologic: Eosinophilia, neutropenia, leukopenia, thrombocytopenia

Hepatic: Elevated liver enzymes

Miscellaneous: Serum sickness-like reaction

Drug Interactions Oral contraceptives (decreased effectiveness), probenecid (increase serum concentration of dicloxacillin)

Food Interactions Food decreases the rate and extent of absorption

Stability Reconstituted dicloxacillin suspension is stable for 7 days at room temperature or 14 days if refrigerated

Mechanism of Action Inhibits bacterial cell wall synthesis by binding to one or more of the penicillin-binding proteins and interfering with the final transpeptidation step of peptidoglycan synthesis

Pharmacokinetics

Absorption: 35% to 76% absorbed from the GI tract

Distribution: Into bone, bile, pleural fluid, synovial fluid, and amniotic fluid; appears in breast milk

Protein binding: 96% to 98%

Half-life: Adults: 0.6-0.8 hours; slightly prolonged in patients with renal impairment

Time to peak serum concentration: Within 0.5-2 hours

Elimination: Partially eliminated by the liver and excreted in bile; 31% to 65% eliminated in urine as unchanged drug and active metabolite

Neonates: Prolonged

CF patients: More rapid elimination than healthy patients

Dialysis: Not dialyzable (0% to 5%)

Usual Dosage Oral:

Children <40 kg: 25-50 mg/kg/day divided every 6 hours; doses of 50-100 mg/kg/day in divided doses every 6 hours have been used for follow-up therapy of osteomyelitis; maximum dose: 2 g/day

Children >40 kg and Adults: 125-500 mg every 6 hours; maximum dose: 2 g/day

Administration Oral: Administer with water 1 hour before or 2 hours after meals on an empty stomach

Monitoring Parameters Periodic monitoring of CBC, BUN, serum creatinine, urinalysis, and liver enzymes during prolonged therapy

Additional Information

Sodium content of 250 mg capsule: 0.6 mEq

Sodium content of 5 mL suspension: 2.9 mEq

Dosage Forms

Capsule, as sodium: 125 mg, 250 mg, 500 mg

Powder for oral suspension, as sodium: 62.5 mg/5 mL (80 mL, 100 mL, 200 mL)

Dicyclomine (dye SYE kloe meen)

Related Information

Carbohydrate and Alcohol Content of Liquid Medications for Use in Patients Receiving Ketogenic Diets *on page 1258*

Overdose and Toxicology *on page 1222*

U.S. Brand Names Bentyl®

Canadian Brand Names Bentylol; Formulex; Lomine; Protylol

Synonyms Dicycloverine

Therapeutic Category Anticholinergic Agent; Antispasmodic Agent, Gastrointestinal

Generic Available Yes

Use Treatment of functional disturbances of GI motility such as irritable bowel syndrome

Pregnancy Risk Factor B

Contraindications Hypersensitivity to any anticholinergic drug; narrow-angle glaucoma, tachycardia, GI obstruction, obstruction of the urinary tract, myasthenia gravis; should not be used in infants <6 months of age due to reports of respiratory distress, seizures, syncope, asphyxia, pulse rate fluctuations, muscular hypotonia, and coma

Precautions Use with caution in patients with hepatic or renal disease, ulcerative colitis, hyperthyroidism, cardiovascular disease, hypertension, hiatal hernia, autonomic neuropathy

Adverse Reactions Children with Down's syndrome, spastic paralysis, or brain damage are more sensitive to toxic effects than adults

Cardiovascular: Tachycardia, palpitations, orthostatic hypotension

Central nervous system: Seizures, coma, nervousness, excitement, confusion, insomnia, headache

Dermatologic: Urticaria, pruritus, dry skin, photosensitivity

Gastrointestinal: Nausea, vomiting, constipation, xerostomia, dry throat, dysphagia

Genitourinary: Urinary retention

Local: Injection site reactions

Neuromuscular & skeletal: Muscular hypotonia, weakness

Ocular: Blurred vision, photophobia

Respiratory: Respiratory distress, asphyxia, dry nose

Miscellaneous: Decreased diaphoresis

Drug Interactions Additive adverse effects when given with medications with anticholinergic activity; may alter GI absorption of various drugs due to prolonged GI transit time; antacids; antagonizes effects of antiglaucoma agents

Stability Protect from light

Mechanism of Action Blocks the action of acetylcholine at parasympathetic sites in smooth muscle, secretory glands and the CNS

Pharmacodynamics

Onset of effects: 1-2 hours

Duration: Up to 4 hours

Pharmacokinetics

Absorption: Oral: Well absorbed

Distribution: V_d: 3.65 L/kg

Bioavailability: 67%

Half-life:

Initial phase: 1.8 hours

Terminal phase: 9-10 hours

Time to peak serum concentration: Oral: 1-1.5 hours

Elimination: 80% in urine; 10% in feces

Usual Dosage

Infants >6 months: Oral: 5 mg/dose 3-4 times/day

Children: Oral: 10 mg/dose 3-4 times/day

Adults:

Oral: Initial: 20 mg 4 times/day, then increase up to 40 mg 4 times/day

I.M.: 20 mg/dose 4 times/day; oral therapy should replace I.M. therapy as soon as possible

Administration

Oral: Administer 30 minutes before eating

Parenteral: I.M. only; not for I.V. use

Patient Information Limit alcohol

Dosage Forms

Capsule, as hydrochloride: 10 mg

Injection, as hydrochloride: 10 mg/mL (2 mL, 10 mL)

Syrup, as hydrochloride: 10 mg/5 mL (118 mL, 473 mL)

Tablet, as hydrochloride: 20 mg

♦ **Dicycloverine** see Dicyclomine on page 326

Didanosine (dye DAN oh seen)

Related Information

Adult and Adolescent HIV on page 1166

(Continued)

Didanosine *(Continued)*

U.S. Brand Names Videx® Oral

Synonyms DDI; Dideoxyinosine

Therapeutic Category Antiretroviral Agent; HIV Agents (Anti-HIV Agents); Nucleoside Reverse Transcriptase Inhibitor (NRTI)

Generic Available No

Use Treatment of HIV infection in combination with other antiretroviral agents; (**Note:** HIV regimens consisting of **three** antiretroviral agents are strongly recommended)

Pregnancy Risk Factor B (Fatal lactic acidosis/severe hepatomegaly with steatosis has been reported in pregnant women who received the combination of didanosine and stavudine with other antiretroviral agents)

Contraindications Hypersensitivity to didanosine or any component

Warnings Major clinical toxicities of didanosine include pancreatitis and peripheral neuropathy; fatal and nonfatal pancreatitis has been reported during therapy; risk factors for developing pancreatitis include a previous history of the condition, didanosine dosage >10 mg/kg/day, concurrent cytomegalovirus or *Mycobacterium avium-intracellulare* infection, and concomitant use of stavudine with or without hydroxyurea, pentamidine, or co-trimoxazole. Dose-related (treatment-limiting) peripheral neuropathy occurs most often after 2-6 months of continuous didanosine administration; may cause retinal depigmentation in children receiving doses >300 mg/m^2/day. Fatal cases of lactic acidosis and severe hepatomegaly with steatosis have been reported with use of didanosine and other NRTIs; obesity and prolonged nucleoside exposure may be risk factors

Precautions Use with caution in patients with phenylketonuria (tablets contain aspartame which is metabolized to phenylalanine), patients on sodium-restricted diets, patients with history of pancreatitis, and patients with renal or hepatic impairment; adjust dosage in patients with renal impairment or peripheral neuropathy; discontinue didanosine if clinical signs of pancreatitis occur; only after pancreatitis has been ruled out should dosing be resumed

Adverse Reactions

    Central nervous system: Headache (32% to 36%), insomnia, malaise, CNS depression, fever

    Dermatologic: Rash, pruritus, alopecia

    Endocrine & metabolic: Hypokalemia, hyperuricemia, increased triglycerides, hyperglycemia, lactic acidosis

    Gastrointestinal: Diarrhea (18%), nausea, vomiting, anorexia, stomatitis, pancreatitis (9%, dose-related, less common in children than adults), abdominal pain

    Hepatic: Elevated liver enzymes, hepatic failure, elevated amylase

    Neuromuscular & skeletal: Peripheral neuropathy (dose-related), myalgia, arthritis, weakness

    Ocular: Retinal depigmentation, optic neuritis

    Respiratory: Cough, dyspnea

Drug Interactions Antacids, allopurinol, omeprazole, ganciclovir, cimetidine, and ranitidine may increase absorption of didanosine; methadone decreases didanosine concentration; decreases absorption of ketoconazole, itraconazole, indinavir, ganciclovir, dapsone, ciprofloxacin, tetracyclines (administer at least 2 hours before or 2 hours after didanosine); drugs associated with peripheral neuropathy (cisplatin, isoniazid, metronidazole, phenytoin, vincristine, stavudine, zalcitabine, dapsone, ethambutol, ethionamide, hydralazine, and nitrofurantoin) may increase the risk for didanosine peripheral neuropathy; drugs associated with pancreatitis (alcohol, I.V. pentamidine) may increase the risk of pancreatitis; concomitant administration of didanosine and delavirdine may decrease absorption of both drugs (separate dosing by at least 2 hours); concomitant administration of didanosine and ritonavir may decrease AUC of didanosine

Food Interactions Food decreases oral bioavailability by as much as 50%; do not mix with fruit juice or other acid-containing liquid since didanosine is unstable in acidic solutions

Stability Undergoes rapid degradation when exposed to an acidic environment; tablets dispersed in water are stable for 1 hour at room temperature; reconstituted buffered solution is stable for 4 hours at room temperature; reconstituted unbuffered solution is stable for 30 days if refrigerated; unbuffered powder for oral solution must be reconstituted with water and mixed with an equal volume of double strength antacid at time of preparation; when unbuffered powder for oral solution is reconstituted and admixed with a double-strength antacid to make a 20 mg/mL solution for adult once-daily dosing, the admixture is stable for 24 hours at room temperature and for 30 days if refrigerated

Mechanism of Action A purine dideoxynucleoside analog converted within the cell to an active metabolite, dideoxyadenosine triphosphate which serves as a substrate and inhibitor of viral RNA-directed DNA polymerase resulting in premature termination of viral DNA synthesis

Pharmacokinetics

Distribution: Extensive intracellular distribution; low penetration into CNS; crosses the placenta

V_d:

Children: 35.6 L/m^2; range: 18.4-61 L/m^2

Adults: 18.4-60.7 L/m^2

Protein binding: <5%

Metabolism: Converted intracellularly to active triphosphate form

Bioavailability: Variable and affected by the presence of food in the GI tract, gastric pH, and the dosage form administered

Children and Adolescents: 32% to 42% (ranges from 13% to 78%)

Adults:

Tablet: 40%

Powder: 30%

Half-life:

Plasma:

Children and Adolescents: 0.8 hour

Adults: 1.3-1.6 hours

Intracellular: Adults: 25-40 hours

Elimination: Unchanged drug excreted in urine

Children: 6% to 30%

Adults: 20% to 55%

Usual Dosage Oral: (Use in combination with other antiretroviral agents):

Neonates <90 days: Based on clinical study data from PACTG 239: 50 mg/m^2/dose every 12 hours

Children <13 years: Dosing is based on body surface area (m^2): 180-300 mg/m^2/day divided every 12 hours. **Note:** Use lower dosage range for patients on combination therapy with other antiretrovirals; may need higher dose in patients with central nervous system disease.

Children ≥13 years and Adults: **Note:** Although once-daily dosing is available, it should only be considered for adult patients whose management requires once-daily administration (eg, in renal impairment); the preferred dosing frequency of didanosine is twice daily because there is more evidence to support the effectiveness of this dosing frequency (BMS study AI454-148)

<60 kg: 125 mg every 12 hours using 2 tablets/dose **or** 250 mg once daily using 2 tablets/dose

Buffered powder for oral solution: 167 mg every 12 hours

Delayed-release capsule: 250 mg once daily

≥60 kg: 200 mg every 12 hours using 2 tablets/dose **or** 400 mg once daily using 2 tablets/dose or a special Videx® solution in double-strength antacid which provides 400 mg/20 mL for once-daily dosing

Buffered powder for oral solution: 250 mg every 12 hours

Delayed-release capsule: 400 mg once daily

Dosing adjustment in renal impairment: Adults: Dosing based on patient weight, creatinine clearance, and dosage form:

Dosing for patients <60 kg:

Cl_{cr} 30-59 mL/minute:

Tablet: 75 mg twice daily

Buffered powder for oral solution: 100 mg twice daily

Delayed-release capsule: 125 mg once daily

Cl_{cr} 10-29 mL/minute:

Tablet: 100 mg once daily

Buffered powder for oral solution: 100 mg once daily

Delayed-release capsule: 125 mg once daily

Cl_{cr} <10 mL/minute:

Tablet: 75 mg once daily

Buffered powder for oral solution: 100 mg once daily

Delayed-release capsule: Use alternate formulation

Dosing for patients ≥60 kg:

Cl_{cr} 30-59 mL/minute:

Tablet: 100 mg twice daily

Buffered powder for oral solution: 100 mg twice daily

Delayed-release capsule: 200 mg once daily

Cl_{cr} 10-29 mL/minute:

Tablet: 150 mg once daily

Buffered powder for oral solution: 167 mg once daily

Delayed-release capsule: 125 mg once daily

(Continued)

Didanosine *(Continued)*

Cl_{cr} <10 mL/minute:
Tablet: 100 mg once daily
Buffered powder for oral solution: 100 mg once daily
Delayed-release capsule: 125 mg once daily

Administration Oral: Administer on an empty stomach 1 hour before or at least 2 hours after a meal; tablets should be chewed, crushed, or dispersed in water for oral administration; tablets dispersed in water must be administered within 1 hour; unbuffered pediatric powder should be reconstituted with water and admixed in equal parts with a double-strength antacid to provide a final concentration of 10 mg/mL; unbuffered pediatric powder has also been reconstituted and admixed with a double-strength antacid to provide a final concentration of 20 mg/mL to be used for once-daily dosing in adults; shake oral solution well before use; administer at least 1 hour apart from indinavir or 2 hours apart from ritonavir; didanosine should be given at least 1 hour before or 2 hours after lopinavir/ritonavir; when administering chewable tablets, at least 2 tablets should be taken per dose to ensure adequate buffering capacity

Monitoring Parameters Serum potassium, uric acid, lactic acid, creatinine; hemoglobin, CBC with neutrophil and platelet count, CD4 cells; HIV RNA plasma level; liver function tests, serum amylase and triglyceride levels; weight gain; perform dilated retinal exam every 6 months; signs and symptoms of peripheral neuropathy

Patient Information The buffered powder vehicle may contribute to the development of diarrhea; inform physician if numbness, tingling, persistent severe abdominal pain, nausea, or vomiting occurs; shake oral solution well before use and keep refrigerated; discard solution after 30 days and obtain new supply

Additional Information
Contents of each tablet: 11.5 mEq of sodium, 15.7 mEq of magnesium, along with phenylalanine; tablets are buffered with dihydroxyaluminum sodium carbonate, magnesium hydroxide, and sodium citrate
Sodium content of each packet of buffered powder for oral solution: 60 mEq

Dosage Forms
Capsule, delayed-release: 125 mg, 200 mg, 250 mg, 400 mg
Powder for oral solution:
Buffered (single dose packet): 100 mg, 167 mg, 250 mg
Pediatric (for 10 mg/mL solution): 2 g, 4 g
Tablet, buffered, chewable: 25 mg, 50 mg, 100 mg, 150 mg, 200 mg [mint flavor]

References

Balis FM, Pizzo PA, Butler KM, et al, "Clinical Pharmacology of 2', 3'-Dideoxyinosine in Human Immunodeficiency Virus-Infected Children," *J Infect Dis*, 1992, 165(1):99-104.
Butler KM, Husson RN, Balis FM, et al, "Dideoxyinosine in Children With Symptomatic Human Immunodeficiency Virus Infection," *N Engl J Med*, 1991, 324(3):137-44.
Panel on Clinical Practices for Treatment of HIV Infection, "Guidelines for the Use of Antiretroviral Agents in HIV-Infected Adults and Adolescents," January 28, 2000, http://www.hivatis.org.
Working Group on Antiretroviral Therapy and Medical Management of HIV-Infected Children, "Guidelines for the Use of Antiretroviral Agents in Pediatric HIV Infection," January 7, 2000, http://www.hivatis.org.

♦ **2',3'-didehydro-3'-deoxythymidine** *see* Stavudine *on page 913*

♦ **Dideoxycytidine** *see* Zalcitabine *on page 1020*

♦ **Dideoxyinosine** *see* Didanosine *on page 327*

♦ **Didronel®** *see* Etidronate Disodium *on page 411*

♦ **Diflucan®** *see* Fluconazole *on page 430*

♦ **Digestive Enzymes [OTC]** *see* Pancrelipase *on page 755*

♦ **Digibind®** *see* Digoxin Immune Fab *on page 333*

♦ **Digitek®** *see* Digoxin *on page 330*

Digoxin *(di JOKS in)*

Related Information
Adult ACLS Algorithm, Narrow-Complex Supraventricular Tachycardia *on page 1046*
Blood Level Sampling Time Guidelines *on page 1220*
Carbohydrate and Alcohol Content of Liquid Medications for Use in Patients Receiving Ketogenic Diets *on page 1258*
Overdose and Toxicology *on page 1222*

U.S. Brand Names Digitek®; Lanoxicaps®; Lanoxin®

Canadian Brand Names Novo-Digoxin

Therapeutic Category Antiarrhythmic Agent, Miscellaneous; Cardiac Glycoside

Generic Available Yes: Tablet

Use Treatment of CHF; slows the ventricular rate in tachyarrhythmias such as atrial fibrillation, atrial flutter, supraventricular tachycardia

Pregnancy Risk Factor C

Contraindications Hypersensitivity to digoxin, other digitalis preparations, or any component; ventricular fibrillation, A-V block, idiopathic hypertrophic subaortic stenosis, or constrictive pericarditis

Warnings Use with extreme caution in patients with hypoxia, hypothyroidism, acute myocarditis, electrolyte disorders, acute MI

Precautions Use with caution and reduce dosage in patients with renal impairment

Adverse Reactions

Cardiovascular: Sinus bradycardia, A-V block, S-A block, atrial or nodal ectopic beats, ventricular arrhythmias, bigeminy, trigeminy, atrial tachycardia with A-V block

Central nervous system: Drowsiness, fatigue, headache, lethargy, vertigo, disorientation

Endocrine & metabolic: Hyperkalemia with acute toxicity

Gastrointestinal: Vomiting, nausea, feeding intolerance, abdominal pain, diarrhea

Neuromuscular & skeletal: Neuralgia

Ocular: Blurred vision, halos, yellow or green vision, diplopia, photophobia, flashing lights

Drug Interactions Antacids, kaolin-pectin, cholestyramine, cisapride, colestipol, sucralfate, and metoclopramide may decrease absorption of digoxin; quinidine, nifedipine, itraconazole, indomethacin, verapamil, amiodarone, erythromycin, propafenone, tetracycline, and spironolactone may increase digoxin serum concentration; penicillamine may decrease digoxin's pharmacologic effects; calcium (especially rapid I.V. use) may cause severe arrhythmias; paroxetine may decrease the AUC of digoxin by 15%; ritonavir may increase or decrease digoxin levels, close monitoring of digoxin levels is recommended; suspected interaction with nevirapine, careful monitoring is recommended

Food Interactions Meals containing increased fiber (bran) or foods high in pectin, may decrease oral absorption of digoxin; avoid natural licorice (causes sodium and water retention and increases potassium loss); maintain adequate amounts of potassium in diet to decrease risk of hypokalemia (hypokalemia may increase risk of digoxin toxicity)

Stability I.V. solution compatibility: D_5W, $D_{10}W$, NS, SWI (when diluted fourfold or greater); do not mix with other drugs; store at room temperature; protect from light

Mechanism of Action Increases the influx of calcium ions, from extracellular to intracellular cytoplasm by inhibition of sodium and potassium ion movement across the myocardial membranes; this increase in calcium ions results in a potentiation of the activity of the contractile heart muscle fibers and an increase in the force of myocardial contraction (positive inotropic effect); inhibits adenosine triphosphatase (ATPase); decreases conduction through the S-A and A-V nodes

Pharmacodynamics

Onset of effects:

Oral: 0.5-2 hours

I.V.: 5-30 minutes

Maximum effect:

Oral: 2-8 hours

I.V.: 1-4 hours

Duration (adults): 3-4 days

Pharmacokinetics

Distribution: Distribution phase: 6-8 hours

V_d:

Neonates, full-term: 7.5-10 L/kg

Children: 16 L/kg

Adults: 7 L/kg

Renal disease: Decreased V_d

Protein binding: 20% to 25%

Bioavailability (dependent upon formulation):

Capsules: 90% to 100%

Elixir: 70% to 85%

Tablets: 60% to 80%

Half-life, elimination (dependent upon age, renal and cardiac function):

Premature: 61-170 hours

Neonates, full-term: 35-45 hours

Infants: 18-25 hours

Children: 35 hours

Adults: 38-48 hours

Anephric adults: >4.5 days

Anuric adults: 3.5-5 days

(Continued)

Digoxin *(Continued)*

Elimination: 50% to 70% excreted unchanged in urine
Dialysis: Nondialyzable (0% to 5%)

Usual Dosage Dosage must be individualized due to substantial individual variation; table lists dose based on average patient response.

Dosage Recommendations for Digoxin*

Age	Total Digitalizing Dose† (mcg/kg)		Daily Maintenance Dose‡ (mcg/kg)	
	P.O.	I.V. or I.M.	P.O.	I.V. or I.M.
Neonates				
Preterm	20-30	15-25	5-7.5	4-6
Full-term	25-35	20-30	6-10	5-8
Infants and Children				
1 mo - 2 y	35-60	30-50	10-15	7.5-12
2-5 y	30-40	25-35	7.5-10	6-9
5-10 y	20-35	15-30	5-10	4-8
>10 y	10-15	8-12	2.5-5	2-3
Adults	0.75-1.5 mg	0.5-1 mg	0.125-0.5 mg	0.1-0.4 mg

*Based on lean body weight and normal renal function for age. Decrease maintenance dose in patients with decreased renal function and decrease total digitalizing dose by 50% in end-stage renal disease.

†Give one-half of the total digitalizing dose (TDD) in the initial dose, then give one-quarter of the TDD in each of two subsequent doses at 6- to 12-hour intervals. Obtain EKG 6 hours after each dose to assess potential toxicity.

‡Divided every 12 hours in infants and children <10 years of age. Given once daily to children >10 years of age and adults.

Dosing adjustment in renal impairment: (Monitor patient closely):
Total digitalizing dose: Reduce by 50% in end stage renal disease
Maintenance dose:
Cl_{cr} 10-50 mL/minute: Administer 25% to 75% of normal daily dose (divided and given at normal intervals) or administer normal dose every 36 hours
Cl_{cr} <10 mL/minute: Administer 10% to 25% of normal daily dose (divided and given at normal intervals) or give normal dose every 48 hours

Administration

Oral: Administer consistently with relationship to meals; avoid concurrent administration (ie, administer digoxin 1 hour before or 2 hours after) with meals high in fiber or pectin and with drugs that decrease oral absorption of digoxin
Parenteral: Administer I.V. doses (undiluted or diluted at least fourfold) slowly over 5-10 minutes; I.M. route not usually recommended due to local irritation, pain, and tissue damage

Monitoring Parameters Heart rate and rhythm, periodic EKG; follow serum potassium, magnesium, and calcium closely (especially in patients receiving diuretics or amphotericin); decreased serum potassium and magnesium, or increased serum magnesium and calcium may increase digoxin toxicity; assess renal function (serum BUN, S_{cr}) in order to adjust dose; obtain serum drug concentrations at least 8-12 hours after a dose, preferably prior to next scheduled dose

Reference Range Therapeutic: 0.8-2 ng/mL (SI: 1.0-2.6 nmol/L); Adults: <0.5 ng/mL (SI: <0.6 nmol/L) probably indicates underdigitalization unless there are special circumstances. Toxicity usually associated with levels >2 ng/mL (SI: >2.6 nmol/L). **Note:** Serum concentration must be used in conjunction with clinical symptoms and EKG to confirm diagnosis of digoxin intoxication.

Test Interactions Spironolactone may interfere with radioimmunoassay

Patient Information Notify physician if decreased appetite, nausea, vomiting, diarrhea, or visual changes occur

Additional Information Digoxin-like immunoreactive substance (DLIS) may cross-react with digoxin immunoassay and falsely increase serum concentrations; DLIS has been found in patients with renal dysfunction, liver disease, CHF, neonates, and pregnant women (third trimester)

Dosage Forms

Capsule (Lanoxicaps®): 50 mcg, 100 mcg, 200 mcg
Elixir, pediatric (Lanoxin®): 50 mcg/mL with alcohol 10% [lime flavor] (2.5 mL, 5 mL, 60 mL)
Injection (Lanoxin®): 250 mcg/mL (1 mL, 2 mL)
Injection, pediatric (Lanoxin®): 100 mcg/mL (1 mL)

Tablet:
Digitek®: 125 mcg, 250 mcg
Lanoxin®: 125 mcg, 250 mcg, 500 mcg

References

Bakir M and Bilgic A, "Single Daily Dose of Digoxin for Maintenance Therapy of Infants and Children With Cardiac Disease: Is It Reliable?" *Pediatr Cardiol*, 1994, 15(5):229-32.

Bendayan R and McKenzie MW, "Digoxin Pharmacokinetics and Dosage Requirements in Pediatric Patients," *Clin Pharm*, 1983, 2(3):224-35.

Park MK, "Use of Digoxin in Infants and Children With Specific Emphasis on Dosage," *J Pediatr*, 1986, 108(6):871-7.

Digoxin Immune Fab (di JOKS in i MYUN fab)

U.S. Brand Names Digibind®

Synonyms Antidigoxin Fab Fragments

Therapeutic Category Antidote, Digoxin

Generic Available No

Use Treatment of potentially life-threatening digoxin or digitoxin intoxication in carefully selected patients; use in life-threatening ventricular arrhythmias secondary to digoxin, acute digoxin ingestion (ie, >10 mg in adults or >4 mg in children), hyperkalemia (serum potassium >5 mEq/L) in the setting of digoxin toxicity

Pregnancy Risk Factor C

Contraindications Hypersensitivity to ovine (sheep) proteins; renal or cardiac failure

Warnings Hypokalemia has been reported to occur following reversal of digitalis intoxication; monitor serum potassium levels closely; Fab fragments may be eliminated more slowly in patients with renal failure; heart failure may be exacerbated as digoxin level is reduced; total serum digoxin concentration may rise precipitously following administration of Digibind®, but this will be almost entirely bound to the Fab fragment and not able to react with receptors in the body; Digibind® will interfere with digitalis immunoassay measurements - this will result in clinically misleading serum digoxin concentrations until the Fab fragment is eliminated from the body (several days to >1 week after Digibind® administration); serum digoxin levels drawn prior to therapy may be difficult to evaluate if 6-8 hours have not elapsed after the last dose of digoxin (time to equilibration between serum and tissue); redigitalization should not be initiated until Fab fragments have been eliminated from the body, which may occur over several days or greater than a week in patients with impaired renal function

Precautions Use with caution in renal or cardiac failure; allergic reactions possible; epinephrine should be immediately available; patients may deteriorate due to withdrawal of digoxin and may require I.V. inotropic support (eg, dobutamine) or vasodilators

Adverse Reactions
Cardiovascular: Worsening of low cardiac output or CHF, rapid ventricular response in patients with atrial fibrillation as digoxin is withdrawn
Dermatologic: Urticarial rash
Endocrine & metabolic: Hypokalemia
Miscellaneous: Facial edema and redness, allergic reactions

Stability Reconstituted solutions are stable 4 hours at 2°C to 8°C

Mechanism of Action Binds with molecules of free (unbound) digoxin or digitoxin and then is removed from the body by renal excretion

Pharmacodynamics Onset of action: Improvement in signs and symptoms occurs within 2-30 minutes following I.V. infusion

Pharmacokinetics
Half-life: 15-20 hours, prolonged in patients with renal impairment
Elimination: Renal with levels declining to undetectable amounts within 5-7 days

Usual Dosage To determine the dose of digoxin immune Fab, first determine the total body load of digoxin (TBL) or digitoxin (depending upon which product was ingested) as follows (using either an approximation of the amount ingested or a postdistribution serum digoxin/digitoxin concentration (C)):

TBL of **digoxin** (in mg) = C (in ng/mL) x 5.6 x body weight (in kg)/1000
or
TBL = mg of **digoxin** ingested (as tablets or elixir) x 0.8

TBL of **digitoxin** (mg) = C (in ng/mL) x 0.56 x body weight (in kg)/1000
or
TBL of **digitoxin** (in mg) = mg digitoxin ingested
Dose of digoxin immune Fab **(in mg)** I.V. = TBL x 76
Dose of digoxin immune Fab **(# vials)** I.V. = TBL/0.5
See tables on next page.
(Continued)

Digoxin Immune Fab *(Continued)*

Infants and Children Dose Estimates of Digibind® (in mg) From Serum Digoxin Concentration

Patient Weight (kg)	Serum Digoxin Concentration (ng/mL)						
	1	2	4	8	12	16	20
1	0.4 mg*	1 mg*	1.5 mg*	3 mg	5 mg	6 mg	8 mg
3	1 mg*	2 mg*	5 mg	9 mg	14 mg	18 mg	23 mg
5	2 mg*	4 mg	8 mg	15 mg	23 mg	30 mg	38 mg
10	4 mg	8 mg	15 mg	30 mg	46 mg	61 mg	76 mg
20	8 mg	15 mg	30 mg	61 mg	91 mg	122 mg	152 mg

*Dilution of reconstituted vial to 1 mg/mL may be desirable.

Adult Dose Estimate of Digibind® (in # of Vials) From Serum Digoxin Concentration

Patient Weight (kg)	Serum Digoxin Concentration (ng/mL)						
	1	2	4	8	12	16	20
40	0.5 v*	1 v	2 v	3 v	5 v	7 v	8 v
60	0.5 v	1 v	3 v	5 v	7 v	10 v	12 v
70	1 v	2 v	3 v	6 v	9 v	11 v	14 v
80	1 v	2 v	3 v	7 v	10 v	13 v	16 v
100	1 v	2 v	4 v	8 v	12 v	16 v	20 v

* v = vials

Administration Parenteral: I.V.: Digoxin immune Fab is reconstituted by adding 4 mL sterile water, resulting in a 9.5 mg/mL concentration for I.V. infusion; the reconstituted solution may be further diluted with NS to a convenient volume (eg, 1 mg/mL); infuse over 15-30 minutes; to remove protein aggregates, 0.22 micron in-line filter is needed

Monitoring Parameters Serum potassium; serum digoxin/digitoxin level prior to first dose of digoxin immune Fab; (digoxin levels will greatly increase with Digibind® use and are not an accurate determination of body stores); continuous EKG monitoring

Additional Information Each 38 mg vial will bind approximately 0.5 mg digoxin or digitoxin; for individuals at increased risk of sensitivity (see Contraindications) an intradermal or scratch technique skin test using a 1:100 dilution of reconstituted digoxin immune Fab diluted in NS has been used. Skin test volume is 0.1 mL of 1:100 dilution; evaluate after 20 minutes.

Dosage Forms Powder for injection, lyophilized: 38 mg

References

Hickey AR, Wenger TL, Carpenter VP, et al, "Digoxin Immune Fab Therapy in the Management of Digitalis Intoxication: Safety and Efficacy Results of an Observational Surveillance Study," *J Am Coll Cardiol,* 1991, 17(3):590-8.

Dihydroergotamine *(dye hye droe er GOT a meen)*

U.S. Brand Names D.H.E. 45® Injection; Migranal® Nasal Spray

Synonyms DHE

Therapeutic Category Alpha-Adrenergc Blocking Agent, Intranasal; Alpha-Adrenergic Blocking Agent, Parenteral; Antimigraine Agent; Ergot Alkaloid and Derivative

Generic Available Yes

Use Treatment of migraine headache with or without aura; injection also indicated for treatment of cluster headaches

Pregnancy Risk Factor X

Contraindications Hypersensitivity to dihydroergotamine, other ergot alkaloid, or any component; pregnancy; patients with uncontrolled hypertension, ischemic heart disease, angina pectoris, history of MI, silent ischemia, or coronary artery vasospasm including Prinzmetal's angina; patients with hemiplegic or basilar migraine; patients with peripheral vascular disease, sepsis, severe hepatic or renal dysfunction, and following vascular surgery; **do not** coadminister with ritonavir, nelfinavir, and amprenavir; do not use within 24 hours of sumatriptan, zolmitriptan, other serotonin agonists, or ergot-like agents; do not use during or within 2 weeks of discontinuing MAO inhibitors

Warnings May cause vasospastic reactions; persistent vasospasm may lead to gangrene or death in patients with compromised circulation; discontinue if signs of vasoconstriction develop; rare reports of increased blood pressure in patients without history of hypertension; rare reports of adverse cardiac events (acute MI, life-threatening arrhythmias, death) have been reported following use of the injection; cerebral hemorrhage, subarachnoid hemorrhage, and stroke have also occurred following use of the injection

Precautions Not for prolonged use; use with caution and only after a satisfactory cardiovascular evaluation has been performed in patients with risk factors for CAD; it is also recommended in these patients that the healthcare provider should administer the first dose; cardiovascular status should be periodically evaluated

Adverse Reactions

Cardiovascular: Cerebral hemorrhage, coronary artery vasospasm, edema, flushing, hypertension, myocardial infarction, myocardial ischemia, palpitations, subarachnoid hemorrhage, transient ventricular tachycardia, ventricular fibrillation, tachycardia, bradycardia

Central nervous system: Dizziness, somnolence, anxiety, headache, stroke

Dermatologic: Rash, pruritus

Endocrine & metabolic: Hot flashes

Gastrointestinal: Nausea, taste disturbance, vomiting, diarrhea, abdominal pain, cramps, diarrhea, dry mouth

Local: Application site reaction

Neuromuscular & skeletal: Asthenia, stiffness, hyperkinesis, muscular weakness, myalgia, paresthesia, tremor

Respiratory:

Nasal spray: Pharyngitis, rhinitis, nasal congestion, rhinorrhea, sneezing, nasal edema

Injection: Pleural fibrosis

Miscellaneous: Retroperitoneal fibrosis (injection), increased sweating

Drug Interactions CYP3A inhibitor

May increase serum levels of cyclosporine and tacrolimus; increased serum levels of dihydroergotamine with macrolide antibiotics (eg, erythromycin, clarithromycin, and troleandomycin), ritonavir, amprenavir, and nelfinavir; MAO inhibitors; propranolol may potentiate the vasoconstrictive action of ergotamine; nicotine may increase ischemic response by provoking vasoconstriction; nitroglycerin may increase bioavailability of dihydroergotamine; dihydroergotamine decreases antianginal effects of nitrate; sumatriptan and other serotonin 5-HT$_1$ receptor agonists may prolong vasospastic reactions (see Contraindications); concomitant use with peripheral vasoconstrictors may cause synergistic elevation of blood pressure; use with a selective serotonin reuptake inhibitor (SSRI) (eg, dexfenfluramine, fluoxetine, paroxetine), may result in a condition known as serotonin syndrome (confusion, mental status change, diaphoresis, tremor, myoclonus, shivering, hyper-reflexia, weakness, incoordination, hypertension)

Stability Store below 25°C (77°F); do not refrigerate or freeze; protect from heat and light; once the nasal spray applicator has been prepared, use within 8 hours; discard any unused solution

Mechanism of Action Ergot alkaloid alpha-adrenergic blocker which aborts vascular headaches by direct vasoconstriction of vascular smooth muscle, particularly of the carotid artery bed but also peripheral and cerebral vessels, which reduces the amplitude of pulsation in the cranial arteries; it also has partial agonist or antagonist activity against tryptaminergic and dopaminergic receptors; it is less active than ergotamine

Pharmacodynamics

Onset of action:

I.M.: 15-30 minutes

Intranasal: 30 minutes

I.V.: Immediate

Duration: I.M.: 3-4 hours

Pharmacokinetics

Distribution: V$_d$: 14.5 L/kg (~800 L)

Bioavailability: Intranasal: 32%

Protein binding: 93%

Metabolism: Extensively in the liver; one active metabolite

Half-life: Distribution phase: 0.9-2.1 hours; terminal elimination phase: 7-32 hours

Time to peak serum concentration: I.M.: Within 15-30 minutes; intranasal: 0.5-1 hour; I.V.: 15 minutes; S.C.: 15-45 minutes

Elimination: Predominately into bile and feces and 10% excreted in urine, mostly as metabolites

Usual Dosage Adolescents and Adults: Treatment should be initiated at the first symptom or sign of an attack; nasal spray may be used at any stage of a migraine attack

(Continued)

Dihydroergotamine *(Continued)*

I.M., S.C.: 1 mg at first sign of headache; repeat hourly to a maximum total dose of 3 mg/day; do not exceed 6 mg/week

I.V.: 1 mg at first sign of headache; repeat hourly up to a maximum total dose of 2 mg/day; do not exceed 6 mg/week

Intranasal: 1 spray (0.5 mg) of nasal spray into each nostril (total: 1 mg); repeat if needed within 15 minutes; maximum: 4 sprays (2 mg/day); do not exceed 8 sprays (4 mg)/week

Dosing adjustment in renal impairment: Contraindicated in severe renal impairment

Dosing adjustment in hepatic impairment: Dosage reductions are probably necessary but specific guidelines are not available; contraindicated in severe hepatic dysfunction

Administration

Intranasal (For complete directions, see patient instruction booklet): Prior to administration, the nasal spray applicator must be primed (pumped 4 times); spray once into each nostril; avoid deep inhalation through the nose while spraying or immediately after spraying; do not tilt head back

I.M., S.C.: Administer without dilution

I.V.: Administer without dilution slowly over 2-3 minutes

Patient Information Take this drug as rapidly as possible when first symptoms occur; may cause drowsiness and impair ability to perform hazardous activities which require mental alertness or physical coordination; report heart palpitations, severe nausea or vomiting, or severe numbness of fingers or toes; do not assemble nasal spray until needed for use

Additional Information Nasal spray contains caffeine.

Dosage Forms

Injection, as mesylate: 1 mg/mL (1 mL)

Spray, nasal, as mesylate: 4 mg/mL [0.5 mg/spray] (1 mL)

Dihydrotachysterol (dye hye droe tak IS ter ole)

U.S. Brand Names DHT™; Hytakerol®

Synonyms Dichysterol

Therapeutic Category Nutritional Supplement; Vitamin D Analog; Vitamin, Fat Soluble

Generic Available Yes

Use Treatment of hypocalcemia associated with hypoparathyroidism; prophylaxis of hypocalcemic tetany following thyroid surgery; suppression of hyperparathyroidism and treatment of renal osteodystrophy in patients with chronic renal failure

Pregnancy Risk Factor C

Contraindications Hypercalcemia; hypersensitivity to dihydrotachysterol or any component

Warnings Use cautiously in patients with renal stones, renal failure, and heart disease; calcium phosphate may precipitate if the product of serum calcium multiplied by phosphate (Ca x P) >70; adequate dietary calcium is necessary for a clinical response to therapy

Adverse Reactions Related to accompanying hypercalcemia

Central nervous system: Convulsions

Endocrine & metabolic: Hypercalcemia, metastatic calcification, polydipsia

Gastrointestinal: Nausea, vomiting, anorexia, weight loss

Hematologic: Anemia

Neuromuscular & skeletal: Weakness

Renal: Renal damage, polyuria

Drug Interactions Cholestyramine may reduce absorption; clofibrate, thiazides, phenobarbital, and phenytoin decrease the half-life of dihydrotachysterol; potential dihydrotachysterol-induced hypercalcemia may precipitate arrhythmias with cardiac glycosides

Mechanism of Action A synthetic reduction product of tachysterol, a close isomer of vitamin D; stimulates calcium and phosphate absorption from the small intestine, promotes secretion of calcium from bone to blood

Pharmacodynamics

Maximum hypercalcemic effects: Within 2 weeks

Duration: As long as 9 weeks

Pharmacokinetics

Absorption: Well absorbed from the GI tract

Metabolism: Hydroxylated in liver to 25-hydroxy-dihydrotachysterol

Usual Dosage Oral:
Hypoparathyroidism:
Neonates: 0.05-0.1 mg/day
Infants and young Children: Initial: 1-5 mg/day for 4 days, then 0.5-1.5 mg/day
Older Children and Adults: Initial: 0.75-2.5 mg/day for 4 days, then 0.2-1 mg/day; maximum dose: 1.5 mg/day
Nutritional rickets: 0.5 mg as a single dose or 13-50 mcg/day until healing occurs
Renal osteodystrophy:
Children and Adolescents: 0.1-0.5 mg/day
Adults: 0.1-0.6 mg/day
Administration Oral: May administer without regard to meals
Monitoring Parameters Serum calcium and phosphate, renal function, alkaline phosphatase, 24-hour urinary calcium
Additional Information 1 mg is approximately equivalent to 120,000 international units vitamin D_2
Dosage Forms
Capsule (Hytakerol®): 0.125 mg
Solution, oral concentrate (DHT™): 0.2 mg/mL (30 mL)
Tablet (DHT™): 0.125 mg, 0.2 mg, 0.4 mg

♦ **1,25 dihydroxycholecalciferol** *see* Calcitriol *on page 166*
♦ **Diiodohydroxyquin** *see* Iodoquinol *on page 546*
♦ **Dilacor® XR** *see* Diltiazem *on page 337*
♦ **Dilantin®** *see* Phenytoin *on page 791*
♦ **Dilaudid®** *see* Hydromorphone *on page 510*
♦ **Dilaudid® Cough Syrup** *see* Hydromorphone *on page 510*
♦ **Dilaudid-HP®** *see* Hydromorphone *on page 510*

Diltiazem (dil TYE a zem)

Related Information
Adult ACLS Algorithm, Narrow-Complex Supraventricular Tachycardia *on page 1046*
U.S. Brand Names Cardizem®; Cardizem® CD; Cardizem® SR; Cartia XT™; Dilacor® XR; Tiazac®
Canadian Brand Names Alti-Diltiazem; Apo-Diltiaz; Gen-Diltiazem; Novo-Diltiazem; Nu-Diltiaz
Therapeutic Category Antianginal Agent; Antihypertensive Agent; Calcium Channel Blocker
Generic Available Yes
Use
Oral: Hypertension; chronic stable angina or angina from coronary artery spasm
Injection: Atrial fibrillation or atrial flutter; paroxysmal supraventricular tachycardias (PSVT)
Pregnancy Risk Factor C
Contraindications Hypersensitivity to diltiazem or any component; severe hypotension; second or third degree heart block; sick-sinus syndrome; acute MI with pulmonary congestion
Warnings May cause bradycardia, second or third degree heart block, hypotension, hepatic injury; may worsen CHF; use with certain medications may result in additive effects on cardiac condition (see Drug Interactions)
Precautions Use with caution in patients with CHF or impaired renal or hepatic function
Adverse Reactions
Cardiovascular: Arrhythmia, bradycardia, hypotension, A-V block, tachycardia (rare), flushing, peripheral edema, CHF
Central nervous system: Headache, dizziness, insomnia, nervousness
Dermatologic: Urticaria, rash; erythema multiforme, exfoliative dermatitis (rare)
Gastrointestinal: Nausea, vomiting, constipation, dyspepsia, dysgeusia
Hematologic: Leukopenia (rare), thrombocytopenia (rare)
Hepatic: Mild to marked elevations in liver enzyme tests (rare)
Neuromuscular & skeletal: Gait abnormality, tremor, paresthesia, weakness
Drug Interactions Cytochrome P-450 isoenzyme CYP3A3/4 substrate; isoenzyme CYP1A2, CYP2D6, and CYP3A3/4 inhibitor
Cimetidine may increase diltiazem serum concentration; digoxin, beta-adrenergic blocking agents may increase risk of bradycardia or heart block; diltiazem may decrease metabolism and increase concentrations of cyclosporine, carbamazepine, digoxin, midazolam; diltiazem may increase the effect/toxicity of digitalis
(Continued)

Diltiazem *(Continued)*

glycosides, encainide, fentanyl; rifampin may decrease diltiazem serum concentrations

Food Interactions Food may increase absorption of diltiazem from sustained-release preparation; high fat meal does not effect extent of absorption of Cardizem® CD or Tiazac®; avoid natural licorice (causes sodium and water retention and increases potassium loss)

Stability Injection: Refrigerate vials; do not freeze; may store at room temperature for up to 1 month; may dilute with NS, D_5W or $D_5^1/_2NS$ for continuous infusion; not compatible with furosemide

Mechanism of Action Inhibits calcium ion from entering the "slow channels" or select voltage-sensitive areas of vascular smooth muscle and myocardium during depolarization; produces a relaxation of coronary vascular smooth muscle and coronary vasodilation; increases myocardial oxygen delivery in patients with vasospastic angina

Pharmacodynamics

Onset:

Oral:

Tablet: 30-60 minutes

Sustained release: 2-3 hours

Parenteral: I.V. (bolus): Within 3 minutes

Maximum effect:

Antiarrhythmic (I.V. bolus): 2-7 minutes

Antihypertensive (Oral): Within 2 weeks

Pharmacokinetics

Absorption: 80%

Distribution: V_d: 1.7 L/kg; appears in breast milk

Protein binding: 70% to 80%

Metabolism: Extensive first-pass effect; metabolized in the liver; desacetyldiltiazem is an active metabolite (25% to 50% as potent as diltiazem based on coronary vasodilation effects); desacetyldiltiazem may accumulate with plasma concentrations 10% to 20% of diltiazem levels

Bioavailability: ~40%

Half-life: 3-4.5 hours, up to 8 hours with chronic high dosing

Time to peak serum concentration:

Tablet: 2-3 hours

Cardizem® CD: 10-14 hours

Cardizem® SR: 6-11 hours

Elimination: In urine and bile mostly as metabolites; 2% to 4% excreted as unchanged drug in urine

Dialysis: Not dialyzable

Usual Dosage

Children: Minimal information available; some centers use the following:

Hypertension: Oral: Initial: 1.5-2 mg/kg/day in 3-4 divided doses; maximum dose: 3.5 mg/kg/day

Note: Doses up to 8 mg/kg/day given in 4 divided doses have been used for investigational therapy of Duchenne muscular dystrophy

Adolescents and Adults:

Oral: Hypertension:

Capsule, sustained release:

Cardizem® CD: 180-300 mg once daily; maximum: 480 mg once daily

Cardizem® SR: 60-120 mg twice daily

Dilacor® XR: 180-240 mg once daily

Tiazac®: 120-240 mg once daily; maximum: 540 mg once daily

Tablet: 30-120 mg 3-4 times/day; dosage should be increased gradually, at 1- to 2-day intervals until optimum response is obtained; usual maintenance dose: 180-360 mg/day

I.V. (antiarrhythmic): Initial: 0.25 mg/kg as a bolus over 2 minutes, if response is inadequate a second bolus dose (0.35 mg/kg) may be administered after 15 minutes; further bolus doses should be individualized

I.V. continuous infusion (start after I.V. bolus doses): 5-15 mg/hour for up to 24 hours

Conversion from I.V. diltiazem to oral diltiazem: Start first oral dose approximately 3 hours after bolus dose

Oral dose (mg/day) is approximately equal to [rate (mg/hour) x 3 + 3] x 10;

Note: Dose per day may need to be divided depending on formulation used (see Usual Dosage above)

3 mg/hour = 120 mg/day

5 mg/hour = 180 mg/day
7 mg/hour = 240 mg/day
11 mg/hour = 360 mg/day (maximum recommended dose)

Administration
Oral: May be administered with or without food, but should be administered consistently with relation to meals; administer with a full glass of water; swallow sustained release preparation (CD, SR, XR, Tiazac®) whole, do not chew, break, or crush

Tiazac® capsules (extended release) may be opened and sprinkled on applesauce; swallow applesauce immediately, do not chew; follow with some cool water (adults: 1 glass) to ensure complete swallowing; do not divide capsule contents (ie, do not administer partial doses); do not store mixture of applesauce and capsule contents, use immediately

Parenteral:
I.V. bolus: Adults: Infuse over 2 minutes
I.V. continuous: Maximum final concentration: 1 mg/mL

Monitoring Parameters Blood pressure, renal function, liver enzymes

Patient Information Do not discontinue abruptly; report any dizziness, shortness of breath, palpitations, or edema; avoid alcohol

Nursing Implications Do not crush sustained release capsules (CD, SR, XR, Tiazac®)

Dosage Forms
Capsule, sustained release, as hydrochloride:
Cardizem® CD: 120 mg, 180 mg, 240 mg, 300 mg, 360 mg
Cardizem® SR: 60 mg, 90 mg, 120 mg
Cartia XT™: 120 mg, 180 mg, 240 mg, 300 mg
Dilacor® XR: 120 mg, 180 mg, 240 mg
Tiazac®: 120 mg, 180 mg, 240 mg, 300 mg, 360 mg, 420 mg
Injection, as hydrochloride: 5 mg/mL (5 mL, 10 mL)
Cardizem®: 5 mg/mL (5 mL, 10 mL)
Tablet, as hydrochloride (Cardizem®): 30 mg, 60 mg, 90 mg, 120 mg

Extemporaneous Preparations A 12 mg/mL oral liquid preparation made from tablets (regular, not sustained release) and 3 different vehicles (cherry syrup, a 1:1 mixture of Ora-Sweet® and Ora-Plus®, or a 1:1 mixture of Ora-Sweet® SF and Ora-Plus®) was stable for 60 days when stored in amber plastic prescription bottles in the dark at room temperature (25°C) or under refrigeration (5°C); grind sixteen 90 mg tablets in a mortar into a fine powder; add 10 mL of the vehicle and mix well to form a uniform paste; mix while adding the vehicle in geometric proportions to **almost** 120 mL; transfer to a calibrated bottle and qsad with vehicle to 120 mL; label "shake well" and "protect from light"

Allen LV and Erickson MA, "Stability of Baclofen, Captopril, Diltiazem Hydrochloride, Dipyridamole, and Flecainide Acetate in Extemporaneously Compounded Oral Liquids," *Am J Health Sys Pharm*, 1996, 53(18):2179-84.

References
Bertorini TE, Palmieri GMA, Griffin JW, et al, "Effect of Chronic Treatment With the Calcium Antagonist Diltiazem in Duchenne Muscular Dystrophy," *Neurology*, 1988, 38(4):609-13.

♦ **Dimedrine (Can)** *see* Brompheniramine and Pseudoephedrine *on page 153*

Dimenhydrinate (dye men HYE dri nate)

Related Information
Overdose and Toxicology *on page 1222*

U.S. Brand Names Calm-X® [OTC]; Dramamine®; Hydrate®

Canadian Brand Names Anti-Nauseant; Apo-Dimenhydrinate; Childrens Motion Sickness Liquid; Gravol; Nauseatol; Novo-Dimenate; Travamine; Travel Aid; Traveltabs

Therapeutic Category Antiemetic; Antihistamine

Generic Available Yes

Use Treatment and prevention of nausea, vertigo, and vomiting associated with motion sickness

Pregnancy Risk Factor B

Contraindications Hypersensitivity to dimenhydrinate or any component

Warnings Parenteral product contains benzyl alcohol which has been associated with a fatal "gasping syndrome" in premature infants; chewable tablets contain the dye tartrazine which may cause allergic reactions in sensitive individuals (particularly if sensitive to aspirin)

Precautions Use with caution in patients with a history of seizure disorder; may produce excitation in the young child; use with caution in any condition which may
(Continued)

Dimenhydrinate *(Continued)*

be aggravated by anticholinergic symptoms such as prostatic hypertrophy, asthma, bladder neck obstruction, narrow-angle glaucoma, etc

Adverse Reactions
Cardiovascular: Hypotension, palpitations, tachycardia
Central nervous system: Drowsiness, headache, paradoxical CNS stimulation, dizziness
Dermatologic: Photosensitivity, urticaria, rash
Gastrointestinal: Anorexia, xerostomia, dry mucous membranes, constipation
Genitourinary: Urinary frequency, dysuria
Hematologic: Hemolytic anemia
Local: Pain at the injection site
Ocular: Blurred vision, diplopia
Otic: Tinnitus
Respiratory: Chest tightness, wheezing, thickened secretions

Drug Interactions Enhances sedative effects of other CNS depressants, may potentiate anticholinergic effects; may mask early signs and symptoms of ototoxicity in patients on aminoglycosides, furosemide, etc

Mechanism of Action Competes with histamine for H_1-receptor sites on effector cells in the GI tract, blood vessels, and respiratory tract; diminishes vestibular stimulation and depresses labyrinthine function through its central anticholinergic activity; consists of equimolar proportions of diphenhydramine and chlorotheophylline

Pharmacodynamics
Onset of action:
Oral: Within 15-30 minutes
I.M.: 20-30 minutes
I.V.: Immediate
Duration: ~3-6 hours

Pharmacokinetics
Absorption: Well absorbed from the GI tract
Metabolism: Extensive in the liver

Usual Dosage Oral, I.M., I.V.:
Children:
2-5 years: 12.5-25 mg every 6-8 hours, maximum dose: 75 mg/day
6-12 years: 25-50 mg every 6-8 hours, maximum dose: 150 mg/day
or
Alternately: 5 mg/kg/day or 150 mg/m²/day in 4 divided doses, not to exceed 300 mg/day
Children ≥12 years and Adults: 50-100 mg every 4-6 hours, not to exceed 400 mg/day

Administration
Oral: Administer with food or water
Parenteral: Dilute to a maximum concentration of 5 mg/mL in NS and infuse over 2 minutes; may be administered I.M.

Patient Information Causes drowsiness and may impair ability to perform hazardous tasks requiring mental alertness

Dosage Forms
Injection (Hydrate®): 50 mg/mL (1 mL, 10 mL)
Liquid (Dramamine®): 12.5 mg/4 mL
Tablet (Dramamine®): 50 mg
Tablet, chewable (Dramamine®): 50 mg [orange flavor, contains tartrazine]

Dimercaprol *(dye mer KAP role)*

U.S. Brand Names BAL in Oil®

Therapeutic Category Antidote, Arsenic Toxicity; Antidote, Gold Toxicity; Antidote, Lead Toxicity; Antidote, Mercury Toxicity; Chelating Agent, Parenteral

Generic Available No

Use Antidote to gold, arsenic, and mercury poisoning; adjunct to edetate calcium disodium in lead poisoning

Pregnancy Risk Factor C

Contraindications Hepatic insufficiency; patients with hypersensitivity reactions to peanuts (injection in peanut oil); do not use in iron, cadmium, or selenium poisoning; do not use iron supplements during therapy

Precautions Use with caution in patients with renal impairment or hypertension; produces hemolysis in persons with G-6-PD deficiency, especially in the presence of infection or other stressful situations; due to increased frequency of histamine-release related side effects, pretreatment with antihistamines is recommended; urine should be kept alkaline to prevent dissociation of chelate

Adverse Reactions
Cardiovascular: Hypertension, tachycardia
Central nervous system: Nervousness, seizures, fever (30% of children), headache, anxiety
Gastrointestinal: Vomiting, nausea, salivation
Hematologic: Transient neutropenia
Local: Pain at the injection site, sterile abscesses
Neuromuscular & skeletal: Paresthesia of hands
Ocular: Blepharospasm, conjunctivitis, lacrimation, burning eyes
Renal: Nephrotoxicity
Respiratory: Rhinorrhea
Miscellaneous: Burning sensation of the lips, mouth, throat, and penis

Drug Interactions Iron (chelation product toxic to kidneys)

Stability Do not mix in the same syringe with edetate calcium disodium

Mechanism of Action Sulfhydryl group combines with ions of various heavy metals (arsenic, gold, mercury, lead) to form relatively stable, nontoxic, soluble chelates which are excreted in the urine

Pharmacokinetics
Distribution: To all tissues including the brain
Metabolism: Rapid to inactive products
Time to peak serum concentration: 30-60 minutes
Elimination: In urine and feces via bile

Usual Dosage Children and Adults: I.M.:
Mild arsenic and gold poisoning: 2.5 mg/kg/dose every 6 hours for 2 days, then every 12 hours on the third day, and once daily thereafter for 10 days
Severe arsenic and gold poisoning: 3 mg/kg/dose every 4 hours for 2 days then every 6 hours on the third day, then every 12 hours thereafter for 10 days
Mercury poisoning: 5 mg/kg initially followed by 2.5 mg/kg/dose 1-2 times/day for 10 days
Lead poisoning: (use with edetate calcium disodium):
Mild: 4 mg/kg/dose for one dose then 3 mg/kg/dose every 4 hours for 2-7 days
Severe and acute encephalopathy: (**blood levels >70 mcg/dL**): 4 mg/kg/dose every 4 hours in combination with edetate calcium disodium for at least 72 hours; may use for up to 5 days; if additional days of therapy (>5 days) are indicated, a minimum of 2 days without treatment should elapse before considering another treatment course

Administration Parenteral: Administer undiluted, deep I.M.

Monitoring Parameters Specific heavy metal levels, urine pH

Dosage Forms Injection: 100 mg/mL (3 mL)

References
"Treatment Guidelines for Lead Exposure in Children. American Academy of Pediatrics Committee on Drugs," *Pediatrics*, 1995, 96(1 Pt 1):155-60.

♦ **Diotrope (Can)** *see* Tropicamide *on page 991*

♦ **Dipalmitoylphosphatidylcholine** *see* Colfosceril *on page 265*

♦ **Dipentum®** *see* Olsalazine *on page 732*

♦ **Diphen® AF [OTC]** *see* Diphenhydramine *on page 342*

♦ **Diphen® Cough [OTC]** *see* Diphenhydramine *on page 342*

♦ **Diphenhist [OTC]** *see* Diphenhydramine *on page 342*

Diphenhydramine (dye fen HYE dra meen)

Related Information
Carbohydrate and Alcohol Content of Liquid Medications for Use in Patients Receiving Ketogenic Diets *on page 1258*
Compatibility of Medications Mixed in a Syringe *on page 1238*
OTC Cough & Cold Preparations, Pediatric *on page 1072*
Overdose and Toxicology *on page 1222*

U.S. Brand Names
AllerMax® [OTC]; Banophen® [OTC]; Benadryl® [OTC]; Benadryl® Allergy [OTC]; Benadryl® Injection; Compoz® Nighttime Sleep Aid [OTC]; Diphen® AF [OTC]; Diphen® Cough [OTC]; Diphenhist [OTC]; Dormin® [OTC]; Genahist® [OTC]; Hyrexin-50® Injection; Miles Nervine® [OTC]; Nytol® [OTC]; Scot-Tussin® Allergy Relief [OTC]; Siladryl® [OTC]; Simply Allergy® [OTC]; Simply Sleep® [OTC]; Sleepinal® [OTC]; Sominex® [OTC]; Tusstat®; Unisom® Maximum Strength [OTC]

Canadian Brand Names
Aller-Aide; Allerdryl; Allergy Elixir; Allergy Formula; Allergy Tablets; Allernix; Calmex; Dormiphen; Dormox Extra Fort; Insomnal; Nytol Extra Strength; PMS-Diphenhydramine; Sleep Aid; Sleep-Eze D

Therapeutic Category
Antidote, Drug-induced Dystonic Reactions; Antidote, Hypersensitivity Reactions; Antihistamine; Sedative

Generic Available
Yes

Use
Symptomatic relief of allergic symptoms caused by histamine release which include nasal allergies and allergic dermatosis; mild nighttime sedation, prevention of motion sickness, as an antitussive; treatment of phenothiazine-induced dystonic reactions

Pregnancy Risk Factor
B

Contraindications
Hypersensitivity to diphenhydramine or any component; should not be used in acute attacks of asthma

Warnings
Topical diphenhydramine should not be used to treat chickenpox, poison ivy, or sunburn, on large areas of the body, or on blistered or oozing skin, due to potential for causing toxic psychosis, particularly in children

Precautions
Use with caution in patients with angle-closure glaucoma, peptic ulcer, urinary tract obstruction, hyperthyroidism; may cause paradoxical excitation in young children

Adverse Reactions
Cardiovascular: Hypotension, palpitations, tachycardia
Central nervous system: Sedation, dizziness, paradoxical excitement, fatigue, insomnia
Dermatologic: Photosensitivity, rash, urticaria
Gastrointestinal: Nausea, vomiting, xerostomia, dry mucous membranes, anorexia, constipation, epigastric distress
Genitourinary: Urinary retention, dysuria
Hematologic: Rare: Hemolytic anemia, aplastic anemia, thrombocytopenia
Neuromuscular & skeletal: Paresthesia of hands, tremor
Ocular: Blurred vision
Respiratory: Chest tightness, thickened bronchial secretions, wheezing

Drug Interactions
Cytochrome P-450 isoenzyme CYP2D6 substrate
Additive sedation when given with drugs which depress the CNS; may impair absorption of aminosalicylic acid

Stability
Compatible when mixed in the same syringe: atropine, chlorpromazine, cimetidine, droperidol, fentanyl, glycopyrrolate, hydromorphone, meperidine, metoclopramide, midazolam, morphine, promethazine, and ranitidine

Mechanism of Action
Competes with histamine for H_1-receptor sites on effector cells in the GI tract, blood vessels, and respiratory tract

Pharmacodynamics
Maximum sedative effect: 1-3 hours after administration
Duration of action: 4-7 hours

Pharmacokinetics
Absorption: Oral: Well absorbed but 40% to 60% of an oral dose reaches the systemic circulation due to first-pass metabolism
Protein-binding: 78%

Metabolism: Extensive in the liver

Half-life: 2-8 hours

Time to peak serum concentration: 2-4 hours

Usual Dosage

Oral, I.M., I.V.:

Treatment of phenothiazine dystonic reactions and moderate to severe allergic reactions:

Children: 5 mg/kg/day or 150 mg/m^2/day in divided doses every 6-8 hours, not to exceed 300 mg/day

Adults: 25-50 mg every 4 hours, not to exceed 400 mg/day

Minor allergic rhinitis or motion sickness:

Children 2 to <6 years: 6.25 mg every 4-6 hours; maximum: 37.5 mg/day

Children 6 to <12 years: 12.5-25 mg every 4-6 hours; maximum: 150 mg/day

Children ≥12 years and Adults: 25-50 mg every 4-6 hours; maximum: 300 mg/day

Antitussive: Oral:

Children 2 to <6 years: 6.25 mg every 4 hours; maximum 37.5 mg/day

Children 6 to <12 years: 12.5 mg every 4 hours; maximum 75 mg/day

Children ≥12 years and Adults: 25 mg every 4 hours; maximum 150 mg/day

Night-time sleep aid: 30 minutes before bedtime:

Children 2 to <12 years: 1 mg/kg/dose; maximum: 50 mg/dose

Children ≥12 years and Adults: 50 mg

Topical cream, gel, or stick:

Children ≥2 to 12 years: Apply 1% concentration not more than 3-4 times/day

Children ≥12 years and Adults: Apply 1% or 2% concentration not more than 3-4 times/day

Administration

Oral: Administer with food to avoid GI distress

Parenteral: I.V.: Dilute with compatible I.V. fluid to a maximum concentration of 25 mg/mL and infuse over 10-15 minutes (maximum rate of infusion: 25 mg/minute)

Topical: Shake well (gel); apply thin coat to affected area (see Warnings)

Test Interactions May suppress the wheal and flare reactions to skin test antigens; discontinue 4 days prior to skin testing procedures

Patient Information May cause drowsiness and impair ability to perform hazardous activities which require mental alertness or physical coordination

Dosage Forms

Capsule, as hydrochloride: 25 mg, 50 mg

Cream, as hydrochloride: 2%

Elixir, as hydrochloride: 12.5 mg/5 mL (5 mL, 10 mL, 20 mL, 60 mL, 120 mL, 180 mL, 240 mL, 480 mL, 3780 mL)

Gel, as hydrochloride: 1% (118 g); 2% (118 g)

Injection, as hydrochloride: 50 mg/mL (1 mL, 10 mL)

Solution, topical spray, as hydrochloride: 2% (60 mL)

Stick, as hydrochloride: 2% (14 mL)

Syrup, as hydrochloride: 12.5 mg/5 mL (120 mL, 480 mL, 3780 mL)

Tablet, as hydrochloride: 25 mg, 50 mg

Tablet, chewable, as hydrochloride: 12.5 mg

Diphenoxylate and Atropine (dye fen OKS i late & A troe peen)

U.S. Brand Names Lomotil®; Lonox®

Synonyms Atropine and Diphenoxylate

Therapeutic Category Antidiarrheal

Generic Available Yes

Use Treatment of diarrhea

Restrictions C-V

Pregnancy Risk Factor C

Contraindications Hypersensitivity to diphenoxylate, atropine, or any component; severe liver disease, jaundice, dehydration, and narrow-angle glaucoma; do not use in children <2 years of age

Warnings Reduction of intestinal motility may be deleterious in diarrhea resulting from *Shigella*, *Salmonella*, toxigenic strains of *E. coli* and from pseudomembranous enterocolitis associated with broad spectrum antibiotics; children (especially those with Down syndrome) may develop signs of atropinism (dry skin and mucous membranes, thirst, hyperthermia, tachycardia, urinary retention, flushing) even at the recommended dosages

Precautions Use with extreme caution in patients with dehydration, cirrhosis, hepatorenal disease, renal dysfunction, and acute ulcerative colitis

(Continued)

Diphenoxylate and Atropine *(Continued)*

Adverse Reactions

Cardiovascular: Tachycardia

Central nervous system: Sedation, dizziness, euphoria, headache, hyperthermia

Dermatologic: Pruritus, urticaria

Gastrointestinal: Nausea, vomiting, abdominal discomfort, paralytic ileus, pancreatitis, xerostomia

Genitourinary: Urinary retention

Neuromuscular & skeletal: Weakness

Ocular: Blurred vision

Respiratory: Respiratory depression (young children may be at greater risk)

Miscellaneous: Physical and psychological dependence with prolonged use

Drug Interactions
MAO inhibitors (hypertensive crisis), CNS depressants, alcohol, anticholinergic agents, naltrexone; the herbal medicine St John's wort (*Hypericum perforatum*) may increase serious side effects, its use is **not** recommended

Stability
Protect from light

Mechanism of Action
Diphenoxylate inhibits excessive GI motility and GI propulsion; commercial preparations contain a subtherapeutic amount of atropine to discourage abuse

Pharmacodynamics

Onset of action: Within 45-60 minutes

Peak effect: Within 2 hours

Duration: 3-4 hours

Tolerance to antidiarrheal effects may occur with prolonged use

Pharmacokinetics

Absorption: Oral: Well absorbed

Metabolism: Extensive in the liver to diphenoxylic acid (active)

Half-life:

Diphenoxylate: 2.5 hours

Diphenoxylic acid: 12-24 hours

Time to peak serum concentration: ~2 hours

Elimination: Primarily in feces (via bile); ~14% is excreted in urine as metabolites; <1% excreted unchanged in urine

Usual Dosage
Oral (as diphenoxylate):

Children: **Liquid: Note:** Only the liquid product is recommended for children under 13 years of age; do not exceed recommended doses; reduce dose as soon as symptoms are initially controlled; maintenance doses may be as low as 25% of initial dose; if no improvement within 48 hours of therapy, diphenoxylate is not likely to be effective

Initial: 0.3-0.4 mg/kg/day in 4 divided doses **or**

Manufacturer's recommendations: Initial:

<2 years: Not recommended

2 years (11-14 kg): 1.5-3 mL 4 times/day

3 years (12-16 kg): 2-3 mL 4 times/day

4 years (14-20 kg): 2-4 mL 4 times/day

5 years (16-23 kg): 2.5-4.5 mL 4 times/day

6-8 years (17-32 kg): 2.5-5 mL 4 times/day

9-12 years (23-55 kg): 3.5-5 mL 4 times/day

13-16 years: 5 mg (either 2 tablets or 10 mL) 3 times/day

Alternative pediatric dosing: Initial:

<2 years: Not recommended

2-5 years: 2 mg 3 times/day

5-8 years: 2 mg 4 times/day

8-12 years: 2 mg 5 times/day

Adults: Initial: 15-20 mg/day in 3-4 divided doses; maintenance: 5-15 mg/day in 2-3 divided doses

Note: Do not exceed recommended doses; reduce dose once symptoms are initially controlled; acute diarrhea usually improves within 48 hours; if chronic diarrhea dose not improve within 10 days at maximum daily doses of 20 mg, diphenoxylate is not likely to be effective.

Administration
Oral: May be administered with food to decrease GI upset; **Note:** Dropper has a 2 mL (1 mg) capacity and is calibrated in increments of 1/2 mL (0.25 mg)

Monitoring Parameters
Bowel frequency, signs and symptoms of atropinism, fluid and electrolytes

Patient Information
Avoid alcohol and the herbal medicine St John's wort; may cause drowsiness or dizziness and impair ability to perform activities requiring

mental alertness or physical coordination; may cause dry mouth; may be habit forming

Additional Information Naloxone reverses toxicity due to diphenoxylate; Lomotil® solution also contains sorbitol, cherry flavoring, and yellow dye 6

Dosage Forms

Solution, oral: Diphenoxylate hydrochloride 2.5 mg and atropine sulfate 0.025 mg per 5 mL (4 mL, 10 mL, 60 mL)

Tablet: Diphenoxylate hydrochloride 2.5 mg and atropine sulfate 0.025 mg

♦ **Diphenylhydantoin** *see* Phenytoin *on page 791*

♦ **Diphtheria and Tetanus Toxoids** *see page 1172*

♦ **Diphtheria, Tetanus, and Acellular Pertussis Vaccine** *see page 1172*

♦ **Diphtheria, Tetanus Toxoids, and Whole-Cell Pertussis Vaccine** *see page 1172*

♦ **Dipivalyl Epinephrine** *see* Dipivefrin *on page 345*

Dipivefrin (dye PI ve frin)

U.S. Brand Names Propine®

Canadian Brand Names PMS-Dipivefrin

Synonyms Dipivalyl Epinephrine; DPE

Therapeutic Category Adrenergic Agonist Agent, Ophthalmic; Ophthalmic Agent, Vasoconstrictor

Generic Available Yes

Use Reduces elevated IOP in chronic open-angle glaucoma; treatment of ocular hypertension

Pregnancy Risk Factor B

Contraindications Hypersensitivity to dipivefrin, any component, sulfites (commercial preparation contains sodium metabisulfite), or epinephrine; contraindicated in patients with angle-closure glaucoma

Precautions Use with caution in patients with vascular hypertension or cardiac disorders and in aphakic patients (dipivefrin may cause cystoid macular edema in aphakic patients)

Adverse Reactions

Central nervous system: Headache

Local: Burning, stinging

Ocular: Ocular congestion, photophobia, mydriasis, blurred vision, ocular pain, bulbar conjunctival follicles, blepharoconjunctivitis, cystoid macular edema

Drug Interactions Effects of lowering IOP may be additive when used with topical miotics, timolol, betaxolol, or carbonic anhydrase inhibitors

Stability Protect from light and avoid exposure to air; discolored or darkened solutions indicate loss of potency

Mechanism of Action Dipivefrin is a prodrug of epinephrine which is the active agent that stimulates alpha- and/or beta-adrenergic receptors increasing aqueous humor outflow

Pharmacodynamics

Onset of action:

Ocular pressure effects: Within 30 minutes

Mydriasis: Within 30 minutes

Peak effect: Ocular pressure effects: Within 1 hour

Duration:

Ocular pressure effects: 12 hours or longer

Mydriasis: Several hours

Pharmacokinetics Absorption: Rapid into the aqueous humor; converted to epinephrine

Usual Dosage Children and Adults: Ophthalmic: Initial: Instill 1 drop every 12 hours

Administration Ophthalmic: Instill drop into eye; apply finger pressure to lacrimal sac during and for 1-2 minutes after instillation to decrease risk of absorption and systemic effects; avoid contacting bottle tip with skin or eye

Monitoring Parameters IOP

Patient Information Discolored solutions should be discarded; may cause burning or stinging, blurred vision, and sensitivity to light

Additional Information Contains sodium metabisulfite

Dosage Forms Solution, ophthalmic, as hydrochloride: 0.1% (5 mL, 10 mL, 15 mL)

♦ **Diprivan®** *see* Propofol *on page 842*

♦ **Diprolene®** *see* Betamethasone *on page 140*

♦ **Diprolene® AF** *see* Betamethasone *on page 140*

♦ **Diprolene Glycol (Can)** *see* Betamethasone *on page 140*

♦ **Dipropylacetic Acid** see Valproic Acid and Derivatives on page 998

♦ **Diprosone**® see Betamethasone on page 140

Dipyridamole (dye peer ID a mole)

U.S. Brand Names Persantine®

Canadian Brand Names Apo-Dipyridamole FC; Apo-Dipyridamole SC; Novo-Dipiradol

Therapeutic Category Antiplatelet Agent; Vasodilator, Coronary

Generic Available Yes

Use Maintain patency after surgical grafting procedures including coronary artery bypass; with warfarin to decrease thrombosis in patients after artificial heart valve replacement; for chronic management of angina pectoris; with aspirin to prevent coronary artery thrombosis; in combination with aspirin or warfarin to prevent other thromboembolic disorders; dipyridamole may also be given 2 days prior to open heart surgery to prevent platelet activation by extracorporeal bypass pump; diagnostic agent I.V. (dipyridamole stress test) for coronary artery disease

Pregnancy Risk Factor B

Contraindications Hypersensitivity to dipyridamole or any component

Precautions May further decrease blood pressure in patients with hypotension due to peripheral vasodilation

Adverse Reactions

Cardiovascular: Vasodilatation, flushing, syncope

Central nervous system: Dizziness, headache (dose-related)

Dermatologic: Rash, pruritus

Gastrointestinal: Abdominal distress, nausea, vomiting, diarrhea

Neuromuscular & skeletal: Weakness

Drug Interactions Heparin, warfarin, streptokinase, urokinase, alteplase, aspirin, NSAIDs, cefamandole, cefoperazone, cefotetan, and valproic acid may increase risk of bleeding; decreased coronary artery vasodilation from I.V. dipyridamole may occur in patients receiving theophylline or caffeine

Stability Do not freeze; protect I.V. preparation from light

Mechanism of Action Inhibits the activity of adenosine deaminase and phosphodiesterase, which causes an accumulation of adenosine, adenine nucleotides, and cyclic AMP; these mediators then inhibit platelet aggregation and may cause vasodilation; may also stimulate release of prostacyclin or PGD_2; causes coronary vasodilation

Pharmacokinetics Oral:

Absorption: Slow and variable

Distribution: V_d: Adults: 2-3 L/kg

Protein binding: 91% to 99%

Metabolism: In the liver to glucuronide conjugate

Bioavailability: Ranges from 27% to 66%

Half-life, terminal: 10-12 hours

Time to peak serum concentration: Within 2-2.5 hours

Elimination: In feces via bile as glucuronide conjugates and unchanged drug

Usual Dosage

Children:

Oral: 3-6 mg/kg/day in 3 divided doses

Doses of 4-10 mg/kg/day have been used investigationally to treat proteinuria in pediatric renal disease

Mechanical prosthetic heart valves: 2-5 mg/kg/day [used in combination with an oral anticoagulant in children who have systemic embolism despite adequate oral anticoagulant therapy (INR 2.5-3.5), and used in combination with low-dose oral anticoagulation (INR 2-3) plus aspirin in children in whom full-dose oral anticoagulation is contraindicated]

Adults:

Oral: 75-400 mg/day in 3-4 divided doses

Dipyridamole stress test (for evaluation of myocardial perfusion): I.V.: 0.142 mg/kg/minute for a total of 4 minutes (0.57 mg/kg total); maximum dose: 60 mg; inject thallium 201 within 5 minutes after end of injection of dipyridamole

Platelet aggregation inhibitor: I.V. infusion: 250 mg/day at a rate of 10 mg/hour; maximum dose: 400 mg/day (use lower doses with aspirin)

Administration

Oral: Administer with water on an empty stomach 1 hour before or 2 hours after meals; may take with milk or food to decrease GI upset

Parenteral: I.V.: Dilute in at least a 1:2 ratio with NS, $^1/_2$NS, or D_5W; infusion of undiluted dipyridamole may cause local irritation; see Usual Dosage for infusion rates

Monitoring Parameters Blood pressure, heart rate

Test Interactions Patients on theophylline may show false-negative thallium scan result

Patient Information Notify physician or pharmacist if taking other medications that affect bleeding, such as warfarin or NSAIDs; avoid alcohol

Dosage Forms

Injection: 5 mg/mL (2 mL, 10 mL)

Tablet: 25 mg, 50 mg, 75 mg

Extemporaneous Preparations A 10 mg/mL oral liquid preparation made from tablets and 3 different vehicles (cherry syrup, a 1:1 mixture of Ora-Sweet® and Ora-Plus®, or a 1:1 mixture of Ora-Sweet® SF and Ora-Plus®) was stable for 60 days when stored in amber plastic prescription bottles in the dark, at room temperature (25°C) or under refrigeration (5°C); grind twenty-four 50 mg tablets in a mortar into a fine powder; add 20 mL of the vehicle and mix well to form a uniform paste; mix while adding the vehicle in geometric proportions to **almost** 120 mL; transfer to a calibrated bottle and qsad with vehicle to 120 mL; label "shake well" and "protect from light"

Allen LV and Erickson MA, "Stability of Baclofen, Captopril, Diltiazem Hydrochloride, Dipyridamole, and Flecainide Acetate in Extemporaneously Compounded Oral Liquids," *Am J Health Sys Pharm*, 1996, 53(18):2179-84.

References

Monagle P, Michelson AD, Bovill E, et al, "Antithrombotic Therapy in Children," *Chest*, 2001, 119(1 Suppl):344S-370S.

Rao PS, Solymar L, Mardini MK, et al, "Anticoagulant Therapy in Children With Prosthetic Valves," *Ann Thorac Surg*, 1989, 47(4):589-92.

Ueda N, Kawaguchi S, Niinomi Y, et al, "Effect of Dipyridamole Treatment on Proteinuria in Pediatric Renal Disease," *Nephron*, 1986, 44(3):174-9.

♦ **Disanthrol**® **[OTC]** *see* Docusate and Casanthranol *on page 351*

♦ **Disodium Cromoglycate** *see* Cromolyn *on page 273*

♦ **Disodium Thiosulfate Pentahydrate** *see* Sodium Thiosulfate *on page 909*

♦ **d-Isoephedrine** *see* Pseudoephedrine *on page 852*

♦ **Disonate**® **[OTC]** *see* Docusate *on page 350*

Disopyramide (dye soe PEER a mide)

U.S. Brand Names Norpace®; Norpace® CR

Canadian Brand Names Rythmodan

Therapeutic Category Antiarrhythmic Agent, Class I-A

Generic Available Yes

Use Suppression and prevention of unifocal and multifocal ventricular premature complexes, coupled ventricular premature complexes, and/or paroxysmal ventricular tachycardia; also effective in the conversion and prevention of recurrence of atrial fibrillation, atrial flutter, and paroxysmal atrial tachycardia

Pregnancy Risk Factor C

Contraindications Pre-existing second or third degree A-V block; congenital QT prolongation; cardiogenic shock; hypersensitivity to disopyramide or any component

Precautions Pre-existing urinary retention, existing or family history of angle-closure glaucoma, myasthenia gravis, hypotension during initiation of therapy, CHF unless caused by an arrhythmia, widening of QRS complex during therapy or lengthening of QT interval (>25% to 50% of baseline QRS complex or Q-T interval), sick sinus syndrome, Wolf Parkinson White syndrome (WPW) or bundle-branch block; may increase ventricular rate in patients with atrial flutter who have not received digoxin; use with caution and decrease dose in patients with renal and hepatic impairment; not recommended for use 48 hours before or 24 hours after verapamil; do not administer with clarithromycin or erythromycin (see Drug Interactions)

Adverse Reactions

Cardiovascular: CHF, edema, chest pain, syncope and hypotension, conduction disturbances including A-V block, widening QRS complex and lengthening of QT interval

Central nervous system: Fatigue, headache, malaise, nervousness, acute psychosis, depression, dizziness

Dermatologic: Generalized rashes

Endocrine & metabolic: Hypoglycemia, increased cholesterol and triglycerides; may initiate contractions of pregnant uterus; hyperkalemia may enhance toxicities

Gastrointestinal: Xerostomia, dry throat, constipation, nausea, vomiting, diarrhea, pain, gas, anorexia, weight gain

Genitourinary: Urinary retention/hesitancy

Hepatic: Elevated liver enzymes, hepatic cholestasis

Neuromuscular & skeletal: Weakness

(Continued)

Disopyramide *(Continued)*

Ocular: Blurred vision, dry eyes

Respiratory: Dyspnea (<1%), dry nasal membranes

Drug Interactions Cytochrome P-450 isoenzyme CYP3A4 substrate

Hepatic microsomal enzyme inducing agents (ie, phenytoin, phenobarbital, rifampin) may increase metabolism of disopyramide and lower serum concentrations; clarithromycin and erythromycin may increase disopyramide serum concentrations which can be life-threatening; other antiarrhythmic agents (quinidine, procainamide, lidocaine, propranolol) may increase adverse conduction effects (widening QRS complex, lengthening QT interval); verapamil (disopyramide is not recommended for use 48 hours before or 24 hours after verapamil)

Mechanism of Action Class IA antiarrhythmic: Decreases myocardial excitability and conduction velocity; reduces disparity in refractory period between normal and infarcted myocardium; possesses anticholinergic, peripheral vasoconstrictive and negative inotropic effects

Pharmacodynamics

Capsules, regular:

Onset of action: 30-210 minutes

Duration: 1.5-8.5 hours

Pharmacokinetics

Protein binding: Concentration dependent, stereoselective, and ranges from 20% to 60%

Distribution: V_d: Children: 1 L/kg

Metabolism: In the liver; major metabolite has anticholinergic and antiarrhythmic effects

Bioavailability: 60% to 83%

Half-life:

Children: 3.15 hours

Adults: 4-10 hours (mean: 6.7 hours), increased half-life with hepatic or renal disease

Elimination: 40% to 60% excreted unchanged in urine and 10% to 15% in feces

Clearance is greater and half-life shorter in children vs adults; clearance (children): 3.76 mL/minute/kg

Usual Dosage Oral:

Children (start with lower dose listed):

<1 year: 10-30 mg/kg/day in 4 divided doses

1-4 years: 10-20 mg/kg/day in 4 divided doses

4-12 years: 10-15 mg/kg/day in 4 divided doses

12-18 years: 6-15 mg/kg/day in 4 divided doses

Adults: **Note:** Some patients may require initial loading dose; see product information for details

<50 kg: 100 mg every 6 hours **or** 200 mg every 12 hours (controlled release)

>50 kg: 150 mg every 6 hours **or** 300 mg every 12 hours (controlled release); if no response, may increase to 200 mg every 6 hours; maximum dose required for patients with severe refractory ventricular tachycardia is 400 mg every 6 hours. **Note:** Use lower doses (100 mg of nonsustained release every 6-8 hours) in adults with cardiomyopathy or cardiac decompensation.

Adult dosing adjustment in renal impairment: 100 mg (nonsustained release) given at the following intervals: See table

Creatinine Clearance (mL/min)	Dosage Interval
30-40	Every 8 hours
15-30	Every 12 hours
<15	Every 24 hours

Administration Oral: Administer on an empty stomach; do not crush, break, or chew controlled release capsules, swallow whole

Monitoring Parameters Blood pressure, EKG, drug level; serum potassium, glucose, cholesterol, triglycerides, and liver enzymes; especially important to monitor EKG in patients with hepatic or renal disease, heart disease, or others with increased risk of adverse effects

Reference Range Therapeutic:

Atrial arrhythmias: 2.8-3.2 µg/mL (SI: 8.3-9.4 µmol/L)

Ventricular arrhythmias: 3.3-7.5 µg/mL (SI: 9.7-22 µmol/L)

Toxic: >7 µg/mL (SI: >20.7 µmol/L)

Patient Information Avoid alcohol; notify physician if urinary retention or worsening of CHF occurs; may cause dry mouth

Dosage Forms

Capsule, as phosphate (Norpace®): 100 mg, 150 mg

Capsule, sustained action, as phosphate (Norpace® CR): 100 mg, 150 mg

Extemporaneous Preparations Extemporaneous suspensions in cherry syrup (1 mg/mL and 10 mg/mL) are stable for 4 weeks in amber glass bottles stored at 5°C, 30°C, or at room temperature; shake well before use; do not use extended release capsules for this suspension

Mathur LK, Lai PK, and Shively CD, "Stability of Disopyramide Phosphate in Cherry Syrup," *J Hosp Pharm*, 1982, 39(2):309-10.

References

Chiba K, Koike K, Nakamoto M, et al, "Steady-State Pharmacokinetics and Bioavailability of Total and Unbound Disopyramide in Children With Cardiac Arrhythmias," *Ther Drug Monit*, 1992, 14(2):112-8.

Echizen H, Takahashi H, Nakamura H, et al, "Stereoselective Disposition and Metabolism of Disopyramide in Pediatric Patients," *J Pharmacol Exp Ther*, 1991, 259(3):953-60.

♦ **Ditropan®** *see* Oxybutynin *on page 744*

♦ **Ditropan® XL** *see* Oxybutynin *on page 744*

♦ **Diuril®** *see* Chlorothiazide *on page 224*

♦ **Dixarit (Can)** *see* Clonidine *on page 255*

♦ **dl-Alpha Tocopherol** *see* Vitamin E *on page 1014*

♦ **DM** *see* Dextromethorphan *on page 316*

♦ **D-Mannitol** *see* Mannitol *on page 619*

♦ **DM Cough Syrup (Can)** *see* Dextromethorphan *on page 316*

♦ **DM Cough Syrup Expectorant (Can)** *see* Guaifenesin and Dextromethorphan *on page 487*

♦ **4-DMDR** *see* Idarubicin *on page 523*

♦ **DM Plus Expectorant (Can)** *see* Guaifenesin and Dextromethorphan *on page 487*

♦ **DMSA** *see* Succimer *on page 917*

♦ **DM Sans Sucre (Can)** *see* Dextromethorphan *on page 316*

♦ **DNase** *see* Dornase Alfa *on page 355*

♦ **DNR** *see* Daunorubicin *on page 298*

♦ **Doak-Oil (Can)** *see* Coal Tar *on page 260*

Dobutamine (doe BYOO ta meen)

Related Information

Emergency Pediatric Drip Calculations *on page 1033*

Extravasation Treatment *on page 1085*

U.S. Brand Names Dobutrex®

Therapeutic Category Adrenergic Agonist Agent; Sympathomimetic

Generic Available Yes

Use Short-term management of patients with cardiac decompensation

Pregnancy Risk Factor B

Contraindications Hypersensitivity to sulfites (commercial preparation contains sodium bisulfite); patients with idiopathic hypertrophic subaortic stenosis (IHSS)

Warnings Potent drug; must be diluted prior to use. Patient's hemodynamic status should be monitored.

Precautions Hypovolemia should be corrected prior to use; infiltration causes local inflammatory changes, extravasation may cause dermal necrosis

Adverse Reactions

Cardiovascular: Ectopic heartbeats, increased heart rate, chest pain, palpitations, elevation in blood pressure; in higher doses ventricular tachycardia or arrhythmias may be seen; patients with atrial fibrillation or flutter are at risk of developing a rapid ventricular response

Central nervous system: Headache

Gastrointestinal: Nausea, vomiting

Local: Phlebitis

Neuromuscular & skeletal: Mild leg cramps, paresthesia

Respiratory: Dyspnea

Drug Interactions Beta-adrenergic blocking agents, general anesthetics

Stability Stable in various parenteral solutions for 24 hours; incompatible with alkaline solutions, do not give through same I.V. line as heparin, sodium bicarbonate, ethacrynic acid, cefazolin, or penicillin; compatible when coadministered with dopamine, nitroprusside, potassium chloride, protamine sulfate, tobramycin, epinephrine, (Continued)

Dobutamine *(Continued)*

atracurium, vecuronium, isoproterenol, and lidocaine; pink discoloration of dobutamine hydrochloride indicates slight oxidation, but no significant loss of potency if
administered within the recommended time period

Mechanism of Action Stimulates beta$_1$-adrenergic receptors, causing increased
contractility and heart rate, with little effect on beta$_2$- or alpha-receptors

Pharmacodynamics
Onset of action: I.V.: 1-10 minutes
Peak effect: Within 10-20 minutes

Pharmacokinetics
Metabolism: In tissues and the liver to inactive metabolites
Half-life: 2 minutes

Usual Dosage I.V. continuous infusion:
Neonates: 2-15 mcg/kg/minute, titrate to desired response
Children and Adults: 2.5-15 mcg/kg/minute, titrate to desired response; maximum
dose: 40 mcg/kg/minute

Administration Parenteral: Dilute in dextrose or NS; maximum recommended
concentration: 5000 mcg/mL (5 mg/mL); rate of infusion (mL/hour) = dose (mcg/kg/
minute) x weight (kg) x 60 minutes/hour divided by the concentration (mcg/mL);
administer into large vein; use infusion device to control rate of flow

Monitoring Parameters EKG, heart rate, CVP, MAP, urine output; if pulmonary
artery catheter is in place, monitor CI, PCWP, RAP, and SVR. Dobutamine lowers
central venous pressure and wedge pressure but has little effect on pulmonary
vascular resistance.

Dosage Forms Injection, as hydrochloride: 12.5 mg/mL (20 mL, 100 mL)

♦ **Dobutrex®** *see Dobutamine on page 349*

Docusate *(DOK yoo sate)*

U.S. Brand Names Colace® [OTC]; DC 240® Softgel® [OTC]; Dialose® [OTC];
Diocto® [OTC]; Diocto-K® [OTC]; Dioeze® [OTC]; Disonate® [OTC]; DOK® [OTC];
DOS® Softgel® [OTC]; D-S-S® [OTC]; Kasof® [OTC]; Modane® Soft [OTC]; Pro-Cal-
Sof® [OTC]; Regulax SS® [OTC]; Regutol® [OTC]; Sulfalax® [OTC]; Surfak® [OTC]

Canadian Brand Names Albert Docusate; Calax; Correctol Stool Softener; Ex-Lax
Stool Softener; PMS-Docusate Calcium; PMS-Docusate Sodium; Regulex; Selax;
Silace; SoFlax

Synonyms DOSS; DSS

Therapeutic Category Laxative, Surfactant; Stool Softener

Generic Available Yes

Use Stool softener in patients who should avoid straining during defecation; constipation associated with hard, dry stools; ceruminolytic

Pregnancy Risk Factor C

Contraindications Concomitant use of mineral oil; intestinal obstruction, acute
abdominal pain, nausea, vomiting; hypersensitivity to docusate or any component

Adverse Reactions
Dermatologic: Rash
Gastrointestinal: Intestinal obstruction, diarrhea, abdominal cramping
Local: Throat irritation

Drug Interactions Docusate may increase absorption of mineral oil; docusate may
increase the GI toxicity of aspirin

Mechanism of Action Reduces surface tension of the oil-water interface of the stool
resulting in enhanced incorporation of water and fat allowing for stool softening

Pharmacodynamics Onset of action: 12-72 hours

Usual Dosage
Infants and Children: Oral: 5 mg/kg/day in 1-4 divided doses **or** dose by age:
<3 years: 10-40 mg/day in 1-4 divided doses
3-6 years: 20-60 mg/day in 1-4 divided doses
6-12 years: 40-150 mg/day in 1-4 divided doses
Adolescents and Adults: Oral: 50-400 mg/day in 1-4 divided doses
Older Children and Adults: Rectal: Add 50-100 mg of docusate liquid (not syrup) to
enema fluid (NS or water)

Administration
Oral: Administer docusate liquid (not syrup) with milk, fruit juice, or infant formula to
mask the bitter taste; ensure adequate fluid intake
Rectal: Administer as a retention or flushing enema

Additional Information Docusate sodium 5-10 mg/mL **liquid** instilled in the ear as a
ceruminolytic produces substantial ear wax disintegration within 15 minutes and
complete disintegration after 24 hours

Dosage Forms

Capsule, as calcium: 240 mg

DC 240® Softgel®, Pro-Cal-Sof®, Sulfalax®: 240 mg

Surfak®: 50 mg, 240 mg

Capsule, as potassium:

Diocto-K®: 100 mg

Kasof®: 240 mg

Capsule, as sodium: 50 mg, 100 mg, 250 mg

Colace®: 50 mg, 100 mg

Dioeze®: 250 mg

Disonate®: 100 mg, 240 mg

DOK®: 100 mg, 250 mg

DOS® Softgel®: 100 mg, 250 mg

Doxinate®: 250 mg

D-S-S®: 100 mg

Modane® Soft: 100 mg

Pro-Sof®: 100 mg, 250 mg

Regulax SS®: 100 mg, 250 mg

Liquid, as sodium (Diocto®, Colace®, Disonate®, DOK®): 150 mg/15 mL (30 mL, 60 mL, 480 mL)

Solution, oral, as sodium (Doxinate®): 50 mg/mL with alcohol 5% (60 mL, 3780 mL)

Syrup, as sodium: 50 mg/15 mL (15 mL, 30 mL); 60 mg/15 mL (480 mL, 3780 mL)

Colace®, Diocto®, Disonate®, DOK®, Pro-Sof®: 60 mg/15 mL (240 mL, 480 mL, 3780 mL)

Tablet, as sodium (Dialose®, Regutol®): 100 mg

References

Chen DA and Caparosa RJ, "A Nonprescription Cerumenolytic," *Am J Otol*, 1991, 12(6):475-6.

Docusate and Casanthranol (DOK yoo sate & ka SAN thra nole)

U.S. Brand Names Dialose® Plus Capsule [OTC]; Diocto C® [OTC]; Diocto-K Plus® [OTC]; Dioctolose Plus® [OTC]; Disanthrol® [OTC]; DSMC Plus® [OTC]; D-S-S Plus® [OTC]; Genasoft® Plus [OTC]; Peri-Colace® [OTC]; Pro-Sof® Plus [OTC]; Regulace® [OTC]

Synonyms Casanthranol and Docusate; DSS With Casanthranol

Therapeutic Category Laxative, Stimulant; Laxative, Surfactant; Stool Softener

Generic Available Yes

Use Treatment of constipation generally associated with dry, hard stools and decreased intestinal motility

Pregnancy Risk Factor C

Contraindications Concomitant use of mineral oil; intestinal obstruction; acute abdominal pain; nausea, vomiting; hypersensitivity to docusate, casanthranol, or any component

Warnings Do not use when abdominal pain, nausea, or vomiting are present

Precautions Casanthranol is habit-forming; may result in laxative dependence and loss of normal bowel function with prolonged use

Adverse Reactions

Dermatologic: Rash

Gastrointestinal: Intestinal obstruction, diarrhea, abdominal cramping

Local: Throat irritation

Drug Interactions Docusate may increase absorption of mineral oil; docusate may increase the GI toxicity of aspirin

Mechanism of Action Combination stool softener (docusate) which lowers surface tension of the stool allowing water and lipids to penetrate and a stimulant laxative (casanthranol) which produces a net intestinal fluid accumulation and laxation

Pharmacodynamics Onset of action: 8-12 hours after administration but may require up to 24 hours

Usual Dosage Oral:

Children: 5-15 mL of syrup at bedtime or 1 capsule at bedtime

Adults: 1-2 capsules or 15-30 mL syrup at bedtime, may be increased to 2 capsules or 30 mL twice daily or 3 capsules at bedtime

Administration Oral: Administer with plenty of fluids

Monitoring Parameters Bowel frequency

Dosage Forms

Capsule (Dialose® Plus, Diocto-K Plus®, Dioctolose Plus®, DSMC Plus®): Docusate potassium 100 mg and casanthranol 30 mg

Capsule (Disanthrol®, D-S-S Plus®, Genasoft® Plus, Peri-Colace®, Pro-Sof® Plus, Regulace®): Docusate sodium 100 mg and casanthranol 30 mg

(Continued)

Docusate and Casanthranol *(Continued)*

Syrup (Diocto C®, Peri-Colace®): Docusate sodium 60 mg and casanthranol 30 mg per 15 mL (240 mL, 480 mL, 4000 mL)

♦ **DOK® [OTC]** *see Docusate on page 350*

Dolasetron *(dol A se tron)*

U.S. Brand Names Anzemet®

Synonyms Hydrodolasetron

Therapeutic Category Antiemetic

Generic Available No

Use Prevention of chemotherapy-induced nausea and vomiting; prevention and treatment of postoperative nausea and vomiting

Pregnancy Risk Factor B

Contraindications Hypersensitivity to dolasetron or any component

Warnings Dolasetron may cause EKG interval changes (PR, QT_c, JT prolongation and QRS widening) related in magnitude and frequency to blood levels of the active metabolite, hydrodolasetron; interval prolongation could lead to cardiovascular consequences such as heart block or cardiac arrhythmias

Precautions Use with caution in patients with, or who may develop, prolongation of cardiac conduction intervals, particularly QT_c; conditions include hypokalemia, hypomagnesemia, or congenital QT syndrome; use with caution in patients receiving antiarrhythmic or other medications known to prolong the QT interval (eg, class I or III antiarrhythmic agents) or medications known to reduce potassium or magnesium levels (eg, diuretics)

Adverse Reactions

Cardiovascular: Prolonged QT interval and other EKG changes (see Warnings), hypertension, hypotension, edema, increased sweating

Central nervous system: Headache, fatigue, dizziness, fever, chills, shivering, agitation, sleep disorder, confusion, anxiety, abnormal dreams

Dermatologic: Rash, urticaria

Gastrointestinal: Diarrhea, abdominal pain, constipation, dyspepsia, anorexia, pancreatitis (rarely), taste perversion

Genitourinary: Urinary retention, acute renal failure (rarely), polyuria (rarely), dysuria (rarely)

Hepatic: Transient elevations in liver enzymes

Local: Venous irritation

Neuromuscular & skeletal: Myalgia, arthralgia

Ocular: Photophobia (rarely), abnormal vision

Otic: Tinnitus (rarely)

Miscellaneous: Hypersensitivity reactions

Drug Interactions Cytochrome P-450 isoenzyme CYP2D6 and CYP3A3/4 substrate Increased hydrodolasetron (active metabolite) serum levels with cimetidine; decreased hydrodolasetron serum levels with rifampin; decreased clearance of hydrodolasetron with atenolol; (see Warnings and Precautions)

Stability Injection is stable after dilution in NS, D_5W, $D_5^1/_2NS$, D_5LR, LR, and 10% mannitol injection for 24 hours at room temperature and 48 hours under refrigeration

Mechanism of Action Dolasetron and its major metabolite, hydrodolasetron, are selective 5-HT_3 receptor antagonists, blocking serotonin, both peripherally on vagal nerve terminals and centrally in the chemoreceptor trigger zone

Pharmacokinetics Due to the rapid metabolism of dolasetron to hydrodolasetron (primary active metabolite), the majority of the following pharmacokinetic parameters relate to hydrodolasetron:

Distribution:

Children: 5.9-7.4 L/kg

Adults: 4.15-5.5 L/kg

Metabolism: Rapidly converted by carbonyl reductase to active major metabolite, hydrodolasetron; hydrodolasetron is metabolized by the cytochrome P-450 CYP2D6 and CYP3A enzyme systems and flavin mono-oxygenase

Bioavailability: Oral: Children: 59% (formulation not specified), adults: 70% to 80%

Half-life, elimination:

Dolasetron: <10 minutes

Hydrodolasetron:

Oral: Children: 5.7 hours, adults: 8.1 hours (range: 5-10 hours)

I.V.: Children: 4.8 hours, adults: 7.3 hours (range: 4-8 hours)

Time to peak concentration:

Oral: 1-1.5 hours

I.V.: 0.6 hours

Elimination: Dolasetron: <1% excreted unchanged in urine; hydrodolasetron: 53% to 61% excreted unchanged in urine within 36 hours

Usual Dosage
Prevention of chemotherapy-induced nausea and vomiting: **Oral:** Administered within 1 hour before chemotherapy; or **I.V.:** Administered 30 minutes before chemotherapy:
  Children ≥2 to 16 years:
    Oral, I.V.: 1.8 mg/kg as a single dose (maximum: 100 mg)
  Adults:
    Oral: 100 mg as a single dose
    I.V.: 1.8 mg/kg or alternatively 100 mg as a single dose
Prevention or treatment of postoperative nausea and vomiting: **Oral:** Administered 2 hours before surgery and; **I.V.:** Administered 15 minutes prior to cessation of anaesthesia or as soon as symptoms present
  Children ≥2 to 16 years:
    Oral: 1.2 mg/kg as a single dose (maximum: 100 mg)
    I.V.: 0.35 mg/kg as a single dose (maximum: 12.5 mg)
  Adults:
    Oral: 100 mg as a single dose
    I.V.: 12.5 mg as a single dose

Dosage adjustment in hepatic or renal impairment: No dosage adjustment needed

Administration
Oral: May be administered with or without food; injection may be used orally, dilute injection in apple or apple-grape juice; stable for 2 hours at room temperature
Parenteral: I.V.: Infuse undiluted over 30 seconds or dilute in 50 mL compatible I.V. fluid and infuse over ≤15 minutes; do not mix with other medications

Monitoring Parameters Baseline EKG in high-risk patients (see Warnings and Precautions), emesis episodes

Dosage Forms As mesylate:
  Injection: 20 mg/mL (0.625 mL, 5 mL)
  Tablet: 50 mg, 100 mg

References
"ASHP Therapeutic Guidelines on the Pharmacologic Management of Nausea and Vomiting in Adult and Pediatric Patients Receiving Chemotherapy or Radiation Therapy or Undergoing Surgery," *Am J Health Syst Pharm*, 1999, 56(8):729-64.
Coppes MJ, Lau R, Ingram LC, et al, "Open-Label Comparison of the Antiemetic Efficacy of Single Intravenous Doses of Dolasetron Mesylate in Pediatric Cancer Patients Receiving Moderately to Highly Emetogenic Chemotherapy," *Med Pediatr Oncol*, 1999, 33(2):99-105.

◆ **Dolophine®** *see* Methadone *on page 641*
◆ **Domeboro® [OTC]** *see* Aluminum Acetate *on page 62*
◆ **Donnatal®** *see* Hyoscyamine, Atropine, Scopolamine, and Phenobarbital *on page 519*
◆ **Dopamet (Can)** *see* Methyldopa *on page 651*

Dopamine (DOE pa meen)

Related Information
  Adult ACLS Algorithm, Bradycardia *on page 1044*
  Emergency Pediatric Drip Calculations *on page 1033*
  Extravasation Treatment *on page 1085*

Canadian Brand Names Intropin

Therapeutic Category Adrenergic Agonist Agent; Sympathomimetic

Generic Available Yes

Use Increase cardiac output, blood pressure, and urine flow as an adjunct in the treatment of shock or hypotension which persists after adequate fluid volume replacement; in low dosage to increase renal perfusion

Pregnancy Risk Factor C

Contraindications Hypersensitivity to sulfites (commercial preparation contains sodium bisulfite); pheochromocytoma, or ventricular fibrillation

Warnings Potent drug; must be diluted prior to use. Patient's hemodynamic status should be monitored.

Precautions Blood volume depletion should be corrected, if possible, before starting dopamine therapy. Dopamine must not be used as sole therapy in hypovolemic patients. Extravasation may cause tissue necrosis (treat extravasation with phentolamine; see Extravasation Treatment *on page 1085*); due to potential gangrene of extremities, use with caution in patients with occlusive vascular disease.
(Continued)

Dopamine (Continued)

Adverse Reactions

Cardiovascular: Ectopic heartbeats, tachycardia, vasoconstriction, cardiac conduction abnormalities, widened QRS complex, hypertension, ventricular arrhythmias, gangrene of the extremities (with high doses for prolonged periods or even with low doses in patients with occlusive vascular disease), anginal pain, palpitations

Central nervous system: Anxiety, headache

Gastrointestinal: Nausea, vomiting

Genitourinary: Decreased urine output (high dose)

Neuromuscular & skeletal: Piloerection

Ocular: Dilated pupils

Renal: Azotemia

Respiratory: Dyspnea

Drug Interactions Dopamine's cardiac and pressor response are prolonged and intensified by MAO inhibitors, alpha- and beta-adrenergic agonists, and oxytocic drugs; tricyclic antidepressants may decrease effects; use with phenytoin has resulted in seizures, severe hypotension, and bradycardia; use with halogenated hydrocarbon anesthetics may lead to serious arrhythmias; dopamine's cardiac effects are antagonized by beta-adrenergic blocking agents; vasoconstrictive effects are antagonized by alpha-adrenergic blocking agents

Stability Protect from light; solutions that are darker than slightly yellow should not be used; incompatible with alkaline solutions or iron salts; compatible when coadministered with dobutamine, epinephrine, isoproterenol, lidocaine, atracurium, vecuronium

Mechanism of Action Stimulates both adrenergic and dopaminergic receptors; low doses are mainly dopaminergic which stimulate and produce renal and mesenteric vasodilation; intermediate doses stimulate both dopaminergic and beta$_1$-adrenergic receptors and produce cardiac stimulation (increased heart rate and cardiac index) and increased renal blood flow; high doses stimulate alpha-adrenergic receptors primarily (vasoconstriction and increased blood pressure)

Pharmacodynamics

Onset of action: Adults: 5 minutes

Duration: Due to its short duration of action (<10 minutes) a continuous infusion must be used

Pharmacokinetics

Metabolism: In plasma, kidneys, and liver; 75% to inactive metabolites by monoamine oxidase and catechol-o-methyltransferase and 25% to norepinephrine (active)

Half-life: 2 minutes

Clearance: Neonatal clearance varies and appears to be age related. Clearance is more prolonged with combined hepatic and renal dysfunction. Dopamine has exhibited nonlinear kinetics in children; dose changes in children may not achieve steady-state for approximately 1 hour rather than 20 minutes seen in adults.

Usual Dosage I.V. infusion:

The hemodynamic effects of dopamine are dose-dependent:

Low dosage: 1-5 mcg/kg/minute, increased renal blood flow and urine output

Intermediate dosage: 5-15 mcg/kg/minute, increased renal blood flow, heart rate, cardiac contractility, cardiac output, and blood pressure

High dosage: >15 mcg/kg/minute, alpha-adrenergic effects begin to predominate, vasoconstriction, increased blood pressure

Neonates: 1-20 mcg/kg/minute continuous infusion, titrate to desired response

Children: 1-20 mcg/kg/minute, maximum dose: 50 mcg/kg/minute continuous infusion, titrate to desired response

Adults: 1 mcg/kg/minute up to 50 mcg/kg/minute, titrate to desired response

If dosages >20-30 mcg/kg/minute are needed, a more direct-acting pressor may be beneficial (ie, epinephrine, norepinephrine)

Administration Parenteral: Must be diluted prior to administration; maximum concentration: 3200 mcg/mL (3.2 mg/mL); (concentrations as high as 6000 mcg/mL have been infused into large veins, safely and with efficacy, in cases of extreme fluid restriction); rate of infusion (mL/hour) = dose (mcg/kg/minute) x weight (kg) x 60 minutes/hour divided by concentration (mcg/mL); administer into large vein to prevent the possibility of extravasation; use infusion device to control rate of flow; administration into an umbilical arterial catheter is **not** recommended

Monitoring Parameters EKG, heart rate, CVP, MAP, urine output; if pulmonary artery catheter is in place, monitor CI, PWCP, SVR, RAP, and PVR

Dosage Forms

Infusion, as hydrochloride, in D$_5$W: 0.8 mg/mL (250 mL, 500 mL); 1.6 mg/mL (250 mL, 500 mL); 3.2 mg/mL (250 mL)

Injection, as hydrochloride: 40 mg/mL (5 mL, 10 mL, 20 mL); 80 mg/mL (5 mL, 10 mL, 20 mL); 160 mg/mL (5 mL)

References
Banner W, Jr, Vernon DD, Dean JM, et al, "Nonlinear Dopamine Pharmacokinetics in Pediatric Patients," *J Pharmacol Exp Ther*, 1989, 249(1):131-3.

♦ **Dopram®** *see* Doxapram *on page 357*
♦ **Dormin® [OTC]** *see* Diphenhydramine *on page 342*
♦ **Dormiphen (Can)** *see* Diphenhydramine *on page 342*
♦ **Dormox Extra Fort (Can)** *see* Diphenhydramine *on page 342*

Dornase Alfa (DOOR nase AL fa)

U.S. Brand Names Pulmozyme®
Synonyms DNase; Recombinant Human Deoxyribonuclease
Therapeutic Category Enzyme, Inhalant; Mucolytic Agent
Generic Available No
Use Management of cystic fibrosis patients to reduce the frequency of respiratory infections and to improve pulmonary function
Pregnancy Risk Factor B
Contraindications Hypersensitivity to dornase alfa, Chinese hamster ovary cell products (eg, epoetin alfa), or any component
Warnings Safety and efficacy has not been established in children <5 years of age or in patients with forced vital capacity <40% of normal; no data exists regarding safety during lactation
Adverse Reactions
Cardiovascular: Chest pain
Dermatologic: Skin rash
Gastrointestinal: Sore throat
Hepatic: Liver disease
Ocular: Conjunctivitis
Respiratory: Increased cough, dyspnea, hemoptysis, wheezing, laryngitis, rhinitis, pharyngitis
Miscellaneous: Voice alteration, hoarseness
Drug Interactions None known at this time
Stability Must be stored in the refrigerator at 2°C to 8°C (36°F to 46°F) and protected from strong light; unopened vials left at room temperature for a total time of 24 hours should be discarded; discard solution if cloudy or discolored
Mechanism of Action Dornase alfa is a deoxyribonuclease (DNA) enzyme produced by recombinant gene technology. Dornase selectively cleaves DNA, thus reducing mucous viscosity seen in the pulmonary secretions of cystic fibrosis patients. As a result, airflow in the lung is improved and the risk of bacterial infection may be decreased.
Pharmacodynamics Onset of improved pulmonary function tests (PFTs): 3-8 days; PFTs will return to baseline 2-3 weeks after discontinuation of therapy
Pharmacokinetics Following nebulization, enzyme levels are measurable in the sputum within 15 minutes and decline rapidly thereafter
Usual Dosage
Infants and Children ≤5 years: Not approved for use, however studies using this therapy in small numbers of children as young as 3 months of age have reported efficacy and similar side effects. See References.
Children >5 years and Adults: Inhalation: 2.5 mg/day through selected nebulizers in conjunction with a Pulmo-Aide® or a Pari-Proneb® compressor; some patients, especially older than 21 years of age or with forced vital capacity (FVC) >85%, may benefit from twice daily administration
Administration Nebulization: Should not be diluted or mixed with any other drugs in the nebulizer, this may inactivate the drug
Dosage Forms Solution, inhalation: 1 mg/mL (2.5 mL)
References
Fuchs HJ, Borowitz DS, Christiansen DH, et al, "Effect of Aerosolized Recombinant Human DNase on Exacerbations of Respiratory Symptoms and on Pulmonary Function in Patients With Cystic Fibrosis," *N Engl J Med*, 1994, 331(10):637-42.
Mueller GA, Rubins G, Wessel D, et al, "Effects of Dornase Alfa on Pulmonary Function Tests in Infants with Cystic Fibrosis," *Am J Respir Crit Care Med*, 1996, 153:A70.
Rose M, Kirchner K, McCubbin M, et al, "Aerosol Delivery and Safety of rhDNASE in Young Children With Cystic Fibrosis: A Bronchoscopic Study," *Pediatr Pulmonol*, 1996, 13(Suppl):A268.

♦ **Doryx®** *see* Doxycycline *on page 362*
♦ **DOSS** *see* Docusate *on page 350*
♦ **DOS® Softgel® [OTC]** *see* Docusate *on page 350*

Doxacurium (doks a KYOO ri um)

U.S. Brand Names Nuromax®

Therapeutic Category Neuromuscular Blocker Agent, Nondepolarizing; Skeletal Muscle Relaxant, Paralytic

Generic Available No

Use Doxacurium is indicated for use as an adjunct to general anesthesia. It provides skeletal muscle relaxation during surgery or endotracheal intubation; increases pulmonary compliance during mechanical ventilation

Pregnancy Risk Factor C

Contraindications Hypersensitivity to doxacurium or any component

Warnings Ventilation must be supported during neuromuscular blockade

Precautions Contains benzyl alcohol; avoid use in neonates; use with caution in patients with neuromuscular disease such as myasthenia gravis, cardiovascular disease; use with caution and reduce dosage in patients with renal or hepatic impairment; certain clinical conditions may result in potentiation or antagonism of neuromuscular blockade, see table.

Clinical Conditions Affecting Neuromuscular Blockade

Potentiation	Antagonism
Electrolyte abnormalities	Alkalosis
Severe hyponatremia	Hypercalcemia
Severe hypocalcemia	Demyelinating lesions
Severe hypokalemia	Peripheral neuropathies
Hypermagnesemia	Diabetes mellitus
Neuromuscular diseases	
Acidosis	
Acute intermittent porphyria	
Renal failure	
Hepatic failure	

Potential Drug Interactions

Potentiation	Antagonism
Inhalation anesthetics	Calcium
Desflurane, sevoflurane, enflurane and	Carbamazepine
isoflurane > halothane > nitrous	Phenytoin
oxide	Steroids (chronic administration)
Antibiotics	Theophylline
Aminoglycosides, polymyxins,	Anticholinesterases*
clindamycin, vancomycin	Neostigmine, pyridostigmine,
Magnesium	edrophonium, echothiophate
Antiarrhythmics	ophthalmic solution
Quinidine, procainamide, bretylium, and	Caffeine
possibly lidocaine	Azathioprine
Diuretics	
Furosemide, mannitol, thiazides	
Amphotericin B (secondary to hypokalemia)	
Local anesthetics	
Dantrolene (directly depresses skeletal muscle)	
Beta blockers	
Calcium channel blockers	
Ketamine	
Lithium	
Succinylcholine (when administered prior to nondepolarizing neuromuscular-blocking agent)	
Cyclosporine	

*Can prolong the effects of acetylcholine

Adverse Reactions The most frequent adverse reactions appear as an extension of the agent's neuromuscular blocking actions

Cardiovascular: Hypotension (rare), bradycardia (rare)

Central nervous system: Fever

Dermatologic: Cutaneous flushing, urticaria

Neuromuscular & skeletal: Muscle weakness

Ocular: Diplopia

Respiratory: Respiratory insufficiency and apnea, bronchospasm, wheezing

Drug Interactions See table on previous page.

Stability Stable for 24 hours at room temperature when diluted in concentrations up to 0.1 mg/mL in D_5W or NS; compatible with sufentanil, alfentanil, and fentanyl; incompatible with alkaline solutions

Mechanism of Action Doxacurium is a long-acting nondepolarizing skeletal muscle relaxant. The drug is a bis-quaternary benzylisoquinolinium diester, with a chemical structure similar to that of atracurium. Similar to other nondepolarizing neuromuscular blocking agents, doxacurium produces muscle relaxation by competing with acetylcholine for cholinergic receptor sites on the postjunctional membrane; significant presynaptic depressant activity is also observed.

Pharmacodynamics

Onset of effects: 5-11 minutes

Duration: 30 minutes (range: 12-54 minutes)

Pharmacokinetics

Distribution: V_d: Adults: 0.22 L/kg

Protein binding: 30%

Half-life:

Normal: 1.5 hours

Renal dysfunction: 3.7 hours

Liver dysfunction: 1.9 hours

Elimination: Primarily as unchanged drug via the kidneys (80%) and biliary tract (20%)

Usual Dosage I.V. (in obese patients, use ideal body weight):

Children 2-12 years: Initial: 0.03-0.05 mg/kg/dose (30-50 mcg/kg/dose); maintenance: 0.005-0.01 mg/kg (5-10 mcg/kg/dose) every 30-45 minutes, or as needed depending upon individual patient response

Continuous infusion: 0.1-0.2 mcg/kg/minute or 6-12 mcg/kg/hour

Children >12 years and Adults: Initial: 0.025-0.05 mg/kg/dose (25-50 mcg/kg/dose); maintenance: 0.005-0.01 mg/kg/dose (5-10 mcg/kg/dose) every 60-100 minutes

Continuous infusion: 0.1-0.2 mcg/kg/minute or 6-12 mcg/kg/hour

Dosing adjustment in renal or hepatic impairment: Reduce initial dose and titrate carefully as duration may be prolonged

Administration Parenteral: I.V.: May be administered by rapid I.V. injection undiluted

Monitoring Parameters Peripheral nerve stimulation testing (measures twitch response), heart rate, blood pressure, assisted ventilation status

Additional Information Doxacurium is a long-acting nondepolarizing neuromuscular blocker with virtually no cardiovascular side effects. The characteristics of this agent make it especially useful in procedures requiring careful maintenance of hemodynamic stability for prolonged periods

Dosage Forms Injection, as chloride: 1 mg/mL (5 mL)

References

Martin LD, Bratton SL, and O'Rourke PP, "Clinical Uses and Controversies of Neuromuscular Blocking Agents in Infants and Children," *Crit Care Med*, 1999, 27(7):1358-68.

Doxapram (DOKS a pram)

U.S. Brand Names Dopram®

Therapeutic Category Central Nervous System Stimulant, Nonamphetamine; Respiratory Stimulant

Generic Available No

Use Respiratory and CNS stimulant; idiopathic apnea of prematurity refractory to xanthines

Pregnancy Risk Factor B

Contraindications Hypersensitivity to doxapram or any component; epilepsy, cerebral edema, head injury, asthma or restrictive pulmonary disease, pheochromocytoma, cardiovascular or coronary artery disease, hypertension, hyperthyroidism, cardiac arrhythmias

Warnings Should be used with caution in newborns as the U.S. product contains benzyl alcohol (0.9%); recommended doses of doxapram for neonates will deliver 5.4-27 mg/kg/day of benzyl alcohol; large amounts of benzyl alcohol (>100 mg/kg/day) have been associated with fatal toxicity (gasping syndrome); the use of doxa-
(Continued)

Doxapram *(Continued)*

pram in newborns should be reserved for neonates who are unresponsive to the treatment of apnea with therapeutic serum concentrations of theophylline or caffeine; not an antagonist to muscle relaxant drugs nor a specific narcotic antagonist; doxapram alone may not stimulate adequate spontaneous breathing or provide sufficient arousal in patients who are severely depressed; use as an adjunct to establish supportive measures

Adverse Reactions

Cardiovascular: Hypertension (dose-related), tachycardia, arrhythmias, hypotension, flushing

Central nervous system: CNS stimulation, restlessness, lightheadedness, jitters, hallucinations, irritability, seizures, headache, fever, hypothermia

Hematologic: Hemolysis

Gastrointestinal: Abdominal distension, nausea, vomiting, retching, increased gastric residuals

Local: Phlebitis

Metabolic: Hyperglycemia

Neuromuscular & skeletal: Tremor, hyper-reflexia

Ocular: Lacrimation, mydriasis

Renal: Glucosuria

Respiratory: Coughing, laryngospasm, dyspnea

Miscellaneous: Diaphoresis

Drug Interactions Sympathomimetic drugs and MAO inhibitors may cause significant increase in blood pressure; general anesthetics

Stability Stable at room temperature; incompatible with aminophylline, sodium bicarbonate, thiopental sodium, and other alkaline solutions

Mechanism of Action Stimulates respiration through action on respiratory center in medulla or through reflex stimulation of carotid, aortic, or other peripheral chemoreceptors; antagonizes opiate-induced respiratory depression, but does not affect analgesia

Pharmacodynamics Following I.V. injection:

Onset of respiratory stimulation: Within 20-40 seconds

Peak effect: Within 1-2 minutes

Duration: 5-12 minutes

Pharmacokinetics

Metabolism: Extensive in the liver

Distribution: V_d: Neonates: 4-7.3 L/kg

Half-life:

Neonates, premature: 6.6-8.2 hours

Adults: Mean: 3.4 hours (range: 2.4-4.1 hours)

Clearance: Neonates, premature: 0.44-0.7 L/hour/kg

Usual Dosage I.V.:

Neonatal apnea (apnea of prematurity): Initial loading dose: 2.5-3 mg/kg followed by a continuous infusion of 1 mg/kg/hour; titrate to the lowest rate at which apnea is controlled (maximum dose: 2.5 mg/kg/hour)

Adults: Respiratory depression following anesthesia:

Initial: 0.5-1 mg/kg; may repeat at 5-minute intervals; maximum total dose: 2 mg/kg

I.V. infusion: Initial: 5 mg/minute until adequate response or adverse effects seen; decrease to 1-3 mg/minute; usual total dose: 0.5-4 mg/kg or 300 mg

Administration Parenteral: I.V. use only: Dilute loading dose to a maximum concentration of 2 mg/mL and infuse over 15-30 minutes; for infusion, dilute in NS or dextrose to 1 mg/mL (maximum concentration: 2 mg/mL); irritating to tissues; avoid extravasation

Monitoring Parameters Blood pressure, heart rate, deep tendon reflexes; for apnea: number, duration, and severity of apneic episodes

Reference Range Initial studies suggest a therapeutic serum level of at least 1.5 mg/L; toxicity becomes frequent at serum levels >5 mg/L

Dosage Forms Injection, as hydrochloride: 20 mg/mL (20 mL)

References
Barrington KJ, Finer NN, Torok-Both G, et al, "Dose-Response Relationship of Doxapram in the Therapy for Refractory Idiopathic Apnea of Prematurity," *Pediatrics*, 1987, 80(1):22-7.

Doxepin *(DOKS e pin)*

Related Information

Comparison of Adverse Effects of Antidepressants *on page 1066*

Comparison of Usual Adult Dosage and Mechanism of Action of Antidepressants *on page 1065*

Drugs and Breast-Feeding *on page 1243*

Overdose and Toxicology *on page 1222*

U.S. Brand Names Prudoxin™; Sinequan®; Zonalon®

Canadian Brand Names Alti-Doxepin; Apo-Doxepin; Novo-Doxepin; Triadapin

Therapeutic Category Antianxiety Agent; Antidepressant, Tricyclic

Generic Available Yes

Use

Oral: Treatment of various forms of depression, usually in conjunction with psychotherapy; treatment of anxiety disorders; analgesic for certain chronic and neuropathic pain

Topical: Adults: Short-term (<8 days) therapy of moderate pruritus due to atopic dermatitis or lichen simplex chronicus

Pregnancy Risk Factor C (Topical: B)

Contraindications Hypersensitivity to doxepin or any component (cross-sensitivity with other tricyclic antidepressants may occur); narrow-angle glaucoma; patients with urinary retention

Warnings Do not discontinue abruptly in patients receiving chronic high dose therapy

Precautions Use with caution in patients with cardiovascular disease, conduction disturbances, seizure disorders, urinary retention, hyperthyroidism or those receiving thyroid replacement; avoid use during lactation; use with caution in pregnancy

Adverse Reactions Pronounced sedation and anticholinergic adverse effects may occur

Cardiovascular: Hypotension, arrhythmias

Central nervous system: Sedation, confusion, dizziness, headache; drowsiness occurs in 20% of patients receiving topical cream especially if applied to >10% of body surface area; reduction in area treated, number of applications per day, amount of cream used, or discontinuation of cream may be needed if excessive drowsiness occurs

Dermatologic: Photosensitivity

Endocrine & metabolic: SIADH (rare)

Gastrointestinal: Constipation, nausea, vomiting, xerostomia, increased appetite, weight gain

Genitourinary: Urinary retention

Hematologic: Blood dyscrasias (rare)

Hepatic: Hepatitis

Local: Stinging and burning at application site; exacerbation of pruritus or eczema; allergic contact dermatitis

Neuromuscular & skeletal: Fine tremor

Ocular: Blurred vision

Otic: Tinnitus

Miscellaneous: Hypersensitivity reactions

Drug Interactions Cytochrome P-450 isoenzyme CYP2D6 substrate

CNS depressants, alcohol, MAO inhibitors (serious side effects including death have been reported; use within 14 days is not recommended), guanethidine, clonidine, antithyroid agents, cimetidine, carbamazepine; tolazamide (severe hypoglycemia may occur); the herbal medicine St John's wort (*Hypericum perforatum*) may increase serious side effects, its use is **not** recommended

Food Interactions Oral solution is physically incompatible with carbonated beverages and grape juice; diets rich in fiber may decrease drug effects

Stability Protect from light; store cream at ≤80°F (27°C)

Mechanism of Action Increases the synaptic concentration of serotonin and/or norepinephrine in the central nervous system by inhibition of their reuptake by the presynaptic neuronal membrane

Pharmacodynamics Maximum antidepressant effects: Usually occur after >2 weeks; anxiolytic effects may occur sooner

Pharmacokinetics

Distribution: Crosses the placenta; appears in breast milk

Protein binding: 80% to 85%

Metabolism: Hepatic to metabolites, including desmethyldoxepin (active)

Half-life, adults: 6-8 hours

Elimination: Renal

Usual Dosage

Oral:

Children: 1-3 mg/kg/day in single or divided doses

(Continued)

Doxepin *(Continued)*

Adolescents: Initial: 25-50 mg/day in single or divided doses; gradually increase to 100 mg/day

Adults: Initial: 30-150 mg/day at bedtime or in 2-3 divided doses; may increase up to 300 mg/day; single dose should not exceed 150 mg; select patients may respond to 25-50 mg/day

Topical: Adults: Apply to affected area 4 times/day

Administration

Oral: Administer with food to decrease GI upset; oral concentrate should be diluted in water, milk, or juice (but not grape juice) prior to administration (use 120 mL for adults); do not mix with carbonated beverages

Topical: Apply cream to affected area with at least 3-4 hours between applications; do not use occlusive dressings; avoid contact with eyes

Monitoring Parameters Blood pressure, heart rate, mental status, weight, liver enzymes, CBC with differential

Reference Range Utility of serum level monitoring controversial

Therapeutic concentration: Doxepin plus desmethyldoxepin: 110-250 ng/mL (SI: 4-9 nmol/L)

Toxic concentration: >300 ng/mL (SI: >11 nmol/L)

Patient Information May cause drowsiness and impair ability to perform activities requiring mental alertness or physical coordination; may cause dry mouth; avoid alcohol and the herbal medicine St John's wort; limit caffeine; may increase appetite; do not discontinue abruptly; avoid unnecessary exposure to sunlight

Nursing Implications Do not use occlusive dressings with cream (increases dermal absorption)

Additional Information Safety and effectiveness of topical cream when used for >8 days has not been established; use >8 days may result in an increase in serum concentrations and systemic effects

Dosage Forms

Capsule, as hydrochloride (Sinequan®): 10 mg, 25 mg, 50 mg, 75 mg, 100 mg, 150 mg

Concentrate, oral, as hydrochloride (Sinequan®): 10 mg/mL (120 mL)

Cream:

Prudoxin™: 5% (45 g)

Zonalon®: 5% (30 g)

References

Levy HB, Harper CR, and Weinberg WA, " A Practical Approach to Children Failing in School," *Pediatr Clin North Am*, 1992, 39(4):895-928.

Doxorubicin (doks oh ROO bi sin)

Related Information

Drugs and Breast-Feeding *on page 1243*

Emetogenic Potential of Single Chemotherapeutic Agents *on page 1129*

Extravasation Treatment *on page 1085*

U.S. Brand Names Adriamycin PFS™; Adriamycin RDF™; Rubex®

Canadian Brand Names Caelyx

Synonyms ADR; Hydroxydaunomycin

Therapeutic Category Antineoplastic Agent, Anthracycline; Antineoplastic Agent, Antibiotic

Generic Available Yes

Use Treatment of various solid tumors including ovarian, breast, and bladder tumors; various lymphomas and leukemias (AML, ALL), soft tissue sarcomas, neuroblastoma, osteosarcoma

Pregnancy Risk Factor D

Contraindications Hypersensitivity to doxorubicin or any component; severe CHF, cardiomyopathy, pre-existing myelosuppression; patients who have received a total dose of 550 mg/m^2 of doxorubicin or 400 mg/m^2 in patients with previous or concomitant treatment with daunorubicin, idarubicin, mitoxantrone, cyclophosphamide, or irradiation of the cardiac region

Warnings The FDA currently recommends that procedures for proper handling and disposal of antineoplastic agents be considered. **I.V. use only**; severe local tissue necrosis will result if extravasation occurs; irreversible myocardial toxicity may occur if the total cumulative dose approaches 450 mg/m^2 in adults with normal cardiac function or 300 mg/m^2 in adults with prior mediastinal irradiation, concurrent cyclophosphamide therapy, or pre-existing heart disease; severe myelosuppression is also possible. Pediatric patients are at increased risk for developing delayed cardiac toxicity and CHF during early adulthood due to an increasing census of long-term survivors; periodic long-term monitoring of cardiac function is recommended. Pediatric patients are at risk of developing secondary acute myeloid leukemia.

Precautions Modify dosage in patients with impaired hepatic function

Adverse Reactions

Cardiovascular: CHF, cardiomyopathy, cardiotoxicity (transient type with abnormal EKG and arrhythmias, or a chronic, cumulative, dose-dependent type which progresses to CHF), cardiorespiratory decompensation, facial flushing

Dermatologic: Alopecia, hyperpigmentation of nail beds, urticaria

Endocrine & metabolic: Hyperuricemia, infertility, prepubertal growth failure

Gastrointestinal: Stomatitis, esophagitis, nausea, vomiting, mucositis, anorexia, diarrhea, ulceration and necrosis of the colon

Genitourinary: Discoloration of urine (red/orange), cystitis

Hematologic: Leukopenia (nadir: 10-14 days), thrombocytopenia, anemia

Hepatic: Transient elevation of liver function tests

Local: Tissue necrosis upon extravasation, erythematous streaking along the vein if administered too rapidly, phlebitis

Ocular: Lacrimation

Miscellaneous: Anaphylaxis

Drug Interactions Cytochrome P-450 isoenzyme CYP3A3/4 substrate; isoenzyme CYP2D6 inhibitor

May potentiate the toxicity of cyclophosphamide, mercaptopurine; ritonavir and cyclosporine decrease doxorubicin metabolism; doxorubicin decreases carbamazepine, digoxin, and phenytoin levels

Stability Protect from light; store vials containing powder at room temperature, refrigerate vials containing liquid; reconstituted vials stable for 24 hours at room temperature and 48 hours if refrigerated. Discard unused portion of preservative free injection vial. Incompatible with hydrocortisone, fluorouracil, furosemide, sodium bicarbonate, aminophylline, heparin, cephalothin, dexamethasone; unstable in solutions with a pH <3 or >7. Color change from red to purple indicates decomposition of drug.

Mechanism of Action Inhibits DNA and RNA synthesis by intercalating between DNA base pairs and by steric obstruction; produces oxygen-free radicals which cause DNA denaturation; inhibits DNA topoisomerase I resulting in DNA strand breaks

Pharmacokinetics

Distribution: Into breast milk; does not penetrate into CSF; distributes into cells rapidly with high concentrations in lung, kidney, muscle, spleen, and liver

Protein binding: 75%

Metabolism: In both the liver and in plasma to both active and inactive metabolites

Half-life, triphasic:

Primary: 30 minutes

Secondary: 3-3.5 hours for its metabolites

Terminal: 17-30 hours for doxorubicin and its metabolites

Elimination: Undergoes triphasic elimination; 40% to 60% eventually excreted in bile and feces; <5% excreted in urine, primarily as unchanged drug and metabolites

Clearance:

Infants <2 years: 813 mL/minute/m^2

Children >2 years: 1540 mL/minute/m^2

Usual Dosage Patient's ideal weight should be used to calculate body surface area. Lower dose regimens should be given to patients with decreased bone marrow reserve, prior radiation therapy, or marrow infiltration with malignant cells.

I.V. (refer to individual protocols):

Children: 35-75 mg/m^2 as a single dose, repeat every 21 days; or 20-30 mg/m^2 once weekly; or 60-90 mg/m^2 given as a continuous infusion over 96 hours every 3-4 weeks

Adults: 60-75 mg/m^2 as a single dose, repeat every 21 days; or 20-30 mg/m^2/day for 2-3 days, repeat in 4 weeks or 20 mg/m^2 once weekly

Dosing adjustment in hepatic impairment:

Bilirubin 1.2-3 mg/dL: Reduce dose by 50%

Bilirubin >3 mg/dL: Reduce dose by 75%

Administration Parenteral: I.V. use only; reconstitute IVP doses with D$_5$W or NS to ensure isotonicity of the final solution; administer slow IVP at a rate no faster than over 3-5 minutes or by I.V. infusion over 1-4 hours at a concentration not to exceed 2 mg/mL, or by I.V. continuous infusion

Monitoring Parameters CBC with differential, erythrocyte and platelet count; echocardiogram, liver function tests including AST, ALT, alkaline phosphatase, and bilirubin; observe I.V. injection site for infiltration and vein irritation

(Continued)

Doxorubicin (Continued)

Patient Information Transient red-orange discoloration of urine can occur for up to 48 hours after a dose; avoid unnecessary exposure to sunlight; notify physician if fever, sore throat, bleeding, or bruising occurs; report any stinging sensation at the injection site during infusion

Nursing Implications Local erythematous streaking along the vein and/or facial flushing may indicate too rapid a rate of administration; drug is very irritating; avoid extravasation; if extravasation occurs, apply cold packs immediately for 30-60 minutes, then alternate off/on every 15 minutes for 1 day; apply 1.5 mL of dimethyl-sulfoxide 99% (w/v) solution to the site every 6 hours for 14 days; allow to air-dry; do not cover. Take precautions to prevent contact with the patient's urine and other body fluids for at least 5 days after each treatment.

Additional Information Myelosuppressive effects:
WBC: Moderate
Platelets: Moderate
Onset (days): 7
Nadir (days): 10-14
Recovery (days): 21-28

Dosage Forms
Injection, as hydrochloride:
Aqueous, with NS: 2 mg/mL (5 mL, 10 mL, 25 mL)
Preservative free (Adriamycin PFS™): 2 mg/mL (5 mL, 10 mL, 25 mL, 100 mL)
Powder for injection, as hydrochloride, lyophilized: 10 mg, 20 mg, 50 mg
Rubex®: 10 mg, 50 mg, 100 mg
Powder for injection, as hydrochloride, lyophilized, rapid dissolution formula (Adriamycin RDF™): 10 mg, 20 mg, 50 mg, 150 mg

References
Berg SL, Grisell DL, DeLaney TF, et al, "Principles of Treatment of Pediatric Solid Tumors," *Pediatr Clin North Am*, 1991, 38(2):249-67.

Ishii E, Hara T, Ohkubo K, et al, "Treatment of Childhood Acute Lymphoblastic Leukemia With Intermediate Dose Cytosine Arabinoside and Adriamycin," *Med Pediatr Oncol*, 1986, 14(2):73-7.

Legha SS, Benjamin RS, Mackay B, et al, "Reduction of Doxorubicin Cardiotoxicity by Prolonged Continuous Intravenous Infusion," *Ann Intern Med*, 1982, 96(2):133-9.

♦ **Doxy-200®** see Doxycycline on page 362
♦ **Doxy-Caps®** see Doxycycline on page 362
♦ **Doxychel®** see Doxycycline on page 362
♦ **Doxycin (Can)** see Doxycycline on page 362

Doxycycline (doks i SYE kleen)

U.S. Brand Names Bio-Tab®; Doryx®; Doxy-200®; Doxy-Caps®; Doxychel®; Doxy-Tabs®; Dynacin®; Monodox®; Vibramycin®; Vibra-Tabs®

Canadian Brand Names Apo-Doxy; Doxycin; Doxytec; Novo-Doxylin; Nu-Doxycycline

Therapeutic Category Antibiotic, Tetracycline Derivative

Generic Available Yes

Use
Children, Adolescents, Adults: Treatment of Rocky Mountain spotted fever caused by susceptible *Rickettsia*; treatment of ehrlichiosis

Older Children, Adolescents, Adults: Treatment of Lyme disease, *Mycoplasma* infection, or *Legionella*; management of malignant pleural effusions when intrapleural therapy is indicated

Adolescents and Adults: Treatment of nongonococcal pelvic inflammatory disease and urethritis due to *Chlamydia*; treatment for victims of sexual assault

Pregnancy Risk Factor D

Contraindications Hypersensitivity to doxycycline, tetracycline, or any component; children <8 years; severe hepatic dysfunction

Warnings Photosensitivity reaction may occur with this drug; avoid prolonged exposure to sunlight or tanning equipment. Do not administer to children <8 years of age due to associated retardation in skeletal development; use of tetracyclines during tooth development may cause permanent discoloration of the teeth and enamel hypoplasia; staining of teeth is dose-related so that duration of therapy should be minimized; doxycycline may be less likely to stain developing teeth than tetracycline since it binds less strongly to calcium; prolonged use may result in superinfection.

Adverse Reactions
Central nervous system: Increased intracranial pressure, bulging fontanels in infants
Dermatologic: Rash, photosensitivity, discoloration of nails
Gastrointestinal: Nausea, diarrhea, esophagitis and esophageal ulceration with the hyclate salt formulation; anorexia, pseudomembranous colitis, oral candidiasis

Hematologic: Neutropenia, eosinophilia

Hepatic: Hepatotoxicity

Local: Phlebitis, pain at the injection site

Neuromuscular & skeletal: Retardation of skeletal development in infants

Miscellaneous: May cause discoloration of teeth in children <8 years of age

Drug Interactions Cytochrome P-450 isoenzyme CYP3A3/4 substrate

Antacids containing aluminum, calcium, or magnesium; zinc, kaolin, pectin, iron, and bismuth subsalicylate may decrease doxycycline bioavailability; rifampin, barbiturates, phenytoin, and carbamazepine decrease doxycycline's half-life; doxycycline enhances the hypoprothrombinemic effect of warfarin

Food Interactions Administration with iron, calcium, milk or dairy products may decrease doxycycline absorption; may decrease absorption of calcium, iron, magnesium, zinc and amino acids

Stability Reconstituted oral doxycycline suspension is stable for 2 weeks at room temperature; I.V. doxycycline solutions must be protected from direct sunlight

Mechanism of Action Inhibits protein synthesis by binding to the 30S and possibly the 50S ribosomal subunit(s) of susceptible bacteria preventing additions of amino acids to the growing peptide chain; may also cause alterations in the cytoplasmic membrane

Pharmacokinetics

Absorption: Almost completely from the GI tract; absorption can be reduced by food or milk by 20%

Distribution: Widely distributed into body tissues and fluids including synovial and pleural fluid, bile, bronchial secretions; poor penetration into the CSF; appears in breast milk

Protein binding: 80% to 85%

Metabolism: Not metabolized in the liver; partially inactivated in the GI tract by chelate formation

Bioavailability: 90% to 100%

Half-life: 12-15 hours (usually increases to 22-24 hours with multiple dosing)

Time to peak serum concentration: Oral: Within 1.5-4 hours

Elimination: In the urine (23%) and feces (30%)

Dialysis: Not dialyzable (0% to 5%)

Usual Dosage

Children ≥8 years: Oral, I.V.: 2-4 mg/kg/day divided every 12-24 hours, not to exceed 200 mg/day

Lyme disease: Oral: 100 mg/dose twice daily for 14-21 days

Chlamydial infections: Oral: 100 mg/dose twice daily for 7-10 days

Adolescents and Adults: Oral, I.V.: 100-200 mg/day in 1-2 divided doses

Lyme disease: Oral: 100 mg/dose twice daily for 14-21 days

Pelvic inflammatory disease:

Hospitalized regimen: Oral, I.V.: 100 mg every 12 hours for 14 days administered with cefoxitin or cefotetan

Outpatient regimen: Oral: 100 mg every 12 hours for 14 days plus single dose ceftriaxone

Sclerosing agent for pleural effusion: 500 mg in 25-30 mL of NS instilled into the pleural space to control pleural effusions associated with metastatic tumors; or for recurrent malignant pleural effusions: 500 mg in 250 mL NS

Administration

Oral: Administer capsules or tablets with adequate amounts of fluid; avoid antacids, infant formula, milk, dairy products, and iron for 1 hour before or 2 hours after administration of doxycycline; may be administered with food to decrease GI upset; shake suspension well before use

Parenteral: For I.V. use only; administer by slow I.V. intermittent infusion over a minimum of 1-2 hours at a concentration not to exceed 1 mg/mL (may be infused over 1-4 hours); concentrations <0.1 mg/mL are not recommended

Sclerosing agent:

To control pleural effusions associated with metastatic tumors: Instill into the pleural space through a thoracostomy tube following drainage of the accumulated pleural fluid; clamp the tube then remove the fluid

For recurrent malignant pleural effusions: Administer via chest tube lavage, clamp tube for 24 hours then drain

Monitoring Parameters Periodic monitoring of renal, hematologic, and hepatic function tests; observe for changes in bowel frequency

Test Interactions False-negative urine glucose using Clinistix®, Tes-Tape®

Patient Information Avoid unnecessary exposure to sunlight or tanning equipment; may discolor teeth if <8 years of age; may discolor fingernails

(Continued)

Doxycycline *(Continued)*

Nursing Implications Check for signs of phlebitis; I.V. doxycycline should not be given I.M. or S.C.; avoid extravasation

Dosage Forms

Capsule, as hyclate: 50 mg, 100 mg

Doxychel®, Monodox®, Vibramycin®: 50 mg

Doxy®, Doxychel®, Monodox®, Vibramycin®: 100 mg

Capsule, coated pellets, as hyclate (Doryx®): 100 mg

Powder for injection, as hyclate: 100 mg, 200 mg

Doxy®, Doxychel®, Vibramycin® IV: 100 mg, 200 mg

Powder for oral suspension, as monohydrate (Vibramycin®): 25 mg/5 mL [raspberry flavor] (60 mL)

Syrup, as calcium (Vibramycin®): 50 mg/5 mL [raspberry-apple flavor] (30 mL, 473 mL)

Tablet, as hyclate

Doxychel®: 50 mg

Bio-Tab®, Doxychel®, Vibra-Tabs®: 100 mg

References

Centers for Disease Control and Prevention, "1998 Guidelines for Treatment of Sexually Transmitted Diseases," *MMWR Morb Mortal Wkly Rep*, 1998, 47(RR-1):1-111.

♦ **Doxy-Tabs®** *see Doxycycline on page 362*

♦ **Doxytec (Can)** *see Doxycycline on page 362*

♦ **DPA** *see Valproic Acid and Derivatives on page 998*

♦ **DPE** *see Dipivefrin on page 345*

♦ **D-Penicillamine** *see Penicillamine on page 769*

♦ **DPH** *see Phenytoin on page 791*

♦ **DPPC** *see Colfosceril on page 265*

♦ **Dramamine®** *see Dimenhydrinate on page 339*

♦ **Dramamine® II [OTC]** *see Meclizine on page 622*

♦ **Drisdol®** *see Ergocalciferol on page 392*

♦ **Dristan Long-Lasting Nasal (Can)** *see Oxymetazoline on page 749*

♦ **Drixoral Decongestant Nasal (Can)** *see Oxymetazoline on page 749*

♦ **Drixoral ND (Can)** *see Pseudoephedrine on page 852*

Dronabinol *(droe NAB i nol)*

U.S. Brand Names Marinol®

Synonyms Tetrahydrocannabinol; THC

Therapeutic Category Antiemetic

Generic Available Yes

Use Treatment of nausea and vomiting secondary to cancer chemotherapy in patients who have not responded to conventional antiemetics; treatment of anorexia associated with weight loss in AIDS patients

Restrictions C-III

Pregnancy Risk Factor C

Contraindications Should not be used in patients with a history of schizophrenia; hypersensitivity to dronabinol, any component, marijuana, or sesame oil

Warnings Dronabinol has a high potential for abuse; limit antiemetic therapy availability to current cycle of chemotherapy

Precautions Use with caution in patients with heart disease, hepatic disease, or seizure disorders; reduce dosage in patients with severe hepatic impairment

Adverse Reactions

Cardiovascular: Orthostatic hypotension, tachycardia, palpitations, vasodilation, hypotension

Central nervous system: Drowsiness, dizziness, vertigo, difficulty in concentrating, mood change, euphoria, detachment, depression, anxiety, paranoia, hallucinations, nervousness, ataxia, headache, memory lapse

Gastrointestinal: Xerostomia, diarrhea

Hepatic: Elevated liver enzymes

Neuromuscular & skeletal: Myalgia, tremor, paresthesia, weakness

Ocular: Vision difficulties

Respiratory: Sinusitis, cough, rhinitis

Miscellaneous: Diaphoresis

Drug Interactions Cytochrome P-450 isoenzyme CYP2C18 and CYP3A3/4 substrate

Additive tachycardia, hypertension with amphetamines, cocaine, sympathomimetics, tricyclic antidepressants; additive CNS effects with sedatives, antihistamines, hypnotics, psychomimetics, tricyclic antidepressants, alcohol; hypomanic state with disulfiram, fluoxetine; increases theophylline metabolism; decreases barbiturate clearance

Stability Store in a cool place

Mechanism of Action Dronabinol is the principal psychoactive substance found in *Cannabis sativa* (marijuana); its mechanism of action as an antiemetic is not well defined, it probably inhibits the vomiting center in the medulla oblongata

Pharmacodynamics
Onset of action: 30 minutes to 1 hour
Peak effect: 2-4 hours
Duration: 4-6 hours

Pharmacokinetics
Absorption: Oral: 90% to 95%; first-pass metabolism results in low systemic bioavailability
Distribution: V_d: ~10L/kg
Protein binding: 97% to 99%
Metabolism: Extensive first-pass; metabolized in the liver to several metabolites some of which are active
Bioavailability: 10% to 20%
Half-life:
Biphasic: Alpha: 4 hours
Terminal: 25-36 hours
Time to peak serum concentration: Within 2-3 hours
Elimination: Biliary excretion is the major route of elimination

Usual Dosage Oral:
Antiemetic: Children and Adults: 5 mg/m^2 1-3 hours before chemotherapy, then give 5 mg/m^2/dose every 2-4 hours after chemotherapy for a total of 4-6 doses/day; dose may be increased up to a maximum of 15 mg/m^2 per dose if needed (dosage may be increased in 2.5 mg/m^2 increments)
Appetite stimulant: Adults: 2.5 mg twice daily before lunch and dinner; if intolerant, a dosage of 2.5 mg once daily at night may be tried; maximum dosage (escalating): 5 mg 4 times/day (20 mg/day)

Administration May be administered without regard to meals; take before meals if used to stimulate appetite

Monitoring Parameters Heart rate, blood pressure

Patient Information Causes drowsiness and may impair ability to perform hazardous tasks requiring mental alertness or physical coordination

Dosage Forms Capsule, gelatin: 2.5 mg, 5 mg, 10 mg

References
Lane M, Smith FE, Sullivan RA, et al, "Dronabinol and Prochlorperazine Alone and in Combination as Antiemetic Agents for Cancer Chemotherapy," *Am J Clin Oncol*, 1990, 13(6):480-4.

Droperidol (droe PER i dole)

Related Information
Compatibility of Medications Mixed in a Syringe *on page 1238*

U.S. Brand Names Inapsine®

Therapeutic Category Antiemetic; Antipsychotic Agent

Generic Available Yes

Use Tranquilizer and antiemetic in surgical and diagnostic procedures; antiemetic for cancer chemotherapy and postoperative patients; preoperative medication

Pregnancy Risk Factor C

Contraindications Hypersensitivity to droperidol or any component

Precautions Use with caution in patients with impaired hepatic or renal function

Adverse Reactions
Cardiovascular: Hypotension (especially in hypovolemic patients), tachycardia
Central nervous system: Extrapyramidal reactions such as dystonic reactions, akathisia, and oculogyric crisis; anxiety, hyperactivity, drowsiness, dizziness, hallucinations, chills
Respiratory: Laryngospasm, bronchospasm

Drug Interactions Use with other CNS depressants may have additive effects (CNS, respiratory depression, etc); droperidol plus fentanyl or other analgesics may increase blood pressure; conduction anesthesia may increase hypotension; droperidol plus epinephrine may decrease blood pressure due to alpha-adrenergic blockade effects of droperidol; droperidol plus atropine may cause tachycardia

Stability Physically compatible and chemically stable with D_5W, LR, NS at a concentration of 20 mg/L
(Continued)

Droperidol *(Continued)*

Mechanism of Action Alters the action of dopamine in the CNS, at subcortical levels, to produce sedation and a dissociative state; also possesses alpha-adrenergic blockade effects

Pharmacodynamics
Onset of action: 3-10 minutes
Peak effects: Within 30 minutes
Duration: 2-4 hours (up to 12 hours)

Pharmacokinetics
Metabolism: In the liver
Half-life, adults: 2.3 hours
Elimination: In urine (75%) and feces (22%)

Usual Dosage Titrate carefully to desired effect
Children 2-12 years:
Premedication: I.M.: 0.088-0.165 mg/kg
Adjunct to general anesthesia: I.V. induction: 0.088-0.165 mg/kg
Nausea and vomiting: I.M., I.V.: 0.05-0.06 mg/kg/dose every 4-6 hours as needed
Postop antiemetic: I.V.: 0.01-0.03 mg/kg/dose every 6-8 hours as needed
Adults:
Premedication: I.M.: 2.5-10 mg 30-60 minutes preoperatively
Adjunct to general anesthesia: I.V. induction: 0.22-0.275 mg/kg; maintenance: 1.25-2.5 mg/dose
Alone in diagnostic procedures: I.M.: Initial: 2.5-10 mg 30-60 minutes before, then 1.25-2.5 mg if needed
Nausea and vomiting: I.M., I.V.: 2.5-5 mg/dose every 3-4 hours as needed

Administration Parenteral: Administer by slow I.V. injection over 2-5 minutes

Monitoring Parameters Blood pressure, heart rate, respiratory rate

Additional Information Does not possess analgesic effects; has little or no amnesic properties

Dosage Forms Injection: 2.5 mg/mL (1 mL, 2 mL)

References
Yaster M, Sola JE, Pegoli W Jr, et al, "The Night After Surgery: Postoperative Management of the Pediatric Outpatient - Surgical and Anesthetic Aspects," *Pediatr Clin North Am*, 1994, 41(1):199-220.

Droperidol and Fentanyl *(droe PER i dole & FEN ta nil)*

Related Information
Overdose and Toxicology *on page 1222*

Synonyms Fentanyl and Droperidol

Therapeutic Category Analgesic, Narcotic

Generic Available Yes

Use To produce and maintain analgesia and sedation during diagnostic or surgical procedures (neuroleptanalgesia and neuroleptanesthesia); adjunct to general anesthesia

Restrictions C-II

Pregnancy Risk Factor C

Contraindications Hypersensitivity to droperidol, any component, or fentanyl; patients who have taken MAO inhibitors within 14 days

Warnings Rapid I.V. injection can cause muscle rigidity, particularly involving the muscles of respiration

Precautions Use with caution in patients with impaired hepatic, renal, or respiratory function and those with pre-existing cardiac bradyarrhythmias

Adverse Reactions
Cardiovascular: Hypotension, hypertension, bradycardia
Central nervous system: Postoperative drowsiness, dysphoria, disorientation, restlessness, delirium, extrapyramidal symptoms, hypothermia
Endocrine & metabolic: Hyperglycemia
Gastrointestinal: Nausea, vomiting
Neuromuscular & skeletal: Muscular rigidity
Ocular: Miosis
Respiratory: Respiratory depression, apnea, laryngospasm, bronchospasm
Miscellaneous: Shivering

Drug Interactions Fentanyl is a cytochrome P-450 isoenzyme CYP3A3/4 substrate CNS depressant drugs may have additive effects; MAO inhibitors may cause hypertensive crisis

Mechanism of Action See individual monographs for Droperidol *on page 365* and Fentanyl *on page 422*

Usual Dosage

Children:

Premedication: I.M.: 0.03 mL/kg (maximum dose: 2 mL) 30-60 minutes prior to procedure

Adjunct to general anesthesia: I.V.: Total dose: 0.05 mL/kg as slow infusion (1 mL/ 1-2 minutes) until sleep occurs

Adults:

Premedication: I.M.: 0.5-2 mL 30-60 minutes prior to surgery

Adjunct to general anesthesia: I.V.: 0.09-0.11 mL/kg as slow infusion (1 mL/1-2 minutes) until sleep occurs

Administration Parenteral: I.V.: Infuse slowly at a rate of 1 mL per 1-2 minutes

Monitoring Parameters Vital signs, oxygen saturation, blood pressure

Nursing Implications An opioid antagonist, resuscitative and intubation equipment, and oxygen should be available

Dosage Forms Injection: Droperidol 2.5 mg and fentanyl 50 mcg per mL (2 mL, 5 mL)

♦ **Drotic® Otic** see Neomycin, (Bacitracin) Polymyxin B, and Hydrocortisone on page 705

♦ **Droxia™** see Hydroxyurea on page 514

♦ **Dr. Scholl's® Callus Remover [OTC]** see Salicylic Acid on page 886

♦ **Dr. Scholl's® Clear Away [OTC]** see Salicylic Acid on page 886

♦ **Dr. Scholl's® Corn Remover [OTC]** see Salicylic Acid on page 886

♦ **Drugs and Breast-Feeding** see page 1243

♦ **Dryox® Gel [OTC]** see Benzoyl Peroxide on page 136

♦ **Dryox® Wash [OTC]** see Benzoyl Peroxide on page 136

♦ **DSCG** see Cromolyn on page 273

♦ **DSMC Plus® [OTC]** see Docusate and Casanthranol on page 351

♦ **D-S-S® [OTC]** see Docusate on page 350

♦ **D-S-S Plus® [OTC]** see Docusate and Casanthranol on page 351

♦ **DSS With Casanthranol** see Docusate and Casanthranol on page 351

♦ **DTIC (Can)** see Dacarbazine on page 292

♦ **DTIC-Dome®** see Dacarbazine on page 292

♦ **DTO** see Opium Tincture on page 737

♦ **d-Tubocurarine** see Tubocurarine on page 992

♦ **Dulcolax® [OTC]** see Bisacodyl on page 143

♦ **Dull-C® [OTC]** see Ascorbic Acid on page 106

♦ **Duofilm® [OTC]** see Salicylic Acid on page 886

♦ **Duoforte (Can)** see Salicylic Acid on page 886

♦ **Duonalc-E (Can)** see Ethyl Alcohol on page 409

♦ **Duoplant® [OTC]** see Salicylic Acid on page 886

♦ **Duplex® T [OTC]** see Coal Tar on page 260

♦ **Duraclon™** see Clonidine on page 255

♦ **Duragesic®** see Fentanyl on page 422

♦ **Duralith (Can)** see Lithium on page 600

♦ **Duramist Plus® [OTC]** see Oxymetazoline on page 749

♦ **Duramorph®** see Morphine Sulfate on page 683

♦ **Duratears® [OTC]** see Ocular Lubricant on page 732

♦ **Duration® [OTC]** see Oxymetazoline on page 749

♦ **Duratuss® DM** see Guaifenesin and Dextromethorphan on page 487

♦ **Duratuss-G®** see Guaifenesin on page 485

♦ **Duricef®** see Cefadroxil Monohydrate on page 188

♦ **Duvoid (Can)** see Bethanechol on page 142

d-Xylose (dee ZYE lose)

U.S. Brand Names Xylo-Pfan® [OTC]

Synonyms Wood Sugar; Xylose

Therapeutic Category Diagnostic Agent, Intestinal Absorption

Generic Available No

Use Diagnostic agent used in the determination of intestinal disorders due to disease or injury, which result in carbohydrate malabsorption, such as celiac disease, malabsorptive enteropathy, giardiasis, and food- or protein-induced enterocolitis

Pregnancy Risk Factor Unknown

Contraindications Hypersensitivity to d-xylose or any component

(Continued)

367

d-Xylose *(Continued)*

Warnings False-positive results may occur in patients with renal impairment, dehydration, edema, massive ascites, iron deficiency, inadequate circulating blood volume, anemia, pernicious anemia, severe diarrhea, vomiting, gastric stasis, thyroid dysfunction, and massive overgrowth of intestinal bacteria due to abnormally low excretion of d-xylose

Adverse Reactions Gastrointestinal: Nausea, intestinal bloating, vomiting, cramping, abdominal discomfort, diarrhea

Drug Interactions Indomethacin and neomycin inhibit the intestinal absorption of d-xylose; aspirin inhibits the urinary excretion of d-xylose

Stability Store powder at room temperature in an airtight container

Mechanism of Action D-xylose is a 5 carbon monosaccharide which is absorbed from the small intestine; its mechanism of absorption is not completely understood, however, a small portion is absorbed via an active transport system as seen with glucose; it does not depend upon bile or pancreatic juices for absorption; measurement of d-xylose blood or urinary concentrations evaluates the extent of carbohydrate absorption

Pharmacokinetics

Absorption: Oral: 35% in the small intestine; absorption is dose-dependent (eg, 5 g doses are absorbed more readily than 25 g doses)

Distribution: 0.21-0.32 L/kg

Metabolism: Via Krebs cycle and phosphoglucuronic pathways to carbon dioxide, water, and unidentified metabolites

Elimination: 25% of 25 g dose or 35% of 5 g dose is excreted unchanged in urine within 5 hours; decreased rate of elimination and renal clearance may be observed in geriatric patients

Usual Dosage Oral: Give after fasting at least 4 hours in infants and overnight in children and adults (see Administration):

Infants and Children: 500 mg/kg or 14.5 g/m^2 or 5 g as a single dose; maximum dose: 25 g

Adults: 5 g or 25 g as a single dose

Administration Oral:

Infants and Children: Dissolve powder in sufficient water to result in 5% to 10% solution (50-100 mg/mL; eg, 25 g in 250-500 mL water)

Adults: Dissolve 5 g or 25 g in 200-300 mL water, then after the dose is taken, administer 200-400 mL water

Monitoring Parameters Blood and urinary d-xylose concentrations

Reference Range The following peak blood d-xylose concentration and urinary excretion values indicate **NORMAL** absorption of d-xylose: See tables

Patient Information Do not eat for at least 5 hours after the test; fluids may be consumed after the test; contact your physician if abdominal pain or discomfort is severe or continues for >5 hours

Dosage Forms Powder for oral solution: 25 g

References

Buts JP, Morin CL, Roy CC, et al, "One-Hour Blood Xylose Test: A Reliable Index of Small Bowel Function," *J Pediatr*, 1978, 92(5):729-33.

Peak Blood d-Xylose Concentration (mg/dL)

Time After Dose (minutes)	Infants/Children	Adults (after 5 g or 25 g dose)
30	≥15	–
60	≥20	≥30
120	≥20	≥30

ALTERNATIVE METHOD: If using 5 g dosage instead of dosage per weight: Measure blood d-xylose concentration (mg/dL) prior to administration (baseline) and 60 minutes after administration. Calculate corrected d-xylose blood value as follows:

$$\text{Corrected d-xylose blood value} = \frac{(\text{value at 60 min} - \text{baseline value}) \times \text{actual surface area}}{1.73}$$

NORMAL CORRECTED BLOOD VALUE = 9.8-20 mg/dL

Urinary Excretion

	Mean 5-hour excretion expressed as a percentage of ingested d-xylose*	
Infants/Children		Adults (after 25 g dose)
<6 mo	11% to 30%	
6-12 mo	20% to 32%	
1-3 y	20% to 42%	
3-10 y	25% to 45%	4.5 g total urinary excretion
>10 y	25% to 50%	
or % excretion > (0.2 x age/months) + 12		

*The lower the d-xylose blood or urine concentration findings, the greater the chance of intestinal disease or abnormal condition.

♦ **Dycill®** see Dicloxacillin on page 326

♦ **Dyclone®** see Dyclonine on page 369

Dyclonine (DYE kloe neen)

U.S. Brand Names Dyclone®; Sucrets® [OTC]

Canadian Brand Names Sucrets; Sucrets for Kids

Therapeutic Category Local Anesthetic, Oral

Generic Available No

Use As a local anesthetic prior to laryngoscopy, bronchoscopy, or endotracheal intubation; used topically for temporary relief of pain associated with oral mucosa, skin, episiotomy, or anogenital lesions; the 0.5% topical solution may be used to block the gag reflex, and to relieve the pain of oral ulcers or stomatitis; the lozenge is used for temporary relief of sore throat pain and gum irritation

Pregnancy Risk Factor C

Contraindications Hypersensitivity to chlorobutanol (preservative used in dyclonine), dyclonine, or any component

Warnings Resuscitative equipment, oxygen and resuscitative drugs should be immediately available when dyclonine topical solution is administered to mucous membranes; may impair swallowing and enhance the danger of aspiration

Precautions Use with caution in patients with sepsis or traumatized mucosa in the area of application to avoid rapid systemic absorption; use with caution in patients with shock or heart block

Adverse Reactions Excessive dosage and rapid absorption may result in adverse CNS and cardiovascular effects

Cardiovascular: Hypotension, bradycardia, cardiac arrest, edema

Central nervous system: Excitation, drowsiness, nervousness, dizziness, seizures

Dermatologic: Rash, urticaria

Local: Slight irritation and stinging may occur when applied

Ocular: Blurred vision

Respiratory: Respiratory arrest

Miscellaneous: Allergic reactions

Stability Store in tight, light-resistant container; avoid freezing

Mechanism of Action Blocks impulses at peripheral nerve endings in skin and mucous membranes by altering cell membrane permeability to ionic transfer

Pharmacodynamics

Onset of local anesthesia: 2-10 minutes

Duration: 30-60 minutes

Usual Dosage

Children and Adults:

Topical solution: Mouth sores: 5-10 mL of 0.5% or 1% to oral mucosa (swab or swish and then spit) 3-4 times/day as needed; maximum single dose: 200 mg (40 mL of 0.5% solution or 20 mL of 1% solution); solution may be diluted 1:1 with water

Bronchoscopy: Use 2 mL of the 1% solution or 4 mL of the 0.5% solution sprayed onto the larynx and trachea every 5 minutes for 2-3 applications until the reflex has been abolished

Children >3 years: Topical: Slowly dissolve 1 lozenge (1.2 mg) in mouth every 2 hours, if necessary

Children >12 years and Adults: Topical: Slowly dissolve 1 lozenge (3 mg) in mouth every 2 hours, if necessary

(Continued)

Dyclonine *(Continued)*

Administration Topical: Apply to mucous membranes of the mouth or throat area: food should not be ingested for 60 minutes following application in the mouth or throat area

Patient Information Do not chew lozenge; numbness of the tongue and buccal mucosa may result in increased risk of biting trauma; may impair swallowing

Nursing Implications Use the lowest dose needed to provide effective anesthesia; not for injection; do not apply nasally or to the eye

Dosage Forms

Lozenges, as hydrochloride: 1.2 mg, 3 mg

Solution, topical, as hydrochloride: 0.5% (30 mL); 1% (30 mL)

References

Carnel SB, Blakeslee DB, Oswald SG, et al, "Treatment of Radiation- and Chemotherapy-Induced Stomatitis," *Otolaryngol Head Neck Surg,* 1990, 102(4):326-30.

♦ **Dynacin®** *see* Doxycycline *on page 362*

♦ **Dyna-Hex® [OTC]** *see* Chlorhexidine Gluconate *on page 220*

♦ **Dynapen®** *see* Dicloxacillin *on page 326*

♦ **Dyrenium®** *see* Triamterene *on page 981*

♦ **EarSol® HC** *see* Hydrocortisone *on page 506*

♦ **Easprin®** *see* Aspirin *on page 109*

♦ **EC-Naprosyn®** *see* Naproxen *on page 699*

Econazole *(e KONE a zole)*

U.S. Brand Names Spectazole™

Canadian Brand Names Ecostatin

Therapeutic Category Antifungal Agent, Topical

Generic Available No

Use Topical treatment of tinea pedis, tinea cruris, tinea corporis, tinea versicolor, and cutaneous candidiasis

Pregnancy Risk Factor C

Contraindications Hypersensitivity to econazole or any component

Warnings Not for ophthalmic or intravaginal use

Precautions Discontinue the drug if sensitivity or chemical irritation occurs; cross-sensitization may occur with other imidazole derivatives (ie, clotrimazole, miconazole)

Adverse Reactions

Dermatologic: Pruritus, erythema, contact dermatitis

Local: Burning, stinging

Mechanism of Action Alters fungal cell wall membrane permeability; may interfere with RNA and protein synthesis, and lipid metabolism

Pharmacokinetics

Absorption: Following topical administration, <10% is percutaneously absorbed

Metabolism: In the liver to >20 metabolites

Elimination: <1% of an applied dose recovered in urine or feces

Usual Dosage Children and Adults: Topical:

Tinea cruris, corporis, pedis, and tinea versicolor: Apply once daily

Cutaneous candidiasis: Apply twice daily

Administration Topical: Apply a sufficient amount of cream to cover affected areas; do not apply to the eye or intravaginally

Patient Information For external use only

Additional Information Candidal infections and tinea cruris, versicolor, and corporis should be treated for 2 weeks and tinea pedis for 1 month; occasionally, longer treatment periods may be required

Dosage Forms Cream, as nitrate: 1% (15 g, 30 g, 85 g)

♦ **Econopred®** *see* Prednisolone *on page 821*

♦ **Econopred® Plus** *see* Prednisolone *on page 821*

♦ **Ecostatin (Can)** *see* Econazole *on page 370*

♦ **Ecotrin® [OTC]** *see* Aspirin *on page 109*

♦ **Ectosone (Can)** *see* Betamethasone *on page 140*

♦ **Edathamil Disodium** *see* Edetate Disodium *on page 372*

♦ **Edecrin®** *see* Ethacrynic Acid *on page 404*

Edetate Calcium Disodium (ED e tate KAL see um dye SOW dee um)

U.S. Brand Names Calcium Disodium Versenate®

Synonyms Calcium Disodium Edathamil; Calcium Disodium Edetate; Calcium Edetate; Calcium EDTA

Therapeutic Category Antidote, Lead Toxicity; Chelating Agent, Parenteral

Generic Available No

Use Treatment of acute and chronic lead poisoning; also used as an aid in the diagnosis of lead poisoning

Pregnancy Risk Factor B

Contraindications Severe renal disease, anuria

Warnings Do not exceed recommended daily dose; avoid rapid I.V. infusion in the management of lead encephalopathy, intracranial pressure may be increased to lethal levels; I.M. administration is the preferred route in these patients; if anuria, increasing proteinuria, or hematuria occurs during therapy, discontinue calcium EDTA

Precautions Renal tubular necrosis and fatal nephrosis may occur, especially with high doses; establish urine flow prior to administration

Adverse Reactions

Cardiovascular: Hypotension, arrhythmias, EKG changes

Central nervous system: Fever, headache, chills

Dermatologic: Skin lesions, cheilosis

Endocrine & metabolic: Hypercalcemia, zinc deficiency

Gastrointestinal: GI upset, anorexia, nausea, vomiting

Hematologic: Transient marrow suppression, anemia

Hepatic: Mild elevation in liver function tests

Local: Pain at injection site following I.M. injection, thrombophlebitis following I.V. infusion (when concentration >5 mg/mL)

Neuromuscular & skeletal: Arthralgia, tremor, numbness, paresthesia

Ocular: Lacrimation

Renal: Renal tubular necrosis, proteinuria, microscopic hematuria

Respiratory: Sneezing, nasal congestion

Drug Interactions Do not use simultaneously with zinc insulin preparations

Stability Dilute with NS or D_5W; physically incompatible with $D_{10}W$, LR; do not mix in the same syringe with dimercaprol

Mechanism of Action Calcium is displaced by divalent and trivalent heavy metals, forming a nonionizing soluble complex that is excreted in the urine

Pharmacodynamics

Onset of chelation with I.V. administration: 1 hour

Peak excretion of chelated lead with I.V. administration: 24-48 hours

Pharmacokinetics

Absorption: I.M., S.C.: Well absorbed

Distribution: Into extracellular fluid; minimal CSF penetration

Half-life, plasma:

I.M.: 1.5 hours

I.V.: 20 minutes

Elimination: Rapid in urine as metal chelates or unchanged drug

Usual Dosage Several regimens have been recommended:

Diagnosis of lead poisoning: Mobilization test (not recommended by AAP guidelines): I.M., I.V.:

Children: 500 mg/m²/dose, (maximum dose: 1 g) as a single dose or divided into 2 doses

Adults: 500 mg/m²/dose

Note: Urine is collected for 24 hours after first EDTA dose and analyzed for lead content; if the ratio of mcg of lead in urine to mg calcium EDTA given is >1, then test is considered positive; for convenience, an 8-hour urine collection may be done after a single 50 mg/kg I.M. (maximum dose: 1 g) or 500 mg/m² I.V. dose; a positive test occurs if the ratio of lead excretion to mg calcium EDTA >0.5-0.6.

Treatment of lead poisoning: Children and Adults (each regimen is specific for route):

Symptoms of lead encephalopathy and/or blood lead level >70 mcg/dL: Treat 5 days; give in conjunction with dimercaprol; wait a minimum of 2 days with no treatment before considering a repeat course:

I.M.: 250 mg/m²/dose every 4 hours

I.V.: 50 mg/kg/day as 24-hour continuous I.V. infusion **or** 1-1.5 g/m² I.V. as either an 8- to 24-hour infusion or divided into 2 doses every 12 hours

(Continued)

Edetate Calcium Disodium *(Continued)*

Symptomatic lead poisoning **without** encephalopathy **or** asymptomatic with blood lead level >70 mcg/dL: Treat 3-5 days; treatment with dimercaprol is recommended until the blood lead level concentration <50 mcg/dL:

I.M.: 167 mg/m^2 every 4 hours

I.V.: 1 g/m^2 as an 8- to 24-hour infusion or divided every 12 hours

Asymptomatic **children** with blood lead level 45-69 mcg/dL: I.V.: 25 mg/kg/day for 5 days as an 8- to 24-hour infusion or divided into 2 doses every 12 hours

Depending upon the blood lead level, additional courses may be necessary; repeat at least 2-4 days and preferably 2-4 weeks apart

Adults with lead nephropathy: An alternative dosing regimen reflecting the reduction in renal clearance is based upon the serum creatinine (see table):

Alternative Dosing Regimen for Adults With Lead Nephropathy

Serum Creatinine (mg/dL)	Ca EDTA dosage
≤2	1 g/m^2/day for 5 days
>2-3	500 mg/m^2/day for 5 days
>3-4	500 mg/m^2/dose every 48 hours for 3 doses
>4	500 mg/m^2/week

Repeat these regimens monthly until lead excretion is reduced toward normal.

Administration Parenteral:

Intermittent I.V. infusion: Administer the dose I.V. over at least 1 hour in asymptomatic patients, 2 hours in symptomatic patients

Single daily I.V. continuous infusion: Dilute to 2-4 mg/mL in D$_5$W or NS and infuse over at least 8 hours, usually over 12-24 hours

I.M. injection: To minimize pain at the injection site, 1.67 mL of 2% procaine may be added to 5 mL calcium EDTA, resulting in 150 mg/mL concentration with 0.5% procaine (stable 3 months; see Nahata, 1997)

Monitoring Parameters BUN, serum creatinine, urinalysis, fluid balance, EKG, blood and urine lead concentrations

Test Interactions If calcium EDTA is given as a continuous I.V. infusion, stop the infusion for at least 1 hour before blood is drawn for lead concentration to avoid a falsely elevated value

Dosage Forms Injection: 200 mg/mL (5 mL)

References

American Academy of Pediatrics Committee on Drugs, "Treatment Guidelines for Lead Exposure in Children," *Pediatrics*, 1995, 96(1 Pt 1):155-60.

Nahata MC and Hipple TF, *Pediatric Drug Formulations*, 3rd ed, Cincinnati, OH: Harvey Whitney Books Co, 1997.

Edetate Disodium *(ED e tate dye SOW dee um)*

U.S. Brand Names Endrate®

Synonyms Edathamil Disodium; EDTA; Sodium Edetate

Therapeutic Category Antidote, Hypercalcemia; Chelating Agent, Parenteral

Generic Available Yes

Use Emergency treatment of hypercalcemia; control digitalis-induced cardiac dysrhythmias (ventricular arrhythmias)

Pregnancy Risk Factor C

Contraindications Severe renal failure or anuria, hypocalcemia, patients with active tuberculosis or healed calcified tubercular lesions

Warnings Use of this drug is recommended only when the severity of the clinical condition justifies the aggressive measures associated with this type of therapy. Use with caution in patients with intracranial lesions, seizure disorders, coronary or peripheral vascular disease; cardiac function should be evaluated prior to therapy

Precautions Sudden, precipitous decreases of serum calcium may occur, a source of I.V. calcium replacement should be readily available; blood sugar and insulin requirements may be lower when used in insulin-dependent diabetics

Adverse Reactions

Cardiovascular: Arrhythmias, hypotension

Central nervous system: Seizures, headache, chills, fever

Dermatologic: Skin eruptions

Endocrine/metabolic: Hypomagnesemia, hypokalemia, hypocalcemia, hyperuricemia

Gastrointestinal: Vomiting, diarrhea, abdominal cramps

Genitourinary: Urinary urgency, dysuria

Hematologic: Anemia

Local: Thrombophlebitis, pain at injection site

Neuromuscular & skeletal: Back pain, muscle cramps, paresthesia, tetany

Renal: Nephrotoxicity, acute tubular necrosis, polyuria, oliguria, glucosuria

Respiratory: Respiratory arrest

Drug Interactions May reduce insulin requirements in diabetic patients treated with insulin

Stability Physically compatible with dextrose and saline I.V. solutions

Mechanism of Action Chelates with divalent or trivalent metals to form a soluble complex that is then eliminated in urine

Pharmacokinetics

Metabolism: Not metabolized

Half-life: 20-60 minutes

Elimination: Following chelation, 95% excreted in urine as chelates within 24-48 hours

Usual Dosage I.V.:

Hypercalcemia:

Children: 40-70 mg/kg/day slow infusion over 3-4 hours or more to a maximum of 3 g/24 hours; administer for 5 days and allow 5 days between courses of therapy **or** 50 mg/kg **or** 1.5 g/m^2 as a single dose

Adults: 50 mg/kg/day over 3 or more hours to a maximum of 3 g/24 hours; administer for 5 days followed by 2 days without drug and repeat course up to 15 total doses

Digitalis-induced arrhythmias: Children and Adults: 15 mg/kg/hour (maximum dose: 60 mg/kg/day) as continuous infusion

Administration Parenteral: I.V.: Must be diluted before I.V. use in D$_5$W or NS to a maximum concentration of 30 mg/mL (3%) and infused over at least 3 hours; avoid extravasation; **not for I.M. use**

Monitoring Parameters Serum and urine electrolytes (including calcium and magnesium), blood pressure (during infusion), renal function (before and during therapy), liver function, EKG

Test Interactions Colorimetric, oxalate, or other precipitation methods for measuring serum calcium

Nursing Implications Patient should remain supine for a short period after infusion

Additional Information Sodium content of 1 g: 5.4 mEq

Dosage Forms Injection: 150 mg/mL (20 mL)

♦ **Edex® Injection** see Alprostadil on page 56

♦ **Ed-In-SOL® [OTC]** see Iron Supplements (Oral/Enteral) on page 548

Edrophonium (ed roe FOE nee um)

Related Information

Overdose and Toxicology on page 1222

U.S. Brand Names Enlon®; Reversol®; Tensilon®

Therapeutic Category Antidote, Neuromuscular Blocking Agent; Cholinergic Agent; Diagnostic Agent, Myasthenia Gravis

Generic Available No

Use Diagnosis of myasthenia gravis; differentiation of cholinergic crises from myasthenia crises; reversal of nondepolarizing neuromuscular blockers; treatment of paroxysmal atrial tachycardia

Pregnancy Risk Factor C

Contraindications Hypersensitivity to edrophonium or any component (injection contains sodium sulfite and phenol); GI or GU mechanical obstruction

Warnings Overdosage can cause cholinergic crisis which may be fatal; I.V. atropine should be readily available for treatment of cholinergic reactions; contains sodium sulfite; avoid use in sensitive individuals

Precautions Use with caution in asthmatic patients and those receiving a cardiac glycoside

Adverse Reactions

Cardiovascular: Arrhythmias (especially bradycardia), hypotension, A-V block

Central nervous system: Seizures, drowsiness, headache, dysphoria

Gastrointestinal: Nausea, vomiting, diarrhea, excessive salivation, stomach cramps

Genitourinary: Urinary frequency

Local: Thrombophlebitis

Neuromuscular & skeletal: Weakness, muscle cramps, muscle spasms

Ocular: Diplopia, miosis, lacrimation

Respiratory: Laryngospasm, bronchospasm, respiratory paralysis, increased bronchial secretions

(Continued)

Edrophonium *(Continued)*

Miscellaneous: Diaphoresis, hypersensitivity reactions

Drug Interactions Digoxin may enhance bradycardia potential of edrophonium; succinylcholine and decamethonium effects are prolonged by edrophonium; quinidine may antagonize effects of edrophonium; antagonizes effects of nondepolarizing muscle relaxants (eg, pancuronium, vecuronium)

Mechanism of Action Inhibits destruction of acetylcholine by acetylcholinesterase. This facilitates transmission of impulses across myoneural junction and results in increased cholinergic responses such as miosis, increased tonus of intestinal and skeletal muscles, bronchial and ureteral constriction, bradycardia, and increased salivary and sweat gland secretions

Pharmacodynamics
Onset:
I.M.: 2-10 minutes
I.V.: 30-60 seconds
Duration:
I.M.: 5-30 minutes
I.V.: 5-10 minutes

Usual Dosage Usually administered I.V., however, if not possible, I.M. or S.C. may be used

Infants: Diagnosis of myasthenia gravis: Initial:
I.M.: 0.5-1 mg
I.V.: Initial: 0.1 mg, followed by 0.4 mg (if no response); total dose = 0.5 mg
Children:
Diagnosis of myasthenia gravis: Initial:
I.M.: ≤34 kg: 2 mg; >34 kg: 5 mg
I.V.: 0.04 mg/kg given over 1 minute followed by 0.16 mg/kg given within 45 seconds (if no response) (maximum dose: 10 mg total)
Titration of oral anticholinesterase therapy: I.V.: 0.04 mg/kg once given 1 hour after oral intake of the drug being used in treatment; if strength improves, an increase in neostigmine or pyridostigmine dose is indicated
Adults:
Diagnosis of myasthenia gravis: Initial:
I.M.: Initial: 10 mg; if no cholinergic reaction occurs, administer 2 mg 30 minutes later to rule out false-negative reaction
I.V.: 2 mg test dose administered over 15-30 seconds; 8 mg given 45 seconds later (if no response is seen); test dose may be repeated after 30 minutes.
Titration of oral anticholinesterase therapy: I.V.: 1-2 mg given 1 hour after oral dose of anticholinesterase; if strength improves, an increase in neostigmine or pyridostigmine dose is indicated
Differentiation of cholinergic from myasthenic crisis: I.V.: 1 mg, may repeat after 1 minute (**Note:** Intubation and controlled ventilation may be required if patient has cholinergic crises.)
Reversal of nondepolarizing neuromuscular blocking agents (neostigmine with atropine usually preferred): I.V.: 10 mg over 30-45 seconds, may repeat every 5-10 minutes up to 40 mg total dose
Termination of paroxysmal atrial tachycardia: I.V.: 5-10 mg
Dosing adjustment in renal impairment: Dose may need to be reduced in patients with chronic renal failure

Administration Parenteral: Edrophonium is administered by direct I.V. or I.M. injection; see Usual Dosage

Monitoring Parameters Pre-. and postinjection strength (cranial musculature is most useful); heart rate, respiratory rate, blood pressure, changes in fasciculations

Dosage Forms Injection, as chloride: 10 mg/mL (1 mL, 10 mL, 15 mL)

♦ **ED-SPAZ®** *see* Hyoscyamine *on page 517*
♦ **EDTA** *see* Edetate Disodium *on page 372*
♦ **E.E.S.®** *see* Erythromycin *on page 394*
♦ **E.E.S. 400®** *see* Erythromycin *on page 394*
♦ **E.E.S.® Chewable** *see* Erythromycin *on page 394*
♦ **E.E.S.® Granules** *see* Erythromycin *on page 394*
♦ **EFA Steri (Can)** *see* Sodium Chloride *on page 906*

Efavirenz *(eh FAH vih rehnz)*

Related Information
Adult and Adolescent HIV *on page 1166*
Pediatric HIV *on page 1162*

U.S. Brand Names Sustiva™

Therapeutic Category Antiretroviral Agent; HIV Agents (Anti-HIV Agents); Non-nucleoside Reverse Transcriptase Inhibitor (NNRTI)

Generic Available No

Use Treatment of HIV-1 infection in combination with other antiretroviral agents. (**Note:** HIV regimens consisting of **three** antiretroviral agents are strongly recommended)

Pregnancy Risk Factor C

Contraindications Hypersensitivity to efavirenz or any component; concurrent therapy with astemizole, cisapride, midazolam, triazolam, or ergot derivatives

Warnings Efavirenz is a mixed inducer/inhibitor of CYP450 enzymes and numerous drug interactions occur. Due to potential serious and/or life-threatening drug interactions, certain drugs are contraindicated (see Contraindications and Drug Interactions). Resistance emerges rapidly if administered as monotherapy; always use efavirenz in combination with at least two other antiretroviral agents; do not add efavirenz as a single agent to antiretroviral regimens that are failing; initiate in combination with at least one other antiretroviral agent to which the patient is naive.

Precautions Use with caution in patients with a history of mental illness or substance abuse (delusions, inappropriate behavior, and severe acute depression may occur); serious CNS and psychiatric symptoms may occur (see Adverse Effects); discontinue if severe rash (involving blistering, desquamation, mucosal involvement, or fever) occurs; rash is more common and more severe in children versus adults, **consider prophylaxis with antihistamines in children**; use with caution in patients with known or suspected hepatitis B or C, those receiving other hepatotoxic medications, and those with hepatic impairment; weigh risk versus benefit in patients with persistent elevations of serum transaminases (ie, >5 times normal); cross resistance with other non-nucleoside reverse transcriptase inhibitors may occur

Adverse Reactions

Central nervous system: (Note: Overall incidence of CNS adverse effects was 53% versus 25% in controls; CNS effects in children have been reported in one study to be 9%) somnolence, dizziness, drowsiness, abnormal dreams, insomnia, confusion, headache, hypoesthesia, impaired concentration, abnormal thinking, agitation, amnesia, depersonalization, euphoria, hallucinations, delusions, inappropriate behavior; fever (children 26%); anxiety, nervousness; serious psychiatric adverse effects (patients with history of psychiatric disorders may be at greater risk): Suicidal ideation/attempts, severe acute depression, aggressive behavior, paranoid reactions, manic reactions

Dermatologic: Rash, usually pruritic maculopapular skin eruptions (incidence: children 40%, adults 26%; median onset, adults: 11 days, children: 9 days [range 6-205 days], **Note:** Most rashes in children appeared within 14 days after starting therapy; median duration, adults: 16 days, children: 6 days [range 2-37 days], **Note:** Median duration of rash in children who continued therapy was 9 days; rash may be treated with antihistamines and corticosteroids and usually resolves within one month while continuing therapy; **Note:** Blistering, desquamation, fever, mucosal involvement, or ulceration may occur and requires discontinuation of drug, see Precautions); pruritus, increased sweating

Endocrine & metabolic: Hypercholesterolemia, hypertriglyceridemia

Gastrointestinal: Nausea or vomiting (children 16%), diarrhea/loose stools (children 39%), abdominal pain, asymptomatic elevations in serum amylase, pancreatitis (several cases)

Hepatic: Elevated liver enzymes (patients with hepatitis B or C may be at greater risk)

Respiratory: Cough (children 25%)

Miscellaneous: Alcohol intolerance

Drug Interactions Cytochrome P-450 isoenzyme CYP3A4 and CYP2B6 substrate; mixed inducer/inhibitor of CYP450 enzymes: Induces CYP3A4 and inhibits isoenzymes CYP2C9, 2C19, and 3A4

Concurrent use of efavirenz with astemizole, cisapride, midazolam, triazolam, or ergot derivatives is contraindicated (efavirenz may inhibit the metabolism of these drugs and result in serious or life-threatening effects); efavirenz decreases serum concentrations of indinavir (indinavir dosage increase is recommended), saquinavir (use of saquinavir as sole protease inhibitor with efavirenz is not recommended), amprenavir, and clarithromycin; efavirenz increases serum concentrations of nelfinavir, ritonavir, ethinyl estradiol, and 14-hydroxy metabolite of clarithromycin; efavirenz may increase or decrease the effects of warfarin

Saquinavir, rifampin, rifabutin, phenobarbital and other enzyme inducing agents may decrease efavirenz serum concentrations; the herbal medicine, St John's wort

(Continued)

Efavirenz *(Continued)*

(*Hypericum perforatum*) may significantly decrease concentrations of efavirenz and is not recommended for concurrent use; ritonavir may increase efavirenz AUC by 20%; alcohol or other CNS depressants may increase adverse effects; rash may be more common when efavirenz is used with clarithromycin (consider azithromycin use); interaction with oral contraceptives is not fully characterized (use reliable barrier method)

Food Interactions Food does not usually effect bioavailability; high fat meals increase bioavailability by 50%

Stability Store at room temperature

Mechanism of Action A non-nucleoside reverse transcriptase inhibitor which specifically binds to HIV-1 reverse transcriptase and blocks RNA-dependent and DNA-dependent DNA polymerase activity including HIV-1 replication; does not require intracellular phosphorylation for antiviral activity

Pharmacokinetics Note: Pharmacokinetics in children ≥3 years of age are thought to be similar to adults

Distribution: CSF concentrations are 0.69% of plasma (range 0.26% to 1.2%); however, CSF: Plasma concentration ratio is 3 times higher than free fraction in plasma

Protein binding: 99.5% to 99.8%, primarily to albumin

Metabolism: In the liver, primarily by cytochrome P-450 enzymes (mainly isoenzymes CYP3A4 and CYP2B6) to hydroxylated metabolites which then undergo glucuronidation; induces P-450 enzymes and it's own metabolism

Bioavailability: 42% (increased with fatty meal)

Half-life, adults:

Single dose: 52-76 hours

Multiple dose: 40-55 hours

Time to peak concentration: 3-5 hours

Elimination: <1% excreted unchanged in the urine; 14% to 34% excreted as metabolites in the urine and 16% to 61% in feces (primarily as unchanged drug)

Usual Dosage Oral: (use in combination with other antiretroviral agents)

Neonates, Infants, and Children <3 years: Not approved for use (no information available)

Children ≥3 years: Dose according to body weight:

10 kg to <15 kg: 200 mg once daily

15 kg to <20 kg: 250 mg once daily

20 kg to <25 kg: 300 mg once daily

25 kg to <32.5 kg: 350 mg once daily

32.5 kg to <40 kg: 400 mg once daily

≥40 kg: 600 mg once daily

Adults: 600 mg once daily

Administration Administer dose at bedtime to decrease CNS adverse effects (especially during the first 2-4 weeks of therapy); may be administered without regard to food; avoid administration with high fat meals; capsules may be opened and added to food or liquids, but efavirenz tastes peppery (grape jelly may be used to improve taste)

Monitoring Parameters Signs and symptoms of rash; viral load; CD4 counts; serum amylase; liver enzymes in patients with known or suspected hepatitis B or C, those receiving concomitant ritonavir, and those receiving other hepatotoxic medications; serum cholesterol, triglycerides

Test Interactions False positive test for cannabinoids using the CEDIA DAU Multilevel THC assay

Patient Information May cause drowsiness and impair ability to perform activities requiring mental alertness or physical coordination; avoid alcohol; efavirenz is not a cure for HIV; notify physician immediately if rash develops; report the use of other medications, nonprescription medications and herbal or natural products to your physician and pharmacist; take efavirenz everyday as prescribed; do not change dose or discontinue without physician's advice; if a dose is missed, take it as soon as possible, then return to normal dosing schedule; if a dose is skipped, do **not** double the next dose

Additional Information An oral liquid formulation of efavirenz (strawberry/mint-flavored solution) is available on an investigational basis from DuPont Pharmaceuticals Company as part of an expanded access program for HIV-infected children and adolescents 3-16 years of age.

Dosage Forms Capsule: 50 mg, 100 mg, 200 mg

References

Adkins JC and Noble S, "Efavirenz," *Drugs*, 1998, 56(6):1055-64.

Collura JM and Kraus DM, "New Pediatric Antiretroviral Agents," *J Pediatr Health Care*, 2000, 14(4):183-90.

Panel on Clinical Practices for Treatment of HIV Infection, "Guidelines for the Use of Antiretroviral Agents in HIV-Infected Adults and Adolescents," April 23, 2001, http://www.hivatis.org.

Piscitelli SC, Burstein AH, Chaitt D, et al, "Indinavir Concentrations and St John's Wort," *Lancet*, 2000, 355(9203):547-8.

Starr SE, Fletcher CV, Spector SA, et al, "Combination Therapy With Efavirenz, Nelfinavir, and Nucleoside Reverse-transcriptase Inhibitors in Children Infected with Human Immunodeficiency Virus Type 1. Pediatric AIDS Clinical Trials Group 382 Team," *N Engl J Med* 1999, 341(25):1874-81.

Working Group on Antiretroviral Therapy and Medical Management of HIV-Infected Children, "Guidelines for the Use of Antiretroviral Agents in Pediatric HIV Infection," January 7, 2000, http://www.hivatis.org.

♦ **Effer-K**™ *see* Potassium Supplements *on page 816*

♦ **Efidac/24® [OTC]** *see* Pseudoephedrine *on page 852*

♦ **Eflone**™ *see* Fluorometholone *on page 443*

♦ **Efudex®** *see* Fluorouracil *on page 444*

♦ **Egozinc (Can)** *see* Zinc Oxide *on page 1026*

♦ **EHDP** *see* Etidronate Disodium *on page 411*

♦ **ELA-Max® [OTC]** *see* Lidocaine *on page 590*

♦ **ELA-Max® 5 [OTC]** *see* Lidocaine *on page 590*

♦ **Elavil®** *see* Amitriptyline *on page 77*

♦ **Electrolyte Lavage Solution** *see* Polyethylene Glycol-Electrolyte Solution *on page 811*

♦ **Elimite**™ **Cream** *see* Permethrin *on page 783*

♦ **Elixophyllin®** *see* Theophylline *on page 943*

♦ **Elspar®** *see* Asparaginase *on page 107*

♦ **Eltor 120 (Can)** *see* Pseudoephedrine *on page 852*

♦ **Eltroxin (Can)** *see* Levothyroxine *on page 588*

♦ **Emergency Pediatric Drip Calculations** *see page 1033*

♦ **Emetogenic Potential of Single Chemotherapeutic Agents** *see page 1129*

♦ **Emgel®** *see* Erythromycin *on page 394*

♦ **EMLA®** *see* Lidocaine and Prilocaine *on page 594*

♦ **Emo-Cort (Can)** *see* Hydrocortisone *on page 506*

♦ **Empirin® [OTC]** *see* Aspirin *on page 109*

♦ **Empracet (Can)** *see* Acetaminophen and Codeine *on page 31*

♦ **Empracet® 30, 60 (Can)** *see* Acetaminophen and Codeine *on page 31*

♦ **Emtec-30 (Can)** *see* Acetaminophen and Codeine *on page 31*

♦ **Emulsoil® [OTC]** *see* Castor Oil *on page 186*

♦ **E-Mycin®** *see* Erythromycin *on page 394*

♦ **E-Mycin-E®** *see* Erythromycin *on page 394*

Enalapril/Enalaprilat (e NAL a pril/e NAL a pril at)

U.S. Brand Names Vasotec®; Vasotec® I.V.

Canadian Brand Names Apo-Enalapril

Therapeutic Category Angiotensin-Converting Enzyme (ACE) Inhibitor; Antihypertensive Agent

Generic Available Yes

Use Management of mild to severe hypertension, CHF, and asymptomatic left ventricular dysfunction; has also been used to treat proteinuria in steroid-resistant nephrotic syndrome patients (see Additional Information)

Pregnancy Risk Factor C (1st trimester); D (may cause injury and death to the developing fetus when used during the 2nd and 3rd trimesters of pregnancy)

Contraindications Hypersensitivity to enalapril, enalaprilat, any component, or other ACE inhibitors; patients with idiopathic or hereditary angioedema or a history of angioedema with ACE inhibitors

Warnings Serious adverse effects including angioedema, anaphylactoid reactions, neutropenia, agranulocytosis, hypotension, and hepatic failure may occur (see Adverse Reactions); risk of neutropenia may be increased in patients with renal dysfunction and especially in patients with both collagen vascular disease and renal dysfunction

Precautions Use with caution and modify dosage in patients with renal impairment, especially renal artery stenosis; elevated BUN and S_{cr} may occur in these patients; dosage reduction or discontinuation of enalapril or discontinuation of concomitant diuretic may be needed; use with caution and modify dosage in patients with hyponatremia, hypovolemia, severe CHF, left ventricular outflow tract obstruction, or with coadministered diuretic therapy; experience in children is limited; severe hypotension may occur in patients who are sodium and/or volume depleted, initiate lower doses and monitor closely when starting therapy in these patients; use with caution (Continued)

Enalapril/Enalaprilat (Continued)

in neonates; injectable product contains benzyl alcohol 9 mg/mL (benzyl alcohol is converted to benzoic acid which may displace bilirubin from protein binding sites and at larger doses can cause the gasping syndrome in neonates)

Adverse Reactions

Cardiovascular: Hypotension, syncope

Central nervous system: Fatigue, vertigo, insomnia, dizziness, headache

Dermatologic: Rash, angioedema. **Note:** The relative risk of angioedema with ACE inhibitors is higher within the first 30 days of use (compared to >1 year of use), for Black Americans (compared to Whites), for lisinopril or enalapril (compared to captopril), and for patients previously hospitalized within 30 days (Brown, 1996).

Endocrine & metabolic: Hypoglycemia, hyperkalemia

Gastrointestinal: Nausea, diarrhea, ageusia

Genitourinary: Impotence

Hematologic: Agranulocytosis, neutropenia, anemia

Hepatic: Cholestatic jaundice, fulminant hepatic necrosis (rare, but potentially fatal)

Neuromuscular & skeletal: Muscle cramps

Renal: Deterioration in renal function

Respiratory: Cough, dyspnea, eosinophilic pneumonitis; **Note:** An isolated dry cough lasting >3 weeks was reported in 7 of 42 pediatric patients (17%) receiving ACE inhibitors (see von Vigier, 2000)

Drug Interactions Cytochrome P-450 isoenzyme CYP3A3/4 substrate

Use with potassium-sparing diuretics may result in an additive hyperkalemic effect; diuretics or other antihypertensive agents may increase hypotensive effect; indomethacin or NSAIDs may decrease hypotensive effect; enalapril may increase lithium levels; use with NSAIDs in patients with compromised renal function may increase renal dysfunction (usually reversible)

Food Interactions Food does not affect absorption; limit salt substitutes or potassium-rich diet; avoid natural licorice (causes sodium and water retention and increases potassium loss)

Stability Store vials below 86°F (30°C); solutions for I.V. infusion mixed in NS, D_5W, D_5NS, or D_5LR are stable for 24 hours at room temperature

Mechanism of Action Competitive inhibitor of angiotensin-converting enzyme (ACE); prevents conversion of angiotensin I to angiotensin II, a potent vasoconstrictor; results in lower levels of angiotensin II which causes an increase in plasma renin activity and a reduction in aldosterone secretion

Pharmacodynamics (Antihypertensive effect)

Onset of action:

Oral: Within 1 hour

I.V.: Within 15 minutes

Maximum effect:

Oral: Within 4-8 hours

I.V.: Within 1-4 hour

Duration:

Oral: 12-24 hours

I.V.: Dose dependent, usually 4-6 hours

Pharmacokinetics

Absorption: Oral: 55% to 75% (enalapril)

Protein binding: 50% to 60%

Metabolism: Enalapril is a prodrug (inactive) and undergoes biotransformation to enalaprilat (active) in the liver

Half-life:

Enalapril:

CHF neonates 10-19 days of age (n=3): 10.3 hours (range: 4.2-13.4 hours)

CHF: Infants >27 days and Children ≤6.5 years of age (n=11): 2.7 hours (range: 1.3-6.3 hours)

Healthy adults: 2 hours

CHF adults: 3.4-5.8 hours

Enalaprilat:

CHF neonates 10-19 days of age (n=3): 11.9 hours (range 5.9-15.6 hours)

CHF: Infants >27 days and Children ≤6.5 years of age (n=11): 11.1 hours (range: 5.1-20.8 hours)

Infants 6 weeks to 8 months: 6-10 hours

Adults: 35-38 hours

Time to peak serum concentration: Oral:

Enalapril: Within 0.5-1.5 hours

Enalaprilat (active): Within 3-4.5 hours

Elimination: Principally in urine (60% to 80%) with some fecal excretion

Usual Dosage Use lower listed initial dose in patients with hyponatremia, hypovolemia, severe CHF, decreased renal function, or in those receiving diuretics

Manufacturer's recommendations: Pediatric hypertensive patients: Oral: **Enalapril:** Initial: 0.08 mg/kg once daily (maximum dose: 5 mg); adjust dose according to blood pressure readings; doses >0.58 mg/kg (or >40 mg) have not been studied

Alternative pediatric dosing:

Neonates:

Oral: **Enalapril:** Initial: 0.1 mg/kg/day given every 24 hours; increase dose and interval as required every few days (see Additional Information)

I.V.: **Enalaprilat:** 5-10 mcg/kg/dose administered every 8-24 hours (as determined by blood pressure readings) has been used for the treatment of neonatal hypertension; monitor patients carefully; select patients may require higher doses

Infants and Children:

Oral: **Enalapril:** Initial: 0.1 mg/kg/day in 1-2 divided doses; increase as required over 2 weeks to maximum of 0.5 mg/kg/day; mean dose required for CHF improvement in 39 children (9 days to 17 years of age) was 0.36 mg/kg/day; investigationally, select individuals have been treated with doses up to 0.94 mg/kg/day (Leversha, 1994)

I.V.: **Enalaprilat:** 5-10 mcg/kg/dose administered every 8-24 hours (as determined by blood pressure readings); monitor patients carefully; select patients may require higher doses

Adolescents and Adults:

Oral: **Enalapril:** Initial: 2.5-5 mg/day then increase as required; usual dose for hypertension: 10-40 mg/day in 1-2 divided doses; usual dose for CHF: 5-20 mg/day in 2 divided doses; maximum dose: 40 mg/day

Asymptomatic left ventricular dysfunction: Initial: 2.5 mg twice daily; increase as tolerated; usual dose: 20 mg/day in 2 divided doses

I.V.: **Enalaprilat:** 0.625-1.25 mg/dose every 6 hours; doses as high as 5 mg/dose every 6 hours have been tolerated for up to 36 hours; little experience with doses >20 mg/day

Dosing adjustment in renal impairment: Note: Use in neonates and children ≤16 years of age with GFR <30 mL/min/1.73 m^2 is not recommended (no dosing data exists)

Cl_{cr} 10-50 mL/minute: Administer 75% to 100% of dose

Cl_{cr} <10 mL/minute: Administer 50% of dose

Administration

Oral: May administer without regard to food

Parenteral: I.V.: Administer as I.V. infusion (undiluted solution or further diluted) over 5 minutes; to deliver small I.V. doses, a dilution with NS to a final concentration of 25 mcg/mL can be made

Monitoring Parameters Blood pressure, renal function, WBC, serum potassium, serum glucose

Patient Information Limit alcohol; notify physician if vomiting, diarrhea, excessive perspiration, or dehydration occurs, or if swelling of face, lips, tongue, or difficulty in breathing occurs; do not use a salt substitute (potassium-containing) without physician advice

Nursing Implications Discontinue if angioedema occurs; observe closely for hypotension within 1-3 hours of first dose or with new higher dose

Additional Information Severe hypotension was reported in a **preterm** neonate (birth weight 835 g, gestational age 26 weeks, postnatal age 9 days) who was treated with enalapril 0.1 mg/kg orally; hypotension responded to I.V. plasma and dopamine; the authors suggest starting enalapril in preterm infants at 0.01 mg/kg and increasing upwards in a stepwise fashion with very close monitoring of blood pressure and urine output. However, in this case report, oral enalapril at doses of 0.01 mg/kg to 0.04 mg/kg did not adequately control blood pressure. Further studies are needed. (Schilder, 1995)

Over the years, several pediatric studies have examined the effects of ACE inhibitors on proteinuria. In a more recent retrospective study, enalapril (in doses of 2.5-5 mg/day) administered either as monotherapy (n=17; mean age: 13.7 years; range 8-17 years) or with prednisone (n=11; mean age: 12.6 years; range: 7-16 years), significantly decreased proteinuria in normotensive proteinuric children (with or without nephrotic syndrome); no significant change in blood pressure was observed (Sasinka, 1999). In a smaller study of children with persistent proteinuria (n=7; 6 with steroid resistant nephrotic syndrome; mean age: 13.5 years; range: 7-18 years), enalapril (at mean oral doses of 0.3 mg/kg/day) significantly reduced proteinuria in 5 of the 7 patients (Lama, 2000). Another recent study assessed the effects (Continued)

Enalapril/Enalaprilat *(Continued)*

of enalapril on urinary protein electrophoretic patterns in 13 children (mean age: 8 years; range: 1.8-12 years) with steroid resistant nephrotic syndrome; oral enalapril was initially dosed at 0.2 mg/kg/day (with a maximum dose of 30 mg/day); doses were increased each month by 0.1 mg/kg/day until the patients' urinary protein decreased by 50% from baseline; prednisone was added after 2 months in 11 of the 13 children at doses of 30 mg/m² given every other day; four patients had a complete remission of proteinuria after 4-12 months; an 80% decrease in urinary total protein and a 70% decrease in urinary albumin was observed in the other patients; the pattern of urinary protein shifted from a nonselective to an albumin-selective urinary protein loss in all patients; significant increases in plasma total protein and albumin occurred; it is important to note that 3 of the 13 patients (23%) required interruption of enalapril during transient acute renal failure due to an infectious disease (Delucchi, 2000). Further pediatric studies are needed to identify optimal enalapril oral doses and to establish safety and efficacy for this use.

Dosage Forms

Injection, as enalaprilat: 1.25 mg/mL (1 mL, 2 mL)

Tablet, as maleate: 2.5 mg, 5 mg, 10 mg, 20 mg

Extemporaneous Preparations

A 1 mg/mL oral suspension made from tablets, Bicitra®, and Ora-Sweet® SF is stable for 30 days when stored in a polyethylene terephthalate bottle under refrigeration (2°C to 8°C); place ten 20 mg tablets in a 200 mL polyethylene terephthalate bottle; add 50 mL of Bicitra®; shake well for at least 2 minutes; let stand for 1 hour then shake for one additional minute; add 150 mL of Ora-Sweet® SF and shake well; label "shake well" [Vasotec® tablets (package insert), 2001].

A 1 mg/mL oral liquid preparation made from tablets and 3 different vehicles (cherry syrup, a 1:1 mixture of Ora-Sweet® and Ora-Plus®, or a 1:1 mixture of Ora-Sweet® SF and Ora-Plus®) was stable for 60 days when stored in amber plastic prescription bottles in the dark at room temperature (25°C) or under refrigeration (5°C); grind six 20 mg tablets in a mortar into a fine powder; add 15 mL of the vehicle and mix well to form a uniform paste; mix while adding the vehicle in geometric proportions to **almost** 120 mL; transfer to a calibrated bottle and qsad with vehicle to 120 mL; label "shake well" and "protect from light" (Allen, 1998).

A 1 mg/mL oral liquid preparation made from tablets and 3 different vehicles (deionized water, citrate buffer solution at pH 5.0, or a 1:1 mixture of Ora-Sweet® and Ora-Plus®) was stable for 91 days when stored in plastic prescription bottles in the dark under refrigeration (4°C). When stored at room temperature (25°C), the preparations made in citrate buffer solution at pH 5.0 and the 1:1 mixture of Ora-Sweet® and Ora-Plus® were also stable for 91 days, but the preparation made in deionized water was stable for only 56 days. Grind twenty 10 mg tablets in a mortar; add a small amount of vehicle and mix well to form a smooth paste; mix while adding increasing amounts of the vehicle to make the mixture pourable; transfer to a graduated cylinder and qsad to 200 mL; **Note:** To prepare the isotonic citrate buffer solution (pH 5.0), see reference; label "shake well" and "protect from light" (Nahata, 1998).

A more dilute oral liquid preparation of 0.1 mg/mL made from tablets and an isotonic buffer solution at pH 5.0 was stable for 90 days when stored in amber, high density polyethylene bottles under refrigeration (5°C); grind one 20 mg tablet in a glass mortar into a fine powder; triturate with isotonic citrate buffer (pH 5.0) and filter; qsad to 200 mL with buffer solution; label "shake well" and "protect from light" (Boulton, 1994).

Allen LV and Erickson MA, "Stability of Alprazolam, Chloroquine Phosphate, Cisapride, Enalapril Maleate, and Hydralazine Hydrochloride in Extemporaneously Compounded Oral Liquids," *Am J Health Syst Pharm,* 1998, 55(18):1915-20.

Boulton DW, Woods DJ, Fawcett JP, et al, "The Stability of an Enalapril Maleate Oral Solution Prepared From Tablets," *Aust J Hosp Pharm,* 1994, 24(2):151-6.

Nahata MC, Morosco RS, and Hipple TF, "Stability of Enalapril Maleate in Three Extemporaneously Prepared Oral Liquids," *Am J Health Syst Pharm,* 1998, 55(11):1155-7.

Vasotec® (package insert), West Point, PA: Merck & Co., Inc; 2001.

References

Brown NJ, Ray WA, Snowden M, et al, "Black Americans Have an Increased Rate of Angiotensin-Converting Enzyme Inhibitor-Associated Angioedema," *Clin Pharmacol Ther,* 1996, 60(1):8-13.

Bult Y and van den Anker J, "Hypertension in a Preterm Infant Treated With Enalapril," *J Pediatr Pharm Pract,* 1997, 2(4):229-31.

Delucchi A, Cano F, Rodriguez E, et al, "Enalapril and Prednisone in Children With Nephrotic-Range Proteinuria," *Pediatr Nephrol,* 2000, 14(12):1088-91.

Frenneaux M, Stewart RA, Newman CM, et al, "Enalapril for Severe Heart Failure in Infancy," *Arch Dis Child,* 1989, 64(2):219-23.

Lama G, Luongo I, Piscitelli A, et al, "Enalapril: Antiproteinuric Effect in Children With Nephrotic Syndrome," *Clin Nephrol*, 2000, 53(6):432-6.

Leversha AM, Wilson NJ, Clarkson PM, et al, "Efficacy and Dosage of Enalapril in Congenital and Acquired Heart Disease," *Arch Dis Child*, 1994, 70(1):35-9.

Lloyd TR, Mahoney LT, Knoedel D, et al, "Orally Administered Enalapril for Infants With Congestive Heart Failure: A Dose Finding Study," *J Pediatr*, 1989, 114(4 Pt 1):650-4.

Marcadis ML, Kraus DM, Hatzopoulos FK, et al, "Use of Enalaprilat for Neonatal Hypertension," *J Pediatr*, 1991, 119(3):505-6.

Nakamura H, Ishii M, Sugimura T, et al, "The Kinetic Profiles of Enalapril and Enalaprilat and Their Possible Developmental Changes in Pediatric Patients With Congestive Heart Failure," *Clin Pharmacol Ther*, 1994, 56(2):160-8.

Sasinka MA, Podracka L, Boor A, et al, "Enalapril Treatment of Proteinuria in Normotensive Children," *Bratisl Lek Listy*, 1999, 100(9):476-80.

Schilder JL and Van den Anker JN, "Use of Enalapril in Neonatal Hypertension," *Acta Paediatr*, 1995, 84(12):1426-8.

von Vigier RO, Mozzettini S, Truttmann AC, et al, "Cough is Common in Children Prescribed Converting Enzyme Inhibitors," *Nephron*, 2000, 84(1):98.

Wells TG, Bunchman TE, Kearns GL, "Treatment of Neonatal Hypertension With Enalaprilat," *J Pediatr*, 1990, 117(4):664-7.

- **Enbrel®** *see* Etanercept *on page 403*
- **Endantadine (Can)** *see* Amantadine *on page 62*
- **Endocarditis Prophylaxis** *see page 1160*
- **Endocet (Can)** *see* Oxycodone and Acetaminophen *on page 747*
- **Endodan (Can)** *see* Oxycodone and Aspirin *on page 748*
- **Endrate®** *see* Edetate Disodium *on page 372*
- **Enlon®** *see* Edrophonium *on page 373*

Enoxaparin (e noks ah PAIR in)

U.S. Brand Names Lovenox®

Therapeutic Category Anticoagulant; Low Molecular Weight Heparin (LMWH)

Generic Available No

Use Prophylaxis and treatment of thromboembolic disorders, specifically: (in adults) prevention of DVT following hip or knee replacement surgery, abdominal surgery in patients at thromboembolic risk (ie, >40 years of age, obese, general anesthesia >30 minutes, malignancy, history of DVT or pulmonary embolism) and in medical patients at thromboembolic risk due to severely restricted mobility during acute illness; administered with warfarin: For inpatient treatment of acute DVT (with or without pulmonary embolism) and outpatient treatment of acute DVT (without pulmonary embolism); administered with aspirin: For prevention of ischemic complications of non-Q-wave MI and unstable angina

Pregnancy Risk Factor B

Contraindications Active major bleeding; hypersensitivity to enoxaparin, heparin, any component, or pork products (enoxaparin is derived from porcine intestinal mucosa); acute heparin-induced or low molecular weight heparin-induced thrombocytopenia

Warnings Bleeding or thrombocytopenia may occur; major hemorrhages (eg, intracranial and retroperitoneal bleeding) may be fatal; thrombocytopenia with thrombosis may occur and may be complicated by limb ischemia, organ infarction, or death. Use with extreme caution in patients with an increased risk of hemorrhage (eg, active GI ulceration or bleeding, angiodysplastic GI disease, bacterial endocarditis, bleeding disorders, hemorrhagic stroke); recent brain, spinal, or ophthalmological surgery; concomitant platelet inhibitor therapy (see Drug Interactions); or a history of heparin-induced thrombocytopenia. Do not use unit-for-unit in place of heparin or other low molecular weight heparins (units are not equivalent).

Epidural or spinal hematoma resulting in long-term or permanent paralysis may occur in patients receiving low molecular weight heparins or heparinoids during epidural/spinal anesthesia or spinal puncture; these patients must be monitored frequently for neurological impairment and treated immediately if compromised; the use of indwelling spinal catheters for analgesia, concomitant use of platelet inhibitors, NSAIDs, or other anticoagulants, and repeated or traumatic epidural/spinal puncture increase the risk for epidural/spinal hematoma; potential benefits must be weighed against the risks. Enoxaparin should be withheld (at least 2 doses) and antifactor Xa activity should be determined (if possible), prior to lumbar or epidural procedures.

Precautions Use with caution in patients with uncontrolled arterial hypertension, bleeding diathesis, history of recent GI ulceration, diabetic retinopathy, and hemorrhage; use with caution and consider dosage decrease in patients with severe renal dysfunction (Cl_{cr} <30 mL/minute); institute appropriate therapy if thromboembolism occurs despite enoxaparin prophylaxis

(Continued)

Enoxaparin *(Continued)*

Adverse Reactions
Cardiovascular: Edema

Central nervous system: Fever

Endocrine & metabolic: Hyperlipidemia (very rare)

Gastrointestinal: Nausea

Hematologic: Hemorrhage, thrombocytopenia (incidence of heparin-induced thrombocytopenia is less than with heparin therapy)

Hepatic: Elevated SGOT and SGPT (asymptomatic, fully reversible, rarely associated with elevated bilirubin levels)

Local: Irritation, pain, hematoma, ecchymosis, erythema at S.C. injection site

Drug Interactions Anticoagulants, thrombolytic agents (alteplase, streptokinase, urokinase), platelet inhibitors (aspirin, salicylates, NSAIDs including ketorolac, dipyridamole, and sulfinpyrazone) may increase the risk of bleeding

Stability Store at room temperature; does not contain preservatives, discard unused portions; do not mix with other injections or infusions

Mechanism of Action Potentiates the action of antithrombin III and inactivates coagulation factor Xa; also inactivates factor IIa (thrombin), but to a much lesser degree; ratio of antifactor Xa to antifactor IIa activity is ~4:1 (ratio for unfractionated heparin is 1:1)

Pharmacodynamics Antifactor Xa and antithrombin (antifactor IIa) activities:

Maximum effect: S.C.: 3-5 hours

Duration: ~12 hours following a 40 mg daily dose given S.C.

Pharmacokinetics Based on antifactor Xa activity

Distribution: Does not cross the placental barrier

Mean V_d: Adults: 6 L

Protein binding: Does not bind to most heparin binding proteins

Bioavailability: S.C.: 92%

Half-life: S.C.: Adults: 4.5 hours (range 2.2-6 hours)

Elimination: 40% of I.V. dose is excreted in urine as active and inactive fragments; 8% to 20% of antifactor Xa activity is recovered within 24 hours in the urine

Clearance: Decreased by 30% in patients with Cl_{cr} <30 mL/minute

Usual Dosage S.C.:
Neonates, Infants, and Children: *Chest*, 2001 Recommendations:

Initial:

Infants <2 months:

Prophylaxis: 0.75 mg/kg every 12 hours

Treatment: 1.5 mg/kg every 12 hours

Infants >2 months and Children ≤18 years:

Prophylaxis: 0.5 mg/kg every 12 hours

Treatment: 1 mg/kg every 12 hours

Maintenance: See **Dosage Titration** table: **Note:** In a recent prospective study of 177 courses of enoxaparin in pediatric patients (146 treatment courses; 31 prophylactic courses) considerable variation in maintenance dosage requirements was observed (see Dix, 2000)

Enoxaparin Dosage Titration

Antifactor Xa	Dose Titration	Time to Repeat Antifactor Xa Level
<0.35 units/mL	Increase dose by 25%	4 h after next dose
0.35-0.49 units/mL	Increase dose by 10%	4 h after next dose
0.5-1 unit/mL	Keep same dosage	Next day, then 1 wk later, then monthly (4 h after dose)
1.1-1.5 units/mL	Decrease dose by 20%	Before next dose
1.6-2 units/mL	Hold dose for 3 h and decrease dose by 30%	Before next dose, then 4 h after next dose
>2 units/mL	Hold all doses until antifactor Xa is 0.5 units/mL, then decrease dose by 40%	Before next dose and every 12 h until antifactor Xa <0.5 units/mL

Modified from Monagle P, Michelson AD, Bovill E, et al, "Antithrombotic Therapy in Children," *Chest*, 2001, 119:344S-70S.

Adults: **Note:** Consider lower doses for patients <45 kg

Prevention of DVT:

Knee replacement surgery: 30 mg every 12 hours; give first dose 12-24 hours after surgery (provided hemostasis has been established); average duration 7-10 days, up to 14 days

Hip replacement surgery: Initial phase: 30 mg every 12 hours with first dose 12-24 hours after surgery (provided hemostasis has been established) or consider 40 mg once daily with first dose given 12 ± 3 hours prior to surgery; average duration of initial phase: 7-10 days, up to 14 days; after initial phase, give 40 mg once daily for 3 weeks

Abdominal surgery in patients at risk: 40 mg once daily; give first dose 2 hours prior to surgery; average duration: 7-10 days, up to 12 days

Medical patients at risk due to severely restricted mobility during acute illness: 40 mg once daily; average duration: 6-11 days, up to 14 days

Treatment of acute DVT and pulmonary embolism: Note: Initiate warfarin therapy when appropriate (usually within 72 hours of starting enoxaparin), continue enoxaparin for a minimum of 5 days (average 7 days) until INR is therapeutic

Inpatient treatment of acute DVT with or without pulmonary embolism: 1 mg/kg every 12 hours or 1.5 mg/kg once daily

Outpatient treatment of acute DVT without pulmonary embolism: 1 mg/kg every 12 hours

Dosage adjustment in renal impairment: No specific guidelines are available, but clearance is decreased when Cl_{cr} <30 mL/minute; monitor antifactor Xa activity to adjust dosage

Administration Parenteral: For S.C. use only; do not administer I.M. or I.V.; administer by deep S.C. injection; do not rub injection site after S.C. administration as bruising may occur

Monitoring Parameters CBC with platelets, stool occult blood tests; antifactor Xa activity in select patients (eg, neonates, infants, and children, and patients with significant renal impairment, active bleeding, or abnormal coagulation parameters); **Note**: Routine monitoring of PT and APTT is not warranted since PT and APTT are relatively insensitive measures of low molecular weight heparin activity; consider monitoring bone density in infants and children with long-term use

Reference Range Antifactor Xa level of 0.5-1 unit/mL measured 4-6 hours after S.C. administration

Nursing Implications Instruct patients on proper S.C. injection technique if patient will self-inject.

Additional Information Discontinue therapy if platelets fall <100,000/mm³; each 10 mg of enoxaparin sodium equals ~1000 international units of antifactor Xa activity.

Enoxaparin contains fragments of unfractionated heparin produced by alkaline degradation (depolymerization) of heparin benzyl ester; enoxaparin has mean molecular weights of 3500-5600 daltons, which are much lower than mean molecular weights of unfractionated heparin (12,000-15,000 daltons). Low molecular weight heparins (LMWH) have several advantages over unfractionated heparin: better S.C. bioavailability, more convenient administration (S.C. versus I.V.), longer half-life (longer dosing interval), more predictable pharmacokinetics and pharmacodynamic (anticoagulant) effect, less intensive laboratory monitoring, reduced risk of heparin-induced thrombocytopenia, potential for outpatient use, and probable reduced risk of osteoporosis (further studies are needed).

Accidental overdosage may be treated with protamine sulfate; 1 mg protamine sulfate neutralizes 1 mg enoxaparin; first dose of protamine sulfate should equal the dose of enoxaparin injected, a second dose of 0.5 mg protamine sulfate per 1 mg enoxaparin may be given if APTT remains prolonged 2-4 hours after first dose (see Protamine *on page 850*)

Dosage Forms Injection, as sodium, preservative free:

Prefilled syringe: 30 mg/0.3 mL; 40 mg/0.4 mL

Graduated prefilled syringe: 60 mg/0.6 mL, 80 mg/0.8 mL, 100 mg/1 mL

Ampul: 30 mg/0.3 mL

References

deVeber G, Chan A, Monagle P, et al, "Anticoagulation Therapy in Pediatric Patients With Sinovenous Thrombosis: A Cohort Study," *Arch Neurol*, 1998, 55(12):1533-7.

Dix D, Andrew M, Marzinotto V, et al, "The Use of Low Molecular Weight Heparin in Pediatric Patients: A Prospective Cohort Study," *J Pediatr*, 2000, 136(4):439-45.

Hirsh J, Warkentin TE, Shaughnessy SG, et al, "Heparin and Low-Molecular-Weight Heparin: Mechanisms of Action, Pharmacokinetics, Dosing, Monitoring, Efficacy, and Safety," *Chest*, 2001, 119:64S-94S.

Martineau P and Tawil N, "Low-Molecular-Weight Heparins in the Treatment of Deep-Vein Thrombosis," *Ann Pharmacother*, 1998, 32(5):588-98, 601.

(Continued)

Enoxaparin *(Continued)*

Massicotte P, Adams M, Marzinotto V, et al, "Low-Molecular-Weight Heparin in Pediatric Patients With Thrombotic Disease: A Dose Finding Study," *J Pediatr*, 1996, 128(3):313-8.

Monagle P, Michelson AD, Bovill E, et al, "Antithrombotic Therapy in Children," *Chest*, 2001, 119:344S-70S.

♦ **Entacyl (Can)** *see* Piperazine *on page 804*
♦ **Entocort (Can)** *see* Budesonide *on page 154*
♦ **Entrophen (Can)** *see* Aspirin *on page 109*
♦ **Entsol™ [OTC]** *see* Sodium Chloride *on page 906*
♦ **Enulose®** *see* Lactulose *on page 571*
♦ **E Pam (Can)** *see* Diazepam *on page 320*
♦ **Ephedra** *see* Ephedrine *on page 384*

Ephedrine *(e FED rin)*

U.S. Brand Names Pretz-D® [OTC]
Synonyms Ephedra; Ephedrinum; Ma Huang
Therapeutic Category Adrenergic Agonist Agent; Antiasthmatic; Bronchodilator; Sympathomimetic
Generic Available Yes
Use Treatment of mild asthma, nasal congestion, acute bronchospasm, idiopathic orthostatic hypotension; adjunctive agent for treatment of shock
Pregnancy Risk Factor C
Contraindications Hypersensitivity to ephedrine or any component; patients with hypertension, cardiac arrhythmias, angle-closure glaucoma, and psychoneurosis; use during halothane or cyclopropane anesthesia (see Drug Interactions)
Warnings Use of ephedrine as a pressor is not a substitute for replacement of blood, plasma, fluids, and electrolytes; blood volume should be corrected as fully as possible before ephedrine therapy; must not be used as sole therapy in hypovolemic patients; hypoxia, hypercapnia, and acidosis may reduce the effectiveness and increase the incidence of side effects of ephedrine; may cause hypertension which may result in intracranial hemorrhage; long-term use may cause anxiety and symptoms of paranoid schizophrenia; the FDA has issued warnings concerning ephedrine-containing nonprescription products with claims of producing such effects as euphoria, increased sexual sensation, increased energy, and weight loss; healthcare professionals are urged to be aware of these products and counsel patients, when appropriate, about the potential adverse effects of ephedrine such as headache, dizziness, heart irregularities, seizures, and possibly death
Precautions Use with caution in patients with hyperthyroidism, diabetes mellitus, prostatic hypertrophy, coronary insufficiency, and angina
Adverse Reactions
  Cardiovascular: Hypertension, precordial pain, edema, palpitations, tachycardia, arrhythmias
  Central nervous system: Nervousness, anxiety, apprehension, fear, tension, agitation, excitation, restlessness, irritability, insomnia, dizziness, vertigo, confusion, delirium, hallucinations, euphoria, paranoid psychosis, headache
  Dermatologic: Rash
  Gastrointestinal: Nausea, vomiting, xerostomia, mild epigastric distress, anorexia
  Genitourinary: Urinary retention
  Neuromuscular & skeletal: Tremors, hyperactive reflexes, weakness
Drug Interactions Increased effects with other sympathomimetic agents; reduced pressor response to ephedrine with alpha-adrenergic blocking agents and methyldopa; increased cardiac irritability and arrhythmias with halothane and cyclopropane anesthesia; increased pressor effects with MAO inhibitors; cardiac glycosides may increase cardiac stimulation; medications which alkalinize or acidify the urine may result in increased or decreased ephedrine effects (see Pharmacokinetics); increased CNS and GI effects when used with theophylline
Stability Protect from light
Mechanism of Action Stimulates both alpha- and beta-adrenergic receptors and also stimulates the release of norepinephrine from storage sites resulting in bronchodilation, cardiac stimulation, and increased systolic and diastolic blood pressure; tachyphylaxis may occur
Pharmacodynamics
  Bronchodilation:
    Onset of effect: Oral: 15-60 minutes
    Duration: Oral: 2-4 hours
  Pressor/cardiac effects: Duration:
    Oral: 4 hours

I.M., S.C.: 1 hour
Pharmacokinetics
Absorption: Oral: Complete
Metabolism: Liver by oxidative deamination, demethylation, aromatic hydroxylation, and conjugation
Bioavailability: Oral: 85%
Half-life: 4.9-6.5 hours
Elimination: Dependent upon urinary pH with greatest excretion in acid pH; urine pH 5: 74% to 99% excreted unchanged; urine pH 8: 22% to 25% excreted unchanged

Usual Dosage
Bronchodilation and nasal decongestion:
  Oral:
    Children >2-6 years: 2-3 mg/kg/day or 100 mg/m^2/day in 4-6 divided doses
    Children 7-11 years: 6.25-12.5 mg every 4 hours; not to exceed 75 mg/day
    Children ≥12 years and Adults: 12.5-50 mg every 3-4 hours; not to exceed 150 mg/day
  Spray:
    Children 6-12 years: 1-2 sprays in each nostril not more than every 4 hours; do not exceed 3 days of therapy
    Children >12 years and Adults: 2-3 sprays in each nostril not more than every 4 hours; do not exceed 3 days of therapy

Orthostatic hypotension: Oral: Adults: 25 mg 1-4 times/day

Adjunctive agent in the treatment of shock: Use the smallest effective dose for the shortest time:
  Children <12 years: I.M., I.V., S.C.: 3 mg/kg/day in 4-6 divided doses
  Children ≥12 years and Adults:
    I.M., S.C.: 25-50 mg (range: 10-50 mg); may repeat with a second dose of 50 mg; not to exceed 150 mg/24 hours
    I.V.: 10-25 mg; may repeat with a second dose in 5-10 minutes of 25 mg; not to exceed 150 mg/24 hours

Administration
Oral: May be administered without regard to food
Parenteral:
  I.M., S.C.: May be administered undiluted
  I.V.: May be administered by slow I.V. push
Spray: Spray into each nostril while gently occluding the other

Monitoring Parameters Vital signs, pulmonary function tests, respiratory rate (when applicable)

Test Interactions May cause a false-positive test for amphetamine (by EMIT assay)

Patient Information Use for self-medication for asthma only under physician's direction; contact your physician if nervousness, tremor, insomnia, nausea, or loss of appetite occur; see Warnings

Additional Information Because ephedrine has been used to synthesize methamphetamine, restrictions are in place to reduce the potential for misuse (diversion) and abuse; 24 g of ephedrine (in terms of base) is the limit for a single transaction for drug products containing ephedrine regardless of the form in which these drugs are packaged

Dosage Forms As sulfate:
Capsule: 25 mg
Injection: 50 mg/mL (1 mL)
Spray, nasal (Pretz-D®): 0.25% (50 mL)

- ◆ **Ephedrinum** *see* Ephedrine *on page 384*
- ◆ **Epidermal Thymocyte Activating Factor** *see* Aldesleukin *on page 47*
- ◆ **Epi EZ (Can)** *see* Epinephrine *on page 385*
- ◆ **Epifrin®** *see* Epinephrine *on page 385*
- ◆ **Epiject (Can)** *see* Valproic Acid and Derivatives *on page 998*

Epinephrine (ep i NEF rin)
Related Information
Adult ACLS Algorithm, Asystole *on page 1043*
Adult ACLS Algorithm, Bradycardia *on page 1044*
Adult ACLS Algorithm, Cardiac Arrest *on page 1039*
Adult ACLS Algorithm, Comprehensive ECC *on page 1040*
Adult ACLS Algorithm, Pulseless Electrical Activity *on page 1042*
Adult ACLS Algorithm, V. Fib and Pulseless VT *on page 1041*
Asthma Guidelines *on page 1210*
CPR Pediatric Drug Dosages *on page 1031*
(Continued)

Epinephrine *(Continued)*

Emergency Pediatric Drip Calculations *on page 1033*
Extravasation Treatment *on page 1085*
Neonatal Resuscitation Algorithm *on page 1034*
Pediatric ALS Algorithm, Bradycardia *on page 1035*
Pediatric ALS Algorithm, Pulseless Arrest *on page 1036*

U.S. Brand Names Adrenalin®; AsthmaHaler® Mist [OTC]; Epifrin®; EpiPen®; EpiPen® Jr; Glaucon®; Primatene® Mist [OTC]; S₂® [OTC]

Canadian Brand Names Epi EZ

Synonyms Adrenaline; Racemic Epinephrine

Therapeutic Category Adrenergic Agonist Agent; Antiasthmatic; Antidote, Hypersensitivity Reactions; Bronchodilator; Decongestant, Nasal; Sympathomimetic

Generic Available Yes

Use Treatment of bronchospasm, anaphylactic reactions, cardiac arrest, and management of open-angle (chronic simple) glaucoma; nasal decongestant (topical nasal formulation); upper airway obstruction and croup (racemic epinephrine)

Pregnancy Risk Factor C

Contraindications Hypersensitivity to epinephrine or any component; cardiac arrhythmias, angle-closure glaucoma

Precautions Patients with diabetes mellitus, cardiovascular disease (angina, tachycardia, MI), thyroid disease, or cerebral arteriosclerosis; rebound nasal congestion may occur after frequent nasal use

Adverse Reactions

Cardiovascular: Pallor, tachycardia, hypertension, increased myocardial oxygen consumption, cardiac arrhythmias, sudden death

Central nervous system: Anxiety, headache

Gastrointestinal: Nausea

Genitourinary: Acute urinary retention in patients with bladder outflow obstruction

Neuromuscular & skeletal: Weakness, tremor

Ocular: Precipitation of or exacerbation of narrow-angle glaucoma

Renal: Decreased renal and splanchnic blood flow

Drug Interactions Increased cardiac irritability if administered concurrently with halogenated inhalational anesthetics; beta-blocking agents (ie, propranolol); alpha-blocking agents (eg, phentolamine); alpha- and beta-blocking agents (labetalol); phenothiazines with alpha-blocking activity; tricyclic antidepressants enhance pressor response to epinephrine

Stability Protect from light; incompatible with alkaline solutions (sodium bicarbonate); compatible when coadministered with dopamine, dobutamine, inamrinone (amrinone), atracurium, pancuronium, and vecuronium

Mechanism of Action Stimulates alpha-, beta₁- and beta₂-adrenergic receptors resulting in relaxation of smooth muscle of the bronchial tree, cardiac stimulation, and dilation of skeletal muscle vasculature; small doses can cause vasodilation via beta₂-vascular receptors; large doses may produce constriction of skeletal and vascular smooth muscle; decreases production of aqueous humor and increases aqueous outflow; dilates the pupil by contracting the dilator muscle

Pharmacodynamics

Local vasoconstriction (topical):

Onset: 5 minutes

Duration: <1 hour

Onset of bronchodilation:

Inhalation: Within 1 minute

S.C.: Within 5-10 minutes

Peak ocular effect: Following conjunctival instillation intraocular pressures fall within 1 hour with a maximal response occurring within 4-8 hours

Duration: Ocular effects persist for 12-24 hours

Pharmacokinetics

Absorption: Orally ingested doses are rapidly metabolized in GI tract and liver; pharmacologically active concentrations are **not** achieved

Distribution: Crosses placenta but not blood-brain barrier

Metabolism: Extensive in the liver and other tissues by the enzymes catechol-o-methyltransferase and monoamine oxidase

Usual Dosage

Neonates: I.V., Intratracheal: 0.01-0.03 mg/kg (0.1-0.3 mL/kg of **1:10,000** solution) every 3-5 minutes as needed

Infants and Children:

I.M.: EpiPen® and EpiPen® Jr: 0.01 mg/kg

or as alternative

<30 kg: 0.15 mg; >30 kg: 0.3 mg

S.C.: 0.01 mg/kg (0.01 mL/kg/dose of **1:1000** solution) not to exceed 0.5 mg **or**
  Suspension: 0.005 mL/kg/dose (1:200); not to exceed 0.15 mL every 8-12 hours
Bradycardia:
  I.V.: 0.01 mg/kg (0.1 mL/kg) of **1:10,000** solution (maximum dose: 1 mg or 10
    mL); may repeat every 3-5 minutes as needed
  Intratracheal: 0.1 mg/kg (0.1 mL/kg) of **1:1000** solution; doses as high as 0.2
    mg/kg may be effective; may repeat every 3-5 minutes as needed
Asystole or pulseless arrest:
  I.V. or I.O.: 0.01 mg/kg (0.1 mL/kg) of **1:10,000** solution; may repeat every 3-5
    minutes as needed; if ineffective, may increase dosage to 0.1 mg/kg (0.1 mL/
    kg of **1:1000** solution; doses as high as 0.2 mg/kg may be effective); repeat
    every 3-5 minutes as needed [increased dosage no longer routinely recom-
    mended by the American Heart Association (see References)]
  Intratracheal: 0.1 mg/kg (0.1 mL/kg) of **1:1000** solution (doses as high as 0.2
    mg/kg may be effective)
Continuous I.V. infusion rate: 0.1-1 mcg/kg/minute; titrate dosage to desired effect
Nebulization: 0.25-0.5 mL of 2.25% **racemic epinephrine** solution diluted in 3 mL
  NS, or L-epinephrine at an equivalent dose; racemic epinephrine 10 mg = 5 mg
  L-epinephrine; use lower end of dosing range for younger infants
Ophthalmic: Instill 1-2 drops in eye(s) once or twice daily
Nasal: Children ≥6 years and Adults: Apply drops locally as needed; do not
  exceed 1 mL every 15 minutes

Adults:
  Asystole: I.V.: 1 mg every 3-5 minutes; if this approach fails, alternative regimens
    include:
    Intermediate: 2-5 mg every 3-5 minutes
    Escalating: 1 mg, 3 mg, 5 mg at 3-minute intervals
    High: 0.1 mg/kg every 3-5 minutes
  Intratracheal: 1 mg (although the optimal dose is unknown, doses of 2-2.5 times
    the I.V. dose may be needed)
  I.M., S.C.: 0.1-0.5 mg every 10-15 minutes
  Continuous I.V. infusion rate: Initial: 1 mcg/minute (range: 1-10 mcg/minute);
    titrate dosage to desired effect
  Ophthalmic: Instill 1-2 drops in eye(s) once or twice daily; when treating open-
    angle glaucoma, the concentration and dosage must be adjusted to the
    response of the patient
Administration
  Inhalation: Nebulization: Dilute in 3 mL NS
  Intratracheal: Dilute with normal saline to a total volume of 3-5 mL and follow with
    several positive pressure ventilations
  Nasal: Apply as drops or with sterile swab
  Ophthalmic: Instill drops into affected eye(s); avoid contacting bottle tip with skin or
    eye; apply finger pressure to lacrimal sac during and for 1-2 minutes after instilla-
    tion to decrease risk of absorption and systemic effects
  Oral inhalation: Shake well before use; use spacer in children <8 years of age
  Parenteral:
    Direct I.V. or I.O. administration: Dilute to a maximum concentration of 100 mcg/
      mL (if using 1:10,000 concentration, no dilution is necessary)
    Continuous I.V. infusion: Rate of infusion (mL/hour) = dose (mcg/kg/minute) x
      weight (kg) x 60 minutes/hour divided by the concentration (mcg/mL); maximum
      concentration: 64 mcg/mL
    I.M. (EpiPen® and EpiPen® Jr): Intramuscularly into anterolateral aspect of thigh
    S.C.: Use only 1:1000 solution or 1:200 suspension
Monitoring Parameters EKG, heart rate, blood pressure, site of infusion for exces-
sive blanching/extravasation
Nursing Implications Tissue irritant; extravasation may be treated by local small
injections of a diluted phentolamine solution (mix 5 mg with 9 mL NS)
Dosage Forms
  Aerosol, oral:
    Primatene® Mist: 0.2 mg/spray (15 mL, 22.5 mL)
    As Bitartrate (AsthmaHaler® Mist): 0.3 mg/spray [epinephrine base 0.16 mg/spray]
      (15 mL)
  Emergency kit, auto-injector:
    EpiPen®: Delivers 0.3 mg I.M. of epinephrine 1:1000 (2 mL)
    EpiPen® Jr.: Delivers 0.15 mg I.M. of epinephrine 1:2000 (2 mL)
  Solution, as hydrochloride:
    Oral inhalation:
      Adrenalin®: 1% [10 mg/mL - 1:100] (7.5 mL)
(Continued)

Epinephrine (Continued)

S₂®: Racepinephrine 2.25% [contains d-epinephrine 1.1125% and l-epinephrine 1.25%] (0.5 mL, 15 mL)

Injection: 0.1 mg/mL [1:10,000] (10 mL); 1 mg/mL [1:1000] (1 mL, 2 mL, 30 mL)
  Adrenalin®: 1 mg/mL [1:1000] (1 mL, 30 mL)
  Nasal (Adrenalin®): 0.1% [1 mg/mL - 1:1000] (30 mL)
  Ophthalmic, as hydrochloride:
    Epifrin®: 0.5% (15 mL)
    Epifrin®, Glaucon®: 1% (10 mL, 15 mL); 2% (10 mL, 15mL)

References

American College of Cardiology, American Heart Association Task Force, "Adult Advanced Cardiac Life Support" and "Pediatric Advanced Life Support Guidelines," *JAMA*, 1992, 268(16):2199-241 and 2262-75.

"Guidelines 2000 for Cardiopulmonary Resuscitation and Emergency Cardiovascular Care. Part 10: Pediatric Advanced Life Support. The American Heart Association in Collaboration With the International Liaison Committee on Resuscitation," *Circulation*, 2000, 102(8 Suppl):I291-342.

"Guidelines 2000 for Cardiopulmonary Resuscitation and Emergency Cardiovascular Care. Part 11: Neonatal Resuscitation. The American Heart Association in Collaboration With the International Liaison Committee on Resuscitation," *Circulation*, 2000, 102(8 Suppl):I343-57.

Waisman Y, Klein BL, Boenning DA, et al, "Prospective Randomized Double-Blind Study Comparing L-Epinephrine and Racemic Epinephrine Aerosols in the Treatment of Laryngotracheitis (Croup)," *Pediatrics*, 1992, 89(2):302-6.

- ◆ **Epinephrine and Lidocaine** *see* Lidocaine and Epinephrine *on page 593*
- ◆ **EpiPen®** *see* Epinephrine *on page 385*
- ◆ **EpiPen® Jr** *see* Epinephrine *on page 385*
- ◆ **Epitol®** *see* Carbamazepine *on page 175*
- ◆ **Epival (Can)** *see* Valproic Acid and Derivatives *on page 998*
- ◆ **Epivir®** *see* Lamivudine *on page 572*
- ◆ **Epivir-HBV®** *see* Lamivudine *on page 572*
- ◆ **EPO** *see* Epoetin Alfa *on page 388*

Epoetin Alfa (e POE e tin AL fa)

U.S. Brand Names Epogen®; Procrit®

Canadian Brand Names Eprex

Synonyms EPO; Erythropoietin; rHuEPO; rHuEPO-α

Therapeutic Category Colony-Stimulating Factor; Recombinant Human Erythropoietin

Generic Available No

Use Anemia associated with end-stage renal disease; anemia in cancer patients with nonmyeloid malignancies on chemotherapy; anemia related to AIDS and therapy with zidovudine-treated, HIV-infected patients; endogenous serum erythropoietin (EPO) levels which are inappropriately low for hemoglobin level (eg, anemia of neoplasia); anemia of prematurity; patients undergoing autologous blood donation prior to surgery (EPO may accelerate recovery of hemoglobin level and, in some cases, permit more units of blood to be donated)

Pregnancy Risk Factor C

Contraindications Hypersensitivity to albumin (human) or mammalian cell-derived products; uncontrolled hypertension; neutropenia in newborns

Factors Limiting Response to Epoetin Alfa

Factor	Mechanism
Iron deficiency	Limits hemoglobin synthesis
Blood loss/hemolysis	Counteracts epoetin alfa-stimulated erythropoiesis
Infection/inflammation	Inhibits iron transfer from storage to bone marrow
	Suppresses erythropoiesis through activated macrophages
Aluminum overload	Inhibits iron incorporation into heme protein
Bone marrow replacement Hyperparathyroidism Metastatic, neoplastic	Limits bone marrow volume
Folic acid/vitamin B_{12} deficiency	Limits hemoglobin synthesis
Patient compliance	Self-administered epoetin alfa or iron therapy

Warnings The multidose formulation contains benzyl alcohol; avoid use in neonates. Pooled use of unused portions of preservative-free EPO has resulted in microbial contamination, bacteremia, and pyrogenic reactions. Preservative-free formulations are intended for single use only.

Precautions Use with caution in patients with porphyria or a history of seizures. Decrease the EPO dose if an increase in hematocrit exceeds 4 points in any 2-week period. EPO is not intended for patients who require acute corrections of anemia and is not a substitute for emergency blood transfusion.

Assessment of iron stores and therapeutic iron supplementation is essential to optimal EPO therapy. Iron supplementation is necessary to provide for increased requirements during expansion of the red cell mass secondary to marrow stimulation by EPO, unless iron stores are already in excess.

Adverse Reactions

Cardiovascular: Hypertension, edema, chest pain, myocardial infarction, CVA/TIA

Central nervous system: Fatigue, dizziness, headache, seizure, fever

Dermatologic: Rash, urticaria

Local: Pain, irritation at injection site (S.C. injection)

Gastrointestinal: Nausea, diarrhea, vomiting

Hematologic: Neutropenia

Neuromuscular & skeletal: Arthralgias, weakness

Respiratory: Cough

Miscellaneous: Hypersensitivity reactions

Stability Refrigerate; single-dose vials contain no preservatives; discard after entry (see Warnings). Multiple-dose vials contain benzyl alcohol preservative and are stable 2 weeks at room temperature and when refrigerated, may be used up to 21 days after initial entry. EPO is stable for 24 hours when diluted in dextrose I.V. fluid which contains at least 0.05% human albumin or parenteral nutrition solutions containing at least 0.5% amino acids. EPO may be diluted with NS or bacteriostatic NS in a 1:1 ratio at the time of S.C. administration.

Mechanism of Action Epoetin alfa, a glycoprotein manufactured by recombinant DNA technology, has the same effects as endogenous erythropoietin. EPO induces erythropoiesis by stimulating the division and differentiation of committed erythroid progenitor cells. It induces the release of reticulocytes from the bone marrow into the bloodstream, where they mature to erythrocytes (dose response relationship) resulting in an increase in reticulocyte counts followed by a rise in hematocrit and hemoglobin levels. There is normally an inverse correlation between the plasma EPO level and the hemoglobin concentration (only when the hemoglobin concentration is <10.5 g/dL).

Pharmacodynamics

Onset of action: Several days

Peak effect: 2-6 weeks

Pharmacokinetics

Absorption: S.C.: 31.9%

Distribution: Adults: V_d: 9 L; rapid in the plasma compartment; majority of drug is taken up by the liver, kidneys, and bone marrow

Bioavailability: S.C.: ~21% to 31%

Half-life:

Neonates: S.C.: 17.6 hours on day 3 of therapy, 11.2 hours on day 10 of therapy

Adults: 4-13 hours in patients with chronic renal failure (CRF); half-life is 20% shorter in patients with normal renal function

Time to peak serum concentration: S.C.: 5-24 hours

Elimination: Some metabolic degradation does occur with small amounts recovered in the urine

Clearance: Neonates: S.C. or continuous I.V. infusion: 26-35 mL/hour/kg on day 3 of therapy and 65-87 mL/hour/kg on day 10 of therapy

Note: While a much higher peak plasma concentration is achieved after I.V. bolus administration, it declines at a more rapid rate (over 2-3 days) than after subcutaneous administration (plasma concentrations greater than endogenous are maintained for at least 4 days). Subcutaneous administration is associated with a 30% to 50% lower EPO dose requirement.

Usual Dosage Dosing schedules need to be individualized and careful monitoring of patients receiving the drug is recommended. EPO may be ineffective if other factors such as iron or B_{12}/folate deficiency limit marrow response. Dosage based upon S.C. administration; use of I.V. administration may result in the need to increase doses by as much as 30% to 50% to achieve the same outcome: I.V., S.C.:

Neonates: Anemia of prematurity: Variable regimens: 25-100 units/kg/dose 3 times/ week **or** 100 units/kg/dose 5 times/week **or** 200 units/kg/dose every other day for 10 doses

(Continued)

Epoetin Alfa *(Continued)*

Children and Adults:

Anemia in cancer patients: 150 units/kg/dose 3 times/week; maximum 1200 units/kg/week

Anemia in chronic renal failure: 50-150 units/kg/dose 3 times/week

Note: Once weekly dosage has been studied in chronic renal failure patients. When transitioning from multiple doses/week to once weekly, begin with a weekly dosage equal to the current total dose per week. Allow at least 4 weeks to determine full effects of the new regimen.

Epoetin Alfa Dosage Adjustments

Target hematocrit range	30% to 33% (maximum 36%)
Reduce dose when	Target range is reached **or** hematocrit increases >4 points in any 2-week period
Increase dose when	Hematocrit does not increase by 5-6 points after 8 weeks of therapy **and** hematocrit is below target range
Stop therapy when	Hematocrit ≥40%; reinstate therapy at a lower dose after the hematocrit decreases to 36%
Maintenance dose (chronic renal failure)	Individualize: General dosage range: 25 units/kg 3 times/week

Zidovudine-treated, HIV-infected patients: Initial: 100 units/kg/dose 3 times/week for 8 weeks; after 8 weeks of therapy the dose may be adjusted by 50-100 units/kg increments 3 times/week to a maximum dose of 300 units/kg 3 times/week

Presurgery, autologous blood donation: Adults: 300 units/kg/day for 10 days before surgery, the day of surgery, and 4 days after surgery **or as an alternative**, 600 units/kg/week at 21-, 14-, and 7 days before surgery and on the day of surgery

Administration Parenteral: Do not shake as this may denature the glycoprotein rendering the drug biologically inactive

S.C. is the preferred route of administration; 1:1 dilution with bacteriostatic NS (containing benzyl alcohol) acts as a local anesthetic to reduce pain at the injection site. Multiple-dose vials already contain benzyl alcohol.

I.V.: Dilute with an equal volume of NS and infuse over 1-3 minutes; it may be administered into the venous line at the end of the dialysis procedure

Monitoring Parameters

Careful monitoring of blood pressure is indicated; problems with hypertension have been noted especially in renal failure patients treated with EPO. Other patients are less likely to develop this complication. See table.

Test	Initial Phase Frequency	Maintenance Phase Frequency
Hematocrit/hemoglobin	2 times/week	2-4 times/month
Blood pressure	3 times/week	3 times/week
Serum ferritin	Monthly	Quarterly
Transferrin saturation	Monthly	Quarterly
Serum chemistries including CBC with differential, creatinine, blood urea nitrogen, potassium, phosphorous	Regularly per routine	Regularly per routine
Reticulocyte count	Baseline prior to starting therapy	After 10 days of therapy

Hematocrit should be determined twice weekly until stabilization within the target range (30% to 36%), and twice weekly for at least 2-6 weeks after a dose increase.

Reference Range The decision to initiate EPO therapy may be made by utilizing an endogenous erythropoietin serum level measurement. Endogenous erythropoietin levels are inversely related to the hemoglobin (and hematocrit) level in anemias that are not attributed to impaired erythropoietin production (eg, iron deficiency anemia). A normal erythropoietin level, for subjects with normal hemoglobin and hematocrit, is 4.1-22.2 mIU/mL. Baseline erythropoietin levels in anemic patients may increase up to 100-1000 fold in untreated patients with a normal release of erythropoietin. The following table illustrates the "normal" response to anemia. EPO is indicated in patients who do not exhibit a normal response to anemia (eg, the measurement of endogenous erythropoietin is low relative to a normal response). If the patient has exhibited a normal response, addition of exogenous EPO may not be beneficial. Clinical studies involving the following disease states have established criteria for assessment of endogenous erythropoietin levels prior to initiating EPO therapy:

Zidovudine-treated HIV patients: Available evidence indicates patients with endogenous serum erythropoietin levels >500 mIU/mL are unlikely to respond

Cancer chemotherapy patients: Treatment of patients with endogenous serum erythropoietin levels >200 mIU/mL is not recommended.

Inverse Relationship of Endogenous Erythropoietin to Hemoglobin

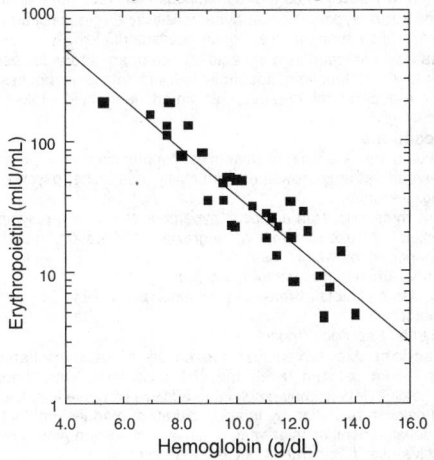

Patient Information Frequent blood tests are needed to determine the correct dose; notify physician if any severe headache develops; due to increased risk of seizure activity in CRF patients during the first 90 days of therapy, avoid potentially hazardous activities (eg, driving during this period)

Additional Information Optimal response is achieved when iron stores are maintained with supplemental iron if necessary; evaluate iron stores prior to and during therapy

Reimbursement Hotline (Epogen®): 1-800-272-9376
Professional Services [Amgen]: 1-800-77-AMGEN
Reimbursement Hotline (Procrit®): 1-800-553-3851
Professional Services [Ortho Biotech]: 1-800-325-7504

Dosage Forms

Injection, preservative free: 2000 units/mL (1 mL); 3000 units/mL (1 mL); 4000 units/mL (1 mL); 10,000 units/mL (1 mL)

Injection, with preservative: 10,000 units/mL (2 mL); 20,000 units/mL (1 mL); 40,000 units/mL (1 mL)

References

Blanche S, Caniglia M, Fischer A, et al, "Zidovudine Therapy in Children With Acquired Immunodeficiency Syndrome," *Am J Med*, 1988, 85(2A):203-7.

Halperin DS, Wacker P, Lacourt G, et al, "Effects of Recombinant Human Erythropoietin in Infants With the Anemia of Prematurity: A Pilot Study," *J Pediatr*, 1990, 116(5):779-86.

Ohls RK and Christensen, RD, "Stability of Human Recombinant Epoetin Alfa in Commonly Used Neonatal Intravenous Solutions," *Ann Pharmacother*, 1996, 30(5):466-468.

Ohls RK, Veerman MW, and Christensen RD, "Pharmacokinetics and Effectiveness of Recombinant Erythropoietin Administered to Preterm Infants by Continuous Infusion in Total Parenteral Nutrition Solution," *J Pediatr*, 1996, 128(4):518-23.

Rhondeau SM, Christensen RD, Ross MP, et al, "Responsiveness to Recombinant Human Erythropoietin of Marrow Erythroid Progenitors From Infants With the Anemia of Prematurity," *J Pediatr*, 1988, 112(6):935-40.

Shannon KM, Keith JF 3rd, Mentzer WC, et al, "Recombinant Human Erythropoietin Stimulates Erythropoiesis and Reduces Erythrocyte Transfusions in Very Low Birth Weight Preterm Infants," *Pediatrics*, 1995, 95(1):1-8.

Sinai-Trieman L, Salusky IB, and Fine RN, "Use of Subcutaneous Recombinant Human Erythropoietin in Children Undergoing Continuous Cycling Peritoneal Dialysis," *J Pediatr*, 1989, 114(4 Pt 1):550-4.

♦ **Epogen®** *see* Epoetin Alfa *on page 388*

♦ **Eprex (Can)** *see* Epoetin Alfa *on page 388*

♦ **Epsom Salts (Magnesium Sulfate)** *see* Magnesium Supplements *on page 614*

Ergocalciferol (er goe kal SIF e role)

U.S. Brand Names Calciferol™; Drisdol®

Canadian Brand Names Ostoforte; Radiostol

Synonyms Activated Ergosterol; Viosterol; Vitamin D_2

Therapeutic Category Nutritional Supplement; Vitamin D Analog; Vitamin, Fat Soluble

Generic Available Yes

Use Refractory rickets; hypophosphatemia; hypoparathyroidism

Pregnancy Risk Factor A (C if dose exceeds RDA recommendation)

Contraindications Hypercalcemia; hypersensitivity to ergocalciferol or any component; malabsorption syndrome; evidence of vitamin D toxicity

Precautions Use with caution in patients with coronary artery disease, renal stones, and impaired renal function; adequate calcium intake is necessary for clinical response to ergocalciferol therapy; maintain adequate fluid intake; avoid hypercalcemia

Adverse Reactions

Cardiovascular: Hypertension, arrhythmias, hypotension

Central nervous system: Drowsiness, irritability, headache, psychosis

Dermatologic: Pruritus

Endocrine & metabolic: Mild acidosis, hypercholesterolemia, polydipsia

Gastrointestinal: Nausea, vomiting, anorexia, constipation, metallic taste, xerostomia, pancreatitis, weight loss

Genitourinary: Albuminuria, nocturia, polyuria

Neuromuscular & skeletal: Weakness, myalgia, bone pain

Ocular: Photophobia

Renal: Polyuria, nephrocalcinosis

Drug Interactions May antagonize the effects of calcium channel blockers by increasing serum calcium level; may be associated with digoxin toxicity by increasing calcium levels; may result in an additive increase in calcium levels due to decreased calcium excretion by thiazide diuretics; magnesium-containing antacids (potential development of hypermagnesemia); cholestyramine, colestipol, orlistat, and excessive use of mineral oil decrease absorption

Stability Protect from light

Mechanism of Action Vitamin D stimulates calcium and phosphate absorption from the small intestine; promotes secretion of calcium from bone to blood; promotes renal tubule phosphate resorption; acts directly on bone cells (osteoblasts) to stimulate skeletal growth and on the parathyroid glands to suppress parathyroid hormone synthesis and secretion

Pharmacodynamics Peak effect occurs in ~1 month following daily doses

Pharmacokinetics

Absorption: Readily absorbed from GI tract; absorption requires intestinal presence of bile

Metabolism: Inactive until hydroxylated in the liver and the kidney to calcifediol and then to calcitriol (most active form)

Usual Dosage Oral dosing is preferred; use I.M. only in patients with GI, liver, or biliary disease associated with malabsorption of vitamin D:

Adequate Intake (AI) (1997 National Academy of Science Recommendations):

Neonates, Children and Adults: 200 international units/day

Dietary supplementation (each mcg = 40 USP units):

Premature infants: 10-20 mcg/day (400-800 units), up to 750 mcg/day (30,000 units)

Infants and healthy Children: 10 mcg/day (400 units)

Adults: 10 mcg/day (400 units)

Renal failure:

Children: 100-1000 mcg/day (4000-40,000 units)

Adults: 500 mcg/day (20,000 units)

Hypoparathyroidism:

Children: 1.25-5 mg/day (50,000-200,000 units) with calcium supplements

Adults: 625 mcg to 5 mg/day (25,000-200,000 units) with calcium supplements

Vitamin D-dependent rickets:

Children: 75-125 mcg/day (3000-5000 units); maximum dose: 1500 mcg/day

Adults: 250 mcg to 1.5 mg/day (10,000-60,000 units)

Nutritional rickets and osteomalacia:

Children and Adults (with normal absorption): 25-125 mcg/day (1000-5000 units) for 6-12 weeks

Children with malabsorption: 250-625 mcg/day (10,000-25,000 units)

Adults with malabsorption: 250-7500 mcg/day (10,000-300,000 units)

Vitamin D-resistant rickets:
Children: Initial: 1000-2000 mcg/day (40,000-80,000 units) with phosphate supplements; daily dosage is increased at 3- to 4-month intervals in 250-500 mcg (10,000-20,000 units) increments
Adults: 250-1500 mcg/day (10,000-60,000 units) with phosphate supplements

Administration
Oral: May be administered without regard to meals; for oral liquid, use accompanying dropper for dosage measurements
Parenteral: Injection for I.M. use only

Monitoring Parameters Serum calcium and phosphorus levels; alkaline phosphatase, BUN; bone x-ray (hypophosphatemia or hypoparathyroidism)

Reference Range Serum calcium times serum phosphorus should not exceed 70 mg/dL to avoid ectopic calcification; ergocalciferol levels: 10-60 ng/mL

Additional Information 1.25 mg ergocalciferol provides 50,000 units of vitamin D activity; 1 drop of 8000 units/mL = 200 units (40 drops = 1 mL)

Dosage Forms
Capsule (Drisdol®): 50,000 units [1.25 mg]
Injection (Calciferol™): 500,000 units/mL [12.5 mg/mL] (1 mL)
Liquid (Calciferol™, Drisdol®): 8000 units/mL [200 mcg/mL] (60 mL) [OTC]

References
"Dietary Reference Intakes for Calcium, Phosphorus, Magnesium, Vitamin D, and Fluoride. Standing Committee on the Scientific Evaluation of Dietary Reference Intakes, Food and Nutrition Board, Institute of Medicine," National Academy of Sciences, Washington, DC: National Academy Press, 1997.

♦ **Ergomar®** *see* Ergotamine *on page 393*

Ergotamine (er GOT a meen)

Related Information
Drugs and Breast-Feeding *on page 1243*
Overdose and Toxicology *on page 1222*

U.S. Brand Names Cafergot®; Ergomar®; Wigraine®

Synonyms Ergotamine and Caffeine

Therapeutic Category Alpha-Adrenergic Blocking Agent, Oral; Antimigraine Agent; Ergot Alkaloid and Derivative

Generic Available Yes

Use Prevent or abort vascular headaches, such as migraine or cluster

Pregnancy Risk Factor X

Contraindications Hypersensitivity to ergotamine, caffeine, or any component; peripheral vascular disease, hepatic or renal disease, hypertension, peptic ulcer disease, sepsis, coronary heart disease

Warnings Avoid during pregnancy; patients who take ergotamine for extended periods of time may become dependent on it; may be harmful due to reduction in cerebral blood flow; may precipitate angina, MI, or aggravate intermittent claudication

Precautions Avoid prolonged administration or excessive dosage because of the danger of ergotism and gangrene

Adverse Reactions
Cardiovascular: Angina-like precordial pain, transient tachycardia or bradycardia, vasospasm, vasoconstriction, claudication
Central nervous system: Rebound headaches (with abrupt withdrawal), drowsiness, dizziness
Dermatologic: Pruritus
Gastrointestinal: Nausea, vomiting, diarrhea, xerostomia
Local: Edema
Neuromuscular & skeletal: Leg cramps, myalgia, weakness, paresthesia of the extremities

Drug Interactions Increased peripheral ischemia with macrolides, enhanced vasoconstriction with beta-blocking agents; increased vasoconstrictor effects with methysergide

Food Interactions Caffeine may increase GI absorption of ergotamine

Mechanism of Action Ergot alkaloid alpha-adrenergic blocker directly stimulates vascular smooth muscle to vasoconstrict peripheral and cerebral vessels; may also have antagonist effects on serotonin

Pharmacokinetics
Absorption: Oral, rectal: Erratic; absorption is enhanced by caffeine coadministration
Metabolism: Extensive in the liver
Bioavailability: Poor overall (<5%)
Time to peak serum concentration: Oral: Within 0.5-3 hours
(Continued)

Ergotamine *(Continued)*

Elimination: In bile as metabolites (90%)

Usual Dosage

Older Children and Adolescents: Oral, S.L.: 1 mg at onset of attack; then 1 mg every 30 minutes as needed, up to a maximum of 3 mg per attack

Adults:

Oral:

Cafergot®: 2 mg at onset of attack; then 1-2 mg every 30 minutes as needed; maximum dose: 6 mg per attack; do not exceed 10 mg/week

Ergomar®: 1 tablet under tongue at first sign, then 1 tablet every 30 minutes; maximum: 3 tablets/24 hours, 5 tablets/week

Rectal, suppositories (Cafergot®, Wigraine®, Cafatine®): 1 suppository at first sign of an attack; follow with second dose after 1 hour, if needed; maximum dose: 2 per attack; do not exceed 5/week

Administration Place sublingual tablets under tongue; oral tablets may be taken without regard to meals

Patient Information Any symptoms such as nausea, vomiting, numbness or tingling, and chest, muscle, or abdominal pain should be reported to the physician at the first sign of an attack; do **not** exceed recommended dosage; avoid coffee, tea, and cola

Dosage Forms

Suppository, rectal (Cafergot®): Ergotamine tartrate 2 mg and caffeine 100 mg (12s)

Tablet (Wigraine®): Ergotamine tartrate 1 mg and caffeine 100 mg

Tablet, sublingual (Ergomar®): Ergotamine tartrate 2 mg

- ♦ **Ergotamine and Caffeine** *see Ergotamine on page 393*
- ♦ **E•R•O [OTC]** *see Carbamide Peroxide on page 178*
- ♦ **Erybid (Can)** *see Erythromycin on page 394*
- ♦ **Eryc®** *see Erythromycin on page 394*
- ♦ **Erycette®** *see Erythromycin on page 394*
- ♦ **EryDerm®** *see Erythromycin on page 394*
- ♦ **Erygel®** *see Erythromycin on page 394*
- ♦ **Erymax®** *see Erythromycin on page 394*
- ♦ **Ery-Tab®** *see Erythromycin on page 394*
- ♦ **Erythro Base (Can)** *see Erythromycin on page 394*
- ♦ **Erythrocin®** *see Erythromycin on page 394*
- ♦ **Erythromid (Can)** *see Erythromycin on page 394*

Erythromycin *(er ith roe MYE sin)*

Related Information

Carbohydrate and Alcohol Content of Liquid Medications for Use in Patients Receiving Ketogenic Diets *on page 1258*

U.S. Brand Names AK-Mycin®; Akne-Mycin®; A/T/S®; C-Solve-2®; E.E.S.®; E.E.S. 400®; E.E.S.® Chewable; E.E.S.® Granules; Emgel®; E-Mycin®; E-Mycin-E®; Eryc®; Erycette®; EryDerm®; Erygel®; Erymax®; Ery-Tab®; Erythrocin®; E-Solve-2®; ETS-2%®; Ilosone®; Ilosone® Pulvules®; Ilotycin®; PCE®; Staticin®; T-Stat®; Wyamycin® S

Canadian Brand Names Apo-Erythro Base; Apo-Erythro E-C; Apo-Erythro ES; Apo-Erythro S; Diomycin; Erybid; Erythro Base; Erythromid; Novo-Rythro Encap; Nu-Erythromycin; PMS-Erythromycin

Synonyms Erythromycin Base

Therapeutic Category Antibiotic, Macrolide; Antibiotic, Ophthalmic

Generic Available Yes

Use Treatment of mild to moderately severe infections of the upper and lower respiratory tract, pharyngitis and skin infections due to susceptible streptococci and staphylococci; other susceptible bacterial infections including *Mycoplasma pneumoniae*, *Legionella* pneumonia, Lyme disease, diphtheria, pertussis, chancroid, *Chlamydia*, and *Campylobacter* gastroenteritis; used in conjunction with neomycin for decontaminating the bowel for surgery; ophthalmic ointment used to prevent gonococcal ophthalmia neonatorum

Pregnancy Risk Factor B

Contraindications Hepatic impairment; concomitant administration with astemizole, terfenadine, or cisapride; hypersensitivity to erythromycin or any component

Warnings Hepatic impairment with or without jaundice has occurred primarily in older children and adults; it may be accompanied by malaise, nausea, vomiting, abdominal colic, and fever; discontinue use if these occur; avoid using erythromycin lactobionate in neonates since formulation may contain benzyl alcohol which is associated with a fatal gasping syndrome in neonates; risk of serious cardiac arrhythmias exist in patients receiving erythromycin and astemizole, terfenadine, or cisapride (do not use concurrently with erythromycin)

Adverse Reactions

Cardiovascular: Ventricular arrhythmias, prolongation of the QT interval; bradycardia, hypotension with I.V. administration

Central nervous system: Fever, dizziness

Dermatologic: Skin rash, pruritus

Gastrointestinal: Abdominal pain, cramping, nausea, vomiting, diarrhea, stomatitis

Hematologic: Eosinophilia

Hepatic: Cholestatic hepatitis, jaundice; (incidence of erythromycin-associated hepatotoxicity is ~0.1% in children and 0.25% in adults)

Local: Thrombophlebitis (I.V. form)

Otic: Ototoxicity (after I.V. use)

Miscellaneous: Allergic reactions, anaphylaxis

Drug Interactions Cytochrome P-450 isoenzyme CYP3A3/4 substrate; isoenzyme CYP1A2 and CYP3A3/4 inhibitor

Erythromycin decreases clearance of astemizole, terfenadine, carbamazepine, cisapride, cyclosporine, protease inhibitors, lovastatin, simvastatin, midazolam, phenytoin, alfentanil, and triazolam; erythromycin may decrease theophylline clearance, increase theophylline's half-life by up to 60%, and result in theophylline toxicity (patients on high dose theophylline and erythromycin or who have received erythromycin for >5 days may be at higher risk); may potentiate anticoagulant effect of warfarin; may increase toxicity of ergotamine; may increase serum levels of digoxin, disopyramide, and quinidine

Stability Erythromycin lactobionate should be reconstituted with SWI without preservatives to avoid gel formation; the reconstituted solution is stable for 2 weeks when refrigerated or 24 hours at room temperature. Erythromycin I.V. infusion solution is stable at pH 6-8.

Mechanism of Action Inhibits bacterial RNA-dependent protein synthesis at the chain elongation step; binds to the 50S ribosomal subunit resulting in blockage of transpeptidation

Pharmacokinetics

Absorption: Variable but better with salt forms like the estolate than with base form; 18% to 45% absorbed orally; ethylsuccinate may be better absorbed with food

Distribution: Crosses the placenta; distributes into body tissues, fluids, and breast milk with poor penetration into the CSF

V_d: 0.64 L/kg

Protein binding: 75% to 90%

Metabolism: In the liver by demethylation

Half-life:

Neonates (≤15 days of age): 2.1 hours

Adults: 1.5-2 hours

Time to peak serum concentration: Oral:

Base: 4 hours

Stearate: 3 hours

Ethylsuccinate: 0.5-2.5 hours

Estolate: 2-4 hours (time to peak is delayed in the presence of food except when using estolate)

Elimination: 2% to 5% unchanged drug excreted in urine, major excretion in feces (via bile)

Dialysis: Not removed by peritoneal dialysis or hemodialysis

Usual Dosage

Neonates:

Oral: Ethylsuccinate: Postnatal age:

≤7 days: 20 mg/kg/day in divided doses every 12 hours

>7 days, <1200 g: 20 mg/kg/day in divided doses every 12 hours

>7 days, 1200-2000 g: 30 mg/kg/day in divided doses every 8 hours

>7 days, >2000 g: 30-40 mg/kg/day in divided doses every 6-8 hours

Ophthalmic: Prophylaxis of neonatal gonococcal ophthalmia: 0.5-1 cm ribbon of ointment should be instilled into each conjunctival sac once

I.V.: One study (n=14, ≤15 days of age, birth weight ≤1500 g) used erythromycin lactobionate in doses of 25 or 40 mg/kg/day divided every 6 hours for treatment of *Ureaplasma urealyticum* infection

Chlamydial conjunctivitis and pneumonia: Oral: Ethylsuccinate: 50 mg/kg/day divided every 6 hours for 14 days

Infants and Children:

Oral:

Base and ethylsuccinate: 30-50 mg/kg/day divided every 6-8 hours; do not exceed 2 g/day (as base) or 3.2 g/day (as ethylsuccinate); (**Note:** Due to

(Continued)

Erythromycin *(Continued)*

differences in absorption, 200 mg erythromycin ethylsuccinate produces the same serum levels as 125 mg erythromycin base or estolate)

Estolate: 30-50 mg/kg/day divided every 6-12 hours; do not exceed 2 g/day

Stearate: 30-50 mg/kg/day divided every 6 hours; do not exceed 2 g/day

Chlamydia trachomatis: Oral: 50 mg/kg/day divided every 6 hours for 10-14 days

Pertussis: Oral: 40-50 mg/kg/day divided every 6 hours for 14 days (some experts recommend using the estolate salt)

Preop bowel preparation: Oral: 20 mg/kg erythromycin base at 1, 2, and 11 PM on the day before surgery combined with mechanical cleansing of the large intestine and oral neomycin

I.V.:

Lactobionate: 15-50 mg/kg/day divided every 6 hours, not to exceed 4 g/day

Glucepate: 15-50 mg/kg/day divided every 6 hours, not to exceed 4 g/day

Children and Adults:

Ophthalmic: Instill ointment one or more times daily depending on the severity of the infection

Topical: Apply 2% solution over the affected area twice daily after the skin has been thoroughly washed and patted dry

Adults:

Oral:

Base, delayed release: 333 mg every 8 hours

Estolate, stearate or base: 250-500 mg every 6-12 hours

Ethylsuccinate: 400-800 mg every 6-12 hours

Chancroid: Oral: Base: 500 mg 4 times/day for 7 days

Chlamydia trachomatis: Oral:

Base: 500 mg 4 times/day for 7 days **or**

Ethylsuccinate: 800 mg 4 times/day for 7 days

Preop bowel preparation: Oral: 1 g erythromycin base at 1, 2, and 11 PM on the day before surgery combined with mechanical cleansing of the large intestine and oral neomycin

I.V.: Lactobionate or glucepate: 15-20 mg/kg/day divided every 6 hours or given as a continuous infusion over 24 hours, not to exceed 4 g/day

Prokinetic agent (to improve gastric emptying time and intestinal motility):

Children: Lactobionate or glucepate: Initial: 3 mg/kg I.V. infused over 60 minutes followed by 20 mg/kg/day orally in 3-4 divided doses before meals, or before meals and at bedtime

Adults: Lactobionate or glucepate: Initial: 200 mg I.V. followed by 250 mg orally 3 times/day 30 minutes before meals

Administration

Ophthalmic ointment for prevention of neonatal ophthalmia: Wipe each eyelid gently with sterile cotton; instill 0.5-1 cm ribbon of ointment in each lower conjunctival sac; massage eyelids gently to spread the ointment; after 1 minute, excess ointment can be wiped away with sterile cotton

Oral: Avoid milk and acidic beverages 1 hour before or after a dose; administer after food to decrease GI discomfort; ethylsuccinate chewable tablets should not be swallowed whole; do not chew or break delayed release capsule or enteric coated tablets, swallow whole

Parenteral: Administer by I.V. intermittent or continuous infusion diluted in either dextrose or saline solutions to a concentration of 1-2.5 mg/mL; maximum concentration: 5 mg/mL; I.V. intermittent infusions may be administered over 20-60 minutes; to decrease vein irritation, administer as a continuous infusion at a concentration ≤1 mg/mL; prolonging the infusion duration over 60 minutes or longer has been recommended to decrease the cardiotoxic effects of erythromycin

Monitoring Parameters Liver function tests

Test Interactions False-positive urinary catecholamines, 17-hydroxycorticosteroids and 17-ketosteroids

Nursing Implications Do not crush enteric coated or delayed release drug products

Additional Information Treatment of erythromycin-associated cardiac toxicity with prolongation of the QT interval and ventricular tachydysrhythmias includes discontinuing erythromycin and administering magnesium.

Dosage Forms

Capsule, as estolate: 125 mg, 250 mg

Capsule, delayed release, as base: 250 mg

Injection, glucepate: 1 g (30 mL)

Injection, lactobionate: 500 mg, 1 g

Gel, topical: 2% (30 g)

Ointment, ophthalmic: 5 mg/g (3.5 g)
  Ointment, topical: 2% (25 g)
Solution, topical: 1.5% (60 mL); 2% (60 mL)
Suspension:
  Oral, as estolate: 125 mg/5 mL (480 mL); 250 mg/5 mL (480 mL)
  Oral, as ethylsuccinate: 200 mg/5 mL (480 mL); 400 mg/5 mL (480 mL)
  Oral drops, as estolate: 100 mg/mL (10 mL)
  Oral drops, as ethylsuccinate: 100 mg/2.5 mL (30 mL)
Swab: 2% (60s)
Tablet:
  Chewable, as estolate: 125 mg, 250 mg
  Chewable, as ethylsuccinate: 200 mg
  Delayed release, as base: 250 mg, 333 mg, 500 mg
  Film coated, as base: 250 mg, 500 mg
  Film coated, as ethylsuccinate: 400 mg
  Film coated, as stearate: 250 mg, 500 mg
  Polymer coated particles, as base: 333 mg
  Polymer coated particles, as estolate: 500 mg

References
Di Lorenzo C, Lachman R, and Hyman PE, "Intravenous Erythromycin for Postpyloric Intubation," *J Pediatr Gastroenterol Nutr*, 1990, 11(1):45-7.

Janssens J, Peeters TL, Vantrappen G, et al, "Improvement of Gastric Emptying in Diabetic Gastroparesis by Erythromycin," *N Engl J Med*, 1990, 322(15):1028-31.

Reid B, DiLorenzo C, Travis L, et al, "Diabetic Gastroparesis Due to Postprandial Antral Hypomotility in Childhood," *Pediatrics*, 1992, 90(1 Pt 1):43-6.

Thoene DE and Johnson CE, "Pharmacotherapy of Otitis Media," *Pharmacotherapy*, 1991, 11(3):212-21.

Waites KB, Sims PJ, Crouse DT, et al, "Serum Concentrations of Erythromycin After Intravenous Infusion in Preterm Neonates Treated for *Ureaplasma urealyticum* Infection," *Pediatr Infect Dis J*, 1994, 13(4):287-93.

Erythromycin and Sulfisoxazole
(er ith roe MYE sin & sul fi SOKS a zole)

Related Information
  Carbohydrate and Alcohol Content of Liquid Medications for Use in Patients Receiving Ketogenic Diets *on page 1258*

U.S. Brand Names Eryzole®; Pediazole®; Sulfimycin®

Synonyms Sulfisoxazole and Erythromycin

Therapeutic Category Antibiotic, Macrolide; Antibiotic, Sulfonamide Derivative

Generic Available Yes

Use Treatment of susceptible bacterial infections of the upper and lower respiratory tract; otitis media in children caused by susceptible strains of *Haemophilus influenzae*; other infections in patients allergic to penicillin

Pregnancy Risk Factor C

Contraindications Hepatic dysfunction; hypersensitivity to erythromycin, any component, or sulfonamides; infants <2 months of age (sulfas compete with bilirubin for binding sites which may result in kernicterus in newborns); patients with porphyria; pregnant women at term; mothers nursing infants <2 months of age; concomitant administration of astemizole, terfenadine, or cisapride

Warnings Risk of serious cardiac arrhythmias exist in patients receiving erythromycin, astemizole, terfenadine, or cisapride (do not use concurrently); fatalities due to Stevens-Johnson syndrome, toxic epidermal necrolysis, fulminant hepatic necrosis, agranulocytosis, and aplastic anemia have occurred with the administration of sulfonamides; prolonged use may result in superinfection or pseudomembranous colitis

Precautions Use with caution in patients with impaired renal or hepatic function, G-6-PD deficiency (hemolysis may occur)

Adverse Reactions
  Cardiovascular: Tachycardia, palpitations, syncope
  Central nervous system: Headache, disorientation, fever, dizziness
  Dermatologic: Rash, photosensitivity, Stevens-Johnson syndrome, toxic epidermal necrolysis, pruritus, urticaria
  Gastrointestinal: Abdominal cramping, nausea, vomiting, diarrhea, pseudomembranous colitis, anorexia, stomatitis, pancreatitis
  Genitourinary: Crystalluria, hematuria
  Hematologic: Agranulocytosis, aplastic anemia, leukopenia, eosinophilia, thrombocytopenia
  Hepatic: Hepatic necrosis, jaundice
  Renal: Toxic nephrosis, elevated BUN and serum creatinine, acute renal failure
  Respiratory: Cough, shortness of breath, pulmonary infiltrates
  Miscellaneous: Anaphylaxis
(Continued)

Erythromycin and Sulfisoxazole *(Continued)*

Drug Interactions Erythromycin is a cytochrome P-450 isoenzyme CYP3A3/4 substrate; isoenzyme CYP1A2 and CYP3A3/4 inhibitor

Erythromycin decreases clearance of astemizole, terfenadine, carbamazepine, cisapride, cyclosporine, protease inhibitors, lovastatin, simvastatin, midazolam, phenytoin, alfentanil, and triazolam; erythromycin may decrease theophylline clearance, increase theophylline's half-life by up to 60%, and result in theophylline toxicity (patients on high dose theophylline and erythromycin or who have received erythromycin for >5 days may be at higher risk); may potentiate anticoagulant effect of warfarin; may increase toxicity of ergotamine; may increase serum levels of digoxin, disopyramide, and quinidine

Sulfisoxazole may decrease the amount of thiopental needed for anesthesia; sulfisoxazole may displace methotrexate from plasma protein-binding sites increasing free methotrexate concentrations; displaces tolbutamide, chlorpropamide, oral anticoagulants from protein binding sites; PABA (antagonizes the antibacterial activity of sulfas)

Stability Reconstituted suspension is stable for 14 days when refrigerated

Mechanism of Action Erythromycin inhibits bacterial protein synthesis by binding to the 50S ribosomal subunit; sulfisoxazole competitively inhibits bacterial synthesis of folic acid from para-aminobenzoic acid

Pharmacokinetics

Erythromycin ethylsuccinate:

Absorption: Well absorbed from the GI tract

Distribution: Widely distributed into most body tissues and fluids; poor penetration into CSF; crosses the placenta; excreted in breast milk

Protein binding: 75% to 90%

Metabolism: In the liver by demethylation

Half-life: 1-1.5 hours

Elimination: Unchanged drug is excreted and concentrated in bile; <5% of dose eliminated in urine

Dialysis: Not removed by peritoneal dialysis or hemodialysis

Sulfisoxazole acetyl:

Absorption: Hydrolyzed in the GI tract to sulfisoxazole which is rapidly and completely absorbed; the small intestine is the major site of absorption

Distribution: Into extracellular space; CSF concentration ranges from 8% to 57% of blood concentration in patients with normal meninges; crosses the placenta, excreted in breast milk

Protein binding: 85%

Metabolism: Undergoes N-acetylation and N-glucuronide conjugation in the liver

Half-life: 4.6-7.8 hours, prolonged in renal impairment

Elimination: 50% in urine as unchanged drug

Dialysis: >50% removed by hemodialysis

Usual Dosage Oral (dosage recommendation is based on the product's erythromycin content):

Children ≥2 months: 40-50 mg/kg/day in divided doses every 6-8 hours; not to exceed 2 g erythromycin or 6 g sulfisoxazole/day

Adults: 400 mg erythromycin and 1200 mg sulfisoxazole every 6 hours

Administration Oral: Administer with or without food; shake suspension well before use; maintain adequate fluid intake to prevent crystalluria and kidney stone formation

Monitoring Parameters CBC, urinalysis; periodic liver function and renal function tests; observe patient for diarrhea

Test Interactions False-positive urinary protein; false-positive urinary catecholamines, 17-hydroxycorticosteroids and 17-ketosteroids

Patient Information Avoid prolonged exposure to sunlight

Dosage Forms Suspension, oral: Erythromycin ethylsuccinate 200 mg and sulfisoxazole acetyl 600 mg per 5 mL (100 mL, 150 mL, 200 mL, 250 mL)

References

Rodriguez WJ, Schwartz RH, Sait T, et al, "Erythromycin-Sulfisoxazole vs Amoxicillin in the Treatment of Acute Otitis Media in Children," *Am J Dis Child*, 1985, 139(8):766-70.

♦ **Eskalith® CR** *see* Lithium *on page 600*

Esmolol (ES moe lol)

Related Information
Overdose and Toxicology *on page 1222*

U.S. Brand Names Brevibloc®

Therapeutic Category Antiarrhythmic Agent, Class II; Antihypertensive Agent; Beta-Adrenergic Blocker

Generic Available No

Use Supraventricular tachycardia (primarily to control ventricular rate) and hypertension (especially perioperatively)

Pregnancy Risk Factor C

Contraindications Sinus bradycardia or heart block, uncompensated CHF, cardiogenic shock; hypersensitivity to esmolol, any component, or other beta-blockers

Warnings Caution should be exercised when discontinuing esmolol infusions to avoid withdrawal effects

Precautions Use with extreme caution in patients with hyper-reactive airway disease; use lowest dose possible and discontinue infusion if bronchospasm occurs; use with caution in diabetes mellitus, hypoglycemia, renal failure; avoid extravasation

Adverse Reactions

Cardiovascular: Hypotension (especially with doses >200 mcg/kg/minute), bradycardia, Raynaud's phenomena

Central nervous system: Dizziness, somnolence, confusion, lethargy, depression, headache

Gastrointestinal: Nausea, vomiting

Local: Phlebitis, skin necrosis after extravasation

Respiratory: Bronchoconstriction (less than propranolol, but more likely with higher doses)

Miscellaneous: Diaphoresis, adverse reactions similar to other beta-blockers may occur

Drug Interactions Esmolol may increase digoxin or theophylline serum concentrations; morphine may increase esmolol blood concentrations; xanthines (eg, theophylline, caffeine) may decrease effects of esmolol

Food Interactions Avoid xanthine-containing foods or beverages

Mechanism of Action Class II antiarrhythmic: Competitively blocks response to beta$_1$-adrenergic stimulation with little or no effect on beta$_2$-receptors except at high doses (ie, cardioselective at lower doses); no intrinsic sympathomimetic activity; no membrane-stabilizing activity; ultrashort-acting

Pharmacodynamics

Onset of action: I.V.: Beta blockade occurs within 2-10 minutes (onset of effects is quickest when loading doses are administered)

Duration: Short (10-30 minutes)

Pharmacokinetics

Protein binding: 55%

Distribution: V$_d$:
Children: 2 L/kg
Adults: 3.5 L/kg (range: 2-5 L/kg)

Metabolism: In blood by esterases

Half-life, elimination:
Children:
18 months to 14 years (n=12): 2.88 ± 2.67 minutes
2.5-16 years (n=20): 4.5 ± 2.1 minutes
Adults: 9 minutes

Elimination: ~69% of dose excreted in urine as metabolites and 2% as unchanged drug

Usual Dosage Must be adjusted to individual response and tolerance

Children: I.V.: Limited information available

Supraventricular tachycardia (SVT): Some centers have utilized initial doses of 100-500 mcg/kg given over 1 minute followed by a continuous infusion for control of SVT. One electrophysiologic study assessing esmolol-induced beta-blockade (n=20, 2-16 years of age) used an initial dose of 600 mcg/kg over 2 minutes followed by an infusion of 200 mcg/kg/minute; the infusion was titrated upward by 50-100 mcg/kg/minute every 5-10 minutes until a reduction >10% in heart rate or mean blood pressure occurred. Mean dose required: 550 mcg/kg/minute with a range of 300-1000 mcg/kg/minute.

Postoperative hypertension: Loading doses of 500 mcg/kg/minute over 1 minute with doses of 50-250 mcg/kg/minute (mean 173) have been used in addition to

(Continued)

Esmolol *(Continued)*

nitroprusside in a small number of patients (7 patients, 7-19 years of age, median age 13 years) after coarctation of aorta repair.

Adults: I.V.: Loading dose: 500 mcg/kg over 1 minute; follow with a 50 mcg/kg/minute infusion for 4 minutes; if response is inadequate, rebolus with another 500 mcg/kg loading dose over 1 minute, and increase the maintenance infusion to 100 mcg/kg/minute. Repeat this process until a therapeutic effect has been achieved or to a maximum recommended maintenance dose of 200 mcg/kg/minute. Usual dosage range: 50-200 mcg/kg/minute with average dose = 100 mcg/kg/minute.

Administration Parenteral: I.V.: The 250 mg/mL ampul is **not** for direct I.V. injection, but must first be diluted to a final concentration not to exceed 10 mg/mL (ie, 2.5 g in 250 mL or 5 g in 500 mL); infuse I.V. loading dose over 1-2 minutes

Monitoring Parameters Blood pressure, EKG, heart rate, respiratory rate, I.V. site

Nursing Implications Decrease infusion rate or discontinue if hypotension, CHF, etc occur

Dosage Forms Injection, as hydrochloride: 10 mg/mL (10 mL); 250 mg/mL (10 mL)

References

Cuneo BF, Zales VR, Blahunka PC, et al, "Pharmacodynamics and Pharmacokinetics of Esmolol, A Short-Acting Beta-Blocking Agent in Children," *Pediatr Cardiol*, 1994, 15(6):296-301.

Trippel DL, Wiest DB, and Gillette PC, "Cardiovascular and Antiarrhythmic Effects of Esmolol in Children," *J Pediatr*, 1991, 119(1):142-7.

Vincent RN, Click LA, Williams HM, et al, "Esmolol As an Adjunct in the Treatment of Systemic Hypertension After Operative Repair of Coarctation of the Aorta," *Am J Cardiol*, 1990, 65(13):941-3.

Wiest DB, Trippel DL, Gillette PC, et al, "Pharmacokinetics of Esmolol in Children," *Clin Pharmacol Ther*, 1991, 49(6):618-23.

♦ **E-Solve-2**® *see Erythromycin on page 394*

♦ **Estar**® **[OTC]** *see Coal Tar on page 260*

♦ **Estimated Comparative Daily Dosages for Inhaled Corticosteroids** *see page 1216*

♦ **Estrace**® *see Estradiol on page 400*

♦ **Estraderm**® *see Estradiol on page 400*

Estradiol *(es tra DYE ole)*

U.S. Brand Names Alora®; Climara®; Delestrogen®; Depo®-Estradiol; Depogen®; Esclim®; Estrace®; Estraderm®; Estro-Cyp®; Gynodiol™; Vagifem®; Valergen®; Vivelle®; Vivelle® Dot

Canadian Brand Names Estrogel; Oesclim

Therapeutic Category Estrogen Derivative; Estrogen Derivative, Vaginal

Generic Available Yes

Use Atrophic vaginitis, atrophic dystrophy of vulva, menopausal symptoms, female hypogonadism; prevention of postmenopausal osteoporosis

Pregnancy Risk Factor X

Contraindications Thromboembolic disorders, active arterial thrombosis, thyroid dysfunction, blood dyscrasias; hypersensitivity to estradiol or any component; known or suspected pregnancy

Warnings Estrogens have been reported to increase the risk of endometrial carcinoma; do not use estrogens during pregnancy

Precautions Use with caution in patients with renal or hepatic insufficiency, or diseases that may be exacerbated by fluid retention; estrogens may cause premature closure of the epiphyses in young individuals

Adverse Reactions

Cardiovascular: Hypertension, edema, thromboembolic disorders

Central nervous system: Depression, headache, dizziness

Dermatologic: Chloasma, melasma

Endocrine & metabolic: Breast enlargement, breast tenderness, changes in libido, impaired glucose tolerance, hypercalcemia, folate deficiency; increased risk of endometrial hyperplasia

Gastrointestinal: Nausea, vomiting, bloating, abdominal cramps, pancreatitis, weight gain or weight loss, gall bladder disease

Genitourinary: Changes in menstrual flow

Hepatic: Cholestatic jaundice

Local: Pain at injection site; topical may cause burning or irritation

Neuromuscular & skeletal: Premature closure of epiphyses in young patients (large and repeated doses over an extended period of time)

Drug Interactions Cytochrome P-450 isoenzyme CYP1A2 and CYP3A3/4 substrate Rifampin (decreased effect of estrogens); anticoagulants, bromocriptine, dantrolene (increased risk of hepatotoxicity); estrogens may decrease the clearance and increase serum concentrations and toxic effects of corticosteroids and cyclo-sporine

Food Interactions Larger doses of vitamin C (eg, 1 g/day in adults) may increase the serum concentrations and adverse effects of estradiol; vitamin C supplements are not recommended, but this effect may be decreased if vitamin C supplement is given 2-3 hours after estrogen; dietary intake of folate and pyridoxine may need to be increased

Mechanism of Action Increases the synthesis of DNA, RNA, and various proteins in target tissues; reduces the release of gonadotropin-releasing hormone from the hypothalamus; reduces FSH and LH release from the pituitary

Usual Dosage Adolescents and Adults: All dosage needs to be adjusted based upon the patient's response

Female hypogonadism:
  I.M.:
    Cypionate: 1.5-2 mg given once each month
    Valerate: 10-20 mg given once each month
  Oral: 0.5-2 mg/day in a cyclic regimen (3 weeks on drug, 1 week off)
  Transdermal:
    Once-weekly patch (Climara®): Initial: 0.025-0.05 mg/day patch applied once weekly (titrate dosage to response)
    Twice-weekly patch (Alora®, Esclim®, Estraderm®, Vivelle®): Initial: 0.05 mg patch (titrate dosage to response) applied twice weekly in a cyclic regimen (3 weeks on drug, 1 week off) in patients with intact uterus and continuously in patients without a uterus
  Vaginal and vulval atrophy: Intravaginal: Initial: 200-400 mcg of estradiol once daily for 1-2 weeks; taper dose gradually to 100-200 mcg of estradiol once daily for 1-2 weeks; maintenance, cyclic regimen (after vaginal mucosa restored): 100 mcg of estradiol 1-3 times/week for 3 weeks, then no drug for the 4th week per cycle

Administration
  Oral: Administer with food or after a meal to reduce GI upset
  Parenteral: Injection for I.M. use only
  Transdermal: Apply to clean dry area; do not apply to breasts; do not apply to waistline (may loosen patch); rotate application sites

Monitoring Parameters Blood pressure, serum calcium, glucose, liver enzymes; bone maturation and epiphyseal effects in young patients in whom bone growth is not complete

Test Interactions Thyroid function tests: Estrogens may increase thyroid binding globulin and circulating total thyroid hormone (when measured by T_4 RIA, T_4 by column, or by PBI); decreases free T_3 resin uptake; concentration of free T_4 is not altered

Patient Information Limit alcohol; limit caffeine; notify physician if sudden severe headache or vomiting, disturbance of vision or speech, numbness or weakness of extremity, sharp or crushing chest pain, calf pain, shortness of breath, severe abdominal pain or mass, mental depression, or unusual bleeding occurs

Dosage Forms
  Cream, vaginal, as base (Estrace®): 0.1 mg/g (42.5 g)
  Injection, as **cypionate** (Depo®-Estradiol, Depogen®): 5 mg/mL (5 mL, 10 mL)
  Injection, as **valerate**:
    Delestrogen®: 10 mg/mL (5 mL); 20 mg/mL (5 mL, 10 mL); 40 mg/mL (5 mL, 10 mL)
    Valergen®: 20 mg/mL (5 mL, 10 mL); 40 mg/mL (5 mL, 10 mL)
  Tablet, micronized, as base:
    Estrace®: 0.5 mg, 1 mg, 2 mg
    Gynodiol™: 0.5 mg, 1 mg, 1.5 mg, 2 mg
  Tablet, vaginal, as base (Vagifem®): 25 mcg
  Transdermal system, as base:
    Alora® [twice weekly patch]:
      0.05 mg/24 hours [18 cm²]
      0.075 mg/24 hours [27 cm²]
      0.1 mg/24 hours [36 cm²]
    Climara® [once weekly patch]:
      0.025 mg/24 hours [6.5 cm²]
      0.05 mg/24 hours [12.5 cm²]
      0.075 mg/24 hours [18.75 cm²]
      0.1 mg/24 hours [25 cm²]
    Esclim® [twice weekly patch]:
      0.025 mg/24 hours [11 cm²]
      0.0375 mg/24 hours [16.5 cm²]
(Continued)

Estradiol *(Continued)*

    0.05 mg/24 hours [22 cm^2]
    0.075 mg/24 hours [33 cm^2]
    0.1 mg/24 hours [44 cm^2]
  Estraderm® [twice weekly patch]:
    0.05 mg/24 hours [10 cm^2]
    0.1 mg/24 hours [20 cm^2]
  Vivelle® [twice weekly patch]:
    0.025 mg/24 hours [7.25 cm^2]
    0.0375 mg/24 hours [11 cm^2]
    0.05 mg/24 hours [14.5 cm^2]
    0.075 mg/24 hours [22 cm^2]
    0.1 mg/24 hours [29 cm^2]
  Vivelle® Dot [twice weekly patch]:
    0.0375 mg/24 hours [3.75 cm^2]
    0.05 mg/24 hours [5 cm^2]
    0.075 mg/24 hours [7.5 cm^2]
    0.1 mg/24 hours [10 cm^2]

♦ **Estro-Cyp®** *see Estradiol on page 400*
♦ **Estrogel (Can)** *see Estradiol on page 400*
♦ **Estrogenic Substances, Conjugated** *see Estrogens (Conjugated) on page 402*

Estrogens (Conjugated) (ES troe jenz KON joo gate ed)

U.S. Brand Names Premarin®
Canadian Brand Names C.E.S.; Congest; PMS-Conjugated Estrogens
Synonyms C.E.S.; Conjugated Estrogens; Estrogenic Substances, Conjugated
Therapeutic Category Estrogen Derivative; Estrogen Derivative, Vaginal
Generic Available No

Use Dysfunctional uterine bleeding, hypogonadism, atrophic vaginitis, vasomotor symptoms of menopause; postmenopausal hormonal replacement therapy

Pregnancy Risk Factor X

Contraindications Undiagnosed vaginal bleeding; hypersensitivity to estrogens or any component; thrombophlebitis or thromboembolic disorders; pregnancy; known or suspected breast cancer (except in select patients being treated for metastatic disease); estrogen-dependent neoplasia

Warnings Estrogens have been reported to increase the risk of endometrial carcinoma; do not use estrogens during pregnancy

Precautions Use with caution in patients with asthma, epilepsy, migraine, diabetes, hypercalcemia, cardiac, liver, or renal dysfunction; estrogens may cause premature closure of the epiphyses in young individuals; may greatly increase triglycerides and lead to pancreatitis and other problems in patients with familial defects of lipoprotein

Adverse Reactions
  Cardiovascular: Hypertension, edema, thromboembolic disorder
  Central nervous system: Depression, headache, dizziness
  Dermatologic: Chloasma, melasma
  Endocrine & metabolic: Breast enlargement, breast tenderness, changes in libido, impaired glucose tolerance, hypercalcemia, folate deficiency; increased risk of endometrial hyperplasia
  Gastrointestinal: Nausea, vomiting, bloating, abdominal cramps, pancreatitis, weight gain or weight loss, gall bladder disease
  Genitourinary: Changes in menstrual flow
  Hepatic: Cholestatic jaundice
  Local: Pain at injection site
  Neuromuscular & skeletal: Premature closure of epiphyses in young patients

Drug Interactions Rifampin (decreased effect of estrogens), anticoagulants, bromocriptine, dantrolene (increased risk of hepatotoxicity); estrogens may decrease the clearance and increase the serum concentrations and toxic effects of corticosteroids and cyclosporine

Food Interactions Larger doses of vitamin C (eg, 1 g/day in adults) may increase the serum concentrations and adverse effects of estrogens; vitamin C supplements are not recommended, but this effect may be decreased if vitamin C supplement is given 2-3 hours after estrogen; dietary intake of folate and pyridoxine may need to be increased

Stability Injection: Store in the refrigerator; compatible with NS, dextrose, and invert sugar solutions; not compatible with ascorbic acid, protein hydrolysate, or acidic pH

Mechanism of Action Increases the synthesis of DNA, RNA, and various proteins in target tissues; reduces the release of gonadotropin-releasing hormone from the hypothalamus; reduces FSH and LH release from the pituitary

Usual Dosage Adolescents and Adults:

Hypogonadism: Oral: 2.5-7.5 mg/day in divided doses for 20 days, off 10 days and repeat until menses occur

Dysfunctional uterine bleeding:

Stable hematocrit: Oral: 1.25 mg twice daily for 21 days; if bleeding persists after 48 hours, increase to 2.5 mg twice daily; if bleeding persists after 48 more hours, increase to 2.5 mg 4 times/day; some recommend starting at 2.5 mg 4 times/day (**Note:** Medroxyprogesterone acetate 10 mg/day is also given on days 17-21; see Neistein, 1991)

Alternatively: Oral: 2.5-5 mg/day for 7-10 days; then decrease to 1.25 mg/day for 2 weeks

Unstable hematocrit: Oral, I.V.: 5 mg 2-4 times/day; if bleeding is profuse, 20-40 mg every 4 hours up to 24 hours may be used; **Note:** A progestational-weighted contraception pill should also be given (eg, Ovral® 2 tablets stat and 1 tablet 4 times/day or medroxyprogesterone acetate 5-10 mg 4 times/day; see Neistein, 1991)

Alternatively: I.M., I.V.: 25 mg every 6-12 hours until bleeding stops

Vaginal and vulval atrophy: Intravaginal or topical: Cyclic regimen: 1.25-2.5 mg/day of conjugated estrogens for 3 weeks, then no drug for the 4th week per cycle; repeat as clinically needed

Administration

Oral: Administer with food or after eating to reduce GI upset; administration of dose at bedtime may decrease adverse effects

Parenteral: Add sterile diluent provided by manufacturer and shake gently; I.V.: Administer slow I.V. avoid vascular flushing; I.M.: may be administered I.M. for dysfunctional uterine bleeding, but I.V. use is preferred (more rapid response)

Monitoring Parameters Blood pressure, serum calcium, glucose, liver enzymes; dysfunctional uterine bleeding: Hematocrit, hemoglobin, PT; bone maturation and epiphyseal effects in young patients in whom bone growth is not complete

Test Interactions Thyroid function tests: Estrogens may increase thyroid binding globulin and circulating total thyroid hormone (when measured by T_4 RIA, T_4 by column, or by PBI); decreases free T_3 resin uptake; concentration of free T_4 is not altered

Patient Information Limit caffeine; notify physician if sudden severe headache, vomiting, disturbance of vision or speech, numbness or weakness of extremity, sharp or crushing chest pain, calf pain, shortness of breath, severe abdominal pain or mass, mental depression, or unusual bleeding occurs

Dosage Forms

Cream, vaginal: 0.625 mg/g (42.5 g)

Powder for injection: 25 mg

Tablet: 0.3 mg, 0.625 mg, 0.9 mg, 1.25 mg, 2.5 mg

References

Neistein LS, *Adolescent Health Care - A Practical Guide*, 2nd ed, Baltimore: Urban & Schwarzenberg, 1991, 661-6.

♦ **ETAF** see Aldesleukin on page 47

Etanercept (et a NER cept)

U.S. Brand Names Enbrel®

Therapeutic Category Antirheumatic, Disease Modifying

Generic Available No

Use Treatment of polyarticular-course juvenile rheumatoid arthritis in patients who have had an inadequate response to one or more disease-modifying antirheumatic drugs; treatment of signs and symptoms of moderately to severely active rheumatoid arthritis in patients who have had an inadequate response to one or more disease-modifying antirheumatic drugs or in combination with methotrexate in patients who do not respond adequately to methotrexate alone

Pregnancy Risk Factor B

Contraindications Hypersensitivity to etanercept or any component (ie, mannitol, sucrose, tromethamine, and benzyl alcohol); patients with any serious active infection or sepsis

Warnings Some patients have developed serious infections and several have died from their infections while taking etanercept; patients who develop a new infection while being treated with etanercept should be monitored closely. Rare cases of CNS demyelinating disorders, such as multiple sclerosis, myelitis, and optic neuritis, have been reported in patients undergoing etanercept therapy.

(Continued)

Etanercept *(Continued)*

Precautions Use with caution in patients with a history of recurrent infections or illnesses such as poorly controlled diabetes which predisposes the patient to infection; discontinue etanercept in a child who develops varicella infection or who has a significant exposure to varicella virus and consider prophylactic treatment with varicella-zoster immune globulin; patients with latex allergy should not handle the needle cover of the diluent syringe since it contains latex; anti-TNF therapies such as etanercept may affect host defenses against infections and malignancies

Adverse Reactions

Central nervous system: Headache (19%), depression, personality disorder, dizziness

Dermatologic: Rash

Gastrointestinal: Nausea (9%), abdominal pain (19%), vomiting (13%), esophagitis/gastritis

Hematologic: Pancytopenia, aplastic anemia

Local: Injection site reactions (erythema, discomfort, itching, swelling)

Respiratory: Respiratory tract infection, rhinitis

Miscellaneous: Allergic reaction (hives, difficulty breathing), positive antinuclear antibodies, positive antidouble-stranded DNA antibodies

Drug Interactions Live vaccines (unknown whether secondary transmission of infection in live vaccines can occur)

Stability Store vial in the refrigerator; do not freeze; etanercept solution should be used within 6 hours of reconstitution; do not shake or agitate vigorously; do not use if discolored or cloudy; do not filter reconstituted solution; do not add or mix with other medications

Mechanism of Action Binds to tumor necrosis factor (TNF) and blocks its interaction with cell surface TNF receptors rendering TNF biologically inactive; modulates biological responses that are induced or regulated by TNF

Pharmacodynamics

Onset of action: One week of treatment

Peak effect: Full effect is usually seen within 3 months

Pharmacokinetics

Absorption: Absorbed slowly after S.C. injection

Distribution: V_d: 1.78-3.39 L/m^2

Bioavailability: S.C.: 60%

Half-life: Adults: 115 hours (range: 98-300 hours)

Time to peak serum concentration: S.C.: 72 hours (range: 48-96 hours)

Elimination: Clearance:

Children 4-17 years: 46 mL/hour/m^2

Adults: 52 mL/hour/m^2

Usual Dosage S.C.:

Children 4-17 years: 0.4 mg/kg/dose twice weekly given 72-96 hours apart; maximum dose: 25 mg

Adult: 25 mg twice weekly given 72-96 hours apart

Administration Parenteral: Administer by S.C. injection into thigh, abdomen, or upper arm; injection sites should be rotated with subsequent doses given at least 1 inch from an old site; do not inject into areas where the skin is tender, bruised, red, or hard

Monitoring Parameters Assess for joint swelling, pain, and tenderness; ESR or C-reactive protein level

Patient Information Notify physician if persistent fever, bruising, bleeding, or pallor occurs.

Dosage Forms Powder for injection: 25 mg vial

References

Lovell DJ, Giannini EH, Whitmore JB, et al, "Safety and Efficacy of Tumor Necrosis Factor Receptor P75Fc Fusion Protein (TNFR:Fc, ENBREL) in Polyarticular Course Juvenile Rheumatoid Arthritis," Presented at American College of Rheumatology National Meeting, San Diego, CA, 1998.

Moreland LW, Baumgartner SW, Schiff MH, et al, "Treatment of Rheumatoid Arthritis With a Recombinant Human Tumor Necrosis Factor Receptor (p75)-Fc Fusion Protein," *N Engl J Med*, 1997, 337(3):141-7.

Ethacrynic Acid *(eth a KRIN ik AS id)*

U.S. Brand Names Edecrin®

Therapeutic Category Antihypertensive Agent; Diuretic, Loop

Generic Available No

Use Management of edema secondary to CHF, hepatic or renal disease; hypertension

Pregnancy Risk Factor B

Contraindications Hypersensitivity to ethacrynic acid or any component; hypotension, hyponatremic dehydration, metabolic alkalosis with hypokalemia, or anuria

Warnings Loop diuretics are potent diuretics; excess amounts can lead to profound diuresis with fluid and electrolyte loss; close medical supervision and dose evaluation is required; may increase risk of gastric hemorrhage associated with corticosteroid treatment

Precautions Avoid use in patients with severe renal dysfunction (Cl_{cr} <10 mL/minute)

Adverse Reactions
  Cardiovascular: Hypotension
  Central nervous system: Headache, fatigue, mental confusion, vertigo
  Dermatologic: Rash, photosensitivity
  Endocrine & metabolic: Hyperglycemia, fluid and electrolyte imbalances (fluid depletion, hypokalemia, hyponatremia, hypomagnesemia, hypocalcemia), hyperuricemia
  Gastrointestinal: GI irritation, diarrhea, anorexia, abdominal pain, dysphagia, GI bleed
  Hematologic: Thrombocytopenia, neutropenia, agranulocytosis
  Hepatic: Abnormal liver function tests, jaundice, hepatocellular damage
  Local: Local irritation, pain at injection site
  Otic: Ototoxicity, tinnitus
  Renal: Renal injury, hematuria

Drug Interactions Additive potassium depletion with drugs which cause potassium depletion: amphotericin, steroids, corticotropin; decreased renal clearance of lithium; decreased hypoglycemic effect of insulin or oral antidiabetic agents; decreased excretion of ethacrynic acid by probenecid; increased risk of ototoxicity with aminoglycosides; increased warfarin activity due to displacement from protein-binding sites

Food Interactions Need diet rich in potassium and magnesium

Stability When reconstituted with 50 mL D_5W or NS, resultant solution (1 mg/mL) is stable for 24 hours at room temperature

Mechanism of Action Inhibits reabsorption of sodium and chloride in the ascending loop of Henle and distal renal tubule, interfering with the chloride-binding cotransport system, thus causing increased excretion of water, sodium, chloride, magnesium, and calcium

Pharmacodynamics
  Onset of action:
    Oral: Within 30 minutes
    I.V.: 5 minutes
  Peak effect:
    Oral: 2 hours
    I.V.: 15-30 minutes
  Duration:
    Oral: 6-8 hours
    I.V.: 2 hours

Pharmacokinetics
  Absorption: Oral: Rapid
  Protein binding: >90%
  Metabolism: In the liver to active cysteine conjugate (35% to 40%)
  Elimination: In bile, 30% to 60% excreted unchanged in urine

Usual Dosage
  Children:
    Oral: 1 mg/kg/dose once daily, increase at intervals of 2-3 days to a maximum of 3 mg/kg/day
    I.V.: 1 mg/kg/dose; repeat doses are not routinely recommended, however if indicated, repeat doses every 8-12 hours
  Adults:
    Oral: 25-400 mg/day in 1-2 divided doses
    I.V.: 0.5-1 mg/kg/dose (maximum dose: 100 mg/dose); repeat doses not routinely recommended, however if indicated, repeat every 8-12 hours

Administration
  Oral: Administer with food or milk
  Parenteral: Dilute injection with 50 mL D_5W or NS (1 mg/mL concentration resulting); maximum concentration 2 mg/mL; may be injected without further dilution over a period of several minutes or infused over 20-30 minutes; tissue irritant; not to be administered I.M. or S.C.

Monitoring Parameters Serum electrolytes, blood pressure, renal function, hearing

Additional Information Injection contains thimerosal
  (Continued)

Ethacrynic Acid *(Continued)*

Dosage Forms
Powder for injection, as ethacrynate sodium: 50 mg
Tablet: 25 mg, 50 mg

Extemporaneous Preparations To make a 1 mg/mL suspension: Dissolve 120 mg ethacrynic acid powder in 13 mL alcohol, USP; add a small amount of methylparaben 0.005% and propylparaben 0.002% (final concentrations); adjust pH to 7 with 0.1N sodium hydroxide solution; add sufficient 50% sorbitol solution to make a final volume of 120 mL. Stable 220 days at room temperature. Shake well before use.

Das Gupta V, Gibbs CW Jr, and Ghanekar AG, "Stability of Pediatric Liquid Dosage Forms of Ethacrynic Acid, Indomethacin, Methyldopa Hydrochloride, Prednisone and Spironolactone," *Am J Hosp Pharm*, 1978, 35(11):1382-5.

Ethambutol *(e THAM byoo tole)*

U.S. Brand Names Myambutol®
Canadian Brand Names Etibi
Therapeutic Category Antitubercular Agent
Generic Available No
Use Treatment of tuberculosis and other mycobacterial diseases in conjunction with other antimycobacterial agents
Pregnancy Risk Factor B
Contraindications Hypersensitivity to ethambutol or any component; optic neuritis
Warnings Use only in children whose visual acuity can accurately be determined and monitored; not recommended for use in children <13 years of age unless benefit outweighs risk of therapy
Precautions Use with caution in patients with ocular defects or impaired renal function; modify dose in patients with renal impairment
Adverse Reactions
Central nervous system: Malaise, mental confusion, fever, headache, dizziness
Dermatologic: Rash, pruritus
Endocrine & metabolic: Elevated uric acid levels
Gastrointestinal: Nausea, vomiting, anorexia, abdominal pain
Hepatic: Abnormal liver function tests
Neuromuscular & skeletal: Peripheral neuropathy, arthralgia
Ocular: Optic neuritis, decreased visual acuity, decreased red-green color discrimination
Miscellaneous: Anaphylaxis
Mechanism of Action Suppresses mycobacterial multiplication by interfering with RNA synthesis
Pharmacokinetics
Absorption: Oral: ~80%
Distribution: Well distributed throughout the body with high concentrations in kidneys, lungs, saliva, CSF, and red blood cells; crosses the placenta; excreted into breast milk
Protein binding: 20% to 30%
Metabolism: 20% by the liver to inactive metabolite
Half-life: 2.5-3.6 hours (up to 7 hours or longer with renal impairment)
Time to peak serum concentration: Within 2-4 hours
Elimination: ~50% in urine and 20% excreted in feces as unchanged drug
Dialysis: Slightly dialyzable (5% to 20%)
Usual Dosage Oral:
Tuberculosis: Infants, Children, Adolescents, and Adults: 15-25 mg/kg/day once daily **or** 50 mg/kg/dose twice weekly, not to exceed 2.5 g/dose
Nontuberculous mycobacterial infection: Children, Adolescents, and Adults: 15 mg/kg/day, not to exceed 1 g/day
Dosing interval in renal impairment:
Cl_{cr} 10-50 mL/minute: Administer every 24-36 hours
Cl_{cr} <10 mL/minute: Administer every 48 hours and/or reduce usual dose
Administration Oral: Administer with or without food; if GI upset occurs, administer with food
Monitoring Parameters Monthly examination of visual acuity and color discrimination in patients receiving >15 mg/kg/day; periodic renal, hepatic, and hematologic function tests
Patient Information Report to physician any visual changes, numbness or tingling in hands or feet, rash, fever, and chills
Dosage Forms Tablet, as hydrochloride: 100 mg, 400 mg

References

American Academy of Pediatrics, Committee on Infectious Diseases, "Chemotherapy for Tuberculosis in Infants and Children," *Pediatrics*, 1992, 89(1):161-5.

Starke JR and Correa AG, "Management of Mycobacterial Infection and Disease in Children," *Pediatr Infect Dis J*, 1995, 14:455-70.

♦ **Ethanol** *see Ethyl Alcohol on page 409*

Ethionamide (e thye on AM ide)
U.S. Brand Names Trecator®-SC
Therapeutic Category Antitubercular Agent
Generic Available No
Use In conjunction with other antituberculosis agents in the treatment of tuberculosis and other mycobacterial diseases
Pregnancy Risk Factor C
Contraindications Severe hepatic impairment; hypersensitivity to ethionamide or any component
Precautions Use with caution in patients receiving cycloserine or isoniazid or in diabetic patients
Adverse Reactions
  Cardiovascular: Postural hypotension
  Central nervous system: Drowsiness, dizziness, seizures, headache, encephalopathy, depression
  Dermatologic: Rash
  Endocrine & metabolic: Hypoglycemia, goiter, gynecomastia
  Gastrointestinal: Nausea, vomiting, abdominal pain, diarrhea, anorexia, stomatitis, metallic taste, weight loss
  Hematologic: Thrombocytopenia
  Hepatic: Hepatitis; jaundice; elevated AST, ALT, and serum bilirubin
  Neuromuscular & skeletal: Peripheral neuropathy, tremor
  Ocular: Optic neuritis
  Miscellaneous: Excessive salivation
Food Interactions Increase dietary intake of pyridoxine to prevent neurotoxic effects of ethionamide
Mechanism of Action Inhibits peptide synthesis in susceptible organisms
Pharmacokinetics
  Absorption: ~80% is rapidly absorbed from the GI tract
  Distribution: Crosses the placenta; widely distributed into body tissues and fluids including liver, kidneys, and CSF
  Protein binding: 10%
  Metabolism: In the liver to active and inactive metabolites
  Bioavailability: 80%
  Half-life: 2-3 hours
  Time to peak serum concentration: Oral: Within 3 hours
  Elimination: As metabolites (active and inactive) and parent drug in the urine
Usual Dosage Oral:
  Children: 15-20 mg/kg/day in 2-3 divided doses, not to exceed 1 g/day
  Adults: 500-1000 mg/day in 1-3 divided doses
Administration Oral: Administer with meals to decrease GI distress
Monitoring Parameters Initial and periodic serum AST and ALT, blood glucose
Nursing Implications Neurotoxic effects may be relieved by the administration of pyridoxine
Dosage Forms Tablet: 250 mg
References

Donald PR and Seifart HI,"Cerebrospinal Fluid Concentrations of Ethionamide in Children With Tuberculous Meningitis," *J Pediatr*, 1989, 115(3):483-6.

Starke JR and Correa AG, "Management of Mycobacterial Infection and Disease in Children," *Pediatr Infect Dis J*, 1995, 14(6):455-69.

Ethosuximide (eth oh SUKS i mide)
Related Information
  Antiepileptic Drugs *on page 1208*
  Blood Level Sampling Time Guidelines *on page 1220*
  Carbohydrate and Alcohol Content of Liquid Medications for Use in Patients Receiving Ketogenic Diets *on page 1258*
U.S. Brand Names Zarontin®
Therapeutic Category Anticonvulsant, Succinimide
Generic Available Yes
Use Management of absence (petit mal) seizures, myoclonic seizures, and akinetic epilepsy
(Continued)

Ethosuximide *(Continued)*

Pregnancy Risk Factor C

Contraindications Hypersensitivity to ethosuximide or any component

Warnings Ethosuximide may increase tonic-clonic seizures in patients with mixed seizure disorders; ethosuximide must be used in combination with other anticonvulsants in patients with both absence and tonic-clonic seizures

Precautions Use with caution in patients with hepatic or renal disease; abrupt withdrawal of the drug may precipitate absence status

Adverse Reactions

Central nervous system: Sedation, dizziness, lethargy, euphoria, hallucinations, insomnia, agitation, behavioral changes, headache; increase in tonic-clonic seizures (see Warnings)

Dermatologic: Rashes, urticaria

Gastrointestinal: Nausea, vomiting, anorexia, abdominal pain

Hematologic: Rare: Leukopenia, aplastic anemia, thrombocytopenia

Miscellaneous: Hiccups, rarely systemic lupus erythematosus

Drug Interactions Cytochrome P-450 isoenzyme CYP3A3/4 substrate

Phenytoin, carbamazepine, primidone, phenobarbital may increase the hepatic metabolism of ethosuximide; isoniazid may inhibit hepatic metabolism with a resultant increase in ethosuximide serum concentrations; CNS depressants, alcohol may increase adverse effects; haloperidol may change the frequency or pattern of seizure activity; valproic acid (increases or decreases ethosuximide serum concentrations)

Food Interactions Folate requirements may be increased

Mechanism of Action Increases the seizure threshold and suppresses paroxysmal spike-and-wave pattern in absence seizures; depresses nerve transmission in the motor cortex

Pharmacokinetics

Distribution: V_d: Adults: 0.62-0.72 L/kg

Protein binding: <10%

Metabolism: ~80% metabolized in the liver to three inactive metabolites

Half-life:

Children: 30 hours

Adults: 50-60 hours

Time to peak serum concentration:

Capsule: Within 2-4 hours

Syrup: <2-4 hours

Elimination: Slow in urine as metabolites (50%) and as unchanged drug (10% to 20%); small amounts excreted in feces

Dialysis: Removed by hemodialysis and peritoneal dialysis

Usual Dosage Oral:

Children <6 years: Initial: 15 mg/kg/day in 2 divided doses (maximum dose: 250 mg/dose); increase every 4-7 days; usual maintenance dose: 15-40 mg/kg/day in 2 divided doses; maximum dose: 1.5 g/day

Children >6 years and Adults: Initial: 250 mg twice daily; increase by 250 mg/day as needed every 4-7 days up to 1.5 g/day in 2 divided doses; usual maintenance dose: 20-40 mg/kg/day in 2 divided doses

Administration Oral: Administer with food or milk to decrease GI upset

Monitoring Parameters Seizure frequency, trough serum concentrations; CBC with differential, platelets, liver enzymes, urinalysis

Reference Range

Therapeutic: 40-100 µg/mL (SI: 280-710 µmol/L)

Toxic: >150 µg/mL (SI: >1062 µmol/L)

Patient Information Avoid alcohol; causes drowsiness and may impair ability to perform hazardous activities requiring mental alertness and coordination; do not discontinue abruptly

Additional Information Considered to be drug of choice for simple absence seizures

Dosage Forms

Capsule: 250 mg

Syrup: 250 mg/5 mL [raspberry flavor] (473 mL)

References

Marquardt ED, Ishisaka DY, Batra KK, et al, "Removal of Ethosuximide and Phenobarbital by Peritoneal Dialysis in a Child," *Clin Pharm*, 1992, 11(12):1030-1.

♦ **Ethoxynaphthamido Penicillin** *see* Nafcillin *on page 693*

Ethyl Alcohol (ETH il AL koe hol)

U.S. Brand Names Lavacol® [OTC]

Canadian Brand Names Biobase; Duonalc-E

Synonyms Alcohol; Dehydrated Alcohol Injection; Ethanol; EtOH

Therapeutic Category Antidote, Ethylene Glycol Toxicity; Antidote, Methanol Toxicity; Anti-infective Agent, Topical; Fat Occlusion (Central Venous Catheter), Treatment Agent; Neurolytic

Generic Available Yes

Use Antidote for the treatment of methanol and ethylene glycol intoxication; neurolysis of nerves or ganglia for the relief of intractable, chronic pain in such conditions as inoperable cancer and trigeminal neuralgia (dehydrated alcohol injection); topical anti-infective; treatment of occluded central venous catheters due to lipid deposition from fat emulsion infusion (particularly 3-in-1 admixture)

Pregnancy Risk Factor D (X if used for prolonged periods or in high doses at term)

Contraindications Hypersensitivity to ethyl alcohol; seizure disorder and diabetic coma; subarachnoid injection of dehydrated alcohol in patients receiving anticoagulants

Warnings Ethanol is a flammable liquid and should be kept cool and away from any heat source; proper positioning of the patient for neurolytic administration is essential to control localization of the injection of dehydrated alcohol (which is hypobaric) into the subarachnoid space; avoid extravasation; not for S.C. administration; do not administer simultaneously with blood due to the possibility of pseudoagglutination or hemolysis; may potentiate severe hypoprothrombic bleeding; clinical evaluation and periodic lab determinations, including serum ethanol levels, are necessary to monitor effectiveness, changes in electrolyte concentrations, and acid-base balance (when used as an antidote)

Precautions Use with caution in diabetics (alcohol decreases blood sugar), patients with gout, shock, following cranial surgery, and in anticipated postpartum hemorrhage; monitor blood glucose closely, particularly in children as treatment of ingestions is associated with hypoglycemia; avoid extravasation during I.V. administration; ethanol passes freely into breast milk at a level approximately equivalent to maternal serum level; effects on the infant are insignificant until maternal blood level reaches 300 mg/dL; minimize dermal exposure of ethanol in infants as significant systemic absorption and toxicity can occur

Adverse Reactions

Cardiovascular: Tachycardia, hypertension, hypotension, arrhythmias, cardiomegaly, angina, CHF, vasodilation, flushing, hypothermia

Central nervous system: Ataxia, dementia, Wernicke-Korsakoff syndrome, amnesia, paranoia, hyperthermia, vertigo, lethargy, sedation, coma, seizures, hallucinations

Endocrine & metabolic: Hypoglycemia, acidosis, hypokalemia, hypomagnesemia, increased serum osmolality

Dermatologic: Dry skin, irritation

Gastrointestinal: Nausea, diarrhea, abdominal pain, dyspepsia, vomiting, GI hemorrhage, anorexia, pancreatitis, hiccups

Hematologic: Porphyria, megaloblastic anemia

Hepatic: Hepatic cirrhosis, fatty degeneration of liver, hepatic steatosis

Local: Phlebitis

Neuromuscular & skeletal: Hypotonia, dysarthria, myopathy, neuropathy (peripheral); postinjection neuritis with persistent pain, hyperesthesia, and paresthesia (after neurolytic use)

Ophthalmic: Eye stinging (from vapors)

Respiratory: Respiratory depression, tachypnea, bronchial irritation

Drug Interactions Increased CNS depressant effects with sedative hypnotic agents, antihistamines, antidepressants, narcotic analgesics, dronabinol, phenothiazines, benzodiazepines, and metoclopramide; disulfiram-like reaction with cephalosporins, chlorpropamide, disulfiram, furazolidone, metronidazole, and procarbazine; increased GI blood loss and bleeding time with aspirin and salicylates; altered glucose metabolism resulting in either hypoglycemic or hyperglycemic effects with insulin, phenformin, and sulfonylureas; increases phenytoin serum levels; increased oral bioavailability of ethyl alcohol with aspirin, ranitidine, cimetidine, and nizatidine; increases theophylline levels

Stability Store at room temperature (see Warnings); do not use unless solution is clear and container is intact

Mechanism of Action Competitively inhibits the oxidation of methanol and ethylene oxide by alcohol dehydrogenase to their more toxic metabolites; as a neurolytic, ethyl alcohol produces injury to tissue cells by producing dehydration and precipitation of protoplasm; when injected in close proximity to nerve cells, it produces neuritis and nerve degeneration

(Continued)

Ethyl Alcohol *(Continued)*

Pharmacokinetics

Distribution: V_d: 0.6 L/kg

Metabolism: Hepatic to acetaldehyde or acetate by alcohol dehydrogenase

Clearance: 10-20 mL/hour

Hemodialysis clearance: 300-400 mL/minute with an ethanol removal rate of 280 mg/minute

Usual Dosage

Absolute ethanol/ethyl alcohol (EtOH):

Treatment of methanol or ethylene glycol ingestion: Children, Adolescents, and Adults:

Loading dose (LD):

Oral: 0.8-1 mL/kg of 95% EtOH or 2 mL/kg of 40% EtOH

I.V.: 8-10 mL/kg of 10% EtOH solution (see Administration), not to exceed 200 mL

Modified loading dose (if ingestion consists of both EtOH **and** methanol or ethylene glycol): The loading dose is reduced in a proportional manner related to the measured EtOH blood level by multiplying the calculated loading dose described above by the following factor:

$$LD \times \left[\frac{100 - (\text{patient's serum ethanol level in mg/dL})}{100} \right]$$

Maintenance dose:

	Non-Drinker	Average Drinker	Chronic Drinker
EtOH dosage by weight	66 mg/kg/h	110 mg/kg/h	154 mg/kg/h
Oral: 40% EtOH	0.2 mL/kg/h	0.3 mL/kg/h	0.4 mL/kg/h
Oral: 95% EtOH	0.1 mL/kg/h	0.15 mL/kg/h	0.2 mL/kg/h
I.V.: 10% EtOH	0.8 mL/kg/h	1.4 mL/kg/h	2 mL/kg/h

Note: Continue therapy until methanol or ethylene glycol blood level <10 mg/dL

Dosage adjustment for hemodialysis: Increase maintenance dosage by 150 mg/kg/h during hemodialysis

Treatment of fat occlusion of central venous catheters: Children and Adults: I.V. (see institutional-based protocol for catheter clearance assessment, the following assessment is a general methodology): Up to 3 mL of 70% ethanol (maximum 0.55 mL/kg); instill a volume equal to the internal volume of the catheter; may repeat if patency not restored after 30- minute dwell time; if dose repeated, reassess after 4-hour dwell time

Dehydrated alcohol injection: Therapeutic neurolysis (nerve or ganglion block): Adults: Intraneural: Dosage variable depending upon the site of injection, eg, trigeminal neuralgia: 0.05-0.5 mL as a single injection per interspace vs subarachnoid injection: 0.5-1 mL as a single injection per interspace; single doses >1.5 mL are seldom required

Liquid denatured alcohol: Topical: Children and Adults: Apply as needed

Administration

Oral: Dilute ethanol in 6 ounces orange juice and give over 30 minutes

Parenteral: Not for S.C. administration; I.V.: Dilute absolute alcohol for I.V. administration to a final concentration of 5% to 10% v/v in D_5W or $D_{10}W$ (I.V. ethanol is also available commercially in both 5% and 10% solutions; see Dosage Forms); infuse loading dose plus 1 hour of maintenance dosage over 60 minutes; for treatment of occluded central venous catheter, a 70% dilution of ethanol may be made by adding 0.8 mL sterile water to 2 mL 98% ethanol; instill with a volume equal to the internal volume of the catheter; assess patency at 30 minutes (or per institutional protocol); may repeat (see Usual Dosage)

Intraneural: Separate needles should be used for each of multiple injections or sites to prevent residual alcohol deposition at sites not intended for tissue destruction; inject slowly after determining proper placement of needle; since dehydrated alcohol is hypobaric when compared with spinal fluid, proper positioning of the patient is essential to control localization of injections into the subarachnoid space

Monitoring Parameters Antidotal therapy: Blood ethanol levels (at the end of the loading dose, every hour until stabilized, and then every 8-12 hours thereafter); blood glucose, electrolytes, arterial pH, blood gases, methanol or ethylene glycol blood levels

Reference Range

Symptoms associated with serum ethanol levels:

Nausea and vomiting: Serum level >100 mg/dL

Coma: Serum level >300 mg/dL

Antidote for methanol/ethylene glycol: Goal range: Blood ethanol level: 100-130 mg/dL (22-28 mmol/liter)

Patient Information May cause drowsiness and impair ability to perform hazardous activities which require mental alertness or physical coordination

Additional Information Eighty-proof spirits contain 40% ethanol

Dosage Forms

Infusion, in D_5W: 5% alcohol (1000 mL)

Infusion, in D_5W: 10% alcohol (1000 mL)

Injection, absolute: 98% (1 mL, 5 mL)

Injection, dehydrated: 98% (1 mL, 5 mL)

Liquid, topical, denatured: 70% (473 mL, 960 mL)

References

Chernow B, ed, "Poisoning", *Essentials of Critical Care Pharmacology*, 2nd ed, Baltimore: Williams & Wilkins, 1994, 501-29.

Pennington CR and Pithie AD, "Ethanol Lock in the Management of Catheter Occlusion", *JPEN J Parenter Enteral Nutr*, 1987, 11(5):507-8.

Poisoning and Drug Overdose, 2nd ed, Olson KR, ed, Norwalk, Connecticut: Appleton and Lange, 1994, 339-40.

Werlin SL, Lausten T, Jessens, et al, "Treatment of Central Venous Catheter Occlusions With Ethanol and Hydrochloric Acid", *JPEN J Parenter Enteral Nutr*, 1995, 19(5):416-8.

♦ **Ethyl Aminobenzoate** *see* Benzocaine *on page 135*

♦ **Ethyol**® *see* Amifostine *on page 63*

♦ **Etibi (Can)** *see* Ethambutol *on page 406*

Etidronate Disodium (e ti DROE nate dye SOW dee um)

U.S. Brand Names Didronel®

Synonyms EHDP; Sodium Etidronate

Therapeutic Category Antidote, Hypercalcemia; Bisphosphonate Derivative

Generic Available No

Use Symptomatic treatment of Paget's disease and heterotopic ossification due to spinal cord injury; hypercalcemia associated with malignancy

Pregnancy Risk Factor B (oral), C (parenteral)

Contraindications Patients with serum creatinine >5 mg/dL; clinically overt osteomalacia; hypersensitivity to biphosphonates or any component

Precautions Use with caution in patients with restricted calcium and vitamin D intake; I.V. form may be nephrotoxic and should be used with caution, if at all, in patients with impaired renal function; dosage modification required in renal impairment

Adverse Reactions Generally dose-related and most significant when taking oral doses >5 mg/kg/day

Central nervous system: Fever, convulsions, pain

Dermatologic: Angioedema, rash

Endocrine & metabolic: Hyperphosphatemia, hypocalcemia, hypomagnesemia, fluid overload

Gastrointestinal: Diarrhea, nausea, vomiting, occult blood in stools, dysgeusia

Neuromuscular & skeletal: Bone pain, increased risk of fractures, rachitic syndrome (found in children taking dosage >10 mg/kg/day over 1 year or longer)

Renal: Nephrotoxicity

Miscellaneous: Hypersensitivity reactions

Stability When diluted in 250 mL NS, solutions are stable 48 hours at room temperature

Mechanism of Action Decreases bone resorption by inhibiting osteocystic osteolysis; decreases mineral release and matrix or collagen breakdown in bone

Pharmacodynamics

Onset of therapeutic effects: Within 1-3 months of therapy

Duration: Persists for 12 months without continuous therapy

Pharmacokinetics

Absorption: Dependent upon dose administered

Half-life: 8.7 hours (range: 6.9-10 hours)

(Continued)

Etidronate Disodium (Continued)

Elimination: Primarily as unchanged drug in urine with unabsorbed drug eliminated in feces

Usual Dosage

Children and Adults: Heterotopic ossification with spinal cord injury: Oral: 20 mg/kg once daily (or in divided doses if GI discomfort occurs) for 2 weeks, then 10 mg/kg/day for 10 weeks (**Note:** This dosage has been used in children, however, treatment >1 year has been associated with a rachitic syndrome)

Adults:

Paget's disease: Oral: 5-10 mg/kg once daily for no more than 6 months; may give 11-20 mg/kg/day for up to 3 months. Daily dose may be divided if adverse GI effects occur; courses of therapy should be separated by drug-free periods of at least 3 months.

Hypercalcemia associated with malignancy:

I.V.: 7.5 mg/kg once daily for 3 days, may be continued up to 7 days if necessary; courses of therapy should be separated by at least 7 drug-free days

Oral: Start 20 mg/kg once daily (or in divided doses if GI discomfort occurs) on the last day of infusion and continue for 30-90 days

Dosing adjustment in renal impairment:

S_{cr} 2.5-4.9 mg/dL: Use with caution

S_{cr} ≥5 mg/dL: **Not recommended**

Administration

Oral: Administer on an empty stomach, 2 hours before meals; avoid giving foods/supplements with calcium, iron, or magnesium within 2 hours of drug

Parenteral: I.V.: Dilute in a minimum volume of 250 mL NS; infuse over at least 2 hours

Monitoring Parameters Serum calcium, phosphate, creatinine, BUN

Patient Information Maintain adequate intake of calcium and vitamin D

Dosage Forms

Injection: 50 mg/mL (6 mL)

Tablet: 200 mg, 400 mg

♦ **EtOH** see Ethyl Alcohol on page 409

Etoposide (e toe POE side)

Related Information

Emetogenic Potential of Single Chemotherapeutic Agents on page 1129

U.S. Brand Names VePesid®

Synonyms VP-16; VP-16-213

Therapeutic Category Antineoplastic Agent, Mitotic Inhibitor

Generic Available Yes

Use Treatment of testicular and lung carcinomas, malignant lymphoma, Hodgkin's disease, leukemias (ALL, ANLL, AML), neuroblastoma; treatment of Ewing's sarcoma, rhabdomyosarcoma, osteosarcoma, Wilms' tumor, brain tumors; conditioning regimen with hematopoietic stem cell support

Pregnancy Risk Factor D

Contraindications Hypersensitivity to etoposide or any component

Warnings The FDA currently recommends that procedures for proper handling and disposal of antineoplastic agents be considered. Severe myelosuppression with resulting infection or bleeding may occur; injectable etoposide contains polysorbate 80 (polysorbate 80 has caused thrombocytopenia, ascites, and renal, pulmonary, and hepatic failure in premature infants who received an injectable vitamin E product containing polysorbate 80). Higher rates of anaphylactoid reactions have been reported in children who received I.V. infusions of etoposide at higher than recommended concentrations; injection contains benzyl alcohol as a preservative; use with caution in neonates

Precautions Use with caution and consider dosage reduction in patients with hepatic impairment, bone marrow suppression, and renal impairment

Adverse Reactions

Cardiovascular: Hypotension, tachycardia, facial flushing

Central nervous system: Somnolence, fatigue, fever, headache, chills

Dermatologic: Alopecia, rash, urticaria, angioedema

Gastrointestinal: Nausea, vomiting, diarrhea, mucositis, anorexia, constipation

Hematologic: Myelosuppression, anemia (granulocyte nadir: ~7-14 days, platelet nadir: ~9-16 days)

Hepatic: Hepatotoxicity

Local: Thrombophlebitis

Neuromuscular & skeletal: Peripheral neuropathy, weakness

Respiratory: Bronchospasm

Miscellaneous: Anaphylactoid reactions

Food Interactions Administration of food does not affect GI absorption with doses ≤200 mg

Stability Stability of diluted injection is concentration dependent (ie, 0.2 mg/mL: 96 hours; 0.4 mg/mL: 48 hours; 1 mg/mL: 2 hours; 2 mg/mL: 1 hour); at a concentration of 1 mg/mL in NS or D_5W, crystallization has occurred within 30 minutes; **incidence of precipitation increases when final infusion concentration is >0.4 mg/mL;** intact vials remain stable for 2 years at room temperature; refrigerate capsules

Mechanism of Action Inhibits mitotic activity; inhibits DNA type II topoisomerase producing single- and double-strand DNA breaks

Pharmacokinetics

Absorption: Oral: Large variability

Distribution: CSF concentration is <5% of plasma concentration

Children V_{dss}: 10 L/m^2

Adults: V_{dss}: 7-17 L/m^2

Protein binding: 94% to 97%

Metabolism: In the liver (with a biphasic decay)

Bioavailability: Averages 50% (range: 10% to 80%, dose-dependent)

Half-life, terminal:

Children: 6-8 hours

Adults: 4-15 hours with normal renal and hepatic function

Time to peak serum concentration: Oral: Within 1-1.5 hours

Elimination: Both unchanged drug and metabolites are excreted in urine and a small amount (2% to 16%) in feces; up to 55% of an I.V. dose is excreted unchanged in urine in children

Usual Dosage Refer to individual protocols

Children: I.V.: 60-150 mg/m^2/day for 2-5 days every 3-6 weeks

AML:

Remission induction: 150 mg/m^2/day for 2-3 days for 2-3 cycles

Intensification or consolidation: 250 mg/m^2/day for 3 days, on courses 2-5

Brain tumor: 150 mg/m^2/day on days 2 and 3 of treatment course

Neuroblastoma: 100 mg/m^2/day over 1 hour on days 1-5 of cycle; repeat cycle every 4 weeks

High-dose conditioning regimen for allogeneic BMT: 60 mg/kg/dose as a single dose

BMT conditioning regimen used in patients with rhabdomyosarcoma or neuroblastoma: I.V. continuous infusion: 160 mg/m^2/day for 4 days

Adults:

Testicular cancer: I.V.: 50-100 mg/m^2/day on days 1-5 or 100 mg/m^2/day on days 1, 3 and 5 every 3-4 weeks for 3-4 courses

Small cell lung cancer:

Oral: Twice the I.V. dose rounded to the nearest 50 mg given once daily if total dose ≤400 mg/day or in divided doses if >400 mg/day

I.V.: 35 mg/m^2/day for 4 days or 50 mg/m^2/day for 5 days every 3-4 weeks

Dosing adjustment in renal impairment:

Cl_{cr} 10-50 mL/minute: Administer 75% of normal dose

Cl_{cr} <10 mL/minute: Administer 50% of normal dose

Dosing adjustment in patients with elevated serum bilirubin: Reduce dose by 50% for bilirubin 1.5-3 mg/dL; reduce dose by 75% for bilirubin >3 mg/dL

Administration

Oral: If necessary, the injection may be used for oral administration. Mix with orange juice, apple juice, or lemonade at a final concentration not to exceed 0.4 mg/mL to prevent precipitation. Etoposide has been found to be stable with no loss of potency over 3 hours when administered in apple juice or lemonade at concentrations of 1 mg/mL.

Parenteral: I.V.: Do not administer by rapid I.V. injection or by intrathecal, intraperitoneal, or intrapleural routes due to possible severe toxicity. Administer I.V. infusion via an in-line 0.22 micron filter over at least 60 minutes at a rate not to exceed 100 mg/m^2/hour (or 3.3 mg/kg/hour) to minimize the risk of hypotensive reactions at a final concentration for administration of 0.2-0.4 mg/mL in NS or D_5W. More concentrated I.V. solutions (0.6-1 mg/mL) can be infused but have shorter stability times (see Stability). For high-dose etoposide infusions, undiluted etoposide (20 mg/mL) has been infused as a single dose from a glass syringe via syringe pump through a central venous catheter over 1-4 hours. Problems associated with higher than recommended concentrations of etoposide infusions include cracking of hard plastic in chemo venting pins and infusion lines; inspect infusion solution for particulate matter and plastic devices for cracks and leaks.

(Continued)

Etoposide (Continued)

Monitoring Parameters CBC with differential and platelet count, hemoglobin, vital signs (blood pressure), bilirubin, and renal function tests; inspect solution and tubing for precipitation before and during infusion

Patient Information Notify physician if fever, sore throat, painful/burning urination, bruising, bleeding or shortness of breath occurs

Nursing Implications Adequate airway and other supportive measures and agents for treating hypotension or anaphylactoid reactions should be present when I.V. etoposide is given

Dosage Forms

Capsule: 50 mg

Injection: 20 mg/mL (5 mL, 25 mL)

References

Berg SL, Grisell DL, DeLaney TF, et al, "Principles of Treatment of Pediatric Solid Tumors," *Pediatr Clin North Am,* 1991, 38(2):249-67.

Boos J, Krümpelmann S, Schulze-Westhoff P, et al, "Steady-State Levels and Bone Marrow Toxicity of Etoposide in Children and Infants: Does Etoposide Require Age-Dependent Dose Calculation?" *J Clin Oncol,* 1995, 13(12):2954-60.

Clark PL and Slevin ML, "The Clinical Pharmacology of Etoposide and Teniposide," *Clin Pharmacokinet,* 1987, 12(4):223-52.

Lazarus HM, Creger RJ, and Diaz D, "Simple Method for the Administration of High-Dose Etoposide During Autologous Bone Marrow Transplantation," *Cancer Treat Rep,* 1985, 70(6):819-20.

Nishikawa A, Nakamura Y, Nobori U, et al, "Acute Monocytic Leukemia in Children. Response to VP-16-213 as a Single Agent," *Cancer,* 1987, 60(9):2146-9.

O'Dwyer PJ, Leyland-Jones B, Alonso MT, et al, "Etoposide (VP-16-213): Current Status of an Active Anticancer Drug," *N Engl J Med,* 1985, 312(11):692-700.

♦ **ETS-2%**® *see* Erythromycin *on page 394*

♦ **Euglucon (Can)** *see* Glyburide *on page 476*

♦ **Eurax**® *see* Crotamiton *on page 275*

♦ **Eutectic Mixture of Lidocaine and Prilocaine** *see* Lidocaine and Prilocaine *on page 594*

♦ **Exact**® **Cream [OTC]** *see* Benzoyl Peroxide *on page 136*

♦ **Ex-Lax Chocolated (Can)** *see* Senna *on page 896*

♦ **Ex-Lax Extra Strength (Can)** *see* Senna *on page 896*

♦ **Ex-Lax Stool Softener (Can)** *see* Docusate *on page 350*

♦ **Ex-Lax Sugar Coated (Can)** *see* Senna *on page 896*

♦ **Exosurf**® **Neonatal** *see* Colfosceril *on page 265*

♦ **Expectorant Cough Formula (Can)** *see* Guaifenesin *on page 485*

♦ **Expectorant Cough Syrup (Can)** *see* Guaifenesin *on page 485*

♦ **Expectorant Syrup (Can)** *see* Guaifenesin *on page 485*

♦ **Exsel**® *see* Selenium Sulfide *on page 896*

♦ **Extravasation Treatment** *see page 1085*

♦ **Ezide**® *see* Hydrochlorothiazide *on page 503*

♦ **F₃T** *see* Trifluridine *on page 984*

Factor IX Complex (Human) (FAK ter nyne KOM pleks HYU man)

U.S. Brand Names Bebulin® VH; Konÿne® 80; Profilnine® SD; Proplex® T

Canadian Brand Names Immunine VH

Therapeutic Category Antihemophilic Agent; Blood Product Derivative

Generic Available No

Use To control bleeding in patients with factor IX deficiency (hemophilia B or Christmas disease); prevention/control of bleeding in hemophilia A patients with inhibitors to factor VIII; Proplex® T is indicated to prevent or control bleeding due to factor VII deficiency

Pregnancy Risk Factor C

Contraindications Liver disease, intravascular coagulation or fibrinolysis

Precautions Use with caution in patients with liver dysfunction; risk of viral transmission is not totally eradicated, prepared from pooled human plasma

Adverse Reactions

Cardiovascular: Flushing

Central nervous system: Somnolence, fever, headache, chills

Dermatologic: Urticaria

Gastrointestinal: Nausea, vomiting

Hematologic: Disseminated intravascular coagulation, thrombosis following high dosages in hemophilia B patients

Neuromuscular & skeletal: Paresthesia

Miscellaneous: Tightness in chest and neck

Drug Interactions Increased risk of thrombosis with aminocaproic acid (some recommend to delay the administration of aminocaproic acid 8 hours after factor IX complex administration)

Stability Store unopened vials in refrigerator; do not freeze; administer within 3 hours after reconstitution; **do not refrigerate after reconstitution**; Profilnine® SD: May store unopened vials at room temperature (<30°C) for up to 3 months; Konyne® 80: May store unopened vials at <25°C for up to 1 month

Mechanism of Action Replaces deficient clotting factors including factors II, VII, IX, and X

Pharmacokinetics Cleared rapidly from the serum in two phases
Half-life:
First phase: 4-6 hours
Terminal: 22.5 hours

Usual Dosage Dose is expressed in terms of factor IX units; dose must be individualized; **Note:** 1 unit/kg raises factor IX levels 1%

Children and Adults: I.V.:
Factor IX deficiency: Hospitalized patients: 20-50 international units/kg/dose; may be higher in special cases; may be given every 24 hours or more often in special cases
Factor VIII inhibitor patients: 75-100 international units/kg/dose; may be given every 6-12 hours

Administration Parenteral: I.V. administration only; rate of administration should be individualized for patient's comfort; maximum rates of administration: Bebulin® VH: 2 mL/minute; Konyne® 80: 100 international units/minute; Profilnine® SD: 10 mL/minute; Proplex® T: 3 mL/minute; use filter needle to draw product into syringe; visually inspect for particulate matter and discoloration prior to administration whenever permitted by solution or container

Monitoring Parameters Levels of factors II, IX, and X; signs/symptoms of bleeding; hemoglobin, hematocrit

Reference Range Patients with severe hemophilia will have factor IX levels <1%, often undetectable. Moderate forms of the disease have levels of 1% to 10% while some mild cases may have 11% to 49% of normal factor IX. Plasma concentration is about 4 mg/L.

Additional Information AlphaNine® SD and Mononine® contain only factor IX and should not be confused with factor IX **complex**

Dosage Forms Injection: (**Note:** Exact potency labeled on each vial)
Bebulin® VH: Single dose vial
Konyne® 80: ~500 international units (20 mL); ~1000 international units (40 mL) [single use vials]
Profilnine® SD: Single dose vial
Proplex® T: Single dose vial

References
Lusher JM, "Thrombogenicity Associated With Factor IX Complex Concentrates," *Semin Hematol*, 1991, 28(3 Suppl 6):3-5.

♦ **Factor VIII** *see* Antihemophilic Factor (Human) *on page 98*
♦ **Factrel®** *see* Gonadorelin *on page 482*

Famciclovir (fam SYE kloe veer)

U.S. Brand Names Famvir®
Therapeutic Category Antiviral Agent, Oral
Generic Available No
Use Management of acute herpes zoster (shingles); treatment or suppression of recurrent genital herpes in the immunocompetent; treatment of recurrent mucocutaneous herpes simplex infections in HIV patients
Pregnancy Risk Factor B
Contraindications Hypersensitivity to famciclovir, penciclovir, or any component
Precautions Use with caution and decrease dose in patients with renal dysfunction; dosage adjustment may be needed in patients with poorly compensated hepatic impairment
Adverse Reactions
Central nervous system: Headache, fatigue, dizziness, fever, somnolence
Dermatologic: Pruritus, rash
Gastrointestinal: Nausea, diarrhea, vomiting, constipation, anorexia, abdominal pain
Neuromuscular & skeletal: Rigors, paresthesia
Drug Interactions Probenecid may increase penciclovir serum concentrations
Food Interactions Rate of absorption and/or conversion to penciclovir and peak concentration are reduced with food, but bioavailability is not affected
(Continued)

Famciclovir *(Continued)*

Mechanism of Action Synthetic guanine derivative, prodrug for penciclovir; penciclovir has inhibitory activity against varicella zoster virus (VZV) and herpes simplex virus type 1 and 2 (HSV 1 and HSV 2); penciclovir is converted to penciclovir monophosphate (by viral thymidine kinase in VZV-, HSV 1-, and HSV 2-infected cells), then to penciclovir triphosphate which competes with deoxyguanosine triphosphate for viral DNA polymerase and incorporation into viral DNA; therefore, inhibits DNA synthesis and viral replication

Pharmacokinetics Penciclovir:

Absorption: Rapid

Distribution: V_{dss}: Healthy adults: 73-85 L

Protein binding: <20%

Metabolism: Famciclovir is a prodrug which is metabolized via deacetylation and oxidation in the intestinal wall and liver to penciclovir (active) during extensive first-pass metabolism

Bioavailability: 72% to 83%

Half-life:

Serum: 2-3 hours; increased with renal dysfunction

Mean half-life, terminal:

Cl_{cr} >80 mL/minute: 2.15 hours

Cl_{cr} 60-80 mL/minute: 2.47 hours

Cl_{cr} 30-59 mL/minute: 3.87 hours

Cl_{cr} <29 mL/minute: 9.85 hours

Intracellular penciclovir triphosphate: HSV 1: 10 hours; HSV 2: 20 hours; VZV: 7 hours

Time to peak serum concentration: ~1 hour

Elimination: Primary route is the kidney with 73% excreted in urine (predominantly as penciclovir) and 27% in feces; penciclovir undergoes tubular secretion; requires dosage adjustment with renal impairment

Usual Dosage Oral:

Adolescents (AAP, 2000):

Genital herpes infection: 750 mg/day in 3 divided doses for 7-10 days

Episodic recurrent genital herpes infection: 250 mg/day in 2 divided doses for 5 days

Daily suppressive therapy: 250-500 mg/day in 2 divided doses for 1 year; then reassess for recurrence of herpes infection

Adults:

Herpes zoster: 500 mg every 8 hours for 7 days; initiate as soon as diagnosed; initiation of therapy within 48 hours of rash onset may be more beneficial; no efficacy data available for treatment initiated >72 hours after onset of rash

Recurrent genital herpes: 125 mg twice daily for 5 days; initiate at first sign or symptom; efficacy is not established if treatment is started >6 hours after onset of lesions or symptoms

Suppression of recurrent genital herpes: 250 mg twice daily for up to 1 year

HIV patients with recurrent orolabial or genital herpes: 500 mg twice daily for 7 days

Dosing interval in renal impairment: Adults:

Herpes zoster:

Cl_{cr} ≥60 mL/minute: Administer 500 mg every 8 hours

Cl_{cr} 40-59 mL/minute: Administer 500 mg every 12 hours

Cl_{cr} 20-39 mL/minute: Administer 500 mg every 24 hours

Cl_{cr} <20 mL/minute: Administer 250 mg every 24 hours

Patients on hemodialysis: Administer 250 mg after each dialysis

Recurrent genital herpes:

Cl_{cr} ≥40 mL/minute: Administer 125 mg every 12 hours

Cl_{cr} 20-39 mL/minute: Administer 125 mg every 24 hours

Cl_{cr} <20 mL/minute: Administer 125 mg every 48 hours

Patients on hemodialysis: Administer 125 mg after each dialysis

Suppression of recurrent genital herpes:

Cl_{cr} ≥40 mL/minute: Administer 250 mg every 12 hours

Cl_{cr} 20-39 mL/minute: Administer 125 mg every 12 hours

Cl_{cr} <20 mL/minute: Administer 125 mg every 24 hours

Patients on hemodialysis: Administer 125 mg after each dialysis

Recurrent orolabial or genital herpes in HIV infected patients:

Cl_{cr} ≥40 mL/minute: Administer 500 mg every 12 hours

Cl_{cr} 20-39 mL/minute: Administer 500 mg every 24 hours

Cl_{cr} <20 mL/minute: Administer 250 mg every 24 hours

Patients on hemodialysis: Administer 250 mg after each dialysis

Administration Oral: May be administered without regard to meals; may be administered with food to decrease GI upset

Monitoring Parameters Resolution of rash

Patient Information Famciclovir is not a cure for genital herpes

Dosage Forms Tablet: 125 mg, 250 mg, 500 mg

References

Boike SC, Pue MA, and Freed MI, "Pharmacokinetics of Famciclovir in Subjects With Varying Degrees of Renal Impairment," *Clin Pharmacol Ther*, 1994, 55(4):418-26.

Pickering LK, ed, *2000 Red Book, Report of the Committee on Infectious Diseases*, 25th ed, Elk Grove Village IL: American Academy of Pediatrics, 2000, 676.

Famotidine (fa MOE ti deen)

Related Information

Carbohydrate and Alcohol Content of Liquid Medications for Use in Patients Receiving Ketogenic Diets *on page 1258*

U.S. Brand Names Pepcid®; Pepcid® AC [OTC]; Pepcid RPD®

Canadian Brand Names Acid Control; Acid Halt; Alti-Famotidine; Apo-Famotidine; Gen-Famotidine; Novo-Famotidine; Nu-Famotidine; Peptic Guard; Rhoxal-Famotidine; Ulcidine

Therapeutic Category Gastrointestinal Agent, Gastric or Duodenal Ulcer Treatment; Histamine H_2 Antagonist

Generic Available No

Use Short-term therapy and treatment of duodenal ulcer, gastric ulcer, control gastric pH in critically ill patients, symptomatic relief in gastritis, gastroesophageal reflux disease (GERD), active benign ulcer, and pathological hypersecretory conditions; over-the-counter (OTC) formulation for use in the relief of heartburn, acid indigestion, and sour stomach

Pregnancy Risk Factor B

Contraindications Hypersensitivity to famotidine, any component, or other H_2 antagonists

Warnings Use with caution and modify dose in patients with renal impairment

Precautions Pepcid RPD® tablets contain phenylalanine; avoid use in phenylketonurics

Adverse Reactions

Cardiovascular: Bradycardia, tachycardia, palpitations, hypertension

Central nervous system: Headache, vertigo, anxiety, dizziness, seizures, depression, insomnia, drowsiness, confusion, fever

Dermatologic: Acne, pruritus, urticaria, dry skin, alopecia

Gastrointestinal: Constipation, nausea, vomiting, diarrhea, abdominal discomfort, flatulence, belching, dysgeusia, dry mouth, anorexia

Genitourinary: Impotence

Hematologic: Thrombocytopenia, pancytopenia, leukopenia (rare)

Hepatic: Elevated liver enzymes, hepatomegaly, cholestatic jaundice

Neuromuscular & skeletal: Weakness, arthralgias, paresthesia, muscle cramps

Ocular: Orbital edema

Otic: Ototoxicity, tinnitus

Renal: Elevated BUN and serum creatinine, proteinuria

Respiratory: Bronchospasm

Drug Interactions Decreased absorption of ketoconazole, triamterene, delavirdine, itraconazole, cefpodoxime, cyanocobalamin, indomethacin, melphalan; decreased effect of tolazoline

Food Interactions Limit xanthine-containing foods and beverages

Stability Concentrate for injection must be refrigerated but is stable for 48 hours at room temperature; if concentrated injection is diluted in D_5W or NS it is stable 48 hours at room temperature; commercially available diluted solution in NS is stable at room temperature for 15 months; injection is also compatible with $D_{10}W$, LR injection, 5% bicarbonate injection, and standard parenteral nutrition solutions with electrolytes, multivitamins, and trace minerals; reconstituted oral solution is stable for 30 days at room temperature

Mechanism of Action Competitive inhibition of histamine at H_2-receptors of the gastric parietal cells, which results in inhibition of gastric acid secretion

Pharmacodynamics

Onset of GI effect: Oral, I.V.: Within 1 hour

Peak effect:

Oral: 1-4 hours

I.V.: 30 minutes to 3 hours

Duration: 10-12 hours

(Continued)

Famotidine *(Continued)*

Pharmacokinetics
Distribution: V_d:
 Children: 2 ±1.5 L/kg
 Adults: 0.94-1.33 L/kg
Protein binding: 15% to 20%
Metabolism: 30% to 35% liver metabolism
Bioavailability: Oral: 40% to 45%
Half-life:
 Children: 3.3 ±2.5 hours
 Adults: 2.5-3.5 hours; increases with renal impairment; if Cl_{cr} <10 mL/minute, half-life ≥20 hours
 Anuria: 24 hours
Elimination: 65% to 70% unchanged drug in urine

Usual Dosage
Infants and Children <16 years: Oral, I.V.:
 Peptic ulcer: 0.5 mg/kg/day at bedtime or divided twice daily (maximum: 40 mg/day)
 GERD: 1 mg/kg/day divided twice daily (maximum: 80 mg/day)
Adults:
 Oral:
  Duodenal ulcer, gastric ulcer: 20 mg/day at bedtime for 4-8 weeks (a regimen of 10 mg twice daily is also effective); maximum: 40 mg/day
  Hypersecretory conditions: Initial: 20 mg every 6 hours, may increase up to 160 mg every 6 hours
  Esophagitis: 20-40 mg twice daily for up to 12 weeks
  GERD: 20 mg twice daily for 6 weeks
  Acid indigestion, heartburn, or sour stomach (OTC use): 10 mg 15-60 minutes before eating; not more than 2 tablets per day
 I.V.: 20 mg every 12 hours

Dosing adjustment in renal impairment:
Cl_{cr} 10-50 mL/minute: Administer normal dose every 24 hours or 50% of dose at normal dosing interval
Cl_{cr} <10 mL/minute: Administer normal dose every 36-48 hours

Administration
Oral: May administer with food and antacids; shake suspension vigorously for 10-15 seconds prior to each use; Pepcid RPD® tablets should be placed on the tongue to disintegrate and be swallowed with saliva
Parenteral: I.V.: Dilute to a maximum concentration of 4 mg/mL; may be administered I.V. push at 10 mg/minute over 2 minutes or as an infusion over 15-30 minutes

Patient Information
Avoid excessive amounts of coffee and aspirin; when self medicating, if the symptoms of heartburn, acid indigestion, or sour stomach persist after 2 weeks of continuous use of the drug, consult a clinician.

Dosage Forms
Capsule, gelatin (Pepcid® AC): 10 mg
Infusion, premixed in NS (Pepcid®): 20 mg (50 mL)
Injection (Pepcid®): 10 mg/mL (2 mL, 4 mL, 20 mL)
Powder for oral suspension (Pepcid®): 40 mg/5 mL [cherry-banana-mint flavor] (50 mL)
Tablet, chewable (Pepcid® AC): 10 mg [contains 1.4 mg phenylalanine]
Tablet, film coated (Pepcid®): 20 mg, 40 mg
 Pepcid® AC: 10 mg
Tablet, orally disintegrating (Pepcid RPD®): 20 mg [contains 1.05 mg phenylalanine], 40 mg [contains 2.1 mg phenylalanine]

Extemporaneous Preparations
An 8 mg/mL suspension may be made by crushing seventy 40 mg tablets; work into a paste with a small amount of sterile water; add a 1:1 mixture of Ora-Plus® and Ora-Sweet® to a total volume of 350 mL; stable 95 days at 23°C to 35°C
 Dentinger PJ, Swenson CF, and Anaizi NH, "Stability of Famotidine in an Extemporaneously Compounded Oral Liquid," *Am J Health Syst Pharm*, 2000, 57(14):1340-2.

References
James LP and Kearns GL, "Pharmacokinetics and Pharmacodynamics of Famotidine in Paediatric Patients," *Clin Pharmacokinet*, 1996, 31(2):103-10.
Treem WR, Davis PM, and Hyams JS, "Suppression of Gastric Acid Secretion by Intravenous Administration of Famotidine in Children," *J Pediatr*, 1991, 118(5):812-6.

♦ **FAMP** *see* Fludarabine *on page 433*

♦ **Famvir®** *see Famciclovir on page 415*

♦ **Fansidar®** *see Sulfadoxine and Pyrimethamine on page 924*

♦ **F-ara-AMP** *see Fludarabine on page 433*

Fat Emulsion (fat e MUL shun)

Related Information
Parenteral Nutrition (PN) *on page 1106*

U.S. Brand Names Intralipid®; Liposyn® II

Synonyms Intravenous Fat Emulsion; Lipid Emulsion

Therapeutic Category Caloric Agent; Intravenous Nutritional Therapy

Generic Available Yes

Use Source of calories and essential fatty acids for patients requiring parenteral nutrition of extended duration

Pregnancy Risk Factor C

Contraindications Pathologic hyperlipidemia; lipoid nephrosis; hypersensitivity to fat emulsion and severe egg or legume (soybean) allergies; pancreatitis with hyperlipemia

Precautions Use with caution in patients with severe liver damage, pulmonary disease, anemia, or blood coagulation disorder, and in jaundiced or premature infants

Adverse Reactions
Cardiovascular: Cyanosis, flushing, chest pain
Hepatic: Hyperlipemia, hepatomegaly
Local: Thrombophlebitis
Respiratory: Dyspnea
Miscellaneous: Sepsis

Stability May be stored at room temperature; do not use if emulsion appears to be layering out; exposure to light, particularly phototherapy light, used in treatment or prevention of hyperbilirubinemia has been associated with increased lipid oxidation; the clinical significance remains to be established

Mechanism of Action Essential for normal structure and function of cell membranes

Usual Dosage I.V. infusion: Fat emulsion should not exceed 60% of the total daily calories

> **Note:** At the onset of therapy, the patient should be observed for any immediate allergic reactions such as dyspnea, cyanosis, and fever. Slower initial rates of infusion may be used for the first 10-15 minutes of the infusion (eg, 0.1 mL/minute of 10% or 0.05 mL/minute of 20% solution).

> Premature infants: Initial dose: 0.25-0.5 g/kg/day, increase by 0.25-0.5 g/kg/day to a maximum of 3-4 g/kg/day; maximum rate of infusion: 0.15 g/kg/hour (0.75 mL/kg/hour of 20% solution)

> Infants and Children: Initial dose: 0.5-1 g/kg/day, increase by 0.5 g/kg/day to a maximum of 3-4 g/kg/day; maximum rate of infusion: 0.25 g/kg/hour (1.25 mL/kg/hour of 20% solution)

> Adolescents and Adults: Initial dose: 1 g/kg/day, increase by 0.5-1 g/kg/day to a maximum of 2.5 g/kg/day; maximum rate of infusion: 0.25 g/kg/hour (1.25 mL/kg/hour of 20% solution); do not exceed 50 mL/hour (20%) or 100 mL/hour (10%)

> Children and Adults: Fatty acid deficiency: 8% to 10% of total caloric intake; infuse once or twice weekly

Administration Parenteral: May be simultaneously infused with amino acid, dextrose mixtures by means of Y-connector located near infusion site into either central or peripheral line

Monitoring Parameters Serum triglycerides, free fatty acids

Additional Information 10% = 1.1 Kcal/mL, 20% = 2 Kcal/mL; both solutions are isotonic and may be administered peripherally; avoid use of 10% fat emulsion in preterm infants; a greater accumulation of plasma lipids occurs due to the greater phospholipid load of the 10% fat emulsion

Dosage Forms Injection: 10% [100 mg/mL] (50 mL, 250 mL, 500 mL); 20% [200 mg/mL] (50 mL, 250 mL, 500 mL)

References
Haumont D, Richelle M, Deckelbaum RJ, et al, "Effect of Liposomal Content of Lipid Emulsions of Plasma Lipid Concentrations in Low Birth Weight Infants Receiving Parenteral Nutrition," *J Pediatr*, 1992, 121(5 Pt 1):759-63.

Neuzil J, Darlow BA, Inder TE, et al, "Oxidation of Parenteral Lipid Emulsion by Ambient and Phototherapy Lights: Potential Toxicity of Routine Parenteral Feeding," *J Pediatr*, 1995, 126(5 Pt 1):785-90.

♦ **5-FC** *see Flucytosine on page 432*

♦ **Feen-A-Mint (Can)** *see Bisacodyl on page 143*

Felbamate (FEL ba mate)

Related Information

Antiepileptic Drugs *on page 1208*

Carbohydrate and Alcohol Content of Liquid Medications for Use in Patients Receiving Ketogenic Diets *on page 1258*

U.S. Brand Names Felbatol®

Therapeutic Category Anticonvulsant, Miscellaneous

Generic Available No

Use Not a first-line agent, see Warnings; reserved for patients who do not adequately respond to alternative agents and whose epilepsy is so severe that the benefit outweighs the risk of liver failure or aplastic anemia; used as monotherapy and adjunctive therapy in patients ≥14 years of age with partial seizures with and without secondary generalization; adjunctive therapy in children ≥2 years of age who have partial and generalized seizures associated with Lennox-Gastaut syndrome

Pregnancy Risk Factor C

Contraindications History of or current blood dyscrasia or hepatic dysfunction; hypersensitivity to felbamate, any component, or other carbamates (eg, meprobamate)

Warnings Thirty-three cases of aplastic anemia (with 8 deaths) and 14 cases of hepatic failure (with 8 deaths) have been reported in patients who received felbamate. The manufacturer (Carter Wallace) and the FDA recommend the use of this agent be suspended unless withdrawal of the product would place a patient at greater risk.

Aplastic anemia: Of the 27 cases analyzed by the manufacturer, 26 occurred in adult patients (mean age: 42 years) exposed to felbamate for a mean of 170 days at a mean dose of 3168 mg/day. One case occurred in a 13-year old exposed to felbamate for 276 days at a dose of ~69 mg/kg/day. Twenty-three of 27 patients received other antiepileptic drugs (AEDs) and 9 received drugs associated with blood dyscrasias. The 8 deaths occurred in adults (mean age: 47 years). Six of the 8 patients had a history of blood dyscrasias and 6 had allergies to medications (3 to AEDs). The onset of aplastic anemia ranged from 5-30 weeks.

Hepatic failure: Of the 14 cases, 6 cases occurred in children 3-12 years of age (mean: 6 years) exposed to felbamate for 30-218 days (mean: 115 days) at a mean dose of 1520 mg/day

All patients receiving felbamate **must** be monitored closely; in addition, a CBC with differential and platelet count should be taken before, during, and for a significant time after discontinuing felbamate therapy; liver enzyme tests and bilirubin should be obtained before initiation and every 1-2 weeks during therapy. Felbamate should be immediately withdrawn if abnormal liver function tests or bone marrow suppression occur.

The FDA and the manufacturer strongly recommend that physicians discuss the risks of felbamate with each patient and a written informed consent be obtained from the patient prior to starting therapy or before continuing therapy. A patient information consent form is included as part of the package insert and is available from the local Wallace representative or by calling 609-655-6147.

Precautions Use with caution in patients concurrently receiving other antiepileptic drugs due to the potential for drug interactions; decrease dosage of phenytoin, carbamazepine, or valproic acid by 20% to 30% when felbamate is added to the regimen and when felbamate doses are titrated upwards; monitor serum levels of concomitant antiepileptic drug therapy

Adverse Reactions

Central nervous system: Headache, insomnia, somnolence, fatigue, dizziness, anxiety, drowsiness, depression, behavior changes, ataxia

Dermatologic: Acne, rash, pruritus

Gastrointestinal: Anorexia, vomiting, nausea, diarrhea, constipation, dyspepsia, gum bleeding or hyperplasia, weight loss

Hematologic: Thrombocytopenia, granulocytopenia, agranulocytosis, purpura, leukopenia, aplastic anemia (100-fold increase in risk; see Warnings)

Hepatic: Elevated liver enzymes, hepatitis, acute liver failure, may be associated with death (see Warnings)

Drug Interactions Cytochrome P-450 isoenzyme CYP2C19 inhibitor

Phenytoin, carbamazepine may increase and valproic acid may decrease the clearance of felbamate; felbamate increases the concentrations of phenytoin and valproic acid; felbamate decreases carbamazepine concentrations but increases the concentration of carbamazepine epoxide (active metabolite)

Food Interactions Food does **not** affect absorption

Stability Store in tightly closed container at room temperature away from excessive heat, moisture, or direct sunlight

Mechanism of Action Mechanism of action is unknown but may be similar to other anticonvulsants; has weak inhibitory effects on GABA and benzodiazepine receptor binding; does not have activity at the MK-801 receptor binding site of the NMDA receptor-ionophore complex.

Pharmacokinetics

Absorption: Oral: Rapid and almost complete

Distribution: V_d: Adults: Mean: 0.75 L/kg; range: 0.7-1.1 L/kg

Protein binding: 20% to 25%, primarily to albumin

Metabolism: In the liver via hydroxylation and conjugation

Bioavailability: >90%

Half-life: Adults: Mean: 20-30 hours, shorter (ie, 14 hours) with concomitant enzyme-inducing drugs

Time to peak serum concentration: 1-4 hours

Elimination: 40% to 50% excreted as unchanged drug and 40% as inactive metabolites in urine

Clearance, apparent:

Children 2-9 years: 61.3 ±8.2 mL/kg/hour

Children 10-12 years: 34.3 ±4.3 mL/kg/hour

Usual Dosage See Precautions regarding concomitant antiepileptic drugs

Children 2-14 years with Lennox-Gastaut: Adjunctive therapy: Initial: 15 mg/kg/day in 3-4 divided doses; increase dose by 15 mg/kg/day increments at weekly intervals; maximum dose: 45 mg/kg/day or 3600 mg/day (whichever is less)

Children ≥14 years and Adults:

Adjunctive therapy: Initial: 1200 mg/day in 3-4 divided doses; increase daily dose by 1200 mg increments every week to a maximum dose of 3600 mg/day

Conversion to monotherapy: Initial: 1200 mg/day in 3 or 4 divided doses; at week 2, increase daily dose by 1200 mg increments every week to a maximum dose of 3600 mg/day. Decrease dose of other anticonvulsants by 1/3 their original dose at initiation of felbamate, and when felbamate dose is increased at week 2; continue to reduce other anticonvulsants as clinically needed.

Monotherapy: Initial: 1200 mg/day in 3 or 4 divided doses; titrate dosage upward according to clinical response and monitor patients closely; increase daily dose in 600 mg increments every 2 weeks to 2400 mg/day; maximum dose: 3600 mg/day

Administration Oral: May be administered without regard to meals; shake suspension well before use

Monitoring Parameters Serum concentrations of concomitant anticonvulsant therapy; liver enzymes, bilirubin, CBC with differential, platelet count prior to therapy and every 1-2 weeks

Reference Range Not necessary to routinely monitor serum drug levels; dose should be titrated to clinical response; therapeutic range not fully determined; proposed 30-100 µg/mL

Patient Information Do not abruptly discontinue, an increase in seizure activity may result; report any unusual symptoms, such as a rash, bruises, bleeding, sore throat, fever, and/or dark urine to physician immediately

Additional Information Monotherapy has not been associated with gingival hyperplasia, impaired concentration, weight gain, or abnormal thinking; felbamate has also been used in a small number of patients with infantile spasms (see Pellock, 1999); an open-label study in children with refractory partial seizures (n=30; mean age: 9 years; range: 2-17 years) found that children >10 years of age had a more favorable response; this was thought to be related to the higher felbamate serum concentrations (and lower apparent clearance) in children >10 years of age compared to those <10 years; the faster apparent clearance in children <10 years of age should be considered when using this agent (Carmant, 1994)

Dosage Forms

Suspension, oral: 600 mg/5 mL (240 mL, 960 mL)

Tablet: 400 mg, 600 mg

References

Carmant L, Holmes GL, Sawyer S, et al, "Efficacy of Felbamate in Therapy for Partial Epilepsy in Children," *J Pediatr*, 1994, 125(3):481-6.

Dodson WE, "Felbamate in the Treatment of Lennox-Gastaut Syndrome: Results of a 12-Month Open-Label Study Following a Randomized Clinical Trial," *Epilepsia*, 1993, 34(Suppl 7):S18-24.

Leppik IE, "Felbamate," *Epilepsia*, 1995, 36(Suppl 2):S66-72.

Pellock JM, "Managing Pediatric Epilepsy Syndromes With New Antiepileptic Drugs," *Pediatrics*, 1999, 104(5 Pt 1):1106-16.

The Felbamate Study Group in Lennox-Gastaut Syndrome, "Efficacy of Felbamate in Childhood Epileptic Encephalopathy (Lennox-Gastaut Syndrome)," *N Engl J Med*, 1993, 328(1):29-33.

(Continued)

Felbamate (Continued)

Written Communication, Elisabeth Neumann, Director Medical Services, Wallace Laboratories, June 13, 1995.

♦ **Felbatol®** see Felbamate on page 420
♦ **Feldene®** see Piroxicam on page 806
♦ **Fenesin™ [OTC]** see Guaifenesin on page 485
♦ **Fenesin DM®** see Guaifenesin and Dextromethorphan on page 487

Fentanyl (FEN ta nil)

Related Information

Adult ACLS Algorithm, Synchronized Cardioversion on page 1048
Compatibility of Medications Mixed in a Syringe on page 1238
Narcotic Analgesics Comparison on page 1070
Overdose and Toxicology on page 1222
Preprocedure Sedatives in Children on page 1201
Serotonin Syndrome on page 1247

U.S. Brand Names Actiq®; Duragesic®; Sublimaze®

Therapeutic Category Analgesic, Narcotic; General Anesthetic

Generic Available Injection: Yes

Use Sedation; relief of pain; preoperative medication; adjunct to general or regional anesthesia; management of chronic pain (transdermal product)

Oral transmucosal: Actiq®: Breakthrough cancer pain in adult patients tolerant to opioid therapy and who are currently receiving opiates for persistent cancer pain. Patients are considered opioid tolerant if they are receiving at least 60 mg/day of morphine, 50 mcg/hour of transdermal fentanyl, or an equivalent dose of another opioid for 1 week or longer.

Restrictions C-II

Pregnancy Risk Factor C (D if used for prolonged periods or in high doses at term)

Contraindications Hypersensitivity or intolerance to fentanyl or any component; transdermal system is contraindicated in patients with hypersensitivity to contact adhesives; increased intracranial pressure; severe respiratory depression; severe liver or renal insufficiency; Actiq® is contraindicated in patients who are not opioid tolerant and in the treatment of acute or postoperative pain.

Warnings Physical and psychological dependence may occur with prolonged use.

I.V. use: Rapid I.V. infusion may result in skeletal muscle and chest wall rigidity → impaired ventilation → respiratory distress → apnea, bronchoconstriction, laryngospasm; inject slowly over 3-5 minutes; nondepolarizing skeletal muscle relaxant may be required

Actiq®: Use only for the care of cancer patients; should be used only by specialists who are knowledgeable in treating cancer pain; keep out of the reach of children and discard any open units properly; contains an amount of medication that can be fatal to children

Precautions Use with caution in patients with bradycardia, hepatic, renal, or respiratory disease or those with increased ICP, head injuries, or impaired consciousness; patients must be monitored until fully recovered; decrease dose in patients with hepatic and/or renal disease; not recommended if patient received MAO inhibitors within 14 days; use of transdermal system is not recommended in children <12 years or those <18 years and <50 kg

Adverse Reactions

Cardiovascular: Hypotension, bradycardia, flushing

Central nervous system: CNS depression, drowsiness, dizziness, sedation, euphoria

Dermatologic: Erythema, pruritus, facial pruritus with oral transmucosal product

Endocrine & metabolic: ADH release

Gastrointestinal: Nausea, vomiting, constipation, biliary tract spasm

Genitourinary: Urinary tract spasm

Local: Transdermal system: Edema, erythema, pruritus

Neuromuscular & skeletal: Skeletal and thoracic muscle rigidity especially following rapid I.V. administration

Ocular: Miosis

Respiratory: Respiratory depression, apnea

Miscellaneous: Physical and psychological dependence with prolonged use. **Note:** Neonates who receive a total fentanyl dose >1.6 mg/kg or continuous infusion duration >5 days are more likely to develop narcotic withdrawal symptoms; children 1 week to 22 months: those who receive a total dose of 1.5 mg/kg or duration >5 days have a 50% chance of developing narcotic withdrawal and those receiving a total dose >2.5 mg/kg or duration of infusion >9 days have a 100%

chance of developing withdrawal. Doses should be tapered to prevent withdrawal symptoms.

Drug Interactions Cytochrome P-450 isoenzyme CYP3A3/4 substrate

CNS depressants, alcohol, phenothiazines, MAO inhibitors, tricyclic antidepressants may potentiate fentanyl's adverse effects; the herbal medicine St John's wort (*Hypericum perforatum*) may increase serious side effects, its use is **not** recommended

Stability Protect from light

Mechanism of Action Binds with stereospecific opioid mu receptors at many sites within the CNS, increases pain threshold, alters pain reception, inhibits ascending pain pathways

Pharmacodynamics Respiratory depressant effect may last longer than analgesic effect

Onset of analgesia:
  I.M.: 7-15 minutes
  I.V.: Almost immediate
  Transdermal: 6-8 hours
  Transmucosal: 5-15 minutes
Maximum effect:
  Transdermal: 24 hours
  Transmucosal: 20-30 minutes
Duration:
  I.M.: 1-2 hours
  I.V.: 30-60 minutes
  Transdermal: 72 hours
  Transmucosal: 1-2 hours

Pharmacokinetics

Absorption: Transmucosal: Rapid; ~25% absorbed from buccal mucosa; 75% swallowed with saliva and slowly absorbed from GI tract

Distribution: Highly lipophilic, redistributes into muscle and fat
  V_d: Adults: 4 L/kg
  V_{dss}: Children: 0.05-14 years of age (after long-term continuous infusion): ~15 L/kg (range: 5-30 L/kg)

Protein binding: 80% to 85%, primarily to alpha-1-acid glycoprotein

Metabolism: >90% metabolized in the liver via N-dealkylation and hydroxylation to inactive metabolites

Bioavailability: Transmucosal: ~50% (range: 36% to 71%)

Half-life:
  Children 5 months to 4.5 years: Mean: 2.4 hours
  Children 0.5-14 years (after long-term continuous infusion): ~21 hours (range: 11-36 hours)
  Adults: I.V.: 2-4 hours
    Transdermal: 17 hours (range: 13-22); apparent half-life increased with transdermal due to continued absorption
    Transmucosal: 6.6 hours (range: 5-15 hours)

Elimination: In urine primarily as metabolites and <10% as unchanged drug

  Clearance: Newborn infants: Clearance may be significantly correlated to gestational age and birth weight (see Saarenmaa, 2000)

Usual Dosage Doses should be titrated to appropriate effects; wide range of doses, dependent upon desired degree of analgesia/anesthesia, clinical environment, and patient's status

Neonates and younger Infants:
  Sedation/analgesia: Slow I.V. push: 1-4 mcg/kg/dose; may repeat every 2-4 hours
  Continuous sedation/analgesia: Initial I.V. bolus: 1-2 mcg/kg, then 0.5-1 mcg/kg/hour; titrate upward
    Mean required dose: Neonates with gestational age <34 weeks: 0.64 mcg/kg/hour; neonates with gestational age ≥34 weeks: 0.75 mcg/kg/hour
  Continuous sedation/analgesia during ECMO: Initial I.V. bolus: 5-10 mcg/kg slow I.V. push over 10 minutes, then 1-5 mcg/kg/hour; titrate upward; tolerance may develop; higher doses (up to 20 mcg/kg/hour) may be needed by day 6 of ECMO

Older Infants and Children 1-12 years:
  Sedation for minor procedures/analgesia: I.M., I.V.: 1-2 mcg/kg/dose; may repeat at 30- to 60-minute intervals. **Note:** Children 18-36 months of age may require 2-3 mcg/kg/dose.
  Continuous sedation/analgesia: Initial I.V. bolus: 1-2 mcg/kg then 1 mcg/kg/hour; titrate upward; usual: 1-3 mcg/kg/hour; some require 5 mcg/kg/hour
  Transdermal: Not recommended

(Continued)

Fentanyl *(Continued)*

Children >12 years and Adults:

Sedation for minor procedures/analgesia: I.V.: 0.5-1 mcg/kg/dose; may repeat after 30-60 minutes; **or** 25-50 mcg, repeat full dose in 5 minutes if needed, may repeat 4-5 times with 25 mcg at 5-minute intervals if needed. **Note:** Higher doses are used for major procedures.

Preoperative sedation, adjunct to regional anesthesia, postoperative pain: I.M., I.V.: 50-100 mcg/dose

Adjunct to general anesthesia: I.M., I.V.: 2-50 mcg/kg

General anesthesia without additional anesthetic agents: I.V. 50-100 mcg/kg with O_2 and skeletal muscle relaxant

Transdermal: Initial: 25 mcg/hour system; use short-acting analgesics for first 24 hours with supplemental PRN doses thereafter; dose may be increased after 3 days; if currently receiving opiates, convert to fentanyl equivalent and administer equianalgesic dosage; (see package insert for further information); transdermal patch is usually administered every 72 hours but select patients may require every 48-hour administration; dosage increase should be tried before 48-hour schedule is used

Actiq®: Breakthrough cancer pain: Transmucosal: Adults: Titrate dose to provide adequate analgesia: Initial: 200 mcg; may redose 15 minutes after completion of first dose if needed; no more than 2 units are recommended for each break-through cancer pain episode; titrate dose up to next higher strength if treatment of several consecutive breakthrough episodes requires >1 Actiq® per episode; evaluate each new dose over several breakthrough cancer pain episodes (generally 1-2 days) to determine proper dose of analgesia with acceptable side effects. Once dose has been determined, consumption should be limited to ≤4 units per day. Re-evaluate long-acting opioid dose if patient requires >4 units/day. If signs of excessive opioid effects occur before a dose is complete, the unit should be removed from the mouth immediately, and subsequent doses decreased.

Dosing adjustment in renal impairment:

Cl_{cr} 10-50 mL/minute: Administer 75% of dose

Cl_{cr} <10 mL/minute: Administer 50% of dose

Administration

Transdermal: Apply to nonhairy, dry, nonirritated flat area of front or back of upper torso; do **not** shave area; do not apply new patch to same place as old patch; **Note:** Transdermal patch is a membrane-controlled system; do **not** cut the patch to deliver partial doses; rate of drug delivery, reservoir contents, and adhesion may be affected if cut; if partial dose is needed, surface area of patch can be blocked proportionally using adhesive bandage (see Lee, 1997); do **not** use soap, alcohol, or other solvents to remove transdermal gel if it accidentally touches skin as they may increase transdermal absorption, use copious amounts of water

Transmucosal: Foil overwrap should be removed just prior to administration; once removed, patient should place the unit in mouth and suck (not chew) it

Actiq®: Place in mouth between cheek and lower gum; occasionally move unit from one side of the mouth to the other; consume unit over 15 minutes; remove unit from mouth if signs of excessive opioid effects appear before unit is totally consumed

Parenteral: I.V.: Administer by slow I.V. push over 3-5 minutes or by continuous infusion; larger bolus doses (>5 mcg/kg) should be given slow I.V. push over 5-10 minutes

Monitoring Parameters Respiratory rate, blood pressure, heart rate, oxygen saturation, bowel sounds, abdominal distention

Patient Information Avoid alcohol; may cause drowsiness and impair ability to perform activities requiring mental alertness or physical coordination; an Actiq® Welcome Kit, containing educational materials and safe storage containers (to keep medication away from children), as well as a patient safety video, is available from the manufacturer; these can be obtained by healthcare professionals who call 1-888-818-4113; dispose of transmucosal and transdermal products properly; keep all products (even if used) out of the reach of children; see Actiq® Patient Leaflet for details on proper storage, administration, and disposal of Actiq®, as well as, instructions about overdose management.

Nursing Implications Patients with elevated temperature may have increased fentanyl absorption transdermally, observe for adverse effects, dosage adjustment may be needed; pharmacologic and adverse effects can be seen after discontinuation of transdermal system, observe patients for at least 12 hours after transdermal product removed; destroy unused portion of fentanyl Oralet® and Actiq® according to hospital policy on controlled substances; partial unused doses of Actiq® can be dissolved under hot running tap water; dispose of handle properly; keep out of the reach of children

Additional Information An opioid antagonist, resuscitative and intubation equipment, and oxygen should be available; fentanyl is 50-100 times as potent as morphine; morphine 10 mg I.M. = fentanyl 0.1-0.2 mg I.M.; fentanyl has less hypotensive effects than morphine or meperidine due to minimal or no histamine release; keep transmucosal and transdermal products (both used and unused) out of the reach of children; special child-resistant containers are available to temporarily store partially-consumed units that cannot be disposed of immediately

Dosage Forms

Injection, preservative free, as citrate: 0.05 mg/mL (2 mL, 5 mL, 10 mL, 20 mL, 30 mL, 50 mL)

Sublimaze®: 2 mL, 5 mL, 10 mL, 20 mL

Lozenge, oral transmucosal, as citrate mounted on a plastic radiopaque handle (Actiq®): 200 mcg, 400 mcg, 600 mcg, 800 mcg, 1200 mcg, 1600 mcg [raspberry flavor]

Transdermal system (Duragesic®): 25 mcg/hour [10 cm^2]; 50 mcg/hour [20 cm^2]; 75 mcg/hour [30 cm^2]; 100 mcg/hour [40 cm^2] (all available in 5s)

References
Billmire DA, Neale HW, and Gregory RO, "Use of I.V. Fentanyl in the Outpatient Treatment of Pediatric Facial Trauma," J Trauma, 1985, 25(11):1079-80.

Katz R, Kelly HW, and Hsi A, "Prospective Study on the Occurrence of Withdrawal in Critically Ill Children Who Receive Fentanyl by Continuous Infusion," Crit Care Med, 1994, 22(5):763-7.

Lee NA and Anderson PO, "Giving Partial Doses of Transdermal Patches," Am J Health Syst Pharm, 1997, 54(15):1759-60.

Leuschen MP, Willett LD, Hoie EB, et al, "Plasma Fentanyl Levels in Infants Undergoing Extracorporeal Membrane Oxygenation," J Thorac Cardiovasc Surg, 1993, 105(5):885-91.

Roth B, Schlunder C, Houben F, et al, "Analgesia and Sedation in Neonatal Intensive Care Using Fentanyl by Continuous Infusion," Dev Pharmacol Ther, 1991, 17(3-4):121-7.

Saarenmaa E, Neuvonen PJ, and Fellman V, "Gestational Age and Birth Weight Effects on Plasma Clearance of Fentanyl in Newborn Infants," J Pediatr, 2000, 136(6):767-70.

Schechter NL, Weisman SJ, Rosenblum M, et al, "The Use of Oral Transmucosal Fentanyl Citrate for Painful Procedures in Children," Pediatrics, 1995, 95(3):335-9.

Zeltzer LK, Altman A, Cohen D, et al, "Report of the Subcommittee on the Management of Pain Associated With Procedures in Children With Cancer," Pediatrics, 1990, 86(5 Pt 2):826-31.

Filgrastim (fil GRA stim)

U.S. Brand Names Neupogen®
Synonyms G-CSF; Granulocyte Colony Stimulating Factor
Therapeutic Category Colony-Stimulating Factor
Generic Available No
Use Reduction of the duration of neutropenia and the associated risk of infection in patients with malignancies receiving myelosuppressive chemotherapeutic regimens associated with a significant incidence of severe neutropenia with fever; cancer patients receiving bone marrow transplant; severe chronic neutropenia which includes patients with congenital neutropenia, cyclic neutropenia, or idiopathic neutropenia; mobilization of peripheral blood progenitor cells into the peripheral blood for collection by leukapheresis; AIDS patients receiving zidovudine; neonatal neutropenia

Pregnancy Risk Factor C
(Continued)

425

Filgrastim *(Continued)*

Contraindications Hypersensitivity to *E. coli*-derived proteins, G-CSF, or any component; use in patients receiving concomitant chemotherapy and radiation therapy

Warnings Leukocytosis (white blood cell counts ≥100,000/mm³) has been observed in approximately 2% of patients receiving G-CSF at doses >5 mcg/kg/day

Precautions Do not administer 24 hours prior to or within 24 hours following the administration of chemotherapy; use with caution in any malignancy with myeloid characteristics due to G-CSF's potential to act as a growth factor; use with caution in patients with gout, psoriasis; monitor patients with pre-existing cardiac conditions as cardiac events (MIs, arrhythmias) have been reported in premarketing clinical studies. Be alert to the possibility of ARDS in septic patients.

Premature discontinuation of G-CSF therapy prior to the time of recovery from the expected neutrophil nadir are generally not recommended. A transient increase in neutrophil counts is typically seen 1-2 days after initiation of therapy. For a sustained therapeutic response, G-CSF should be continued until the post nadir absolute neutrophil count (ANC) reaches:

10,000/mm³ in chemotherapy treated patients, or

>1000/mm³ for 3 consecutive days in bone marrow transplant patients

Most patients experience a 30% to 50% decrease in circulating leukocytes within 1-2 days following discontinuation of G-CSF

Adverse Reactions

Cardiovascular: Transient decrease in blood pressure, vasculitis, chest pain

Central nervous system: Fever, headache

Dermatologic: Exacerbation of pre-existing skin disorders, alopecia

Endocrine & metabolic: Reversible increase in uric acid, lactate dehydrogenase

Gastrointestinal: Splenomegaly, nausea, vomiting, diarrhea, mucositis

Hematologic: Thrombocytopenia, leukocytosis

Hepatic: Elevated alkaline phosphatase

Neuromuscular & skeletal: Medullary bone pain (24% incidence) is generally dose-related, localized to the lower back, posterior iliac crests, and sternum; osteoporosis

Renal: Hematuria, proteinuria

Stability Store in refrigerator; do not freeze; stable for 24 hours at room temperature; solutions with concentration ≥15 mcg/mL in D_5W are stable for 24 hours; incompatible with salt solutions

Mechanism of Action Stimulates the production, maturation, and activation of neutrophils; G-CSF activates neutrophils to increase both their migration and cytotoxicity

Pharmacodynamics

Onset of action: Immediate transient leukopenia with the nadir occurring 5-15 minutes after an I.V. dose or 30-60 minutes after a S.C. dose followed by a sustained elevation in neutrophil levels within the first 24 hours reaching a plateau in 3-5 days

Duration: Upon discontinuation of G-CSF, ANC decreases by 50% within 2 days and returns to pretreatment levels within 1 week; WBC counts return to normal range in 4-7 days

Pharmacokinetics

Distribution: V_d: 150 mL/kg

Bioavailability: Not bioavailable after oral administration

Half-life: Neonates: 4.4 hours; Adults: 1.8-3.5 hours

Time to peak serum concentration: S.C.: Within 2-6 hours

Elimination: No evidence of drug accumulation over a 11- to 20-day period

Usual Dosage I.V., S.C. (refer to individual protocols):

Neonates: 5-10 mcg/kg/day once daily for 3-5 days has been administered to neutropenic neonates with sepsis. There was a rapid and significant increase in peripheral neutrophil counts and the neutrophil storage pool.

Children and Adults: 5-10 mcg/kg/day (~150-300 mcg/m²/day) once daily for up to 14 days until ANC = 10,000/mm³; dose escalations at 5 mcg/kg/day may be required in some individuals when response at 5 mcg/kg/day is not adequate; in phase 3 trials, efficacy was observed at dosages of 4-8 mcg/kg/day with myelosuppressive chemotherapy

Peripheral blood progenitor cell (PBPC) mobilization: S.C.: 10 mcg/kg/day given for 4 days before the first leukapheresis procedure and continued until the last leukapheresis

Patients with congenital neutropenia: S.C.: Initial: 6 mcg/kg/dose twice daily; dosages of 2-60 mcg/kg/day individualized according to neutrophil count have been administered to children and adults

Patients with idiopathic or cyclic neutropenia: S.C.: 5 mcg/kg/day once daily

Cancer patients receiving bone marrow transplant: I.V. infusion, S.C.: 5-10 mcg/kg/day administered ≥24 hours after cytotoxic chemotherapy and ≥24 hours after bone marrow infusion

Dosage adjustment during neutrophil recovery period: see table

Filgrastim Dose Based on Neutrophil Response

Absolute Neutrophil Count (ANC)	Filgrastim Dose Adjustment
When ANC >1000/mm³ for 3 consecutive days	Reduce to 5 mcg/kg/day
If ANC remains >1000/mm³ for 3 more consecutive days	Discontinue filgrastim
If ANC decreases to <1000/mm³	Resume at 5 mcg/kg/day

If ANC decreases <1000/mm³ during the 5 mcg/kg/day dose, increase dose to 10 mcg/kg/day and follow the above steps in the table.

Administration Parenteral:
S.C.: Administer undiluted solution
S.C. continuous infusion: Dilute dose in 10 mL D₅W and infuse at a rate of 10 mL/24 hours
I.V. continuous infusion; Administer over 15-60 minutes or as a continuous I.V. infusion at a final concentration of at least 15 mcg/mL in D₅W. If the final concentration of G-CSF in D₅W is <15 mcg/mL, then add 2 mg albumin/mL to I.V. fluid; the solution is stable for 24 hours; albumin acts as a carrier molecule to prevent drug adsorption to the I.V. tubing. Albumin should be added to the D₅W prior to addition of G-CSF; final concentration of G-CSF for administration <5 mcg/mL is not recommended; do not shake solution to avoid foaming.

Monitoring Parameters CBC with differential and platelet count, hematocrit, uric acid, urinalysis, liver function tests

Reference Range Blood samples for monitoring the hematologic effects of G-CSF should be drawn just before the next dose at least twice weekly

Patient Information Possible bone pain

Nursing Implications Bone pain management is usually successful with non-narcotic analgesic therapy

Dosage Forms Injection, preservative free: 300 mcg/mL (1 mL, 1.6 mL), produced by recombinant DNA technology using an *E. coli* expression system

References
"Update of Recommendations for the Use of Hematopoietic Colony-Stimulating Factors: Evidence-based Clinical Practice Guidelines. American Society of Clinical Oncology," *J Clin Oncol*, 1996, 14(6):1957-60.
Bonilla MA, Gillio AP, Ruggeiro M, et al, "Effects of Recombinant Human Granulocyte Colony-Stimulating Factor on Neutropenia in Patients With Congenital Agranulocytosis," *N Engl J Med*, 1989, 320(24):1574-80.
Gilmore MM, Stroncek DF, and Korones DN, "Treatment of Alloimmune Neonatal Neutropenia With Granulocyte Colony-Stimulating Factor," *J Pediatr*, 1994, 125(6 Pt 1):948-51
Hollingshead LM, Goa KL, "Recombinant Granulocyte Colony-Stimulating Factor (rG-CSF). A Review of Its Pharmacological Properties and Prospective Role in Neutropenic Conditions," *Drugs*, 1991, 42(2):300-30.
Morstyn G, Campbell L, Lieschke G, et al, "Treatment of Chemotherapy-Induced Neutropenia by Subcutaneously Administered Granulocyte Colony-Stimulating Factor With Optimization of Dose and Duration of Therapy," *J Clin Oncol*, 1989, 7(10):1554-62.
Wolach B, "Neonatal Sepsis: Pathogenesis and Supportive Therapy," *Semin Perinatol*, 1997, 21(1):28-38.

♦ **Fisalamine** *see* Mesalamine *on page 634*
♦ **FK506** *see* Tacrolimus *on page 934*
♦ **Flagyl® Oral** *see* Metronidazole *on page 662*
♦ **Flamazine (Can)** *see* Silver Sulfadiazine *on page 901*
♦ **Flarex®** *see* Fluorometholone *on page 443*
♦ **Flatulex® [OTC]** *see* Simethicone *on page 902*

Flecainide (fle KAY nide)
U.S. Brand Names Tambocor®
Therapeutic Category Antiarrhythmic Agent, Class I-C
Generic Available No
Use Prevention and suppression of documented life-threatening ventricular arrhythmias (ie, sustained ventricular tachycardia); prevention of symptomatic, disabling supraventricular tachycardias in patients without structural heart disease
Pregnancy Risk Factor C
(Continued)

Flecainide *(Continued)*

Contraindications Hypersensitivity to flecainide or any component; pre-existing second or third degree A-V block; right bundle-branch block associated with left hemiblock (bifascicular block) or trifascicular block; cardiogenic shock, myocardial depression

Warnings The manufacturer and FDA recommend that this drug be reserved for life-threatening ventricular arrhythmias unresponsive to conventional therapy. Its use for symptomatic nonsustained ventricular tachycardia, frequent premature ventricular complexes (PVCs), uniform and multiform PVCs and/or coupled PVCs is no longer recommended. Flecainide can worsen or cause arrhythmias with an associated risk of death. Proarrhythmic effects range from an increased number of PVCs to more severe ventricular tachycardias (ie, tachycardias that are more sustained or more resistant to conversion to sinus rhythm).

Precautions Use with caution in patients with pacemakers, sick sinus syndrome, CHF, myocardial dysfunction, and renal and/or hepatic impairment; use decreased doses and cautiously titrate dose according to serum concentrations and clinical effects in patients with CHF, or myocardial, liver or renal dysfunction. Flecainide may cause increases in PR, QRS, and QT intervals and new first degree or bundle branch block; use with caution and consider dosing reduction when increases in such intervals occur.

Adverse Reactions
Cardiovascular: Bradycardia, heart block, worsening ventricular arrhythmias, CHF, palpitations, chest pain, edema; increased P-R interval and QRS duration
Central nervous system: Dizziness, fatigue, nervousness, hypoesthesia, headache
Dermatologic: Rash
Gastrointestinal: Nausea
Hematologic: Blood dyscrasias
Hepatic: Hepatic dysfunction
Neuromuscular & skeletal: Paresthesia, tremor
Ocular: Blurred vision
Respiratory: Dyspnea

Drug Interactions Cytochrome P-450 isoenzyme CYP2D6 substrate
Other antiarrhythmic agents may increase adverse cardiac effects; flecainide may increase plasma digoxin concentrations; use with beta-blockers, disopyramide, or verapamil may result in possible additive negative inotropic effects; alkalinizing agents (high-dose antacids, carbonic anhydrase inhibitors or sodium bicarbonate) may decrease flecainide's clearance; urinary acidifiers may increase flecainide's clearance; amiodarone and cimetidine increase flecainide serum concentrations; concurrent use of flecainide with ritonavir or lopinavir is not recommended

Food Interactions Dairy products (milk, infant formula, yogurt) may interfere with the absorption of flecainide in infants; there is one case report of a neonate (GA 34 weeks PNA >6 days) who required extremely large doses of oral flecainide when administered every 8 hours with feedings ("milk feeds"); changing the feedings from "milk feeds" to 5% glucose feeds alone resulted in a doubling of the flecainide serum concentration and toxicity (see Russell, 1989); clearance of flecainide may be decreased in patients with strict vegetarian diets due to urinary pH ≥8

Mechanism of Action Class IC antiarrhythmic; slows conduction in cardiac tissue by altering transport of ions across cell membranes; causes slight prolongation of refractory periods; decreases the rate of rise of the action potential without affecting its duration; increases electrical stimulation threshold of ventricle, HIS-Purkinje system; possesses local anesthetic and moderate negative inotropic effects

Pharmacokinetics
Absorption: Oral: Rapid and nearly complete
Distribution: V_d: Adults: 5-13.4 L/kg
Protein binding: 40% to 50% (alpha$_1$ glycoprotein)
Metabolism: In the liver
Bioavailability: 85% to 90%
Half-life, elimination: Increased half-life with CHF or renal dysfunction
Newborns: ~29 hours
Infants: 11-12 hours
Children: 8 hours
Adults: ~20 hours (range: 12-27 hours)
Time to peak serum concentration: ~3 hours (range 1-6 hours)
Elimination: In urine as unchanged drug (10% to 50%) and metabolites
Dialysis: Not dialyzable

Usual Dosage Oral:
Children: Initial: 1-3 mg/kg/day or 50-100 mg/m²/day in 3 divided doses; usual: 3-6 mg/kg/day or 100-150 mg/m²/day in 3 divided doses; up to 8 mg/kg/day or 200

mg/m^2/day for uncontrolled patients with subtherapeutic levels; higher doses have been reported, however they may be associated with an increased risk of proar-rhythmias; a review of world literature reports the average effective dose to be 4 mg/kg/day or 140 mg/m^2/day

Adults: Life-threatening ventricular arrhythmias: Initial: 100 mg every 12 hours, increase by 100 mg/day (given in 2 doses/day) every 4 days; usual: ≤300 mg/day; maximum: 400 mg/day; for patients receiving 400 mg/day who are not controlled and have trough concentrations <0.6 mcg/mL, dosage may be increased to 600 mg/day

Prevention of paroxysmal supraventricular arrhythmias in patients with disabling symptoms but no structural heart disease: Initial: 50 mg every 12 hours; maximum dose: 300 mg/day

Dosing adjustment in renal failure:

Manufacturer recommendations: Adults: Cl$_{cr}$ ≤35 mL/minute/1.73 m^2: Initial: 50 mg every 12 hours or 100 mg once daily; increase dose slowly at intervals >4 days; monitor plasma levels closely

Alternative adjustment: Children and Adults Cl$_{cr}$ ≤20 mL/minute: Decrease the usual dose by 25% to 50%

Administration Oral: May be administered in children and adults without regard to food; in infants receiving milk or milk based formulas, avoid concurrent administration with feedings; monitor serum concentrations and decrease the dose when the diet changes to a decreased consumption of milk

Monitoring Parameters EKG, serum concentrations; **Note**: Obtain serum trough concentrations at steady state (after at least 3 days when doses are started or changed) or when dietary changes due to maturation or concurrent illness occur

Reference Range Therapeutic: 0.2-1 μg/mL (SI: 0.4-2 μmol/L). **Note**: Pediatric patients may respond at the lower end of the recommended therapeutic range (0.2-0.5 μg/mL) but up to 0.8 μg/mL may be required.

Patient Information May cause dizziness; notify physician if chest pain, faintness, palpitations, dizziness or visual disturbances occur

Additional Information Single oral dose flecainide for termination of PSVT in children and young adults (n=25) and combination therapy of flecainide with amiodarone for refractory tachyarrhythmias in infancy (n=9) have been reported (See References)

Dosage Forms Tablet, as acetate: 50 mg, 100 mg, 150 mg

Extemporaneous Preparations

A 5 mg/mL suspension compounded from tablets and an oral flavored commercially available diluent (Roxane®) was stable for up to 45 days when stored at 5°C or 25°C in amber glass bottles (Wiest, 1992)

A 20 mg/mL oral liquid preparation made from tablets and 3 different vehicles (cherry syrup, a 1:1 mixture of Ora-Sweet® and Ora-Plus®, or a 1:1 mixture of Ora-Sweet® SF and Ora-Plus®) was stable for 60 days when stored in amber plastic prescription bottles in the dark at room temperature (25°C) or under refrigeration (5°C); grind twenty-four 100 mg tablets in a mortar into a fine powder; add 20 mL of the vehicle and mix well to form a uniform paste; mix while adding the vehicle in geometric proportions to **almost** 120 mL; transfer to a calibrated bottle and qsad with vehicle to 120 mL; label "shake well" and "protect from light" (Allen, 1996).

Allen LV and Erickson MA, "Stability of Baclofen, Captopril, Diltiazem Hydrochloride, Dipyridamole, and Flecainide Acetate in Extemporaneously Compounded Oral Liquids," *Am J Health Syst Pharm*, 1996, 53(18):2179-84.

Wiest DB, Garner SS, and Pagacz LR, "Stability of Flecainide Acetate in an Extemporaneously Compounded Oral Suspension," *Am J Hosp Pharm*, 1992, 49(6):1467-70.

References

Fenrich AL Jr, Perry JC, and Friedman RA, "Flecainide and Amiodarone: Combined Therapy for Refractory Tachyarrhythmias in Infants," *J Am Coll Cardiol*, 1995, 25(5):1195-8.

Musto B, Cavallaro C, Musto A, et al, "Flecainide Single Oral Dose for Management of Paroxysmal Supraventricular Tachycardia in Children and Young Adults," *Am Heart J*, 1992, 124(1):110-5.

Perry JC and Garson A Jr, "Flecainide Acetate for Treatment of Tachyarrhythmias in Children: Review of World Literature on Efficacy, Safety, and Dosing," *Am Heart J*, 1992, 124(6):1614-21.

Perry JC, McQuinn RL, Smith RT Jr, et al, "Flecainide Acetate for Resistant Arrhythmias in the Young: Efficacy and Pharmacokinetics," *J Am Coll Cardiol*, 1989, 14(1):185-91.

Priestley KA, Ladusans EJ, Rosenthal E, et al, "Experience With Flecainide for the Treatment of Cardiac Arrhythmias in Children," *Eur Heart J*, 1988, 9(12):1284-90.

Russell GA and Martin RP, "Flecainide Toxicity," *Arch Dis Child*, 1989, 64(6):860-2.

Zeigler V, Gillette PC, Ross BA, et al, "Flecainide for Supraventricular and Ventricular Arrhythmias in Children and Young Adults," *Am J Cardiol*, 1988, 62(10 Pt 1):818-20.

♦ **Fleet® Babylax® [OTC]** *see Glycerin on page 478*

♦ **Fleet® Enema [OTC]** *see Phosphate Supplements on page 794*

♦ **Fleet® Laxative [OTC]** *see Bisacodyl on page 143*

- ◆ **Fleet® Mineral Oil Enema [OTC]** *see* Mineral Oil *on page 675*
- ◆ **Fleet® Phospho®-Soda [OTC]** *see* Phosphate Supplements *on page 794*
- ◆ **Fleet® Relief®** *see* Hemorrhoidal Preparations *on page 490*
- ◆ **Flexeril®** *see* Cyclobenzaprine *on page 278*
- ◆ **Flexitec (Can)** *see* Cyclobenzaprine *on page 278*
- ◆ **Flonase®** *see* Fluticasone *on page 451*
- ◆ **Florical® [OTC]** *see* Calcium Supplements *on page 167*
- ◆ **Florinef (Can)** *see* Fludrocortisone *on page 435*
- ◆ **Florinef® Acetate** *see* Fludrocortisone *on page 435*
- ◆ **Flovent®** *see* Fluticasone *on page 451*
- ◆ **Flovent® Diskus®** *see* Fluticasone *on page 451*
- ◆ **Flovent® Rotadisk®** *see* Fluticasone *on page 451*
- ◆ **Flubenisolone** *see* Betamethasone *on page 140*

Fluconazole (floo KOE na zole)

Related Information
Carbohydrate and Alcohol Content of Liquid Medications for Use in Patients Receiving Ketogenic Diets *on page 1258*

U.S. Brand Names Diflucan®

Canadian Brand Names Apo-Fluconazole

Therapeutic Category Antifungal Agent, Systemic

Generic Available No

Use Treatment of susceptible fungal infections including oropharyngeal, esophageal, and vaginal candidiasis; treatment of systemic candidal infections including urinary tract infection, peritonitis, cystitis, and pneumonia; strains of *Candida* with decreased *in vitro* susceptibility to fluconazole are being isolated with increasing frequency; fluconazole is more active against *C. albicans* than other candidal strains like *C. parapsilosis*, *C. glabrata*, and *C. tropicalis*; treatment and suppression of cryptococcal meningitis; prophylaxis of candidiasis in patients undergoing bone marrow transplantation; alternative to amphotericin B in patients with pre-existing renal impairment or when requiring concomitant therapy with other potentially nephrotoxic drugs

Pregnancy Risk Factor C

Contraindications Hypersensitivity to fluconazole, other azoles, or any component; concurrent use with astemizole, cisapride, and terfenadine

Warnings Patients who develop abnormal liver function tests during fluconazole therapy should be monitored closely for the development of more severe hepatic injury; if clinical signs and symptoms consistent with liver disease develop that may be attributable to fluconazole, fluconazole should be discontinued

Precautions Use with caution and modify dosage in patients with impaired renal function; oral suspension contains sodium benzoate, use with caution in neonates

Adverse Reactions
Cardiovascular: Pallor

Central nervous system: Dizziness, headache (1.9%), seizures

Dermatologic: Skin rash (1.8%), exfoliative skin disorders, Stevens-Johnson syndrome

Endocrine & metabolic: Hypokalemia, hypercholesterolemia, hypertriglyceridemia

Gastrointestinal: Nausea (2%), abdominal pain (3%), vomiting (5%), diarrhea (2%)

Hematologic: Eosinophilia, leukopenia, thrombocytopenia

Hepatic: Elevated AST, ALT, or alkaline phosphatase; hepatitis; cholestasis

Miscellaneous: Anaphylaxis

Drug Interactions Cytochrome P-450 isoenzyme CYP2CP substrate; CYP2C19 and CYP3A3/4 (weak) isoenzyme inhibitor

Oral antidiabetic agents (fluconazole reduces the metabolism and increases the concentration of tolbutamide, glyburide, and glipizide); hydrochlorothiazide (increases fluconazole AUC); warfarin (increased prothrombin time); fluconazole increases plasma cyclosporine, zidovudine, cisapride, (fatal arrhythmias including ventricular tachycardia, ventricular fibrillation, torsade de pointes, and QT prolongation have been reported in patients taking cisapride concurrently with fluconazole), astemizole, terfenadine, rifabutin, and phenytoin concentrations; rifampin increases fluconazole metabolism; antagonism may occur if amphotericin B and fluconazole are used concomitantly

Food Interactions Food decreases the rate but not the extent of absorption

Stability Incompatible with ampicillin, calcium gluconate, ceftazidime, cefotaxime, cefuroxime, ceftriaxone, clindamycin, furosemide, imipenem, ticarcillin, and piperacillin; reconstituted oral suspension is stable for 14 days at room temperature or if refrigerated

Mechanism of Action Interferes with fungal cytochrome P-450 sterol C-14 alpha-demethylation activity, decreasing ergosterol synthesis (principal sterol in fungal cell membrane) and inhibiting cell membrane formation

Pharmacokinetics

Absorption: Oral: Well absorbed; food does not affect extent of absorption

Distribution: Distributes widely into body tissues and fluids including the CSF, saliva, sputum, vaginal fluid, skin, eye; excreted in breast milk

Protein binding: 11% to 12%

Bioavailability: Oral: >90%

Half-life:

Premature newborns: 73.6 hours; 6 days PNA: 53.2 hours; 12 days PNA: 46.6 hours

Children:

9 months to 13 years: 19.5-25 hours (with oral dose)

5-15 years: 15.2-17.6 hours (with multiple I.V. dosing)

Adults: 25-30 hours with normal renal function

Time to peak serum concentration: Oral: Within 2-4 hours (1-2 hours in fasted patients)

Elimination: 80% of dose excreted unchanged in urine; 11% of dose excreted in urine as metabolites

Dialysis: Hemodialysis: 3-hour session decreases plasma concentration 50%

Usual Dosage Daily dose of fluconazole is the same for oral and I.V. administration:

Oral, I.V.:

Premature neonates:

≤29 weeks gestation:

Postnatal age 0-14 days: 5-6 mg/kg/dose every 72 hours

Postnatal age >14 days: 5-6 mg/kg/dose every 48 hours

30-36 weeks gestation: Postnatal age 0-14 days: 3-6 mg/kg/dose every 48 hours

Neonates >14 days, Infants, Children: Once daily: See table

Safety profile of fluconazole has been studied in 577 children ages 1 day to 17 years. Doses as high as 12 mg/kg/day once daily (equivalent to adult doses of 400 mg/day) have been used to treat candidiasis in immunocompromised children; 10-12 mg/kg/day doses once daily have been used prophylactically against fungal infections in pediatric bone marrow transplantation patients. Do not exceed 600 mg/day.

Adults: Oral, I.V.: Once daily: See table

Indication	Day 1	Daily Therapy	Minimum Duration of Therapy
Neonates 0-14 days: Same dosage as older children but administered every 24-72 h			
Neonates >14 days, infants, and children			
Oropharyngeal candidiasis	6 mg/kg	3 mg/kg	14 d
Esophageal candidiasis	6 mg/kg	3 mg/kg up to 12 mg/kg/d	21 d
Systemic candidiasis	6-12 mg/kg/d		28 d
Cryptococcal meningitis			
acute	12 mg/kg	6 mg/kg up to 12 mg/kg/d	10-12 wk after CSF culture becomes negative
relapse	6 mg/kg		
Adults			
Oropharyngeal candidiasis	200 mg	100 mg	14 d
Esophageal candidiasis	200 mg	100-400 mg	21 d
Systemic candidiasis	400 mg	200-800 mg	28 d
Cryptococcal meningitis			
acute	400 mg	200-800 mg	10-12 wk after CSF culture becomes negative
relapse	200 mg	200 mg	

Vaginal candidiasis: Oral: 150 mg single dose

Prophylaxis against fungal infections in bone marrow transplantation patients: Oral, I.V.: 400 mg/day once daily

Dosing adjustment in renal impairment:

Cl_{cr} 21-50 mL/minute: Administer 50% of recommended dose

Cl_{cr} <20 mL/minute: Administer 25% of recommended dose

Patients receiving hemodialysis: One recommended dose after each dialysis

(Continued)

Fluconazole *(Continued)*

Administration
Oral: Administer with or without food; shake suspension well before use

Parenteral: Fluconazole must be administered by I.V. infusion over approximately 1-2 hours at a rate not to exceed 200 mg/hour and a final concentration for administration of 2 mg/mL; for pediatric patients receiving doses ≥6 mg/kg/day, administer I.V. infusion over 2 hours

Monitoring Parameters Periodic liver function and renal function tests

Patient Information Notify physician of unusual bleeding or bruising, yellowing of skin and eyes, or severe skin rash

Dosage Forms
Injection: 2 mg/mL (100 mL, 200 mL)

Suspension, oral: 10 mg/mL (35 mL), 40 mg/mL (35 mL)

Tablet: 50 mg, 100 mg, 150 mg, 200 mg

References
Como JA and Dismukes WE, "Oral Azole Drugs as Systemic Antifungal Therapy," *N Engl J Med*, 1993, 330(4):263-72.

Goodman JL, Winston DJ, Greenfield RA, et al, "A Controlled Trial of Fluconazole to Prevent Fungal Infections in Patients Undergoing Bone Marrow Transplantation," *N Engl J Med*, 1992, 326(13):845-51.

Lee JW, Seibel NL, Amantea M, et al, "Safety and Pharmacokinetics of Fluconazole in Children With Neoplastic Diseases," *J Pediatr*, 1992, 120(6):987-93.

Moncino MD and Gutman LT, "Severe Systemic Cryptococcal Disease in a Child: Review of Prognostic Indicators Predicting Treatment Failure and an Approach to Maintenance Therapy With Oral Fluconazole," *Pediatr Infect Dis J*, 1990, 9(5):363-8.

Viscoli C, Castagnola E, Fioredda F, et al, "Fluconazole in the Treatment of Candidiasis in Immunocompromised Children," *Antimicrob Agents Chemother*, 1991, 35(2):365-7.

Flucytosine *(floo SYE toe seen)*

Related Information
Blood Level Sampling Time Guidelines on page 1220

U.S. Brand Names Ancobon®

Synonyms 5-FC; 5-Flurocytosine

Therapeutic Category Antifungal Agent, Systemic

Generic Available No

Use In combination with amphotericin B in the treatment of serious *Candida*, *Aspergillus*, *Cryptococcus*, and *Torulopsis* infections (resistance emerges if flucytosine is used as a single agent)

Pregnancy Risk Factor C

Contraindications Hypersensitivity to flucytosine or any component

Precautions Use with extreme caution in patients with renal impairment, bone marrow suppression, patients with AIDS; dosage modification required in patients with impaired renal function; monitor serum concentration

Adverse Reactions
Central nervous system: Confusion, headache, sedation, hallucinations, vertigo, ataxia

Dermatologic: Rash

Endocrine & metabolic: Temporary growth failure

Gastrointestinal: Nausea, vomiting, diarrhea, enterocolitis

Hematologic: Bone marrow suppression (often observed after 10-26 days of therapy and occurs more frequently with sustained concentrations >100 mcg/mL), anemia, leukopenia, thrombocytopenia

Hepatic: Elevated liver enzymes, hepatitis

Neuromuscular & skeletal: Neuropathy

Renal: Elevated BUN and serum creatinine

Miscellaneous: Anaphylaxis

Drug Interactions Increased efficacy as well as toxicity (enterocolitis, myelosuppression) with concurrent amphotericin administration; antacids and aluminum or magnesium salts delay the rate of absorption

Food Interactions Food decreases the rate, but not the extent of absorption

Mechanism of Action Penetrates fungal cells and is converted to fluorouracil which competes with uracil interfering with fungal RNA and protein synthesis

Pharmacokinetics
Absorption: Oral: 75% to 90%; rate of absorption is delayed in patients with renal impairment

Distribution: Widely distributed into body tissues and fluids including CSF, aqueous humor, peritoneal fluid, bronchial secretions, liver, kidney, heart, and joints

Protein binding: 2% to 4%

Metabolism: Minimal

Bioavailability: Decreased in neonates

Half-life:
  Neonates: 4-34 hours
  Adults: 3-8 hours (prolonged as high as 200 hours in anuria)
  Time to peak serum concentration: Oral: Within 2-6 hours
  Elimination: 75% to 90% excreted unchanged in urine by glomerular filtration
  Dialysis: Dialyzable (50% to 100%)

Usual Dosage Oral:
  Neonates: Initial: 50-100 mg/kg/day in divided doses every 12-24 hours
  Infants, Children, Adults: 100-150 mg/kg/day in divided doses every 6 hours
  Dosing adjustment in renal impairment:
    Cl$_{cr}$ 10-50 mL/minute: Administer every 12 hours
    Cl$_{cr}$ <10 mL/minute: Administer every 24 hours

Administration Oral: Administer with food over a 15-minute period to decrease nausea and vomiting

Monitoring Parameters Serum creatinine, BUN, alkaline phosphatase, AST, ALT, CBC, platelet count; serum flucytosine concentrations

Reference Range Therapeutic levels: 25-100 µg/mL; with invasive candidiasis, maintain peak plasma concentration between 40-60 mcg/mL; increased bone marrow suppression with sustained serum flucytosine concentration >100 µg/mL; obtain flucytosine concentration 60 minutes after an oral dose; obtain trough level immediately before the next dose; maintain trough ≥25 mcg/mL to prevent emergence of resistant strains

Test Interactions Flucytosine causes markedly false elevations in serum creatinine values when the Ektachem® analyzer is used

Additional Information Resistance develops rapidly if used alone; more rapid emergence of fungal resistance may occur when lower doses are used

Dosage Forms Capsule: 250 mg, 500 mg

Extemporaneous Preparations Flucytosine oral liquid has been prepared by using the contents of ten 500 mg capsules triturated in a mortar and pestle with a small amount of distilled water; the mixture was transferred to a 500 mL volumetric flask; the mortar was rinsed several times with a small amount of distilled water and the fluid added to the flask; sufficient distilled water was added to make a total volume of 500 mL of a 10 mg/mL liquid; oral liquid was stable for 70 days when stored in glass or plastic prescription bottles at 4°C or for up to 14 days at room temperature.

  Wintermeyer SM and Nahata MC, "Stability of Flucytosine in an Extemporaneously Compounded Oral Liquid," *Am J Health-Syst Pharm*, 1996, 53:407-9.

References
Baley JE, Meyers C, Kliegman RM, et al, "Pharmacokinetics, Outcome of Treatment, and Toxic Effects of Amphotericin B and 5-Fluorocytosine in Neonates," *J Pediatr*, 1990, 116(5):791-7.

♦ **Fludara**® *see* Fludarabine *on page 433*

Fludarabine (floo DARE a been)

Related Information
  Emetogenic Potential of Single Chemotherapeutic Agents *on page 1129*

U.S. Brand Names Fludara®

Synonyms FAMP; F-ara-AMP

Therapeutic Category Antineoplastic Agent, Antimetabolite

Generic Available No

Use Treatment of B-cell chronic lymphocytic leukemia unresponsive to previous therapy with an alkylating agent containing regimen; non-Hodgkin's lymphoma. Fludarabine has been tested in patients with refractory acute lymphocytic leukemia and acute nonlymphocytic leukemia, but required a highly toxic dose to achieve response.

Pregnancy Risk Factor D

Contraindications Hypersensitivity to fludarabine phosphate or any component

Warnings The FDA currently recommends that procedures for proper handling and disposal of antineoplastic agents be considered; doses ≥77 mg/m²/day for 5-7 days were associated with severe neurotoxicity. Neurotoxicity can occur 21-60 days after completing a course of fludarabine and appears to be dose related. Severe bone marrow suppression has been observed at therapeutic doses. Hematologic function must be frequently monitored. Concomitant therapy with pentostatin may be associated with severe pulmonary toxicity.

Precautions Use with caution in patients with pre-existing neurologic problems and in patients with renal insufficiency; dosage adjustment may be needed in patients with impaired renal function or bone marrow suppression

Adverse Reactions
  Cardiovascular: Edema
  (Continued)

Fludarabine *(Continued)*

Central nervous system: Neurotoxicity (primarily progressive demyelinating enceph-alopathy with mental status deterioration), somnolence, seizures, fever, agitation, confusion, depression, chills, fatigue, headache

Dermatologic: Pruritus, rash, alopecia

Endocrine & metabolic: Metabolic acidosis, tumor lysis syndrome, (hyperuricemia, hyperphosphatemia, hypocalcemia, hyperkalemia), hyperglycemia

Gastrointestinal: Nausea, vomiting, diarrhea, stomatitis, metallic taste, GI bleeding, anorexia

Hematologic: Leukopenia, neutropenia, thrombocytopenia, lymphocytopenia, auto-immune hemolytic anemia, anemia

Hepatic: Elevated transaminase levels

Neuromuscular & skeletal: Myalgia, peripheral neuropathy, weakness, blurred vision, photophobia

Ocular: Blindness, blurred vision, photophobia

Renal: Hematuria, renal failure

Respiratory: Interstitial pneumonitis

Drug Interactions Cytarabine when administered with or prior to a fludarabine dose competes for deoxycytidine kinase decreasing the phosphorylation of fludarabine to the active F-ara-ATP (inhibits the antineoplastic effect of fludarabine); however, administering fludarabine prior to cytarabine may stimulate activation of cytarabine; pentostatin (increased pulmonary toxicity)

Stability Store vial in refrigerator; reconstituted 25 mg/mL fludarabine solution should be used within 8 hours after preparation since it contains no preservatives. When fludarabine is diluted in D_5W or NS to a final concentration of 1 mg/mL, the solution is stable for 24 hours at room temperature. Discard solution if a slight haze develops.

Mechanism of Action F-ara-AMP is dephosphorylated to 2-fluoro-ara-A which enters the cell by a carrier mediated transport process; it is phosphorylated intracel-lularly to the active metabolite F-ara-ATP. F-ara-ATP competes with deoxyadeno-sine triphosphate for incorporation into the A-sites of the DNA strand inhibiting DNA synthesis in the S-phase via inhibition of DNA polymerases and RNA reductase.

Pharmacokinetics

Distribution: Widely distributed with extensive tissue binding

Half-life: Terminal:

Children: 12.4-19 hours

Adults: 7-20 hours

Elimination: Fludarabine clearance appears to be inversely correlated with serum creatinine; at a dose of 25 mg/m^2/day for 5 days, 24% of dose excreted in urine; at higher doses, 41% to 60% of dose renally excreted

Usual Dosage Not currently FDA approved for use in children (refer to individual protocols): I.V.:

Children:

Acute leukemia: 10 mg/m^2 bolus over 15 minutes followed by a continuous infu-sion of 30.5 mg/m^2/day over 5 days; or 10.5 mg/m^2 bolus over 15 minutes followed by a continuous infusion of 30.5 mg/m^2/day over 48 hours followed by cytarabine has been used in clinical trials

Solid tumors: 9 mg/m^2 bolus followed by 27 mg/m^2/day continuous infusion over 5 days

Adults: Chronic lymphocytic leukemia: 20-25 mg/m^2/day over 30 minutes for 5 days; doses up to 30 mg/m^2/day as single daily doses for 5 days have also been used; courses are usually repeated every 28 days

Dosing adjustment in renal impairment: Cl_{cr} <50 mL/minute: Dose reduction is indicated in patients with renal failure; no specific guidelines are available; monitor closely for toxicity

Administration Parenteral: Fludarabine phosphate has been administered by inter-mittent I.V. infusion over 15-30 minutes and by continuous infusion; in clinical trials the loading dose has been diluted in 20 mL D_5W and administered over 15 minutes and the continuous infusion diluted to 240 mL in D_5W and administered at a constant rate of 10 mL/hour; in other clinical studies fludarabine has been diluted to a concentration of 0.25-1 mg/mL in D_5W or NS

Monitoring Parameters CBC with differential, platelet count, AST, ALT, creatinine, serum albumin, uric acid, and examination for visual changes

Patient Information Notify physician if fever, sore throat, bleeding, bruising, tach-ypnea, respiratory distress, or neurologic changes occur

Nursing Implications Prophylactic allopurinol, adequate hydration, and urinary alkalinization should be considered for patients with large initial tumor burdens

Additional Information Myelosuppressive effects:
Granulocyte nadir: 13 days (3-25)
Platelet nadir: 16 days (2-32)
Recovery: 5-7 weeks
Dosage Forms Powder for injection, as phosphate, lyophilized: 50 mg
References
Avramis VI, Champagne J, Sato J, et al, "Pharmacology of Fludarabine Phosphate After a Phase I/II Trial by a Loading Bolus and Continuous Infusion in Pediatric Patients," *Cancer Res*, 1990, 50(22):7226-31.
Von Hoff DD, "Phase I Clinical Trials With Fludarabine Phosphate," *Semin Oncol*, 1990, 17(5 Suppl 8):33-8.

Fludrocortisone (floo droe KOR ti sone)

Related Information
Corticosteroids Comparison, Systemic *on page 1067*
U.S. Brand Names Florinef® Acetate
Canadian Brand Names Florinef
Synonyms Fluohydrisone; Fluohydrocortisone; 9α-Fluorohydrocortisone
Therapeutic Category Adrenal Corticosteroid; Corticosteroid, Systemic; Glucocorticoid; Mineralocorticoid
Generic Available No
Use Addison's disease; partial replacement therapy for adrenal insufficiency; treatment of salt-losing forms of congenital adrenogenital syndrome; has been used with increased sodium intake for the treatment of idiopathic orthostatic hypotension
Pregnancy Risk Factor C
Contraindications Hypersensitivity to fludrocortisone or any component; CHF, systemic fungal infections
Precautions Dosage should be tapered gradually if therapy is discontinued; use with caution in patients with hypertension, edema, or renal dysfunction
Adverse Reactions
Cardiovascular: Hypertension, edema, CHF
Central nervous system: Convulsions, headache
Dermatologic: Acne, rash, bruising
Endocrine & metabolic: Hypokalemic alkalosis, suppression of growth, hyperglycemia, hypothalamic-pituitary-adrenal suppression
Gastrointestinal: Peptic ulcer
Neuromuscular & skeletal: Muscle weakness
Ocular: Cataracts
Drug Interactions Digoxin (fludrocortisone-induced hypokalemia may increase digoxin toxicity); phenytoin and rifampin may increase metabolism of fludrocortisone; hypokalemia-causing medications may increase risk of hypokalemia
Food Interactions Systemic use of mineralocorticoids/corticosteroids may require a diet with increased potassium, vitamins A, B_6, C, D, folate, calcium, zinc, and phosphorus, and decreased sodium; with fludrocortisone a decrease in dietary sodium is often not required as the increased retention of sodium is usually the desired therapeutic effect
Mechanism of Action Potent mineralocorticoid with glucocorticoid activity; promotes increased reabsorption of sodium and loss of potassium from distal tubules
Pharmacodynamics Duration: 1-2 days
Pharmacokinetics
Absorption: Rapid and complete from GI tract
Protein binding: 42%
Metabolism: In the liver
Half-life:
Plasma: ~3.5 hours
Biological: 18-36 hours
Usual Dosage Oral:
Infants and Children: 0.05-0.1 mg/day
Congenital adrenal hyperplasia (salt losers): Maintenance: Range: 0.05-0.3 mg/day (AAP, 2000)
Adults: 0.05-0.2 mg/day
Administration Oral: May administer with food to decrease GI upset
Monitoring Parameters Serum electrolytes, blood pressure, serum renin
Patient Information Notify physician if dizziness, severe or continuing headache, swelling of feet or lower legs, or unusual weight gain occurs
Additional Information In patients with salt-losing forms of congenital adrenogenital syndrome, use along with cortisone or hydrocortisone; fludrocortisone 0.1 mg has sodium retention activity equal to DOCA® 1 mg
(Continued)

Fludrocortisone *(Continued)*

Dosage Forms Tablet, as acetate: 0.1 mg

References

American Academy of Pediatrics, Section on Endocrinology and Committee on Genetics, "Technical Report: Congenital Adrenal Hyperplasia," *Pediatrics*, 2000, 106(6):1511-8.

♦ **Fluid and Electrolyte Requirements in Children** *see page 1102*

♦ **Flumadine**® *see* Rimantadine *on page 878*

Flumazenil *(FLO may ze nil)*

U.S. Brand Names Romazicon®

Canadian Brand Names Anexate

Therapeutic Category Antidote, Benzodiazepine

Generic Available No

Use Benzodiazepine antagonist; reverses sedative effects of benzodiazepines used in general anesthesia or conscious sedation; management of benzodiazepine overdose; **not indicated** for ethanol, barbiturate, general anesthetic or narcotic overdose

Pregnancy Risk Factor C

Contraindications Hypersensitivity to flumazenil, any component, or benzodiazepines; patients given benzodiazepines for control of potentially life-threatening conditions (eg, control of intracranial pressure or status epilepticus); patients with signs of serious cyclic-antidepressant overdosage

Warnings Seizures may occur in patients physically dependent on benzodiazepines, in patients treated with benzodiazepines for seizure disorders or other reasons, in overdose patients with seizure activity prior to flumazenil, or in patients with serious cyclic antidepressant overdoses; higher than normal doses of benzodiazepines may be required to treat these seizures; mixed drug overdose patients who have ingested drugs that increase the likelihood of seizures (eg, cocaine, lithium, cyclosporine, cyclic antidepressants, bupropion, methylxanthines, MAO inhibitors, isoniazid, or propoxyphene) are at extremely high risk for seizures (flumazenil may be contraindicated in these patients)

Precautions Resedation may occur with flumazenil use (due to its short half-life in comparison to some benzodiazepines); pediatric patients (especially 1-5 years of age) may experience resedation; these patients may require repeat bolus doses or continuous infusion; monitor patients for return of sedation and respiratory depression. Flumazenil should be used with caution in the intensive care unit because of increased risk of unrecognized benzodiazepine dependence in such settings. Flumazenil may provoke panic attacks in patients with panic disorder. Do not use flumazenil until effects of neuromuscular blockers have been fully reversed.

Adverse Reactions

Cardiovascular: Arrhythmias, bradycardia, tachycardia, chest pain, hypertension, hypotension

Central nervous system: Seizures (more common in patients physically dependent on benzodiazepines or with cyclic antidepressant overdoses, see Warnings), fatigue, dizziness, headache, agitation, emotional lability, anxiety, euphoria, depression, abnormal crying

Endocrine & metabolic: Hot flashes

Gastrointestinal: Nausea, vomiting, xerostomia

Local: Pain at injection site

Ocular: Blurred vision

Miscellaneous: Increased diaphoresis, shivering, hiccups, sensation of coldness; can precipitate acute withdrawal symptoms in patients physically dependent on benzodiazepines

Drug Interactions Use with caution in mixed drug overdose; toxic effects of other drugs (especially with cyclic antidepressants) may occur with reversal of benzodiazepine effects

Stability Compatible with D_5W, LR, or NS for 24 hours; discard any unused solution after 24 hours

Mechanism of Action Antagonizes the effect of benzodiazepines on the GABA/benzodiazepine receptor complex. Flumazenil is benzodiazepine specific and does not antagonize other nonbenzodiazepine GABA agonists (including ethanol, barbiturates, general anesthetics); does not reverse the effects of opiates.

Pharmacodynamics

Onset of benzodiazepine reversal: Within 1-3 minutes

Peak effect: 6-10 minutes

Duration: Usually <1 hour; duration is related to dose given and benzodiazepine plasma concentrations; reversal effects of flumazenil may wear off before effects of benzodiazepine and resedation may occur

Pharmacokinetics Follows a two compartment open model; **Note:** Clearance and V_d per kg are similar for children and adults, but children display more variability

Distribution: Adults:

Initial V_d: 0.5 L/kg

V_{dss} 0.77-1.6 L/kg

Protein binding: ~50%

Metabolism: In the liver to the de-ethylated free acid and its glucuronide conjugate

Half-life

Children: Terminal: 20-75 minutes (mean: 40 minutes)

Adults:

Alpha: 7-15 minutes

Terminal: 41-79 minutes

Elimination: Clearance dependent upon hepatic blood flow, hepatically eliminated; <1% excreted unchanged in urine

Usual Dosage I.V.:

Children:

Reversal of benzodiazepine when used in conscious sedation or general anesthesia: Initial dose: 0.01 mg/kg (maximum dose: 0.2 mg) given over 15 seconds; may repeat 0.01 mg/kg (maximum dose: 0.2 mg) after 45 seconds, and then every minute to a maximum total cumulative dose of 0.05 mg/kg or 1 mg, whichever is lower; usual total dose: 0.08-1 mg (mean: 0.65 mg)

Management of benzodiazepine overdose: Minimal information available; initial dose: 0.01 mg/kg (maximum dose: 0.2 mg) with repeat doses of 0.01 mg/kg (maximum dose: 0.2 mg) given every minute to a maximum total cumulative dose of 1 mg; as an alternative to repeat bolus doses, follow up continuous infusions of 0.005-0.01 mg/kg/hour have been used; further studies are needed

Adults:

Reversal of benzodiazepine when used in conscious sedation or general anesthesia: 0.2 mg given over 15 seconds; may repeat 0.2 mg after 45 seconds and then every 60 seconds up to a total of 1 mg, usual total dose: 0.6-1 mg. In event of resedation, may repeat doses at 20-minute intervals with maximum of 1 mg/dose (given at 0.2 mg/minute); maximum dose: 3 mg in 1 hour.

Management of benzodiazepine overdose: 0.2 mg over 30 seconds; may give 0.3 mg dose after 30 seconds if desired level of consciousness is not obtained; additional doses of 0.5 mg can be given over 30 seconds at 1-minute intervals up to a cumulative dose of 3 mg; usual cumulative dose: 1-3 mg; rarely, patients with partial response at 3 mg may require additional titration up to total dose of 5 mg; if patient has not responded 5 minutes after cumulative dose of 5 mg, the major cause of sedation is not likely due to benzodiazepines. In the event of resedation, may repeat doses at 20-minute intervals with maximum of 1 mg/dose (given at 0.5 mg/minute); maximum dose: 3 mg in 1 hour.

Dosing adjustment in hepatic impairment: Initial dose: Use normal dose; repeat doses should be decreased in size or frequency

Administration Parenteral: For I.V. use only; administer by rapid I.V. injection over 15-30 seconds via a freely running I.V. infusion into larger vein (to decrease chance of pain, phlebitis). Children: Do not exceed 0. 2 mg/minute. Adults: Repeat doses: Do not exceed 0.2 mg/minute for reversal of general anesthesia and do not exceed 0.5 mg/minute for reversal of benzodiazepine overdose.

Monitoring Parameters Level of consciousness and resedation, blood pressure, heart rate, respiratory rate, continuous pulse oximetry; monitor for resedation for 1-2 hours after reversal of sedation in patients who receive benzodiazepine sedation

Patient Information Flumazenil does not consistently reverse amnesia; do not engage in activities requiring alertness for 18-24 hours after discharge; resedation may occur in patients on long-acting benzodiazepines (such as diazepam); avoid alcohol or OTC medications for 18-24 hours after flumazenil is used or if benzodiazepine effects persist

Nursing Implications Flumazenil does not effectively reverse hypoventilation, even in alert patients

Additional Information In one study of conscious sedation reversal in 107 pediatric patients (1-17 years of age), resedation occurred between 19-50 minutes after the start of flumazenil. Flumazenil has been used to successfully treat paradoxical reactions in children associated with midazolam use (eg, agitation, restlessness, combativeness) (see Massanari, 1997).

Dosage Forms Injection: 0.1 mg/mL (5 mL, 10 mL)

(Continued)

Flumazenil (Continued)

References

Baktai G, Szekely E, Marialigeti T, et al, "Use of Midazolam (Dormicum) and Flumazenil (Anexate) in Paediatric Bronchology," Curr Med Res Opin, 1992, 12(9):552-9.

Clark RF, Sage TA, Tunget C, et al, "Delayed Onset Lorazepam Poisoning Successfully Reversed By Flumazenil in a Child: Case Report and Review of the Literature," Pediatr Emerg Care, 1995, 11(1):32-4.

Jones RD, Lawson AD, Andrew LJ, et al, "Antagonism of the Hypnotic Effect of Midazolam in Children: A Randomized, Double Blind Study of Placebo and Flumazenil Administered After Midazolam-Induced Anaesthesia," Br J Anaesth, 1991, 66(6):660-6.

Massanari M, Novitsky J, and Reinstein LJ, "Paradoxical Reactions in Children Associated With Midazolam Use During Endoscopy," Clin Pediatr, 1997, 36(12):681-4.

Richard P, Autret E, Bardol J, et al, "The Use of Flumazenil in a Neonate," J Toxicol Clin Toxicol, 1991, 29(1):137-40.

Roald OK and Dahl V, "Flunitrazepam Intoxication in a Child Successfully Treated With the Benzodiazepine Antagonist Flumazenil," Crit Care Med, 1989, 17(12):1355-6.

Shannon M, Albers G, Burkhart K, et al, "Safety and Efficacy of Flumazenil in the Reversal of Benzodiazepine-Induced Conscious Sedation. The Flumazenil Pediatric Study Group," J Pediatr, 1997, 131(4):582-6.

Sugarman JM and Paul RI, "Flumazenil: A Review," Pediatr Emerg Care, 1994, 10(1):37-43.

Flunisolide (floo NIS oh lide)

Related Information

Asthma Guidelines on page 1210
Estimated Comparative Daily Dosages for Inhaled Corticosteroids on page 1216

U.S. Brand Names AeroBid®; AeroBid®-M; Nasalide®; Nasarel®

Canadian Brand Names Alti-Flunisolide; Apo-Flunisolide; Rhinalar

Therapeutic Category Adrenal Corticosteroid; Antiasthmatic; Anti-inflammatory Agent; Corticosteroid, Inhalant (Oral); Corticosteroid, Intranasal; Glucocorticoid

Generic Available No

Use

Oral inhalation: Long-term (chronic) control of persistent bronchial asthma; **NOT** indicated for the relief of acute bronchospasm. Also used to help reduce or discontinue oral corticosteroid therapy for asthma.

Intranasal: Management of seasonal or perennial rhinitis

Pregnancy Risk Factor C

Contraindications Hypersensitivity to flunisolide or any component; primary treatment of status asthmaticus; untreated nasal mucosa infection

Warnings Fatalities have occurred due to adrenal insufficiency in asthmatic patients during and after switching from systemic corticosteroids to aerosol steroids; several months may be required for full recovery of the adrenal glands; during this period, aerosol steroids do **not** provide the systemic corticosteroid needed to treat patients requiring stress doses (ie, patients with major stress such as trauma, surgery, or infections); when used at high doses, hypothalamic-pituitary-adrenal (HPA) suppression may occur; use with inhaled or systemic corticosteroids (even alternate-day dosing) may increase risk of HPA suppression; withdrawal and discontinuation of corticosteroids should be done carefully; immunosuppression may occur

Precautions Avoid using higher than recommended doses; suppression of HPA function, suppression of linear growth, or hypercorticism (Cushing's syndrome) may occur; use with extreme caution in patients with respiratory tuberculosis, untreated systemic infections, or ocular herpes simplex

Adverse Reactions

Cardiovascular: Palpitations (oral inhalation), hypertension (oral inhalation)

Central nervous system: Dizziness, headache, nervousness

Dermatologic: Rash, itching, eczema

Endocrine & metabolic: Adrenal suppression, potential growth suppression

Gastrointestinal: Nausea, vomiting, diarrhea, upset stomach, sore throat, bitter taste, aftertaste

Genitourinary: Menstrual disturbances (oral inhalation)

Local: Nasal burning

Respiratory: Sneezing, nasal congestion, nasal dryness, pharyngitis, epistaxis, Candida infections of the nose or pharynx, atrophic rhinitis, upper respiratory infections

Drug Interactions Expected interactions similar to other corticosteroids

Stability Store intranasal solutions at 59°F to 86°F

Mechanism of Action Controls the rate of protein synthesis, depresses the migration of polymorphonuclear leukocytes and fibroblasts, reverses capillary permeability, and stabilizes lysosomal membranes at the cellular level to prevent or control inflammation

Pharmacodynamics Clinical effects are due to a direct local effect rather than systemic absorption

Onset of action: Intranasal: Within a few days
Maximum effects: Intranasal: 1-2 weeks

Pharmacokinetics
Absorption: Nasal inhalation: ~50%; oral inhalation: ~40%
Metabolism: Rapid in the liver to a less active metabolite, followed by glucuronide and sulfate conjugation
Half-life: 1.8 hours
Elimination: Excreted in urine and feces

Usual Dosage Manufacturer recommendation:
Intranasal:
Children 6-14 years: Initial: 1 spray to each nostril 3 times/day or 2 sprays to each nostril 2 times/day; maximum dose: 4 sprays to each nostril per day; after symptoms are controlled, dose should be reduced to lowest effective amount; maintenance: 1 spray each nostril once daily
Adults: Initial: 2 sprays to each nostril twice daily; may increase in 4-7 days if needed to 2 sprays to each nostril 3 times/day; maximum dose: 8 sprays to each nostril per day; after symptoms are controlled, dose should be reduced to lowest effective amount; maintenance: 1 spray to each nostril once daily
Oral inhalation: Doses should be titrated to the lowest dose once asthma is controlled:
Children: 6-15 years: 2 inhalations twice daily
Adults: 2 inhalations twice daily; maximum dose: 8 inhalations/day
NIH Guidelines (NIH, 1997) [give in divided doses twice daily]
Children:
"Low" dose: 500-750 mcg/day (2-3 puffs/day)
"Medium" dose: 1000-1250 mcg/day (4-5 puffs/day)
"High" dose: >1250 mcg/day (>5 puffs/day)
Adults:
"Low" dose: 500-1000 mcg/day (2-4 puffs/day)
"Medium" dose: 1000-2000 mcg/day (4-8 puffs/day)
"High" dose: >2000 mcg/day (>8 puffs/day)

Administration Do not spray in eyes
Oral inhalant: Use a spacer for children <8 years of age; shake well before use; rinse mouth after inhalation to decrease chance of oral candidiasis
Intranasal: Clear nasal passages by blowing nose prior to use; shake well before use

Monitoring Parameters Check mucus membranes for signs of fungal infection; monitor growth in pediatric patients

Patient Information Notify physician if condition being treated persists or worsens; do not decrease dose or discontinue without physician approval
Oral inhalant: Report sore mouth or mouth lesions to physician

Additional Information Nasalide® and Nasarel® do not contain fluorocarbons. AeroBid® and AeroBid-M® contain fluorocarbon propellants. The efficacy of Nasalide® and Nasarel® are similar; however, more nasal burning and stinging were reported with Nasalide®, and more taste problems (eg, aftertaste) were reported with Nasarel®. These differences are due to the different vehicles of the two products. If bronchospasm with wheezing occurs after use of oral inhalation, a fast-acting bronchodilator may be used.

Dosage Forms Inhalant:
Oral:
AeroBid®: 250 mcg/actuation [100 metered doses] (7 g)
AeroBid-M® (menthol flavor): 250 mcg/actuation [100 metered doses] (7 g)
Nasal (Nasalide®, Nasarel®): 25 mcg/actuation [200 sprays] (25 mL)

References
Expert Panel Report 2, "Guidelines for the Diagnosis and Management of Asthma," *Clinical Practice Guidelines*, National Institutes of Health, National Heart, Lung, and Blood Institute, NIH Publication No. 94-4051, April, 1997.

Fluocinolone (floo oh SIN oh lone)

Related Information
Corticosteroids Comparison, Topical *on page 1068*

U.S. Brand Names Capex®; Derma-Smoothe/FS®; Synalar®; Synemol®

Canadian Brand Names Fluoderm®; Lidemol

Therapeutic Category Adrenal Corticosteroid; Anti-inflammatory Agent; Corticosteroid, Topical; Glucocorticoid

Generic Available Yes

Use Relief of susceptible inflammatory dermatosis
Derma-Smoothe/FS®: Children ≥6 years: Moderate to severe atopic dermatitis (for use ≤4 weeks); Adults: Atopic dermatitis or psoriasis of the scalp
(Continued)

Fluocinolone *(Continued)*

Pregnancy Risk Factor C

Contraindications Fungal infection, hypersensitivity to fluocinolone or any component, TB of skin, herpes (including varicella)

Warnings Infants and small children may be more susceptible to adrenal axis suppression from topical corticosteroid therapy; systemic effects may occur when used on large areas of the body, denuded areas, for prolonged periods of time, or with an occlusive dressing; Derma-Smoothe/FS® contains peanut oil, use with caution in patients with peanut hypersensitivity

Adverse Reactions

Dermatologic: Acne, hypopigmentation, allergic dermatitis, maceration of the skin, skin atrophy, folliculitis, hypertrichosis

Endocrine & metabolic: Hypothalamic-pituitary-adrenal suppression, Cushing's syndrome, growth retardation

Local: Burning, itching, irritation, dryness

Miscellaneous: Secondary infection

Mechanism of Action Not well defined topically; possesses anti-inflammatory, antiproliferative, and immunosuppressive properties

Usual Dosage

Children and Adults: Topical: Apply thin layer 2-4 times/day

Derma-Smoothe/FS®:

Children ≥6 years: Atopic dermatitis: Apply in a thin layer to moistened skin of affected area twice daily for ≤4 weeks

Adults:

Atopic dermatitis: Apply a thin layer to affected area 3 times/day

Scalp psoriasis: Thoroughly wet or dampen hair and scalp; apply to scalp in a thin layer, massage well, cover scalp with shower cap (supplied); leave for a minimum of 4 hours or overnight, then wash hair and rinse thoroughly

Administration Topical: Apply sparingly in a thin film; rub in lightly; Derma-Smoothe/FS®: Do not apply to face or diaper area; avoid application to intertriginous areas (may increase local adverse effects)

Patient Information Avoid contact with eyes; do not use for longer than directed; do not overuse; notify physician if condition being treated persists or worsens

Nursing Implications Do not use tight fitting diapers or plastic pants on a child being treated in diaper area; Derma-Smoothe/FS® is not recommended for diaper dermatitis

Additional Information Considered a moderate-potency steroid; the high potency cream (0.2%) is not recommended for use in children <2 years of age; Derma-Smoothe/FS® is made with 48% peanut oil, NF

Dosage Forms

Cream, as acetonide:

Synalar®: 0.01% (15 g, 60 g)

Synalar®, Synemol®: 0.025% (15 g, 60 g, 425 g)

Ointment, topical, as acetonide (Synalar®): 0.025% (15 g, 30 g, 60 g)

Oil, as acetonide (Derma-Smoothe/FS®): 0.01% (120 mL) [contains peanut oil]

Atopic pak: 0.01% with moisturizer (360 mL) [contains peanut oil]

Shampoo, as acetonide (Capex®): 0.01% (180 mL)

Solution, topical, as acetonide (Synalar®): 0.01% (20 mL, 60 mL)

Fluocinonide (floo oh SIN oh nide)

Related Information

Corticosteroids Comparison, Topical *on page 1068*

U.S. Brand Names Lidex®; Lidex-E®

Canadian Brand Names Lidemol; Lyderm; Lydonide; Tiamol; Topactin; Topsyn

Therapeutic Category Adrenal Corticosteroid; Anti-inflammatory Agent; Corticosteroid, Topical; Glucocorticoid

Generic Available Yes

Use Inflammation of corticosteroid-responsive dermatoses

Pregnancy Risk Factor C

Contraindications Hypersensitivity to fluocinonide or any component; viral, fungal, or tubercular skin lesions; herpes (including varicella)

Warnings Infants and small children may be more susceptible to adrenal axis suppression from topical corticosteroid therapy; systemic effects may occur when used on large areas of the body, denuded areas, for prolonged periods of time, or with occlusive dressings

Adverse Reactions
    Dermatologic: Acne, hypopigmentation, allergic dermatitis, maceration of the skin, skin atrophy, folliculitis, hypertrichosis
    Endocrine & metabolic: Hypothalamic-pituitary-adrenal suppression, Cushing's syndrome, growth retardation
    Local: Burning, itching, irritation, dryness
    Miscellaneous: Secondary infection

Mechanism of Action Not well defined topically; possesses anti-inflammatory, antiproliferative, and immunosuppressive properties

Usual Dosage Children and Adults: Topical: Apply thin layer to affected area 2-4 times/day depending on the severity of the condition

Administration Topical: Apply sparingly in a thin film; rub in lightly

Patient Information Do not overuse; avoid contact with eyes; do not use for longer than directed; avoid use on face; notify physician if condition being treated persists or worsens

Nursing Implications Do not use tight fitting diapers or plastic pants on a child being treated in the diaper area

Additional Information Considered to be a high potency steroid

Dosage Forms
    Cream:
        Anhydrous, emollient (Lidex®): 0.05% (15 g, 30 g, 60 g, 120 g)
        Aqueous, emollient (Lidex-E®): 0.05% (15 g, 30 g, 60 g, 120 g)
    Gel, topical (Lidex®): 0.05% (15 g, 30 g, 60 g)
    Ointment, topical (Lidex®): 0.05% (15 g, 30 g, 60 g, 120 g)
    Solution, topical (Lidex®): 0.05% (20 mL, 60 mL)

♦ **Fluoderm (Can)** *see Fluocinolone on page 439*
♦ **Fluohydrisone** *see Fludrocortisone on page 435*
♦ **Fluohydrocortisone** *see Fludrocortisone on page 435*
♦ **FluorCare® Neutral** *see Fluoride on page 441*

Fluoride (FLOR ide)

U.S. Brand Names ACT® [OTC]; FluorCare® Neutral; Fluorigard® [OTC]; Fluorinse®; Fluoritab®; FluoroFoam™; Flura-Drops®; Flura-Loz®; Flura®-Tab; Gel-Kam®; Luride®; Luride® Lozi-Tab®; Pediaflor®; Pharmaflur®; Phos-Flur®; Phos-Flur® Rinse [OTC]; PreviDent®; PreviDent® 5000 Plus™; Thera-Flur®; Thera-Flur-N®

Therapeutic Category Mineral, Oral; Mineral, Oral Topical

Generic Available Yes

Use Prevention of dental caries

Pregnancy Risk Factor C

Contraindications Hypersensitivity to fluoride, tartrazine, or any component; when fluoride content of drinking water exceeds 0.7 ppm; low sodium or sodium-free diets; do not use 1 mg tablets in children <3 years of age or when drinking water fluoride content is ≥0.3 ppm; do not use 1 mg/5 mL rinse (as supplement) in children <6 years of age

Precautions Prolonged ingestion with excessive doses may result in dental fluorosis and osseous changes; dosage should be adjusted in proportion to the amount of fluoride in the drinking water; do **not** exceed recommended dosage

Adverse Reactions
    Central nervous system: Headache
    Dermatologic: Rash, eczema, atopic dermatitis, urticaria
    Gastrointestinal: GI upset, nausea, vomiting
    Miscellaneous: Products containing stannous fluoride may stain the teeth

Drug Interactions Magnesium-, aluminum-, and calcium-containing products may decrease absorption of fluoride

Food Interactions Do not administer with milk

Stability Sodium fluoride solutions decompose in glass containers; store only in tightly closed plastic containers; aqueous solutions of stannous fluoride decompose within hours of preparation; prepare solutions immediately before use

Mechanism of Action Promotes remineralization of decalcified enamel; inhibits the cariogenic microbial process in dental plaque; increases tooth resistance to acid dissolution

Pharmacokinetics
    Absorption: Via GI tract, lungs, and skin
    Distribution: 50% of fluoride is deposited in teeth and bone after ingestion; crosses placenta; appears in breast milk; topical application works superficially on enamel and plaque
    Elimination: In urine and feces

(Continued)

Fluoride *(Continued)*

Usual Dosage Oral:

Adequate Intake (AI) (1997 National Academy of Science Recommendations):

Children:

0-6 months: 0.01 mg/day

7-12 months: 0.5 mg/day

1-3 years: 0.7 mg/day

4-8 years: 1 mg/day

9-13 years: 2 mg/day

14-18 years: 3 mg/day

Children >19 and Adults:

Males: 4 mg/day

Females: 3 mg/day

The recommended daily fluoride intake is adjusted in proportion to the fluoride content of available drinking water; see **Recommended Daily Fluoride Dose** table

Recommended Daily Fluoride Dose

Fluoride Content of Drinking Water	Daily Dose, Oral Fluoride (mg)
<0.3 ppm	
Birth - 6 mo	0
6 mo to 3 y	0.25
3-6 y	0.5
6-16 y	1
0.3-0.6 ppm	
Birth - 3 y	0
3-6 y	0.25
6-16 y	0.5
>0.6 ppm	
All ages	0

Adapted from *AAP News*, 1995, 11(2):18.

Dental rinse: See **Sodium Fluoride Dental Rinse Dosing** table

Sodium fluoride (dosage based upon concentration of solution):

Note: 2% concentrations are administered by dental personnel only

Sodium Fluoride Dental Rinse Dosing

Age	% Solution	Dosage
6 y	0.05%	10 mL daily
6-12 y	0.02%	10 mL twice daily
	0.2%	5 mL once weekly
>12 y	0.02%	10 mL twice daily
	0.2%	10 mL once weekly

Acidulated phosphate fluoride rinse: Children 6 years and Adults: 5-10 mL of 0.02% daily at bedtime

Gel:

Acidulated phosphate fluoride: Adults: 4-8 drops of 0.5% gel daily or for desensitizing exposed root surfaces, use a few drops of 0.5% to 1.2% gel applied and brushed onto affected area each night

Stannous fluoride: Children >6 years and Adults: Apply 0.4% gel to teeth once daily

Administration Oral:

Dental gel: Do **not** swallow; gel drops are placed in trough of applicator; applicator is applied over upper and lower teeth at same time; bite down for 6 minutes

Dental rinse: Swish or rinse in mouth then expectorate; do not swallow

Tablet: Dissolve in mouth, chew, swallow whole, or add to drinking water or fruit juice; administer with food (but not milk) to eliminate GI upset

Reference Range Total plasma fluoride: 0.14-0.19 µg/mL

Dosage Forms Fluoride ion content listed in brackets

Cream, topical, as sodium fluoride (PreviDent® 5000 Plus™): 1.1% [2.5 mg/dose] (51 g)

Foam, topical, as acidulated phosphate fluoride (FluoroFoam™): 1.2%

Gel-drops, neutral (Thera-Flur®-N): 0.5% [3 mg/0.6 mL] (24 mL)

Gel, topical:
  Acidulated phosphate fluoride: Phos-Flur® Gel: 1.1% [0.5%] (54 g)
  Sodium fluoride (FluoroCare® Neutral): 2%
  Sodium fluoride (PreviDent®): 1.1% [0.5%] (60 g, 250 g)
  Stannous fluoride (Gel Kam®): 0.4% [0.1%] (120 g)

Rinse, topical, as sodium:
  ACT®, Fluorigard®: 0.05% [0.02%] (480 mL)
  Fluorinse® (alcohol free), PreviDent® Rinse: 0.2% [0.09%] (240 mL, 480 mL)
  As stannous fluoride concentrate (Gel-Kam®): 0.63% (75 mL)

Solution, oral, as sodium:
  Phos-Flur®: 0.044% [0.02% mg/mL] (500 mL)
  Flura-Drops®: 0.55 mg/drop [0.25 mg/drop] (24 mL)
  Luride®, Pediaflor®: 1.1 mg/mL [0.5 mg/mL] (50 mL) (sugar free)
  Fluoritab® Liquid: 11 mg/mL [5 mg/mL]

Tablet, as sodium:
  Chewable:
    Fluoritab®, Luride® 0.25 mg F Lozi-Tabs® Quarter-Strength: 0.55 mg (sugar free) [0.25 mg]
    Fluoritab® (sugar free), Luride® 0.5 mg F Lozi-Tab® Half-Strength (sugar free), Pharmaflur®: 1.1 mg [0.5 mg]
    Flura-Loz® (sugar free), Luride® 1 mg F Lozi-Tab® Full-Strength (sugar free), Pharmaflur®: 2.2 mg [1 mg]
    Fluoritab® (sugar free), Flura® Tab® (sugar free): 2.2 mg [1 mg]

References
"Dietary Reference Intakes for Calcium, Phosphorus, Magnesium, Vitamin D, and Fluoride. Standing Committee on the Scientific Evaluation of Dietary Reference Intakes, Food and Nutrition Board, Institute of Medicine," National Academy of Sciences, Washington, DC: National Academy Press, 1997.

♦ **Fluorigard® [OTC]** *see* Fluoride *on page 441*

♦ **Fluorinse®** *see* Fluoride *on page 441*

♦ **Fluoritab®** *see* Fluoride *on page 441*

♦ **FluoroFoam™** *see* Fluoride *on page 441*

♦ **9α-Fluorohydrocortisone** *see* Fludrocortisone *on page 435*

Fluorometholone (flure oh METH oh lone)

U.S. Brand Names Eflone™; Flarex®; Fluor-Op®; FML®; FML® Forte; FML® S.O.P

Therapeutic Category Adrenal Corticosteroid; Anti-inflammatory Agent, Ophthalmic; Corticosteroid, Ophthalmic; Glucocorticoid

Generic Available No

Use Inflammatory conditions of the eye, including keratitis, iritis, cyclitis, and conjunctivitis

Pregnancy Risk Factor C

Contraindications Herpes simplex, fungal diseases, most viral diseases

Warnings Not recommended for children <2 years of age; some products contain sulfites

Precautions Prolonged use may result in glaucoma, increased intraocular pressure, or other ocular damage

Adverse Reactions
Local: Stinging, burning
Ocular: Increased intraocular pressure, open-angle glaucoma, defect in visual acuity and field of vision, cataracts, photosensitivity

Mechanism of Action Decreases inflammation by suppression of migration of polymorphonuclear leukocytes and reversal of increased capillary permeability

Pharmacokinetics Absorption: Into aqueous humor with slight systemic absorption

Usual Dosage Children >2 years and Adults: Ophthalmic:
Ointment: May be applied every 4 hours in severe cases or 1-3 times/day in mild to moderate cases.
Drops: Instill 1-2 drops into conjunctival sac every hour during day, every 2 hours at night until favorable response is obtained, then use 1 drop every 4 hours; in mild or moderate inflammation: 1-2 drops into conjunctival sac 2-4 times/day.

Administration Ophthalmic: Avoid contact of medication tube or bottle tip with skin or eye; shake suspension well before use; suspension: Apply finger pressure to lacrimal sac during and for 1-2 minutes after instillation to decrease risk of absorption and systemic effects
(Continued)

Fluorometholone *(Continued)*

Patient Information May cause blurring of vision and photosensitivity; do not discontinue without consulting physician; notify physician if improvement does not occur after 7-8 days

Dosage Forms Ophthalmic:
Ointment (FML® S.O.P.): 0.1% (3.5 g)
Suspension:
Fluor-Op®, FML®: 0.1% (5 mL, 10 mL, 15 mL)
FML® Forte: 0.25% (2 mL, 5 mL, 10 mL, 15 mL)
Suspension, as acetate (Eflone™, Flarex®): 0.1% (5 mL, 10 mL)

♦ **Fluor-Op®** *see Fluorometholone on page 443*

♦ **Fluoroplex®** *see Fluorouracil on page 444*

Fluorouracil *(flure oh YOOR a sil)*

Related Information
Emetogenic Potential of Single Chemotherapeutic Agents *on page 1129*

U.S. Brand Names Adrucil®; Efudex®; Fluoroplex®

Synonyms 5-Fluorouracil; 5-FU

Therapeutic Category Antineoplastic Agent, Antimetabolite

Generic Available Yes: Injection

Use Treatment of carcinoma of stomach, colon, rectum, breast, and pancreas; topically for management of multiple actinic keratoses and superficial basal cell carcinomas

Pregnancy Risk Factor D

Contraindications Hypersensitivity to fluorouracil or any component; patients with poor nutritional status, bone marrow suppression, thrombocytopenia; pregnancy

Warnings The FDA currently recommends that procedures for proper handling and disposal of antineoplastic agents be considered; if intractable vomiting, diarrhea, or hemorrhage occurs, discontinue fluorouracil immediately

Precautions Use with caution and modify dosage in patients with renal or hepatic impairment

Adverse Reactions
Cardiovascular: Cardiac arrhythmias, heart failure, hypotension
Central nervous system: Headache, cerebellar ataxia (gait and speech abnormalities), somnolence, dizziness
Dermatologic: Alopecia, skin pigmentation, pruritic maculopapular rash, partial loss of nails or hyperpigmentation of nail bed, photosensitivity
Gastrointestinal: Nausea, vomiting, diarrhea, anorexia, GI hemorrhage, stomatitis, esophagitis
Hematologic: Myelosuppression, granulocytopenia, thrombocytopenia
Hepatic: Hepatotoxicity
Ocular: Visual disturbances, nystagmus, conjunctivitis
Miscellaneous: Palmar-plantar erythrodysesthesias (erythematous, desquamative rash involving hands and feet accompanied by pain, tingling, and swollen palms; this adverse effect may be treated with oral pyridoxine)

Drug Interactions Cimetidine (increases 5-FU concentration); leucovorin may potentiate the antitumor activity of 5-FU

Food Interactions Use of acidic solutions such as orange juice or other fruit juices to dilute 5-FU for oral administration may result in precipitation of the drug and decreased absorption; increase dietary intake of thiamine

Stability Store at room temperature; protect from light; slight discoloration of injection during storage does not affect potency; if precipitate forms, redissolve drug by heating to 140°F, shake well; allow to cool to body temperature before administration; incompatible with cytarabine, diazepam, doxorubicin, methotrexate

Mechanism of Action A pyrimidine antimetabolite that inhibits thymidylate synthase leading to depletion of the DNA precursor thymidine; incorporated into RNA, DNA

Pharmacokinetics
Absorption: Oral: Erratic
Distribution: Into tumors, intestinal mucosa, liver, bone marrow, and CSF
Protein binding: <10%
Metabolism: Inactive metabolites are formed following metabolism in the liver
Bioavailability: 50% to 80%; variable due to saturable first-pass elimination process
Half-life, biphasic:
Alpha: 10-20 minutes
Terminal: 15-19 hours
Elimination: Biphasic elimination with <10% of dose excreted unchanged in the urine

Usual Dosage Children and Adults (refer to individual protocols with dose based on lean body weight):

I.V.:

  Initial: 400-500 mg/m^2/day (12 mg/kg/day; maximum dose: 800 mg/day) for 4-5 days

  Maintenance: 200-250 mg/m^2/dose (6 mg/kg) every other day for 4 doses; repeat in 4 weeks

  Single weekly bolus dose of 15 mg/kg or 500 mg/m^2 can be administered depending on the patient's reaction to the previous course of treatment; maintenance dose of 5-15 mg/kg/week as a single dose not to exceed 1 g/week

I.V. infusion: 15 mg/kg/day or 500 mg/m^2/day (maximum daily dose: 1 g) has been given by I.V. infusion over 4 hours for 5 days; **or** 800-1200 mg/m^2 for continuous infusion over 24-120 hours

Oral: 15-20 mg/kg/day for 5-8 days has been used for colorectal carcinoma; 15 mg/kg/week for hepatoma

Dosing adjustment in hepatic impairment: Bilirubin >5 mg/dL: Not recommended for use

Topical: Cream or solution: Apply twice daily

Administration

Oral: Administer in early morning on an empty stomach; do not eat for 2 hours before and after dosage administration; dilute injectable fluorouracil solution dose in 4 oz of water or a diluted bicarbonate buffer solution to increase absorption; do not mix with orange juice or other fruit juices

Parenteral: Administer by direct I.V. injection (50 mg/mL solution needs no further dilution) over several minutes or by I.V. intermittent or continuous infusion diluted in saline or dextrose solutions; toxicity (eg, myelosuppression) may be reduced by giving the drug as a continuous infusion. Doses >750-800 mg/m^2 should be administered as a continuous infusion, **not** by bolus injection; dose-limiting toxicity with continuous infusion is mucous membrane toxicity (ie, stomatitis, diarrhea)

Topical: Apply with a nonmetallic applicator or gloved fingers in a sufficient amount to cover affected area

  1% or 2%: Apply to lesions on the head and neck for the treatment of multiple actinic keratoses

  5%: Use on lesions in areas other than the head and neck for multiple actinic keratoses; only 5% preparations are used for the treatment of superficial basal cell carcinoma

Monitoring Parameters CBC with differential and platelet count, renal function tests, liver function tests

Patient Information Avoid unnecessary exposure to sunlight; maintain adequate hydration; report signs and symptoms of infection, bleeding, bruising, vision changes; unremitting nausea, vomiting, or diarrhea; chest pain or palpitations; or CNS changes

Nursing Implications Wash hands immediately after topical application of the cream or solution

Additional Information Myelosuppressive effects:

WBC: Mild

Platelets: Mild

Onset (days): 7-10

Nadir (days): 9-14

Recovery (days): 21

Dosage Forms

Cream, topical:

  Efudex®: 5% (25 g)

  Fluoroplex®: 1% (30 g)

Injection (Adrucil®): 50 mg/mL (10 mL, 20 mL, 50 mL, 100 mL)

Solution, topical:

  Efudex®: 2% (10 mL); 5% (10 mL)

  Fluoroplex®: 1% (30 mL)

References

Balis FM, Holcenberg JS and Bleyer WA, "Clinical Pharmacokinetics of Commonly Used Anticancer Drugs," *Clin Pharmacokinet*, 1983, 8(3):202-32.

♦ **5-Fluorouracil** *see* Fluorouracil *on page 444*

Fluoxetine (floo OKS e teen)

Related Information

Carbohydrate and Alcohol Content of Liquid Medications for Use in Patients Receiving Ketogenic Diets *on page 1258*

Comparison of Adverse Effects of Antidepressants *on page 1066*

(Continued)

Fluoxetine *(Continued)*

Comparison of Usual Adult Dosage and Mechanism of Action of Antidepressants *on page 1065*

Drugs and Breast-Feeding *on page 1243*

Serotonin Syndrome *on page 1247*

U.S. Brand Names Prozac®; Prozac® Weekly™; Sarafem™

Canadian Brand Names Alti-Fluoxetine; Apo-Fluoxetine; Gen-Fluoxetine; Novo-Fluoxetine; Nu-Fluoxetine; PMS-Fluoxetine

Therapeutic Category Antidepressant, Selective Serotonin Reuptake Inhibitor (SSRI)

Generic Available No

Use Treatment of depression, obsessive-compulsive disorder, bulimia nervosa, premenstrual dysphoric disorder (PMDD)

Pregnancy Risk Factor C

Contraindications Hypersensitivity to fluoxetine or any component; use of MAO inhibitors within 14 days (potentially fatal reactions may occur, see Drug Interactions); concurrent use of thioridazine or use within 5 weeks after fluoxetine is discontinued (see Drug Interactions)

Warnings Rash or urticaria may occur along with leukocytosis, fever, edema, arthralgia, lymphadenopathy, respiratory distress, and other symptoms; rare cases of vasculitis and lupus-like syndrome have been reported; anaphylactoid reactions including laryngospasm, bronchospasm, angioedema, and urticaria may occur; discontinue use if rash or other allergic reaction occurs

Precautions Due to limited experience, use with caution in patients with renal or hepatic impairment, seizure disorders, cardiac dysfunction, diabetes mellitus; decrease dose in liver dysfunction; use with caution in patients at high risk for suicide; add or initiate other antidepressants with caution for up to 5 weeks after stopping fluoxetine

Adverse Reactions Predominant adverse effects are CNS and GI:

Central nervous system: Headache, nervousness, insomnia, drowsiness, anxiety, dizziness, fatigue, sedation, mania, irritability, suicidal ideation, extrapyramidal reactions (rare); difficulty concentrating

Dermatologic: Rash, urticaria (7%), pruritus

Endocrine & metabolic: Hypoglycemia, hyponatremia (elderly or volume-depleted patients), sexual dysfunction, decreased libido

Gastrointestinal: Nausea, diarrhea, xerostomia, anorexia, dyspepsia, constipation, weight loss

Hematologic: Altered platelet function (rare)

Neuromuscular & skeletal: Tremor

Ocular: Visual disturbances

Miscellaneous: Anaphylactoid reactions, allergies, diaphoresis

Drug Interactions Cytochrome P-450 isoenzyme CYP2D6 substrate (minor pathway), CYP3A3/4 substrate; CYP2C9 isoenzyme inducer; CYP1A2 (at higher doses), CYP2C9, CYP2C19, CYP2D6, CYP3A3/4 isoenzyme inhibitor (extent of CYP3A4 inhibition may not be clinically significant; however, the metabolite norfluoxetine is a more potent CYP3A inhibitor)

With MAO inhibitors, fever, tremors, seizures, delirium, coma may occur (use of MAO inhibitors within 14 days of fluoxetine use is contraindicated); tryptophan (which can be metabolized to serotonin) may increase CNS and GI toxic effects and the herbal medicine St John's wort (*Hypericum perforatum*) may increase serious side effects (the use of these agents is **not** recommended). Fluoxetine may inhibit metabolism and increase effects of tricyclic antidepressants, trazodone, phenytoin, carbamazepine, haloperidol, clozapine, alprazolam, and diazepam; fluoxetine may inhibit the metabolism of thioridazine and increase the risk of serious adverse effects, such as QT_c prolongation, serious ventricular arrhythmias (eg, torsade de pointes) and sudden death (concurrent use of thioridazine or use within 5 weeks of discontinuation of fluoxetine is contraindicated); may antagonize buspirone effects; may displace highly protein bound drugs and cause adverse effects; may increase prothrombin time in patients receiving warfarin; use with sumatriptan may cause weakness, incoordination, and hyper-reflexia; may increase or decrease serum lithium levels (monitor levels closely)

Food Interactions Tryptophan supplements may increase CNS and GI adverse effects (eg, restlessness, agitation, GI problems); food does not affect bioavailability, but may delay absorption by 1-2 hours

Stability Store at room temperature; protect tablets, immediate release capsules, and solution from light

Mechanism of Action Inhibits CNS neuron serotonin uptake; minimal or no effect on reuptake of norepinephrine or dopamine; does not significantly bind to alpha-adrenergic, histamine or cholinergic receptors; may therefore be useful in patients at risk from sedation, hypotension and anticholinergic effects of tricyclic antidepressants

Pharmacodynamics Peak effect: Maximum antidepressant effects usually occur after more than 4 weeks; due to long half-life, resolution of adverse reactions after discontinuation may be slow

Pharmacokinetics

Absorption: Oral: Well absorbed; enteric-coated pellets contained in Prozac® Weekly™ resist dissolution until GI pH >5.5 and therefore delay onset of absorption 1-2 hours compared to immediate release formulations

Distribution: Adults: V_d: 20-45 L/kg; widely distributed

Protein binding: ~95% (albumin and alpha$_1$-glycoprotein)

Metabolism: In the liver to norfluoxetine (active) and other metabolites

Bioavailability: Capsules, tablets, solution, and weekly capsules are bioequivalent

Half-life: Adults:

Fluoxetine: Acute dosing: 1-3 days; chronic dosing: 4-6 days

Norfluoxetine: Acute and chronic dosing: 4-16 days

Time to peak serum concentration: Immediate release formulation: After 6-8 hours

Elimination: In urine as fluoxetine (2.5% to 5%) and norfluoxetine (10%)

Usual Dosage Oral:

Children <5 years: No dosing information available

Children 5-18 years: Dose and safety not established; initial doses of 5-10 mg/day (or even 10 mg given 3 times a week) may result in less adverse effects; dose is titrated upwards as needed; usual dose: 20 mg/day; **Note:** A double-blind, placebo-controlled, randomized trial of fluoxetine in 96 children and adolescents with depression (mean age: ~12 years; range: 7-17 years) used a fixed dose of 20 mg/day administered in the morning (Emslie, 1994); a study in children 8-15 years of age with obsessive compulsive disorder (n=14) used a fixed dose of 20 mg/day (Riddle, 1992); a study of children 10-18 years of age with obsessive compulsive symptoms and Tourette's syndrome (n=5) used 20-40 mg/day dose (Kurlan, 1993); 6 children 6-12 years of age with elective mutism were treated with initial doses of 0.2 mg/kg/day for 1 week, then 0.4 mg/kg/day for 1 week, then 0.6 mg/kg/day for 10 weeks (Black,1994); further studies are needed

Adults:

Depression or obsessive-compulsive disorder: Initial dose: 20 mg/day administered in the morning; may increase after several weeks by 20 mg/day increments; maximum dose: 80 mg/day; doses >20 mg/day can be given either once daily (in the morning) or divided into morning or noon doses

Depression: Weekly dosing: Patients maintained on 20 mg/day may be changed to Prozac® Weekly™ 90 mg/week, starting 7 days after the last 20 mg/day dose

Bulimia nervosa: 60 mg/day administered in the morning; may need to titrate up to this dose over several days in some patients; higher doses have not been well studied

Premenstrual dysphoric disorder: 20 mg/day; doses >60 mg/day have not been studied; maximum dose: 80 mg/day

Dosage adjustment in renal impairment: Adjustment not routinely needed

Dosage adjustment in hepatic impairment: Lower doses or less frequent administration are recommended

Administration Oral: May be administered without regard to food

Monitoring Parameters Liver function, weight; monitor for rash and signs or symptoms of anaphylactoid reactions

Reference Range

Therapeutic: Fluoxetine 100-800 ng/mL (SI: 289-2314 nmol/L); norfluoxetine 100-600 ng/mL (SI: 289-1735 nmol/L)

Toxic: (Fluoxetine plus norfluoxetine): >2000 ng/mL (SI: >5784 nmol/L)

Patient Information Avoid alcohol, tryptophan supplements, and the herbal medicine St John's wort; may cause dizziness or drowsiness and impair ability to perform activities requiring mental alertness or physical coordination; may cause dry mouth

Nursing Implications Last dose of the day should be given before 4 PM (to avoid insomnia)

Additional Information Oral solution contains benzoic acid; a recent report describes 5 children (age: 8-15 years) who developed epistaxis (n=4) or bruising (n=1) while receiving SSRI therapy (sertraline) (Lake, 2000)

Dosage Forms Available as fluoxetine hydrochloride; mg strength refers to fluoxetine

(Continued)

Fluoxetine *(Continued)*

Capsule:
Prozac®: 10 mg, 20 mg, 40 mg
Sarafem™: 10 mg, 20 mg
Capsule, delayed release (Prozac® Weekly™): 90 mg
Solution, oral (Prozac®): 20 mg/5 mL [mint flavor; contains 0.23% alcohol] (120 mL)
Tablet (Prozac®): 10 mg

Extemporaneous Preparations Dilutions of the commercially available oral solution may be made; 1 mg/mL and 2 mg/mL dilutions in Simple Syrup USP, Simple Syrup - British Pharmacopoeia, Aromatic Elixir USP, grape-cranberry drink (Ocean Spray® Cran-Grape), and deionized water were stable for 8 weeks when stored in amber glass bottles at 5°C and 30°C (Peterson, 1994).

Peterson JA, Risley DS, Anderson PN, et al, "Stability of Fluoxetine Hydrochloride in Fluoxetine Solution Diluted With Common Pharmaceutical Diluents," *Am J Hosp Pharm*, 1994, 51(10):1342-5.

References

Black B and Uhde TW, "Treatment of Elective Mutism With Fluoxetine: A Double Blind, Placebo-Controlled Study," *J Am Acad Child Adolesc Psychiatry*, 1994, 33(7):1000-6.

Como PG and Kurlan R, "An Open-Label Trial of Fluoxetine for Obsessive-Compulsive Disorder in Gilles de la Tourette's Syndrome," *Neurology*, 1991, 41(6):872-4.

Emslie GJ, Rush AJ, Weinberg WA, et al, "A Double-Blind, Randomized, Placebo-Controlled Trial of Fluoxetine in Children and Adolescents With Depression," *Arch Gen Psychiatry*, 1997, 54(11):1031-7.

Findling RL, Reed MD, and Blumer JL, "Pharmacological Treatment of Depression in Children and Adolescents," *Paediatr Drugs*, 1999, 1(3):161-82.

Kurlan R, Como PG, Deeley C, et al, "A Pilot Controlled Study of Fluoxetine for Obsessive-Compulsive Symptoms in Children With Tourette's Syndrome," *Clin Neuropharmacol*, 1993, 16(2):167-72.

Lake MB, Birmaher B, Wassick S, et al, "Bleeding and Selective Serotonin Reuptake Inhibitors in Childhood and Adolescence," *J Child Adolesc Psychopharmacol*, 2000, 10(1):35-8.

Riddle MA, Hardin MT, King R, et al, "Fluoxetine Treatment of Children and Adolescents With Tourette's and Obsessive-Compulsive Disorders: Preliminary Clinical Experience," *J Am Acad Child Adolesc Psychiatry*, 1990, 29(1):45-8.

Riddle MA, Scahill L, King RA, et al, "Double-Blind, Crossover Trial of Fluoxetine and Placebo in Children and Adolescents With Obsessive-Compulsive Disorder," *J Am Acad Child Adolesc Psychiatry*, 1992, 31(6):1062-9.

Thomsen PH, "Obsessive-Complusive Disorder: Pharmacological Treatment," *Eur Child Adolesc Psychiatry*, 2000, 9 Suppl 1:I76-84.

Fluoxymesterone *(floo oks i MES te rone)*

U.S. Brand Names Halotestin®
Therapeutic Category Androgen
Generic Available Yes
Use Replacement of endogenous testicular hormone; in females used as palliative treatment of breast cancer, postpartum breast engorgement
Restrictions C-III
Pregnancy Risk Factor X
Contraindications Serious cardiac disease, liver or kidney disease; hypersensitivity to fluoxymesterone or any component
Precautions May accelerate bone maturation without producing compensatory gain in linear growth; in prepubertal children perform radiographic examination of the hand and wrist every 6 months to determine the rate of bone maturation and to assess the effect of treatment on the epiphyseal centers

Adverse Reactions

Cardiovascular: Edema
Central nervous system: Anxiety, mental depression, headache
Dermatologic: Acne, hirsutism
Endocrine & metabolic: Gynecomastia, amenorrhea, hypercalcemia, female virilization
Gastrointestinal: Nausea
Genitourinary: Priapism
Hematologic: Polycythemia, suppression of clotting factors II, VII, IX, X
Hepatic: Cholestatic hepatitis
Neuromuscular & skeletal: Paresthesia
Miscellaneous: Hypersensitivity reactions

Drug Interactions May potentiate the action of oral anticoagulants; may decrease blood glucose concentrations and insulin requirements in patients with diabetes; may elevate cyclosporin levels; may increase extrapyramidal side effects and other CNS effects when coadministered with lithium; may potentiate respiratory depressant effects of narcotics

Mechanism of Action Synthetic androgenic anabolic steroid hormone responsible for the normal growth and development of male sex organs and maintenance of secondary sex characteristics; synthetic testosterone derivative with significant androgen activity; stimulates RNA polymerase activity resulting in an increase in protein production; increases bone development

Pharmacokinetics
Absorption: Oral: Rapid
Protein binding: 98%
Metabolism: In the liver
Half-life: 10-100 minutes
Elimination: Enterohepatic circulation and urinary excretion (90%)
Halogenated derivative of testosterone with up to 5 times the activity of methyltestosterone

Usual Dosage Adults: Oral:
Male:
Hypogonadism: 5-20 mg/day
Delayed puberty: 2.5-20 mg/day for 4-6 months
Female:
Inoperable breast carcinoma: 10-40 mg/day in divided doses for 1-3 months
Breast engorgement: 2.5 mg after delivery, 5-10 mg/day in divided doses for 4-5 days

Monitoring Parameters Periodic radiographic exams of hand and wrist (when used in children); hemoglobin, hematocrit (if receiving high dosages or long-term therapy)

Dosage Forms Tablet: 2 mg, 5 mg, 10 mg

- ♦ **Flura-Drops**® *see* Fluoride *on page 441*
- ♦ **Flura-Loz**® *see* Fluoride *on page 441*
- ♦ **Flura**®**-Tab** *see* Fluoride *on page 441*

Flurazepam (flure AZ e pam)

Related Information
Overdose and Toxicology *on page 1222*

U.S. Brand Names Dalmane®

Canadian Brand Names Apo-Flurazepam; Novo-Flupam; PMS-Flurazepam; Somnol; Som Pam

Therapeutic Category Benzodiazepine; Hypnotic; Sedative

Generic Available Yes

Use Short-term treatment of insomnia

Restrictions C-IV

Pregnancy Risk Factor X

Contraindications Hypersensitivity to flurazepam or any component (there may be cross-sensitivity with other benzodiazepines), pregnancy, pre-existing CNS depression, respiratory depression, narrow-angle glaucoma

Precautions Use with caution in patients receiving other CNS depressants, patients with low albumin, hepatic dysfunction and in the elderly

Adverse Reactions
Central nervous system: Drowsiness, dizziness, confusion; residual daytime sedation; paradoxical reactions, hyperactivity, and excitement (rare), ataxia
Miscellaneous: Physical and psychological dependence with prolonged use

Drug Interactions Cytochrome P-450 isoenzyme CYP3A3/4 substrate
Additive CNS depression with other CNS depressants, alcohol; cimetidine may decrease and enzyme inducers may increase metabolism of flurazepam; concurrent use of flurazepam with ritonavir is not recommended

Mechanism of Action Depresses all levels of the CNS, including the limbic and reticular formation, by binding to the benzodiazepine site on the gamma-aminobutyric acid (GABA) receptor complex and modulating GABA, which is a major inhibitory neurotransmitter in the brain

Pharmacodynamics Hypnotic effects:
Onset of action: 15-20 minutes
Peak: 3-6 hours
Duration: 7-8 hours

Pharmacokinetics
Metabolism: In the liver to N-desalkylflurazepam (active)
Half-life, metabolite (adults): 40-114 hours

Usual Dosage Oral:
Children:
<15 years: Dose not established
>15 years: 15 mg at bedtime
Adults: 15-30 mg at bedtime

Administration May be administered without regard to meals; administer dose at bedtime

(Continued)

449

Flurazepam *(Continued)*

Patient Information Avoid alcohol and other CNS depressants; may be habit-forming; avoid abrupt discontinuation after prolonged use

Dosage Forms Capsule, as hydrochloride: 15 mg, 30 mg

Flurbiprofen *(flure BI proe fen)*

U.S. Brand Names Ansaid®; Ocufen®

Canadian Brand Names Alti-Flurbiprofen; Apo-Flurbiprofen; Froben; Froben-SR; Novo-Flurprofen; Nu-Flurprofen; Ocufen

Therapeutic Category Analgesic, Non-narcotic; Anti-inflammatory Agent; Anti-inflammatory Agent, Ophthalmic; Nonsteroidal Anti-inflammatory Drug (NSAID), Ophthalmic; Nonsteroidal Anti-inflammatory Drug (NSAID), Oral

Generic Available Tablet: Yes

Use

Ophthalmic: For inhibition of intraoperative trauma-induced miosis; the value of flurbiprofen for the prevention and management of postoperative ocular inflammation and postoperative cystoid macular edema remains to be determined

Systemic: Management of inflammatory disease and rheumatoid disorders; dysmenorrhea; pain

Pregnancy Risk Factor B (D in 3rd trimester)

Contraindications Dendritic keratitis; hypersensitivity to flurbiprofen, any component, aspirin, or other NSAIDs

Warnings Use with caution in patients with history of herpes simplex, keratitis, and patients who might be affected by inhibition of platelet aggregation; use with caution in patients in whom asthma, rhinitis, or urticaria is precipitated by aspirin or other NSAIDs

Precautions Use oral form with caution in renal or hepatic impairment, GI disease, cardiac disease, and patients receiving anticoagulants

Adverse Reactions

Cardiovascular: Edema

Central nervous system: Headache, fatigue, drowsiness, vertigo

Dermatologic: Pruritus, rash

Gastrointestinal: Abdominal discomfort, nausea, heartburn, constipation, vomiting, GI bleeding, ulcers, perforation

Hematologic: Thrombocytopenia, inhibits platelet aggregation; prolongs bleeding time; agranulocytosis

Hepatic: Hepatitis

Ocular: Slowing of corneal wound healing, mild ocular stinging, itching, burning, ocular irritation

Otic: Tinnitus

Renal: Renal dysfunction

Drug Interactions Cytochrome P-450 isoenzyme CYP2C9 substrate and inhibitor

Oral: May decrease antihypertensive effects of ACE inhibitors or angiotensin II antagonists; drug interactions similar to other NSAIDs may occur

Ophthalmic: Carbachol and acetylcholine chloride may not be effective when used concurrently with flurbiprofen

Food Interactions Food may decrease the rate but not the extent of absorption

Mechanism of Action Inhibits prostaglandin synthesis by decreasing the activity of the enzyme, cyclo-oxygenase, which results in decreased formation of prostaglandin precursors

Pharmacokinetics Oral:

Time to peak serum concentration: Within 1.5-2 hours

Elimination: 95% in urine

Usual Dosage

Children and Adults: Ophthalmic: Instill 1 drop every 30 minutes starting 2 hours prior to surgery (total of 4 drops to each affected eye)

Adults: Oral:

Arthritis: 200-300 mg/day in 2-4 divided doses; maximum dose: 100 mg/dose; maximum: 300 mg/day

Dysmenorrhea: 50 mg 4 times/day

Administration

Oral: Administer with food, milk, or antacid to decrease GI effects

Ophthalmic: Instill drops into affected eye(s); avoid contact of container tip with skin or eye; apply finger pressure to lacrimal sac during and for 1-2 minutes after instillation to decrease risk of absorption and systemic effects

Monitoring Parameters Systemic use: CBC, platelets, BUN, serum creatinine, liver enzymes, occult blood loss, periodic eye exams

Patient Information Ophthalmic solution may cause mild burning or stinging, notify physician if this becomes severe or is persistent

Dosage Forms
Solution, ophthalmic, as sodium (Ocufen®): 0.03% (2.5 mL)
Tablet (Ansaid®): 50 mg, 100 mg

♦ **5-Flurocytosine** *see* Flucytosine *on page 432*

Fluticasone (floo TIK a sone)

Related Information
Asthma Guidelines *on page 1210*
Estimated Comparative Daily Dosages for Inhaled Corticosteroids *on page 1216*
U.S. Brand Names Cutivate™; Flonase®; Flovent®; Flovent® Diskus®; Flovent® Rotadisk®
Therapeutic Category Adrenal Corticosteroid; Antiasthmatic; Anti-inflammatory Agent; Corticosteroid, Inhalant (Oral); Corticosteroid, Intranasal; Corticosteroid, Topical; Glucocorticoid
Generic Available No
Use
Oral inhalation: Long-term (chronic) control of persistent bronchial asthma; NOT indicated for the relief of acute bronchospasm. Also used to help reduce or discontinue oral corticosteroid therapy for asthma (see Additional Information)
Intranasal: Management of seasonal and perennial allergic and nonallergic rhinitis
Topical: Relief of inflammation and pruritus associated with corticosteroid-responsive dermatoses [medium potency topical corticosteroid]
Pregnancy Risk Factor C
Contraindications Hypersensitivity to fluticasone or any component; primary treatment of status asthmaticus
Warnings Fatalities have occurred due to adrenal insufficiency in asthmatic patients during and after switching from systemic corticosteroids to aerosol steroids (see Additional Information); several months may be required for full recovery of the adrenal glands; patients receiving higher doses of systemic corticosteroids (eg, adults receiving ≥20 mg of prednisone per day) may be at greater risk; during this period of adrenal suppression, aerosol steroids do **not** provide the systemic corticosteroid needed to treat patients requiring stress doses (ie, patients with major stress such as trauma, surgery, or infections); when used at high doses, hypothalamic-pituitary-adrenal (HPA) suppression may occur; use with inhaled or systemic corticosteroids (even alternate-day dosing) may increase risk of HPA suppression; withdrawal and discontinuation of corticosteroids should be done carefully; immunosuppression may occur

Topical use: Adverse systemic effects may occur when used on large areas of the body, denuded areas, for prolonged periods of time, with an occlusive dressing, and/or in infants or small children; use with caution in pediatric patients
Precautions Avoid using higher than recommended doses; suppression of HPA function, suppression of linear growth, or hypercorticism (Cushing's syndrome) may occur; these adverse effects (as well as intracranial hypertension) may occur with topical use and have been reported in pediatric patients (see also Additional Information); use with extreme caution in patients with respiratory tuberculosis, untreated systemic infections, or ocular herpes simplex; use with caution and monitor patients closely with hepatic dysfunction. Eosinophilic conditions (eosinophilia, vasculitic rash, cardiac complications, worsening pulmonary symptoms, and/or neuropathy) may occur and are usually associated with withdrawal or decrease of oral corticosteroids after the initiation of fluticasone (oral inhalation); a causal relationship by fluticasone has not been established
Adverse Reactions
Central nervous system: Headache, dizziness, malaise, fatigue, insomnia
Dermatologic:
Inhalational use: Dermatitis, rash
Topical use: Pruritus, dry skin, numbness of fingers, acne, hypopigmentation, allergic dermatitis, maceration of the skin, skin atrophy, folliculitis, hypertrichosis, itching
Endocrine & metabolic: HPA suppression, Cushing's syndrome, growth suppression
Gastrointestinal: Oral candidiasis, nausea, vomiting, diarrhea, dyspepsia
Local: Burning, irritation
Neuromuscular & skeletal: Muscular soreness
Ocular: Eye pain
Respiratory: Respiratory infection, pharyngitis, nasal congestion, sinusitis, nasal discharge, rhinitis, epistaxis (intranasal), dysphonia (oral inhalation),
Miscellaneous: Secondary infection, eosinophilic conditions (see Precautions)
(Continued)

Fluticasone *(Continued)*

Drug Interactions Cytochrome P-450 isoenzyme CYP3A3/4 substrate

Ketoconazole and other P-450 3A4 isoenzyme inhibitors may increase fluticasone serum concentrations

Stability

Oral inhalation: Aerosol canister: Store between 36°F to 86°F with nozzle end down; do not store at >120°F; protect from freezing and direct sunlight; Rotadisk®: Store at controlled room temperature; keep dry; discard Rotadisk® blisters 2 months after opening moisture-proof foil overwrap (or before expiration date); Diskus®: Store at controlled room temperature; keep dry; protect from direct heat or sunlight; discard Diskus® 6 weeks (for 50 mcg strength) or 2 months (for 100 mcg and 250 mcg strengths) after opening moisture-proof foil overwrap or when dose indicator reads "0" (whichever comes first); **Note:** Diskus® device is not reusable

Intranasal: Store nasal spray between 39°F to 86°F

Mechanism of Action Controls the rate of protein synthesis, depresses the migration of polymorphonuclear leukocytes and fibroblasts, reverses capillary permeability, and stabilizes lysosomal membranes at the cellular level to prevent or control inflammation

Pharmacodynamics

Oral inhalation: Clinical effects are due to direct local effect rather than systemic absorption

Onset of action: Within 24 hours

Maximum effect: 1-2 weeks or more

Duration after discontinuation: Several days or more

Pharmacokinetics

Distribution: V_d: Adults: 4.2 L/kg

Protein binding: 91%

Metabolism: Via cytochrome P-450 3A4 pathway

Bioavailability: Oral inhalation: 30% of dose delivered from activator; Diskus®: 18%

Half-life: 7.8 hours

Usual Dosage

Intranasal:

Children <4 years: Not recommended

Children ≥4 years and Adolescents: Initial: 1 spray (50 mcg/spray) to each nostril daily (100 mcg/day); if response is inadequate, give 2 sprays to each nostril daily (200 mcg/day); once symptoms are controlled, reduce dose to 100 mcg/day (1 spray to each nostril daily); maximum dose: 200 mcg/day (4 sprays/day)

Adults: Initial: 200 mcg/day given as 2 sprays (50 mcg/spray) to each nostril daily or 1 spray to each nostril twice daily; dosage may be reduced to 100 mcg/day (1 spray to each nostril daily) after the first few days if symptoms are controlled; maximum dose: 200 mcg/day (4 sprays/day)

Oral inhalation: If adequate response is not seen after 2 weeks of initial dosage, increase dosage; doses should be titrated to the lowest effective dose once asthma is controlled; Manufacturer recommendations:

Inhalation aerosol (Flovent®): Children ≥12 years and Adults:

Patients previously treated with bronchodilators only: Initial: 88 mcg twice daily; maximum dose: 440 mcg twice daily

Patients treated with an inhaled corticosteroid: Initial: 88-220 mcg twice daily; maximum dose: 440 mcg twice daily; may start doses above 88 mcg twice daily in poorly controlled patients or in those who previously required higher doses of inhaled corticosteroids

Patients previously treated with oral corticosteroids: Initial: 880 mcg twice daily; maximum dose: 880 mcg twice daily

NIH Guidelines (NIH, 1997) [give in divided doses twice daily]:

Children:

"Low" dose: 88-176 mcg/day (44 mcg/puff: 2-4 puffs/day)

"Medium" dose: 176-440 mcg/day (44 mcg/puff: 4-10 puffs/day or 110 mcg/puff: 2-4 puffs/day)

"High" dose: >440 mcg/day (110 mcg/puff: >4 puffs/day or 220 mcg/puff: >2 puffs/day)

Adults:

"Low" dose: 88-264 mcg/day (44 mcg/puff: 2-6 puffs/day or 110 mcg/puff: 2 puffs/day)

"Medium" dose: 264-660 mcg/day (110 mcg/puff: 2-6 puffs/day)

"High" dose: >660 mcg/day (110 mcg/puff: >6 puffs/day or 220 mcg/puff: >3 puffs/day)

FLUTICASONE

Inhalation powder (Flovent® Diskus® and Flovent® Rotadisk®): **Note:** Children maintained on Flovent® Rotadisk® who are switched to Flovent® Diskus® may require dosage adjustment

Children 4-11 years: Patients previously treated with bronchodilators alone or inhaled corticosteroids: Initial: 50 mcg twice daily; maximum dose: 100 mcg twice daily; may start higher initial dose in poorly controlled patients or in those who previously required higher doses of inhaled corticosteroids

Adolescents and Adults:

Patients previously treated with bronchodilators alone: Initial: 100 mcg twice daily; maximum dose: 500 mcg twice daily

Patients previously treated with inhaled corticosteroids: Initial: 100-250 mcg twice daily; maximum dose: 500 mcg twice daily; may start doses above 100 mcg twice daily in poorly controlled patients or in those who previously required higher doses of inhaled corticosteroids

Patients previously treated with oral corticosteroids: Initial: Diskus®: 500-1000 mcg twice daily (select dose based on assessment of individual patient); Rotadisk®: 1000 mcg twice daily (this dose is based on clinical data using Flovent® inhalation aerosol); maximum dose: 1000 mcg twice daily; **Note:** Inability to reduce oral corticosteroid therapy (see Additional Information) may indicate need for maximum fluticasone dose

Topical:

Cream:

Infants <3 months: Not approved for use

Infants ≥3 months, Children, and Adults: **Note:** Safety and efficacy of use >4 weeks in pediatric patients have not been established:

Atopic dermatitis: Apply a thin film to affected area once or twice daily

Other dermatoses: Apply a thin film to affected area twice daily

Ointment: Adolescents and Adults: Apply sparingly in a thin film twice daily

Administration

Intranasal spray: Shake bottle gently before use; clear nasal passages by blowing nose prior to use; nasal spray pump must be primed (6 actuations) before first use or after ≥1 week of non-use; discard unit after 120 metered sprays are used

Oral inhalation: Rinse mouth after inhalation to decrease chance of oral candidiasis

Aerosol inhalation: Shake canister well before use; use a spacer device for children <8 years of age

Powder for oral inhalation:

Diskus®: Do not use with spacer device; do not exhale into Diskus®; do not wash or take apart; activate and use Diskus® in horizontal position

Rotadisk®: Do not puncture blister until taking dose with Diskhaler®; do not use with a spacer device

Topical: Apply sparingly to affected area, gently rub in until disappears; do not use on open skin; avoid application on face, underarms, or groin area unless directed by physician; avoid contact with eyes; do not occlude area unless directed; do not apply to diaper area

Monitoring Parameters Oral inhalation: Check mucus membranes for signs of fungal infection; monitor growth in pediatric patients

Patient Information Notify physician if condition being treated persists or worsens; do not decrease dose or discontinue without physician approval; avoid exposure to chicken pox or measles; if exposed, seek medical advice without delay

Oral inhalation: Report sore mouth or mouth lesions to physician

Additional Information When using fluticasone oral inhalation to help reduce or discontinue oral corticosteroid therapy, begin prednisone taper after at least 1 week of fluticasone inhalation therapy; do not decrease prednisone faster than 2.5 mg/day on a weekly basis; monitor patients for signs of asthma instability and adrenal insufficiency (see Warnings); decrease fluticasone to lowest effective dose **after** prednisone reduction is complete. If bronchospasm with wheezing occurs after oral inhalation use, a fast-acting bronchodilator may be used.

Topical: HPA axis suppression occurred in 2 children (2 and 5 years old) of 43 pediatric patients treated topically for 4 weeks; application covered at least 35% of body surface area

Dosage Forms

Powder, oral inhalation, as propionate

Flovent® Diskus® [approved by FDA October, 2000; projected availability December, 2001]:

50 mcg [delivers 47 mcg/inhalation] (28 doses, 60 doses)

100 mcg [delivers 94 mcg/inhalation] (28 doses, 60 doses)

250 mcg [delivers 235 mcg/inhalation] (28 doses, 60 doses)

Flovent® Rotadisk® (4 blisters of the drug per Rotadisk®, 15 Rotadisks® per pack):

50 mcg [delivers 44 mcg/inhalation]

(Continued)

Fluticasone *(Continued)*

   100 mcg [delivers 88 mcg/inhalation]
   250 mcg [delivers 220 mcg/inhalation]
  Spray, aerosol, oral inhalation, as propionate (Flovent®):
   44 mcg/actuation [7.9 g = 60 actuations or 13 g = 120 actuations]
   110 mcg/actuation [7.9 g = 60 actuations or 13 g = 120 actuations]
   220 mcg/actuation [7.9 g = 60 actuations or 13 g = 120 actuations]
  Spray, intranasal, as propionate (Flonase®): 50 mcg/actuation [16 g = 120 actuations]
  Topical, as propionate (Cutivate™):
   Cream: 0.05% (15 g, 30 g, 60 g)
   Ointment: 0.005% (15 g, 30 g, 60 g)

References
Expert Panel Report 2, "Guidelines for the Diagnosis and Management of Asthma," *Clinical Practice Guidelines,* National Institutes of Health, National Heart, Lung, and Blood Institute, NIH Publication No. 94-4051, April, 1997.

♦ **FML®** *see* Fluorometholone *on page 443*
♦ **FML® Forte** *see* Fluorometholone *on page 443*
♦ **FML® S.O.P** *see* Fluorometholone *on page 443*
♦ **Foille® [OTC]** *see* Benzocaine *on page 135*
♦ **Foille® Medicated First Aid [OTC]** *see* Benzocaine *on page 135*
♦ **Folacin** *see* Folic Acid *on page 454*
♦ **Folate** *see* Folic Acid *on page 454*

Folic Acid *(FOE lik AS id)*

U.S. Brand Names Folvite®
Canadian Brand Names Apo-Folic; Novo-Folacid
Synonyms Folacin; Folate; Pteroylglutamic Acid
Therapeutic Category Nutritional Supplement; Vitamin, Water Soluble
Generic Available Yes
Use Treatment of megaloblastic and macrocytic anemias due to folate deficiency; dietary supplement to prevent neural tube defects
Pregnancy Risk Factor A (C if dose exceeds RDA recommendation)
Contraindications Pernicious, aplastic, or normocytic anemias
Warnings Large doses may mask the hematologic effects of B_{12} deficiency, thus obscuring the diagnosis of pernicious anemia while allowing the neurologic complications due to B_{12} deficiency to progress; injection contains benzyl alcohol (1.5%) as preservative, therefore, avoid use in neonates
Adverse Reactions
 Cardiovascular: Slight flushing
 Central nervous system: Irritability, difficulty sleeping, confusion, malaise
 Dermatologic: Pruritus, rash
 Gastrointestinal: GI upset
 Miscellaneous: Hypersensitivity reactions
Drug Interactions May decrease phenytoin serum concentration; hematologic response antagonized by chloramphenicol; folic acid antagonists (ie, methotrexate, pyrimethamine, trimethoprim) prevent the formation of tetrahydrofolic acid (active metabolite), therefore, folic acid is not effective for the treatment of overdosage of these drugs (leucovorin must be used); decreased folic acid absorption with sulfasalazine and aminosalicylic acid; decreased folic acid concentration with phenytoin, primidone, para-aminosalicylic acid
Mechanism of Action Folic acid is necessary for formation of a number of coenzymes in many metabolic systems, particularly for purine and pyrimidine synthesis; required for nucleoprotein synthesis and maintenance in erythropoiesis; stimulates WBC and platelet production in folate deficiency anemia
Pharmacodynamics Peak effect: Oral: Within 30-60 minutes
Pharmacokinetics
 Absorption: In the proximal part of the small intestine
 Time to peak serum concentration: Oral: 1 hour
 Elimination: Primarily via liver metabolism
Usual Dosage
 Recommended daily allowance (RDA): Oral:*
  Premature neonates: 50 mcg (~15 mcg/kg/day)
  Neonates to 6 months: 25-35 mcg
  Children:
   6 months to 3 years: 50 mcg
   4-6 years: 75 mcg

7-10 years: 100 mcg
11-14 years: 150 mcg
Children >15 years and Adults: 200 mcg
Pregnant women: 400 mcg
Folic acid deficiency: Oral, I.M., I.V., S.C.:
Infants: 15 mcg/kg/dose daily or 50 mcg/day
Children: 1 mg/kg/dose initial dosage; maintenance dose: 1-10 years: 0.1-0.4 mg/day
Children >11 years and Adults: 1 mg/day initial dosage; maintenance dose: 0.5 mg/day

Administration
Oral: May be administered without regard to meals
Parenteral: I.V.: Dilute with sterile water, dextrose or saline solution to 0.1 mg/mL; if I.M. route used, administer deep I.M.; may also administer S.C.

Monitoring Parameters CBC with differential

Reference Range Total folate: Normal: 5-15 ng/mL; folate deficiency: <5 ng/mL; megaloblastic anemia: <2 ng/mL

Additional Information Oral liquid vitamin drops (eg, Vi-Daylin®) do not contain folic acid due to the instability of folic acid in the pH of these formulations.

Dosage Forms
Injection, as sodium folate: 5 mg/mL (10 mL)
Tablet: 0.1 mg, 0.4 mg, 0.8 mg, 1 mg

Extemporaneous Preparations A 50 mcg/mL solution may be made by mixing 1 mL (5 mg) folic acid injection in 90 mL purified water; adjust pH to 9 with sodium hydroxide 0.1 N (approximately 2.8 mL), then add purified water to make a total volume of 100 mL; stable 30 days at room temperature
Smith SG, "A Folic Acid Solution for Oral Use," *Pharm J*, 1976, 216:108.

♦ **Folinic Acid** *see* Leucovorin *on page 580*
♦ **Folvite®** *see* Folic Acid *on page 454*

Fomepizole (foe ME pi zole)

U.S. Brand Names Antizol®

Synonyms 4-Methylpyrazole; 4-MP

Therapeutic Category Antidote, Ethylene Glycol Toxicity; Antidote, Methanol Toxicity

Generic Available No

Use Antidote for ethylene glycol (antifreeze) or methanol toxicity; may be useful in propylene glycol toxicity

Pregnancy Risk Factor C

Contraindications Hypersensitivity to fomepizole, other pyrazoles, or any component

Warnings By inhibiting the action of alcohol dehydrogenase, fomepizole reduces the elimination of alcohol; this must be considered when using fomepizole, as alcohol is often ingested concomitantly by patients with ethylene glycol intoxication; likewise, alcohol may reduce the elimination of fomepizole by the same mechanism; safety and efficacy in pediatric patients has not been established

Precautions Management of ethylene glycol ingestion may require treatment of metabolic acidosis, acute renal failure, adult respiratory distress syndrome, and hypocalcemia; dialysis should be considered, in addition to fomepizole therapy, in patients with acute renal failure, severe metabolic acidosis, or a serum ethylene glycol concentration >50 mg/dL; adjust dosage for renal dysfunction (see Usual Dosage)

Adverse Reactions
Cardiovascular: Bradycardia, tachycardia, hypotension
Central nervous system: Headache, dizziness, seizure, slurred speech, fever, somnolence
Dermatologic: Rash
Gastrointestinal: Nausea, vomiting, diarrhea, anorexia, heartburn, metallic taste, abdominal pain
Hematologic: Eosinophilia, anemia
Hepatic: Transient elevations in transaminase levels
Local: Phlebosclerosis, vein irritation
Ocular: Nystagmus, blurred vision
Respiratory: Pharyngitis, hiccups
Miscellaneous: Hypersensitivity reactions

Drug Interactions Alcohol (see Warnings)

Stability Store at room temperature; fomepizole solidifies at temperatures <25°C (77°F); if solidification occurs, liquefy by running the vial under warm water or by
(Continued)

Fomepizole *(Continued)*

holding in the hand; solidification does not affect the efficacy, safety, or stability of fomepizole; stabile diluted in NS or D_5W for 48 hours; does not contain a preservative; use within 24 hours of dilution

Mechanism of Action A competitive alcohol dehydrogenase inhibitor, fomepizole complexes and inactivates alcohol dehydrogenase thus preventing formation of the toxic metabolites of the alcohols

Pharmacokinetics

Distribution: V_d: 0.6-1.02 L/kg; rapidly distributes into total body water

Protein binding: Negligible

Metabolism: Liver; primarily to 4-carboxypyrazole; after single doses, exhibits saturable, Michaelis-Menton kinetics; with multiple dosing, fomepizole induces its own metabolism via the cytochrome P-450 system; after enzyme induction elimination follows first order kinetics

Elimination: 1% to 3.5% excreted unchanged in the urine

Dialyzable

Usual Dosage I.V.:

Children: Has not been studied

Adults **not requiring** hemodialysis: Initial: 15 mg/kg loading dose; followed by 10 mg/kg every 12 hours for 4 doses; then 15 mg/kg every 12 hours until ethylene glycol or methanol levels have been reduced to <20 mg/dL

Adults **requiring** hemodialysis: Since fomepizole is dialyzable, follow the above dose recommendations at intervals related to institution of hemodialysis and its duration:

Dose at the beginning of hemodialysis:

If <6 hours since last fomepizole dose: Do **not** administer dose

If ≥6 hours since last fomepizole dose: Administer next scheduled dose

Dose during hemodialysis: Administer every 4 hours

Dose at the time hemodialysis is completed (dependent upon the time between the last dose and the end of hemodialysis):

<1 hour: Do **not** administer at the end of hemodialysis

1-3 hours: Administer $1/2$ of the next scheduled dose

>3 hours: Administer the next scheduled dose

Maintenance dose off hemodialysis: Give next scheduled dose 12 hours from last dose administered

Dosage adjustment in renal impairment: Fomepizole is substantially excreted by the kidney and the risk of toxic reactions to this drug may be increased in patients with impaired renal function; no dosage recommendations for patients with impaired renal function have been established

Administration Parenteral: I.V. Dilute in at least 100 mL NS or D_5W (<25 mg/mL); infuse over 30 minutes; rapid infusion of concentrations ≥25 mg/mL has been associated with vein irritation and phlebosclerosis

Monitoring Parameters Vital signs, arterial blood gases, acid-base status, urinary oxalate, anion and osmolar gaps, clinical signs and symptoms of toxicity (arrhythmias, seizures, coma); serum and urinary ethylene glycol or serum methanol level depending upon the agent ingested; formic acid level (methanol ingestion)

Reference Range Ethylene glycol or methanol serum concentration: Goal: <20 mg/dL; therapeutic plasma fomepizole level: 0.8 mcg/mL

Additional Information If ethylene glycol poisoning is left untreated, the natural progression of the poisoning leads to accumulation of toxic metabolites, including glycolic and oxalic acids; these metabolites can induce metabolic acidosis, seizures, stupor, coma, calcium oxaluria, acute tubular necrosis and death; as ethylene glycol levels diminish in the blood when metabolized to glycolate, the diagnosis of this poisoning may be difficult

Dosage Forms Injection, concentrate: 1 g/mL (1.5 mL)

♦ **Formula 44 (Can)** *see* Dextromethorphan *on page 316*
♦ **Formula 44E (Can)** *see* Guaifenesin and Dextromethorphan *on page 487*
♦ **Formulex (Can)** *see* Dicyclomine *on page 326*
♦ **5-Formyl Tetrahydrofolate** *see* Leucovorin *on page 580*
♦ **Fortaz®** *see* Ceftazidime *on page 201*
♦ **Fortovase®** *see* Saquinavir *on page 889*

Foscarnet *(fos KAR net)*

U.S. Brand Names Foscavir®

Synonyms PFA; Phosphonoformate

Therapeutic Category Antiviral Agent, Parenteral

Generic Available No

Use Alternative to ganciclovir for treatment of CMV infections; treatment of CMV retinitis in patients with acquired immunodeficiency syndrome; treatment of acyclovir-resistant mucocutaneous herpes simplex virus infections in immunocompromised patients and acyclovir-resistant herpes zoster infections

Pregnancy Risk Factor C

Contraindications Hypersensitivity to foscarnet or any component; Cl_{cr} <0.4 mL/minute/kg

Warnings Renal impairment occurs to some degree in the majority of patients treated with foscarnet; renal impairment may occur at any time and is usually reversible within 1 week following dose adjustment or discontinuation of therapy; however, several patients have died with renal failure within 4 weeks of stopping foscarnet; foscarnet is deposited in teeth and bone of young, growing animals; it has adversely affected tooth enamel development in rats; safety and effectiveness in children has not been studied

Patients with a low ionized calcium may experience perioral tingling, numbness, parasthesia, tetany, and seizures. Risk factor for seizures include a low baseline ANC, impaired renal function, and low total serum calcium.

Precautions Use with caution in patients with renal impairment, patients with altered electrolyte levels, and patients with neurologic or cardiac abnormalities; adjust dose for patients with impaired renal function; discontinue treatment in adults if serum creatinine ≥2.9 mg/dL; therapy can be restarted if serum creatinine ≤2 mg/dL

Adverse Reactions
Cardiovascular: Hypertension, palpitations, chest pain, EKG abnormalities
Central nervous system: Fatigue, fever, headache, seizures, hallucinations, dizziness, agitation, amnesia
Endocrine & metabolic: Hypocalcemia, hypomagnesemia, hypokalemia, hypo- or hyperphosphatemia
Gastrointestinal: Nausea, diarrhea, vomiting, weight loss, pancreatitis
Genitourinary: Vulvovaginal ulceration, penile epithelium ulceration, dysuria, urethral disorder
Hematologic: Decreases in hemoglobin and hematocrit
Hepatic: Elevated liver enzymes, cholecystitis, hepatitis
Local: Thrombophlebitis
Neuromuscular & skeletal: Peripheral neuropathy, paresthesia, tremor
Renal: Elevated BUN and serum creatinine, polyuria, oliguria, renal failure, proteinuria
Respiratory: Coughing, dyspnea, bronchospasm

Drug Interactions Pentamidine (additive hypocalcemia); aminoglycosides, amphotericin B (additive nephrotoxicity)

Stability Store at room temperature; refrigeration may result in crystallization of the drug; incompatible with dextrose ≥30%, I.V. solutions containing calcium, magnesium, vancomycin, TPN

Mechanism of Action Pyrophosphate analog which inhibits DNA synthesis by interfering with viral DNA polymerase and reverse transcriptase

Induction Treatment

Cl_{cr} (mL/min/kg)	mg/kg/8h
≥1.6	60
1.5	56.5
1.4	53
1.3	49.4
1.2	45.9
1.1	42.4
1	38.9
0.9	35.3
0.8	31.8
0.7	28.3
0.6	24.8
0.5	21.2
0.4	17.7

Pharmacokinetics
Distribution: V_d: Adults: 0.74 L/kg; minimal penetration of the drug across the blood-brain barrier
(Continued)

Foscarnet *(Continued)*

Protein binding: 14% to 17%

Half-life, plasma: Adults with normal renal function: 3-4.5 hours
Terminal: 18-42 hours

Elimination: 80% to 90% excreted unchanged in urine

Usual Dosage Children and Adults: I.V.:

CMV retinitis: Induction treatment: 180 mg/kg/day divided every 8 hours for 14-21 days
Maintenance therapy: 90-120 mg/kg/day as a single infusion once daily

Acyclovir-resistant herpes simplex virus infection: 40 mg/kg/dose every 8 hours or 40-60 mg/kg/dose every 12 hours for up to 3 weeks or until lesions heal; repeat treatment may lead to the development of resistance

Dosing interval in renal impairment: See tables on previous page and below.

Maintenance Therapy

Cl$_{cr}$ (mL/min/kg)	mg/kg
≥1.4	90-120 q24h
1-1.4	70-90 q24h
0.8-1.	50-65 q24h
0.6-0.8	80-105 q48h
0.5-0.6	60-80 q48h
0.4-0.5	50-65 q48h
<0.4	not recommended

Administration Parenteral: 24 mg/mL solution may be administered without further dilution when using a central venous catheter for infusion; for peripheral vein administration, the solution **must** be diluted to a final concentration **not to exceed** 12 mg/mL with either NS or D$_5$W; administer by I.V. infusion at a rate **not to exceed** 60 mg/kg/dose over 1 hour or 120 mg/kg/dose over 2 hours

Monitoring Parameters Serum creatinine, calcium, phosphorus, potassium, magnesium; hemoglobin, ophthalmologic exams

Reference Range Therapeutic for CMV: 150 µg/mL

Patient Information Report any numbness in the extremities, paresthesias, or perioral tingling

Nursing Implications Provide adequate hydration with I.V. NS or D$_5$W prior to and during treatment to minimize nephrotoxicity

Dosage Forms Injection: 24 mg/mL (250 mL, 500 mL)

References

Butler KM, DeSmet MD, Husson RN, et al, "Treatment of Aggressive Cytomegalovirus Retinitis With Ganciclovir in Combination With Foscarnet in a Child Infected With Human Immunodeficiency Virus," *J Pediatr*, 1992, 120(3):483-6.

"1999 USPHS/IDSA Guidelines for the Prevention of Opportunistic Infections in Persons Infected With Human Immunodeficiency Virus. U.S. Public Health Service (USPHS) and Infectious Diseases Society of America (IDSA)," *MMWR*, 1999, 48(RR-10):1-66.

♦ **Foscavir®** *see Foscarnet on page 456*

Fosphenytoin *(FOS fen i toyn)*

Related Information

Blood Level Sampling Time Guidelines *on page 1220*

U.S. Brand Names Cerebyx®

Synonyms 3-Phosphoryloxymethyl Phenytoin Disodium

Therapeutic Category Anticonvulsant, Hydantoin

Generic Available No

Use Management of generalized convulsive status epilepticus; used for short-term parenteral administration of phenytoin; prevention and management of seizures responsive to phenytoin

Pregnancy Risk Factor D

Contraindications Hypersensitivity to fosphenytoin, phenytoin, or any other component; heart block, sinus bradycardia

Warnings Abrupt withdrawal may precipitate status epilepticus; monitor blood pressure and EKG with I.V. loading doses; use with caution in patients with severe myocardial insufficiency and hypotension; discontinue if skin rash develops, do not resume drug if rash is exfoliative, purpuric, bullous, or if SLE, Stevens-Johnson syndrome, or toxic epidermal necrolysis is suspected; discontinue if acute hepatotoxicity occurs

Precautions Use with caution in patients with porphyria; consider the amount of phosphate delivered by fosphenytoin in patients who require phosphate restriction; use with caution and modify dosage in patients with hepatic or renal dysfunction

Adverse Reactions

Cardiovascular: Hypotension (with rapid I.V. administration), vasodilation, tachycardia, bradycardia

Central nervous system: Slurred speech, dizziness, drowsiness, headache, somnolence, ataxia, fever

Dermatologic: Rash, exfoliative dermatitis, facial edema

Endocrine & metabolic: Folic acid depletion, hyperglycemia

Gastrointestinal: Nausea, vomiting, taste perversion

Genitourinary: Pelvic pain

Hematologic: Neutropenia, thrombocytopenia, anemia (megaloblastic)

Local: Pain on injection; since fosphenytoin is water soluble and has a lower pH (8.8) than phenytoin (12), irritation at injection site or phlebitis is reduced; I.M.: Local itching

Neuromuscular & skeletal: Osteomalacia

Ocular: Nystagmus, blurred vision, diplopia

Otic: Tinnitus

Miscellaneous: Lymphadenopathy; sensory disturbances (burning, pruritus, tingling, paresthesia) occur predominantly in the groin area, but may occur in the lower back, abdomen, head or neck (these effects may be related to the phosphate load); paresthesia and pruritus are more common with I.V. vs I.M. administration and are dose and infusion rate related

Drug Interactions No drugs are known to interfere with the conversion of fosphenytoin to phenytoin; see Phenytoin *on page 791* for phenytoin interactions

Stability Store unopened vials in the refrigerator; fosphenytoin at concentrations of 1, 8, and 20 mg phenytoin sodium equivalents (**PE**)/mL in D_5W or NS is stable for 30 days when stored at 25°C or 4°C in glass bottles or polyvinyl chloride infusion bags, and when frozen at -20°C in polyvinyl chloride infusion bags. After removal from the freezer, these solutions are stable for 7 days at 25°C or 4°C.

Undiluted fosphenytoin injection (50 mg **PE**/mL) is stable in polypropylene syringes for 30 days at 25°C, 4°C, or frozen at -20°C.

Fosphenytoin at concentrations of 1, 8, and 20 mg **PE**/mL prepared in D_5/$\frac{1}{2}$NS, D_5/$\frac{1}{2}$NS with KCl 20 mEq/L, D_5/$\frac{1}{2}$NS with 40 mEq/L, LR, D_5/LR, D_{10}W, amino acid 10%, mannitol 20%, hetastarch 6% in NS or Plasma-Lyte® A injection is stable in polyvinyl chloride bags for 7 days when stored at 25°C (room temperature).

Mechanism of Action Diphosphate ester salt of phenytoin which acts as a water soluble prodrug of phenytoin; after administration, plasma and tissue esterases convert fosphenytoin to phosphate, formaldehyde and phenytoin (as the active moiety); phenytoin works by stabilizing neuronal membranes and decreasing seizure activity by increasing efflux or decreasing influx of sodium ions across cell membranes in the motor cortex during generation of nerve impulses

Pharmacokinetics The pharmacokinetics of fosphenytoin-derived phenytoin are the same as those for phenytoin (see Phenytoin *on page 791*). Parameters listed below are for fosphenytoin (the prodrug) unless otherwise noted. **Note:** The pharmacokinetics of fosphenytoin have been studied in a limited number of children 5-18 years of age and have been found to be similar to the pharmacokinetics observed in young adults (see Pellock, 1996).

Bioavailability: I.M., I.V.: 100%

Distribution: Adults: V_d: 4.3-10.8 L; V_d of fosphenytoin increases with dose and rate of administration

Protein binding: 95% to 99% primarily to albumin; binding of fosphenytoin to protein is saturable (the percent bound decreases as total concentration increases); fosphenytoin displaces phenytoin from protein binding sites; during the time fosphenytoin is being converted to phenytoin, fosphenytoin may temporarily increase the free fraction of phenytoin up to 30% unbound

Metabolism: Each millimole of fosphenytoin is metabolized to 1 millimole of phenytoin, phosphate, and formaldehyde; formaldehyde is converted to formate, which is then metabolized by a folate-dependent mechanism; conversion of fosphenytoin to phenytoin increases with increasing dose and infusion rate, most likely due to a decrease in fosphenytoin protein binding

Conversion of fosphenytoin to phenytoin: Half-life: 15 minutes

Time for complete conversion to phenytoin:

I.M.: 4 hours after injection

I.V.: 2 hours after the end of infusion

Elimination: 0% fosphenytoin excreted in urine

(Continued)

Fosphenytoin (Continued)

Usual Dosage

The dose, concentration in solutions, and infusion rates for fosphenytoin are expressed as PHENYTOIN SODIUM EQUIVALENTS (PE)

Fosphenytoin should ALWAYS be prescribed and dispensed in mg of PE; otherwise significant medication errors may occur

Children 5-18 years: I.V.: A limited number of children have been studied. Seven children received a single I.V. loading dose of fosphenytoin 10-20 mg **PE**/kg for the treatment of acute generalized convulsive status epilepticus (Pellock, 1996). Some centers are using the phenytoin dosing guidelines in children and dosing fosphenytoin using **PE** doses equal to the phenytoin doses (ie, phenytoin 1 mg = fosphenytoin 1 mg **PE**). Further pediatric studies are needed.

Adults:
Loading dose:
Status epilepticus: I.V.: 15-20 mg **PE**/kg
Nonemergent loading: I.M., I.V.: 10-20 mg **PE**/kg
Initial daily maintenance dose: I.M., I.V.: 4-6 mg **PE**/kg; I.M. dose may be administered as a single daily dose using 1 or 2 injection sites; some patients may require more frequent dosing

I.M. or I.V. substitution for oral phenytoin: Initial: Use the same total daily dose in **PE** of fosphenytoin (ie, phenytoin 1 mg = fosphenytoin 1 mg **PE**); plasma concentrations may increase slightly with this method because oral phenytoin sodium is 90% bioavailable and phenytoin derived from I.M. or I.V. fosphenytoin is 100% bioavailable. Monitor clinical response and phenytoin concentrations to further guide dosage adjustments after 3-4 days

Dosing adjustments in renal/hepatic impairment:
Cirrhosis: Phenytoin clearance may be substantially reduced and monitoring of plasma concentrations with dosage adjustments is advisable
Renal or hepatic disease and patients with hypoalbuminemia: Fosphenytoin conversion to phenytoin may be increased (due to lower protein binding) without a similar increase in phenytoin clearance, leading to a potential increase in the frequency and severity of adverse effects

Administration Dilute with D_5W or NS to 1.5-25 mg **PE**/mL
Children 5-18 years: An administration rate of 3 mg **PE**/kg/minute with a maximum of 150 mg **PE**/minute was used in 7 patients (see Pellock, 1996)
Adults: Administer at a rate of 100-150 mg **PE**/minute with a maximum infusion rate of 150 mg **PE**/minute

Monitoring Parameters Serum phenytoin concentrations, CBC with differential, liver enzymes; blood pressure, vital signs (with I.V. use); free (unbound) and total serum phenytoin concentrations in patients with hyperbilirubinemia, hypoalbuminemia, renal dysfunction, uremia, or hepatic disease

Reference Range Monitor **phenytoin** serum concentrations; obtain phenytoin concentrations 2 hours after the end of an I.V. infusion or 4 hours after an I.M. injection of fosphenytoin; see Phenytoin *on page 791* for phenytoin reference range

Additional Information Dosing equivalency: Fosphenytoin sodium 1.5 mg is equivalent to phenytoin sodium 1 mg which is equivalent to fosphenytoin 1 mg **PE**

Phosphate load: Each mg **PE** of fosphenytoin delivers 0.0037 mmol of phosphate

Formaldehyde production from fosphenytoin is not expected to be clinically significant in adults with short-term use (eg, 1 week); potentially harmful amounts of phosphate and formaldehyde could occur with an overdose of fosphenytoin; fosphenytoin is more water soluble than phenytoin and, therefore, the injection does not contain propylene glycol; antiarrhythmic effects should be similar to phenytoin

Dosage Forms Injection, as sodium: 75 mg/mL [equivalent to 50 mg/mL phenytoin sodium (ie, 50 mg **PE**/mL)] (2 mL, 10 mL)

References

Boucher BA, Feler CA, Dean JC, et al, "The Safety, Tolerability, and Pharmacokinetics of Fosphenytoin After Intramuscular and Intravenous Administration in Neurosurgery Patients," *Pharmacotherapy*, 1996, 16(4):638-45.

Boucher BA, "Fosphenytoin: A Novel Phenytoin Prodrug," *Pharmacotherapy*, 1996, 16(5):777-91.

Fischer JH, Cwik MS, Luer MS, et al, "Stability of Fosphenytoin Sodium With Intravenous Solutions in Glass Bottles, Polyvinyl Chloride Bags, and Polypropylene Syringes," *Ann Pharmacother*, 1997, 31(5):553-9.

Pellock JM, "Fosphenytoin Use in Children," *Neurology*, 1996, 46(6 Suppl 1):S14-6.

Wilder BJ, Campbell K, Ramsay RE, et al, "Safety and Tolerance of Multiple Doses of Intramuscular Fosphenytoin Substituted for Oral Phenytoin in Epilepsy or Neurosurgery," *Arch Neurol*, 1996, 53(8):764-8.

- **Fostex® 10% BPO Gel [OTC]** *see* Benzoyl Peroxide *on page 136*
- **Fostex® 10% Wash [OTC]** *see* Benzoyl Peroxide *on page 136*
- **Fostex® Bar [OTC]** *see* Benzoyl Peroxide *on page 136*
- **Fostex® Medicated Cleansing [OTC] Freezone® [OTC]** *see* Salicylic Acid *on page 886*
- **Fototar® [OTC]** *see* Coal Tar *on page 260*
- **Fowlers (Can)** *see* Attapulgite *on page 118*
- **Freeda® Vitamin E** *see* Vitamin E *on page 1014*
- **Froben (Can)** *see* Flurbiprofen *on page 450*
- **Froben-SR (Can)** *see* Flurbiprofen *on page 450*
- **5-FU** *see* Fluorouracil *on page 444*
- **Fulvicin® P/G** *see* Griseofulvin *on page 484*
- **Fulvicin-U/F®** *see* Griseofulvin *on page 484*
- **Fungizone®** *see* Amphotericin B (Conventional) *on page 83*
- **Fung-O® [OTC]** *see* Salicylic Acid *on page 886*
- **Fungoid® Creme** *see* Miconazole *on page 668*
- **Fungoid® Tincture** *see* Miconazole *on page 668*
- **Fungoid® Topical Solution** *see* Undecylenic Acid and Derivatives *on page 994*
- **Furadantin®** *see* Nitrofurantoin *on page 716*
- **Furalan®** *see* Nitrofurantoin *on page 716*
- **Furan®** *see* Nitrofurantoin *on page 716*
- **Furanite®** *see* Nitrofurantoin *on page 716*

Furazolidone (fyoor a ZOE li done)

U.S. Brand Names Furoxone®

Therapeutic Category Antibiotic, Miscellaneous; Antiprotozoal

Generic Available No

Use Treatment of bacterial or protozoal diarrhea and enteritis caused by susceptible organisms: *Giardia lamblia* and *Vibrio cholerae*

Pregnancy Risk Factor C

Contraindications Hypersensitivity to furazolidone or any component; concurrent use of alcohol; infants <1 month of age because of the possibility of producing hemolytic anemia; MAO inhibitors, tyramine-containing foods

Precautions Use with caution in patients with G-6-PD deficiency

Adverse Reactions

Cardiovascular: Hypotension

Central nervous system: Dizziness, drowsiness, malaise, fever, headache, polyneuritis

Dermatologic: Rash

Endocrine & metabolic: Hypoglycemia, disulfiram-like reaction after alcohol ingestion

Gastrointestinal: Nausea, vomiting, diarrhea

Genitourinary: Discoloration of urine (brown)

Hematologic: Agranulocytosis, hemolysis in patients with G-6-PD deficiency and neonates, leukopenia

Respiratory: Pulmonary infiltration

Miscellaneous: Hypersensitivity reactions including angioedema, hypotension, fever, urticaria, arthralgia

Drug Interactions Adrenergic agents, tricyclic antidepressants, MAO inhibitors (may increase hypertensive effect); alcohol (may cause disulfiram-like reactions)

Food Interactions Avoid tyramine-containing foods (cheese, broad beans, dry or aged sausage, nonfresh meat, liver, salami, mortadella, concentrated yeast extracts, liquid and powdered protein supplements, fermented bean curd and soya bean, meat extract and hydrolyzed protein extracts, raspberries, Chianti wine, Kimchee, or sauerkraut)

Stability Protect from light

Mechanism of Action Inhibits several vital enzymatic reactions causing antibacterial and antiprotozoal action; acts as a monoamine oxidase inhibitor and may prevent acetylation of coenzyme A

Pharmacokinetics

Absorption: Oral: Poor

Metabolism: Inactivated in the intestine

Elimination: 5% of oral dose excreted in urine as active drug and metabolites

Usual Dosage Oral:

Children >1 month: 5-8.8 mg/kg/day divided every 6 hours, not to exceed 400 mg/day

(Continued)

Furazolidone (Continued)

Adults: 100 mg 4 times/day

Administration Oral: May be administered without regard to food

Monitoring Parameters CBC

Test Interactions False-positive results for urine glucose with Clinitest®

Patient Information May discolor urine to a brown tint; avoid alcohol during treatment and for 4 days after discontinuing furazolidone; avoid tyramine-containing foods (see Food Interactions)

Dosage Forms

Suspension: 50 mg/15 mL (60 mL, 473 mL)

Tablet: 100 mg

References

Murphy TV and Nelson JD, "Five vs Ten Days' Therapy With Furazolidone for Giardiasis," *Am J Dis Child*, 1983, 137(3):267-70.

Turner JA, "Giardiasis and Infections With Dientamoeba Fragilis," *Pediatr Clin North Am*, 1985, 32(4):865-80.

♦ **Furazosin** see Prazosin on page 820

Furosemide (fyoor OH se mide)

Related Information

Carbohydrate and Alcohol Content of Liquid Medications for Use in Patients Receiving Ketogenic Diets on page 1258

U.S. Brand Names Lasix®

Canadian Brand Names Apo-Furosemide; Furoside; Lasix Special; Novo-Semide

Therapeutic Category Antihypertensive Agent; Diuretic, Loop

Generic Available Yes

Use Management of edema associated with CHF and hepatic or renal disease; used alone or in combination with antihypertensives in treatment of hypertension

Pregnancy Risk Factor C

Contraindications Hypersensitivity to furosemide or any component; anuria

Warnings Loop diuretics are potent diuretics; excess amounts can lead to profound diuresis with fluid and electrolyte loss

Precautions Hepatic cirrhosis (rapid alterations in fluid/electrolytes may precipitate coma)

Adverse Reactions

Cardiovascular: Orthostatic hypotension

Central nervous system: Dizziness, vertigo, headache

Dermatologic: Urticaria, photosensitivity

Endocrine & metabolic: Hypokalemia, hyponatremia, hypomagnesemia, hypocalcemia, hyperglycemia, hypochloremia, alkalosis, dehydration, hyperuricemia

Gastrointestinal: Pancreatitis, nausea; oral solutions may cause diarrhea due to sorbitol content; anorexia, vomiting, constipation, abdominal cramping

Hematologic: Agranulocytosis, anemia, thrombocytopenia

Hepatic: Ischemic hepatitis, jaundice

Otic: Potential ototoxicity

Renal: Nephrocalcinosis, prerenal azotemia, interstitial nephritis, hypercalciuria

Drug Interactions Indomethacin decreases the effect of furosemide; decreased lithium excretion; decreased glucose tolerance with antidiabetic agents; increased ototoxicity with aminoglycosides and ethacrynic acid; drugs affected by potassium depletion (ie, digoxin); increased anticoagulant activity of warfarin; increased salicylate toxicity due to decreased excretion; decreased furosemide effects when administered at the same time as sucralfate

Food Interactions Do not mix with acidic solutions; limit intake of natural licorice (causes sodium and water retention and increases potassium loss)

Stability Furosemide injection should be stored at controlled room temperature and protected from light; exposure to light may cause discoloration; do not use furosemide solutions if they have a yellow color; refrigeration may result in precipitation or crystallization, however, resolubilization at room temperature or warming may be performed without affecting the stability; furosemide solutions are unstable in acidic media but very stable in basic media; I.V. infusion solution mixed in NS or D_5W solution is stable for 24 hours at room temperature

Mechanism of Action Inhibits reabsorption of sodium and chloride in the ascending loop of Henle and distal renal tubule, interfering with the chloride-binding cotransport system, thus causing increased excretion of water, potassium, sodium, chloride, magnesium, and calcium

Pharmacodynamics

Onset of action:
Oral: Within 30-60 minutes
I.M.: 30 minutes
I.V.: 5 minutes
Peak effect: Oral: Within 1-2 hours
Duration:
Oral: 6-8 hours
I.V.: 2 hours

Pharmacokinetics

Absorption: 65% in patients with normal renal function, decreases to 45% in patients with renal failure
Protein binding: 98%
Half-life: Adults:
Normal renal function: 30 minutes
Renal failure: 9 hours
Elimination: 50% of oral dose and 80% of I.V. dose excreted unchanged in the urine within 24 hours; the remainder is eliminated by other nonrenal pathways including liver metabolism and excretion of unchanged drug in feces

Usual Dosage

Neonates, premature: (see Additional Information)
Oral: Bioavailability is poor by this route; doses of 1-4 mg/kg/dose 1-2 times/day have been used
I.M., I.V.: 1-2 mg/kg/dose given every 12-24 hours
Infants and Children:
Oral: 1-6 mg/kg/day divided every 6-12 hours
I.M., I.V.: 1-2 mg/kg/dose every 6-12 hours
Continuous infusion: 0.05 mg/kg/hour; titrate dosage to clinical effect
Adults:
Oral: Initial: 20-80 mg/dose; increase in increments of 20-40 mg/dose at intervals of 6-8 hours; usual maintenance dose interval is twice daily or every day; may be titrated up to 600 mg/day with severe edematous states
I.M., I.V.: 20-40 mg/dose; repeat in 1-2 hours as needed and increase by 20 mg/dose until the desired effect has been obtained; usual dosing interval: 6-12 hours; for acute pulmonary edema, the usual dose is 40 mg I.V.; if not adequate, may increase dose to 80 mg
Continuous I.V. infusion: Initial I.V. bolus dose of 0.1 mg/kg followed by continuous I.V. infusion doses of 0.1 mg/kg/hour doubled every 2 hours to a maximum of 0.4 mg/kg/hour

Dosing adjustment in renal impairment: Adults: Acute renal failure: High doses (up to 1-3 g/day - oral/I.V.) have been used to initiate desired response; avoid use in oliguric states
Dialysis: Not removed by hemo- or peritoneal dialysis; supplemental dose is not necessary

Dosing adjustment in hepatic disease: Diminished natriuretic effect with increased sensitivity to hypokalemia and volume depletion in cirrhosis; monitor effects, particularly with high doses

Administration

Oral: May administer with food or milk to decrease GI distress
Parenteral: I.V.: May be administered undiluted direct I.V. at a maximum rate of 0.5 mg/kg/minute for doses <120 mg and 4 mg/minute for doses >120 mg; may also be diluted for infusion 1-2 mg/mL (maximum concentration: 10 mg/mL) over 10-15 minutes (following maximum rate as above)

Monitoring Parameters Serum electrolytes, renal function, blood pressure, hearing (if high dosages used)

Additional Information Single dose studies utilizing nebulized furosemide at 1-2 mg/kg/dose (diluted to a final volume of 2 mL with NS) have been shown to be effective in improving pulmonary function in preterm infants with bronchopulmonary dysplasia undergoing mechanical ventilation; no diuresis or systemic side effects were noted

Dosage Forms

Injection: 10 mg/mL (2 mL, 4 mL, 8 mL, 10 mL)
Solution, oral: 10 mg/mL (60 mL, 120 mL); 40 mg/5 mL (5 mL, 500 mL)
Tablet: 20 mg, 40 mg, 80 mg

References

Copeland JG, Campbell DW, Plachetka JR, et al, "Diuresis With Continuous Infusion of Furosemide After Cardiac Surgery," *Am J Surg*, 1983, 146(6):796-9.
Pai VB and Nahata MC, "Aerosolized Furosemide in the Treatment of Acute Respiratory Distress and Possible Bronchopulmonary Dysplasia in Preterm Neonates," *Ann Pharmacother*, 2000, 34(3):386-92.

(Continued)

Furosemide *(Continued)*

Rastogi A, Luayon M, Ajayi OA, et al, "Nebulized Furosemide in Infants With Bronchopulmonary Dysplasia," *J Pediatr*, 1994, 125(6 Pt 1):976-9.

Rudy DW, Voelker JR, Greene PK, et al, "Loop Diuretics for Chronic Renal Insufficiency: A Continuous Infusion Is More Efficacious Than Bolus Therapy," *Ann Intern Med*, 1991, 115(5):360-6.

♦ **Furoside (Can)** *see* Furosemide *on page 462*

♦ **Furoxone**® *see* Furazolidone *on page 461*

Gabapentin (GA ba pen tin)

Related Information
Antiepileptic Drugs *on page 1208*

U.S. Brand Names Neurontin®

Therapeutic Category Anticonvulsant, Miscellaneous

Generic Available No

Use Adjunct for treatment of partial seizures in children >12 years and adults (with or without secondary generalized seizures); adjunct for treatment of partial seizures in children 3-12 years of age

Pregnancy Risk Factor C

Contraindications Hypersensitivity to gabapentin or any component

Warnings Neuropsychiatric adverse events, such as emotional lability (eg, behavioral problems), hostility, aggressive behaviors, thought disorder (eg, problems with concentration and school performance) and hyperkinesia (eg, hyperactivity and restlessness), have been reported in pediatric patients (see Adverse Reactions); abrupt withdrawal may precipitate status epilepticus or increase in seizures; decrease dose gradually over at least 1 week

Precautions Use with caution and decrease the dose in patients with renal dysfunction; in male (but not female) rats receiving gabapentin, a high incidence of pancreatic acinar adenocarcinoma was noted, the clinical significance in humans is unknown; effectiveness in children <3 years is not established

Adverse Reactions

Central nervous system: Somnolence, dizziness, ataxia, fatigue, depression, nervousness, fever; neuropsychiatric adverse events in children 3-12 years of age: Emotional lability (behavioral problems): 6% incidence; hostility (including aggressive behaviors): 5.2%; hyperkinesia (hyperactivity, restlessness): 4.7%; thought disorder (problems with concentration and school performance): 1.7%; **Note:** Most of these pediatric neuropsychiatric adverse events are mild to moderate in terms of intensity but discontinuation of gabapentin may be required; children with mental retardation and attention deficit disorders may be at increased risk for behavioral side effects

Dermatologic: Pruritus

Gastrointestinal: Dyspepsia, constipation, nausea, vomiting, weight gain

Genitourinary: Impotence

Hematologic: Leukopenia

Neuromuscular & skeletal: Back pain, dysarthria, tremor, myalgia

Ocular: Nystagmus, diplopia

Drug Interactions Antacids reduce the bioavailability of gabapentin by 20% (separate administration times by at least 2 hours); cimetidine may decrease the clearance of gabapentin (minor effect); gabapentin may increase levels of norethindrone (minor effect); gabapentin does not alter the pharmacokinetics of other antiepileptic drugs

Food Interactions Food slightly increases rate and extent of absorption (AUC and peak increase by 14%)

Stability Refrigerate oral solution

Mechanism of Action Not fully elucidated, most likely binds to an undefined neuroreceptor in the brain that is possibly linked with, or identical to a site resembling the L-system amino acid carrier protein; although structurally similar to the inhibitory neurotransmitter, gamma-aminobutyric acid (GABA), gabapentin does not significantly affect the GABA system; it does **not** bind to GABA receptors, affect GABA neuronal uptake nor mimic GABA effects

Pharmacokinetics

Absorption: Very rapid; via an active (ie, facilitated transport) saturable process; dose-dependent

Distribution: V_d: Adults: 50-60 L or 0.65-1.04 L/kg; CSF concentrations are ~20% of plasma concentrations; distributes to breast milk

Protein binding: <3% (not clinically significant)

Metabolism: Not metabolized

Bioavailability: ~60% (300 mg dose); bioavailability decreases with increasing doses

Time to peak serum concentration: Infants 1 month to Children 12 years and Adults: 2-3 hours

Half-life, elimination:

Infants 1 month to Children 12 years: 4.7 hours

Adults, normal: 5.3 hours (range: 5-9); increased half-life with decreased renal function; anuric adult patients: 132 hours; adults on hemodialysis: 51 hours

Elimination: Excreted unchanged in the urine (75% to 80%) and feces (10% to 20%)

Clearance: (**Note:** Apparent oral clearance is directly proportional to Cl$_{cr}$): Clearance in infants is highly variable; oral clearance (per kg) in children <5 years of age is higher than in children ≥5 years of age

Usual Dosage Oral: **Note:** Do not exceed 12 hours between doses with 3 times/day dosing:

Children 3-12 years: Initial: 10-15 mg/kg/day divided in 3 doses/day; titrate dose upward over ~3 days; usual dose: Children 3-4 years: 40 mg/kg/day divided into 3 doses/day; children ≥5 to 12 years: 25-35 mg/kg/day divided into 3 doses/day; doses up to 50 mg/kg/day were well tolerated in one long-term study

Children >12 years and Adults: Initial: 300 mg 3 times/day; titrate dose upward if needed; usual dose: 900-1800 mg/day divided in 3 doses/day; doses up to 2400 mg/day divided in 3 doses/day are well tolerated long-term; maximum dose: 3600 mg/day

Dosing adjustment in renal impairment: Children ≥12 years and Adults:

Cl$_{cr}$ >60 mL/minute: Administer 400 mg 3 times daily

Cl$_{cr}$ 30-60 mL/minute: 300 mg twice daily

Cl$_{cr}$ 15-30 mL/minute: 300 mg/day

Cl$_{cr}$ <15 mL/minute: 150 mg/day or 300 mg every other day

Hemodialysis patients ≥12 years of age: Initial: Loading dose of 300-400 mg; give 200-300 mg after each 4-hour dialysis

Administration Oral: May be administered without regard to meals; administration with meals may decrease adverse GI effects; dose may be administered as combination of dosage forms; do not administer within 2 hours of magnesium- or aluminum-containing antacids

One pediatric study (Khurana, 1996) mixed the contents of the capsule in drinks (eg, orange juice) or food (eg, applesauce) for patients who could not swallow the capsule; oral solution is now available

Monitoring Parameters Seizure frequency and duration; renal function; weight; behavior in children

Reference Range Minimum effective serum concentration may be 2 µg/mL; **routine monitoring of drug levels is not required**

Test Interactions False positive urinary protein with N-Multistix SG® test

Patient Information Take only as prescribed; may cause dizziness and impair the ability to perform activities requiring mental alertness or physical coordination; may cause somnolence, and other symptoms and signs of CNS depression; do not operate machinery or drive a car until you have experience with the drug

Nursing Implications Doses should be titrated based on clinical response; content of capsule is bitter tasting

Additional Information Gabapentin is not effective for absence seizures; gabapentin does not induce liver enzymes

Dosage Forms

Capsule: 100 mg, 300 mg, 400 mg

Solution, oral: 250 mg/5 mL [cool strawberry anise flavor] (480 mL)

Tablet, film-coated: 600 mg, 800 mg

References

Andrews CO and Fischer JH, "Gabapentin: A New Agent for the Management of Epilepsy," *Ann Pharmacother*, 1994, 28(10):1188-96.

Bourgeois BF, "Antiepileptic Drugs in Pediatric Practice," *Epilepsia*, 1995, 36(Suppl 2):S34-45.

Khurana DS, Riviello J, Helmers S, et al, "Efficacy of Gabapentin Therapy in Children With Refractory Partial Seizures," *J Pediatr*, 1996, 128(6):829-33.

Lee DO, Steingard RJ, Cesena M, et al, "Behavioral Side Effects of Gabapentin in Children," *Epilepsia*, 1996, 37(1):87-90.

Leiderman D, Garofalo E, and LaMoreaux L, "Gabapentin Patients With Absence Seizures: Two Double-Blind, Placebo Controlled Studies," *Epilepsia*, 1993, 34(Suppl 6):45 (abstract).

Pellock JM, "Managing Pediatric Epilepsy Syndromes With New Antiepileptic Drugs," *Pediatrics*, 1999, 104(5 Pt 1):1106-16.

Pressler KL, Jabbour JT, Rose DF, et al, "Gabapentin and Aggression in Pediatric Patients: A Review of the Literature," *Journal of Pediatric Pharmacy Practice*, 1998, 3(2):100-5.

♦ **Gabitril**® *see* Tiagabine *on page 957*

♦ **Galzin**™ *see* Zinc Supplements *on page 1026*

♦ **Gamimune**® **N** *see* Immune Globulin (Intravenous) *on page 529*

♦ **Gamma Benzene Hexachloride** *see* Lindane *on page 595*

♦ **Gammagard**® *see* Immune Globulin (Intravenous) *on page 529*

♦ **Gammagard® S/D** *see* Immune Globulin (Intravenous) *on page 529*

♦ **Gammar®-P I.V.** *see* Immune Globulin (Intravenous) *on page 529*

Ganciclovir (gan SYE kloe veer)

U.S. Brand Names Cytovene®; Vitrasert®

Synonyms DHPG; GCV; Nordeoxyguanosine

Therapeutic Category Antiviral Agent, Oral; Antiviral Agent, Parenteral

Generic Available No

Use Treatment of cytomegalovirus (CMV) retinitis in immunocompromised patients, as well as CMV GI infections and pneumonitis; prevention of CMV disease in transplant patients who have been diagnosed with latent or active CMV; ganciclovir also has antiviral activity against herpes simplex virus types 1 and 2

Pregnancy Risk Factor C

Contraindications Absolute neutrophil count <500/mm^3; platelet count <25,000/mm^3; hypersensitivity to ganciclovir, acyclovir, or any component

Warnings Ganciclovir may adversely affect spermatogenesis and fertility; due to its mutagenic potential, contraceptive precautions for female and male patients need to be followed during and for at least 90 days after therapy with the drug; ganciclovir is potentially carcinogenic

Precautions Dosage adjustment or interruption of ganciclovir therapy may be necessary in patients with neutropenia and/or thrombocytopenia and patients with impaired renal function; use with extreme caution in children since long-term safety has not been determined and due to ganciclovir's potential for long-term carcinogenic and adverse reproductive effects

Adverse Reactions

Cardiovascular: Edema, arrhythmias, hypertension

Central nervous system: Headaches, seizure, confusion, nervousness, dizziness, hallucinations, coma, fever, encephalopathy, malaise

Dermatologic: Rash, pruritus, urticaria, acne

Gastrointestinal: Nausea, vomiting, diarrhea, pancreatitis

Hematologic: Neutropenia (oral ganciclovir is associated with less neutropenia and fewer bacterial infections than I.V. ganciclovir), thrombocytopenia, leukopenia, anemia, eosinophilia

Hepatic: Elevated liver function tests

Local: Phlebitis

Ocular: Retinal detachment, photophobia, abnormal vision, loss of vision

Renal: Hematuria, elevated BUN and serum creatinine

Respiratory: Dyspnea

Drug Interactions Zidovudine (pancytopenia), imipenem/cilastatin (seizures), immunosuppressive agents increase suppression of bone marrow; amphotericin B, tacrolimus, cyclosporine increase nephrotoxicity; probenecid decreases renal clearance of ganciclovir; increases didanosine AUC (increases risk of peripheral neuropathy, pancreatitis)

Food Interactions High fat meal may increase AUC by 22%

Stability Reconstituted solution is stable for 12 hours at room temperature; **do not refrigerate**; reconstitute with sterile water **not** bacteriostatic water because parabens may cause precipitation; diluted I.V. ganciclovir solutions in D$_5$W or NS with a concentration <10 mg/mL are stable for 24 hours

Mechanism of Action Ganciclovir is phosphorylated to a substrate which competitively inhibits the binding of deoxyguanosine triphosphate to DNA polymerase; ganciclovir triphosphate competes with deoxyguanosine triphosphate for incorporation into viral DNA and interferes with viral DNA chain elongation resulting in inhibition of viral replication

Pharmacokinetics

Absorption: Oral: Poor

Distribution: Distributes to most body fluids, tissues, and organs including the eyes and brain

Protein binding: 1% to 2%

Bioavailability: Fasting: 5%; following food: 6% to 9%

Half-life (prolonged with impaired renal function):

Neonates 2-49 days of age: 2.4 hours

Adults: Mean: 2.5-3.6 hours (range: 1.7-5.8 hours)

Time to peak serum concentration: Oral: 2-2.5 hours

Elimination: Majority (80% to 99%) excreted as unchanged drug in the urine

Dialysis: 40% to 50% removed by a 4-hour hemodialysis

Usual Dosage

Slow I.V. infusion:

Retinitis: Children >3 months and Adults:

Induction therapy: 10 mg/kg/day divided every 12 hours as a 1- to 2-hour infusion for 14-21 days

Maintenance therapy: 5 mg/kg/day as a single daily dose for 7 days/week or 6 mg/kg/day for 5 days/week

Prevention of CMV disease in transplant recipients: Children and Adults:

Initial: 10 mg/kg/day divided every 12 hours for 7-14 days, followed by 5 mg/kg/day once daily 7 days/week or 6 mg/kg/day once daily 5 days/week for 100 days

Lung/heart-lung transplant patients (CMV + donor with CMV + recipient): 6 mg/kg/day once daily for 28 days

Other CMV infections: Children and Adults: Initial: 10 mg/kg/day divided every 12 hours for 14-21 days or 7.5 mg/kg/day divided every 8 hours; maintenance therapy: 5 mg/kg/day as a single daily dose for 7 days/week or 6 mg/kg/day for 5 days/week

Note: Preliminary data indicates that a higher initial dose of 15 mg/kg/day divided every 12 hours and more prolonged treatment may be more effective in infants with symptomatic congenital CMV infection

Oral (following induction treatment with I.V. ganciclovir):

Children: Maintenance dose, prophylaxis of CMV disease: In a study of 36 children 6 months to 16 years of age, 30 mg/kg/dose every 8 hours with food produced serum levels similar to the 1000 mg 3 times/day dose that is effective for maintenance treatment of CMV retinitis in adults (see Frenkel, 2000).

Adults: Maintenance: 1000 mg 3 times/day **or** 500 mg 6 times/day every 3 hours during waking hours

Sustained release intravitreal implant: CMV retinitis:

Children ≥9 years: One implant every 6-9 months plus ganciclovir 30 mg/kg/dose orally 3 times/day

Adults: One implant every 6-9 months plus ganciclovir 1-1.5 g orally 3 times/day

Dosing interval in renal impairment:

Oral: Adults:

Cl_{cr} 50-69 mL/minute: Administer 1500 mg/day or 500 mg 3 times/day

Cl_{cr} 25-49 mL/minute: Administer 1000 mg/day or 500 mg twice daily

Cl_{cr} 10-24 mL/minute: Administer 500 mg/day

Cl_{cr} <10 mL/minute: Administer 500 mg 3 times/week following hemodialysis

I.V. induction:

Cl_{cr} 50-69 mL/minute: Administer 2.5 mg/kg every 12 hours

Cl_{cr} 25-49 mL/minute: Administer 2.5 mg/kg every 24 hours

Cl_{cr} 10-24 mL/minute: Administer 1.25 mg/kg every 24 hours

Cl_{cr} <10 mL/minute: Administer 1.25 mg/kg/dose 3 times/week following hemodialysis

I.V. maintenance:

Cl_{cr} 50-69 mL/minute: Administer 2.5 mg/kg/dose every 24 hours

Cl_{cr} 25-49 mL/minute: Administer 1.25 mg/kg/dose every 24 hours

Cl_{cr} 10-24 mL/minute: Administer 0.625 mg/kg/dose every 24 hours

Cl_{cr} <10 mL/minute: Administer 0.625 mg/kg/dose 3 times/week following hemodialysis

Administration Follow same precautions utilized with antineoplastic agents when preparing and administering ganciclovir

Oral: Do not open or crush ganciclovir capsules; administer with food

Parenteral: Do not administer I.M. or S.C. since the reconstituted ganciclovir injection may cause severe tissue irritation due to its high pH; administer by slow I.V. infusion over at least 1 hour at a final concentration for administration not to exceed 10 mg/mL; infuse through a 0.22-5 micron in-line filter

Monitoring Parameters CBC with differential and platelet count, urine output, serum creatinine, ophthalmologic exams, liver function tests

Nursing Implications Handle and dispose according to guidelines issued for cytotoxic drugs; avoid direct contact of skin or mucous membranes with the powder contained in capsules or the I.V. solution; to minimize the risk of phlebitis, infuse through a large vein with adequate blood flow; maintain adequate patient hydration

Additional Information Sodium content of 1 g: 4 mEq

Dosage Forms

Capsule: 250 mg

Implant, intravitreal: 4.5 mg (released gradually over 5-8 months)

Powder for injection, lyophilized, as sodium: 500 mg

Extemporaneous Preparations A 100 mg/mL suspension can be prepared in a vertical flow hood by emptying eighty 250 mg capsules of ganciclovir into a glass *(Continued)*

Ganciclovir *(Continued)*

mortar wetted and triturated with Ora-Sweet® to a smooth paste. Add 50 mL of Ora-Sweet® to the paste, mix, and transfer contents to an amber polyethylene terephthate bottle. Rinse the mortar with 50 mL of Ora-Sweet® and transfer contents to the bottle. Rinse the mortar with the last third of the vehicle and transfer contents to the bottle. Add enough vehicle to make a final volume of 200 mL. The suspension is stable for 123 days when stored at 23°C to 25°C.

Anaizi NH, Swenson CF, and Dentinger PJ, "Stability of Ganciclovir in Extemporaneously Compounded Oral Liquids," *Am J Health Syst Pharm*, 1999, 56(17):1738-41.

References

Fletcher C, Sawchuk R, Chinnock B, et al, "Human Pharmacokinetics of the Antiviral Drug DHPG," *Clin Pharmacol Ther*, 1986, 40(3):281-6.

Frenkel LM, Capparelli EV, Dankner WM, et al, "Oral Ganciclovir in Children: Pharmacokinetics, Safety, Tolerance, and Antiviral Effects," *J Infect Dis*, 2000, 182(6):1616-24.

Goodrich JM, Bowden RA, Fisher L, et al, "Ganciclovir Prophylaxis to Prevent Cytomegalovirus Disease After Allogeneic Marrow Transplant," *Ann Intern Med*, 1993, 118(3):173-8.

Gudnason T, Belani KK, and Balfour HH Jr, "Ganciclovir Treatment of Cytomegalovirus Disease in Immunocompromised Children," *Pediatr Infect Dis J*, 1989, 8(7):436-40.

Merigan TC, Renlund DG, Keay S, et al, "A Controlled Trial of Ganciclovir to Prevent Cytomegalovirus Disease After Heart Transplantation," *N Engl J Med*, 1992, 326(18):1182-6.

"1999 USPHS/IDSA Guidelines for the Prevention of Opportunistic Infections in Persons Infected With Human Immunodeficiency Virus. U.S. Public Health Service (USPHS) and Infectious Diseases Society of America (IDSA)," *MMWR*, 1999, 48(RR-10):66.

- ◆ **Gani-Tuss® NR** *see* Guaifenesin and Codeine *on page 486*
- ◆ **Gantanol®** *see* Sulfamethoxazole *on page 925*
- ◆ **Gantrisin®** *see* Sulfisoxazole *on page 928*
- ◆ **Garamycin®** *see* Gentamicin *on page 469*
- ◆ **Garatec (Can)** *see* Gentamicin *on page 469*
- ◆ **Gastrocrom®** *see* Cromolyn *on page 273*
- ◆ **Gas-X® [OTC]** *see* Simethicone *on page 902*
- ◆ **Gas-X® Maximum Strength [OTC]** *see* Simethicone *on page 902*
- ◆ **Gaviscon® [OTC]** *see* Antacid Preparations *on page 95*
- ◆ **G-CSF** *see* Filgrastim *on page 425*
- ◆ **GCV** *see* Ganciclovir *on page 466*
- ◆ **Gel-Kam®** *see* Fluoride *on page 441*
- ◆ **Genac® [OTC]** *see* Triprolidine and Pseudoephedrine *on page 989*
- ◆ **Genahist® [OTC]** *see* Diphenhydramine *on page 342*
- ◆ **Gen-Alprazolam (Can)** *see* Alprazolam *on page 55*
- ◆ **Gen-Amantadine (Can)** *see* Amantadine *on page 62*
- ◆ **Gen-Amiodarone (Can)** *see* Amiodarone *on page 72*
- ◆ **Gen-Amoxicillin (Can)** *see* Amoxicillin *on page 80*
- ◆ **Genapap® [OTC]** *see* Acetaminophen *on page 29*
- ◆ **Genaphed® [OTC]** *see* Pseudoephedrine *on page 852*
- ◆ **Genasal® [OTC]** *see* Oxymetazoline *on page 749*
- ◆ **Genasoft® Plus [OTC]** *see* Docusate and Casanthranol *on page 351*
- ◆ **Genasyme® [OTC]** *see* Simethicone *on page 902*
- ◆ **Gen-Atenolol (Can)** *see* Atenolol *on page 111*
- ◆ **Genatuss® [OTC]** *see* Guaifenesin *on page 485*
- ◆ **Genatuss DM® [OTC]** *see* Guaifenesin and Dextromethorphan *on page 487*
- ◆ **Gen-Azathioprine (Can)** *see* Azathioprine *on page 121*
- ◆ **Gen-Baclofen (Can)** *see* Baclofen *on page 129*
- ◆ **Gen-Beclo AQ (Can)** *see* Beclomethasone *on page 131*
- ◆ **Gen-Budesonide (Can)** *see* Budesonide *on page 154*
- ◆ **Gen-Captopril (Can)** *see* Captopril *on page 173*
- ◆ **Gen-Carbamazepine (Can)** *see* Carbamazepine *on page 175*
- ◆ **Gen-Cimetidine (Can)** *see* Cimetidine *on page 234*
- ◆ **Gen-Cyclobenzaprine (Can)** *see* Cyclobenzaprine *on page 278*
- ◆ **Gen-Diltiazem (Can)** *see* Diltiazem *on page 337*
- ◆ **Genebs® [OTC]** *see* Acetaminophen *on page 29*
- ◆ **Gen-Famotidine (Can)** *see* Famotidine *on page 417*
- ◆ **Genfiber® [OTC]** *see* Psyllium *on page 853*
- ◆ **Gen-Fluoxetine (Can)** *see* Fluoxetine *on page 445*
- ◆ **Gen-Glybe (Can)** *see* Glyburide *on page 476*
- ◆ **Gen-Ipratropium (Can)** *see* Ipratropium *on page 547*

♦ **Gen-Medroxy (Can)** *see* Medroxyprogesterone *on page 624*
♦ **Gen-Metformin (Can)** *see* Metformin *on page 639*
♦ **Gen-Metoprolol (Type L) (Can)** *see* Metoprolol *on page 660*
♦ **Gen-Nifedipine (Can)** *see* Nifedipine *on page 714*
♦ **Gen-Nortriptyline (Can)** *see* Nortriptyline *on page 724*
♦ **Genoptic®** *see* Gentamicin *on page 469*
♦ **Genotropin® Injection** *see* Human Growth Hormone *on page 498*
♦ **Gen-Oxybutynin (Can)** *see* Oxybutynin *on page 744*
♦ **Gen-Piroxicam (Can)** *see* Piroxicam *on page 806*
♦ **Genpril® [OTC]** *see* Ibuprofen *on page 520*
♦ **Gen-Ranitidine (Can)** *see* Ranitidine *on page 865*
♦ **Gen-Salbutamol (Can)** *see* Albuterol *on page 45*
♦ **Gentacidin®** *see* Gentamicin *on page 469*
♦ **Gent-AK®** *see* Gentamicin *on page 469*

Gentamicin (jen ta MYE sin)

Related Information
Blood Level Sampling Time Guidelines *on page 1220*
Endocarditis Prophylaxis *on page 1160*
Overdose and Toxicology *on page 1222*

U.S. Brand Names Garamycin®; Genoptic®; Gentacidin®; Gent-AK®; Gentrasul®; G-myticin®; Jenamicin®

Canadian Brand Names Alcomicin; Diogent; Garatec; Minims-Gentamicin

Therapeutic Category Antibiotic, Aminoglycoside; Antibiotic, Ophthalmic; Antibiotic, Topical

Generic Available Yes

Use Treatment of susceptible bacterial infections, normally gram-negative organisms including *Pseudomonas, E. coli, Proteus, Serratia,* and gram-positive *Staphylococcus;* treatment of bone infections, CNS infections, respiratory tract infections, skin and soft tissue infections, as well as abdominal and urinary tract infections, endocarditis, and septicemia; used in combination with ampicillin as empiric therapy for sepsis in newborns; used topically to treat superficial infections of the skin or ophthalmic infections caused by susceptible bacteria

Pregnancy Risk Factor D

Contraindications Hypersensitivity to gentamicin, any component, or other aminoglycosides

Warnings Parenteral aminoglycosides are associated with significant nephrotoxicity or ototoxicity; the ototoxicity is directly proportional to the amount of drug given and the duration of treatment; tinnitus or vertigo are indications of vestibular injury and impending irreversible bilateral deafness; renal damage is usually reversible and is associated with decreased creatinine clearance and urine specific gravity, elevated BUN and serum creatinine, casts in the urine, oliguria, and proteinuria; some formulations contain sulfites which may cause allergic reactions. Aminoglycosides can cause fetal harm when administered to a pregnant woman; aminoglycosides have been associated with several reports of total irreversible bilateral congenital deafness in pediatric patients exposed *in utero.*

Precautions Use with caution in neonates due to renal immaturity that results in a prolonged gentamicin half-life and in patients with pre-existing renal impairment, auditory or vestibular impairment, hypocalcemia, myasthenia gravis, and in conditions which depress neuromuscular transmission; modify dosage in patients with renal impairment and in neonates on extracorporeal membrane oxygenation (ECMO)

Adverse Reactions
Central nervous system: Vertigo, ataxia, gait instability, dizziness, headache, fever
Dermatologic: Rash, pruritus, erythema
Endocrine & metabolic: Hypomagnesemia
Gastrointestinal: Nausea, vomiting, anorexia
Genitourinary: Decrease in urine specific gravity, casts in urine, possible electrolyte wasting
Hematologic: Granulocytopenia, thrombocytopenia, eosinophilia
Hepatic: Elevated AST and ALT
Local: Thrombophlebitis
Neuromuscular & skeletal: Neuromuscular blockade, muscle cramps, tremor, weakness
Ocular: Optic neuritis; ophthalmic use: burning, stinging, redness, lacrimation

(Continued)

Gentamicin *(Continued)*

Otic: Ototoxicity (may be associated with high serum aminoglycoside concentrations persisting for prolonged periods) with tinnitus, hearing loss; early toxicity usually affects high-pitched sound

Renal: Nephrotoxicity (high trough levels) with proteinuria, reduction in glomerular filtration rate, elevated serum creatinine

Drug Interactions Increased toxicity: Concurrent use of amphotericin B, magnesium, cephalosporins, penicillins, loop diuretics, vancomycin, cisplatin, indomethacin; potentiates effect of neuromuscular blocking agents and botulinum toxin

Stability Incompatible with penicillins, cephalosporins, heparin

Mechanism of Action Inhibits initiation of cellular bacterial protein synthesis by binding to 30S and 50S ribosomal subunits resulting in a defective bacterial cell membrane

Pharmacokinetics

Absorption: Oral: Poorly absorbed (<2%)

Distribution: Crosses the placenta; distributes primarily in the extracellular fluid volume and in most tissues; poor penetration into CSF; drug accumulates in the renal cortex; small amounts distribute into bile, sputum, saliva, tears, and breast milk

V_d: Increased in neonates and with fever, edema, ascites, fluid overload; V_d is decreased in patients with dehydration

Neonates: 0.45 ± 0.1 L/kg

Infants: 0.4 ± 0.1 L/kg

Children: 0.35 ± 0.15 L/kg

Adolescents: 0.3 ± 0.1 L/kg

Adults: 0.2-0.3 L/kg

Protein binding: <30%

Half-life:

Neonates:

<1 week: 3-11.5 hours

1 week to 1 month: 3-6 hours

Infants: 4 ± 1 hour

Children: 2 ± 1 hour

Adolescents: 1.5 ± 1 hour

Adults with normal renal function: 1.5-3 hours

Anuria: 36-70 hours

Time to peak serum concentration:

I.M.: Within 30-90 minutes

I.V.: 30 minutes after 30-minute infusion

Elimination: Clearance is directly related to renal function; eliminated almost completely by glomerular filtration of unchanged drug with excretion into urine

Clearance:

Neonates: 0.045 ± 0.01 L/hour/kg

Infants: 0.1 ± 0.05 L/hour/kg

Children: 0.1 ± 0.03 L/hour/kg

Adolescents: 0.09 ± 0.03 L/hour/kg

Dialysis: Dialyzable (50% to 100%)

Usual Dosage Dosage should be based on an estimate of ideal body weight, except in neonates (neonatal dosage should be based on actual weight unless the patient has hydrocephalus or hydrops fetalis):

Neonates: I.M., I.V.:

Premature neonate, <1000 g: 3.5 mg/kg/dose every 24 hours

0-4 weeks, <1200 g: 2.5 mg/kg/dose every 18-24 hours

Postnatal age ≤7 days: 2.5 mg/kg/dose every 12 hours

Postnatal age >7 days:

1200-2000 g: 2.5 mg/kg/dose every 8-12 hours

>2000 g: 2.5 mg/kg/dose every 8 hours

Initial dose for term neonates receiving ECMO: I.V.: 2.5 mg/kg/dose every 18 hours; subsequent doses should be individualized by monitoring serum drug concentrations; when ECMO is discontinued, dosage may require readjustment due to large shifts in body water

Infants and Children <5 years: I.M., I.V.: 2.5 mg/kg/dose every 8 hours*

Endocarditis prophylaxis (high-risk patients): 1.5 mg/kg (maximum: 120 mg) within 30 minutes of starting the procedure plus ampicillin or vancomycin (in patients allergic to ampicillin)

Pulmonary infection in cystic fibrosis: 2.5-3.3 mg/kg/dose every 6-8 hours

Patients on hemodialysis: 1.25-1.75 mg/kg/dose postdialysis

Children ≥5 years: I.M., I.V.: 2-2.5 mg/kg/dose every 8 hours*

Once daily dosing (investigational): 5-6 mg/kg/dose every 24 hours

Endocarditis prophylaxis (high-risk patients): 1.5 mg/kg (maximum: 120 mg) within 30 minutes of starting the procedure plus ampicillin or vancomycin (in patients allergic to ampicillin)

Pulmonary infection in cystic fibrosis: 2.5-3.3 mg/kg/dose every 6-8 hours

Patients on hemodialysis: 1.25-1.75 mg/kg/dose postdialysis

*Some patients may require larger or more frequent doses (eg, every 6 hours) if serum levels document the need (ie, cystic fibrosis, patients with major burns, or febrile granulocytopenic patients); modify dose based on individual patient requirements as determined by renal function, serum drug concentrations, and patient-specific clinical parameters

Intraventricular/intrathecal **(use a preservative free preparation)**:

Newborns: 1 mg/day

Infants >3 months and Children: 1-2 mg/day

Adults: 4-8 mg/day

Infants, Children, and Adults:

Topical: Apply 3-4 times/day

Ophthalmic:

Ointment: Apply 2-3 times/day

Solution: Instill 1-2 drops every 2-4 hours, up to 2 drops every hour for severe infections

Adults: I.M., I.V.: 3-6 mg/kg/day in divided doses every 8 hours; studies of once daily dosing have used I.V. doses of 4-6.6 mg/kg once daily

Endocarditis prophylaxis (high-risk patients): 1.5 mg/kg (maximum: 120 mg) within 30 minutes of starting the procedure plus ampicillin or vancomycin (in patients allergic to ampicillin)

Patients on hemodialysis: 0.5-0.7 mg/kg/dose postdialysis

Dosing adjustment in renal impairment: I.M., I.V.: 2.5 mg/kg** (Cl_{cr} <60 mL/minute/1.73 m^2)

**2-3 serum level measurements should be obtained after the initial dose to measure the patient's pharmacokinetic parameters (eg, half-life, V_d) in order to determine the frequency and amount of subsequent doses

Administration

Ophthalmic: Gentamicin solution is not for subconjunctival injection. Solution may be instilled into the affected eye or a small amount of ointment may be placed into the conjunctival sac. Avoid contaminating tip of the solution bottle or ointment tube. Solution: Apply finger pressure to lacrimal sac during and for 1-2 minutes after instillation to decrease risk of absorption and systemic effects.

Parenteral: Administer by I.M., I.V. slow intermittent infusion over 30-60 minutes or by direct injection over 15 minutes; final concentration for I.V. administration should not exceed 10 mg/mL; administer other antibiotics, such as penicillins and cephalosporins, at least 1 hour before or after gentamicin

Topical: Apply a small amount gently to the cleansed affected area

Monitoring Parameters Urinalysis, urine output, BUN, serum creatinine, peak and trough serum gentamicin concentrations, hearing test

Not all infants and children who receive aminoglycosides require monitoring of serum aminoglycoside concentrations. Indications for use of aminoglycoside serum concentration monitoring include:

Treatment course >5 days

Patients with decreased or changing renal function

Patients with poor therapeutic response

Infants <3 months of age

Atypical body constituency (obesity, expanded extracellular fluid volume)

Clinical need for higher doses or shorter intervals (eg, cystic fibrosis, burns, endocarditis, meningitis, critically ill patients, relatively resistant organism)

Patients on hemodialysis or chronic ambulatory peritoneal dialysis

Signs of nephrotoxicity or ototoxicity

Concomitant use of other nephrotoxic agents

Reference Range

Peak: 4-12 μg/mL; peak values are 2-3 times greater with once daily dosing regimens

Trough: 0.5-2 μg/mL

Test Interactions Aminoglycoside levels measured in blood taken from Silastic® central line catheters can sometimes give falsely high readings

Patient Information Report any dizziness or sensations of ringing or fullness in ears to the physician

Nursing Implications Obtain drug levels after the third or fourth dose except in neonates and patients with rapidly changing renal function in whom levels need to

(Continued)

Gentamicin *(Continued)*

be measured sooner; peak gentamicin serum concentrations are drawn 30 minutes after the end of a 30-minute I.V. infusion, immediately on completion of a 1-hour I.V. infusion, or 1 hour after an intramuscular injection; trough levels are drawn within 30 minutes before the next dose; provide adequate patient hydration and perfusion

Dosage Forms
Cream, topical, as sulfate: 0.1% (15 g)
Infusion, in D₅W, as sulfate: 60 mg, 80 mg, 100 mg
Infusion, in NS, as sulfate: 40 mg, 60 mg, 80 mg, 90 mg, 100 mg, 120 mg
Injection, as sulfate: 40 mg/mL (1 mL, 1.5 mL, 2 mL)
  Pediatric, as sulfate: 10 mg/mL (2 mL)
Ointment:
  Ophthalmic, as sulfate: 0.3% (3.5 g)
  Topical, as sulfate: 0.1% (15 g)
Solution, ophthalmic, as sulfate: 0.3% (1 mL, 5 mL, 15 mL)

References
Bhatt-Mehta V, Johnson CE and Schumacher RE, "Gentamicin Pharmacokinetics in Term Neonates Receiving Extracorporeal Membrane Oxygenation," *Pharmacotherapy*, 1992, 12(1):28-32.
Gilbert DN, "Once-Daily Aminoglycoside Therapy," *Antimicrob Agents Chemother*, 1991, 35(3):399-405.
Reimche LD, Rooney, ME, Hindmarsh KW, et al, "An Evaluation of Gentamicin Dosing According to Renal Function in Neonates With Suspected Sepsis," *Am J Perinatol*, 1987, 4(3):262-5.
Shevchuk YM and Taylor DM, "Aminoglycoside Volume of Distribution in Pediatric Patients," *DICP*, 1990, 24(3):273-6.

♦ **Gentamicin and Prednisolone** *see* Prednisolone and Gentamicin *on page 823*

Gentian Violet *(JEN shun VYE oh let)*

Synonyms Crystal Violet; Methylrosaniline Chloride
Therapeutic Category Antibacterial, Topical; Antifungal Agent, Topical
Generic Available Yes
Use Treatment of cutaneous or mucocutaneous infections caused by *Candida albicans* and other superficial skin infections refractory to topical nystatin, clotrimazole, miconazole, or econazole
Pregnancy Risk Factor C
Contraindications Hypersensitivity to gentian violet; ulcerated areas; patients with porphyria
Warnings May result in tattooing of the skin when applied to granulation tissue
Adverse Reactions
Dermatological: Staining of skin (purple), vesicle formation
Gastrointestinal: Esophagitis
Local: Burning, irritation, vesicle formation, sensitivity reactions, ulceration of mucous membranes
Respiratory: Laryngitis, tracheitis may result from swallowing gentian violet solution, laryngeal obstruction following frequent or prolonged use
Mechanism of Action Topical antiseptic/germicide effective against some vegetative gram-positive bacteria, particularly *Staphylococcus* species, and some yeast; it is much less effective against gram-negative bacteria and is ineffective against acid-fast bacteria
Usual Dosage Topical:
Infants: Apply 3-4 drops of a 0.5% solution under the tongue or on lesion after feedings
Children and Adults: Apply 1% to 2% solution to lesion 2-3 times/day for 3 days, do not swallow
Administration Topical: Apply to lesions with cotton; do not apply to ulcerative lesions on the face
Patient Information Drug stains skin and clothing purple; proper hygiene and skin care need to be used to prevent spread of infection and reinfection
Nursing Implications Keep affected area dry and exposed to air
Additional Information 0.25% or 0.5% solution is less irritating than a 1% to 2% solution and is reported to be as effective
Dosage Forms Solution, topical: 1% (30 mL); 2% (30 mL)

♦ **Gen-Timolol (Can)** *see* Timolol *on page 962*
♦ **Gentran®** *see* Dextran *on page 311*
♦ **Gentrasul®** *see* Gentamicin *on page 469*
♦ **Gen-Trazodone (Can)** *see* Trazodone *on page 977*
♦ **Gen-Triazolam (Can)** *see* Triazolam *on page 982*
♦ **Gen-Valproic (Can)** *see* Valproic Acid and Derivatives *on page 998*
♦ **Gen-Verapamil (Can)** *see* Verapamil *on page 1007*

♦ **Gen-XENE®** *see* Clorazepate *on page 257*

♦ **Geocillin®** *see* Carbenicillin *on page 179*

♦ **GG** *see* Guaifenesin *on page 485*

♦ **Glaucon®** *see* Epinephrine *on page 385*

♦ **Glibenclamide** *see* Glyburide *on page 476*

Glipizide (GLIP i zide)

U.S. Brand Names Glucotrol®; Glucotrol® XL

Synonyms Glydiazinamide

Therapeutic Category Antidiabetic Agent, Oral; Antidiabetic Agent, Sulfonylurea; Hypoglycemic Agent, Oral

Generic Available Yes

Use Management of type II diabetes mellitus (noninsulin-dependent, NIDDM) when hyperglycemia cannot be managed by diet alone; may be used concomitantly with metformin or insulin to improve glycemic control

Pregnancy Risk Factor C

Contraindications Hypersensitivity to glipizide, any component, or other sulfonamides; type 1 diabetes mellitus (insulin-dependent, IDDM), diabetic ketoacidosis with or without coma

Warnings Chemical similarities are present among sulfonamides, sulfonylureas, carbonic anhydrase inhibitors, thiazides, and loop diuretics (except ethacrynic acid), and although only glipizide use in patients with sulfonamide allergy is specifically contraindicated in product labeling, there is a risk of cross-reaction in patients with allergies to any of these compounds; use caution when the previous reaction has been severe; product labeling states oral hypoglycemic drugs may be associated with an increased cardiovascular mortality as compared to treatment with diet alone or diet plus insulin; data to support this association are limited, and several studies, including a large prospective trial (UKPDS) have not supported an association

Precautions Use with caution in patients with adrenal or pituitary insufficiency; hypoglycemic reactions are more prevalent in debilitated, malnourished patients, patients with mild disease or impaired hepatic or renal function; hypoglycemia may also occur with inadequate caloric intake, strenuous exercise, or concurrent use with other hypoglycemic drugs

Adverse Reactions

Cardiovascular: Edema, flushing, hypertension, arrhythmias

Central nervous system: Headache, dizziness, drowsiness, insomnia, anxiety, depression, migraine

Dermatologic: Rash, urticaria, photosensitivity

Endocrine & metabolic: Hypoglycemia, hyponatremia, weight gain

Gastrointestinal: Anorexia, nausea, vomiting, diarrhea, epigastric fullness, flatulence, constipation, heartburn

Genitourinary: Dysuria

Hematologic: Blood dyscrasias, aplastic anemia, hemolytic anemia, bone marrow suppression, thrombocytopenia, agranulocytosis

Hepatic: Cholestatic jaundice, elevated liver enzymes

Neuromuscular & skeletal: Arthralgia, leg cramps, myalgia

Ocular: Blurred vision, ocular pain, conjunctivitis

Renal: Diuretic effect (mild), SIADH, urolithiasis

Respiratory: Rhinitis, dyspnea

Drug Interactions Drugs which tend to produce hyperglycemia (eg, diuretics, corticosteroids, phenothiazines, thyroid products, estrogens, oral contraceptives, phenytoin, nicotinic acid, sympathomimetics, calcium channel-blocking drugs, rifampin, and isoniazid) may lead to a loss of glycemic control; disulfiram-like reactions with alcohol; drugs which produce an increase in glipizide's hypoglycemic effects: ACE inhibitors, cimetidine, chloramphenicol, anabolic steroids, monoamine oxidase inhibitors, fluoroquinolone antibiotics, and probencid; since this agent is highly protein bound, use of other protein-bound drugs may result in adverse effects when glipizide therapy is initiated or discontinued; beta-adrenergic blocking agents may impair glucose tolerance, increase the frequency or severity of hypoglycemia, block hypoglycemia-induced tachycardia, delay the rate of recovery of blood glucose concentration following drug-induced hypoglycemia, and may alter the hemodynamic response to hypoglycemia; glipizide may increase cyclosporine and tacrolimus serum concentrations; cholestyramine decreases glipizide absorption

Food Interactions Food delays absorption but does not affect the extent of absorption or peak levels achieved

Stability Store at room temperature; protect from light

(Continued)

Glipizide *(Continued)*

Mechanism of Action Stimulates insulin release from the pancreatic beta cells, reduces glucose output from the liver, and increases insulin sensitivity at peripheral target sites

Pharmacodynamics

Onset of action: Immediate release formulation: 15-30 minutes; extended release formulation: 2-3 hours

Peak response: Immediate release formulation: Within 2-3 hours; extended release formulation: 6-12 hours

Duration of action: Immediate release formulation: 12-24 hours; extended release formulation: 24 hours

Average decrease in fasting blood glucose (when used as monotherapy): 60-70 mg/dL

Pharmacokinetics

Absorption: Rapid and complete

Protein binding: 92% to 99%

Distribution: V_d: Adults: 11-25 L

Bioavailability: 80% to 100%

Time to peak serum concentration: Immediate release formulation: 1-3 hours

Metabolism: Extensive liver metabolism to inactive metabolites

Half-life: 2-4 hours

Elimination: 60% to 90% of drug excreted into urine within 24-72 hours as unchanged drug and metabolites; 5% to 20% excreted in feces within 24-96 hours

Usual Dosage Adults: Oral:

Management of noninsulin-dependent diabetes mellitus in patients **previously untreated:** Initial: 5 mg/day immediate release or extended release tablets; adjust dosage in 2.5-5 mg daily increments in intervals of 3-7 days for immediate release tablets or 5 mg daily increments in intervals of at least 7 days for extended release tablets; if total daily dose for immediate release tablets is >15 mg, divide into twice daily dosage; maximum daily dose for immediate release tablets: 40 mg; maximum daily dose for extended release tablets: 20 mg

Note: patients may be converted from immediate release tablets to extended release tablets by giving the nearest equivalent total daily dose once daily

Management of noninsulin-dependent diabetes mellitus in patients **previously maintained on insulin:** Initial dose dependent upon previous insulin dosage:

Insulin dosage ≤20 units/day: Use recommended initial dose and abruptly discontinue insulin

Insulin dosage >20 units/day: Use recommended initial dose and reduce daily insulin dosage by 50%; continue to withdraw daily insulin dosage gradually over several days as tolerated with incremental increases of glipizide

Dosing adjustment/comments in renal impairment: Cl_{cr} <10 mL/minute: Some investigators recommend not using

Dosing adjustment in hepatic impairment: Reduce initial dosage to 2.5 mg/day

Administration Oral: Administer 30 minutes before a meal; extended release tablets should be swallowed whole; do not cut, crush, or chew

Monitoring Parameters Signs and symptoms of hypoglycemia, fasting blood glucose, glycosylated hemoglobin (hemoglobin A_{1c})

Reference Range Target range:

Blood glucose: Fasting and preprandial: 80-120 mg/dL; bedtime: 100-140 mg/dL

Glycosylated hemoglobin (hemoglobin A_{1c}): <7%

Patient Information Do not change dose or discontinue without consulting prescriber; avoid alcohol while taking this medication, may cause severe reaction; maintain regular dietary intake and exercise routine; always carry quick source of sugar; if experiencing a hypoglycemic reaction, contact prescriber immediately; use sunscreen, wear protective clothing and eyewear, and avoid direct sunlight; report severe or persistent side effects, extended vomiting or flu-like symptoms, skin rash, easy bruising or bleeding, or change in color of urine or stool.

Additional Information When transferring from other sulfonylurea antidiabetic agents to glyburide, with the exception of chlorpropamide, the administration of the other agent may be abruptly discontinued; due to the prolonged elimination half-life of chlorpropamide, a 2- to 3-day drug-free interval may be advisable before glipizide therapy is begun

Dosage Forms

Tablet: 5 mg, 10 mg

Tablet, extended release: 2.5 mg, 5 mg, 10 mg

References

DeFronzo RA, "Pharmacologic Therapy for Type 2 Diabetes Mellitus," *Ann Intern Med*, 1999, 131(4):281-303.

"Intensive Blood-Glucose Control With Sulphonylureas or Insulin Compared With Conventional Treatment and Risk of Complications in Patients With Type 2 Diabetes (UKPDS 33) UK Prospective Diabetes Study (UKPDS) Group," *Lancet*, 1998, 352(9131):837-53.

♦ **GlucaGen®** *see* Glucagon (rDNA Origin) *on page 475*

♦ **Glucagon Diagnostic Kit** *see* Glucagon (rDNA Origin) *on page 475*

♦ **Glucagon Emergency Kit** *see* Glucagon (rDNA Origin) *on page 475*

Glucagon (rDNA Origin) (GLOO ka gon)

U.S. Brand Names GlucaGen®; Glucagon Diagnostic Kit; Glucagon Emergency Kit

Therapeutic Category Antihypoglycemic Agent

Generic Available No

Use Management of hypoglycemia; diagnostic aid in the radiologic examination of GI tract when a hypotonic state is needed; used with some success as a cardiac stimulant in management of severe cases of beta-adrenergic blocking agent overdosage

Pregnancy Risk Factor B

Contraindications Hypersensitivity to glucagon or any component

Warnings Use with caution in patients with a history of insulinoma and/or pheochromocytoma; because glucagon depletes glycogen stores, the patient should be given supplemental carbohydrates as soon as physically possible

Adverse Reactions
Cardiovascular: Hypotension
Dermatologic: Urticaria
Gastrointestinal: Nausea, vomiting
Respiratory: Respiratory distress
Miscellaneous: Hypersensitivity reactions

Drug Interactions Enhances anticoagulant effect of warfarin; phenytoin inhibits the stimulant effect of glucagon on insulin release by the islet cells; propranolol partially inhibits the hyperglycemic effect of glucagon

Stability Glucagon (rDNA origin) for injection (Lilly) should be stored at controlled room temperature; glucagon (rDNA origin) for injection (GlucaGen®) should be refrigerated; both injections should be used immediately after reconstitution

Mechanism of Action Glucagon (rDNA origin) is genetically engineered and identical to human glucagon. It stimulates adenylate cyclase to produce increased cyclic AMP. It promotes hepatic glycogenolysis and gluconeogenesis, causing an increase in blood glucose levels; produces both positive inotropic and chronotropic effects.

Pharmacodynamics
Blood glucose effect (after 1 mg dosage):
Onset of action: I.M.: 8-10 minutes; I.V.: 1 minute
Duration: I.M.: 12-27 minutes; I.V.: 9-17 minutes

GI tract effect:
Onset of action: Within 1-10 minutes
Duration: 12-30 minutes

Pharmacokinetics
Distribution: V_d: 0.25 L/kg
Metabolism: Extensively degraded in liver and kidneys
Half-life, plasma: 8-18 minutes
Clearance: 13.5 mL/minute/kg

Usual Dosage
Hypoglycemia or insulin shock therapy: I.M., I.V., S.C. (may repeat in 20 minutes as needed):
Neonates, Infants and Children ≤20 kg: 0.02-0.03 mg/kg or 0.5 mg
Children >20 kg and Adults: 1 mg
Diagnostic aid: Adults: I.M., I.V.: 0.25-2 mg 10 minutes prior to procedure

Administration Parenteral: Dilute with manufacturer provided diluent resulting in 1 mg/mL; if doses exceeding 2 mg are used, dilute with sterile water instead of diluent; administer by direct I.V. injection, I.M., or S.C.

Monitoring Parameters Blood glucose, blood pressure

Additional Information 1 unit = 1 mg

Dosage Forms
Powder for injection, lyophilized, as hydrochloride (Glucagon Diagnostic Kit, Glucagon Emergency Kit): 1 mg [1 unit] (diluent available in disposable syringe)
Powder for injection, lyophilized, as hydrochloride (GlucaGen®, Glucagon): 1 mg [1 unit]

♦ **Glucocerebrosidase** *see* Alglucerase *on page 52*

♦ **Glucodex (Can)** *see* Dextrose *on page 317*

♦ **Glucophage®** *see* Metformin *on page 639*

- **Glucophage® XR** *see* Metformin *on page 639*
- **Glucose** *see* Dextrose *on page 317*
- **Glucose Monohydrate** *see* Dextrose *on page 317*
- **Glucotrol®** *see* Glipizide *on page 473*
- **Glucotrol® XL** *see* Glipizide *on page 473*
- **Glutose® [OTC]** *see* Dextrose *on page 317*
- **Glybenclamide** *see* Glyburide *on page 476*
- **Glybenzcyclamide** *see* Glyburide *on page 476*

Glyburide (GLYE byoor ide)

U.S. Brand Names Diaβeta®; Glynase™ PresTab™; Micronase®

Canadian Brand Names Albert Glyburide; Apo-Glyburide; Euglucon; Gen-Glybe; Novo-Glyburide; Nu-Glyburide; PMS-Glyburide

Synonyms Glibenclamide; Glybenclamide; Glybenzcyclamide

Therapeutic Category Antidiabetic Agent, Oral; Antidiabetic Agent, Sulfonylurea; Hypoglycemic Agent, Oral

Generic Available Yes

Use Management of type II diabetes mellitus (noninsulin-dependent, NIDDM) when hyperglycemia cannot be managed by diet alone; may be used concomitantly with metformin or insulin to improve glycemic control

Pregnancy Risk Factor C

Contraindications Hypersensitivity to glyburide, any component, or other sulfonamides; type 1 diabetes mellitus (insulin-dependent, IDDM), diabetic ketoacidosis with or without coma

Warnings Chemical similarities are present among sulfonamides, sulfonylureas, carbonic anhydrase inhibitors, thiazides, and loop diuretics (except ethacrynic acid), and although only glyburide use in patients with sulfonamide allergy is specifically contraindicated in product labeling, there is a risk of cross-reaction in patients with allergies to any of these compounds; avoid use when the previous reaction has been severe; product labeling states oral hypoglycemic drugs may be associated with an increased cardiovascular mortality as compared to treatment with diet alone or diet plus insulin; data to support this association are limited, and several studies, including a large prospective trial (UKPDS) have not supported an association.

Precautions Use with caution in patients with adrenal or pituitary insufficiency; hypoglycemic reactions are more prevalent in debilitated, malnourished patients, patients with mild disease or impaired hepatic or renal function; hypoglycemia may also occur with inadequate caloric intake, strenuous exercise, or concurrent use with other hypoglycemic drugs

Adverse Reactions

Central nervous system: Headache, dizziness

Dermatologic: Pruritus, rash, urticaria, photosensitivity reaction

Endocrine & metabolic: Hypoglycemia, weight gain

Gastrointestinal: Nausea, epigastric fullness, heartburn, constipation, diarrhea, anorexia

Genitourinary: Nocturia

Hematologic: Leukopenia, thrombocytopenia, hemolytic anemia, aplastic anemia, bone marrow suppression, agranulocytosis

Hepatic: Cholestatic jaundice, elevated liver enzymes

Neuromuscular & skeletal: Arthralgia, paresthesia

Ocular: Blurred vision

Renal: Diuretic effect (minor), urolithiasis

Drug Interactions Cytochrome P-450 isoenzyme CYP3A3/4 enzyme substrate

Drugs which tend to produce hyperglycemia (eg, diuretics, corticosteroids, phenothiazines, thyroid products, estrogens, oral contraceptives, phenytoin, nicotinic acid, sympathomimetics, calcium channel-blocking drugs, rifampin, and isoniazid) may lead to a loss of glycemic control; disulfiram-like reactions with alcohol; drugs which produce an increase in glyburide's hypoglycemic effects: chloramphenicol, monoamine oxidase inhibitors, fluoroquinolone antibiotics, and probencid; since this agent is highly protein bound, use of other protein-bound drugs may result in adverse effects when glyburide therapy is initiated or discontinued; beta-adrenergic blocking agents may impair glucose tolerance, increase the frequency or severity of hypoglycemia, block hypoglycemia-induced tachycardia, delay the rate of recovery of blood glucose concentration following drug-induced hypoglycemia, and may alter the hemodynamic response to hypoglycemia

Food Interactions Food does not affect absorption.

Mechanism of Action Stimulates insulin release from the pancreatic beta cells, reduces glucose output from the liver, and increases insulin sensitivity at peripheral target sites

Pharmacodynamics

Onset of action: 45-60 minutes

Maximum effects: 1.5-3 hours

Duration: Conventional formulations: 16-24 hours; micronized formulations: 12-24 hours

Average decrease in fasting blood glucose (when used as monotherapy): 60-70 mg/dL

Pharmacokinetics

Absorption: Reliably and almost completely absorbed

Distribution: V_d: 0.125 L/kg

Metabolism: Completely metabolized to one moderately active and several inactive metabolites

Plasma protein binding: High (>99%)

Half-life: Biphasic: Terminal elimination half-life: Average: 1.4-1.8 hours (range: 0.7-3 hours); may be prolonged with renal or hepatic insufficiency

Time to peak serum concentration: Conventional formulation: 4 hours; micronized formulation: 2-3 hours

Elimination: 30% to 50% of dose excreted in the urine as metabolites in first 24 hours; the remainder of the metabolite via biliary excretion

Dialysis: Not dialyzable

Usual Dosage Adults: Oral: Formulations of micronized glyburide (Glynase™ PresTab™) are **not** bioequivalent with conventional formulations (Diaβeta®, Micronase®) and dosage should be retitrated when transferring patients from one formulation to the other

Management of noninsulin-dependent diabetes mellitus in patients **previously untreated**:

Tablet (Diaβeta®, Micronase®):

Initial: 2.5-5 mg/day; in patients who are more sensitive to hypoglycemic drugs (see Precautions), start at 1.25 mg/day; increase in increments of no more than 2.5 mg/day at weekly intervals

Maintenance: 1.25-20 mg/day given as single or divided doses; maximum: 20 mg/day; doses >10 mg should be divided into twice daily doses

Micronized tablets (Glynase™ PresTab™):

Initial: 1.5-3 mg/day; in patients who are more sensitive to hypoglycemic drugs (see Precautions), start at 0.75 mg/day; increase in increments of no more than 1.5 mg/day at weekly intervals

Maintenance: 0.75-12 mg/day given as a single dose or in divided doses; doses >6 mg/day should be divided into twice daily doses

Management of noninsulin-dependent diabetes mellitus in patients **previously maintained on insulin**: Initial dosage dependent upon previous insulin dosage, see table

Previous Daily Insulin Dosage (units)	Initial Glyburide Dosage (mg conventional formulation)	Initial Glyburide Dosage (mg micronized formulation)	Insulin Dosage Change (after glyburide started)
<20	2.5-5	1.5-3	Discontinue
20-40	5	3	Discontinue
>40	5 (increase in increments of 1.25-2.5 mg every 2-10 days)	3 (increase in increments of 0.75-1.5 mg every 2-10 days)	Reduce insulin dosage by 50% (gradually taper off insulin as glyburide dosage increased)

Dosing adjustment in renal impairment: Cl_{cr} <50 mL/minute: Not recommended

Dosing adjustment in hepatic impairment: Use conservative initial and maintenance doses and avoid use in severe disease

Administration Oral: May administer with food every morning 30 minutes before breakfast or the first main meal

Monitoring Parameters Signs and symptoms of hypoglycemia, fasting blood glucose, hemoglobin A_{1c}

Reference Range Target range:

Blood glucose: Fasting and preprandial: 80-120 mg/dL; bedtime: 100-140 mg/dL

Glycosylated hemoglobin (hemoglobin A_{1c}): <7%

(Continued)

Glyburide *(Continued)*

Patient Information Do not change dose or discontinue without consulting prescriber; avoid alcohol while taking this medication, may cause severe reaction; maintain regular dietary intake and exercise routine; always carry quick source of sugar; if experiencing a hypoglycemic reaction, contact prescriber immediately; use sunscreen, wear protective clothing and eyewear, and avoid direct sunlight; report severe or persistent side effects, extended vomiting or flu-like symptoms, skin rash, easy bruising or bleeding, or change in color of urine or stool

Additional Information When transferring from other sulfonylurea antidiabetic agents to glyburide, with the exception of chlorpropamide, the administration of the other agent may be abruptly discontinued; due to the prolonged elimination half-life of chlorpropamide, a 2- to 3-day drug-free interval may be advisable before glyburide therapy is begun

Dosage Forms

Tablet (Diaβeta®, Micronase®): 1.25 mg, 2.5 mg, 5 mg

Tablet, micronized: 1.5 mg, 3 mg, 4.5 mg, 6 mg

Tablet, micronized (Glynase™ PresTab™): 1.5 mg, 3 mg, 6 mg

References

DeFronzo RA, "Pharmacologic Therapy for Type 2 Diabetes Mellitus," *Ann Intern Med*, 1999, 131(4):281-303.

"Intensive Blood-Glucose Control With Sulphonylureas or Insulin Compared With Conventional Treatment and Risk of Complications in Patients With Type 2 Diabetes (UKPDS 33) UK Prospective Diabetes Study (UKPDS) Group," *Lancet*, 1998, 352(9131):837-53.

Glycerin (GLIS er in)

U.S. Brand Names Fleet® Babylax® [OTC]; Ophthalgan®; Osmoglyn®; Sani-Supp® Suppository [OTC]

Synonyms Glycerol

Therapeutic Category Laxative, Osmotic

Generic Available Yes

Use Constipation; reduction of intraocular pressure; reduction of corneal edema; glycerin has been administered orally to reduce intracranial pressure; laxative used in newborns to promote bilirubin excretion by reducing enterohepatic circulation, decreasing gastrointestinal transit time, and stimulating passage of meconium

Pregnancy Risk Factor C

Contraindications Hypersensitivity to glycerin or any component; severe dehydration, anuria

Precautions Use oral glycerin with caution in patients with cardiac, renal or hepatic disease and in diabetics

Adverse Reactions

Central nervous system: Dizziness, headache, confusion, disorientation

Endocrine & metabolic: Hyperglycemia, dehydration

Gastrointestinal: Diarrhea, nausea, tenesmus, thirst, cramping pain, vomiting, rectal irritation

Local: Pain/irritation with ophthalmic solution (may need to apply a topical ophthalmic anesthetic before glycerin administration)

Stability Protect from heat; freezing should be avoided

Mechanism of Action Osmotic dehydrating agent which increases osmotic pressure; draws fluid into colon and thus stimulates evacuation; glycerin ophthalmic solution's osmotic action reduces edema and causes clearing of corneal haze; when given orally, glycerin increases osmotic pressure of the plasma drawing water from the extravascular spaces into the blood producing a decrease in intraocular pressure

Pharmacodynamics

Onset of action for glycerin suppository or enema: 15-30 minutes

Onset of action in decreasing intraocular pressure: Within 10-30 minutes

Duration: 4-8 hours

Increased intracranial pressure decreases within 10-60 minutes following an oral dose

Duration: ~2-3 hours

Pharmacokinetics

Absorption:

Oral: Well absorbed

Rectal: Poorly absorbed

Metabolism: Primarily in the liver with 20% metabolized in the kidney

Half-life: 30-45 minutes

Time to peak serum concentration: Oral: Within 60-90 minutes

Elimination: Only a small percentage of drug is excreted unchanged in urine

Usual Dosage

Constipation: Rectal: Administered in single doses only at infrequent intervals

Neonates: 0.5 mL/kg/dose of rectal solution as an enema

Children <6 years: 1 infant suppository as needed or 2-5 mL of rectal solution as an enema

Children ≥6 years and Adults: 1 adult suppository as needed or 5-15 mL of rectal solution as an enema

Children and Adults:

Reduction of intraocular pressure: Oral: 1-1.8 g/kg 1-1½ hours preoperatively; additional doses may be administered at 5-hour intervals

Reduction of intracranial pressure: Oral: 1.5 g/kg/day divided every 4 hours; 1 g/kg/dose every 6 hours has also been used

Reduction of corneal edema: Ophthalmic: Instill 1-2 drops in eye(s) every 3-4 hours

Administration

Oral: Orange or lemon juice may be added to unflavored 50% oral solution; pour solution over crushed ice and drink through a straw to improve palatability

Ophthalmic: Instill drops onto the eye; avoid contaminating tip of the solution bottle

Rectal: Insert suppository in the rectum and retain 15 minutes

Monitoring Parameters Blood glucose, intraocular pressure, evacuation of stool

Patient Information Do not use if experiencing abdominal pain, nausea, or vomiting

Nursing Implications Use caution during insertion of suppository to avoid intestinal perforation, especially in neonates; instruct patient to lie down after oral glycerin administration to prevent or relieve headaches

Dosage Forms

Solution:

Ophthalmic, sterile (Ophthalgan®): Glycerin with chlorobutanol 0.55% (7.5 mL)

Oral (Osmoglyn®): 50% [lime flavor] (220 mL)

Rectal (Fleet® Babylax®): 4 mL/applicator (6s)

Suppository, rectal (Sani-Supp®): Glycerin with sodium stearate (infant and adult sizes)

References

Heinemeyer G, "Clinical Pharmacokinetic Considerations in the Treatment of Increased Intracranial Pressure," *Clin Pharmacokinet*, 1987, 13(1):1-25.

Rottenberg DA, Hurwitz BJ, and Posner JB, "The Effect of Oral Glycerol on Intraventricular Pressure in Man," *Neurology*, 1977, 27(7):600-8.

Zenk KE, Koeppel RM, and Liem LA, "Comparative Efficacy of Glycerin Enemas and Suppository Chips in Neonates," *Clin Pharm*, 1993, 12(11):846-8.

♦ **Glycerol** *see* Glycerin *on page 478*

♦ **Glycerol Guaiacolate** *see* Guaifenesin *on page 485*

♦ **Glycerol Guaiacolate and Codeine** *see* Guaifenesin and Codeine *on page 486*

♦ **Glyceryl Trinitrate** *see* Nitroglycerin *on page 717*

♦ **Glycon (Can)** *see* Metformin *on page 639*

Glycopyrrolate (glye koe PYE roe late)

Related Information

Compatibility of Medications Mixed in a Syringe *on page 1238*

Overdose and Toxicology *on page 1222*

U.S. Brand Names Robinul®; Robinul® Forte

Synonyms Glycopyrronium

Therapeutic Category Anticholinergic Agent; Antispasmodic Agent, Gastrointestinal

Generic Available Yes

Use Adjunct in treatment of peptic ulcer disease; inhibition of salivation and excessive secretions of the respiratory tract; reversal of the muscarinic effects of cholinergic agents such as neostigmine and pyridostigmine during reversal of neuromuscular blockade

Pregnancy Risk Factor B

Contraindications Narrow-angle glaucoma; acute hemorrhage; tachycardia; hypersensitivity to glycopyrrolate or any component; ulcerative colitis; obstructive uropathy; paralytic ileus; myasthenia gravis

Warnings Infants, patients with Down syndrome, and children with spastic paralysis or brain damage may be hypersensitive to antimuscarinic effects

Precautions Use with caution in patients with fever, hyperthyroidism, hepatic or renal disease, hypertension, CHF, GI infections, diarrhea, reflux esophagitis

Adverse Reactions

Cardiovascular: Tachycardia, orthostatic hypotension, ventricular fibrillation, palpitations

(Continued)

479

Glycopyrrolate *(Continued)*

Central nervous system: Drowsiness, nervousness, headache, insomnia, confusion, loss of memory, fatigue, ataxia

Dermatologic: Rash, dry skin

Gastrointestinal: Xerostomia, constipation, nausea, vomiting, dry throat, dysphagia

Genitourinary: Urinary retention, dysuria

Local: Irritation at injection site

Neuromuscular & skeletal: Weakness

Ocular: Blurred vision

Respiratory: Dry nose

Miscellaneous: Decreased diaphoresis

Drug Interactions Phenothiazines, meperidine, amantadine, tricyclic antidepressants, and quinidine (additive anticholinergic effect); wax-matrix potassium chloride (increased severity of potassium-induced GI mucosal lesions); antacids (decreased absorption); decreased effect of levodopa

Stability Unstable at pH >6; compatible in the same syringe with atropine, benzquinamide, chlorpromazine, codeine, diphenhydramine, droperidol, fentanyl, hydromorphone, hydroxyzine, lidocaine, meperidine, promethazine, morphine, neostigmine, oxymorphone, procaine, prochlorperazine, promazine, pyridostigmine, scopolamine, triflupromazine, and trimethobenzamide

Mechanism of Action Inhibits the muscarinic action of acetylcholine at postganglionic parasympathetic neuroeffector sites in smooth muscle, secretory glands, and CNS

Pharmacodynamics

Onset of action:

Oral: Within 1 hour

I.M., S.C.: 15-30 minutes

I.V.: 1-10 minutes

Peak effect: I.M., S.C.: 30-45 minutes

Duration of effect (anticholinergic effects):

Oral: 8-12 hours

Parenteral: 7 hours

Pharmacokinetics

Absorption: Oral: Poor and erratic; 10% absorption

Distribution: Does not adequately penetrate into CNS

Elimination: Primarily unchanged via biliary elimination (70% to 90%)

Usual Dosage

Children:

Control of secretions:

Oral: 40-100 mcg/kg/dose 3-4 times/day

I.M., I.V.: 4-10 mcg/kg/dose every 3-4 hours

Preoperative: I.M.:

<2 years: 4.4-8.8 mcg/kg 30-60 minutes before procedure

>2 years: 4.4 mcg/kg 30-60 minutes before procedure

Children and Adults: Reversal of muscarinic effects of cholinergic agents: I.V.: 0.2 mg for each 1 mg of neostigmine or 5 mg of pyridostigmine administered

Adults:

Peptic ulcer:

Oral: 1-2 mg 2-3 times/day

I.M., I.V.: 0.1-0.2 mg 3-4 times/day

Preoperative: I.M.: 4.4 mcg/kg 30-60 minutes before procedure

Administration

Oral: May be administered without regard to meals

Parenteral: Dilute to a concentration of 2 mcg/mL (maximum concentration: 200 mcg/mL); infuse over 15-20 minutes; may be administered direct I.V. at a maximum rate of 20 mcg/minute; may be administered I.M.

Monitoring Parameters Heart rate

Dosage Forms

Injection: 0.2 mg/mL (1 mL, 2 mL, 5 mL, 20 mL)

Robinul®: 0.2 mg/mL (1 mL, 2 mL, 5 mL, 20 mL)

Tablet:

Robinul®: 1 mg

Robinul® Forte: 2 mg

♦ **Glycopyrronium** *see Glycopyrrolate on page 479*

♦ **Glycosum** *see Dextrose on page 317*

♦ **Glydiazinamide** *see Glipizide on page 473*

♦ **Glynase™ PresTab™** *see Glyburide on page 476*

♦ **Gly-Oxide**® **[OTC]** *see* Carbamide Peroxide *on page 178*
♦ **Glytuss**® **[OTC]** *see* Guaifenesin *on page 485*
♦ **GM-CSF** *see* Sargramostim *on page 890*
♦ **G-myticin**® *see* Gentamicin *on page 469*

Gold Sodium Thiomalate (gold SOW dee um thye oh MAL ate)

U.S. Brand Names Aurolate®
Therapeutic Category Gold Compound
Generic Available Yes
Use Treatment of progressive rheumatoid arthritis
Pregnancy Risk Factor C
Contraindications Severe hepatic or renal dysfunction; hypersensitivity to gold compounds or other heavy metals; systemic lupus erythematosus; history of blood dyscrasias; CHF, exfoliative dermatitis, or colitis; avoid concomitant use of antimalarials, immunosuppressive agents, penicillamine, or phenylbutazone
Warnings Explain the possibility of adverse reactions before initiating therapy; signs of gold toxicity include: decrease in hemoglobin, leukocytes, granulocytes and platelets, proteinuria, hematuria, pigmentation, pruritus, stomatitis or persistent diarrhea, rash, metallic taste; advise patient to report any symptoms of toxicity
Precautions Frequent monitoring of patients for signs and symptoms of toxicity will prevent serious adverse reactions; NSAIDs and corticosteroids may be discontinued after initiating gold therapy; must not be injected I.V.
Adverse Reactions
    Cardiovascular: Flushing
    Central nervous system: Seizures, headache
    Dermatologic: Exfoliative urticaria, dermatitis, erythema nodosum, alopecia, shedding of nails, pruritus, gray-to-blue pigmentation of skin and mucous membranes
    Gastrointestinal: Stomatitis, nausea, diarrhea, abdominal cramps, metallic taste, gingivitis, glossitis, ulcerative enterocolitis, GI hemorrhage, dysphagia
    Genitourinary: Vaginitis
    Hematologic: Eosinophilia, leukopenia, agranulocytosis, thrombocytopenia
    Hepatic: Hepatitis
    Neuromuscular & skeletal: Arthralgias, peripheral neuropathy
    Ocular: Blurred vision, conjunctivitis, corneal ulcers, iritis
    Renal: Hematuria, proteinuria, nephrotic syndrome
    Respiratory: Interstitial pneumonitis and fibrosis
    Miscellaneous: Hypersensitivity reactions including anaphylaxis (rare)
Drug Interactions Decreased effect with penicillamine, acetylcysteine
Mechanism of Action Unknown, may decrease prostaglandin synthesis or may alter cellular mechanisms by inhibiting sulfhydryl systems
Pharmacokinetics
    Distribution: Breast milk to plasma ratio: 0.02-0.3
    Half-life: 3-27 days (may lengthen with multiple doses)
    Time to peak serum concentration: I.M.: Within 3-6 hours
    Elimination: Majority (50% to 90%) excreted in urine with smaller amounts (10% to 50%) excreted in feces (via bile)
Usual Dosage I.M.:
    Children: Initial: Test dose of 10 mg I.M. is recommended, followed by 1 mg/kg I.M. weekly for 20 weeks (maximum dose: 50 mg); maintenance: 1 mg/kg/dose at 2- to 4-week intervals thereafter for as long as therapy is clinically beneficial and toxicity does not develop. Administration for 2-4 months is usually required before clinical improvement is observed.
    Adults: 10 mg first week; 25 mg second week; then 25-50 mg/week until clinical improvement or a 1 g cumulative dose has been given. If improvement occurs without adverse reactions, give 25-50 mg every 2 weeks for 2-20 weeks; if it continues stable, give 25-50 mg every 3-4 weeks indefinitely.
    Dosage adjustment in renal impairment:
        Cl_{cr} 50-80 mL/minute: Administer 50% of dose
        Cl_{cr} <50 mL/minute: Avoid use
Administration Parenteral: Administer I.M. only, preferably intragluteally; addition of 0.1 mL of 1% lidocaine to each injection may reduce the discomfort associated with I.M. administration; patients should be recumbent during injection and for 10 minutes afterwards; observe closely for 15 minutes after injection
Monitoring Parameters CBC, platelets, hemoglobin, urinalysis, renal and liver function tests
Reference Range Gold: Normal: 0-0.1 µg/mL (SI: 0-0.0064 µmol/L); Therapeutic: 1-3 µg/mL (SI: 0.06-0.18 µmol/L); Urine <0.1 µg/24 hours
Dosage Forms Injection: 50 mg/mL (1 mL, 10 mL)

♦ **GoLYTELY®** see Polyethylene Glycol-Electrolyte Solution on page 811

Gonadorelin (goe nad oh REL in)

U.S. Brand Names Factrel®; Lutrepulse®
Canadian Brand Names Relisorm
Synonyms LH-RH; LRH
Therapeutic Category Diagnostic Agent, Gonadotrophic Hormone; Gonadotropin
Generic Available No
Use Evaluation of hypothalamic-pituitary gonadotropic function; used to evaluate abnormal gonadotropin regulation as in precocious puberty and delayed puberty; treatment of primary hypothalamic amenorrhea
Pregnancy Risk Factor B
Contraindications Hypersensitivity to gonadorelin or any component
Warnings Anaphylactic reactions have occurred following multiple-dose administration; multiple pregnancy is a possibility with Lutrepulse®
Adverse Reactions
  Cardiovascular: Flushing
  Central nervous system: Lightheadedness, headache
  Dermatologic: Skin rash
  Gastrointestinal: Nausea, abdominal discomfort
  Local: Pain, pruritus, edema
  Miscellaneous: Hypersensitivity reactions
Drug Interactions Androgens, estrogens, progestins, glucocorticoids affect pituitary secretion of gonadotropins; spironolactone, levodopa may increase gonadotropin levels; oral contraceptives, digoxin may suppress gonadotropin levels; phenothiazines, dopamine antagonists may blunt response to gonadorelin
Stability Prepare immediately prior to use; after reconstitution, store at room temperature and use within 1 day; discard unused portion
Mechanism of Action Stimulates the release of luteinizing hormone (LH) from the anterior pituitary gland
Pharmacodynamics
  Onset of action: Following administration maximal LH release occurs within 20 minutes
  Duration: 3-5 hours
Pharmacokinetics Half-life: 4 minutes
Usual Dosage
  Children: I.V. **(as hydrochloride salt)**: 100 mcg to evaluate abnormal gonadotropin regulation
  Children >12 years and Adults: I.V., S.C. **(as hydrochloride salt)**: 100 mcg; administer to women during early phase of menstrual cycle (day 1-7)
  Adults: I.V. **(as acetate salt)**: 5 mcg (range: 1-20 mcg) every 90 minutes for 7 days via the Lutrepulse® pump; recommended treatment interval: 21 days
Administration Parenteral:
  Hydrochloride salt: Dilute in 3 mL of NS; administer I.V. push over 30 seconds
  Acetate salt (Lutrepulse®): Fill presterilized reservoir bag with reconstituted solution; administer I.V. using the Lutrepulse® pump
Monitoring Parameters Plasma LH and FSH
  Hypothalamic/pituitary function evaluation: Draw blood samples for LH 15 minutes before and immediately before gonadorelin dose, then at 15, 30, 45, 60, and 120 minutes after dose
Dosage Forms
  Injection, as acetate (Lutrepulse®): 0.8 mg, 3.2 mg
  Injection, as hydrochloride (Factrel®): 100 mcg, 500 mcg
References
  Pescovitz OH, Comite F, Hench K, et al, "The NIH Experience With Precocious Puberty: Diagnostic Subgroups and Response to Short-Term Luteinizing Hormone-Releasing Hormone Analogue Therapy," J Pediatr, 1986, 108(1):47-54.

♦ **Gordofilm® [OTC]** see Salicylic Acid on page 886

Granisetron (gra NI se tron)

U.S. Brand Names Kytril™
Therapeutic Category Antiemetic
Generic Available No
Use Prophylaxis and treatment of chemotherapy and radiation-related nausea and emesis; prevention of postoperative nausea and vomiting
Pregnancy Risk Factor B
Contraindications Hypersensitivity to granisetron or any component

Warnings Use with caution in patients with liver disease or in pregnant patients

Precautions Some injectable products contain benzyl alcohol, avoid use in neonates

Adverse Reactions

Cardiovascular: Hypertension, hypotension, arrhythmias such as bradycardia, atrial fibrillation, A-V block

Central nervous system: Agitation, anxiety, CNS stimulation, headache, insomnia, somnolence, fever

Dermatologic: Skin rashes

Gastrointestinal: Constipation, diarrhea, dysgeusia, abdominal pain

Hepatic: Elevated liver enzymes

Drug Interactions Cytochrome P-450 isoenzyme CYP3A3/4 substrate

Because granisetron is metabolized by hepatic cytochrome P-450 drug metabolizing enzymes, inducers or inhibitors of this system may change the clearance and half-life

Stability Stable when mixed in NS, D_5W for at least 24 hours

Mechanism of Action Selective 5-HT$_3$ receptor antagonist, blocking serotonin, both peripherally on vagal nerve terminals and centrally in the chemoreceptor trigger zone

Pharmacodynamics

Onset of action: I.V.: 1-3 minutes

Duration: I.V.: ≤24 hours

Pharmacokinetics

Distribution: V_d: 2-3 L/kg; widely distributed throughout the body

Half-life:

Cancer patients: 10-12 hours

Healthy volunteers: 3-4 hours

Elimination: Primarily nonrenal, 8% to 15% of dose excreted unchanged in urine

Usual Dosage

Treatment of chemotherapy-induced emesis: Initial dose given just prior to chemo-therapy (15-60 minutes before)

Children ≥2 years: I.V.: Manufacturer's recommendation: 10 mcg/kg; or as an alternative based on clinical research: 20-40 mcg/kg

As intervention therapy for breakthrough nausea and vomiting, during the first 24 hours following chemotherapy, 2 or 3 repeat infusions (same dose) have been administered

Adults:

Oral: 2 mg once daily or 1 mg twice daily

I.V.: 10 mcg/kg or 1 mg

Treatment of postoperative nausea and vomiting: Children ≥4 years and Adults: 20-40 mcg/kg as a single dose postoperatively

Administration

Oral: Given at least 1 hour prior to chemotherapy and then 12 hours later; shake oral suspension well before use

Parenteral: I.V.: Infuse over 30 seconds undiluted **or** dilute in small volume NS or D_5W and administer over 5 minutes **or** dilute in 20-50 mL of NS or D_5W and infuse over 30 minutes to 1 hour

Dosage Forms

Injection, preservative free, as hydrochloride: 1 mg/mL (1 mL)

Injection, with benzyl alcohol, as hydrochloride: 1 mg/mL (4 mL)

Tablet, as hydrochloride: 1 mg

Extemporaneous Preparations

A 0.2 mg/mL suspension may be made by crushing twelve 1 mg tablets. Add 30 mL distilled water, mix well, and transfer to a bottle. Rinse the mortar with 10 mL cherry syrup and add to bottle. Add enough cherry syrup to make a final volume of 60 mL. Label "shake well"; stable 14 days at room temperature or refrigerated (Quercia, 1997).

A 50 mcg/mL suspension may be made by crushing one 1 mg tablet. Add 1% methylcellulose and syrup NF to a total volume of 20 mL (may also use Ora-Sweet® or Ora-Plus® instead of methylcellulose and syrup); shake well; stable 91 days refrigerated (Nahata, 1998).

Nahata MC, Morosco RS, and Hipple TF, "Stability of Granisetron Hydrochloride in Two Oral Suspensions," *Am J Health Syst Pharm*, 1998, 55(23):2511-3.

Quercia RA, Zhang J, Fan C, et al, "Stability of Granisetron Hydrochloride in an Extemporaneously Prepared Oral Liquid," *Am J Health-Syst Pharm*, 1997, 54(12):1404-6.

References

"ASHP Therapeutic Guidelines on the Pharmacologic Management of Nausea and Vomiting in Adult and Pediatric Patients Receiving Chemotherapy or Radiation Therapy or Undergoing Surgery," *Am J Health Syst Pharm*, 1999, 56(8):729-64.

(Continued)

Granisetron *(Continued)*

Hahlen K, Quintana E, Pinkerton CR, et al, "A Randomized Comparison of Intravenously Administered Granisetron Versus Chlorpromazine Plus Dexamethasone in the Prevention of Ifosfamide-Induced Emesis in Children," *J Pediatr*, 1995, 126(2):309-13.

Lemerle J, Amaral D, Southall DP, et al, "Efficacy and Safety of Granisetron in the Prevention of Chemotherapy-Induced Emesis in Paediatric Patients," *Eur J Cancer*, 1991, 27(9):1081-3.

♦ **Granulocyte Colony Stimulating Factor** *see* Filgrastim *on page 425*

♦ **Granulocyte Macrophage Colony Stimulating Factor** *see* Sargramostim *on page 890*

♦ **Gravol (Can)** *see* Dimenhydrinate *on page 339*

♦ **Grifulvin® V** *see* Griseofulvin *on page 484*

♦ **Grisactin®** *see* Griseofulvin *on page 484*

♦ **Grisactin® Ultra** *see* Griseofulvin *on page 484*

Griseofulvin *(gri see oh FUL vin)*

Related Information

Carbohydrate and Alcohol Content of Liquid Medications for Use in Patients Receiving Ketogenic Diets *on page 1258*

U.S. Brand Names Fulvicin® P/G; Fulvicin-U/F®; Grifulvin® V; Grisactin®; Grisactin® Ultra; Gris-PEG®

Synonyms Griseofulvin Microsize; Griseofulvin Ultramicrosize

Therapeutic Category Antifungal Agent, Systemic

Generic Available Yes

Use Treatment of tinea infections of the skin, hair, and nails caused by susceptible species of *Microsporum*, *Epidermophyton*, or *Trichophyton*

Pregnancy Risk Factor C

Contraindications Hypersensitivity to griseofulvin or any component; severe liver disease, porphyria (interferes with porphyrin metabolism); pregnant women

Precautions Avoid exposure to intense sunlight to prevent photosensitivity reactions; use with caution in patients with penicillin hypersensitivity

Adverse Reactions

Central nervous system: Fatigue, confusion, impaired judgment, insomnia, headache, incoordination, dizziness

Dermatologic: Rash, urticaria, photosensitivity reaction

Endocrine & metabolic: Estrogen-like effects in children

Gastrointestinal: Nausea, vomiting, diarrhea, oral thrush

Hematologic: Leukopenia, granulocytopenia

Hepatic: Hepatotoxicity

Neuromuscular & skeletal: Paresthesia

Renal: Proteinuria

Miscellaneous: Lupus-like syndrome

Drug Interactions Phenobarbital decreases griseofulvin concentrations; griseofulvin decreases warfarin effectiveness; griseofulvin decreases oral contraceptive efficacy; griseofulvin potentiates the effects of alcohol and causes flushing and tachycardia

Food Interactions Fatty meal will increase griseofulvin absorption

Mechanism of Action Inhibits fungal cell mitosis at metaphase by disrupting the cell's mitotic spindle structure; binds to human keratin making it resistant to fungal invasion

Pharmacokinetics

Absorption: Ultramicrosize griseofulvin absorption is almost complete; absorption of microsize griseofulvin is variable (25% to 70% of an oral dose); absorbed from the duodenum

Distribution: Deposited in the keratin layer of skin, hair, and nails; concentrates in liver, fat, and skeletal muscles; crosses the placenta

Metabolism: Extensive in the liver

Half-life: 9-22 hours

Elimination: <1% excreted unchanged in urine; also excreted in feces and perspiration

Usual Dosage Oral:

Children:

Microsize: 10-20 mg/kg/day in single or 2 divided doses

Ultramicrosize: >2 years: 5-10 mg/kg/day in single or 2 divided doses

Adults:

Microsize: 500-1000 mg/day in single or divided doses

Ultramicrosize: 330-375 mg/day in single or divided doses; doses up to 750 mg/day have been used for infections more difficult to eradicate such as tinea unguium

Duration of therapy depends on the site of infection:
Tinea corporis: 2-4 weeks
Tinea capitis: 4-6 weeks or longer
Tinea pedis: 4-8 weeks
Tinea unguium: 3-6 months or longer

Administration Oral: Administer with a fatty meal (peanuts or ice cream to increase absorption), or with food or milk to avoid GI upset

Monitoring Parameters Periodic renal, hepatic, and hematopoietic function tests

Test Interactions False-positive urinary VMA levels

Patient Information Avoid exposure to sunlight; avoid alcohol

Dosage Forms
Microsize:
Capsule (Grisactin®): 125 mg, 250 mg
Suspension, oral (Grifulvin® V): 125 mg/5 mL with alcohol 0.2% (120 mL)
Tablet:
Fulvicin-U/F®, Grifulvin® V: 250 mg
Fulvicin-U/F®, Grifulvin® V, Grisactin-500®: 500 mg
Ultramicrosize:
Tablet:
Fulvicin® P/G: 165 mg, 330 mg
Fulvicin® P/G, Grisactin® Ultra, Gris-PEG®: 125 mg, 250 mg
Grisactin® Ultra: 330 mg

References
Ginsburg CM, McCracken GH Jr, Petruska M, et al, "Effect of Feeding on Bioavailability of Griseofulvin in Children," *J Pediatr*, 1983, 102(2):309-11.

♦ **Griseofulvin Microsize** *see Griseofulvin on page 484*
♦ **Griseofulvin Ultramicrosize** *see Griseofulvin on page 484*
♦ **Gris-PEG®** *see Griseofulvin on page 484*
♦ **Growth Hormone** *see Human Growth Hormone on page 498*

Guaifenesin (gwye FEN e sin)

Related Information
OTC Cough & Cold Preparations, Pediatric *on page 1072*

U.S. Brand Names Breonesin® [OTC]; Diabetic Tussin EX® [OTC]; Duratuss-G®; Fenesin™ [OTC]; Genatuss® [OTC]; Glytuss® [OTC]; Guaifenex LA®; Guiatuss® [OTC]; Humibid® L.A. [OTC]; Humibid® Sprinkle [OTC]; Hytuss® [OTC]; Hytuss-2X® [OTC]; Liquibid® [OTC]; Muco-Fen-LA®; Mytussin® [OTC]; Naldecon® Senior EX [OTC]; Organidin NR®; Respa-GF; Robitussin® [OTC]; Scot-Tussin® [OTC]; Siltussin® SA [OTC]; Touro Ex®; Tussin® [OTC]

Canadian Brand Names Balminil Expectorant; Benylin-E; Calmylin Expectorant; Cough Syrup Expectorant; Expectorant Cough Formula; Expectorant Cough Syrup; Expectorant Syrup; Koffex Expectorant; Sirop Expectorant; Tussin GF Expectorant

Synonyms GG; Glyceryl Guaiacolate

Therapeutic Category Expectorant

Generic Available Yes

Use Temporary control of cough due to minor throat and bronchial irritation

Pregnancy Risk Factor C

Contraindications Hypersensitivity to guaifenesin or any component

Adverse Reactions
Central nervous system: Drowsiness, headache
Dermatologic: Rash
Gastrointestinal: Nausea, vomiting

Mechanism of Action Thought to act as an expectorant by irritating the gastric mucosa and stimulating respiratory tract secretions, thereby increasing respiratory fluid volumes and decreasing phlegm viscosity

Usual Dosage Oral:
Children:
<2 years: 12 mg/kg/day in 6 divided doses
2-5 years: 50-100 mg every 4 hours, not to exceed 600 mg/day
6-11 years: 100-200 mg every 4 hours, not to exceed 1.2 g/day
Children >12 years and Adults: 200-400 mg every 4 hours to a maximum of 2.4 g/day

Administration Oral: Administer with a large quantity of fluid to ensure proper action

Test Interactions May cause a colorimetric interference with certain laboratory determinations of 5-hydroxyindoleacetic acid (5-HIAA) and vanillylmandelic acid (VMA)

(Continued)

Guaifenesin *(Continued)*

Dosage Forms
Capsule (Breonesin®, Hytuss-2X®): 200 mg
Capsule, sustained release (Humibid® Sprinkle): 300 mg
Liquid:
Diabetic Tussin EX®, Organidin® NR: 100 mg/5 mL (30 mL, 118 mL, 240 mL, 480 mL, 3840 mL)
Naldecon® Senior EX: 200 mg/5 mL (118 mL)
Syrup:
Genatuss®, Halotussin®, Mytussin®, Robitussin®: 100 mg/5 mL with alcohol 3.5% (5 mL, 10 mL, 15 mL, 30 mL, 120 mL, 240 mL, 473 mL, 3840 mL)
Guiatuss®, Siltussin® SA, Tussin®: 100 mg/5 mL (120 mL, 240 mL, 480 mL, 3840 mL)
Tablet:
Glytuss®, Organidin NR®: 200 mg
Hytuss®: 100 mg
Tablet, sustained release:
Duratuss-G®: 1200 mg
Fenesin™, Guaifenex LA®, Humibid® L.A., Liquibid®, Muco-Fen-LA®, Respa-GF®: 600 mg
Touro Ex®: 575 mg

Guaifenesin and Codeine (gwye FEN e sin & KOE deen)

Related Information
OTC Cough & Cold Preparations, Pediatric *on page 1072*

U.S. Brand Names Brontex®; Cheracol® With Codeine; Gani-Tuss® NR; Guaituss AC®; Halotussin® AC; Mytussin® AC; Robitussin® A-C; Romilar® AC; Tussi-Organidin® NR; Tussi-Organidin® S-NR

Synonyms Codeine and Glycerol Guaiacolate; Codeine and Guaifenesin; Glycerol Guaiacolate and Codeine

Therapeutic Category Antitussive; Cough Preparation; Expectorant

Generic Available Yes

Use Temporary control of cough due to minor throat and bronchial irritation

Restrictions C-V

Pregnancy Risk Factor C

Contraindications Hypersensitivity to guaifenesin, codeine, or any component

Precautions Use with caution in patients with hypersensitivity reactions to other phenanthrene derivative opioid agonists (morphine, hydrocodone, hydromorphone, levorphanol, oxycodone, oxymorphone)

Adverse Reactions
Codeine:
Cardiovascular: Palpitations, bradycardia, peripheral vasodilation
Central nervous system: CNS depression, dizziness, drowsiness, sedation, increased intracranial pressure
Dermatologic: Pruritus from histamine release
Endocrine & metabolic: Antidiuretic hormone release
Gastrointestinal: Nausea, vomiting, constipation, biliary tract spasm
Genitourinary: Urinary tract spasm
Ocular: Miosis
Respiratory: Respiratory depression
Miscellaneous: Histamine release, physical and psychological dependence with prolonged use
Guaifenesin:
Central nervous system: Drowsiness, headache
Dermatologic: Rash
Gastrointestinal: Nausea, vomiting

Drug Interactions CNS depressant medications produce additive sedative properties

Mechanism of Action See individual monographs for Guaifenesin *on page 485* and Codeine *on page 262*

Usual Dosage Oral:
Children:
2-6 years: 1-1.5 mg/kg codeine/day divided into 4 doses administered every 4-6 hours (maximum dose: 30 mg/24 hours)
6-12 years: 5 mL every 4 hours, not to exceed 30 mL/24 hours
>12 years: 10 mL every 4 hours, up to 60 mL/24 hours

Adults: 5-10 mL or 1 tablet every 4-6 hours; not to exceed 120 mg (60 mL) codeine/day or 6 tablets/day

Administration Oral: Administer with a large quantity of fluid to ensure proper action

Test Interactions May cause a colorimetric interference with certain laboratory determinations of 5-hydroxy indoleacetic acid (5-HIAA) and vanillylmandelic acid (VMA)

Dosage Forms
Syrup:
Brontex®: Guaifensin 75 mg and codeine phosphate 2.5 mg per 5 mL (480 mL)
Gani-Tuss® NR, Guiatuss® AC, Halotussin® AC, Mytussin® AC, Robitussin® AC, Romilar® AC, Tussi-Organidin® NR, Tussi-Organidin® S-NR: Guaifenesin 100 mg and codeine phosphate 10 mg per 5 mL (60 mL, 120 mL, 480 mL, 3840 mL)
Tablet (Brontex®): Guaifenesin 300 mg and codeine phosphate 10 mg

Guaifenesin and Dextromethorphan
(gwye FEN e sin & deks troe meth OR fan)

Related Information
OTC Cough & Cold Preparations, Pediatric on page 1072

U.S. Brand Names Aquatab® DM; Benylin® Expectorant [OTC]; Cheracol D® [OTC]; Diabetic Tussin DM [OTC]; Duratuss® DM; Fenesin DM®; Genatuss DM® [OTC]; Guiatuss DM® [OTC]; Halotussin® DM [OTC]; Humibid® DM; Iobid DM®; Kolephrin® GG/DM [OTC]; Muco-Fen-DM®; Mytussin® DM [OTC]; Naldecon® Senior DX [OTC]; Phanatuss® [OTC]; Respa-DM®; Rhinosyn-DMX® [OTC]; Robafen DM® [OTC]; Robitussin®-DM [OTC]; Safe Tussin® 30 [OTC]; Scot-Tussin® Senior Clear [OTC]; Siltussin DM® [OTC]; Syracol-CF® [OTC]; Tolu-Sed® DM [OTC]; Touro® DM; Tuss-DM® [OTC]; Tussin® DM [OTC]; Tussi-Organidin® DM NR; Vicks® 44E [OTC]; Vicks® Pediatric Formula 44E [OTC]

Canadian Brand Names Balminil DM E; Benylin DM-E; Cough Syrup DM-E; Cough Syrup DM Expectorant; Cough Syrup with Guaifenesin & Dextromethorphan; DM Cough Syrup Expectorant; DM Plus Expectorant; Formula 44E; Koffex DM-E; Syrup DM-E

Synonyms Dextromethorphan and Glycerol Guaiacolate; Dextromethorphan and Guaifenesin

Therapeutic Category Antitussive; Cough Preparation; Expectorant

Generic Available Yes

Use Temporary control of cough due to minor throat and bronchial irritation

Pregnancy Risk Factor C

Contraindications Hypersensitivity to guaifenesin, dextromethorphan, or any component

Adverse Reactions
Central nervous system: Drowsiness, dizziness, headache
Dermatologic: Rash
Gastrointestinal: Nausea

Mechanism of Action See individual monographs for Guaifenesin on page 485 and Dextromethorphan on page 316

Pharmacodynamics Onset of action: Antitussive effect: Oral: 15-30 minutes

Pharmacokinetics Absorption: Dextromethorphan is rapidly absorbed from the GI tract

Usual Dosage Oral (dose expressed in mg of dextromethorphan):
Children: 1-2 mg/kg/day every 6-8 hours
Adults: 60-120 mg/day divided every 6-8 hours

Administration Oral: Administer with a large quantity of fluid to ensure proper effect

Test Interactions May cause a colorimetric interference with certain laboratory determinations of 5-hydroxy indoleacetic acid (5-HIAA) and vanillylmandelic acid (VMA)

Dosage Forms
Syrup:
Benylin® Expectorant: Guaifenesin 100 mg and dextromethorphan hydrobromide 5 mg per 5 mL (118 mL)
Cheracol D®, Diabetic Tussin DM®, Genatuss DM®, Guiatuss DM®, Halotussin® DM, Mytussin® DM, Phanatuss®, Robafen DM®, Robitussin®-DM, Siltussin DM®, Tolu-Sed® DM, Tussin® DM, Tussi-Organidin® DM NR: Guaifenesin 100 mg and dextromethorphan hydrobromide 10 mg per 5 mL (5 mL, 120 mL, 180 mL, 240 mL, 360 mL, 480 mL, 3780 mL)
Duratuss® DM: Guaifenesin 200 mg and dextromethorphan hydrobromide 20 mg per 5 mL (480 mL, 3840 mL)
Kolephrin® GG/DM: Guaifenesin 150 mg and dextromethorphan hydrobromide 10 mg per 5 mL (120 mL)

(Continued)

Guaifenesin and Dextromethorphan *(Continued)*

Naldecon® Senior DX: Guaifenesin 200 mg and dextromethorphan hydrobromide 10 mg per 5 mL (118 mL)

Rhinosyn-DMX®, Safe Tussin® 30: Guaifenesin 100 mg and dextromethorphan hydrobromide 15 mg per 5 mL (120 mL)

Scot-Tussin® Senior: Guaifenesin 200 mg and dextromethorphan hydrobromide 15 mg per 5 mL (30 mL, 120 mL, 240 mL, 480 mL, 3875 mL)

Vicks® 44E: Guaifenesin 66.7 mg and dextromethorphan hydrobromide 6.7 mg per 5 mL (120 mL, 240 mL)

Vicks® Pediatric Formula 44E: Guaifenesin 33.3 mg and dextromethorphan hydrobromide 3.3 mg per 5 mL (120 mL)

Tablet, extended release:

Aquatab® DM: Guaifenesin 1200 mg and dextromethorphan hydrobromide 60 mg

Guaifenex DM®, Iobid DM®, Fenesin DM®, Humibid® DM, Muco-Fen-DM®, Respa-DM®: Guaifenesin 600 mg and dextromethorphan hydrobromide 30 mg

Syracol-CF®: Guaifenesin 200 mg and dextromethorphan hydrobromide 15 mg

Touro® DM: Guaifenesin 575 mg and dextromethorphan hydrobromide 30 mg

Tuss-DM®: Guaifenesin 200 mg and dextromethorphan hydrobromide 10 mg

♦ **Guaifenex LA®** *see* Guaifenesin *on page 485*

♦ **Guaituss AC®** *see* Guaifenesin and Codeine *on page 486*

♦ **Guiatuss® [OTC]** *see* Guaifenesin *on page 485*

♦ **Guiatuss DM® [OTC]** *see* Guaifenesin and Dextromethorphan *on page 487*

♦ **G-well®** *see* Lindane *on page 595*

♦ **Gyne-Lotrimin® Vaginal [OTC]** *see* Clotrimazole *on page 259*

♦ **Gynodiol™** *see* Estradiol *on page 400*

♦ **H₂O₂** *see* Hydrogen Peroxide *on page 509*

♦ **Haemophilus b Oligosaccharide Conjugate Vaccine** *see page 1172*

♦ **Halcion®** *see* Triazolam *on page 982*

♦ **Haldol®** *see* Haloperidol *on page 488*

♦ **Haldol® Decanoate** *see* Haloperidol *on page 488*

♦ **Halenol® [OTC]** *see* Acetaminophen *on page 29*

♦ **Halfprin® [OTC]** *see* Aspirin *on page 109*

Haloperidol (ha loe PER i dole)

Related Information

Carbohydrate and Alcohol Content of Liquid Medications for Use in Patients Receiving Ketogenic Diets *on page 1258*

Drugs and Breast-Feeding *on page 1243*

U.S. Brand Names Haldol®; Haldol® Decanoate

Canadian Brand Names Apo-Haloperidol; Novo-Peridol; Peridol; PMS-Haloperidol; Rho-Haloperidol

Therapeutic Category Antipsychotic Agent; Phenothiazine Derivative

Generic Available Yes

Use Treatment of psychoses, Tourette's disorder, and severe behavioral problems in children; emergency sedation of severely agitated or delirious patients

Pregnancy Risk Factor C

Contraindications Hypersensitivity to haloperidol or any component; narrow-angle glaucoma, bone marrow suppression, CNS depression, severe liver or cardiac disease, parkinsonism

Warnings Safety and efficacy have not been established in children <3 years of age

Precautions Use with caution in patients with renal or hepatic dysfunction, thyrotoxicosis, cardiovascular disease, or history of seizures

Adverse Reactions

Cardiovascular: Tachycardia, hypotension

Central nervous system: Extrapyramidal reactions, neuroleptic malignant syndrome, tardive dyskinesia, drowsiness

Dermatologic: Rash, contact dermatitis

Endocrine & metabolic: Galactorrhea, gynecomastia, hyperglycemia, hypoglycemia, hyponatremia, hypomagnesemia

Gastrointestinal: Xerostomia, constipation

Genitourinary: Urinary retention

Hematologic: Leukopenia, leukocytosis, anemia

Hepatic: Hepatotoxicity (rare)

Ocular: Blurred vision

Drug Interactions Cytochrome P-450 isoenzyme CYP1A2, CYP2D6 (minor), and CYP3A3/4 substrate; CYP2D6 and CYP3A3/4 isoenzyme inhibitor

CNS depressants may increase adverse effects; epinephrine may cause hypotension; carbamazepine and phenobarbital may increase metabolism and decrease effectiveness of haloperidol; use of haloperidol with anticholinergic agents may increase intraocular pressure; concurrent use with lithium has occasionally caused acute encephalopathy-like syndrome

Food Interactions Drug may precipitate if oral concentrate is mixed with coffee or tea

Mechanism of Action Competitive blockade of postsynaptic dopamine receptors in the mesolimbic dopaminergic system; depresses cerebral cortex and hypothalamus; exhibits a strong alpha-adrenergic and anticholinergic blocking activity

Pharmacokinetics

Absorption: Oral: Well absorbed, undergoes first-pass metabolism in the liver

Distribution: Crosses the placenta; appears in breast milk

Protein binding: 92%

Metabolism: In the liver, hydroxy-metabolite is active

Bioavailability: Oral: 60%

Half-life: Adults: 20 hours; range: 13-35 hours

Elimination: Excreted in urine and feces as drug and metabolites

Usual Dosage

Children:

3-12 years (15-40 kg): Oral: Initial: 0.25-0.5 mg/day given in 2-3 divided doses; increase by 0.25-0.5 mg every 5-7 days; maximum dose: 0.15 mg/kg/day; usual maintenance:

Agitation or hyperkinesia: 0.01-0.03 mg/kg/day once daily

Tourette's disorder: 0.05-0.075 mg/kg/day in 2-3 divided doses

Psychotic disorders: 0.05-0.15 mg/kg/day in 2-3 divided doses

Note: Preliminary findings of a double-blind, placebo controlled study reported the mean optimal dose in 12 schizophrenic children 5-12 years to be ~2 mg/day (range: 0.5-3.5 mg/day or 0.02-0.12 mg/kg/day) given in 3 divided doses

6-12 years: I.M. **(as lactate)**: 1-3 mg/dose every 4-8 hours to a maximum of 0.15 mg/kg/day; switch to oral therapy as soon as able

Adults:

Oral: 0.5-5 mg 2-3 times/day; usual maximum dose: 30 mg/day; some patients may require 100 mg/day

I.M.:

As **lactate**: 2-5 mg every 4-8 hours as needed

As **decanoate**: Initial: 10-15 times the individual patients' stabilized oral dose, given at 3- to 4-week intervals

Administration

Oral: Administer with food or milk to decrease GI distress; prior to administration, dilute oral concentrate with ≥2 ounces of water or acidic beverage; do not mix oral concentrate with coffee or tea

Parenteral: **Decanoate** product is for I.M. use only, do not give I.V.; although not FDA-approved, haloperidol **lactate** has been administered I.V.

Monitoring Parameters Blood pressure, CBC with differential, liver enzymes with long-term use; serum glucose, sodium, magnesium

Patient Information Avoid alcohol; may cause drowsiness and impair ability to perform activities requiring mental alertness or physical coordination; may cause dry mouth

Nursing Implications Observe for extrapyramidal effects

Dosage Forms

Concentrate, oral, as lactate: 2 mg/mL (5 mL, 10 mL, 15 mL, 120 mL)

Injection, as decanoate: 50 mg/mL (1 mL, 5 mL); 100 mg/mL (1 mL, 5 mL)

Injection, as lactate: 5 mg/mL (1 mL, 10 mL)

Tablet: 0.5 mg, 1 mg, 2 mg, 5 mg, 10 mg, 20 mg

References

Serrano AC, "Haloperidol - Its Use in Children," *J Clin Psychiatry*, 1981, 42(4):154-6.

Spencer EK, Kafantaris V, Padron-Gayol MV, et al, "Haloperidol in Schizophrenic Children: Early Findings From a Study in Progress," *Psychopharmacol Bull*, 1992, 28(2):183-6.

Haloprogin (ha loe PROE jin)

U.S. Brand Names Halotex®

Therapeutic Category Antifungal Agent, Topical

Generic Available No

Use Topical treatment of tinea pedis, tinea cruris, tinea corporis, tinea manuum caused by *Trichophyton rubrum*, *Trichophyton tonsurans*, *Trichophyton mentagrophytes*, *Microsporum canis*, or *Epidermophyton floccosum*

(Continued)

Haloprogin *(Continued)*

Pregnancy Risk Factor C

Contraindications Hypersensitivity to haloprogin or any component

Warnings Safety and efficacy have not been established in children

Adverse Reactions

Dermatologic: Pruritus, folliculitis, vesicle formation, erythema, scaling

Local: Irritation, burning sensation

Mechanism of Action Inhibits yeast cell respiration and disrupts its cell membrane

Pharmacokinetics Absorption: Poor through the skin ($\sim$11%)

Usual Dosage Children and Adults: Topical: Twice daily for 2-3 weeks; intertriginous areas may require up to 4 weeks of treatment

Administration Topical: A small amount of cream or 2-3 drops of the solution should be rubbed gently into the affected area

Patient Information Avoid contact with eyes, for topical use only; contact physician if increased irritation occurs

Dosage Forms

Cream: 1% (15 g, 30 g)

Solution, topical: 1% with alcohol 75% (10 mL, 30 mL)

- ◆ **Halotestin**® *see* Fluoxymesterone *on page 448*
- ◆ **Halotex**® *see* Haloprogin *on page 489*
- ◆ **Halotussin**® **AC** *see* Guaifenesin and Codeine *on page 486*
- ◆ **Halotussin**® **DM [OTC]** *see* Guaifenesin and Dextromethorphan *on page 487*
- ◆ **Haltran**® **[OTC]** *see* Ibuprofen *on page 520*
- ◆ **HAT Antibody** *see* Daclizumab *on page 293*
- ◆ **hCG** *see* Chorionic Gonadotropin *on page 232*
- ◆ **HCTZ** *see* Hydrochlorothiazide *on page 503*
- ◆ **HDA Toothache**® **[OTC]** *see* Benzocaine *on page 135*
- ◆ **Heavy Mineral Oil** *see* Mineral Oil *on page 675*
- ◆ **Hemet**® **Rectal [OTC]** *see* Hemorrhoidal Preparations *on page 490*
- ◆ **Hemocaine**® **[OTC]** *see* Hemorrhoidal Preparations *on page 490*
- ◆ **Hemocyte**® **[OTC]** *see* Iron Supplements (Oral/Enteral) *on page 548*
- ◆ **Hemofil**® **M** *see* Antihemophilic Factor (Human) *on page 98*

Hemorrhoidal Preparations *(HEM or oyd al prep a RAY shuns)*

U.S. Brand Names A-Caine® Rectal [OTC]; Anumed® [OTC]; Anusol® [OTC]; Calmol 4®; CPI® [OTC]; Fleet® Relief®; Hemet® Rectal [OTC]; Hemocaine® [OTC]; Hem-Prep® [OTC]; Nupercainal®; Pazo® Hemorrhoid [OTC]; Perifoam® [OTC]; Posterisan® [OTC]; Preparation H® [OTC]; ProctoFoam® [OTC]; Rectal Medicone® [OTC]; Tronolane®

Therapeutic Category Topical Skin Product

Generic Available Yes

Use Symptomatic relief of pain and discomfort in external and internal hemorrhoids, proctitis, papillitis, cryptitis, anal fissures, incomplete fistulas and relief of local pain following anorectal surgery

Contraindications Hypersensitivity to any component

Warnings Some preparations contain a sulfite which may cause allergic-type reactions

Adverse Reactions

Dermatologic: Rash

Local: Irritation, burning, itching

Mechanism of Action

Dibucaine, benzocaine, pramoxine: Temporarily relieves pain, itching, and irritation by blocking nerve impulses at the sensory nerve endings in the skin and mucous membranes

Emollient/protectant (glycerin, lanolin, mineral oil, petrolatum, zinc oxide, cocoa butter, shark liver oil): Form a physical barrier and lubricate tissues preventing irritation of the anorectal area and water loss

Pharmacodynamics

Onset of effect: Topical:

Pramoxine: 3-5 minutes

Dibucaine: <15 minutes

Benzocaine: 1 minute

Usual Dosage

Children and Adults: Topical: Apply ointment as a thin layer to the perianal area and the anal canal 3-6 times/day

Benzocaine-containing preparations: Apply up to 6 times/day

Dibucaine-containing preparations: Apply ointment into the rectum each morning and evening and after each bowel movement; ointment may be applied topically to anal tissues; apply up to 3-4 times/day

    Children: No more than 7.5 g in a 24-hour period

    Adults: No more than 30 g in a 24-hour period

Pramoxine-containing preparations: Apply up to 5 times/day (2-3 times/day and after bowel movements)

Adults: Rectal: Insert 1 suppository in the morning and at bedtime and after each bowel movement

Administration

Rectal: Foam, ointment, and cream for rectal use are instilled using a rectal applicator. The aerosol should not be inserted into the anus.

Topical: Apply cream or ointment to affected areas and rub in gently. A small amount of foam may be applied to the affected area using a cleansing tissue or pad.

Patient Information If anorectal symptoms do not improve in 7 days, or if bleeding, protrusion or seepage occurs, consult physician; avoid contact of topical preparations to the eyes

Dosage Forms

Dibucaine: 1%: Nupercainal® hemorrhoidal and anesthetic ointment

Pramoxine:

    Cream: 1%: Tronolane®

    Foam: 1%: ProctoFoam®: 15 g, 45 g

    Ointment: 1%: Fleet Relief®; Anusol®

    Rectal suppository: 1%: Americaine® hemorrhoidal ointment

Benzocaine: 20%: Americaine® hemorrhoidal ointment

Emollient/protectants (glycerin, lanolin, mineral oil, petrolatum, zinc oxide, cocoa butter, shark liver oil):

    Cream: Preparation H®

    Ointment: Preparation H®

    Suppository: Preparation H®, Calmol 4®; Wyanoids® Relief Factor; Nupercainal®

♦ **Hem-Prep® [OTC]** see Hemorrhoidal Preparations on page 490

♦ **Hemril®-HC** see Hydrocortisone on page 506

♦ **Hepalean (Can)** see Heparin on page 491

♦ **Hepalean-Lok (Can)** see Heparin on page 491

Heparin (HEP a rin)

Related Information

Overdose and Toxicology on page 1222

U.S. Brand Names Hep-Lock®

Canadian Brand Names Hepalean; Hepalean-Lok

Synonyms Heparin Lock Flush

Therapeutic Category Anticoagulant

Generic Available Yes

Use Prophylaxis and treatment of thromboembolic disorders

Pregnancy Risk Factor C

Contraindications Hypersensitivity to heparin or any component; severe thrombocytopenia, subacute bacterial endocarditis, suspected intracranial hemorrhage, shock, severe hypotension, uncontrollable bleeding (unless secondary to disseminated intravascular coagulation)

Warnings Some preparations contain benzyl alcohol as a preservative. In neonates, large amounts of benzyl alcohol (>100 mg/kg/day) have been associated with fatal toxicity (gasping syndrome); the use of preservative free heparin is, therefore, recommended in neonates. Some preparations contain sulfites which may cause allergic reactions.

Precautions Use with caution as hemorrhage may occur; risk factors for hemorrhage include: I.M. injections; peptic ulcer disease; intermittent I.V. injections (vs continuous I.V. infusion); increased capillary permeability; menstruation; recent surgery or invasive procedures; severe renal, hepatic, or biliary disease; and indwelling catheters

Heparin does not possess fibrinolytic activity and, therefore, cannot lyse established thrombi; discontinue heparin if hemorrhage occurs; severe hemorrhage or overdosage may require protamine

Adverse Reactions

Central nervous system: Fever, headache, chills

Dermatologic: Urticaria, alopecia

(Continued)

Heparin *(Continued)*

Gastrointestinal: Nausea, vomiting

Hematologic: Hemorrhage, thrombocytopenia (may be more common with beef lung heparin vs porcine mucosa heparin; however, if a patient receiving beef lung heparin experiences severe thrombocytopenia it is **not** recommended to switch to porcine mucosa heparin because a similar reaction may occur)

Hepatic: Elevated liver enzymes

Local: Irritation, ulceration, cutaneous necrosis has been rarely reported with deep S.C. injections

Neuromuscular & skeletal: Osteoporosis (with long-term use)

Drug Interactions Thrombolytic agents (urokinase, streptokinase, alteplase) and drugs which affect platelet function (eg, aspirin, NSAIDs, dipyridamole) may potentiate the risk of hemorrhage; digoxin, tetracycline, nicotine, antihistamines, and I.V. nitroglycerin may decrease heparin's anticoagulant effect.

Mechanism of Action Potentiates the action of antithrombin III and thereby inactivates thrombin (as well as activated coagulation factors IX, X, XI, XII, and plasmin) and prevents the conversion of fibrinogen to fibrin; heparin also stimulates release of lipoprotein lipase (lipoprotein lipase hydrolyzes triglycerides to glycerol and free fatty acids)

Pharmacodynamics Onset of anticoagulation effect:

S.C.: 20-60 minutes

I.V.: Immediate

Pharmacokinetics

Absorption: S.C., I.M.: Erratic

Distribution: Does not cross the placenta; does not appear in breast milk

Metabolism: Believed to be partially metabolized in the reticuloendothelial system

Half-life: Mean: 90 minutes (range: 1-2 hours); affected by obesity, renal function, hepatic function, malignancy, presence of pulmonary embolism, and infections

Elimination: Renal; small amount excreted unchanged in urine

Usual Dosage

Line flushing: When using daily flushes of heparin to maintain patency of single and double lumen central catheters, 10 units/mL is commonly used for younger infants (eg, <10 kg) while 100 units/mL is used for older infants, children, and adults. Capped polyvinyl chloride catheters and peripheral heparin locks require flushing more frequently (eg, every 6-8 hours). Volume of heparin flush is usually similar to volume of catheter (or slightly greater) or may be standardized according to specific hospital's policy (eg, 2-5 mL/flush). Dose of heparin flush used should not approach therapeutic unit per kg dose. Additional flushes should be given when stagnant blood is observed in catheter, after catheter is used for drug or blood administration, and after blood withdrawal from catheter.

TPN: Heparin 1 unit/mL (final concentration) may be added to TPN solutions, both central and peripheral. (Addition of heparin to peripheral TPN has been shown to increase duration of line patency.) The final concentration of heparin used for TPN solutions may need to be decreased to 0.5 units/mL in small infants receiving larger TPN volumes in order to avoid approaching therapeutic amounts.

Arterial lines: Heparinize with a usual final concentration of 1 unit/mL; range: 0.5-2 units/mL; in order to avoid large total doses and systemic effects, use 0.5 unit/mL in low birth weight/premature newborns and in other patients receiving multiple lines containing heparin

Prophylaxis for cardiac catheterization via an artery: Newborns and Children: I.V.: Bolus: 100-150 units/kg (see Monagle, 2001)

Systemic heparinization:

Neonates and Infants <1 year: I.V. infusion: Initial loading dose: 75 units/kg given over 10 minutes; then initial maintenance dose: 28 units/kg/hour; adjust dose to maintain APTT of 60-85 seconds (assuming this reflects an antifactor Xa level of 0.3-0.7); see table.

Children >1 year:

Intermittent I.V.: Initial: 50-100 units/kg, then 50-100 units/kg every 4 hours (**Note:** Continuous I.V. infusion is preferred):

I.V. infusion: Initial loading dose: 75 units/kg given over 10 minutes, then initial maintenance dose: 20 units/kg/hour; adjust dose to maintain APTT of 60-85 seconds (assuming this reflects an antifactor Xa level of 0.3-0.7); see table.

PEDIATRIC PROTOCOL FOR SYSTEMIC HEPARIN ADJUSTMENT

To be used after initial loading dose and maintenance I.V. infusion dose (see Usual Dosage listed above) to maintain APTT of 60-85 seconds (assuming this reflects antifactor Xa level of 0.3-0.7)

Obtain blood for APTT 4 hours after heparin loading dose and 4 hours after every infusion rate change

Obtain daily CBC and APTT after APTT is therapeutic

APTT (seconds)	Dosage Adjustment	Time to Repeat APTT
<50	Give 50 units/kg bolus and increase infusion rate by 10%	4 h after rate change
50-59	Increase infusion rate by 10%	4 h after rate change
60-85	Keep rate the same	Next day
86-95	Decrease infusion rate by 10%	4 h after rate change
96-120	Hold infusion for 30 minutes and decrease infusion rate by 10%	4 h after rate change
>120	Hold infusion for 60 minutes and decrease infusion rate by 15%	4 h after rate change

Modified from Monagle P, Michelson AD, Bovill E, et al, "Antithrombotic Therapy in Children," *Chest*, 2001, 119:344S-70S.

Adults:
  Prophylaxis (low dose heparin): S.C.: 5000 units every 8-12 hours
  Intermittent I.V.: Initial: 10,000 units, then 50-70 units/kg (5000-10,000 units) every 4-6 hours
  I.V. infusion: Initial loading dose: 80 units/kg; initial maintenance dose: 18 units/kg/hour with dose adjusted according to APTT; usual range: 10-30 units/kg/hour
Adults: *Chest* 2001 Recommendations (see Hirsh, 2001):
  Prophylaxis of DVT and PE: S.C.: 5000 units every 8 or 12 hours or adjusted low-dose heparin
  Treatment of DVT: Initial loading dose: I.V. bolus: 5000 units, then initial maintenance dose: I.V. infusion: 32,000 units/day (1333 units/hour); adjust dose to maintain therapeutic APTT; recommendations also list S.C. 35,000-40,000 units/day (**Note:** S.C. dose which was divided into 2 daily doses, is no longer used clinically)
  Unstable angina or acute MI without thrombolytic therapy: Initial loading dose: I.V. bolus: 5000 units, then initial maintenance dose: I.V. infusion: 32,000 units/day (1333 units/hour); adjust dose to maintain therapeutic APTT
  Acute MI after thrombolytic therapy (role of heparin unproven): Initial loading dose: I.V. bolus: 5000 units, then initial maintenance dose: I.V. infusion: 24,000 units/day (1000 units/hour); adjust dose to maintain therapeutic APTT
Administration Parenteral: Continuous I.V. infusion is preferred vs I.V. intermittent injections; heparin lock flush solutions are intended only to maintain patency of I.V. devices and are **not** for systemic anticoagulation
Monitoring Parameters Platelet counts, signs of bleeding, hemoglobin, hematocrit, APTT; for full-dose heparin (ie, nonlow dose), the dose should be titrated according to APTT (see table). For intermittent I.V. injections, APTT is measured 3.5-4 hours after I.V. injection.
Reference Range Treatment of venous thrombotic disease: Recommended APTT should reflect a heparin level by protamine titration of 0.2-0.4 units/mL or an antifactor Xa level of 0.3-0.7 units/mL; this usually reflects an APTT of 60-85 seconds or a ratio (patient/control APTT) of 1.5-2.5; a lower therapeutic range (corresponding to antifactor Xa level of 0.14-0.34 units/mL) is recommended for patients with acute MI who received thrombolytic therapy
Test Interactions ↑ thyroxine (S) (competitive protein binding methods)
Patient Information Limit alcohol
Nursing Implications Do not administer I.M. due to pain, irritation, and hematoma formation
Additional Information To reverse the effects of heparin, use protamine (see Protamine *on page 850* for specifics); heparin is available from beef lung and from porcine intestinal mucosa sources
  Duration of heparin therapy (pediatric):
    DVT: At least 5 days
    Extensive DVT or pulmonary embolism (PE): 7-10 days
    Note: Oral anticoagulation can be started on day 1 of heparin, except for extensive DVT or PE, when it should be delayed; oral anticoagulation should be overlapped with heparin for 5 days
Dosage Forms
  Heparin sodium:
    Lock flush injection:
      Beef lung source: 10 units/mL (1 mL, 2 mL, 2.5 mL, 3 mL, 5 mL, 10 mL, 30 mL); 100 units/mL (1 mL, 2 mL, 2.5 mL, 3 mL, 5 mL, 10 mL, 30 mL)
  (Continued)

Heparin *(Continued)*

Porcine intestinal mucosa source: 10 units/mL (1 mL, 2 mL, 10 mL, 30 mL); 100 units/mL (1 mL, 2 mL, 10 mL, 30 mL)

Porcine intestinal mucosa source, preservative free: 10 units/mL (1 mL); 100 units/mL (1 mL)

Multiple-dose vial injection:

Beef lung source, with preservative: 1000 units/mL (5 mL, 10 mL, 30 mL); 5000 units/mL (10 mL); 10,000 units/mL (4 mL, 5 mL, 10 mL); 20,000 units/mL (2 mL, 5 mL, 10 mL); 40,000 units/mL (5 mL)

Porcine intestinal mucosa source, with preservative: 1000 units/mL (10 mL, 30 mL); 5000 units/mL (10 mL); 10,000 units/mL (4 mL, 5 mL); 20,000 units/mL (2 mL, 5 mL)

Single-dose vial injection:

Beef lung source: 1000 units/mL (1 mL); 5000 units/mL (1 mL); 10,000 units/mL (1 mL); 20,000 units/mL (1 mL); 40,000 units/mL (1 mL)

Porcine intestinal mucosa: 1000 units/mL (1 mL); 5000 units/mL (1 mL); 10,000 units/mL (1 mL); 20,000 units/mL (1 mL); 40,000 units/mL (1 mL)

Unit dose injection:

Porcine intestinal mucosa source, with preservative: 1000 units/dose (1 mL, 2 mL); 2500 units/dose (1 mL); 5000 units/dose (0.5 mL, 1 mL); 7500 units/dose (1 mL); 10,000 units/dose (1 mL); 15,000 units/dose (1 mL); 20,000 units/dose (1 mL)

Heparin sodium infusion, porcine intestinal mucosa source:

D_5W: 40 units/mL (500 mL); 50 units/mL (250 mL, 500 mL); 100 units/mL (100 mL, 250 mL)

NaCl 0.45%: 2 units/mL (500 mL, 1000 mL); 50 units/mL (250 mL, 500 mL); 100 units/mL (250 mL)

NaCl 0.9%: 2 units/mL (500 mL, 1000 mL); 5 units/mL (1000 mL); 50 units/mL (250 mL, 500 mL, 1000 mL)

References

Andrew M, Marzinotto V, Massicotte P, et al, "Heparin Therapy in Pediatric Patients: A Prospective Cohort Study," *Pediatr Res*, 1994, 35(1):78-83.

Hirsh J, Warkentin TE, Shaughnessy SG, et al, "Heparin and Low-Molecular Weight-Heparin: Mechanisms of Action, Pharmacokinetics, Dosing, Monitoring, Efficacy and Safety," *Chest*, 2001, 119:64S-94S.

Monagle P, Michelson AD, Bovill E, et al, "Antithrombotic Therapy in Children," *Chest*, 2001, 119:344S-70S.

- ◆ **Heparin Lock Flush** *see Heparin on page 491*
- ◆ **Hepatitis A Vaccine** *see page 1172*
- ◆ **Hepatitis B Immune Globulin** *see page 1172*
- ◆ **Hepatitis B Vaccine** *see page 1172*
- ◆ **Hep-Lock®** *see Heparin on page 491*
- ◆ **Heptovir (Can)** *see Lamivudine on page 572*
- ◆ **HES** *see Hetastarch on page 494*
- ◆ **Hespan®** *see Hetastarch on page 494*

Hetastarch *(HET a starch)*

U.S. Brand Names Hespan®

Synonyms HES; Hydroxyethyl Starch

Therapeutic Category Plasma Volume Expander

Generic Available No

Use Blood volume expander used in treatment of shock or impending shock when blood or blood products are not available; does not have oxygen-carrying capacity and is not a substitute for blood or plasma

Pregnancy Risk Factor C

Contraindications Severe bleeding disorders, renal failure with oliguria or anuria, or severe CHF; management of cerebral vasospasm associated with subarachnoid hemorrhage or for conditions other than leukapheresis which necessitate repeated use of the drug over several days

Warnings Anaphylactoid reactions have occurred; use with caution in patients with thrombocytopenia (may interfere with platelet function); large volume may cause drops in hemoglobin concentrations; use with caution in patients at risk from overexpansion of blood volume, including the very young or aged patients, those with CHF or pulmonary edema; large volumes may interfere with platelet function and prolong PT and PTT times; use with caution in patients with a history of liver disease

Adverse Reactions

Cardiovascular: Heart failure, circulatory overload, peripheral edema

Central nervous system: Headache, fever, chills

Dermatologic: Urticaria, pruritus

Endocrine & metabolic: Parotid gland enlargement, hyperchloremic metabolic acidosis, hypernatremia

Gastrointestinal: Vomiting, increased amylase levels

Hematologic: Thrombocytopenia, transient prolongation of PT, PTT, clotting time, and bleeding time

Hepatic: Increased indirect bilirubin

Neuromuscular & skeletal: Myalgia

Ocular: Periorbital edema

Respiratory: Wheezing

Miscellaneous: Anaphylactoid reactions

Stability Do not use if crystalline precipitate forms or is turbid deep brown

Mechanism of Action Hetastarch. a synthetic polymer, produces plasma volume expansion by virtue of its highly colloidal starch structure

Pharmacodynamics

Onset of volume expansion: I.V.: Within 30 minutes

Duration: 24-36 hours

Pharmacokinetics

Metabolism: Molecules >50,000 daltons require enzymatic degradation by the reticuloendothelial system or amylases in the blood prior to urinary and fecal excretion

Elimination: Smaller molecular weight molecules are readily excreted in urine; approximately 40% of dose excreted in first 24 hours in patients with normal renal function

Usual Dosage I.V. infusion:

Children: 10 mL/kg/dose; the total daily dose should not exceed 20 mL/kg

Adults: 500-1000 mL (30-60 g) per dose; the total daily dose should not exceed 1.2 g/kg or 90 g (1500 mL)

Dosing adjustment in renal impairment: Cl_{cr} <10 mL/minute: Initial dose is the same but subsequent doses should be reduced by 20% to 50% of normal

Administration Parenteral: I.V.: Maximum rate of infusion: 1.2 g/kg/hour (20 mL/kg/hour)

Monitoring Parameters Volume expansion: capillary refill time, CVP, RAP, MAP, urine output, heart rate, if pulmonary artery catheter in place, monitor PWCP, SVR, and PVR; hemoglobin, hematocrit; for leukapheresis, monitor CBC, total leukocyte and platelet counts, leukocyte differential count, hemoglobin, hematocrit, prothrombin time, and partial thromboplastin time

Additional Information Each 500 mL provides 77 mEq sodium chloride; currently available product in the United States is high molecular weight (HMW); low molecular weight (LMW) products available in Europe may have an improved adverse reaction profile

Dosage Forms Infusion, in sodium chloride 0.9%: 6% (500 mL)

References

Brutocao D, Bratton SL, Thomas JR, et al, "Comparison of Hetastarch With Albumin for Postoperative Volume Expansion in Children After Cardiopulmonary Bypass," *J Cardiothoracic Vasc Anesth*, 1996, 10(3):348-51.

♦ **Hexachlorocyclohexane** *see* Lindane *on page 595*

Hexachlorophene (heks a KLOR oh feen)

U.S. Brand Names pHisoHex®; Septisol®

Therapeutic Category Antibacterial, Topical; Soap

Generic Available Yes

Use Surgical scrub and as a bacteriostatic skin cleanser; to control an outbreak of gram-positive staphylococcal infection when other infection control procedures have been unsuccessful

Pregnancy Risk Factor C

Contraindications Hypersensitivity to halogenated phenol derivatives or hexachlorophene; use in premature infants; use on burned or denuded skin; use with an occlusive dressing; application to mucous membranes

Warnings Do not use for bathing infants; do not apply to mucous membranes; premature and low birth weight infants are particularly susceptible to hexachlorophene topical absorption; irritability, generalized clonic muscular contractions, decerebrate rigidity, and brain lesions in the white matter have occurred in infants following topical use of 6% hexachlorophene; exposure of preterm infants or patients with extensive burns has been associated with apnea, convulsions, agitation, and coma

Adverse Reactions

Central nervous system: CNS injury, seizures, irritability

(Continued)

Hexachlorophene *(Continued)*

Dermatologic: Dermatitis, erythema, dry skin, photosensitivity

Drug Interactions Polysorbate 80, nonionic detergents with concentration >8% may decrease antibacterial activity of hexachlorophene

Stability Store in nonmetallic container (incompatible with many metals); protect from light

Mechanism of Action Bacteriostatic polychlorinated biphenol which inhibits membrane-bound enzymes and disrupts the cell membrane

Pharmacokinetics

Absorption: Percutaneously through inflamed, excoriated and intact skin

Distribution: Crosses the placenta

Half-life, infants: 6.1-44.2 hours

Usual Dosage Children and Adults: Topical: Apply 5 mL cleanser and water to area to be cleansed; lather and rinse thoroughly under running water; for use as a surgical scrub, a second application of 5 mL cleanser should be made and the hands and forearms scrubbed for an additional 3 minutes, rinsed thoroughly with running water and dried

Administration Topical: For external use only; rinse thoroughly after each use

Patient Information Avoid prolonged contact with skin

Dosage Forms

Foam (Septisol®): 0.23% with alcohol 56% (180 mL, 600 mL)

Liquid, topical (pHisoHex®): 3% (8 mL, 150 mL, 500 mL, 3840 mL)

References

Lester RS, "Topical Formulary for the Pediatrician," *Pediatr Clin North Am*, 1983, 30(4):749-65.

♦ **Hexadrol Phosphate (Can)** *see* Dexamethasone *on page 307*

♦ **Hexamethylenetetramine** *see* Methenamine *on page 643*

♦ **Hexit (Can)** *see* Lindane *on page 595*

♦ **Hiclens® [OTC]** *see* Chlorhexidine Gluconate *on page 220*

♦ **Hibidil (Can)** *see* Chlorhexidine Gluconate *on page 220*

♦ **Hibitane (Can)** *see* Chlorhexidine Gluconate *on page 220*

♦ **Hiprex®** *see* Methenamine *on page 643*

♦ **Histantil (Can)** *see* Promethazine *on page 836*

Histrelin *(his TREL in)*

U.S. Brand Names Supprelin™

Synonyms ORF17070; RWJ17070

Therapeutic Category Gonadotropin Releasing Hormone Analog

Generic Available No

Use Central idiopathic precocious puberty; also used to treat estrogen-associated gynecological disorders [ie, endometriosis, intermittent porphyria, possibly premenstrual syndrome, leiomyomata uteri (uterine fibroids)]

Pregnancy Risk Factor X

Contraindications Hypersensitivity to histrelin or any component; pregnancy or expected pregnancy, breast-feeding

Precautions Inadequate control of pubertal process may occur with noncompliance or changes in the dosing schedule

Adverse Reactions

Central nervous system: Anxiety, depression, irritability, insomnia, headaches, rarely increase in seizure frequency

Endocrine & metabolic: Prevention of ovulation and menses, inhibition of spermatogenesis, breast tenderness, amenorrhea, transient testicular enlargement

Gastrointestinal: Nausea, vomiting

Genitourinary: Vaginal dryness, dyspareunia, increase in urinary calcium excretion

Local: Irritation at injection site

Neuromuscular & skeletal: Joint stiffness, possible osteoporosis

Miscellaneous: Severe hypersensitivity reactions (ie, angioedema, urticaria, hypotension, etc)

Stability Protect from light, store in refrigerator, discard unused portion

Mechanism of Action Central idiopathic precocious puberty: Histrelin is a synthetic long-acting gonadotropin-releasing hormone analog; with daily administration, it desensitizes the pituitary to endogenous gonadotropin-releasing hormone (ie, suppresses gonadotropin release by causing down regulation of the pituitary); this results in a decrease in gonadal sex steroid production which stops the secondary sexual development

Pharmacodynamics Precocious puberty: Onset of hormonal response: Physical evidence of reduction in secretion of sex steroids within 3 months

Usual Dosage S.C.:
Children ≥2 years: Central idiopathic precocious puberty: 10 mcg/kg/day; give as a single daily injection
Adult female:
Acute intermittent porphyria: 5 mcg/day
Endometriosis: 100 mcg/day
Leiomyomata uteri: 20-50 mcg/day or 4 mcg/kg/day

Administration Parenteral: S.C.: Vary the injection site daily; administer dose at the same time each day; allow vial to warm to room temperature before giving dose

Monitoring Parameters Precocious puberty: Prior to initiating therapy: Height and weight, hand and wrist x-rays, total sex steroid levels, beta-hCG level, adrenal steroid level, gonadotropin-releasing hormone stimulation test, pelvic/adrenal/testicular ultrasound/head CT; during therapy monitor 3 months after initiation and then every 6-12 months; serial levels of sex steroids and gonadotropin-releasing hormone testing; physical exam; secondary sexual development

Additional Information Noncompliance or changing the dosage schedule may result in inadequate control; histrelin may be discontinued when the patient reaches the appropriate age for puberty

Dosage Forms Injection: 7-day kits of single use: 120 mcg/0.6 mL; 300 mcg/0.6 mL; 600 mcg/0.6 mL

♦ **Hi-Vegi-LIP [OTC]** *see Pancrelipase on page 755*
♦ **Hivid®** *see Zalcitabine on page 1020*
♦ **HMS Liquifilm®** *see Medrysone on page 625*
♦ **HN₂** *see Mechlorethamine on page 621*
♦ **Hold® DM [OTC]** *see Dextromethorphan on page 316*

Homatropine (hoe MA troe peen)
U.S. Brand Names Isopto® Homatropine
Canadian Brand Names Minims-Homatropine
Therapeutic Category Anticholinergic Agent, Ophthalmic; Ophthalmic Agent, Mydriatic
Generic Available Yes
Use Producing cycloplegia and mydriasis for refraction; treatment of acute inflammatory conditions of the uveal tract
Pregnancy Risk Factor C
Contraindications Hypersensitivity to homatropine or any component; narrow-angle glaucoma, acute hemorrhage
Precautions Use with caution in patients with hypertension, cardiac disease, increased intraocular pressure, obstructive uropathy, paralytic ileus, or ulcerative colitis
Adverse Reactions
Cardiovascular: Vascular congestion, edema
Central nervous system: Drowsiness
Dermatologic: Eczematoid dermatitis
Ocular: Follicular conjunctivitis, blurred vision, increased intraocular pressure, stinging, exudate
Mechanism of Action Blocks response of iris sphincter muscle and the accommodative muscle of the ciliary body to cholinergic stimulation resulting in dilation and loss of accommodation
Pharmacodynamics Ophthalmic:
Onset of accommodation and pupil effect:
Maximum mydriatic effect: Within 10-30 minutes
Maximum cycloplegic effect: Within 30-90 minutes
Duration:
Mydriasis: Persists for 6 hours to 4 days
Cycloplegia: 10-48 hours
Usual Dosage Ophthalmic:
Children:
Mydriasis and cycloplegia for refraction: Instill 1 drop of 2% solution immediately before the procedure; repeat at 10-minute intervals as needed
Uveitis: Instill 1 drop of 2% solution 2-3 times/day
Adults:
Mydriasis and cycloplegia for refraction: Instill 1-2 drops of 2% solution or 1 drop of 5% solution before the procedure; repeat at 5- to 10-minute intervals as needed
Uveitis: Instill 1-2 drops of either 2% or 5% solution 2-3 times/day up to every 3-4 hours as needed
(Continued)

Homatropine *(Continued)*

Administration Ophthalmic: Finger pressure should be applied to lacrimal sac for 1-2 minutes after instillation to decrease risk of absorption and systemic effects

Dosage Forms Solution, ophthalmic, as hydrobromide: 2% (1 mL, 5 mL); 5% (1 mL, 5 mL)

Isopto® Homatropine 2% (5 mL); 5% (5 mL, 15 mL)

♦ **Horse Antihuman Thymocyte Gamma Globulin** *see* Lymphocyte Immune Globulin *on page 612*

♦ **12-Hour Nasal® [OTC]** *see* Oxymetazoline *on page 749*

♦ **H.P. Acthar® Gel** *see* Corticotropin *on page 267*

♦ **HPMPC** *see* Cidofovir *on page 233*

♦ **Humalog®** *see* Insulin Preparations *on page 538*

♦ **Humalog® Mix 75/25™** *see* Insulin Preparations *on page 538*

Human Growth Hormone *(HYU man grothe HOR mone)*

U.S. Brand Names Genotropin® Injection; Humatrope® Injection; Norditropin® Injection; Nutropin® AQ Injection; Nutropin® Depot™; Nutropin® Injection; Protropin® Injection; Saizen® Injection; Serostim® Injection

Synonyms Growth Hormone; Somatrem; Somatropin

Therapeutic Category Growth Hormone

Generic Available No

Use Long-term treatment of growth failure from lack of or inadequate endogenous growth hormone secretion; Nutropin®: Treatment of children who have growth failure associated with chronic renal insufficiency up until the time of renal transplantation; short stature associated with Turner syndrome in patients whose epiphyses are not closed; adults with growth hormone deficiency as a result of pituitary disease, hypothalamic disease, surgery, radiation, or trauma; Serostim®: AIDS-related wasting or cachexia

Pregnancy Risk Factor C; Serostim® (only): B

Contraindications Do not use for growth promotion in pediatric patients with closed epiphyses; hypersensitivity to human growth hormone, benzyl alcohol (sometrem), M-cresol, or glycerin (somatropin) or any component; evidence of active malignancy; progression of any underlying intracranial lesion or actively growing intracranial tumor; patients with acute critical illness due to complications following open heart or abdominal surgery, multiple accidental trauma, or acute respiratory failure

Precautions Use with caution in patients with diabetes or family history of diabetes; somatrem contains benzyl alcohol, use with caution in neonates; insulin dosage may require adjustment when growth hormone therapy is instituted; patients with hypopituitarism may develop hypothyroidism during growth hormone therapy; children may develop slipped capital epiphyses during therapy; progression of scoliosis may occur in patients with a history of scoliosis

Adverse Reactions

Cardiovascular: Mild transient edema

Central nervous system: Headache, intracranial hypertension

Dermatologic: Increased growth of pre-existing nevi; local lipoatrophy or lipodystrophy (S.C. administration)

Endocrine & metabolic: Reversible hypothyroidism (reported in pituitary-derived growth hormone), mild hyperglycemia; gynecomastia (rare)

Gastrointestinal: Pancreatitis (rare)

Hematologic: Small risk for developing leukemia

Local: Pain at injection site

Neuromuscular & skeletal: Carpal tunnel syndrome (rare), pain in hip/knee

Renal: Glucosuria

Drug Interactions Corticosteroids may inhibit growth hormone activity

Stability Refrigerate once reconstituted (all products except Nutropin® Depot™); stable for 14 days after reconstitution when refrigerated; Nutropin® AQ (aqueous form) is stable for 28 days after initial entry; Nutropin® Depot™ must be used immediately after reconstitution

Mechanism of Action Somatropin and somatrem are purified polypeptide hormones of recombinant DNA origin; somatropin contains the identical sequence of amino acids found in human growth hormone while somatrem's amino acid sequence is identical plus an additional amino acid, methionine; human growth hormone stimulates growth of linear bone, skeletal muscle, and organs; stimulates erythropoietin which increases red blood cell mass; exerts both insulin-like and diabetogenic effects

Pharmacokinetics Somatrem and somatropin have equivalent pharmacokinetic profiles

Absorption: I.M.: Well absorbed

Distribution: V_d: 50 mL/kg

Metabolism: ~90% of dose metabolized in the liver and kidney cells

Bioavailability: S.C.: 81 ± 20%

Half-life: S.C.: 2.3 ± 0.42 hours

Elimination: 0.1% of dose excreted in urine unchanged

Usual Dosage

Children: I.M., S.C.:

Growth hormone inadequacy:

Somatrem: 0.3 mg/kg (0.9 international units/kg) **weekly** divided into daily doses

Somatropin:

Humatrope®: 0.18 mg/kg (0.54 international units/kg) **weekly** divided into equal doses given either on alternate days or 6 times per week; maximum **weekly** dosage: 0.3 mg/kg (0.9 international units/kg)

Norditropin®: 0.024-0.034 mg/kg/dose (0.07-0.1 international units/kg/dose) 6-7 times per week

Nutropin®: 0.3 mg/kg (0.9 international units/kg) **weekly** divided into daily doses; in pubertal patients, dosage may be increased to 0.7 mg/kg (2.1 international units/kg) **weekly** divided into daily doses

Saizen®: 0.06 mg/kg (0.18 international units/kg) 3 times per week

Nutropin® Depot™: S.C. only:

Once-monthly injection: 1.5 mg/kg body weight administered on the same day of each month; patients >15 kg will require more than one injection per dose

Twice-monthly injection: 0.75 mg/kg body weight administered twice each month on the same days of each month (eg, days 1 and 15 of each month); patients >30 kg will require more than one injection per dose; twice monthly dosing is recommended in patients >45 kg

Note: Human growth hormone therapy should be discontinued when the patient has reached satisfactory adult height, when epiphyses have fused, or when the patient ceases to respond. Growth of ≥5 cm/year is expected, if growth rate does not exceed 2.5 cm in a 6-month period, double the dose for the next 6 months, if there is still no satisfactory response, discontinue therapy

Chronic renal insufficiency: Nutropin®: Weekly dosage of 0.35 mg/kg (approximately 1.05 international units/kg); may be continued until time of transplantation

Turner syndrome: Weekly dosage ≤0.375 mg/kg (1.125 international units/kg) divided into equal doses daily or on 3 alternate days

Adults: Growth hormone deficiency: 0.006 mg/kg/day (0.018 international units/kg/day) once daily; may be increased to a maximum of 0.025 mg/kg/day (0.075 international units/kg) in patients <35 years of age and to a maximum of 0.0125 mg/kg/day (0.0375 international units/kg/day) in patients >35 years of age

AIDS-related wasting or cachexia: Serostim®:

Children (limited information): 0.04-0.07 mg/kg/day for 4 weeks

Adults: Administered once daily at bedtime:

<35 kg: 0.1 mg/kg

35-44 kg: 4 mg

45-55 kg: 5 mg

>55 kg: 6 mg

Administration Parenteral: Administer S.C. or I.M.; do not shake; rotate injection site

Somatrem: Reconstitute each 5 mg vial with 1-5 mL bacteriostatic water for injection, USP (benzyl alcohol preserved) only; when using in newborns, reconstitute with preservative free sterile water

Somatropin: Reconstitute each 5 mg vial with 1.5-5 mL diluent; when using in newborns, reconstitute with preservative free sterile water

Norditropin® Cartridges: Must be used with the NordiPen® injection pen (each cartridge has a color-coded injection pen which is graduated to deliver the appropriate dose); do not interchange

Nutropin® Depot™: Reconstitute vials with provided diluent only, resulting in 19 mg/mL concentration; swirl vigorously for 2 minutes until all the powder is fully dispersed; withdraw measured dose, change to a new needle, and administer immediately to avoid settling of the suspension in the syringe; inject S.C. at a continuous rate over no more than 5 seconds

Note: When treating chronic renal insufficiency patients, growth hormone should be administered as follows: in hemodialysis patients, administer injection at night just prior to sleeping and at least 3-4 hours after dialysis; in chronic cycling peritoneal dialysis patients, administer injection in the morning after dialysis; in chronic

(Continued)

Human Growth Hormone *(Continued)*

ambulatory peritoneal dialysis patients administer injection in the evening at the time of the overnight exchange.

Monitoring Parameters Growth curve, periodic thyroid function tests, bone age (annually), periodical urine testing for glucose, somatomedin C levels

Patient Information Report the development of a severe headache, acute visual changes, a limp or complaints of hip or knee pain to your physician

Additional Information S.C. administration can cause local lipoatrophy or lipodystrophy and may enhance the development of neutralizing antibodies

Dosage Forms Powder for injection (lyophilized):

Somatropin:

Genotropin®: 1.5 mg [1.3 mg/mL (4 international units/mL)]; 5.8 mg [5 mg/mL (15 international units/mL)]; 13.8 mg [12 mg/mL (36 international units/mL)]

Humatrope®: 5 mg ~15 international units

Norditropin®: 4 mg ~12 international units; 8 mg ~24 international units

Norditropin® Cartridges: 5 mg (1.5 mL); 10 mg (1.5 mL); 15 mg (1.5 mL)

Nutropin® (rDNA origin): 5 mg ~15 international units (10 mL); 10 mg ~30 international units (10 mL)

Nutropin® AQ (rDNA origin): 10 mg ~30 international units (2 mL)

Nutropin® Depot™ (rDNA origin): 13.5 mg (3 mL); 18 mg (3 mL); 22.5 mg (3 mL)

Saizen® (rDNA origin): 5 mg ~15 international units

Serostim®: 4 mg (12 international units); 5 mg (15 international units); 10 mg (30 international units)

Somatrem, Protropin®: 5 mg ~15 international units (10 mL); 10 mg ~30 international units (10 mL)

References

Howrie DL, "Growth Hormone for the Treatment of Growth Failure in Children," *Clin Pharm*, 1987, 6(4):283-91.

- ◆ **Humanized Anti-CD25 mo Ab** *see* Daclizumab *on page 293*
- ◆ **Humanized Anti-interleukin-2 Receptor mo Ab** *see* Daclizumab *on page 293*
- ◆ **Humanized Anti-Tac mo Ab** *see* Daclizumab *on page 293*
- ◆ **Humate-P®** *see* Antihemophilic Factor (Human) *on page 98*
- ◆ **Humatin®** *see* Paromomycin *on page 762*
- ◆ **Humatrope® Injection** *see* Human Growth Hormone *on page 498*
- ◆ **Humibid® DM** *see* Guaifenesin and Dextromethorphan *on page 487*
- ◆ **Humibid® L.A. [OTC]** *see* Guaifenesin *on page 485*
- ◆ **Humibid® Sprinkle [OTC]** *see* Guaifenesin *on page 485*
- ◆ **HuMIST® [OTC]** *see* Sodium Chloride *on page 906*
- ◆ **Humulin 10/90, 20/80, 30/70, 40/60, 50/50 (Can)** *see* Insulin Preparations *on page 538*
- ◆ **Humulin® 50/50** *see* Insulin Preparations *on page 538*
- ◆ **Humulin® 70/30** *see* Insulin Preparations *on page 538*
- ◆ **Humulin® L** *see* Insulin Preparations *on page 538*
- ◆ **Humulin® N** *see* Insulin Preparations *on page 538*
- ◆ **Humulin® R** *see* Insulin Preparations *on page 538*
- ◆ **Humulin® R (Concentrated)** *see* Insulin Preparations *on page 538*
- ◆ **Humulin® U** *see* Insulin Preparations *on page 538*
- ◆ **Hurricaine®** *see* Benzocaine *on page 135*

Hyaluronidase *(hye al yoor ON i dase)*

Related Information

Extravasation Treatment *on page 1085*

U.S. Brand Names Wydase®

Therapeutic Category Antidote, Extravasation

Generic Available No

Use Increase the dispersion and absorption of other drugs; increase rate of absorption of parenteral fluids given by hypodermoclysis; management of I.V. extravasations

Pregnancy Risk Factor C

Contraindications Hypersensitivity to hyaluronidase or any component; do not inject in or around infected, inflamed, or cancerous areas

Warnings Drug infiltrates in which hyaluronidase is **not** the extravasation management of choice include dopamine and alpha agonists

Precautions Hypersensitivity reactions may occur; a preliminary intradermal skin test should be performed utilizing 0.02 mL of a 150 units/mL solution

Adverse Reactions
 Cardiovascular: Tachycardia, hypotension
 Central nervous system: Dizziness, chills
 Dermatologic: Urticaria, erythema
 Gastrointestinal: Nausea, vomiting

Drug Interactions Salicylates, cortisone, ACTH, estrogens, antihistamines (decrease effectiveness of hyaluronidase)

Stability Reconstituted hyaluronidase solution prepared from a 150 unit vial of lyophilized powder for injection is stable for 24 hours; refrigerate the stabilized hyaluronidase solution for injection

Mechanism of Action Modifies the permeability of connective tissue through hydrolysis of hyaluronic acid, one of the chief ingredients of tissue cement which offers resistance to diffusion of liquids through tissues; hyaluronidase increases both the distribution and absorption of locally injected substances

Pharmacodynamics
 Onset by the S.C. or intradermal routes for the treatment of extravasation: Immediate
 Duration: 24-48 hours

Usual Dosage
 Infants and Children: Management of I.V. extravasation: S.C., intradermal: Reconstitute the 150 unit vial of lyophilized powder with 1 mL NS; take 0.1 mL of this solution and dilute with 0.9 mL NS to yield 15 units/mL; using a 25- or 26-gauge needle, five 0.2 mL injections are made subcutaneously or intradermally into the extravasation site at the leading edge, changing the needle after each injection; **Note:** Some centers utilize a 150 units/mL hyaluronidase solution and, without further dilution, administer 0.2 mL injections subcutaneously or intradermally into the extravasation site at the leading edge

 Adults: Absorption and dispersion of drugs: I.M., S.C.: 150 units is added to the vehicle containing the drug

 Hypodermoclysis: S.C.: 15 units is added to each 100 mL of I.V. fluid to be administered
  Premature Infants and Neonates: Volume of a single clysis should not exceed 25 mL/kg and the rate of administration should not exceed 2 mL/minute
  Children <3 years: Volume of a single clysis should not exceed 200 mL
  Children ≥3 years and Adults: Rate and volume of administration should not exceed those used for I.V. infusion

Administration Management of intravenous extravasations: Do not administer I.V.; stop the infusion and remove needle; elevate extremity; administer hyaluronidase within the first few minutes to 1 hour after the extravasation is recognized

Monitoring Parameters Observe appearance of lesion for induration, swelling, discoloration, blanching, and blister formation every 15 minutes for ~2 hours

Dosage Forms
 Injection, stabilized solution: 150 units/mL (1 mL, 10 mL)
 Powder for injection, lyophilized: 150 units, 1500 units

References
 Raszka WV, Keuser TK, Smith FR, et al, "The Use of Hyaluronidase in the Treatment of Intravenous Extravasation Injuries," *J Perinatol,* 1990, 10(2):146-9.
 Zenk KE, "Hyaluronidase: An Antidote for Intravenous Extravasations," *CSHP Voice,* 1981, 66-8.
 Zenk KE, Dungy CI, and Greene GR, "Nafcillin Extravasation Injury: Use of Hyaluronidase as an Antidote," *Am J Dis Child,* 1981, 135(12):1113-4.

♦ **Hycort (Can)** *see* Hydrocortisone *on page 506*
♦ **Hyderm (Can)** *see* Hydrocortisone *on page 506*

Hydralazine (hye DRAL a zeen)

 U.S. Brand Names Apresoline®
 Canadian Brand Names Apo-Hydralazine; Novo-Hylazin; Nu-Hydral
 Therapeutic Category Antihypertensive Agent; Vasodilator
 Generic Available Yes
 Use Management of moderate to severe hypertension, CHF, hypertension secondary to pre-eclampsia/eclampsia, primary pulmonary hypertension
 Pregnancy Risk Factor C
 Contraindications Hypersensitivity to hydralazine or any component; dissecting aortic aneurysm, mitral valve rheumatic heart disease, coronary artery disease
 Warnings Monitor blood pressure closely with I.V. use; modify dosage in patients with severe renal impairment; some formulations may contain tartrazines or sulfites
 Precautions Discontinue hydralazine in patients who develop SLE-like syndrome or positive ANA; use with caution in patients with severe renal disease or cerebral vascular accidents
 (Continued)

Hydralazine *(Continued)*

Adverse Reactions
Cardiovascular: Palpitations, flushing, tachycardia, edema, orthostatic hypotension (rare)

Central nervous system: Malaise, fever, headache, dizziness

Dermatologic: Rash

Gastrointestinal: Anorexia, nausea, vomiting, diarrhea

Neuromuscular & skeletal: Arthralgias, weakness, pyridoxine deficiency-induced peripheral neuropathy (paresthesia, numbness)

Miscellaneous: Positive ANA, positive LE cells, SLE-like syndrome

Drug Interactions MAO inhibitors may cause a significant decrease in blood pressure; indomethacin may decrease hypotensive effects

Food Interactions Avoid natural licorice (causes sodium and water retention and increases potassium loss); long-term use of hydralazine may cause pyridoxine deficiency resulting in numbness, tingling, and paresthesias; if symptoms develop, pyridoxine supplements may be needed

Stability Changes color after contact with a metal filter; do not store intact ampuls in refrigerator

Mechanism of Action Direct vasodilation of arterioles (with little effect on veins) which results in decreased systemic resistance

Pharmacodynamics
Onset of action:
- Oral: 20-30 minutes
- I.V.: 5-20 minutes

Duration:
- Oral: 2-4 hours
- I.V.: 2-6 hours

Pharmacokinetics
Distribution: Crosses placenta; appears in breast milk

Protein-binding: 85% to 90%

Metabolism: Acetylated in the liver

Bioavailability: 30% to 50%; large first-pass effect orally

Half-life, adults: 2-8 hours; half-life varies with genetically determined acetylation rates

Elimination: 14% excreted unchanged in urine

Usual Dosage
Infants and Children:
- Oral: Initial: 0.75-1 mg/kg/day in 2-4 divided doses, not to exceed 25 mg/dose; increase over 3-4 weeks to maximum of 5 mg/kg/day in infants over 7.5 mg/kg/day in children, given in 2-4 divided doses; maximum daily dose: 200 mg/day
- I.M., I.V.: Initial: 0.1-0.2 mg/kg/dose (not to exceed 20 mg) every 4-6 hours as needed; up to 1.7-3.5 mg/kg/day divided in 4-6 doses

Adults:
- Oral: Initial: 10 mg 4 times/day, increase by 10-25 mg/dose every 2-5 days to maximum of 300 mg/day
- I.M., I.V.: Hypertension: Initial: 10-20 mg/dose every 4-6 hours as needed, may increase to 40 mg/dose
- I.M., I.V.: Pre-eclampsia/eclampsia: 5 mg/dose then 5-10 mg every 20-30 minutes as needed

Dosing interval in renal impairment:
- Cl_{cr} 10-50 mL/minute: Administer every 8 hours
- Cl_{cr} <10 mL/minute: Administer every 8-16 hours in fast acetylators and every 12-24 hours in slow acetylators

Administration
Oral: Administer with food

Parenteral: I.V.: Do not exceed rate of 0.2 mg/kg/minute; maximum concentration for I.V. use: 20 mg/mL

Monitoring Parameters Heart rate, blood pressure, ANA titer

Patient Information Limit alcohol; notify physician if flu-like symptoms occur

Nursing Implications I.V. use: Monitor blood pressure closely

Additional Information Slow acetylators, patients with decreased renal function and patients receiving >200 mg/day (chronically) are at higher risk for SLE. Titrate dosage to patient's response. Usually administered with diuretic and a beta-blocker to counteract hydralazine's side effects of sodium and water retention and reflex tachycardia.

Dosage Forms
Injection, as hydrochloride: 20 mg/mL (1 mL)

Tablet, as hydrochloride: 10 mg, 25 mg, 50 mg, 100 mg

Extemporaneous Preparations

A flavored syrup (1.25 mg/mL) has been made using seventy-five hydralazine hydrochloride 50 mg tablets, dissolved in 250 mL of distilled water with 2250 g of Lycasin® (75% w/w maltitol syrup vehicle); edetate disodium 3 g and sodium saccharin 3 g dissolved in 50 mL distilled water was added; solution was preserved with 30 mL of a solution containing methylparaben 10% (w/v) and propylparaben 2% (w/v) in propylene glycol; flavored with 3 mL orange flavoring; qsad to 3 L with distilled water and then pH adjusted to pH of 3.7 using glacial acetic acid; measured stability was 5 days at room temperature (25°C); less than 2% loss of hydralazine occurred at 2 weeks when syrup was stored at 5°C (Alexander, 1993)

A 4 mg/mL oral liquid preparation made from tablets was **not** stable for very long; preparation made in cherry syrup was not even stable for 1 day; preparation made in a 1:1 mixture of Ora-Sweet® and Ora-Plus® was stable for only 1 day under refrigeration (5°C) and not even 1 day at room temperature (25°C); preparation made in a 1:1 mixture of Ora-Sweet® SF and Ora-Plus® was stable for only 2 days under refrigeration (5°C), but not even 1 day at room temperature (25°C) (Allen, 1998).

Alexander KS, Pudipeddi M, and Parker GA, "Stability of Hydralazine Hydrochloride Syrup Compounded From Tablets," *Am J Hosp Pharm*, 1993, 50(4):683-6.

Allen LV and Erickson MA, "Stability of Alprazolam, Chloroquine Phosphate, Cisapride, Enalapril Maleate, and Hydralazine Hydrochloride in Extemporaneously Compounded Oral Liquids," *Am J Health Syst Pharm*, 1998, 55(18):1915-20.

- ♦ **Hydrate**® *see* Dimenhydrinate *on page 339*
- ♦ **Hydrated Chloral** *see* Chloral Hydrate *on page 215*
- ♦ **Hydrea**® *see* Hydroxyurea *on page 514*
- ♦ **Hydrisalic**™ **[OTC]** *see* Salicylic Acid *on page 886*
- ♦ **Hydrocet**® *see* Hydrocodone and Acetaminophen *on page 505*

Hydrochlorothiazide (hye droe klor oh THYE a zide)

Related Information

Carbohydrate and Alcohol Content of Liquid Medications for Use in Patients Receiving Ketogenic Diets *on page 1258*

U.S. Brand Names Ezide®; HydroDIURIL®; Microzide™; Oretic®

Canadian Brand Names Apo-Hydro; Novo-Hydrazide; Urozide

Synonyms HCTZ

Therapeutic Category Antihypertensive Agent; Diuretic, Thiazide

Generic Available Yes: Tablet

Use Management of mild to moderate hypertension; treatment of edema in CHF and nephrotic syndrome

Pregnancy Risk Factor B

Contraindications Hypersensitivity to hydrochlorothiazide or any component; cross-sensitivity with other thiazides or sulfonamides; anuria

Precautions Use with caution in patients with severe renal disease (Cl_{cr} <10 mL/minute), impaired hepatic function, hepatic disease, gout, lupus erythematosus, diabetes mellitus; some products may contain tartrazine

Adverse Reactions

Cardiovascular: Hypotension

Central nervous system: Drowsiness, vertigo, headache

Dermatologic: Photosensitivity

Endocrine & metabolic: Hypokalemia, hyperglycemia, hypochloremic metabolic alkalosis, hyperlipidemia, hyperuricemia

Gastrointestinal: Nausea, vomiting, anorexia, diarrhea, cramping, pancreatitis

Hematologic: Aplastic anemia, hemolytic anemia, leukopenia, agranulocytosis, thrombocytopenia

Hepatic: Hepatitis, intrahepatic cholestasis

Neuromuscular & skeletal: Muscle weakness, paresthesia

Renal: Polyuria, prerenal azotemia

Drug Interactions NSAIDs decrease antihypertensive effect; steroids, amphotericin B increase potassium losses; hydrochlorothiazide increases hypersensitivity reactions to allopurinol; decreased clearance of lithium; increased hyperglycemia with diazoxide; hydrochlorothiazide decreases effectiveness of antidiabetic agents in blood sugar control; cholestyramine decreases hydrochlorothiazide absorption

Food Interactions Avoid natural licorice (causes sodium and water retention and increases potassium loss); may need to decrease sodium and calcium and increase potassium, zinc, magnesium, and riboflavin in diet

(Continued)

Hydrochlorothiazide *(Continued)*

Mechanism of Action Inhibits sodium reabsorption in the distal tubules causing increased excretion of sodium and water as well as potassium, hydrogen, magnesium, phosphate, calcium, and bicarbonate ions

Pharmacodynamics
Onset of diuretic action: Oral: Within 2 hours
Peak effects: Within 3-6 hours
Duration: 6-12 hours

Pharmacokinetics
Absorption: Oral: ~60% to 80%
Distribution: Breast milk to plasma ratio: 0.25
Half-life: 5.6-14.8 hours
Elimination: Unchanged in urine

Usual Dosage Oral: (daily dosages should be decreased if used with other antihypertensives):

Neonates and Infants <6 months: 2-4 mg/kg/day in 2 divided doses; maximum daily dosage: 37.5 mg

Infants >6 months and Children: 2 mg/kg/day in 2 divided doses; maximum daily dosage: 200 mg

Adults: 12.5-100 mg/day in 1-2 doses; maximum dose: 200 mg/day

Dosage adjustment in renal impairment: Cl_{cr} <25-50 mL/minute: May not be effective

Administration Oral: Administer with food or milk

Monitoring Parameters Serum electrolytes, BUN, creatinine, blood pressure, fluid balance, body weight

Dosage Forms
Capsule: 12.5 mg
Solution, oral: 50 mg/5 mL [mint flavor] (500 mL)
Tablet: 25 mg, 50 mg, 100 mg

Hydrochlorothiazide and Spironolactone

(hye droe klor oh THYE a zide & speer on oh LAK tone)

U.S. Brand Names Aldactazide®

Canadian Brand Names Apo-Spirozide; Novo-Spirozine

Synonyms Spironolactone and Hydrochlorothiazide

Therapeutic Category Antihypertensive Agent, Combination; Diuretic, Combination

Generic Available Yes

Use Management of mild to moderate hypertension; treatment of edema in CHF and nephrotic syndrome

Pregnancy Risk Factor C

Contraindications Anuria, hyperkalemia, renal or hepatic failure; hypersensitivity to hydrochlorothiazide, spironolactone, or any component; cross-sensitivity with other thiazides or sulfonamides; patients receiving triamterene or amiloride

Warnings This fixed combination is not indicated for initial therapy of hypertension; therapy requires titration to the individual patient; if dosage so determined represents this fixed combination, its use may be more convenient

Adverse Reactions See individual components, Hydrochlorothiazide *on page 503* and Spironolactone *on page 911*, for full adverse drug reaction information

Drug Interactions Drugs that increase serum potassium (amiloride, triamterene, indomethacin, ACE inhibitors); digoxin decreases renal clearance; see individual components, Hydrochlorothiazide *on page 503* and Spironolactone *on page 911*, for complete drug interaction information

Food Interactions Avoid food with high potassium content, natural licorice (causes sodium and water retention and increases potassium loss), and salt substitutes

Usual Dosage Oral: As the product is in a fixed combination of equal mg doses, the following dosages represent mg of either spironolactone **or** hydrochlorothiazide

Children: 1.5-3 mg/kg/day in 2-4 divided doses; maximum daily dosage: 200 mg
Adults: 12.5-200 mg in 1-2 divided doses

Administration Oral: Administer in the morning; administer the last dose of multiple doses before 6 PM unless instructed otherwise; administer with food or milk

Monitoring Parameters Blood pressure, serum electrolytes, renal function

Test Interactions Spironolactone may interfere with plasma and urinary cortisol levels and the radioimmunoassay for digoxin

Dosage Forms Tablet:
25/25: Hydrochlorothiazide 25 mg and spironolactone 25 mg

50/50: Hydrochlorothiazide 50 mg and spironolactone 50 mg

Extemporaneous Preparations A 5 mg/mL oral suspension may be compounded by crushing twenty-four 25 mg (spironolactone/HCTZ) Aldactazide® tablets; add geometric amounts of a 1:1 mixture of Ora-Sweet® and Ora-Plus®, or Ora-Sweet® SF and Ora-Plus®, or cherry syrup alone to a final volume of 120 mL; shake well, refrigerate; stable 60 days

Allen LV and Erickson MA, "Stability of Labetalol Hydrochloride, Metoprolol Tartrate, Verapamil Hydrochloride, and Spironolactone With Hydrochlorothiazide in Extemporaneously Compounded Oral Liquids," *Am J Health Syst Pharm*, 1996, 53(19):2304-9.

♦ **Hydrocil® [OTC]** *see* Psyllium *on page 853*

Hydrocodone and Acetaminophen
(hye droe KOE done & a seet a MIN oh fen)

Related Information
Narcotic Analgesics Comparison *on page 1070*
Overdose and Toxicology *on page 1222*

U.S. Brand Names Anexsia®; Bancap HC®; Ceta-Plus®; Co-Gesic®; Hydrocet®; Hydrogesic®; Hy-Phen®; Lorcet® 10/650; Lorcet®-HD; Lorcet® Plus; Lortab®; Margesic® H; Norco®; Stagesic®; T-Gesic®; Vicodin®; Vicodin® ES; Zydone®

Synonyms Acetaminophen and Hydrocodone

Therapeutic Category Analgesic, Narcotic; Antitussive; Cough Preparation

Generic Available Yes

Use Relief of moderate to severe pain; antitussive (hydrocodone)

Restrictions C-III

Pregnancy Risk Factor C

Contraindications CNS depression; hypersensitivity to hydrocodone, acetaminophen, or any component; severe respiratory depression

Warnings Some tablets contain sulfites which may cause allergic reactions

Precautions Use with caution in patients with hypersensitivity reactions to other phenanthrene derivative opioid agonists (morphine, codeine, hydromorphone, oxycodone, oxymorphone, levorphanol)

Adverse Reactions
Cardiovascular: Hypotension, bradycardia, peripheral vasodilation
Central nervous system: CNS depression, drowsiness, dizziness, sedation, increased intracranial pressure
Endocrine & metabolic: Antidiuretic hormone release
Gastrointestinal: Nausea, vomiting, constipation, biliary tract spasm
Genitourinary: Urinary tract spasm
Ocular: Miosis
Respiratory: Respiratory depression
Miscellaneous: Histamine release, physical and psychological dependence with prolonged use

Drug Interactions CNS depressants, alcohol, phenothiazines, tricyclic antidepressants may potentiate the adverse effects of hydrocodone

Food Interactions Rate of absorption of acetaminophen may be decreased when given with food high in carbohydrates

Mechanism of Action Inhibits the synthesis of prostaglandins in the central nervous system and peripherally blocks pain impulse generation; produces antipyresis from inhibition of hypothalamic heat-regulating center

Pharmacodynamics Narcotic analgesia: Oral:
Onset of action: Within 10-20 minutes
Duration: 3-6 hours

Usual Dosage Oral:
Antitussive (doses based on hydrocodone):
Children: 0.6 mg/kg/day or 20 mg/m²/day divided in 3-4 doses/day
<2 years: Do not exceed 1.25 mg/single dose
2-12 years: Do not exceed 5 mg/single dose
>12 years: Do not exceed 10 mg/single dose
Analgesic: **Doses should be titrated to appropriate analgesic effect**
Children: Dose has not been well established
Adults: 1-2 tablets or capsules every 4-6 hours as needed
AHCPR dosing guidelines (doses based on hydrocodone): Opioid naive patients: (See Carr, 1992 and Jacox, 1994)
Children and Adults <50 kg: Moderate to severe pain: Usual initial dose: 0.2 mg/kg every 3-4 hours

(Continued)

Hydrocodone and Acetaminophen *(Continued)*

Children and Adults ≥50 kg: Moderate to severe pain: Usual initial dose: 10 mg every 3-4 hours

Administration Oral: May administer with food or milk to decrease GI distress

Monitoring Parameters Pain relief, respiratory rate, blood pressure

Patient Information Avoid alcohol; may cause drowsiness and impair ability to perform hazardous activities requiring mental alertness; may be habit-forming

Dosage Forms

Capsule (Bancap HC®, Ceta-Plus®, Hydrocet®, Hydrogesic®, Lorcet®-HD, Margesic® H, Stagesic®, T-Gesic®): Hydrocodone bitartrate 5 mg and acetaminophen 500 mg

Elixir, oral (Lortab®): Hydrocodone bitartrate 2.5 mg and acetaminophen 167 mg per 5 mL [tropical fruit punch flavor; contains alcohol 7%] (480 mL)

Tablet: Hydrocodone bitartrate 5 mg and acetaminophen 400 mg; hydrocodone bitartrate 7.5 mg and acetaminophen 400 mg; hydrocodone bitartrate 10 mg and acetaminophen 400 mg; hydrocodone bitartrate 5 mg and acetaminophen 500 mg; hydrocodone bitartrate 7.5 mg and acetaminophen 500 mg; hydrocodone bitartrate 7.5 mg and acetaminophen 650 mg; hydrocodone bitartrate 7.5 mg and acetaminophen 750 mg; hydrocodone bitartrate 10 mg and acetaminophen 325 mg; hydrocodone bitartrate 10 mg and acetaminophen 650 mg; hydrocodone bitartrate 10 mg and acetaminophen 660 mg

Lortab® 2.5/500: Hydrocodone bitartrate 2.5 mg and acetaminophen 500 mg

Anexsia® 5/500, Co-Gesic®, Hy-Phen®, Lortab® 5/500, Vicodin®: Hydrocodone bitartrate 5 mg and acetaminophen 500 mg

Lortab® 7.5/500: Hydrocodone bitartrate 7.5 mg and acetaminophen 500 mg

Anexsia® 7.5/650, Lorcet® Plus: Hydrocodone bitartrate 7.5 mg and acetaminophen 650 mg

Vicodin® ES: Hydrocodone bitartrate 7.5 mg and acetaminophen 750 mg

Norco®: Hydrocodone bitartrate 10 mg and acetaminophen 325 mg

Lortab® 10/500: Hydrocodone bitartrate 10 mg and acetaminophen 500 mg

Lorcet® 10/650: Hydrocodone bitartrate 10 mg and acetaminophen 650 mg

Anexsia® 10/660, Vicodin® HP: Hydrocodone bitartrate 10 mg and acetaminophen 660 mg

Zydone®: Hydrocodone bitartrate 5 mg and acetaminophen 400 mg; hydrocodone bitartrate 7.5 mg and acetaminophen 400 mg; Hydrocodone bitartrate 10 mg and acetaminophen 400 mg

References

Carr D, Jacox A, Chapman CR, et al, "Clinical Practice Guideline Number 1: Acute Pain Management: Operative or Medical Procedures and Trauma," Rockville, Maryland: U.S. Department of Health and Human Services, Public Health Service, Agency for Health Care Policy and Research, AHCPR Publication No 92-0032, 1992.

Jacox A, Carr D, Payne R, et al, "Clinical Practice Guideline Number 9: Management of Cancer Pain," Rockville, Maryland: U.S. Department of Health and Human Services, Public Health Service, Agency for Health Care Policy and Research, AHCPR Publication No. 94-0592, 1994.

♦ **Hydrocort®** [OTC] *see* Hydrocortisone *on page 506*

Hydrocortisone *(hye droe KOR ti sone)*

Related Information

Carbohydrate and Alcohol Content of Liquid Medications for Use in Patients Receiving Ketogenic Diets *on page 1258*

Corticosteroids Comparison, Systemic *on page 1067*

Corticosteroids Comparison, Topical *on page 1068*

U.S. Brand Names A-hydroCort®; Ala-Cort®; Ala-Scalp®; Anucort™ HC; Anusol-HC®; Anusol® HC-1 [OTC]; CaldeCORT® [OTC]; Cetacort®; Colocort™; CortaGel® Extra Strength [OTC]; Cortaid® Intensive Therapy [OTC]; Cortaid® Maximum Strength [OTC]; Cortef®; Cortenema®; Cortifoam®; Cortisone® 10 Quick Shot; Cortizone®-5 [OTC]; Cortizone®-10 [OTC]; Cortizone® for Kids [OTC]; Delacort®; Dermarest Dricort® [OTC]; Dermtex® HC [OTC]; EarSol® HC; Hemril®-HC; Hydrocort® [OTC]; Hydrocortone®; Hydrocortone® Phosphate; Hytone®; LactiCare-HC®; Locoid®; Nupercainal® Hydrocortisone Cream [OTC]; Nutracort®; Pandel®; Preparation H® Hydrocortisone [OTC]; Proctocort™; ProctoCream® HC; Solu-Cortef®; Texacort®; T/Scalp® [OTC]; Westcort®

Canadian Brand Names Aquacort; Barriere-HC; Cortacet; Cortamed; Cortate; Cortifoam; Cortoderm; Emo-Cort; Hycort; Hyderm; Hydrosone; Novo-Hydrocort; Prevex HC; Sarna HC

Synonyms Compound F; Cortisol

Therapeutic Category Adrenal Corticosteroid; Antiasthmatic; Anti-inflammatory Agent; Anti-inflammatory Agent, Rectal; Corticosteroid, Rectal; Corticosteroid, Systemic; Corticosteroid, Topical; Glucocorticoid

Generic Available Yes

Use Management of adrenocortical insufficiency; relief of inflammation of corticosteroid-responsive dermatoses; adjunctive treatment of ulcerative colitis

Pregnancy Risk Factor C

Contraindications Serious infections, except septic shock or tuberculous meningitis; hypersensitivity to hydrocortisone or any component; viral, fungal, or tubercular skin lesions

Warnings Acute adrenal insufficiency may occur with abrupt withdrawal after long-term therapy or with stress; infants and small children may be more susceptible to hypothalamic-pituitary-adrenal (HPA) suppression from topical therapy; some preparations and manufacturer supplied diluents contain benzyl alcohol (eg, Act-o-vial®, A-hydroCort®)

Precautions Use with caution in patients with hyperthyroidism, cirrhosis, nonspecific ulcerative colitis, hypertension, osteoporosis, thromboembolic tendencies, CHF, convulsive disorders, myasthenia gravis, thrombophlebitis, peptic ulcer, diabetes; suppression of HPA function, suppression of linear growth, or hypercorticism (Cushing's syndrome) may occur

Adverse Reactions

Cardiovascular: Hypertension, edema

Central nervous system: Euphoria, insomnia, headache

Dermatologic: Acne, dermatitis, skin atrophy

Endocrine & metabolic: Hypokalemia, hyperglycemia, Cushing's syndrome, growth suppression; suppression of HPA function

Gastrointestinal: Peptic ulcer

Ocular: Cataracts

Miscellaneous: Immunosuppression

Drug Interactions Cytochrome P-450 isoenzyme CYP2D6 and CYP3A3/4 substrate Barbiturates, phenytoin, rifampin, salicylates, NSAIDs, diuretics (potassium depleting), warfarin; caffeine and alcohol may increase risk for GI ulcer; live virus vaccines (increase risk of viral infection); vaccines may have decreased effects

Food Interactions Systemic use of corticosteroids may require a diet with increased potassium, vitamins A, B_6, C, D, folate, calcium, zinc, phosphorus, and decreased sodium

Mechanism of Action Decreases inflammation by suppression of migration of polymorphonuclear leukocytes and reversal of increased capillary permeability

Pharmacodynamics Anti-inflammatory effects:

Peak effect:

Oral: 12-24 hours

I.V.: 4-6 hours

Duration: 8-12 hours

Pharmacokinetics

Absorption: Rapid by all routes, except rectally

Metabolism: In the liver

Half-life, biologic: 8-12 hours

Elimination: Renally, mainly as 17-hydroxysteroids and 17-ketosteroids

Usual Dosage Dose should be based on severity of disease and patient response;

Note: A variety of salt forms are available and can lead to confusion in prescribing, dispensing, and administration; use the appropriate salt/dosage form for the following indications:

Acetate: For intra-articular, intrasynovial, intrabursal, intralesional, or soft tissue injection only

Cypionate: Oral suspension

Sodium phosphate: For general I.V. use

Sodium succinate: For general I.V. use, I.V. use in patients allergic to sodium phosphate salt, I.V. for shock and for intrathecal use (must reconstitute with a preservative free diluent or use a preservative free product)

Acute adrenal insufficiency: I.M., I.V.:

Infants and young Children: 1-2 mg/kg/dose I.V. bolus, then 25-150 mg/day in divided doses every 6-8 hours

Older Children: 1-2 mg/kg I.V. bolus, then 150-250 mg/day in divided doses every 6-8 hours

Adults: 100 mg I.V. bolus, then 300 mg/day in divided doses every 8 hours or as a continuous infusion for 48 hours; once patient is stable change to oral, 50 mg every 8 hours for 6 doses, then taper to 30-50 mg/day in divided doses

Anti-inflammatory or immunosuppressive:

Infants and Children:

Oral: 2.5-10 mg/kg/day or 75-300 mg/m²/day divided every 6-8 hours

I.M., I.V.: 1-5 mg/kg/day or 30-150 mg/m²/day divided every 12-24 hours

(Continued)

Hydrocortisone *(Continued)*

Adolescents and Adults: Oral, I.M., I.V., S.C.: 15-240 mg every 12 hours

Congenital adrenal hyperplasia: AAP Recommendations: Oral: Initial: 10-20 mg/m²/day in 3 divided doses; usual requirement: Infants: 2.5-5 mg 3 times/day; Children: 5-10 mg 3 times/day; **Note:** Administer morning dose as early as possible; tablets may result in more reliable serum concentrations than oral liquid formulations; individualize dose by monitoring growth, hormone levels, and bone age; mineralcorticoid (eg, fludrocortisone) and sodium supplement may be required in salt losers

Physiologic replacement: Children:

Oral: 0.5-0.75 mg/kg/day or 20-25 mg/m²/day divided every 8 hours

I.M.: 0.25-0.35 mg/kg/day or 12-15 mg/m²/day once daily

Shock: I.V.: **Sodium succinate:**

Children: Initial: 50 mg/kg then repeated in 4 hours and/or every 24 hours if needed

Adolescents and Adults: 500 mg to 2 g every 2-6 hours

Status asthmaticus:

Children: I.V.: Optional loading dose: 4-8 mg/kg; maximum: 250 mg; then maintenance: 2 mg/kg/dose every 6 hours

Adults: 100-500 mg every 6 hours

Adolescents and Adults: Rectal: Insert 1 application 1-2 times/day for 2-3 weeks

Ulcerative colitis: One enema nightly for 21 days, or until remission occurs; clinical symptoms should subside within 3-5 days; discontinue use if no improvement within 2-3 weeks; some patients may require 2-3 months of therapy; if therapy lasts >21 days, discontinue slowly by decreasing use to every other night for 2-3 weeks

Children and Adults: Topical: Apply 3-4 times/day

Administration

Oral: Administer with food or milk to decrease GI upset

Parenteral:

I.V. bolus: Dilute to 50 mg/mL and administer over 3-5 minutes

I.V. intermittent infusion: Dilute to 1 mg/mL and administer over 20-30 minutes; maximum concentration: 5 mg/mL

Rectal: Patient should lie on left side during administration and for 30 minutes after; retain enema for at least 1 hour, preferably all night

Topical: Apply a thin film to clean, dry skin and rub in gently

Monitoring Parameters Blood pressure, weight, serum glucose, electrolytes; growth in pediatric patients

Reference Range Hydrocortisone (normal endogenous morning levels) 4-30 μg/mL

Test Interactions Skin tests

Patient Information Limit caffeine; avoid alcohol; do not decrease dose or discontinue without physician's approval; avoid exposure to measles or chicken pox, advise physician immediately if exposed

Additional Information To facilitate retention of enema, prior antidiarrheal medication or sedation may be required (especially when beginning therapy)

Dosage Forms

Hydrocortisone **acetate**:

Aerosol, rectal

Cortifoam®: 10% [90 mg/applicatorful] 20 g

CaldeCORT®: 1% (15 g, 30 g)

Cream, rectal (Nupercainal® Hydrocortisone Cream): 1% (30 g)

Cream, topical (Hydrocort® Acetate With Aloe): 0.5% (30 g)

Injection, suspension: 25 mg/mL (10 mL)

Ointment, rectal (Anusol® HC-1): 1% (21 g)

Ointment, topical:

Cortaid® Maximum Strength: 1% (15 g, 30 g)

Hydrocort® With Aloe: 0.5% (30 g)

Suppository, rectal

Anucort™ HC, Anusol-HC®, Hemril® HC: 25 mg

Proctocort™: 30 mg

Hydrocortisone **base**:

Aerosol, topical:

Cortizone® 10 Quick Shot, Dermtex® HC: 1% (45 mL, 52 mL)

Cream: 0.5% (15 g, 30 g, 454 g); 1% (15 g, 20 g, 30 g, 120 g, 454 g); 2.5% (20 g, 30 g, 454 g)

Cortizone®-5, Cortizone® for Kids: 0.5% (15 g, 30 g, 60 g)

Ala-Cort®, Cortaid® Intensive Therapy, Cortaid® Maximum Strength, Cortizone®-10 Maximum Strength, Dermarest Dricort®, Dermtex® HC: 1% (15 g, 30 g, 60 g, 90 g)

Hydrocort®, Hytone®: 2.5% (20 g, 30 g, 60 g)

Rectal

Anusol® HC, Proctocort™: 2.5% (30 g)

Preparation H® Hydrocortisone, Proctocort™: 1% (30 g)

Gel (CortaGel® Extra Strength): 1% (15 g, 30 g)

Liquid (T/Scalp®): 1% (60 mL)

Lotion: 0.5% (60 mL); 1% (60 mL, 120 mL); 2.5% (60 mL)

Ala-Cort®, Cetacort®, Delacort®, Hytone®, LactiCare-HC®, Nutracort®: 1% (30 mL, 60 mL, 120 mL)

Ala-Scalp®: 2% (30 mL)

Hytone®, LactiCare-HC®, Nutracort®: 2.5% (60 mL, 120 mL)

Ointment, topical: 0.5% (30 g); 1% (15 g, 20 g, 30 g, 60 g, 454 g); 2.5% (20 g, 30 g, 454 g)

Cortizone®-5: 0.5% (30 g)

Cortizone®-10: 1% (30 g, 60 g)

Hytone®: 2.5% (30 g)

Solution, otic (EarSol® HC): 1% (30 mL)

Solution, rectal (Colocort™): 100 mg/60 mL (7s)

Solution, topical (Texacort®): 1% (30 mL)

Spray: 1% (45 mL)

Stick, roll-on (Cortaid® Maximum Strength): 1% (14 g)

Suspension, rectal (Cortenema®): 100 mg/60 mL (7s)

Tablet: 20 mg

Cortef®: 5 mg, 10 mg, 20 mg

Hydrocortone®: 10 mg

Hydrocortisone **butyrate** (Locoid®):

Cream: 0.1% (15 g, 45 g)

Ointment, topical: 0.1% (15 g, 45 g)

Solution, topical: 0.1% (20 mL, 60 mL)

Hydrocortisone **cypionate**:

Suspension, oral (Cortef®): 10 mg/5 mL (120 mL)

Hydrocortisone **probutate**:

Cream (Pandel®): 0.1% (15 g, 45 g, 80 g)

Hydrocortisone **sodium phosphate**:

Injection (Hydrocortone® Phosphate): 50 mg/mL (2 mL)

Hydrocortisone **sodium succinate**:

Powder for injection (A-hydroCort®, Solu-Cortef®): 100 mg, 250 mg, 500 mg, 1000 mg

Hydrocortisone **valerate** (Westcort®):

Cream: 0.2% (15 g, 45 g, 60 g)

Ointment, topical: 0.2% (15 g, 45 g, 60 g)

Extemporaneous Preparations A 2.5 mg/mL oral suspension prepared from tablets (with a vehicle containing sodium carboxymethylcellulose, syrup, hydroxybenzoate 0.1% preservatives, polysorbate 80, and citric acid) and stored in the dark in amber high density polyethylene bottles was stable for 90 days when stored at 5°C or 25°C and stable for 30 days when stored at 40°C; a 2.5 mg/mL oral suspension prepared from powder and the same vehicle was stable for 90 days when stored in the dark in amber polyethylene bottles at 40°C (Fawcett, 1995).

Fawcett JP, Boulton DW, Jiang R, et al, "Stability of Hydrocortisone Oral Suspensions Prepared From Tablets and Powder," *Ann Pharmacother*, 1995, 29(10):987-90.

References

American Academy of Pediatrics, Section on Endocrinology and Committee on Genetics, "Technical Report: Congenital Adrenal Hyperplasia," *Pediatrics*, 2000, 106(6):1511-8.

♦ **Hydrocortisone, Neomycin, (Bacitracin), and Polymyxin B** *see* Neomycin, (Bacitracin) Polymyxin B, and Hydrocortisone *on page 705*

♦ **Hydrocortone®** *see* Hydrocortisone *on page 506*

♦ **Hydrocortone® Phosphate** *see* Hydrocortisone *on page 506*

♦ **HydroDIURIL®** *see* Hydrochlorothiazide *on page 503*

♦ **Hydrodolasetron** *see* Dolasetron *on page 352*

♦ **Hydrogen Dioxide** *see* Hydrogen Peroxide *on page 509*

Hydrogen Peroxide (HYE droe jen per OKS ide)

U.S. Brand Names Peroxyl®

Synonyms H_2O_2; Hydrogen Dioxide; Peroxide

(Continued)

Hydrogen Peroxide *(Continued)*

Therapeutic Category Antibacterial, Otic; Antibacterial, Topical; Antibiotic, Oral Rinse

Generic Available Yes

Use Cleanse wounds, suppurating ulcers, and local infections; used in the treatment of inflammatory conditions of the external auditory canal and as a mouthwash or gargle; hydrogen peroxide concentrate (30%) has been used as a hair bleach and as a tooth bleaching agent

Contraindications Should not be used in abscesses

Warnings Hydrogen peroxide concentrate (30%) is a caustic liquid; it should not be tasted since it is strongly irritating to skin or mucous membranes

Precautions Repeat use as a mouthwash or gargle may produce irritation of the buccal mucous membrane or "hairy tongue"; bandages should not be applied too quickly after its use

Adverse Reactions
Dermatologic: Bleaching effect on hair, irritating burn
Gastrointestinal: Rupture of the colon, proctitis, ulcerative colitis, gas embolism, hairy tongue
Local: Irritation of the buccal mucous membrane

Stability Protect from light and heat; decomposes upon standing, upon repeated agitation, or when in contact with oxidizing or reducing substances

Mechanism of Action Antiseptic oxidant that slowly releases oxygen and water upon contact with serum or tissue catalase

Pharmacodynamics Duration of action: Only while bubbling action occurs

Usual Dosage Children and Adults:
Mouthwash or gargle: Dilute the 3% solution with an equal volume of water; swish around in the mouth over the affected area for at least 1 minute and then expel; use up to 4 times/day (after meals and at bedtime)
Topical:
1.5% to 3% solution for cleansing wounds
1.5% gel for cleansing wounds or mouth/gum irritations: Apply a small amount to the affected area for at least 1 minute, then expectorate; use up to 4 times/day (after meals and at bedtime)

Administration Topical: Do not inject or instill into closed body cavities from which released oxygen cannot escape; strong solutions (30.5%) of hydrogen peroxide should not be applied undiluted to tissues

Dosage Forms
Gel, oral: 1.5% (15 g)
Solution:
Concentrate: 30.5% (480 mL)
Topical: 3% (120 mL, 480 mL)

◆ **Hydrogesic®** *see Hydrocodone and Acetaminophen on page 505*
◆ **Hydromorph (Can)** *see Hydromorphone on page 510*
◆ **Hydromorph Contin (Can)** *see Hydromorphone on page 510*

Hydromorphone *(hye droe MOR fone)*

Related Information
Laboratory Detection of Drugs in Urine *on page 1234*
Narcotic Analgesics Comparison *on page 1070*
Overdose and Toxicology *on page 1222*

U.S. Brand Names Dilaudid®; Dilaudid® Cough Syrup; Dilaudid-HP®

Canadian Brand Names Hydromorph; Hydromorph Contin; PMS-Hydromorphone

Therapeutic Category Analgesic, Narcotic; Antitussive; Cough Preparation

Generic Available Yes

Use Management of moderate to severe pain; antitussive at lower doses

Restrictions C-II

Pregnancy Risk Factor C

Contraindications Hypersensitivity to hydromorphone or any component

Warnings Syrup contains tartrazine which may cause allergic reactions

Precautions Use with caution in patients with hypersensitivity reactions to other phenanthrene derivative opioid agonists (morphine, hydrocodone, levorphanol, oxycodone, oxymorphone, codeine) or significant respiratory disease

Adverse Reactions
Cardiovascular: Palpitations, hypotension, bradycardia, peripheral vasodilation
Central nervous system: CNS depression, increased intracranial pressure, drowsiness, dizziness, sedation

Dermatologic: Pruritus
Endocrine & metabolic: Antidiuretic hormone release
Gastrointestinal: Nausea, vomiting, constipation, biliary tract spasm
Genitourinary: Urinary tract spasm
Ocular: Miosis
Respiratory: Respiratory depression
Miscellaneous: Histamine release, physical and psychological dependence with prolonged use

Drug Interactions CNS depressants, alcohol, phenothiazines, tricyclic antidepressants may potentiate the adverse effects of hydromorphone

Stability Protect tablets from light; do not store intact ampuls in refrigerator; a slight yellow discoloration has not been associated with a loss of potency

Mechanism of Action Binds to opiate receptors in the CNS, causing inhibition of ascending pain pathways, altering the perception of and response to pain; causes cough suppression by direct central action in the medulla; produces generalized CNS depression

Pharmacodynamics Analgesic effects: Oral:
Onset of action: Within 15-30 minutes
Peak effect: Within 30-90 minutes
Duration: 4-5 hours; suppository may provide longer duration of effect

Pharmacokinetics
Metabolism: Primarily in the liver
Bioavailability: Oral: 62%
Half-life: 1-3 hours
Elimination: In urine, principally as glucuronide conjugates

Usual Dosage
Antitussive: Oral:
Children 6-12 years: 0.5 mg every 3-4 hours as needed
Children >12 years and Adults: 1 mg every 3-4 hours as needed
Pain: Doses should be titrated to appropriate analgesic effects; when changing routes of administration, note that oral doses are less than one-half as effective as parenteral doses (may be only $\frac{1}{5}$ as effective):
Young children:
Oral: 0.03-0.08 mg/kg/dose every 4-6 hours as needed; maximum dose: 5 mg/dose
I.V.: 0.015 mg/kg/dose every 4-6 hours as needed
Older Children and Adults: Oral, I.M., I.V., S.C.: 1-4 mg/dose every 4-6 hours as needed; usual adult dose: 2 mg/dose
Adults: Rectal: 3 mg (1 suppository) every 6-8 hours as needed
AHCPR dosing guidelines: Opioid naive patients: (See Carr, 1992 and Jacox, 1994)
Children and Adults <50 kg: Moderate to severe pain: Usual initial dose:
Oral: 0.06 mg/kg every 3-4 hours
I.V.: 0.015 mg/kg every 3-4 hours
Children and Adults ≥50 kg: Moderate to severe pain: Usual initial dose:
Oral: 6 mg every 3-4 hours
I.M., I.V., S.C.: 1.5 mg every 3-4 hours

Administration
Oral: Administer with food or milk to decrease GI upset
Parenteral: I.V.: Administer via slow I.V. injection over at least 2-3 minutes
Rectal: Insert suppository rectally and retain

Monitoring Parameters Pain relief, respiratory rate, blood pressure

Patient Information Avoid alcohol; may cause drowsiness and impair ability to perform hazardous activities requiring mental alertness; may be habit-forming; do not abruptly discontinue with long-term use

Additional Information Equianalgesic doses: Morphine 10 mg I.M. = hydromorphone 1.5 mg I.M.

Dosage Forms
Injection, as hydrochloride: 1 mg/mL (1 mL); 2 mg/mL (1 mL, 20 mL); 4 mg/mL (1 mL)
Dilaudid-HP®: 10 mg/mL (1 mL, 5 mL)
Powder for injection, as hydrochloride (Dilaudid-HP®): 250 mg
Solution, as hydrochloride: 5 mg/5 mL (480 mL)
Suppository, rectal, as hydrochloride: 3 mg (6s)
Syrup (Dilaudid® Cough Syrup): Hydromorphone 1 mg with guaifenesin 100 mg per 5 mL [contains 5% alcohol and tartrazine] (480 mL)
Tablet, as hydrochloride: 2 mg, 4 mg, 8 mg
(Continued)

Hydromorphone *(Continued)*

References

Carr D, Jacox A, Chapman CR, et al, "Clinical Practice Guideline Number 1: Acute Pain Management: Operative or Medical Procedures and Trauma," Rockville, Maryland: U.S. Department of Health and Human Services, Public Health Service, Agency for Health Care Policy and Research, AHCPR Publication No 92-0032, 1992.

Jacox A, Carr D, Payne R, et al, "Clinical Practice Guideline Number 9: Management of Cancer Pain," Rockville, Maryland: U.S. Department of Health and Human Services, Public Health Service, Agency for Health Care Policy and Research, AHCPR Publication No. 94-0592, 1994.

◆ **Hydrosone (Can)** *see* Hydrocortisone *on page 506*

◆ **Hydroxide and Magnesium Carbonate** *see* Antacid Preparations *on page 95*

Hydroxocobalamin (hye droks oh koe BAL a min)

U.S. Brand Names LA-12®

Canadian Brand Names Acti-B$_{12}$

Synonyms Vitamin B$_{12}$

Therapeutic Category Nutritional Supplement; Vitamin, Water Soluble

Generic Available No

Use Treatment of pernicious anemia and other vitamin B$_{12}$ deficiency states; dietary supplement particularly in conditions of increased requirements (eg, pregnancy, thyrotoxicosis, hemorrhage, malignancy, liver or kidney disease)

Pregnancy Risk Factor C

Contraindications Hypersensitivity to cyanocobalamin or any component, cobalt

Warnings Parenteral injections may contain preservatives, avoid use in neonates; anaphylactic shock has occurred after parenteral vitamin B$_{12}$ administration; intradermal skin testing may be used prior to administration in individuals sensitive to cobalt

Precautions Serum potassium concentrations should be monitored early as severe hypokalemia has occurred after the conversion of megaloblastic anemia to normal erythropoiesis; the increase in nucleic acid degradation produced by administration of hydroxocobalamin to deficient patients may result in gout in susceptible individuals; use of hydroxocobalamin in folic acid deficient individuals may improve folate-deficient megaloblastic anemia and obscure the true diagnosis

Adverse Reactions

Cardiovascular: Peripheral vascular thrombosis

Dermatologic: Itching, exanthema, urticaria

Endocrine & metabolic: Hypokalemia

Gastrointestinal: Diarrhea

Local: Pain at injection site

Miscellaneous: Hypersensitivity reactions

Drug Interactions Decreased absorption of hydroxocobalamin from GI tract by aminoglycoside antibiotics, colchicine, extended release potassium products, aminosalicylic acid, excessive alcohol use, phenytoin, and phenobarbital; antagonism of hematopoietic response to hydroxocobalamin when administered with chloramphenicol

Stability Protect from light

Mechanism of Action Coenzyme for various metabolic functions, including fat and carbohydrate metabolism and protein synthesis, used in cell replication and hematopoiesis

Pharmacodynamics

Onset: I.M.:

Megaloblastic anemia:

Conversion of megaloblastic to normoblastic erythroid hyperplasia within bone marrow: 8 hours

Increased reticulocytes: 2-5 days

Complicated vitamin B$_{12}$ deficiency:

Psychiatric sequelae: 24 hours

Thrombocytopenia: 10 days

Granulocytopenia: 2 weeks

Pharmacokinetics

Distribution: Principally stored in the liver; also stored in the kidneys and adrenals

Protein binding: Bound to transcobalamin II

Metabolism: Converted in the tissues to active coenzymes methylcobalamin and deoxyadenosylcobalamin

Time to peak serum concentration: 2 hours

Elimination: 50% to 98% unchanged in the urine

Usual Dosage I.M.:

Schilling test (diagnostic for vitamin B_{12} deficiency): Children and Adults: 1000 mcg once

Congenital transcobalamin deficiency: Neonates: 1000 mcg twice weekly

Vitamin B_{12} deficiency or pernicious anemia: Varying regimens:

Uncomplicated disease:

Children: Initial: 100 mcg/day for 10-15 days (total dose: 1-5 mg); maintenance: 60 mcg/month

or as an alternative: 30-50 mcg/day for at least 2 weeks (total dose: 1-5 mg); maintenance: 100 mcg/month

Adults: Initial: 30 mcg/day for 5-10 days; maintenance: 100-200 mcg/monthly

or as an alternative: 1000 mcg/day for 5-10 days, followed by 100-200 mcg/month

or as an alternative: 100 mcg/day for 1 week, followed by 100 mcg every other day for 2 weeks; maintenance: 100 mcg/month

Complicated disease (eg, severe anemia with heart failure, thrombocytopenia with bleeding, granulocytopenia with infection, severe neurologic damage): Adults: 1000 mcg plus folic acid 15 mg once, followed by 100 mcg/day plus oral folic acid 5 mg/day for 1 week; maintenance dosing as above

Dosage interval in hepatic or renal impairment: A decrease in the interval between injections may be required

Administration Parenteral: I.M. injection only; do not administer S.C.

Monitoring Parameters Serum potassium, erythrocyte and reticulocyte counts, hemoglobin, hematocrit

Reference Range Normal: 200-900 pg/mL; vitamin B_{12} deficiency: <200 pg/mL; megaloblastic anemia: <100 pg/mL

Patient Information Life-long therapy is required in patients with pernicious anemia or other absorption defects; do not discontinue therapy without consulting your physician

Additional Information Cyanocobalamin is preferred over hydroxocobalamin due to reports of antibody formation to the hydroxocobalamin-transcobalamin complex

Dosage Forms Injection: 1000 mcg/mL (10 mL, 30 mL)

♦ **Hydroxy-1,4-naphthoquinone** *see* Atovaquone *on page 113*

Hydroxychloroquine (hye droks ee KLOR oh kwin)

U.S. Brand Names Plaquenil® Sulfate

Therapeutic Category Antimalarial Agent; Antirheumatic, Disease Modifying

Generic Available No

Use Suppression or chemoprophylaxis of malaria caused by susceptible *P. vivax*, *P. ovale*, *P. malariae*, and some strains of *P. falciparum* (not active against pre-erythrocytic or exoerythrocytic tissue stages of *Plasmodium*); treatment of systemic lupus erythematosus (SLE) and rheumatoid arthritis

Pregnancy Risk Factor C

Contraindications Retinal or visual field changes; hypersensitivity to hydroxychloroquine, 4-aminoquinoline derivatives, or any component; patients with porphyria or psoriasis

Warnings Long-term use in children is **not** recommended; daily dose >6-6.5 mg/kg/day in patients with abnormal hepatic or renal function may be associated with an increased risk of retinal toxicity

Precautions Use with caution in patients with hepatic disease and G-6-PD deficiency

Adverse Reactions

Central nervous system: Insomnia, nervousness, nightmares, psychosis, headache, confusion, agitation, ataxia

Dermatologic: Lichenoid dermatitis, bleaching of the hair, pruritus, hyperpigmentation

Gastrointestinal: GI irritation, anorexia, nausea, vomiting, diarrhea

Hematologic: Bone marrow suppression, thrombocytopenia

Hepatic: Hepatic failure

Neuromuscular & skeletal: Muscle weakness, peripheral neuropathy

Ocular: Visual field defects, blindness, retinitis, macular degeneration, decreased night vision

Drug Interactions Increases digoxin serum levels

Food Interactions Food increases bioavailability

Stability Protect from light

Mechanism of Action Interferes with digestive vacuole function within sensitive malarial parasites by increasing the pH and interfering with lysosomal degradation

(Continued)

Hydroxychloroquine *(Continued)*

of hemoglobin; inhibits locomotion of neutrophils and chemotaxis of eosinophils; impairs complement-dependent antigen-antibody reactions

Pharmacodynamics Onset of action for JRA: 2-4 months, up to 6 months

Pharmacokinetics

Absorption: Highly variable (31% to 100%)

Distribution: Extensive distribution to most body fluids and tissues; excreted into breast milk; crosses the placenta

Metabolism: In the liver

Bioavailability: Increased when administered with food

Elimination: Metabolites and unchanged drug slowly excreted in the urine

Usual Dosage Oral:

Children:

Chemoprophylaxis of malaria: 5 mg/kg **(base)** once weekly; should not exceed the recommended adult dose; begin 1-2 weeks before exposure; continue for 4 weeks after leaving endemic area

Uncomplicated acute attack of malaria: 10 mg/kg **(base)** initial dose; followed by 5 mg/kg **(base)** in 6-8 hours on day 1; 5 mg/kg **(base)** as a single dose on day 2 and on day 3

JRA or SLE: 3-5 mg/kg/day **(as sulfate)** divided 1-2 times/day to a maximum of 400 mg/day **(as sulfate)**; not to exceed 7 mg/kg/day

Adults:

Chemoprophylaxis of malaria: 310 mg **(base)** once weekly on same day each week; begin 1-2 weeks before exposure; continue for 4 weeks after leaving endemic area

Uncomplicated acute attack of malaria: 620 mg **(base)** first dose day 1; 310 mg **(base)** in 6-8 hours day 1; 310 mg **(base)** as a single dose day 2; and 310 mg **(base)** as a single dose on day 3

Rheumatoid arthritis: 400-600 mg/day **(as sulfate)** once daily to start; increase dose until optimum response level is reached; usually after 4-12 weeks dose should be reduced by 50% and a maintenance dose given of 200-400 mg/day **(as sulfate)** divided 1-2 times/day

Lupus erythematosus: 400 mg **(as sulfate)** every day or twice daily for several weeks depending on response; 200-400 mg/day **(as sulfate)** for prolonged maintenance therapy

Administration Oral: Administer with food or milk to decrease GI distress

Monitoring Parameters Ophthalmologic examination, CBC; check for muscular weakness with prolonged therapy

Patient Information Wear sunglasses in bright sunlight; notify physician if blurring of vision, vision change, emotional change, or unusual skin rashes occur; may cause dizziness and vision changes, so exercise caution when driving; avoid alcohol; contraindicated during breast-feeding

Dosage Forms Tablet, as sulfate: 200 mg [base 155 mg]

Extemporaneous Preparations A 25 mg/mL hydroxychloroquine sulfate suspension is made by removing the coating off of fifteen 200 mg hydroxychloroquine sulfate tablets with a towel moistened with alcohol; tablets are ground to a fine powder and levigated to a paste with 15 mL of Ora-Plus® suspending agent; add an additional 45 mL of suspending agent and levigate until a uniform mixture is obtained; qs ad to 120 mL with sterile water for irrigation; a 30 day expiration date is recommended, although stability testing has not been performed

Pesko LJ, "Compounding: Hydroxychloroquine," *Am Druggist*, 1993, 207:57.

References

Emery H, "Clinical Aspects of Systemic Lupus Erythematosus in Childhood," *Pediatr Clin North Am*, 1986, 33(5):1177-90.

Giannini EH and Cawkwell GD, "Drug Treatment in Children With Juvenile Rheumatoid Arthritis. Past, Present, and Future," *Pediatr Clin North Am*, 1995, 42(5):1099-125.

"Guidelines for the Management of Rheumatoid Arthritis. American College of Rheumatology Ad Hoc Committee on Clinical Guidelines," *Arthritis Rheum*, 1996, 39(5):713-22.

- ♦ **Hydroxydaunomycin** *see* Doxorubicin *on page 360*
- ♦ **Hydroxyethyl Starch** *see* Hetastarch *on page 494*
- ♦ **Hydroxynorephedrine** *see* Metaraminol *on page 638*

Hydroxyurea *(hye droks ee yoor EE a)*

Related Information

Adult and Adolescent HIV *on page 1166*

Emetogenic Potential of Single Chemotherapeutic Agents *on page 1129*

U.S. Brand Names Droxia™; Hydrea®

Therapeutic Category Antineoplastic Agent, Miscellaneous

Generic Available Yes

Use Treatment of chronic myelocytic leukemia (CML), melanoma, and ovarian carcinoma; used with radiation in treatment of tumors of the head and neck; adjunct in the management of sickle cell patients; combination therapy with didanosine for treatment of HIV infection

Pregnancy Risk Factor D

Contraindications Severe anemia, severe bone marrow suppression; WBC <2500/mm^3 or platelet count <100,000/mm^3; hypersensitivity to hydroxyurea or any component

Warnings The FDA currently recommends that procedures for proper handling and disposal of antineoplastic agents be considered; hydroxyurea is presumed to be a human carcinogen; secondary leukemia and skin cancer have been reported in patients receiving long-term hydroxyurea therapy. Hydroxyurea is embryotoxic and causes fetal malformations.

Precautions Use with caution and modify dose in patients with renal impairment

Adverse Reactions

Central nervous system: Dizziness, disorientation, hallucinations, seizures, headache, fever

Dermatologic: Maculopapular rash, facial erythema, thinning of the skin

Endocrine & metabolic: Hyperuricemia

Gastrointestinal: Nausea, vomiting, diarrhea, constipation, anorexia, stomatitis

Genitourinary: Dysuria

Hematologic: Myelosuppression (leukopenia, thrombocytopenia), megaloblastic anemia,

Hepatic: Elevated hepatic enzymes

Renal: Renal tubular function impairment, elevated BUN, elevated serum creatinine

Drug Interactions Fluorouracil, cytarabine (increases cytarabine activity)

Stability Store in a tightly sealed container since the drug is degraded by moisture; store at room temperature

Mechanism of Action Interferes with synthesis of DNA during the S-phase of cell division without interfering with RNA synthesis; inhibits ribonucleoside diphosphate reductase preventing conversion of ribonucleotides to deoxyribonucleotides; hydroxyurea also inhibits the incorporation of thymidine into DNA; in sickle cell patients, hydroxyurea increases the production of fetal hemoglobin

Pharmacodynamics Peak response for sickle cell disease: 6-18 months

Pharmacokinetics

Absorption: Readily from the GI tract

Distribution: Readily crosses the blood-brain barrier and the placenta; distributes into peritoneal or pleural effusions; excreted in breast milk

Metabolism: In the liver

Half-life: 3-4 hours

Time to peak serum concentration: Within 2 hours

Elimination: 50% of drug excreted unchanged in urine; renal excretion of urea (metabolite) and respiratory excretion of CO_2 (metabolic end product)

Usual Dosage Oral (refer to individual protocols): Base dosage on ideal body weight:

Children:

Treatment of pediatric astrocytoma, medulloblastoma, and primitive neuroectodermal tumors: No FDA approved dosage regimens have been established. Dosages of 1500-3000 mg/m^2 as a single dose in combination with other agents, followed by a second course 2 weeks later with subsequent courses every 4-6 weeks have been used (eight-in-1 regimen).

CML: Initial: 10-20 mg/kg/day once daily; adjust dose according to hematologic response

Children and Adults: Sickle cell anemia: Initial dose: 15 mg/kg/day (range: 10-20 mg/kg/day) once daily; increase dose in increments of 5 mg/kg/day every 12 weeks to a maximum dose of 35 mg/kg/day; reduced dosage of hydroxyurea alternating with erythropoietin may decrease myelotoxicity and increase levels of fetal hemoglobin in patients who have not been helped by hydroxyurea alone

Adults:

Solid tumors:

Intermittent therapy: 80 mg/kg as a single dose every third day

Continuous therapy: 20-30 mg/kg/day given as a single dose/day

Concomitant therapy with irradiation: 80 mg/kg as a single dose every third day starting at least 7 days before initiation of irradiation

Resistant chronic myelocytic leukemia: 20-30 mg/kg/day once daily

HIV infection: 500 mg twice daily (15 mg/kg/day divided twice daily) in combination with didanosine 200 mg twice daily

(Continued)

Hydroxyurea *(Continued)*

Dosing adjustment in renal impairment: Dose should be reduced 50% in patients with a GFR <10 mL/minute

Administration Oral: Administer with water on an empty stomach; for patients unable to swallow capsules, contents of capsule may be emptied into a glass of water if administered immediately

Monitoring Parameters CBC with differential and platelet count, hemoglobin, renal function and liver function tests, serum uric acid

Test Interactions False-negative triglyceride measurement by a glycerol oxidase method

Patient Information Inform physician if fever, sore throat, bruising, or bleeding develops; advise women of childbearing potential to avoid becoming pregnant while taking hydroxyurea

Additional Information Myelosuppressive effects:
WBC: Moderate
Platelets: Moderate
Onset (days): 7
Nadir (days): 10
Recovery (days): 21

Dosage Forms Capsule: 200 mg, 300 mg, 400 mg, 500 mg

References

Geyer JR, Finlay JL, Boyett JM, et al, "Survival of Infants With Malignant Astrocytomas. A Report From the Childrens Cancer Group," *Cancer*, 1995, 75(4):1045-50.

Geyer JR, Pendergrass TW, Milstein JM, et al, "Eight Drugs in One Day Chemotherapy in Children With Brain Tumors: A Critical Toxicity Appraisal," *J Clin Oncol*, 1988, 6(6):996-1000.

Maier-Redelsperger M, de Montalembert M, Flahault A, et al, "Fetal Hemoglobin and F-Cell Responses to Long-Term Hydroxyurea Treatment in Young Sickle Cell Patients. The French Study Group on Sickle Cell Disease," *Blood*, 1998, 91(12):4472-9.

Montaner JS, Zala C, Conway B, et al, "A Pilot Study of Hydroxyurea Among Patients With Advanced Human Immunodeficiency Virus (HIV) Disease Receiving Chronic Didanosine Therapy: Canadian HIV Trials Network Protocol 080," *J Infect Dis*, 1997, 175(4):801-6.

Rodgers GP, Dover GJ, Noguchi CT, et al, "Hematologic Responses of Patients With Sickle Cell Disease to Treatment With Hydroxyurea," *N Engl J Med*, 1990, 322(15):1037-45.

Rodgers GP, Dover GJ, Uyesaka N, et al, "Augmentation by Erythropoietin of the Fetal-Hemoglobin Response to Hydroxyurea in Sickle Cell Disease," *N Engl J Med*, 1993, 328(2):73-80.

Hydroxyzine *(hye DROKS i zeen)*

Related Information
Carbohydrate and Alcohol Content of Liquid Medications for Use in Patients Receiving Ketogenic Diets *on page 1258*
Compatibility of Medications Mixed in a Syringe *on page 1238*

U.S. Brand Names Atarax®; Vistaril®

Canadian Brand Names Apo-Hydroxyzine; Novo-Hydroxyzin; PMS-Hydroxyzine

Therapeutic Category Antianxiety Agent; Antiemetic; Antihistamine; Sedative

Generic Available Yes

Use Treatment of anxiety; preoperative sedative; antipruritic; antiemetic

Pregnancy Risk Factor C

Contraindications Hypersensitivity to hydroxyzine or any component

Warnings Subcutaneous, intra-arterial and I.V. administration **not** recommended since thrombosis and digital gangrene can occur; extravasation can result in sterile abscess and marked tissue induration

Precautions Injection may contain benzyl alcohol (avoid use in neonates); use with caution in patients with narrow-angle glaucoma, prostatic hypertrophy, bladder neck obstruction, asthma, or COPD

Adverse Reactions
Cardiovascular: Hypotension
Central nervous system: Drowsiness, dizziness, headache, ataxia
Gastrointestinal: Xerostomia
Genitourinary: Urinary retention
Local: Pain at injection site
Neuromuscular & skeletal: Weakness
Miscellaneous: Anticholinergic effects

Drug Interactions Hydroxyzine may potentiate other CNS depressants, alcohol, or anticholinergics, and can antagonize the vasopressor effects of epinephrine

Stability Protect from light

Mechanism of Action Competes with histamine for H_1-receptor sites on effector cells in the gastrointestinal tract, blood vessels, and respiratory tract

Pharmacodynamics
Onset of effects: Within 15-30 minutes

Duration: 4-6 hours

Usual Dosage
Children:
Oral: 2 mg/kg/day divided every 6-8 hours
I.M.: 0.5-1 mg/kg/dose every 4-6 hours as needed
Adults:
Antiemetic: I.M.: 25-100 mg/dose every 4-6 hours as needed
Anxiety: Oral: 25-100 mg 4 times/day; maximum dose: 600 mg/day
Preoperative sedation:
Oral: 50-100 mg
I.M.: 25-100 mg
Management of pruritus: Oral: 25 mg 3-4 times/day

Administration
Oral: May be administered without regard to food; shake suspension well before use
Parenteral: For I.M. administration in children, injections should be made into the midlateral muscles of the thigh; hydroxyzine has been administered slow I.V. to oncology patients via central venous lines without problems

Monitoring Parameters Relief of symptoms, mental status

Patient Information Avoid alcohol; may cause dry mouth; may cause drowsiness and impair ability to perform hazardous activities requiring mental alertness

Additional Information Atarax® syrup contains sucrose, peppermint oil, spearmint oil, menthol, alcohol, and sodium benzoate; Vistaril® oral suspension contains sorbitol, carboxymethylcellulose sodium, propylene glycol, lemon flavor, and sorbic acid

Dosage Forms
Hydroxyzine **hydrochloride**:
Injection: 25 mg/mL (1 mL, 10 mL)
Vistaril®: 25 mg/mL (10 mL); 50 mg/mL (1 mL, 2 mL, 10 mL)
Syrup (Atarax®): 10 mg/5 mL [contains 0.5% alcohol] (120 mL, 480 mL, 4000 mL)
Tablet (Atarax®): 10 mg, 25 mg, 50 mg, 100 mg
Hydroxyzine **pamoate**:
Capsule (Vistaril®): 25 mg, 50 mg, 100 mg
Suspension, oral (Vistaril®:) 25 mg/5 mL [lemon flavor] (120 mL, 480 mL)

References
Berde C, Ablin A, Glazer J, et al, "American Academy of Pediatrics Report of the Subcommittee on Disease-Related Pain in Childhood Cancer," *Pediatrics*, 1990, 86(5 Pt 2):818-25.

♦ **Hyoscine** *see* Scopolamine *on page 892*

Hyoscyamine (hye oh SYE a meen)

U.S. Brand Names Anaspaz®; A-Spas® S/L; Cystospaz®; Cystospaz-M®; ED-SPAZ®; Levbid®; Levsin®; Levsinex®; Levsin/SL®; NuLev™

Therapeutic Category Anticholinergic Agent; Antispasmodic Agent, Gastrointestinal

Generic Available Yes

Use Treatment of GI tract disorders caused by spasm; adjunctive therapy for peptic ulcers and hypermotility disorders of lower urinary tract; infant colic

Pregnancy Risk Factor C

Contraindications Hypersensitivity to hyoscyamine or any component; narrow-angle glaucoma, GI and GU obstruction, paralytic ileus, severe ulcerative colitis, myasthenia gravis

Warnings Low doses may cause a paradoxical decrease in heart rate; some commercial products contain sodium metabisulfite which may cause allergic reactions in susceptible individuals; heat prostration may occur in hot weather

Precautions Use with caution in patients with hyperthyroidism, CHF, cardiac arrhythmias, prostatic hypertrophy, autonomic neuropathy, chronic lung disease, biliary tract disease, children with spastic paralysis

Adverse Reactions
Cardiovascular: Tachycardia or palpitations, bradycardia (with very low doses), orthostatic hypotension
Central nervous system: Headache, lightheadedness, short-term memory loss, fatigue, delirium, restlessness, ataxia, dizziness, insomnia, psychosis, euphoria, nervousness, confusion, insomnia, fever
Dermatologic: Dry skin, photosensitivity, rash, urticaria
Gastrointestinal: Xerostomia, nausea, vomiting, constipation, dysphagia, dysgeusia, dry throat
Genitourinary: Difficult urination, urinary retention
Local: Irritation at injection site
Neuromuscular & skeletal: Weakness, tremor
(Continued)

Hyoscyamine *(Continued)*

Ocular: Blurred vision, photophobia, mydriasis, anisocoria, cycloplegia, increased intraocular pressure

Respiratory: Dry nose

Miscellaneous: Decreased diaphoresis

Drug Interactions Decreased absorption when given with antacids; increased anticholinergic activity with amantadine, antimuscarinics, haloperidol, phenothiazines, tricyclic antidepressants, antihistamines; MAO inhibitors

Mechanism of Action Blocks the action of acetylcholine at parasympathetic sites in smooth muscle, secretory glands, and the CNS; specific anticholinergic responses are dose-related; increases cardiac output, dries secretions, antagonizes histamine and serotonin

Pharmacodynamics

Onset of action:

Oral: 20-30 minutes

Sublingual: 5-20 minutes

I.V.: 2-3 minutes

Duration: 4-6 hours

Pharmacokinetics

Absorption: Well absorbed from the GI tract

Distribution: Crosses the placenta; small amounts appear in breast milk

Protein binding: 50%

Metabolism: In the liver

Half-life: 3.5 hours

Elimination: 30% to 50% eliminated unchanged in urine within 12 hours

Usual Dosage

GI tract disorders:

Infants <2 years: Oral: The following table lists the hyoscyamine dosage using the drop formulation; hyoscyamine drops are dosed every 4 hours as needed

Hyoscyamine Drops Dosage

Weight (kg)	Dose (drops)	Maximum Daily Dose (drops)
2.3	3	18
3.4	4	24
5	5	30
7	6	36
10	8	48
15	11	66

Oral, S.L.:

Children 2-12 years: 0.0625-0.125 mg every 4 hours as needed; maximum daily dosage 0.75 mg

Children >12 years to Adults: 0.125-0.25 mg every 4 hours as needed; maximum daily dosage 1.5 mg **or** using timed release 0.375-0.75 mg every 12 hours; maximum daily dosage 1.5 mg

I.V., I.M., S.C.: Children >12 years to Adults: 0.25-0.5 mg at 4-hour intervals for 1-4 doses

Adjunct to anesthesia: I.M., I.V., S.C.: Children >2 years to Adults: 5 mcg/kg given 30-60 minutes prior to induction of anesthesia

Hypermotility of lower urinary tract: Oral, S.L.: Adults: 0.15-0.3 mg four times daily; using timed release formulation: 0.375 mg every 12 hours

Reversal of neuromuscular blockage: I.V., I.M., S.C.: 0.2 mg for every 1 mg neostigmine or equivalent dose of physostigmine

Administration

Oral: Administer before meals; timed release tablets are scored and may be cut for easier dosage titration; S.L.: Place under the tongue

Parenteral: May be administered I.M., I.V., and S.C.; no information is available for I.V. administration rate or dilution

Monitoring Parameters Pulse, anticholinergic effects, urine output, GI symptoms

Patient Information Maintain good oral hygiene habits, because lack of saliva may increase chance of cavities; notify physician if skin rash, flushing or eye pain occurs, or if difficulty in urinating, constipation, or sensitivity to light becomes severe or persists; may cause dizziness or blurred vision; may cause drowsiness and impair ability to perform hazardous activities requiring mental alertness or physical coordination

Dosage Forms
Capsule, timed release, as sulfate (Cystospaz-M®, Levsinex®): 0.375 mg
Elixir, as sulfate (Levsin®): 0.125 mg/5 mL with alcohol 20% (480 mL)
Injection, as sulfate (Levsin®): 0.5 mg/mL (1 mL)
Solution, oral drops, as sulfate (Levsin®): 0.125 mg/mL with 5% alcohol (15 mL)
Tablet (Cystospaz®): 0.15 mg
Tablet, as sulfate: (Anaspaz®, Levsin®) 0.125 mg
Tablet, extended release, as sulfate (Levbid®): 0.375 mg
Tablet, orally disintegrating, as sulfate (NuLev™): 0.125 mg
Tablet, sublingual, as sulfate (A-Spas® S/L, Levsin/SL®): 0.125 mg

Hyoscyamine, Atropine, Scopolamine, and Phenobarbital

(hye oh SYE a meen, A troe peen, skoe POL a meen & fee noe BAR bi tal)

U.S. Brand Names Donnatal®

Synonyms Atropine, Hyoscyamine, Scopolamine, and Phenobarbital; Phenobarbital, Hyoscyamine, Atropine, and Scopolamine; Scopolamine, Hyoscyamine, Atropine, and Phenobarbital

Therapeutic Category Anticholinergic Agent; Antispasmodic Agent, Gastrointestinal

Generic Available Yes

Use Adjunct in treatment of peptic ulcer disease, irritable bowel, spastic colitis, spastic bladder, and renal colic

Pregnancy Risk Factor C

Contraindications Hypersensitivity to hyoscyamine, atropine, scopolamine, phenobarbital, or any component; narrow-angle glaucoma, tachycardia, GI and GU obstruction, myasthenia gravis, asthma

Warnings Heat prostration can occur in the presence of high environmental temperature

Precautions Use with caution in patients with hepatic or renal disease, hyperthyroidism, cardiovascular disease, hypertension, prostatic hypertrophy, autonomic neuropathy

Adverse Reactions
Cardiovascular: Tachycardia, palpitations, bradycardia (with very low doses of atropine)
Central nervous system: Headache, drowsiness, nervousness, confusion, insomnia, fever
Gastrointestinal: Xerostomia, nausea, vomiting, constipation, dysphagia, paralytic ileus, dysgeusia
Genitourinary: Impotence, urinary retention
Neuromuscular & skeletal: Weakness
Ocular: Blurred vision, photophobia, mydriasis, cycloplegia, increased intraocular pressure
Respiratory: Nasal congestion
Miscellaneous: Hypersensitivity reactions, decreased diaphoresis

Drug Interactions Additive CNS depression with CNS depressants, antihistamines, phenothiazines, tricyclic antidepressants; additive anticholinergic activity with antihistamines, phenothiazines, amantadine

Mechanism of Action Anticholinergic agents (hyoscyamine, atropine, and scopolamine) inhibit the muscarinic actions of acetylcholine at the postganglionic parasympathetic neuroeffector sites including smooth muscle, secretory glands, and CNS sites; specific anticholinergic responses are dose-related

Pharmacokinetics Absorption: Well absorbed from the GI tract

Donnatal® Dosage

Weight (kg)	Dose (mL)	
	Every 4 Hours	Every 6 Hours
4.5	0.5	0.75
10	1	1.5
14	1.5	2
23	2.5	3.8
34	3.8	5
≥45	5	7.5

(Continued)

Hyoscyamine, Atropine, Scopolamine, and Phenobarbital
(Continued)

Usual Dosage Oral:

Children: Donnatal®: 0.1 mL/kg/dose every 4 hours; maximum dose: 5 mL **or** see table on previous page for alternative.

Adults: Donnatal®: 1-2 tablets or capsules 3-4 times/day **or** 5-10 mL 3-4 times/day

Administration Oral: Do not crush or chew extended release tablets

Patient Information Maintain good oral hygiene habits because lack of saliva may increase chance of cavities. Notify physician if skin rash, flushing or eye pain occurs, or if difficulty in urinating, constipation, or sensitivity to light becomes severe or persists; observe caution while driving or performing other tasks requiring alertness, as may cause drowsiness, dizziness, or blurred vision

Dosage Forms

Capsule (Donnatal®): Hyoscyamine sulfate 0.1037 mg, atropine sulfate 0.0194 mg, scopolamine hydrobromide 0.0065 mg, and phenobarbital 16.2 mg

Elixir (Donnatal®): Hyoscyamine sulfate 0.1037 mg, atropine sulfate 0.0194 mg, scopolamine hydrobromide 0.0065 mg, and phenobarbital 16.2 mg per 5 mL (5 mL, 120 mL, 480 mL, 4000 mL)

Tablet (Donnatal®): Hyoscyamine sulfate 0.1037 mg, atropine sulfate 0.0194 mg, scopolamine hydrobromide 0.0065 mg, and phenobarbital 16.2 mg

- ◆ **Hyperstat®** *see* Diazoxide *on page 323*
- ◆ **Hy-Phen®** *see* Hydrocodone and Acetaminophen *on page 505*
- ◆ **HypRho®-D** *see* Rh₀(D) Immune Globulin (Intramuscular) *on page 869*
- ◆ **HypRho®-D Mini-Dose** *see* Rh₀(D) Immune Globulin (Intramuscular) *on page 869*
- ◆ **Hyrexin-50® Injection** *see* Diphenhydramine *on page 342*
- ◆ **Hytakerol®** *see* Dihydrotachysterol *on page 336*
- ◆ **Hytinic® [OTC]** *see* Iron Supplements (Oral/Enteral) *on page 548*
- ◆ **Hytone®** *see* Hydrocortisone *on page 506*
- ◆ **Hytuss® [OTC]** *see* Guaifenesin *on page 485*
- ◆ **Hytuss-2X® [OTC]** *see* Guaifenesin *on page 485*
- ◆ **Ibenzmethyzin** *see* Procarbazine *on page 832*
- ◆ **Ibidomide** *see* Labetalol *on page 568*

Ibuprofen (eye byoo PROE fen)

Related Information

Carbohydrate and Alcohol Content of Liquid Medications for Use in Patients Receiving Ketogenic Diets *on page 1258*

Overdose and Toxicology *on page 1222*

U.S. Brand Names Advil® [OTC]; Advil® Migraine [OTC]; Children's Advil® [OTC]; Children's Advil® Suspension; Children's Motrin® [OTC]; Genpril® [OTC]; Haltran® [OTC]; Ibu-Tab®; Infants' Advil® Concentrated Drops [OTC]; Infants' Motrin [OTC]; Junior Strength Advil® [OTC]; Junior Strength Motrin® [OTC]; Menadol® [OTC]; Midol® Maximum Strength Cramp Formula [OTC]; Motrin®; Motrin® IB [OTC]; Motrin® Migraine Pain [OTC]; Nuprin® [OTC]; Uni-Pro® [OTC]

Canadian Brand Names Apo-Ibuprofen; Novo-Profen; Nu-Ibuprofen

Synonyms *p*-Isobutylhydratropic Acid

Therapeutic Category Analgesic, Non-narcotic; Anti-inflammatory Agent; Antipyretic; Nonsteroidal Anti-inflammatory Drug (NSAID), Oral

Generic Available Yes

Use Inflammatory diseases and rheumatoid disorders including juvenile rheumatoid arthritis (JRA); mild to moderate pain; migraine pain; fever; dysmenorrhea; gout

Pregnancy Risk Factor B (D if used in the 3rd trimester)

Contraindications Hypersensitivity to ibuprofen, any component, aspirin, or other NSAIDs; active GI bleeding, ulcer disease

Precautions Use with caution in patients with CHF, hypertension, decreased renal or hepatic function, dehydration, history of GI disease (bleeding or ulcers), or those receiving anticoagulants; chewable tablets contain phenylalanine, use with caution in patients with phenylketonuria

Adverse Reactions

Cardiovascular: Edema

Central nervous system: Dizziness, drowsiness, fatigue, headache

Dermatologic: Rash, urticaria

Gastrointestinal: Dyspepsia, heartburn, nausea, vomiting, abdominal pain, peptic ulcer, GI bleed, GI perforation

Hematologic: Neutropenia, anemia, agranulocytosis, inhibition of platelet aggregation

Hepatic: Hepatitis

Ocular: Vision changes

Otic: Tinnitus

Renal: Acute renal failure

Drug Interactions Cytochrome P-450 isoenzyme CYP2C8 and CYP2C9 substrate

May increase digoxin, methotrexate and lithium serum concentrations; may decrease antihypertensive effects of ACE inhibitors or angiotensin II antagonists (monitor blood pressure); may decrease effects of other antihypertensive agents, furosemide, and thiazides; aspirin may decrease ibuprofen serum concentrations; other GI irritants (eg, NSAIDs, oral potassium) may increase adverse GI effects

Food Interactions Food may decrease the rate but not the extent of oral absorption

Mechanism of Action Inhibits prostaglandin synthesis by decreasing the activity of the enzyme, cyclo-oxygenase, which results in decreased formation of prostaglandin precursors

Pharmacodynamics

Fever reduction:

Onset (single dose 8 mg/kg):

Infants ≤1 year: Mean ± SD: 69 ± 22 minutes

Children ≥6 years: 109 ± 64 minutes

Peak effect: 2-4 hours

Duration: 6-8 hours (dose-related)

Pharmacokinetics

Absorption: Oral: Rapid (80%)

Protein binding: 90% to 99%

Metabolism: Oxidized in the liver

Half-life:

Children: 1-2 hours; children 3 months to 10 years: Mean: 1.6 hours

Adults: 2-4 hours

Time to peak serum concentration: Tablets: 2 hours; suspension: 1 hour

Children with cystic fibrosis:

Suspension (n=22): 0.74 ±0.43 hours (median: 30 minutes)

Chewable tablet (n=4): 1.5 ±0.58 hours (median: 1.5 hours)

Tablet (n=12): 1.33 ±0.95 hours (median: 1 hour)

Elimination: ~1% excreted as unchanged drug and 14% as conjugated ibuprofen in urine; 45% to 80% eliminated in urine as metabolites; some biliary excretion

Usual Dosage Oral:

Infants and Children:

Analgesic: 4-10 mg/kg/dose every 6-8 hours

Antipyretic: 6 months to 12 years: Temperature <102.5°F (39°C): 5 mg/kg/dose; temperature ≥102.5°F: 10 mg/kg/dose; give every 6-8 hours; maximum daily dose: 40 mg/kg/day

Juvenile rheumatoid arthritis: 6 months to 12 years: 30-50 mg/kg/day in 4 divided doses; start at lower end of dosing range and titrate; maximum dose: 2.4 g/day

OTC pediatric labeling (analgesic, antipyretic): 2-11 years: 7.5 mg/kg/dose every 6-8 hours; maximum daily dose: 30 mg/kg

Cystic fibrosis: Ibuprofen when taken chronically (for 4 years) in doses to achieve peak plasma concentrations of 50-100 mcg/mL has been shown to slow the progression of lung disease in mild cystic fibrosis patients >5 years of age, and especially in patients who started therapy when <13 years of age. Doses administered twice daily ranged from 16.2-31.6 mg/kg/dose with 90% of patients requiring 20-30 mg/kg/dose (mean dose: ~25 mg/kg/dose), but individual patient's dose requirements were not predictable. Patients did not take pancreatic enzymes nor eat for 2 hours after the dose (Konstan, 1995). In children with cystic fibrosis, an initial ibuprofen pharmacokinetic analyses is recommended using tablet doses of 20-30 mg/kg to optimize concentrations in the therapeutic range; blood sampling is recommended at 1, 2, and 3 hours postdose. A recent pharmacokinetic study in children with cystic fibrosis demonstrated that ibuprofen oral suspension also delivers therapeutic plasma concentrations; this study recommends using a 20 mg/kg dose of ibuprofen suspension for the initial pharmacokinetic analyses and obtaining blood samples at 30, 45, and 60 minutes postdose (Scott, 1999); further studies are needed

Adolescents and Adults:

Inflammatory disease: 400-800 mg/dose 3-4 times/day; maximum dose: 3.2 g/day

Pain/fever/dysmenorrhea: 200-400 mg/dose every 4-6 hours; maximum daily dose: 1.2 g

(Continued)

Ibuprofen *(Continued)*

Administration Oral: Administer with food or milk to decrease GI upset; shake suspension well before use

Monitoring Parameters CBC, occult blood loss, liver enzymes; urine output, serum BUN, and creatinine in patients receiving diuretics, those with decreased renal function, or in patients on chronic therapy; patients receiving long-term therapy for JRA should receive periodic ophthalmological exams

Reference Range Plasma concentrations >200 µg/mL may be associated with severe toxicity; cystic fibrosis: therapeutic peak plasma concentration: 50-100 mcg/mL

Patient Information Avoid alcohol; may cause dizziness or drowsiness and impair ability to perform tasks requiring mental alertness; notify physician if changes in vision occur

OTC (pediatrics): Do not administer to children for >3 days unless recommended by physician or other health care professional; notify physician if child's condition does not improve or if worsens within 24 hours

Additional Information Nystagmus, dizziness, hypotension, apnea and coma have been reported with overdose.

Note: A study comparing the short-term use of acetaminophen and ibuprofen in 84,192 children (6 months to 12 years of age) found no significant difference in the rates of hospitalization for acute GI bleeding, acute renal failure, anaphylaxis or Reye's syndrome. (Four of 55,785 children in the ibuprofen group and zero of 28,130 children in the acetaminophen group were hospitalized with acute GI bleeding). A low WBC occurred more frequently in the ibuprofen group (8 vs 0) (see Lesko, 1995).

There is currently no scientific evidence to support alternating acetaminophen with ibuprofen in the treatment of fever (see Mayoral, 2000)

I.V. ibuprofen was shown to be as effective as I.V. indomethacin for the treatment of PDA in preterm infants with RDS; in addition, ibuprofen was significantly less likely to cause oliguria (Van Overmeire, 2000); further studies are needed; **Note:** I.V. ibuprofen is not commercially available in the USA, but has FDA orphan drug status and may be obtained (as ibuprofen lysine) only through a compassionate-use program (sponsored by Farmacon-IL, L.L.C. of Westport, Connecticut)

Dosage Forms

Caplet: 200 mg [OTC]

Advil®, Motrin® IB, Motrin® Migraine Pain, Nuprin®: 200 mg

Capsule, liqui-gel: 200 mg [OTC]

Advil® Migraine (solubolized ibuprofen), Advil®: 200 mg

Drops, oral (Infants' Motrin®): 40 mg/mL [berry flavor] (15 mL) [OTC]

Gelcap: 200 mg [OTC]

Advil®: 200 mg

Suspension, oral: 100 mg/5 mL (60 mL, 120 mL, 240 mL, 480 mL)

Children's Motrin®: 100 mg/5 mL [berry, grape, and bubble gum flavors] (60 mL, 120 mL) [OTC]

Children's Advil®, Motrin®: 100 mg/5 mL (60 mL, 120 mL, 480 mL)

Suspension, oral, **drops**: 40 mg/mL [OTC]

Infants' Advil® Concentrated Drops: 40 mg/mL (15 mL)

Tablet: 100 mg [OTC], 200 mg [OTC], 300 mg, 400 mg, 600 mg, 800 mg

Junior Strength Motrin®: 100 mg [OTC]

Advil®, Genpril®, Haltran®, Midol® Maximum Strength Cramp Formula, Menadol®, Motrin® IB, Nuprin®, Uni-Pro®: 200 mg [OTC]

Ibu-Tab®, Motrin®: 400 mg, 600 mg, 800 mg

Tablet, chewable: 50 mg [OTC], 100 mg [OTC]

Children's Advil®: 50 mg [fruit and grape flavors; with 2.1 mg phenylalanine] [OTC]

Children's Motrin®: 50 mg [orange flavor; with 3 mg phenylalanine] [OTC]

Junior Strength Advil®: 100 mg [fruit and grape flavors; with 4.2 mg phenylalanine] [OTC]

Junior Strength Motrin®: 100 mg [orange flavor; with 6 mg phenylalanine] [OTC]

References

Berde C, Ablin A, Glazer J, et al, "American Academy of Pediatrics Report of the Subcommittee on Disease-Related Pain in Childhood Cancer," *Pediatrics*, 1990, 86(5 Pt 2):818-25.

Brewer EJ, "Nonsteroidal Anti-inflammatory Agents," *Arthritis Rheum*, 1977, 20(2):513-25.

Kauffman RE and Nelson MV, "Effect of Age on Ibuprofen Pharmacokinetics and Antipyretic Response," *J Pediatr*, 1992, 121(6):969-73.

Konstan MW, Byard PJ, Hoppel CL, et al, "Effect of High-Dose Ibuprofen in Patients With Cystic Fibrosis," *N Engl J Med*, 1995, 332(13):848-54.

Lesko SM and Mitchell AA, "An Assessment of the Safety of Pediatric Ibuprofen. A Practitioner-Based Randomized Clinical Trial," *JAMA*, 1995, 273(12):929-33.

Mayoral CE, Marino RV, Rosenfeld, W, et al, "Alternating Antipyretics: Is This an Alternative?" *Pediatrics*, 2000, 105(5):1009-12.

Scott CS, Retsch-Bogart GZ, Kustra RP, et al, "The Pharmacokinetics of Ibuprofen Suspension, Chewable Tablets, and Tablets in Children With Cystic Fibrosis," *J Pediatr*, 1999, 134(1):58-63.

Van Overmeire B, Smets K, Lecoutere D, et al, "A Comparison of Ibuprofen and Indomethacin for Closure of Patent Ductus Arteriosus," *N Engl J Med*, 2000, 343(10):674-81.

♦ **Ibu-Tab**® *see* Ibuprofen *on page 520*
♦ **ICN-1299** *see* Ribavirin *on page 872*
♦ **IDA** *see* Idarubicin *on page 523*
♦ **Idamycin**® *see* Idarubicin *on page 523*

Idarubicin (eye da ROO bi sin)

Related Information
Emetogenic Potential of Single Chemotherapeutic Agents *on page 1129*

U.S. Brand Names Idamycin®

Synonyms 4-Demethoxydaunorubicin; 4-DMDR; IDA

Therapeutic Category Antineoplastic Agent, Anthracycline; Antineoplastic Agent, Antibiotic

Generic Available No

Use Used in combination with other antineoplastic agents for treatment of acute leukemias (AML, ANLL, ALL)

Pregnancy Risk Factor D

Contraindications Hypersensitivity to idarubicin or any component; patients with pre-existing bone marrow suppression unless the benefit warrants the risk; severe CHF, cardiomyopathy, or arrhythmias

Warnings The FDA currently recommends that procedures for proper handling and disposal of antineoplastic agents be considered; I.V. use only, severe local tissue necrosis will result if extravasation occurs; pre-existing heart disease, chest radiation, and previous therapy with anthracyclines at high cumulative doses increase risk of idarubicin-induced cardiac toxicity (manifested by potentially fatal CHF, life-threatening arrhythmias, or cardiomyopathies); the maximum lifetime anthracycline dose for idarubicin is approximately 137.5 mg/m^2; severe myelosuppression occurs in all patients given a therapeutic dose and is the dose-limiting adverse effect associated with idarubicin

Precautions Use with caution and reduce dose in patients with impaired hepatic or renal function and patients receiving concurrent radiation therapy

Adverse Reactions
Cardiovascular: Arrhythmias, EKG changes, cardiomyopathy, CHF
Dermatologic: Alopecia, rash, urticaria
Endocrine & metabolic: Hyperuricemia
Gastrointestinal: Nausea, vomiting, diarrhea, stomatitis, anorexia, mucositis
Genitourinary: Discoloration of urine (pink or red)
Hematologic: Leukopenia (nadir: 8-29 days), thrombocytopenia (nadir: 10-15 days), anemia
Hepatic: Elevated liver enzymes or bilirubin
Local: Tissue necrosis upon extravasation, erythematous streaking
Miscellaneous: Anaphylaxis

Stability Store vials under refrigeration and protect from light; incompatible with acyclovir, ceftazidime, furosemide, hydrocortisone, sodium bicarbonate and heparin; inactivated by alkaline solutions

Mechanism of Action Intercalates with DNA causing strand breakage and affects topoisomerase II activity resulting in inhibition of chain elongation and inhibition of DNA and RNA synthesis

Pharmacokinetics
Distribution:
V_d: Large volume of distribution due to extensive tissue binding; distributes into CSF
V_{dss}: 1700 L/m^2
Protein binding:
Idarubicin: 97%
Idarubicinol: 94%
Metabolism: In the liver to idarubicinol (active metabolite)
Half-life:
Children: 18.7 hours (range: 2.5-22.4 hours)
Adults: 19 hours (range: 10.5-34.7 hours)
Idarubicinol: 45-56.8 hours
Elimination: Primarily by biliary excretion; 2.3% to 6.5% of a dose is eliminated renally
(Continued)

Idarubicin *(Continued)*

Usual Dosage I.V. (refer to individual protocols):
  Children:
    Leukemia: 10-12 mg/m^2 once daily for 3 days of treatment course
    Solid tumors: 5 mg/m^2 once daily for 3 days of treatment course
  Adults: 8-12 mg/m^2 once daily for 3 days of treatment course in combination with Ara-C; reduce dose by 25% if severe mucositis is present
  Dosing adjustment in hepatic and/or renal impairment:
    Serum creatinine ≥2 mg/dL: Reduce dose by 25%
    Bilirubin >2.5 mg/dL: Reduce dose by 50%
    Bilirubin >5 mg/dL: **Do not administer**

Administration Do not administer I.M. or S.C.
  Parenteral: I.V.: Administer by I.V. intermittent infusion over 10-30 minutes into a free flowing I.V. solution of NS or D$_5$W; administer at a final concentration of 1 mg/mL

Monitoring Parameters CBC with differential, platelet count, ECHO, EKG, serum electrolytes, creatinine, uric acid, ALT, AST, bilirubin, signs of extravasation

Patient Information Notify physician if fever, sore throat, bleeding, or bruising occur

Nursing Implications Maintain adequate patient hydration; local erythematous streaking along the vein may indicate too rapid a rate of administration; care should be taken to avoid extravasation; if extravasation occurs, the manufacturer recommends that the affected extremity be elevated and that topical ice packs be placed over the affected area immediately for 30 minutes, then apply for 30 minutes 4 times/day for 3 days; alternative therapy includes topical application of dimethylsulfoxide

Dosage Forms Solution for injection, as hydrochloride: 1 mg/mL (5 mL, 10 mL, 20 mL)

References

Dinndorf PA, Avramis VI, Wiersma S, et al, "Phase I/II Study of Idarubicin Given With Continuous Infusion Fludarabine Followed by Continuous Infusion Cytarabine in Children With Acute Leukemia: A Report From the Children's Cancer Group," *J Clin Oncol*, 1997, 15(8):2780-5.

Leahey A, Kelly K, Rorke LB, et al, "A Phase I/II Study of Idarubicin (Ida) With Continuous Infusion Fludarabine (F-ara-A) and Cytarabine (ara-C) for Refractory or Recurrent Pediatric Acute Myeloid Leukemia (AML)," *J Pediatr Hematol Oncol*, 1997, 19(4):304-8.

Reid JM, Pendergrass TW, Krailo MD, et al, "Plasma Pharmacokinetics and Cerebrospinal Fluid Concentrations of Idarubicin and Idarubicinol in Pediatric Leukemia Patients: A Children's Cancer Study Group Report," *Cancer Res*, 1990, 50(20):6525-8.

♦ **Ifex®** *see Ifosfamide on page 524*
♦ **IFLrA** *see Interferon Alfa-2a on page 542*
♦ **IFN** *see Interferon Alfa-2a on page 542*
♦ **IFN-α-2** *see Interferon Alfa-2b on page 544*

Ifosfamide *(eye FOSS fa mide)*

Related Information
  Emetogenic Potential of Single Chemotherapeutic Agents *on page 1129*

U.S. Brand Names Ifex®

Therapeutic Category Antineoplastic Agent, Alkylating Agent

Generic Available No

Use In combination with other antineoplastics in treatment of lung cancer, Hodgkin's and non-Hodgkin's lymphoma, breast cancer, acute and chronic lymphocytic leukemia, ovarian cancer, testicular cancer, and sarcomas

Pregnancy Risk Factor D

Contraindications Hypersensitivity to ifosfamide or any component; patients with severely depressed bone marrow function

Warnings The FDA currently recommends that procedures for proper handling and disposal of antineoplastic agents be considered. May require therapy cessation if confusion or coma occurs; monitor for hemorrhagic cystitis and severe myelosuppression; carcinogenic in rats

Precautions Use with caution in patients with impaired renal function or those with compromised bone marrow reserve

Adverse Reactions
  Cardiovascular: Cardiotoxicity
  Central nervous system: Somnolence, lethargy, confusion, depressive psychoses, hallucinations, dizziness, seizures, fever, ataxia
  Dermatologic: Alopecia
  Gastrointestinal: Nausea, vomiting, stomatitis, diarrhea
  Genitourinary: Dysuria, hemorrhagic cystitis
  Hematologic: Myelosuppression (leukocyte nadir: 7-14 days)

Hepatic: Elevated liver enzymes

Local: Phlebitis

Neuromuscular & skeletal: Polyneuropathy

Renal: Renal tubular acidosis, hematuria, elevated BUN and serum creatinine

Drug Interactions Cytochrome P-450 isoenzyme CYP2B6 and CYP3A3/4 substrate
Phenobarbital, phenytoin, chloral hydrate may increase the conversion of ifosfamide
to active metabolites and increase toxicity; cisplatin may increase ifosfamide renal
damage

Stability Reconstituted solution is stable for 7 days at room temperature and 21 days
when refrigerated

Mechanism of Action Causes cross-linking of DNA strands by binding with nucleic
acids and other intracellular structures; inhibits protein synthesis and DNA synthesis

Pharmacokinetics Dose-dependent pharmacokinetics

Distribution: Unchanged ifosfamide penetrates the blood-brain barrier

Metabolism: Requires biotransformation by the cytochrome P-450 enzyme system
in the liver before it can act as an alkylating agent; following hydroxylation, the
metabolite breaks down to acrolein (bladder irritant) and ifosfamide mustard
(active drug)

Half-life: Terminal:

Low dose (1800 mg/m^2): 4-7 hours

High dose ($3800-5000 \text{ mg/m}^2$): 11-15 hours

Elimination: 60% to 80% of a dose is excreted in urine as unchanged drug and
metabolites

Usual Dosage I.V. (refer to individual protocols):

Children: $1200-1800 \text{ mg/m}^2$/day for 5 days every 21-28 days or 5000 mg/m^2 as a
single 24-hour infusion or 3 g/m^2/day for 2 days

Adults: $700-2000 \text{ mg/m}^2$/day for 5 days or 2400 mg/m^2/day for 3 days every 21-28
days; 5000 mg/m^2 as a single dose over 24 hours

Administration Parenteral: Administer as a slow I.V. intermittent infusion over at
least 30 minutes at a final concentration for administration not to exceed 40 mg/mL
(usual concentration for administration is between 0.6-20 mg/mL), or administer as a
24-hour infusion

Monitoring Parameters CBC with differential and platelet count, urine output,
urinalysis, liver function and renal function tests

Nursing Implications Maintain adequate patient hydration

Additional Information Usually used in combination with mesna, an agent used to
prevent hemorrhagic cystitis

Dosage Forms Powder for injection: 1 g, 3 g

References

Ninane J, Baurain R, and de Kraker J, "Alkylating Activity in Serum, Urine, and CSF Following High-Dose
Ifosfamide in Children," *Cancer Chemother Pharmacol*, 1989, 24(Suppl 1):S2-6.

Pinkerton CR, Rogers H, James C, et al, "A Phase II Study of Ifosfamide in Children With Recurrent Solid
Tumors," *Cancer Chemother Pharmacol*, 1985, 15(3):258-62.

♦ **IGIV** see Immune Globulin (Intravenous) on page 529

♦ **IL-2** see Aldesleukin on page 47

♦ **Iletin II Pork NPH (Can)** see Insulin Preparations on page 538

♦ **Iletin II Pork Regular (Can)** see Insulin Preparations on page 538

♦ **Ilosone®** see Erythromycin on page 394

♦ **Ilosone® Pulvules®** see Erythromycin on page 394

♦ **Ilotycin®** see Erythromycin on page 394

♦ **Imidazole Carboxamide** see Dacarbazine on page 292

Imiglucerase (imi GLOO ser ase)

U.S. Brand Names Cerezyme®

Therapeutic Category Enzyme, Glucocerebrosidase; Gaucher's Disease, Treatment Agent

Generic Available No

Use Long-term enzyme replacement therapy for patients with Type 1 Gaucher's
disease

Pregnancy Risk Factor C

Contraindications Hypersensitivity to imiglucerase or any component

Warnings During clinical trials, 16% of patients developed IgG antibodies reactive
with imiglucerase; no serious symptoms of hypersensitivity were reported, however,
close observation for hypersensitivity reactions over long-term usage is recommended

Adverse Reactions

Cardiovascular: Hypertension (mild)

(Continued)

Imiglucerase *(Continued)*

Central nervous system: Headache, dizziness
Dermatologic: Rash, pruritus
Gastrointestinal: Nausea, abdominal discomfort
Genitourinary: Decreased urinary frequency

Drug Interactions No information available at this time

Stability Store in refrigerator 2°C to 8°C (36°F to 46°F); after reconstitution, stable for 24 hours refrigerated

Mechanism of Action Imiglucerase, produced by recombinant DNA technology, is an analog of glucocerebrosidase; it acts by replacing the missing enzyme associated with Gaucher's disease; Gaucher's disease is an inherited metabolic disorder caused by the defective activity of beta-glucosidase and the resultant accumulation of glucosyl ceramide laden macrophages in the liver, bone, and spleen; this results in one or more of the following conditions: anemia, thrombocytopenia, bone disease, hepatomegaly, splenomegaly

Pharmacodynamics

Onset of significant improvement in symptoms:
  Hepatosplenomegaly and hematologic abnormalities: Within 6 months
  Improvement in bone mineralization: Noted at 80-104 weeks of therapy

Pharmacokinetics

Distribution: V_d: 0.09-0.15 L/kg
Half-life, elimination: 3.6-10.4 minutes
Clearance: 9.8-20.3 mL/minute/kg

Usual Dosage I.V.: Children and Adults:

Initial: Dosage dependent upon disease severity: Usual: 60 units/kg every 2 weeks; range in dosage: 2.5 units/kg 3 times/week to 60 units/kg once weekly to every 4 weeks

Maintenance: After patient response is well established a reduction in dosage may be attempted; progressive reductions may be made at intervals of 3-6 months

Administration Parenteral: Reconstitution with 5.1 mL sterile water results in 40 units/mL concentration; further dilute 5 mL (200 units) in 100-200 mL NS; infuse over 1-2 hours or a maximum of 1 unit/kg/minute

Monitoring Parameters CBC, platelets, liver function tests

Dosage Forms Powder for injection, preservative free (lyophilized): 212 units [equivalent to a withdrawal dose of 200 units]; 424 units [equivalent to a withdrawal dose of 400 units]

♦ **Imipemide** *see* Imipenem and Cilastatin *on page 526*

Imipenem and Cilastatin *(i mi PEN em & sye la STAT in)*

U.S. Brand Names Primaxin®

Synonyms Cilastatin and Imipenem; Imipemide

Therapeutic Category Antibiotic, Carbapenem

Generic Available No

Use Treatment of documented multidrug-resistant gram-negative infection due to organisms proven or suspected to be susceptible to imipenem/cilastatin; treatment of multiple organism infection in which other agents have an insufficient spectrum of activity or are contraindicated due to toxic potential; therapeutic alternative for treatment of gram-negative sepsis in immunocompromised patients

Pregnancy Risk Factor C

Contraindications Hypersensitivity to imipenem/cilastatin or any component

Warnings Serious and occasionally fatal hypersensitivity reactions have been reported in patients receiving beta-lactam therapy; careful inquiry should be made concerning previous hypersensitivity reactions to penicillins, cephalosporins, or other beta-lactams before initiating imipenem. Seizures have been reported with imipenem therapy in children with meningitis. Pseudomembranous colitis has been reported in patients receiving imipenem; prolonged use may result in superinfection.

Precautions Use with caution in patients with history of seizures or who are predisposed and in patients with a history of hypersensitivity to penicillins; use with caution and adjust dose in patients with impaired renal function

Adverse Reactions

Cardiovascular: Hypotension, tachycardia
Central nervous system: Seizures, hallucinations, altered effect, confusion, fever, dizziness
Dermatologic: Rash, pruritus
Gastrointestinal: Nausea, vomiting, diarrhea, pseudomembranous colitis
Genitourinary: Discoloration of urine, anuria, oliguria
Hematologic: Eosinophilia, neutropenia

Hepatic: Transient elevation in liver enzymes

Local: Phlebitis, irritation at injection site

Miscellaneous: Emergence of resistant strains of *P. aeruginosa*

Drug Interactions Beta-lactam antibiotics, probenecid; ganciclovir (increased risk of seizures)

Stability When reconstituted suspension is further diluted with NS, it is stable for 10 hours at room temperature or 48 hours under refrigeration; when reconstituted suspension is further diluted with a compatible solution other than NS, it is stable for 4 hours at room temperature and 24 hours under refrigeration; incompatible with TPN; inactivated at alkaline or acidic pH

Mechanism of Action Inhibits cell wall synthesis by binding to all of the penicillin-binding proteins with greatest affinity for PBP 1 and PBP 2; cilastatin prevents renal metabolism of imipenem by competitive inhibition of dehydropeptidase along the brush border of the proximal renal tubules

Pharmacokinetics

Distribution: Imipenem appears in breast milk; crosses the placenta; only low concentrations penetrate into CSF

Protein binding:

Imipenem: 13% to 21%

Cilastatin: 40%

Metabolism: Imipenem is metabolized in the kidney by dehydropeptidase; cilastatin is partially metabolized in the kidneys

Half-life, both: Prolonged with renal insufficiency

Neonates: 1.5-3 hours

Infants and Children: 1-1.4 hours

Adults: 1 hour

Elimination: When imipenem is given with cilastatin, urinary excretion of unchanged imipenem increases to 70%; 70% to 80% of a cilastatin dose is excreted unchanged in the urine

Moderately dialyzable (20% to 50%)

Usual Dosage Dosage recommendation based on imipenem component for non-CNS infections: I.V. infusion: (I.M. is limited to mild-moderate infections):

Neonates:

0-4 weeks, <1200 g: 20 mg/kg/dose every 18-24 hours

Postnatal age ≤7 days, 1200-1500 g: 40 mg/kg/day divided every 12 hours

Postnatal age ≤7 days, >1500 g: 50 mg/kg/day divided every 12 hours

Postnatal age >7 days, 1200-1500 g: 40 mg/kg/day divided every 12 hours

Postnatal age >7 days, >1500 g: 75 mg/kg/day divided every 8 hours

Infants 4 weeks to 3 months: 100 mg/kg/day divided every 6 hours

Infants ≥3 months and Children: 60-100 mg/kg/day divided every 6 hours; maximum dose: 4 g/day

Adults:

Serious infections: 2-4 g/day divided every 6 hours

Mild to moderate infections: 1-2 g/day in 3-4 divided doses

Dosing adjustment in renal impairment: Imipenem doses should be reduced in patients with Cl_{cr} <30-70 mL/minute/1.73 m^2: See table.

Creatinine Clearance (mL/min/1.73 m^2)	Frequency	% Decrease in Daily Maximum Dose
30-70	Every 6 hours	50
20-30	Every 8 hours	63
<20	Every 12 hours	75

Administration

I.M.: Administer suspension by deep I.M. injection into a large muscle mass; the I.M. powder for suspension should be reconstituted with lidocaine hydrochloride 1% injection (without epinephrine)

I.V.: Administer by I.V. intermittent infusion; final concentration should not exceed 5 mg/mL; in fluid-restricted patients, a final concentration of 7 mg/mL has been administered; doses ≤500 mg may be infused over 15-30 minutes; doses >500 mg should be infused over 40-60 minutes

Monitoring Parameters Periodic renal, hepatic, and hematologic function tests

Test Interactions Interferes with urinary glucose determination using Clinitest®; Positive Coombs' [direct]

Nursing Implications If nausea and/or vomiting occur during administration, decrease the rate of I.V. infusion

Additional Information Sodium content of 1 g: 3.2 mEq

(Continued)

Imipenem and Cilastatin (Continued)

Dosage Forms Powder for injection, as sodium:

I.M.:
  Imipenem 500 mg and cilastatin 500 mg
  Imipenem 750 mg and cilastatin 750 mg
I.V.:
  Imipenem 250 mg and cilastatin 250 mg
  Imipenem 500 mg and cilastatin 500 mg

References

Ahonkhai VI, Cyhan GM, Wilson SE, et al, "Imipenem-Cilastatin in Pediatric Patients: An Overview of Safety and Efficacy in Studies Conducted in the United States," *Pediatr Infect Dis J*, 1989, 8(11):740-4.

Overturf GD, "Use of Imipenem-Cilastatin in Pediatrics," *Pediatr Infect Dis J*, 1989, 8(11):792-4.

Wong VK, Wright HT Jr, Ross LA, et al, "Imipenem/Cilastatin Treatment of Bacterial Meningitis in Children," *Pediatr Infect Dis J*, 1991, 10(2):122-5.

Imipramine (im IP ra meen)

Related Information

Comparison of Adverse Effects of Antidepressants *on page 1066*

Comparison of Usual Adult Dosage and Mechanism of Action of Antidepressants *on page 1065*

Drugs and Breast-Feeding *on page 1243*

Overdose and Toxicology *on page 1222*

U.S. Brand Names Tofranil®; Tofranil-PM®

Canadian Brand Names Apo-Imipramine; Impril; Novo-Pramine; PMS-Imipramine

Therapeutic Category Antidepressant, Tricyclic

Generic Available Yes: Tablet

Use Treatment of various forms of depression, often in conjunction with psychotherapy; enuresis in children; analgesic for certain chronic and neuropathic pain

Pregnancy Risk Factor D

Contraindications Hypersensitivity to imipramine (cross-sensitivity with other tricyclics may occur) or any component; use of MAO inhibitors within 14 days (potentially fatal reactions may occur, see Drug Interactions); narrow-angle glaucoma

Warnings Do not discontinue abruptly in patients receiving long-term high-dose therapy; some oral preparations contain tartrazine and injection contains sulfites both of which can cause allergic reactions

Precautions Use with caution in patients with cardiovascular disease, conduction disturbances, seizure disorders, urinary retention, anorexia, hyperthyroidism or those receiving thyroid replacement

Adverse Reactions Less sedation and anticholinergic effects than amitriptyline

Cardiovascular: Arrhythmias, hypotension (especially orthostatic)

Central nervous system: Drowsiness, sedation, confusion, dizziness, fatigue, anxiety, nervousness, sleep disorders, seizures

Dermatologic: Rash, photosensitivity

Gastrointestinal: Nausea, vomiting, constipation, xerostomia, decreased appetite

Genitourinary: Urinary retention

Hematologic: Blood dyscrasias

Hepatic: Hepatitis

Ocular: Blurred vision, increased intraocular pressure

Neuromuscular & skeletal: Weakness

Miscellaneous: Hypersensitivity reactions

Drug Interactions Cytochrome P-450 isoenzyme CYP1A2 (demethylation), CYP2C9 (demethylation), CYP2C19 (demethylation), CYP2D6 (hydroxylation), and CYP3A3/4 substrate

May decrease or reverse effects of guanethidine and clonidine; may increase effects of CNS depressants, alcohol, adrenergic agents, anticholinergic agents; with MAO inhibitors, fever, tachycardia, hypertension, seizures, and death may occur (do not use MAO inhibitors within 14 days of imipramine); the herbal medicine St John's wort (*Hypericum perforatum*) may increase serious side effects, its use is **not** recommended; similar interactions as with other tricyclics may occur

Food Interactions Riboflavin dietary requirements may be increased; food does not alter bioavailability

Mechanism of Action Increases the synaptic concentration of serotonin and/or norepinephrine in the central nervous system by inhibition of their reuptake by the presynaptic neuronal membrane

Pharmacodynamics Maximum antidepressant effects usually occur after ≥2 weeks

Pharmacokinetics

Absorption: Oral: Well absorbed

Distribution: Crosses the placenta; distributes into breast milk
V_d: Children: 14.5 L/kg; Adults: ~17 L/kg
Protein binding: >90% (primarily to alpha$_1$ acid glycoprotein and lipoproteins; to a lesser extent albumin)
Metabolism: In the liver by microsomal enzymes to desipramine (active) and other metabolites; significant first-pass effect
Bioavailability: 20% to 80%
Half-life: Adults: Range: 6-18 hours
  Mean: Children: 11 hours; Adults: 16-17 hours
  Desipramine (active metabolite): Adults: 22-28 hours
Time to peak serum concentration: Within 1-2 hours
Elimination: In the urine

Usual Dosage
Children: Oral:
  Depression: 1.5 mg/kg/day with dosage increments of 1 mg/kg every 3-4 days to a maximum dose of 5 mg/kg/day in 1-4 divided doses; monitor carefully especially with doses ≥3.5 mg/kg/day
  Enuresis: ≥6 years: Initial: 10-25 mg at bedtime, if inadequate response still seen after 1 week of therapy, increase by 25 mg/day; dose should not exceed 2.5 mg/kg/day or 50 mg at bedtime if 6-12 years of age or 75 mg at bedtime if ≥12 years of age
  Adjunct in the treatment of cancer pain: Initial: 0.2-0.4 mg/kg at bedtime; dose may be increased by 50% every 2-3 days up to 1-3 mg/kg/dose at bedtime
Adolescents: Oral: Initial: 25-50 mg/day; increase gradually; maximum dose: 200 mg/day in single or divided doses
Adults:
  Oral: Initial: 25 mg 3-4 times/day, increase dose gradually, total dose may be given at bedtime; maximum dose: 300 mg/day
  I.M.: Initial: Up to 100 mg/day in divided doses; change to oral as soon as possible

Administration Oral: May administer with food to decrease GI distress

Monitoring Parameters EKG, CBC, supine and standing blood pressure (especially in children), liver enzymes

Reference Range
Therapeutic: Imipramine and desipramine 150-250 ng/mL (SI: 530-890 nmol/L); desipramine 150-300 ng/mL (SI: 560-1125 nmol/L)
Potentially toxic: >300 ng/mL (SI: >1070 nmol/L)
Toxic: >1000 ng/mL (SI: >3570 nmol/L)

Patient Information Limit caffeine; avoid alcohol and the herbal medicine St. John's wort; may cause drowsiness and impair ability to perform hazardous activities requiring mental alertness; may cause dry mouth

Dosage Forms
Capsule, as pamoate (Tofranil-PM®): 75 mg, 100 mg, 125 mg, 150 mg
Injection, as hydrochloride (Tofranil®): 12.5 mg/mL (2 mL)
Tablet, as hydrochloride (Tofranil®): 10 mg, 25 mg, 50 mg

References
Berde C, Ablin A, Glazer J, et al, "American Academy of Pediatrics Report of the Subcommittee on Disease-Related Pain in Childhood Cancer," Pediatrics, 1990, 86(5 Pt 2):818-25.
Levy HB, Harper CR, and Weinberg WA, "A Practical Approach to Children Failing in School," Pediatr Clin North Am, 1992, 39(4):895-928.

♦ **Imitrex®** see Sumatriptan on page 931
♦ **Immune Globulin, Intramuscular** see page 1172

Immune Globulin (Intravenous)
(i MYUN GLOB yoo lin, IN tra VEE nus)

U.S. Brand Names Gamimune® N; Gammagard®; Gammagard® S/D; Gammar®-P I.V.; Panglobulin™; Polygam® S/D; Sandoglobulin®; Venoglobulin®-I; Venoglobulin®-S

Synonyms IGIV; IVIG

Therapeutic Category Immune Globulin

Generic Available Yes

Use Immunodeficiency syndrome, idiopathic thrombocytopenic purpura (ITP) and B-cell chronic lymphocytic leukemia (CLL); used in conjunction with appropriate anti-infective therapy to prevent or modify acute bacterial or viral infections in patients with iatrogenically-induced or disease-associated immunodepression; autoimmune neutropenia, bone marrow transplantation patients, Kawasaki disease, pediatric HIV infection, HIV-associated thrombocytopenia, Guillain-Barré syndrome, dermatomyositis, polymyositis, demyelinating polyneuropathies
(Continued)

Immune Globulin (Intravenous) *(Continued)*

FDA and NIH Recommendations for the use of IGIV:
Primary immunodeficiencies
Kawasaki disease
Pediatric HIV infection
Chronic B-cell lymphocytic leukemia
Recent bone marrow transplantation
Immune-mediated thrombocytopenia
Chronic inflammatory demyelinating polyneuropathy

Pregnancy Risk Factor C

Contraindications Hypersensitivity to immune globulin, blood products, or any component, IgA deficiency (except with the use of Gammagard® S/D or Polygam® S/D)

Warnings Renal dysfunction and/or acute renal failure has been reported with the administration of IVIG; 88% of the cases were associated with the administration of sucrose-containing IVIG products (Sandoglobulin®, Panglobulin™, Gammar®-P I.V.)

Precautions Use with caution in patients at increased risk for developing acute renal failure (patients with pre-existing renal insufficiency, diabetes mellitus, volume depletion, sepsis, paraproteinemia, and concomitant nephrotoxic drugs). Assure that patients are not volume depleted prior to the initiation of an IVIG infusion.

Adverse Reactions
Cardiovascular: Flushing of the face, hypotension, tachycardia
Central nervous system: Dizziness, fever, headache, chills, anxiety, lightheadedness
Gastrointestinal: Nausea, vomiting
Neuromuscular & skeletal: Myalgia
Renal: Acute renal failure
Respiratory: Tightness in the chest
Miscellaneous: Hypersensitivity reactions, diaphoresis, aseptic meningitis

Drug Interactions Live virus vaccines (measles, mumps, rubella)

Stability Do not mix with other drugs or I.V. infusion fluids; see table for storage

Mechanism of Action Replacement therapy for primary and secondary immunodeficiencies; interference with F_c receptors on the cells of the reticuloendothelial system for autoimmune cytopenias and ITP

Pharmacokinetics Half-life: 21-29 days

Usual Dosage Children and Adults: I.V.:
Immunodeficiency syndrome: 300-400 mg/kg/dose once a month; maintain trough IgG concentration of 500 mg/dL
Chronic lymphocytic leukemia (CLL): 400 mg/kg/dose every 3 weeks
Idiopathic thrombocytopenic purpura: 400-1000 mg/kg/day for 2-5 consecutive days; maintenance dose: 400-1000 mg/kg/dose every 3-6 weeks based on clinical response and platelet count
Pediatric HIV infection: 400 mg/kg/dose every 4 weeks in those patients with hypogammaglobulinemia (IgG concentration <250 mg/dL), those with recurrent serious bacterial infections (2 or more infections in a 1-year period), those who fail to form antibodies to common antigens such as measles vaccine, and those living in areas where measles is prevalent and have not developed an antibody response after 2 doses of MMR
HIV-associated thrombocytopenia: 500-1000 mg/kg/day for 3-5 days
Kawasaki disease: 2 g/kg as a single dose, given over 10-12 hours; if signs and symptoms persist, retreatment with a second 2 g/kg infusion should be considered
Congenital and acquired immunodeficiency syndrome: 100-400 mg/kg/dose every 3-4 weeks
Adjuvant in severe cytomegalovirus infection: 500 mg/kg/dose every other day for 7 doses
Bone marrow transplant: 400-500 mg/kg/dose every week for 3 months and then once every month
Guillain-Barré syndrome: 400 mg/kg/day for 4 days **or** 1 g/kg/day for 2 days **or** 2 g/kg as a single dose
Refractory dermatomyositis: 2 g/kg/dose every month for 3-4 doses
Refractory polymyositis: 1 g/kg/day for 2 days every month for 4 doses
Chronic inflammatory demyelinating polyneuropathy: 400 mg/kg/day for 5 days once each month **or** 1 g/kg/day for 2 days once each month
Severe systemic viral and bacterial infections:
Neonates: 500 mg/kg/day for 2 days then once weekly
Children: 500-1000 mg/kg/week
Prevention of gastroenteritis: Infants and Children: Oral: 50 mg/kg/day divided every 6 hours

Administration Do not administer I.M. or S.C.

I.V. infusion: For initial treatment, a lower concentration and/or administer at the slowest infusion rate (see recommended initial infusion rate in tables) for the first 30 minutes. Titrate rate up gradually to the maximum infusion rate. If an adverse reaction occurs, reduce I.V. infusion rate to previously tolerated rate. See tables.

Intravenous Immune Globulin Product Comparison

	Gamimune® N	Gammagard® S/D	Gammar-P® IV	Iveegam®
FDA indication	Primary immuno-deficiency, ITP, bone marrow transplantation, pediatric HIV infection	Primary immuno-deficiency, ITP, CLL prophylaxis, Kawasaki disease	Primary immuno-deficiency	Primary immuno-deficiency, Kawasaki syndrome
Contraindication	IgA deficiency	None (caution with IgA deficiency)	IgA deficiency	IgA deficiency
IgA content	270 mcg/mL	1.2 mcg/mL	<25 mcg/mL	<10 mcg/mL
g sucrose/g Ig	0	0	1.0	0
Adverse reactions	3.5% to 14.3%	6%	16%	1%
Plasma source	>2000 paid donors	10,000 paid donors	>1000 paid donors	>6000 paid donors
Half-life	21 d	24 d	21-24 d	26-29 d
IgG subclass (%)				
IgG$_1$ (60-70)	61.3	67 (66.8)[1]	69	64.1[2]
IgG$_2$ (19-31)	27.6	25 (25.4)	23	30.3
IgG$_3$ (5-8.4)	6.8	5 (7.4)	6	4
IgG$_4$ (0.7-4)	4.3	3 (0.3)	2	1.5
Monomers	>90%	>96.4%	>98%	93.8%
Gammaglobulin	>98%	>90%	>98%	100%
Storage	Refrigerate	Room temp	Room temp	Refrigerate
Recommended initial infusion rate	0.01-0.02 mL/kg/min	0.5 mL/kg/h	0.01-0.02 mL/kg/min	1 mL/min
Maximum infusion rate	0.08 mL/kg/min	4 mL/kg/h	0.06 mL/kg/min	2 mL/min
Maximum concentration for infusion	10%	10%	10%	5%

	Polygam® S/D	Sandoglobulin® or Panglobulin™	Venoglobulin®-S
FDA indication	Primary immuno-deficiency, ITP, CLL, Kawasaki disease	Primary immuno-deficiency, ITP	Primary immuno-deficiency, ITP, Kawasaki disease
Contraindication	None (caution with IgA deficiency)	IgA deficiency	IgA deficiency
IgA content	1.2 mcg/mL	720 mcg/mL	5% (15.1 mcg/mL) 10% (20-50 mcg/mL)
g sucrose/g Ig	0	1.67	0
Adverse reactions	6%	2.9%-10%	5.8%-14.8%
Plasma source	50,000 voluntary donors	>16,000 voluntary donors	>10,000 paid donors
Half-life	24 d	23 d	33.5 d
IgG subclass (%)			
IgG$_1$ (60-70)	67	60.5 (55.3)[1]	65.7-67.2
IgG$_2$ (19-31)	25	30.2 (35.7)	23.7-25.3
IgG$_3$ (5-8.4)	5	6.6 (6.3)	5.7-5.9
IgG$_4$ (0.7-4)	3	2.6 (2.6)	3-3.4
Monomers	>96.4%	92%	>95%
Gammaglobulin	>90%	>96%	>99%
Storage	Room temp	Room temp	5% Room temp 10% Refrigerate
Recommended initial infusion rate	0.5 mL/kg/h	0.01-0.03 mL/kg/min	0.01-0.02 mL/kg/min
Maximum infusion rate	4 mL/kg/h	2.5 mL/min	0.04 mL/kg/min
Maximum concentration for infusion	10%	12%	10%

[1]Skvaril F and Gardi A, "Differences Among Available Immunoglobulin Preparations for Intravenous Use," *Pediatr Infect Dis J*, 1988, 7:543-48.

[2]Roomer J, Morgenthaler JJ, Scherz R, et al, "Characterization of Various Immunoglobulin Preparations for Intravenous Application," *Vox Sang*, 1982, 42:62-73.

Reference: ASHP Commission on Therapeutics, "ASHP Therapeutic Guidelines for Intravenous Immune Globulin," *Clin Pharm*, 1992, 11:117-36.

(Continued)

Immune Globulin (Intravenous) (Continued)

Monitoring Parameters Platelet count, blood pressure, vital signs, Quantitative Immunoglobulins (QUIGS), trough IgG concentration; periodic monitoring of renal function tests and urine output in patients with an increased risk for developing acute renal failure

Patient Information Notify physician of any sudden weight gain, fluid retention/edema, decreased urine output, and/or shortness of breath

Nursing Implications Appropriate agents for treatment of a hypersensitivity reaction (eg, epinephrine) should be readily available; patients may need to be pretreated with an antipyretic, antihistamine, and/or corticosteroid to prevent chills and fever; adverse reactions may also be alleviated by decreasing the rate or the concentration of infusion or utilizing a different IGIV preparation

Dosage Forms
Injection: Gamimune® N:
    5% [50 mg/mL] with maltose 10% (0.5 g, 2.5 g, 5 g, 10 g)
    10% (1 g, 2.5 g, 5 g, 10 g, 20 g)
Powder for injection, lyophilized:
    Gammagard® S/D: 0.5 g, 2.5 g, 5 g, 10 g
    Gammar®-P IV: 1 g, 2.5 g, 5 g, 10 g
    Iveegam®: 0.5 g, 1 g, 2.5 g, 5 g
    Polygam® S/D: 2.5 g, 5 g, 10 g
    Sandoglobulin®: 1 g, 3 g, 6 g, 12 g
    Venoglobulin®-S:
      5%: 2.5 g, 5 g, 10 g
      10%: 5 g, 10 g, 20 g

References
"Antiretroviral Therapy and Medical Management of Pediatric HIV Infection and 1997 USPHS/IDSA Report on the Prevention of Opportunistic Infections in Persons Infected With Human Immunodeficiency Virus," *Pediatrics*, 1998, 102(Suppl):999-1085.
ASHP Commission on Therapeutics, "ASHP Therapeutic Guidelines for Intravenous Immune Globulin," *Am J Hosp Pharm*, 1992, 49(3):652-4.
Blanchette VS, Luke B, Andrew M, et al, "A Prospective Randomized Trial of High-Dose Intravenous Immune Globulin G Therapy, Oral Prednisone Therapy, and No Therapy in Childhood Acute Immune Thrombocytopenic Purpura," *J Pediatr*, 1993, 123(6):989-95.
NIH Consensus Conference, "Intravenous Immunoglobulin, Prevention and Treatment of Disease," *JAMA*, 1990, 264(24):3189-93.
"University Hospital Consortium Expert Panel for Off-Label Use of Polyvalent Intravenously Administered Immunoglobulin Preparations Consensus Statement," *JAMA*, 1995, 273(23):1865-70.

♦ **Immunine VH (Can)** *see* Factor IX Complex (Human) *on page 414*
♦ **Immunization Guidelines** *see page 1172*
♦ **Imodium® A-D [OTC]** *see* Loperamide *on page 603*
♦ **Imodium® Advanced** *see* Loperamide *on page 603*
♦ **Impril (Can)** *see* Imipramine *on page 528*
♦ **Imuran®** *see* Azathioprine *on page 121*

Inamrinone (eye NAM ri none)

U.S. Brand Names Inocor®
Synonyms Amrinone
Therapeutic Category Phosphodiesterase Enzyme Inhibitor
Generic Available Yes

Use Short-term treatment of low cardiac output states (sepsis, CHF); reserved for patients who have not responded adequately to therapy with digitalis, diuretics, and vasodilators; adjunctive therapy of pulmonary hypertension

Pregnancy Risk Factor C

Contraindications Hypersensitivity to inamrinone lactate, any component, or sulfites (contains sodium metabisulfite); valvular obstructive disease

Precautions Monitor for hypotension, thrombocytopenia, hepatotoxicity, and GI effects; discontinue inamrinone if significant increase in liver enzymes with symptoms of idiosyncratic hypersensitivity reaction (ie, eosinophilia) occurs; monitor fluids and electrolytes. Diuresis may result from improvement in cardiac output and may require dosage reduction of diuretics. Inamrinone may exacerbate myocardial ischemia or worsen ventricular ectopy.

Adverse Reactions
Cardiovascular: Hypotension (1.3% incidence), ventricular and supraventricular arrhythmias (3% incidence); may be related to infusion rate

Gastrointestinal: Nausea (1.7%), vomiting (0.9%), abdominal pain (0.4%), anorexia (0.4%); GI effects may be due to an increase in gastric acid secretion and intestinal motility, secondary to phosphodiesterase inhibition

Hematologic: Thrombocytopenia (2.4% incidence), may be dose-related; in one study, 8 of 16 children (1.5 months to 11.2 years of age) developed thrombocytopenia (mean count 66 x 10^9 platelets/L). Inamrinone bolus doses ranged from 1.2-3 mg/kg given in 4 divided doses over 1 hour and were followed by continuous infusions of 5-10 mcg/kg/minute. Thrombocytopenia developed 19-71 hours after starting inamrinone (mean $\pm$ SD = 51 $\pm$ 25 hours). Resolution of thrombocytopenia occurred 54 $\pm$ 15 hours after therapy was discontinued; thrombocytopenia developed in patients with a higher total dose, longer duration of infusion, higher plasma concentrations of N-acetylamrinone (major metabolite of inamrinone), and higher plasma ratios of N-acetylamrinone to inamrinone.

Hepatic: Hepatotoxicity (0.2% incidence)

Drug Interactions Disopyramide may increase hypotension (one case report; use with caution); diuretics may cause significant hypovolemia (dosage reduction of diuretic may be required)

Stability Dilute only with NS or ½NS; do not directly dilute with dextrose-containing solutions, chemical interaction occurs; may be administered I.V. (via Y-site) into running dextrose infusions. Furosemide forms a precipitate when injected in I.V. lines containing inamrinone; incompatible with sodium bicarbonate; use diluted solutions of inamrinone (1-3 mg/mL) within 24 hours.

Mechanism of Action Inhibits phosphodiesterase III (PDE III), the major PDE in cardiac and vascular tissues. Inhibition of PDE III increases cyclic adenosine monophosphate (cAMP) which potentiates the delivery of calcium to myocardial contractile systems and results in a positive inotropic effect. Inhibition of PDE III in vascular tissue results in relaxation of vascular muscle and vasodilatation.

Pharmacodynamics

Onset of action: I.V.: Within 2-5 minutes

Peak effect: Within 10 minutes

Duration: Dose dependent with low doses lasting ~30 minutes and higher doses lasting ~2 hours

Pharmacokinetics

Distribution: V_d:

Neonates: 1.8 L/kg

Infants: 1.6 L/kg

Adults: 1.2 L/kg

Protein binding: 10% to 49%

Metabolism: In the liver to several metabolites (N-acetate, N-glycolyl, N-glucuronide, and O-glucuronide)

Half-life:

Neonates, 1-2 weeks of age: 22.2 hours

Infants 6-38 weeks of age: 6.8 hours; negative correlation of age with half-life in infants 4-38 weeks of age

Infants and Children (1 month to 15 years of age): 2.2-10.5 hours

Adults, normal volunteers: 3.6 hours

Adults with CHF: 5.8 hours

Elimination: Excreted in urine as metabolites and unchanged drug; 10% to 40% as unchanged drug in the urine within 24 hours

Usual Dosage I.V.: **Note:** Dose should not exceed 10 mg/kg/24 hours; doses of 18 mg/kg/day have been used in adults for a short duration; titrate infusion based on patient clinical response and adverse effects

Neonates: 0.75 mg/kg I.V. bolus over 2-3 minutes followed by maintenance infusion 3-5 mcg/kg/minute; I.V. bolus may need to be repeated in 30 minutes; see Additional Information

Infants and Children: 0.75 mg/kg I.V. bolus over 2-3 minutes followed by maintenance infusion 5-10 mcg/kg/minute; I.V. bolus may need to be repeated in 30 minutes; see Additional Information

Adults: 0.75 mg/kg I.V. bolus over 2-3 minutes followed by maintenance infusion of 5-10 mcg/kg/minute; I.V. bolus may need to be repeated in 30 minutes

PALS Guidelines 2000: I.V., I.O.: Loading dose: 0.75-1 mg/kg over 5 minutes; if tolerated, loading dose may be repeated up to 2 times; maximum total loading dose: 3 mg/kg; follow with maintenance infusion of 5-10 mcg/kg/minute; **Note:** If hypotension occurs during loading dose, administer 5-10 mL/kg of NS or other appropriate fluid and position patient flat or with head down (if patient can tolerate); if hypotension continues after fluid loading, administer a vasopressor agent and do not administer further inamrinone loading doses

(Continued)

Inamrinone *(Continued)*

ACLS Guidelines 2000: Adults: 0.75 mg/kg I.V. bolus over 2-3 minutes followed by maintenance infusion of 5-15 mcg/kg/minute; I.V. bolus may need to be repeated in 30 minutes

Administration Parenteral:

I.V. bolus: Infuse over 2-3 minutes; may be administered undiluted

Continuous infusion: Dilute with NS or $\frac{1}{2}$NS to final concentration of 1-3 mg/mL; use controlled infusion device (eg, I.V. pump)

Monitoring Parameters Blood pressure, heart rate, platelet count, liver enzymes, fluid status, intake and output, body weight, serum electrolytes; if Swan-Ganz catheter is present, monitor cardiac index, stroke volume, systemic vascular resistance, pulmonary vascular resistance

Reference Range Proposed: Adults: 3 µg/mL; linear correlation with cardiac index observed from 0.5-7 µg/mL

Nursing Implications Do **not** administer furosemide I.V. push via "Y" site into inamrinone solutions as precipitate will occur; monitor patients closely (see Monitoring Parameters)

Additional Information Preliminary pharmacokinetic studies estimate that total initial bolus doses of 3-4.5 mg/kg given in divided doses to neonates and infants are required to obtain serum concentrations similar to therapeutic adult levels. The use of these higher doses has been reported in a small number of infants and children. Some centers use a total loading dose of 3 mg/kg (administered as 4 doses of 0.75 mg/kg/dose given every 15 minutes); each of the 0.75 mg/kg doses is given over 5 minutes. Further pharmacodynamic studies are needed to define pediatric inamrinone dosing guidelines.

Use of inamrinone in controlled trials did not extend beyond 48 hours; due to potential serious adverse effects and limited experience, inamrinone should only be used in patients who have not responded to other therapies (ie, digoxin, diuretics, vasodilators). Inamrinone has not been shown to be safe or effective for long-term treatment of CHF.

Effective July 1, 2000, the nonproprietary name of the drug (amrinone) was officially changed by the U.S. Pharmacopeia (USP) Nomenclature Committee and the U.S. Adopted Names (USAN) Council to inamrinone to prevent confusion with amiodarone; other countries will still use the name amrinone

Dosage Forms Injection, as lactate: 5 mg/mL (20 mL)

References

Allen-Webb EM, Ross MP, Pappas JB, et al, "Age-Related Amrinone Pharmacokinetics in a Pediatric Population," *Crit Care Med*, 1994, 22(6):1016-24.

"Guidelines 2000 for Cardiopulmonary Resuscitation and Emergency Cardiovascular Care, Part 6: Advanced Cardiovascular Life Support, The American Heart Association in Collaboration With the International Liaison Committee on Resuscitation," *Circulation*, 2000, 102(8 Suppl):I86-171.

"Guidelines 2000 for Cardiopulmonary Resuscitation and Emergency Cardiovascular Care, Part 10: Pediatric Advanced Life Support, The American Heart Association in Collaboration With the International Liaison Committee on Resuscitation," *Circulation*, 2000, 102(8 Suppl): I291-342.

Lawless S, Burckart G, Diven W, et al, "Amrinone in Neonates and Infants After Cardiac Surgery," *Crit Care Med*, 1989, 17(8):751-4.

Lawless ST, Zaritsky A, and Miles MV, "The Acute Pharmacokinetics and Pharmacodynamics of Amrinone in Pediatric Patients," *J Clin Pharmacol*, 1991, 31(9):800-3.

Lynn AM, Sorensen GK, and Williams GD, "Hemodynamic Effects of Amrinone and Colloid Administration in Children Following Cardiac Surgery," *J Cardiothorac Vasc Anesth*, 1993, 7(5):560-5.

Ross MP, Allen-Webb EM, Pappas JB, et al, "Amrinone-Associated Thrombocytopenia: Pharmacokinetic Analysis," *Clin Pharmacol Ther*, 1993, 53(6):661-7.

♦ **Inapsine®** *see* Droperidol *on page 365*

♦ **Inderal®** *see* Propranolol *on page 847*

♦ **Inderal® LA** *see* Propranolol *on page 847*

Indinavir *(in DIN a veer)*

Related Information

Adult and Adolescent HIV *on page 1166*

Pediatric HIV *on page 1162*

U.S. Brand Names Crixivan®

Synonyms L-735,524; MK-639

Therapeutic Category Antiretroviral Agent; HIV Agents (Anti-HIV Agents); Protease Inhibitor

Use Treatment of HIV infection in combination with other antiretroviral agents; (**Note:** Current preferred HIV regimens consist of three antiretroviral agents); postexposure chemoprophylaxis following occupational exposure to HIV

Pregnancy Risk Factor C

Contraindications Hypersensitivity to indinavir or any component

Warnings Cases of nephrolithiasis and nephrolithiasis associated with renal insufficiency or acute renal failure have been reported. If signs and symptoms of nephrolithiasis occur (flank pain with or without hematuria), interrupt or discontinue therapy.
Due to potential serious and life-threatening drug interactions, the following drugs
should not be coadministered with indinavir: terfenadine, astemizole, cisapride,
ergot alkaloid derivatives, triazolam, and midazolam. Concomitant use with rifampin
is contraindicated since rifampin may markedly reduce indinavir concentrations.
Spontaneous bleeding episodes have been reported in patients with hemophilia A
and B. New onset diabetes mellitus, exacerbation of diabetes and hyperglycemia
have been reported in HIV-infected patients receiving protease inhibitors. Redistribution or accumulation of body fat may occur in patients taking protease inhibitors.

Precautions Use with caution in patients with hepatic impairment; modify dose in
patients with impaired liver function

Adverse Reactions

    Central nervous system: Insomnia, dizziness, headache, somnolence, asthenia,
      depression

    Dermatologic: Rash, dry skin, urticaria, pruritus, paronychia

    Endocrine & metabolic: Rare: Hyperglycemia, diabetes, ketoacidosis; elevated
      serum cholesterol and triglycerides

    Gastrointestinal: Nausea (10%), vomiting, diarrhea, abdominal pain, dyspepsia,
      metallic taste, pancreatitis

    Genitourinary: Dysuria

    Hematologic: Hemolytic anemia, spontaneous bleeding episodes in hemophiliacs
      (rare)

    Hepatic: Hyperbilirubinemia (10%), elevated liver function tests, jaundice, liver
      cirrhosis

    Neuromuscular & skeletal: Arthralgia

    Renal: Nephrolithiasis (4%), hematuria, proteinuria, renal failure, interstitial nephritis

    Respiratory: Dry throat, pharyngitis

    Miscellaneous: Redistribution of body fat to cause protease paunch, buffalo hump,
      facial atrophy, and breast enlargement

Drug Interactions Cytochrome P-450 isoenzyme CYP3A3/4 substrate; isoenzyme
CYP3A3/4 inhibitor

    Coadministration with didanosine will decrease indinavir absorption; coadministra-
    tion with rifampin or rifabutin will greatly reduce indinavir levels; indinavir
    increases rifabutin concentrations (decrease daily rifabutin dose by 50%); keto-
    conazole and itraconazole increase indinavir concentrations (dosage reduction of
    indinavir is recommended); ritonavir and nelfinavir decrease the metabolism of
    indinavir; coadministration with nevirapine may decrease indinavir concentrations;
    efavirenz decreases indinavir concentrations (indinavir dosage increase is recom-
    mended); delavirdine increases indinavir concentrations (dosage reduction of
    indinavir is recommended); indinavir inhibits the metabolism of HMG-CoA reduc-
    tase inhibitors (atorvastatin, lovastatin, simvastatin) which increases the risk of
    myopathy; avoid concurrent use of astemizole or cisapride with indinavir due to
    potential for life-threatening cardiotoxicity; coadministration of benzodiazepines
    with indinavir may result in prolonged sedation and respiratory depression;
    indinavir increases the AUC of amprenavir; St John's wort induces CYP3A
    enzymes and has lead to 57% reductions in indinavir AUC's and 81% reductions
    in serum trough concentrations, which may lead to treatment failures; (see Warn-
    ings related to potentially serious and life-threatening drug interactions)

Food Interactions Decreased absorption when administered with high amounts of
protein or fatty foods; 26% decrease in AUC when administered with grapefruit juice

Stability Store capsules at room temperature in original container with desiccant
since capsules are sensitive to moisture

Mechanism of Action A protease inhibitor which acts on an enzyme late in the HIV
replication process after the virus has entered into the cell's nucleus preventing
cleavage of the gag-pol protein precursors resulting in the production of immature,
noninfectious virions; cross-resistance with other protease inhibitors is possible

Pharmacokinetics

    Absorption: Rapid; presence of food decreases the extent of absorption

    Protein binding: 60%

    Metabolism: In the liver by CYP3A4 system to inactive metabolites

    Bioavailability: Wide interpatient variability in children: 15% to 50%

    Half-life: 1.8-2 hours

    Time to peak serum concentration: 0.8-1 hour

    Elimination: 83% in feces as unabsorbed drug and metabolites; 10% excreted in
      urine as unchanged drug

(Continued)

Indinavir *(Continued)*

Usual Dosage Oral:

Neonates: Should not be administered to neonates until further studies are performed due to side effect of hyperbilirubinemia

Children: Under study in clinical trials: 500 mg/m^2/dose every 8 hours; maximum dose: 800 mg/dose every 8 hours

Adolescents and Adults: 800 mg/dose every 8 hours

Chemoprophylaxis after high-risk occupational exposure to HIV: 800 mg/dose every 8 hours in combination with zidovudine and lamivudine; start treatment as soon as possible (within a few hours following exposure) and continue for 4 weeks

Dosage adjustment in mild to moderate hepatic impairment: Reduce dose by 25%

Administration Administer with water on an empty stomach or with a light snack 1 hour before or 2 hours after a meal; may administer with other liquids (ie, skim milk, apple juice) or a light snack (ie, dry toast or cornflakes with skim milk); if coadministered with didanosine, give at least 1 hour apart on an empty stomach

Monitoring Parameters Serum bilirubin, liver function tests, urinalysis, blood glucose levels, CD4 cell count, plasma levels of HIV RNA

Patient Information If dose is missed, the dose should be omitted and the next dose taken at the usual scheduled time; do not double the next dose

Nursing Implications Ensure adequate patient hydration to minimize the risk of nephrolithiasis

Dosage Forms Capsule: 200 mg, 333 mg, 400 mg

References

CDC and the National Foundation for Infectious Disease, "Update: Provisional Public Health Service Recommendations for Chemoprophylaxis After Occupational Exposure to HIV," *MMWR Morb Mortal Wkly Rep*, 1996, 45(22):468-80.

Mueller BU, Smith S, Sleasman J, et al, "A Phase I/II Study of the Protease Inhibitor Indinavir (MK-0639) in Children With HIV Infection," *Eleventh International Conference on AIDS*, Vancouver, Canada, 1996.

Stein DS, Fish DG, Bilello JA, et al, "A 24-Week Open-Label Phase I/II Evaluation of the HIV Protease Inhibitor MK-639 (Indinavir)," *AIDS*, 1996, 10(5):485-92.

Working Group on Antiretroviral Therapy and Medical Management of HIV-Infected Children, "Guidelines for the Use of Antiretroviral Agents in Pediatric HIV Infection," January 7, 2000, http://www.hivatis.org.

♦ **Indocid (Can)** *see* Indomethacin *on page 536*

♦ **Indocid PDA (Can)** *see* Indomethacin *on page 536*

♦ **Indocin®** *see* Indomethacin *on page 536*

♦ **Indocin® I.V.** *see* Indomethacin *on page 536*

♦ **Indocin® SR** *see* Indomethacin *on page 536*

Indomethacin *(in doe METH a sin)*

Related Information

Overdose and Toxicology *on page 1222*

U.S. Brand Names Indocin®; Indocin® I.V.; Indocin® SR

Canadian Brand Names Apo-Indomethacin; Indocid; Indocid PDA; Indotec; Novo-Methacin; Nu-Indo; Pro-Indo; Rhodacine

Therapeutic Category Analgesic, Non-narcotic; Anti-inflammatory Agent; Antipyretic; Nonsteroidal Anti-inflammatory Drug (NSAID), Oral; Nonsteroidal Anti-inflammatory Drug (NSAID), Parenteral

Generic Available Yes, except injection

Use Management of inflammatory diseases and rheumatoid disorders; moderate pain; acute gouty arthritis; I.V. form used as alternative to surgery for closure of patent ductus arteriosus (PDA) in neonates

Pregnancy Risk Factor B (D if used longer than 48 hours or after 34 weeks gestation)

Contraindications Hypersensitivity to indomethacin, any component, aspirin, or other NSAIDs; active GI bleeding, ulcer disease; premature neonates with necrotizing enterocolitis, impaired renal function (eg, neonates with urine output <0.6 mL/kg/hour or serum creatinine ≥1.8 mg/dL), IVH, active bleeding, thrombocytopenia

Precautions Use with caution in patients with cardiac dysfunction, hypertension, renal or hepatic impairment, epilepsy, patients receiving anticoagulants and for treatment of JRA in children (fatal hepatitis has been reported)

Adverse Reactions

Cardiovascular: Hypertension, edema

Central nervous system: Somnolence, fatigue, depression, confusion, dizziness, headache

Dermatologic: Rash

Endocrine & metabolic: Hyperkalemia, dilutional hyponatremia (I.V.), hypoglycemia (I.V.)

Gastrointestinal: Nausea, vomiting, epigastric pain, abdominal pain, anorexia, GI bleeding, ulcers, perforation

Hematologic: Hemolytic anemia, bone marrow suppression, agranulocytosis, thrombocytopenia, inhibition of platelet aggregation

Hepatic: Hepatitis

Ocular: Corneal opacities

Otic: Tinnitus

Renal: Renal failure, oliguria

Miscellaneous: Hypersensitivity reactions

Drug Interactions Cytochrome P-450 isoenzyme CYP2C9 substrate

Indomethacin may increase serum concentrations of digoxin, methotrexate, lithium, and aminoglycosides (reported with I.V. use in neonates); may increase nephrotoxicity of cyclosporine; may decrease antihypertensive and diuretic effects of furosemide and thiazides; may increase serum potassium with potassium-sparing diuretics; may decrease antihypertensive effects of beta-blockers, hydralazine, ACE inhibitors and angiotensin II antagonists; aspirin may decrease and probenecid may increase indomethacin serum concentrations; other GI irritants (eg, potassium supplements, NSAIDs) may increase GI adverse effects

Food Interactions Food may decrease the rate but not the extent of absorption

Stability

Oral suspension: Store below 86°F; do not freeze

I.V. product: Protect from light; not stable in alkaline solution; reconstitute just prior to administration; discard any unused portion; do not use preservative-containing diluents for reconstitution; will precipitate if reconstituted with solutions at pH <6 (product is not buffered)

Mechanism of Action Inhibits prostaglandin synthesis by decreasing the activity of the enzyme, cyclo-oxygenase, which results in decreased formation of prostaglandin precursors

Pharmacokinetics

Absorption: Oral:

Neonates: Incomplete, nonuniform

Adults: Rapid and well absorbed

Distribution:

Neonates: PDA: 0.36 L/kg

Post-PDA closure: 0.26 L/kg

Adults: 0.34-1.57 L/kg

Protein binding: 99%

Metabolism: In the liver via glucuronide conjugation and other pathways

Bioavailability: Oral:

Neonates, premature: 13% to 20%

Adults: ~100%

Half-life:

Neonates:

Postnatal age (PNA) <2 weeks: ~20 hours

PNA >2 weeks: ~11 hours

Adults: 2.6-11.2 hours

Elimination: Significant enterohepatic recycling; 33% excreted in feces as demethylated metabolites with 1.5% as unchanged drug; 60% eliminated in urine as drug and metabolites

Usual Dosage

Patent ductus arteriosus:

Neonates: I.V.: Initial: 0.2 mg/kg, followed by 2 doses depending on postnatal age (PNA):

PNA **at time of first dose** <48 hours: 0.1 mg/kg at 12- to 24-hour intervals

PNA **at time of first dose** 2-7 days: 0.2 mg/kg at 12- to 24-hour intervals

PNA **at time of first dose** >7 days: 0.25 mg/kg at 12- to 24-hour intervals

In general, may use 12-hour dosing interval if urine output >1 mL/kg/hour after prior dose; use 24-hour dosing interval if urine output is <1 mL/kg/hour but >0.6 mL/kg/hour; doses should be withheld if patient has oliguria (urine output <0.6 mL/kg/hour) or anuria

Inflammatory/rheumatoid disorders:

Oral:

Children: 1-2 mg/kg/day in 2-4 divided doses; maximum dose: 4 mg/kg/day; not to exceed 150-200 mg/day

Adults: 25-50 mg/dose 2-3 times/day; maximum dose: 200 mg/day; extended release capsule should be given on a 1-2 times/day schedule

(Continued)

Indomethacin *(Continued)*

Rectal: Adults: Persistent night pain and/or morning stiffness: 50-100 mg at bedtime (as part of total daily dose maximum of 200 mg/day)

Administration

Oral: Administer with food, milk, or antacids to decrease GI adverse effects; extended release capsules must be swallowed whole, do not crush or chew

Parenteral: I.V.: Administer over 20-30 minutes at a concentration of 0.5-1 mg/mL in preservative free sterile water for injection or preservative free NS

Note: Do **not** administer via I.V. bolus or I.V. infusion via an umbilical catheter into vessels near the superior mesenteric artery, as these may cause vasoconstriction and can compromise blood flow to the intestines. Do not administer intra-arterially.

Rectal: Insert into rectum and retain

Monitoring Parameters BUN, serum creatinine, liver enzymes, CBC with differential; in addition, in neonates treated for PDA: heart rate, heart murmur, blood pressure, urine output, echocardiogram, serum sodium, platelet count, and serum concentrations of concomitantly administered drugs which are renally eliminated (eg, aminoglycosides, digoxin); periodic ophthalmic exams with chronic use

Patient Information Avoid alcohol; may cause dizziness

Additional Information Indomethacin may mask signs and symptoms of infections; fatalities in children have been reported, due to unrecognized overwhelming sepsis; drowsiness, lethargy, nausea, vomiting, seizures, paresthesia, headache, dizziness, tinnitus, GI bleeding, cerebral edema, and cardiac arrest have been reported with overdoses

Dosage Forms

Capsule: 25 mg, 50 mg

Capsule, sustained release (Indocin® SR): 75 mg

Powder for injection, as sodium trihydrate: 1 mg

Suppository, rectal: 50 mg

Suspension, oral: 25 mg/5 mL [pineapple-coconut-mint flavor] (237 mL)

References

Coombs RC, Morgan ME, Durbin GM, et al, "Gut Blood Flow Velocities in the Newborn: Effects of Patent Ductus Arteriosus and Parenteral Indomethacin," *Arch Dis Child*, 1990, 65(10 Spec No):1067-71.

Gersony WM, Peckham GJ, Ellison RC, et al, "Effects of Indomethacin in Premature Infants With Patent Ductus Arteriosus: Results of a National Collaborative Study," *J Pediatr*, 1983, 102(6):895-906.

Kraus DM and Pham JT, "Neonatal Therapy," *Applied Therapeutics: The Clinical Use of Drugs*, 7th ed, Koda-Kimble MA, Young LY, eds, Baltimore, MD: Lippincott Williams & Wilkins, 2001.

♦ **Indotec (Can)** *see* Indomethacin *on page 536*

♦ **Infants' Advil® Concentrated Drops [OTC]** *see* Ibuprofen *on page 520*

♦ **Infants' Motrin [OTC]** *see* Ibuprofen *on page 520*

♦ **Infasurf®** *see* Calfactant *on page 171*

♦ **Infazinc (Can)** *see* Zinc Oxide *on page 1026*

♦ **Infectrol®** *see* Dexamethasone, Neomycin, and Polymyxin B *on page 309*

♦ **InFed®** *see* Iron Supplements (Parenteral) *on page 551*

♦ **Inflamase® Forte** *see* Prednisolone *on page 821*

♦ **Inflamase® Mild** *see* Prednisolone *on page 821*

♦ **Influenza Virus Vaccine** *see page 1172*

♦ **Infumorph™** *see* Morphine Sulfate *on page 683*

♦ **INH** *see* Isoniazid *on page 554*

♦ **Inocor®** *see* Inamrinone *on page 532*

♦ **Insomnal (Can)** *see* Diphenhydramine *on page 342*

♦ **Insta-Glucose® [OTC]** *see* Dextrose *on page 317*

Insulin Preparations *(IN su lin prep a RAY shuns)*

U.S. Brand Names Humalog®; Humalog® Mix 75/25™; Humulin® 50/50; Humulin® 70/30; Humulin® L; Humulin® N; Humulin® R; Humulin® R (Concentrated); Humulin® U; Lantus®; Lente® Iletin® II; Novolin® 70/30; Novolin® L; Novolin® N; Novolin® R; NovoLog™; NPH Iletin® II; Pork Regular Iletin® II; Velosulin® BR Human (Buffered)

Canadian Brand Names Humulin 10/90, 20/80, 30/70, 40/60, 50/50; Iletin II Pork NPH; Iletin II Pork Regular; Novolin 10/90, 20/80, 30/70, 40/60, 50/50; Novolin Lente; Novolin NPH; Novolin Toronto; Novolin Ultralente

Therapeutic Category Antidiabetic Agent, Parenteral

Generic Available Yes

Use Treatment of insulin-dependent diabetes mellitus, also noninsulin-dependent diabetes mellitus unresponsive to treatment with diet and/or oral hypoglycemics; to assure proper utilization of glucose and reduce glucosuria in nondiabetic patients receiving parenteral nutrition whose glucosuria cannot be adequately controlled with infusion rate adjustments or those who require assistance in achieving optimal caloric intakes; treatment of hyperkalemia (use with glucose to shift potassium into cells to lower serum potassium levels)

Pregnancy Risk Factor B

Contraindications Hypoglycemia; only regular insulin may be given intravenously; hypersensitivity to the insulin source (eg, beef or pork) or any components

Warnings Any change of insulin should be made cautiously; changing manufacturers, type and/or method of manufacture, may result in the need for a change of dosage; human insulin differs from animal-source insulin; hypoglycemia may result from increased work or exercise without eating

Adverse Reactions Primarily symptoms of hypoglycemia

Cardiovascular: Palpitations, tachycardia, pallor

Central nervous system: Fatigue, mental confusion, loss of consciousness, headache, hypothermia

Dermatologic: Urticaria, redness

Endocrine & metabolic: Hypoglycemia, hypokalemia

Gastrointestinal: Hunger, nausea, numbness of mouth

Local: Itching, redness, edema, stinging, or warmth at injection site, atrophy or hypertrophy of S.C. fat tissue

Neuromuscular & skeletal: Muscle weakness, tremors, tingling of fingers

Ocular: Transient presbyopia or blurred vision

Miscellaneous: Diaphoresis, anaphylaxis

Drug Interactions See table.

Drug Interactions With Insulin

Decrease Hypoglycemic Effects	Increase Hypoglycemic Effects
Acetazolamide	ACE inhibitors
Antiretrovirals	Alcohol
Asparaginase	Alpha-blockers
Calcitonin	Anabolic steroids
Contraceptives, oral	Beta blockers, nonselective
Corticosteroids	Calcium
Cyclophosphamide	Chloroquine
Diazoxide	Clofibrate
Diltiazem	Guanethidine
Dobutamine	Lithium
Epinephrine	MAO inhibitors
Estrogens	Mebendazole
Ethacrynic acid	Octreotide
Isoniazid	Oral antidiabetic agents
Lithium	(oral hypoglycemic agents)
Morphine	Pentamidine
Niacin	Phenylbutazone
Phenothiazines	Pyridoxine
Phenytoin	Salicylates
Nicotine	Sulfinpyrazone
Thiazide diuretics	Sulfonamides
Thyroid hormone	Tetracyclines

Stability

Newer neutral formulations of insulin are stable at room temperature up to 1 month and 3 months refrigerated; cold (freezing) causes more damage to insulin than room temperatures up to 100°F; avoid direct sunlight; cold injections should be avoided

Insulin Mixture Compatibility

Insulin Preparations	Compatible Mixed With
Insulin injection (regular)	All (except Velosulin® BR and Lantus®)
Prompt insulin zinc suspension (Semilente®)	Lente®
Lispro insulin solution (Humalog®)	Ultralente®, NPH
Isophane insulin suspension (NPH)	Regular and Humalog®
Insulin zinc suspension (Lente®)	Regular and Semilente®
Extended insulin zinc suspension (Ultralente®)	Regular, Semilente®, Humalog®

(Continued)

Insulin Preparations *(Continued)*

When mixing with NPH insulin in any proportion, the excess protamine may combine with regular insulin and may reduce or delay activity of regular insulin (does not appear to be clinically significant); phosphate-buffered regular insulins bind with Lente® insulins forming short-acting insulin

Stability of parenteral admixture of regular insulin in NS or 1/2 NS at room temperature (25°C) and at refrigeration temperature (4°C): 24 hours; all bags should be prepared fresh; tubing should be flushed 30 minutes prior to administration to allow adsorption as time permits

Mechanism of Action The principal hormone required for proper glucose utilization in normal metabolic processes; it is obtained from beef or pork pancreas or a biosynthetic process converting pork insulin to human insulin; insulins are categorized into 3 groups related to promptness, duration, and intensity of action

Pharmacodynamics Onset and duration of hypoglycemic effects depend upon the route of administration, site of injection, volume and concentration of injection, and the preparation administered; see table.

Pharmacodynamics of Insulin Preparations

Insulin Preparations	Onset (h)	Peak (h)	Duration (h)
Rapid-Acting			
Insulin aspart (NovoLog™)	0.25	1-3	3-5
Insulin injection (regular)	0.5-1	2-3	5-7
Prompt insulin zinc suspension (Semilente®)	1-1.5	5-10	12-16
Lispro insulin (Humalog®)	0.25	0.5-1.5	6-8
Intermediate-Acting			
Isophane insulin suspension (NPH)	1-1.5	4-12	24
Insulin zinc suspension (Lente®)	1-2.5	7-15	24
Long-Acting			
Extended insulin zinc suspension (Ultralente®)	4-8	10-30	>36
Insulin glargine (Lantus®)	5	*	>24

*Has no pronounced peak

Usual Dosage Dose requires continuous medical supervision; only regular insulin may be given I.V. The daily dose should be divided up depending upon the product used and the patient's response (see table) (eg, regular insulin every 4-6 hours; NPH insulin every 8-12 hours).

Children and Adults: S.C.: 0.5-1 unit/kg/day in divided doses

Adolescents (during growth spurt) S.C.: 0.8-1.2 units/kg/day in divided doses

Diabetic ketoacidosis: Children: I.V. loading dose: 0.1 unit/kg, then maintenance continuous infusion: 0.1 unit/kg/hour (range: 0.05-0.2 unit/kg/hour depending upon the rate of decrease of serum glucose). Decreasing the serum glucose level too rapidly may lead to cerebral edema; optimum rate of decrease (serum glucose): 80-100 mg/dL/hour

Insulin Dosing Sliding Scale

Urine Glucose	Insulin Dose (units/kg)	
	Urine Ketones (-)	Urine Ketones (+)
0-1/2%	0	0
3/4%	0.03-0.1	0.05-0.12
1%	0.07-0.2	0.1-0.25
2%	0.15-0.4	0.2-0.5

Note: Newly diagnosed patients with juvenile onset diabetes mellitus presenting in DKA and patients with blood sugars <800 mg/dL may be relatively "sensitive" to insulin and should receive loading and initial maintenance doses approximately $\frac{1}{2}$ of those indicated above.

Sliding scale: Use only for brief transitional periods of treatment; newly diagnosed patients with juvenile onset diabetes may be "sensitive" to exogenous insulin and should be treated with the lower end of these ranges; see table.

To optimize caloric intake in neonates while on parenteral nutrition:

Continuous infusion: I.V.: Neonates: 0.01-0.1 unit/kg/hour; neonates are very sensitive to insulin; start at low end of infusion rate and monitor closely

Treatment of hyperkalemia (after treatment with I.V. calcium gluconate and $NaHCO_3$):

Children: Dextrose 0.5-1 g/kg (using 25% or 50%) combined with insulin 1 unit for every 4-5 g dextrose; infuse over 2 hours **or** dextrose 0.5-1 g/kg infused over 15-30 minutes followed by 0.1 unit/kg insulin S.C. or I.V.

Adults: 50% dextrose at 0.5-1 mL/kg and insulin 1 unit for every 4-5 g dextrose given

Dosing adjustment in renal impairment: Children and Adults:

Cl_{cr} 10-50 mL/minute: Administer 75% of recommended dose

Cl_{cr} <10 mL/minute: Administer 25% to 50% of recommended dose (follow blood sugar closely)

Administration

Parenteral: S.C., I.M. S.C.: Administration is usually made into the thighs, arms, buttocks, or abdomen, with sites rotated; when mixing regular insulin with other preparations of insulin, regular insulin should be drawn into syringe first; insulin lispro and insulin aspart (when used as "meal-time" insulin, due to a rapid onset of effect) should be administered 15 minutes before meals; regular insulin should be administered 30-60 minutes before meals; insulin glargine (Lantus®) should be administered once daily at bedtime; do not mix Velosulin® BR or Lantus® with other insulins; to achieve complete suspension, insulin pens should be tipped at least 20 times before injection

I.V. (**only regular insulin** may be administered I.V.) infusion (requires use of an infusion pump): To minimize adsorption problems to I.V. solution bag and tubing:

If new tubing is **not** needed: Wait a minimum of 30 minutes between the preparation of the solution and the initiation of the infusion

If new tubing is needed: After receiving the insulin drip solution, the administration set should be attached to the I.V. container and the line should be flushed with the insulin solution. The nurse should then wait 30 minutes, then flush the line again with the insulin solution prior to initiating the infusion.

Because of adsorption, the actual amount of insulin being administered could be substantially less than the apparent amount. Therefore, adjustment of the insulin drip rate should be based on effect and not solely on the apparent insulin dose. Furthermore, the apparent I.V. infusion dose should not be used as the basis for determining the subsequent insulin dose upon discontinuing the insulin drip. Dosage adjustment requires continuous medical supervision.

Monitoring Parameters Urine sugar and acetone, blood sugar, serum electrolytes, hemoglobin A_{1c}

Reference Range Target range:

Blood glucose: Fasting and preprandial: 80-120 mg/dL; bedtime: 100-140 mg/dL

Glycosolated hemoglobin (hemoglobin A_{1c}): <7%

Patient Information Do not change insulins without physician's approval; patients should be counseled by someone experienced in diabetes education regarding signs and symptoms of hyper- and hypoglycemia, exercise and diet, blood glucose monitoring, and other related topics

Additional Information The term "purified" refers to insulin preparations containing no more than 10 ppm proinsulin (purified and human insulins are less immunogenic); buffering agent in Velosulin® BR may alter the activity of other insulin products

Dosage Forms All insulins are 100 units/mL (10 mL) except where indicated:

RAPID-ACTING:

Insulin aspart (rDNA origin): NovoLog™ (10 mL; 3 mL PenFill cartridges)

Insulin lispro rDNA origin: Humalog® [*Lilly*] (1.5 mL cartridge, 3 mL disposable pen, 10 mL vial)

Insulin Injection (Regular Insulin)

Human:

rDNA: Humulin® R [*Lilly*] (1.5 mL cartridges, 10 mL vials), Novolin® R [*Novo Nordisk*] (10 mL), Novolin® R PenFill [*Novo Nordisk*] (1.5 mL, 3 mL), Novolin® R Prefilled [*Novo Nordisk*] (1.5 mL)

rDNA, Buffered: Velosulin® BR (10 mL)

(Continued)

Insulin Preparations *(Continued)*

rDNA (concentrated): Humulin® U-500 [*Lilly*] (500 units/mL, 20 mL vial)
Pork: Regular Insulin [*Novo Nordisk*]
Purified pork: Pork Regular Iletin® II [*Lilly*] (10 mL)

INTERMEDIATE-ACTING:
Insulin Zinc Suspension (Lente)
Human, rDNA: Humulin® L [*Lilly*] (10 mL), Novolin® L [*Novo Nordisk*] (10 mL)
Purified pork: Lente® Iletin® II [*Lilly*] (10 mL)

Isophane Insulin Suspension (NPH)
Human, rDNA: Humulin® N [*Lilly*] (1.5 mL cartridges, 3 mL disposable pen, 10 mL
vial), Novolin® N [*Novo Nordisk*] (10 mL), Novolin® N PenFill [*Novo Nordisk*] (1.5
ml, 3 mL) Novolin® N Prefilled [*Novo Nordisk*] (1.5 mL)
Purified pork: Pork NPH Iletin® II [*Lilly*] (10 mL)

LONG-ACTING:
Insulin zinc suspension, extended (Ultralente®)
Human, rDNA: Humulin® U [Lilly] (10 mL)
Insulin glargine, rDNA: Lantus® [*Avantis Pharmaceuticals Inc*] (3 mL cartridge, 5 mL
vial, 10 mL vial)

COMBINATIONS:

Isophane Insulin Suspension and Insulin Injection
Isophane insulin suspension (50%) and insulin injection (50%) human (rDNA):
Humulin® 50/50 [*Lilly*] (10 mL)
Isophane insulin suspension (70%) and insulin injection (30%) human (rDNA):
Humulin® 70/30 [*Lilly*] (1.5 mL cartridge, 3 mL disposable Pen, 10 mL vial),
Novolin® 70/30 [*Novo Nordisk*] (10 mL), Novolin® 70/30 PenFill [*Novo Nordisk*]
(1.5 mL, 3 mL), Novolin® 70/30 Prefilled [*Novo Nordisk*] (1.5 mL)

Insulin Lispro Protamine Suspension and Insulin Lispro Injection
Insulin lispro protamine suspension (75%) and insulin lispro injection (25%)
Humalog® Mix 75/25™ [*Lilly*] (3 mL disposable pen, 10 mL vial)

HIGH POTENCY:
Insulin injection, concentrated, rDNA human: Humulin® R U-500 [*Lilly*] (500 units/
mL, 20 mL vial)

References
Simeon PS, Geffner ME, Levin SR, et al, "Continuous Insulin Infusions in Neonates: Pharmacologic
Availability of Insulin in Intravenous Solutions," *J Pediatr*, 1994, 124(5 Pt 1):818-20.

♦ **Insulin Reaction [OTC]** *see* Dextrose *on page 317*
♦ **Intal**® *see* Cromolyn *on page 273*
♦ **α-2-interferon** *see* Interferon Alfa-2b *on page 544*

Interferon Alfa-2a (in ter FEER on AL fa too aye)

U.S. Brand Names Roferon-A®
Synonyms IFLrA; IFN; rIFN-α
Therapeutic Category Antineoplastic Agent, Miscellaneous; Biological Response
Modulator; Interferon
Generic Available No
Use FDA approved in patients >18 years of age: Hairy cell leukemia, AIDS-related
Kaposi's sarcoma, Philadelphia chromosome-positive chronic myelogenous
leukemia, hemangiomas of infancy; multiple unlabeled uses
Pregnancy Risk Factor C
Contraindications Hypersensitivity to alpha interferon or any component
Warnings The FDA currently recommends that procedures for proper handling and
disposal of antineoplastic agents be considered; safety and efficacy in children <18
years of age have not been established; injection contains benzyl alcohol which may
be toxic to newborns in high doses, use with caution in newborns
Precautions Use with caution in patients with seizure disorders, brain metastases,
multiple sclerosis, compromised CNS, and patients with pre-existing cardiac
disease, myelosuppression, or severe renal/hepatic impairment
Adverse Reactions Flu-like symptoms (fever, fatigue/malaise, myalgia, chills, headache, arthralgia, rigors) begin about 2-6 hours after the dose is given and may
persist as long as 24 hours; usually patient can build up a tolerance to side effects

Cardiovascular: Tachycardia, arrhythmias, hypotension, edema, chest pain
Central nervous system: Fatigue/malaise, dizziness, depression, confusion, sensory
neuropathy, psychiatric symptoms (psychosis, mania, depression, suicidal
behavior), fever, headache, EEG abnormalities, chills

Dermatologic: Partial alopecia, rash, dry skin

Endocrine & metabolic: Increased uric acid level, thyroid dysfunction, hyperglycemia, hypertriglyceridemia

Gastrointestinal: Anorexia, xerostomia, nausea, vomiting, diarrhea, abdominal cramps, dysgeusia, weight loss, stomatitis

Hematologic: Leukopenia (mainly neutropenia); anemia; thrombocytopenia; decreased hemoglobin, hematocrit, platelets; neutralizing antibodies

Hepatic: Elevated ALT and AST

Local: Burning, pain, erythema, rash at the site of injection

Neuromuscular & skeletal: Myalgia, arthralgia, rigors, leg cramps

Ocular: Blurred vision

Renal: Proteinuria, elevated BUN and serum creatinine

Respiratory: Coughing, nasal congestion

Miscellaneous: Diaphoresis

Drug Interactions

Interferon Alfa-2b: Possible competitive binding to same receptors

Acyclovir: Possible synergistic effects

Theophylline: Clearance of theophylline is reduced

Vinblastine: May increase interferon toxicity; increased neurotoxicity

Zidovudine: Possible additive myelosuppression

Stability Store in refrigerator; do not shake; after reconstitution stable at room temperature for 24 hours; do not store in syringes for prolonged periods

Mechanism of Action Inhibits cellular growth, alters the state of cellular differentiation, interferes with oncogene expression, alters cell surface antigen expression, increases phagocytic activity of macrophages and augments cytotoxicity of lymphocytes for target cells

Pharmacokinetics

Absorption: I.M., S.C.: >80%

Metabolism: In the kidney, filtered, and absorbed at the renal tubule

Half-life:

I.M., I.V.: 2 hours

S.C.: 3 hours

Time to peak serum concentration: Within 3-8 hours

Usual Dosage Refer to individual protocols

Infants and Children:

Hemangiomas of infancy, pulmonary hemangiomatosis: S.C.: 1-3 million units/m^2/day once daily

Philadelphia chromosome-positive CML: I.M., S.C.: 2.5-5 million units/m^2 daily

Children >18 years and Adults: I.M., S.C.:

Hairy cell leukemia: Induction dose is 3 million units/day for 16-24 weeks; maintenance: 3 million units 3 times/week

AIDS-related Kaposi's sarcoma: Induction dose: 36 million units/day for 10-12 weeks; maintenance: 36 million units 3 times/week (may begin with dose escalation from 3 to 9 to 18 million units each day over 3 consecutive days followed by 36 million units/day for the remainder of the 10-12 weeks of induction); or 20 million units/m^2 daily for 4 weeks, then if responding, 20 million units/m^2 3 times/week

CML: 9 million units daily

Hepatitis C: Initial: 6 million units once daily for 3 weeks followed by 3 million units 3 times/week for 6 months

Melanoma: 12 million units/m^2 3 times/week for 3 months

Administration Parenteral: S.C. (rather than I.M.) administration is suggested for those patients who are at risk for bleeding or are thrombocytopenic; rotate S.C. injection site

Monitoring Parameters Baseline EKG, CBC with differential and platelet count, electrolytes, liver and renal function tests, weight

Patient Information Do not change dosage as changes in dosage may result; possible mental status changes may occur while on therapy

Nursing Implications Patient should be well hydrated; pretreatment with NSAIDs or acetaminophen can decrease fever and its severity and alleviate headache

Additional Information Indications and dosage regimens are specific for a particular brand of interferon; other brands of interferon (ie, Intron® A) have different indications and dosage guidelines; do not change brands of interferon as changes in dosage may result

Dosage Forms

Injection: 3 million units/mL (1 mL); 6 million units/mL (3 mL); 36 million units/mL (1 mL)

Powder for injection: 6 million units/mL when reconstituted

(Continued)

Interferon Alfa-2a *(Continued)*

References

Ezekowitz RAB, Mulliken JB, and Folkman J, "Interferon Alfa-2a Therapy for Life-Threatening Hemangiomas of Infancy," *N Engl J Med*, 1992, 326(22):1456-63.

White CW, Sondheimer HM, Crouch EC, et al, "Treatment of Pulmonary Hemangiomatosis With Recombinant Interferon Alfa-2a," *N Engl J Med*, 1989, 320(18):1197-200.

Interferon Alfa-2b *(in ter FEER on AL fa too bee)*

U.S. Brand Names Intron® A

Synonyms IFN-α-2; α-2-interferon; rIFN-α2

Therapeutic Category Antineoplastic Agent, Miscellaneous; Biological Response Modulator; Interferon

Generic Available No

Use Induce hairy cell leukemia remission; treatment of AIDS-related Kaposi's sarcoma; condylomata acuminata; chronic hepatitis C; chronic hepatitis B

Pregnancy Risk Factor C

Contraindications Hypersensitivity to interferon alfa-2b or any component

Warnings The FDA currently recommends that procedures for proper handling and disposal of antineoplastic agents be considered; safety and efficacy in children <18 years of age have not been established; injection contains benzyl alcohol which may be toxic to newborns in high doses, use with caution in newborns

Precautions Use with caution in patients with seizure disorders, brain metastases, compromised CNS, multiple sclerosis, and patients with pre-existing cardiac disease, severe renal or hepatic impairment, or myelosuppression

Adverse Reactions Flu-like symptoms (fever, fatigue/malaise, myalgia, chills, headache, arthralgia, rigors) begin about 2-6 hours after the dose is given and may persist as long as 24 hours; usually patient can build up a tolerance to side effects

Cardiovascular: Tachycardia, arrhythmias, hypotension, edema, chest pain

Central nervous system: Fatigue/malaise, dizziness, depression, confusion, sensory neuropathy, psychiatric symptoms (psychosis, mania, depression, suicidal behavior), fever, headache, EEG abnormalities, chills

Dermatologic: Partial alopecia, rash

Endocrine & metabolic: Elevated uric acid level, thyroid dysfunction, hyperglycemia, hypertriglyceridemia

Gastrointestinal: Anorexia, xerostomia, nausea, vomiting, diarrhea, abdominal cramps, dysgeusia, weight loss

Hematologic: Leukopenia (mainly neutropenia); anemia; thrombocytopenia; decreased hemoglobin, hematocrit, platelets; neutralizing antibodies

Hepatic: Elevated ALT and AST

Local: Burning, pain, erythema, rash at the site of injection

Neuromuscular & skeletal: Myalgia, arthralgia, rigors

Ocular: Blurred vision

Renal: Proteinuria, elevated BUN and serum creatinine

Respiratory: Coughing, nasal congestion

Miscellaneous: Diaphoresis

Drug Interactions

Interferon Alfa-2a: May competitively bind to same receptors

Acyclovir: Possible synergistic effect

Theophylline: Clearance of theophylline is reduced

Vinblastine: May increase interferon toxicity; increased neurotoxicity

Zidovudine: Possible additive myelosuppression

Stability Refrigerate; reconstituted solution is stable for 1 month when refrigerated

Mechanism of Action Inhibits cellular growth, alters the state of cellular differentiation, interferes with oncogene expression, alters cell surface antigen expression, increases phagocytic activity of macrophages, and augments cytotoxicity of lymphocytes for target cells

Pharmacokinetics

Metabolism: Majority of dose is thought to be metabolized in the kidney, filtered and absorbed at the renal tubule

Half-life, elimination:

I.M., I.V.: 2 hours

S.C.: 3 hours

Time to peak serum concentration: I.M., S.C.: ~6-8 hours

Usual Dosage Adults (refer to individual protocols):

Hairy cell leukemia: I.M., S.C.: 2 million units/m² 3 times/week

AIDS-related Kaposi's sarcoma: I.M., S.C.: 30 million units/m² 3 times/week or 50 million units/m² I.V. 5 days/week every other week

Condylomata acuminata: Intralesionally: 1 million units/lesion 3 times/week for 3 weeks; not to exceed 5 million units per treatment (maximum dose: 5 lesions at one time) (use only the 10 million units vial)

Chronic hepatitis B: I.M., S.C.: 5 million units given once daily **or** 10 million units given 3 times/week for 4 months

Chronic hepatitis C: I.M., S.C.: 3 million units 3 times/week for approximately a 6-month course; relapse of hepatitis has occurred after treatment was stopped

Administration Parenteral: S.C. (rather than I.M.) administration is suggested for those patients who are at risk for bleeding or are thrombocytopenic; rotate S.C. injection site

Monitoring Parameters Baseline EKG, CBC with differential and platelet count, liver function tests, electrolytes, weight, chest x-ray

Patient Information Do not change brands of interferon as changes in dosage may result; do not operate heavy machinery while on therapy since changes in mental status may occur

Nursing Implications Patient should be well hydrated; may pretreat with NSAID or acetaminophen to decrease fever and its severity and to alleviate headache

Additional Information Myelosuppressive effects:

WBC: Mild

Platelets: Mild

Onset (days): 7-10

Nadir (days): 14

Recovery (days): 21

Dosage Forms Powder for injection, lyophilized: 3 million units, 5 million units, 10 million units, 18 million units, 25 million units, 50 million units

References

Davis GL, Balart LA, Schiff ER, et al, "Treatment of Chronic Hepatitis C With Recombinant Interferon Alfa. A Multicenter Randomized, Controlled Trial. Hepatitis Interventional Therapy Group," *N Engl J Med*, 1989; 321(22):1501-6.

Perrillo RP, "Interferon in the Management of Chronic Hepatitis B," *Dig Dis Sci*, 1993, 38(4):577-93.

- ♦ **Interleukin-2** *see Aldesleukin on page 47*
- ♦ **Intralipid**® *see Fat Emulsion on page 419*
- ♦ **Intravenous Fat Emulsion** *see Fat Emulsion on page 419*
- ♦ **Intron**® **A** *see Interferon Alfa-2b on page 544*
- ♦ **Intropin (Can)** *see Dopamine on page 353*
- ♦ **Invirase**® *see Saquinavir on page 889*
- ♦ **Iobid DM**® *see Guaifenesin and Dextromethorphan on page 487*

Iodine (EYE oh dyne)

Related Information

Drugs and Breast-Feeding *on page 1243*

Therapeutic Category Topical Skin Product

Generic Available Yes

Use Used topically as an antiseptic in the management of minor, superficial skin wounds and has been used to disinfect the skin preoperatively

Pregnancy Risk Factor D

Contraindications Hypersensitivity to iodide preparations or any component; neonates

Warnings May be highly toxic if ingested

Adverse Reactions

Local: Skin irritation, discoloration, and burns

Miscellaneous: Hypersensitivity, allergic reactions

Mechanism of Action Free iodine oxidizes microbial protoplasm making it effective against bacteria, fungi, yeasts, protozoa, and viruses; complexes with amino groups in tissue compounds to form iodophors from which the iodine is slowly released causing a sustained action

Usual Dosage Apply topically as necessary to affected areas of skin

Administration Topical: Apply to affected areas; avoid tight bandages because iodine may cause burns on occluded skin

Patient Information May stain skin and clothing

Additional Information Sodium thiosulfate inactivates iodine and is an effective chemical antidote for iodine poisoning; solutions of sodium thiosulfate may be used to remove iodine stains from skin and clothing

Dosage Forms

Solution: 2% (500 mL); 5% (500 mL, 4000 mL)

Tincture: 2% (500 mL, 4000 mL); 7% (500 mL, 4000 mL)

- ♦ **Iodine Sodium** *see Trace Metals on page 972*

♦ **Iodochlorhydroxyquin** *see* Clioquinol *on page 252*
♦ **Iodopen**® *see* Trace Metals *on page 972*

Iodoquinol (eye oh doe KWIN ole)

U.S. Brand Names Yodoxin®
Canadian Brand Names Diodoquin
Synonyms Diiodohydroxyquin
Therapeutic Category Amebicide
Generic Available No
Use Treatment of acute and chronic intestinal amebiasis due to *Entamoeba histolytica*; asymptomatic cyst passers; *Blastocystis hominis* infections; iodoquinol alone is ineffective for amebic hepatitis or hepatic abscess
Pregnancy Risk Factor C
Contraindications Hypersensitivity to iodine, iodoquinol, or any component; hepatic or renal damage; pre-existing optic neuropathy
Precautions Use with caution in patients with thyroid disease or neurological disorders
Adverse Reactions
Central nervous system: Agitation, retrograde amnesia, fever, chills, headache, ataxia
Dermatologic: Anal pruritus, rash, acne
Endocrine & metabolic: Enlargement of the thyroid
Gastrointestinal: Nausea, vomiting, diarrhea, gastritis, anorexia, constipation
Neuromuscular & skeletal: Weakness, peripheral neuropathy, myalgia
Ocular: Optic neuritis, optic atrophy, visual impairment
Mechanism of Action Contact amebicide that works in the lumen of the intestine by an unknown mechanism
Pharmacokinetics
Absorption: Oral: Poor and irregular
Metabolism: In the liver
Elimination: In feces; metabolites appear in urine
Usual Dosage Oral:
Children: 30-40 mg/kg/day in 3 divided doses for 20 days; not to exceed 1.95 g/day
Adults: 650 mg 3 times/day after meals for 20 days; not to exceed 2 g/day
Administration Oral: Administer medication after meals; tablets may be crushed and mixed with applesauce or chocolate syrup
Monitoring Parameters Ophthalmologic exam
Test Interactions May increase protein-bound serum iodine concentrations reflecting a decrease in iodine 131 uptake; false-positive ferric chloride test for phenylketonuria
Patient Information Notify physician if rash occurs
Dosage Forms
Powder: 25 g
Tablet: 210 mg, 650 mg

♦ **Ionil**® **[OTC]** *see* Salicylic Acid *on page 886*
♦ **Ionil**® **Plus [OTC]** *see* Salicylic Acid *on page 886*

Ipecac Syrup (IP e kak SIR up)

Therapeutic Category Antidote, Emetic
Generic Available Yes
Use Treatment of acute oral drug overdosage and certain poisonings; use only in alert conscious patients who have ingested potentially toxic amounts of substance
Pregnancy Risk Factor C
Contraindications Do not use in unconscious patients, patients with absent gag reflex or seizures; ingestion of strong bases or acids, other corrosive substances, volatile oils, hydrocarbons with high potential for aspiration
Warnings Avoid use in patients with coagulopathy or bleeding problems (risk of gastroesophageal hemorrhage) and in patients receiving calcium channel blockers, beta-blockers, clonidine, or digitalis glycosides (risk of exaggerated vagal stimulation with gagging, resulting in severe bradycardia); do not confuse ipecac syrup with ipecac fluid extract; fluid extract is 14 times more potent than syrup
Precautions Use with caution in patients with cardiovascular disease and bulimics
Adverse Reactions
Cardiovascular: Cardiotoxicity
Central nervous system: Lethargy, drowsiness
Gastrointestinal: Protracted vomiting, diarrhea; Mallory-Weiss syndrome, gastric rupture

Neuromuscular & skeletal: Myopathy
Respiratory: Aspiration (can be fatal)

Drug Interactions Activated charcoal may decrease effectiveness

Food Interactions Milk, carbonated beverages may decrease effectiveness

Mechanism of Action Irritates the gastric mucosa and stimulates the medullary chemoreceptor trigger zone to induce vomiting

Pharmacodynamics

Onset of vomiting after oral dose: Within 15-30 minutes; usual: 20 minutes
Duration: 20-25 minutes; can last longer, up to 1-2 hours

Usual Dosage Oral:

Children:
<6 months: Not recommended
6-12 months: 5-10 mL followed by 10-20 mL/kg or 120-240 mL of water; repeat dose one time if vomiting does not occur within 20-30 minutes
1-12 years: 15 mL followed by 10-20 mL/kg or 120-240 mL of water; repeat dose one time if vomiting does not occur within 20-30 minutes
Adolescents and Adults: 30 mL followed by 240 mL of water; repeat dose one time if vomiting does not occur within 20-30 minutes

Administration Oral: Administer within 60 minutes of ingestion; follow administration with water; do not administer with milk or carbonated beverages

Nursing Implications Do **not** administer to unconscious patients

Additional Information Patients should be kept active and moving following administration of ipecac; if vomiting does not occur after second dose, gastric lavage may be considered to remove ingested substance

The Position Statement of The American Academy of Clinical Toxicology and The European Association of Poisons Centres and Clinical Toxicologists does not recommend routine administration of ipecac syrup to poisoned patients; scientific literature does not support that ipecac improves patient outcome; this paper states that the **routine** administration of ipecac syrup in the emergency room should be abandoned. Also, scientific literature cannot support or exclude giving ipecac syrup soon after toxic ingestions; administration of ipecac syrup may delay the administration or decrease the effectiveness of activated charcoal, oral antidotes, or whole bowel irrigation; its use should be considered only if it can be given within 60 minutes after ingestion of poison.

Dosage Forms Syrup: 70 mg/mL (15 mL, 30 mL, 473 mL, 4000 mL)

References

"Position Statement: Ipecac Syrup. American Academy of Clinical Toxicology; European Association of Poisons Centres and Clinical Toxicologists," *J Toxicol Clin Toxicol*, 1997, 35(7):699-709.
Shannon M, "Ingestion of Toxic Substances by Children," *N Engl J Med*, 2000, 342(3):186-91.

Ipratropium (i pra TROE pee um)

Related Information

Asthma Guidelines *on page 1210*

U.S. Brand Names Atrovent®

Canadian Brand Names Alti-Ipratropium; Apo-Ipravent; Gen-Ipratropium; Novo-Ipramide; Nu-Ipratropium; PMS-Ipratropium

Therapeutic Category Antiasthmatic; Anticholinergic Agent; Bronchodilator

Generic Available No

Use Anticholinergic bronchodilator used in bronchospasm associated with asthma, COPD, bronchitis, and emphysema; symptomatic relief of rhinorrhea associated with allergic and nonallergic rhinitis

Pregnancy Risk Factor B

Contraindications Hypersensitivity to ipratropium, atropine, or its derivatives; history of hypersensitivity to soya lecithin or related food products such as soy bean and peanut

Warnings Not indicated for the initial treatment of acute episodes of bronchospasm

Precautions Use with caution in patients with narrow-angle glaucoma, bladder neck obstruction, or prostatic hypertrophy

Adverse Reactions

Note: Ipratropium is poorly absorbed from the lung, so systemic effects are rare

Cardiovascular: Palpitations, tachycardia, flushing, hypotension, hypertension
Central nervous system: Nervousness, dizziness, headache, fatigue, drowsiness, insomnia
Dermatologic: Rash, pruritus, alopecia
Gastrointestinal: Nausea, xerostomia, constipation
Genitourinary: Dysuria
Ocular: Blurred vision
(Continued)

Ipratropium (Continued)

Respiratory: Cough, hoarseness, dry secretions, epistaxis (with nasal spray)

Drug Interactions Additive effects with anticholinergics or drugs with anticholinergic properties

Stability Compatible for 1 hour when mixed with albuterol or metaproterenol in a nebulizer

Mechanism of Action Blocks the action of acetylcholine at parasympathetic sites in bronchial smooth muscle causing bronchodilation; inhibits secretions from the serous and seromucous glands lining the nasal mucosa

Pharmacodynamics

Onset of bronchodilation: 1-3 minutes after administration

Peak effect: Maximal effect within 1.5-2 hours

Duration: Bronchodilation persists for up to 4-6 hours

Pharmacokinetics

Absorption: Not readily absorbed into the systemic circulation from the surface of the lung or from the GI tract

Distribution: Following inhalation, 15% of dose reaches the lower airways

Half-life: 2 hours

Usual Dosage

Neonates: Nebulization: 25 mcg/kg/dose 3 times/day

Infants and Children: Nebulization: 125-250 mcg 3 times/day

Children 3-12 years: Metered inhaler: 1-2 inhalations 3 times/day, up to 6 inhalations/24 hours

Children ≥12 years and Adults:

Nebulization: 500 mcg 3-4 times/day

Metered inhaler: 2 inhalations 4 times/day, up to 12 inhalations/24 hours

Nasal spray:

Children >6 years and Adults: 0.03%: 2 sprays in each nostril 2-3 times/day

Children >5 years and Adults: 0.06%: 2 sprays in each nostril 3-4 times/day

Administration

Nasal spray: Pump must be primed before usage by 7 actuations into the air away from the face; if not used for >24 hours, pump must be reprimed with 2 actuations; if not used >7 days, reprime with 7 actuations

Nebulization: May be administered with or without dilution in NS

Oral Inhalation: Shake well before use; use spacer device in children <8 years

Dosage Forms Solution, as bromide:

Inhalation, oral: 18 mcg/actuation (14 g)

Nasal spray: 0.03% (30 mL); 0.06% (15 mL)

Nebulizing: 0.02% (2.5 mL)

References

Henry RI, Hiller EG, Milner AD, et al, "Nebulised Ipratropium Bromide and Sodium Cromoglycate in the First 2 Years of Life," *Arch Dis Child*, 1984, 59(1):54-7.

Mann NP and Hiller RG, "Ipratropium Bromide in Children With Asthma," *Thorax*, 1982, 37(1):72-4.

Schuh S, Johnson DW, Callahan S, et al, "Efficacy of Frequent Nebulized Ipratropium Added to Frequent High-Dose Albuterol Therapy in Severe Childhood Asthma," *J Pediatr*, 1995, 126(4):639-45.

Schuh S, Johnson D, Canny G, et al, "Efficacy of Adding Nebulized Ipratropium Bromide to Nebulized Albuterol Therapy in Acute Bronchiolitis," *Pediatrics*, 1992, 90(6): 920-3.

Wang EE, Milner R, Allen U, et al, "Bronchodilators for Treatment of Mild Bronchiolitis: A Factorial Randomized Trial," *Arch Dis Child*, 1992, 67(3):289-93.

Wilkie RA and Bryan MH, "Effect of Bronchodilators on Airway Resistance in Ventilator-dependent Neonates With Chronic Lung Disease," *J Pediatr*, 1987, 111(2):278-82.

♦ **Iproveratril** see Verapamil on page 1007

♦ **Ircon® [OTC]** see Iron Supplements (Oral/Enteral) on page 548

♦ **Iron Dextran** see Iron Supplements (Parenteral) on page 551

♦ **Iron Sucrose** see Iron Supplements (Parenteral) on page 551

♦ **Iron Sulfate (Ferrous Sulfate)** see Iron Supplements (Oral/Enteral) on page 548

Iron Supplements (Oral/Enteral) (EYE ern SUP la ments)

Related Information

Carbohydrate and Alcohol Content of Liquid Medications for Use in Patients Receiving Ketogenic Diets on page 1258

Overdose and Toxicology on page 1222

U.S. Brand Names Ed-In-SOL® [OTC]; Feosol® [OTC]; Feostat® [OTC]; Feratab® [OTC]; Fergon® [OTC]; Fer-In-Sol® [OTC]; Fer-Iron® [OTC]; Ferrex 150® [OTC]; Ferro-Sequels® [OTC]; Hemocyte® [OTC]; Hytinic® [OTC]; Ircon® [OTC]; Mol-Iron® [OTC]; Nephro-Fer™ [OTC]; Niferex® [OTC]; Niferex® 150 [OTC]; Nu-Iron® [OTC]; Nu-Iron® 150 [OTC]; Slow FE® [OTC]

Synonyms $FeSO_4$ (Ferrous Sulfate); Iron Sulfate (Ferrous Sulfate)

Available Salts Ferrous Fumarate; Ferrous Gluconate; Ferrous Sulfate

Therapeutic Category Iron Salt; Mineral, Oral

Generic Available Yes

Use Prevention and treatment of iron deficiency anemias; supplemental therapy for patients receiving epoetin alfa

Pregnancy Risk Factor A

Contraindications Hemochromatosis, hemolytic anemia; hypersensitivity to iron salts

Warnings Avoid use in premature infants until the vitamin E stores, deficient at birth, are replenished

Precautions Avoid using for longer than 6 months, except in patients with conditions that require prolonged therapy; avoid in patients with peptic ulcer, enteritis, or ulcerative colitis; avoid in patients receiving frequent blood transfusions

Adverse Reactions

Gastrointestinal: GI irritation, epigastric pain, nausea, diarrhea, dark stools, constipation

Genitourinary: Discoloration of urine (black or dark)

Miscellaneous: Liquid preparations may temporarily stain the teeth

Drug Interactions Absorption of oral preparation of iron and tetracyclines are decreased when both of these drugs are given together; concurrent administration of antacids and cimetidine may decrease iron absorption; iron may decrease absorption of penicillamine, levothyroxine, methyldopa, and levodopa when given at the same time; response to iron therapy may be delayed in patients receiving chloramphenicol; concurrent administration ≥200 mg vitamin C per 30 mg elemental iron increases absorption of oral iron; absorption of quinolones may be decreased due to formation of a ferric ion-quinolone complex

Food Interactions Milk, cereals, dietary fiber, tea, coffee, or eggs decrease absorption of iron

Mechanism of Action Iron is released from the plasma and eventually replenishes the depleted iron stores in the bone marrow where it is incorporated into hemoglobin

Pharmacodynamics

Onset of action: Hematologic response to either oral or parenteral iron salts is essentially the same; red blood cell form and color changes within 3-10 days

Peak effect: Peak reticulocytosis occurs in 5-10 days, and hemoglobin values increase within 2-4 weeks

Pharmacokinetics

Absorption: Oral: Iron is absorbed in the duodenum and upper jejunum; in persons with normal iron stores 10% of an oral dose is absorbed, this is increased to 20% to 30% in persons with inadequate iron stores; food and achlorhydria will decrease absorption

Elimination: Iron is largely bound to serum transferrin and excreted in the urine, sweat, sloughing of intestinal mucosa, and by menses

Usual Dosage Note: Multiple salt forms of iron exist; close attention must be paid to the salt form when ordering and administering iron; incorrect selection or substitution of one salt for another without proper dosage adjustment may result in serious over- or underdosing.

Oral (dose expressed in terms of **elemental** iron):

Recommended Daily Allowance, see table

Recommended Daily Allowance of Iron (dosage expressed as elemental iron)

Age	RDA (mg)
<5 mo	5
5 mo to 10 y	10
Male	
11-18 y	12
>18 y	10
Female	
11-50 y	15
>50 y	10

Premature neonates: 2-4 mg elemental iron/kg/day divided every 12-24 hours (maximum dose: 15 mg/day)

(Continued)

Iron Supplements (Oral/Enteral) *(Continued)*

Infants and Children:
Severe iron deficiency anemia: 4-6 mg elemental iron/kg/day in 3 divided doses
Mild to moderate iron deficiency anemia: 3 mg elemental iron/kg/day in 1-2 divided doses
Prophylaxis: 1-2 mg elemental iron/kg/day up to a maximum of 15 mg elemental iron/day

Adults:
Iron deficiency: 2-3 mg/kg/day or 60-100 mg elemental iron twice daily up to 60 mg elemental iron 4 times/day, or 50 mg elemental iron (extended release) 1-2 times/day
Prophylaxis: 60-100 mg elemental iron/day; see table

Elemental Iron Content of Iron Salts

Iron Salt	Elemental Iron Content (% of salt form)	Approximate Equivalent Doses (mg of iron salt)
Ferrous fumarate	33	197
Ferrous gluconate	11.6	560
Ferrous sulfate	20	324
Ferrous sulfate, exsiccated	30	217

Administration Oral: Do not chew or crush sustained release preparations; administer with water or juice between meals for maximum absorption; may administer with food if GI upset occurs; do not administer with milk or milk products

Monitoring Parameters Serum iron, total iron binding capacity, reticulocyte count, hemoglobin, ferritin

Reference Range
Serum iron:
Newborns: 110-270 µg/dL
Infants: 30-70 µg/dL
Children: 55-120 µg/dL
Adults: Male: 75-175 µg/dL; Female: 65-165 µg/dL
Total iron binding capacity:
Newborns: 59-175 µg/dL
Infants: 100-400 µg/dL
Children and Adults: 230-430 µg/dL
Transferrin: 204-360 mg/dL
Percent transferrin saturation: 20% to 50%
Iron levels >300 µg/dL may be considered toxic; should be treated as an overdosage
Ferritin: 13-300 ng/mL

Test Interactions False-positive for blood in stool by the guaiac test

Patient Information May color the stools and urine black; do not take within 2 hours of tetracyclines or fluoroquinolones, do not take with milk or antacids; keep out of reach of children

Additional Information When treating iron deficiency anemias, treat for 3-4 months after hemoglobin/hematocrit return to normal in order to replenish total body stores; elemental iron dosages as high as 15 mg/kg/day have been used to supplement neonates receiving concomitant epoetin alpha in the treatment of anemia of prematurity

Dosage Forms Amount of **elemental** iron is listed in brackets
Ferrous fumarate:
Suspension, oral (Feostat®): 100 mg/5 mL [33 mg/5 mL] (240 mL)
Tablet: 325 mg [106 mg]
Hemocyte®: 324 mg [106 mg]
Ircon®: 200 mg [66 mg]
Nephro-Fer™: 350 mg [115 mg]
Tablet, chewable (chocolate flavor): Feostat®: 100 mg [33 mg]
Tablet, timed release:
Ferro-Sequels®: 150 mg [50 mg] with docusate sodium 100 mg
Ferrous gluconate:
Tablet: 300 mg [34 mg]; 325 mg [38 mg]
Fergon®: 240 mg [27 mg]
Ferrous sulfate:
Capsule, exsiccated, timed release: 159 mg [50 mg]

Drops, oral: (Ed-In-Sol®, Fer-Iron®, Fer-In-Sol®): 75 mg/0.6 mL [15 mg/0.6 mL] (50 mL)

Elixir (Feosol®): 220 mg/5 mL [44 mg/5 mL] with alcohol 5% (473 mL)

Syrup (Fer-In-Sol®): 90 mg/5 mL [18 mg/5 mL] with alcohol 5% (480 mL)

Tablet: 324 mg [65 mg]

Exsiccated (Feosol®) 200 mg [65 mg]

Exsiccated, timed release (Slow FE®): 160 mg [50 mg]

Feratab®: 300 mg [60 mg]

Mol-Iron®: 195 mg [39 mg]

Lysaccharide - iron complex:

Capsule (Ferrex 150®, Hytinic®, Niferex®-150, Nu-Iron®-150): 150 mg

Elixir (Niferex®, Nu-Iron®): 100 mg/5 mL (240 mL)

Tablet (Niferex®): 50 mg

Iron Supplements (Parenteral) (EYE ern SUP la ments)

U.S. Brand Names Dexferrum®; Ferrlecit®; InFed®; Venofer®

Synonyms Iron Dextran; Iron Sucrose

Available Salts Sodium Ferric Gluconate

Therapeutic Category Iron Salt, Parenteral; Mineral, Parenteral

Generic Available Yes (iron dextran only)

Use

Iron dextran: Treatment of microcytic, hypochromic anemia resulting from iron deficiency when oral iron administration is infeasible or ineffective

Ferric gluconate and iron sucrose: Treatment of microcytic, hypochromic anemia in combination with erythropoietin in hemodialysis patients when iron administration is not feasible or ineffective

Pregnancy Risk Factor B (ferric gluconate, iron sucrose); C (iron dextran)

Contraindications Hypersensitivity to the iron formulation or any component; anemias that are not associated with iron deficiency; hemochromatosis; hemolytic anemia; iron overload

Warnings Deaths associated with parenteral iron administration following anaphylactic-type reactions have been reported; treatment agents for anaphylactic reactions (eg, epinephrine, steroids, diphenhydramine) should be immediately available; a test dose is recommended prior to initial therapy; rapid I.V. administration is associated with flushing, fatigue, weakness, chest, back, groin, or flank pain, and hypotension; ferric gluconate formulation contains benzyl alcohol - avoid use in neonates; use only in patients where the iron deficient state is not amenable to oral iron therapy; only iron dextran is approved for I.M. administration

Precautions Use with caution in patients with histories of significant allergies, asthma, hepatic impairment, rheumatoid arthritis

Adverse Reactions Anaphylactoid reactions: Respiratory difficulties and cardiovascular collapse have been reported and occur most frequently within the first several minutes of administration

Cardiovascular: Cardiovascular collapse, hypotension, flushing, chest pain, syncope, tachycardia, MI, hypovolemia

Central nervous system: Dizziness, fever, headache, chills, shivering, malaise, insomnia, agitation, somnolence

Dermatologic: Urticaria, pruritus, rash

Gastrointestinal: Nausea, vomiting, diarrhea, metallic taste, abdominal pain, dyspepsia, flatulence, eructation, melena

Genitourinary: Discoloration of urine

Hematologic: Leukocytosis

Hepatic: Elevated liver enzymes

Local: Pain, staining of skin at the site of I.M. injection, phlebitis

Neuromuscular & skeletal: Arthralgia, arthritic reactivation in patients with quiescent arthritis, backache, paresthesia, leg cramps, weakness

Ocular: Blurred vision, conjunctivitis

Renal: Hematuria

Respiratory: Dyspnea, cough, rhinitis, upper respiratory infection, pulmonary edema, pneumonia

Miscellaneous: Lymphadenopathy, diaphoresis

Note: Sweating, urticaria, arthralgia, fever, chills, dizziness, headache, and nausea may be delayed 24-48 hours after I.V. administration or 3-4 days after I.M. administration

Stability Store at room temperature; use immediately after dilution in NS; product literature states parenteral iron formulations should not be mixed with other medications or in parenteral nutrition solutions

(Continued)

Iron Supplements (Parenteral) *(Continued)*

Mechanism of Action Replaces iron found in hemoglobin, myoglobin, and specific enzymes; allows transportation of oxygen via hemoglobin

Pharmacodynamics

Onset of action: Hematologic response to either oral or parenteral iron salts is essentially the same; red blood cell form and color changes within 3-10 days

Peak effect: Peak reticulocytosis occurs in 5-10 days, and hemoglobin values increase within 2-4 weeks

Pharmacokinetics

Absorption: I.M.: 60% absorbed after 3 days; 90% after 1-3 weeks, the balance is slowly absorbed over months

Following I.V. doses, the uptake of iron by the reticuloendothelial system appears to be constant at about 10-20 mg/hour

Elimination: By the reticuloendothelial system and excreted in urine and feces (via bile)

Not dialyzable

Usual Dosage Multiple forms for parenteral iron exist; close attention must be paid to the specific product when ordering and administering; test doses are recommended before starting therapy

Ferric gluconate: Adults: I.V.: **Dosage expressed in mg elemental iron:** Test dose: 25 mg (2 mL); repletion dose: 125 mg (10 mL) during hemodialysis; most patients will require a cumulative dose of 1 g over ~8 sequential dialysis treatments to achieve a favorable response

Iron dextran:

I.M., I.V.: Test dose (given 1 hour prior to starting iron dextran therapy):

Infants: 12.5 mg (0.25 mL)

Children, Adolescents, and Adults: 25 mg (0.5 mL)

Total replacement dosage of iron dextran for iron deficiency anemia:

$(mL) = 0.0476 \times LBW\ (kg) \times (Hb_n - Hb_o) + 1\ mL/per\ 5\ kg\ LBW$ (up to maximum of 14 mL)

LBW = lean body weight

Hb_n = desired hemoglobin (g/dL) = 12 if <15 kg or 14.8 if >15 kg

Hb_o = measured hemoglobin (g/dL)

Total iron replacement dosage for acute blood loss: Assumes 1 mL of normocytic, normochromic red cells = 1 mg elemental iron: Iron dextran (mL) = 0.02 x blood loss (mL) x hematocrit (expressed as a decimal fraction)

Note: Total dose infusions have been used safely and are the preferred method of administration

I.M.: Maximum daily dose: Injected in daily or less frequent increments:

Infants <5 kg: 25 mg

Children 5-10 kg: 50 mg

Children >10 kg and Adults: 100 mg

Iron sucrose: Adults: I.V. **(doses expressed in mg of elemental iron):**

Test dose: 50 mg (while product labeling does not indicate need for a test dose in product-naive patients, test doses were administered in some clinical trials); 100 mg (5 mL) administered 1-3 times/week during dialysis, for a total dose of 1000 mg (10 doses); administer no more than 3 times/week; may continue to administer at lowest dose necessary to maintain target hemoglobin, hematocrit, and iron storage parameters

Administration Parenteral: Avoid dilution in dextrose due to an increased incidence of local pain and phlebitis

Iron dextran:

I.M.: Use Z-track technique for I.M. administration (deep into the upper outer quadrant of buttock)

I.V.: Infuse test dose over at least 5 minutes; dilute replacement dose in NS (50-100 mL), maximum concentration 50 mg/mL and infuse over 1-6 hours at a maximum rate of 50 mg/minute

Ferric gluconate: Dilute test dose in 50 mL NS and infuse over 1 hour; dilute repletion dose (125 mg) in 100 mL NS and infuse over at least 1 hour; do not exceed 2.1 mg/minute; **not for I.M. administration**

Iron sucrose:

Slow I.V. injection: 1 mL (20 mg iron) of undiluted solution per minute (5 minutes/vial)

Infusion: Dilute 1 vial (5 mL) in maximum of 100 mL 0.9% NaCl; infuse over at least 15 minutes; **not for I.M. administration**

Monitoring Parameters Reticulocyte count, serum ferritin, hemoglobin, serum iron concentrations, and TIBC may not be meaningful for 3 weeks after administration, especially after large I.V. doses

Reference Range

Serum iron:
Newborns: 110-270 µg/dL
Infants: 30-70 µg/dL
Children: 55-120 µg/dL
Adults: Male: 75-175 µg/dL; female: 65-165 µg/dL

Total iron binding capacity:
Newborns: 59-175 µg/dL
Infants: 100-400 µg/dL
Children and Adults: 230-430 µg/dL

Transferrin: 204-360 mg/dL

Percent transferrin saturation: 20% to 50%

Iron levels >300 µg/dL may be considered toxic; should be treated as an overdosage

Ferritin: 13-300 ng/mL

Test Interactions May cause falsely elevated values of serum bilirubin and falsely decreased values of serum calcium

Nursing Implications Only iron dextran is approved for I.M. administration

Additional Information Iron storage may lag behind the appearance of normal red blood cell morphology; use periodic hematologic determination to assess therapy; VLBW infants receiving I.V. iron sucrose 2 mg/kg/day with erythropoietin showed improved erythropoiesis when compared with oral iron supplementation and erythropoietin (Pollak, et al)

Dosage Forms Expressed as mg of **elemental iron:**

Ferric gluconate injection: 12.5 mg/mL (5 mL) [with 9 mg benzyl alcohol/mL]
Iron dextran injection: 50 mg/mL (1 mL, 2 mL)
Iron sucrose injection: 20 mg/mL (5 mL)

References

Auerbach M, Witt D, Toler W, et al, "Clinical Use of the Total Dose Intravenous Infusion of Iron Dextran," *J Lab Clin Med*, 1988, 111(5):566-70.

Benito RP and Guerrero TC, "Response to a Single Intravenous Dose Versus Multiple Intramuscular Administration of Iron-Dextran Complex: A Comparative Study," *Curr Ther Res Clin Exp*, 1973, 15(7):373-82.

Pollak A, Hayde M, Hayn M, et al, "Effect of Intravenous Iron Supplementation on Erythropoiesis in Erythropoietin-Treated Premature Infants," *Pediatrics*, 2001, 107(1):78-85.

♦ **Isoamyl Nitrite** *see* Amyl Nitrite *on page 94*

Isoetharine (eye soe ETH a reen)

Related Information
Asthma Guidelines *on page 1210*

Therapeutic Category Adrenergic Agonist Agent; Antiasthmatic; Bronchodilator; Sympathomimetic

Generic Available Yes

Use Bronchodilator used in asthma and for the reversible bronchospasm occurring with bronchitis and emphysema

Pregnancy Risk Factor C

Contraindications Hypersensitivity to isoetharine, any component, or other sympathomimetics

Warnings Isoetharine hydrochloride solution contains sulfites which may cause allergic reactions in some patients

Precautions Excessive, prolonged use may lead to decreased effectiveness; use with caution in patients with hyperthyroidism, hypertension, acute coronary artery disease, cerebral arteriosclerosis

Adverse Reactions

Cardiovascular: Tachycardia, hypertension, palpitations

Central nervous system: Anxiety, dizziness, restlessness, excitement, headache, nervousness, insomnia, lightheadedness

Gastrointestinal: Nausea, vomiting, xerostomia

Neuromuscular & skeletal: Tremor, weakness

Drug Interactions Additive effects when used in combination with other sympathomimetics; decreased effect with beta-blocking agents

Mechanism of Action Relaxes bronchial smooth muscle and peripheral vasculature by action on beta$_2$-receptors with little effect on heart rate

Pharmacodynamics

Peak effect: Following oral inhalation: Within 5-15 minutes

Duration: 1-4 hours

(Continued)

Isoetharine *(Continued)*

Pharmacokinetics
Metabolism: In many tissues including the liver and lungs

Elimination: Renal, primarily (90%) as metabolites

Usual Dosage Treatments are usually not repeated more often than every 4 hours, except in severe cases

Nebulizer:
Children: 0.01 mL/kg (0.1 mg/kg) of 1% solution; minimum dose 0.1 mL (1 mg); maximum dose: 0.5 mL (5 mg)

Adults: 0.5-1 mL (2.5-5 mg) of a 0.5% solution or equivalent dosages using 0.125%, 0.2%, 0.25%, or 1% solutions

Inhalation: Adults: 1-2 inhalations every 4 hours as needed

Administration
Nebulization: Dilute dosage of 0.5% or 1% solutions in 2-3 mL NS; 0.125%, 0.2%, and 0.25% solutions may be administered without dilution

Oral inhalation: Shake well before use; use spacer device in children <8 years of age

Monitoring Parameters Heart rate, blood pressure, respiratory rate

Dosage Forms Solution, inhalation, as hydrochloride: 1% (10 mL, 30 mL)

References
Rachelefsky GS and Siegel SC, "Asthma in Infants and Children - Treatment of Childhood Asthma: Part 11," *J Allergy Clin Immunol*, 1985, 76(3):409-25.

Isoniazid *(eye soe NYE a zid)*

Related Information
Overdose and Toxicology *on page 1222*

U.S. Brand Names Laniazid® Oral; Nydrazid® Injection

Canadian Brand Names Isotamine; PMS-Isoniazid

Synonyms INH; Isonicotinic Acid Hydrazide

Therapeutic Category Antitubercular Agent

Generic Available Yes

Use Treatment of susceptible mycobacterial infection due to *M. tuberculosis* and prophylactically to those individuals exposed to tuberculosis

Pregnancy Risk Factor C

Contraindications Acute liver disease; hypersensitivity to isoniazid or any component; previous history of hepatic damage during isoniazid therapy

Warnings Severe and sometimes fatal hepatitis may occur or develop even after many months of treatment; the administration of isoniazid in combination with rifampin is associated with an increased incidence of hepatotoxicity if isoniazid dose is >10 mg/kg/day; patients must report any prodromal symptoms of hepatitis such as fatigue, weakness, malaise, anorexia, nausea, vomiting, dark urine, or yellowing of eyes

Precautions Use with caution in patients with renal impairment and chronic liver disease

Adverse Reactions
Central nervous system: Seizure, stupor, dizziness, agitation, euphoria, psychosis, fever, ataxia

Dermatologic: Skin eruptions, rash, acne

Endocrine & metabolic: Hyperglycemia, metabolic acidosis, pellagra

Gastrointestinal: Nausea, vomiting, epigastric distress; diarrhea (associated with administration of syrup formulation)

Hematologic: Agranulocytosis, hemolytic anemia, aplastic anemia, thrombocytopenia, eosinophilia, leukopenia

Hepatic: Hepatitis, 3% to 10% of children experience transient elevated liver transaminase levels

Local: Irritation at I.M. injection site

Neuromuscular & skeletal: Peripheral neuropathy

Ocular: Optic neuritis

Otic: Tinnitus

Miscellaneous: Hypersensitivity reaction

Drug Interactions Cytochrome P-450 isoenzyme CYP2E1 substrate; isoenzyme CYP2E1 inducer; isoenzyme CYP1A2, CYP2C, CYP2C9, CYP2C19, and CYP3A3/4 inhibitor

May increase serum concentrations of phenytoin, carbamazepine, diazepam; aluminum salts may decrease isoniazid absorption; prednisolone may increase isoniazid metabolism; cycloserine, ethionamide (additive CNS toxicity); disulfiram (coordination difficulty, psychotic episode); meperidine (serotonin syndrome); rifampin (increased hepatotoxicity)

Food Interactions Rate and extent of isoniazid absorption may be reduced when administered with food; avoid foods with histamine or tyramine (cheese, broad beans, dry sausage, salami, nonfresh meat, liver pate, soya bean, liquid and powdered protein supplements, wine); increase dietary intake of folate, niacin, magnesium, and pyridoxine; the American Academy of Pediatrics recommends that pyridoxine supplementation (1-2 mg/kg/day) should be administered to patients with nutritional deficiencies including all symptomatic HIV-infected children, children or adolescents on meat or milk-deficient diets, breast-feeding infants and their mothers, pregnant adolescents and women, and those predisposed to neuritis to prevent peripheral neuropathy

Stability Protect from light and excessive heat; avoid freezing

Mechanism of Action Inhibits mycolic acid synthesis resulting in disruption of the bacterial cell wall

Pharmacokinetics

Absorption: Oral, I.M.: Rapid and complete

Distribution: Crosses the placenta; appears in breast milk; distributes into most body tissues and fluids including the CSF

Protein binding: 10% to 15%

Metabolism: By the liver to acetylisoniazid with decay rate determined genetically by acetylation phenotype; undergoes further hydrolysis to isonicotinic acid and acetylhydrazine

Half-life: May be prolonged in patients with impaired hepatic function or severe renal impairment

Fast acetylators: 30-100 minutes

Slow acetylators: 2-5 hours

Time to peak serum concentration: Oral: Within 1-2 hours

Elimination: 75% to 95% excreted in urine as unchanged drug and metabolites; small amounts excreted in feces and saliva

Dialysis: Dialyzable (50% to 100%)

Usual Dosage Oral, I.M.:

Infants and Children:

Treatment: 10-15 mg/kg/day in 1-2 divided doses; maximum dose: 300 mg/day

Prophylaxis: 10 mg/kg/day given once daily, not to exceed 300 mg/day

Adults:

Treatment: 5 mg/kg/day given daily (usual dose: 300 mg)

Disseminated disease: 10 mg/kg/day in 1-2 divided doses

Prophylaxis: 300 mg/day given daily

American Thoracic Society and CDC currently recommend twice weekly therapy as part of a short-course regimen which follows 1-2 months of daily treatment for uncomplicated pulmonary tuberculosis in **compliant** patients

Children: 20-30 mg/kg/dose (up to 900 mg/dose) twice weekly

Adults: 15 mg/kg/dose (up to 900 mg/dose) twice weekly

Duration of therapy:

Asymptomatic infection (positive skin test):

Isoniazid susceptible: 9 months of isoniazid

Isoniazid resistant: 9 months of rifampin

Pulmonary, hilar adenopathy, and extrapulmonary infection other than meningitis, bone/joint, or disseminated infection:

6 months which includes 2-month therapy of isoniazid, rifampin, and pyrazinamide daily followed by 4 months of isoniazid and rifampin daily **or** 2 months of isoniazid, rifampin, and pyrazinamide daily, followed by 4 months of isoniazid and rifampin twice weekly under direct observation

alternatively

9 months of isoniazid and rifampin daily **or** 1 month of isoniazid and rifampin daily followed by 8 months of isoniazid and rifampin twice weekly under direct observation; if isoniazid resistance is identified, rifampin and ethambutol should be continued for a maximum of 12 months

Note: If drug resistance is possible, ethambutol or streptomycin should be added to the initial therapy regimen until susceptibility is determined

Meningitis, bone/joint, and disseminated infection:

12 months which includes 2 months of isoniazid, rifampin, pyrazinamide, and streptomycin daily followed by 10 months of isoniazid and rifampin daily **or** 2 months of isoniazid, rifampin, pyrazinamide, and streptomycin daily followed by 10 months of isoniazid and rifampin twice weekly under direct observation

Administration

Oral: Administer 1 hour before or 2 hours after meals with water; administration of isoniazid syrup has been associated with diarrhea

(Continued)

Isoniazid *(Continued)*

Parenteral: I.M.: Administer I.M. when oral therapy is not possible

Monitoring Parameters Periodic liver function tests; monitoring for prodromal signs of hepatitis; ophthalmologic exam; chest x-ray

Test Interactions False-positive urinary glucose with Clinitest®

Patient Information Report any prodromal symptoms of hepatitis (fatigue, weakness, nausea, vomiting, dark urine, or yellowing of eyes) or any burning, tingling, or numbness in the extremities; avoid alcohol

Dosage Forms

Injection: 100 mg/mL (10 mL)

Syrup: 50 mg/5 mL [orange flavor] (473 mL)

Tablet: 50 mg, 100 mg, 300 mg

References

Ad Hoc Committee of the Scientific Assembly on Microbiology, Tuberculosis, and Pulmonary Infections, "Treatment of Tuberculosis and Tuberculosis Infection in Adults and Children," *Clin Infect Dis*, 1995, 21:9-27.

American Academy of Pediatrics, Committee on Infectious Diseases, "Chemotherapy for Tuberculosis in Infants and Children," *Pediatrics*, 1992, 89(1):161-5.

Starke JR, "Modern Approach to the Diagnosis and Treatment of Tuberculosis in Children," *Pediatr Clin North Am*, 1988, 35(3):441-64.

Starke JR, "Multidrug Therapy for Tuberculosis in Children," *Pediatr Infect Dis J*, 1990, 9(11):785-93.

Van Scoy RE and Wilkowske CJ, "Antituberculous Agents: Isoniazid, Rifampin, Streptomycin, Ethambutol, and Pyrazinamide," *Mayo Clin Proc*, 1983, 58(4):233-40.

♦ **Isonicotinic Acid Hydrazide** *see* Isoniazid *on page 554*

♦ **Isonipecaine** *see* Meperidine *on page 628*

♦ **Isoprenaline** *see* Isoproterenol *on page 556*

Isoproterenol *(eye soe proe TER e nole)*

Related Information

Adult ACLS Algorithm, Stable Ventricular Tachycardia *on page 1047*

Asthma Guidelines *on page 1210*

Emergency Pediatric Drip Calculations *on page 1033*

U.S. Brand Names Isuprel®

Synonyms Isoprenaline

Therapeutic Category Adrenergic Agonist Agent; Antiasthmatic; Beta$_1$ & Beta$_2$-Adrenergic Agonist Agent; Bronchodilator; Sympathomimetic

Generic Available Yes

Use Asthma or COPD (reversible airway obstruction); ventricular arrhythmias due to A-V nodal block; hemodynamically compromised bradyarrhythmias or atropine-resistant bradyarrhythmias, temporary use in third degree A-V block until pacemaker insertion; low cardiac output or vasoconstrictive shock states

Pregnancy Risk Factor C

Contraindications Angina, pre-existing cardiac arrhythmias (ventricular); tachycardia or A-V block caused by cardiac glycoside intoxication; allergy to sulfites or isoproterenol or other sympathomimetic amines; narrow-angle glaucoma

Warnings Tolerance may occur with prolonged use; when discontinuing an isoproterenol continuous infusion used for bronchodilation, the infusion **must** be gradually tapered over a 24- to 48-hour period to prevent rebound bronchospasm

Precautions Use with caution in diabetics, renal or cardiovascular disease, hyperthyroidism, prostatic hypertrophy

Adverse Reactions

Cardiovascular: Flushing of the face or skin, ventricular arrhythmias, tachycardia, hypotension, chest pain, palpitations, hypertension

Central nervous system: Nervousness, restlessness, anxiety, dizziness, headache, vertigo, insomnia

Endocrine & metabolic: Parotid glands swelling

Gastrointestinal: Heartburn, GI distress, nausea, vomiting, dry throat, pinkish-red saliva (after inhalation), xerostomia

Neuromuscular & skeletal: Tremor, weakness, trembling

Respiratory: Cough, dyspnea, bronchitis (after inhalation therapy)

Miscellaneous: Diaphoresis

Drug Interactions Additive effects and increased cardiotoxicity when administered concomitantly with other sympathomimetic amines; beta-adrenergic blocking agents may decrease effectiveness due to beta blockade; may increase theophylline elimination

Mechanism of Action Stimulates beta$_1$- and beta$_2$-receptors resulting in relaxation of bronchial, GI, and uterine smooth muscle; increased heart rate and contractility; vasodilation of peripheral vasculature

Pharmacodynamics

Onset of action:
    Oral inhalation: 2-5 minutes
    I.V.: Immediately
    S.L.: ~30 minutes

Duration:
    Oral inhalation: 30 minutes to 2 hours
    I.V. (single dose): Few minutes
    S.L. or S.C.: Up to 2 hours

Pharmacokinetics

Metabolism: By conjugation in many tissues including the liver and lungs

Half-life: 2.5-5 minutes

Elimination: In urine principally as sulfate conjugates

Usual Dosage

Neonates, Infants, and Children: I.V. infusion: 0.05-2 mcg/kg/minute; rate (mL/hour) = dose (mcg/kg/minute) x weight (kg) x 60 minutes/hour divided by concentration (mcg/mL)

Children:
    Oral inhalation: 1-2 metered doses up to 6 times/day
    Nebulization: 0.01 mL/kg (0.1 mg/kg) of 1% solution; minimum dose: 0.1 mL (1 mg); maximum dose: 0.5 mL (5 mg); or equivalent doses using 0.25% and 0.5% solutions
    S.L.: 5-10 mg every 3-4 hours (maximum dose: 30 mg/day)

Adults:
    Oral inhalation: 1-2 metered doses 4-6 times/day
    Nebulization: 0.25-0.5 mL (2.5-5 mg) of a 1% solution or equivalent doses using 0.25% or 0.5% solutions
    S.L.: 10-20 mg every 3-4 hours (maximum dose: 60 mg/day)
    I.V. infusion: 2-20 mcg/minute

Administration

Nebulization: Dilute dosage from 1% solution in 2-3 mL NS; other solutions at concentrations <1% may be administered without dilution

Oral: Do not swallow sublingual tablets, allow to dissolve under the tongue

Oral inhalation: Shake well before use; use spacer device in children <8 years of age

Parenteral: May be administered undiluted by direct I.V. injection; for continuous infusions, dilute in dextrose or NS to a maximum concentration of 20 mcg/mL; concentrations as high as 64 mcg/mL have been used safely and with efficacy in situations of extreme fluid restriction

Monitoring Parameters Heart rate, blood pressure, respiratory rate, arterial blood gases, central venous pressure, EKG

Patient Information After inhalation therapy, may cause saliva to turn pinkish-red; do not exceed recommended dosage; wait at least 3-5 minutes between metered dose inhalations (if more than 1 inhalation per dose)

Additional Information Hypotension is more common in hypovolemic patients

Dosage Forms Injection, as hydrochloride: 0.02% [0.2 mg/mL = 1:5000] (1 mL, 5 mL, 10 mL)

References

Rachelefsky GS and Siegel SC, "Asthma in Infants and Children - Treatment of Childhood Asthma: Part 1I," *J Allergy Clin Immunol*, 1985, 76(3):409-25.

♦ **Isoptin®** *see* Verapamil *on page 1007*

♦ **Isoptin® SR** *see* Verapamil *on page 1007*

♦ **Isopto® Atropine** *see* Atropine *on page 116*

♦ **Isopto® Carpine** *see* Pilocarpine *on page 800*

♦ **Isopto® Homatropine** *see* Homatropine *on page 497*

♦ **Isopto® Hyoscine** *see* Scopolamine *on page 892*

♦ **Isotamine (Can)** *see* Isoniazid *on page 554*

Isotretinoin (eye soe TRET i noyn)

U.S. Brand Names Accutane®

Canadian Brand Names Isotrex

Synonyms 13-*cis*-Retinoic Acid

Therapeutic Category Acne Products; Retinoic Acid Derivative; Vitamin A Derivative

Generic Available No

(Continued)

Isotretinoin *(Continued)*

Use Treatment of severe recalcitrant cystic and/or conglobate acne unresponsive to conventional therapy; used investigationally for the treatment of children with high-risk neuroblastoma that does not respond to conventional therapy

Pregnancy Risk Factor X

Contraindications Hypersensitivity to isotretinoin, parabens, vitamin A or other retinoids; patients who are pregnant or intend to become pregnant during treatment; nursing mothers

Warnings Major human fetal abnormalities to isotretinoin administration have been documented; during pregnancy, it can cause fetal defects in the CNS (cerebral abnormalities, hydrocephalus, microcephaly, cranial nerve deficit, cerebellar malformation), skull, ear, eye, and cardiovascular systems, cleft palate, and parathyroid hormone deficiency; not to be used in women of childbearing potential unless woman is capable of complying with effective contraceptive measures. Prescription for isotretinoin should not be issued until a female patient has had negative results from 2 urine or serum pregnancy tests, one performed in the prescriber's office when the patient is qualified for therapy, the second one performed on the second day of next normal menstrual period or 11 days after the last unprotected act of sexual intercourse, whichever is later; prescriber should prescribe no more than a 1-month supply of drug and no automatic refills; effective contraception must be used for at least 1 month before beginning therapy, during therapy, and for 1 month after discontinuation of therapy. Isotretinoin may cause depression, psychosis, and suicidal ideations; concomitant use with tetracyclines has been associated with cases of pseudotumor cerebri; avoid concomitant treatment with tetracyclines

Precautions Use with caution in patients with diabetes mellitus or hypertriglyceridemia

Adverse Reactions

Cardiovascular: Palpitations, tachycardia, vascular thrombotic stroke, edema, vasculitis

Central nervous system: Fatigue, headache, dizziness, pseudotumor cerebri, psychosis, mental depression, suicidal ideation, seizures, insomnia

Dermatologic: Pruritus, alopecia, cheilitis, photosensitivity, rash

Endocrine & metabolic: Hypertriglyceridemia, hyperuricemia, hyperglycemia, hypercalcemia

Gastrointestinal: Xerostomia, anorexia, nausea, vomiting, inflammatory bowel syndrome, acute pancreatitis

Hematologic: Increase in erythrocyte sedimentation rate, decrease in hemoglobin and hematocrit, neutropenia

Hepatic: Hepatitis; elevated AST, ALT, and alkaline phosphatase

Neuromuscular & skeletal: Bone pain, arthralgia, myalgia, skeletal hyperostosis, premature epiphyseal closure

Ocular: Conjunctivitis, corneal opacities, cataracts, blurred vision

Renal: Hematuria, proteinuria

Respiratory: Epistaxis, bronchospasm

Miscellaneous: Hypersensitivity reactions

Drug Interactions Increased clearance of carbamazepine; vitamin A supplements increase toxic effects; alcohol may potentiate an increase in serum triglycerides; concomitant use with tetracyclines has been associated with cases of pseudotumor cerebri

Food Interactions Food or milk increases isotretinoin bioavailability

Stability Protect from light

Mechanism of Action Reduces sebaceous gland size and reduces sebum production; regulates cell proliferation and differentiation

Pharmacokinetics

Absorption: Oral: Demonstrates biphasic absorption

Distribution: Crosses the placenta; appears in breast milk, bile

Protein binding: 99% to 100%

Metabolism: In the liver; major metabolite: 4-oxo-isotretinoin (active); undergoes enterohepatic circulation

Half-life, terminal: 10-20 hours for isotretinoin, and 17-50 hours for its metabolite

Time to peak serum concentration: Within 3 hours

Elimination: Excreted in feces as unchanged drug and in urine as metabolites

Usual Dosage Oral:

Children: Maintenance therapy for neuroblastoma: 160 mg/m^2/day in 2 divided doses for 14 consecutive days in a 28-day cycle has been used investigationally

Children and Adults: Acne: 0.5-2 mg/kg/day in 2 divided doses (dosages as low as 0.05 mg/kg/day have been reported to be beneficial) for 15-20 weeks or until the total cyst count decreases by 70%, whichever is sooner

Administration Oral: Capsules can be swallowed or chewed and swallowed; the capsule may be opened with a large needle and the contents placed on apple sauce or ice cream for patients unable to swallow the capsule; administer with meals

Monitoring Parameters CBC with differential, platelet count, baseline ESR, serum triglyceride, liver enzymes, ophthalmologic exam, blood glucose, pregnancy test in female patients of childbearing potential

Patient Information Do not take vitamin supplements containing vitamin A; use caution when driving at night since decreased night vision can develop suddenly; patients who wear contact lenses may experience decreased tolerance to the lenses; avoid alcohol; avoid exposure to direct sunlight; notify physician of any abdominal pain, rectal bleeding, or severe diarrhea; female patients of childbearing potential must be counseled to use 2 effective forms of contraception simultaneously, unless absolute abstinence is the chosen method; provide female patients instruction to join the Accutane® survey and watch a videotape that provides information about contraceptive methods; inform patients not to donate blood during therapy and for 1 month following discontinuation of therapy

Dosage Forms Capsule: 10 mg, 20 mg, 40 mg

References

American Academy of Pediatrics Committee on Drugs, "Retinoid Therapy for Severe Dermatological Disorders," *Pediatrics*, 1992, 90(1 Pt 1):119-20.

DiGiovanna JJ and Peck GL, "Oral Synthetic Retinoid Treatment in Children," *Pediatr Dermatol*, 1983, 1(1):77-88.

Matthay KK, Villablanca JG, Seeger RC, et al, "Treatment of High-Risk Neuroblastoma With Intensive Chemotherapy, Radiotherapy, Autologous Bone Marrow Transplantation, and 13-cis-Retinoic Acid. Children's Cancer Group," *N Engl J Med*, 1999, 341:1165-73.

Reynolds CP, Kane DJ, Einhorn PA, et al, "Response of Neuroblastoma to Retinoic Acid *In Vitro*, and *In Vivo*," *Prog Clin Biol Res*, 1991, 366:203-11

♦ **Isotrex (Can)** see Isotretinoin *on page 557*

♦ **Isoxazolyl Penicillin** see Oxacillin *on page 740*

♦ **I-Sulfacet®** see Sulfacetamide *on page 922*

♦ **Isuprel®** see Isoproterenol *on page 556*

Itraconazole (i tra KOE na zole)

U.S. Brand Names Sporanox®

Therapeutic Category Antifungal Agent, Systemic

Generic Available No

Use Treatment of susceptible systemic fungal infections in immunocompromised and nonimmunocompromised patients including blastomycosis, coccidioidomycosis, paracoccidioidomycosis, histoplasmosis, and aspergillosis in patients who do not respond to or cannot tolerate amphotericin B; treatment of oropharyngeal or esophageal candidiasis (oral solution only)

Pregnancy Risk Factor C

Contraindications Hypersensitivity to itraconazole or any component; concomitant administration with terfenadine, astemizole, cisapride, alprazolam, triazolam, or HMG-CoA reductase inhibitors metabolized by CYP3A4 isoenzyme (ie, lovastatin, simvastatin)

Warnings Itraconazole has induced bone defects (decreased bone plate activity, thinning of the zona compacta of large bones, increased bone fragility) and change in tooth appearance in rats; severe cardiovascular effects including QT interval prolongation, ventricular tachycardia, ventricular fibrillation, cardiac arrest, palpitations, syncope, and death have occurred in patients receiving itraconazole concomitantly with terfenadine, astemizole, or cisapride; do not use concurrently with terfenadine, astemizole, cisapride, alprazolam, triazolam, lovastatin, or simvastatin; **itraconazole solution and capsules should not be used interchangeably**

Precautions Use with caution in patients with hypersensitivity to other azole antifungal agents and in patients with hepatic impairment; discontinue if signs and symptoms of liver disease develop

Adverse Reactions

Cardiovascular: Hypertension, ventricular fibrillation, edema

Central nervous system: Headache, dizziness, somnolence, fever, fatigue

Dermatologic: Rash, pruritus, urticaria, angioedema, toxic epidermal necrolysis

Endocrine & metabolic: Hypokalemia, adrenal insufficiency, gynecomastia

Gastrointestinal: Nausea, vomiting, diarrhea, abdominal pain, anorexia

Hematologic: Thrombocytopenia, leukopenia

Hepatic: Elevated liver enzymes, hepatitis

Otic: Tinnitus

Renal: Albuminuria

Drug Interactions Cytochrome P-450 isoenzyme CYP3A3/4 substrate; isoenzyme CYP3A3/4 inhibitor

(Continued)

Itraconazole *(Continued)*

Decreased effect of itraconazole with rifampin, rifabutin, carbamazepine, isoniazid, phenytoin, and phenobarbital (increases itraconazole's metabolism); H₂ antagonists, omeprazole, antacids, didanosine (decreases absorption)

Increased effect of cyclosporine, tacrolimus (interferes with clearance); digoxin, warfarin, amlodipine, buspirone, corticosteroids, protease inhibitors (ie, indinavir), and hypoglycemic agents (decreased metabolism)

Increased toxicity of terfenadine, astemizole, alprazolam, triazolam, oral midazolam, cisapride, lovastatin, simvastatin, vinca alkaloids; see Warnings

Food Interactions Grapefruit juice decreases itraconazole AUC by 30%; avoid drinking grapefruit juice while taking oral itraconazole; absorption of capsule and oral solution are increased when taken with a cola beverage

Capsule: Food increases bioavailability

Solution: 31% increase in AUC if taken without food

Stability Store at room temperature; protect from light. Avoid freezing. Following dilution of itraconazole injection in NS, the solution is stable for up to 48 hours when refrigerated and protected from light.

Mechanism of Action Inhibits ergosterol synthesis in fungal cell membranes by inhibiting fungal cytochrome P-450

Pharmacokinetics

Absorption:

Capsule: Rapid and complete when capsule is given immediately after a meal (bioavailability: 100%); decreased absorption reported when administered via nasogastric tube

Oral solution: Solution better absorbed on empty stomach

Distribution: High affinity for tissues (liver, lung, kidney, adipose tissue, brain, vagina, dermis, epidermis); poor penetration into CSF, eye fluid, saliva; distributes into breast milk, bronchial exudate, and sputum

Protein binding: 99%

Metabolism: Saturable hepatic metabolism to active and inactive metabolites

Bioavailability: Capsules:

Fasted state: 40%

Fed state: Dose administered immediately after a meal: 100%

Half-life: 17-30 hours

Elimination: Metabolites are excreted in urine (35%) and bile (55%)

Dialysis: Nondialyzable

Usual Dosage

Oral:

Children: Efficacy of itraconazole has not been established; a limited number of children have been treated with itraconazole using doses of 3-5 mg/kg/day once daily; doses as high as 5-10 mg/kg/day divided every 12-24 hours have been used in 32 patients with chronic granulomatous disease for prophylaxis against *Aspergillus* infection; doses of 6-8 mg/kg/day have been used in the treatment of disseminated histoplasmosis

Prophylaxis for first episode of *Cryptococcus neoformans* or *Histoplasma capsulatum* in HIV-infected infants and children: 2-5 mg/kg/dose every 12-24 hours

Prophylaxis for recurrence of opportunistic disease in HIV-infected infants and children:

Cryptococcus neoformans: 2-5 mg/kg/dose every 12-24 hours

Histoplasma capsulatum: 2-5 mg/kg/dose every 12-48 hours

Adults:

Blastomycosis and nonmeningeal histoplasmosis: Initial: 200 mg once daily; if poor response, increase dose in 100 mg increments to a maximum of 400 mg/day in 2 divided doses

Life-threatening infection and aspergillosis: Initial loading dose can be administered as follows: 600 mg/day in 3 divided doses for the first 3-4 days; maintenance: 200-400 mg/day in 2 divided doses; maximum dose: 600 mg/day in 3 divided doses

Esophageal candidiasis: Vigorously swish 10 mL in the mouth for several seconds and then swallow daily; maximum dose: 200 mg/day

Oropharyngeal candidiasis: Vigorously swish 10 mL in the mouth for several seconds at a time once daily (20 mL total daily dose), or 10 mL twice daily in patients refractory to oral fluconazole

I.V.: Adults: Blastomycosis, aspergillosis, or histoplasmosis: 200 mg twice daily for 4 doses then decrease dose to 200 mg once daily. Safety and efficacy of I.V. itraconazole administered for longer than 14 days has not been established; therapy should be completed using oral itraconazole

Administration

Oral: Avoid grapefruit juice

    Capsules: Administer with food

    Solution: Administer on an empty stomach

Parenteral I.V. infusion: Dilute entire contents of an ampul (250 mg) in 50 mL of NS diluent provided by the manufacturer to provide a solution with a final concentration of 3.33 mg/mL. Calculate itraconazole dosage volume needed and infuse over 60 minutes using the infusion set provided by the manufacturer and a dedicated I.V. line. Do not mix with other drugs. After completion of infusion, flush infusion set with 15-20 mL NS over 5-15 minutes, then discard the entire I.V. line.

Monitoring Parameters Periodic liver function tests, serum potassium; monitor for prodromal signs of hepatitis

Reference Range Therapeutic blood level: >250 ng/mL

Patient Information Report any prodromal symptoms of hepatitis (fatigue, weakness, nausea, vomiting, dark urine, or yellowing of eyes); avoid grapefruit juice

Nursing Implications Do not administer with antacids or H_2 antagonists

Dosage Forms

Capsule: 100 mg

Injection, kit: 10 mg/mL (25 mL)

Solution, oral: 100 mg/10 mL (150 mL)

References

Cowie F, Meller ST, Cushing P, et al, "Chemoprophylaxis for Pulmonary Aspergillosis During Intensive Chemotherapy," *Arch Dis Child*, 1994, 70(2):136-8.

Mouy R, Veber F, Blanche S, et al, "Long-Term Itraconazole Prophylaxis Against *Aspergillus* Infections in Thirty-Two Patients With Chronic Granulomatous Disease," *J Pediatr*, 1994, 125(6 Pt 1):998-1003.

Tobon AM, Franco L, Espinal D, et al, "Disseminated Histoplasmosis in Children: The Role of Itraconazole Therapy," *Pediatr Infect Dis J*, 1996; 15:1002-8.

"1999 USPHS/IDSA Guidelines for the Prevention of Opportunistic Infections in Persons Infected With Human Immunodeficiency Virus. USPHS/IDSA Prevention of Opportunistic Infections Working Group," *MMWR Morb Mortal Wkly Rep*, 1999, 48 (RR-10):1-66.

Kaolin and Pectin (KAY oh lin & PEK tin)

Related Information

Carbohydrate and Alcohol Content of Liquid Medications for Use in Patients Receiving Ketogenic Diets *on page 1258*

U.S. Brand Names Kaodene® NN [OTC]; Kao-Spen® [OTC]; Kapectolin® [OTC]

Synonyms Pectin and Kaolin

Therapeutic Category Antidiarrheal

Generic Available Yes

Use Treatment of uncomplicated diarrhea

Pregnancy Risk Factor C

Contraindications Hypersensitivity to kaolin, pectin, or any component

Warnings Not to be used for self-medication of diarrhea for >48 hours or in presence of high fever in infants and children <3 years of age; do not use for diarrhea associated with pseudomembraneous enterocolitis or in diarrhea caused by toxigenic bacteria

Precautions Some products have added bismuth subsalicylate; use these products with caution in patients with bleeding disorders, salicylate sensitivity; do not use the subsalicylate-containing products in children <16 years of age who have chickenpox or flu symptoms due to the association with Reye's syndrome

(Continued)

Kaolin and Pectin (Continued)

Drug Interactions Kaolin and pectin may decrease absorption of quinidine, chloroquine, lincomycin, and digoxin (tablets only)

Usual Dosage Adequate controlled clinical studies documenting the efficacy of these combination products are lacking. Their usage and dosage have been primarily empiric; the table lists the manufacturer's recommended dosage.

Kaolin and Pectin Dosage*
(*mL/dose after each bowel movement)

Product	Dosage (by age)		
	3-6 y	6-12 y	>12 y to adult
Kao-Spen®	—	—	60-120 mL
Kaolin w/pectin (Kapectolin®)	15-30 mL	30-60 mL	60-120 mL
Kaodene® NN	15 mL	22.5 mL	45 mL

Administration May be administered without regard to meals

Dosage Forms Suspension, oral:
Kaodene® NN: Kaolin 650 mg and pectin 32.4 mg per 5 mL (120 mL)
Kao-Spen®: Kaolin 866 mg and pectin 43.3 mg per 5 mL (3780 mL)
Kapectolin®: Kaolin 15 g and pectin 333 mg per 5 mL (120 mL, 240 mL, 480 mL)

Ketamine (KEET a meen)

Related Information
Adult ACLS Algorithm, Synchronized Cardioversion on page 1048
Preprocedure Sedatives in Children on page 1201

U.S. Brand Names Ketalar®

Therapeutic Category General Anesthetic

Generic Available No

Use Anesthesia, short surgical procedures, dressing changes

Restrictions C-III

Pregnancy Risk Factor D

Contraindications Elevated intracranial pressure; patients with hypertension, aneurysms, thyrotoxicosis, CHF, angina, psychotic disorders; hypersensitivity to ketamine or any component

Warnings Use only by or under the direct supervision of physicians experienced in administering general anesthetics. Resuscitative equipment should be available for use. Postanesthetic emergence reactions which can manifest as vivid dreams, hallucinations and/or frank delirium occur in 12% of patients; these reactions are less common in pediatric patients; emergence reactions may occur up to 24 hours postoperatively and may be reduced by minimization of verbal, tactile, and visual patient stimulation during recovery, or by pretreatment with a benzodiazepine.

Precautions Use with caution in patients with gastroesophageal reflux; use with caution and decrease the dose in patients with hepatic dysfunction; use with caution in patients with a full stomach, patients should fast (ie, be NPO) for an appropriate time before being sedated for elective procedures

Adverse Reactions

Cardiovascular: Hypertension, tachycardia, increased cardiac output, paradoxical direct myocardial depression, hypotension, bradycardia, increases cerebral blood flow

Central nervous system: Tonic-clonic movements, increased intracranial pressure, hallucinations

Endocrine & metabolic: Increased metabolic rate

Gastrointestinal: Hypersalivation, vomiting, postoperative nausea

Neuromuscular & skeletal: Increased skeletal muscle tone, tremor, purposeless movement, fasciculations

Ocular: Diplopia, nystagmus, increased intraocular pressure

Respiratory: Increased airway resistance, cough reflex may be depressed, decreased bronchospasm; respiratory depression or apnea with large doses or rapid infusions, laryngospasm; increased bronchial mucous gland secretion

Miscellaneous: Emergence reactions

Drug Interactions Cytochrome P-450 isoenzyme CYP3A substrate

Barbiturates, narcotics, hydroxyzine prolong recovery from anesthesia

Stability Do not mix with barbiturates or diazepam as precipitation may occur

Mechanism of Action Produces dissociative anesthesia by direct action on the cortex and limbic system

Pharmacodynamics

Duration of action: Following single dose:

Anesthesia:

I.M.: 12-25 minutes

I.V.: 5-10 minutes

Analgesia: I.M.: 15-30 minutes

Recovery:

I.M.: 3-4 hours

I.V.: 1-2 hours

Usual Dosage

Children:

Oral: 6-10 mg/kg for 1 dose (mixed in cola or other beverage) given 30 minutes before the procedure

I.M.: 3-7 mg/kg

I.V.: Range: 0.5-2 mg/kg, use smaller doses (0.5-1 mg/kg) for sedation for minor procedures; usual induction dosage: 1-2 mg/kg

Continuous I.V. infusion: Sedation: 5-20 mcg/kg/minute; start at lower dosage listed and titrate to effect

Adults:

I.M.: 3-8 mg/kg

I.V.: Range: 1-4.5 mg/kg; usual induction dosage: 1-2 mg/kg

Children and Adults: Maintenance: Supplemental doses of $1/3$ to $1/2$ of initial dose

Administration

Oral: Use 100 mg/mL I.V. solution and mix the appropriate dose in 0.2-0.3 mL/kg of cola or other beverage

Parenteral: I.V.: Administer slowly, do not exceed 0.5 mg/kg/minute; do not administer faster than 60 seconds; do not exceed final concentration of 2 mg/mL

Monitoring Parameters Cardiovascular effects, heart rate, blood pressure, respiratory rate, transcutaneous O_2 saturation

Nursing Implications Resuscitative equipment should be available for use

Additional Information Used in combination with anticholinergic agents to decrease hypersalivation; should not be used for sedation for procedures that require a total lack of movement (eg, MRI, radiation therapy) due to association with purposeless movements

Dosage Forms Injection, as hydrochloride: 10 mg/mL (20 mL); 50 mg/mL (10 mL); 100 mg/mL (5 mL)

References

Cote CJ, "Sedation for the Pediatric Patient: A Review," *Pediatr Clin North Am*, 1994, 41(1):31-58.

Gutstein HB, Johnson KL, Heard MN, et al, "Oral Ketamine Premedication in Children," *Anesthesiology*, 1992, 76(1):28-33.

(Continued)

Ketamine *(Continued)*

Tobias JD, Phipps S, Smith B, et al, "Oral Ketamine Premedication to Alleviate the Distress of Invasive Procedures in Pediatric Oncology Patients," *Pediatrics*, 1992, 90(4):537-41.

Tobias JD and Rasmussen GE, "Pain Management and Sedation in the Pediatric Intensive Care Unit," *Pediatr Clin North Am*, 1994, 41(6):1269-92.

Ketoconazole (kee toe KOE na zole)

U.S. Brand Names Nizoral®

Canadian Brand Names Apo-Ketoconazole

Therapeutic Category Antifungal Agent, Systemic; Antifungal Agent, Topical

Generic Available No

Use Treatment of susceptible fungal infections, including candidiasis, oral thrush, blastomycosis, histoplasmosis, paracoccidioidomycosis, chronic mucocutaneous candidiasis, as well as certain recalcitrant cutaneous dermatophytes; used topically for treatment of tinea corporis, tinea cruris, tinea versicolor, and cutaneous candidiasis; shampoo is used for dandruff

Pregnancy Risk Factor C

Contraindications Hypersensitivity to ketoconazole or any component; single agent in the treatment of CNS fungal infections (due to poor CNS penetration); concomitant administration of astemizole, terfenadine, or cisapride

Warnings Has been associated with hepatotoxicity, including some fatalities; perform periodic liver function tests; high doses of ketoconazole may depress adrenocortical function and decrease serum testosterone concentrations; risk of serious cardiac arrhythmias in patients receiving ketoconazole and astemizole, terfenadine, or cisapride; do not use concurrently with astemizole, terfenadine, or cisapride

Precautions Gastric acidity is necessary for the dissolution and absorption of ketoconazole; avoid concomitant (within 2 hours) administration of antacids, H_2-blockers, anticholinergics; use with caution in patients with impaired hepatic function

Adverse Reactions

Central nervous system: Lethargy, nervousness, headache, dizziness, somnolence, fever, chills, bulging fontanelles

Dermatologic: Pruritus, rash, dry skin

Endocrine & metabolic: Adrenocortical insufficiency, gynecomastia, decreased libido

Gastrointestinal: Nausea, vomiting, abdominal discomfort, GI bleeding, diarrhea

Genitourinary: Oligospermia

Hematologic: Leukopenia, thrombocytopenia, hemolytic anemia

Hepatic: Hepatotoxicity; elevated AST, ALT, and alkaline phosphatase; jaundice

Local: Irritation, stinging

Miscellaneous: Anaphylaxis

Drug Interactions Cytochrome P-450 isoenzyme CYP3A3/4 substrate; CYP1A2, CYP2C, CYP2C9 (weak), CYP2C19 (weak), CYP3A3/4, and CYP3A5-7 isoenzyme inhibitor

Drugs that decrease ketoconazole absorption (raise gastric pH) such as antacids, didanosine, sodium bicarbonate, omeprazole, H_2-receptor blockers; sucralfate decreases absorption of ketoconazole by 20%; drugs that decrease serum concentrations of ketoconazole (rifampin, isoniazid, phenytoin); drug concentrations that are increased by ketoconazole (phenytoin, astemizole, cisapride, digoxin, cyclosporine, triazolam, midazolam, HMC-CoA reductase inhibitors, corticosteroids, terfenadine, indinavir, saquinavir, warfarin); drugs that cause hepatotoxicity; alcohol may cause disulfiram-like reactions; increased trough concentrations of delavirdine if given with ketoconazole (see Warnings)

Food Interactions Food may increase ketoconazole absorption; administration with an acidic beverage (eg, Coca-Cola, Pepsi, citrus juice) increases ketoconazole absorption

Mechanism of Action Alters the permeability of the cell wall; inhibits fungal biosynthesis of triglycerides and phospholipids; inhibits several fungal enzymes that results in a build-up of toxic concentrations of hydrogen peroxide

Pharmacokinetics

Absorption: Oral: Rapid (~75%)

Distribution: Minimal penetration into the CNS; distributes to bile, saliva, urine, sweat, synovial fluid, lungs, liver, kidney and bone marrow

Protein binding: 84% to 99%

Metabolism: Partially in the liver by enzymes to inactive compounds

Bioavailability: Decreases as pH of the gastric contents increase

Half-life, biphasic:

Alpha: 2 hours

Terminal: 8 hours

Time to peak serum concentration: Oral: Within 1-2 hours

Elimination: Primarily in feces (57%) with smaller amounts excreted in urine (~13%)

Dialysis: Not dialyzable (0% to 5%)

Usual Dosage

Infants and Children: Oral: 3.3-6.6 mg/kg/day once daily

Prophylaxis for recurrence of mucocutaneous candidiasis with HIV infection: 5-10 mg/kg/day divided every 12-24 hours; maximum: 800 mg/day divided twice daily

Adults: Oral: 200-400 mg/day as a single daily dose; maximum: 800 mg/day divided twice daily

Children and Adults:

Shampoo: Shampoo twice weekly (at least 3 days should elapse between each shampoo) for 4 weeks

Topical: Apply once daily to twice daily

Administration

Oral: May administer with or without food or with juice; administer with food to decrease nausea and vomiting; administer 2 hours prior to antacids, didanosine, proton pump inhibitors, or H_2-receptor antagonists to prevent decreased ketoconazole absorption; shake suspension well before use

Shampoo: Apply to wet hair and massage over entire scalp for 1 minute; rinse hair thoroughly and reapply shampoo for 3 minutes; rinse

Topical: Apply a sufficient amount and rub gently into the affected and surrounding area

Monitoring Parameters Liver function tests, signs of adrenal dysfunction

Patient Information Cream is for topical application to the skin only; avoid contact with the eye; notify physician of unusual fatigue, weakness, vomiting, dark urine, or yellowing of eyes; avoid alcohol

Additional Information Cream contains sodium sulfite

Dosage Forms

Cream: 2% (15 g, 30 g, 60 g)

Shampoo: 2% (120 mL)

Tablet: 200 mg

Extemporaneous Preparations A 20 mg/mL suspension may be made by pulverizing twelve 200 mg ketoconazole tablets to a fine powder; add 40 mL Ora-Plus® in small portions with thorough mixing; incorporate Ora-Sweet® to make a final volume of 120 mL and mix thoroughly; shake well before using; protect from light; stable for 60 days when stored without light at 5°C and 25°C

Allen LV and Erickson MA, "Stability of Ketoconazole, Metolazone, Metronidazole, Procainamide, Hydrochloride, and Spironolactone in Extemporaneously Compounded Oral Liquids," *AM J Health-Syst Pharm*, 1996, 53:2073-8.

References

Como JA and Dismukes WE, "Oral Azole Drugs as Systemic Antifungal Therapy," *N Engl J Med*, 1994, 330(4):263-72.

Ginsburg AM, McCracken GH Jr, and Olsen K, "Pharmacology of Ketoconazole Suspension in Infants and Children," *Antimicrob Agents Chemother*, 1983, 23(5):787-9.

Herrod HG, "Chronic Mucocutaneous Candidiasis in Childhood and Complications of non-*Candida* Infection: A Report of the Pediatric Immunodeficiency Collaborative Study Group," *J Pediatr*, 1990, 116(3):377-82.

Ketorolac (KEE toe role ak)

U.S. Brand Names Acular®; Acular® P.F.; Toradol®

Canadian Brand Names Apo-Ketorolac; Novo-Ketorolac

Therapeutic Category Analgesic, Non-narcotic; Anti-inflammatory Agent; Antipyretic; Nonsteroidal Anti-inflammatory Drug (NSAID), Ophthalmic; Nonsteroidal Anti-inflammatory Drug (NSAID), Oral; Nonsteroidal Anti-inflammatory Drug (NSAID), Parenteral

Generic Available Yes: Injection, tablet

Use

Oral, I.M., I.V.,: Short-term (≤5 days) management of moderate to severe pain, including postoperative pain, visceral pain associated with cancer, pain associated with trauma, acute renal colic

Ophthalmic: Ocular itch associated with seasonal allergic conjunctivitis

Pregnancy Risk Factor C (D if used in 3rd trimester)

Contraindications Hypersensitivity to ketorolac, any component, or in patients with nasal polyps, angioedema, or bronchospastic reactions to aspirin or other NSAIDs; patients with active peptic ulcer disease (PUD), recent GI bleeding or perforation, or history of PUD or GI bleeding; advanced renal dysfunction; patients at risk for renal failure due to hypovolemia; women in labor and delivery or breast-feeding; preoperative or intraoperative use; patients with cerebrovascular bleeding, incomplete hemostasis, hemorrhagic diathesis, or at high risk of bleeding; contraindicated for (Continued)

Ketorolac *(Continued)*

epidural or intrathecal use due to alcohol content; do not administer with aspirin, NSAIDs, or probenecid

Precautions Use with caution and reduce dose in patients with decreased renal function; hepatic impairment; CHF; patients in whom prolongation of bleeding time would cause adverse effects; not recommended after plastic or neurosurgery due to increased risk of bleeding

Adverse Reactions

Cardiovascular: Edema (4%)

Central nervous system: Somnolence, drowsiness (6%), dizziness (7%), headache (17%), insomnia, euphoria, hallucinations, malaise (<1%)

Dermatologic: Purpura, urticaria

Gastrointestinal: Dyspepsia (12%), nausea (12%), diarrhea (7%), GI pain, peptic ulcer, melena, rectal bleeding, constipation (<1%)

Genitourinary: Urinary frequency

Hematologic: Inhibits platelet aggregation, may prolong bleeding time

Hepatic: Elevated liver enzymes

Local: Pain at injection site (2%)

Ocular: Blurred vision

Renal: Oliguria, interstitial nephritis, acute renal failure (rare)

Respiratory: Dyspnea, wheezing

Miscellaneous: Anaphylaxis, hypersensitivity reactions

Drug Interactions Warfarin, heparin, lithium, methotrexate, salicylates, NSAIDs, GI irritants (eg, potassium supplements), probenecid (significantly increases ketorolac half-life and plasma levels), furosemide, phenytoin, carbamazepine; ketorolac may decrease antihypertensive effects of ACE inhibitors and angiotensin II antagonists

Food Interactions High-fat meals may delay time to peak (by ~1 hour) and decrease peak concentrations

Stability Protect from light; color change indicates degradation; do not administer in same syringe with narcotics; ketorolac will precipitate if mixed with morphine, meperidine, promethazine, or hydroxyzine

Mechanism of Action Inhibits prostaglandin synthesis by decreasing the activity of the enzyme, cyclo-oxygenase, which results in decreased formation of prostaglandin precursors

Pharmacodynamics Analgesia:

Onset:

Oral: 30-60 minutes

I.M., I.V.: ~30 minutes

Peak:

Oral: 1.5-4 hours

I.M., I.V.: 1-2 hours

Duration: 4-6 hours

Pharmacokinetics

Absorption:

Oral: Well absorbed

I.M.: Rapid and complete

Distribution: Crosses placenta, crosses into breast milk, poor penetration into CSF; follows two-compartment model

V_d beta: Adults: 0.11-0.33 L/kg (mean: 0.18 L/kg)

Protein binding: 99%

Metabolism: In the liver; undergoes hydroxylation and glucuronide conjugation; in children 4-8 years, V_{dss} and plasma clearance were twice as high as adults, but terminal half-life was similar

Bioavailability: Oral, I.M.: 100%

Half-life, terminal:

Children 4-8 years: ~6 hours; range: 3.5-10 (n=10)

Adults: Mean: ~5 hours; range: 4-9 hours

With renal impairment: S_{cr} 1.9-5 mg/dL: Mean: ~11 hours; range: 4-19 hours

Renal dialysis patients: Mean: ~14 hours; range: 8-40 hours

Time to peak serum concentration:

Oral: ~45 minutes

I.M.: 30-45 minutes

I.V.: 1-3 minutes

Elimination: Renal excretion, 58% to 61% in urine as unchanged drug

Usual Dosage Note: The use of ketorolac in children <16 years of age is outside of product labeling

Children 2-16 years: Dosing guidelines are not established; **do not exceed adult doses**; see Additional Information

Single-dose treatment:

I.M., I.V.: 0.4-1 mg/kg as a single dose; **Note:** Limited information exists. Single I.V. doses of 0.5 mg/kg, 0.75 mg/kg, 0.9 mg/kg and 1 mg/kg have been studied in children 2-16 years of age for postoperative analgesia. One study (Maunuksela, 1992) used a titrating dose starting with 0.2 mg/kg up to a total of 0.5 mg/kg (median dose required: 0.4 mg/kg).

Oral: One study used 1 mg/kg as a single dose for analgesia in 30 children (mean ± SD age: 3 ± 2.5 years) undergoing bilateral myringotomy

Multiple-dose treatment: I.M., I.V., Oral: No pediatric studies exist; one report (Buck, 1994) of the clinical experience with ketorolac in 112 children, 6 months to 19 years of age (mean: 9 years), described usual I.V. maintenance doses of 0.5 mg/kg every 6 hours (mean dose: 0.52 mg/kg; range: 0.17-1 mg/kg)

Children >16 years and >50 kg and Adults <65 years:

Single-dose treatment:

I.M.: 60 mg as a single dose

I.V.: 30 mg as a single dose

Multiple-dose treatment:

I.M., I.V.: 30 mg every 6 hours; maximum dose: 120 mg/day

Oral: Initial: 20 mg, then 10 mg every 4-6 hours; maximum dose: 40 mg/day

Adults ≥65 years, renally impaired, or <50 kg:

Single-dose treatment:

I.M.: 30 mg as a single dose

I.V.: 15 mg as a single dose

Multiple-dose treatment:

I.M., I.V.: 15 mg every 6 hours; maximum dose: 60 mg/day

Oral: 10 mg every 4-6 hours; maximum dose: 40 mg/day

Adults: Ophthalmic: Instill 1 drop in eye(s) 4 times/day for up to 7 days

Administration

Ophthalmic: Instill drops into affected eye(s); avoid contact of container tip with skin or eyes; apply finger pressure to lacrimal sac during and for 1-2 minutes after instillation to decrease risk of absorption and systemic effects

Oral: May administer with food or milk to decrease GI upset

Parenteral:

I.M.: Administer slowly and deeply into muscle; 60 mg/2 mL Tubex® is for I.M. use only

I.V. bolus: Administer over at least 15 seconds; I.V. ketorolac has been infused over 1-5 minutes in children

Monitoring Parameters Signs of pain relief (eg, increased appetite and activity); BUN, serum creatinine, liver enzymes, occult blood loss, urinalysis

Reference Range Serum concentration:

Therapeutic: 0.3-5 µg/mL

Toxic: >5 µg/mL

Patient Information Avoid alcohol; may cause drowsiness or dizziness and may impair ability to perform activities requiring mental alertness or physical coordination; do not exceed 5 days total use (I.M., I.V., oral)

Additional Information 30 mg provides analgesia comparable to 12 mg of morphine or 100 mg of meperidine; ketorolac may possess an opioid-sparing effect; diarrhea, pallor, vomiting, and labored breathing may occur with overdose

Note: A single I.V. dose of ketorolac (0.75 mg/kg) in 21 children (2.5-9 years of age) undergoing outpatient strabismus surgery was associated with less postoperative emesis than morphine plus metoclopramide (Munro, 1994). However, a single dose of I.V. ketorolac (1 mg/kg) in 25 children (2-15 years of age) undergoing tonsillectomy was associated with an increase in surgical bleeding, more patients requiring extra hemostatic measures (eg, synthetic collagen, extra Neo-Synephrine® packing), and a higher estimated blood loss compared to rectal acetaminophen (Rusy, 1995); further studies are needed.

Dosage Forms

Injection, as tromethamine (Toradol®): 15 mg/mL (1 mL); 30 mg/mL (1 mL, 2 mL)

Solution, ophthalmic, as tromethamine

Acular®: 0.5% [contains benzalkonium chloride] (3 mL, 5 mL, 10 mL)

Acular® P.F.: 0.5% [preservative free] (0.4 mL)

Tablet, as tromethamine (Toradol®): 10 mg

References

Buck ML, "Clinical Experience With Ketorolac in Children," *Ann Pharmacother*, 1994, 28(9):1009-13.

Maunuksela E, Kokki H, and Bullingham RES, "Comparison of Intravenous Ketorolac With Morphine for Postoperative Pain in Children," *Clin Pharmacol Ther*, 1992, 52(4):436-43.

(Continued)

Ketorolac *(Continued)*

Munro HM, Reigger LQ, Reynolds PI, et al, "Comparison of the Analgesic and Emetic Properties of Ketorolac and Morphine for Paediatric Outpatient Strabismus Surgery," *Br J Anaesth*, 1994, 72(6):624-8.

Rusy LM, Houck CS, Sullivan LJ, et al, "A Double-Blind Evaluation of Ketorolac Tromethamine Versus Acetaminophen in Pediatric Tonsillectomy: Analgesia and Bleeding," *Anesth Analg*, 1995, 80(2):226-9.

Watcha MF, Jones MB, Lagueruela RG, et al, "Comparison of Ketorolac and Morphine as Adjuvants During Pediatric Surgery," *Anesthesiology*, 1992, 76(3):368-72.

- **K-Exit (Can)** *see* Sodium Polystyrene Sulfonate *on page 908*
- **K-Gen®** *see* Potassium Supplements *on page 816*
- **KI** *see* Potassium Iodide *on page 815*
- **Kidrolase (Can)** *see* Asparaginase *on page 107*
- **Kionex™** *see* Sodium Polystyrene Sulfonate *on page 908*
- **Klean-Prep (Can)** *see* Polyethylene Glycol-Electrolyte Solution *on page 811*
- **Klonopin™** *see* Clonazepam *on page 254*
- **K-Lor™** *see* Potassium Supplements *on page 816*
- **Klor-Con® 8** *see* Potassium Supplements *on page 816*
- **Klor-Con® 10** *see* Potassium Supplements *on page 816*
- **Klor-Con/25®** *see* Potassium Supplements *on page 816*
- **Klor-Con® EF** *see* Potassium Supplements *on page 816*
- **Klorvess® Effervescent** *see* Potassium Supplements *on page 816*
- **Klotrix®** *see* Potassium Supplements *on page 816*
- **K-Lyte®** *see* Potassium Supplements *on page 816*
- **K-Lyte/Cl®** *see* Potassium Supplements *on page 816*
- **K-lyte DS** *see* Potassium Supplements *on page 816*
- **Koate®-DVI** *see* Antihemophilic Factor (Human) *on page 98*
- **Koffex DM (Can)** *see* Dextromethorphan *on page 316*
- **Koffex DM-E (Can)** *see* Guaifenesin and Dextromethorphan *on page 487*
- **Koffex Expectorant (Can)** *see* Guaifenesin *on page 485*
- **Kolephrin® GG/DM [OTC]** *see* Guaifenesin and Dextromethorphan *on page 487*
- **Kondremul® [OTC]** *see* Mineral Oil *on page 675*
- **Konsyl® [OTC]** *see* Psyllium *on page 853*
- **Konsyl-D® [OTC]** *see* Psyllium *on page 853*
- **Konȳne® 80** *see* Factor IX Complex (Human) *on page 414*
- **K-Pek® [OTC]** *see* Attapulgite *on page 118*
- **K-Phos® M.F.** *see* Phosphate Supplements *on page 794*
- **K-Phos® Neutral** *see* Phosphate Supplements *on page 794*
- **K-Phos® No. 2** *see* Phosphate Supplements *on page 794*
- **K-Phos® Original** *see* Phosphate Supplements *on page 794*
- **Kristalose®** *see* Lactulose *on page 571*
- **K-Tab®** *see* Potassium Supplements *on page 816*
- **Kutrase®** *see* Pancrelipase *on page 755*
- **Ku-Zyme®** *see* Pancrelipase *on page 755*
- **Ku-Zyme® HP** *see* Pancrelipase *on page 755*
- **K-Vescent® Potassium Chloride** *see* Potassium Supplements *on page 816*
- **Kwell®** *see* Lindane *on page 595*
- **Kwellada-P (Can)** *see* Permethrin *on page 783*
- **Kytril™** *see* Granisetron *on page 482*
- **L-3-Hydroxytyramine** *see* Levodopa *on page 585*
- **L-735,524** *see* Indinavir *on page 534*
- **LA-12®** *see* Cyanocobalamin *on page 277*
- **LA-12®** *see* Hydroxocobalamin *on page 512*

Labetalol *(la BET a lole)*

Related Information
Overdose and Toxicology *on page 1222*
U.S. Brand Names Normodyne®; Trandate®
Synonyms Ibidomide
Therapeutic Category Alpha-/Beta- Adrenergic Blocker; Antihypertensive Agent
Generic Available Yes
Use Treatment of mild to severe hypertension; I.V. for hypertensive emergencies
Pregnancy Risk Factor C

Contraindications Asthma, obstructive airway disease, cardiogenic shock, uncompensated CHF, bradycardia, pulmonary edema, or heart block; history of asthma or obstructive airway disease

Warnings Orthostatic hypotension may occur with I.V. administration; patient should remain supine during and for up to 3 hours after I.V. administration; use with extreme caution when reducing severely elevated blood pressure; cerebral and cardiac adverse effects (infarction/ischemia) may occur if blood pressure is decreased too rapidly; blood pressure should be lowered over as long a period of time that is compatible with the status of the patient

Precautions Paradoxical increase in blood pressure has been reported with treatment of pheochromocytoma or clonidine withdrawal syndrome; use with extreme caution in patients with hyper-reactive airway disease, CHF, diabetes mellitus, hepatic dysfunction

Adverse Reactions
Cardiovascular: Orthostatic hypotension especially with I.V. administration, edema, CHF, A-V conduction disturbances (but less than with propranolol), bradycardia

Central nervous system: Drowsiness, fatigue, dizziness, behavior disorders, headache

Dermatologic: Rash, tingling in scalp or skin (transient with initiation of therapy)

Gastrointestinal: Nausea, xerostomia

Genitourinary: Sexual dysfunction, urinary problems

Neuromuscular & skeletal: Reversible myopathy has been reported in 2 children, paresthesia

Respiratory: Bronchospasm, nasal congestion

Drug Interactions Cytochrome P-450 isoenzyme CYP2D6 substrate and inhibitor
Cimetidine may potentiate labetalol action; additive hypotensive effects with other hypotensive drugs; halothane may cause synergistic hypotension; tricyclic antidepressants; beta agonists; nitroglycerin; calcium antagonists

Food Interactions Avoid natural licorice (causes sodium and water retention and increases potassium loss); food may increase bioavailability

Stability
Injection: Store at room temperature; do not freeze; protect from light; stable in D_5W, saline for 24 hours; incompatible with sodium bicarbonate, furosemide; most stable in pH of 2-4

Tablets: Store at room temperature; protect unit dose boxes from excessive moisture

Mechanism of Action Blocks alpha-, beta$_1$- and beta$_2$-adrenergic receptor sites; elevated renins are reduced

Pharmacodynamics
Onset of action:
Oral: 20 minutes to 2 hours
I.V.: 2-5 minutes

Peak effect:
Oral: 1-4 hours
I.V.: 5-15 minutes

Duration:
Oral: 8-24 hours (dose dependent)
I.V.: 2-4 hours

Pharmacokinetics
Distribution: Crosses the placenta; small amounts in breast milk
V_d: Adults: 3-16 L/kg; mean: 9.4 L/kg

Protein-binding: 50%

Metabolism: In the liver primarily via glucuronide conjugation; extensive first-pass effect

Bioavailability: Oral: 25%; increased bioavailability with liver disease, elderly

Half-life: 5-8 hours

Elimination: Possible decreased clearance in neonates/infants; <5% excreted in urine unchanged

Usual Dosage
Children: **Note:** Limited information regarding labetalol use in pediatric patients is currently available in the literature; labetalol should be initiated cautiously in pediatric patients (using the lower doses listed) with careful dosage adjustment and blood pressure monitoring

Oral: Some centers recommend initial oral doses of 4 mg/kg/day in 2 divided doses. (Reported oral doses have started at 3 mg/kg/day and 20 mg/kg/day and have increased up to 40 mg/kg/day.)

I.V., intermittent bolus doses: Initial doses of 0.2-0.5 mg/kg/dose with a range of 0.2-1 mg/kg/dose have been suggested; maximum dose: 20 mg/dose

(Continued)

Labetalol *(Continued)*

Treatment of pediatric hypertensive emergencies: Initial continuous infusions of 0.4-1 mg/kg/hour with a maximum of 3 mg/kg/hour have been used; one study used initial bolus dose of 0.2-1 mg/kg (maximum dose: 20 mg, mean: 0.5 mg/kg) followed by a continuous infusion of 0.25-1.5 mg/kg/hour (mean: 0.78 mg/kg/hour)

Adults:

Oral: Initial: 100 mg twice daily, may increase as needed every 2-3 days by 100 mg until desired response is obtained; usual dose: 200-400 mg twice daily; not to exceed 2.4 g/day

I.V.: Initial: 20 mg; may give 40-80 mg at 10-minute intervals, up to 300 mg total dose

I.V. infusion: Initial: 2 mg/minute; titrate to response

Administration

Oral: May administer with food but should be administered in a consistent manner with regards to meals

Parenteral:

I.V. bolus: Administer over 2-3 minutes; do not administer faster than 2 mg/minute; maximum concentration: 5 mg/mL

I.V. continuous infusion: Dilute to 1 mg/mL; undiluted labetalol injection (5 mg/mL) has been administered to a very small number of adult patients who were extremely fluid restricted

Monitoring Parameters Blood pressure, heart rate, pulse, EKG

Test Interactions False-positive urine catecholamines, VMA if measured by fluorometric or photometric methods; use HPLC or specific catecholamine radioenzymatic technique

Patient Information Limit alcohol; may cause drowsiness, dizziness and impair ability to perform activities requiring mental alertness; do not stop medication abruptly

Nursing Implications Instruct patient regarding compliance; do **not** abruptly withdraw medication in patients with ischemic heart disease; labetalol may mask other signs and symptoms of diabetes mellitus, but sweating can still occur

Dosage Forms

Injection, as hydrochloride: 5 mg/mL (20 mL, 40 mL, 60 mL)

Prefilled syringes: 5 mg/mL (4 mL, 8 mL)

Tablet, as hydrochloride: 100 mg, 200 mg, 300 mg

Extemporaneous Preparations

A 40 mg/mL oral liquid preparation made from tablets and 3 different vehicles (cherry syrup, a 1:1 mixture of Ora-Sweet® and Ora-Plus®, or a 1:1 mixture of Ora-Sweet® SF and Ora-Plus®) was stable for 60 days when stored in amber plastic prescription bottles in the dark at room temperature (25°C) or under refrigeration (5°C); grind sixteen 30 mg tablets in a mortar into a fine powder; add 20 mL of the vehicle and mix well to form a uniform paste; mix while adding the vehicle in geometric proportions to **almost** 120 mL; transfer to a calibrated bottle and qsad with vehicle to make 120 mL; label "shake well" and "protect from light" (Allen, 1996).

Extemporaneously prepared solutions (approximate concentrations 7-10 mg/mL) prepared in distilled water, simple syrup, apple juice, grape juice, and orange juice were stable for 4 weeks when stored in amber glass or plastic prescription bottles at 23°C and 4°C (Nahata, 1991).

Allen LV and Erickson MA, "Stability of Labetalol Hydrochloride, Metoprolol Tartrate, Verapamil Hydrochloride, and Spironolactone With Hydrochlorothiazide in Extemporaneously Compounded Oral Liquids," *Am J Health Syst Pharm*, 1996, 53(19):2304-9.

Nahata MC, "Stability of Labetolol Hydrochloride in Distilled Water, Simple Syrup, and Three Fruit Juices," *DICP*, 1991, 25(5):465-9.

References

Bunchman TE, Lynch RE, and Wood EG, "Intravenously Administered Labetalol for Treatment of Hypertension in Children," *J Pediatr*, 1992, 120(1):140-4.

Farine M, and Arbus GS, "Management of Hypertensive Emergencies in Children," *Pediatr Emerg Care*, 1989, 5(1):51-5.

Ishisaka DY, Yonan CD, Housel BF, "Labetalol for Treatment of Hypertension in a Child," *Clin Pharm*, 1991, 10(7):500-1 (case report).

Jones SE, "Coarctation in Children. Controlled Hypotension Using Labetalol and Halothane," *Anaesthesia*, 1979, 34(10):1052-5.

Jureidini KF, "Oral Labetalol in a Child With Phaeochromocytoma and Five Children With Renal Hypertension," *N Z Med J*, 1980, 10:479 (abstract).

Mueller JB and Solhaug MJ, "Labetalol in Pediatric Hypertensive Emergencies," *Pediatr Res*, 1988, 23(Pt 2):543A (abstract).

Wesley AG, Hariparsad D, Pather M, et al, "Labetalol in Tetanus. The Treatment of Sympathetic Nervous System Overactivity," *Anaesthesia*, 1983, 38(3):243-9.

♦ **Laboratory Detection of Drugs in Urine** *see page 1234*
♦ **Lacri-Lube**® **SOP [OTC]** *see Ocular Lubricant on page 732*
♦ **LactiCare-HC**® *see Hydrocortisone on page 506*
♦ **Lactinex**® **[OTC]** *see Lactobacillus acidophilus and Lactobacillus bulgaricus on page 571*

Lactobacillus acidophilus and *Lactobacillus bulgaricus*

(lak toe ba SIL us as i DOF fil us & lak toe ba SIL us bul GAR i cus)

U.S. Brand Names Bacid® [OTC]; Kala [OTC]; Lactinex® [OTC]; More-Dophilus® [OTC]; Superdophilus® [OTC]

Canadian Brand Names Fermalac

Therapeutic Category Antidiarrheal

Generic Available No

Use Uncomplicated diarrhea particularly that caused by antibiotic therapy; re-establish normal physiologic and bacterial flora of the intestinal tract

Contraindications Allergy to milk or lactose

Warnings Discontinue if high fever present

Adverse Reactions Gastrointestinal: Intestinal flatus

Stability Store in the refrigerator

Mechanism of Action Creates an environment unfavorable to potentially pathogenic fungi or bacteria through the production of lactic acid, and favors establishment of an aciduric flora, thereby suppressing the growth of pathogenic microorganisms; helps re-establish normal intestinal flora

Pharmacokinetics
　Absorption: Not orally absorbed
　Distribution: Locally, primarily in the colon
　Elimination: In feces

Usual Dosage Children and Adults: Oral:
　Capsule: 1-2 capsules 2-4 times/day
　Granules: 1 packet added to or taken with cereal, food, milk, fruit juice, or water, 3-4 times/day
　Powder: $^1/_4$-1 teaspoon 1-3 times/day with liquid
　Tablet, chewable: 4 tablets 3-4 times/day; may follow each dose with a small amount of milk, fruit juice, or water
　Recontamination protocol for BMT unit: 1 packet 3 times/day for 6 doses for those patients who refuse yogurt

Administration Oral: Granules, powder, or contents of capsules may be added to or administered with cereal, food, milk, fruit juice, or water

Dosage Forms
　Capsule (Bacid®): *Lactobacillus acidophilus* 500 million units
　Powder for suspension:
　　More-Dophilus®: *Lactobacillus acidophilus* 12.4 billion units/5 mL [carrot derived] (30 g, 120 g)
　　Superdophilus®: *Lactobacillus acidophilus* 2 billion units/g (49 g)
　Tablet (Kala): *Lactobacillus acidophilus* 200 million units [soy based]

♦ **Lactoflavin** *see Riboflavin on page 874*

Lactulose (LAK tyoo lose)

Related Information
　Carbohydrate and Alcohol Content of Liquid Medications for Use in Patients Receiving Ketogenic Diets *on page 1258*

U.S. Brand Names Cephulac®; Cholac®; Chronulac®; Constilac®; Constulose®; Enulose®; Kristalose®

Canadian Brand Names Acilac; Laxilose; PMS-Lactulose

Therapeutic Category Ammonium Detoxicant; Hyperammonemia Agent; Laxative, Miscellaneous

Generic Available Yes

Use Adjunct in the prevention and treatment of portal-systemic encephalopathy (PSE); treatment of chronic constipation

Pregnancy Risk Factor B

Contraindications Patients with galactosemia

Warnings Accumulation of hydrogen gas in intestine could result in an explosion if the patient were to undergo electrocautery procedure

(Continued)

Lactulose *(Continued)*

Precautions Use with caution in patients with diabetes mellitus; do not use with other laxatives especially when initiating PSE treatment as increased loose stools may falsely suggest adequate lactulose dosage

Adverse Reactions Gastrointestinal: Flatulence, abdominal discomfort, diarrhea, nausea, vomiting

Drug Interactions Oral antibiotics may interfere with desired degradation of lactulose by eliminating key GI bacteria; nonsorbable antacids may eliminate desired lactulose-induced decreased GI tract pH

Food Interactions Contraindicated in patients on galactose-restricted diet

Mechanism of Action The bacterial degradation of lactulose resulting in an acidic pH inhibits the diffusion of NH_3 into the blood by causing the conversion of NH_3 to NH_4+; also enhances the diffusion of NH_3 from the blood into the gut where conversion to NH_4+ occurs; produces an osmotic effect in the colon with resultant distention promoting peristalsis and elimination of NH_4+ from the body

Pharmacokinetics

Absorption: Oral: Not absorbed appreciably

Metabolism: By colonic flora to lactic acid and acetic acid

Elimination: Primarily in feces and urine ($\sim$3%)

Usual Dosage

Prevention and treatment of portal systemic encephalopathy (PSE): Oral:

Infants: 2.5-10 mL/day divided 3-4 times/day, adjust dosage to produce 2-3 soft stools per day

Children: 40-90 mL/day divided 3-4 times/day, adjust dosage to produce 2-3 soft stools per day

Adults:

Oral:

Acute episodes of PSE: 30-45 mL (20-30 g) at 1- to 2-hour intervals until laxative effect observed, then adjust dosage to produce 2-3 soft stools per day

Chronic therapy: 30-45 mL/dose (20-30 g/dose) 3-4 times/day; titrate dose every 1-2 days to produce 2-3 soft stools per day

Rectal: 300 mL diluted with 700 mL of water or NS, and given via a rectal balloon catheter and retained for 30-60 minutes; may give every 4-6 hours

Constipation: Oral:

Children: 7.5 mL/day (5 g/day) after breakfast

Adults: 15-30 mL/day (10-20 g/day); increase to a maximum of 60 mL/day (40 g/day) if needed

Administration

Oral: Administer with juice, milk, or water; dissolve crystals in 4 ounces of water or juice

Rectal: See Usual Dosage

Monitoring Parameters Serum ammonia, serum potassium, fluid status, stool output

Additional Information Upon discontinuation of therapy, allow 24-48 hours for resumption of normal bowel movements

Dosage Forms

Crystals (Kristalose®): 10 g, 20 g (packets)

Syrup: 10 g/15 mL (15 mL, 30 mL, 237 mL, 473 mL, 946 mL, 1890 mL)

♦ **L-AmB** *see* Amphotericin B Liposome *on page 87*

♦ **Lamictal**® *see* Lamotrigine *on page 575*

Lamivudine *(la MI vyoo deen)*

Related Information

Adult and Adolescent HIV *on page 1166*

Pediatric HIV *on page 1162*

U.S. Brand Names Epivir®; Epivir-HBV®

Canadian Brand Names Heptovir; 3TC

Synonyms 2'-Deoxy-3'-Thiacytidine; 3TC

Therapeutic Category Antiretroviral Agent; HIV Agents (Anti-HIV Agents); Nucleoside Reverse Transcriptase Inhibitor (NRTI)

Generic Available No

Use Treatment of HIV infection in combination with other antiretroviral agents. (**Note:** HIV regimens consisting of **three** antiretroviral agents are strongly recommended); chemoprophylaxis after occupational exposure to HIV; management of chronic hepatitis B infection associated with evidence of hepatitis B viral replication and active liver inflammation

Pregnancy Risk Factor C

Contraindications Hypersensitivity to lamivudine or any component

Warnings The major clinical toxicity of lamivudine in pediatric patients is pancreatitis which has occurred in 14% of patients in one open-label, uncontrolled study; discontinue lamivudine therapy if clinical signs, symptoms, or laboratory abnormalities suggestive of pancreatitis occur. Lactic acidosis and severe hepatomegaly with steatosis have been reported with the use of lamivudine. A majority of these cases have been in women. Obesity and prolonged nucleoside exposure may be risk factors. Discontinue lamivudine if clinical or laboratory abnormalities suggestive of lactic acidosis or pronounced hepatotoxicity occur.

Precautions Use with extreme caution and only if there is no satisfactory alternative therapy in pediatric patients with a history of pancreatitis or other significant risk factors for the development of pancreatitis; reduce dosage in patients with impaired renal function; mothers should not breast-feed if they are receiving lamivudine

Adverse Reactions

Central nervous system: Headache (6% to 11%), fatigue, insomnia, psychomotor disorders (11% to 15%)

Dermatologic: Rash, pruritus, urticaria, alopecia

Endocrine & metabolic: Lactic acidosis, hyperglycemia

Gastrointestinal: Nausea, feeding problem (12% to 19%), abdominal discomfort (10% to 12%), pancreatitis (14%), diarrhea, vomiting, anorexia

Hematologic: Neutropenia

Hepatic: Elevated ALT, AST, bilirubin, and amylase; hepatic steatosis, severe hepatomegaly

Neuromuscular & skeletal: Paresthesias, peripheral neuropathy, musculoskeletal pain (8% to 11%), gait disorder, myalgia, muscle weakness, rhabdomyolysis, elevated CPK

Respiratory: Cough

Drug Interactions Coadministration with trimethoprim/sulfamethoxazole increases the AUC of lamivudine (significance is unknown); when used with zidovudine, may prevent emergence of zidovudine resistance

Stability Store tablets and oral solution at room temperature in tightly closed bottles

Mechanism of Action A synthetic nucleoside analogue that is converted intracellularly to the active triphosphate metabolite which inhibits reverse transcription via viral DNA chain termination after incorporation of the nucleoside analogue. Lamivudine triphosphate is a weak inhibitor of DNA polymerase alpha- and beta-mitochondrial DNA polymerase.

Pharmacokinetics

Distribution: Into extravascular spaces; CSF concentration ranged from 5.6% to 30.9% of the simultaneous serum concentration

Protein binding: <36%

Metabolism: Converted intracellularly to the active triphosphate form

Bioavailability:

Children 4.8 months to 16 years: 70%

Adolescents and Adults: 82%

Half-life, elimination:

Children 4 months to 14 years: 1.7 hours

Adults with normal renal function: 2.5 hours

Time to peak serum concentration:

Fasting state: 0.9 hours

Fed state: 3.2 hours

Elimination: 70% of dose eliminated unchanged in urine

Usual Dosage Oral:

Neonates <30 days: 2 mg/kg/dose twice daily is being studied in clinical trials

Children: 4 mg/kg/dose twice daily; maximum dose: 150 mg/dose every 12 hours

Adolescents and Adults, body weight <50 kg: 2 mg/kg/dose twice daily

Adolescents (in later puberty: Tanner V) and Adults, body weight ≥50 kg: 150 mg/dose twice daily

Chemoprophylaxis after occupational exposure to HIV: 150 mg/dose twice daily in combination with zidovudine 200 mg 3 times/day and indinavir 800 mg 3 times/day are first-line agents after exposures for which prophylaxis is recommended.

Adolescents ≥16 years and Adults: Chronic hepatitis B infection: 100 mg/dose once daily

Dosing adjustment in renal impairment for HIV: Adults:

Cl_{cr} 30-49 mL/minute: 150 mg once daily

Cl_{cr} 15-29 mL/minute: 150 mg first dose, then 100 mg once daily

Cl_{cr} 5-14 mL/minute: 150 mg first dose, then 50 mg once daily

Cl_{cr} <5 mL/minute: 50 mg first dose, then 25 mg once daily

(Continued)

Lamivudine *(Continued)*

Dosing adjustment in renal impairment for chronic hepatitis B: Adults:
Cl$_{cr}$ 30-49 mL/minute: 100 mg first dose, then 50 mg once daily
Cl$_{cr}$ 15-29 mL/minute: 100 mg first dose, then 25 mg once daily
Cl$_{cr}$ 5-14 mL/minute: 35 mg first dose, then 15 mg once daily
Cl$_{cr}$ <5 mL/minute: 35 mg first dose, then 10 mg once daily
Dosing adjustment in hepatic impairment: No data

Administration Oral: Administer with or without food

Monitoring Parameters CBC with differential, hemoglobin, ALT, AST, serum amylase, bilirubin, CD4 cell count, HIV RNA plasma levels; signs and symptoms of pancreatitis, lactic acidosis, and pronounced hepatotoxicity

Patient Information Lamivudine is not a cure; notify physician if persistent severe abdominal pain, nausea, vomiting, numbness, or tingling occur; avoid alcohol

Dosage Forms
Solution: 5 mg/mL (240 mL); 10 mg/mL (240 mL)
Tablet: 100 mg, 150 mg

References
CDC and the National Foundation for Infectious Disease, "Update: Provisional Public Health Service Recommendations for Chemoprophylaxis After Occupational Exposure to HIV," *MMWR Morb Mortal Wkly Rep*, 1996, 45(22):468-80.

Eron JJ, Benoit SL, Jemsek J, et al, "Treatment With Lamivudine, Zidovudine, or Both in HIV-Positive Patients With 200 to 500 CD4+ Cells Per Cubic Millimeter," *N Engl J Med*, 1995, 333(25):1662-9.

Lai CL, Chien RN, Leung NW, et al, "A One-Year Trial of Lamivudine for Chronic Hepatitis B," *N Engl J Med*, 1998, 339(2):61-8.

Lewis LL, Mueller B, Schock R, et al, "A Phase I/II Study to Evaluate the Safety, Toxicity, and Preliminary Efficacy of Combinations of Lamivudine (3TC), Zidovudine (AZT) and Didanosine (ddl) in Children With HIV Infection," *Natl Conf Hum Retroviruses Relat Infect* (2nd), 1995, Jan 29-Feb 2:103.

Lewis LL, Venzon D, Church J, et al, "Lamivudine in Children With Human Immunodeficiency Virus Infection: A Phase I/II Study," *J Infect Dis*, 1996, 174(1):16-25.

Working Group on Antiretroviral Therapy and Medical Management of HIV-Infected Children, "Guidelines for the Use of Antiretroviral Agents in Pediatric HIV Infection," January 7, 2000, http://www.hivatis.org.

♦ **Lamivudine, Abacavir, and Zidovudine** *see* Abacavir, Lamivudine, and Zidovudine *on page 26*

Lamivudine and Zidovudine *(la MI vyoo deen & zye DOE vyoo deen)*

U.S. Brand Names Combivir®

Synonyms AZT and 3TC; 3TC and AZT; 3TC and ZDV; Zidovudine and Lamivudine; ZVD and 3TC

Therapeutic Category Antiretroviral Agent; HIV Agents (Anti-HIV Agents); Nucleoside Reverse Transcriptase Inhibitor (NRTI)

Generic Available No

Use Treatment of HIV-1 infection in combination with at least one other antiretroviral agent; (**Note:** HIV regimens consisting of **three** antiretroviral agents are strongly recommended)

Pregnancy Risk Factor C

Contraindications Hypersensitivity to lamivudine, zidovudine, or any component

Warnings This product contains lamivudine and zidovudine as a fixed-dose combination; ordinarily, concomitant use of Combivir® with either lamivudine or zidovudine is not recommended. The major clinical toxicity of lamivudine in pediatric patients is pancreatitis; discontinue therapy if clinical signs, symptoms, or laboratory abnormalities suggestive of pancreatitis occur. Zidovudine is associated with hematologic toxicity including granulocytopenia and severe anemia requiring transfusions; use with caution in patients with ANC <1000 cells/mm³ or hemoglobin <9.5 g/dL; discontinue treatment in children with an ANC <500 cells/mm³ until marrow recovery is observed; use of erythropoietin, filgrastim, or reduced zidovudine dosage may be necessary in some patients; prolonged use of zidovudine may cause myositis and myopathy; zidovudine has been shown to be carcinogenic in rats and mice.

Cases of lactic acidosis, severe hepatomegaly with steatosis, and death have been reported with the use of lamivudine, zidovudine and other antiretroviral agents; most of these cases have been in women; prolonged nucleoside use, obesity, and prior liver disease may be risk factors; use with extreme caution in patients with other risk factors for liver disease; discontinue therapy in patients who develop laboratory or clinical evidence of lactic acidosis or pronounced hepatotoxicity.

Precautions Always use Combivir® in combination with another antiretroviral agent; use with extreme caution and only if there is no satisfactory alternative therapy in pediatric patients with a history of pancreatitis or other significant risk factors for pancreatitis; use with caution in patients with bone marrow compromise or in patients with impaired renal or hepatic function. The dose of lamivudine should be reduced in patients with renal dysfunction; the dose of zidovudine should be reduced or therapy interrupted in patients with anemia, granulocytopenia, myopathy, renal or hepatic impairment; use of the fixed-dose combination product (Combivir®) is not recommended for patients who need a dosage reduction (use individual antiretroviral agents to appropriately adjust dosages).

Adverse Reactions See Lamivudine *on page 572* and Zidovudine *on page 1022*

Drug Interactions See Lamivudine *on page 572* and Zidovudine *on page 1022*

Food Interactions Food does not affect the extent of of absorption

Mechanism of Action See Lamivudine *on page 572* and Zidovudine *on page 1022*

Pharmacokinetics One Combivir® tablet is bioequivalent to one lamivudine 150 mg tablet plus one zidovudine 300 mg tablet; see Lamivudine *on page 572* and Zidovudine *on page 1022*

Usual Dosage Oral: Adolescents ≥12 years and Adults: One tablet twice daily
   Dosage adjustment in renal impairment: Cl_{cr} ≤50 mL/minute: Not recommended (use individual antiretroviral agents to reduce dosage)

Administration Oral: May be administered without regard to meals

Monitoring Parameters CBC with differential, hemoglobin, MCV, reticulocyte count, liver enzymes, serum amylase, bilirubin, CD4 cell count, HIV RNA plasma levels, renal and hepatic function tests; signs and symptoms of pancreatitis, lactic acidosis, pronounced hepatotoxicity, anemia, and bone marrow suppression

Patient Information Avoid alcohol; Combivir® is not a cure; notify physician if persistent severe abdominal pain, nausea, or vomiting occurs; take Combivir® every day as prescribed; do not change dose or discontinue without physician's advice. If a dose is missed, take it as soon as possible, then return to normal dosing schedule; if a dose is skipped, do **not** double the next dose

Dosage Forms Tablet: Lamivudine 150 mg and zidovudine 300 mg

♦ **Lamivudine, Zidovudine, and Abacavir** *see* Abacavir, Lamivudine, and Zidovudine *on page 26*

Lamotrigine (la MOE tri jeen)

Related Information
   Antiepileptic Drugs *on page 1208*
   Carbohydrate and Alcohol Content of Liquid Medications for Use in Patients Receiving Ketogenic Diets *on page 1258*

U.S. Brand Names Lamictal®

Synonyms BW-430C; LTG

Therapeutic Category Anticonvulsant, Miscellaneous

Generic Available No

Use Adjunctive treatment of partial seizures in adults (with or without secondary generalized seizures) and generalized seizures of Lennox-Gastaut syndrome in pediatric and adult patients; monotherapy of partial seizures in adults who are converted from a single enzyme-inducing AED
   Note: Preliminary investigations have shown potential efficacy as add-on therapy for absence, atypical absence, generalized tonic-clonic, atonic, tonic, and myoclonic seizures; and as monotherapy in adults and adolescents for partial seizures and idiopathic generalized tonic-clonic seizures; additional studies are underway

Pregnancy Risk Factor C

Contraindications Hypersensitivity to lamotrigine or any component

Warnings Skin rash may occur (10%) and can be serious enough to require hospitalization or discontinuation of drug; serious skin rashes (including Stevens-Johnson syndrome) occur in ~1% of pediatric patients and in 0.3% of adults; in addition to pediatric age, the risk of rash may be increased in patients receiving valproic acid, high initial doses, or with rapid dosage increases; rash usually appears in the first 2-8 weeks of therapy, but may occur after prolonged treatment (eg, 6 months). Benign rashes may occur, but one cannot predict which rashes will become serious or life-threatening; the manufacturer recommends (ordinarily) discontinuation of lamotrigine at the first sign of rash (unless rash is clearly not drug related); discontinuation of lamotrigine may not prevent rash from becoming life-threatening or permanently disfiguring or disabling

Precautions Use with caution and decrease the dose in patients with renal or moderate to severe hepatic dysfunction; do not abruptly discontinue; when discontinuing therapy, gradually reduce the dose by ~50% per week and taper over at least 2 weeks unless safety concerns require a more rapid withdrawal. Lamotrigine binds to melanin and may possibly accumulate in the eye and other tissues rich in melanin; long-term ophthalmologic effects are unknown.

Adverse Reactions
   Central nervous system: Dizziness, sedation, headache, agitation, ataxia, fever; exacerbation of seizures has been reported
   (Continued)

Lamotrigine *(Continued)*

Dermatologic: Rash (higher incidence in children and in patients receiving valproic acid, high initial lamotrigine doses, or rapid dosage increases), angioedema, Stevens-Johnson syndrome, photosensitivity

Gastrointestinal: Nausea, vomiting

Ocular: Diplopia, amblyopia, nystagmus

Drug Interactions Acetaminophen may increase the clearance of lamotrigine; carbamazepine, when administered at the same time as lamotrigine, may increase adverse effects such as dizziness, diplopia, ataxia (space administration of drugs by at least 1 hour); valproic acid may increase incidence of rash and increases half-life and serum concentrations of lamotrigine; enzyme-inducing drugs (eg, carbamazepine, phenytoin) decrease lamotrigine's half-life by ~50%; lamotrigine may increase the clearance of valproic acid

Food Interactions Absorption is not affected by food

Stability Store at room temperature in a dry place away from heat and light

Mechanism of Action A triazine derivative which affects voltage-sensitive sodium channels and inhibits presynaptic release of glutamate and aspartate (excitatory amino acid CNS neurotransmitters)

Pharmacokinetics

Absorption: Oral: Rapid, 97.6% absorbed

Distribution: V_d: Adults: 1.1 L/kg; range: 0.9-1.3 L/kg; crosses into breast milk

Protein binding: 55% (primarily albumin)

Metabolism: >75% metabolized in the liver via glucuronidation; autoinduction may occur

Bioavailability: 98%

Half-life:

Children:

With enzyme-inducing AEDs (eg, phenytoin, carbamazepine): ~7-10 hours

With enzyme inducer and valproic acid (VPA): ~15-27 hours

With VPA: ~44-94 hours

Adults:

Normal: Single dose: 33 hours; multiple dose: ~25 hours

With enzyme-inducing AEDs: ~13-14 hours (range: 8-33 hours)

With enzyme inducer and VPA: ~27 hours

With VPA: 59 hours (range: 30-89 hours)

Hepatic dysfunction: Child-Pugh classification:

Grade A: 36 hours

Grade B: 60 hours

Grade C: 110 hours

Renal dysfunction (Cl_{cr} 13 mL/minute): ~43 hours

Severe renal dysfunction (Cl_{cr} <10 mL/minute): 57.4 hours

During dialysis: 13 hours

Time to peak serum concentration: Oral: ~2 hours (range: 1.4-4.8 hours); select patients may have second peak at 4-6 hours due to enterohepatic recirculation

Elimination: 75% to 90% excreted as glucuronide metabolites and 10% as unchanged drug

Dialysis: ~20% is removed during 4-hour hemodialysis period

Usual Dosage Note: Dosage depends on patient's concomitant medications, ie, valproic acid and enzyme-inducing AEDs (such as phenytoin, phenobarbital, carbamazepine, and primidone) (see Additional Information)

Adjunctive (add-on) therapy:

Children 2-12 years: **Note: Only whole tablets should be used for dosing**; children 2-6 years will likely require maintenance doses at the higher end of recommended range

Patients receiving AED regimens containing valproic acid:

Weeks 1 and 2: 0.15 mg/kg/day in 1-2 divided doses; round dose down to the nearest whole tablet; use 2 mg every other day for patients weighing >6.7 kg and <14 kg

Weeks 3 and 4: 0.3 mg/kg/day in 1-2 divided doses; round dose down to the nearest whole tablet

Maintenance dose: Titrate dose to effect; after week 4, increase dose every 1-2 weeks by a calculated increment; calculate increment as 0.3 mg/kg/day rounded down to the nearest whole tablet; add this amount to the previously administered daily dose; usual maintenance: 1-5 mg/kg/day in 1-2 divided doses; maximum: 200 mg/day

Patients receiving **enzyme-inducing** AED regimens **without** valproic acid:

Weeks 1 and 2: 0.6 mg/kg/day in 2 divided doses; round dose down to the nearest whole tablet

Weeks 3 and 4: 1.2 mg/kg/day in 2 divided doses; round dose down to the nearest whole tablet

Maintenance dose: Titrate dose to effect; after week 4, increase dose every 1-2 weeks by a calculated increment; calculate increment as 1.2 mg/kg/day rounded down to the nearest whole tablet; add this amount to the previously administered daily dose; usual maintenance: 5-15 mg/kg/day in 2 divided doses; maximum: 400 mg/day

Children >12 years and Adults:

Patients receiving AED regimens containing valproic acid:

Weeks 1 and 2: 25 mg every other day

Weeks 3 and 4: 25 mg every day

Maintenance dose: Titrate dose to effect; after week 4, increase dose every 1-2 weeks by 25-50 mg/day; usual maintenance: 100-400 mg/day in 1-2 divided doses; usual maintenance in patients adding lamotrigine to valproic acid **alone**: 100-200 mg/day

Patients receiving **enzyme-inducing** AED regimens **without** valproic acid:

Weeks 1 and 2: 50 mg/day

Weeks 3 and 4: 100 mg/day in 2 divided doses

Maintenance dose: Titrate dose to effect; after week 4, increase dose every 1-2 weeks by 100 mg/day; usual maintenance: 300-500 mg/day in 2 divided doses; doses as high as 700 mg/day in 2 divided doses have been used

Conversion from single enzyme-inducing AED to lamotrigine monotherapy: **Note**: First add lamotrigine and titrate it to the recommended maintenance monotherapy dose, while maintaining the enzyme-inducing AED at a fixed level; then gradually withdraw the enzyme-inducing AED over a 4-week period

Children ≥16 years and Adults:

Weeks 1 and 2: 50 mg/day

Weeks 3 and 4: 100 mg/day in 2 divided doses

Maintenance dose: After week 4, increase dose every 1-2 weeks by 100 mg/day; recommended maintenance monotherapy dose: 500 mg/day in 2 divided doses

Dosage adjustment in hepatic impairment:

Moderate impairment, Child-Pugh Grade B: Reduce initial, escalation, and maintenance doses by ~50%

Severe impairment , Child-Pugh Grade C: Reduce initial, escalation, and maintenance doses by ~75%

Note: Adjust escalation and maintenance doses by clinical response

Administration Oral: May be administered without regard to food

Regular tablet: Do not chew, as a bitter taste may result

Chewable, dispersible tablet: Only whole tablets should be administered; may swallow whole, chew, or disperse in water or diluted fruit juice; if chewed, administer a small amount of water or diluted fruit juice to help in swallowing. To disperse, add tablets to a small amount of liquid (~1 teaspoon or enough to cover the medication); when the tablets are completely dispersed (in about 1 minute), swirl the solution and administer the entire amount immediately. Do not attempt to administer partial quantities of dispersed tablets.

Monitoring Parameters Seizure frequency, duration, and severity

Reference Range Clinical value of serum concentrations not well established; proposed therapeutic range: 1-5 µg/mL

Patient Information Report any rash, fever, or swelling of glands to the physician immediately

Additional Information Low water solubility. Does **not** induce P-450 microsomal enzymes. The effect of AEDs (other than enzyme-inducing AEDs and valproic acid) on the metabolism of lamotrigine is not known and no specific dosing guidelines are recommended. Prudence dictates conservative initial doses and titration (as with regimens containing valproic acid); expected maintenance dosing would fall between maintenance doses with valproic acid and maintenance doses of enzyme-inducing AED regimens without valproic acid.

Dosage Forms

Tablet: 25 mg, 100 mg, 150 mg, 200 mg

Tablet, chewable, dispersible: 2 mg, 5 mg, 25 mg

Extemporaneous Preparations A 1 mg/mL oral suspension made from tablets and 2 different vehicles (a 1:1 mixture of Ora-Sweet® and Ora-Plus®, or a 1:1 mixture of Ora-Sweet® SF and Ora-Plus®) was stable for 91 days when stored in amber plastic prescription bottles at room temperature (25°C) or under refrigeration (4°C); grind one 100 mg tablet in a mortar into a fine powder; add a small amount of the vehicle and mix well to form a uniform paste; mix while adding the vehicle in geometric proportions to **almost** 100 mL; transfer the mixture to a graduated (Continued)

Lamotrigine *(Continued)*

cylinder and qsad with vehicle to make 100 mL; label "shake well" and "protect from light" (Nahata, 1999)

> Nahata MC, Morosco RS, and Hipple TF, "Stability of Lamotrigine in Two Extemporaneously Prepared Oral Suspensions at 4°C and 25°C," *Am J Health Syst Pharm*, 1999, 56(3):240-2.

References

Battino D, Estienne M, and Avanzini G, "Clinical Pharmacokinetics of Antiepileptic Drugs in Paediatric Patients: Part II. Phenytoin, Carbamazepine, Sulthiame, Lamotrigine, Vigabatrin, Oxcarbazepine, and Felbamate," *Clin Pharmacokinet*, 1995, 29(5):341-69.

Besag FM, Wallace SJ, Dulac O, et al, "Lamotrigine for the Treatment of Epilepsy in Childhood," *J Pediatr*, 1995, 127(6):991-7.

Burstein AH, "Lamotrigine," *Pharmacotherapy*, 1995, 15(2):129-43.

Dooley J, Camfield P, Gordon K, et al, "Lamotrigine-Induced Rash in Children," *Neurology*, 1996, 46(1):240-2.

Fitton A, and Goa KL, "Lamotrigine: An Update of its Pharmacology and Therapeutic Use in Epilepsy," *Drugs*, 1995, 50(4):691-713.

Messenheimer JA, "Lamotrigine," *Epilepsia*, 1995, 36(Suppl 2):S87-94.

Messenheimer JA, Giorgi L, and Risner ME, "The Tolerability of Lamotrigine in Children," *Drug Saf*, 2000, 22(4):303-12.

Nahata MC, Morosco RS, and Hipple RT, "Stability of Lamotrigine in Two Extemporaneously Prepared Oral Suspensions at 4°C and 25°C," *Am J Health Syst Pharm*, 1999, 56(93):240-2.

♦ **Lamprene**® *see* Clofazimine *on page 253*

♦ **Lanacane**® **[OTC]** *see* Benzocaine *on page 135*

♦ **Laniazid**® **Oral** *see* Isoniazid *on page 554*

♦ **Lanoxicaps**® *see* Digoxin *on page 330*

♦ **Lanoxin**® *see* Digoxin *on page 330*

Lansoprazole *(lan SOE pra zole)*

U.S. Brand Names Prevacid®

Therapeutic Category Gastric Acid Secretion Inhibitor; Gastrointestinal Agent, Gastric or Duodenal Ulcer Treatment; Proton Pump Inhibitor

Generic Available No

Use Short-term treatment (up to 4 weeks) for healing and symptomatic relief of active duodenal ulcer; short-term treatment (up to 8 weeks) for healing and symptomatic relief of all grades of erosive esophagitis; maintenance of healed erosive esophagitis; pathological hypersecretory conditions, including Zollinger-Ellison syndrome; adjuvant therapy in the treatment of *Helicobacter pylori*-associated antral gastritis; short-term treatment of symptomatic gastroesophageal reflux disease (GERD); prevention and treatment of NSAID-associated gastric ulcers

Pregnancy Risk Factor B

Contraindications Hypersensitivity to lansoprazole or any component

Warnings Long-term effects are not known; enterochromaffin (ECF)-like hyperplasia and subsequent carcinoids have developed in rats following lifetime exposure to high doses (150 mg/kg/day)

Precautions Symptomatic response to therapy does not preclude the presence of gastric malignancy; use with caution in patients with liver disease, dosage reduction should be considered

Adverse Reactions

Cardiovascular: Angina, hypertension, hypotension, palpitations

Central nervous system: Fatigue, dizziness, headache

Dermatologic: Rash

Gastrointestinal: Abdominal pain, nausea, melena, anorexia, cholelithiasis, xerostomia, dyspepsia, eructation, discoloration of feces, flatulence, hypergastrinemia, increased appetite, diarrhea

Hepatic: Elevated serum transaminases

Otic: Tinnitus

Renal: Proteinuria

Drug Interactions Cytochrome P-450 isoenzyme CYP2C19 and CYP3A3/4 substrate

Due to profound and long-lasting inhibition of gastric acid secretion, potential for interfering with the absorption of drugs where acid pH is important exists (such as ketoconazole, ampicillin, iron salts, and digoxin); sucralfate delays and decreases lansoprazole absorption by 30%; lansoprazole increases theophylline clearance mildly (~10%)

Food Interactions Food decreases lansoprazole's bioavailability by 50%

Stability Lansoprazole is unstable in acidic media (eg, stomach contents) and is, therefore, administered as enteric coated granules in capsule form

Mechanism of Action Suppresses gastric acid secretion by selectively inhibiting the parietal cell membrane enzyme (H+, K+)-ATPase or proton pump; demonstrates antimicrobial activity against *Helicobacter pylori*

Pharmacodynamics

Duration of antisecretory activity: >24 hours

Relief of symptoms:

Gastric or duodenal ulcers: 1 week

Reflux esophagitis: 1-4 weeks

Ulcer healing:

Duodenal: 2 weeks

Gastric: 4 weeks

Pharmacokinetics

Absorption: Extremely acid labile and will degrade in acid pH of stomach; enteric coated granules improve bioavailability (80%)

Protein binding: 97%

Metabolism: Extensive by the liver to inactive metabolites; in acid media of gastric parietal cell, lansoprazole is transformed to active sulfanilamide metabolite

Half-life: Plasma: 1.3-1.7 hours

Time to peak serum concentration: 1.7 hours

Elimination: 14% to 25% in urine as metabolites; <1% as unchanged drug; biliary excretion is major route of elimination

Usual Dosage Oral:

Children: Limited data in single dose studies in children 3 months to 14 years; dosing range used: 0.5-1.6 mg/kg:

<10 kg: 7.5 mg

10-20 kg: 15 mg

≥20 kg: 30 mg

Children ≥12 years and Adults:

Duodenal ulcer: 15 mg once daily for 4 weeks; maintenance therapy: 15 mg once daily

Primary gastric ulcer (and also associated with NSAID use): 30 mg once daily for up to 8 weeks

Erosive esophagitis: 30 mg once daily for up to 8 weeks; additional 8 weeks may be tried in those patients who failed to respond or for a recurrence of esophagitis; maintenance: 15 mg once daily

GERD: 15 mg once daily for up to 8 weeks

Pathological hypersecretory conditions: Initial: 60 mg daily; adjust dosage based upon patient response; doses of 90 mg twice daily have been used; administer doses >120 mg/day in divided doses

Reflux esophagitis: 30-60 mg daily for 8 weeks

Helicobacter pylori-associated antral gastritis: 30 mg twice daily for 2 weeks (in combination with 1 g amoxicillin and 500 mg clarithromycin given twice daily for 14 days). Alternatively, in patients allergic to or intolerant of clarithromycin or in whom resistance to clarithromycin is known or suspected, lansoprazole 30 mg every 8 hours and amoxicillin 1 g every 8 hours may be given for 2 weeks

Prevention of NSAID-associated gastric ulcer: 15 mg daily for up to 12 weeks

Administration Oral: Administer before eating; capsules may be opened and mixed with small amount of applesauce prior to administration without affecting the bioavailability; do not chew granules; for nasogastric tube administration, the capsules can be opened, the granules mixed (not crushed) with 40 mL of apple, cranberry, grape, orange, pineapple, prune, tomato, and V-8® vegetable juice, and then injected through the NG tube into the stomach; granules remain intact when mixed and stored for up to 30 minutes

Monitoring Parameters Patients with Zollinger-Ellison syndrome should be monitored for gastric acid output, which should be maintained at 10 mEq/hour or less during the last hour before the next lansoprazole dose; lab monitoring should include CBC, liver function, renal function, and serum gastrin levels

Reference Range Plasma levels do not correlate with pharmacologic activity

Dosage Forms Capsule, delayed release: 15 mg, 30 mg

Extemporaneous Preparations A 3 mg/mL suspension of lansoprazole is prepared by emptying the contents of ten 30 mg capsules and adding 100 mL 8.4% sodium bicarbonate solution; stir for 30 minutes; protect from light; stable for 8 hours at room temperature and for 14 days refrigerated (DiGiacinto, 2000). **Note:** The same formulation was studied by Phillips, et al. A 2-week stability at room temperature and 4-week stability under refrigeration were reported.

DiGiacinto JL, Olsen KM, Bergman KL, et al, "Stability of Suspension Formulations of Lansoprazole and Omeprazole Stored in Amber-Colored Plastic Oral Syringes," *Ann Pharmacother*, 2000, 34(5):600-4.

(Continued)

Lansoprazole *(Continued)*

Phillips JO, Metzler MH, and Olsen K, "The Stability of SImplified Lansoprazole Suspension (SLS)," *Gastroen*, 1999, 116:A89.

References

Chun AH, Eason CJ, Shi HH, et al, "Lansoprazole: An Alternative Method of Administration of a Capsule Dosage Formulation," *Clin Ther*, 1995, 17(3):441-7.

Oderda G, Chiorboli E, Haitink AR, "Inhibition of Hastric ACidity in Children by Lansoprazole Granules," *Gastroent*, 1998, 114(4pt2):A295.

Tran A, et al, "Pharmacokinetics/Pharmacodynamics Study of Oral Lansoprazole in Children," *Fundam Clin Pharmacol*, 1996, 10:A221.

- ♦ **Lantus®** *see* Insulin Preparations *on page 538*
- ♦ **Lanvis (Can)** *see* Thioguanine *on page 950*
- ♦ **Largactil (Can)** *see* Chlorpromazine *on page 226*
- ♦ **Larodopa®** *see* Levodopa *on page 585*
- ♦ **Lasix®** *see* Furosemide *on page 462*
- ♦ **Lasix Special (Can)** *see* Furosemide *on page 462*
- ♦ **Lassar's Zinc Paste** *see* Zinc Oxide *on page 1026*
- ♦ **Lavacol®** [OTC] *see* Ethyl Alcohol *on page 409*
- ♦ **Laxative Pills (Can)** *see* Senna *on page 896*
- ♦ **Laxilose (Can)** *see* Lactulose *on page 571*
- ♦ **LazerSporin-C® Otic** *see* Neomycin, (Bacitracin) Polymyxin B, and Hydrocortisone *on page 705*
- ♦ *L*-Bunolol *see* Levobunolol *on page 584*
- ♦ **L-carnitine** *see* Carnitine *on page 184*
- ♦ **LCD** *see* Coal Tar *on page 260*
- ♦ **LCR** *see* Vincristine *on page 1011*
- ♦ *L*-Dopa *see* Levodopa *on page 585*
- ♦ **Le 500 D (Can)** *see* Cascara Sagrada *on page 185*
- ♦ **Ledercillin® VK** *see* Penicillin V Potassium *on page 774*
- ♦ **Legatrin® [OTC]** *see* Quinine *on page 862*
- ♦ **Lenoltec No 4 (Can)** *see* Acetaminophen and Codeine *on page 31*
- ♦ **Lente® Iletin® II** *see* Insulin Preparations *on page 538*

Leucovorin *(loo koe VOR in)*

Synonyms Citrovorum Factor; Folinic Acid; 5-Formyl Tetrahydrofolate

Therapeutic Category Antidote, Methotrexate; Folic Acid Derivative

Generic Available Yes

Use Diminish toxicity and counteract the effects of impaired methotrexate elimination and of inadvertent overdosages of folic acid antagonists; treatment of folate deficient megaloblastic anemias of infancy, sprue, pregnancy; nutritional deficiency when oral folate therapy is not possible; adjunctive treatment with sulfadiazine and pyrethamine to prevent hematologic toxicity

Pregnancy Risk Factor C

Contraindications Pernicious anemia and other megaloblastic anemias secondary to the lack of vitamin B_{12}

Warnings Administer promptly; when the time interval between administration of folic acid antagonists and leucovorin rescue increases, its effectiveness in treatment of toxicity diminishes

Adverse Reactions

Dermatologic: Rash, pruritus, erythema, urticaria

Hematologic: Thrombocytosis

Respiratory: Wheezing

Miscellaneous: Anaphylactoid reactions

Drug Interactions Leucovorin enhances the toxicity of fluorouracil; high doses of leucovorin may reduce the efficacy of intrathecally administered methotrexate

Stability When powder for injection is reconstituted with bacteriostatic water for injection, stability is 7 days at room temperature; protect from light; when doses >10 mg/m^2 are used, prepare leucovorin with preservative free sterile water to decrease the amount of benzyl alcohol intake; do not mix in the same solution with 5-fluorouracil as precipitation occurs

Mechanism of Action A derivative of tetrahydrofolic acid, a reduced form of folic acid; does not require a reduction by dihydrofolate reductase for activation; allows for purine and thymidine synthesis, a necessity for normal erythropoiesis; leucovorin supplies the necessary cofactor blocked by methotrexate, enters the cells via the same active transport system as methotrexate

Pharmacodynamics Onset of action:
Oral: Within 30 minutes
I.V.: Within 5 minutes

Pharmacokinetics
Absorption: Oral, I.M.: Rapid
Metabolism: Rapidly converted to (5MTHF) 5-methyl-tetrahydrofolate (active) in the intestinal mucosa and by the liver
Bioavailability:
Oral absorption is saturable in doses >25 mg; apparent bioavailability:
Tablet, 25 mg: 97%
Tablet, 50 mg: 75%
Tablet, 100 mg: 37%
Injection solution, when administered orally, provides equivalent bioavailability
Half-life:
Leucovorin: 15 minutes
5MTHF: 33-35 minutes
Elimination: Primarily in urine (80% to 90%) with small losses appearing in feces (5% to 8%)

Usual Dosage Children and Adults:
Treatment of folic acid antagonist overdosage (eg, pyrimethamine, trimethoprim): Oral: 2-15 mg/day for 3 days or until blood counts are normal or 5 mg every 3 days; doses of 6 mg/day are needed for patients with platelet counts <100,000/mm³
Folate deficient megaloblastic anemia: I.M.: 1 mg/day
Megaloblastic anemia secondary to congenital deficiency of dihydrofolate reductase: I.M.: 3-6 mg/day
Rescue dose: I.V.: 10 mg/m² to start, then 10 mg/m² every 6 hours orally for 72 hours; if serum creatinine 24 hours after methotrexate is elevated ≥50% **or** the serum methotrexate concentration is >5 x 10⁻⁶ M (see graph), increase dose to 100 mg/m²/dose every 3 hours until serum methotrexate level is less than 1 x 10⁻⁸ M

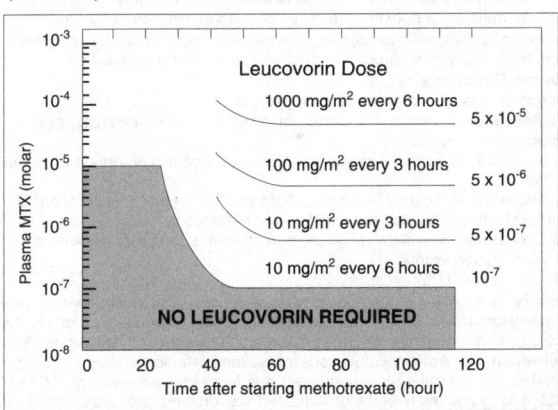

LEUCOVORIN RESCUE DOSE
(Determined by Plasma Methotrexate Level and Time After Start of Methotrexate Infusion)

Adjunctive treatment with sulfadiazine to prevent hematologic toxicity (for toxoplasmosis): Infants, Children, and Adults: Oral, I.V.: 5-10 mg every 3 days (see Sulfadiazine *on page 923*)
Adjunctive treatment with pyrimethamine to prevent hematologic toxicity (*Pneumocystis carinii*): Adolescents and Adults: Oral, I.V.: 25 mg once weekly
Investigational: Post I.T. methotrexate: Oral, I.V.: 12 mg/m² as a single dose; post high-dose methotrexate: 100-1000 mg/m²/dose until the serum methotrexate level is less than 1 x 10⁻⁷ molar

Administration
Oral: **This drug should be given parenterally instead of orally in patients with GI toxicity, nausea, vomiting, and when individual doses are >25 mg.**
(Continued)

Leucovorin *(Continued)*

Parenteral: Reconstitute 50 mg or 100 mg powder for injection vials with 5-10 mL sterile water (350 mg vial requires 17 mL diluent resulting in 20 mg/mL final concentration); infuse at a maximum rate of 160 mg/minute.

Monitoring Parameters CBC with differential; plasma methotrexate concentration as a therapeutic guide to high-dose methotrexate therapy with leucovorin factor rescue. Leucovorin is continued until the plasma methotrexate level is less than 1 x 10^{-7} molar. Each dose of leucovorin is increased if the plasma methotrexate concentration is excessively high (see graph). With 4- to 6-hour high-dose methotrexate infusions, plasma drug values in excess of 5 x 10^{-5} and 10^{-6} molar at 24 and 48 hours after starting the infusion, respectively, are often predictive of delayed methotrexate clearance; see graph.

Dosage Forms

Injection, as calcium: 10 mg/mL (10 mL, 25 mL, 50 mL)

Powder for injection, as calcium: 50 mg, 100 mg, 200 mg, 350 mg, 500 mg

Tablet, as calcium: 5 mg, 10 mg, 15 mg, 25 mg

♦ **Leukeran**® *see* Chlorambucil *on page 217*

♦ **Leukine**® *see* Sargramostim *on page 890*

Leuprolide *(loo PROE lide)*

U.S. Brand Names Lupron®; Lupron Depot®; Lupron Depot-3® Month; Lupron Depot-4® Month; Lupron Depot-Ped™

Synonyms Leuprorelin

Therapeutic Category Antineoplastic Agent, Hormone (Gonadotropin Hormone-Releasing Antigen); Luteinizing Hormone-Releasing Hormone Analog

Generic Available No

Use Treatment of precocious puberty; palliative treatment of advanced prostate carcinoma

Pregnancy Risk Factor X

Contraindications Pernicious anemia; hypersensitivity to leuprolide or any component; pregnancy

Warnings The FDA currently recommends that procedures for proper handling and disposal of antineoplastic agents be considered; gonadotropin-releasing hormone (GnRH) analog treatment of rodents has shown an increased incidence of pituitary tumors; urinary tract obstruction may occur upon initiation of therapy

Precautions Use with caution in patients with hypersensitivity to benzyl alcohol; long-term safety of leuprolide in children has not been established

Adverse Reactions

Cardiovascular: Edema, cardiac arrhythmias

Central nervous system: Dizziness, lethargy, insomnia, headache, pain

Dermatologic: Rash

Endocrine & metabolic: Estrogenic effects (gynecomastia, breast tenderness), hot flashes

Gastrointestinal: Nausea, vomiting, diarrhea, GI bleeding, constipation, anorexia

Hematologic: Decreased hemoglobin and hematocrit

Neuromuscular & skeletal: Myalgia, paresthesia, bone pain, weakness

Ocular: Blurred vision

Miscellaneous: Diaphoresis

Stability Refrigerate leuprolide acetate injection; leuprolide (Depot®) powder for suspension and its diluent may be stored at room temperature; upon reconstitution, the suspension is stable for 24 hours; protect from light and heat; do not freeze vials

Mechanism of Action Continuous daily administration results in suppression of ovarian and testicular steroidogenesis due to decreased levels of LH and FSH so that puberty and the pubertal growth spurt are arrested; produces a "medical castration" in prostate cancer patients

Pharmacokinetics

Serum testosterone levels first increase within 3 days of therapy, then decrease after 2-4 weeks with continued therapy; requires parenteral administration since it is rapidly destroyed within the GI tract

Protein binding: 7% to 15%

Bioavailability:

Oral: 0%

S.C.: 94%

Half-life: 3 hours

Elimination: Not well defined

Usual Dosage Refer to individual protocol

Children: Precocious puberty:
  I.M. (Depot®) formulation: 0.15-0.3 mg/kg/dose given every 28 days; minimum dose: 7.5 mg; younger children generally require higher dosages on a mg/kg basis than older children
    Initial dose for girls <8 years or boys <9 years (titrate dose in 3.75 mg increments every 4 weeks until clinical or laboratory tests indicate no disease progression):
      <25 kg: 7.5 mg every 4 weeks
      25-37.5 kg: 11.25 mg every 4 weeks
      >37.5 kg: 15 mg every 4 weeks
  S.C.: 35-50 mcg/kg once daily
Adults: Advanced prostatic carcinoma:
  I.M. (Depot® formulation): 7.5 mg/dose given monthly **or** 22.5 mg once every 3 months
  S.C.: 1 mg/day

Administration
Parenteral: Do not administer I.V.:
  I.M.: For the Depot® formulation, diluent is added to the vial to form a milky suspension
  S.C.: 5 mg/mL solution is administered undiluted into areas on the arm, thigh, or abdomen

Monitoring Parameters Precocious puberty: Height, weight, bone age, Tanner staging test, GnRH testing (blood LH and FSH levels), testosterone in males and estradiol in females; closely monitor patients with prostatic carcinoma for plasma testosterone, acid phosphatase, and signs of weakness, paresthesias, and urinary tract obstruction during the first few weeks of therapy

Patient Information Female patients should be informed that menstruation or spotting may occur for the first 2 months of therapy; notify physician if vaginal bleeding continues after 2 months of drug therapy

Nursing Implications Rotate S.C. and I.M. injection sites periodically

Dosage Forms
Injection, as acetate: 5 mg/mL (2.8 mL)
Powder for injection (depot), as acetate:
  Depot®: 3.75 mg, 7.5 mg
  Depot-3® Month: 11.25 mg, 22.5 mg
  Depot-4® Month: 30 mg
  Depot-Ped™: 7.5 mg, 11.25 mg, 15 mg

References
Kappy MS, Stuart T, and Perelman A, "Efficacy of Leuprolide Therapy in Children With Central Precocious Puberty," *Am J Dis Child*, 1988, 142(10):1061-4.
Lee PA and Page JG, "Effects of Leuprolide in the Treatment of Central Precocious Puberty," *J Pediatr*, 1989, 114(2):321-4.

♦ **Leuprorelin** *see* Leuprolide *on page 582*
♦ **Leurocristine** *see* Vincristine *on page 1011*
♦ **Leustatin**™ *see* Cladribine *on page 245*

Levalbuterol (leve al BYOO ter ole)

U.S. Brand Names Xopenex™
Synonyms Levosalbutamol; R-albuterol; R-salbutamol
Therapeutic Category Adrenergic Agonist Agent; Antiasthmatic; Beta$_2$-Adrenergic Agonist Agent; Bronchodilator; Sympathomimetic
Generic Available No
Use Treatment and prevention of bronchospasm in patients with reversible obstructive airway disease
Pregnancy Risk Factor C
Contraindications Hypersensitivity to levalbuterol, any component, albuterol, or adrenergic amine
Warnings Paradoxical bronchospasm may occur, especially with the first use
Precautions Use with caution in patients with hyperthyroidism, hypokalemia, diabetes mellitus, cardiovascular disorders including coronary insufficiency, hypertension, or history of arrhythmias; excessive or prolonged use can lead to tolerance
Adverse Reactions
Cardiovascular: Tachycardia, hypertension, hypotension, syncope, EKG abnormalities, chest pain
Central nervous system: Nervousness, dizziness, anxiety, headache, insomnia
Endocrine & metabolic: Hyperglycemia, hypokalemia
Gastrointestinal: Dyspepsia, diarrhea, xerostomia, dry throat, gastroenteritis, nausea
(Continued)

Levalbuterol *(Continued)*

Neuromuscular & skeletal: Leg cramps, pain, tremor

Ocular: Eye itching

Respiratory: Cough, rhinitis, sinusitis, turbinate edema, paradoxical bronchospasm

Miscellaneous: Hypersensitivity reactions, flu-like syndrome

Drug Interactions Action of levalbuterol is antagonized by beta-adrenergic blocking agents such as propranolol; cardiovascular effects are potentiated in patients also receiving MAO inhibitors or tricyclic antidepressants; concomitant administration of sympathomimetics may result in enhanced cardiovascular effects

Food Interactions Caffeinated beverages may increase side effects of levalbuterol

Stability Store at room temperature; protect from light; after the foil covering is removed, use within 2 weeks; discard vial if solution is not colorless

Mechanism of Action R-enantiomer of racemic albuterol; relaxes bronchial smooth muscle by action on $beta_2$-receptors with little effect on heart rate

Pharmacodynamics

Onset of action: 10-17 minutes

Peak effect: 1.5 hours

Duration of action: 5-6 hours

Pharmacokinetics Nebulization:

Distribution: V_d: Adults: 1900 L

Metabolism: In the liver to an inactive sulfate

Half-life: 3.3-4.0 hours

Time to peak serum concentration: 0.2-1.8 hours

Elimination: 3% to 6% excreted unchanged in urine

Usual Dosage Inhalation by nebulization (**dosage expressed in terms of mg levalbuterol**):

Children 2-11 years: Limited data; in a randomized, double-blind, single dose, crossover study (Gawchik, 1999), doses ranging from 0.16-1.25 mg were used safely with clinically significant improvements in pulmonary function tests

Children ≥12 years and Adults: 0.63 mg 3 times/day, every 6-8 hours; may be increased to 1.25 mg 3 times/day

Administration Inhalation: By nebulization only; no dilution required

Monitoring Parameters Serum potassium, heart rate, asthma symptoms, pulmonary function tests, respiratory rate; arterial or capillary blood gases (if patient's condition warrants)

Patient Information Do not exceed recommended dosage; rinse mouth with water following each inhalation to help with dry throat and mouth; if more than one inhalation is necessary, wait at least 1 full minute between inhalations; notify physician if palpitations, tachycardia, chest pain, muscle tremors, dizziness, or headache occur, or if breathing difficulty persists; limit caffeinated beverages

Additional Information 0.63 mg levalbuterol comparable to 2.5 mg albuterol

Dosage Forms Solution, for inhalation: 0.63 mg/3 mL [0.73 mg levalbuterol hydrochloride] (3 mL); 1.25 mg/3 mL [1.44 mg levalbuterol hydrochloride] (3 mL)

References

Gawchik SM, Saccar CL, Noonan M, et al, "The Safety and Efficacy of Nebulized Levalbuterol Compared With Racemic Albuterol and Placebo in the Treatment of Asthma in Pediatric Patients," *J Allergy Clin Immunol*, 1999, 103(4):615-21.

♦ **Levaquin**™ *see* Levofloxacin *on page 586*

♦ **Levarterenol** *see* Norepinephrine *on page 722*

♦ **Levate (Can)** *see* Amitriptyline *on page 77*

♦ **Levbid**® *see* Hyoscyamine *on page 517*

Levobunolol *(lee voe BYOO noe lole)*

U.S. Brand Names AKBeta®; Betagan® Liquifilm®

Canadian Brand Names Novo-Levobunolol; Ophtho-Bunolol; PMS-Levobunolol

Synonyms *L*-Bunolol

Therapeutic Category Beta-Adrenergic Blocker, Ophthalmic

Generic Available Yes

Use To lower intraocular pressure in chronic open-angle glaucoma or ocular hypertension

Pregnancy Risk Factor C

Contraindications Hypersensitivity to levobunolol or any component; asthma, severe COPD, sinus bradycardia, second or third degree A-V block, cardiogenic shock

Warnings Contains metabisulfite; avoid use in susceptible individuals; use only in combination with miotic for patients with angle closure glaucoma

Precautions Use with caution in patients with CHF, diabetes mellitus, hyperthyroidism, myasthenia gravis

Adverse Reactions
Cardiovascular: Bradycardia, arrhythmias, hypotension, palpitations, cerebral ischemia, cerebral vascular accident, syncope, heart block, CHF
Central nervous system: Dizziness, headache, depression, ataxia, cerebral ischemia
Dermatologic: Rash, alopecia, itching
Endocrine & metabolic: Masked symptoms of hypoglycemia in diabetics
Gastrointestinal: Nausea, heartburn, diarrhea
Ocular: Stinging, burning, erythema, itching, blepharoconjunctivitis, keratitis, ptosis, decreased visual acuity, conjunctivitis, tearing
Respiratory: Bronchospasm

Drug Interactions May have additive toxicity with systemic beta-adrenergic blocking drugs; ophthalmic epinephrine decreases effectiveness

Mechanism of Action A nonselective beta-adrenergic blocking agent that lowers intraocular pressure by reducing aqueous humor production

Pharmacodynamics
Onset of action: Following ophthalmic instillation, decreases in intraocular pressure can be noted within 1 hour
Peak effect: Within 2-6 hours
Maximal effectiveness: 2-3 weeks
Duration: 1-7 days

Pharmacokinetics
Absorption: May be absorbed systemically and produce systemic side effects
Metabolism: Extensively metabolized into several metabolites; primary metabolite (active) dihydrolevobunolol
Elimination: Not well defined

Usual Dosage Adults: 1-2 drops of 0.5% solution in eye(s) once daily or 1-2 drops of 0.25% solution twice daily; may increase to 1 drop of 0.5% solution twice daily

Administration Intraocular: Apply drops into conjunctival sac of affected eye(s); avoid contacting bottle tip with skin; apply gentle pressure to lacrimal sac during and immediately following instillation (1-2 minutes) to decrease systemic absorption; see manufacturer's information regarding proper usage of C Cap (compliance cap)

Monitoring Parameters Intraocular pressure

Dosage Forms Solution, ophthalmic, as hydrochloride:
Betagan®: 0.25% [2.5 mg/mL] (5 mL, 10 mL, 15 mL)
AKBeta®, Betagan®: 0.5% [5 mg/mL] (2 mL, 5 mL, 10 mL, 15 mL)

♦ **Levocarnitine** see Carnitine on page 184

Levodopa (lee voe DOE pa)

Related Information
Serotonin Syndrome on page 1247

U.S. Brand Names Larodopa®

Synonyms L-3-Hydroxytyramine; L-Dopa

Therapeutic Category Anti-Parkinson's Agent; Diagnostic Agent, Growth Hormone Function

Generic Available No

Use Diagnostic agent for growth hormone deficiency; treatment of Parkinson's disease

Pregnancy Risk Factor C

Contraindications Hypersensitivity to levodopa or any component; narrow-angle glaucoma, MAO inhibitor therapy, melanomas, or any undiagnosed skin lesions

Warnings GI hemorrhage has occurred in patients with a history of peptic ulcer disease; some products contain tartrazine which may cause hypersensitivity reactions in susceptible individuals

Precautions Use cautiously in patients with severe cardiovascular disease or pulmonary disease, asthma, occlusive cerebrovascular disease, renal, hepatic, or endocrine disease, affective disorders, major psychoses, cardiac arrhythmias, and chronic wide-angle glaucoma

Adverse Reactions
Cardiovascular: Orthostatic hypotension, palpitations, cardiac arrhythmias, hypertension
Central nervous system: Memory loss, nervousness, anxiety, insomnia, fatigue, hallucinations, dystonic movements, ataxia, headache, confusion
Gastrointestinal: Nausea, vomiting, GI bleeding, constipation, anorexia, xerostomia
Hematologic: Hemolytic anemia
(Continued)

Levodopa *(Continued)*

Neuromuscular & skeletal: Muscle twitching
Ocular: Blurred vision, eyelid spasms
Miscellaneous: Discoloration of sweat

Drug Interactions Antacids increase bioavailability of levodopa; benzodiazepines, hydantoins, methionine, papaverine, and pyridoxine decrease levodopa's effectiveness; iron salts and anticholinergics decrease GI absorption of levodopa; MAO inhibitors may increase hypertensive reaction; levodopa may decrease metoclopramide's effects; methyldopa may have additive hypotensive effects

Food Interactions High protein diets may decrease the efficacy of levodopa when used for parkinsonism via competition with amino acids in crossing the blood-brain barrier; avoid foods high in pyridoxine content such as liver, fish, whole grain cereals, peas, and beans

Mechanism of Action Increases dopamine levels in the brain; stimulates dopaminergic receptors in the basal ganglia to improve the balance between cholinergic and dopaminergic activity

Pharmacokinetics

Metabolism: Majority of drug is peripherally decarboxylated to dopamine; small amounts of levodopa reach the brain where it is also decarboxylated to active dopamine

Half-life: 1.2-2.3 hours

Time to peak serum concentration: Oral: Within 1-2 hours

Elimination: Primarily in urine (80%) as dopamine, norepinephrine, and homovanillic acid

Usual Dosage

Children: Oral (given as a single dose to evaluate growth hormone deficiency)

0.5 g/m^2 **or**

<30 lb: 125 mg

30-70 lb: 250 mg

>70 lb: 500 mg

Adults: Parkinson's disease: 500-1000 mg/day in divided doses every 6-12 hours; increase by 100-750 mg/day every 3-7 days until response or total dose of 8000 mg is reached

Administration Oral: Administer with food

Monitoring Parameters Growth hormone level

Test Interactions False-positive reaction for urinary glucose with Clinitest®; false-negative reaction using Clinistix®; false-positive urine ketones with Acetest®, Ketostix®, Labstix®; false-positive Coombs' test; false increase in uric acid with colorimetric method

Dosage Forms Tablet: 250 mg

References

Cara JF and Johanson HJ, "Growth Hormone for Short Stature Not Due to Classic Growth Hormone Deficiency," *Pediatr Clin North Am*, 1990, 37(6):1229-54.

Levofloxacin *(lee voe FLOKS a sin)*

U.S. Brand Names Levaquin™; Quixin™ Ophthalmic

Therapeutic Category Antibiotic, Ophthalmic; Antibiotic, Quinolone

Generic Available No

Use Treatment of acute maxillary sinusitis, lower respiratory tract infections, skin and skin structure infections, complicated urinary tract infections and acute pyelonephritis due to multidrug-resistant organisms susceptible to levofloxacin including *Streptococcus pneumoniae* (including penicillin-resistant strains), *S. aureus*, *Haemophilus influenzae*, *H. parainfluenzae*, *Moraxella catarrhalis*, *Klebsiella pneumoniae*, *Legionella pneumophila*, *Chlamydia pneumoniae*, *Mycoplasma pneumoniae*, *E. coli*, *Enterococcus fecalis*, *S. pyogenes*, *Proteus mirabilis*, *Enterobacter cloacae*, (Less active than ciprofloxacin against *Pseudomonas aeruginosa*); infectious diarrhea due to enterotoxigenic *E. coli*, *Shigella*, *Salmonella*, *Campylobacter* spp, *Vibrio parahaemolyticus*. Used ophthalmically for treatment of bacterial conjunctivitis due to *S. aureus* (methicillin-susceptible strains), *S. epidermidis*, *S. pneumoniae*, *Streptococcus* (groups C/F), *Streptococcus* (group G), Viridans group *Streptococci*, *Corynebacterium* spp, *H. influenzae*, *Acinetobacter iwoffii*, or *Serratia marcescens*.

Pregnancy Risk Factor C

Contraindications Hypersensitivity to levofloxacin, any component, or other quinolones. Not recommended for use in pregnant women or during breast-feeding

Warnings Not recommended in children <18 years of age; levofloxacin increased the incidence and severity of osteochondrosis in immature rats and dogs. Fluoroquinolones have caused arthropathy with erosions of the cartilage in weight-bearing joints of immature animals; Achilles tendonitis and tendon rupture have been reported with fluoroquinolones; prolonged use may result in superinfection; CNS stimulation and increased intracranial pressure may occur resulting in tremors, restlessness, confusion, and rarely hallucinations or convulsive seizures; serious and occasionally fatal hypersensitivity and/or anaphylactic reactions have been reported often following the first dose

Precautions Use with caution in patients with known or suspected CNS disorders, seizure disorders, or renal impairment; modify dosage in patients with renal impairment. Rare cases of torsade de pointes have been reported in patients taking levofloxacin so use with caution in patients on concurrent therapy with Class Ia or Class III antiarrhythmics or in patients with bradycardia, hypokalemia, or hypomagnesemia

Adverse Reactions

Cardiovascular: Cardiac failure, hypertension, hypotension, bradycardia, tachycardia, edema, torsade de pointes (rare)

Central nervous system: Dizziness, fever, headache, insomnia, seizures, fatigue, nervousness, restlessness, confusion, hallucinations, anxiety, lightheadedness,

Dermatologic: Photosensitivity, pruritus, urticaria, rash, Stevens-Johnson syndrome

Gastrointestinal: Nausea, vomiting, diarrhea, constipation, anorexia, abdominal pain, pseudomembranous colitis

Genitourinary: Vaginitis

Hematologic: Granulocytopenia, leukopenia, thrombocytopenia

Hepatic: Elevated liver enzymes

Local: With I.V.: Phlebitis, burning, pain, erythema, swelling

Neuromuscular & skeletal: Tremor, arthralgia, tendonitis

Ocular: Ophthalmic solution: Foreign body sensation, transient decreased vision; ocular pain, burning, itching, dryness, discomfort, photophobia

Miscellaneous: Anaphylaxis

Drug Interactions Cytochrome P-450 isoenzyme CYP1A2 enzyme inhibitor (minor) Decreased absorption with antacids containing aluminum, magnesium, and/or calcium, sucralfate, metal cations (ie, zinc, iron, copper, magnesium), and didanosine; may decrease serum levels of phenytoin; cimetidine and probenecid increase serum levels and half-life of levofloxacin; concomitant use with foscarnet or NSAIDs may increase risk of seizures

Food Interactions Iron and mineral supplements decrease levofloxacin concentrations

Stability Injection is stable for 72 hours when diluted to 5 mg/mL in a compatible I.V. fluid (ie, D_5W, NS, D_5W with NaCl and KCl, D_5LR) and stored at room temperature; stable for 14 days when stored under refrigeration; incompatible with mannitol, sodium bicarbonate, multivalent cations (eg, magnesium)

Mechanism of Action L-isomer of the racemate, ofloxacin, levofloxacin inhibits DNA gyrase (bacterial topoisomerase II) thereby inhibiting relaxation of supercoiled DNA and promoting breakage of DNA strands. DNA gyrase maintains the superhelical structure of DNA and is required for DNA replication, transcription, repair, recombination and transposition.

Pharmacokinetics

Absorption: Well absorbed

Distribution: Widely distributed in the body including blister fluid, macrophages, lung tissue; excreted in breast milk

V_d: Adults: 89-112

Protein binding: 24% to 38%

Bioavailability: Oral: 99%

Half-life: 6-8 hours

Time to peak serum concentration: Oral: Within 1-2 hours; food prolongs the time to peak by approximately 1 hour and decreases the peak concentration by 14%

Elimination: 87% excreted unchanged in urine over 48 hours by tubular secretion and glomerular filtration

Dialysis: Not removed by hemodialysis or peritoneal dialysis

Usual Dosage

Oral, I.V.:

Children: **Note:** Limited information regarding levofloxacin use in pediatric patients is currently available in the literature; some centers recommend initial doses of 5-10 mg/kg/dose every 24 hours; maximum dose: 500 mg

Adults:

Chronic bronchitis: 500 mg every 24 hours for 7 days

Community-acquired pneumonia: 500 mg every 24 hours for 7-14 days

Acute maxillary sinusitis: 500 mg every 24 hours for 10-14 days

Uncomplicated skin infections: 500 mg every 24 hours for 7-10 days

Complicated UTI or acute pyelonephritis: 250 mg every 24 hours for 10 days

(Continued)

Levofloxacin *(Continued)*

Drug-resistant tuberculosis: 500-1000 mg every 24 hours (maximum dose: 1 g)
Travelers' diarrhea: 500 mg every 24 hours for up to 3 days

Children ≥1 year and Adults: Ophthalmic:
Treatment day 1 and day 2: Instill 1-2 drops into affected eye(s) every 2 hours while awake, up to 8 times/day
Treatment day 3 through 7: Instill 1-2 drops into affected eye(s) every 4 hours while awake, up to 4 times/day

Dosing interval in renal impairment:
Cl_{cr} 20-49 mL/minute: Administer 250 mg every 24 hours (initial dose: 500 mg)
Cl_{cr} 10-19 mL/minute: Administer 250 mg every 48 hours (initial dose: 500 mg for most infections; 250 mg for UTI or pyelonephritis)

Administration
Oral: May administer with or without food; avoid antacid use; drink plenty of fluids to maintain proper hydration and urine output
Parenteral: Final concentration for administration should not exceed 5 mg/mL; administer by slow I.V. infusion over 60 minutes; avoid rapid or bolus I.V. infusion due to risk of hypotension
Ophthalmic: Not for subconjunctival injection or for use into anterior chamber of the eye. Contact lenses should not be worn during treatment; instill drops into conjunctival sac of affected eye(s); avoid contacting bottle tip with skin

Monitoring Parameters Patient receiving concurrent levofloxacin and theophylline should have serum levels of theophylline monitored; monitor INR in patients receiving warfarin; monitor blood glucose in patients receiving antidiabetic agents; monitor renal and hematopoietic function periodically; number and type of stools/day for diarrhea

Patient Information Avoid exposure to direct sunlight; drink plenty of fluids; may cause dizziness or lightheadedness and impair ability to perform activities which require mental alertness; notify physician if tendon pain or swelling occurs, palpitations or chest pain, signs of allergy, or if persistent diarrhea occurs

Nursing Implications Do not administer antacids with or within 2 hours before or 2 hours after a levofloxacin dose; ensure adequate patient hydration

Dosage Forms
Infusion, in D_5W: 5 mg/mL (50 mL, 100 mL)
Injection: 25 mg/mL (20 mL)
Solution, ophthalmic: 0.5% (2.5 mL, 5 mL)
Tablet: 250 mg, 500 mg

Extemporaneous Preparations A 50 mg/mL oral suspension made from six 500 mg tablets and two different vehicles (a 1:1 mixture of Ora-Plus® and strawberry syrup NF) was stable for 57 days when stored in amber plastic prescription bottles at room temperature (23°C to 25°C) or under refrigeration (3°C to 5°C); crush six 500 mg tablets in a mortar into a fine powder; add a small amount of the vehicle and mix well to form a uniform paste; mix while adding the vehicle in geometric proportions to almost 60 mL; transfer the mixture to a graduated cylinder and qsad with vehicle to make 60 mL; label "shake well."

VandenBussche HL, Johnson CE, Fontana EM, et al, "Stability of Levofloxacin in an Extemporaneously Compounded Oral Liquid," *Am J Health Syst Pharm*, 1999, 56(22):2316-8.

References
Ernst ME, Ernst EJ, and Klepser ME, "Levofloxacin and Trovafloxacin: The Next Generation of Fluoroquinolones?" *Am J Health Syst Pharm*, 1997, 54(22):2569-84.
Schaad UB, "Role of the New Quinolones in Pediatric Practice," *Pediatr Infect Dis J*, 1992, 11(12):1043-6.

♦ **Levophed®** *see* Norepinephrine *on page 722*
♦ **Levosalbutamol** *see* Levalbuterol *on page 583*
♦ **Levo-T (Can)** *see* Levothyroxine *on page 588*
♦ **Levotec (Can)** *see* Levothyroxine *on page 588*
♦ **Levothroid®** *see* Levothyroxine *on page 588*

Levothyroxine *(lee voe thye ROKS een)*

U.S. Brand Names Levothroid®; Levoxyl®; Synthroid®; Unithroid®
Canadian Brand Names Eltroxin; Levo-T; Levotec
Synonyms *L*-Thyroxine; T_4 Thyroxine
Therapeutic Category Thyroid Product
Generic Available Yes
Use Replacement or supplemental therapy in hypothyroidism; management of nontoxic goiter, chronic lymphocytic thyroiditis, as adjunctive therapy with antithyroid agents in thyrotoxicosis to prevent goitrogenesis and hypothyroidism

Pregnancy Risk Factor A

Contraindications Hypersensitivity to levothyroxine sodium or any component; recent MI or thyrotoxicosis; uncorrected adrenal insufficiency

Warnings High doses may produce serious or even life-threatening toxic effects particularly when used with some anorectic drugs; use with extreme caution in patients with cardiovascular disease, adrenal insufficiency, hypertension or coronary artery disease; patients with diabetes mellitus and insipidus may have their symptoms exaggerated or aggravated

Adverse Reactions

Cardiovascular: Palpitations, tachycardia, cardiac arrhythmias, angina, CHF, hypertension

Central nervous system: Nervousness, insomnia, fever, headache

Dermatologic: Alopecia

Gastrointestinal: Diarrhea, abdominal cramps, increased appetite, weight loss

Neuromuscular & skeletal: Tremor

Miscellaneous: Diaphoresis

Drug Interactions Cholestyramine resin, iron salts, sodium polystyrene sulfonate, aluminum hydroxide, and sucralfate decrease absorption; antidiabetic drug requirements are increased; estrogens increase thyroid requirements; levothyroxine increases effect of oral anticoagulants; phenytoin may decrease levothyroxine levels

Food Interactions Limit intake of goitrogenic foods (asparagus, cabbage, peas, turnip greens, broccoli, spinach, brussel sprouts, lettuce, soybeans); soybean-based formulas may decrease absorption

Stability I.V. form must be prepared immediately prior to administration

Mechanism of Action Primary active compound is T_3 (triiodothyronine), which may be converted from T_4 (thyroxine); exact mechanism of action is unknown; however, it is believed the thyroid hormone exerts its many metabolic effects through control of DNA transcription and protein synthesis; involved in normal metabolism, growth, and development; promotes gluconeogenesis, increases utilization and mobilization of glycogen stores, and stimulates protein synthesis, increases basal metabolic rate

Pharmacodynamics

Onset of action:

Oral: 3-5 days for therapeutic effects

I.V.: Within 6-8 hours

Pharmacokinetics

Absorption: Oral: Erratic (48% to 79%)

Metabolism: In the liver to triiodothyronine (active)

Half-life: 6-7 days

Time to peak serum concentration: Within 2-4 hours

Elimination: In feces and urine

Usual Dosage

Neonates, Infants, and Children: Daily dosage:

Oral:

0-6 months: 8-10 mcg/kg or 25-50 mcg

6-12 months: 6-8 mcg/kg or 50-75 mcg

1-5 years: 5-6 mcg/kg or 75-100 mcg

6-12 years: 4-5 mcg/kg or 100-150 mcg

>12 years: 2-3 mcg/kg or ≥150 mcg

Growth and puberty complete: 1.6 mcg/kg

I.V., I.M.: 50% to 75% of the oral dose

Adults:

Oral: 12.5-50 mcg/day to start, then increase by 25-50 mcg/day at intervals of 2-4 weeks; average adult dose: 100-200 mcg/day

I.V., I.M.: 50% of the oral dose

Myxedema coma or stupor: I.V.: 300-500 mcg one time, then 75-100 mcg daily; begin oral therapy as soon as tolerated

Thyroid suppression therapy: Oral: 2-6 mcg/kg/day for 7-10 days

Administration

Oral: Administer on an empty stomach

Parenteral: Dilute vial with 5 mL NS; use immediately after reconstitution; administer by direct I.V. infusion over 2- to 3-minute period; may administer I.M.

Monitoring Parameters T_4, TSH, heart rate, blood pressure, clinical signs of hypo- and hyperthyroidism; TSH is the most reliable guide for evaluating adequacy of thyroid replacement dosage. TSH may be elevated during the first few months of thyroid replacement despite patients being clinically euthyroid. In cases where T_4 remains low and TSH is within normal limits, an evaluation of "free" (unbound) T_4 is needed to evaluate further increase in dosage

(Continued)

Levothyroxine (Continued)

Reference Range See normal values in Normal Laboratory Values for Children *on page 1187*

Test Interactions Many drugs may have effects on thyroid function tests: para-aminosalicylic acid, aminoglutethimide, amiodarone, barbiturates, carbamazepine, chloral hydrate, clofibrate, colestipol, corticosteroids, danazol, diazepam, estrogens, ethionamide, fluorouracil, I.V. heparin, insulin, lithium, methadone, methimazole, mitotane, nitroprusside, oxyphenbutazone, phenylbutazone, PTU, perphenazine, phenytoin, propranolol, salicylates, sulfonylureas, and thiazides

Patient Information Do not change brands without physician's knowledge; report immediately to physician any chest pain, increased pulse, palpitations, heat intolerances, excessive sweating; do not discontinue without notifying physician

Additional Information Levothroid® tablets contain lactose; 15-37.5 mcg liothyronine = 50-60 mcg levothyroxine = 60 mg thyroid USP = 45 mg Thyroid Strong® = 60 mg thyroglobulin = 50-60 mcg liotrix

Dosage Forms

Powder for injection, as sodium, lyophilized (Synthroid®): 0.2 mg/vial; 0.5 mg/vial

Tablet, as sodium: 0.025 mg, 0.05 mg, 0.075 mg, 0.088 mg, 0.1 mg, 0.112 mg, 0.125 mg, 0.15 mg, 0.137 mg, 0.175 mg, 0.2 mg, 0.3 mg

Extemporaneous Preparations A 25 mcg/mL extemporaneous suspension may be compounded by crushing twenty-five 0.1 mg tablets; measure 40 mL glycerol; triturate powder into a pourable suspension with a small amount of glycerol and transfer to a calibrated 100 mL amber bottle; rinse the mortar with about 10 mL of the glycerol and pour into the bottle; repeat until the glycerol is used up; add water to bring the oral liquid to a total volume of 100 mL; label "shake well" and "refrigerate". The suspension is stable 8 days refrigerated.

Boulton DV, Fawcett JP, and Woods DJ, "Stability of an Extemporaneously Compounded Levothyroxine Sodium Oral Liquid," *Am J Health-Syst Pharm*, 1996; 53:1157-61.

- ♦ **Levoxyl®** *see Levothyroxine on page 588*
- ♦ **Levsin®** *see Hyoscyamine on page 517*
- ♦ **Levsinex®** *see Hyoscyamine on page 517*
- ♦ **Levsin/SL®** *see Hyoscyamine on page 517*
- ♦ **LH-RH** *see Gonadorelin on page 482*
- ♦ **Lidemol (Can)** *see Fluocinolone on page 439*
- ♦ **Lidemol (Can)** *see Fluocinonide on page 440*
- ♦ **Lidex®** *see Fluocinonide on page 440*
- ♦ **Lidex-E®** *see Fluocinonide on page 440*

Lidocaine (LYE doe kane)

Related Information

Adult ACLS Algorithm, Stable Ventricular Tachycardia *on page 1047*
Adult ACLS Algorithm, V. Fib and Pulseless VT *on page 1041*
CPR Pediatric Drug Dosages *on page 1031*
Emergency Pediatric Drip Calculations *on page 1033*
Pediatric ALS Algorithm, Pulseless Arrest *on page 1036*
Pediatric ALS Algorithm, Tachycardia - Rapid Rhythm and Adequate Perfusion *on page 1037*
Pediatric ALS Algorithm, Tachycardia - Rapid Rhythm and Evidence of Poor Perfusion *on page 1038*

U.S. Brand Names Anestacon®; ELA-Max® [OTC]; ELA-Max® 5 [OTC]; Lidoderm®; Solarcaine® Aloe Extra Burn Relief [OTC]; Xylocaine®; Xylocaine® MPF; Xylocaine® Viscous; Zilactin®-L [OTC]

Canadian Brand Names Afterburn; Lidodan; PMS-Lidocaine Viscous; Solarcaine Lidocaine; Xylocaine; Xylocard; Zilactin-L

Synonyms Lignocaine

Therapeutic Category Analgesic, Topical; Antiarrhythmic Agent, Class I-B; Local Anesthetic, Injectable; Local Anesthetic, Topical

Generic Available Yes

Use Ventricular ectopy, ventricular tachycardia (VT), ventricular fibrillation (VF); for pulseless VT or VF **after** defibrillation and epinephrine; control of hemodynamically compromising premature ventricular contractions; stable, monomorphic VT (with normal or impaired cardiac function); stable, polymorphic VT (with normal baseline or prolonged QT interval); local anesthetic; pain relief of postherpetic neuralgia

Pregnancy Risk Factor B

Contraindications Hypersensitivity to lidocaine, amide-type local anesthetics, or any component; patients with Adams-Stokes syndrome or with severe degree of S-A, A-V, or intraventricular heart block (without a pacemaker)

Warnings Decrease dose in patients with decreased cardiac output or hepatic disease; do not use lidocaine solutions containing epinephrine for treatment of arrhythmias; do not use preservative-containing solution for I.V. use; do not apply patch to larger areas or for longer than recommended (toxicities may result)

Precautions Hepatic disease, heart failure, marked hypoxia, severe respiratory depression, hypovolemia or shock; incomplete heart block or bradycardia, atrial fibrillation

Adverse Reactions

Cardiovascular: Bradycardia, hypotension, heart block, arrhythmias, cardiovascular collapse

Central nervous system: Lethargy, coma, agitation, slurred speech, seizures, anxiety, euphoria, hallucinations

Gastrointestinal: Nausea, vomiting

Local: Thrombophlebitis; with patch: Erythema, edema, abnormal sensation

Neuromuscular & skeletal: Paresthesia, muscle twitching

Ocular: Blurred vision, diplopia

Respiratory: Respiratory depression or arrest

Miscellaneous: Allergic and anaphylactoid reactions (rare)

Drug Interactions Cytochrome P-450 isoenzyme CYP 3A3/4 substrate

Cimetidine or beta-blockers may increase lidocaine serum concentration and toxicity; Class I antiarrhythmic agents (mexiletine, tocainide) may increase adverse or toxic effects

Mechanism of Action Class IB antiarrhythmic; suppresses automaticity of conduction tissue by increasing electrical stimulation threshold of ventricle, HIS-Purkinje system, and spontaneous depolarization of the ventricles during diastole by a direct action on the tissues; blocks both the initiation and conduction of nerve impulses by decreasing the neuronal membrane's permeability to sodium ions, which results in inhibition of depolarization with resultant blockade of conduction

Pharmacodynamics

Antiarrhythmic effect:

Onset of action (single I.V. bolus dose): 45-90 seconds

Duration: 10-20 minutes

Local anesthetic effect: Duration: 1-2 hours

Pharmacokinetics

Distribution: V_d alterable by many patient factors; decreased V_d in CHF and liver disease

Protein binding: 60% to 80%; binds to alpha$_1$-acid glycoprotein

Metabolism: 90% in the liver; active metabolites monoethylglycinexylidide (MEGX) and glycinexylidide (GX) can accumulate and may cause CNS toxicity

Half-life, biphasic:

Alpha: 7-30 minutes

Beta, terminal:

Infants, premature: 3.2 hours

Adults: 1.5-2 hours

CHF, liver disease, shock, severe renal disease: Prolonged half-life

Elimination: <10% excreted unchanged in urine

Dialysis: Dialyzable (0% to 5%)

Usual Dosage

Children and Adults:

Topical: Apply to affected area as needed; maximum dose: 3 mg/kg/dose; do not repeat within 2 hours

Injectable local anesthetic: Dose varies with procedure, degree of anesthesia needed, vascularity of tissue, duration of anesthesia required, and physical condition of patient; maximum dose: 4.5 mg/kg/dose; do not repeat within 2 hours

Children:

I.V., I.O.: (**Note:** For use in pulseless VT or VF, give after defibrillation and epinephrine): Loading dose: 1 mg/kg; follow with continuous infusion; may administer second bolus of 0.5-1 mg/kg if delay between bolus and start of infusion is >15 minutes; continuous infusion: 20-50 mcg/kg/minute. Use 20 mcg/kg/minute in patients with shock, hepatic disease, cardiac arrest, mild CHF; moderate to severe CHF may require ½ loading dose and lower infusion rates to avoid toxicity.

E.T.: 2-10 times the I.V. bolus dose

(Continued)

Lidocaine *(Continued)*

Adults (decrease the dose in patients with CHF, acute MI with hypotension, shock, poor peripheral perfusion states, or hepatic disease; usual bolus dose, but ½ of normal maintenance infusion should be used in these patients):

I.V.:

Antiarrhythmic: Initial bolus: 1-1.5 mg/kg; may repeat doses of 0.5-0.75 mg/kg every 5-10 minutes if needed to a total of 3 mg/kg; continuous infusion: Initial: 1-4 mg/minute

Ventricular fibrillation or pulseless VT (after defibrillation and epinephrine or vasopressin): Initial dose: 1-1.5 mg/kg IVP; may repeat 0.5-0.75 mg in 3-5 minutes; maximum total dose: 3 mg/kg; follow with continuous infusion after return of perfusion; continuous infusion: 1-4 mg/min; **Note:** Use only bolus doses for cardiac arrest caused by VF or pulseless VT

Patients with impaired cardiac function: Initial bolus: 0.5-0.75 mg/kg IVP; may repeat every 5-10 minutes; follow with continuous infusion: Initial: 1-4 mg/min; maximum total dose: 3 mg/kg (administered over 1 hour)

Prevention of ventricular fibrillation: I.V.: Initial bolus: 0.5 mg/kg; repeat every 5-10 minutes to a total dose of 2 mg/kg

Refractory ventricular fibrillation: Repeat 1.5 mg/kg bolus may be given 3-5 minutes after initial dose

E.T.: 2-2.5 times the I.V. bolus dose

I.M.: Prehospital post-MI antiarrhythmic prophylaxis: 300 mg

Lidoderm® patch: Postherpetic neuralgia: Apply patch to most painful areas; up to 3 patches may be applied per application; patch may remain in place for up to 12 hours in any 24-hour period

Administration

Endotracheal:

Children: Dilute to 5 mL with NS prior to E.T. administration; follow ET administration with 5 manual ventilations

Adults: Dilute in 10 mL NS or distilled water prior to E.T. administration (**Note:** Use of distilled water results in greater absorption, but a greater adverse effect on PaO_2)

Parenteral: I.V.: Solutions of 40-200 mg/mL must be diluted for I.V. use; final concentration not to exceed 20 mg/mL for I.V. push or 8 mg/mL for I.V. infusion; I.V. push rate of administration should not exceed 0.7 mg/kg/minute or 50 mg/minute, whichever is less; I.V. continuous infusion must be administered with a calibrated infusion device

Transdermal: Apply patch to intact skin so most painful area is covered; do not apply to broken or inflamed skin; patch may be cut to appropriate size; remove immediately if burning sensation occurs; wash hands after applying patch; avoid eye contact; keep out of the reach of children; dispose of used patch properly (see Additional Information)

Monitoring Parameters Monitor EKG continuously; serum concentrations with continuous infusion; I.V. site (local thrombophlebitis may occur with prolonged infusions)

Reference Range

Therapeutic: 1.5-5 µg/mL (SI: 6-21 µmol/L)

Potentially toxic: >6 µg/mL (SI: >26 µmol/L)

Toxic: >9 µg/mL (SI: >38 µmol/L)

Nursing Implications Multiple products and concentrations exist; use of an I.V. fluid filter is recommended where possible

Additional Information Transdermal patches (both used and unused) may cause toxicities in children; used patches still contain large amounts of lidocaine; store and dispose patches out of the reach of children

Dosage Forms

Cream, rectal, as hydrochloride (ELA-Max® 5): 5% (30 g)

Cream, topical, as hydrochloride (ELA-Max®): 4% (5 g, 30 g)

Gel, topical, as hydrochloride (Solarcaine® Extra Burn Relief): 0.5% (120 g)

Injection, as hydrochloride: 0.5% [5 mg/mL] (50 mL); 1% [10 mg/mL] (2 mL, 5 mL, 10 mL, 20 mL, 30 mL, 50 mL); 1.5% [15 mg/mL] (20 mL); 2% [20 mg/mL] (2 mL, 5 mL, 10 mL, 20 mL, 30 mL, 50 mL); 4% [40 mg/mL] (5 mL, 50 mL); 10% [100 mg/mL] (10 mL); 20% [200 mg/mL] (10 mL)

Xylocaine®: 0.5% [5 mg/mL] (50 mL); 1% [10 mg/mL] (2 mL, 5 mL, 10 mL, 20 mL, 30 mL, 50 mL); 2% [20 mg/mL] (2 mL, 5 mL, 10 mL, 20 mL, 30 mL, 50 mL); 4% [40 mg/mL] (5 mL, 50 mL)

Injection, preservative free, as hydrochloride (Xylocaine® MPF): 0.5% [5 mg/mL] (50 mL); 1% [10 mg/mL] (2 mL, 5 mL, 10 mL, 20 mL, 30 mL, 50 mL); 2% [20 mg/mL] (2 mL, 5 mL, 10 mL, 20 mL, 30 mL, 50 mL); 4% [40 mg/mL] (5 mL, 50 mL)

Injection, as hydrochloride:
Direct I.V.: 1% [10 mg/mL] (5 mL); 2% [20 mg/mL] (5 mL)
I.V. admixture, preservative free: 4% [40 mg/mL] (25 mL); 10% [100 mg/mL] (10 mL); 20% [200 mg/mL] (5 mL, 10 mL)
I.V. infusion, in D$_5$W: 0.2% [2 mg/mL] (500 mL); 0.4% [4 mg/mL] (250 mL, 500 mL); 0.8% [8 mg/mL] (250 mL, 500 mL)
Jelly, topical, as hydrochloride (Anestacon®, Xylocaine®): 2% (15 mL, 30 mL)
Liquid, topical, as hydrochloride (Zilactin®-L): 2.5% (10 mL) [OTC]
Liquid, viscous, as hydrochloride (Xylocaine® Viscous): 2% (20 mL, 100 mL, 450 mL)
Ointment, topical, as hydrochloride (Xylocaine®): 2.5% [OTC], 5% (3.5 g, 35 g)
Solution, topical, as hydrochloride: 2% [20 mg/mL] (15 mL, 240 mL)
Xylocaine®: 4% [40 mg/mL] (50 mL)
Spray, topical, as hydrochloride (Solarcaine® Extra Burn Relief): 0.5% (135 g)
Transdermal patch (Lidoderm®): 5% (30s)

References
"Guidelines 2000 for Cardiopulmonary Resuscitation and Emergency Cardiovascular Care, Part 6: Advanced Cardiovascular Life Support, The American Heart Association in Collaboration With the International Liaison Committee on Resuscitation," *Circulation*, 2000, 102(8 Suppl):I86-171.
"Guidelines 2000 for Cardiopulmonary Resuscitation and Emergency Cardiovascular Care, Part 10: Pediatric Advanced Life Support, The American Heart Association in Collaboration With the International Liaison Committee on Resuscitation," *Circulation*, 2000, 102(8 Suppl): I291-342.

Lidocaine and Epinephrine (LYE doe kane & ep i NEF rin)

U.S. Brand Names Xylocaine® MPF With Epinephrine; Xylocaine® With Epinephrine
Synonyms Epinephrine and Lidocaine
Therapeutic Category Local Anesthetic, Injectable
Generic Available Yes
Use Local infiltration anesthesia
Pregnancy Risk Factor B
Contraindications Hypersensitivity to epinephrine, lidocaine, amide-type local anesthetics, or any component
Warnings Some products contain sulfites which may cause allergic reactions
Precautions Do not use solutions in distal portions of the body (digits, nose, ears, penis); do not use large doses in patients with conduction defects (ie, heart block)
Adverse Reactions
Cardiovascular: Hypotension, bradycardia
Central nervous system: Lightheadedness, nervousness, confusion, dizziness, drowsiness, convulsions
Dermatologic: Urticaria
Neuromuscular & skeletal: Tremor
Ocular: Blurred vision
Otic: Tinnitus
Mechanism of Action Lidocaine blocks both the initiation and conduction of nerve impulses via decreased permeability of sodium ions; epinephrine increases the duration of action of lidocaine by causing vasoconstriction (via alpha effects) which slows the vascular absorption of lidocaine
Pharmacodynamics
Peak effect: Within 5 minutes
Duration: 2-6 hours, dependent on dose and anesthetic procedure
Usual Dosage Dosage varies with the anesthetic procedure
Children: Use lidocaine concentrations of 0.5% or 1% (or even more dilute) to decrease possibility of toxicity; lidocaine dose (when using combination product of lidocaine and epinephrine) should not exceed 7 mg/kg/dose; do not repeat within 2 hours
Administration Local injection: Before injecting, withdraw syringe plunger to make sure that injection is not into vein or artery; do not administer I.V. or intra-arterially
Additional Information Use preservative free solutions for epidural or caudal use
Dosage Forms Injection:
Xylocaine® With Epinephrine:
Epinephrine 1:200,000 and lidocaine hydrochloride 0.5% [5 mg/mL] (50 mL)
Epinephrine 1:200,000 and lidocaine hydrochloride 1% [10 mg/mL] (30 mL)
Epinephrine 1:200,000 and lidocaine hydrochloride 1.5% [15 mg/mL] (5 mL, 10 mL, 30 mL)
Epinephrine 1:200,000 and lidocaine hydrochloride 2% [20 mg/mL] (20 mL)
Epinephrine 1:100,000 and lidocaine hydrochloride 1% [10 mg/mL] (20 mL, 50 mL)
Epinephrine 1:100,000 and lidocaine hydrochloride 2% [20 mg/mL] (1.8 mL, 20 mL, 50 mL)
(Continued)

593

Lidocaine and Epinephrine *(Continued)*

Xylocaine® MPF With Epinephrine [preservative free]:

Epinephrine 1:200,000 and lidocaine hydrochloride 1% [10 mg/mL] (10 mL, 30 mL)

Epinephrine 1:200,000 and lidocaine hydrochloride 1.5% [15 mg/mL] (10 mL, 30 mL)

Epinephrine 1:200,000 and lidocaine hydrochloride 2% [20 mg/mL] (20 mL)

Lidocaine and Prilocaine (LYE doe kane & PRIL oh kane)

U.S. Brand Names EMLA®

Synonyms Eutectic Mixture of Lidocaine and Prilocaine; Prilocaine and Lidocaine

Therapeutic Category Analgesic, Topical; Antipruritic, Topical; Local Anesthetic, Topical

Generic Available No

Use Topical anesthetic for use on normal intact skin to provide local analgesia for minor procedures such as I.V. cannulation or venipuncture; topical anesthetic for superficial minor surgery of genital mucous membranes and as an adjunct for local infiltration anesthesia in genital mucous membranes; has also been used for painful procedures such as lumbar puncture and skin graft harvesting

Pregnancy Risk Factor B

Contraindications Hypersensitivity to lidocaine, prilocaine, amide-type local anesthetics, or any component; patients with congenital or idiopathic methemoglobinemia, neonates <37 weeks gestation, infants <12 months of age who are receiving concurrent treatment with methemoglobin-inducing agents (ie, sulfas, acetaminophen, benzocaine, chloroquine, dapsone, nitrofurantoin, nitroglycerin, nitroprusside, phenobarbital, phenytoin, primaquine, quinine)

Precautions Use with caution in patients with severe hepatic disease, patients with G-6-PD deficiency, and patients taking drugs associated with drug-induced methemoglobinemia; adjust dosage by using smaller areas for application in small children (especially infants <3 months of age) or patients with impaired renal or hepatic function

Adverse Reactions

Cardiovascular: Bradycardia, hypotension, shock, angioedema

Central nervous system: Nervousness, euphoria, confusion, dizziness, drowsiness, convulsions, CNS excitation, alteration in temperature sensation

Dermatologic: Rash, urticaria

Hematologic: Methemoglobinemia

Local: Blanching, itching, erythema, edema

Neuromuscular & skeletal: Tremor

Ocular: Blurred vision

Otic: Tinnitus

Respiratory: Respiratory depression, bronchospasm

Drug Interactions Class IB antiarrhythmic drugs (tocainide, mexiletine): toxic effects are additive; drugs known to induce methemoglobinemia (see Contraindications)

Stability Store at room temperature

Mechanism of Action Local anesthetic action occurs by stabilization of neuronal membranes and inhibiting the ionic fluxes required for the initiation and conduction of impulses

Pharmacodynamics

Onset of action: 1 hour for sufficient dermal analgesia

Peak effect: 2-3 hours

Duration: 1-2 hours after removal of the cream

Pharmacokinetics

Absorption: Topical: Related to the duration of application and to the area over which it is applied

3-hour application: 3.6% lidocaine and 6.1% prilocaine were absorbed

24-hour application: 16.2% lidocaine and 33.5% prilocaine were absorbed

Distribution: Both cross the blood-brain barrier; lidocaine and probably prilocaine are excreted in breast milk; V_d:

Lidocaine: 1.1-2.1 L/kg

Prilocaine: 0.7-4.4 L/kg

Protein binding:

Lidocaine: 70%

Prilocaine: 55%

Metabolism:

Lidocaine: Metabolized by the liver to inactive and active metabolites

Prilocaine: Metabolized in both the liver and kidneys

Half-life:
    Lidocaine: 65-150 minutes, prolonged with cardiac or hepatic dysfunction
    Prilocaine: 10-150 minutes, prolonged in hepatic or renal dysfunction
Usual Dosage Topical:
    Newborns ≥37 weeks gestation, Children, and Adults: For minor procedures, apply
    2.5 g/site for at least 60 minutes; for painful procedures, apply 2 g/10 cm² of skin
    and leave on for at least 2 hours; see table.

**EMLA® Cream Maximum Recommended Dose and Application Area* for
Infants and Children Based on Application to Intact Skin**

Age and Body Weight Requirements	Maximum Total Dose of EMLA®	Maximum Application Area	Maximum Application Time
Birth to 3 mo or <5 kg	1g	10 cm²	1 h
3-12 mo and >5 kg	2 g	20 cm²	4 h
1-6 y and >10 kg	10 g	100 cm²	4 h
7-12 y and >20 kg	20 g	200 cm²	4 h

    Adult male genital skin as an adjunct prior to local anesthetic infiltration: Apply 1 g/
    10 cm² to skin surface for 15 minutes followed immediately by local anesthetic
    infiltration after removal of EMLA® cream
    Preliminary results in a study of 30 preterm neonates (n=30) using a single 0.5 g
    dose of EMLA® applied to the heel for 1 hour resulted in no measurable
    changes in methemoglobin levels
Administration Topical: Do not use on mucous membranes or the eyes; apply a
thick layer of cream to intact skin and cover with an occlusive dressing
Patient Information Not for ophthalmic use; for external use only. EMLA® may block
sensation in the treated skin.
Nursing Implications In small infants and children, an occlusive bandage should be
placed over the EMLA® cream to prevent the child from placing the cream in his/her
mouth or smearing the cream on the eyes
Dosage Forms
    Cream: Lidocaine 2.5% and prilocaine 2.5% [2 Tegaderm® dressings] (5 g, 30 g)
    Disc, anesthetic: 1 g
References
    Broadman LM, Soliman IE, Hannallah RS, et al, "Analgesic Efficacy of Eutectic Mixture of Local Anesthetics (EMLA®) vs Intradermal Infiltration Prior to Venous Cannulation in Children," *Am J Anaesth*, 1987, 34:S56.
    Halperin DL, Koren G, Attias D, et al, "Topical Skin Anesthesia for Venous Subcutaneous Drug Reservoir and Lumbar Puncture in Children," *Pediatrics*, 1989, 84(2):281-4.
    Robieux I, Kumar R, Radhakrishnan S, et al, "Assessing Pain and Analgesia With a Lidocaine-Prilocaine Emulsion in Infants and Toddlers During Venipuncture," *J Pediatr*, 1991, 118(6):971-3.
    Taddio A, Shennan AT, Stevens B, et al, "Safety of Lidocaine-Prilocaine Cream in the Treatment of Preterm Neonates," *J Pediatr*, 1995, 127(6):1002-5.

♦ **Lidodan (Can)** *see* Lidocaine *on page 590*
♦ **Lidoderm**® *see* Lidocaine *on page 590*
♦ **Lid-Pack (Can)** *see* Bacitracin and Polymyxin B *on page 129*
♦ **Lignocaine** *see* Lidocaine *on page 590*
♦ **Lin-Amox (Can)** *see* Amoxicillin *on page 80*
♦ **Lin-Buspirone (Can)** *see* Buspirone *on page 159*
♦ **Linctus Codeine Blac (Can)** *see* Codeine *on page 262*

Lindane (LIN dane)
U.S. Brand Names G-well®; Kwell®; Scabene®
Canadian Brand Names Hexit; PMS-Lindane
Synonyms Benzene Hexachloride; Gamma Benzene Hexachloride; Hexachlorocyclohexane
Therapeutic Category Antiparasitic Agent, Topical; Pediculocide; Scabicidal Agent; Shampoos
Generic Available Yes
Use Alternative treatment of scabies (*Sarcoptes scabiei*), *Pediculus capitis* (head lice), and *Pediculus pubis* (crab lice); (the AAP and CDC consider permethrin 5% to be the scabicide of choice due to its safety and efficacy profile; many clinicians no longer recommend lindane as initial therapy for pediculosis due to reports of resistance and neurotoxicity)
Pregnancy Risk Factor B
(Continued)

Lindane (Continued)

Contraindications Hypersensitivity to lindane or any component; premature neonates; pregnant or lactating women; acutely inflamed skin or raw, weeping surfaces

Warnings Avoid contact with the face, eyes, mucous membranes, and urethral meatus

Precautions Use with caution in infants, small children and patients with pre-existing seizure disorders due to its potential for neurologic toxicity; if used in young children, cover hands to prevent accidental lindane ingestion from thumbsucking; **consider alternative therapy for the treatment of scabies in infants and young children <2 years of age (ie, permethrin)**

Adverse Reactions

Cardiovascular: Cardiac arrhythmia

Central nervous system: Dizziness, restlessness, seizures, headache, ataxia

Dermatologic: Eczematous eruptions, contact dermatitis, rash

Gastrointestinal: Nausea, vomiting

Hematologic: Aplastic anemia

Hepatic: Hepatitis

Local: Burning and stinging

Ocular: Conjunctivitis

Renal: Hematuria

Respiratory: Pulmonary edema

Mechanism of Action Directly absorbed by parasites and ova through the exoskeleton; stimulates the nervous system resulting in seizures and death of parasitic arthropods

Pharmacokinetics

Absorption: Topical: Up to 13% absorbed systemically (absorption is greater when applied to damaged skin, face, scalp, neck, or scrotum)

Distribution: Stored in body fat and accumulates in the brain; skin and adipose tissue may act as repositories

Metabolism: By the liver

Half-life, children: 17-22 hours

Time to peak serum concentration: Children: Topical: 6 hours

Elimination: In urine and feces

Usual Dosage Children and Adults: Topical:

Scabies: Apply a thin layer of lotion and massage it on skin from the neck to the toes (head to toe in infants).

Infants: Wash off 6 hours after application

Children: Wash off 6-8 hours after application

Adults: Bathe and remove drug 8-12 hours after application

Do not reapply sooner than 1 week later if live mites appear

Pediculosis: 15-30 mL of shampoo is applied and lathered for 4 minutes; rinse hair thoroughly and comb with a fine tooth comb to remove nits; repeat treatment in 7 days if lice or nits are still present

Pediculosis of the eyelashes: Do not treat with lindane; instead, apply an occlusive ophthalmic ointment like petrolatum to the eyelid margins twice daily for 10 days

Administration

For topical use only; do not apply to face; avoid getting in eyes; do **not** apply lotion immediately after a hot, soapy bath; lotion should be applied to dry, cool skin

Before applying lindane shampoo, wash hair with a plain shampoo, then dry

Patient Information Clothing and bedding should be washed in hot water or by dry cleaning to kill the scabies mite; combs and brushes may be washed with lindane shampoo then thoroughly rinsed with water

Nursing Implications

Children <6 years: ~30 mL lotion is sufficient volume for one application

Children ≥6 years and Adults: ~30-60 mL lotion is sufficient volume for one application

Pruritus associated with scabies or pediculosis may persist for longer than 1 week following treatment with drug. Oral antihistamine and/or topical corticosteroid may be used to help relieve pruritus.

Additional Information Excessive absorption may result in overdose with signs and symptoms which include nausea, vomiting, seizures, headaches, arrhythmias, apnea, pulmonary edema, hematuria, hepatitis, coma, and even death

Dosage Forms

Lotion: 1% (60 mL, 473 mL, 4000 mL)

Shampoo: 1% (60 mL, 473 mL, 4000 mL)

References

Eichenfield LF, Honig PJ, "Blistering Disorders in Childhood," *Pediatr Clin North Am*, 1991, 38(4):959-76.

Hogan DJ, Schachner L, Tanglertsampan C, "Diagnosis and Treatment of Childhood Scabies and Pediculosis," *Pediatr Clin North Am*, 1991, 38(4):941-57.

Pramanik AK and Hansen RC, "Transcutaneous Gamma Benzene Hexachloride Absorption and Toxicity in Infants and Children," *Arch Dermatol*, 1979, 115(10):1224-5.

♦ **Lioresal®** *see* Baclofen *on page 129*

♦ **Liotec (Can)** *see* Baclofen *on page 129*

Liothyronine (lye oh THYE roe neen)

U.S. Brand Names Cytomel®; Triostat™

Synonyms *L*-Triiodothyronine; T_3

Therapeutic Category Thyroid Product

Generic Available Yes

Use Replacement or supplemental therapy in hypothyroidism, management of nontoxic goiter, chronic lymphocytic thyroiditis, as an adjunct in thyrotoxicosis and as a diagnostic aid; levothyroxine is recommended for chronic therapy; (if rapid correction of thyroid is needed, T_3 is preferred, but use cautiously and with lower recommended doses)

Pregnancy Risk Factor A

Contraindications Recent MI or thyrotoxicosis; hypersensitivity to liothyronine sodium or any component; uncorrected adrenal insufficiency

Warnings Patients with diabetes mellitus and insipidus may have their symptoms exaggerated or aggravated. Ineffective for weight reduction; high doses may produce serious or even life-threatening toxic effects particularly when used with some anorectic drugs. Short duration of action permits more rapid assessment of dosage changes and rapid diminution of adverse effects upon discontinuation.

Precautions Use with extreme caution in patients with cardiovascular disease, adrenal insufficiency, or coronary artery disease

Adverse Reactions

Cardiovascular: Palpitations, tachycardia, cardiac arrhythmias, angina, CHF, hypertension

Central nervous system: Nervousness, insomnia, fever, headache

Dermatologic: Alopecia, dermatitis herpetiformis

Gastrointestinal: Diarrhea, abdominal cramps, increased appetite, weight loss

Local: Phlebitis with parenteral form

Neuromuscular & skeletal: Tremor

Miscellaneous: Diaphoresis

Drug Interactions

Cholestyramine resin, iron salts, sodium polystyrene sulfonate, aluminum hydroxide, and sucralfate decrease absorption; antidiabetic drug requirements are increased; estrogens increase thyroid requirements; liothyronine increases effect of oral anticoagulants

Food Interactions Limit intake of goitrogenic foods (asparagus, cabbage, peas, turnip greens, broccoli, spinach, brussel sprouts, lettuce, soybeans)

Stability Store parenteral solution at temperatures between 2°C and 8°C (36°F to 46°F); I.V. form must be prepared immediately prior to administration

Mechanism of Action Primary active compound is T_3 (triiodothyronine), which may be converted from T_4 (thyroxine); exact mechanism of action is unknown, however it is believed the thyroid hormone exerts its many metabolic effects through control of DNA transcription and protein synthesis; involved in normal metabolism, growth, and development; promotes gluconeogenesis, increases utilization and mobilization of glycogen stores, and stimulates protein synthesis; increases basal metabolic rate

Pharmacodynamics

Onset of effect: Within a few hours

Maximum effect: Within 48-72 hours

Duration: Up to 72 hours

Pharmacokinetics

Absorption: Oral: Well absorbed (~85% to 90%)

Metabolism: In the liver to inactive compounds

Half-life: 25 hours (range: 16-49 hours); hypothyroid 1.4 days; hyperthyroid 0.6 days

Elimination: 76% to 83% In urine

Usual Dosage

Congenital hypothyroidism (Cretinism): Neonates, Infants, and Children <3 years: Oral: 5 mcg/day; increase by 5 mcg every 3 days to a maximum dosage of 20 mcg/day for neonates and infants, 50 mcg/day for children 1-3 years of age

(Continued)

Liothyronine *(Continued)*

Hypothyroidism:

Children: Oral: 5 mcg/day increase by 5 mcg increments every 1-2 weeks; usual maintenance dose 15-20 mcg/day

Adults: Oral: 25 mcg/day increase by 12.5-25 mcg/day every 1-2 weeks to a maximum of 100 mcg/day

Goiter, nontoxic:

Children: Oral: 5 mcg/day increase by 5 mcg increments every 1-2 weeks; usual maintenance dose 15-20 mcg/day

Adults: Oral: 5 mcg/day; increase by 5-10 mcg/day every 1-2 weeks; when 25 mcg is reached, increase dosage by 12.5-25 mcg every 1-2 weeks; usual maintenance dosage: 75 mcg/day

T_3 suppression test: Adults: Oral: 75-100 mcg/day for 7 days

Myxedema coma: Adults: I.V.: 25-50 mcg

Patients with known or suspected cardiovascular disease: 10-20 mcg

Note: Normally, at least 4 hours should be allowed between I.V. doses to adequately assess therapeutic response and no more than 12 hours should elapse between doses to avoid fluctuations in hormone levels. Oral therapy should be resumed as soon as the clinical situation has been stabilized and the patient is able to take oral medication. If levothyroxine rather than liothyronine sodium is used in initiating oral therapy, there is a delay of several days before the onset of levothyroxine activity and I.V. liothyronine sodium therapy should be discontinued gradually.

Administration

Oral: Administer on an empty stomach

Parenteral: I.V.: Dilute 200 mcg/mL vial with 2 mL of NS injection and shake well until a clear solution is obtained; use immediately after reconstitution; should not be admixed with other solutions

Monitoring Parameters T_3, TSH, heart rate, blood pressure, clinical signs of hypo- and hyperthyroidism; TSH is the most reliable guide for evaluating adequacy of thyroid replacement dosage. TSH may be elevated during the first few months of thyroid replacement despite patients being clinically euthyroid.

Reference Range See normal values in Normal Laboratory Values for Children *on page 1187*

Test Interactions Many drugs may have effects on thyroid function tests (ie, para-aminosalicylic acid, aminoglutethimide, amiodarone, barbiturates, carbamazepine, chloral hydrate, clofibrate, colestipol, corticosteroids, danazol, diazepam, estrogens, ethionamide, fluorouracil, I.V. heparin, insulin, lithium, methadone, methimazole, mitotane, nitroprusside, oxyphenbutazone, phenylbutazone, PTU, perphenazine, phenytoin, propranolol, salicylates, sulfonylureas, and thiazides)

Patient Information Do not change brands without physician's knowledge; report immediately to physician any chest pain, increased pulse, palpitations, heat intolerance, excessive sweating; do not discontinue without notifying physician

Additional Information 15-37.5 mcg liothyronine = 50-60 mcg levothyroxine = 60 mg thyroid USP = 45 mg Thyroid Strong® = 60 mg thyroglobulin = 50-60 mcg liotrix

Dosage Forms

Injection, as sodium (Triostat™): 10 mcg/mL (1 mL)

Tablet, as sodium (Cytomel®): 5 mcg, 25 mcg, 50 mcg

♦ **Lipancreatin** *see* Pancrelipase *on page 755*

♦ **Lipid Emulsion** *see* Fat Emulsion *on page 419*

♦ **Liposyn® II** *see* Fat Emulsion *on page 419*

♦ **Lipram®** *see* Pancrelipase *on page 755*

♦ **Liquibid® [OTC]** *see* Guaifenesin *on page 485*

♦ **Liqui-Char® [OTC]** *see* Charcoal *on page 213*

♦ **Liquid Antidote** *see* Charcoal *on page 213*

♦ **Liquid Paraffin** *see* Mineral Oil *on page 675*

Lisinopril *(lyse IN oh pril)*

Related Information

Carbohydrate and Alcohol Content of Liquid Medications for Use in Patients Receiving Ketogenic Diets *on page 1258*

U.S. Brand Names Prinivil®; Zestril®

Canadian Brand Names Apo-Lisinopril

Therapeutic Category Angiotensin-Converting Enzyme (ACE) Inhibitor; Antihypertensive Agent

Generic Available No

Use Management of hypertension; adjunctive treatment of CHF; adjunctive therapy in hemodynamically stable post MI patients to improve survival

Pregnancy Risk Factor C (1st trimester); D (may cause injury and death to the developing fetus when used during the 2nd and 3rd trimesters of pregnancy)

Contraindications Hypersensitivity to lisinopril, any component, or other ACE inhibitors; patients with idiopathic or hereditary angioedema or a history of angioedema with previous ACE inhibitor use

Warnings Serious adverse effects including angioedema, anaphylactoid reactions, neutropenia, agranulocytosis, hypotension, and hepatic failure may occur (see Adverse Reactions); risk of neutropenia may be increased in patients with renal dysfunction, especially if the patients have collagen vascular diseases

Precautions Use with caution and modify dosage in patients with renal impairment, especially renal artery stenosis; elevated BUN and S_{cr} may occur in these patients; discontinuation of concomitant diuretic or lisinopril may be needed; use with caution and modify dosage in patients with hyponatremia, hypovolemia, severe CHF, left ventricular outflow tract obstruction, or with coadministered diuretic therapy. Severe hypotension may occur in patients who are sodium and/or volume depleted; initiate lower doses and monitor closely when starting therapy in these patients.

Adverse Reactions
Cardiovascular: Hypotension, chest discomfort, orthostatic hypotension
Central nervous system: Dizziness, headache, fatigue
Dermatologic: Rash, angioedema. **Note:** The relative risk of angioedema with ACE inhibitors is higher within the first 30 days of use (compared to >1 year of use), for Black Americans (compared to Whites), for lisinopril or enalapril (compared to captopril), and for patients previously hospitalized within 30 days (Brown, 1996).
Endocrine & metabolic: Hyperkalemia
Gastrointestinal: Diarrhea, nausea, vomiting, ageusia
Hematologic: Neutropenia, agranulocytosis
Hepatic: Cholestatic jaundice, fulminant hepatic necrosis (rare, but potentially fatal)
Renal: Elevated BUN, elevated serum creatinine
Respiratory: Cough, dyspnea, eosinophilic pneumonitis; **Note:** An isolated dry cough lasting >3 weeks was reported in 7 of 42 pediatric patients (17%) receiving ACE inhibitors (see von Vigier, 2000)
Neuromuscular & skeletal: Weakness

Drug Interactions Use with potassium-sparing diuretics may result in an additive hyperkalemic effect; diuretics and other antihypertensive agents may increase hypotensive effect; indomethacin or NSAIDs may decrease hypotensive effect; lisinopril may increase lithium levels; use with NSAIDs in patients with renal impairment may further decrease renal function (usually reversible)

Food Interactions Food does not effect oral absorption; limit salt substitutes or potassium-rich diet; avoid natural licorice (causes sodium and water retention and increases potassium loss)

Mechanism of Action Competitive inhibitor of angiotensin-converting enzyme (ACE); prevents conversion of angiotensin I to angiotensin II, a potent vasoconstrictor; results in lower levels of angiotensin II which causes an increase in plasma renin activity and a reduction in aldosterone secretion

Pharmacodynamics
Onset of action (decrease in blood pressure): 1 hour
Peak effect: 6-8 hours
Duration of action: 24 hours

Pharmacokinetics
Absorption: Oral: 25%
Protein binding: 25%
Half-life: 11-13 hours; half-life increases with renal dysfunction
Elimination: Excreted in urine as unchanged drug

Usual Dosage Oral: Dosage must be titrated according to patient's response; use lower doses (~1/2 of those listed) for patients with hyponatremia, hypovolemia, severe CHF, decreased renal function, or in those receiving diuretics:

Children: Currently, no pediatric dosing information is available
Adults:
Hypertension (**Note:** If possible, discontinue diuretics 2-3 days prior to initiating lisinopril; restart diuretic, if needed, after blood pressure is stable): Initial: 10 mg/day given once daily; increase dose by 5-10 mg/day at 1- to 2-week intervals; usual dose: 20-40 mg/day given once daily; doses up to 80 mg/day have been used, but do not appear to have a greater effect
CHF: Initial: 5 mg once daily (with diuretics and digitalis); increase dose by ≤10 mg/day at ≥2 week intervals based on clinical response; usual dose: 5-40 mg/day given once daily; maximum dose: 40 mg/day
(Continued)

Lisinopril *(Continued)*

Dosing adjustment in renal impairment:
Cl_{cr} 10-30 mL/minute: Administer 50% of normal dose
Cl_{cr} <10 mL/minute: Administer 25% of normal dose

Administration Oral: May be administered without regard to food

Monitoring Parameters Blood pressure, BUN, serum creatinine, renal function, WBC, and serum potassium

Patient Information Limit alcohol; notify physician if vomiting, diarrhea, excessive perspiration, or dehydration occurs or if swelling of face, lips, tongue or difficulty in breathing occurs; do not use a salt substitute (potassium-containing) without physician advice

Nursing Implications Discontinue if angioedema occurs; observe closely for hypotension after the first dose or initiation of a new higher dose (keep in mind that maximum effect on blood pressure occurs at 6-8 hours)

Dosage Forms Tablet: 2.5 mg, 5 mg, 10 mg, 20 mg, 30 mg, 40 mg

References

Brown NJ, Ray WA, Snowden M, et al, "Black Americans Have an Increased Rate of Angiotensin-Converting Enzyme Inhibitor-Associated Angioedema," *Clin Pharmacol Ther*, 1996, 60(1):8-13.

Chase SL and Sutton JD, "Lisinopril: A New Angiotensin-Converting Enzyme Inhibitor," *Pharmacotherapy*, 1989, 9(3):120-30.

Raia JJ Jr, Barone JA, Byerly WG, et al, "Angiotensin-Converting Enzymes Inhibitors: A Comparative Review," *DICP*, 1990, 24(5):506-25.

von Vigier RO, Mozzettini S, Truttmann AC, et al, "Cough is Common in Children Prescribed Converting Enzyme Inhibitors," *Nephron*, 2000, 84(1):98.

Lithium *(LITH ee um)*

Related Information
Carbohydrate and Alcohol Content of Liquid Medications for Use in Patients Receiving Ketogenic Diets *on page 1258*
Drugs and Breast-Feeding *on page 1243*
Serotonin Syndrome *on page 1247*

U.S. Brand Names Eskalith®; Eskalith® CR; Lithobid®

Canadian Brand Names Duralith; PMS-Lithium Carbonate

Therapeutic Category Antidepressant, Miscellaneous; Antimanic Agent

Generic Available Yes

Use Management of acute manic episodes, bipolar disorders, and depression

Pregnancy Risk Factor D

Contraindications Hypersensitivity to lithium or any component; severe cardiovascular or renal disease

Warnings Lithium toxicity is closely related to serum levels and can occur at therapeutic doses; serum lithium determinations are required to monitor therapy

Precautions Use with caution in patients with cardiovascular or thyroid disease, patients receiving thiazide diuretics (monitor lithium levels, lithium dosage reduction may be required)

Adverse Reactions
Cardiovascular: Arrhythmias, sinus node dysfunction
Central nervous system: Sedation, confusion, somnolence, seizures, fatigue, headache, vertigo
Dermatologic: Rash
Endocrine & metabolic: Nephrogenic diabetes insipidus (thirst, polyuria, polydipsia), goiter, hypothyroidism
Gastrointestinal: Nausea, diarrhea, vomiting, xerostomia
Hematologic: Leukocytosis
Neuromuscular & skeletal: Muscle hyperirritability, muscle weakness, tremor

Drug Interactions Thiazide diuretics or NSAIDs may decrease lithium renal excretion and enhance lithium toxicity; iodide salts (or iodine) may increase hypothyroid effects

Food Interactions Avoid changes in sodium content of diet (reduction in sodium intake can increase lithium toxicity); syrup may precipitate in tube feedings

Mechanism of Action Alters cation transport across cell membrane in nerve and muscle cells and influences reuptake of serotonin and/or norepinephrine

Pharmacokinetics
Distribution: Crosses the placenta; appears in breast milk at 35% to 50% of the concentrations in serum
Adults:
V_d: Initial: 0.3-0.4 L/kg
V_{dss}: 0.7-1 L/kg

Half-life, terminal: Adults: 18-24 hours, can increase to more than 36 hours in elderly or patients with renal impairment

Time to peak serum concentration (nonsustained release product): Within 0.5-2 hours

Elimination: 90% to 98% of a dose is excreted in the urine as unchanged drug; other excretory routes include feces (1%) and sweat (4% to 5%)

Dialysis: Dialyzable (50% to 100%)

Usual Dosage Oral: Monitor serum concentrations and clinical response (efficacy and toxicity) to determine proper dose

Children: 15-60 mg/kg/day in 3-4 divided doses; dose not to exceed usual adult dosage; initiate at lower dose and adjust dose weekly based on levels

Adolescents: 600-1800 mg/day in 3-4 divided doses for regular tablets or 2 divided doses for sustained release tablets

Adults: 300 mg 3-4 times/day; usual maximum maintenance dose: 2.4 g/day or 450-900 mg of sustained release tablets twice daily

Dosing adjustment in renal impairment:
Cl$_{cr}$ 10-50 mL/minute: Administer 50% to 75% of normal dose
Cl$_{cr}$ <10 mL/minute: Administer 25% to 50% of normal dose

Administration Oral: Administer with meals to decrease GI upset; do not crush or chew slow- or extended-release dosage form, swallow whole

Monitoring Parameters Serum lithium every 3-4 days during initial therapy; obtain lithium serum concentrations 8-12 hours postdose; renal, hepatic, thyroid and cardiovascular function; CBC with differential, urinalysis, serum sodium, calcium, potassium

Reference Range
Therapeutic: Acute mania: 0.6-1.5 mEq/L (SI: 0.6-1.5 mmol/L); protection against future episodes in most patients with bipolar disorder: 0.8-1 mEq/L (SI: 0.8-1 mmol/L). A higher rate of relapse is described in subjects who are maintained <0.4 mEq/L (SI: <0.4 mmol/L)
Toxic: >2 mEq/L (SI: >2 mmol/L)

Patient Information Limit caffeine; limit alcohol; avoid tasks requiring psychomotor coordination until CNS effects are known; may cause dry mouth

Nursing Implications Avoid dehydration

Dosage Forms
Capsule, as carbonate: 150 mg, 300 mg, 600 mg
Eskalith®: 300 mg
Syrup, as citrate: 300 mg/5 mL (5 mL, 10 mL, 480 mL)
Tablet, as carbonate: 300 mg
Tablet:
Controlled release, as carbonate (Eskalith® CR): 450 mg
Slow release, as carbonate (Lithobid®): 300 mg

References
Levy HB, Harper CR, and Weinberg WA, "A Practical Approach to Children Failing in School," *Pediatr Clin North Am*, 1992, 39(4):895-928.

- ◆ **Lithobid®** *see Lithium on page 600*
- ◆ **LMD®** *see Dextran on page 311*
- ◆ **LoCHOLEST®** *see Cholestyramine Resin on page 229*
- ◆ **LoCHOLEST® Light** *see Cholestyramine Resin on page 229*
- ◆ **Locoid®** *see Hydrocortisone on page 506*
- ◆ **Lomine (Can)** *see Dicyclomine on page 326*
- ◆ **Lomotil®** *see Diphenoxylate and Atropine on page 343*

Lomustine (loe MUS teen)

Related Information
Emetogenic Potential of Single Chemotherapeutic Agents *on page 1129*

U.S. Brand Names CeeNU®

Synonyms CCNU

Therapeutic Category Antineoplastic Agent, Alkylating Agent (Nitrosourea)

Generic Available No

Use Treatment of brain tumors, Hodgkin's and non-Hodgkin's lymphomas, melanoma, renal carcinoma, lung cancer, colon cancer

Pregnancy Risk Factor D

Contraindications Hypersensitivity to lomustine or any component

Warnings The FDA currently recommends that procedures for proper handling and disposal of antineoplastic agents be considered. Bone marrow suppression, notably thrombocytopenia and leukopenia, may lead to bleeding and overwhelming infections in an already compromised patient; nadir: ~6 weeks; do not give courses more
(Continued)

Lomustine *(Continued)*

frequently than every 6 weeks because the toxicity is cumulative; lomustine has been found to be mutagenic, teratogenic, and carcinogenic in animals.

Precautions Use with caution in patients with depressed platelet, leukocyte or erythrocyte counts; reduce dosage by 25% when platelet nadirs are 50,000-74,999/mm³; reduce dosage by 50% when platelet nadirs are 25,000-49,999/mm³; reduce dosage by 75% when platelet nadirs are <25,000/mm³

Adverse Reactions

Central nervous system: Disorientation, lethargy, ataxia

Dermatologic: Alopecia

Gastrointestinal: Nausea, vomiting, stomatitis, anorexia, diarrhea

Hematologic: Anemia, thrombocytopenia, leukopenia, myelosuppression (occurs 4-6 weeks after a dose and may persist 1-2 weeks)

Hepatic: Hepatotoxicity, elevation of hepatic enzymes

Neuromuscular & skeletal: Dysarthria

Ocular: Blindness

Renal: Renal failure, interstitial nephritis

Respiratory: Pulmonary fibrosis with total cumulative dose >1 g/m²

Drug Interactions Phenobarbital may increase metabolism and reduce activity of lomustine; cimetidine may decrease metabolism and increase myelotoxicity of lomustine

Food Interactions Avoid concurrent administration of food/drugs that cause vomiting

Stability Avoid exposure to excessive heat (>40°C) and prolonged exposure to moisture

Mechanism of Action Inhibits DNA and RNA synthesis through DNA alkylation and DNA cross-linking; carbamoylates amine groups on proteins; inhibits DNA polymerase activity, RNA and protein synthesis

Pharmacokinetics

Absorption: Rapid and complete absorption from the GI tract (30-60 minutes)

Distribution: Lomustine and/or its metabolites penetrate into the CNS; metabolites are present in breast milk

Protein binding: >90%

Metabolism: Rapid conversion to 4-hydroxy metabolites (active) partially by liver microsomal enzymes during first pass through the liver

Half-life, terminal (active metabolite): 1.3-2 days

Time to peak serum concentration (of active metabolite): Within 3 hours

Elimination: Excreted primarily in urine as metabolites; <5% fecal excretion

Usual Dosage Oral (refer to individual protocol):

Children: 75-150 mg/m² as a single dose every 6 weeks; subsequent doses are readjusted after initial treatment according to platelet and leukocyte counts (see Precautions)

Adults: 100-130 mg/m² as a single dose every 6 weeks; readjust after initial treatment according to platelet and leukocyte counts (see Precautions)

With compromised marrow function: Initial dose: 100 mg/m² as a single dose every 6 weeks

Administration Oral: Administer with fluids on an empty stomach; do not administer food or drink for 2 hours after lomustine administration to decrease incidence of nausea and vomiting

Monitoring Parameters CBC with differential and platelet count, hepatic and renal function tests, pulmonary function tests

Patient Information Notify physician if fever, sore throat, bleeding, or bruising occur; avoid alcohol for short periods after taking lomustine

Dosage Forms

Capsule: 10 mg, 40 mg, 100 mg

Dose Pack: 10 mg (2s); 100 mg (2s); 40 mg (2s)

References

Berg SL, Grisell DL, DeLaney TF, et al, "Principles of Treatment of Pediatric Solid Tumors," *Pediatr Clin North Am*, 1991, 38(2):249-67.

Pendergrass TW, Milstein JM, Geyer JR, et al, "Eight Drugs in One Day Chemotherapy for Brain Tumors: Experience in 107 Children and Rationale for Preradiation Chemotherapy," *J Clin Oncol*, 1987, 5(8):1221-31.

♦ **Loniten**® *see* Minoxidil *on page 676*

♦ **Lonox**® *see* Diphenoxylate and Atropine *on page 343*

♦ **Loperacap (Can)** *see* Loperamide *on page 603*

Loperamide (loe PER a mide)

Related Information

Carbohydrate and Alcohol Content of Liquid Medications for Use in Patients Receiving Ketogenic Diets *on page 1258*

U.S. Brand Names Imodium® A-D [OTC]; Imodium® Advanced

Canadian Brand Names Anti-Diarrheal; Apo-Loperamide; Diahalt; Diarr-Eze; Diarrhea Relief; Loperacap; Novo-Loperamide; PMS-Loperamine; Riva-Loperamide

Therapeutic Category Antidiarrheal

Generic Available Yes

Use Treatment of acute diarrhea and chronic diarrhea associated with inflammatory bowel disease; chronic functional diarrhea (idiopathic), chronic diarrhea caused by bowel resection or organic lesions; to decrease the volume of ileostomy discharge

Pregnancy Risk Factor B

Contraindications Hypersensitivity to loperamide or any component; patients who must avoid constipation; infectious diarrhea resulting from organisms that penetrate the intestinal mucosa (eg, *Shigella, Salmonella*); patients with pseudomembranous colitis; bloody diarrhea

Precautions If clinical improvement in acute diarrhea is not observed in 48 hours, discontinue use; monitor patients with hepatic dysfunction closely for CNS toxicity

Adverse Reactions

Central nervous system: Sedation, fatigue, dizziness

Dermatologic: Rash

Gastrointestinal: Nausea, vomiting, constipation, abdominal cramping, xerostomia

Miscellaneous: Hypersensitivity reactions

Drug Interactions Additive CNS toxicity with CNS depressants, phenothiazines, tricyclic antidepressants, alcohol

Mechanism of Action Acts directly on intestinal muscles to inhibit peristalsis and prolong transit time

Pharmacodynamics Onset of action: Within 30-60 minutes

Pharmacokinetics

Absorption: Oral: 40%

Protein binding: 97%

Metabolism: Hepatic (>50%) to inactive compounds

Half-life: 9-14 hours

Time to peak serum concentration:

Capsules: 5 hours

Liquid: 2.5 hours

Elimination: Fecal and urinary (1%) excretion of metabolites and unchanged drug (30% to 40%)

Usual Dosage Oral:

Acute diarrhea:

Children: Initial doses (in first 24 hours):

2-5 years: 1 mg 3 times/day

6-8 years: 2 mg twice daily

8-12 years: 2 mg 3 times/day

After initial dosing, 0.1 mg/kg doses after each loose stool but not exceeding initial dosage

Adults: 4 mg (2 capsules) initially, followed by 2 mg after each loose stool, up to 16 mg/day (8 capsules)

Traveler's diarrhea: Treat for no more than 2 days

6-8 years: 1 mg after first loose stool followed by 1 mg after each subsequent stool; maximum dose: 4 mg/day

9-11 years: 2 mg after first loose stool followed by 1 mg after each subsequent stool; maximum dose: 6 mg/day

12 years to Adults: 4 mg after first loose stool followed by 2 mg after each subsequent stool; maximum dose: 8 mg/day

Chronic diarrhea: Children: 0.08-0.24 mg/kg/day divided 2-3 times/day, maximum dose: 2 mg/dose

Administration Oral: Drink plenty of fluids to help prevent dehydration

Patient Information Do not exceed maximum daily dosage; may cause drowsiness and impair ability to perform hazardous tasks requiring mental alertness; if acute diarrhea lasts longer than 48 hours; consult physician

Dosage Forms

Caplet, as hydrochloride (Imodium® A-D): 2 mg

Capsule, as hydrochloride: 2 mg

Liquid, oral, as hydrochloride (Imodium® A-D): 1 mg/5 mL (60 mL, 90 mL, 120 mL)

Tablet, as hydrochloride: 2 mg

(Continued)

Loperamide *(Continued)*

Tablet, chewable, as hydrochloride (Imodium® Advanced): 2 mg with simethicone 125 mg

Lopinavir and Ritonavir (lop IN uh veer & rit ON uh veer)

U.S. Brand Names Kaletra™

Synonyms ABT-378/Ritonavir; Ritonavir and Lopinavir

Therapeutic Category Antiretroviral Agent; HIV Agents (Anti-HIV Agents); Protease Inhibitor

Generic Available No

Use Treatment of HIV infection in combination with other antiretroviral agents **(Note:** HIV regimens consisting of three antiretroviral agents are strongly recommended)

Pregnancy Risk Factor C

Contraindications Hypersensitivity to lopinavir, ritonavir, or any component; concurrent therapy with medications that largely rely on cytochrome P-450 isoenzymes CYP3A or CYP2D6 for clearance and that have an association between increased plasma concentrations and serious or life-threatening effects (eg, astemizole, cisapride, dihydroergotamine, ergonovine, ergotamine, flecainide, methylergonovine, midazolam, pimozide, propafenone, terfenadine, triazolam)

Warnings Lopinavir and ritonavir are potent CYP3A isoenzyme inhibitors that interact with numerous drugs. Due to potential serious and/or life-threatening drug interactions, some drugs are contraindicated (see Contraindications and Drug Interactions) and other medications may require concentration monitoring or dosage adjustment if coadministered with lopinavir and ritonavir (see Drug Interactions). Concomitant use with certain medications may require dosage adjustment of lopinavir and ritonavir (see Drug Interactions).

Potentially fatal pancreatitis may occur; markedly elevated serum triglycerides is a risk factor for developing pancreatitis; advanced HIV disease or a history of pancreatitis may also place patients at increased risk; discontinue lopinavir and ritonavir therapy if clinical signs, symptoms, or laboratory abnormalities suggestive of pancreatitis occur. New onset diabetes mellitus, exacerbations of diabetes, and hyperglycemia have been reported in HIV-infected patients receiving protease inhibitors.

Precautions Use with caution in patients with hepatic impairment (lopinavir and ritonavir are primarily metabolized by the liver); hepatitis or markedly elevated transaminases prior to therapy may increase risk for further elevations in liver enzymes. Spontaneous bleeding episodes have been reported in patients with hemophilia type A and B receiving protease inhibitors. Large increases in total cholesterol and triglycerides have been reported; patients should be monitored prior to therapy and periodically during treatment. Redistribution or accumulation of body fat has been observed in patients using antiretroviral therapy.

Adverse Reactions

Central nervous system: Headache (2% to 7%), insomnia (1% to 2%), pain

Dermatologic: Rash (1% to 4%; children 2%)

Endocrine & metabolic: Hyperglycemia (2% to 4%), hypertriglyceridemia (5% to 26%), hypercholesterolemia (7% to 26%), hyperuricemia (up to 4%); new onset diabetes, exacerbation of diabetes mellitus; central redistribution of body fat: Central obesity, buffalo hump, facial atrophy, and breast enlargement; decreased serum sodium (children 3%), decreased serum phosphorus (up to 2%)

Gastrointestinal: Nausea (2% to 16%), vomiting (2% to 5%), diarrhea (14% to 24%), abnormal stools (up to 6%), abdominal pain (1% to 5%), elevated amylase (2% to 5%)

Hematologic: Decreased platelets (4% children), decreased neutrophils (1% to 3%), possible spontaneous bleeding in hemophiliacs

Hepatic: Elevated liver enzymes, elevated bilirubin (children 3%)

Neuromuscular & skeletal: Asthenia (3% to 7%)

Drug Interactions Cytochrome P-450 isoenzyme CYP3A substrate and inhibitor; CYP2D6 isoenzyme inhibitor (to a lesser degree than CYP3A); may induce glucuronidation; does not inhibit CYP1A2, CYP2B6, CYP2C9, CYP2C19, or CYP2E1 at clinically obtained concentrations

Lopinavir/ritonavir may inhibit the metabolism of the following drugs and cause serious or life-threatening adverse effects: Astemizole, cisapride, dihydroergotamine, ergonovine, ergotamine, flecainide, methylergonovine, midazolam, pimozide, propafenone, terfenadine, triazolam (concurrent therapy with these drugs and lopinavir/ritonavir is contraindicated). Lopinavir/ritonavir may increase the toxic effects of amiodarone, bepridil, systemic lidocaine, quinidine, warfarin, cyclosporine, tacrolimus, rapamycin (serum concentration monitoring of these drugs is necessary). Lopinavir/ritonavir may increase the concentrations of the following drugs: Clarithromycin (decrease clarithromycin dosage in patients with renal impairment), ketoconazole (high dose ketoconazole is not recommended), itraconazole (high dose itraconazole is not recommended), rifabutin and rifabutin metabolite (rifabutin dose should be decreased by at least 75% of the normal dose; further reduction in dosage may be needed, monitor closely for adverse effects). Lopinavir/ritonavir may also increase serum concentrations or toxicity of lovastatin or simvastatin (concurrent use of these agents is not recommended), atorvastatin or cerivastatin (use lowest possible dose of these agents, monitor closely; consider use of pravastatin, fluvastatin), nifedipine, felodipine, nicardipine, sildenafil. When given with reduced doses of concurrent protease inhibitors, lopinavir/ritonavir may increase the trough concentrations of amprenavir, indinavir, and saquinavir, but AUCs may be similar (appropriate doses of combination protease inhibitors have not been established).

Lopinavir/ritonavir may decrease the concentrations of atovaquone and methadone (increased doses of these agents may be needed). Lopinavir/ritonavir may decrease the efficacy of estrogen-based oral contraceptives (additional or alternative contraceptive methods should be used). Lopinavir/ritonavir may potentially decrease abacavir and zidovudine concentrations through induction of glucuronidation (clinical significance unknown).

Rifampin may significantly reduce lopinavir/ritonavir plasma concentrations and should not be used concurrently. The herbal medicine, St John's wort (*Hypericum perforatum*), may significantly decrease concentrations of lopinavir/ritonavir and is not recommended for concurrent use. Efavirenz and nevirapine decrease lopinavir concentrations (an increased dose of lopinavir/ritonavir should be considered). Phenobarbital, phenytoin, carbamazepine, dexamethasone may decrease lopinavir concentrations (these agents may decrease effectiveness of lopinavir/ritonavir, use with caution). Delavirdine and ritonavir may increase lopinavir concentrations.

Oral solution contains alcohol and may produce disulfiram-like reaction when coadministered with disulfiram or metronidazole. Didanosine should be given at least 1 hour before or 2 hours after lopinavir/ritonavir.

Food Interactions Compared to fasting, a moderate fat meal increased lopinavir AUC by 48% (capsules) and 80% (oral solution); a high fat meal increased lopinavir AUC by 97% (capsules) and 130% (oral solution)

Stability Capsules and oral solution: Store at 2°C to 8°C (36°F to 46°F) until dispensed; refrigerated products are stable until labeled expiration date; stability at room temperature: 2 months; avoid exposure to excessive heat

Mechanism of Action This product is a fixed-dose combination of lopinavir and ritonavir; antiretroviral effects are due to lopinavir, a protease inhibitor; lopinavir acts on an enzyme (protease) late in the HIV replication process after the virus has entered into the cell's nucleus. Lopinavir binds to the protease activity site and inhibits the activity of the enzyme, thus preventing cleavage of viral polyprotein precursors (gag-pol protein precursors) into individual functional proteins found in infectious HIV. This results in the formation of immature, noninfectious viral particles. Ritonavir inhibits the metabolism of lopinavir via the cytochrome P-450 CYP3A isoenzyme pathway and significantly increases plasma concentrations of lopinavir.

Pharmacokinetics Information below refers to Lopinavir; see Ritonavir *on page 879* for additional information.

Protein binding: 98% to 99%; binds to both alpha$_1$ - acid glycoprotein and albumin; higher affinity for alpha$_1$-acid glycoprotein

Metabolism: Primarily oxidative, via cytochrome P-450 CYP3A isoenzyme; 13 oxidative metabolites identified; may induce its own metabolism

Bioavailability: Absolute bioavailability not established; AUC for oral solution was 22% lower than capsule when given under fasting conditions; concentrations were similar under nonfasting conditions

Half-life: Adults: Mean: 5-6 hours

Elimination: 2.2% of dose eliminated unchanged in urine; 83% of dose eliminated in feces

Clearance: (Apparent oral): Adults: 6-7 L/hour

Dialysis: Unlikely to remove significant amounts of drug (due to high protein binding)

Usual Dosage Oral:

Patients receiving concomitant antiretroviral therapy **without** efavirenz or nevirapine:

Children 6 months to 12 years: Dosage based on weight and lopinavir component:

7 to <15 kg: Lopinavir 12 mg/kg twice daily

15-40 kg: Lopinavir 10 mg/kg twice daily

>40 kg: Lopinavir 400 mg (3 capsules or 5 mL) twice daily

(Continued)

Lopinavir and Ritonavir *(Continued)*

Children >12 years and Adults: Lopinavir 400 mg/ritonavir 100 mg (3 capsules or 5 mL) twice daily

Treatment of experienced patients with suspected reduced susceptibility to lopinavir who are receiving concomitant antiretroviral therapy **with efavirenz or nevirapine**:

Children 6 months to 12 years: Dosage based on weight and lopinavir component:
7 to <15 kg: Lopinavir 13 mg/kg twice daily
15-45 kg: Lopinavir 11 mg/kg twice daily
>45 kg: Lopinavir 533 mg (4 capsules or 6.5 mL) twice daily

Children >12 years and Adults: Lopinavir 533 mg/ritonavir 133 mg (4 capsules or 6.5 mL) twice daily

Dosing adjustment in renal impairment: Has not been studied in patients with renal impairment; however, a decrease in clearance is not expected

Dosing adjustment in hepatic impairment: Plasma levels may be increased in patients with hepatic impairment

Administration Oral: Administer with food to enhance bioavailability and decrease kinetic variability

Monitoring Parameters Signs and symptoms of pancreatitis; serum glucose, triglycerides, cholesterol, liver enzyme tests, amylase, CBC with differential, CD4 cell count, viral load

Patient Information Lopinavir and ritonavir is not a cure for HIV; notify physician if symptoms of pancreatitis occur (nausea, vomiting, abdominal pain); report the use of other medications, nonprescription medications and herbal or natural products to your physician and pharmacist; take lopinavir and ritonavir everyday as prescribed; do not change dose or discontinue without physician's advice; if a dose is missed, take it as soon as possible, then return to normal dosing schedule; if a dose is skipped, do not double the next dose

Additional Information Oral solution contains 42.4% alcohol (v/v); overdose in a child may cause potentially lethal alcohol toxicity; treatment should be supportive and include general poisoning management; activated charcoal may help remove unabsorbed medication; dialysis unlikely to be of benefit

Preliminary studies have reported response rates (defined as viral loads <400 copies/mL) of 91%, 81%, and 33% for patients with 0-5, 6-7, and 8-10 protease mutations at baseline, respectively (see Hurst, 2000)

Dosage Forms

Capsule: Lopinavir 133.3 mg and ritonavir 33.3 mg

Solution, oral: Lopinavir 80 mg and ritonavir 20 mg per mL (160 mL) [contains 42.4% alcohol]

References

Hurst M and Faulds D, "Lopinavir," *Drugs*, 2000, 60(6):1371-9.

Panel on Clinical Practices for Treatment of HIV Infection, "Guidelines for the Use of Antiretroviral Agents in HIV-Infected Adults and Adolescents," April 23, 2001, http://www.hivatis.org.

Piscitelli SC, Burstein AH, Chaitt D, et al, "Indinavir Concentrations and St John's Wort," *Lancet*, 2000, 355(9203):547-8.

♦ **Lopremone** *see* Protirelin *on page 851*
♦ **Lopresor (Can)** *see* Metoprolol *on page 660*
♦ **Lopressor®** *see* Metoprolol *on page 660*
♦ **Lorabid™** *see* Loracarbef *on page 606*

Loracarbef (lor a KAR bef)

Related Information

Carbohydrate and Alcohol Content of Liquid Medications for Use in Patients Receiving Ketogenic Diets *on page 1258*

U.S. Brand Names Lorabid™

Therapeutic Category Antibiotic, Carbacephem

Generic Available No

Use Treatment of mild to moderate community-acquired infections of the respiratory tract, skin and skin structure, and urinary tract that are caused by susceptible *S. pneumoniae, H. influenzae, M. catarrhalis, S. aureus, S. pyogenes,* and *E. coli*

Pregnancy Risk Factor B

Contraindications Hypersensitivity to loracarbef, any component, or cephalosporins

Warnings Prolonged use may result in superinfection or pseudomembranous colitis

Precautions Use with caution in patients with a previous history of hypersensitivity to other beta-lactam antibiotics (eg, penicillins); use with caution in patients with impaired renal function and patients with a history of colitis; modify dosage in patients with renal impairment

Adverse Reactions

Cardiovascular: Vasodilation

Central nervous system: Headache, somnolence, nervousness, dizziness, insomnia

Gastrointestinal: Diarrhea, nausea, vomiting, abdominal pain, anorexia, pseudo-membranous colitis

Dermatologic: Skin rashes, urticaria, pruritus, erythema multiforme, Stevens-Johnson syndrome

Genitourinary: Candidal vaginitis

Hematologic: Transient thrombocytopenia, leukopenia, eosinophilia, prolongation of prothrombin time

Hepatic: Transient elevations of ALT, AST, alkaline phosphatase; cholestasis

Renal: Transient elevation of BUN and serum creatinine

Respiratory: Rhinitis

Miscellaneous: Anaphylaxis, superinfection

Drug Interactions Probenecid inhibits renal excretion and increases the serum concentration of loracarbef

Food Interactions Administration with food decreases and delays the peak plasma concentration

Stability After reconstitution, suspension may be stored at room temperature for 14 days

Mechanism of Action Inhibits bacterial cell wall synthesis by binding to one or more of the penicillin binding proteins; inhibits the final transpeptidation step of peptidoglycan synthesis in bacterial cell walls, thus inhibiting cell wall biosynthesis. Upon exposure to beta-lactam antibiotics, bacteria eventually lyse due to ongoing activity of cell wall autolytic enzymes (autolysins and murein hydrolases) while cell wall assembly is arrested.

Pharmacokinetics

Absorption: Oral: Rapid; 90% absorbed from the GI tract

Distribution: Loracarbef middle-ear fluid concentration approximates 48% of the plasma concentration 2 hours after a dose in pediatric patients

Protein binding: 25%

Bioavailability: 90%

Half-life, elimination:

Children (suspension): ~0.78-0.85 hours

Adults, normal renal function: ~1 hour

Time to peak serum concentration: 0.5-1 hour after administration

Elimination: Primarily by the kidneys as unchanged drug in the urine

Usual Dosage Oral:

Children 6 months to 12 years:

Acute otitis media: 30 mg/kg/day divided every 12 hours for 10 days (should be treated with the **suspension** which results in higher peak plasma concentrations than the capsule)

Acute maxillary sinusitis: 30 mg/kg/day divided every 12 hours for 10 days

Pharyngitis/tonsillitis/skin and skin structure infections: 15 mg/kg/day divided every 12 hours

Adults:

Pneumonia, chronic bacterial bronchitis, sinusitis: 400 mg every 12 hours

Acute bacterial bronchitis: 200-400 mg every 12 hours

Uncomplicated urinary tract infections: 200 mg once daily for 7 days

Skin and skin structure: 200 mg every 12 hours

Uncomplicated pyelonephritis: 400 mg every 12 hours for 14 days

Dosing adjustment in renal impairment:

Cl$_{cr}$ 10-49 mL/minute: 50% of usual dose at usual interval or usual dose given half as often

Cl$_{cr}$ <10 mL/minute: Give usual dose every 3-5 days

Hemodialysis: Removed by hemodialysis; postdialysis dose should be administered when appropriate

Administration Oral: Administer on an empty stomach at least 1 hour before or 2 hours after meals; shake suspension well before use

Monitoring Parameters Observe patient for diarrhea; with prolonged therapy, monitor renal function periodically

Dosage Forms

Capsule: 200 mg, 400 mg

Suspension, oral: 100 mg/5 mL (50 mL, 100 mL); 200 mg/5 mL (50 mL, 75 mL, 100 mL)

References

Force RW and Nahata MC, "Loracarbef: A New Orally Administered Carbacephem Antibiotic," *Ann Pharmacother*, 1993, 27(3):321-9.

(Continued)

Loracarbef *(Continued)*

Foshee WS, "Loracarbef (LY163892) Versus Amoxicillin-Clavulanate in the Treatment of Acute Otitis Media With Effusion," *J Pediatr*, 1992, 120(6):980-6.

Nelson JD, Shelton S, and Kusmiesz H, "Pharmacokinetics of LY163892 in Infants and Children," *Antimicrob Agents Chemother*, 1988, 32(11):1738-9.

Loratadine (lor AT a deen)

U.S. Brand Names Claritin®; Claritin® RediTab®

Therapeutic Category Antihistamine

Generic Available No

Use Symptomatic relief of nasal and non-nasal symptoms of allergic rhinitis; treatment of chronic idiopathic urticaria

Pregnancy Risk Factor B

Contraindications Hypersensitivity to loratadine or any component

Warnings Use with caution and adjust dosage in patients with severe liver impairment or renal impairment

Precautions Use cautiously in patients who are also taking ketoconazole, itraconazole, fluconazole, erythromycin, clarithromycin, or other drugs which may impair loratadine's hepatic metabolism; although increased plasma levels of loratadine have been observed, no adverse effects with concomitant administration have been reported including QT interval prolongation which has occurred when similar antihistamines, terfenadine and astemizole, were combined with these agents; while less sedating than other antihistamines, loratadine may cause drowsiness and impair ability to perform hazardous activities requiring mental alertness. Use cautiously in breast-feeding women as breast milk levels of loratadine are equivalent to serum levels

Adverse Reactions

Cardiovascular: Hypotension, hypertension, palpitations, tachycardia, chest pain, syncope

Central nervous system: Headache, somnolence, fatigue, anxiety, depression, dizziness, fever, migraine, agitation, nervousness

Dermatologic: Alopecia, dermatitis, dry skin, rash, pruritus, photosensitivity

Gastrointestinal: Xerostomia, nausea, vomiting, gastritis, abdominal pain

Endocrine & metabolic: Breast pain and enlargement (rare), menorrhagia, dysmenorrhea

Neuromuscular & skeletal: Hyperkinesia, arthralgias, myalgias, leg cramps

Ophthalmic: Blurred vision, altered lacrimation, eye pain, conjunctivitis

Genitourinary: Discoloration of urine

Respiratory: Nasal dryness, pharyngitis, dyspnea, nasal congestion, wheezing

Miscellaneous: Diaphoresis

Drug Interactions Cytochrome P-450 isoenzyme CYP2D6 and CYP3A3/4 substrate

Increased plasma concentrations and AUC of loratadine and its active metabolite with ketoconazole, erythromycin, and cimetidine; no change in QT_c interval or cardiac arrhythmias have been seen (see Warnings); a prolonged QT interval was reported in one patient who was receiving quinidine and loratadine; additive CNS depression with other CNS depressants, alcohol, and procarbazine; prolonged anticholinergic effects with MAO inhibitors

Food Interactions Administration with food increases loratadine's bioavailability by 40%

Mechanism of Action Long-acting tricyclic antihistamine with selective peripheral histamine H_1 receptor antagonistic properties

Pharmacodynamics

Onset of Action: Within 1-3 hours

Peak effect: 8-12 hours

Duration: >24 hours

Pharmacokinetics

Absorption: Rapid; food increases total bioavailability (AUC) by 40%

Distribution: Binds preferentially to peripheral nervous system H1 receptors; no appreciable entry into CNS; loratadine and metabolite pass easily into breast milk and achieve concentrations equivalent to plasma levels; breast milk to plasma ratio: 1.17

Protein binding: 97% (loratadine), 73% to 77% (metabolite)

Metabolism: Extensive first-pass metabolism by cytochrome P-450 system to an active metabolite (descarboethoxyloratadine)

Half-life: 8.4 hours (loratadine), 28 hours (metabolite)

Time to peak serum concentration: 1-2 hours

Elimination: 80% eliminated via urine & feces as metabolic products

Usual Dosage Oral:
Children 2-5 years: 5 mg once daily
Children ≥6 years and Adults: 10 mg once daily
Dosing interval in renal (GFR <30 mL/minute) or hepatic impairment: Administer dosage every other day
Administration Oral: Administer on an empty stomach or before meals; place Claritin® RediTab® (rapidly disintegrating tablet) on the tongue; tablet disintegration occurs rapidly; may administer with or without water
Monitoring Parameters Improvement in signs and symptoms of allergic rhinitis or chronic idiopathic urticaria
Reference Range Therapeutic serum levels (not used clinically): Loratadine: 2.5-100 ng/mL; active metabolite: 0.5-100 ng/mL
Test Interactions Antigen skin testing
Patient Information Drink plenty of water; may cause dry mouth; may color urine; may cause drowsiness and impair ability to perform hazardous tasks requiring mental alertness or physical coordination; avoid prolonged exposure to sunlight; notify physician if fainting episode occurs
Dosage Forms
Syrup: 1 mg/mL (16 oz)
Tablet: 10 mg
Tablet, rapid-disintegrating (Claritin® RediTab®): 10 mg
References
Lin CC, Radwanski E, Affrime M, et al, "Pharmacokinetics of Loratadine in Pediatric Subjects," *Am J Therapeut*, 1995, 2:504-8.
Luck JC and Evrard HM, "Atrial Fibrillation Associated With Loratadine Use," *J Allergy Clin Immunol*, 1995, 95(2):282.
Lutsky BN, Klose P, Melon J, et al, "A Comparative Study of the Efficacy and Safety of Loratadine Syrup and Terfenadine Suspension in the Treatment of 3 to 6 Year Old Children With Seasonal Allergic Rhinitis," *Clin Ther*, 1993, 15(5):855-65.
Salmun LM, Herron JM, Banfield C, et al, "The Pharmacokinetics, Electrocardiographic Effects, and Tolerability of Loratadine Syrup in Children Aged 2 to 5 Years," *Clin Ther*, 2000, 22(5):613-21.

Lorazepam (lor A ze pam)

Related Information
Carbohydrate and Alcohol Content of Liquid Medications for Use in Patients Receiving Ketogenic Diets *on page 1258*
Drugs and Breast-Feeding *on page 1243*
Overdose and Toxicology *on page 1222*
Preprocedure Sedatives in Children *on page 1201*
U.S. Brand Names Ativan®; Lorazepam Intensol®
Canadian Brand Names Apo-Lorazepam; Novo-Lorazem; Nu-Loraz; PMS-Lorazepam; Pro-Lorazepam; Riva-Lorazepam
Therapeutic Category Antianxiety Agent; Anticonvulsant; Benzodiazepine; Antiemetic; Benzodiazepine; Hypnotic; Sedative
Generic Available Yes
Use Management of anxiety; status epilepticus; preoperative sedation and amnesia
Restrictions C-IV
Pregnancy Risk Factor D
Contraindications Hypersensitivity to lorazepam or any component; there may be a cross-sensitivity with other benzodiazepines; do not use in a comatose patient, those with pre-existing CNS depression, narrow-angle glaucoma, severe uncontrolled pain, severe hypotension
Warnings Dilute injection prior to I.V. use with equal volume of compatible diluent; do not inject intra-arterially, arteriospasm and gangrene may occur; injection contains benzyl alcohol 2%, polyethylene glycol and propylene glycol, which may be toxic to newborns in high doses
Precautions Use with caution in neonates, especially in preterm infants (several cases of neurotoxicity and myoclonus have been reported); use with caution in patients with renal or hepatic impairment, compromised pulmonary function, or those receiving other CNS depressants
Adverse Reactions
Cardiovascular: Bradycardia, circulatory collapse, hypertension, or hypotension
Central nervous system: Confusion, CNS depression, sedation, drowsiness, lethargy, hangover effect, dizziness, transitory hallucinations, ataxia, rhythmic myoclonic jerking in preterm infants
Gastrointestinal: Constipation, xerostomia, nausea, vomiting
Genitourinary: Urinary incontinence or retention
Local: Pain with injection
Ocular: Diplopia, nystagmus
(Continued)

Lorazepam *(Continued)*

Respiratory: Respiratory depression, apnea

Miscellaneous: Physical and psychological dependence with prolonged use

Drug Interactions Cytochrome P-450 isoenzyme CYP3A3/4 substrate

Other CNS or respiratory depressants may increase adverse effects

Stability Do not use if injection is discolored or contains precipitate; protect from light; refrigerate injectable form and oral solution; injection is stable at room temperature for 8 weeks

Mechanism of Action Depresses all levels of the CNS, including the limbic and reticular formation, by binding to the benzodiazepine site on the gamma-aminobutyric acid (GABA) receptor complex and modulating GABA, which is a major inhibitory neurotransmitter in the brain

Pharmacodynamics Sedation:

Onset of effect:

Oral: Within 60 minutes

I.M.: 30-60 minutes

I.V.: 15-30 minutes

Duration: 8-12 hours

Pharmacokinetics

Absorption: Oral, I.M.: Rapid, complete

Distribution: Crosses into placenta; crosses into breast milk

V_d:

Neonates: 0.76 L/kg

Adults: 1.3 L/kg

Protein binding: ~85%

Metabolism: Primarily by glucuronide conjugation in the liver

Bioavailability: Oral: 90% to 93%

Half-life:

Full-term neonates: 40.2 hours; range: 18-73 hours

Older Children: 10.5 hours; range: 6-17 hours

Adults: 12.9 hours; range: 10-16 hours

Elimination: In urine primarily as the glucuronide conjugate

Usual Dosage

Adjunct to antiemetic therapy: Children: I.V.: 0.04-0.08 mg/kg/dose (maximum dose: 4 mg) every 6 hours as needed

Anxiety/sedation:

Infants and Children: Oral, I.V.: Usual: 0.05 mg/kg/dose (maximum dose: 2 mg/dose) every 4-8 hours; range: 0.02-0.1 mg/kg

Adults: Oral: 1-10 mg/day in 2-3 divided doses; usual dose: 2-6 mg/day in divided doses

Insomnia: Adults: Oral: 2-4 mg at bedtime

Operative amnesia: Adults: I.V.: up to 0.05 mg/kg; maximum dose: 4 mg/dose

Preoperative: Adults: I.M.: 0.05 mg/kg administered 2 hours before surgery; maximum dose: 4 mg/dose; I.V.: 0.044 mg/kg 15-20 minutes before surgery; usual maximum dose: 2 mg/dose

Sedation (preprocedure): Infants and Children:

Oral, I.M., I.V.: Usual: 0.05 mg/kg; range: 0.02-0.09 mg/kg

I.V.: may use smaller doses (eg, 0.01-0.03 mg/kg) and repeat every 20 minutes, as needed to titrate to effect

Status epilepticus: I.V.:

Neonates: 0.05 mg/kg over 2-5 minutes; may repeat in 10-15 minutes (see warning regarding benzyl alcohol)

Infants and Children: 0.1 mg/kg slow I.V. over 2-5 minutes, do not exceed 4 mg/single dose; may repeat second dose of 0.05 mg/kg slow I.V. in 10-15 minutes if needed

Adolescents: 0.07 mg/kg slow I.V. over 2-5 minutes; maximum dose: 4 mg/dose; may repeat in 10-15 minutes

Adults: 4 mg/dose given slowly over 2-5 minutes; may repeat in 10-15 minutes; usual total maximum dose per 12-hour period: 8 mg

Administration

Oral: May administer with food to decrease GI distress; dilute oral solution in water, juice, soda, or semisolid food (eg, applesauce, pudding)

Parenteral: I.V.: Do not exceed 2 mg/minute or 0.05 mg/kg over 2-5 minutes; dilute I.V. dose with equal volume of compatible diluent (D_5W, NS, SWI); administer I.V. using repeated aspiration with slow I.V. injection, to make sure the injection is not intra-arterial and that perivascular extravasation has not occurred

Monitoring Parameters Respiratory rate, blood pressure, heart rate; CBC with differential and liver function with long-term use

Patient Information Avoid alcohol; limit caffeine; may be habit-forming; may cause drowsiness and impair ability to perform activities requiring mental alertness or physical coordination; may cause dry mouth

Additional Information Single oral doses >0.09 mg/kg produced increased ataxia without increasing sedative benefit vs lower doses; since both strengths of injection contain 2% benzyl alcohol, Neofax® recommends using the 4 mg/mL strength for dilution with preservative free sterile water to make a 0.4 mg/mL dilution for I.V. use in neonates (in order to decrease the amount of benzyl alcohol delivered to the neonate); however, the stability of this dilution has not been studied. Diarrhea in a 9 month old infant receiving high-dose oral lorazepam was attributed to the lorazepam oral solution that contained polyethylene glycol and propylene glycol (both are osmotically active); diarrhea resolved when crushed tablets were substituted for the oral solution (see Marshall, 1995).

Dosage Forms

Injection: 2 mg/mL (1 mL, 10 mL); 4 mg/mL (1 mL, 10 mL)

Solution, oral concentrate, (Lorazepam Intensol®): 2 mg/mL [alcohol and dye free] (30 mL)

Tablet: 0.5 mg, 1 mg, 2 mg

References

Crawford TO, Mitchell WG, and Snodgrass SR, "Lorazepam in Childhood Status Epilepticus and Serial Seizures: Effectiveness and Tachyphylaxis," *Neurology*, 1987, 37(2):190-5.

Deshmukh A, Wittert W, Schnitzler E, et al, "Lorazepam in the Treatment of Refractory Neonatal Seizures: A Pilot Study," *Am J Dis Child*, 1986, 140(10):1042-4.

Henry DW, Burwinkle JW, and Klutman NE, "Determination of Sedative and Amnestic Doses of Lorazepam in Children," *Clin Pharm*, 1991, 10(8):625-9.

Lee DS, Wong HA, and Knoppert DC, "Myoclonus Associated With Lorazepam Therapy in Very-Low-Birth-Weight Infants," *Biol Neonate*, 1994, 66(6):311-5.

Marshall JD, Farrar HC, and Kearns GL, "Diarrhea Associated With Enteral Benzodiazepine Solutions," *J Pediatr*, 1995, 126(4):657-9.

McDermott CA, Kowalczyk AL, Schnitzler ER, et al, "Pharmacokinetics of Lorazepam in Critically Ill Neonates With Seizures," *J Pediatr*, 1992, 120(3):479-83.

- **Lorazepam Intensol®** *see* Lorazepam *on page 609*
- **Lorcet® 10/650** *see* Hydrocodone and Acetaminophen *on page 505*
- **Lorcet®-HD** *see* Hydrocodone and Acetaminophen *on page 505*
- **Lorcet® Plus** *see* Hydrocodone and Acetaminophen *on page 505*
- **Loroxide® [OTC]** *see* Benzoyl Peroxide *on page 136*
- **Lortab®** *see* Hydrocodone and Acetaminophen *on page 505*
- **Losec (Can)** *see* Omeprazole *on page 733*
- **Lotrimin AF® Topical [OTC]** *see* Clotrimazole *on page 259*
- **Lotrimin® Topical** *see* Clotrimazole *on page 259*
- **Lovenox®** *see* Enoxaparin *on page 381*
- **L-PAM** *see* Melphalan *on page 626*
- **LRH** *see* Gonadorelin *on page 482*
- **L-Sarcolysin** *see* Melphalan *on page 626*
- **LTG** *see* Lamotrigine *on page 575*
- **L-Thyroxine** *see* Levothyroxine *on page 588*
- **L-Triiodothyronine** *see* Liothyronine *on page 597*
- **Lugol's Solution** *see* Potassium Iodide *on page 815*
- **Luminal®** *see* Phenobarbital *on page 785*
- **Lupicare™ Dandruff [OTC]** *see* Salicylic Acid *on page 886*
- **Lupicare™ Psoriasis [OTC]** *see* Salicylic Acid *on page 886*
- **Lupron®** *see* Leuprolide *on page 582*
- **Lupron Depot®** *see* Leuprolide *on page 582*
- **Lupron Depot-3® Month** *see* Leuprolide *on page 582*
- **Lupron Depot-4® Month** *see* Leuprolide *on page 582*
- **Lupron Depot-Ped™** *see* Leuprolide *on page 582*
- **Luride®** *see* Fluoride *on page 441*
- **Luride® Lozi-Tab®** *see* Fluoride *on page 441*
- **Lutrepulse®** *see* Gonadorelin *on page 482*
- **Luxiq™** *see* Betamethasone *on page 140*
- **Lyderm (Can)** *see* Fluocinonide *on page 440*
- **Lydonide (Can)** *see* Fluocinonide *on page 440*

Lymphocyte Immune Globulin (LIM foe site i MYUN GLOB yoo lin)

U.S. Brand Names Atgam®

Synonyms Antithymocyte Globulin (equine); ATG; Horse Antihuman Thymocyte Gamma Globulin

Therapeutic Category Immunosuppressant Agent

Generic Available No

Use Prevention and/or treatment of allograft rejection; treatment of moderate to severe aplastic anemia in patients not considered suitable candidates for bone marrow transplantation; prevention of graft-vs-host disease following bone marrow transplantation

Pregnancy Risk Factor C

Contraindications Hypersensitivity to ATG, thimerosal, any component, or other equine gamma globulins; severe, unremitting leukopenia and/or thrombocytopenia

Warnings Should only be used by physicians experienced in immunosuppressive therapy or management of renal transplant patients; adequate laboratory and supportive medical resources must be readily available in the facility for patient management

Adverse Reactions
Cardiovascular: Hypotension, hypertension, tachycardia, edema
Central nervous system: Seizures, fever, headache, chills
Dermatologic: Rash, pruritus, urticaria
Gastrointestinal: Diarrhea, nausea, stomatitis
Hematologic: Leukopenia, thrombocytopenia, hemolysis, anemia
Local: Thrombophlebitis
Neuromuscular & skeletal: Arthralgia; pain in the chest, flank, or back; weakness
Renal: Acute renal failure
Respiratory: Dyspnea
Miscellaneous: Lymphadenopathy, serum sickness, night sweats; anaphylaxis may be indicated by hypotension or respiratory distress

Stability Store in refrigerator; dilute in $\frac{1}{2}$NS or NS; when diluted to concentrations up to 4 mg/mL, ATG infusion solution is stable for 24 hours; use of dextrose solutions is not recommended; precipitation can occur in solutions with a low salt concentration (ie, D_5W)

Mechanism of Action May involve elimination of antigen-reactive T-lymphocytes (killer cells) in peripheral blood or alteration of T-cell function

Pharmacokinetics
Distribution: Poor into lymphoid tissues; binds to circulating lymphocytes, granulocytes, platelets, bone marrow cells
Half-life, plasma: 1.5-12 days
Elimination: ~1% of dose excreted in urine

Usual Dosage Intradermal skin test is recommended prior to administration of the initial dose of ATG; use 0.1 mL of a 1:1000 dilution of ATG in NS; observe the skin test every 15 minutes for 1 hour; a local reaction ≥10 mm diameter with a wheal or erythema or both should be considered a positive skin test

I.V.:
Children:
Aplastic anemia protocol: 10-20 mg/kg/day for 8-14 days, or 40 mg/kg/day once daily over 4 hours for 4 days; then give 10-30 mg/kg/dose every other day for 7 more doses
Cardiac allograft: 10 mg/kg/day for 7 days or as per protocol
Renal allograft: 5-25 mg/kg/day or as per protocol
Children and Adults:
Rejection prevention: 15 mg/kg/day for 14 days, then give every other day for 7 more doses; initial dose should be administered within 24 hours before or after transplantation
Rejection treatment: 10-15 mg/kg/day for 14 days, then give every other day for 7 more doses

Administration Parenteral: Administer via central line; use of high flow veins will minimize the occurrence of phlebitis and thrombosis; administer by slow I.V. infusion through a 0.2-1 micron in-line filter over 4-8 hours at a final concentration not to exceed 4 mg ATG/mL

Monitoring Parameters Lymphocyte profile; CBC with differential and platelet count, vital signs during administration, renal function test

Nursing Implications Patient may need to be pretreated with an antipyretic, antihistamine, and/or corticosteroid to prevent chills and fever

Dosage Forms Injection: 50 mg/mL (5 mL)

References
Rosenfeld SJ, Kimball J, Vining D, et al, "Intensive Immunosuppression With Antithymocyte Globulin and Cyclosporine as Treatment for Severe Acquired Aplastic Anemia," *Blood*, 1995, 85(11):3058-65.

Whitehead B, James I, Helms P, et al, "Intensive Care Management of Children Following Heart and Heart-Lung Transplantation," *Intensive Care Med*, 1990, 16(7):426-30.

♦ **Lymphocyte Mitogenic Factor** *see* Aldesleukin *on page 47*

♦ **Lyphocin**® *see* Vancomycin *on page 1001*

♦ **Lysatec-rt-PA (Can)** *see* Alteplase *on page 58*

♦ **Maalox® [OTC]** *see* Antacid Preparations *on page 95*

♦ **Maalox Anti-Gas® [OTC]** *see* Simethicone *on page 902*

♦ **Maalox Anti-Gas® Extra Strength** *see* Simethicone *on page 902*

♦ **Maalox® Plus Extra Strength [OTC]** *see* Antacid Preparations *on page 95*

♦ **Macrobid**® *see* Nitrofurantoin *on page 716*

♦ **Macrodantin**® *see* Nitrofurantoin *on page 716*

♦ **Macrodex**® *see* Dextran *on page 311*

Mafenide (MA fe nide)

U.S. Brand Names Sulfamylon®

Therapeutic Category Antibiotic, Topical

Generic Available No

Use Adjunct in the treatment of second and third degree burns to prevent septicemia caused by susceptible organisms such as *Pseudomonas aeruginosa*

Pregnancy Risk Factor C

Contraindications Hypersensitivity to mafenide, sulfites, or any component

Warnings Superinfection with nonsusceptible organisms has occurred in burn wounds treated with mafenide

Precautions Use with caution in patients with renal impairment and in patients with G-6-PD deficiency

Adverse Reactions

Dermatologic: Erythema, rash, pruritus, urticaria

Endocrine & metabolic: Hyperchloremia, metabolic acidosis

Hematologic: Bone marrow suppression, hemolytic anemia, bleeding, porphyria, eosinophilia

Local: Burning sensation, excoriation, pain, swelling

Respiratory: Hyperventilation, tachypnea

Miscellaneous: Hypersensitivity reactions, facial edema

Stability Prepared topical solution is stable for 48 hours at room temperature

Mechanism of Action Interferes with bacterial cellular metabolism and bacterial folic acid synthesis through competitive inhibition of para-aminobenzoic acid

Pharmacokinetics

Absorption: Diffuses through devascularized areas and is rapidly absorbed from burned surface

Metabolism: To para-carboxybenzene sulfonamide which is a carbonic anhydrase inhibitor

Time to peak serum concentration: Topical: 2-4 hours

Elimination: In urine as metabolites

Usual Dosage Children ≥3 months and Adults: Topical

Cream: Apply once or twice daily; apply to a thickness of approximately 16 mm; the burned area should be covered with cream at all times

Solution: Irrigate dressing every 4 hours or as needed to keep gauze moistened

Administration Topical:

Cream: Apply to cleansed, debrided, burned area with a sterile-gloved hand

Solution: Reconstitute 50 g powder by adding to 1 liter sterile water or 1 liter NS for irrigation; mix until completely dissolved; filter solution through a 0.22 micron filter before use; cover area with gauze and the dressing wetted with mafenide solution; wound dressing may be left undisturbed for up to 5 days

Monitoring Parameters Acid base balance, improvement of wound healing

Patient Information Inform physician if rash, blisters, or swelling appear

Nursing Implications For external use only

Dosage Forms

Cream, topical, as acetate: 85 mg/g (56.7 g, 113.4 g, 411 g)

Powder, topical: 5% (50 g)

♦ **Mag-200 [OTC]** *see* Magnesium Supplements *on page 614*

♦ **Mag-Carb™ [OTC]** *see* Magnesium Supplements *on page 614*

♦ **Mag G® [OTC]** *see* Magnesium Supplements *on page 614*

- **Magnesia Magma (Magnesium Hydroxide)** *see* Magnesium Supplements *on page 614*
- **Magnesium Carbonate** *see* Magnesium Supplements *on page 614*
- **Magnesium Chloride** *see* Magnesium Supplements *on page 614*
- **Magnesium Citrate** *see* Magnesium Supplements *on page 614*
- **Magnesium Gluconate** *see* Magnesium Supplements *on page 614*
- **Magnesium Hydroxide** *see* Magnesium Supplements *on page 614*
- **Magnesium Hydroxide and Mineral Oil Emulsion** *see* Magnesium Supplements *on page 614*
- **Magnesium Lactate** *see* Magnesium Supplements *on page 614*
- **Magnesium Oxide** *see* Magnesium Supplements *on page 614*
- **Magnesium Sulfate** *see* Magnesium Supplements *on page 614*

Magnesium Supplements (mag NEE zee um SUP la ments)

Related Information

Adult ACLS Algorithm, Stable Ventricular Tachycardia *on page 1047*
Adult ACLS Algorithm, V. Fib and Pulseless VT *on page 1041*
CPR Pediatric Drug Dosages *on page 1031*
Pediatric ALS Algorithm, Pulseless Arrest *on page 1036*

U.S. Brand Names Almora® [OTC]; Mag-200 [OTC]; Mag-Carb™ [OTC]; Mag G® [OTC]; Magonate® [OTC]; Mag-Ox 400® [OTC]; Mag-Tab SR® [OTC]; Magtrate [OTC]; Phillips'® Milk of Magnesia [OTC]; Phillips'® M-O [OTC]; Slow-Mag® [OTC]; Uro-Mag® [OTC]

Synonyms Citrate of Magnesia (Magnesium Citrate); Epsom Salts (Magnesium Sulfate); Magnesia Magma (Magnesium Hydroxide); Milk of Magnesia (Magnesium Hydroxide); MOM (Magnesium Hydroxide)

Available Salts Magnesium Carbonate; Magnesium Chloride; Magnesium Citrate; Magnesium Gluconate; Magnesium Hydroxide; Magnesium Hydroxide and Mineral Oil Emulsion; Magnesium Lactate; Magnesium Oxide; Magnesium Sulfate

Therapeutic Category Antacid; Anticonvulsant, Miscellaneous; Electrolyte Supplement, Oral; Electrolyte Supplement, Parenteral; Laxative, Osmotic; Magnesium Salt

Generic Available Yes

Use

Treatment and prevention of hypomagnesemia **(magnesium chloride, magnesium lactate, magnesium carbonate, magnesium sulfate, magnesium gluconate, and magnesium oxide)**

Treatment of hypertension **(magnesium sulfate)**

Treatment of torsade de pointes **(magnesium sulfate)**

Treatment of encephalopathy and seizures associated with acute nephritis **(magnesium sulfate)**

Short-term treatment of constipation **(magnesium citrate, magnesium hydroxide, magnesium sulfate, and magnesium oxide)**

Treatment of hyperacidity symptoms **(magnesium hydroxide and magnesium oxide)**

Unlabeled use: Adjunctive treatment for bronchodilation in moderate to severe acute asthma **(magnesium sulfate)**

Pregnancy Risk Factor B

Contraindications Serious renal impairment, myocardial damage, heart block; patients with colostomy or ileostomy, intestinal obstruction, impaction, or perforation, appendicitis, abdominal pain

Precautions Use with caution in patients with impaired renal function (accumulation of magnesium may lead to magnesium intoxication); use with caution in digitalized patients (may alter cardiac conduction leading to heart block)

Adverse Reactions Adverse effects with magnesium therapy are related to the magnesium serum level

>3 mg/dL: Depressed CNS, blocked peripheral neuromuscular transmission leading to anticonvulsant effects

>5 mg/dL: Depressed deep tendon reflexes, flushing, somnolence

>12 mg/dL: Respiratory paralysis, complete heart block

Other effects:

Cardiovascular: Hypotension

Endocrine & metabolic: Hypermagnesemia

Gastrointestinal: Diarrhea, abdominal cramps, gas formation

Neuromuscular & skeletal: Muscle weakness

Drug Interactions Magnesium salts, when given orally, may decrease the absorption of the following: H_2 antagonists, phenytoin, iron salts, penicillamine, tetracycline, ciprofloxacin, benzodiazepines, chloroquine, steroids, and glyburide; systemic magnesium may enhance the effects of calcium channel blockers and neuromuscular blockers; may share additive CNS depressant effects with CNS depressants; if sufficient alkalinization of the urine by magnesium salts occurs, the excretion of salicylates is enhanced and the tubular reabsorption of quinidine is enhanced (increased effect)

Mechanism of Action Magnesium is important as a cofactor in many enzymatic reactions in the body. There are at least 300 enzymes which are dependent upon magnesium for normal functioning. Actions on lipoprotein lipase have been found to be important in reducing serum cholesterol. Magnesium is necessary for the maintaining of serum potassium and calcium levels due to its effect on the renal tubule. In the heart, magnesium acts as a calcium channel blocker. It also activates sodium potassium ATPase in the cell membrane to promote resting polarization and produce arrhythmias. Promotes bowel evacuation by causing osmotic retention of fluid which distends the colon and produces increased peristaltic activity when taken orally. To reduce stomach acidity, it reacts with hydrochloric acid in the stomach to form magnesium chloride.

Pharmacodynamics
Onset of action:
Anticonvulsant:
I.M.: 60 minutes
I.V.: Immediately
Laxative: Oral: 4-8 hours
Duration: Anticonvulsant:
I.M.: 3-4 hours
I.V.: 30 minutes

Pharmacokinetics
Absorption: Oral: Up to 30%
Elimination: Renal with unabsorbed drug excreted in feces

Usual Dosage Note: Multiple salt forms of magnesium exist; close attention must be paid to the salt form when ordering and administering magnesium; incorrect selection or substitution of one salt for another without proper dosage adjustment may result in serious over- or underdosing.

Recommended daily allowance of magnesium: See table.

**Magnesium - Recommended Daily Allowance (RDA)
and Estimated Average Requirement (EAR)
(in terms of elemental magnesium)**

Age	RDA (mg/day)	EAR (mg/day)
<6 mo	40	30
6-12 mo	60	75
1-3 y	80	65
4-8 y	130	110
Male		
9-13 y	240	200
14-18 y	410	340
19-30 y	400	330
Female		
9-13 y	240	200
14-18 y	360	300
19-30 y	310	255

HYPOMAGNESEMIA:
Neonates: I.V.:
Magnesium sulfate: 25-50 mg/kg/dose (0.2-0.4 mEq/kg/dose) every 8-12 hours for 2-3 doses
Magnesium chloride: 0.2-0.4 mEq/kg/dose every 8-12 hours for 2-3 doses
Children:
I.M., I.V.:
Magnesium sulfate: 25-50 mg/kg/dose (0.2-0.4 mEq/kg/dose) every 4-6 hours for 3-4 doses; maximum single dose: 2000 mg (16 mEq)
Magnesium chloride: 0.2-0.4 mEq/kg/dose every 4-6 hours for 3-4 doses; maximum single dose 16 mEq
(Continued)

Magnesium Supplements *(Continued)*

Oral:

Magnesium chloride, gluconate, lactate, carbonate, oxide, or sulfate salts: 10-20 mg/kg **elemental magnesium** per dose 4 times/day

Adults:

Magnesium gluconate: Oral: 500-1000 mg 3 times/day

Magnesium sulfate:

I.M., I.V.: 1 g every 6 hours for 4 doses, or 250 mg/kg over a 4-hour period; for severe hypomagnesemia: 8-12 g/day in divided doses has been used

Oral: 3 g every 6 hours for 4 doses

DAILY MAINTENANCE MAGNESIUM: I.V.:

Magnesium sulfate or magnesium chloride:

Neonates, Infants, and Children ≤45 kg: 0.25-0.5 mEq/kg/day

Adolescents >45 kg and Adults: 0.2-0.5 mEq/kg/day or 3-10 mEq/1000 kcal/day (maximum 8-16 mEq/day)

MANAGEMENT OF SEIZURES AND HYPERTENSION: I.M., I.V.:

Magnesium sulfate:

Children: 20-100 mg/kg/dose every 4-6 hours as needed; in severe cases doses as high as 200 mg/kg/dose have been used

Adults: 1 g every 6 hours for 4 doses as needed

TREATMENT OF TORSADE DE POINTES VT: I.V.:

Magnesium sulfate: Infants and Children: 25-50 mg/kg/dose; not to exceed 2 g/dose

BRONCHODILATION (adjunctive treatment in moderate to severe acute asthma): I.V.:

Magnesium sulfate:

Children: 25 mg/kg/dose (maximum dose 2 g) as a single dose

Adults: 2 g as a single dose

Note: Literature evaluating magnesium sulfate's efficacy in the relief of bronchospasm has utilized single dosages in patient's with acute symptomatology who have received aerosol β-agonist therapy (see References). A recent study (Ciarallo, 2000) showed significant improvement in pulmonary function in children who received a single dose of 40 mg/kg magnesium sulfate vs. placebo

CATHARTIC: Oral:

Magnesium citrate (Citrate of magnesia):

<6 years: 2-4 mL/kg given once or in divided doses

6-12 years: 100-150 mL

≥12 years and Adults: 150-300 mL

Magnesium hydroxide (Milk of magnesia, MOM):

<2 years: 0.5 mL/kg/dose

2-5 years: 5-15 mL/day once or in divided doses

6-11 years: 15-30 mL/day once or in divided doses

≥12 years and adults: 30-60 mL/day once or in divided doses

Magnesium hydroxide and mineral oil (Haley's M-O®) (pediatric dosage to provide equivalent dosage of magnesium hydroxide)

<2 years: 0.6 mL/kg/dose

2-5 years: 6-18 mL/day once or in divided doses

6-11 years: 18-36 mL/day once or in divided doses

≥12 years and Adults: 30-45 mL once or in divided doses

Magnesium sulfate:

Children: 0.25 g/kg/dose once or in divided doses

Adults: 10-30 g

Magnesium oxide: Adults: 2-4 g at bedtime with full glass of water

Elemental Magnesium Content of Magnesium Salts

Magnesium Salt	Elemental Magnesium (mg per 500 mg salt)	mEq Magnesium per 500 mg salt
Magnesium carbonate	140	11.7
Magnesium chloride	59	4.9
Magnesium gluconate	27	2.4
Magnesium lactate	50	4.2
Magnesium oxide	302	25
Magnesium sulfate	49.3	4.1

ANTACID Oral:

Magnesium hydroxide:

Children: Liquid: 2.5-5 mL/dose, up to 4 times/day

Adults:

Liquid: 5-15 mL/dose, up to 4 times/day

Liquid concentrate: 2.5-7.5 mL/dose, up to 4 times/day

Tablet: 622-1244 mg/dose, up to 4 times/day

Magnesium oxide: Adults: 140 mg 3-4 times/day or 400-840 mg/day

Dosing in renal impairment: Patients in severe renal failure should not receive magnesium due to toxicity from accumulation. Patients with a Cl_{cr} <25 mL/minute receiving magnesium should have serum magnesium levels monitored.

Administration

Oral:

Solution: Mix with water and administer on an empty stomach; chill **magnesium citrate** prior to administration to improve palatability

Tablet: Take with full glass of water; chew **magnesium hydroxide** chewable tablets thoroughly; do not chew or crush sustained release formulations

Parenteral: Intermittent infusion: Dilute to a concentration of 0.5 mEq/mL (60 mg/mL of **magnesium sulfate**) (maximum concentration: 1.6 mEq/mL, 200 mg/mL of **magnesium sulfate**) and infuse over 2-4 hours; do not exceed 1 mEq/kg/hour (125 mg/kg/hour of **magnesium sulfate**); in severe circumstances, half of the dosage to be administered may be infused over the first 15-20 minutes; for I.M. administration, dilute **magnesium sulfate** to a maximum concentration of 200 mg/mL prior to injection; rapid infusions (utilized for treatment of severe asthma or torsade de pointes VT) over 10-20 minutes may be used **(magnesium sulfate)**

Monitoring Parameters Serum magnesium, deep tendon reflexes, respiratory rate, renal function, blood pressure, stool output (laxative use)

Reference Range

Neonates and Infants: 1.5-2.3 mEq/L

Children: 1.5-2.0 mEq/L

Adults: 1.4-2.0 mEq/L

Additional Information 1 g elemental magnesium = 83.3 mEq = 41.1 mmol

Dosage Forms Amount of magnesium salt is listed with **elemental** magnesium content in brackets

Magnesium, amino acid chelate: Tablet: 500 mg [100 mg]

Magnesium carbonate: Capsule, gelatin (Mag-Carb™): 250 mg [5.8 mEq; 70 mg]

Magnesium chloride:

Injection: 20% [1.97 mEq/mL] (50 mL)

Tablet, sustained release (Slow-Mag®): 535 mg [5.2 mEq; 63 mg]

Magnesium citrate: Solution: 290 mg/5 mL (300 mL)

Magnesium gluconate:

Solution (Magonate®): 1000 mg/5 mL [4.8 mEq; 54 mg] (480 mL)

Tablet (Almora®, Mag G®, Magonate®, Magtrate®): 500 mg [2.4 mEq; 27 mg]

Magnesium hydroxide:

Liquid (Phillips'® Milk of Magnesia): 400 mg/5 mL (10 mL, 30 mL, 145 mL, 360 mL, 480 mL, 960 mL, 3780 mL)

Liquid, concentrate: 10 mL equivalent to 30 mL milk of magnesia USP

Concentrated Phillips'® Milk of Magnesia: 800 mg/5 mL [strawberry flavor] (240 mL)

Tablet, chewable (Phillips'® Milk of Magnesia): 311 mg

Magnesium hydroxide and mineral oil:

Suspension (Phillips'® M-O): Magnesium hydroxide 300 mg and mineral oil 1.25 mL per 5 mL

Magnesium lactate: Caplet, sustained release (Mag-Tab SR®): 835 mg [7 mEq; 84 mg]

Magnesium oxide:

Capsule (Uro-Mag®): 140 mg [7 mEq; 84 mg]

Tablet (Mag-Ox 400®): 400 mg [20 mEq; 242 mg], 420 mg [21 mEq; 254 mg]

Magnesium sulfate:

Injection: 125 mg/mL (8 mL); 500 mg/mL (2 mL, 5 mL, 10 mL, 20 mL, 50 mL)

Injection, premixed: 10 mg/mL [in D_5W] (100 mL, 1000 mL); 20 mg/mL [in D_5W] (500 mL, 1000 mL); 40 mg/mL [in water for injection] (100 mL, 500 mL, 1000 mL); 80 mg/mL [in water for injection] (500 mL)

References

Bloch H, Silverman R, Mancherje N, et al, "Intravenous Magnesium Sulfate as an Adjunct in the Treatment of Acute Asthma," *Chest*, 1995, 107(6):1576-81.

Chernow B, Smith J, Rainey TG, et al, "Hypomagnesemia: Implications for the Critical Care Specialist," *Crit Care Med*, 1982, 10(3):193-6.

Ciarallo L, Brousseau D, and Reinert S, "Higher-Dose Intravenous Magnesium Therapy for Children With Moderate to Severe Acute Asthma," *Arch Pediatr Adolesc Med*, 2000, 154(10):979-83.

(Continued)

Magnesium Supplements *(Continued)*

Ciarallo L, Sauer AH, and Shannon MW, "Intravenous Magnesium Therapy for Moderate to Severe Pediatric Asthma: Results of a Randomized, Placebo-Controlled Trial," *J Pediatr*, 1996, 129(6):809-14.

"Dietary Reference Intakes for Calcium, Phosphorus, Magnesium, Vitamin D, and Fluoride. Standing Committee on the Scientific Evaluation of Dietary Reference Intakes, Food and Nutrition Board, Institute of Medicine," National Academy of Sciences, Washington, DC: National Academy Press, 1997.

Engel J, "Normal Laboratory Values," *Pocket Guide to Pediatric Assessment*, St Louis, MO: CV Mosby, 1989, 259.

"Guidelines 2000 for Cardiopulmonary Resuscitation and Emergency Cardiovascular Care. Part 10: Pediatric Advanced Life Support. The American Heart Association in Collaboration With the International Liaison Committee on Resuscitation," *Circulation*, 2000, 102(8 Suppl):I291-342.

- ♦ **Magonate®** [OTC] *see* Magnesium Supplements *on page 614*
- ♦ **Mag-Ox 400®** [OTC] *see* Magnesium Supplements *on page 614*
- ♦ **Mag-Tab SR®** [OTC] *see* Magnesium Supplements *on page 614*
- ♦ **Magtrate** [OTC] *see* Magnesium Supplements *on page 614*
- ♦ **Ma Huang** *see* Ephedrine *on page 384*
- ♦ **Mallamint®** [OTC] *see* Calcium Supplements *on page 167*
- ♦ **Mallergan-VC® With Codeine** *see* Promethazine, Phenylephrine, and Codeine *on page 840*

Malt Soup Extract *(malt soop EKS trakt)*

U.S. Brand Names Maltsupex® [OTC]

Therapeutic Category Laxative, Bulk-Producing

Generic Available No

Use Short-term treatment of constipation

Contraindications Hypersensitivity to barley malt extract or any component

Warnings Do not use when abdominal pain, nausea, or vomiting are present

Adverse Reactions Gastrointestinal: Abdominal cramps, diarrhea, rectal obstruction

Mechanism of Action Holds water in stool, reduces fecal pH

Pharmacodynamics Onset of action: Effect is usually apparent in 12-24 hours

Pharmacokinetics Hydrolyzed in the colon, metabolized by the liver

Usual Dosage Oral:

Infants >1 month:

Breast-fed:

Liquid: 1-2 teaspoonfuls in 2-4 oz of water or fruit juice 1-2 times/day for 3-4 days

Powder: 4 g in 2-4 oz of water or fruit juice daily for 3-4 days

Bottle-fed:

Liquid: $\frac{1}{2}$ to 2 tablespoonfuls/day in formula for 3-4 days, then 1-2 teaspoonfuls/day

Powder: 8-16 g/day in formula for 3-4 days, then 4-8 g/day

Children:

2-6 years:

Liquid: 7.5 mL 1-2 times/day for 3-4 days

Powder: 8 g twice daily for 3-4 days

6-12 years:

Liquid: 15-30 mL 1-2 times/day for 3-4 days

Powder: Up to 16 g/day for 3-4 days

Children ≥12 years and Adults:

Liquid: 30 mL twice daily for 3-4 days, then 15-30 mL at bedtime

Powder: Up to 32 g twice daily for 3-4 days, then 16-32 g at bedtime

Tablets: 4 tablets 4 times/day (maximum dose: 64 g/day)

Administration Oral: Add to warm water and stir; then add milk, formula, water, or fruit juice until dissolved

Dosage Forms

Liquid: Nondiastatic barley malt extract 16 g/15 mL (240 mL, 480 mL)

Powder: Nondiastatic barley malt extract 16 g/tablespoonful (240 g, 480 g)

Tablet: Nondiastatic barley malt extract 750 mg

- ♦ **Maltsupex®** [OTC] *see* Malt Soup Extract *on page 618*
- ♦ **Mandelamine®** *see* Methenamine *on page 643*
- ♦ **Manganese Chloride** *see* Trace Metals *on page 972*
- ♦ **Manganese Sulfate** *see* Trace Metals *on page 972*

Mannitol (MAN i tole)

U.S. Brand Names Osmitrol®; Resectisol®

Synonyms D-Mannitol

Therapeutic Category Diuretic, Osmotic

Generic Available Yes

Use Reduction of increased intracranial pressure (ICP) associated with cerebral edema; promotion of diuresis in the prevention and/or treatment of oliguria or anuria due to acute renal failure; reduction of increased intraocular pressure; promotion of urinary excretion of toxic substances

Pregnancy Risk Factor C

Contraindications Hypersensitivity to mannitol or any component; severe renal disease, dehydration, active intracranial bleeding, severe pulmonary edema, or congestion

Adverse Reactions

Cardiovascular: Circulatory overload, CHF (due to inadequate urine output and overexpansion of extracellular fluid)

Central nervous system: Convulsions, headache

Endocrine & metabolic: Fluid and electrolyte imbalance, hyponatremia or hypernatremia, hypokalemia or hyperkalemia, water intoxication, dehydration and hypovolemia secondary to rapid diuresis

Gastrointestinal: Xerostomia

Local: Tissue necrosis

Respiratory: Pulmonary edema

Miscellaneous: Allergic reactions

Drug Interactions Lithium

Stability Store at room temperature (15°C to 30°C); protect from freezing; crystallization may occur at low temperatures; do not use solutions that contain crystals; heating in a hot water bath and vigorous shaking may be utilized for resolubilization of crystals; cool solutions to body temperature before using; incompatible with strongly acidic or alkaline solutions; potassium chloride or sodium chloride may cause precipitation of mannitol 20% or 25% solution

Mechanism of Action Increases the osmotic pressure of glomerular filtrate, which inhibits tubular reabsorption of water and electrolytes and increases urinary output

Pharmacodynamics After I.V. injection:

Diuresis: Onset of action: Within 1-3 hours

Reduction in ICP:

Onset of action: Within 15 minutes

Duration: 3-6 hours

Pharmacokinetics

Distribution: Remains confined to extracellular space; does not penetrate blood-brain barrier (except in very high concentrations or with acidosis)

Metabolism: Minimal amounts in the liver to glycogen

Half-life: 1.1-1.6 hours

Elimination: Primarily unchanged in urine by glomerular filtration

Usual Dosage I.V.:

Children:

Test dose (to assess adequate renal function): 200 mg/kg (maximum dose: 12.5 g) over 3-5 minutes to produce a urine flow of at least 1 mL/kg/hour for 1-3 hours

Initial: 0.5-1 g/kg

Maintenance: 0.25-0.5 g/kg every 4-6 hours

Adults:

Test dose: 12.5 g (200 mg/kg) over 3-5 minutes to produce a urine flow of at least 30-50 mL of urine per hour over the next 2-3 hours

Initial: 0.5-1 g/kg

Maintenance: 0.25-0.5 g/kg every 4-6 hours

Administration Parenteral: In-line filter set (≤5 micron) should always be used for mannitol infusion with concentrations ≥20%; administer test dose (for oliguria) I.V. push over 3-5 minutes; for cerebral edema or elevated ICP, administer over 20-30 minutes

Monitoring Parameters Renal function, daily fluid intake and output, serum electrolytes, serum and urine osmolality; for treatment of elevated intracranial pressure, maintain serum osmolality 310-320 mOsm/kg

Nursing Implications Avoid extravasation; crenation and agglutination of red blood cells may occur if administered with whole blood

Additional Information Approximate osmolarity: Mannitol 20%: 1100 mOsm/L; mannitol 25%: 1375 mOsm/L

(Continued)

Mannitol *(Continued)*

Dosage Forms

Injection (Osmitrol®): 5% [50 mg/mL] (1000 mL); 10% [100 mg/mL] (500 mL, 1000 mL); 15% [150 mg/mL] (500 mL); 20% [200 mg/mL] (150 mL, 250 mL, 500 mL); 25% [250 mg/mL] (50 mL)

Solution, urogenital (Resectisol®): 5% [50 mg/mL] (2000 mL, 4000 mL)

- ♦ **Mapap® [OTC]**   *see* Acetaminophen *on page 29*
- ♦ **Marcaine®**   *see* Bupivacaine *on page 158*
- ♦ **Marcillin®**   *see* Ampicillin *on page 88*
- ♦ **Margesic® H**   *see* Hydrocodone and Acetaminophen *on page 505*
- ♦ **Marinol®**   *see* Dronabinol *on page 364*
- ♦ **Matulane®**   *see* Procarbazine *on page 832*
- ♦ **Maxair™**   *see* Pirbuterol *on page 805*
- ♦ **Maxair™ Autohaler™**   *see* Pirbuterol *on page 805*
- ♦ **Maxenal (Can)** *see* Pseudoephedrine *on page 852*
- ♦ **Maxidex®**   *see* Dexamethasone *on page 307*
- ♦ **Maxipime®**   *see* Cefepime *on page 191*
- ♦ **Maxi-Strength Wart Remover [OTC]**   *see* Salicylic Acid *on page 886*
- ♦ **Maxitrol®**   *see* Dexamethasone, Neomycin, and Polymyxin B *on page 309*
- ♦ **Maxivate®**   *see* Betamethasone *on page 140*
- ♦ **Mazepine (Can)** *see* Carbamazepine *on page 175*
- ♦ **Mazon Medicated Soap (Can)** *see* Coal Tar *on page 260*
- ♦ **MCT Oil® [OTC]**   *see* Medium Chain Triglycerides *on page 623*
- ♦ **Measles and Rubella Vaccines, Combined** *see page 1172*
- ♦ **Measles, Mumps, and Rubella Vaccines, Combined** *see page 1172*
- ♦ **Measles Virus Vaccine, Live, Attenuated** *see page 1172*
- ♦ **Measurin® [OTC]**   *see* Aspirin *on page 109*
- ♦ **Mebaral®**   *see* Mephobarbital *on page 631*

Mebendazole *(me BEN da zole)*

U.S. Brand Names Vermox®

Therapeutic Category Anthelmintic

Generic Available Yes

Use Treatment of enterobiasis (pinworm infection), trichuriasis (whipworm infection), ascariasis (roundworm infection), and hookworm infections caused by *Necator americanus* or *Ancylostoma duodenale*; drug of choice in the treatment of capillariasis

Pregnancy Risk Factor C

Contraindications Hypersensitivity to mebendazole or any component

Warnings Pregnancy and children <2 years of age are relative contraindications since safety has not been established

Adverse Reactions

Central nervous system: Dizziness, fever, headache

Dermatologic: Rash, pruritus, alopecia

Gastrointestinal: Diarrhea, abdominal pain, nausea, vomiting

Hematologic: Neutropenia, anemia, leukopenia

Hepatic: Transient abnormalities in liver function tests

Otic: Tinnitus

Renal: Hematuria

Drug Interactions Anticonvulsants such as carbamazepine and phenytoin may increase metabolism of mebendazole

Food Interactions Food increases mebendazole absorption

Mechanism of Action Selectively and irreversibly blocks uptake of glucose and other nutrients in susceptible intestine-dwelling helminths

Pharmacokinetics

Absorption: Oral: 2% to 10%

Distribution: To Liver, fat, muscle, plasma, and hepatic cysts

Protein binding: 95%

Metabolism: Extensive in the liver

Half-life: 2.8-9 hours

Time to peak serum concentration: Variable (0.5-7 hours)

Elimination: Primarily in feces as inactive metabolites with 5% to 10% eliminated in urine

Dialysis: Not dialyzable

Usual Dosage Children and Adults: Oral:
  Pinworms: Single chewable tablet (100 mg); may need to repeat after 2 weeks
  Whipworms, roundworms, hookworms: 100 mg twice daily, morning and evening on 3 consecutive days; if patient is not cured within 3-4 weeks, a second course of treatment may be administered
  Capillariasis: 200 mg twice daily for 20 days

Administration Oral: Administer with food; tablet can be crushed and mixed with food, swallowed whole, or chewed

Monitoring Parameters For treatment of trichuriasis, ascariasis, hookworm, or mixed infections, check for helminth ova in the feces within 3-4 weeks following the initial therapy

Dosage Forms Tablet, chewable: 100 mg

References
  Hotez PJ, "Hookworm Disease in Children," *Pediatr Infect Dis J*, 1989, 8(8):516-20.

Mechlorethamine (me klor ETH a meen)

Related Information
  Emetogenic Potential of Single Chemotherapeutic Agents *on page 1129*
  Extravasation Treatment *on page 1085*

U.S. Brand Names Mustargen® Hydrochloride

Synonyms HN₂; Mustine; Nitrogen Mustard

Therapeutic Category Antineoplastic Agent, Alkylating Agent (Nitrogen Mustard)

Generic Available No

Use Combination therapy of Hodgkin's disease, brain tumors, non-Hodgkin's lymphoma, and malignant lymphomas; palliative treatment of lung, breast, and ovarian carcinoma; sclerosing agent in intracavitary therapy of pleural, pericardial, and other malignant effusions

Pregnancy Risk Factor D

Contraindications Hypersensitivity to mechlorethamine or any component; pre-existing profound myelosuppression

Warnings The FDA currently recommends that procedures for proper handling, administration, and disposal of mechlorethamine powder and solution be followed. Avoid inhalation of dust or vapors and contact with skin or mucous membranes. Mechlorethamine is potentially carcinogenic, teratogenic, and mutagenic. It may cause permanent sterility and birth defects. Extravasation of the drug into subcutaneous tissues results in painful inflammation, erythema, and induration; sloughing may occur; promptly infiltrate the area with sterile isotonic sodium thiosulfate ($^1/_6$ molar) and apply a cold compress for 6-12 hours. See Extravasation Treatment *on page 1085*

Precautions Use with caution in patients with myelosuppression; patients with lymphoma should receive adequate hydration, alkalinization of the urine and/or prophylactic allopurinol to prevent complications such as uric acid nephropathy and hyperuricemia

Adverse Reactions
  Cardiovascular: Thrombosis
  Central nervous system: Vertigo, fever, headache, drowsiness, lethargy, encephalopathy (high dose)
  Dermatologic: Rash, alopecia
  Endocrine & metabolic: Amenorrhea, impaired spermatogenesis, hyperuricemia
  Gastrointestinal: Nausea, vomiting, anorexia, diarrhea, metallic taste, mucositis
  Hematologic: Myelosuppression (leukopenia, thrombocytopenia), hemolytic anemia
  Local: Thrombophlebitis, tissue necrosis upon extravasation
  Neuromuscular & skeletal: Weakness
  Ocular: Lacrimation
  Otic: Tinnitus, deafness
  Miscellaneous: Hypersensitivity reactions, diaphoresis, anaphylaxis

Stability Highly unstable in neutral or alkaline solutions; use immediately after reconstitution; discard any unused drug after 60 minutes (although manufacturer reports only 15 minutes of stability after reconstitution, other studies indicate it is stable longer)

Mechanism of Action Alkylating agent that inhibits DNA and RNA synthesis via formation of carbonium ions which can attach to nucleic acids at the N^7 position of guanine; cross-links strands of DNA causing miscoding, breakage, and failure of replication

Pharmacokinetics
  Absorption: Incomplete after intracavitary administration secondary to rapid deactivation by body fluids
  (Continued)

Mechlorethamine *(Continued)*

Distribution: Following I.V. administration, drug undergoes rapid hydrolysis to a highly reactive alkylating intermediate; unchanged drug is undetectable in the blood within a few minutes

Half-life: <1 minute

Elimination: <0.01% of unchanged drug is recovered in urine

Usual Dosage Refer to individual protocols

Children:

Lymphoma: MOPP regimen: Mustargen® (mechlorethamine), Oncovin® (vincristine), procarbazine, and prednisone: I.V.: 6 mg/m² on days 1 and 8 of a 28-day cycle

Brain tumors: MOPP regimen: I.V.: 3 mg/m² on days 1 and 8 of a 28-day cycle

Adults:

I.V.: 0.4 mg/kg or 12-16 mg/m² as a single monthly dose or divided into 0.1 mg/kg/day once daily for 4 days, repeated at 4- to 6-week intervals

Intracavitary: 10-30 mg or 0.2-0.4 mg/kg

Administration

Intracavitary: Dilute dose in up to 100 mL NS; paracentesis is performed to remove most of the fluid from the cavity prior to administration; inject drug slowly with frequent aspiration to ensure that a free flow of fluid is present; change patient's position every 5-10 minutes for 1 hour following injection to distribute drug uniformly throughout the cavity

Parenteral: **DO NOT ADMINISTER I.M. or SUBCUTANEOUSLY.** Administer I.V. push through a side port of an established I.V. line over 1-5 minutes at a concentration not to exceed 1 mg/mL

Monitoring Parameters CBC with differential and platelet count, hemoglobin

Patient Information Report to physician any pain or irritation at the site of injection, fever, sore throat, bruising, bleeding, shortness of breath, itching, or wheezing

Nursing Implications Avoid extravasation, inhalation of vapors, or contact with skin, mucous membranes, and eyes since mechlorethamine is a potent vesicant. If accidental eye contact occurs, copious irrigation for at least 15 minutes with NS or a balanced salt ophthalmic irrigating solution should be instituted immediately followed by prompt ophthalmologic consultation. If accidental skin contact occurs, irrigate the affected area with copious amounts of water for at least 15 minutes while removing contaminated clothing, followed by application of a 2% sodium thiosulfate solution; contaminated clothing should be destroyed. Medical attention should be sought immediately. For nitrogen mustard extravasations, infiltrate area with a 1/6 molar sodium thiosulfate solution and apply cold compresses for 6-12 hours; 1/6 molar sodium thiosulfate solution can be prepared by diluting 4 mL of 10% sodium thiosulfate injection with 6 mL of sterile water for injection; Dorr recommends to inject 2 mL of the 1/6 molar solution into site for each milligram of mechlorethamine extravasated

Additional Information Myelosuppressive effects:

WBC: Severe

Platelets: Severe

Onset (days): 4-7

Nadir (days): 14

Recovery (days): 21

Dosage Forms Powder for injection, as hydrochloride: 10 mg

References

Ater JL, van Eys J, Woo SY, et al, "MOPP Chemotherapy Without Irradiation as Primary Postsurgical Therapy for Brain Tumors in Infants and Young Children," *J Neurooncol*, 1997, 32(3):243-52.

Berg SL, Grisell DL, DeLaney TF, et al, "Principles of Treatment of Pediatric Solid Tumors," *Pediatr Clin North Am*, 1991, 38(2):249-67.

Dorr RT, Soble M, and Alberts DS, "Efficacy of Sodium Thiosulfate as a Local Antidote to Mechlorethamine Skin Toxicity in the Mouse," *Cancer Chemother Pharmacol*, 1988, 22(4):299-302.

Krischer JP, Ragab AH, Kun L, et al, "Nitrogen Mustard, Vincristine, Procarbazine, and Prednisone as Adjuvant Chemotherapy in the Treatment of Medulloblastoma. A Pediatric Oncology Group Study," *J Neurosurg*, 1991, 74(6):905-9.

♦ Meclastine *see* Clemastine *on page 249*

Meclizine *(MEK li zeen)*

Related Information

Overdose and Toxicology *on page 1222*

U.S. Brand Names Antivert®; Bonine® [OTC]; Dramamine® II [OTC]

Canadian Brand Names Bonamine

Synonyms Meclozine

Therapeutic Category Antiemetic; Antihistamine

Generic Available Yes

Use Prevention and treatment of motion sickness; management of vertigo

Pregnancy Risk Factor B

Contraindications Hypersensitivity to meclizine or any component

Precautions Use with caution in patients with angle-closure glaucoma or obstructive diseases of the GI or GU tract

Adverse Reactions

Cardiovascular: Hypotension, palpitations, tachycardia

Central nervous system: Drowsiness, fatigue, auditory and visual hallucinations, restlessness, excitation, insomnia, nervousness

Dermatologic: Urticaria, rash

Gastrointestinal: Xerostomia, anorexia, nausea, vomiting, diarrhea, constipation, appetite increase, weight gain

Hepatic: Cholestatic jaundice, hepatitis

Neuromuscular & skeletal: Myalgia, tremor, paresthesia

Ocular: Blurred vision, diplopia

Otic: Tinnitus

Respiratory: Bronchospasm, epistaxis

Drug Interactions Additive sedation with CNS depressants (eg, sedatives, alcohol, antihistamines)

Mechanism of Action Has central anticholinergic action and CNS depressant activity; decreases excitability of the middle ear labyrinth and blocks conduction in the middle ear vestibular-cerebellar pathways

Pharmacodynamics

Onset of action: Oral: 30-60 minutes

Duration: 12-24 hours

Pharmacokinetics

Metabolism: In the liver

Half-life: 6 hours

Elimination: As metabolites in urine and as unchanged drug in feces

Usual Dosage Children >12 years and Adults: Oral:

Motion sickness: 25-50 mg 1 hour before travel, repeat dose every 24 hours if needed

Vertigo: 25-100 mg/day in divided doses

Administration Oral: Administer with food to decrease GI distress

Patient Information May cause drowsiness and impair ability to perform hazardous activities requiring mental alertness or physical coordination

Dosage Forms

Capsule, as hydrochloride (Meni-D®): 25 mg, 30 mg

Tablet, as hydrochloride: 12.5 mg, 25 mg, 50 mg

Antivert®: 12.5 mg, 25 mg, 50 mg

Dramamine® II: 25 mg

Tablet, chewable, as hydrochloride (Bonine®): 25 mg

♦ **Mecloprodin** *see* Clemastine *on page 249*

♦ **Meclozine** *see* Meclizine *on page 622*

♦ **Meda-Cap® [OTC]** *see* Acetaminophen *on page 29*

♦ **Meda® Tab [OTC]** *see* Acetaminophen *on page 29*

♦ **Medicinal Carbon** *see* Charcoal *on page 213*

♦ **Medicinal Charcoal** *see* Charcoal *on page 213*

♦ **Medicone® [OTC]** *see* Phenylephrine *on page 789*

♦ **Mediplast® [OTC]** *see* Salicylic Acid *on page 886*

♦ **Medi-Quick® Ointment [OTC]** *see* Neomycin, Polymyxin B, and Bacitracin *on page 707*

Medium Chain Triglycerides (mee DEE um chane trye GLIS er ides)

U.S. Brand Names MCT Oil® [OTC]

Synonyms Triglycerides, Medium Chain

Therapeutic Category Caloric Agent; Nutritional Supplement

Generic Available No

Use Nutritional supplement for those who cannot digest long chain fats; malabsorption associated with disorders such as pancreatic insufficiency, bile salt deficiency, and bacterial overgrowth of the small bowel; induce ketosis as a prevention for seizures (akinetic, clonic, and petit mal)

Pregnancy Risk Factor C

Contraindications Hypersensitivity to any component; should not be used in patients with hepatic encephalopathy due to earlier observations which report that

(Continued)

Medium Chain Triglycerides *(Continued)*

short chain fatty acids may have a narcotic effect on the CNS and inhibit oxidative phosphorylation

Warnings Patients with cirrhosis demonstrate higher concentrations of medium chain fatty acids in the serum and CSF than normal individuals; impaired hepatic clearance of medium chain fatty acids due to parenchymal dysfunction of medium chain fatty acid oxidation, portal systemic shunt, and impaired protein binding of fatty acid enhance the passive diffusion of medium chain fatty acids into the CSF

Precautions Use with caution in patients with hepatic cirrhosis and complications such as portacaval shunts or encephalopathy

Adverse Reactions
Central nervous system: Sedation, narcosis, coma (cirrhotics)
Endocrine & metabolic: Ketosis
Gastrointestinal: Nausea, vomiting, abdominal pain, diarrhea, borborygmi

Mechanism of Action A semisynthetic class of lipids; medium chain triglycerides (MCT) are composed of fatty acids with chain length varying from 6-12 carbon atoms; preparations contain approximately 75% octanoic (caprylic), 20% to 25% decanoic (capric); 1% hexanoic (caproic), and 1% dodecanoic (lauric) acids

MCT are hydrolyzed in the stomach and in the small intestine by pancreatic lipase to form medium chain fatty acids; the medium chain fatty acids are incorporated into bile salts for more rapid solubilization and entrance into the mucosal cell and into the portal venous blood; MCT can also be absorbed unchanged as a triglyceride into the mucosal cell; medium chain fatty acids presented to the liver are minimally converted to hepatic lipid and are rapidly oxidized to carbon dioxide, ketones, and acetate; the medium chain fatty acids are also esterified to long chain triglycerides

Pharmacodynamics Onset of action: Octanoic acid appeared in each subject by 30 minutes following ingestion; effect on seizures in children: Within 6 weeks

Pharmacokinetics
Absorption: Up to 30% of dose can be absorbed unchanged as a triglyceride in the mucosal cell
Metabolism: Almost entirely oxidized by the liver to acetyl CoA fragments and to carbon dioxide; little deposited in adipose tissue or elsewhere
Elimination: As much as 20% of oral dose of MCT, recovered in expired CO_2 in 50 minutes; <10% elimination of medium chain fatty acids in feces

Usual Dosage Oral:
Infants: Nutritional supplement: Initial: 0.5 mL every other feeding, then advance to every feeding, then increase in increments of 0.25-0.5 mL/feeding at intervals of 2-3 days as tolerated
Children: Seizures: About 40 mL with each meal or 50% to 70% (800-1120 kcal) of total calories (1600 kcal) as the oil will induce the ketosis necessary for seizure control
Children and Adults: Cystic fibrosis: 3 tablespoons/day in divided doses
Adults: Malabsorption syndromes: 15 mL 3-4 times/day

Administration Oral:
Dilute with at least an equal volume of water or mix with some other vehicle such as fruit juice (should not be cold; flavoring may be added); mixture should be sipped slowly; administer no more than 15-20 mL at any one time (up to 100 mL may be administered in divided doses in a 24-hour period)
Possible GI side effects from medication can be prevented if therapy is initiated with small supplements at meals and gradually increased according to patient's tolerance

Patient Information GI symptoms may occur during the first few days of administration and then disappear; it is important to continue therapy with at least the smallest dose

Additional Information Does not provide any essential fatty acids; contains only saturated fats; supplementation with safflower, corn oil, or other polyunsaturated vegetable oil must be given to provide the patient with the essential fatty acids; caloric content: 8.3 calories/g; 115 calories/15 mL

Dosage Forms Oil: 14 g/15 mL (960 mL)

♦ **Medrol**® *see Methylprednisolone on page 655*

Medroxyprogesterone *(me DROKS ee proe JES te rone)*

U.S. Brand Names Depo-Provera®; Provera®
Canadian Brand Names Alti-MPA; Gen-Medroxy; Novo-Medrone
Synonyms Acetoxymethylprogesterone; Methylacetoxyprogesterone
Therapeutic Category Contraceptive, Progestin Only; Progestin
Generic Available Yes

Use Secondary amenorrhea or abnormal uterine bleeding due to hormonal imbalance; prevention of pregnancy

Pregnancy Risk Factor X

Contraindications Thrombophlebitis; hypersensitivity to medroxyprogesterone or any component; cerebral apoplexy, undiagnosed vaginal bleeding, liver dysfunction, thromboembolic disorders, breast cancer, pregnancy (known or suspected)

Warnings Discontinue if there is a sudden partial or complete loss of vision, proptosis, diplopia, migraine, if papilledema or retinal vascular lesions are present, or any other symptom of a thromboembolic event

Precautions Use with caution in patients with mental depression, diabetes, epilepsy, asthma, migraines, renal or cardiac dysfunction

Adverse Reactions
Cardiovascular: Edema, thromboembolic disorders
Central nervous system: Depression, dizziness, nervousness, fever, insomnia
Dermatologic: Melasma, chloasma, urticaria, acne, photosensitivity, alopecia, hirsutism
Endocrine & metabolic: Menstrual irregularities, amenorrhea, breakthrough bleeding, breast tenderness
Gastrointestinal: Weight gain or loss, anorexia
Hepatic: Cholestatic jaundice
Local: Pain at injection site, thrombophlebitis
Neuromuscular & skeletal: Weakness

Drug Interactions Aminoglutethimide depresses serum concentrations of medroxyprogesterone acetate

Mechanism of Action Inhibits secretion of pituitary gonadotropins, which prevents follicular maturation and ovulation, transforms a proliferative endometrium into a secretory one

Pharmacokinetics
Absorption: I.M.: Slow
Bioavailability: 0.6% to 10%
Protein binding: 90%
Metabolism: In the liver
Half-life: 30 days
Elimination: Oral: In urine and feces

Usual Dosage Adolescents and Adults:
Amenorrhea: Oral: 5-10 mg/day for 5-10 days or 2.5 mg/day
Abnormal uterine bleeding: Oral: 5-10 mg for 5-10 days starting on day 16 or day 21 of menstrual cycle
Contraception: I.M.: 150 mg every 3 months; first dose to be given only during first 5 days of normal menstrual period; only within 5 days postpartum if not breast-feeding, or only at sixth postpartum week if exclusively breast-feeding

Administration
Oral: Administer with food
Parenteral: I.M. only; not for I.V. use; shake well before drawing into syringe

Test Interactions Altered thyroid and liver function tests, prothrombin time, factors VII, VIII, IX, X, metyrapone test

Patient Information Notify physician if sudden loss of vision or migraine headache occurs; may cause photosensitivity, wear protective clothing or sunscreen

Additional Information I.M. dosing is recommended only for contraceptive purposes or in the treatment of endometrial or renal carcinoma

Dosage Forms
Injection, suspension, as acetate (Depo-Provera®): 150 mg/mL (1 mL); 400 mg/mL (2.5 mL, 10 mL)
Tablet, as acetate (Provera®): 2.5 mg, 5 mg, 10 mg

Medrysone (ME dri sone)

U.S. Brand Names HMS Liquifilm®

Therapeutic Category Anti-inflammatory Agent, Ophthalmic; Corticosteroid, Ophthalmic

Generic Available No

Use Treatment of allergic conjunctivitis, vernal conjunctivitis, episcleritis, ophthalmic epinephrine sensitivity reaction

Pregnancy Risk Factor C

Contraindications Hypersensitivity to medrysone or any component; ocular fungal, viral, or tuberculosis infections; acute superficial herpes simplex

Warnings Effectiveness and safety have not been established in children

Precautions Prolonged use has been associated with the development of corneal or scleral perforation and posterior subcapsular cataracts; may mask or enhance the (Continued)

Medrysone *(Continued)*

establishment of acute purulent untreated infections of the eye; dose should be tapered to avoid disease exacerbation

Adverse Reactions
Local: Stinging, burning
Ocular: Corneal thinning, increased intraocular pressure, glaucoma, damage to the optic nerve, defects in visual activity, cataracts
Miscellaneous: Hypersensitivity reactions

Mechanism of Action Inhibits inflammatory response by suppression of migration of polymorphonuclear leukocytes and reversal of increased capillary permeability

Pharmacokinetics
Absorption: Through aqueous humor
Metabolism: In the liver
Elimination: By the kidneys and feces

Usual Dosage Children and Adults: Ophthalmic: Instill 1 drop in conjunctival sac 2-4 times/day up to every 4 hours; may use every 1-2 hours during first 1-2 days

Administration Ophthalmic: Shake well before use; do not touch dropper to the eye or skin; finger pressure should be applied to lacrimal sac during and for 1-2 minutes after instillation to decrease risk of absorption and systemic reactions

Monitoring Parameters With prolonged use monitor intraocular pressure and periodic examination of lens

Additional Information Medrysone is a synthetic corticosteroid; structurally related to progesterone; if no improvement after several days of treatment, discontinue medrysone and institute other therapy; duration of therapy: 3-4 days to several weeks dependent on type and severity of disease

Dosage Forms Solution, ophthalmic: 1% (5 mL, 10 mL)

♦ **Mefoxin®** *see* Cefoxitin *on page 198*
♦ **Mellaril®** *see* Thioridazine *on page 953*
♦ **Mellaril-S®** *see* Thioridazine *on page 953*

Melphalan (MEL fa lan)

Related Information
Emetogenic Potential of Single Chemotherapeutic Agents *on page 1129*

U.S. Brand Names Alkeran®

Synonyms L-PAM; L-Sarcolysin; Phenylalanine Mustard

Therapeutic Category Antineoplastic Agent, Alkylating Agent (Nitrogen Mustard)

Generic Available No

Use Palliative treatment of multiple myeloma and nonresectable epithelial ovarian carcinoma; neuroblastoma, rhabdomyosarcoma, breast cancer, sarcoma; I.V. formulation: Use in patients in whom oral therapy is not appropriate

Pregnancy Risk Factor D

Contraindications Hypersensitivity to melphalan or any component; severe bone marrow suppression; patients whose disease was resistant to prior therapy

Warnings The FDA currently recommends that procedures for proper handling and disposal of antineoplastic agents be considered; potentially mutagenic, carcinogenic, and teratogenic; long-term oral dosing can increase the chance of developing secondary leukemia; produces amenorrhea

Precautions Cross-sensitivity may exist between melphalan and chlorambucil; reduce dosage or discontinue therapy if leukocyte count is <3000/mm³ or platelet count is <100,000/mm³; use with caution in patients with bone marrow suppression and impaired renal function; dosage reduction may be necessary in patients with impaired renal function

Adverse Reactions
Cardiovascular: Vasculitis, chest pain; hypotension, diaphoresis, and cardiac arrest have been reported following I.V. administration
Dermatologic: Alopecia, rash, pruritus, vesiculation of skin
Endocrine & metabolic: Amenorrhea, sterility
Gastrointestinal: Nausea, vomiting, diarrhea, stomatitis, mucositis, anorexia
Hematologic: Leukopenia, thrombocytopenia, anemia, agranulocytosis, hemolytic anemia
Hepatic: Hepatic veno-occlusive disease
Local: Burning, discomfort, skin ulceration at injection site, tissue necrosis
Respiratory: Pulmonary fibrosis, interstitial pneumonitis
Miscellaneous: Hypersensitivity reaction

MELPHALAN

Drug Interactions Cyclosporine (development of severe renal failure); cimetidine and other H_2 antagonists decrease bioavailability of oral melphalan; nalidixic acid may increase incidence of severe hemorrhagic necrotic enterocolitis

Food Interactions Food interferes with oral absorption

Stability Protect from light and store at room temperature; reconstituted 5 mg/mL solution for injection is stable 90 minutes at room temperature; do not refrigerate since it may precipitate; once reconstituted solution is further diluted for I.V. infusion with NS, administration must be completed within 1 hour

Mechanism of Action Alkylating agent that inhibits DNA and RNA synthesis via formation of carbonium ions; cross-links strands of DNA

Pharmacokinetics
Absorption: Oral: Variable and incomplete
Distribution: Distributes throughout total body water; V_{dss}: 0.5 L/kg
Protein binding: 60% to 90%
Metabolism: Nonenzymatic hydrolysis to mono- or dihydroxy products; some conjugation to glutathione
Bioavailability: Ranges from 49% to 95% depending on the presence of food; average: 60%
Half-life, terminal: 75-120 minutes
Time to peak serum concentration: Oral: Within 2 hours
Elimination: 10% to 15% of dose excreted unchanged in urine; after oral administration, 20% to 50% excreted in stool

Usual Dosage Refer to individual protocols
Children:
I.V.:
Pediatric rhabdomyosarcoma: 10-35 mg/m²/dose every 21-28 days
High-dose melphalan with bone marrow transplantation for neuroblastoma: 70-100 mg/m²/day on day 7 and 6 before BMT; or 140-220 mg/m² single dose before BMT; or 50 mg/m²/day for 4 days; or 70 mg/m²/day for 3 days
Oral: 4-20 mg/m²/day for 1-21 days
Adults:
Multiple myeloma:
Oral: 6 mg/day once daily initially adjusted as indicated or 0.15 mg/kg/day for 7 days or 0.25 mg/kg/day for 4 days, repeat at 4- to 6-week intervals
I.V.: 16 mg/m²/dose every 2 weeks for 4 doses, then repeat monthly as per protocol for multiple myeloma
Ovarian carcinoma: Oral: 0.2 mg/kg/day for 5 days, repeat in 4-5 weeks
Dosing adjustment in renal impairment:
BUN >30 mg/dL: Reduce dose by 50%
Serum creatinine >1.5 mg/dL: Reduce dose by 50%

Administration
Oral: Administer on an empty stomach
Parenteral: I.V.: Reconstitute 50 mg vial for injection with special diluent to yield a 5 mg/mL solution; dilute the reconstituted solution with NS to a final concentration not to exceed 2 mg/mL for I.V. central line administration or 0.45 mg/mL for peripheral I.V. administration; administer by I.V. infusion over 15-30 minutes at a rate not to exceed 10 mg/minute but total infusion should be administered within 1 hour

Monitoring Parameters CBC with differential and platelet count, serum electrolytes, serum uric acid, hemoglobin

Test Interactions Positive Coombs' [direct]

Patient Information Notify physician if fever, shortness of breath, persistent cough, sore throat, bleeding, or bruising occurs

Nursing Implications Ensure adequate patient hydration; care should be taken to avoid extravasation

Additional Information Myelosuppressive effects:
WBC: Moderate
Platelets: Moderate
Onset (days): 7
Nadir (days): 14-21
Recovery (days): 42-50

Dosage Forms
Powder for injection: 50 mg
Tablet: 2 mg

References
Berg SL, Grissell DL, DeLaney TF, et al, "Principles of Treatment of Pediatric Solid Tumors," *Pediatr Clin North Am*, 1991, 38(2):249-67.
Pole JG, Casper J, Elfenbein G, et al, "High-Dose Chemoradiotherapy Supported by Marrow Infusions for Advanced Neuroblastoma: A Pediatric Oncology Group Study," *J Clin Oncol*, 1991, 9(1):152-8.
(Continued)

Melphalan (Continued)

Schroeder H, Pinkerton CR, Powles RL, et al, "High-Dose Melphalan and Total Body Irradiation With Autologous Marrow Rescue in Childhood Acute Lymphoblastic Leukemia After Relapse," *Bone Marrow Transplant*, 1991, 7(1):11-15.

♦ **Menadol® [OTC]** *see* Ibuprofen *on page 520*

♦ **Meningococcal Polysaccharide Vaccine, Groups A, C, Y, and W-135** *see page 1172*

Meperidine (me PER i deen)

Related Information

Adult ACLS Algorithm, Synchronized Cardioversion *on page 1048*
Compatibility of Medications Mixed in a Syringe *on page 1238*
Narcotic Analgesics Comparison *on page 1070*
Overdose and Toxicology *on page 1222*
Preprocedure Sedatives in Children *on page 1201*
Serotonin Syndrome *on page 1247*

U.S. Brand Names Demerol®

Synonyms Isonipecaine; Pethidine

Therapeutic Category Analgesic, Narcotic

Generic Available Yes

Use Management of moderate to severe pain; adjunct to anesthesia and preoperative sedation

Restrictions C-II

Pregnancy Risk Factor B (D if used for prolonged periods or in high doses at term)

Contraindications Hypersensitivity to meperidine or any component; use of MAO inhibitors within 14 days (potentially fatal reactions may occur, see Drug Interactions)

Warnings Some preparations contain sulfites which may cause allergic reactions

Precautions Use with caution in patients with pulmonary, hepatic, or renal disorders; use with caution in patients with tachycardias, biliary colic, increased intracranial pressure, seizure disorders or those receiving high-dose meperidine because normeperidine (an active metabolite and CNS stimulant) may accumulate and precipitate twitches, tremors, or seizures; decrease the dose in patients with renal or hepatic impairment

Adverse Reactions

Cardiovascular: Palpitations, hypotension, bradycardia, peripheral vasodilation, tachycardia

Central nervous system: CNS depression, dizziness, drowsiness, sedation, increased intracranial pressure; active metabolite (normeperidine) may precipitate twitches, tremors, or seizures

Dermatologic: Pruritus

Endocrine & metabolic: Antidiuretic hormone release

Gastrointestinal: Nausea, vomiting, constipation, biliary tract spasm

Genitourinary: Urinary tract spasm

Local: Induration, irritation (repeated S.C. use)

Ocular: Miosis

Respiratory: Respiratory depression

Miscellaneous: Physical and psychological dependence, histamine release

Drug Interactions Cytochrome P-450 isoenzyme CYP2D6 substrate

May aggravate the adverse effects of isoniazid; MAO inhibitors greatly potentiate the effects of meperidine (acute opioid overdosage symptoms can be seen, including severe toxic reactions); the herbal medicine St John's wort (*Hypericum perforatum*) may increase serious side effects, its use is **not** recommended; CNS depressants, alcohol, tricyclic antidepressants, phenothiazines may potentiate the effects of meperidine; phenytoin may decrease the analgesic effects; concurrent use of meperidine with ritonavir is not recommended

Stability Incompatible with aminophylline, heparin, phenobarbital, phenytoin, and sodium bicarbonate

Mechanism of Action Binds to opiate receptors in the CNS, causing inhibition of ascending pain pathways, altering the perception of and response to pain; produces generalized CNS depression

Pharmacodynamics Analgesia:

Onset of action:

Oral, I.M., S.C.: Within 10-15 minutes

I.V.: Within 5 minutes

Peak effect:

Oral, I.M., S.C.: Within 1 hour

I.V.: 5-7 minutes
Duration:
Oral, I.M., S.C.: 2-4 hours
I.V.: 2-3 hours

Pharmacokinetics
Distribution: Crosses the placenta; appears in breast milk
V_{dss}:
Neonates: Preterm 1-7 days: 8.8 L/kg; term 1-7 days: 5.6 L/kg
Infants: 1 week to 2 months: 8 L/kg; 3-18 months: 5 L/kg; 5-8 years: 2.8 L/kg
Adults: 3-4 L/kg
Protein binding: (to alpha$_1$-acid glycoprotein)
Neonates: 52%
Infants: 3-18 months: 85%
Adults: ~60% to 80%
Metabolism: In the liver via hydrolysis and N-demethylation
Bioavailability: ~50% to 60%, increased bioavailability with liver disease
Half-life, terminal:
Preterm infants 3.6-65 days of age: 11.9 hours (range: 3.3-59.4 hours)
Term infants:
0.3-4 days of age: 10.7 hours (range: 4.9-16.8 hours)
26-73 days of age: 8.2 hours (range: 5.7-31.7 hours)
Neonates: 23 hours (range: 12-39 hours)
Infants 3-18 months: 2.3 hours
Children 5-8 years: 3 hours
Adults: 2.5-4 hours
Adults with liver disease: 7-11 hours
Normeperidine (active metabolite): Neonates: 30-85 hours; Adults: 8-16 hours; normeperidine half-life is dependent on renal function and can accumulate with high doses or in patients with decreased renal function; normeperidine may precipitate tremors or seizures
Elimination: ~5% meperidine eliminated unchanged in urine

Usual Dosage Doses should be titrated to appropriate analgesic effect; **when changing route of administration, note that oral doses are about half as effective as parenteral dose**

Children:
Oral, I.M., I.V., S.C.: Usual: 1-1.5 mg/kg/dose every 3-4 hours as needed; 1-2 mg/kg as a single dose preoperative medication may be used; maximum dose: 100 mg/dose
I.V. continuous infusion: Loading dose: 0.5-1 mg/kg followed by initial rate: 0.3 mg/kg/hour; titrate dose to effect; may require 0.5-0.7 mg/kg/hour
Adults: Oral, I.M., I.V.: S.C.: 50-150 mg/dose every 3-4 hours as needed
AHCPR dosing guidelines: Opioid naive patients: **Note:** Oral route not recommended (See Carr, 1992 and Jacox, 1994):
Children and Adults <50 kg: Moderate to severe pain: I.M., I.V., S.C.: Usual initial dose: 0.75 mg/kg every 2-3 hours
Children and Adults ≥50 kg: Moderate to severe pain: I.M., I.V., S.C.: Usual initial dose: 100 mg every 3 hours
Dosing adjustment in renal impairment:
Cl_{cr} 10-50 mL/minute: Administer 75% of normal dose
Cl_{cr} <10 mL/minute: Administer 50% of normal dose

Administration
Oral: Administer with water; dilute syrup in water prior to use (use 4 oz water for adults)
Parenteral:
Slow I.V. push: Do not administer rapid I.V., administer over at least 5 minutes and dilute to ≤10 mg/mL
Intermittent infusion: Dilute to 1 mg/mL and administer over 15-30 minutes

Monitoring Parameters Respiratory and cardiovascular status; relief of pain, level of sedation

Patient Information Avoid alcohol and the herbal medicine St John's wort; may be habit-forming; may cause drowsiness and impair ability to perform activities requiring mental alertness or physical coordination

Additional Information Equianalgesic doses: morphine 10 mg I.M. = meperidine 75-100 mg I.M.; Demerol® syrup also contains glucose, saccharin, artificial banana flavoring, and benzoic acid. **Note:** Although meperidine has been used in combination with chlorpromazine and promethazine as a premedication ("Lytic Cocktail"), this combination may have a higher rate of adverse effects compared to alternative
(Continued)

Meperidine *(Continued)*

sedatives and analgesics (See American Academy of Pediatrics Committee on Drugs, 1995)

Dosage Forms

Injection, as hydrochloride:

Multiple-dose vials: 50 mg/mL (30 mL); 100 mg/mL (20 mL)

Single dose: 10 mg/mL (30 mL); 25 mg/dose (1 mL); 50 mg/dose (1 mL); 75 mg/dose (1 mL, 1.5 mL); 100 mg/dose (1 mL)

Syrup, as hydrochloride: 50 mg/5 mL [banana flavor] (5 mL, 500 mL)

Tablet, as hydrochloride: 50 mg, 100 mg

References

American Academy of Pediatrics Committee on Drugs, "Reappraisal of Lytic Cocktail/Demerol®, Phenergan®, and Thorazine® (DPT) for the Sedation of Children," *Pediatrics*, 1995, 95(4):598-602.

Carr D, Jacox A, Chapman CR, et al, "Clinical Practice Guideline Number 1: Acute Pain Management: Operative or Medical Procedures and Trauma," Rockville, Maryland: U.S. Department of Health and Human Services, Public Health Service, Agency for Health Care Policy and Research, AHCPR Publication No 92-0032, 1992.

Cole TB, Sprinkle RH, Smith SJ, et al, "Intravenous Narcotic Therapy for Children With Severe Sickle Cell Pain Crisis," *Am J Dis Child*, 1986, 140(12):1255-9.

Jacox A, Carr D, Payne R, et al, "Clinical Practice Guideline Number 9: Management of Cancer Pain," Rockville, Maryland: U.S. Department of Health and Human Services, Public Health Service, Agency for Health Care Policy and Research, AHCPR Publication No. 94-0592, 1994.

Olkkola KT, Hamunen K, and Maunuksela EL, "Clinical Pharmacokinetics and Pharmacodynamics of Opioid Analgesics in Infants and Children," *Clin Pharmacokinet*, 1995, 28(5):385-404.

Pokela ML, Olkkola KT, Koivisto ME, et al, "Pharmacokinetics and Pharmacodynamics of Intravenous Meperidine in Neonates and Infants," *Clin Pharmacol Ther*, 1992, 52(4):342-9.

Mephenytoin *(me FEN i toyn)*

Related Information

Overdose and Toxicology *on page 1222*

U.S. Brand Names Mesantoin®

Synonyms Methoin; Methylphenylethylhydantoin; Phenantoin

Therapeutic Category Anticonvulsant, Hydantoin

Generic Available No

Use Treatment of tonic-clonic and partial seizures in patients who are uncontrolled with less toxic anticonvulsants

Pregnancy Risk Factor C

Contraindications Hypersensitivity to mephenytoin or any component

Warnings Fatal irreversible aplastic anemia has occurred

Precautions Abrupt withdrawal may precipitate seizures

Adverse Reactions

Central nervous system: Insomnia, slurred speech, dizziness, lethargy, confusion, coma, sedation, nervousness, ataxia

Dermatologic: Rash, erythema multiforme, alopecia

Gastrointestinal: Nausea, vomiting, weight gain

Hematologic: Neutropenia, leukopenia, thrombocytopenia, agranulocytosis, anemia, Hodgkin's disease-like syndrome; fatal aplastic anemia has occurred

Hepatic: Hepatitis

Neuromuscular & skeletal: Tremor

Ocular: Nystagmus, blurred vision, diplopia, photophobia

Miscellaneous: Serum sickness

Mechanism of Action Stabilizes neuronal membranes and decreases seizure activity by increasing efflux or decreasing influx of sodium ions across cell membranes in the motor cortex during generation of nerve impulses; prolongs effective refractory period and suppresses ventricular pacemaker automaticity, shortens action potential in the heart

Usual Dosage Oral:

Children: 3-15 mg/kg/day in 3 divided doses; usual maintenance dose: 100-400 mg/day in 3 divided doses

Adults: Initial dose: 50-100 mg/day given daily; increase by 50-100 mg at weekly intervals; usual maintenance dose: 200-600 mg/day in 3 divided doses; maximum dose: 800 mg/day

Administration Oral: Administer with food

Monitoring Parameters CBC with differential, platelet count

Reference Range Total mephenytoin (mephenytoin plus 5-ethyl - 5-phenylhydantoin) = 25-40 µg/mL

Patient Information Avoid alcohol; may cause drowsiness and impair ability to perform activities requiring mental alertness or physical coordination

Additional Information Usually used in combination with other anticonvulsants; **Note:** The company that makes Mesantoin® has **discontinued manufacturing**; the drug is currently available from Novartis under a transition program; small quantities may be obtained while transitioning patients to other antiepileptic agents.

Dosage Forms Tablet: 100 mg

Mephobarbital (me foe BAR bi tal)

U.S. Brand Names Mebaral®

Synonyms Methylphenobarbital

Therapeutic Category Anticonvulsant, Barbiturate; Barbiturate; Sedative

Generic Available No

Use Treatment of generalized tonic-clonic and simple partial seizures

Restrictions C-IV

Pregnancy Risk Factor D

Contraindications Hypersensitivity to mephobarbital or any component; pre-existing CNS depression; respiratory depression; severe uncontrolled pain; history of porphyria

Precautions Use with caution in patients with hepatic or renal impairment or respiratory diseases

Adverse Reactions
Central nervous system: Drowsiness, lethargy, paradoxical excitement (especially in children)
Dermatologic: Rash, including Stevens-Johnson syndrome or erythema multiforme
Gastrointestinal: Nausea, vomiting
Hematologic: Agranulocytosis, thrombocytopenic purpura
Miscellaneous: Psychological and physical dependence

Drug Interactions Cytochrome P-450 isoenzyme CYP2C, CYP2C8, and CYP2C19 substrate
Mephobarbital is expected to have similar drug interactions as phenobarbital, since mephobarbital is metabolized in the liver to phenobarbital (see Phenobarbital *on page 785*)

Food Interactions High doses of pyridoxine may decrease drug effect; barbiturates may increase the metabolism of vitamin D & K; dietary requirements of vitamin D, K, C, B$_{12}$, folate and calcium may be increased with long-term use

Mechanism of Action Increases seizure threshold in the motor cortex; depresses monosynaptic and polysynaptic transmission in the CNS; depresses CNS activity by binding to barbiturate site at GABA-receptor complex enhancing GABA activity; depresses reticular activating system; higher doses may be gabamimetic

Pharmacokinetics
Absorption: Oral: ~50%
Protein binding: 58% to 68%
Metabolism: In the liver to phenobarbital
Half-life: 30-70 hours

Usual Dosage Epilepsy: Oral:
Children: 4-10 mg/kg/day in 2-4 divided doses
Adults: 200-600 mg/day in 2-4 divided doses

Administration Oral: Administer with water, milk, or juice

Monitoring Parameters Phenobarbital serum concentrations; CBC with differential, platelet count, hepatic and renal function

Reference Range Phenobarbital level should be in the range of 15-40 µg/mL (SI: 65-172 µmol/L)

Patient Information May cause drowsiness and impair ability to perform activities requiring mental alertness or physical coordination; do not discontinue abruptly; avoid alcohol; limit caffeine

Additional Information Sometimes used in specific patients who have excessive sedation or hyperexcitability from phenobarbital

Dosage Forms Tablet: 32 mg, 50 mg, 100 mg

♦ **Mephyton®** see Phytonadione *on page 798*
♦ **Mepron®** see Atovaquone *on page 113*

Mercaptopurine (mer kap toe PYOOR een)

Related Information
Emetogenic Potential of Single Chemotherapeutic Agents *on page 1129*

U.S. Brand Names Purinethol®

Synonyms 6-Mercaptopurine; 6-MP

Therapeutic Category Antineoplastic Agent, Antimetabolite; Antineoplastic Agent, Purine

Generic Available No

Use Treatment of acute leukemias (ALL, AML, CML); non-Hodgkin's lymphoma

(Continued)

Mercaptopurine *(Continued)*

Pregnancy Risk Factor D

Contraindications Hypersensitivity to mercaptopurine or any component; severe liver disease; severe bone marrow suppression; patients whose disease showed prior resistance to mercaptopurine or thioguanine

Warnings The FDA currently recommends that procedures for proper handling and disposal of antineoplastic agents be considered; mercaptopurine may cause birth defects; potentially carcinogenic

Precautions Use with caution and adjust dosage in patients with renal impairment or hepatic failure; patients who receive allopurinol concurrently should have the mercaptopurine dose reduced by 66% to 75%

Adverse Reactions
Central nervous system: Drug fever
Dermatologic: Rash, hyperpigmentation
Endocrine & metabolic: Hyperuricemia
Gastrointestinal: Mild nausea or vomiting, diarrhea, stomatitis, anorexia
Hematologic: Myelosuppression (leukopenia, thrombocytopenia, anemia), eosinophilia
Hepatic: Hepatotoxicity, hyperbilirubinemia, jaundice, elevation of liver enzymes
Renal: Renal toxicity (oliguria, hematuria)

Drug Interactions Allopurinol may potentiate the effect of bone marrow suppression (blocks metabolism of **orally** administered mercaptopurine by inhibiting xanthine oxidase); mercaptopurine decreases anticoagulant effect of warfarin; doxorubicin, hepatotoxic drugs (may potentiate liver toxicity)

Food Interactions Food decreases bioavailability

Stability Intact vials and tablets should be stored at room temperature and protected from light; reconstitute 500 mg vial with 49.8 mL sterile water; the 10 mg/mL solution is stable for 24 hours

Mechanism of Action Prodrug incorporated into DNA and RNA; blocks purine synthesis and inhibits DNA and RNA synthesis

Pharmacokinetics
Absorption: Oral: Variable and incomplete (16% to 50%)
Distribution: Distributed throughout total body water; penetrates into CSF at low concentrations
Protein binding: 19%
Metabolism: Undergoes first-pass metabolism in the GI mucosa and liver; metabolized in the liver to sulfate conjugates, 6-thiouric acid, and other inactive compounds
Bioavailability: Oral: <20% (variable)
Half-life: Age dependent
Children: <60 minutes
Adults: 36-90 minutes
Time to peak serum concentration: Oral: Within 2 hours
Elimination: 20% excreted unchanged in urine

Usual Dosage Refer to individual protocols
Children:
Oral:
Induction: 2.5-5 mg/kg/day given once daily, or 70-100 mg/m^2/day once daily
Maintenance: 1.5-2.5 mg/kg/day given once daily
I.V. continuous infusion (investigational; distributed under the auspices of the NCI for authorized studies): 50 mg/m^2/hour for 24-48 hours, or 1000 mg/m^2/day for 24 hours
Adults: Oral:
Induction: 2.5-5 mg/kg/day given once daily, or 80-100 mg/m^2/day given once daily
Maintenance: 1.5-2.5 mg/kg/day given once daily
Dosing adjustment in renal impairment: Children and Adults:
Cl_{cr} <50 mL/minute: Administer every 48 hours

Administration
Oral: Do not administer with meals
Parenteral: Administer by slow I.V. push over several minutes or by slow I.V. continuous infusion to reduce the incidence of vein irritation; further dilute the 10 mg/mL reconstituted solution in NS or D_5W to a final concentration for administration of 1-2 mg/mL

Monitoring Parameters CBC with differential and platelet count, liver function tests, uric acid, urinalysis

Patient Information Report to physician if fever, sore throat, bleeding, bruising, shortness of breath, or painful urination occurs; avoid alcohol

Nursing Implications Avoid extravasation
Additional Information Myelosuppressive effects:
WBC: Moderate
Platelets: Moderate
Onset (days): 7-10
Nadir (days): 14
Recovery (days): 21

Dosage Forms
Injection (investigational use only): 500 mg vial
Tablet: 50 mg

Extemporaneous Preparations A 50 mg/mL oral suspension was made by crushing the tablets, mixing with a volume of Cologel® suspending agent equal to $^1/_3$ the final volume, and adding a 2:1 mixture of simple syrup and cherry syrup to make the final volume; stable for 14 days when stored in an amber glass bottle at room temperature

Dressman JB and Poust RI, "Stability of Allopurinol and of Five Antineoplastics in Suspension," *Am J Hosp Pharm*, 1983, 40:616-8.

References
Zimm S, Ettinger LJ, Holcenberg JS, et al, "Phase I and Clinical Pharmacological Study of Mercaptopurine Administered as a Prolonged Intravenous Infusion," *Cancer Res*, 1988, 45(4):1869-73.

♦ **6-Mercaptopurine** *see* Mercaptopurine *on page 631*
♦ **Mercapturic Acid** *see* Acetylcysteine *on page 35*
♦ **Meribin [OTC]** *see* Biotin *on page 143*
♦ **Merlenate® Topical [OTC]** *see* Undecylenic Acid and Derivatives *on page 994*

Meropenem (mer oh PEN em)

U.S. Brand Names Merrem®
Synonyms SM-7338
Therapeutic Category Antibiotic, Carbapenem
Use Treatment of multidrug-resistant gram-negative and gram-positive aerobic and anaerobic pathogens documented or suspected to be susceptible to meropenem; used in treatment of meningitis, lower respiratory tract infections, urinary tract infections, intra-abdominal infections, skin and skin structure infections and sepsis caused by susceptible *S. aureus*, group A *Streptococcus*, *S. pneumoniae*, *H. influenzae*, *N. meningitidis*, *M. catarrhalis*, *E. coli*, *Klebsiella*, *Enterobacter*, *Serratia*, *P. aeruginosa*, *B. cepacia*, and *B. fragilis*

Pregnancy Risk Factor B
Contraindications Hypersensitivity to meropenem, any component, other carbapenems, or in patients who have experienced anaphylactic reactions to beta-lactams
Warnings Safety and efficacy in children <3 months of age have not been established; pseudomembranous colitis has been reported with the use of meropenem; prolonged use may result in superinfection
Precautions Use with caution in patients with a history of seizures, CNS disease, CNS infection, and/or compromised renal function; dosage adjustment required in patients with renal impairment
Adverse Reactions
Cardiovascular: Hypotension
Central nervous system: Seizures (<0.38%), headache, pain, insomnia, dizziness, agitation
Dermatologic: Rash (1.4%), pruritus
Gastrointestinal: Nausea, vomiting (1%), diarrhea (4.3%), melena, constipation, oral moniliasis
Hematologic: Leukopenia, neutropenia
Hepatic: Elevated AST, ALT, alkaline phosphatase, LDH, and bilirubin
Local: Phlebitis (1.2%), inflammation at the injection site
Renal: Elevated BUN and serum creatinine
Respiratory: Dyspnea

Drug Interactions Probenecid inhibits renal excretion of meropenem
Stability Meropenem reconstituted with SWI is stable for up to 2 hours at room temperature or for up to 12 hours when refrigerated; when reconstituted with NS to a final concentration between 2.5-50 mg/mL, the solution is stable for up to 2 hours at room temperature or 18 hours when refrigerated; when reconstituted with D₅W to a final concentration between 2.5-50 mg/mL, the solution is stable for up to 1 hour at room temperature or 8 hours when refrigerated; solutions prepared for infusion in plastic I.V. bags with NS at concentrations ranging from 2.5-20 mg/mL are stable for 4 hours at room temperature or 24 hours when refrigerated
(Continued)

Meropenem *(Continued)*

Mechanism of Action Inhibits cell wall synthesis by binding to penicillin-binding proteins (PBPs) with its strongest affinities for PBPs 2, 3 and 4 of *E. coli* and *P. aeruginosa* and PBPs 1, 2 and 4 of *S. aureus*

Pharmacokinetics

Distribution: Penetrates into most tissues and body fluids including CSF, urinary tract, peritoneal fluid, bile, lung, bronchial mucosa, muscle tissue, and heart valves

Protein binding: 2%

Metabolism: 20% is hydrolyzed in plasma to an inactive metabolite

Half-life:

Premature newborns: 3 hours

Full-term newborns: 2 hours

Infants 3 months to 2 years: 1.4 hours

Children 2-12 years and Adults: 1 hour

Elimination: Cleared by the kidney with 70% excreted unchanged in urine

Usual Dosage I.V.:

Children ≥3 months: 60 mg/kg/day divided every 8 hours; meningitis: 120 mg/kg/day divided every 8 hours; maximum dose: 6 g/day

Adults:

Mild to moderate infection: 1.5-3 g/day divided every 8 hours

Meningitis: 6 g/day divided every 8 hours

Dosage adjustment in renal impairment:

Cl_{cr} 26-50 mL/minute: Standard dose every 12 hours

Cl_{cr} 10-25 mL/minute: One-half dose every 12 hours

Cl_{cr} <10 mL/minute: One-half dose every 24 hours

Administration Administer by I.V. push or I.V. intermittent infusion; final concentration for administration should not exceed 50 mg/mL; infuse I.V. push injection over 3-5 minutes; intermittent infusion dose should be administered over 15-30 minutes

Monitoring Parameters Periodic renal, hepatic, and hematologic function tests

Test Interactions Positive Coombs' [direct]

Additional Information Sodium content 1 g: 3.92 mEq

Dosage Forms Injection, as trihydrate: 500 mg, 1 g

References

Blummer JL, Reed MD, Kearns GL, et al, "Sequential, Single-Dose Pharmacokinetic Evaluation of Meropenem in Hospitalized Infants and Children," *Antimicrob Agents Chemother*, 1995, 39(8):1721-5.

Bradley, JS, "Meropenem: A New, Extremely Broad Spectrum Beta-lactam Antibiotic for Serious Infections in Pediatrics," *Pediatr Infect Dis J*, 1997, 16:263-8.

Odio JM, Puig JR, Feris JM, et al, "Prospective, Randomized, Investigator-Blinded Study of the Efficacy and Safety of Meropenem vs. Cefotaxime Therapy in Bacterial Meningitis in Children. Meropenem Meningitis Study Group," *Pediatr Infect Dis J*, 1999, 18(7):581-90.

Wiseman LR, Wagstaff AJ, Brogden RN, et al, "Meropenem. A Review of its Antibacterial Activity, Pharmacokinetic Properties and Clinical Efficacy," *Drugs*, 1995, 50(1):73-101.

♦ **Merrem**® *see* Meropenem *on page 633*

Mesalamine *(me SAL a meen)*

Related Information

Drugs and Breast-Feeding *on page 1243*

U.S. Brand Names Asacol®; Pentasa®; Rowasa®

Canadian Brand Names Mesasal; Salofalk

Synonyms 5-Aminosalicylic Acid; 5-ASA; Fisalamine; Mesalazine

Therapeutic Category 5-Aminosalicylic Acid Derivative; Anti-inflammatory Agent; Anti-inflammatory Agent, Rectal

Generic Available No

Use Treatment of ulcerative colitis (UC), proctosigmoiditis, and proctitis

Pregnancy Risk Factor B

Contraindications Hypersensitivity to mesalamine, any component, sulfites, or salicylates

Warnings Pericarditis should be considered in patients with chest pain (has occurred rarely with mesalamine containing products); pancreatitis should be considered in any patient with new abdominal complaints; has been implicated in the production of an acute intolerance syndrome or exacerbation of colitis (<3%)

Precautions Use with caution in patients with hypersensitivity to sulfasalazines

Adverse Reactions

Cardiovascular: Pericarditis, chest pain, myocarditis, T-wave abnormalities, edema

Central nervous system: Chills, dizziness, fever, headache, insomnia, malaise, anxiety, depression

Dermatologic: Psoriasis, dry skin, urticaria, pyoderma gangrenosum, erythema nodosum, photosensitivity, lichen planus, alopecia

Endocrine & metabolic: Amenorrhea, menorrhagia, breast pain

Gastrointestinal: Abdominal pain, cramps, flatulence, bloody diarrhea, anal irritation, anorexia, pancreatitis, gastritis, dyspepsia, eructation, vomiting, hemorrhoids, constipation, dysgeusia

Genitourinary: Epididymitis, dysuria, discoloration of urine (yellow-brown)

Hematologic: Agranulocytosis, thrombocytopenia

Hepatic: Elevated liver enzymes, jaundice, cholestatic jaundice, liver necrosis/failure

Neuromuscular & skeletal: Weakness

Renal: Interstitial nephritis, renal papillary necrosis, nephrotic syndrome

Respiratory: Interstitial pneumonitis, pulmonary infiltrates, sinusitis, asthma exacerbation, pleuritis

Miscellaneous: Kawasaki-like syndrome, lupus-like syndrome

Drug Interactions Decreased digoxin bioavailability

Stability Unstable in presence of water or light; once foil has been removed, unopened bottles have an expiration of 1 year following the date of manufacture

Mechanism of Action Mesalamine (5-aminosalicylic acid) is the active component of sulfasalazine; the specific mechanism of action of mesalamine is unknown; however, it is thought that it modulates local chemical mediators of the inflammatory response, especially leukotrienes; action appears topical rather than systemic

Pharmacokinetics

Absorption:

Capsule: 20% to 30%

Rectal: ~15%; variable and dependent upon retention time, underlying GI disease, and colonic pH

Tablet: 28%

Distribution: Breast milk to plasma ratio:

5-ASA: 0.27

Acetyl 5-ASA: 5.1

Metabolism: In the liver by acetylation to acetyl-5-aminosalicylic acid (acetyl-5-ASA-active metabolite) and to glucuronide conjugates; intestinal metabolism may also occur

Half-life:

5-ASA: 0.5-1.5 hours

Acetyl 5-ASA: 5-10 hours

Time to peak serum concentration: Oral, Rectal: Within 4-7 hours

Elimination: Most metabolites are excreted in urine with <2% appearing in feces

Usual Dosage Oral (usual course of therapy is 3-6 weeks):

(Oral products are formulated to slowly release therapeutic quantities of drug throughout the GI tract):

Capsule (ethylcellulose-coated, controlled release):

Children: 50 mg/kg/day divided every 6-12 hours

Adults: 1 g 4 times/day for up to 8 weeks

Tablet (coated with acrylic-based resin; drug released after reaches terminal ileum):

Children: 50 mg/kg/day divided every 8-12 hours

Adults: Treatment: 800 mg 3 times/day; maintenance for remission of UC: 1.6 g daily in divided doses up to 6 months

Retention enema: Adults: 60 mL (4 g) at bedtime, retained overnight, approximately 8 hours for 3-6 weeks

Rectal suppository: Adults: Insert 1 suppository (500 mg) in rectum twice daily, retained for 1-3 hours, for 3-6 weeks

Administration

Oral: Administer with food; swallow tablets whole, do not break outer coating

Rectal: Retain enema for 8 hours or as long as practical; shake rectal suspension well before use

Patient Information May discolor urine yellow-brown

Dosage Forms

Capsule, controlled release (Pentasa®): 250 mg

Suppository, rectal (Rowasa®): 500 mg

Suspension, rectal (Rowasa®): 4 g/60 mL (7s)

Tablet, enteric coated (Asacol®): 400 mg

References

Grand RJ, Ramakrishna J, and Calenda KA, "Inflammatory Bowel Disease in the Pediatric Patient," *Gastroenterol Clin North Am*, 1995, 24(3):613-32.

♦ **Mesalazine** *see* Mesalamine *on page 634*

♦ **Mesantoin®** *see* Mephenytoin *on page 630*

♦ **Mesasal (Can)** *see* Mesalamine *on page 634*
♦ **M-Eslon (Can)** *see* Morphine Sulfate *on page 683*

Mesna (MES na)
U.S. Brand Names Mesnex™
Canadian Brand Names Uromitexan
Synonyms Sodium 2-Mercaptoethane Sulfonate
Therapeutic Category Antidote, Cyclophosphamide-induced Hemorrhagic Cystitis; Antidote, Ifosfamide-induced Hemorrhagic Cystitis
Generic Available No
Use Detoxifying agent used as a protectant against hemorrhagic cystitis induced by ifosfamide and cyclophosphamide
Pregnancy Risk Factor B
Contraindications Hypersensitivity to mesna, other thiol compounds, or any component
Precautions Examine morning urine specimen for hematuria prior to ifosfamide or cyclophosphamide treatment; if hematuria develops, reduce the ifosfamide/cyclophosphamide dose or discontinue the drug and consider increasing the mesna dosage; for children less than 2 years of age, use **preservative free** mesna to decrease the amount of benzyl alcohol delivered to the infant
Adverse Reactions
  Cardiovascular: Hypotension
  Central nervous system: Malaise, headache
  Dermatologic: Skin rash
  Gastrointestinal: Diarrhea, nausea, vomiting, dysgeusia
  Neuromuscular & skeletal: Limb pain
Stability Diluted solutions in D_5W, D_5/NS, NS, or LR are chemically and physically stable for 48 hours at room temperature; compatible with solutions containing ifosfamide or cyclophosphamide; incompatible with cisplatin
Mechanism of Action In the urinary bladder, mesna binds with and detoxifies acrolein and other urotoxic metabolites of ifosfamide and cyclophosphamide via an active sulfhydryl group on mesna
Pharmacokinetics
  Distribution: No tissue penetration; following glomerular filtration, mesna disulfide is reduced in the renal tubules back to mesna and delivered to the bladder in the active form
  Bioavailability: Oral: 50%
  Half-life: 24 minutes (mesna); after I.V. administration, mesna is rapidly oxidized intravascularly to mesna disulfide (half-life: 72 minutes)
  Elimination: Unchanged drug and metabolite are excreted primarily in the urine; time for maximum urinary mesna excretion: 1 hour after I.V. and 2-3 hours after an oral mesna dose
Usual Dosage Children and Adults (refer to individual protocols): **Mesna dose depends on dose of antineoplastic agent used:**

  When used with ifosfamide: I.V.: Mesna dose is 20% w/w of ifosfamide dose 15 minutes before and 4 and 8 hours later or combined with ifosfamide administration; for high-dose ifosfamide, mesna has been administered at a dose of 20% w/w 15 minutes before and every 3 hours for 3-6 doses or combined with ifosfamide administration; (**Note:** In clinical protocols, total daily mesna dose ranged between 60% to 160% w/w of the daily ifosfamide dose)
  When used with cyclophosphamide: I.V.: Mesna dose is 20% w/w of cyclophosphamide dose 15 minutes before and every 3 hours for 3-4 doses or combined with cyclophosphamide administration; (**Note:** In clinical protocols, total daily mesna dose ranged between 60% to 160% w/w of the daily cyclophosphamide dose)
  I.V. continuous infusion: Mesna doses equivalent to 60% to 100% of the ifosfamide or cyclophosphamide dose have been used
  Oral: Mesna dose is 40% w/w of the antineoplastic agent dose in 3 doses at 4-hour intervals or 20 mg/kg/dose every 4 hours x 3 (oral mesna is not recommended for the first dose before ifosfamide or cyclophosphamide)
Administration
  Oral: Dilute mesna solution before oral administration to decrease sulfur odor; mesna can be diluted 1:1 to 1:10 in carbonated cola drinks, fruit juices (grape, apple, tomato, and orange juice) or in plain or chocolate milk (most palatable in chilled grape juice)
  Parenteral: Administer by I.V. infusion over 15-30 minutes, or by continuous I.V. infusion, or per protocol; mesna may be diluted in D_5W or NS to a final concentration of 1-20 mg/mL; may be added to solutions containing ifosfamide or cyclophosphamide

Monitoring Parameters Urinalysis

Test Interactions False-positive urinary ketones with Chemstrip®, Multistix®, or Labstix®

Nursing Implications Used concurrently with and/or following high-dose ifosfamide or cyclophosphamide; ensure adequate patient hydration; report vomiting within 1 hour of an oral mesna dose to physician so that I.V. mesna can be administered

Additional Information pH of the commercial 100 mg/mL solution: 6.5-8.5

Dosage Forms
Injection: 100 mg/mL (10 mL)
Injection, preservative free: 100 mg/mL (2 mL, 4 mL)

References
Ben Yehuda A, Heyman A and Steiner Salz D, "False Positive Reaction for Urinary Ketones With Mesna," *Drug Intell Clin Pharm*, 1987, 21(6): 547-8.
Brock N and Pohl J, "The Development of Mesna for Regional Detoxification," *Cancer Treat Rev*, 1983, 10(Suppl A):33-43.
"Cancer Chemotherapy," *Med Lett Drugs Ther*, 1989, 31(793):49-56.
Schoenike SE and Dana WJ, "Ifosfamide and Mesna," *Clin Pharm*, 1990, 9(3):179-91.

♦ **Mesnex**™ *see* Mesna *on page 636*
♦ **Mestinon**® *see* Pyridostigmine *on page 856*
♦ **Metacortandralone** *see* Prednisolone *on page 821*
♦ **Metadate**® **CD** *see* Methylphenidate *on page 653*
♦ **Metadate**® **ER** *see* Methylphenidate *on page 653*
♦ **Metadol (Can)** *see* Methadone *on page 641*
♦ **Metamucil**® **[OTC]** *see* Psyllium *on page 853*

Metaproterenol (met a proe TER e nol)

Related Information
Asthma Guidelines *on page 1210*
Carbohydrate and Alcohol Content of Liquid Medications for Use in Patients Receiving Ketogenic Diets *on page 1258*

U.S. Brand Names Alupent®

Synonyms Orciprenaline

Therapeutic Category Adrenergic Agonist Agent; Antiasthmatic; Beta$_2$-Adrenergic Agonist Agent; Bronchodilator; Sympathomimetic

Generic Available Yes: Except inhaler

Use Bronchodilator in reversible airway obstruction due to asthma or COPD

Pregnancy Risk Factor C

Contraindications Hypersensitivity to metaproterenol or any component; pre-existing cardiac arrhythmias associated with tachycardia; narrow-angle glaucoma

Warnings Excessive use may result in cardiac arrest and death; do not use concurrently with other sympathomimetic bronchodilators

Precautions Use with caution in patients with ischemic heart disease, hypertension, hyperthyroidism, seizure disorders, CHF, cardiac arrhythmias, and diabetes mellitus

Adverse Reactions
Cardiovascular: Tachycardia, palpitations, hypertension
Central nervous system: Nervousness, dizziness, headache, fatigue, vertigo
Gastrointestinal: Nausea, vomiting, diarrhea, GI distress, xerostomia, dysgeusia, throat irritation
Neuromuscular & skeletal: Tremor, weakness, muscle cramps
Respiratory: Exacerbation of asthma, hoarseness, cough, nasal congestion

Drug Interactions Beta-adrenergic blockers (eg, propranolol) may antagonize metaproterenol's effects; sympathomimetics may increase adverse effects if administered concomitantly; MAO inhibitors may cause hypertensive crisis

Stability Protect from light

Mechanism of Action Relaxes bronchial smooth muscle and peripheral vasculature by action on beta$_2$-receptors

Pharmacodynamics
Onset of bronchodilation:
Oral: Within 30 minutes
Inhalation: Within 60 seconds
Peak effect: Oral: Within 1 hour
Duration: (approximately 1-5 hours) regardless of route administered

Pharmacokinetics
Absorption: Oral: Well absorbed
Metabolism: Extensive first-pass in the liver (~40% of oral dose is available)
Elimination: Mainly as glucuronic acid conjugates
(Continued)

Metaproterenol *(Continued)*

Usual Dosage

Oral:
  Children:
    <2 years: 0.4 mg/kg/dose given 3-4 times/day; in infants, the dose can be given every 8-12 hours
    2-6 years: 1.3-2.6 mg/kg/day divided every 6-8 hours
    6-9 years: 10 mg/dose given 3-4 times/day
  Children >9 years and Adults: 20 mg/dose given 3-4 times/day
Inhalation: Children >12 years and Adults: 2-3 inhalations every 3-4 hours, up to 12 inhalations in 24 hours
Nebulizer:
  Infants and Children: 0.01-0.02 mL/kg (0.5-1 mg/kg) of 5% solution; minimum dose: 0.1 mL (5 mg); maximum dose: 0.3 mL (15 mg) every 4-6 hours (may be given more frequently according to need); equivalent doses using more dilute solutions may be administered at the same frequency
  Adolescents and Adults: 0.2 to 0.3 mL (10-15 mg) of 5% metaproterenol every 4-6 hours (can be given more frequently according to need); equivalent doses using more dilute solutions may be administered at the same frequency

Administration

Nebulization: Dilute 5% solution in 2-3 mL NS; more dilute solutions may be used without dilution
Oral: Administer with food to decrease GI distress

Monitoring Parameters Heart rate, respiratory rate, blood pressure, arterial or capillary blood gases if applicable, pulmonary function tests

Dosage Forms

Aerosol, oral, as sulfate: 0.65 mg/dose (14 g)
Solution for inhalation, preservative free, as sulfate: 0.4% [4 mg/mL] (2.5 mL); 0.6% [6 mg/mL] (2.5 mL); 5% [50 mg/mL] (10 mL, 30 mL)
Syrup, as sulfate: 10 mg/5 mL (120 mL, 480 mL)
Tablet, as sulfate: 10 mg, 20 mg

♦ **Metaradrine** *see* Metaraminol *on page 638*

Metaraminol *(met a RAM i nole)*

U.S. Brand Names Aramine®

Synonyms Hydroxynorephedrine; Metaradrine

Therapeutic Category Adrenergic Agonist Agent; Alpha-Adrenergic Agonist; Sympathomimetic

Generic Available Yes

Use Prevention and treatment of an acute hypotensive state occurring with spinal anesthesia; treatment of shock which persists after adequate fluid volume replacement

Pregnancy Risk Factor C

Contraindications Hypersensitivity to metaraminol or any component; use with cyclopropane or halothane anesthesia

Warnings Contains sulfites, avoid in sensitive individuals; extravasant; may cause tissue necrosis and sloughing of surrounding skin if I.V. infiltration occurs; see Extravasation Treatment *on page 1085*; use of MAO inhibitors may result in potentiation of its pressor effects

Precautions Blood/volume depletion should be corrected, if possible, before metaraminol therapy; use with caution in patients with heart and thyroid disease, hypertension, diabetes mellitus, and cirrhosis; because of its prolonged action, a cumulative effect is possible resulting in a prolonged elevation of blood pressure despite discontinuation of therapy; may provoke a relapse in patients with a history of malaria

Adverse Reactions

Cardiovascular: Tachycardia, bradycardia, hypertension, cardiac arrhythmias, palpitations, cardiac arrest
Central nervous system: Headache, dizziness, apprehension
Gastrointestinal: Nausea
Local: Tissue necrosis, sloughing at injection site, abscess formation
Neuromuscular & skeletal: Tremors
Miscellaneous: Diaphoresis

Drug Interactions Atropine may block the reflex bradycardia caused by metaraminol and enhance the pressor response; tricyclic antidepressants, MAO inhibitors, and ergot alkaloids may potentiate the effects of metaraminol; ectopic arrhythmias with concurrent use of digoxin; phentolamine and other alpha-adrenergic blocking agents will reduce metaraminol's effects

Stability Stable at room temperature; stable when diluted in D_5W, NS, Ringer's injection, LR injection, Normosol®-R, and Normosol®-M in 5% dextrose; use diluted solutions within 24 hours

Mechanism of Action Predominantly stimulates alpha-adrenergic receptors resulting in vasoconstriction and increased systemic blood pressure; it also stimulates beta$_1$-adrenergic receptors causing increased contractility and heart rate; clinically the chronotropic effect (increased heart rate) is overcome by increased vagal activity occurring as a reflex to increased arterial blood pressure; bradycardia usually results; metaraminol also has an indirect effect by releasing norepinephrine from storage sites

Pharmacodynamics
Onset:
I.V.: 1-2 minutes
I.M.: 10 minutes
S.C.: 5-20 minutes
Duration: 20-90 minutes depending upon the route of administration

Usual Dosage Use the lowest effective dosage for the shortest possible time:
Prevention of hypotension: I.M., S.C.:
Children: 0.1 mg/kg or 3 mg/m^2; repeat as needed, after at least 10 minutes
Adults: 2-10 mg; repeat as needed, after at least 10 minutes
Adjunctive treatment of shock: I.V.:
Children: 0.01 mg/kg or 0.3 mg/m^2; may follow with infusion of 0.4 mg/kg or 12 mg/m^2 at a rate adjusted to maintain the desired blood pressure
Adults: 0.5-5 mg; may follow with infusion of 15-100 mg at a rate adjusted to maintain the desired blood pressure

Administration Parenteral: Due to potentially severe tissue irritation, use S.C. route only if other routes are unavailable; may administer single doses without dilution by direct I.V. infusion slowly; for continuous infusion, dilute 15-100 mg in 500 mL of D_5W or NS; concentrations as high as 1 mg/mL have been used; administer I.V. infusions in large peripheral veins or use central venous access

Monitoring Parameters Blood pressure, heart rate, urine output, peripheral perfusion

Nursing Implications Monitor I.V. site closely for signs of infiltration/extravasation

Dosage Forms Injection, as bitartrate: 10 mg/mL (10 mL)

♦ **Meted (Can)** see Sulfur and Salicylic Acid *on page 929*

Metformin (met FOR min)

U.S. Brand Names Glucophage®; Glucophage® XR
Canadian Brand Names Apo-Metformin; Gen-Metformin; Glycon; Novo-Metformin; Nu-Metformin
Synonyms Metformin Hydrochloride
Therapeutic Category Antidiabetic Agent, Oral; Antidiabetic Agent, Biguanide; Hypoglycemic Agent, Oral
Generic Available No
Use Management of type II diabetes mellitus (noninsulin-dependent, NIDDM) as monotherapy when hyperglycemia cannot be managed with diet alone; may be used concomitantly with a sulfonylurea or insulin to improve glycemic control
Pregnancy Risk Factor B
Contraindications Hypersensitivity to metformin or any component; renal disease or renal dysfunction (S_{cr} ≥1.5 mg/dL in males or ≥1.4 mg/dL in females); clinical conditions such as cardiovascular collapse, respiratory failure, acute MI, acute CHF, and septicemia [which may result in decreased renal function (see Warnings)]; acute or chronic metabolic acidosis with or without coma (including diabetic ketoacidosis)
Warnings Lactic acidosis is a rare, but potentially severe consequence of therapy with metformin; withhold therapy in clinical conditions which may predispose to the development of lactic acidosis (eg, hypoxemia, dehydration, hypoperfusion, sepsis) or in any patient with CHF requiring pharmacologic management; the risk of accumulation and lactic acidosis increases with the degree of impairment of renal function and age; avoid use in patients with renal function below the limit of normal for their age; therapy should be suspended for any surgical procedures (resume only after normal intake resumed and normal renal function is verified); temporarily discontinue therapy for 48 hours in patients undergoing radiologic studies involving the intravascular administration of iodinated contrast materials (potential for acute alteration in renal function); avoid use in patients with impaired liver function; avoid excessive acute or chronic ethanol use; lactic acidosis should be suspected in any diabetic patient receiving metformin who has evidence of acidosis when evidence of ketoacidosis is lacking
(Continued)

Metformin *(Continued)*

Precautions Use with caution in patients receiving medications that may affect renal function, particularly tubular secretion, as they may also affect metformin disposition; hypoglycemia (rare with metformin) may occur with inadequate caloric intake, strenuous exercise, or concurrent use with other hypoglycemic drugs

Adverse Reactions

Cardiovascular: Chest discomfort, flushing, palpitation

Central nervous system: Headache, chills, dizziness, lightheadedness

Dermatologic: Rash, urticaria

Endocrine & metabolic: Hypoglycemia (rare), lactic acidosis

Gastrointestinal: Anorexia, nausea, vomiting, diarrhea, flatulence, indigestion, abdominal discomfort, abdominal distention, abnormal stools, constipation, dyspepsia, heartburn, metallic taste

Hematologic: Megaloblastic anemia (rare)

Neuromuscular & skeletal: Weakness, myalgia

Respiratory: Dyspnea, upper respiratory tract infection

Miscellaneous: Decreased vitamin B_{12} levels, increased sweating, flu-like syndrome, nail disorder

Drug Interactions Drugs which tend to produce hyperglycemia (eg, diuretics, corticosteroids, phenothiazines, thyroid products, estrogens, oral contraceptives, phenytoin, nicotinic acid, sympathomimetics, calcium channel blocking drugs, isoniazid) may lead to a loss of glycemic control; alcohol potentiates the effects of metformin on lactate metabolism; cationic drugs (eg, amiloride, digoxin, morphine, procainamide, quinidine, quinine, ranitidine, triamterene, trimethoprim, and vancomycin) which are eliminated by renal tubular secretion have the potential for interaction with metformin by competing for common renal tubular transport systems; cimetidine increases (by 60%) peak metformin blood concentrations; in a single dose study, furosemide increased the metformin blood concentration without altering metformin renal clearance; nifedipine may enhance the absorption of metformin

Food Interactions Food decreases the extent and slightly delays the absorption (clinical significance unknown); may decrease absorption of vitamin B_{12} and folic acid

Stability Store at 20°C to 25°C (68°F to 77°F); protect from light

Mechanism of Action Decreases hepatic glucose production, decreases intestinal absorption of glucose, and improves insulin sensitivity (increases peripheral glucose uptake and utilization)

Pharmacodynamics

Onset of effect: Within days, maximum effects up to 2 weeks

Average decrease in fasting blood glucose: 60-70 mg/dL

Pharmacokinetics

Absorption: Oral: Slowly and incompletely absorbed

Distribution: Adults: V_d: 654 ±358 L

Protein binding, plasma: Negligible

Bioavailability: Oral: 50% to 60% (under fasting conditions)

Half-life, plasma elimination: 3-6 hours

Time to peak serum concentration: 2-4 hours

Elimination: Renal; tubular secretion is major route

Dialysis: Removed by hemodialysis; clearance up to 170 mL/minute

Usual Dosage Oral: **Note:** While significant responses may not be seen at doses <1500 mg daily, a lower recommended starting dose and gradual increase in dosage is recommended to minimize GI symptoms

Treatment of type 2 diabetes mellitus (noninsulin-dependent) in previously untreated patients or patients currently receiving sulfonylurea oral antidiabetic agents:

Children 10-16 years: Initial: 500 mg twice daily; dosage increases should be made weekly, in increments of 500 mg/day in divided doses, up to a maximum of 2000 mg/day.

Children ≥17 years and Adults:

Initial: 500 mg twice daily; dosage increases should be made weekly, in increments of 500 mg/day in 2 divided doses, up to a maximum of 2500 mg/day; doses >2000 mg/day may be better tolerated divided 3 times/day

Alternative dose: Initial: 850 mg once daily; dosage increases should be made in increments of 850 mg every 2 weeks, given in divided doses, up to a maximum of 2550 mg/day

Glucophage® XR (extended release tablets): Initial: 500 mg once daily; dosage may be increased by 500 mg weekly; maximum dose: 2000 mg once daily. If glycemic control is not achieved at maximum dose, may divide dose to 1000 mg twice daily; if doses >2000 mg/day are needed, switch to regular release tablets and titrate to maximum dose of 2550 mg/day

Adjunctive agent to diabetic patient receiving insulin: Children ≥17 years and Adults: Initial: 500 mg metformin or metformin extended release once daily, continue current insulin dose; increase by 500 mg every week; maximum dose: 2500 mg metformin or 2000 mg metformin extended release; decrease insulin dose by 10% to 25% when fasting blood glucose <120 mg/dL

Dosing adjustment in renal impairment: Metformin is contraindicated in the presence of renal dysfunction (see Contraindications)

Dosing adjustment in hepatic impairment: Avoid metformin; liver disease is a risk factor for the development of lactic acidosis during metformin therapy.

Administration Oral:
Glucophage®: Administer in divided doses with meals
Glucophage® XR: Administer with evening meal; extended release tablets should be swallowed whole; do not cut, crush, or chew

Monitoring Parameters Fasting blood glucose, hemoglobin A_{1c}, initial and periodic monitoring of hemoglobin, hematocrit, and red blood cell indices; renal function (baseline and annually)

Reference Range Target range:
Blood glucose: Fasting and preprandial: 80-120 mg/dL; bedtime: 100-140 mg/dL
Glycosylated hemoglobin (hemoglobin A_{1c}): <7%

Patient Information Do not change dose or discontinue without consulting prescriber; avoid alcohol while taking this medication, could cause severe reaction; maintain regular dietary intake and exercise routine; always carry quick source of sugar with you; during the first weeks of therapy, side effects such as headache, nausea, vomiting, or diarrhea may occur; consult prescriber if these persist; report severe or persistent side effects, extended vomiting or flu-like symptoms, skin rash, easy bruising or bleeding, or change in color of urine or stool; contact your healthcare provider immediately if you feel very weak, tired, or uncomfortable, have unusual muscle pain, trouble breathing, unusual stomach discomfort, are dizzy or lightheaded, or suddenly develop a slow or irregular heartbeat; parts of the extended release tablet (which do not contain active ingredient) may be found excreted in the stool

Additional Information When transferring therapy from chlorpropamide to metformin, monitor the patient closely during the first 2 weeks due to the prolonged retention of chlorpropamide in the body, leading to overlapping drug effects and possible hypoglycemia; if the patient has not responded to 4 weeks at the maximum metformin dosage, consider a gradual addition of a sulfonylurea antidiabetic agent, even if prior primary or secondary failure to a sulfonylurea has occurred; continue metformin at the maximum dose

Dosage Forms
Tablet, as hydrochloride: 500 mg, 850 mg, 1000 mg
Tablet, extended release, as hydrochloride: 500 mg

References
DeFronzo RA, "Pharmacologic Therapy for Type 2 Diabetes Mellitus," *Ann Intern Med*, 1999, 131(4):281-303.
Jones K, Arlanian S, McVie R, et al, "Metformin Improves Glycemic Control in Children With Type 2 Diabetes," *Diabetes*, 2000, 49(Suppl 1):A75.
"Type 2 Diabetes in Children and Adolescents. American Diabetes Association," *Diabetes Care*, 2000, 23(3):381-9.

♦ **Metformin Hydrochloride** *see* Metformin *on page 639*

Methadone (METH a done)
Related Information
Narcotic Analgesics Comparison *on page 1070*
Overdose and Toxicology *on page 1222*

U.S. Brand Names Dolophine®
Canadian Brand Names Metadol; Methadose
Therapeutic Category Analgesic, Narcotic
Generic Available Yes
Use Management of severe pain, used in narcotic detoxification maintenance programs and for the treatment of iatrogenic narcotic dependency
Restrictions C-II
Pregnancy Risk Factor B (D if used for prolonged periods or in high doses at term)
Contraindications Hypersensitivity to methadone or any component
Warnings Tablets are to be used only for oral administration and **must not** be used for injection
Precautions Due to the cumulative effects of methadone, the dose and frequency of administration need to be reduced with repeated use; use with caution in patients with respiratory diseases; methadone's effect on respiration lasts longer than analgesic effects
(Continued)

Methadone *(Continued)*

Adverse Reactions

Cardiovascular: Hypotension, bradycardia, peripheral vasodilation

Central nervous system: CNS depression, increased intracranial pressure, drowsiness, dizziness, sedation (marked sedation seen after repeated administration)

Endocrine & metabolic: Antidiuretic hormone release

Gastrointestinal: Nausea, vomiting, constipation, xerostomia, biliary tract spasm

Genitourinary: Urinary tract spasm

Ocular: Miosis

Respiratory: Respiratory depression

Miscellaneous: Histamine release, physical and psychological dependence with prolonged use

Drug Interactions
Cytochrome P-450 isoenzyme CYP1A2, CYP2D6, CYP3A3/4 substrate; CYP2D6 isoenzyme inhibitor

CNS depressants, alcohol, phenothiazines, tricyclic antidepressants may potentiate the adverse effects of methadone; barbiturates, carbamazepine, phenytoin, primidone, efavirenz, nevirapine, ritonavir, lopinavir, and rifampin may increase the metabolism of methadone and may precipitate withdrawal (monitor patients, larger doses of methadone may be required); methadone may decrease stavudine (no dosage adjustment needed) and didanosine concentrations (consider increase in didanosine dose)

Mechanism of Action
Binds to opiate receptors in the CNS, causing inhibition of ascending pain pathways, altering the perception of and response to pain; produces generalized CNS depression

Pharmacodynamics
Analgesia:

Onset of action:

Oral: Within 30-60 minutes

Parenteral: Within 10-20 minutes

Peak action: Parenteral: 1-2 hours

Duration: Oral: 6-8 hours; after repeated doses, duration increases to 22-48 hours

Pharmacokinetics

Distribution: Crosses the placenta; appears in breast milk

V_d: (Mean ± SD)

Children: 7.1 ± 2.5 L/kg

Adults: 6.1 ± 2.4 L/kg

Protein binding: 80% to 85%

Metabolism: N-demethylated in the liver

Half-life: May be prolonged with alkaline pH

Children: 19 ± 14 hours (range: 4-62 hours)

Adults: 35 ± 22 hours (range: 9-87 hours)

Elimination: In urine (<10% as unchanged drug); increased renal excretion with urine pH <6

Usual Dosage
Doses should be titrated to appropriate effects:

Neonatal abstinence syndrome: Oral, I.V.: Initial: 0.05-0.2 mg/kg/dose given every 12-24 hours or 0.5 mg/kg/day divided every 8 hours; individualize dose and tapering schedule to control symptoms of withdrawal; usually taper dose by 10% to 20% per week over 1 to 1½ months. **Note:** Due to long elimination half-life, tapering is difficult; consider alternate agent.

Children:

Analgesia:

I.V.: Initial: 0.1 mg/kg/dose every 4 hours for 2-3 doses, then every 6-12 hours as needed; maximum dose: 10 mg/dose

Oral, I.M., S.C.: Initial: 0.1 mg/kg/dose every 4 hours for 2-3 doses, then every 6-12 hours as needed or 0.7 mg/kg/24 hours divided every 4-6 hours as needed; maximum dose: 10 mg/dose

Iatrogenic narcotic dependency: Oral: Controlled studies have not been conducted; several clinically used dosing regimens have been reported. Methadone dose **must be individualized** and will depend upon patient's previous narcotic dose and severity of opioid withdrawal; patients who have received higher doses of narcotics will require higher methadone doses.

General guidelines: Initial: 0.05-0.1 mg/kg/dose every 6 hours; increase by 0.05 mg/kg/dose until withdrawal symptoms are controlled; after 24-48 hours, the dosing interval can be lengthened to every 12-24 hours; to taper dose, wean by 0.05 mg/kg/day; if withdrawal symptoms recur, taper at a slower rate

Adults:

Analgesia: Oral, I.M., I.V., S.C.: 2.5-10 mg every 3-8 hours as needed, up to 5-20 mg every 6-8 hours

Detoxification: Oral: 15-40 mg/day

Maintenance of opiate dependence: Oral: 20-120 mg/day

Dosing adjustment in renal impairment: Children and Adults:
Cl$_{cr}$ <10 mL/minute: Administer 50% to 75% of normal dose

Administration Oral: Administer with juice or water; dispersible tablet should be completely dissolved before administration; oral dose for detoxification and maintenance may be administered in Tang®, Kool-Aid®, apple juice, grape Crystal Light®

Monitoring Parameters Respiratory, cardiovascular, and mental status, pain relief (if used for analgesia), abstinence scoring system (if used for neonatal abstinence syndrome)

Patient Information Avoid alcohol; may be habit-forming; may cause drowsiness and impair ability to perform activities requiring mental alertness or physical coordination; may cause dry mouth

Additional Information Methadone accumulates with repeated doses and dosage may need to be adjusted downward after 3-5 days to prevent toxic effects. Some patients may benefit from every 8- to 12-hour dosing interval (pain control).

Methadone 10 mg I.M. = morphine 10 mg I.M.

Dosage Forms
Injection, as hydrochloride: 10 mg/mL (1 mL, 10 mL, 20 mL)
Solution, as hydrochloride:
Oral: 5 mg/5 mL (5 mL, 500 mL); 10 mg/5 mL (500 mL)
Oral, concentrate: 10 mg/mL (30 mL)
Tablet, as hydrochloride: 5 mg, 10 mg
Tablet, dispersible, as hydrochloride: 40 mg

References
Anand KJ and Arnold JH, "Opioid Tolerance and Dependence in Infants and Children," *Crit Care Med*, 1994, 22(2):334-42.
Berde C, Ablin A, Glazer J, et al, "American Academy of Pediatrics Report of the Subcommittee on Disease-Related Pain in Childhood Cancer," *Pediatrics*, 1990, 86(5 Pt 2):818-25.
Lauriault G, LeBelle BA, Lodge BA, et al, "Stability of Methadone in Four Vehicles for Oral Administration," *Am J Hosp Pharm*, 1991, 48(6):1252-6.
Olkkola KT, Hamunen K, and Maunuksela EL, "Clinical Pharmacokinetics and Pharmacodynamics of Opioid Analgesics in Infants and Children," *Clin Pharmacokinet*, 1995, 28(5):385-404.

♦ **Methadose (Can)** *see* Methadone *on page 641*

Methenamine (meth EN a meen)

U.S. Brand Names Hiprex®; Mandelamine®; Urex®

Canadian Brand Names Dehydral; Hiprex; Mandelamine; Urasal

Synonyms Hexamethylenetetramine

Therapeutic Category Antibiotic, Miscellaneous

Generic Available Yes

Use Prophylaxis or suppression of recurrent urinary tract infections

Pregnancy Risk Factor C

Contraindications Severe dehydration, renal insufficiency (methenamine is ineffective in patients with renal impairment), hepatic insufficiency in patients receiving hippurate salt; hypersensitivity to methenamine, tartrazine dye (Hiprex® tablets), or any component

Warnings Dosage of 8 g/day has been associated with bladder irritation, albuminuria, and hematuria

Precautions Use with caution in patients with hepatic impairment

Adverse Reactions
Central nervous system: Headache
Dermatologic: Rash, pruritus, urticaria
Gastrointestinal: Nausea, vomiting, diarrhea, abdominal cramping, anorexia, stomatitis
Genitourinary: Bladder irritation, painful and frequent micturition, dysuria, crystalluria
Hepatic: Elevated AST and ALT (with hippurate formulation)
Otic: Tinnitus
Renal: Hematuria
Respiratory: Lipoid pneumonitis (with mandelate suspension), dyspnea

Drug Interactions Sulfamethizole (precipitates in acid urine); sodium bicarbonate, acetazolamide (decrease effect of methenamine)

Food Interactions Foods/diets which alkalinize urine pH >5.5 decrease activity of methenamine; cranberry juice can be used to acidify urine and increase activity of methenamine

Stability Protect from excessive heat

Mechanism of Action Methenamine is hydrolyzed to formaldehyde and ammonia in acidic urine; formaldehyde has nonspecific bactericidal action

(Continued)

Methenamine *(Continued)*

Pharmacokinetics
Absorption: Readily from the GI tract; 10% to 30% of the drug will be hydrolyzed by gastric juices unless it is protected by an enteric coating

Distribution: Distributes into breast milk; crosses the placenta

Metabolism: ~10% to 25% in the liver

Half-life: 3-6 hours

Elimination: Excretion occurs via glomerular filtration and tubular secretion with ~70% to 90% of dose excreted unchanged in urine within 24 hours

Usual Dosage Oral:
Children 6-12 years: Mandelate: 75 mg/kg/day divided every 12 hours or 50-75 mg/kg/day divided every 6-8 hours; maximum dose: 4 g/day

Adults:
Hippurate: 1 g twice daily

Mandelate: 1 g 4 times/day after meals and at bedtime

Administration
Oral: Administer with food to minimize GI upset; shake suspension well before use; patient should drink plenty of fluids to ensure adequate urine flow; administer with cranberry juice, ascorbic acid, or ammonium chloride to acidify urine; avoid intake of alkalinizing agents (sodium bicarbonate, antacids)

Monitoring Parameters
Urinary pH, urinalysis, periodic liver function tests in patients receiving hippurate salt

Test Interactions
Formaldehyde interferes with fluorometric procedures causing falsely increased results for catecholamines and VMA (U); falsely decreased urine estriol concentration with tests using acid hydrolysis

Nursing Implications
Urine should be acidic, pH <5.5 for maximum effect

Additional Information
Should not be used to treat infections outside of the lower urinary tract (ie, pyelonephritis)

Dosage Forms
Suspension, as mandelate: 250 mg/5 mL [coconut flavor]; 500 mg/5 mL [cherry flavor]

Tablet, as hippurate (Hiprex®, Urex®): 1 g [Hiprex® contains tartrazine dye]

Tablet, as mandelate, enteric coated (Mandelamine®): 250 mg, 500 mg, 1 g

References
"Practice Parameter: The Diagnosis, Treatment, and Evaluation of the Initial Urinary Tract Infection in Febrile Infants and Young Children. American Academy of Pediatrics. Committee on Quality Improvement. Subcommittee on Urinary Tract Infection," *Pediatrics*, 1999, 103(4 Pt 1):843-52.

Methimazole *(meth IM a zole)*

U.S. Brand Names Tapazole®

Synonyms Thiamazole

Therapeutic Category Antithyroid Agent

Generic Available No

Use Palliative treatment of hyperthyroidism, to return the hyperthyroid patient to a normal metabolic state prior to thyroidectomy, and to control thyrotoxic crisis that may accompany thyroidectomy

Pregnancy Risk Factor D

Contraindications Hypersensitivity to methimazole or any component, nursing mothers per manufacturer, however, expert analysis and the American Academy of Pediatrics state this drug may be used with caution in nursing mothers (see Drugs and Breast-Feeding *on page 1243*)

Precautions Use with extreme caution in patients receiving other drugs known to cause agranulocytosis

Adverse Reactions
Cardiovascular: Edema, periarteritis

Central nervous system: Drowsiness, vertigo, headache, CNS stimulation, neuropathies, CNS depression, fever, dizziness

Endocrine & metabolic: Goiter

Dermatologic: Rash, urticaria, pruritus, alopecia, skin pigmentation, exfoliative dermatitis

Gastrointestinal: Ageusia, nausea, vomiting, epigastric distress, splenomegaly, constipation, weight gain

Hematologic: Agranulocytosis, hypoprothrombinemia

Hepatic: Cholestatic jaundice, hepatitis

Neuromuscular & skeletal: Arthralgia, myalgia, paresthesia, neuritis

Renal: Nephritis

Respiratory: Interstitial pneumonitis

Miscellaneous: Lupus-like syndrome, lymphadenopathy, insulin autoimmune syndrome

Drug Interactions Lithium and potassium iodide may potentiate hypothyroid effects; potentiates warfarin's anticoagulant effects

Mechanism of Action Inhibits the synthesis of thyroid hormones by blocking the oxidation of iodine in the thyroid gland, blocking iodine's ability to combine with tyrosine to form thyroxine (T_4) and triiodothyronine (T_3)

Pharmacodynamics Antithyroid effect:
Onset: 12-18 hours
Duration: 36-72 hours

Pharmacokinetics
Distribution: Found in high concentrations in breast milk; breast milk to plasma ratio: 1.0
Bioavailability: 80% to 95%
Half-life: 5-13 hours
Time to peak serum concentration: 1 hour
Elimination: <12% excreted in urine

Usual Dosage Oral:
Children:
Initial: 0.4 mg/kg/day in 3 divided doses; maintenance: 0.2 mg/kg/day in 3 divided doses
or
Initial: 0.5-0.7 mg/kg/day or 15-20 mg/m^2/day in 3 divided doses
Maintenance: $^1\!/_3$ to $^2\!/_3$ of initial dose; maximum dose: 30 mg/day
Adults: Initial: 5 mg every 8 hours; 10 mg every 8 hours for moderately severe disease and up to 20 mg every 8 hours for severe hyperthyroidism; maintenance: 5-15 mg/day

Administration Oral: Administer with meals

Monitoring Parameters CBC with differential, liver function (baseline and as needed); serum thyroxine, free thyroxine index, prothrombin time

Patient Information Notify physician of fever, sore throat, unusual bleeding or bruising, headache, rash, or yellowing of skin

Dosage Forms Tablet: 5 mg, 10 mg

References
Raby C, Lagorce JF, Jambut-Absil AC, et al, "The Mechanism of Action of Synthetic Antithyroid Drugs: Iodine Complexation During Oxidation of Iodide," *Endocrinology*, 1990, 126(3):1683-91.

Methocarbamol (meth oh KAR ba mole)

U.S. Brand Names Robaxin®

Therapeutic Category Skeletal Muscle Relaxant, Nonparalytic

Generic Available Yes

Use Treatment of muscle spasm associated with acute painful musculoskeletal conditions; supportive therapy in tetanus

Pregnancy Risk Factor C

Contraindications Hypersensitivity to methocarbamol or any component

Warnings Solution is hypertonic, avoid extravasation; avoid using injection in patients with impaired renal function because the polyethylene glycol vehicle may be irritating to the kidneys

Precautions Use injectable form cautiously in patients with suspected or known seizure disorders

Adverse Reactions
Cardiovascular: Syncope, bradycardia, hypotension
Central nervous system: Drowsiness, dizziness, lightheadedness, headache, fever, vertigo, seizures
Dermatologic: Urticaria, pruritus
Gastrointestinal: Nausea, metallic taste, GI upset, vomiting
Genitourinary: Discoloration of urine (brown, black, or green)
Hematologic: Leukopenia
Local: Pain and phlebitis at injection site, thrombophlebitis
Ocular: Blurred vision, conjunctivitis, nystagmus, diplopia
Respiratory: Nasal congestion
Miscellaneous: Hypersensitivity reactions

Stability Injection when diluted to 4 mg/mL in sterile water, D_5W, or NS is stable for 6 days at room temperature; do **not** refrigerate after dilution

Mechanism of Action CNS depressant with sedative and skeletal muscle relaxant effects; exact mechanism of action is unknown

Pharmacodynamics Onset of action: 30 minutes

Pharmacokinetics Oral:
Metabolism: Extensive in the liver
Half-life: 0.9-1.8 hours
(Continued)

Methocarbamol *(Continued)*

Time to peak serum concentration: Within ~1-2 hours

Usual Dosage

Tetanus: I.V.:

Children (recommended **only** for use in tetanus): 15 mg/kg/dose or 500 mg/m^2/dose, may repeat every 6 hours if needed; maximum dose: 1.8 g/m^2/day for 3 days only

Adults: 1-2 g by direct I.V. injection followed by additional 1-2 g (maximum dose: 3 g total); repeat with 1-2 g every 6 hours until NG tube or oral therapy possible; total daily dose of up to 24 g may be needed

Muscle spasm: Adults:

Oral: 1.5 g 3-4 times/day or 750 mg every 4 hours for 2-3 days, then decrease to 4-4.5 g/day in 3-6 divided doses

I.M., I.V.: 1 g every 8 hours if oral not possible; maximum dose: 3 g/day for 3 consecutive days (except when treating tetanus); may be reinstituted after 2 drug-free days

Dosing adjustment in renal impairment: Do not administer parenteral formulation to patients with renal dysfunction

Administration

Parenteral: I.V.: May be injected directly I.V. without dilution at a maximum rate of 180 mg/m^2/minute but not >3 mL/minute; may also be diluted in NS or D$_5$W to a concentration of 4 mg/mL and infused more slowly; patient should be in the recumbent position during and for 10-15 minutes after I.V. administration

I.M.: Do not inject more than 3 mL per site; not recommended for S.C. administration

Test Interactions 5-hydroxyindoleacetic acid (5-HIAA) and vanillylmandelic acid (VMA)

Patient Information May cause drowsiness and impair ability to perform hazardous activities requiring mental alertness or physical coordination; urine may darken to brown, black, or green

Nursing Implications Avoid infiltration, extremely irritating to tissues

Dosage Forms

Injection: 100 mg/mL in polyethylene glycol 50% (10 mL)

Tablet: 500 mg, 750 mg

Methohexital *(meth oh HEKS i tal)*

Related Information

Adult ACLS Algorithm, Synchronized Cardioversion *on page 1048*
Preprocedure Sedatives in Children *on page 1201*

U.S. Brand Names Brevital® Sodium

Canadian Brand Names Brietal

Therapeutic Category Barbiturate; General Anesthetic; Sedative

Generic Available No

Use Induction and maintenance of general anesthesia for short procedures; induction of hypnotic state

Restrictions C-IV

Pregnancy Risk Factor B

Contraindications Porphyria; hypersensitivity to methohexital, barbiturates, or any component; patients in whom general anesthesia is contraindicated

Warnings Continuously monitor respiratory function, pulse oximetry, and cardiac function. Resuscitative drugs, ventilation and intubation equipment, and trained personnel should be immediately available. For deep sedation, a designated individual (other than the person performing the procedure) should be present to continuously monitor the patient.

Precautions Use with extreme caution in patients with liver impairment, asthma, cardiovascular instability; may precipitate seizures in patients with history of convulsions, especially partial seizure disorders; prolonged administration may result in increased CNS, respiratory, and cardiovascular effects; use with caution in patients with obstructive pulmonary disease, severe hypertension or hypotension, myocardial disease, CHF, severe anemia, extreme obesity, renal impairment, or endocrine disorders

Adverse Reactions

Cardiovascular: Hypotension, peripheral vascular collapse, tachycardia (following induction)

Central nervous system: Seizures, headache, somnolence, unconsciousness

Gastrointestinal: Nausea, vomiting

Local: Pain on I.M. injection, thrombophlebitis

Neuromuscular & skeletal: Twitching, rigidity, tremor, involuntary muscle movement

Respiratory: Apnea, respiratory depression, laryngospasm, coughing

Miscellaneous: Hiccups

Drug Interactions CNS depressants may increase effects; prior chronic use of phenytoin, barbiturates, or other enzyme inducing agents may decrease effect of methohexital; methohexital may affect absorption or elimination of phenytoin, anticoagulants, corticosteroids, halothane, ethanol, propylene glycol containing solutions

Stability Do not dilute with solutions containing bacteriostatic agents; acceptable diluents: D_5W, NS, SWI, or accompanying diluent (for 500 mg vial to make a 1% solution); SWI is the preferred diluent except for making the 0.2% solution for I.V. continuous infusion (use of SWI to make the 0.2% solution will result in extreme hypotonicity; D_5W or NS should be used). Do not use I.V./I.M. solutions if not clear and colorless. Solutions are alkaline (pH 9.5-11) and incompatible with acids (eg, atropine sulfate, succinylcholine chloride); incompatible with phenol-containing solutions, silicone, and LR

Mechanism of Action Ultra short-acting I.V. barbiturate anesthetic; depresses CNS activity by binding to barbiturate site at GABA-receptor complex enhancing GABA activity; depresses reticular activating system; higher doses may be gabamimetic

Pharmacodynamics

Onset of Effect

I.M. (pediatric patients): 2-10 minutes

I.V.: 1 minute

Rectal (pediatric patients): 5-15 minutes

Duration:

I.M.: 1-1.5 hours

I.V.: 7-10 minutes

Rectal: 1-1.5 hours

Pharmacokinetics

Metabolism: In the liver via demethylation and oxidation

Bioavailability: Rectal: 17%

Elimination: Through the kidney via glomerular filtration

Usual Dosage Doses must be titrated to effect

Manufacturer's recommendations:

Infants <1 month: Safety and efficacy not established

Infants ≥1 month and Children:

I.M.: Induction: 6.6-10 mg/kg of a 5% solution

Rectal: Induction: Usual: 25 mg/kg of a 1% solution

Alternative pediatric dosing:

Children 3-12 years:

I.M.: Preoperative: 5-10 mg/kg/dose

I.V.: Induction: 1-2 mg/kg/dose (additional studies are needed)

Rectal: Preoperative/induction: 20-35 mg/kg/dose; usual: 25 mg/kg/dose; maximum dose: 500 mg/dose; give as 10% aqueous solution

Adults: I.V.:

Induction: Range: 50-120 mg or 1-1.5 mg/kg; usual: 70 mg (**Note:** This provides anesthesia for 5-7 minutes)

Maintenance: Intermittent I.V. bolus injection: 20-40 mg (2-4 mL of a 1% solution) every 4-7 minutes **OR** Continuous infusion: Average dose: 6 mg/minute (eg, 3 mL/minute of a 0.2% solution); titrate to effect; reduce administration rate gradually for longer surgical procedures

Administration

Parenteral:

I.M.: Reconstitute with NS to a maximum concentration of 50 mg/mL (5% solution)

I.V.: Adults:

Bolus: Dilute with SWI (preferred), NS, or D_5W to a maximum concentration of 10 mg/mL (1% solution); for induction, infuse a 1% solution at a rate of 1 mL/5 seconds

Continuous infusion: Dilute with D_5W or NS to prepare a 0.2% solution (see Usual Dosage)

Rectal: Dilute with acceptable diluent (see Stability) to a recommended concentration of 10 mg/mL (1% solution)

Monitoring Parameters Blood pressure, heart rate, respiratory rate, oxygen saturation, pulse oximetry

Patient Information May cause drowsiness and impair ability to perform activities requiring mental alertness or physical coordination; do not drive a motor vehicle or operate machinery until 8-12 hours after medication was administered, or until normal functions return (whichever is longer)

(Continued)

Methohexital *(Continued)*

Nursing Implications Check catheter placement prior to I.V. injection; avoid extravasation; avoid intra-arterial administration (thrombosis, necrosis, and gangrene may occur)

Additional Information Does not possess analgesic properties; Brevital® has FDA-approved labeling for I.V. use in adults, and for rectal and I.M. use only in pediatric patients >1 month of age; 100 pediatric patients (3 months to 5 years of age) received rectal methohexital (25 mg/kg) for sedation prior to computed tomography (CT) scan; sedation was adequate in 95% of patients; mean time for full sedation = 8.2 ± 3.9 minutes; mean duration of action = 79.3 ± 30.9 minutes; 10% of patients had transient side effects (see Pomeranz, 2000)

Dosage Forms Powder for injection, as sodium: 500 mg, 2.5 g, 5 g

References

Cote′ CJ, "Sedation for the Pediatric Patient," *Pediatr Clin North Am*, 1994, 41(1):31-58.

Pomeranz ES, Chudnofsky CR, Deegan TJ, et al, "Rectal Methohexital Sedation for Computed Tomography Imaging of Stable Pediatric Emergency Department Patients," *Pediatrics*, 2000, 105(5):1110-4.

♦ **Methoin** *see* Mephenytoin *on page 630*

Methotrexate *(meth oh TREKS ate)*

Related Information

Drugs and Breast-Feeding *on page 1243*
Emetogenic Potential of Single Chemotherapeutic Agents *on page 1129*

U.S. Brand Names Rheumatrex® Oral

Synonyms Amethopterin; MTX

Therapeutic Category Antineoplastic Agent, Antimetabolite; Antirheumatic, Disease Modifying

Generic Available Yes

Use Treatment of trophoblastic neoplasms, leukemias, histiocytoses, osteosarcoma, non-Hodgkin's lymphoma; psoriasis; children with severe polyarticular juvenile rheumatoid arthritis who have failed to respond to other agents

Pregnancy Risk Factor D

Contraindications Hypersensitivity to methotrexate or any component; severe renal or hepatic impairment; pre-existing profound bone marrow suppression; high-dose methotrexate (>1 g/m^2) should not be administered to patients with a creatinine clearance of <50% to 75% of normal

Warnings The FDA currently recommends that procedures for proper handling and disposal of antineoplastic agents be considered. Due to the possibility of severe toxic reactions, fully inform patient of the risks involved; do not use in women of childbearing age unless benefit outweighs risks; may cause hepatotoxicity, fibrosis and cirrhosis, along with marked bone marrow suppression; death from intestinal perforation may occur.

Precautions Use with caution in patients with peptic ulcer disease, ulcerative colitis, pre-existing bone marrow suppression; use with caution and reduce dosage in patients with renal or hepatic impairment, ascites, and pleural effusion

Adverse Reactions

Cardiovascular: Vasculitis

Central nervous system: Malaise, fatigue, dizziness, encephalopathy, seizures, confusion, fever, headache, chills

Dermatitis: Alopecia, rash, depigmentation or hyperpigmentation of skin, photosensitivity, pruritus, urticaria

Endocrine & metabolic: Hyperuricemia

Gastrointestinal: Nausea, vomiting, diarrhea, anorexia, stomatitis, enteritis

Genitourinary: Cystitis

Hematologic: Myelosuppression, leukopenia, thrombocytopenia, anemia, hemorrhage

Hepatic: Hepatotoxicity, elevated liver enzymes, hyperbilirubinemia

Neuromuscular & skeletal: Arthralgia

Ocular: Blurred vision

Renal: Nephropathy (azotemia, hematuria, renal failure)

Respiratory: Interstitial pneumonitis

Miscellaneous: Anaphylaxis

Drug Interactions Salicylates may delay MTX's clearance; sulfonamides, phenytoin displace MTX from protein binding sites; live virus vaccines, pyrimethamine, 5-FU; NSAIDs increase toxicity of MTX by elevating serum MTX concentrations; penicillins may decrease renal clearance of MTX; probenecid decreases the renal elimination of MTX

Food Interactions Milk-rich foods may decrease MTX absorption; folate may decrease drug response

Stability Protect from light; incompatible with fluorouracil, cytarabine, prednisolone, and sodium phosphate

Mechanism of Action An antimetabolite that binds to dihydrofolate reductase blocking the reduction of dihydrofolate to tetrahydrofolic acid; depletion of tetrahydrofolic acid leads to depletion of DNA precursors and inhibition of DNA and purine synthesis

Pharmacodynamics Approximate time to benefit in treatment of rheumatoid arthritis: 1-2 months

Pharmacokinetics

Absorption:

Oral: Average: 30%; variable absorption at low doses (<30 mg/m^2); incomplete absorption after large doses

I.M.: Completely absorbed

Distribution: Small amounts excreted into breast milk; crosses the placenta; does not achieve therapeutic concentrations in the CSF; sustained concentrations are retained in the kidney and liver

Metabolism: In the liver to 7-hydroxymethotrexate

Protein binding: 50% to 60%

Time to peak serum concentration:

Oral: 0.5-4 hours

Parenteral: 0.5-2 hours

Half-life: 8-12 hours

Elimination: Small amounts in feces; primarily excreted unchanged in urine (90%) via glomerular filtration and active secretion by the renal tubule; 1% to 11% of a dose is excreted as the 7-hydroxy metabolite

Usual Dosage Refer to individual protocols:

Children:

Dermatomyositis: Oral: 15-20 mg/m^2/week as a single dose once weekly or 0.3-1 mg/kg/dose once weekly

Juvenile rheumatoid arthritis: Oral, I.M., S.C.: 5-15 mg/m^2/week as a single dose or in 3 divided doses given 12 hours apart; folic acid 1 mg daily or folinic acid ≤5 mg weekly are often used to prevent folate depletion from methotrexate

Antineoplastic dosage range:

Oral:, I.M.: 7.5-30 mg/m^2/week or every 2 weeks

I.V.: 10 mg to 33,000 mg/m^2 bolus dosing or continuous infusion over 6-42 hours

Antineoplastic dosing schedules (adapted from Dorr RT and Von Hoff DD, *Cancer Chemotherapy Handbook*, 2nd ed, 1994): See table

Methotrexate Dosing Schedules

	Dose	Route	Frequency
Conventional dose	15-20 mg/m^2	Oral	Twice weekly
	30-50 mg/m^2	Oral, I.V.	Weekly
	15 mg/day for 5 days	Oral, I.M.	Every 2-3 weeks
Intermediate dose	50-150 mg/m^2	I.V. push	Every 2-3 weeks
	240 mg/m^2*	I.V. infusion	Every 4-7 days
	0.5-1 g/m^2*	I.V. infusion	Every 2-3 weeks
High dose	1-12 g/m^2*	I.V. infusion	Every 1-3 weeks

*Followed with leucovorin rescue

Pediatric solid tumors:

<12 years: 12 g/m^2 (dosage range: 12-18 g)

≥12 years: 8 g/m^2 (maximum dose: 18 g)

Meningeal leukemia: I.T.: 10-15 mg/m^2 (maximum: 15 mg) by protocol **or**

≤3 months: 3 mg dose

4-11 months: 6 mg dose

1 year: 8 mg dose

2 years: 10 mg dose

≥3 years: 12 mg dose

I.T. doses are administered at 2- to 5-day intervals until CSF counts return to normal followed by a dose once weekly for 2 weeks then monthly thereafter

ALL (high dose): I.V.: Loading dose: 200 mg/m^2 followed by a 24-hour infusion of 1200 mg/m^2/day

ANLL: I.V.: 7.5 mg/m^2/day on days 1-5 of treatment course

(Continued)

Methotrexate (Continued)

Resistant ANLL: I.V.: 100 mg/m^2/dose on day 1 of treatment course

Non-Hodgkin's lymphoma: I.V.: 200-500 mg/m^2; repeat every 28 days

Induction of remission in acute lymphoblastic leukemias: Oral: 3.3 mg/m^2/day for 4-6 weeks

Remission maintenance: Oral, I.M.: 20-30 mg/m^2 2 times/week

Adults:

Trophoblastic neoplasms: Oral, I.M.: 15-30 mg/day for 5 days, repeat in 7 days for 3-5 courses

Head and neck cancer: Oral, I.M. I.V.: 25-50 mg/m^2 once weekly

Rheumatoid arthritis: Oral: 7.5 mg once weekly or 2.5 mg every 12 hours for 3 doses/week; not to exceed 20 mg/week

Psoriasis: Oral: 2.5-5 mg/dose every 12 hours for 3 doses/week given once weekly

or

Oral, I.M.: 10-25 mg given once weekly

Dosing adjustment in renal impairment:

Cl$_{cr}$ 61-80 mL/minute: Decrease dose by 25%

Cl$_{cr}$ 51-60 mL/minute: Decrease dose by 33%

Cl$_{cr}$ 10-50 mL/minute: Decrease dose by 50% to 70%

Administration Parenteral:

Methotrexate may be administered I.V. push, I.V. intermittent infusion, or I.V. continuous infusion at a concentration <25 mg/mL; doses >100-300 mg/m^2 are usually administered by I.V. continuous infusion and are followed by a course of leucovorin rescue

For intrathecal use, mix methotrexate without preservatives with NS, Elliotts B solution, or LR to a concentration not greater than 2 mg/mL

Monitoring Parameters CBC with differential and platelet count, creatinine clearance, serum creatinine, BUN, hepatic function tests, serum electrolytes, urinalysis, plasma MTX concentrations (see leucovorin rescue graph *on page 581* to evaluate plasma MTX concentration versus leucovorin rescue dose)

Reference Range Serum levels >1 x 10^{-7} mol/L for more than 40 hours are toxic

Patient Information Report to physician any fever, sore throat, bleeding or bruising, shortness of breath, painful urination; avoid alcohol

Nursing Implications Intensive hydration should be administered and urine should be alkalinized prior to high doses to enhance methotrexate solubility

Additional Information Myelosuppressive effects:

WBC: Mild

Platelets: Moderate

Onset (days): 7

Nadir (days): 10

Recovery (days): 21

Dosage Forms

Injection, as sodium: 2.5 mg/mL (2 mL); 25 mg/mL (2 mL, 4 mL, 8 mL, 10 mL)

Injection, preservative free, as sodium: 25 mg (2 mL, 4 mL, 8 mL, 10 mL)

Powder for injection, as sodium: 20 mg, 25 mg, 50 mg, 100 mg, 250 mg, 1 g

Tablet, as sodium: 2.5 mg

Tablet, as sodium, dose pack: 2.5 mg (4 cards with 2, 3, 4, 5, or 6 tablets each)

References

Berg SL, Grisell DL, DeLaney TF, et al, "Principles of Treatment of Pediatric Solid Tumors," *Pediatr Clin North Am*, 1991, 38(2):249-67.

Bleyer WA, "Clinical Pharmacology of Intrathecal Methotrexate II. An Approved Dosage Regimen Derived From Age-Related Pharmacokinetics," *Cancer Treat Rep*, 1977, 61(8):1419-25.

Crom WR, Glynn-Barnhart AM, Rodman JH, et al, "Pharmacokinetics of Anticancer Drugs in Children," *Clin Pharmacokinet*, 1987, 12(3):168-213.

Giannini EH, Brewer EJ, Kuzmina N, et al, "Methotrexate in Resistant Juvenile Rheumatoid Arthritis. Results of the USA-USSR Double-Blind, Placebo-Controlled Trial," *N Engl J Med*, 1992, 326(16):1043-9.

Greaves MW and Weinstein GD, "Treatment of Psoriasis," *N Engl J Med*, 1995, 332(9):581-8.

Rose CD, Singsen BH, and Eichenfield AH, "Safety and Efficacy of Methotrexate Therapy for Juvenile Rheumatoid Arthritis," *J Pediatr*, 1990, 117(4):653-9.

Methsuximide (meth SUKS i mide)

Related Information

Antiepileptic Drugs *on page 1208*

U.S. Brand Names Celontin®

Therapeutic Category Anticonvulsant, Succinimide

Generic Available No

Use Control of absence (petit mal) seizures; useful adjunct in refractory, partial complex (psychomotor) seizures

Pregnancy Risk Factor C

Contraindications Hypersensitivity to methsuximide or any component

Precautions Use with caution in patients with hepatic or renal disease; avoid abrupt withdrawal

Adverse Reactions

Central nervous system: Dizziness, drowsiness, lethargy, euphoria, nervousness, hallucinations, insomnia, mental confusion, headache, ataxia

Dermatologic: Rash, urticaria, Stevens-Johnson syndrome

Gastrointestinal: Nausea, vomiting, anorexia, diarrhea, abdominal pain

Hematologic: Leukopenia, thrombocytopenia, eosinophilia, pancytopenia, monocytosis

Ocular: Periorbital edema

Miscellaneous: Hiccups

Stability Protect from high temperature

Mechanism of Action Increases the seizure threshold and suppresses paroxysmal spike-and-wave pattern in absence seizures; depresses nerve transmission in the motor cortex

Pharmacokinetics

Metabolism: Rapidly demethylated in the liver to N-desmethylmethsuximide (active metabolite)

Half-life: 2-4 hours

N-desmethylmethsuximide:

Children: 26 hours

Adults: 28-80 hours

Time to peak serum concentration: Within 1-3 hours

Elimination: <1% in urine as unchanged drug

Usual Dosage Oral:

Children: Initial: 10-15 mg/kg/day in 3-4 divided doses; increase weekly up to maximum of 30 mg/kg/day; mean dose required:

<30 kg: 20 mg/kg/day

>30 kg: 14 mg/kg/day

Adults: 300 mg/day for the first week; may increase by 300 mg/day at weekly intervals up to 1.2 g in 2-4 divided doses/day

Administration Oral: Administer with food

Monitoring Parameters CBC with differential, liver enzymes, urinalysis; measure trough serum levels for efficacy and 3-hour postdose concentrations for toxicity

Reference Range Measure N-desmethylmethsuximide concentrations:

Therapeutic: 10-40 µg/mL (SI: 53-212 µmol/L)

Toxic: >40 µg/mL (SI: >212 µmol/L)

Patient Information May cause drowsiness and impair ability to perform activities requiring mental alertness or physical coordination; do not discontinue abruptly

Dosage Forms Capsule: 150 mg, 300 mg

References

Miles MV, Tennison MB, and Greenwood RS, "Pharmacokinetics of N-desmethylmethsuximide in Pediatric Patients," *J Pediatr*, 1989, 114(4 Pt 1):647-50.

Tennison MB, Greenwood RS, Miles MV, "Methsuximide for Intractable Childhood Seizures," *Pediatrics*, 1991, 87(2):186-9.

♦ **Methylacetoxyprogesterone** *see* Medroxyprogesterone *on page 624*

Methyldopa (meth il DOE pa)

U.S. Brand Names Aldomet®

Canadian Brand Names Apo-Methyldopa; Dopamet; Novo-Medopa; Nu-Medopa

Therapeutic Category Alpha-Adrenergic Inhibitors, Central; Antihypertensive Agent

Generic Available Yes

Use Management of moderate to severe hypertension

Pregnancy Risk Factor B

Contraindications Hypersensitivity to methyldopa or any component; liver disease, pheochromocytoma

Warnings Injection contains sodium bisulfite which may cause allergic reactions

Precautions Use with caution and adjust dose in patients with renal dysfunction; active metabolite may accumulate in uremia

Adverse Reactions

Cardiovascular: Orthostatic hypotension, bradycardia, edema

Central nervous system: Drowsiness, sedation, vertigo, headache, depression, memory lapse, fever

Dermatologic: Rash

Endocrine & metabolic: Gynecomastia, sexual dysfunction, sodium retention

(Continued)

Methyldopa *(Continued)*

Gastrointestinal: Nausea, vomiting, diarrhea, xerostomia, "black" tongue

Genitourinary: Discoloration of urine (red or brown)

Hematologic: Hemolytic anemia, positive Coombs' test, leukopenia

Hepatic: Hepatitis, elevated liver enzymes, jaundice, cirrhosis

Neuromuscular & skeletal: Weakness

Respiratory: Nasal congestion

Drug Interactions May increase lithium toxicity; concomitant oral administration of iron salts may decrease oral absorption of methyldopa and result in an increase in blood pressure, spacing drugs 2 hours apart may decrease this effect

Food Interactions Avoid natural licorice (causes sodium and water retention and increases potassium loss); dietary requirements for vitamin B_{12} and folate may be increased with high doses of methyldopa

Mechanism of Action Stimulates inhibitory alpha-adrenergic receptors via alpha-methylnorepinephrine (false transmitter); this results in a decreased sympathetic outflow to the heart, kidneys, and peripheral vasculature; may decrease plasma renin activity

Pharmacodynamics Hypotensive effects:

Peak effect: Oral, I.V.: Single-dose: Within 3-6 hours; multiple-dose: 2-3 days

Duration:

Oral: Single-dose: 12-24 hours; multiple-dose: 1-2 days

I.V.: 10-16 hours

Pharmacokinetics

Absorption: Oral: ~50%

Distribution: Crosses placenta; appears in breast milk

Protein binding: <15%

Metabolism: In the intestine and the liver

Half-life: Elimination:

Neonates: 10-20 hours

Adults: 1-3 hours

Elimination: ~70% of systemic dose eliminated in urine as drug and metabolites

Dialysis: Slightly dialyzable (5% to 20%)

Usual Dosage

Children:

Oral: Initial: 10 mg/kg/day in 2-4 divided doses; increase every 2 days as needed to maximum dose of 65 mg/kg/day; do not exceed 3 g/day

I.V.: Initial: 2-4 mg/kg/dose; if response is not seen within 4-6 hours, may increase to 5-10 mg/kg/dose; administer doses every 6-8 hours; maximum daily dose: 65 mg/kg or 3 g, whichever is less

Adults:

Oral: Initial: 250 mg 2-3 times/day; increase every 2 days as needed; usual dose 500 mg to 2 g daily in 2-4 divided doses; maximum dose: 3 g/day

I.V.: 250-1000 mg every 6-8 hours; maximum dose: 4 g/day

Dosing interval in renal impairment: Children and Adults:

Cl_{cr} >50 mL/minute: Administer normal dose every 8 hours

Cl_{cr} 10-50 mL/minute: Administer normal dose every 8-12 hours

Cl_{cr} <10 mL/minute: Administer normal dose every 12-24 hours

Administration

Oral: May be administered without regard to food; administer new dosage increases in the evening to minimize sedation

Parenteral: I.V.: Infuse I.V. dose slowly over 30-60 minutes at a concentration ≤10 mg/mL

Monitoring Parameters Blood pressure, CBC with differential, hemoglobin, hematocrit, Coombs' test [direct], liver enzymes

Test Interactions Urinary uric acid, serum creatinine (alkaline picrate method), AST (colorimetric method), and urinary catecholamines (falsely high levels)

Patient Information Avoid alcohol; may cause sedation and drowsiness and impair ability to perform activities requiring mental alertness or physical coordination; may cause dry mouth; rise slowly from prolonged sitting or lying position; may cause urine to turn red or brown; notify physician of unexplained prolonged general tiredness, fever, or jaundice

Nursing Implications Transient sedation or depression may occur for first 72 hours of therapy, or when doses are increased

Additional Information Most effective if used with diuretic; titrate dose to optimal blood pressure control with minimal side effects

Dosage Forms

Injection, as methyldopate hydrochloride: 50 mg/mL (5 mL, 10 mL)

Tablet: 125 mg, 250 mg, 500 mg

Methylene Blue (METH i leen bloo)

U.S. Brand Names Urolene Blue®

Therapeutic Category Antidote, Cyanide; Antidote, Drug-induced Methemoglobinemia

Generic Available Yes

Use Antidote for cyanide poisoning and drug-induced methemoglobinemia, indicator dye, bacteriostatic genitourinary antiseptic

Pregnancy Risk Factor C (D if injected intra-amniotically)

Contraindications Renal insufficiency; hypersensitivity to methylene blue or any component

Warnings Do not inject subcutaneously or intrathecally as necrotic abscesses (S.C.) and neural damage (I.T.) including paraplegia have occurred

Precautions Use with caution in patients with G-6-PD deficiency; continued use can cause profound anemia

Adverse Reactions

Cardiovascular: Hypertension, cyanosis, large I.V. doses have been associated with precordial pain

Central nervous system: Dizziness, mental confusion, headache, fever

Dermatologic: Stains skin

Gastrointestinal: Nausea, vomiting, abdominal pain, diarrhea, discoloration of feces (blue-green)

Genitourinary: Bladder irritation, discoloration of urine (blue-green)

Hematologic: Formation of methemoglobin

Miscellaneous: Diaphoresis

Mechanism of Action Weak germicide; in low concentrations hastens the conversion of methemoglobin to hemoglobin; has opposite effect at high concentrations by converting ferrous iron of reduced hemoglobin to ferric iron to form methemoglobin; in cyanide toxicity, it combines with cyanide to form cyanmethemoglobin preventing the interference of cyanide with the cytochrome system

Pharmacokinetics

Absorption: Well absorbed from GI tract

Elimination: In bile, feces, and urine

Usual Dosage

Methemoglobinemia: Children and Adults: I.V.: 1-2 mg/kg or 25-50 mg/m^2; may be repeated after 1 hour if necessary

Chronic methemoglobinemia: Adults: Oral: 100-300 mg/day

NADPH-methemoglobin reductase deficiency: Children: Oral: 1-1.5 mg/kg/day (maximum dose: 300 mg/day) given with 5-8 mg/kg/day ascorbic acid

Genitourinary antiseptic: Adults: Oral: 65-130 mg 3 times/day; maximum dose: 390 mg/day

Chronic urolithiasis: Adults: Oral: 65 mg 3 times/day

Administration

Parenteral: Administer undiluted by direct I.V. injection over several minutes

Oral: Administer after meals with a full glass of water

Patient Information May discolor urine and feces blue-green; may discolor skin on contact

Additional Information Has been used topically (0.1% solutions) in conjunction with polychromatic light to photoinactivate viruses such as herpes simplex (this is an unlabeled indication); has been used alone or in combination with vitamin C for the management of chronic urolithiasis; skin stains may be removed using a hypochlorite solution

Dosage Forms

Injection: 10 mg/mL (1 mL, 10 mL)

Tablet (Urolene Blue®): 65 mg

♦ **Methylin**™ see Methylphenidate *on page 653*

♦ **Methylin**™ **ER** see Methylphenidate *on page 653*

♦ **Methylmorphine** see Codeine *on page 262*

Methylphenidate (meth il FEN i date)

U.S. Brand Names Concerta™; Metadate® CD; Metadate® ER; Methylin™; Methylin™ ER; Ritalin®; Ritalin-SR®

Canadian Brand Names PMS-Methylphenidate; Riphenidate

Therapeutic Category Central Nervous System Stimulant, Nonamphetamine

Generic Available Yes

Use Attention-deficit/hyperactivity disorder (ADHD); narcolepsy

Restrictions C-II

(Continued)

Methylphenidate *(Continued)*

Pregnancy Risk Factor C

Contraindications Hypersensitivity to methylphenidate or any component; glaucoma; motor tics; Tourette's syndrome (diagnosis or family history); patients with marked agitation, tension, and anxiety; use of MAO inhibitors within 14 days (hypertensive crisis may occur)

Warnings Suppression of growth may occur with long-term use in children (monitor carefully); may exacerbate symptoms of thought disorder and behavior disturbance in psychotic children; do not use for severe depression or normal fatigue states; may lower seizure threshold; rare cases of visual disturbances may occur; EKG abnormalities and 4 cases of sudden cardiac death have been reported in children receiving clonidine with methylphenidate; reduce dose of methylphenidate by 40% when used concurrently with clonidine; consider EKG monitoring. A potential for GI obstruction exists with Concerta™ (tablet is nondeformable); do not ordinarily use in patients with severe GI narrowing (eg, small bowel inflammatory disease, short gut syndrome, history of cystic fibrosis, peritonitis, chronic intestinal pseudo-obstruction, or Meckel's diverticulum)

Precautions Use with caution in patients with hypertension, seizures, acute stress reactions, emotional instability, patients with history of drug dependence; hematological monitoring is advised with long term use (see Monitoring Parameters)

Adverse Reactions
Cardiovascular: Tachycardia, hypertension, hypotension, palpitations, cardiac arrhythmias
Central nervous system: Nervousness, insomnia, dizziness, drowsiness, movement disorders, motor tics, precipitation of Tourette's syndrome; fever, headache, toxic psychosis (rare); neuroleptic malignant syndrome (very rare and usually in patients receiving medications associated with the syndrome; one case with concurrent first dose of venlafaxine has been reported)
Dermatologic: Rash
Endocrine & metabolic: Growth retardation
Gastrointestinal: Anorexia, nausea, vomiting, abdominal pain, weight loss, potential for GI obstruction with Concerta™ (see Warnings)
Hematologic: Thrombocytopenia
Ocular: Visual disturbances (rare), blurred vision, problems with accommodation
Miscellaneous: Hypersensitivity reactions; physical and psychological dependence

Drug Interactions Use with clonidine may potentially increase EKG effects (see Warnings); methylphenidate increases serum concentrations of tricyclic antidepressants, selective serotonin reuptake inhibitors, phenylbutazone, warfarin, phenytoin, phenobarbital and primidone (a decrease in the dose of these agents may be required, monitor closely); use of MAO inhibitors within 14 days may result in hypertensive crisis, use of MAOI within 14 days of methylphenidate is contraindicated; the herbal medicine St John's wort (*Hypericum perforatum*) may increase serious side effects, its use is **not** recommended; effects of guanethidine, bretylium may be antagonized by methylphenidate

Food Interactions Food may increase oral absorption
Concerta™: A high fat meal does not alter pharmacokinetics or pharmacodynamics; no evidence of dose dumping occurs when administered with or without food

Stability Dispense in tight, light-resistant container.
Methylin™: Protect from light
Methylin™ ER: Protect from moisture
Concerta™: Protect from humidity

Mechanism of Action Blocks the reuptake mechanism of dopaminergic neurons, appears to act at the cerebral cortex and subcortical structures

Pharmacodynamics Cerebral stimulation:
Peak effect:
Immediate release tablet: Within 2 hours
Sustained release tablet: Within 4-7 hours
Duration:
Immediate release tablet: 3-6 hours
Sustained release tablet: 8 hours
Concerta™: 12 hours

Pharmacokinetics
Absorption: From the GI tract, slow and incomplete
Protein binding: 15%
Metabolism: In the liver via hydroxylation to ritolinic acid
Half-life: 2-4 hours
Elimination: In urine as metabolites and unchanged drug; 45% to 50% excreted in feces via bile

Usual Dosage Oral:

Children ≥6 years: ADHD: Initial: 0.3 mg/kg/dose or 2.5-5 mg/dose given before breakfast and lunch; increase by 0.1 mg/kg/dose or by 5-10 mg/dose at weekly intervals; usual dose: 0.3-1 mg/kg/day; maximum dose: 2 mg/kg/day or 60 mg/day; specific patients may require 3 doses/day (ie, additional dose at 4 PM)

Adults: Narcolepsy: 10 mg 2-3 times/day; maximum dose: 60 mg/day

Methylin™, Metadate® ER, Ritalin-SR®: Children ≥6 years and Adults: Sustained release and extended release tablets (duration of action ~8 hours) may be given in place of regular tablets, once the daily dose is titrated using the regular tablets and the titrated 8-hour dosage corresponds to sustained release tablet size

Concerta™: Children ≥6 years and Adults:

Methylphenidate naive patients: Initial: 18 mg once daily; may increase by 18 mg/day increments at weekly intervals; maximum dose: 54 mg

Switching from methylphenidate immediate release 5 mg 2-3 times/day or sustained release 20 mg daily: Initial: 18 mg once daily; may increase by 18 mg/day increments at weekly intervals; maximum dose: 54 mg

Switching from methylphenidate immediate release 10 mg 2-3 times/day, or sustained release 40 mg daily: Initial: 36 mg once daily; may increase by 18 mg/day increments at weekly intervals; maximum dose: 54 mg

Switching from methylphenidate immediate release 15 mg 2-3 times/day, or sustained release 60 mg daily: Initial: 54 mg once daily; maximum dose: 54 mg

Note: Discontinue medication if no improvement is seen after appropriate dosage adjustment over a one-month period of time

Administration Oral: Immediate and sustained release tablets: Administer on an empty stomach ~30-45 minutes before meals; do not crush, chew, or break sustained or extended release dosage form, swallow whole; to avoid insomnia, last daily dose should be administered several hours before retiring. Concerta™: May be administered without regard to food, but must be taken with water, milk, or juice; administer dose once daily in the morning

Monitoring Parameters CBC with differential, platelet count, blood pressure, height, weight, heart rate

Patient Information Avoid caffeine and the herbal medicine St John's wort; may be habit forming; may cause dizziness or drowsiness and impair ability to perform activities requiring mental alertness or physical coordination; intact Concerta™ tablet shell may appear in stool (this is normal); report the use of other medications and herbal or natural products to your physician and pharmacist.

Additional Information Treatment with methylphenidate should include "drug holidays" or periodic discontinuation in order to assess the patient's requirements, decrease tolerance and limit suppression of linear growth and weight; Concerta™ is an osmotic controlled release formulation, with an immediate release (within 1 hour) outer coating; once daily Concerta™ has been shown to be as effective as immediate release methylphenidate tablets administered 3 times/day (see Pelham, 2001).

Dosage Forms

Capsule, extended release, as hydrochloride (Metadate® CD): 20 mg [approved by FDA April, 2001]

Tablet, as hydrochloride (Methylin™, Ritalin®): 5 mg, 10 mg, 20 mg

Tablet, extended release, as hydrochloride

Concerta™: 18 mg, 36 mg, 54 mg

Metadate® ER, Methylin™ ER: 10 mg, 20 mg

Tablet, sustained release, as hydrochloride (Ritalin-SR®): 20 mg

References

Greenhill LL, "Pharmacologic Treatment of Attention Deficit Hyperactivity Disorder," *Psychiatr Clin North Am*, 1992, 15(1):1-27.

Kelly DP and Aylward GP, "Attention Deficits in School-Aged Children and Adolescents," *Pediatr Clin North Am*, 1992, 39(3):487-512.

Pelham WE, Gnagy EM, Burrows-Maclean L, et al, "Once-a-Day Concerta Methylphenidate Versus Three-Times-Daily Methylphenidate in Laboratory and Natural Settings," *Pediatrics*, 2001, 107(6), http://www.pediatrics.org/cgi/content/full/107/6/e105.

Wilens TE and Biederman J, "The Stimulants," *Psychiatr Clin North Am*, 1992, 15(1):191-222.

♦ **Methylphenobarbital** *see* Mephobarbital *on page 631*
♦ **Methylphenyl** *see* Oxacillin *on page 740*
♦ **Methylphenylethylhydantoin** *see* Mephenytoin *on page 630*
♦ **Methylphytyl Napthoquinone** *see* Phytonadione *on page 798*

Methylprednisolone (meth il pred NIS oh lone)

Related Information

Asthma Guidelines *on page 1210*
Corticosteroids Comparison, Systemic *on page 1067*
(Continued)

Methylprednisolone *(Continued)*

U.S. Brand Names A-methaPred®; Depo-Medrol®; Depopred®; Medrol®; Solu-Medrol®

Synonyms 6-α-Methylprednisolone

Therapeutic Category Adrenal Corticosteroid; Antiasthmatic; Anti-inflammatory Agent; Corticosteroid, Systemic; Glucocorticoid

Generic Available Yes

Use Anti-inflammatory or immunosuppressant agent in the treatment of a variety of diseases including those of hematologic, allergic, inflammatory, neoplastic, and autoimmune origin

Pregnancy Risk Factor C

Contraindications Hypersensitivity to methylprednisolone or any component; administration of live virus vaccines; systemic fungal infections

Warnings May retard bone growth; methylprednisolone **acetate** I.M. injection (multiple-dose vial) and the diluent for methylprednisolone **sodium succinate** injection contain benzyl alcohol as a preservative; avoid use of benzyl alcohol products in neonates, especially premature neonates (benzyl alcohol may cause the gasping syndrome)

Precautions Use with caution in patients with hypothyroidism, cirrhosis, hypertension, CHF, ulcerative colitis, thromboembolic disorders

Adverse Reactions

Cardiovascular: Edema, hypertension

Central nervous system: Vertigo, seizures, psychoses, pseudotumor cerebri, headache

Dermatologic: Acne, skin atrophy, impaired wound healing

Endocrine & metabolic: Cushing's syndrome, pituitary-adrenal axis suppression, growth suppression, glucose intolerance, hypokalemia, alkalosis

Gastrointestinal: Peptic ulcer, nausea, vomiting

Hematologic: Transient leukocytosis

Neuromuscular & skeletal: Muscle weakness, osteoporosis, fractures

Ocular: Cataracts, glaucoma

Miscellaneous: Infections

Drug Interactions Cytochrome P-450 isoenzyme CYP3A3/4 inducer

Barbiturates, phenytoin, rifampin may increase the clearance of methylprednisolone; salicylates; toxoids; methylprednisolone may increase cyclosporine and tacrolimus serum concentrations; live virus vaccines (increase risk of viral infection); vaccines may have decreased effects

Food Interactions Systemic use of corticosteroids may require a diet with increased potassium, vitamins A, B_6, C, D, folate, calcium, zinc and phosphorus and decreased sodium

Mechanism of Action Decreases inflammation by suppression of migration of polymorphonuclear leukocytes and reversal of increased capillary permeability

Pharmacodynamics The time of peak effects and the duration of these effects is dependent upon the route of administration. See table.

Route	Peak Effect	Duration
Oral	1-2 h	30-36 h
I.M. (acetate)	4-8 d	1-4 wk
Intra-articular	1 wk	1-5 wk

Usual Dosage Note: Only sodium succinate salt may be given I.V.

Children:

Anti-inflammatory or immunosuppressive: Oral, I.M., I.V.: 0.5-1.7 mg/kg/day or 5-25 mg/m²/day in divided doses every 6-12 hours

"Pulse" therapy: 15-30 mg/kg/dose over ≥30 minutes given once daily for 3 days

Status asthmaticus: I.V.: Loading dose: 2 mg/kg/dose, then 0.5-1 mg/kg/dose every 6 hours

Lupus nephritis: I.V.: 30 mg/kg over ≥30 minutes every other day for 6 doses

Acute spinal cord injury: I.V.: 30 mg/kg over 15 minutes followed in 45 minutes by a continuous infusion of 5.4 mg/kg/hour for 23 hours

Adults:

Oral: 2-60 mg/day in 1-4 divided doses

High-dose therapy: I.V.: 30 mg/kg over ≥30 minutes; repeat as needed every 4-6 hours for 48-72 hours

I.M. (acetate): 10-80 mg/day once daily

I.V.: 40-250 mg every 4-6 hours

Lupus nephritis: High-dose "pulse" therapy: I.V.: 1 g/day for 3 days

Intra-articular, intralesional: 4-40 mg, up to 80 mg for large joints every 1-5 weeks

Administration

Oral: Administer after meals or with food or milk

Parenteral: I.V.: **Succinate:** Low dose (eg, ≤1.8 mg/kg or ≤125 mg/dose): I.V. push over 3-15 minutes; moderate dose (eg, ≥2 mg/kg or 250 mg/dose): administer over 15-30 minutes; high dose (eg, 15 mg/kg or ≥500 mg/dose): administer over ≥30 minutes; doses >15 mg/kg or ≥1 g: administer over 1 hour. Do **not** administer high-dose I.V. push; hypotension, cardiac arrhythmia, and sudden death have been reported in patients given high-dose methylprednisolone I.V. push over <20 minutes; administer intermittent infusion over 15-60 minutes; maximum concentration: I.V. push: 125 mg/mL; I.V. infusion: 2.5 mg/mL. **Do not give acetate form I.V.**

Monitoring Parameters Blood pressure, serum glucose, and electrolytes

Test Interactions Interferes with skin tests

Patient Information Avoid alcohol; limit caffeine; do not decrease or discontinue dose without physician's approval

Additional Information Sodium content of 1 g sodium succinate injection: 2.01 mEq; methylprednisolone sodium succinate 53 mg = methylprednisolone base 40 mg

Dosage Forms

Injection, as acetate (Depo-Medrol®, Depopred®): 20 mg/mL (5 mL); 40 mg/mL (1 mL, 5 mL, 10 mL); 80 mg/mL (1 mL, 5 mL)

Powder for injection, as sodium succinate (A-methaPred®, Solu-Medrol®): 40 mg, 125 mg, 500 mg, 1000 mg, 2000 mg

Tablet (Medrol®): 2 mg, 4 mg, 8 mg, 16 mg, 24 mg, 32 mg

Tablet, dose pack: 4 mg (21s)

♦ **6-α-Methylprednisolone** *see* Methylprednisolone *on page 655*

♦ **4-Methylpyrazole** *see* Fomepizole *on page 455*

♦ **Methylrosaniline Chloride** *see* Gentian Violet *on page 472*

♦ **Meticorten®** *see* Prednisone *on page 824*

Metoclopramide (met oh kloe PRA mide)

Related Information

Carbohydrate and Alcohol Content of Liquid Medications for Use in Patients Receiving Ketogenic Diets *on page 1258*

Compatibility of Medications Mixed in a Syringe *on page 1238*

Drugs and Breast-Feeding *on page 1243*

U.S. Brand Names Reglan®

Canadian Brand Names Apo-Metoclop; Nu-Metoclopramide

Therapeutic Category Antiemetic; Gastrointestinal Agent, Prokinetic

Generic Available Yes

Use Gastroesophageal reflux; prevention of nausea and vomiting associated with chemotherapy; prevention of postoperative nausea and vomiting; facilitates intubation of the small intestine and symptomatic treatment of diabetic gastric stasis

Pregnancy Risk Factor B

Contraindications Hypersensitivity to metoclopramide or any component; GI obstruction, pheochromocytoma, history of seizure disorder or patients receiving drugs likely to cause extrapyramidal reactions

Warnings Some formulations contain sulfite

Precautions Use with caution and reduce dosage in patients with renal impairment, hypertension, or depression

Adverse Reactions Extrapyramidal reactions occur most frequently in children and young adults and following I.V. administration of high doses, usually within 24-48 hours after starting therapy

Cardiovascular: Hypertension, hypotension, SVT, bradycardia, A-V block

Central nervous system: Drowsiness, fatigue, restlessness, anxiety, agitation, depression, tardive dyskinesia, dystonia, seizures, hallucinations, neuroleptic malignant syndrome

Endocrine & metabolic: Gynecomastia, amenorrhea, galactorrhea, hyperprolactinemia

Gastrointestinal: Constipation, diarrhea

Genitourinary: Urinary frequency, impotence

Hematologic: Methemoglobinemia, neutropenia, leukopenia, agranulocytosis

Hepatic: Porphyria

Ocular: Visual disturbances

Miscellaneous: Hypersensitivity reactions

(Continued)

Metoclopramide *(Continued)*

Drug Interactions Cytochrome P-450 isoenzyme CYP1A2 and CYP2D6 substrate Decreased cimetidine and digoxin GI absorption; increased cyclosporine GI absorption; levodopa decreases metoclopramide effects; increases hypertensive episodes with MAO inhibitors; increased neuromuscular blocking effects of succinylcholine; anticholinergics and narcotic analgesics antagonize GI motility effects of metoclopramide; metoclopramide may increase tacrolimus serum levels

Stability Stable for 48 hours at room temperature when admixed with ascorbic acid, cimetidine (in NS only), cytarabine, dexamethasone sodium phosphate, diphenhydramine, doxorubicin, heparin, benztropine, dexamethasone hydrochloride, hydrocortisone sodium phosphate, lidocaine, magnesium sulfate, mannitol, potassium acetate, potassium chloride, and potassium phosphate; stable for 24 hours at room temperature when admixed with clindamycin (in NS only) and cyclophosphamide; incompatible with cephalothin, chloramphenicol, and sodium bicarbonate

Mechanism of Action Potent dopamine receptor antagonist; blocks dopamine receptors in chemoreceptor trigger zone of the CNS, preventing emesis; accelerates gastric emptying and intestinal transit time without stimulating gastric, biliary, or pancreatic secretions

Pharmacodynamics
Onset of action:
Oral: Within 30-60 minutes
I.M.: Within 10-15 minutes
I.V.: Within 1-3 minutes
Duration: Therapeutic effects persist for 1-2 hours, regardless of route administered

Pharmacokinetics
Distribution: V_d: 3.5 L/kg; crosses the placenta; appears in breast milk; breast milk to plasma ratio: 0.5-4.06
Protein binding: 30%
Bioavailability: Oral: 80 ± 15.5%
Half-life: 2.5-6 hours (half-life and clearance may be dose-dependent)
Elimination: Primarily as unchanged drug in the urine and feces

Usual Dosage
Intubation of small intestine to facilitate radiographic examination of upper GI tract:
I.V.:
Children:
<6 years: 0.1 mg/kg
6-14 years: 2.5-5 mg
Children >14 years and Adults: 10 mg
Gastroesophageal reflux: Oral, I.M., I.V.:
Neonates, Infants and Children: 0.4-0.8 mg/kg/day in 4 divided doses
Adults: 10-15 mg 4 times/day
Postoperative nausea and vomiting: I.V.:
Children: 0.1-0.2 mg/kg/dose; repeat every 6-8 hours as needed
Children >14 years and Adults: 10 mg; repeat every 6-8 hours as needed
Antiemetic **(chemotherapy-induced emesis)**: Oral, I.V.:
Children and Adults: 1-2 mg/kg/dose every 2-4 hours; pretreatment with diphenhydramine will decrease risk of extrapyramidal reactions to this dosage
Diabetic gastroparesis: Adults: Oral, I.V.: 10 mg before each meal and at bedtime for 2-8 weeks
Dosing adjustment in renal impairment: Children and Adults:
Cl_{cr} 40-50 mL/minute: Administer 75% of recommended dose
Cl_{cr} 10-40 mL/minute: Administer 50% of recommended dose
Cl_{cr} <10 mL/minute: Administer 25% to 50% of recommended dose

Administration
Oral: Administer 30 minutes before meals and at bedtime
Parenteral: Dilute to 0.2 mg/mL (maximum concentration: 5 mg/mL) and infuse over 15-30 minutes (maximum rate of infusion: 5 mg/minute); rapid I.V. administration is associated with a transient but intense feeling of anxiety and restlessness, followed by drowsiness

Monitoring Parameters Renal function

Patient Information Causes drowsiness and may impair ability to perform hazardous activities requiring mental alertness or physical coordination

Dosage Forms
Injection, as hydrochloride: 5 mg/mL (2 mL, 10 mL, 30 mL)
Solution, oral, concentrated, as hydrochloride: 10 mg/mL (30 mL)
Syrup, sugar free, as hydrochloride: 5 mg/5 mL (10 mL, 480 mL)
Tablet, as hydrochloride: 5 mg, 10 mg

Metolazone (me TOLE a zone)

U.S. Brand Names Mykrox®; Zaroxolyn®

Therapeutic Category Antihypertensive Agent; Diuretic, Miscellaneous

Generic Available No

Use Management of mild to moderate hypertension (Zaroxolyn® only); treatment of edema in CHF, nephrotic syndrome, and impaired renal function

Pregnancy Risk Factor B

Contraindications Anuria; hypersensitivity to metolazone, any component, other thiazide diuretics, or sulfonamide-derived drugs; patients with hepatic coma

Warnings Mykrox® is **not** therapeutically equivalent to Zaroxolyn® and should not be interchanged for one another

Precautions Use with caution in patients with severe renal disease, impaired hepatic function, gout, lupus erythematosus, diabetes mellitus, moderate-high cholesterol concentrations, and/or high triglycerides

Adverse Reactions

Cardiovascular: Palpitations, chest pain, orthostatic hypotension, precordial pain

Central nervous system: Vertigo, headache, chills, drowsiness

Dermatologic: Rash, dry skin, photosensitivity

Endocrine & metabolic: Hypokalemia, hyponatremia, hypochloremia, metabolic alkalosis, hyperglycemia, hyperuricemia, hypomagnesemia

Gastrointestinal: Abdominal bloating, GI irritation, bitter taste, nausea, vomiting, anorexia

Hematologic: Blood dyscrasias, aplastic anemia, hemolytic anemia, leukopenia, agranulocytosis, thrombocytopenia

Hepatic: Hepatitis

Neuromuscular & skeletal: Arthralgia, back pain, paresthesias

Ocular: Eye itching

Otic: Tinnitus

Renal: Polyuria, prerenal azotemia, uremia

Respiratory: Cough, sinus congestion, epistaxis

Drug Interactions Increased digoxin toxicity (due to potassium and magnesium depletion); increased lithium toxicity; additive potassium losses with amphotericin B and steroids; salicylates and NSAIDs decrease antihypertensive effects; allopurinol increases hypersensitivity reactions; rare occurrence of hemolytic anemia with methyldopa; cholestyramine and colestipol decrease metolazone absorption

Food Interactions Avoid natural licorice (causes sodium and water retention and increases potassium loss)

Mechanism of Action Inhibits sodium reabsorption in the cortical diluting site and proximal convoluted tubules causing increased excretion of sodium and water as well as potassium and hydrogen ions

Pharmacodynamics

Onset of action: 1 hour

Maximal effect (Mykrox®): Hypertension: 2 weeks

Duration: 12-24 hours

Pharmacokinetics

Absorption: Oral: Rate and extent vary with the preparation

Protein binding: 95%

Half-life: 6-20 hours

Elimination: Enterohepatic recycling; 70% to 95% excreted unchanged in urine

Usual Dosage Oral (dosage based on Zaroxolyn®, lower dosages may be used with Mykrox®):

Children: 0.2-0.4 mg/kg/day divided every 12-24 hours

Adults:

Edema: 5-10 mg/dose every 24 hours

Edema associated with renal disease or cardiac failure: 5-20 mg/dose every 24 hours

Hypertension:

Zaroxolyn®: 2.5-5 mg/dose every 24 hours

Mykrox®: 0.5 mg/day; increase to a maximum of 1 mg/day, if needed

Administration Oral: Administer with food to decrease GI distress

Monitoring Parameters Serum electrolytes, renal function, blood pressure

Dosage Forms Tablet:

Zaroxolyn®: 2.5 mg, 5 mg, 10 mg

Mykrox®: 0.5 mg

Extemporaneous Preparations A 1 mg/mL suspension may be made by crushing one 10 mg Zaroxolyn® tablet; add simple syrup to total volume of 10 mL. Label "shake well"; stable 3 months refrigerated

(Continued)

Metolazone (Continued)

Nahata MC, Morosco RS, and Hipple TF, "Stability of Metolazone in an Extemporaneously Prepared Suspension," *Hosp Pharm*, 1997, 32:691-3.

References

Arnold WC, "Efficacy of Metolazone and Furosemide in Children With Furosemide-Resistant Edema," *Pediatrics*, 1984, 74(5):872-5.

Wells TG, "The Pharmacology and Therapeutics of Diuretics in the Pediatric Patient," *Pediatr Clin North Am*, 1990, 37(2):463-504.

♦ Metopirone® *see* Metyrapone *on page 664*

Metoprolol (me toe PROE lole)

U.S. Brand Names Lopressor®; Toprol XL®

Canadian Brand Names Apo-Metoprolol (Type L); Betaloc; Betaloc Durules; Gen-Metoprolol (Type L); Lopresor; Nu-Metop; PMS-Metoprolol (Type B); PMS-Metoprolol (Type L)

Therapeutic Category Antianginal Agent; Antiarrhythmic Agent, Class II; Antihypertensive Agent; Antimigraine Agent; Beta-Adrenergic Blocker

Generic Available Yes: Injection, tablets (nonsustained release)

Use Management of hypertension, angina pectoris, and arrhythmias (such as multifocal atrial tachycardia); prevention of MI and migraine headaches

Pregnancy Risk Factor C (D if used in 2nd of 3rd trimester)

Contraindications Hypersensitivity to metoprolol or any component; sinus bradycardia; heart block greater then first degree (except in patients with a functioning artificial pacemaker); cardiogenic shock; uncompensated CHF

Warnings May depress myocardial activity and precipitate CHF, use with caution and monitor closely, especially in patients with compensated heart failure. In patients with coronary artery disease, exacerbation of angina and, in some cases, MI may occur following abrupt discontinuation of therapy. Beta-blockers should generally be avoided in patients with bronchospastic disease; metoprolol, with relative beta$_1$ selectivity, should be used with caution and closely monitored in patients with bronchospastic disease; beta$_2$ stimulants and the lowest possible dose of metoprolol should be used in these patients. Metoprolol may block hypoglycemia-induced tachycardia and blood pressure changes; use with caution in patients with diabetes mellitus. May mask signs of thyrotoxicosis. Use with caution with verapamil, diltiazem, or anesthetic agents that decrease myocardial function.

Precautions Use with caution in patients with hepatic dysfunction. Patients who have a history of severe anaphylactic hypersensitivity reactions to various substances may be more reactive while receiving beta-blockers; these patients may not be responsive to the normal doses of epinephrine used to treat hypersensitivity reactions

Adverse Reactions

Cardiovascular: Bradycardia, reduced peripheral circulation, palpitations, CHF, hypotension, peripheral edema, worsening of AV conduction disturbances

Central nervous system: Dizziness, tiredness, depression, mental confusion, insomnia

Dermatologic: Rash, pruritus, worsening of psoriasis

Gastrointestinal: Diarrhea, nausea, abdominal pain, dry mouth, constipation

Hematologic (potential): Agranulocytosis, thrombocytopenia

Hepatic: Hepatitis, hepatic dysfunction, jaundice; rare: elevated transaminase, alkaline phosphatase, LDH

Respiratory: Bronchospasm, wheezing, dyspnea

Drug Interactions Cytochrome P-450 isoenzyme CYP 2D6 substrate

Catecholamine-depleting drugs, such as reserpine, may have additive effects (hypotension, bradycardia); hypotensive agents, diuretics, cardiac glycosides, amiodarone, calcium channel blockers, agents that slow AV conduction, and myocardial depressant general anesthetics may have additive effects with beta-blockers; verapamil may significantly increase the oral bioavailability of metoprolol (avoid concomitant use or reduce metoprolol dose and monitor closely); cimetidine, ciprofloxacin, fluoxetine, hydralazine, oral contraceptives, propoxyphene, and quinidine may increase metoprolol serum concentrations and effects. Abrupt withdrawal of clonidine while receiving beta-blockers may result in an exaggerated hypertensive crisis; NSAIDs may decrease the antihypertensive effects of beta-blockers; barbiturates and rifampin may increase the metabolism of metoprolol and decrease metoprolol serum concentrations; metoprolol may increase lidocaine serum concentrations

Food Interactions

Metoprolol tartrate: Food may enhance the extent of oral absorption

Metoprolol succinate (extended release tablets): Food does not significantly affect bioavailability

Stability
Tablets and extended release tablets: Store at controlled room temperature 15°C to 30°C (59°F to 86°F)
Tablets: Protect from moisture and dispense in tight, light-resistant container
Injection: Do not store above 30°C (86°F); protect from light

Mechanism of Action Selective inhibitor of beta$_1$-adrenergic receptors at lower doses; competitively blocks beta$_1$ adrenergic receptors with little or no effect on beta$_2$-receptors at doses in adults <100 mg/day; inhibits beta$_2$- receptors at higher doses; does not exhibit membrane stabilizing or intrinsic sympathomimetic activity

Pharmacodynamics
Beta blockade:
Onset: Oral: Metoprolol tartrate tablets: Within 1 hour
Maximum effect: I.V.: 20 minutes
Duration: Dose dependent
Antihypertensive effect:
Onset: Oral: Metoprolol tartrate tablets: Within 15 minutes
Maximum effect: Oral (multiple dosing): After 1 week
Duration: Oral: Metoprolol tartrate tablets (single dose): 6 hours; metoprolol succinate (extended release tablets): Up to 24 hours

Pharmacokinetics
Absorption: Rapid and complete, with large first-pass effect
Distribution: Crosses the blood brain barrier; CSF concentrations are 78% of plasma concentrations
Protein binding: 12% bound to albumin
Metabolism: Significant first-pass metabolism; extensive metabolism in the liver
Bioavailability: Oral: 50%
Half-Life:
Neonates: 5-10 hours
Adults: 3-7 hours
Adults with chronic renal failure: Similar to normal adults
Elimination: 10% of an I.V. dose and <5% of an oral dose is excreted unchanged in the urine

Usual Dosage (See Additional Information)
Oral: Hypertension:
Children: No pediatric studies are available
Adolescents: Limited information is available. Sixteen hypertensive adolescents (≥13 years of age) were treated with an initial dose of 50 mg twice daily; patients were seen every 4-6 weeks and doses were increased to 100 mg twice daily if blood pressure was not controlled (see Falkner, 1982)
Adults:
Tablets (nonsustained release): Initial: 100 mg/day in single or divided doses, increase at weekly intervals to desired effect; usual dosage range: 100-450 mg/day; doses >450 mg/day have not been studied
Note: Lower once-daily dosing (especially 100 mg/day) may not control blood pressure for 24 hours; larger or more frequent dosing may be needed. Patients with bronchospastic diseases should receive the lowest possible daily dose; dose should initially be divided into 3 doses per day (to avoid high plasma concentrations).
Tablets, extended release: Initial: 50-100 mg/day as a single dose; increase at weekly intervals to desired effect; doses >400 mg/day have not been studied.

Administration Oral:
Metoprolol tartrate tablets: Administer with food or immediately after meals
Metoprolol succinate extended release tablets: May be administered without regard to meals; do not chew, crush, or break extended release tablets

Monitoring Parameters Blood pressure, heart rate, respirations, circulation in extremities

Additional Information Do not abruptly discontinue therapy, taper dosage gradually over 1-2 weeks. Beta-blockers without intrinsic sympathomimetic activity (such as metoprolol) have been shown to decrease morbidity and mortality when initiated in the acute treatment of MI and continued long term; metoprolol injection is used for early treatment of definitive or suspected MI; consult adult reference for further information. Oral to I.V. ratio of approximately 2.5 to 1 provides equivalent maximal beta-blocking activity (ie, 50 mg oral is equivalent to 20 mg I.V.).

Limited pediatric dosing information is available in the literature; in one case report, oral metoprolol (2 mg/kg/day in 3 divided doses) helped control paroxysmal supraventricular tachycardia in a 6 month old infant receiving digoxin (see Hepner, 1983). (Continued)

Metoprolol *(Continued)*

Low dose oral metoprolol (initial: 0.1 mg/kg/dose given twice daily, then increased slowly as needed to a maximum of 0.9 ± 0.7 mg/kg/day) was used to treat severe CHF that failed conventional therapy in 4 children (mean age: 7.8 years) with cardiomyopathy who were under consideration for heart transplantation (see Shaddy, 1998). Two studies (Muller, 1993; O'Marcaigh, 1994) assessed metoprolol for unexplained syncope in children at I.V. doses of 0.1 to 0.2 mg/kg for tilt table testing; in both studies, oral metoprolol was given after tilt table testing to select patients; initial oral doses of 0.8-2.8 mg/kg/day were used in 15 patients (8-20 years of age), but treatment was discontinued in 3 patients receiving 1.8-2.8 mg/kg/day due to adverse effects (Muller, 1993); oral doses of 1 to 2 mg/kg/day, rounded to the nearest 25 mg/day and divided into 2 doses daily were used in 19 patients (7-18 years of age) with unexplained syncope; the mean effective dose was 1.5 mg/kg/day (O'Marcaigh, 1994). High-dose beta-blocker therapy has been recommended to treat childhood hypertrophic cardiomyopathy (see Ostman-Smith 1999). Further pediatric studies are required before these doses can be recommended.

Dosage Forms

Injection, as tartrate (Lopressor®): 1 mg/mL (5 mL)

Tablet, as tartrate (Lopressor®): 50 mg, 100 mg

Tablet, as succinate, extended release (Toprol XL®): 25 mg, 50 mg, 100 mg, 200 mg

Extemporaneous Preparations

A 10 mg/mL metoprolol tartrate oral liquid preparation made with twelve 100 mg tablets and qsad to 120 mL with 3 different vehicles (a 1:1 mixture of Ora-Sweet® and Ora-Plus®, a 1:1 mixture of Ora-sweet® SF and Ora-Plus®, or cherry syrup) was found to be stable for 60 days when stored in amber plastic bottles in the dark at 5°C and 25°C. Microbial growth was not determined. Label "shake well" and "protect from light".

Allen LV and Erickson MA, "Stability of Labetalol Hydrochloride, Metoprolol Tartrate, Verapamil Hydrochloride, and Spironolactone With Hydrochlorothiazide in Extemporaneously Compounded Oral Liquids," *Am J Health Syst Pharm*, 1996, 53(19):2304-9.

References

Falkner B, Lowenthal DT, and Affrime MB, "The Pharmacodynamic Effectiveness of Metoprolol in Adolescent Hypertension," *Pediatr Pharmacol (New York)*, 1982, 2(1):49-55.

Hepner SI, and Davoli E, "Successful Treatment of Supraventricular Tachycardia With Metoprolol, a Cardioselective Beta Blocker," *Clin Pediatr (Phila)*, 1983, 22(7):522-3.

Morselli PL, Boutroy MJ, Bianchetti G, et al, "Pharmacokinetics of Antihypertensive Drugs in the Neonatal Period," *Dev Pharmacol Ther*, 1989, 13(2-4):190-8.

Muller G, Deal BJ, Strasburger JF, et al, "Usefulness of Metoprolol for Unexplained Syncope and Positive Response to Tilt Testing in Young Persons," *Am J Cardiol*, 1993, 71(7):592-5.

O'Marcaigh AS, MacLellan-Tobert SG, and Porter CJ, "Tilt-Table Testing and Oral Metoprolol Therapy in Young Patients With Unexplained Syncope," *Pediatrics*, 1994, 93(2):278-83.

Ostman-Smith I, Wettrell G, and Riesenfield T, "A Cohort Study of Childhood Hypertrophic Cardiomyopathy: Improved Survival Following High-Dose Beta-Adrenoceptor Antagonist Treatment," *J Am Coll Cardiol*, 1999, 34(6):1813-22.

Shaddy RE, "Beta-Blocker Therapy in Young Children With Congestive Heart Failure Under Consideration for Heart Transplantation," *Am Heart J*, 1998, 136(1):19-21.

♦ **MetroGel® Topical** *see* Metronidazole *on page 662*

♦ **MetroGel®-Vaginal** *see* Metronidazole *on page 662*

♦ **Metro I.V.® Injection** *see* Metronidazole *on page 662*

Metronidazole *(me troe NI da zole)*

Related Information

Drugs and Breast-Feeding *on page 1243*

U.S. Brand Names Flagyl® Oral; MetroGel® Topical; MetroGel®-Vaginal; Metro I.V.® Injection; Protostat® Oral

Canadian Brand Names Apo-Metronidazole; NidaGel; Noritate; Novo-Nidazol; Trikacide

Therapeutic Category Amebicide; Antibiotic, Anaerobic; Antibiotic, Topical; Antiprotozoal

Generic Available Yes

Use Treatment of susceptible anaerobic bacterial and protozoal infections in the following conditions: amebiasis (liver abscess, dysentery), giardiasis, symptomatic and asymptomatic trichomoniasis; skin and skin structure infections, CNS infections, intra-abdominal infections, and systemic anaerobic bacterial infections; topically for the treatment of acne rosacea; treatment of antibiotic-associated pseudomembranous colitis (AAPC) caused by *C. difficile*; bacterial vaginosis

Pregnancy Risk Factor B

Contraindications Hypersensitivity to metronidazole or any component; 1st trimester of pregnancy

Warnings Has been shown to be carcinogenic in rodents

Precautions Use with caution in patients with liver impairment, blood dyscrasias, CNS disease; metronidazole injection should be used with caution in patients receiving corticosteroids or patients predisposed to edema (injection contains 28 mEq of sodium/g metronidazole); reduce dosage in patients with severe liver impairment; dosage adjustment is not necessary in patients with moderate to severe renal insufficiency

Adverse Reactions

Central nervous system: Dizziness, confusion, seizures, headache, insomnia, hallucinations, paresthesias

Dermatologic: Rash

Endocrine & Metabolic: Disulfiram-type reaction with alcohol

Gastrointestinal: Metallic taste, nausea, xerostomia, diarrhea, furry tongue, vomiting

Genitourinary: Urethral burning, discoloration of urine (dark or reddish brown)

Hematologic: Leukopenia, neutropenia

Local: Thrombophlebitis

Neuromuscular & skeletal: Peripheral neuropathy

Drug Interactions Disulfiram (psychotic episodes); phenobarbital and rifampin (may increase metabolism of metronidazole); increased levels/toxicity of phenytoin, lithium, warfarin; alcohol may cause disulfiram-like reactions

Food Interactions Peak concentration is decreased and delayed when administered with food

Stability Do not refrigerate neutralized solution because precipitation may occur; reconstituted vials are chemically stable for 96 hours when stored at room temperature; protect from light

Mechanism of Action Reduced to a product which interacts with DNA to cause a loss of helical DNA structure and strand breakage resulting in inhibition of protein synthesis and cell death in susceptible organisms

Pharmacokinetics

Absorption: Oral: Well absorbed

Distribution: Excreted in breast milk; widely distributed into body tissues, fluids including bile, liver, bone, pleural fluid, vaginal secretions, CSF, erythrocytes, and hepatic abscesses

Protein binding: <20%

Metabolism: 30% to 60% in the liver to hydroxylated metabolite (60% to 80% bioactive), acetic acid metabolites, glucuronide, and sulfated conjugates

Half-life (increases with hepatic impairment):

Neonates: 25-75 hours

Children and Adults:

Metronidazole: 6-12 hours

Hydroxymetronidazole: 9.5-20 hours

Time to peak serum concentration: Within 1-2 hours

Elimination: Excreted via the urine (20% as unchanged drug) and feces (6% to 15%)

Dialysis: Extensively removed by hemodialysis and peritoneal dialysis

Usual Dosage

Neonates: Anaerobic infections: Oral, I.V.:

0-4 weeks, <1200 g: 7.5 mg/kg every 48 hours

Postnatal age ≤7 days:

1200-2000 g: 7.5 mg/kg/day given every 24 hours

>2000 g: 15 mg/kg/day in divided doses every 12 hours

Postnatal age >7 days:

1200-2000 g: 15 mg/kg/day in divided doses every 12 hours

>2000 g: 30 mg/kg/day in divided doses every 12 hours

Infants and Children:

Amebiasis: Oral: 35-50 mg/kg/day in divided doses every 8 hours

Other parasitic infections: Oral: 15-30 mg/kg/day in divided doses every 8 hours

Anaerobic infections: Oral, I.V.: 30 mg/kg/day in divided doses every 6 hours; maximum dose: 4 g/day

AAPC: Oral: 30 mg/kg/day divided every 6 hours for 7-10 days

Helicobacter pylori infection (has been used in combination with amoxicillin and bismuth subsalicylate): Oral: 15-20 mg/kg/day in 2 divided doses for 4 weeks

Adults:

Amebiasis: Oral: 500-750 mg every 8 hours

Other parasitic infections: Oral: 250 mg every 8 hours or 2 g as a single dose

Anaerobic infections: Oral, I.V.: 30 mg/kg/day in divided doses every 6 hours; not to exceed 4 g/day

AAPC: Oral: 250-500 mg 3-4 times/day for 10-14 days

Helicobacter pylori infection: Oral: 250-500 mg 3 times/day in combination with at least one other agent active against *H. pylori*

(Continued)

Metronidazole *(Continued)*

STD prophylaxis for acute sexual assault: Oral: 2 g in a single dose in combination with ceftriaxone and doxycycline

Topical: Apply a thin film twice daily to affected areas

Vaginal: One applicatorful (5 g) intravaginally 2 times/day for 5 days

Dosing adjustment in hepatic impairment: 50% to 67% decrease in dosage

Administration

Intravaginal: Use only **vaginal gel** intravaginally; do not apply to the eye

Oral: Administer on an empty stomach; may administer with food if GI upset occurs

Parenteral: Administer I.V. by slow intermittent infusion over 30-60 minutes at a final concentration for administration of 5-8 mg/mL

Topical: Wash affected areas with a mild cleanser; wait 15-20 minutes, then apply a thin film of drug to the affected area and rub in. Do not apply to the eye.

Monitoring Parameters WBC count

Test Interactions May cause falsely decreased AST and ALT levels

Patient Information May discolor urine dark or reddish brown; avoid alcohol; do not take alcohol for at least 48 hours after the last dose

Nursing Implications Avoid contact between the drug and aluminum in the infusion set

Additional Information Sodium content of 500 mg ready-to-use vial: 14 mEq

Dosage Forms

Gel, topical: 0.75% (30 g)

Gel, vaginal: 0.75% (70 g)

Injection, ready to use, in NS: 5 mg/mL (100 mL)

Powder for injection, as hydrochloride: 500 mg

Tablet: 250 mg, 500 mg

Extemporaneous Preparations To prepare metronidazole suspension 50 mg/mL, pulverize ten 250 mg tablets; levigate with a small amount of distilled water; add 10 mL Cologel® and levigate; add sufficient quantity of cherry syrup to total 50 mL and levigate until a uniform mixture is obtained; stable for 30 days if refrigerated

Committee on Extemporaneous Formulations, ASHP Special Interest Group (SIG) on Pediatric Pharmacy Practice, *Handbook on Extemporaneous Formulations*, 1987.

References

Committee on Adolescence, American Academy of Pediatrics, "Sexual Assault and the Adolescent," *Pediatrics*, 1994, 94(5):761-5.

Israel DM and Hassall E, "Treatment and Long-Term Follow-up of *Helicobacter pylori*-Associated Duodenal Ulcer Disease in Children," *J Pediatr*, 1993, 123(1):53-8.

Kelly CP, Pothoulakis C, and LaMont JT, "*Clostridium difficile* Colitis," *N Engl J Med*, 1994, 330(4):257-62.

Oldenburg B and Speck WT, "Metronidazole," *Pediatr Clin North Am*, 1983, 30(1):71-5.

Metyrapone *(me TEER a pone)*

U.S. Brand Names Metopirone®

Therapeutic Category Diagnostic Agent, Hypothalamic-Pituitary ACTH Function

Generic Available No

Use Diagnostic test for hypothalamic-pituitary ACTH function

Pregnancy Risk Factor C

Contraindications Adrenal cortical insufficiency; hypersensitivity to metyrapone or any component

Warnings All corticosteroid therapy should be discontinued prior to and during the metyrapone test

Precautions The test may be abnormal in the presence of thyroid dysfunction; demonstrate the ability of the adrenals to respond to exogenous ACTH before using metyrapone

Adverse Reactions

Cardiovascular: Hypotension, tachycardia

Central nervous system: Dizziness, headache, sedation

Dermatologic: Rash

Gastrointestinal: Abdominal discomfort, nausea

Hematologic: Bone marrow suppression

Drug Interactions Phenytoin, chlorpromazine, amitriptyline, cyproheptadine, estrogens, phenobarbital may reduce test effectiveness

Stability Protect from light

Mechanism of Action Reduces cortisol and corticosterone production by inhibition of 11-beta-hydroxylation of precursors in the adrenal cortex. Continued inhibition stimulates increased ACTH production by the pituitary; increased precursor levels have a weak suppressive activity on ACTH release. Elevated levels of precursor metabolites (17-hydroxycorticosteroids [17-OHCS] or 17-ketogenic steroids [17-

KGS]) appear in the urine which can easily serve as an index of pituitary ACTH responsiveness. Production of aldosterone may also be suppressed by metyrapone. The adrenal cortex must have the ability to respond to ACTH before metyrapone is employed to test the capacity of the pituitary to respond to a decreased concentration of plasma cortisol.

Pharmacodynamics Peak effect: Peak excretion of steroid during the first 24 hours after administration

Pharmacokinetics
Absorption: Oral: Well absorbed
Half-life, elimination: 1-2.5 hours (average)
Elimination: 5.3% of dose excreted in urine unchanged

Usual Dosage Oral:
Children: 15 mg/kg/dose or 300 mg/m²/dose every 4 hours for 6 doses; minimum: 250 mg/dose **or as an alternative** 30 mg/kg as a single dose (maximum: 3 g) given at midnight the night before the test
Adults: 750 mg every 4 hours for 6 doses **or as an alternative** 3 g as a single dose given at midnight the night before the test

Administration Oral: May administer with food or milk to reduce GI irritation

Reference Range Normal response to metyrapone produces a 2-4 times increase in 17-OHCS or 2 times increase in 17-KGS

Patient Information Arise slowly from prolonged sitting or lying position

Dosage Forms Capsule: 250 mg

Mexiletine (MEKS i le teen)

U.S. Brand Names Mexitil®
Canadian Brand Names Novo-Mexiletine
Therapeutic Category Antiarrhythmic Agent, Class I-B
Generic Available Yes
Use Management of serious ventricular arrhythmias; suppression of premature ventricular contractions; diabetic neuropathy
Pregnancy Risk Factor C
Contraindications Cardiogenic shock, second or third degree heart block; hypersensitivity to mexiletine or any component
Warnings Exercise extreme caution in patients with pre-existing sinus node dysfunction; mexiletine can worsen bradycardias and other arrhythmias
Precautions Use with caution in patients with seizure disorders, severe CHF, hypotension

Adverse Reactions
Cardiovascular: Palpitations, bradycardia, chest pain, syncope, hypotension, atrial or ventricular arrhythmias
Central nervous system: Dizziness, confusion, ataxia
Dermatologic: Rash
Gastrointestinal: Nausea, vomiting, diarrhea
Hematologic: Rarely thrombocytopenia
Hepatic: Hepatitis
Neuromuscular & skeletal: Paresthesia, tremor
Ocular: Diplopia
Otic: Tinnitus
Respiratory: Dyspnea
Miscellaneous: Positive antinuclear antibody

Drug Interactions Cytochrome P-450 isoenzyme CYP2D6 substrate; CYP1A2 isoenzyme inhibitor
Phenobarbital, phenytoin, rifampin, and other hepatic enzyme inducers may lower mexiletine plasma levels; cimetidine may increase mexiletine levels; antacids, narcotics, or anticholinergics may decrease rate of absorption; metoclopramide may increase rate of absorption; drugs which affect urine pH can increase or decrease excretion of mexiletine; mexiletine may increase the serum concentrations of theophylline and caffeine

Food Interactions Food may decrease the rate, but not the extent of oral absorption; diets which affect urine pH can increase or decrease excretion of mexiletine; avoid dietary changes that alter urine pH

Mechanism of Action Class IB antiarrhythmic; structurally related to lidocaine; may cause increase in systemic vascular resistance and decrease in cardiac output; no significant negative inotropic effect

Pharmacodynamics Onset after oral dose: 30-120 minutes

Pharmacokinetics
Distribution: V_d: 5-7 L/kg; found in breast milk in similar concentrations as plasma
Protein-binding: 50% to 70%
(Continued)

Mexiletine *(Continued)*

Metabolism: Extensive in the liver (some minor active metabolites)

Bioavailability: Oral: 88%

Half-life, adults: 10-14 hours; increase in half-life with hepatic or heart failure

Elimination: 10% to 15% excreted unchanged in urine; urinary acidification increases excretion

Usual Dosage Oral:

Children: Range: 1.4-5 mg/kg/dose (mean: 3.3 mg/kg/dose) given every 8 hours; start with lower initial dose and increase according to effects and serum concentrations

Adults: Initial: 200 mg every 8 hours (may load with 400 mg if necessary); adjust dose every 2-3 days; usual dose: 200-300 mg every 8 hours; some patients may respond to the same daily dose divided every 12 hours; maximum dose: 1.2 g/day

Dosing adjustment in renal impairment: Children and Adults: Cl_{cr} <10 mL/minute: Administer 50% to 75% of normal dose

Dosing adjustment in hepatic disease: Children and Adults: Administer 25% to 30% of normal dose; patients with severe liver disease may require even lower doses, monitor closely

Administration Oral: Administer with food or milk to decrease GI upset

Monitoring Parameters Liver enzymes, EKG, heart rate, serum concentrations

Reference Range

Therapeutic range: 0.5-2 µg/mL

Potentially toxic: >2 µg/mL

Patient Information Limit caffeine; may cause dizziness; notify physician if persistent abdominal pain, nausea, vomiting, yellowing of the eyes or skin, pale stools, dark urine, fever, sore throat, bleeding, or bruising occurs

Additional Information I.V. form under investigation

Dosage Forms Capsule, as hydrochloride: 150 mg, 200 mg, 250 mg

Extemporaneous Preparations A 10 mg/mL oral suspension can be made using capsules and distilled water or sorbitol USP; grind the contents of eight 150 mg capsules to a powder in a mortar and pestle; then add a small amount of distilled water or sorbitol; mix to make a uniform paste; add distilled water or sorbitol in geometric amounts (while mixing) to **almost** 120 mL; transfer to a graduated cylinder and qsad 120 mL while mixing; suspension made with sorbitol is stable in plastic prescription bottles for 2 weeks at room temperature (25°C) and 4 weeks if refrigerated (4°C); suspension made with distilled water is stable in plastic prescription bottles for 7 weeks at room temperature (25°C) and 13 weeks if refrigerated (4°C); extended storage at 4°C is recommended to minimize microbial contamination; shake well before use

Nahata MC, Morosco RS, and Hipple TF, "Stability of Mexiletine in Two Extemporaneous Liquid Formulations Stored Under Refrigeration and at Room Temperature," *J Am Pharm Assoc*, 2000, 40(2):257-9.

References

Moak JP, Smith RT, and Garson A Jr, "Mexiletine: An Effective Antiarrhythmic Drug for Treatment of Ventricular Arrhythmias in Congenital Heart Disease," *J Am Coll Cardiol*, 1987, 10(4):824-9.

♦ **Mexitil**® *see Mexiletine on page 665*

♦ **Mezlin**® *see Mezlocillin on page 666*

Mezlocillin *(mez loe SIL in)*

U.S. Brand Names Mezlin®

Therapeutic Category Antibiotic, Penicillin (Antipseudomonal)

Generic Available No

Use Treatment of infections caused by susceptible gram-negative aerobic bacilli (*Klebsiella, Proteus, Escherichia coli, Enterobacter, Pseudomonas aeruginosa, Serratia*) involving the skin and skin structure, bone and joint, respiratory tract, urinary tract, gastrointestinal tract, as well as septicemia

Pregnancy Risk Factor B

Contraindications Hypersensitivity to mezlocillin, any component, or penicillins

Warnings If bleeding occurs during therapy, mezlocillin should be discontinued

Precautions Use with caution in patients with renal impairment or biliary obstruction; dosage modification required in patients with impaired renal function

Adverse Reactions

Central nervous system: Seizures, dizziness, fever, headache

Dermatologic: Rash, exfoliative dermatitis

Endocrine & metabolic: Hypokalemia, hypernatremia

Gastrointestinal: Diarrhea

Hematologic: Eosinophilia, hemolytic anemia, neutropenia, leukopenia, thrombocytopenia, prolonged bleeding time

Hepatic: Elevated liver enzymes

Local: Thrombophlebitis

Renal: Interstitial nephritis, elevated BUN, elevated serum creatinine

Miscellaneous: Serum sickness-like reaction

Drug Interactions Aminoglycosides, probenecid (increases serum concentration of mezlocillin), vecuronium (prolongs neuromuscular blockade)

Stability Reconstituted solution is stable for 48 hours at room temperature and 7 days when refrigerated; incompatible with aminoglycosides

Mechanism of Action Inhibits bacterial cell wall synthesis by binding to one or more of the penicillin-binding proteins; inhibits the final transpeptidation step of peptidoglycan synthesis in bacterial cell walls

Pharmacokinetics

Absorption: I.M.: 63%

Distribution: Into bile, heart, peritoneal fluid, sputum, bone; does not cross the blood-brain barrier well unless meninges are inflamed; crosses the placenta; distributes into breast milk at low concentrations

Protein binding: 30%

Metabolism: 5% to 10%

Half-life:

Neonates:

≤7 days: 3.7-4.4 hours

>7 days: 2.5 hours

Infants and Children: 0.5-1 hour

Children 2-19 years: 0.9 hours

Adults: 0.5-0.75 hours (dose dependent); half-life prolonged in renal impairment

Time to peak serum concentration:

I.M.: Within 45-90 minutes

I.V. infusion: Within 5 minutes

Elimination: Principally as unchanged drug in urine, also excreted via bile

Dialysis: Moderately dialyzable (20% to 50%)

Usual Dosage I.M., I.V.:

Neonates:

0-4 weeks, <1200 g: 150 mg/kg/day divided every 12 hours

Postnatal age ≤7 days, ≥1200 g: 150 mg/kg/day divided every 12 hours

Postnatal age >7 days, ≥1200 g: 225 mg/kg/day divided every 8 hours

Children: 200-300 mg/kg/day divided every 4-6 hours; doses as high as 300-450 mg/kg/day divided every 4-6 hours have been used in acute pulmonary exacerbations of cystic fibrosis; maximum dose: 24 g/day

Adults:

Uncomplicated urinary tract infection: 1.5-2 g every 6 hours; serious infections: 3-4 g every 4-6 hours

Dosing interval in renal impairment:

Cl_{cr} 10-30 mL/minute: Administer every 6-8 hours

Cl_{cr} <10 mL/minute: Administer every 8-12 hours

Administration Parenteral:

I.M.: Administer deep I.M. into a large muscle mass (ie, gluteus maximus) over 12-15 seconds

I.V.: Administer IVP over 3-5 minutes at a final concentration for administration not to exceed 100 mg/mL or administer by I.V. intermittent infusion over 15-30 minutes at a concentration of 10-20 mg/mL; maximum concentration for administration in a fluid-restricted patient: 178 mg/mL

Monitoring Parameters Serum electrolytes; periodic renal, hepatic, and hematologic function tests

Test Interactions Positive Coombs' [direct]; false-positive urinary and serum protein

Nursing Implications If the patient is on concurrent aminoglycoside therapy, administration of both agents should be separated by at least 30-60 minutes

Additional Information Sodium content of 1 g: 1.8 mEq

Dosage Forms Powder for injection, as sodium: 1 g, 2 g, 3 g, 4 g, 20 g

References

Odio C, Threlkeld N, Thomas ML, et al, "Pharmacokinetic Properties of Mezlocillin in Newborn Infants," *Antimicrob Agents Chemother*, 1984, 25(5):556-9.

Prober CG, Stevenson DK, and Benitz WE, "The Use of Antibiotics in Neonates Weighing Less Than 1200 Grams," *Pediatr Infect Dis J*, 1990, 9(2):111-21.

♦ **MG217 Medicated Tar-Free [OTC]** *see* Sulfur and Salicylic Acid *on page 929*

♦ **MG217Sal-Acid® [OTC]** *see* Salicylic Acid *on page 886*

♦ **Miacalcin®** *see* Calcitonin *on page 164*

♦ **Micatin® Topical [OTC]** see Miconazole on page 668

Miconazole (mi KON a zole)

U.S. Brand Names Breezee® Mist Antifungal [OTC]; Fungoid® Creme; Fungoid® Tincture; Micatin® Topical [OTC]; Monistat-Derm™ Topical; Monistat™ Vaginal

Canadian Brand Names Micozole; Monazole-7

Therapeutic Category Antifungal Agent, Topical; Antifungal Agent, Vaginal

Generic Available Yes

Use Topical: Treatment of vulvovaginal candidiasis; topical treatment of superficial fungal infections

Pregnancy Risk Factor C

Contraindications Hypersensitivity to miconazole or any component; vaginal preparation should not be used in the first trimester of pregnancy unless the drug is essential to patient's welfare

Warnings The safety of miconazole in infants <1 year of age has not been established

Precautions Use with caution in patients allergic to other imidazole-derivative antifungals (eg, clotrimazole, econazole, ketoconazole)

Adverse Reactions
Central nervous system: Headache
Dermatologic: Maceration, urticaria, rash, pruritus
Genitourinary: Pelvic cramps
Local: Irritation, burning, itching, phlebitis

Drug Interactions Cytochrome P-450 isoenzyme CYP3A3/4 substrate; isoenzyme CYP2C, CYP3A3/4 (moderate), and CYP3A5-7 inhibitor
Enhanced hypoprothrombinemia with warfarin; oral sulfonylureas (severe hypoglycemia); may be antagonistic with amphotericin B; inhibits cisapride metabolism

Stability Store at room temperature

Mechanism of Action Inhibits biosynthesis of ergosterol, damaging the fungal cell wall membrane which increases permeability and causes leaking of nutrients

Pharmacokinetics
Absorption: Vaginal: Small amount absorbed systemically
Distribution: Into body tissues, joints, and fluids; poor penetration into sputum, saliva, urine, and CSF
Protein binding: 91% to 93%
Metabolism: In the liver
Half-life: Multiphasic degradation:
Alpha: 40 minutes
Beta: 126 minutes
Terminal: 24 hours
Elimination: ~50% excreted in feces and <1% in urine as unchanged drug

Usual Dosage
Infants and Children:
Topical: Apply twice daily
Adolescents and Adults:
Vaginal: Insert contents of 1 applicator of vaginal cream or 100 mg vaginal suppository at bedtime for 7 days, or 200 mg vaginal suppository at bedtime for 3 days
Topical: Apply twice daily

Administration
Topical: Apply sparingly to the cleansed, dry affected area; if intertriginous areas are involved, rub cream gently into the skin
Vaginal: Wash hands before using; gently insert tablet or full applicator of cream into vagina at bedtime. Wash applicator with soap and water following use. Remain lying down for 30 minutes following administration.

Monitoring Parameters Hematocrit, hemoglobin, serum electrolytes and lipids

Patient Information Avoid contact with the eyes; do not use vaginal cream or suppositories for self-medication if patient has abdominal pain, fever, or malodorous vaginal discharge; inform physician if vaginal pruritus or discomfort occurs; avoid intercourse during therapy if using vaginal product

Dosage Forms
Cream:
Topical, as nitrate: 2% (15 g, 30 g, 56.7 g, 85 g)
Vaginal, as nitrate: 2% (45 g is equivalent to 7 doses)
Powder, topical, as nitrate: 2% (45 g, 90 g, 113 g)
Solution, topical, as nitrate: 2% with alcohol (7.39 mL, 29.57 mL)
Spray, topical, as nitrate: 2% (105 mL)
Suppository, vaginal, as nitrate: 100 mg (7s); 200 mg (3s)

- **Micozole (Can)** *see* Miconazole *on page 668*
- **MICRhoGAM™** *see* Rh$_o$(D) Immune Globulin (Intramuscular) *on page 869*
- **Micro-K®** *see* Potassium Supplements *on page 816*
- **Micronase®** *see* Glyburide *on page 476*
- **Micronor®** *see* Norethindrone *on page 723*
- **Microzide™** *see* Hydrochlorothiazide *on page 503*
- **Midamor®** *see* Amiloride *on page 67*

Midazolam (MID aye zoe lam)

Related Information

Adult ACLS Algorithm, Synchronized Cardioversion *on page 1048*
Compatibility of Medications Mixed in a Syringe *on page 1238*
Drugs and Breast-Feeding *on page 1243*
Overdose and Toxicology *on page 1222*
Preprocedure Sedatives in Children *on page 1201*

U.S. Brand Names Versed®

Therapeutic Category Anticonvulsant, Benzodiazepine; Benzodiazepine; Hypnotic; Sedative

Generic Available Yes: Injection

Use Sedation, anxiolysis, amnesia prior to procedure or before induction of anesthesia; conscious sedation prior to diagnostic or radiographic procedures; continuous I.V. sedation of intubated and mechanically ventilated patients; status epilepticus

Restrictions C-IV

Pregnancy Risk Factor D

Contraindications Hypersensitivity to midazolam, any component, or cherries (syrup); cross-sensitivity with other benzodiazepines may occur; uncontrolled pain; existing CNS depression; shock; narrow-angle glaucoma

Warnings Midazolam may cause respiratory depression/arrest; deaths and hypoxic encephalopathy have resulted when these were not promptly recognized and treated appropriately; dose must be individualized and patients must be appropriately monitored; serious respiratory adverse events occur most often when midazolam is used in combination with other CNS depressants; personnel and equipment needed for standard respiratory resuscitation should be immediately available during midazolam use; a dedicated individual (other than the one performing the procedure) should monitor the deeply sedated pediatric patient throughout the procedure

Precautions Use with caution in patients with CHF, renal impairment, pulmonary disease, hepatic dysfunction; injection may contain benzyl alcohol and syrup contains sodium benzoate; use with caution in neonates especially premature neonates; several cases of myoclonus have been reported in premature infants; benzodiazepine withdrawal may occur if abruptly discontinued in patients receiving prolonged I.V. continuous infusions; doses should be tapered slowly with prolonged use; do not administer by rapid I.V. injection (especially in neonates where severe hypotension and seizures have occurred after rapid I.V. administration)

Adverse Reactions

Cardiovascular: Cardiac arrest, hypotension, bradycardia

Central nervous system: Drowsiness, sedation, amnesia, dizziness, paradoxical excitement, hyperactivity, combativeness, headache, ataxia, rhythmic myoclonic jerking in preterm infants (~8% incidence), nystagmus

Gastrointestinal: Nausea, vomiting

Local:

I.M., I.V.: Pain and local reactions at injection site (severity less than diazepam)
Nasal: Burning, irritation, discomfort

Neuromuscular & skeletal: Tonic/clonic movements, muscle tremor

Ocular: Blurred vision, diplopia, lacrimation

Respiratory: Respiratory depression, oxygen desaturation, apnea, laryngospasm, bronchospasm, cough

Miscellaneous: Physical and psychological dependence with prolonged use, hiccups

Drug Interactions Cytochrome P-450 isoenzyme CYP3A3/4 substrate

CNS depressants, alcohol may increase sedation and respiratory depression; narcotic agents may increase hypotension (especially in neonates); doses of anesthetic agents should be reduced when used in conjunction with midazolam; cimetidine, ranitidine, erythromycin, diltiazem, verapamil, fluconazole, ketoconazole, itraconazole may increase midazolam serum concentrations; theophylline may antagonize the sedative effects of midazolam; rifampin reduces the plasma concentration of oral midazolam by >90%; carbamazepine and phenytoin may

(Continued)

Midazolam *(Continued)*

increase hepatic metabolism of midazolam; protease inhibitors (indinavir, nelfinavir, ritonavir, saquinavir) and delavirdine may potentially decrease midazolam's metabolism and increase midazolam serum concentrations; concurrent use of midazolam with protease inhibitors or delavirdine is not recommended

Food Interactions Grapefruit juice delays the absorption and significantly increases bioavailability of oral midazolam

Stability Stable at a concentration of 0.5 mg/mL for 24 hours in D_5W or NS and for 4 hours in LR

Mechanism of Action Depresses all levels of the CNS, including the limbic and reticular formation, by binding to the benzodiazepine site on the gamma-aminobutyric acid (GABA) receptor complex and modulating GABA, which is a major inhibitory neurotransmitter in the brain

Pharmacodynamics Sedation:

Onset:
Oral: Children: Within 10-20 minutes
I.M.:
Children: Within 5 minutes
Adults: Within 15 minutes
I.V.: Within 1-5 minutes
Intranasal: Within 5 minutes

Peak:
I.M.:
Children: 15-30 minutes
Adults: 30-60 minutes
I.V.: 5-7 minutes
Intranasal: 10 minutes

Duration:
I.M.: Mean: 2 hours, up to 6 hours
I.V.: 20-30 minutes
Intranasal: 30-60 minutes
Note: Full recovery may take more than 24 hours

Pharmacokinetics

Absorption: Oral, nasal: Rapid

Distribution: V_d:
Infants and Children 6 months to 16 years: 1.24-2.02 L/kg
Adults: 1-3.1 L/kg
Increased V_d with CHF and chronic renal failure; widely distributed in body including CSF and brain; crosses placenta; enters fetal circulation; crosses into breast milk

Protein binding: Children >1 year and Adults: 97%; primarily to albumin

Metabolism: Extensive in the liver via cytochrome P-450 CYP3A4 enzyme; undergoes hydroxylation and then glucuronide conjugation; primary metabolite (alpha-hydroxy-midazolam) is active and equipotent to midazolam

Bioavailability: Oral: 15% to 45% (syrup: 36%); I.M.: >90%; intranasal: ~60%; rectal: ~40% to 50%

Half-life, elimination: Increased half-life with cirrhosis, CHF, obesity, elderly, and acute renal failure
Neonates: 4-12 hours; seriously ill neonates: 6.5-12 hours
Children: I.V.: 2.9-4.5 hours; syrup: 2.2-6.8 hours
Adults: 3 hours (range: 1.8-6.4 hours)

Elimination: 63% to 80% excreted as alpha-hydroxy-midazolam glucuronide in urine; ~2% to 10% in feces, <1% eliminated as unchanged drug in the urine
Mean clearance:
Neonates <39 weeks gestational age (GA): 1.17 mL/minute/kg
Neonates >39 weeks GA: 1.84 mL/minute/kg
Seriously ill neonates: 1.2-2 mL/minute/kg
Infants >3 months: 9.1 mL/minute/kg
Children >1 year: 3.2-13.3 mL/minute/kg
Healthy adults: 4.2-9 mL/minute/kg
Adults with acute renal failure: 1.9 mL/minute/kg

Usual Dosage Dosage must be individualized and based on patient's age, underlying diseases, concurrent medications, and desired effect; decrease dose (by ~30%) if narcotics or other CNS depressants are administered concomitantly; use multiple small doses and titrate to desired sedative effect; allow 3-5 minutes between doses to decrease the chance of oversedation

Neonates:

Conscious sedation during mechanical ventilation: I.V. continuous infusion:

<32 weeks: Initial: 0.03 mg/kg/hour (0.5 mcg/kg/minute)

>32 weeks: Initial: 0.06 mg/kg/hour (1 mcg/kg/minute)

Note: Do not use I.V. loading doses in neonates; for faster achievement of sedation, infuse the continuous infusion at a faster rate for the first several hours; use the smallest dose possible

Infants >2 months and Children:

Status epilepticus refractory to standard therapy: I.V.: Loading dose: 0.15 mg/kg followed by a continuous infusion of 1 mcg/kg/minute; titrate dose upward every 5 minutes until clinical seizure activity is controlled; mean infusion rate required in 24 children was 2.3 mcg/kg/minute with a range of 1-18 mcg/kg/minute (Rivera, 1993)

Infants ≥6 months and Children:

Sedation, anxiolysis, and amnesia prior to procedure or before induction of anesthesia: Oral: Single dose: 0.25-0.5 mg/kg, depending on patient status and desired effect, usual: 0.5 mg/kg; maximum dose: 20 mg;

Patient-specific dosing:

Infants 6 months to <6 years, and less cooperative patients: Higher doses (up to 1 mg/kg) may be required

Children 6 to ≥16 years, or cooperative patients (especially if intensity and duration of sedation is less critical): 0.25 mg/kg may suffice

High risk pediatric patients (respiratory or cardiac compromised, concomitant CNS depressants, higher risk surgical patients): 0.25 mg/kg should be considered

Children:

Preoperative sedation or conscious sedation for procedures:

I.M.: Usual: 0.1-0.15 mg/kg 30-60 minutes before surgery or procedure; range: 0.05-0.15 mg/kg; doses up to 0.5 mg/kg have been used in more anxious patients; maximum total dose: 10 mg

I.V.:

Infants <6 months: Limited information is available in nonintubated infants; dosing recommendations are unclear; infants <6 months are at higher risk for airway obstruction and hypoventilation; titrate dose with small increments to desired clinical effect; monitor carefully

Infants 6 months to Children 5 years: Initial: 0.05-0.1 mg/kg; titrate dose carefully; total dose of 0.6 mg/kg may be required; usual total dose maximum dose: 6 mg

Children 6-12 years: Initial: 0.025-0.05 mg/kg; titrate dose carefully; total doses of 0.4 mg/kg may be required; usual total dose maximum: 10 mg

Children 12-16 years: Dose as adults; usual total dose maximum: 10 mg

Intranasal: Usual: 0.2 mg/kg; may repeat in 5-15 minutes; range: 0.2-0.3 mg/kg/dose

Conscious sedation during mechanical ventilation: I.V.: Continuous infusion: Loading dose: 0.05-0.2 mg/kg given slow I.V. over 2-3 minutes, then follow with initial continuous infusion: 0.06-0.12 mg/kg/hour (1-2 mcg/kg/minute); titrate to the desired effect; range: 0.4-6 mcg/kg/minute

Adults:

Preoperative sedation: I.M.: 0.07-0.08 mg/kg 30-60 minutes presurgery; usual dose: 5 mg

Conscious sedation: I.V.: Titrate dose slowly to desired effect; administer slowly over at least 2 minutes and wait another 2 or more minutes to evaluate effect. Some adults may respond to doses as low as 1 mg; do not give more than 2.5 mg over a period of 2 minutes. Titrate as needed, using small increments every 2-3 minutes. Usual total dose: 2.5-5 mg; total dose >5 mg is generally not needed; maintenance doses may be given by slow titration, if needed, in increments of 25% of the original dose used to reach sedative endpoint.

Conscious sedation during mechanical ventilation: I.V.: Optional loading dose: 0.01-0.05 mg/kg (~0.5-4 mg/dose); may repeat at 10- to 15-minute intervals until patient is adequately sedated, then begin continuous infusion

Continuous infusion: Initial: 0.02-0.1 mg/kg/hour (1-7 mg/hour); use lowest doses listed for patients receiving other sedatives, or opioids, or having residual anesthetic effects; titrate the infusion to achieve adequate level of sedation; use lowest effective dose

Administration

Intranasal: Administer using a 1 mL needleless syringe into the nares over 15 seconds; use the 5 mg/mL injection; 1/2 of the dose may be administered to each nare; **Note:** The 5 mg/mL injection has also been administered as a nasal spray using a graded pump device (see Ljungman, 2000)

(Continued)

Midazolam *(Continued)*

Oral: Administer on empty stomach (feeding is usually contraindicated prior to sedation for procedures)

Parenteral: I.V.: Administer by slow I.V. injection over at least 2-5 minutes at a concentration of 1-5 mg/mL or by I.V. infusion; avoid extravasation; do not administer intra-arterially

Monitoring Parameters Level of sedation, respiratory rate, heart rate, blood pressure, oxygen saturation (ie, pulse oximetry)

Nursing Implications Abrupt discontinuation after prolonged use may result in withdrawal symptoms

Additional Information Sodium content of injection: 0.14 mEq/mL; for Neonates: Since both concentrations of Versed® injection contain 1% benzyl alcohol, use the 5 mg/mL injection and dilute to 0.5 mg/mL with SWI without preservatives to decrease the amount of benzyl alcohol delivered to the neonate, or use preservative free injection; with continuous infusion, midazolam may accumulate in peripheral tissues; use lowest effective infusion rate to reduce accumulation effects; midazolam is 3-4 times as potent as diazepam; paradoxical reactions associated with midazolam use in children (eg, agitation, restlessness, combativeness) have been successfully treated with flumazenil (see Massanari, 1997)

Dosage Forms

Injection, as hydrochloride (Versed®): 1 mg/mL (2 mL, 5 mL, 10 mL); 5 mg/mL (1 mL, 2 mL, 5 mL, 10 mL)

Injection, preservative free, as hydrochloride: 1 mg/mL (2 mL, 5 mL, 10 mL); 5 mg/mL (1 mL, 2 mL, 5 mL, 10 mL)

Syrup, as hydrochloride (Versed®): 2 mg/mL [cherry flavor] (118 mL)

References

Adrian ER, "Intranasal Versed®: The Future of Pediatric Conscious Sedation," *Pediatr Nurs*, 1994, 20(3):287-92.

Booker PD, Beechey A, and Lloyd-Thomas AR, "Sedation of Children Requiring Artificial Ventilation Using an Infusion of Midazolam," *Br J Anaesth*, 1986, 58(10):1104-8.

Burtin P, Jacqz-Aigrain E, Girard P, et al, "Population Pharmacokinetics of Midazolam in Neonates," *Clin Pharmacol Ther*, 1994, 56(6 Pt 1):615-25.

Jacqz-Aigrain E, Daoud P, Burtin P, et al, "Placebo-Controlled Trial of Midazolam Sedation in Mechanically Ventilated Newborn Babies," *Lancet*, 1994, 344(8923):646-50.

Kupietzky A and Houpt MI, "Midazolam: A Review of Its Use for Conscious Sedation of Children," *Pediatr Dent*, 1993, 15(4):237-41.

Ljungman G, Kreuger A, Andreasson S, et al, "Midazolam Nasal Spray Reduces Procedural Anxiety in Children," *Pediatrics*, 2000, 105(1 Pt 1):73-8.

Lugo RA, Fishbein M, Nahata MC, et al, "Complication of Intranasal Midazolam," *Pediatrics*, 1993, 92(4):638.

Magny JF, Zupan V, Dehan M, et al, "Midazolam and Myoclonus in Neonate," *Eur J Pediatr*, 1994, 153(5):389-90.

Malinovsky JM, Populaire C, Cozian A, et al, "Premedication With Midazolam in Children, Effect of Intranasal, Rectal and Oral Routes on Plasma Midazolam Concentrations," *Anaesthesia*, 1995, 50(4):351-4.

Massanari M, Novitsky J, and Reinstein LJ, "Paradoxical Reactions in Children Associated With Midazolam Use During Endoscopy," *Clin Pediatr*, 1997, 36(12):681-4.

Riva J, Lejbusiewicz G, Papa M, et al, "Oral Premedication With Midazolam in Paediatric Anaesthesia. Effects on Sedation and Gastric Contents," *Paediatr Anaesth*, 1997, 7(3):191-6.

Rivera R, Segnini M, Baltodano A, et al, "Midazolam in the Treatment of Status Epilepticus in Children," *Crit Care Med*, 1993, 21(7):991-4.

Silvasi DL, Rosen DA, and Rosen KR, "Continuous Intravenous Midazolam Infusion for Sedation in the Pediatric Intensive Care Unit," *Anesth Analg*, 1988, 67(3):286-8.

◆ **Midol® Maximum Strength Cramp Formula [OTC]** *see* Ibuprofen *on page 520*

◆ **Migranal® Nasal Spray** *see* Dihydroergotamine *on page 334*

◆ **Miles Nervine® [OTC]** *see* Diphenhydramine *on page 342*

◆ **Milkinol® [OTC]** *see* Mineral Oil *on page 675*

◆ **Milk of Magnesia (Magnesium Hydroxide)** *see* Magnesium Supplements *on page 614*

Milrinone *(MIL ri none)*

U.S. Brand Names Primacor®

Therapeutic Category Phosphodiesterase Enzyme Inhibitor

Generic Available No

Use Short-term treatment of acute decompensated heart failure

Pregnancy Risk Factor C

Contraindications Hypersensitivity to milrinone, any component, or inamrinone (amrinone)

Warnings Longer treatment of heart failure (>48 hours) has not been shown to be safe and effective (there are no controlled trials using milrinone infusions for >48 hours); long-term oral use for heart failure was associated with no improvement in symptoms, increased risk of hospitalization, and increased risk of sudden death; monitor EKG continuously to promptly detect and manage ventricular arrhythmias

Precautions Avoid use in patients with severe obstructive aortic or pulmonic valvular disease; use in patients with hypertrophic subaortic stenosis may increase outflow tract obstruction; use with caution in patients with a history of ventricular arrhythmias, atrial fibrillation, or atrial flutter; use with caution and modify dosage in patients with impaired renal function

Adverse Reactions

Central nervous system: Headaches (mild to moderate, 2.9%)

Cardiovascular: Ventricular arrhythmias (12.1%) including ventricular ectopic activity (8.5%), nonsustained ventricular tachycardia (2.8%), sustained ventricular tachycardia (1%), and ventricular fibrillation (0.2%); supraventricular arrhythmias (3.8%); hypotension (2.9%); angina/chest pain (1.2%)

Endocrine & metabolic: Hypokalemia (0.6%)

Hematologic: Thrombocytopenia (0.4%)

Hepatic: Abnormal liver function tests

Neuromuscular & skeletal: Tremor (0.4%)

Respiratory: Bronchospasm (rare)

Stability Incompatible with furosemide (a precipitate forms when furosemide is injected into I.V. lines containing milrinone); compatible with $\frac{1}{2}$NS, NS, and D_5W

Mechanism of Action Inhibits phosphodiesterase III (PDE III), the major PDE in cardiac and vascular tissues. Inhibition of PDE III increases cyclic adenosine monophosphate (cAMP) which potentiates the delivery of calcium to myocardial contractile systems and results in a positive inotropic effect. Inhibition of PDE III in vascular tissue results in relaxation of vascular muscle and vasodilatation.

Pharmacodynamics Onset (improved hemodynamic function): Within 5-15 minutes

Pharmacokinetics

Distribution: V_d beta

Infants (after cardiac surgery): 0.9 ± 0.4 L/kg

Children (after cardiac surgery): 0.7 ± 0.2 L/kg

Adults:

After cardiac surgery: 0.3 ± 0.1 L/kg

CHF (with single injection): 0.38 L/kg

CHF (with infusion): 0.45 L/kg

Protein binding: 70%

Half-life:

Infants (after cardiac surgery): 3.15 ± 2 hours

Children (after cardiac surgery): 1.86 ± 2 hours

Adults:

After cardiac surgery: 1.69 ± 0.18 hours

CHF: 2.3-2.4 hours

Renal impairment: Prolonged half-life

Elimination: Excreted in the urine as unchanged drug (83%) and glucuronide metabolite (12%)

Clearance:

Infants (after cardiac surgery): 3.8 ± 1 mL/kg/minute

Children (after cardiac surgery): 5.9 ± 2 mL/kg/minute

Children (with septic shock): 10.6 ± 5.3 mL/kg/minute

Adults:

After cardiac surgery: 2 ± 0.7 mL/kg/minute

CHF: 2.2-2.3 mL/kg/minute

Renal impairment: Decreased clearance

Usual Dosage

Neonates, Infants, and Children: I.V.: A limited number of studies have used different dosing schemes (see Additional Information). Two recent pharmacokinetic studies propose per kg doses for pediatric patients with septic shock that are greater than those recommended for adults (Lindsay, 1998) and in infants and children after cardiac surgery (Ramamoorthy, 1998). Further pharmacodynamic studies are needed to define pediatric milrinone guidelines. Several centers are using the following guidelines:

Loading dose: 50 mcg/kg administered over 15 minutes followed by a continuous infusion of 0.5 mcg/kg/minute; range: 0.25-0.75 mcg/kg/minute; titrate dose to effect

PALS Guidelines 2000: I.V., I.O.: Loading dose: 50-75 mcg/kg administered over 15 minutes followed by a continuous infusion of 0.5-0.75 mcg/kg/minute

Adults: I.V.: Loading dose: 50 mcg/kg slow I.V. over 10 minutes, followed by a continuous infusion of 0.5 mcg/kg/minute; range: 0.375-0.75 mcg/kg/minute; titrate does to effect; maximum daily dose: 1.13 mg/kg/day

(Continued)

Milrinone *(Continued)*

Dosing adjustment in renal impairment: For continuous infusion:
Cl_{cr} 50 mL/minute/1.73 m^2: Administer 0.43 mcg/kg/minute
Cl_{cr} 40 mL/minute/1.73 m^2: Administer 0.38 mcg/kg/minute
Cl_{cr} 30 mL/minute/1.73 m^2: Administer 0.33 mcg/kg/minute
Cl_{cr} 20 mL/minute/1.73 m^2: Administer 0.28 mcg/kg/minute
Cl_{cr} 10 mL/minute/1.73 m^2: Administer 0.23 mcg/kg/minute
Cl_{cr} 5 mL/minute/1.73 m^2: Administer 0.2 mcg/kg/minute

Administration

Loading dose: Administer slow I.V. push over 15 minutes for pediatric patients and over 10 minutes in adults; loading dose may be given as undiluted solution, but may dilute to 10-20 mL (in adults) for ease of administration.

I.V. continuous infusion: Dilute with $\frac{1}{2}$NS, NS, or D_5W and administer via infusion pump or syringe pump; usual concentration: ≤200 mcg/mL; 250 mcg/mL in NS has been used (see Barton, 1996)

Monitoring Parameters Blood pressure, heart rate, cardiac output, CI, SVR, PVR, CVP, EKG, platelet count, serum potassium, renal function; clinical signs and symptoms of CHF

Nursing Implications Do not administer furosemide I.V. push via "Y" site into milrinone solutions as precipitate will occur; decrease the infusion rate if significant hypotension occurs

Additional Information Dosing schemes and proposed dosing based on pharmacokinetic data:

Neonates: A loading dose of 50 mcg/kg administered over 15 minutes, followed by a continuous infusion of 0.5 mcg/kg/minute for 30 minutes in 10 neonates (3-27 days old, median age 5 days) improved hemodynamic parameters and was well tolerated (see Chang, 1995). Further neonatal studies of longer duration are needed.

Infants and children with septic shock: Twelve patients (9 months to 15 years of age) were administered a loading dose of 50 mcg/kg, followed by a continuous infusion of 0.5 mcg/kg/minute. At 1 hour after the loading dose, if patients did not respond (defined as a ≥20% increase in CI or an improvement in peripheral perfusion), an additional loading dose of 25 mcg/kg was given and the infusion rate was increased to 0.75 mcg/kg/minute. Nine of 12 patients required the additional loading dose and increased rate of infusion (see Barton 1996). A subsequent pharmacokinetic analysis of these patients recommended larger loading doses of 75 mcg/kg and infusion rates of 0.75-1 mcg/kg/minute. However, these doses were based on a one-compartment pharmacokinetic model and are higher then the mean infusion rate of 0.69 mcg/kg/minute used in the study (see Lindsay 1998). Further studies are needed.

Infants and Children after open heart surgery: Group A: Eleven patients received a loading dose of 25 mcg/kg given over 5 minutes followed by an infusion of 0.25 mcg/kg/minute; 30 minutes later, a second 25 mcg/kg loading dose was given and the infusion was increased to 0.5 mcg/kg/minute. Group B: 8 patients received a loading dose of 50 mcg/kg given over 10 minutes followed by an infusion of 0.5 mcg/kg/minute; 30 minutes later, a second loading dose of 25 mcg/kg was given and the infusion was increased to 0.75 mcg/kg/minute. Patients in both groups received a third loading dose of 25 mcg/kg if needed. A two-compartment model and NONMEM pharmacokinetic analyses were performed. Based on the NONMEM analysis, the authors propose the following doses: Infants: Loading dose: 104 mcg/kg and continuous infusion of 0.49 mcg/kg/minute; children: loading dose: 67 mcg/kg and continuous infusion of 0.61 mcg/kg/minute. Further studies are needed before these proposed doses can routinely be used in the pediatric population.

Dosage Forms

Infusion, as lactate, in D_5W: 200 mcg/mL (100 mL, 200 mL)
Injection, as lactate: 1 mg/mL (5 mL, 10 mL, 20 mL)

References

Barton P, Garcia J, Kouatli A, et al, "Hemodynamic Effects of I.V. Milrinone Lactate in Pediatric Patients With Septic Shock. A Prospective Double-Blinded, Randomized, Placebo-Controlled, Interventional Study," *Chest*, 1996, 109(5):1302-12.

Chang AC, Atz AM, Wernovsky G, et al, "Milrinone: Systemic and Pulmonary Hemodynamic Effects in Neonates After Cardiac Surgery," *Crit Care Med*, 1995, 23(11):1907-14.

"Guidelines 2000 for Cardiopulmonary Resuscitation and Emergency Cardiovascular Care, Part 10: Pediatric Advanced Life Support, The American Heart Association in Collaboration With the International Liaison Committee on Resuscitation," *Circulation*, 2000, 102(8 Suppl): I291-342.

Lindsay CA, Barton P, Lawless S, et al, "Pharmacokinetics and Pharmacodynamics of Milrinone Lactate in Pediatric Patients With Septic Shock," *J Pediatr*, 1998, 132(2):329-34.

Ramamoorthy C, Anderson GD, Williams GD, et al, "Pharmacokinetics and Side Effects of Milrinone in Infants and Children After Open Heart Surgery," Anesth Analg, 1998, 86(2):283-9.

Mineral Oil (MIN er al oyl)

U.S. Brand Names Agoral® Plain [OTC]; Fleet® Mineral Oil Enema [OTC]; Kondremul® [OTC]; Milkinol® [OTC]; Neo-Cultol® [OTC]; Zymenol® [OTC]

Synonyms Heavy Mineral Oil; Liquid Paraffin; White Mineral Oil

Therapeutic Category Laxative, Lubricant

Generic Available Yes

Use Temporary relief of constipation, to relieve fecal impaction, preparation for bowel studies or surgery

Pregnancy Risk Factor C

Contraindications Patients with a colostomy or an ileostomy, appendicitis, ulcerative colitis, diverticulitis, dysphagia or hiatal hernia

Warnings Oral form should be avoided in children <4 years of age because of the risk of aspiration

Adverse Reactions

Gastrointestinal: Nausea, vomiting, diarrhea, abdominal cramps, anal itching, anal seepage

Respiratory: Lipid pneumonitis with aspiration

Drug Interactions May impair absorption of fat-soluble vitamins, oral contraceptives, coumarin; increased absorption with docusate

Food Interactions May decrease absorption of fat-soluble vitamins, carotene, calcium, and phosphorus

Mechanism of Action Eases passage of stool by decreasing water absorption, softens stool, and lubricates the intestine

Pharmacodynamics Onset of action: ~6-8 hours

Pharmacokinetics

Absorption: Minimal following oral or rectal administration

Distribution: Into intestinal mucosa, liver, spleen, and mesenteric lymph nodes

Elimination: In feces

Usual Dosage

Children:

Oral: 5-11 years: 5-15 mL once daily or in divided doses; should not be used for longer than 1 week

Rectal: 2-11 years: 30-60 mL as a single dose

Children ≥12 years and Adults:

Oral: 15-45 mL/day once daily or in divided doses; should not be used for longer than 1 week

Rectal: Contents of one retention enema (range 60-150 mL)/day as a single dose

Administration

Oral: Nonemulsified mineral oil may be administered at bedtime on an empty stomach; emulsified mineral oil should be shaken before using; may be administered with meals (more palatable than nonemulsified mineral oil)

Rectal: Gently insert enema tip into rectum with a slight side-to-side movement with tip pointing toward the navel; have patient bear down

Monitoring Parameters Evacuation of stool; anal leakage indicates dose too high or need for disimpaction

Patient Information Do not take if experiencing abdominal pain, nausea, or vomiting. Rectal enema: Do not take if experiencing rectal bleeding

Dosage Forms

Emulsion, oral: Dosage of mineral oil emulsion is expressed in terms of its mineral oil content: 1.4 g/5 mL (480 mL); 2.5 mL/5 mL (420 mL); 2.75 mL/5 mL (480 mL); 4.75 mL/5 mL (240 mL)

Jelly, oral: 2.75 mL/5 mL (180 mL)

Liquid:

Oral: 30 mL, 180 mL, 500 mL, 1000 mL, 4000 mL

Rectal: 133 mL

References

Baker SS, Liptak GS, Colletti RB, et al, "A Medical Position Statement of the North American Society for Pediatric Gastroenterology and Nutrition; Constipation in Infants and Children: Evaluation and treatment," www.naspgn.org/constipation, 2000, 1-34.

♦ **Mini-Gamulin® Rh** see Rh₀(D) Immune Globulin (Intramuscular) on page 869

♦ **Minims-Cyclopentolate (Can)** see Cyclopentolate on page 279

♦ **Minims-Gentamicin (Can)** see Gentamicin on page 469

♦ **Minims-Homatropine (Can)** see Homatropine on page 497

♦ **Minims-Phenylephrine (Can)** see Phenylephrine on page 789

♦ **Minims-Pilocarpine (Can)** see Pilocarpine on page 800

- **Minims-Prednisolone (Can)** *see* Prednisolone *on page 821*
- **Minims-Sodium Chloride (Can)** *see* Sodium Chloride *on page 906*
- **Minims-Tetracaine (Can)** *see* Tetracaine *on page 940*
- **Minims-Tropicamide (Can)** *see* Tropicamide *on page 991*
- **Minipress®** *see* Prazosin *on page 820*
- **Minitran™** *see* Nitroglycerin *on page 717*
- **Minox (Can)** *see* Minoxidil *on page 676*

Minoxidil (mi NOKS i dil)

U.S. Brand Names Loniten®; Rogaine® [OTC]; Rogaine® Extra Strength [OTC]

Canadian Brand Names Apo-Gain; Minox

Therapeutic Category Antihypertensive Agent; Vasodilator

Generic Available Yes

Use Management of severe hypertension; topically for management of alopecia or male pattern alopecia

Pregnancy Risk Factor C

Contraindications Pheochromocytoma; hypersensitivity to minoxidil or any component

Precautions Use with caution in patients with coronary artery disease or with recent MI, pulmonary hypertension, significant renal dysfunction, CHF

Adverse Reactions
    Cardiovascular: Edema, CHF, tachycardia, angina, pericardial effusion and tamponade, EKG changes
    Central nervous system: Dizziness, fatigue, headache
    Dermatologic: Hypertrichosis (commonly occurs within 1-2 months of therapy), coarsening facial features, dermatologic reactions, rash, Stevens-Johnson syndrome, photosensitivity
    Endocrine & metabolic: Sodium and water retention
    Gastrointestinal: Weight gain
    Respiratory: Pulmonary hypertension, pulmonary edema

Drug Interactions Concurrent administration with guanethidine may cause profound orthostatic hypotensive effects; additive hypotensive effects with other hypotensive agents or diuretics

Food Interactions Avoid natural licorice (causes sodium and water retention and increases potassium loss)

Mechanism of Action Produces vasodilation by directly relaxing arteriolar smooth muscle, with little effect on veins; effects may be mediated by cyclic AMP; stimulation of hair growth is secondary to vasodilation, increased cutaneous blood flow and stimulation of resting hair follicles

Pharmacodynamics Hypotensive effects:
    Onset of action: Oral: Within 30 minutes
    Peak effect: Within 2-8 hours
    Duration: Up to 2-5 days

Pharmacokinetics
    Metabolism: 88% primarily via glucuronidation
    Protein-binding: None
    Bioavailability: Oral: 90%
    Half-life, adults: 3.5-4.2 hours
    Elimination: 12% excreted unchanged in urine
    Dialysis: Dialyzable (50% to 100%)

Usual Dosage
    Children <12 years: Hypertension: Oral: Initial: 0.1-0.2 mg/kg once daily; maximum dose: 5 mg/day; increase gradually every 3 days; usual dosage: 0.25-1 mg/kg/day in 1-2 divided doses; maximum dose: 50 mg/day
    Children >12 years and Adults:
        Hypertension: Oral: Initial: 5 mg once daily, increase gradually every 3 days; usual dose: 10-40 mg/day in 1-2 divided doses; maximum dose: 100 mg/day
        Alopecia: Apply twice daily

Administration Oral: May be administered without regard to food

Monitoring Parameters Fluids and electrolytes, body weight, blood pressure

Patient Information May cause dizziness; rise slowly from prolonged lying or sitting position

Additional Information Usually used with a beta-blocker (to treat minoxidil-induced tachycardia) and a diuretic (for treatment of water retention/edema); may take 1-6 months for hypertrichosis to totally reverse after minoxidil therapy is discontinued

Dosage Forms
  Solution, topical:
    Rogaine®: 2% [20 mg/metered dose] (60 mL)
    Rogaine® Extra Strength: 5% [50 mg/metered dose] (60 mL)
  Tablet (Loniten®): 2.5 mg, 10 mg

♦ **Mintezol®** see Thiabendazole on page 947
♦ **Miocarpine (Can)** see Pilocarpine on page 800
♦ **Miochol-E®** see Acetylcholine on page 35
♦ **MiraLax™** see Polyethylene Glycol-Electrolyte Solution on page 811

Misoprostol (mye soe PROST ole)
U.S. Brand Names Cytotec®
Therapeutic Category Gastrointestinal Agent, Gastric or Duodenal Ulcer Treatment; Prostaglandin
Use Prevention of NSAID-induced gastric ulcers; short-term treatment of duodenal and gastric ulcers (up to 8 weeks); improvement in fat absorption in cystic fibrosis patients when used in conjunction with pancreatic enzyme supplements (unlabeled use)
Pregnancy Risk Factor X
Contraindications Hypersensitivity to misoprostol or any component, pregnancy
Warnings Not to be used in pregnant women or women of childbearing potential unless woman is capable of complying with effective contraceptive measures; women should have a negative serum pregnancy test within 2 weeks prior to initiating therapy with therapy begun on the 2nd or 3rd day of next menstrual period
Precautions Use with caution in patients with inflammatory bowel disease and renal impairment
Adverse Reactions
  Central nervous system: Headache
  Gastrointestinal: Nausea, vomiting, constipation, flatulence, diarrhea, abdominal pain
  Genitourinary: Uterine stimulation, vaginal bleeding, menstrual irregularities
Drug Interactions Magnesium containing antacids enhance diarrhea associated with misoprostol
Mechanism of Action Misoprostol, a gastric antisecretory agent, is a synthetic prostaglandin E_1 analog that replaces the protective prostaglandins consumed with prostaglandin-inhibiting therapies (eg, NSAIDs) resulting in reduction of acid secretion from the gastric parietal cell and stimulation of bicarbonate production from the gastric and duodenal mucosa
Pharmacodynamics Inhibition of gastric acid secretion:
  Onset of action: 30 minutes
  Peak effect: 60-90 minutes
  Duration of action: 3 hours
Pharmacokinetics
  Absorption: Rapid
  Protein binding (misoprostol acid): 80% to 90%
  Metabolism: Extensive "first pass" de-esterification to misoprostol acid (active metabolite)
  Bioavailability: 88%
  Half-life (parent and metabolite combined): 1.5 hours
  Time to peak serum concentration (active metabolite): Within 15-30 minutes
  Elimination: In urine (64% to 73% in 24 hours) and feces (15% in 24 hours)
Usual Dosage Oral:
  Prevention of NSAID-induced ulcers: Adults: 200 mcg 4 times/day; if not tolerated, may decrease dose to 100 mcg 4 times/day or 200 mcg twice daily
  Gastric or duodenal ulcers: Adults: 100-200 mcg 4 times/day or 400 mcg twice daily for 4-8 weeks
  Improvement of fat malabsorption in cystic fibrosis (limited data available in children): Children 8-16 years: 100 mcg 4 times/day
Administration Oral: Administer after meals and at bedtime
Patient Information May cause diarrhea when first being used; avoid taking with magnesium-containing antacids
Nursing Implications Incidence of diarrhea may be lessened by having patient take dose right after meals
Dosage Forms Tablet: 100 mcg, 200 mcg
References
  Cleghorn GJ, Shepherd RW, and Holt TL, "The Use of a Synthetic Prostaglandin E1 Analogue (Misoprostol) as an Adjunct to Pancreatic Enzyme Replacement in Cystic Fibrosis," Scand J Gastroenterol Suppl, 1988, 143:142-7.
  (Continued)

Misoprostol *(Continued)*

Robinson PJ, Smith AL, and Sly PD, "Duodenal pH in Cystic Fibrosis and Its Relationship to Fat Malabsorption," *Dig Dis Sci*, 1990, 35(10):1299-304.

♦ **Mithracin®** *see* Plicamycin *on page 807*

♦ **Mithramycin** *see* Plicamycin *on page 807*

Mitomycin *(mye toe MYE sin)*

Related Information
Emetogenic Potential of Single Chemotherapeutic Agents *on page 1129*

U.S. Brand Names Mutamycin®

Synonyms Mitomycin-C; MTC

Therapeutic Category Antineoplastic Agent, Antibiotic

Generic Available No

Use Therapy of disseminated adenocarcinoma of stomach, colon, or pancreas in combination with other approved chemotherapeutic agents; bladder cancer, breast cancer

Pregnancy Risk Factor C

Contraindications Platelet counts <75,000/mm^3; leukocyte counts <3000/mm^3 or serum creatinine >1.7 mg/dL; coagulation disorders; hypersensitivity to mitomycin or any component

Warnings The FDA currently recommends that procedures for proper handling and disposal of antineoplastic agents be considered. Bone marrow suppression, notably thrombocytopenia and leukopenia, may contribute to the development of a secondary infection; hemolytic uremic syndrome, a serious and often fatal syndrome has occurred in patients receiving long-term therapy; the risk of hemolytic uremic syndrome increases with a total cumulative dose >50 mg/m^2; mitomycin is potentially mutagenic and teratogenic.

Precautions Use with caution in patients with myelosuppression, impaired renal or hepatic function; modify dosage in patients with myelosuppression or renal impairment

Adverse Reactions
Central nervous system: Fever
Dermatologic: Alopecia, pruritus
Gastrointestinal: Nausea, vomiting, mouth ulcers, diarrhea, anorexia
Hematologic: Bone marrow suppression (leukopenia, thrombocytopenia), microangiopathic hemolytic anemia
Hepatic: Veno-occlusive disease
Local: Thrombophlebitis
Neuromuscular & skeletal: Paresthesia, weakness
Renal: Hemolytic uremic syndrome, nephrotoxicity
Respiratory: Pulmonary toxicity, interstitial pneumonia

Drug Interactions Anthracyclines (may enhance cardiotoxicity)

Stability Reconstitute solution with sterile water at a concentration of 0.5 mg/mL; the reconstituted solution must be protected from light if not used within 24 hours; stable for 7 days at room temperature and 14 days when refrigerated; I.V. infusion in D$_5$W is stable for 3 hours at room temperature; in NS solution is stable for 12 hours at room temperature; physically compatible with ondansetron for 4 hours

Mechanism of Action Inhibits DNA and RNA synthesis by alkylating and cross-linking the strands of DNA

Pharmacokinetics
Distribution: Into bile and ascites fluid
Half-life, terminal: 50 minutes
Elimination: Primarily by hepatic metabolism followed by urinary excretion (<10% as unchanged drug) and to a small extent biliary excretion

Usual Dosage Children and Adults: I.V. (refer to individual protocols): 10-20 mg/m^2/dose every 6-8 weeks, or 3 mg/m^2/day for 5 days every 4-6 weeks; subsequent doses should be adjusted to platelet and leukocyte response; see table.

Nadir After Prior Dose/mm^3		% of Prior Dose to Be Given
Leukocytes	Platelets	
4000	>100,000	100
3000-3999	75,000-99,999	100
2000-2999	25,000-74,999	70
2000	<25,000	50

Very high doses (40-50 mg/m² as a single dose) have been administered by hepatic artery infusion followed by autologous bone marrow transplantation.

Dosing adjustment in renal impairment: Cl_{cr} <10 mL/minute: Administer 75% of normal dose

Administration Parenteral: Administer by short I.V. infusion over 30-60 minutes or by slow I.V. push over 5-10 minutes through a Y-site of a running I.V.; short I.V. infusions are usually administered at a final concentration of 20-40 mcg/mL (in 50-250 mL of D_5W or NS); I.V. slow push can be administered at a concentration not to exceed 0.5 mg/mL

Monitoring Parameters Platelet count, CBC with differential, hemoglobin, prothrombin time, renal and pulmonary function tests

Patient Information Notify physician if fever, sore throat, bruising, bleeding, shortness of breath, or painful urination occur

Nursing Implications Care should be taken to avoid extravasation since ulceration and tissue sloughing can occur; mitomycin extravasation has been treated using a 99% (w/v) solution of dimethylsulfoxide (DMSO); apply 1.5 mL to the site every 6 hours for 14 days; allow to air-dry; do not cover

Additional Information Myelosuppressive effects:
WBC: Moderate
Platelets: Severe
Onset (days): 21
Nadir (days): 36
Recovery (days): 42-56

Dosage Forms Powder for injection: 5 mg, 20 mg, 40 mg

References
Alberts DS and Dorr RT, "Case Report: Topical DMSO for Mitomycin C-Induced Skin Ulceration," *Oncol Nurs Forum*, 1991, 18(4):693-5.

♦ **Mitomycin-C** *see Mitomycin on page 678*

Mitoxantrone (mye toe ZAN trone)

Related Information
Emetogenic Potential of Single Chemotherapeutic Agents *on page 1129*

U.S. Brand Names Novantrone®

Synonyms DHAD

Therapeutic Category Antineoplastic Agent, Anthracycline; Antineoplastic Agent, Antibiotic

Generic Available No

Use For remission-induction therapy of acute nonlymphocytic leukemia (ANLL) and acute myelogenous leukemia (AML); mitoxantrone is also active against other leukemias, lymphoma, breast cancer, and moderately active against pediatric sarcoma; treatment of patients with pain related to advanced hormone refractory prostate cancer; reducing neurologic disability and/or frequency of clinical relapses in patients with secondary progressive, progressive relapsing, or worsening relapsing-remitting multiple sclerosis

Pregnancy Risk Factor D (may cause fetal harm when administered to a pregnant woman)

Contraindications Hypersensitivity to mitoxantrone or any component; patients with multiple sclerosis who have hepatic impairment; patients with baseline left ventricular ejection fraction <50% or cumulative lifetime dose ≥140 mg/m² should not be treated with mitoxantrone

Warnings Avoid in patients with pre-existing myelosuppression; mitoxantrone is less cardiotoxic than anthracyclines. The predisposing factors for mitoxantrone-induced cardiotoxicity include prior anthracycline therapy, prior cardiovascular disease, and mediastinal irradiation. The risk of developing cardiotoxicity is <3% when the cumulative dose is <140 mg/m²; interstitial pneumonitis has been reported in patients receiving combination chemotherapy that included mitoxantrone; extravasation can result in tissue necrosis with resultant need for debridement and skin grafting; the FDA currently recommends that procedures for proper handling and disposal of antineoplastic agents be considered. Secondary leukemias have been reported in patients treated with mitoxantrone; intrathecal administration is not recommended since local nerve demyelinization, seizures, coma, and paraplegia have been reported with this route.

Precautions Dosage should be reduced in patients with pre-existing bone marrow suppression, previous treatment with cardiotoxic agents, and patients with impaired hepatobiliary function

Adverse Reactions
Cardiovascular: Cardiotoxicity (arrhythmias, CHF), hypotension, tachycardia, cardiomyopathy
(Continued)

Mitoxantrone *(Continued)*

Central nervous system: Seizures, headache

Dermatologic: Alopecia, pruritus, skin desquamation, rash, discoloration of skin (blue-green)

Gastrointestinal: Nausea, diarrhea, vomiting, stomatitis (occurs more frequently with "daily times 3 day" regimens than once every 3 week schedules), mucositis

Genitourinary: Discoloration of urine (blue-green)

Hematologic: Myelosuppression (leukopenia, pancytopenia), mild anemia, thrombocytopenia

Hepatic: Transient elevation of liver enzymes, jaundice

Local: Phlebitis, tissue necrosis with extravasation

Respiratory: Interstitial pneumonitis

Miscellaneous: Anaphylaxis

Drug Interactions Cytochrome P-450 isoenzyme CYP2E1 inducer (weak)

High-dose cytarabine (therapeutic synergy)

Stability After penetration of the stopper, undiluted mitoxantrone solution is stable for 7 days at room temperature or 14 days when refrigerated; incompatible with heparin; physically compatible with ondansetron for at least 4 hours

Mechanism of Action Inhibits DNA and RNA synthesis by intercalating with DNA and causing template disordering and steric obstruction; replication is decreased by binding to DNA topoisomerase II (enzyme responsible for DNA helix supercoiling); active throughout entire cell cycle. Mitoxantrone inhibits B cell, T cell, and macrophage proliferation; impairs antigen presentation and secretion of interferon gamma, TNF_α, IL-2.

Pharmacokinetics

Distribution: Distributes into thyroid, liver, pancreas, spleen, heart, bone marrow, and red blood cells; prolonged retention in tissues; excreted in breast milk

Protein binding: 78%

Half-life, terminal: 23-215 hours and may be prolonged with liver impairment

Elimination: Slowly excreted in urine (6% to 11%) and bile as unchanged drug and metabolites

Usual Dosage I.V. (refer to individual protocols):

Leukemias:

Children ≤2 years: 0.4 mg/kg/day once daily for 3-5 days

Children >2 years and Adults: 12 mg/m^2/day once daily for 2-3 days; acute leukemia in relapse: 8-12 mg/m^2/day once daily for 4-5 days; ANLL: 10 mg/m^2/day once daily for 3-5 days

Solid tumors:

Children: 18-20 mg/m^2 once every 3-4 weeks

Adults: 12-14 mg/m^2 once every 3-4 weeks

Multiple sclerosis: Adults: 12 mg/m^2/dose every 3 months

Dosing adjustment in hepatic impairment: Although official dosage adjustment recommendations have not been established, dosage reduction of 50% in patients with serum bilirubin of 1.5-3 mg/dL and dosage reduction of 75% in patients with serum bilirubin >3 mg/dL have been recommended

Administration Do **not** administer by S.C., I.M., intrathecal, or intra-arterial injection

Parenteral: I.V.: Do **not** administer I.V. push over <3 minutes; may administer by I.V. bolus over >3 minutes, I.V. intermittent infusion over 15-60 minutes or I.V. continuous infusion at a concentration of 0.02-0.5 mg/mL in D$_5$W or NS

Monitoring Parameters CBC with differential, serum uric acid, liver function tests, echocardiogram with monitoring of left ventricular ejection fraction; women of childbearing potential should have a pregnancy test prior to dose

Patient Information May discolor skin, sclera, tears, sweat, and urine to a blue-green color; contraceptive measures are recommended during therapy

Nursing Implications Mitoxantrone is a nonvesicant; if extravasation occurs, the drug should be discontinued and restarted in another vein; extravasation may result in erythema, swelling, pain, burning, and/or a blue discoloration of the skin

Additional Information Myelosuppression (leukocyte nadir: 10-14 days; recovery: 21 days); injection contains 0.14 mEq of sodium/mL

Dosage Forms Injection, as hydrochloride: 2 mg of mitoxantrone base/mL (10 mL, 12.5 mL, 15 mL)

References

Koeller J and Eble M, "Mitoxantrone: A Novel Anthracycline Derivative," *Clin Pharm*, 1988, 7(8):574-81.
LeMaistre CF and Herzig R, "Mitoxantrone: Potential for Use in Intensive Therapy," *Semin Oncol*, 1990, 17(1 Suppl 3):43-8.
Pratt CB, Vietti TJ, Etcubanas E, et al, "Novantrone® for Childhood Malignant Solid Tumors. A Pediatric Oncology Group Phase II Study," *Invest New Drugs*, 1986, 4(1):43-8.

Stevens RF, Hann IM, Wheatley K, et al, "Marked Improvements in Outcome With Chemotherapy Alone in Paediatric Acute Myeloid Leukemia: Results of the United Kingdom Medical Research Council's 10th AML Trial. MRC Childhood Leukaemia Working Party," *Br J Haematol*, 1998, 101(1):130-40.

♦ **Mivacron**® *see* Mivacurium *on page 681*

Mivacurium (mye va KYOO ree um)

U.S. Brand Names Mivacron®

Therapeutic Category Neuromuscular Blocker Agent, Nondepolarizing; Skeletal Muscle Relaxant, Paralytic

Generic Available No

Use Short-acting nondepolarizing neuromuscular blocking agent; an adjunct to general anesthesia; facilitates endotracheal intubation; provides skeletal muscle relaxation during surgery or mechanical ventilation

Pregnancy Risk Factor C

Contraindications Hypersensitivity to mivacurium chloride, any component, or other benzylisoquinolinium agents

Warnings Avoid use of multidose vials in neonates as contains benzyl alcohol

Precautions Use cautiously in patients with reduced plasma cholinesterase activity, asthma, severe cardiovascular disease

Adverse Reactions

Cardiovascular: Hypotension, bradycardia, tachycardia, flushing, cardiac arrhythmias

Central nervous system: Dizziness

Dermatologic: Cutaneous erythema, rash

Neuromuscular & skeletal: Muscle spasms

Local: Injection site reaction

Respiratory: Bronchospasm, wheezing

Miscellaneous: Endogenous histamine release

Drug Interactions See table.

Potential Drug Interactions

Potentiation	Antagonism
Inhalation anesthetics	Calcium
Desflurane, sevoflurane, enflurane and	Carbamazepine
isoflurane > halothane > nitrous	Phenytoin
oxide	Steroids (chronic administration)
Antibiotics	Theophylline
Aminoglycosides, polymyxins,	Anticholinesterases*
clindamycin, vancomycin	Neostigmine, pyridostigmine,
Magnesium	edrophonium, echothiophate
Antiarrhythmics	ophthalmic solution
Quinidine, procainamide, bretylium, and	Caffeine
possibly lidocaine	Azathioprine
Diuretics	
Furosemide, mannitol, thiazides	
Amphotericin B (secondary to hypokalemia)	
Local anesthetics	
Dantrolene (directly depresses skeletal muscle)	
Beta blockers	
Calcium channel blockers	
Ketamine	
Lithium	
Succinylcholine (when administered prior to nondepolarizing neuromuscular-blocking agent)	
Cyclosporine	

*Can prolong the effects of acetylcholine

Stability Store at room temperature; stable in D$_5$W, D$_5$/LR, NS for 24 hours; avoid exposure to direct ultraviolet light; incompatible with alkaline solutions; compatible with Y-site administration with sufentanil, fentanyl, alfentanil, midazolam, droperidol

(Continued)

Mivacurium (Continued)

Mechanism of Action Mivacurium is a short-acting, nondepolarizing, neuromuscular-blocking agent. Like other nondepolarizing drugs, mivacurium antagonizes acetylcholine by competitively binding to cholinergic sites on motor endplates in skeletal muscle.

Pharmacodynamics
Onset of action: 1-3 minutes
Duration of action: Short due to rapid hydrolysis by plasma cholinesterases; recovery from muscular paralysis occurs within 9-20 minutes

Pharmacokinetics Mivacurium exists as a mixture of isomers; the most potent are the *trans-trans* and *cis-trans* isomers
Distribution: V_d: *Trans-trans* isomer: 0.15 L/kg; *cis-trans* isomer: 0.27 L/kg
Metabolism: Enzymatic hydrolysis by plasma cholinesterase
Half-life: *Trans-trans* isomer: 2.3 minutes (range: 1.4-3.6); *cis-trans* isomer: 2.1 minutes (range: 0.8-4.8)
Clearance: *Trans-trans* isomer: 53 mL/minute/kg; *cis-trans* isomer: 99 mL/minute/kg

Usual Dosage Children require higher doses mg/kg than adults and more frequent maintenance doses; I.V.:

Children 2-12 years: 0.2 mg/kg; continuous infusion: 10-14 mcg/kg/minute; doses as high as 31 mcg/kg/minute have been used
Adults: 0.15-0.2 mg/kg; for prolonged neuromuscular block, continuous infusion: 9-10 mcg/kg/minute

Administration Parenteral: Administer undiluted by rapid I.V. injection; infusions diluted in D_5W to a maximum concentration of 0.5 mg/mL

Monitoring Parameters Assisted ventilation status, heart rate, blood pressure, peripheral nerve stimulator measuring twitch response

Nursing Implications Does not alter the patient's state of consciousness; addition of sedation is recommended

Dosage Forms
Infusion, as chloride, in D_5W: 0.5 mg/mL (50 mL, 100 mL)
Injection, as chloride:
Preservative free: 2 mg/mL (5 mL, 10 mL)
With benzyl alcohol: 2 mg/mL (20 mL, 50 mL)

References
Martin LD, Bratton SL, and O'Rourke PP, "Clinical Uses and Controversies of Neuromuscular Blocking Agents in Infants and Children," *Crit Care Med*, 1999, 27(7):1358-68.

- **MK-639** see Indinavir on page 534
- **Modane® Bulk [OTC]** see Psyllium on page 853
- **Modane® Soft [OTC]** see Docusate on page 350
- **Mol-Iron® [OTC]** see Iron Supplements (Oral/Enteral) on page 548
- **Mollifene® Ear Wax Removing Formula [OTC]** see Carbamide Peroxide on page 178
- **Molypen®** see Trace Metals on page 972
- **MOM (Magnesium Hydroxide)** see Magnesium Supplements on page 614
- **Monarc® M** see Antihemophilic Factor (Human) on page 98
- **Monazole-7 (Can)** see Miconazole on page 668
- **Monistat-Derm™ Topical** see Miconazole on page 668
- **Monistat™ Vaginal** see Miconazole on page 668
- **Monoclate-P®** see Antihemophilic Factor (Human) on page 98
- **Monoclonal Antibody** see Muromonab-CD3 on page 688
- **Monodox®** see Doxycycline on page 362

Montelukast (mon te LOO kast)

Related Information
Asthma Guidelines on page 1210

U.S. Brand Names Singulair®

Therapeutic Category Antiasthmatic; Leukotriene Receptor Antagonist

Generic Available No

Use Prophylaxis and chronic treatment of asthma

Pregnancy Risk Factor B

Contraindications Hypersensitivity to montelukast or any component

Warnings Montelukast is not indicated for use in the reversal of bronchospasm in acute asthma attacks, including status asthmaticus; it is not indicated as monotherapy for the treatment and management of exercise-induced bronchospasm; therapy with montelukast can be continued during acute exacerbations of asthma; chewable tablet contains phenylalanine and should be avoided in patients with phenylketonuria

Precautions Phenobarbital reduces the AUC of montelukast ~40% following a single 10 mg dosage; no dosage adjustment of montelukast is indicated, however, appropriate clinical monitoring is indicated when potent cytochrome P-450 enzyme inducers, such as phenobarbital or rifampin, are coadministered with montelukast

Adverse Reactions
Central nervous system: Headache, fever, dizziness, drowsiness, irritability, restlessness, dream abnormalities
Dermatologic: Rash
Gastrointestinal: Diarrhea, nausea, abdominal pain, dyspepsia
Hepatic: Elevated liver enzymes, hepatic eosinophilic infiltration
Otic: Otitis
Respiratory: Sinusitis, laryngitis, nasal congestion, cough
Miscellaneous: Viral infection, influenza, hypersensitivity reactions

Drug Interactions Cytochrome P-450 isoenzyme CYP2A6, CYP2C9, and CYP3A3/4 substrate
Phenobarbital (see Precautions)

Stability Store at room temperature; protect from light

Mechanism of Action Montelukast is a selective leukotriene receptor antagonist that inhibits the cysteinyl leukotriene $CysLT_1$ receptor. This activity produces inhibition of the effects of this leukotriene on bronchial smooth muscle resulting in the attenuation of bronchoconstriction and decreased vascular permeability, mucosal edema, and mucus production.

Pharmacokinetics
Absorption: Rapid
Distribution: V_d: Adults: 8-11 L
Protein binding: 99%
Metabolism: Extensive by cytochrome P-450 3A4 and 2C9
Bioavailability: Tablet:
5 mg: 73%
10 mg: 64%
Time to peak serum concentration: Tablet:
5 mg: 2-2.5 hours
10 mg: 3-4 hours
Elimination: Exclusively via bile; <0.2% excreted in urine

Usual Dosage Oral:
Children
2-5 years: 4 mg/day
6-14 years: 5 mg/day
Adolescents >14 years and Adults: 10 mg/day
Note: None of the clinical trials evaluated the safety and efficacy of therapy with morning dosing; the pharmacokinetics of montelukast are similar whether dosed in the morning or evening

Administration Oral: Administer in the evening without regard to time of meals

Monitoring Parameters Pulmonary function tests (FEV-1), improvement in asthma symptoms

Patient Information Take regularly as prescribed, even during symptom-free periods. Do not use to treat acute episodes of asthma. Do not decrease the dose or stop taking any other asthma medications unless instructed by a physician.

Dosage Forms
Tablet, as sodium: 10 mg
Tablet, chewable (cherry), as sodium: 4 mg, 5 mg

♦ **More-Dophilus® [OTC]** *see Lactobacillus acidophilus and Lactobacillus bulgaricus on page 571*

♦ **Morphine-HP (Can)** *see Morphine Sulfate on page 683*

Morphine Sulfate (MOR feen SUL fate)

Related Information
Compatibility of Medications Mixed in a Syringe *on page 1238*
Laboratory Detection of Drugs in Urine *on page 1234*
Narcotic Analgesics Comparison *on page 1070*
Overdose and Toxicology *on page 1222*
Preprocedure Sedatives in Children *on page 1201*
U.S. Brand Names Astramorph/PF™; Duramorph®; Infumorph™; Kadian™; MS Contin®; MS-IR®; Oramorph SR®; RMS®; Roxanol™
Canadian Brand Names M-Eslon; Morphine-HP; MOS; Statex
Synonyms MS
(Continued)

Morphine Sulfate *(Continued)*

Therapeutic Category Analgesic, Narcotic

Generic Available Yes

Use Relief of moderate to severe acute and chronic pain; pain of MI; relieves dyspnea of acute left ventricular failure and pulmonary edema; preanesthetic medication

Restrictions C-II

Pregnancy Risk Factor B (D if used for prolonged periods or in high doses at term)

Contraindications Hypersensitivity to morphine sulfate or any component; increased intracranial pressure; severe respiratory depression; severe liver or renal insufficiency

Warnings Some preparations contain sulfites which may cause allergic reactions; neonates and infants <3 months of age are more susceptible to respiratory depression, use with caution and in reduced doses in this age group; use only preservative free injections for epidural or intrathecal administration and in neonates

Precautions Use with caution in patients with hypersensitivity reactions to other phenanthrene derivative opioid agonists (codeine, hydrocodone, hydromorphone, levorphanol, oxycodone, oxymorphone)

Adverse Reactions

Cardiovascular: Palpitations, hypotension, bradycardia, peripheral vasodilation

Central nervous system: CNS depression, drowsiness, dizziness, sedation, increased intracranial pressure

Dermatologic: Pruritus (more common with epidural or intrathecal administration)

Endocrine & metabolic: Antidiuretic hormone release

Gastrointestinal: Nausea, vomiting, constipation, biliary tract spasm

Genitourinary: Urinary tract spasm (may be more common with epidural or intrathecal administration), urinary retention

Ocular: Miosis

Respiratory: Respiratory depression

Miscellaneous: Physical and psychological dependence, histamine release

Drug Interactions Cytochrome P-450 isoenzyme CYP2D6 substrate

CNS depressants, alcohol, phenothiazines, tricyclic antidepressants may potentiate the adverse effects of morphine

Food Interactions Food may increase bioavailability of oral morphine solution

Stability Refrigerate suppositories; do not freeze; degradation depends on pH and presence of oxygen; relatively stable in pH ≤4; darkening of solutions indicates degradation

Mechanism of Action Binds to opiate receptors in the CNS, causing inhibition of ascending pain pathways, altering the perception of and response to pain; produces generalized CNS depression

Pharmacodynamics See table.

Dosage Form/Route	Analgesia	
	Peak	Duration
Tablets	1 h	3-5 h
Oral solution	1 h	3-5 h
Epidural	1 h	12-20 h
Extended release tablets	3-4 h	8-12 h
Suppository	20-60 min	3-7 h
Subcutaneous injection	50-90 min	3-5 h
I.M. injection	30-60 min	3-5 h
I.V. injection	20 min	3-5 h

Pharmacokinetics

Absorption: Oral: Variable

Distribution: V_d, apparent: Children 1.7-18.7 years with cancer: Median: 5.2 L/kg; a significantly higher V_d was observed in children <11 years (median: 7.1 L/kg) versus >11 years (median: 4.7 L/kg) (see Hunt, 1999)

Protein binding:

Premature Infants: <20%

Adults: ~35%

Metabolism: In the liver via glucuronide conjugation to morphine-6-glucuronide (active) and morphine-3-glucuronide (inactive)

Half-life:
  Preterm: 10-20 hours
  Neonates: 4.5-13.3 hours (mean: 7.6 hours)
  Infants 1-3 months: 6.2 hours (range: 5-10 hours)
  Children 6 months to 2.5 years: 2.9 hours (range: 1.4-7.8 hours)
  Preschool Children: 1-2 hours
  Children 6-19 years with sickle cell disease: Mean ~1.3 hours
  Adults: 2-4 hours
Elimination: Excreted unchanged in urine
  Neonates: 3% to 15%
  Adults: 6% to 10%
  Clearance:
    Preterm: 0.5-3 mL/minute/kg
    Neonates: 5 mL/minute/kg
    Children 6 months to 2.5 years: 22 mL/minute/kg
    Preschool Children: 20-40 mL/minute/kg
    Children 1.7-18.7 years with cancer: Median: 23.1 mL/minute/kg; a significantly
      higher clearance was observed in children <11 years (median: 37.4 mL/
      minute/kg) versus >11 years (median: 21.9 mL/minute/kg) (see Hunt, 1999)
    Children 6-19 years with sickle cell disease: Mean ~36 mL/minute/kg (range: 6-
      59 mL/minute/kg)
    Adults: 10-20 mL/minute/kg

Usual Dosage Doses should be titrated to appropriate effect; when changing
routes of administration in chronically treated patients, please note that oral doses
are approximately one-half as effective as parenteral dose

Neonates (see Warnings; use preservative free formulation):
  I.M., I.V., S.C.: Initial: 0.05 mg/kg every 4-8 hours; titrate carefully to effect;
    maximum dose: 0.1 mg/kg/dose
  I.V. continuous infusion: Initial: 0.01 mg/kg/hour (10 mcg/kg/hour); do **not** exceed
    infusion rates of 0.015-0.02 mg/kg/hour due to decreased elimination, increased
    CNS sensitivity, and adverse effects
Infants and Children:
  Oral: Tablet and solution (prompt release): 0.2-0.5 mg/kg/dose every 4-6 hours as
    needed; tablet (controlled release): 0.3-0.6 mg/kg/dose every 12 hours
  I.M., I.V., S.C.: 0.1-0.2 mg/kg/dose every 2-4 hours as needed; may initiate at
    0.05 mg/kg/dose; usual maximum dose: 15 mg/dose
  I.V., S.C. continuous infusion:
    Sickle cell or cancer pain: Range: 0.025-2.6 mg/kg/hour (median dose, cancer
      pain: 0.04-0.07 mg/kg/hour)
    Postoperative pain: 0.01-0.04 mg/kg/hour
  Sedation/analgesia for procedures: I.V.: 0.05-0.1 mg/kg 5 minutes before the
    procedure
  Epidural (use preservative free): 0.03-0.05 mg/kg (30-50 mcg/kg); maximum dose:
    0.1 mg/kg (100 mcg/kg) or 5 mg/24 hours
Adolescents >12 years: Sedation/analgesia for procedures: I.V.: 3-4 mg; may repeat
  in 5 minutes if necessary
Adults:
  Oral: Prompt release: 10-30 mg every 4 hours as needed; controlled release: 15-
    30 mg every 8-12 hours
  I.M., I.V., S.C.: 2.5-20 mg/dose every 2-6 hours as needed; usual: 10 mg/dose
    every 4 hours as needed
  I.V., S.C. continuous infusion: 0.8-10 mg/hour; may increase depending on pain
    relief/adverse effects; usual range up to 80 mg/hour
  Epidural (use preservative free): Initial: 5 mg in lumbar region; if inadequate pain
    relief within 1 hour, give 1-2 mg, maximum dose: 10 mg/24 hours
  Intrathecal ($^1/_{10}$ of epidural dose, use preservative free): 0.2-1 mg/dose; repeat
    doses **not** recommended
Dosing adjustment in renal impairment: Children and Adults:
  Cl_{cr} 10-50 mL/minute: Administer 75% of normal dose
  Cl_{cr} <10 mL/minute: Administer 50% of normal dose

Administration
Oral: Administer with food; swallow extended release products whole, do not chew
  or crush
Parenteral:
  I.V. push: Administer over at least 5 minutes at a final concentration of 0.5-5 mg/
    mL (rapid I.V. administration may increase adverse effects)
  Intermittent infusion: Administer over 15-30 minutes
  Continuous I.V. infusion: 0.1-1 mg/mL in D_5W
  Epidural and intrathecal: Use only preservative free injections
(Continued)

Morphine Sulfate *(Continued)*

Monitoring Parameters Respiratory and cardiovascular status, oxygen saturation, pain relief (if used for analgesia), level of sedation

Patient Information Avoid alcohol; may cause drowsiness and impair ability to perform hazardous duties requiring mental alertness or physical coordination; may be habit forming

Nursing Implications Do not administer rapidly I.V.

Additional Information Less adverse effects are associated with epidural compared to intrathecal route of administration; equianalgesic doses: Codeine: 120 mg I.M. = morphine 10 mg I.M. = single dose oral morphine 60 mg **or** chronic dosing oral morphine 15-25 mg

Dosage Forms

Capsule (MSIR®): 15 mg, 30 mg

Capsule, sustained release (Kadian™): 20 mg, 30 mg, 50 mg, 60 mg, 100 mg

Solution for injection: 0.5 mg/mL (30 mL); 1 mg/mL (10 mL, 30 mL, 50 mL, 60 mL); 2 mg/mL (1 mL, 60 mL); 4 mg/mL (1 mL, 30 mL, 50 mL); 5 mg/mL (1 mL, 30 mL, 50 mL); 8 mg/mL (1 mL); 10 mg/mL (1 mL, 10 mL, 20 mL); 15 mg/mL (1 mL, 20 mL); 25 mg/mL (4 mL, 10 mL, 20 mL, 40 mL, 50 mL); 50 mg/mL (10 mL, 20 mL, 40 mL, 50 mL)

Preservative free: 0.5 mg/mL (10 mL); 1 mg/mL (10 mL, 30 mL); 5 mg/mL (30 mL); 10 mg/mL (30 mL); 25 mg/mL (4 mL, 10 mL, 20 mL, 30 mL, 40 mL, 50 mL); 50 mg/mL (10 mL, 20 mL, 30 mL, 40 mL, 50 mL)

Epidural or intrathecal infusion via microinfusion device, preservative free (Infumorph™): 10 mg/mL (20 mL); 25 mg/mL (20 mL)

Epidural, intrathecal, or I.V. infusion, preservative free

Astramorph/PF™: 0.5 mg/mL (2 mL, 10 mL); 1 mg/mL (2 mL, 10 mL)

Duramorph®: 0.5 mg/mL (10 mL); 1 mg/mL (10 mL)

I.V. infusion via PCA pump: 1 mg/mL (10 mL, 30 mL, 50 mL); 5 mg/mL (30 mL, 50 mL)

Premixed I.V. infusion: 0.2 mg/mL in D₅W (250 mL, 500 mL); 1 mg/mL in D₅W (100 mL, 250 mL, 500 mL)

Solution, oral: 10 mg/5 mL (5 mL, 10 mL, 100 mL, 120 mL, 500 mL); 20 mg/5 mL (100 mL, 120 mL, 500 mL); 20 mg/mL (30 mL, 120 mL, 240 mL)

MSIR®: 10 mg/5 mL (120 mL); 20 mg/5 mL (120 mL); 20 mg/mL (30 mL, 120 mL)

Roxanol™: 20 mg/mL (30 mL, 120 mL)

Roxanol™ T: 20 mg/mL [tinted and flavored] (30 mL, 120 mL)

Roxanol™ 100: 100 mg/5 mL [with calibrated spoon] (240 mL)

Suppository, rectal (RMS®): 5 mg, 10 mg, 20 mg, 30 mg

Tablet (MSIR®): 15 mg, 30 mg

Tablet:

Controlled release (MS Contin®): 15 mg, 30 mg, 60 mg, 100 mg, 200 mg

Extended release: 15 mg, 30 mg, 60 mg

Sustained release (Oramorph SR®): 15 mg, 30 mg, 60 mg, 100 mg

References

Berde C, Ablin A, Glazer J, et al, "American Academy of Pediatrics Report of the Subcommittee on Disease-Related Pain in Childhood Cancer," *Pediatrics,* 1990, 86(5 Pt 2):818-25.

Dampier CD, Setty BN, Logan J, et al, "Intravenous Morphine Pharmacokinetics in Pediatric Patients With Sickle Cell Disease," *J Pediatr,* 1995, 126(3):461-7.

Henneberg SW, Hole P, Madsen de Haas I, et al, "Epidural Morphine for Postoperative Pain Relief in Children," *Acta Anaesthesiol Scand,* 1993, 37(7):664-7.

Hunt A, Joel S, Dick G, et al, "Population Pharmacokinetics of Oral Morphine and Its Glucuronides in Children Receiving Morphine as Immediate-Release Liquid or Sustained-Release Tablets for Cancer Pain," *J Pediatr,* 1999, 135(1):47-55.

McRorie TI, Lynn AM, Nespeca MK, et al, "The Maturation of Morphine Clearance and Metabolism," *Am J Dis Child,* 1992, 147(8):972-6.

Olkkola KT, Hamunen K, and Maunuksela EL, "Clinical Pharmacokinetics and Pharmacodynamics of Opioid Analgesics in Infants and Children," *Clin Pharmacokinet,* 1995, 28(5):385-404.

- **M.T.E.-4®** *see* Trace Metals *on page 972*
- **M.T.E.-5®** *see* Trace Metals *on page 972*
- **M.T.E.-6®** *see* Trace Metals *on page 972*
- **M.T.E.-7®** *see* Trace Metals *on page 972*
- **MTX** *see* Methotrexate *on page 648*
- **Muco-Fen-DM®** *see* Guaifenesin and Dextromethorphan *on page 487*
- **Muco-Fen-LA®** *see* Guaifenesin *on page 485*
- **Mucomyst®** *see* Acetylcysteine *on page 35*
- **Mucosil™** *see* Acetylcysteine *on page 35*
- **Multe-Pak-4®** *see* Trace Metals *on page 972*
- **Multiple Trace Metals** *see* Trace Metals *on page 972*
- **Multiple Vitamin Products** *see page 1069*
- **Mumps Virus Vaccine, Live, Attenuated** *see page 1172*

Mupirocin (myoo PEER oh sin)

U.S. Brand Names Bactroban®
Synonyms Pseudomonic Acid A
Therapeutic Category Antibiotic, Topical
Generic Available No
Use Topical treatment of impetigo caused by *Staphylococcus aureus* and *Streptococcus pyogenes*; also effective for the topical treatment of folliculitis, furunculosis, minor wounds, burns, and ulcers caused by susceptible organisms; used as a prophylactic agent applied to intravenous catheter exit sites; used for eradication of *S. aureus* from nasal and perineal carriage sites
Pregnancy Risk Factor B
Contraindications Hypersensitivity to mupirocin, polyethylene glycol, or any component
Warnings Potentially toxic amounts of polyethylene glycol (PEG) contained in the vehicle may be absorbed percutaneously in patients with extensive burns or open wounds; the PEG vehicle may irritate mucous membranes and increase nasal secretions if applied intranasally; prolonged use may result in overgrowth of nonsusceptible organisms
Precautions Use with caution in patients with impaired renal function and in burn patients
Adverse Reactions
  Dermatologic: Pruritus, rash, erythema, dry skin
  Local: Burning, stinging, pain, tenderness, local edema
Stability Do not mix with Aquaphor®, coal tar solution, or salicylic acid
Mechanism of Action Binds to bacterial isoleucyl transfer-RNA synthetase preventing isoleucine incorporation resulting in the inhibition of protein and RNA synthesis
Pharmacokinetics
  Absorption: Following topical administration, penetrates the outer layers of the skin; systemic absorption is minimal through intact skin
  Protein binding: 95%
  Metabolism: Extensive in the liver and skin to monic acid
  Half-life: 17-36 minutes
  Elimination: Metabolite is excreted in urine
Usual Dosage Children and Adults:
  Intranasal (eliminate nasal carriage of *S. aureus*): Apply small amount 2-4 times/day for 5-14 days
  Topical: Apply small amount 3-5 times/day for 5-14 days
Administration For topical use only; do not apply into the eye
Additional Information Contains polyethylene glycol vehicle
Dosage Forms Ointment, topical: 2% (15 g)
References

  Blumer JL, Lemon E, O'Horo J, et al, "Changing Therapy for Skin and Soft Tissue Infections in Children: Have We Come Full Circle?" *Pediatr Infect Dis J*, 1987, 6(1):117-22.
  Britton JW, Fajardo JE, and Krafte-Jacobs B, "Comparison of Mupirocin and Erythromycin in the Treatment of Impetigo," *J Pediatr*, 1990, 117(5):827-9.
  Goldfarb J, Crenshaw D, O'Horo J, et al, "Randomized Clinical Trial of Topical Mupirocin Versus Oral Erythromycin for Impetigo," *Antimicrob Agents Chemother*, 1988, 32(12):1780-3.

- **Murine® Ear [OTC]** *see* Carbamide Peroxide *on page 178*
- **Muro 128® [OTC]** *see* Sodium Chloride *on page 906*

Muromonab-CD3 (myoo roe MOE nab see dee three)

U.S. Brand Names Orthoclone OKT®3

Synonyms Monoclonal Antibody; OKT3

Therapeutic Category Immunosuppressant Agent

Generic Available No

Use Treatment of acute allograft rejection in renal transplant patients; effective in reversing acute hepatic, cardiac, and bone marrow transplant rejection episodes resistant to conventional treatment

Pregnancy Risk Factor C

Contraindications Hypersensitivity to OKT3 or any Murine® product; patients in fluid overload or those with >3% weight gain within 1 week prior to start of OKT3

Warnings May result in an increased susceptibility to infection; severe pulmonary edema has occurred in patients with fluid overload; first-dose effect (flu-like symptoms, anaphylactic-type reaction) may occur within 30 minutes to 6 hours, up to 24 hours after the first dose. Cardiopulmonary resuscitation may be needed. Methylprednisolone sodium succinate given prior to first OKT3 dose and I.V. hydrocortisone sodium succinate given 30 minutes after administration are strongly recommended to decrease the incidence of reactions to the first dose.

Precautions Dosage of concomitant immunosuppressants should be reduced by 50%, and cyclosporine discontinued or decreased by 50% during OKT3 therapy (see Additional Information); maintenance immunosuppression and cyclosporine should be resumed about 3 days before stopping OKT3 to protect against rebound rejection

Adverse Reactions

Cardiovascular: Tachycardia, hypertension, hypotension, perioral and peripheral cyanosis

Central nervous system: Aseptic meningitis, seizures, headache, pyrexia, confusion

Dermatologic: Pruritus, rash

Gastrointestinal: Diarrhea, nausea, vomiting

Neuromuscular & skeletal: Arthralgia, tremor, myalgia

Ocular: Photophobia

Renal: Elevated BUN, elevated serum creatinine

Respiratory: Dyspnea, chest pain, tightness, wheezing, pulmonary edema

Miscellaneous: Flu-like symptoms (ie, fever, chills), anaphylactic-type reactions

Stability Store in refrigerator; do not freeze or shake; OKT3 left out of the refrigerator for more than 4 hours must not be used

Mechanism of Action Coats the circulating T lymphocytes subjecting these cells to opsonization by the reticuloendothelial system; modulates the T lymphocyte antigen receptor CD3 complex which results in the removal of all CD3 molecules from the cell surface so that the cell lacks the ability to function as a T lymphocyte

Pharmacodynamics

Distribution: V_d is closely related to the apparent volume of distribution for albumin

Half-life: 18 hours

Elimination: Binds to T lymphocytes with resultant opsonization and removal by the reticuloendothelial system

Usual Dosage I.V. (refer to individual protocols):

Note: Children and Adults: Methylprednisolone sodium succinate 1 mg/kg I.V. given 2-6 hours prior to first OKT3 administration and I.V. hydrocortisone sodium succinate 50-100 mg given 30 minutes after administration are strongly recommended to decrease the incidence of reactions to the first dose; patient temperature should not exceed 37.8°C (100°F) at time of administration

Children <12 years: 0.1 mg/kg/day once daily for 10-14 days **or** patients ≤30 kg: 2.5 mg once daily for 10-14 days; patients >30 kg: 5 mg once daily for 10-14 days

Children ≥12 years and Adults: 5 mg/day once daily for 10-14 days

Administration Parenteral: Filter each dose through a low protein-binding 0.22 micron filter (Millex GV) before administration; administer I.V. push over 1 minute at a final concentration of 1 mg/mL

Monitoring Parameters Chest x-ray, weight gain, CBC with differential, vital signs (blood pressure, temperature, pulse, respiration) and immunologic monitoring of T cells, serum levels of OKT3, CD3+ cell count

Reference Range Mean serum trough levels rise during the first 3 days, then average 0.9 µg/mL on days 3-14; if serum trough OKT3 concentrations are maintained at 1 µg/mL, then CD3 counts remain low

Nursing Implications Inform patient of expected first dose effects which may include fever, chills, chest tightness, wheezing, nausea, vomiting, and diarrhea; first-dose reaction usually starts 40-60 minutes after the injection and lasts for several hours; first-dose effects are markedly reduced with subsequent doses; monitor patient closely for 48 hours after the first dose; corticosteroids are recommended; acetaminophen and antihistamines can be given concomitantly with OKT3 to reduce early reactions

Additional Information Recommend decreasing dose of prednisone to 0.5 mg/kg, azathioprine to 0.5 mg/kg (approximate 50% decrease in dose), and discontinuing cyclosporine or decreasing cyclosporine dose by 50% while patient is receiving OKT3

Dosage Forms Injection: 5 mg/5 mL

References
Ettenger RB, Marik JL, Rosenthal JT, et al, "OKT₃ for Rejection Reversal in Pediatric Renal Transplantation," *Clin Transpl*, 1988, 2:180-4.

Hooks MA, Wade CS, and Millikan WJ Jr, "Muromonab CD-3: A Review of Its Pharmacology, Pharmacokinetics, and Clinical Use in Transplantation," *Pharmacotherapy*, 1991, 11(1):26-37.

Niaudet P, Murcia I, Jean G, et al, "A Comparative Trial of OKT₃ and Antilymphocyte Serum in the Preventive Treatment of Rejection After Kidney Transplantation in Children," *Ann Pediatr Paris*, 1990, 37(2):83-5.

Todd PA and Brogden RN, "Muromonab CD3 A Review of Its Pharmacology and Therapeutic Potential," *Drugs*, 1989, 37(6):871-99.

♦ **Muse® Pellet** *see* Alprostadil *on page 56*
♦ **Mustargen® Hydrochloride** *see* Mechlorethamine *on page 621*
♦ **Mustine** *see* Mechlorethamine *on page 621*
♦ **Mutamycin®** *see* Mitomycin *on page 678*
♦ **Myambutol®** *see* Ethambutol *on page 406*
♦ **Mycelex®-G Topical** *see* Clotrimazole *on page 259*
♦ **Mycelex®-G Vaginal [OTC]** *see* Clotrimazole *on page 259*
♦ **Mycelex® Troche** *see* Clotrimazole *on page 259*
♦ **Mycifradin® Sulfate** *see* Neomycin *on page 703*
♦ **Mycinettes® [OTC]** *see* Benzocaine *on page 135*
♦ **Mycitracin® [OTC]** *see* Neomycin, Polymyxin B, and Bacitracin *on page 707*
♦ **Mycobutin®** *see* Rifabutin *on page 875*

Mycophenolate (mye koe FEN oh late)

U.S. Brand Names CellCept®
Synonyms RS61443
Therapeutic Category Immunosuppressant Agent
Generic Available No

Use Immunosuppressant agent used in conjunction with other immunosuppressive therapies (eg, cyclosporine and corticosteroids with or without antithymocyte induction) for the prophylaxis of organ rejection in patients receiving allogeneic renal, hepatic, or cardiac transplants; add-on immunosuppressant agent that is typically used in place of azathioprine in combination regimens for the treatment of refractory acute kidney graft rejection; use of mycophenolate is also being studied in bone marrow transplant patients

Pregnancy Risk Factor C

Contraindications Hypersensitivity to mycophenolate mofetil, mycophenolic acid, polysorbate 80 (I.V. formulation), or any component

Warnings Immunosuppression with mycophenolate may result in an increased susceptibility to infection and an increased risk of developing lymphomas and other malignancies, particularly of the skin. Mycophenolate has been shown to have teratogenic effects in animals; in women of childbearing potential, effective contraception must be initiated before starting mycophenolate therapy and continued for 6 weeks after it has been discontinued.

Precautions Use with caution in patients with active serious digestive disease and in patients with renal impairment; modify dosage in patients with severe chronic renal impairment (GFR <25 mL/minute/1.73 m² outside of the immediate post-transplant period) and in patients with neutropenia; the oral suspension contains aspartame which is a source of phenylalanine; use with caution in patients with phenylketonuria

Adverse Reactions
Cardiovascular: Hypertension, chest pain
Central nervous system: Insomnia, dizziness, fever, headache
Dermatologic: Rash, acne
Endocrine & metabolic: Hypercholesterolemia, hypophosphatemia, hypokalemia, hyperkalemia, hyperglycemia
Gastrointestinal: Diarrhea, constipation, nausea, vomiting, oral moniliasis, abdominal pain, dyspepsia, GI tract hemorrhage, colitis, pancreatitis
Genitourinary: Hematuria
Hematologic: Leukopenia, neutropenia, anemia, thrombocytopenia
Local: Phlebitis, thrombosis
(Continued)

Mycophenolate *(Continued)*

Neuromuscular & skeletal: Tremor, back pain, myalgia

Renal: Renal tubular necrosis

Respiratory: Dyspnea, cough, pharyngitis, pulmonary fibrosis

Miscellaneous: 1% incidence of lymphoproliferative disease

Drug Interactions Aluminum- and magnesium-containing antacids decrease mycophenolate absorption; cholestyramine decreases mycophenolate bioavailability by 40% (interrupts enterohepatic recirculation of mycophenolic acid); acyclovir and ganciclovir may compete with mycophenolic acid glucuronide (MPAG) for renal tubular secretion resulting in increased concentrations of both drugs and MPAG; drugs which inhibit renal tubular secretion (probenecid) increase mycophenolate and MPAG concentrations; live vaccines (vaccination may be less effective)

Food Interactions Presence of food decreases mycophenolate peak concentration by 40%

Stability Store at room temperature

Suspension: Store reconstituted suspension in refrigerator or at room temperature; stable for 60 days after reconstitution

Injection: Mycophenolate I.V. infusion solution is stable for 12 hours at room temperature after preparation; administration of the infusion solution should be within 4 hours from reconstitution and dilution of the drug

Mechanism of Action Hydrolyzed to form mycophenolic acid (MPA), the active metabolite, which is a potent, noncompetitive reversible inhibitor of inosine monophosphate dehydrogenase (IMPDH) in the purine biosynthesis pathway; inhibition of IMPDH results in a depletion of guanosine triphosphate and deoxyguanosine triphosphate, thereby inhibiting T- and B-cell proliferation, cytotoxic T-cell generation and antibody secretion.

Pharmacokinetics

Absorption: Rapid and extensive

Distribution: Mean V_d (adults): 4 L/kg

Protein binding:

Mycophenolate: 97%

Mycophenolate glucuronide: 82%

Metabolism: Mycophenolate mofetil undergoes hydrolysis to mycophenolic acid (MPA is the active metabolite); MPA is metabolized to mycophenolic acid glucuronide (MPAG is inactive)

Bioavailability: 94% based on MPA; enterohepatic recirculation contributes to MPA concentration; two 500 mg tablets have been shown to be bioequivalent to four 250 mg capsules or 1000 mg of oral suspension

Half-life: 17.9 hours

Time to peak serum concentration: 0.8-1.3 hours

Elimination: 93% of dose recovered in urine, 6% in feces; 87% of mycophenolic acid dose recovered as MPAG in urine; <1% of dose excreted as MPA in urine

Usual Dosage

Oral:

Children: 600 mg/m²/dose twice daily; maximum dose: 2 g/day; **Note:** Limited information regarding mycophenolate use in pediatric patients is currently available in the literature: 32 pediatric patients (14 underwent living donor and 18 receiving cadaveric donor renal transplants) received mycophenolate 8-30 mg/kg/dose orally twice daily with cyclosporine, prednisone, and Atgam® induction. However, pharmacokinetic studies suggest that doses of mycophenolate adjusted to body surface area resulted in AUCs which better approximated those of adults versus doses adjusted for body weight which resulted in lower AUCs in pediatric patients.

Adults:

Renal transplant: 1 g twice daily in combination with corticosteroids and cyclosporine; dosages as high as 3-3.5 g/day were used in clinical trials, but no efficacy advantage was established

Cardiac transplant: 1.5 g twice daily

Hepatic transplant: 1.5 g twice daily

I.V. infusion (administer within 24 hours following transplantation; can be given for up to 14 days; patients should be switched to oral formulation as soon as oral medication is tolerated):

Adults:

Renal transplant: 1 g twice daily

Cardiac transplant: 1.5 g twice daily

Hepatic transplant: 1 g twice daily

Administration

Oral: Administer on an empty stomach; one center has mixed the contents of the capsule in chocolate syrup; mycophenolate suspension can be administered orally or via a nasogastric tube with a minimum size of 8 French; shake suspension well before use

I.V.: Reconstitute vial with D_5W and further dilute to a final concentration of 6 mg/mL using D_5W. Administer by slow I.V. infusion over a period of no less than 2 hours.

Monitoring Parameters CBC, serum glucose (if diabetic)

Patient Information Do not take within 1 hour before or 2 hours after antacids or cholestyramine; maintain adequate hydration. You will be susceptible to infection (avoid crowds and people with infections). Report to physician any chest pain, acute headache or dizziness, respiratory infection symptoms, difficulty breathing, or unusual bleeding or bruising. You may be at increased risk for skin cancer (wear protective clothing and use sunscreen).

Nursing Implications Mycophenolate capsules should not be opened or crushed; avoid inhalation or direct contact of the capsule contents with skin or mucous membranes

Dosage Forms

Capsule, as mofetil: 250 mg

Powder for injection, as mofetil hydrochloride: 500 mg

Suspension, as mofetil: 200 mg/mL

Tablet, as mofetil: 500 mg

Extemporaneous Preparations A 50 mg/mL suspension can be prepared in a vertical flow hood by emptying six 250 mg mycophenolate mofetil capsules into a mortar wetted and triturated with 7.5 mL Ora-Plus® to a smooth paste. Add 15 mL of cherry syrup and triturate to make a final volume of 30 mL. The suspension is stable for 210 days when stored at 5°C, stable for 28 days when stored at 37°C or 25°C, and stable for 11 days when stored at 45°C.

Venkataramanan R, McCombs JR, Zudarnan S, et al, "Stability of Mycophenolate Mofetil as an Extemporaneous Suspension," *Ann Pharmacother*, 1998, 32:755-7.

References

Ettenger R, Warshaw B, Menster M, et al, "Mycophenolate Mofetil in Pediatric Renal Transplantation: A Report of the Ped MMF Study Group." Abstract: 1996, Annual Meeting, ASTP.

Sollinger HW, "Mycophenolate Mofetil for the Prevention of Acute Rejection in Primary Cadaveric Renal Allograft Recipients. U.S. Renal Transplant Mycophenolate Mofetil Study Group," *Transplantation*, 1995, 60:225-32.

♦ **Mycostatin®** *see* Nystatin *on page 729*

♦ **Mydfrin®** *see* Phenylephrine *on page 789*

♦ **Mydriacyl®** *see* Tropicamide *on page 991*

♦ **Mykrox®** *see* Metolazone *on page 659*

♦ **Mylanta® [OTC]** *see* Antacid Preparations *on page 95*

♦ **Mylanta® Calci Tabs Extra Strength [OTC]** *see* Calcium Supplements *on page 167*

♦ **Mylanta® Calci Tabs Ultra [OTC]** *see* Calcium Supplements *on page 167*

♦ **Mylanta® Children's [OTC]** *see* Calcium Supplements *on page 167*

♦ **Mylanta Gas® [OTC]** *see* Simethicone *on page 902*

♦ **Mylanta Gas® Maximum Strength [OTC]** *see* Simethicone *on page 902*

♦ **Mylanta®-II [OTC]** *see* Antacid Preparations *on page 95*

♦ **Myleran®** *see* Busulfan *on page 161*

♦ **Mylicon® [OTC]** *see* Simethicone *on page 902*

♦ **Myotonachol (Can)** *see* Bethanechol *on page 142*

♦ **Mysoline®** *see* Primidone *on page 827*

♦ **Mytussin® [OTC]** *see* Guaifenesin *on page 485*

♦ **Mytussin® AC** *see* Guaifenesin and Codeine *on page 486*

♦ **Mytussin® DM [OTC]** *see* Guaifenesin and Dextromethorphan *on page 487*

♦ **NAC** *see* Acetylcysteine *on page 35*

♦ ***N*-Acetylcysteine** *see* Acetylcysteine *on page 35*

♦ ***N*-Acetyl-L-Cysteine** *see* Acetylcysteine *on page 35*

♦ **N-Acetyl-P-Aminophenol** *see* Acetaminophen *on page 29*

♦ **NaCl** *see* Sodium Chloride *on page 906*

Nadolol (nay DOE lole)

Related Information

Overdose and Toxicology *on page 1222*

U.S. Brand Names Corgard®

(Continued)

Nadolol *(Continued)*

Canadian Brand Names Alti-Nadolol; Apo-Nadol

Therapeutic Category Antianginal Agent; Antiarrhythmic Agent, Class II; Antihypertensive Agent; Antimigraine Agent; Beta-Adrenergic Blocker

Generic Available Yes

Use Treatment of hypertension and angina pectoris; prophylaxis of migraine headaches

Pregnancy Risk Factor C

Contraindications Uncompensated CHF, cardiogenic shock, bradycardia or heart block, bronchial asthma, bronchospasms

Precautions Therapy should not be discontinued abruptly; reduce dosage gradually over a period of 1-2 weeks; increase dosing interval in patients with renal dysfunction; use with caution in patients with diabetes mellitus

Adverse Reactions

Cardiovascular: Persistent bradycardia, orthostatic hypotension, Raynaud's syndrome, CHF, edema

Central nervous system: Fatigue, dizziness

Dermatological: Rash

Gastrointestinal: GI discomfort

Respiratory: Bronchospasm

Drug Interactions Other hypotensive agents, diuretics and phenothiazines may increase hypotensive effects of nadolol; nadolol may enhance neuromuscular blocking agents and will antagonize beta-sympathomimetic drugs; other drug interactions similar to propranolol may occur

Food Interactions Avoid natural licorice (causes sodium and water retention and increases potassium loss)

Mechanism of Action Competitively blocks response to beta-adrenergic stimulation; nonselective beta-blocker

Pharmacodynamics Duration of effect: 24 hours

Pharmacokinetics

Absorption: Oral: 30% to 40%

Distribution: Concentration in human breast milk is 4.6 times higher than serum

Protein-binding: 28%

Half-life, elimination:

Increased half-life with decreased renal function

Infants 3-22 months (n=3): 3.2-4.3 hours

Children 10 years (n=1): 15.7 hours

Children ~15 years (n=1): 7.3 hours

Adults: 10-24 hours

Dialysis: Moderately dialyzable (20% to 50%)

Usual Dosage Oral:

Children: Very limited information (ie, one study) regarding pediatric dosage currently available in literature: The study used oral nadolol to control supraventricular tachycardia (SVT) in 26 children 3 months to 15 years of age. SVT was well controlled in 23 out of 26 children; recommended initial dose: 0.5-1 mg/kg once daily; monitor carefully, gradually increase dose; median dose required: 1 mg/kg/day; maximum dose: 2.5 mg/kg/day.

Adults: Initial: 40 mg once daily; increase gradually; usual dosage: 40-80 mg/day; may need up to 240-320 mg/day; doses as high as 640 mg/day have been used

Dosage adjustment in adults with renal impairment:

Cl_{cr} 10-50 mL/minute: Administer 50% of normal dose

Cl_{cr} <10 mL/minute: Administer 25% of normal dose

Administration Oral: May administer without regard to meals

Monitoring Parameters Blood pressure, heart rate, fluid intake and output, weight

Patient Information Limit alcohol; do not abruptly discontinue; may mask symptoms of hypoglycemia, but sweating may still occur

Dosage Forms Tablet: 20 mg, 40 mg, 80 mg, 120 mg, 160 mg

References

Devlin RG and Duchin KL, "Nadolol in Human Serum and Breast Milk," *Br J Clin Pharmacol*, 1981, 12(3):393-6.

Mehta AV and Chidambaram B, "Efficacy and Safety of Intravenous and Oral Nadolol for Supraventricular Tachycardia in Children," *J Am Coll Cardiol*, 1992, 19(3):630-5.

Mehta AV and Chidambaram B, and Rice PJ, "Pharmacokinetics of Nadolol in Children With Supraventricular Tachycardia," *J Clin Pharmacol*, 1992, 32(1):1023-7.

♦ **Nadopen-V (Can)** *see* Penicillin V Potassium *on page 774*

♦ **Nadostine (Can)** *see* Nystatin *on page 729*

♦ **Nafcil™ Injection** *see* Nafcillin *on page 693*

Nafcillin (naf SIL in)

Related Information
Extravasation Treatment *on page 1085*

U.S. Brand Names Nafcil™ Injection; Nallpen® Injection; Unipen® Injection; Unipen® Oral

Synonyms Ethoxynaphthamido Penicillin

Therapeutic Category Antibiotic, Penicillin (Antistaphylococcal)

Generic Available Yes

Use Treatment of bacterial infections such as osteomyelitis, septicemia, endocarditis, and CNS infections due to susceptible penicillinase-producing strains of *Staphylococcus*

Pregnancy Risk Factor B

Contraindications Hypersensitivity to nafcillin, any component, or penicillins

Warnings Elimination rate will be decreased in neonates; avoid using in neonates during the first 2 weeks of life

Precautions Extravasation of I.V. infusions should be avoided; modification of dosage is necessary in patients with both severe renal and hepatic impairment; use with caution in patients with cephalosporin hypersensitivity

Adverse Reactions
Central nervous system: Fever
Dermatologic: Skin rash
Endocrine & metabolic: Hypokalemia
Gastrointestinal: Nausea, diarrhea
Hematologic: Neutropenia, anemia, eosinophilia
Hepatic: Elevated AST
Local: Pain, thrombophlebitis
Renal: Acute interstitial nephritis (rare), hematuria
Miscellaneous: Hypersensitivity reactions

Drug Interactions Probenecid (decreases rate of nafcillin elimination), oral anticoagulants (may decrease half-life of warfarin), may increase hepatic metabolism of cyclosporine

Food Interactions Food decreases GI absorption

Stability Refrigerate oral suspension after reconstitution, discard after 7 days. Reconstituted nafcillin 250 mg/mL solution for injection is stable for 3 days at room temperature and 7 days when refrigerated; when diluted for I.V. intermittent infusion in D_5W or NS, solution is stable for 24 hours at room temperature and 96 hours when refrigerated; incompatible with aminoglycosides

Mechanism of Action Interferes with bacterial cell wall synthesis during active multiplication by binding to one or more of the penicillin-binding proteins; inhibits the final transpeptidation step of peptidoglycan synthesis causing cell wall death and resultant bactericidal activity against susceptible bacteria

Pharmacokinetics
Absorption: Oral: Poor and erratic
Distribution: Distributes into bile, synovial, pleural, and pericardial fluids and into bone and liver; CSF penetration is poor unless meninges are inflamed; crosses the placenta
Protein binding: 90%
Metabolism: 70% to 90%
Half-life:
Neonates:
<3 weeks: 2.2-5.5 hours
4-9 weeks: 1.2-2.3 hours
Children 1 month to 14 years: 0.75-1.9 hours
Adults with normal renal and hepatic function: 0.5-1.5 hours
Time to peak serum concentration:
Oral: Within 2 hours
I.M.: Within 30-60 minutes
Elimination: Primarily in bile and 10% to 30% in urine as unchanged drug; undergoes enterohepatic recycling
Dialysis: Not dialyzable (0% to 5%)

Usual Dosage
Neonates: I.M., I.V.:
0-4 weeks, <1200 g: 50 mg/kg/day in divided doses every 12 hours
≤7 days:
1200-2000 g: 50 mg/kg/day in divided doses every 12 hours
>2000 g: 75 mg/kg/day in divided doses every 8 hours
>7 days:
1200-2000 g: 75 mg/kg/day in divided doses every 8 hours
(Continued)

Nafcillin *(Continued)*

>2000 g: 100 mg/kg/day in divided doses every 6 hours
Children:
I.M., I.V.:
Mild to moderate infections: 50-100 mg/kg/day in divided doses every 6 hours
Severe infections: 100-200 mg/kg/day in divided doses every 4-6 hours
Maximum dose: 12 g/day
Oral: 50-100 mg/kg/day divided every 6 hours
Adults:
Oral: 250-500 mg every 4-6 hours, up to 1 g every 4-6 hours for more severe infections
I.M.: 500 mg every 4-6 hours
I.V.: 500-2000 mg every 4-6 hours
Dosing adjustment in patients with both severe renal/hepatic impairment: Use lower range of usual dose or reduce dose 33% to 50%

Administration
Oral: Administer on an empty stomach with water 1 hour before or 2 hours after meals
Parenteral:
I.M.: Administer deep I.M. into a large muscle (ie, gluteus maximus) using a solution containing 250 mg/mL
I.V.: Nafcillin may be administered by I.V. push over 5-10 minutes or by I.V. intermittent infusion over 15-60 minutes at a final concentration not to exceed 40 mg/mL; in fluid-restricted patients, a maximum concentration of 100 mg/mL may be administered

Monitoring Parameters Periodic CBC with differential, urinalysis, BUN, serum creatinine, AST, and ALT

Test Interactions False-positive urinary and serum proteins

Nursing Implications Extravasation may cause tissue sloughing and necrosis; hyaluronidase infiltration may help avoid injury

Additional Information Sodium content of 1 g injection: 2.9 mEq

Dosage Forms
Capsule, as sodium: 250 mg
Powder for injection, as sodium: 500 mg, 1 g, 2 g, 4 g, 10 g
Tablet, as sodium: 500 mg

References
Banner W Jr, Gooch WM 3d, Burckart G, et al, "Pharmacokinetics of Nafcillin in Infants With Low Birth Weights," *Antimicrob Agents Chemother,* 1980, 17(4):691-4.

Zenk KE, Dungy CL, and Greene CR, "Nafcillin Extravasation Injury: Use of Hyaluronidase as an Antidote," *Am J Dis Child,* 1981, 135(12):1113-4.

♦ **Nafrine (Can)** *see* Oxymetazoline *on page 749*

♦ **NaHCO₃** *see* Sodium Bicarbonate *on page 904*

Nalbuphine *(NAL byoo feen)*
U.S. Brand Names Nubain®
Therapeutic Category Analgesic, Narcotic; Opiate Partial Agonist
Generic Available Yes
Use Relief of moderate to severe pain
Pregnancy Risk Factor B (D if used for prolonged periods or in high doses at term)
Contraindications Hypersensitivity to nalbuphine or any component
Warnings Some products may contain sulfites; abrupt discontinuation after prolonged use may result in narcotic withdrawal; administration to patients receiving chronic opiates may precipitate narcotic withdrawal
Precautions Reduce dose with hepatic impairment; use with caution in patients with impaired respiration, recent MI, biliary tract surgery, or sulfite sensitivity; may produce respiratory depression; use with caution in patients with a history of drug dependence, head trauma or increased intracranial pressure, decreased hepatic or renal function, pregnancy, or patients suspected to be opioid dependent
Adverse Reactions
Cardiovascular: Hypotension, tachycardia, bradycardia, peripheral vasodilation
Central nervous system: CNS depression, drowsiness, headache, dizziness, sedation, increased ICP
Dermatologic: Urticaria, pruritus, rash
Gastrointestinal: Anorexia, nausea, vomiting, xerostomia, biliary tract spasm
Genitourinary: Urinary tract spasm, urinary retention
Ocular: Blurred vision, miosis
Respiratory: Respiratory depression

Miscellaneous: Histamine release, physical and psychological dependence, narcotic withdrawal in patients receiving opiate agonists chronically

Drug Interactions CNS depressants, alcohol, phenothiazine, tricyclic antidepressants may potentiate adverse effects

Mechanism of Action Binds to opiate receptors in the CNS, causing inhibition of ascending pain pathways, altering the perception of and response to pain; produces generalized CNS depression; opiate antagonistic effect may result from competitive inhibition at the opiate mu receptor

Pharmacodynamics

Onset of action:
I.M., S.C.: Within 15 minutes
I.V.: 2-3 minutes
Peak effect:
I.M.: 30 minutes
I.V.: 1-3 minutes
Duration: 3-6 hours

Pharmacokinetics

Metabolism: In the liver; extensive first-pass metabolism
Protein binding: ~50%
Half-life, terminal:
Children 1-8 years: 0.9 hours
Adults 23-32 years: ~2 hours; range: 3.5-5 hours
Adults 65-90 years: 2.3 hours
Time to peak serum concentration:
I.M.: 30 minutes
I.V.: 1-3 minutes
Elimination: Metabolites primarily in feces (via bile) and in urine; 4% to 7% eliminated unchanged in the urine

Usual Dosage I.M., I.V., S.C.:
Children 1-14 years: Premedication: 0.2 mg/kg; maximum dose: 20 mg/dose
Children: Analgesia: 0.1-0.15 mg/kg every 3-6 hours as needed
Adults: 10 mg/70 kg every 3-6 hours as needed; maximum single-dose: 20 mg; maximum daily dose: 160 mg

Administration Parenteral: I.V.: Administer over 5-10 minutes; larger doses should be administered over 10-15 minutes

Monitoring Parameters Relief of pain, respiratory and mental status, blood pressure

Patient Information Avoid alcohol; may cause drowsiness and impair ability to perform activities requiring mental alertness or physical coordination; may impair judgment; may be habit-forming; will cause withdrawal in patients currently dependent on narcotics

Nursing Implications Observe patient for excessive sedation, respiratory depression, implement safety measures, assist with ambulation; observe for narcotic withdrawal (nausea, vomiting, abdominal cramps, lacrimation, rhinorrhea, piloerection, anxiety, restlessness, increased temperature)

Additional Information Analgesic potency: 1 mg nalbuphine ~1 mg morphine

Dosage Forms Injection, as hydrochloride: 10 mg/mL (1 mL, 10 mL); 20 mg/mL (1 mL, 10 mL)

References
Jaillon P, Gardin ME, Lecocq B, et al, "Pharmacokinetics of Nalbuphine in Infants, Young Healthy Volunteers, and Elderly Patients," *Clin Pharmacol Ther*, 1989, 46(2):226-33.

♦ **Nalcom (Can)** *see* Cromolyn *on page 273*
♦ **Naldecon® Senior DX [OTC]** *see* Guaifenesin and Dextromethorphan *on page 487*
♦ **Naldecon® Senior EX [OTC]** *see* Guaifenesin *on page 485*

Nalidixic Acid (nal i DIKS ik AS id)

U.S. Brand Names NegGram®

Synonyms Nalidixinic Acid

Therapeutic Category Antibiotic, Quinolone

Generic Available Yes

Use Lower urinary tract infections due to susceptible gram-negative organisms including *E. coli*, *Enterobacter*, *Klebsiella*, and *Proteus* (inactive against *Pseudomonas*)

Pregnancy Risk Factor B

Contraindications History of convulsive disorders; hypersensitivity to nalidixic acid or any component; infants <3 months of age; treatment of UTI in febrile infants and young children in whom renal involvement is likely
(Continued)

Nalidixic Acid *(Continued)*

Warnings Use with caution in prepubertal children since nalidixic acid has been shown to cause cartilage degeneration and arthropathy in immature animals; usefulness may be limited by the emergence of bacterial resistance to nalidixic acid during treatment

Precautions Use with caution in patients with impaired hepatic or renal function, patients with G-6-PD deficiency, severe cerebral arteriosclerosis, or respiratory insufficiency

Adverse Reactions

Central nervous system: Malaise, drowsiness, vertigo, confusion, toxic psychosis, convulsions, fever, headache, increased intracranial pressure, chills, depression, insomnia

Dermatologic: Rash, urticaria, pruritus, photosensitivity

Endocrine & metabolic: Metabolic acidosis (in premature infants)

Gastrointestinal: Nausea, vomiting, diarrhea, abdominal pain

Hematologic: Leukopenia, thrombocytopenia, eosinophilia, hemolytic anemia

Hepatic: Hepatotoxicity, cholestatic jaundice

Neuromuscular & skeletal: Myalgia, weakness, arthralgia with joint stiffness, peripheral neuritis

Ocular: Visual disturbances, nystagmus

Drug Interactions Warfarin (increases anticoagulant effect due to displacement of warfarin from albumin binding sites), antacids (decrease nalidixic acid absorption); may increase incidence of severe hemorrhagic necrotic enterocolitis in patients taking melphalan

Mechanism of Action Inhibits DNA topoisomerase in susceptible organisms resulting in inhibition of DNA polymerization at late stages of chromosomal replication and promotion of double-stranded DNA breakage

Pharmacokinetics

Absorption: Rapid and complete from the GI tract

Distribution: Crosses the placenta; appears in breast milk; negligible amounts enter CSF; achieves significant antibacterial concentrations only in the urinary tract

Protein binding: 90%

Metabolism: Partial in the liver to hydroxynalidixic acid (active metabolite)

Half-life: 6-7 hours (increases significantly with renal impairment)

Time to peak serum concentration: 1-2 hours

Elimination: In urine as unchanged drug and 80% as metabolites; small amounts appear in feces

Usual Dosage Oral:

Children >3 months: 55 mg/kg/day divided every 6 hours

Prophylaxis of UTI: 30 mg/kg/day divided every 12 hours

Adults: Initial: 1 g 4 times/day for 2 weeks; then suppressive therapy of 500 mg 4 times/day

Administration Oral: Administer 1 hour before meals; may administer with food to minimize GI upset; shake suspension well before use

Monitoring Parameters Urinalysis, urine culture; CBC, renal and hepatic function tests

Test Interactions False-positive urine glucose with Clinitest®, false increase in urinary VMA

Patient Information Avoid undue exposure to direct sunlight

Additional Information In a study of 31 case-control pairs, short treatment periods (1-2 weeks) with nalidixic acid in children <15 years of age did not cause arthropathies or hamper growth

Dosage Forms

Suspension, oral: 250 mg/5 mL [raspberry flavor] (473 mL)

Tablet: 250 mg, 500 mg, 1 g

References

Nuutinen M, Turtinen J, and Uhari M, "Growth and Joint Symptoms in Children Treated With Nalidixic Acid," *Pediatr Infect Dis J*, 1994, 13(9):798-800.

"Practice Parameter: The Diagnosis, Treatment, and Evaluation of the Initial Urinary Tract Infection in Febrile Infants and Young Children. American Academy of Pediatrics. Committee on Quality Improvement. Subcommittee on Urinary Tract Infection," *Pediatrics*, 1999, 103(4 Pt 1):843-52.

Stutman HR and Marks MI, "Review of Pediatric Antimicrobial Therapies," *Semin Pediatr Infect Dis*, 1991, 2:3-17.

Naloxone (nal OKS one)

Related Information
CPR Pediatric Drug Dosages *on page 1031*

U.S. Brand Names Narcan®

Synonyms *N*-allylnoroxymorphine

Therapeutic Category Antidote for Narcotic Agonists

Generic Available Yes

Use Reverses CNS and respiratory depression in suspected narcotic overdose; neonatal opiate depression; coma of unknown etiology; used as low dose I.V. continuous infusion for the treatment of narcotic-induced pruritus; used investigationally for shock, phencyclidine, and alcohol ingestion

Pregnancy Risk Factor B

Contraindications Hypersensitivity to naloxone or any component

Warnings May precipitate withdrawal symptoms (hypertension, sweating, agitation, irritability, shrill cry, failure to feed) in patients with physical dependence to opiates (including newborns of narcotic dependent mothers)

Precautions Use with caution in patients with chronic cardiac or pulmonary disease or coronary artery disease. Following the use of narcotics during surgery, naloxone may reverse analgesia and increase blood pressure; use with caution and administer in smaller increments to patients suspected to be opioid dependent and in postoperative patients (to avoid large cardiovascular changes)

Adverse Reactions
Cardiovascular: Hypertension, hypotension, tachycardia, ventricular arrhythmias, cardiac arrest
Gastrointestinal: Nausea, vomiting
Miscellaneous: Increased diaphoresis

Stability Protect from light; stable in NS and D_5W at 4 mcg/mL for 24 hours; do not mix with alkaline solutions

Mechanism of Action Competes and displaces narcotics at narcotic receptor sites

Pharmacodynamics
Onset of action:
E.T., I.M., S.C.: Within 2-5 minutes
I.V.: Within 2 minutes
Duration: (20-60 minutes) is shorter than that of most opioids; therefore, repeated doses are usually needed

Pharmacokinetics
Distribution: Crosses the placenta
Metabolism: Primarily by glucuronidation in the liver
Half-life:
Neonates: 1.2-3 hours
Adults: 0.5-1.5 hours (mean: ~1 hour)
Elimination: In urine as metabolites

Usual Dosage
PALS 2000 Guidelines: I.V. (**Note:** May be administered I.M., S.C., or E.T., but onset of action may be delayed, especially if patient has poor perfusion; recommended PALS E.T. doses are 2-10 times the I.V. dose; see also Administration):
For total reversal of narcotic effect: **Note:** Doses may need to be repeated:
Infants and Children ≤ 5 years or ≤20 kg: 0.1 mg/kg
Children >5 years or >20 kg: 2 mg/dose
Alternative dosing to avoid sudden hemodynamic effects from opioid reversal: Use repeated doses of 0.01-0.03 mg/kg

I.M., I.V. (preferred), E.T. (preferred if I.V. route not available), S.C.: **Note:** The dose for pediatric postoperative narcotic reversal is **one-tenth** of the dose used for opiate intoxication:
Opiate intoxication:
Birth (including premature infants) to 5 years or <20 kg: 0.1 mg/kg; repeat every 2-3 minutes if needed; may need to repeat doses every 20-60 minutes
>5 years or ≥20 kg: 2 mg/dose; if no response, repeat every 2-3 minutes; may need to repeat doses every 20-60 minutes
Children and Adults: I.V. continuous infusion: If continuous infusion is required, calculate the initial dosage/hour based on the effective intermittent dose used and duration of adequate response seen; titrate dose; a range of: 2.5-160 mcg/kg/hour has been reported; taper continuous infusion gradually to avoid relapse
Adults: 0.4-2 mg every 2-3 minutes as needed; may need to repeat doses every 20-60 minutes; **Note:** Use 0.1-0.2 mg increments in patients who are opioid dependent and in postoperative patients to avoid large cardiovascular changes
(Continued)

Naloxone *(Continued)*

Postanesthesia narcotic reversal: Infants and Children: **0.01 mg/kg**; may repeat every 2-3 minutes as needed based on response

Treatment of narcotic-induced pruritus: Limited pediatric information is available; one retrospective study reported the following doses: Children and Adolescents 3-20 years (n=30): I.V.: Continuous infusion: Initial: 2 mcg/kg/hour; **Note:** Most initial nonresponders received antihistamines; may increase by 0.5 mcg/kg/hour every few hours if pruritus continues; mean (±SD) dose: 2.3 ±0.68 mcg/kg/hour; monitor closely; doses ≥3 mcg/kg/hour may increase risk for loss of pain control and patients may require an increase in opioid dose (see Vrchoticky, 2000).

Administration

Endotracheal: Dilute to 1-2 mL with NS; PALS Guidelines 2000 recommendations: Dilute to 3-5 mL with NS; follow with several positive-pressure ventilations

Parenteral:

I.V. continuous infusion: Dilute to 4 mcg/mL in D_5W or NS

I.V. push: Administer over 30 seconds as undiluted preparation

Note: I.M. or S.C. administration in hypotensive patients or patients with peripheral vasoconstriction or hypoperfusion may result in erratic or delayed absorption

Monitoring Parameters Respiratory rate, heart rate, blood pressure

Nursing Implications Use of neonatal naloxone (0.02 mg/mL) is no longer recommended because unacceptably high fluid volumes will result, especially in small neonates; the 0.4 mg/mL preparation is available and can be accurately dosed with appropriately sized syringes (1 mL)

Additional Information Contains methyl and propylparabens

Dosage Forms

Injection, as hydrochloride: 0.4 mg/mL (1 mL, 2 mL, 10 mL); 1 mg/mL (2 mL, 10 mL)

Injection, neonatal, as hydrochloride: 0.02 mg/mL (2 mL)

References

American Academy of Pediatrics Committee on Drugs, "Naloxone Dosage and Route of Administration for Infants and Children: Addendum to Emergency Drug Doses for Infants and Children," *Pediatrics*, 1990, 86(3):484-5.

Chamberlain JM and Klein BL, "A Comprehensive Review of Naloxone for the Emergency Physician," *Am J Emerg Med*, 1994, 12(6):650-60.

"Guidelines 2000 for Cardiopulmonary Resuscitation and Emergency Cardiovascular Care, Part 10: Pediatric Advanced Life Support, The American Heart Association in Collaboration With the International Liaison Committee on Resuscitation," *Circulation*, 2000, 102(8 Suppl): I291-342.

"Guidelines 2000 for Cardiopulmonary Resuscitation and Emergency Cardiovascular Care, Part 11: Neonatal Resuscitation, The American Heart Association in Collaboration With the International Liason Committee on Resuscitation," *Circulation*, 2000, 102(8 Suppl): I343-357.

Vrchoticky T, "Naloxone for the Treatment of Narcotic Indiced Pruritus," *Journal of Pediatric Pharmacy Practice*, 2000, 5(2):92-7.

Naphazoline *(naf AZ oh leen)*

U.S. Brand Names AK-Con®; Albalon® Liquifilm®; Clear Eyes® [OTC]; Clear Eyes® ACR [OTC]; Naphcon® [OTC]; Privine® [OTC]; VasoClear® [OTC]; Vasocon®

Canadian Brand Names Diopticon; Naphcon Forte; Red Away

Therapeutic Category Adrenergic Agonist Agent, Ophthalmic; Decongestant, Nasal; Nasal Agent, Vasoconstrictor; Ophthalmic Agent, Vasoconstrictor

Generic Available Yes

Use Topical ocular vasoconstrictor (to soothe, refresh, moisturize, and relieve redness due to minor eye irritation); temporarily relieves nasal congestion associated with rhinitis, sinusitis, hay fever, or the common cold

Pregnancy Risk Factor C

Contraindications Hypersensitivity to naphazoline or any component; narrow-angle glaucoma; prior to peripheral iridectomy (in patients susceptible to angle block)

Warnings Excessive dosage may cause marked sedation in children, particularly infants; some products contain sulfites which may cause hypersensitivity reactions in susceptible individuals

Precautions Rebound congestion may occur with extended use (use no longer than 3-5 days); use with caution in the presence of hypertension, diabetes mellitus, hyperthyroidism, heart disease, coronary artery disease, cerebral arteriosclerosis, or long-standing asthma

Adverse Reactions

Cardiovascular: Systemic cardiovascular stimulation (rare), pallor

Central nervous system: Dizziness, headache, nervousness, anxiety, tenseness, drowsiness, hallucinations, convulsions, CNS depression, prolonged psychosis

Gastrointestinal: Nausea, vomiting

Local: Transient stinging, nasal mucosa irritation, dryness

Ocular: Mydriasis, increased intraocular pressure, blurring of vision, blepharospasm

Respiratory: Respiratory difficulty, sneezing, rebound nasal congestion

Miscellaneous: Diaphoresis

Drug Interactions Anesthetics (discontinue naphazoline prior to use of anesthetics that sensitize the myocardium to sympathomimetics, ie, cyclopropane, halothane); MAO inhibitors, methyldopa, tricyclic antidepressants increase hypertensive response

Mechanism of Action Stimulates alpha-adrenergic receptors in the arterioles of the conjunctiva and the nasal mucosa to produce vasoconstriction

Pharmacodynamics

Onset of action: Following topical administration, decongestion occurs within 10 minutes

Duration: 2-6 hours

Pharmacokinetics Elimination: Not well defined

Usual Dosage

Nasal: Intranasal not recommended for use in children <6 years of age (especially in infants) due to CNS depression; therapy should not exceed 3-5 days

Children 6-12 years: 0.05%, 1 drop or spray every 6 hours if needed

Children >12 years to Adults: 0.05%, 1-2 drops or sprays every 3-6 hours if needed

Ophthalmic: Therapy should generally not exceed 3-4 days; not recommended for use in children <6 years of age due to CNS depression (especially in infants)

Children >6 years and Adults (0.01% to 0.1%): Instill 1-2 drops every 3-4 hours

Administration

Ophthalmic: Instill drops into conjunctival sac of affected eye; finger pressure should be applied to lacrimal sac during and for 1-2 minutes after instillation to decrease risk of absorption and systemic reactions; avoid contact of bottle tip with skin or eye

Nasal: Spray or drop medication into one nostril while gently occluding the other; then reverse procedure

Patient Information Discontinue eye drops if visual changes or ocular pain occur

Dosage Forms Solution, as hydrochloride:

Nasal:

Drops (Privine®): 0.05% (25 mL)

Spray (Privine®): 0.05% (20 mL, 480 mL)

Ophthalmic:

Clear Eyes®, Clear Eyes® ACR, Naphcon®: 0.012% (6 mL, 15 mL, 30 mL)

VasoClear®: 0.02% (15 mL)

AK-Con®, Albalon®, Vasocon®: 0.1% (15 mL)

♦ **Naphcon® [OTC]** see Naphazoline on page 698

♦ **Naphcon Forte (Can)** see Naphazoline on page 698

♦ **Naprelan®** see Naproxen on page 699

♦ **Naprosyn®** see Naproxen on page 699

Naproxen (na PROKS en)

Related Information

Carbohydrate and Alcohol Content of Liquid Medications for Use in Patients Receiving Ketogenic Diets on page 1258

Overdose and Toxicology on page 1222

U.S. Brand Names Aleve® [OTC]; Anaprox®; Anaprox® DS; EC-Naprosyn®; Naprelan®; Naprosyn®

Canadian Brand Names Apo-Napro-Na; Apo-Naproxen; Naxen; Novo-Naprox; Nu-Naprox; Synflex

Therapeutic Category Analgesic, Non-narcotic; Anti-inflammatory Agent; Antipyretic; Nonsteroidal Anti-inflammatory Drug (NSAID), Oral

Generic Available Yes

Use Management of inflammatory disease and rheumatoid disorders (including juvenile rheumatoid arthritis); acute gout; mild to moderate pain; dysmenorrhea; fever

Pregnancy Risk Factor B (D in 3rd trimester)

Contraindications Hypersensitivity to naproxen, any component, aspirin, or other NSAIDs

Precautions Use with caution in patients with GI disease, cardiac disease, renal or hepatic impairment, and patients receiving anticoagulants

Adverse Reactions

Cardiovascular: Edema

Central nervous system: Fatigue, drowsiness, vertigo, headache

Dermatologic: Pruritus, rash; pseudoporphyria (ie, increased skin fragility and blistering with scarring in sun-exposed skin), incidence: 12% in naproxen-treated children with JRA (discontinue therapy if this occurs)

(Continued)

Naproxen *(Continued)*

Gastrointestinal: Abdominal discomfort, nausea, heartburn, constipation, vomiting, GI bleed, ulcers, perforation

Hematologic: Thrombocytopenia, inhibits platelet aggregation, prolongs bleeding time, agranulocytosis

Hepatic: Hepatitis

Ocular: Visual disturbances

Otic: Tinnitus

Renal: Renal dysfunction

Drug Interactions Cytochrome P-450 isoenzyme CYP2C8 (5-hydroxylation), CYP2C9 (5-hydroxylation), and CYP2C18 substrate

Naproxen may increase serum concentrations of methotrexate and decrease the effects of furosemide; may decrease antihypertensive effects of ACE inhibitors or angiotensin II antagonists; aspirin may decrease and probenecid may increase naproxen serum concentrations; drug interactions similar to other NSAIDs may also occur; other GI irritants (eg, oral potassium supplements) may increase GI adverse effects

Mechanism of Action Inhibits prostaglandin synthesis by decreasing the activity of the enzyme, cyclo-oxygenase, which results in decreased formation of prostaglandin precursors

Pharmacokinetics

Absorption: Oral: Almost 100%

Distribution: Crosses the placenta; ~1% distributed into breast milk

Protein binding: 99%

Metabolism: In the liver

Half-life, elimination: Children: Range: 8-17 hours

Children 8-14 years: 8-10 hours

Adults: 10-20 hours

Time to peak serum concentration: Within 1-2 hours for naproxen sodium; within 2-4 hours for naproxen

Elimination: 10% excreted unchanged in the urine

Usual Dosage Oral as naproxen:

Children >2 years:

Analgesia: 5-7 mg/kg/dose every 8-12 hours

Inflammatory disease: Usual: 10-15 mg/kg/day in 2 divided doses; range: 7-20 mg/kg/day; maximum dose: 1000 mg/day

Adults:

Rheumatoid arthritis, osteoarthritis, and ankylosing spondylitis: 500-1000 mg/day in 2 divided doses

Acute gout: 250 mg every 8 hours

Mild to moderate pain or dysmenorrhea: Initial: 500 mg, then 250 mg every 6-8 hours; maximum dose: 1250 mg/day

Administration Oral: Administer with food, milk, or antacids to decrease GI adverse effects; shake suspension well before use

Monitoring Parameters CBC, BUN, serum creatinine, liver enzymes, occult blood loss, periodic ophthalmologic exams, hemoglobin

Patient Information Avoid alcohol; may cause drowsiness and impair ability to perform activities requiring mental alertness or physical coordination; children with JRA: Protect skin from sun; use sunscreen, wide-brimmed hats, etc

Additional Information Naproxen sodium 220 mg = 200 mg base; naproxen sodium 550 mg = 500 mg base; naproxen sodium 275 mg = 250 mg base

Dosage Forms Sodium content is in brackets

Suspension, oral: 125 mg/5 mL [0.34 mEq/mL] [orange-pineapple flavor] (480 mL)

Tablet (Naprosyn®): 250 mg, 375 mg, 500 mg

Tablet, delayed release, enteric coated (EC-Naprosyn®): 375 mg, 500 mg

Tablet, as sodium

Aleve®: 220 mg [0.87 mEq] (200 mg base)

Anaprox®: 275 mg [1 mEq] (250 mg base)

Anaprox® DS: 550 mg [2 mEq] (500 mg base)

Tablet, as sodium, extended release (Naprelan®): 421.5 mg (375 mg base); 550 mg (500 mg base)

References

Berde C, Ablin A, Glazer J, et al, "American Academy of Pediatrics Report of the Subcommittee on Disease-Related Pain in Childhood Cancer," *Pediatrics*, 1990, 86(5 Pt 2):818-25.

Lang BA and Finlayson LA, "Naproxen-Induced Pseudoporphyria in Patients With Juvenile Rheumatoid Arthritis," *J Pediatr*, 1994, 124(4):639-42.

Wells TG, Mortensen ME, Dietrich A, et al, "Comparison of the Pharmacokinetics of Naproxen Tablets and Suspension in Children," *J Clin Pharmacol*, 1994, 34(1):30-3.

♦ **Narcan**® *see Naloxone on page 697*
♦ **Narcotic Analgesics Comparison** *see page 1070*
♦ **Nasacort**® *see Triamcinolone on page 979*
♦ **Nasacort**® **AQ** *see Triamcinolone on page 979*
♦ **NaSal**™ **[OTC]** *see Sodium Chloride on page 906*
♦ **Nasalcrom**® **[OTC]** *see Cromolyn on page 273*
♦ **Nasalide**® *see Flunisolide on page 438*
♦ **Nasal Moist**® **[OTC]** *see Sodium Chloride on page 906*
♦ **Nasal Relief**® **[OTC]** *see Oxymetazoline on page 749*
♦ **Nasal Sinus Relief (Can)** *see Pseudoephedrine on page 852*
♦ **Nasarel**® *see Flunisolide on page 438*
♦ **Nascobal**® *see Cyanocobalamin on page 277*
♦ **Natulan (Can)** *see Procarbazine on page 832*
♦ **Natural Fiber Laxative**® **[OTC]** *see Psyllium on page 853*
♦ **Natural Lung Surfactant** *see Beractant on page 138*
♦ **Nature's Bounty**® **Vitamin E** *see Vitamin E on page 1014*
♦ **Nauseatol (Can)** *see Dimenhydrinate on page 339*
♦ **Navane**® *see Thiothixene on page 956*
♦ **Naxen (Can)** *see Naproxen on page 699*
♦ **Nebcin**® *see Tobramycin on page 963*
♦ **NebuPent**™ **Inhalation** *see Pentamidine on page 776*

Nedocromil (ne doe KROE mil)

Related Information
Asthma Guidelines *on page 1210*
U.S. Brand Names Alocril™; Tilade®
Therapeutic Category Antiallergic, Ophthalmic; Antiasthmatic; Inhalation, Miscellaneous
Generic Available No
Use
Aerosol: Maintenance therapy in patients with mild to moderate asthma
Ophthalmic: Treatment of itching associated with allergic conjunctivitis
Pregnancy Risk Factor B
Contraindications Hypersensitivity to nedocromil or any component
Warnings If systemic or inhaled steroid therapy is at all reduced, monitor patients carefully; nedocromil is **not** a bronchodilator and, therefore, should not be used for reversal of acute bronchospasm
Precautions Refrain from wearing contact lenses while exhibiting the signs and symptoms of allergic conjunctivitis
Adverse Reactions
Cardiovascular: Chest pain
Central nervous system: Dizziness, dysphonia, headache, fatigue
Dermatologic: Rash
Gastrointestinal: Nausea, vomiting, dyspepsia, diarrhea, abdominal pain, xerostomia, dysgeusia, unpleasant taste
Hepatic: Increased ALT
Neuromuscular and skeletal: Arthritis, tremor
Ocular: Burning, irritation, stinging, conjunctivitis, eye redness, photophobia
Respiratory: Cough, pharyngitis, rhinitis, bronchitis, upper respiratory infection, bronchospasm, increased sputum production, pneumonitis with eosinophilia (PIE syndrome)
Stability Store at room temperature; do not freeze
Mechanism of Action Inhibits the activation of and mediator release from a variety of inflammatory cell types associated with asthma including eosinophils, neutrophils, macrophages, mast cells, monocytes, and platelets; it inhibits the release of histamine, leukotrienes, and slow-reacting substance of anaphylaxis; it inhibits the development of early and late bronchoconstriction responses to inhaled antigen
Pharmacodynamics Inhalation: Duration of effect: 2 hours; maximum therapeutic benefit is seen after at least 1 week of therapy
Pharmacokinetics
Absorption: Systemic: Inhalation: 7% to 9%; ophthalmic: <4%
Protein binding, plasma: 89%
Elimination: Excreted unchanged in urine 70%; feces 30%
(Continued)

Nedocromil *(Continued)*

Usual Dosage

Inhalation: Children ≥6 years and Adults: 2 inhalations 4 times/day; may reduce dosage to 2-3 times/day once desired clinical response to initial dose is observed

Ophthalmic: Children ≥3 years and Adults: 1-2 drops in each eye twice daily throughout the period of exposure to allergen

Administration

Oral inhalation: Shake well before use; must be primed by 3 actuations prior to first use; if canister remains unused for >7 days, reprime with 3 actuations; discard canister after 104 actuations

Ophthalmic: Instill drops into conjunctival sac; avoid contact of bottle tip with skin or eye

Additional Information Has no known therapeutic systemic activity when delivered by inhalation

Dosage Forms

Aerosol, as sodium (Tilade®): 1.75 mg/activation (16.2 g)

Solution as sodium, ophthalmic (Alocril™): 2% (5 mL)

♦ **NegGram®** *see* Nalidixic Acid *on page 695*

Nelfinavir *(nel FIN a veer)*

Related Information

Adult and Adolescent HIV *on page 1166*

Pediatric HIV *on page 1162*

U.S. Brand Names Viracept®

Therapeutic Category Antiretroviral Agent; HIV Agents (Anti-HIV Agents); Protease Inhibitor

Use Treatment of HIV infection in combination with other antiretroviral agents. (**Note:** Current preferred HIV regimens consist of **three** antiretroviral agents)

Pregnancy Risk Factor B

Contraindications Hypersensitivity to nelfinavir or any component

Warnings Avoid use of powder formulation in patients with phenylketonuria since it contains 11.2 mg phenylalanine per gram of powder; due to potential serious and life-threatening drug interactions, the following drugs should not be coadministered with nelfinavir: terfenadine, astemizole, cisapride, triazolam, midazolam, ergot derivatives, amiodarone, or quinidine; concurrent use with some anticonvulsants may significantly limit nelfinavir's effectiveness; spontaneous bleeding episodes have been reported in patients with hemophilia A and B; new onset diabetes mellitus, exacerbations of diabetes and hyperglycemia have been reported in HIV-infected patients receiving protease inhibitors

Precautions Use caution in patients with hepatic insufficiency since nelfinavir is metabolized in the liver and excreted predominantly in the feces

Adverse Reactions

Cardiovascular: Hypertension

Central nervous system: Decreased concentration, anxiety, depression, dizziness, emotional lability, hyperkinesia, insomnia, migraine, seizures, sleep disorder, somnolence, suicide ideation, fever, headache, asthenia, malaise

Dermatologic: Rash, pruritus, urticaria, diaphoresis

Endocrine & metabolic: Hyperlipemia, hyperuricemia; rare: hyperglycemia, diabetes, ketoacidosis; changes in the distribution of body fat

Gastrointestinal: Diarrhea (30%), nausea, flatulence, abdominal pain, anorexia, dyspepsia, epigastric pain, mouth ulceration, GI bleeding, pancreatitis, vomiting

Genitourinary: Kidney calculus, sexual dysfunction

Hematologic: Anemia, leukopenia, thrombocytopenia; rare: spontaneous bleeding episodes in hemophiliacs

Hepatic: Hepatitis, elevated liver function tests

Neuromuscular & skeletal: Weakness, arthralgia, arthritis, cramps, myalgia, myasthenia, myopathy, paresthesia, back pain

Ocular: Acute iritis

Respiratory: Dyspnea, pharyngitis, rhinitis, sinusitis

Drug Interactions Nelfinavir inhibits the metabolism and increases the levels of cisapride, terfenadine, astemizole, amiodarone, quinidine, cyclosporine, tacrolimus, sildenafil, ergot derivatives, midazolam, and triazolam; nelfinavir increases rifabutin plasma AUC by 207% so reduce rifabutin dose by 50% when coadministering with nelfinavir; rifampin decreases nelfinavir plasma AUC by ~82% (concurrent use not recommended); phenobarbital, phenytoin, and carbamazepine decrease nelfinavir concentration; ketoconazole, indinavir, and ritonavir increase nelfinavir concentration; nelfinavir decreases hormone levels of oral contraceptives (ethinyl estradiol, norethindrone); nelfinavir increases levels of saquinavir and indinavir; coadministration with delavirdine increases nelfinavir concentrations by twofold and decreases delavirdine concentrations by 50%; if coadministered with didanosine, administer nelfinavir 2 hours before or 1 hour after didanosine

Food Interactions Administer with food to increase absorption; do not administer with acidic food or juice (ie, orange juice, apple juice, applesauce) since the combination may result in a bitter taste

Stability Store at room temperature

Mechanism of Action A protease inhibitor which acts on an enzyme late in the HIV replication process after the virus has entered into the cell's nucleus preventing cleavage of the gag-pol protein precursors resulting in the production of immature, noninfectious virions; cross-resistance with other protease inhibitors is possible

Pharmacokinetics

Absorption: AUC is two- to threefold higher under fed conditions versus fasting

Distribution: V_d: 2-7 L/kg

Protein binding: 98%

Metabolism: Via multiple cytochrome P-450 isoforms including CYP3A4 to inactive and an active metabolite which has comparable activity to the parent drug

Half-life: 3.5-5 hours

Time to peak serum concentration: 2-4 hours

Elimination: 98% to 99% excreted in feces (78% as metabolites and 22% as unchanged nelfinavir); 1% to 2% excreted in urine

Usual Dosage Oral:

Neonates: Investigational, under study in PACTG 353: 40 mg/kg/dose twice daily

Children and Adolescents (early puberty, Tanner I-II): 20-30 mg/kg/dose 3 times/day (some experts administer a minimum dose of 30 mg/kg/dose 3 times/day); maximum dose: 750 mg/dose 3 times/day

Adolescents (late puberty, Tanner V) and Adults: 750 mg 3 times/day or 1250 mg/dose twice daily

Administration Administer with a meal or light snack to optimize absorption; do not mix with any acidic food or juice because of resulting bitter taste; if patient is unable to swallow tablets, consider using oral powder formulation mixed in small amount of water, milk, formula, dietary supplementation, ice cream, or pudding; do not store mixture for more than 6 hours; tablet can be readily dissolved in water to produce a dispersion that can be mixed with milk or chocolate milk or tablets can be crushed and administered with pudding; if coadministered with didanosine, nelfinavir should be administered 2 hours before or 1 hour after didanosine

Monitoring Parameters Liver function tests, blood glucose levels, CBC with diff, CD4 cell count, plasma levels of HIV RNA

Patient Information Use an alternative method of contraception to birth control pills during nelfinavir therapy. If a nelfinavir dose is missed, take the dose as soon as possible and then return to the normal schedule. However, if a dose is skipped, the patient should not double the next dose.

Nursing Implications Do not add water to bottles of oral powder; a special scoop is provided with powder for measuring purposes. If diarrhea occurs, it may be treated with an antimotility agent like loperamide

Dosage Forms

Powder for oral suspension (200 mg per 1 level teaspoon): 50 mg/g or 50 mg per 1 level scoop (144 g), contains 11.2 mg phenylalanine/g powder

Tablet: 250 mg

References

McDonald CK and Kuritzkes DR, "Human Immunodeficiency Virus Type I Protease Inhibitors," *Arch Intern Med*, 1997, 157(9):951-9.

Working Group on Antiretroviral Therapy and Medical Management of HIV-Infected Children, "Guidelines for the Use of Antiretroviral Agents in Pediatric HIV Infection," January 7, 2000, http://www.hivatis.org.

♦ **Nembutal**® *see* Pentobarbital *on page 779*
♦ **Neo-Calglucon**® **[OTC]** *see* Calcium Supplements *on page 167*
♦ **Neo-Cultol**® **[OTC]** *see* Mineral Oil *on page 675*
♦ **Neo-fradin**® *see* Neomycin *on page 703*
♦ **Neoloid**® **[OTC]** *see* Castor Oil *on page 186*
♦ **Neomixin**® *see* Neomycin, Polymyxin B, and Bacitracin *on page 707*

Neomycin (nee oh MYE sin)

Related Information

Emetogenic Potential of Single Chemotherapeutic Agents *on page 1129*

Overdose and Toxicology *on page 1222*

U.S. Brand Names Mycifradin® Sulfate; Neo-fradin®; Neo-Tabs®

(Continued)

Neomycin *(Continued)*

Therapeutic Category Ammonium Detoxicant; Antibiotic, Aminoglycoside; Antibiotic, Topical; Hyperammonemia Agent

Generic Available Yes

Use Administered orally to prepare GI tract for surgery; treat minor skin infections; treat diarrhea caused by *E. coli*; adjunct in the treatment of hepatic encephalopathy

Pregnancy Risk Factor C

Contraindications Hypersensitivity to neomycin or any component; patients with intestinal obstruction

Warnings Neomycin is more toxic than other aminoglycosides when given parenterally; **do not administer parenterally**; topical neomycin is a contact sensitizer with sensitivity occurring in 5% to 15% of patients treated with the drug; systemic absorption can occur when neomycin is utilized for irrigation of wounds or surgical sites

Precautions Use with caution in patients with renal impairment, pre-existing hearing impairment, neuromuscular disorders; modify dosage in patients with renal impairment

Adverse Reactions

Dermatologic: Contact dermatitis, erythema, rash, urticaria

Gastrointestinal: Nausea, vomiting, diarrhea, colitis, malabsorption

Local: Burning

Neuromuscular & skeletal: Neuromuscular blockade

Ocular: Contact conjunctivitis

Otic: Ototoxicity

Renal: Nephrotoxicity

Miscellaneous: Candidiasis

Drug Interactions Oral neomycin may potentiate the effects of oral anticoagulants; may decrease GI absorption of digoxin and methotrexate; synergistic effects seen with penicillins; increase adverse effects with other neurotoxic, ototoxic or nephrotoxic drugs

Stability Reconstituted neomycin solution is stable for 7 days when refrigerated

Mechanism of Action Interferes with bacterial protein synthesis by binding to 30S ribosomal subunits

Pharmacokinetics

Absorption: Poor orally (3%) or percutaneously; readily absorbed through denuded or abraded skin and body cavities

Distribution: V_d: 0.36 L/kg

Half-life: 2-3 hours (age and renal function dependent)

Time to peak serum concentration:

I.M.: Within 2 hours

Oral: 1-4 hours

Elimination: In urine (30% to 50% as unchanged drug); 97% of an oral dose eliminated unchanged in feces

Dialysis: Dialyzable (50% to 100%)

Usual Dosage

Neonates: Oral: Diarrhea: 50 mg/kg/day divided every 6 hours

Children: Oral: 50-100 mg/kg/day in divided doses every 6-8 hours

Preoperative bowel antisepsis: 90 mg/kg/day divided every 4 hours for 2 days; or 25 mg/kg at 1, 2, and 11 PM on the day preceding surgery as an adjunct to mechanical cleansing of the intestine and in combination with erythromycin base

Hepatic coma: 2.5-7 g/m²/day divided every 4-6 hours for 5-6 days not to exceed 12 g/day

Diarrhea caused by enteropathogenic *E. coli*: 50 mg/kg/day divided every 6 hours for 2-3 days

Children and Adults: Topical: Apply ointment 1-3 times/day; topical solutions containing 0.1% to 1% neomycin have been used for irrigation

Adults: Oral: 500-2000 mg every 6-8 hours

Preoperative bowel antisepsis: 1 g each hour for 4 doses then 1 g every 4 hours for 5 doses; or 1 g at 1 PM, 2 PM, and 11 PM with oral erythromycin on day preceding surgery as an adjunct to mechanical cleansing of the bowel; or 6 g/day divided every 4 hours for 2-3 days

Hepatic coma: 4-12 g/day divided every 4-6 hours

Diarrhea caused by enteropathogenic *E. coli*: 3 g/day divided every 6 hours

Monitoring Parameters Renal function tests

Patient Information Notify physician if ringing in the ears, hearing impairment, or dizziness occurs

Dosage Forms
Cream, as sulfate: 0.5% (15 g)
Ointment, topical, as sulfate: 0.5% (15 g, 30 g, 120 g)
Powder, micronized, as sulfate: For prescription compounding
Solution, oral, as sulfate: 125 mg/5 mL (480 mL)
Tablet, as sulfate: 500 mg

References
Feigin RD and Cherry JD, *Textbook of Pediatric Infectious Diseases*, 4th ed, Philadelphia, PA: WB Saunders Co, 1997.

Neomycin and Polymyxin B (nee oh MYE sin & pol i MIKS in bee)

U.S. Brand Names Neosporin® Cream [OTC]; Neosporin® G.U. Irrigant
Synonyms Polymyxin B and Neomycin
Therapeutic Category Antibiotic, Topical; Antibiotic, Urinary Irrigation; Genitourinary Irrigant
Generic Available Yes
Use Short-term use as a continuous irrigant or rinse in the urinary bladder to prevent bacteriuria and gram-negative rod septicemia associated with the use of indwelling catheters; to help prevent infection in minor cuts, scrapes, and burns
Pregnancy Risk Factor C (D if used as GU irrigant)
Contraindications Hypersensitivity to neomycin, polymyxin B, or any component; ophthalmic use; irrigation should be avoided in patients with defects in the bladder mucosa or wall
Warnings Topical neomycin is a contact sensitizer
Precautions Use with caution in patients with impaired renal function, dehydrated patients, burn patients, and patients receiving a high dose for prolonged treatment; use topical cream with caution in infants with diaper rash involving large area of abraded skin
Adverse Reactions
Dermatologic: Contact dermatitis, erythema, rash, urticaria
Genitourinary: Bladder irritation
Local: Burning
Neuromuscular & skeletal: Neuromuscular blockade
Otic: Ototoxicity
Renal: Nephrotoxicity
Stability Store irrigant solution in the refrigerator
Mechanism of Action Neomycin inhibits bacterial protein synthesis by binding to the 30S ribosomal subunits; polymyxin B interacts with phospholipid components in the cytoplasmic membranes of susceptible bacteria disrupting the osmotic integrity of the cell membrane
Pharmacokinetics Absorption: Not absorbed following topical application to intact skin; absorbed through denuded or abraded skin, peritoneum, wounds, or ulcers
Usual Dosage Children and Adults:
Bladder irrigation: 1 mL is added to 1 L of NS with administration rate adjusted to patient's urine output; usually administered via a 3-way catheter (approximately 40 mL/hour); continuous irrigation or rinse of the urinary bladder should not exceed 10 days
Topical: Apply cream 1-4 times/day
Administration
Bladder irrigant: Do not inject irrigant solution; concentrated irrigant solution must be diluted in 1 liter NS before administration; connect irrigation container to the inflow lumen of a 3-way catheter to permit continuous irrigation of the urinary bladder
Topical: Apply a thin layer to the cleansed, dry affected area; may cover with a sterile bandage
Monitoring Parameters Urinalysis, renal function
Patient Information Notify physician if condition worsens or if rash/irritation develops
Additional Information GU irrigant contains methylparaben
Dosage Forms
Cream: Neomycin sulfate 3.5 mg and polymyxin B sulfate 10,000 units per g (0.94 g, 15 g)
Solution, GU irrigant: Neomycin sulfate 40 mg and polymyxin B sulfate 200,000 units per mL (1 mL, 20 mL)

Neomycin, (Bacitracin) Polymyxin B, and Hydrocortisone

(nee oh MYE sin, bas i TRAY sin, pol i MIKS in bee, & hye droe KOR ti sone)
U.S. Brand Names AK-Spore H.C.® Otic; AntibiOtic® Otic; Bacticort® Otic; Cortatrigen® Otic; Cortisporin® Ophthalmic Suspension; Cortisporin® Otic; Cortisporin®
(Continued)

Neomycin, (Bacitracin) Polymyxin B, and Hydrocortisone
(Continued)

Topical Cream; Drotic® Otic; LazerSporin-C® Otic; Octicair® Otic; Ocutricin® HC Otic; Otocort® Otic; Otomycin-HPN® Otic; Otosporin® Otic; PediOtic® Otic

Canadian Brand Names Cortimyxin

Synonyms Bacitracin, Neomycin, Polymyxin B, and Hydrocortisone; Hydrocortisone, Neomycin, (Bacitracin), and Polymyxin B; Polymyxin B, Neomycin, (Bacitracin), and Hydrocortisone

Therapeutic Category Antibacterial, Otic; Antibiotic, Ophthalmic; Antibiotic, Otic; Antibiotic, Topical; Corticosteroid, Ophthalmic; Corticosteroid, Otic; Corticosteroid, Topical

Generic Available Yes

Use Steroid-responsive inflammatory condition for which a corticosteroid is indicated and where bacterial infection or a risk of bacterial infection exists

Pregnancy Risk Factor C

Contraindications Hypersensitivity to hydrocortisone, polymyxin B sulfate, bacitracin, neomycin sulfate, or any component; herpes simplex, vaccinia and varicella; otic use: perforated tympanic membrane

Warnings Neomycin may cause cutaneous and conjunctival sensitization; children are more susceptible to topical corticosteroid-induced hypothalamic pituitary-adrenal axis suppression and Cushing's syndrome

Precautions Use with caution in patients with chronic otitis media and when the integrity of the tympanic membrane is in question

Adverse Reactions

Dermatologic: Contact dermatitis

Local: Itching, pain, stinging, burning, local edema

Ocular: Elevated intraocular pressure, glaucoma, cataracts, conjunctival erythema; blurring of vision (ophthalmic formulation)

Otic: Ototoxicity

Miscellaneous: Sensitization to neomycin, secondary infections

Usual Dosage

Children: Otic: Solution and suspension: 3 drops into affected ear 3-4 times/day

Adults: Otic: Solution and suspension: 4 drops into affected ear 3-4 times/day

Children and Adults:

Topical ointment: Apply thin layer to affected area 2-4 times/day

Ophthalmic:

Ointment: Apply ½" ribbon to inside of lower lid every 3-4 hours until improvement occurs then 1-3 times/day

Suspension: Instill 1-2 drops in the affected eye every 3-4 hours

Administration Shake ophthalmic and otic suspension well before use

Ophthalmic: Avoid contamination of the tip of the eye dropper or ointment tube; solution and suspension: Apply finger pressure to lacrimal sac during and for 1-2 minutes after instillation to decrease risk of absorption and systemic effects

Otic: Drops can be instilled directly into the affected ear, or a cotton wick may be saturated with suspension and inserted in ear canal. Keep wick moist with suspension every 4 hours; wick should be replaced every 24 hours.

Topical: Apply a thin layer to the cleansed, dry affected area; may cover with a sterile bandage

Patient Information Ophthalmic: May cause sensitivity to bright light; may cause temporary blurring of vision or stinging following administration

Additional Information Otic **suspension** is the preferred otic preparation; otic **suspension** can be used for the treatment of infections of mastoidectomy and fenestration cavities caused by susceptible organisms; otic **solution** is used **only** for superficial infections of the external auditory canal (ie, swimmer's ear)

Dosage Forms

Ointment: Neomycin sulfate 5 mg, bacitracin 400 units, polymyxin B sulfate 5000 units and hydrocortisone 10 mg per g (15 g)

Ointment, ophthalmic: Neomycin sulfate 5 mg, bacitracin 400 units, polymyxin B sulfate and hydrocortisone 10 mg per g (3.5 g)

Solution, otic: Neomycin sulfate 5 mg, polymyxin B sulfate 10,000 units, and hydrocortisone 10 mg per mL (10 mL)

Suspension:

Ophthalmic: Neomycin sulfate 5 mg, polymyxin B sulfate 10,000 units and hydrocortisone 10 mg per mL (7.5 mL)

Otic: Neomycin sulfate 5 mg, polymyxin B sulfate 10,000 units and hydrocortisone 10 mg per mL (10 mL)

♦ **Neomycin, Dexamethasone, and Polymyxin B** Polymyxin B, Dexamethasone, and Neomycin *see* Dexamethasone, Neomycin, and Polymyxin B *on page 309*

Neomycin, Polymyxin B, and Bacitracin
(nee oh MYE sin, pol i MIKS in bee, & bas i TRAY sin)

U.S. Brand Names AK-Spore® Ointment; Medi-Quick® Ointment [OTC]; Mycitracin® [OTC]; Neomixin®; Neosporin® Ophthalmic Ointment; Neosporin® Topical Ointment [OTC]; Ocutricin® Ointment; Septa® Ointment [OTC]; Triple Antibiotic®

Canadian Brand Names Neotopic

Synonyms Bacitracin, Neomycin, and Polymyxin B; Polymyxin B, Neomycin, and Bacitracin

Therapeutic Category Antibiotic, Ophthalmic; Antibiotic, Topical

Generic Available Yes

Use Help prevent infection in minor cuts, scrapes and burns; short-term treatment of superficial external ocular infections caused by susceptible organisms

Pregnancy Risk Factor C

Contraindications Hypersensitivity to neomycin, polymyxin B, zinc bacitracin, or any component

Warnings Symptoms of neomycin sensitization include itching, reddening, edema, failure to heal; ophthalmic ointments may retard corneal healing

Precautions Prolonged use may result in overgrowth of nonsusceptible organisms

Adverse Reactions
Local: Rash and hypersensitivity reactions ranging from generalized itching, local edema, and erythema have been reported; contact dermatitis
Ocular: Conjunctival sensitization, blurring of vision (ophthalmic formulation)

Usual Dosage Children and Adults:
Ophthalmic ointment: Instill into the conjunctival sac 1 or more times daily every 3-4 hours for 7-10 days
Topical: Apply 1-3 times/day

Administration
Ophthalmic: Avoid contamination of the tip of the ointment tube
Topical: Apply a thin layer to the cleansed affected area; may cover with a sterile bandage

Patient Information Ophthalmic: May cause sensitivity to bright light; may cause temporary blurring of vision or stinging following administration

Dosage Forms Ointment:
Ophthalmic: Bacitracin 400 units, neomycin sulfate 3.5 mg, and polymyxin B sulfate 10,000 units per g (3.5 g)
Topical: Bacitracin 400 units, neomycin sulfate 3.5 mg, and polymyxin B sulfate 5000 units per g (0.94 g, 2.4 g, 9.6 g, 14.2 g, 15 g, 28.3 g, 30 g)

Neomycin, Polymyxin B, and Prednisolone
(nee oh MYE sin, pol i MIKS in bee, & pred NIS oh lone)

U.S. Brand Names Poly-Pred® Liquifilm®

Synonyms Polymyxin B, Neomycin, and Prednisolone; Prednisolone, Neomycin, and Polymyxin B

Therapeutic Category Antibiotic, Ophthalmic; Corticosteroid, Ophthalmic

Generic Available Yes

Use Used for steroid-responsive inflammatory ocular condition in which bacterial infection or a risk of bacterial ocular infection exists

Pregnancy Risk Factor C

Contraindications Hypersensitivity to neomycin, polymyxin B, prednisolone, or any component; dendritic keratitis, viral disease of the cornea and conjunctiva, mycobacterial infection of the eye, fungal disease of the ocular structure, or after uncomplicated removal of a corneal foreign body

Warnings Symptoms of neomycin sensitization include itching, reddening, edema, or failure to heal

Precautions Prolonged use may result in overgrowth of nonsusceptible organisms, glaucoma, damage to the optic nerve, defects in visual acuity, and cataract formation

Adverse Reactions
Dermatologic: Cutaneous sensitization, skin rash, delayed wound healing
Ocular: Increased intraocular pressure, glaucoma, optic nerve damage, cataracts, conjunctival sensitization
(Continued)

Neomycin, Polymyxin B, and Prednisolone *(Continued)*

Usual Dosage Children and Adults:

Ophthalmic: Instill 1-2 drops every 3-4 hours; acute infections may require every 30-minute instillation initially with frequency of administration reduced as the infection is brought under control

To treat the eye lids: Instill 1-2 drops every 3-4 hours, close the eye and rub the excess on the lids and lid margins

Administration Ophthalmic: Avoid contamination of the dropper tip; shake suspension well before using; apply finger pressure to lacrimal sac during and for 1-2 minutes after instillation to decrease risk of absorption and systemic effects

Patient Information Ophthalmic: May cause sensitivity to bright light; may cause temporary blurring of vision or stinging following administration

Dosage Forms Suspension, ophthalmic: Neomycin sulfate 0.35%, polymyxin B sulfate 10,000 units and prednisolone acetate 0.5% per mL (5 mL, 10 mL)

◆ **Neonatal Resuscitation Algorithm** *see page 1034*

◆ **Neonatal Trace Metals** *see Trace Metals on page 972*

◆ **Neoral**® *see Cyclosporine on page 284*

◆ **Neosar**® *see Cyclophosphamide on page 281*

◆ **Neosporin**® **Cream [OTC]** *see Neomycin and Polymyxin B on page 705*

◆ **Neosporin**® **G.U. Irrigant** *see Neomycin and Polymyxin B on page 705*

◆ **Neosporin**® **Ophthalmic Ointment** *see Neomycin, Polymyxin B, and Bacitracin on page 707*

◆ **Neosporin**® **Topical Ointment [OTC]** *see Neomycin, Polymyxin B, and Bacitracin on page 707*

Neostigmine *(nee oh STIG meen)*

Related Information

Overdose and Toxicology *on page 1222*

U.S. Brand Names Prostigmin®

Therapeutic Category Antidote, Neuromuscular Blocking Agent; Cholinergic Agent; Diagnostic Agent, Myasthenia Gravis

Generic Available Yes

Use Treatment of myasthenia gravis; prevention and treatment of postoperative bladder distention and urinary retention; reversal of the effects of nondepolarizing neuromuscular blocking agents after surgery

Pregnancy Risk Factor C

Contraindications Hypersensitivity to neostigmine, bromides, or any component; GI or GU obstruction, peritonitis

Warnings Does **not** antagonize, and may prolong the phase I block of depolarizing muscle relaxants (eg, succinylcholine); adequate facilities should be available for cardiopulmonary resuscitation when testing and adjusting dose for myasthenia gravis; have atropine and epinephrine ready to treat hypersensitivity reactions; anticholinesterase insensitivity can develop for brief or prolonged periods

Precautions Use with caution in patients with epilepsy, asthma, bradycardia, hyperthyroidism, cardiac arrhythmias, peptic ulcer, vagotonia, or recent coronary occlusion

Adverse Reactions

Cardiovascular: Bradycardia, hypotension, asystole, A-V block, nodal rhythms, flushing, syncope

Central nervous system: Restlessness, agitation, seizures, dysphonia, dizziness, drowsiness, headache

Dermatologic: Rash, urticaria

Gastrointestinal: Hyperperistalsis, nausea, vomiting, diarrhea, dysphagia, flatulence, abdominal cramps; increased salivary, gastric, and intestinal secretions

Genitourinary: Urinary frequency and incontinence

Local: Thrombophlebitis

Neuromuscular & skeletal: Weakness, muscle cramps, arthralgia, tremor, dysarthria

Ocular: Miosis, lacrimation, diplopia, conjunctival hyperemia

Respiratory: Bronchoconstriction, increased secretions, laryngospasm, dyspnea, respiratory arrest, bronchospasm, respiratory paralysis

Miscellaneous: Allergic reactions, diaphoresis

Drug Interactions Antagonizes effects of nondepolarizing muscle relaxants (eg, pancuronium, tubocurarine); atropine and magnesium antagonize the muscarinic effects of neostigmine; corticosteroids may decrease neostigmine effects; prolongs effects of depolarizing muscle relaxants (eg, succinylcholine)

Mechanism of Action Competitively inhibits the hydrolysis of acetylcholine by acetylcholinesterase facilitating transmission of impulses across the myoneural junction and producing cholinergic activity

Pharmacodynamics
Onset of action:
Oral: 45-75 minutes
I.M.: Within 20-30 minutes
I.V.: Within 1-20 minutes
Duration:
Oral: 2-4 hours
I.M.: 2-4 hours
I.V.: 1-2 hours

Pharmacokinetics
Absorption: Oral: Poor (~1% to 2%)
Metabolism: In the liver
Half-life: 0.5-2.1 hours
Elimination: 50% excreted renally as unchanged drug

Usual Dosage
Myasthenia gravis:
Diagnosis: I.M. (all cholinesterase medications should be discontinued at least 8 hours before; atropine should be administered I.V. immediately prior to or I.M. 30 minutes before neostigmine):
Children: 0.025-0.04 mg/kg as a single dose
Adults: 0.022 mg/kg as a single dose
Treatment (dosage requirements are variable; adjust dosage so patient takes larger doses at times of greatest fatigue):
Children:
Oral: 0.333 mg/kg/dose or 10 mg/m^2/dose 6 times/day
I.M., I.V., S.C.: 0.01-0.04 mg/kg every 2-4 hours
Adults:
Oral: Initial: 15 mg/dose 3 times/day, gradually increase every 1-2 days; usual daily range: 15-375 mg
I.M., I.V., S.C.: 0.5-2.5 mg every 1-3 hours up to 10 mg/24 hours maximum
Reversal of nondepolarizing neuromuscular blockade after surgery in conjunction with atropine or glycopyrrolate: I.V.:
Infants: 0.025-0.1 mg/kg/dose
Children: 0.025-0.08 mg/kg/dose
Adults: 0.5-2 mg; total dose not to exceed 5 mg
Bladder atony: Adults: I.M., S.C.:
Prevention: 0.25 mg every 4-6 hours for 2-3 days
Treatment: 0.5-1 mg every 3 hours for 5 doses after bladder has emptied

Dosing adjustment in renal impairment:
Cl$_{cr}$ 10-50 mL/minute: Administer 50% of normal dose
Cl$_{cr}$ <10 mL/minute: Administer 25% of normal dose

Administration
Parenteral: May be administered undiluted by slow I.V. injection over several minutes; may be administered I.M. or S.C.
Oral: Divide dosages so patient receives larger doses at times of greatest fatigue; may be administered with or without food

Monitoring Parameters Muscle strength, heart rate, respiratory rate

Patient Information The side effects are generally due to exaggerated pharmacologic effects; the most common side effects are salivation and muscle fasciculations; notify physician if nausea, vomiting, muscle weakness, severe abdominal pain, or difficulty breathing occurs

Dosage Forms
Injection, as methylsulfate: 0.5 mg/mL (1 mL, 10 mL); 1 mg/mL (10 mL)
Tablet, as bromide: 15 mg

- **Neostrata Astringent Acne (Can)** see Salicylic Acid on page 886
- **Neo-Synephrine® 12 Hour [OTC]** see Oxymetazoline on page 749
- **Neo-Synephrine® Injectable** see Phenylephrine on page 789
- **Neo-Synephrine® Nasal [OTC]** see Phenylephrine on page 789
- **Neo-Synephrine® Ophthalmic** see Phenylephrine on page 789
- **Neo-Tabs®** see Neomycin on page 703
- **Neotopic (Can)** see Neomycin, Polymyxin B, and Bacitracin on page 707
- **Neotrace-4®** see Trace Metals on page 972
- **Neo-Zol (Can)** see Clotrimazole on page 259
- **Nephro-Calci® [OTC]** see Calcium Supplements on page 167

- **Nephrocaps**® *see page 1069*
- **Nephro-Fer**™ **[OTC]** *see Iron Supplements (Oral/Enteral) on page 548*
- **Nephrovite** *see page 1069*
- **Neupogen**® *see Filgrastim on page 425*
- **Neurontin**® *see Gabapentin on page 464*
- **Neut**® *see Sodium Bicarbonate on page 904*
- **Neutra-Phos**® **[OTC]** *see Phosphate Supplements on page 794*
- **Neutra-Phos**®**-K [OTC]** *see Phosphate Supplements on page 794*
- **Neutrogena**® **Acne Mask [OTC]** *see Benzoyl Peroxide on page 136*
- **Neutrogena**® **Acne Wash [OTC]** *see Salicylic Acid on page 886*
- **Neutrogena**® **Body Clear**™ **[OTC]** *see Salicylic Acid on page 886*
- **Neutrogena**® **Clear Pore [OTC]** *see Salicylic Acid on page 886*
- **Neutrogena**® **Healthy Scalp [OTC]** *see Salicylic Acid on page 886*
- **Neutrogena**® **Maximum Strength T/Sal**® **[OTC]** *see Salicylic Acid on page 886*
- **Neutrogena On-The-Spot Acne Lotion (Can)** *see Benzoyl Peroxide on page 136*
- **Neutrogena**® **On The Spot**® **Acne Patch [OTC]** *see Salicylic Acid on page 886*
- **Neutrogena**® **T/Derm** *see Coal Tar on page 260*

Nevirapine (ne VYE ra peen)

Related Information
Adult and Adolescent HIV *on page 1166*
Pediatric HIV *on page 1162*

U.S. Brand Names Viramune®

Therapeutic Category Antiretroviral Agent; HIV Agents (Anti-HIV Agents); Nonnucleoside Reverse Transcriptase Inhibitor (NNRTI)

Generic Available No

Use Treatment of HIV infection in combination with other antiretroviral agents. (**Note:** Current preferred HIV regimens consist of **three** antiretroviral agents)

Pregnancy Risk Factor C

Contraindications Hypersensitivity to nevirapine or any component

Warnings Severe and life-threatening skin reactions (eg, Stevens-Johnson syndrome) have occurred in patients receiving nevirapine. Discontinue nevirapine in patients who develop a severe rash or rash accompanied by fever, blistering, oral lesions, conjunctivitis, swelling, muscle or joint aches, or malaise. Majority of skin reactions occur within the first 6 weeks of therapy. Initiating therapy at a lower dose for the first 14 days of therapy has been shown to reduce the frequency of rash. Concomitant use of prednisone during the first 6 weeks of therapy was associated with an increase in incidence and severity of rash. Use of prednisone to prevent nevirapine-associated rash is not recommended. Severe, life-threatening, and fatal cases of hepatotoxicity have been reported with the use of nevirapine. Sixty-six percent of serious hepatic events occurred during the first 12 weeks of therapy. Permanently discontinue nevirapine therapy if clinical hepatotoxicity occurs and do not restart after recovery. Nevirapine induces hepatic cytochrome P-450 3A and has the potential for interacting with numerous drugs; drugs having suspected interactions and that should only be used with careful monitoring include rifampin, rifabutin, triazolam, midazolam, oral contraceptives, oral anticoagulants, digoxin, phenytoin, and theophylline.

Precautions Use caution in patients with either renal or hepatic dysfunction; elevated AST or ALT levels and/or a history of chronic hepatitis (B or C) infection are associated with a greater risk of hepatic adverse events

Adverse Reactions
Central nervous system: Headache, fever, sedation
Dermatologic: Rash (usually maculopapular erythematous cutaneous eruptions with or without pruritus, located on the trunk, face, and extremities; 19% of pediatric patients developed rash), Stevens-Johnson syndrome (see Warnings)
Gastrointestinal: Nausea, diarrhea
Hepatic: Elevated liver enzymes, hepatitis (rare), liver failure
Neuromuscular & skeletal: Myalgia

Drug Interactions Cytochrome P-450 isoenzyme CYP3A3/4 substrate, inducer, and inhibitor
Cimetidine, macrolides increase nevirapine plasma concentrations; rifabutin, rifampin decrease nevirapine plasma concentrations; nevirapine decreases indinavir and saquinavir concentrations; may decrease plasma concentration of ritonavir; decreases hormonal contraceptive efficacy; decreases metabolism of triazolam, midazolam, oral anticoagulants, digoxin, phenytoin, theophylline; the

herbal medicine St John's wort (*Hypericum perforatum*) may decrease serum concentration of nevirapine and is not recommended for concurrent use; increased incidence and severity of rash when nevirapine is used with prednisone; nevirapine may reduce plasma concentration of methadone (avoid concurrent use since acute withdrawal symptoms have been reported)

Stability Store at room temperature

Mechanism of Action A non-nucleoside reverse transcriptase inhibitor which specifically binds to HIV-1 reverse transcriptase blocking the RNA-dependent and DNA-dependent DNA polymerase activity and disrupting the virus' life cycle. Nevirapine does not inhibit HIV-2 reverse transcriptase or human DNA polymerase.

Pharmacokinetics

Absorption: Rapid and readily absorbed

Distribution: V_d: 1.21 L/kg; widely distributed; crosses the placenta; excreted in breast milk; 45% of the plasma concentration in CSF

Metabolism: Metabolized by cytochrome P-450 isozymes from the CYP3A family to hydroxylated metabolites; autoinduction of metabolism occurs in 2-4 weeks with a 1.5-2 times increase in clearance; nevirapine is more rapidly metabolized in pediatric patients than in adults

Protein binding, plasma: 60%

Bioavailability: 91% to 93%

Half-life: Single dose (45 hours); multiple dosing (25-30 hours)

Time to peak serum concentration: 4 hours

Elimination: 81.3% in urine as metabolites, 10.1% in feces; <3% of the total dose is eliminated in urine as parent drug

Usual Dosage Oral:

Neonates to 3 months (Investigational, under study in PACTG 365): 5 mg/kg/dose once daily for 14 days, followed by 120 mg/m²/dose every 12 hours for 14 days, followed by 200 mg/m²/dose every 12 hours

Children >3 months: 120 mg/m²/dose once daily for 14 days; increase to 120-200 mg/m²/dose every 12 hours if no rash or other adverse effects occur; maximum dose: 200 mg/dose every 12 hours

Adolescents and Adults: Initial: 200 mg/dose once daily for the first 14 days; increase to full dose if no rash or other adverse effects occur; maintenance dose: 200 mg every 12 hours

Administration Oral: May be administered with or without food; may be administered with an antacid or didanosine; shake suspension gently prior to administration

Monitoring Parameters Clinical chemistry tests, CD4 cell count, plasma levels of HIV RNA; liver function tests at baseline, prior to dose escalation, and at 2 weeks postdose escalation

Patient Information Inform physician immediately of any rash or symptoms of fatigue, malaise, anorexia, or nausea; use an alternative method of contraception from birth control pills during nevirapine therapy; if a dose is missed, take the next dose as soon as possible, however, if a dose is skipped, do not double the next dose

Dosage Forms

Suspension, oral: 10 mg/mL

Tablet: 200 mg

References

D'Aquila RT, Hughes MD, Johnson VA, et al, "Nevirapine, Zidovudine, and Didanosine Compared With Zidovudine and Didanosine in Patients With HIV-1 Infection. A Randomized, Double-Blind, Placebo-Controlled Trial. National Institute of Allergy and Infectious Diseases AIDS Clinical Trials Group Protocol 241 Investigators," *Ann Intern Med*, 1996, 124(12):1019-30.

Mueller BU, Sei S, Anderson B, et al, "Comparison of Virus Burden in Blood and Sequential Lymph Node Biopsy Specimens From Children Infected With Human Immunodeficiency Virus," *J Pediatr*, 1996, 129(3):410-8.

Working Group on Antiretroviral Therapy and Medical Management of HIV-Infected Children, "Guidelines for the Use of Antiretroviral Agents in Pediatric HIV Infection," January 7, 2000, http://www.hivatis.org.

♦ **NH₄Cl** *see* Ammonium Chloride *on page 79*

Niacin (NYE a sin)

U.S. Brand Names Niacor®; Niaspan®; Nicotinex [OTC]; Slo-Niacin® [OTC]

Synonyms Nicotinic Acid; Vitamin B_3

Therapeutic Category Antilipemic Agent; Nutritional Supplement; Vitamin, Water Soluble

Generic Available Yes

Use Adjunctive treatment of hyperlipidemias; peripheral vascular disease and circulatory disorders; treatment of pellagra; dietary supplement

Pregnancy Risk Factor A (C if used in doses greater than RDA suggested doses)

(Continued)

Niacin *(Continued)*

Contraindications Liver disease, peptic ulcer, severe hypotension, arterial hemorrhaging; hypersensitivity to niacin or any component; GERD (relative contraindication)

Warnings Hepatotoxicity may occur and may be more common if extended release product is substituted for immediate release product at same dosage; some products may contain tartrazine

Precautions May elevate uric acid levels, use with caution in patients predisposed to gout; large doses should be administered with caution to patients with gallbladder disease, jaundice, liver disease, diabetes, or renal dysfunction

Adverse Reactions

Cardiovascular: Flushing, hypotension, tachycardia, syncope, vasovagal attacks

Central nervous system: Dizziness, headache

Dermatologic: Pruritus, increased sebaceous gland activity, tingling skin, burning, acanthosis nigricans (reversible)

Endocrine & metabolic: Hyperuricemia, hyperglycemia

Gastrointestinal: GI upset, nausea, vomiting, heartburn, diarrhea, anorexia

Hepatic: Abnormal liver function tests, jaundice, chronic liver damage, hepatitis

Ocular: Blurred vision

Drug Interactions May inhibit uricosuric effects of sulfinpyrazone and probenecid; adrenergic blocking agents may cause additive vasodilating effect and postural hypotension; use with lipid-lowering agents will enhance antilipid effects

Mechanism of Action Component of two coenzymes necessary for tissue respiration, lipid metabolism, and glycogenolysis; inhibits the synthesis of very low density lipoproteins

Pharmacodynamics Vasodilation:

Onset of action: Within 20 minutes

Extended release: Within 1 hour

Duration: 20-60 minutes

Extended release: 8-10 hours

Pharmacokinetics

Distribution: Crosses into breast milk

Metabolism: Niacin in smaller doses is converted to niacinamide which is metabolized in the liver

Half-life: 45 minutes

Elimination: In urine, with ~33% as unchanged drug; with larger doses, a greater percentage is excreted unchanged in urine

Usual Dosage Oral (preferred), I.M., I.V., S.C. (**Note:** Parenteral routes of administration are for treatment of vitamin deficiencies only, not for hyperlipidemia)

Children:

Recommended daily allowances (RDA):

0-0.5 years: 5 mg/day

0.5-1 year: 6 mg/day

1-3 years: 9 mg/day

4-6 years: 12 mg/day

7-10 years: 13 mg/day

Male:

11-14 years: 17 mg/day

15-18 years: 20 mg/day

19-24 years: 19 mg/day

Female: 11-24 years: 15 mg/day

Hyperlipidemia: Initial: 100-250 mg/day (maximum dose: 10 mg/kg/day) in 3 divided doses with meals; increase weekly by 100 mg/day or increase every 2-3 weeks by 250 mg/day as tolerated; evaluate efficacy and adverse effects with laboratory tests at 20 mg/kg/day or 1000 mg/day (whichever is less); continue to increase if needed and as tolerated; re-evaluate at each 500 mg increment; doses up to 2250 mg/day have been used; **Note:** Routine use in children and adolescents is not recommended due to limited safety and efficacy information

Pellagra: 50-100 mg/dose 3 times/day

Adults:

Recommended daily allowances (RDA):

Male:

25-50 years: 19 mg/day

>51 years: 15 mg/day

Female:

25-50 years: 15 mg/day

>51 years: 13 mg/day

Hyperlipidemia:

Immediate release products: Initial: 50-100 mg twice daily for 1 week; increase slowly over 1 month (by doubling daily dose every week) to 1-1.5 g/day divided in 2-3 doses; assess therapy at 4 and 8 weeks of therapy; if needed, dose may be increased slowly to 3 g/day or until desired result is attained; maximum dose: 3 g/day in 3 divided doses; **Note:** Some patients may require a slower dose titration

Extended release products: Initial: 500 mg/day divided in 2 doses for 1 week; increase to 500 mg twice daily for 3 weeks; if needed, dose may be increased to 2 g/day or until desired result is attained; maximum dose: 2 g/day

Niacin deficiency: 10-20 mg/day, maximum dose: 100 mg/day

Pellagra: 50-100 mg 3-4 times/day, maximum dose: 500 mg/day

Administration

Oral: Administer with food or milk to decrease GI upset; swallow timed release tablet and capsule whole; do not chew or crush; to minimize flushing, administer dose at bedtime, take aspirin (adults: 325 mg) 30 minutes before niacin, and avoid alcohol or hot drinks around the time of administration

Parenteral: I.V.: Slow I.V. injection

Monitoring Parameters Blood glucose; serum uric acid, periodic liver function tests (with large doses or prolonged therapy); Treatment of hyperlipidemias: Baseline: Liver enzymes, uric acid, fasting glucose, and minimum of 2 fasting lipid profiles; repeat 4-6 weeks after dose is stabilized; once LDL-C goal is reached, repeat every 2-3 months for first year and then every 6-12 months if no sign of toxicity develops and dose remains stable

Test Interactions False elevations in some fluorometric determinations of urinary catecholamines; false-positive urine glucose (Benedict's reagent)

Patient Information Transient flushing of the skin and a sensation of warmth (especially of face and upper body), itching, tingling or headache may occur; if dizziness occurs, avoid sudden changes in posture and notify physician; notify physician if taking vitamins or other products that contain niacin or nicotinamide; do not change brands once dosage is stabilized; report signs and symptoms of hepatotoxicity (nausea, vomiting, loss of appetite, yellow skin, dark urine, general feeling of weakness) to physician

Additional Information Discontinue use if liver enzymes increase to ≥3 times the upper limit of normal

Dosage Forms

Capsule, timed release: 125 mg, 250 mg, 400 mg, 500 mg

Elixir (Nicotinex®): 50 mg/5 mL (473 mL)

Injection: 100 mg/mL (30 mL)

Tablet: 50 mg, 100 mg, 250 mg, 500 mg

Niacor®: 500 mg

Tablet, extended release: 250 mg, 500 mg, 750 mg, 1000 mg

Niaspan®: 500 mg, 750 mg, 1000 mg

Slo-Niacin®: 250 mg, 500 mg, 750 mg

References

"ASHP Therapeutic Position Statement on the Safe Use of Niacin in the Management of Dyslipidemias. American Society of Health-System Pharmacists," *Am J Health Syst Pharm*, 1997, 54(24):2815-9.

Colletti RB, Neufeld EJ, Roff NK, et al, "Niacin Treatment of Hypercholesterolemia in Children." *Pediatrics*, 1993, 92(1):78-82.

Schuna AA, "Safe Use of Niacin," *Am J Health Syst Pharm*, 1997, 54(24):2803.

♦ **Niacor®** *see* Niacin *on page 711*

♦ **Niaspan®** *see* Niacin *on page 711*

♦ **Niclocide®** *see* Niclosamide *on page 713*

Niclosamide (ni KLOE sa mide)

U.S. Brand Names Niclocide®

Therapeutic Category Anthelmintic

Generic Available No

Use Treatment of *Taenia saginata* (beef tapeworm), *Diphyllobothrium latum* (fish tapeworm), *Dipylidium caninum* (dog and cat tapeworm), and *Hymenolepis nana* (dwarf tapeworm) infections

Pregnancy Risk Factor B

Contraindications Hypersensitivity to niclosamide or any component; treatment of cysticercosis (niclosamide is only active against intestinal cestodes)

Adverse Reactions

Central nervous system: Drowsiness, dizziness, fever, headache

Dermatologic: Rash, pruritus, alopecia

(Continued)

Niclosamide *(Continued)*

Gastrointestinal: Mild abdominal pain, bloating, nausea, vomiting, diarrhea, anorexia, rectal bleeding, dysgeusia, constipation

Miscellaneous: Diaphoresis

Stability Protect from light; avoid freezing

Mechanism of Action Inhibits the synthesis of ATP through inhibition of oxidative phosphorylation in the mitochondria of cestodes

Pharmacokinetics

Absorption: Oral: Unabsorbed from the GI tract

Elimination: In feces

Usual Dosage Oral:

Beef and fish tapeworm:

Children: 40 mg/kg as a single dose one time; maximum dose: 2 g/dose

Adults: 2 g (4 tablets) in a single dose

May repeat treatment 7 days later if proglottids and/or eggs are still present in stool

Dwarf tapeworm:

Children: 40 mg/kg/day once every 24 hours for 7 days, maximum dose: 2 g/day

Adults: 2 g (4 tablets) in a single dose daily for 7 days

Administration Oral: Administer after a light meal (ie, breakfast); have patient chew tablets thoroughly and swallow with a small amount of water; tablets can be pulverized and mixed with water to form a paste for administration to children

Monitoring Parameters Stool for proglottids and eggs

Nursing Implications Can administer laxative 1-4 hours after the niclosamide dose if treating *Taenia solium* infections to prevent the development of cysticercosis

Dosage Forms Tablet, chewable: 500 mg [vanilla flavor]

♦ **Nicotinex [OTC]** *see* Niacin *on page 711*

♦ **Nicotinic Acid** *see* Niacin *on page 711*

♦ **NidaGel (Can)** *see* Metronidazole *on page 662*

Nifedipine *(nye FED i peen)*

U.S. Brand Names Adalat® CC; Procardia®; Procardia XL®

Canadian Brand Names Adalat PA; Apo-Nifed; Gen-Nifedipine; Novo-Nifedin; Nu-Nifed

Therapeutic Category Antianginal Agent; Antihypertensive Agent; Calcium Channel Blocker

Generic Available Yes, except sustained-release tablet

Use Angina, hypertrophic cardiomyopathy, hypertension

Pregnancy Risk Factor C

Contraindications Hypersensitivity to nifedipine or any component

Precautions May increase frequency, duration, and severity of angina during initiation of therapy; use with caution in patients with CHF or aortic stenosis (especially with concomitant beta-blocker)

Adverse Reactions

Cardiovascular: Flushing, hypotension, tachycardia, palpitations, syncope, peripheral edema

Central nervous system: Dizziness, fever, headache, chills

Dermatologic: Dermatitis, urticaria, purpura

Gastrointestinal: Nausea, diarrhea, constipation, gingival hyperplasia

Hematologic: Thrombocytopenia, leukopenia, anemia

Neuromuscular & skeletal: Joint stiffness, arthritis with increased ANA

Ocular: Blurred vision, transient blindness

Respiratory: Shortness of breath

Miscellaneous: Diaphoresis

Drug Interactions Cytochrome P-450 isoenzyme CYP3A3/4 and CYP3A5-7 substrate

Beta-blockers may increase cardiovascular adverse effects; anesthetic doses of fentanyl may cause hypotension; cimetidine may increase nifedipine serum concentration; nifedipine may increase phenytoin, cyclosporine, and possibly digoxin serum concentrations; combined use of nifedipine with cyclosporine may significantly increase gingival hyperplasia; delavirdine may decrease the metabolism of nifedipine and increase nifedipine levels; concurrent use of delavirdine and nifedipine is not recommended; saquinavir may increase nifedipine levels

Food Interactions Capsule is rapidly absorbed orally if it is administered without food but may result in vasodilator side effects; administration with low-fat meals may decrease flushing; grapefruit juice may increase the oral bioavailability of nifedipine tablets; food may decrease the rate but not the extent of absorption of Procardia XL®

Mechanism of Action Inhibits calcium ion from entering the "slow channels" or select voltage-sensitive areas of vascular smooth muscle and myocardium during depolarization, producing a relaxation of coronary vascular smooth muscle and coronary vasodilation; increases myocardial oxygen delivery in patients with vasospastic angina

Pharmacodynamics
Onset:
S.L. or "bite and swallow": Within 1-5 minutes
Oral: Within 20-30 minutes
Duration: 4-6 hours

Pharmacokinetics
Protein-binding: 92% to 98% (concentration-dependent)
Metabolism: In the liver to inactive metabolites
Bioavailability:
Capsules: 45% to 75%
Sustained release: 65% to 86%
Half-life:
Normal adults: 2-5 hours
Cirrhosis: 7 hours
Elimination: In urine

Usual Dosage Oral, S.L. or "bite and swallow" (eg, patient bites capsule to release liquid contents and then swallows): **Note:** Doses are usually titrated upward at 7- to 14-day intervals; may increase every 3 days if clinically necessary:

Children:
Hypertensive emergencies: 0.25-0.5 mg/kg/dose; maximum dose: 10 mg/dose; may repeat if needed every 4-6 hours; monitor carefully; maximum dose: 1-2 mg/kg/day
Hypertrophic cardiomyopathy: 0.6-0.9 mg/kg/24 hours in 3-4 divided doses
Adolescents and Adults: Initial: 10 mg 3 times/day (capsules) or 30-60 mg once daily (sustained release tablet); maintenance: 10-30 mg 3-4 times/day (capsules); maximum dose: 180 mg/24 hours (capsules) or 120 mg/day (sustained release)

Administration Oral: Administer with food; do not administer with grapefruit juice; swallow sustained release tablets whole, do not crush, break, or chew; liquid-filled capsule may be punctured and drug solution administered sublingually or orally; when measuring smaller doses from the liquid-filled capsules, consider the following concentrations (for Procardia®) 10 mg capsule = 10 mg/0.34 mL; 20 mg capsule = 20 mg/0.45 mL
Note: When nifedipine is administered sublingually, only a small amount is absorbed sublingually; the observed effects are actually due to swallowing of the drug with subsequent rapid oral absorption

Monitoring Parameters Blood pressure

Patient Information Avoid alcohol; rise slowly from prolonged sitting or lying position

Dosage Forms
Capsule, liquid-filled (Procardia®): 10 mg, 20 mg
Tablet, extended release (Adalat® CC): 30 mg, 60 mg, 90 mg
Tablet, sustained release (Procardia XL®): 30 mg, 60 mg, 90 mg

References
Dilmen U, Çağlar MK, Senses A, et al, "Nifedipine in Hypertensive Emergencies of Children," *Am J Dis Child*, 1983, 137(12):1162-5.
Lopez-Herce J, Albajara L, Cagigas P, et al, "Treatment of Hypertensive Crisis in Children With Nifedipine," *Intensive Care Med*, 1988, 14(5):519-21.
Rosen WJ and Johnson CE, "Evaluation of Five Procedures for Measuring Nonstandard Doses of Nifedipine Liquid," *Am J Hosp Pharm*, 1989, 46(11):2313-7.

Nitrofurantoin (nye troe fyoor AN toyn)

Related Information

Carbohydrate and Alcohol Content of Liquid Medications for Use in Patients Receiving Ketogenic Diets *on page 1258*

U.S. Brand Names Furadantin®; Furalan®; Furan®; Furanite®; Macrobid®; Macrodantin®

Canadian Brand Names Apo-Nitrofurantoin; Novo-Furan; Novo-Furantoin

Therapeutic Category Antibiotic, Miscellaneous

Generic Available Yes: Tablet and suspension

Use Prevention and treatment of urinary tract infections caused by susceptible gram-negative and some gram-positive organisms including *E. coli, Klebsiella, Enterobacter,* enterococci, and *S. aureus; Pseudomonas, Serratia,* and most species of *Proteus* are generally resistant to nitrofurantoin

Pregnancy Risk Factor B; contraindicated in pregnant women at term and during labor (due to possible hemolytic anemia in the neonate)

Contraindications Hypersensitivity to nitrofurantoin or any component; renal impairment; infants <1 month of age (due to the possibility of hemolytic anemia); pregnant patients at term; should not be used to treat UTI in febrile infants and young children in whom renal involvement is likely

Warnings Therapeutic concentrations of nitrofurantoin are not attained in the urine of patients with renal insufficiency (Cl$_{cr}$ <40 mL/minute, anuria, or oliguria)

Precautions Use with caution in patients with G-6-PD deficiency, patients with anemia, vitamin B deficiency, diabetes mellitus, or electrolyte abnormalities

Adverse Reactions

Central nervous system: Dizziness, headache, chills, fever, vertigo, drowsiness

Dermatologic: Rash, exfoliative dermatitis, urticaria

Gastrointestinal: Nausea, vomiting, anorexia, pancreatitis, pseudomembranous colitis (rare)

Genitourinary: Discoloration of urine (dark yellow or brown)

Hematologic: Hemolytic anemia, eosinophilia, leukopenia, granulocytopenia, thrombocytopenia, megaloblastic anemia

Hepatic: Hepatotoxicity, cholestatic jaundice, hepatitis

Neuromuscular & skeletal: Arthralgia, peripheral neuropathy, muscle weakness, asthenia

Respiratory: Interstitial pneumonitis and/or fibrosis

Miscellaneous: Hypersensitivity reactions

Drug Interactions Probenecid decreases renal excretion of nitrofurantoin, antacids decrease extent and rate of absorption of nitrofurantoin; drugs which delay gastric emptying increase the extent of nitrofurantoin absorption

Food Interactions Food increases the total amount absorbed; cranberry juice and other urinary acidifiers may enhance the action of nitrofurantoin; ensure diet is adequate in protein and vitamin B complex

Stability Protect from light

Mechanism of Action Inhibits several bacterial enzyme systems including acetyl coenzyme A; reduced by bacterial enzymes to active intermediates that may alter ribosomal proteins resulting in inhibition of protein, DNA, RNA, and cell wall synthesis

Pharmacokinetics

Absorption: Well absorbed from the GI tract; macrocrystalline form is absorbed more slowly due to slower dissolution, but causes less GI distress than formulations containing microcrystals of the drug

Distribution: V$_d$: 0.8 L/kg; crosses the placenta; appears in breast milk and bile

Protein binding: ~40%

Metabolism: Partially in the liver

Bioavailability: Presence of food increases bioavailability

Half-life: 20-60 minutes and is prolonged with renal impairment

Elimination: As metabolites and unchanged drug (40%) in the urine and small amounts in the bile; renal excretion is via glomerular filtration and tubular secretion

Usual Dosage Oral:

Children: 5-7 mg/kg/day divided every 6 hours; maximum dose: 400 mg/day

Prophylaxis of UTI: 1-2 mg/kg/day as a single daily dose; maximum dose: 100 mg/day

Adults: 50-100 mg/dose every 6 hours

Prophylaxis of UTI: 50-100 mg/dose at bedtime

Administration Oral: Administer with food or milk; suspension may be mixed with water, milk, fruit juice, or infant formula

Monitoring Parameters Signs of pulmonary reaction; signs of numbness or tingling of the extremities; periodic liver and renal function tests

Test Interactions Causes false-positive urine glucose with Clinitest®

Patient Information May discolor urine to a dark yellow or brown color; avoid alcohol

Dosage Forms
Capsule: 50 mg, 100 mg
Capsule:
Extended release: 100 mg
Macrocrystal: 25 mg, 50 mg, 100 mg
Macrocrystal/monohydrate: 100 mg
Suspension, oral: 25 mg/5 mL (470 mL)

References
Brendstrup L, Hjelt K, Petersen KE, et al, "Nitrofurantoin Versus Trimethoprim Prophylaxis in Recurrent Urinary Tract Infections in Children," *Acta Paediatr Scand*, 1990. 79(12):1225-34.

Coraggio MJ, Gross TP, and Roscelli JD, "Nitrofurantoin Toxicity in Children," *Pediatr Infect Dis J*, 1989, 8(3):163-6.

"Practice Parameter: The Diagnosis, Treatment, and Evaluation of the Initial Urinary Tract Infection in Febrile Infants and Young Children. American Academy of Pediatrics. Committee on Quality Improvement. Subcommittee on Urinary Tract Infection," *Pediatrics*, 1999, 103(4 Pt 1):843-52.

♦ **Nitrogard®** *see* Nitroglycerin *on page 717*

♦ **Nitrogen Mustard** *see* Mechlorethamine *on page 621*

Nitroglycerin (nye troe GLI ser in)

U.S. Brand Names Deponit®; Minitran™; Nitrek®; Nitro-Bid®; Nitro-Dur®; Nitrogard®; Nitroglyn® ER; Nitrolingual®; NitroQuick®; Nitrostat®; Nitro-Tab®; Nitro-Time®; Transderm-Nitro®

Canadian Brand Names Nitroject; Nitrol; Nitrong; Trinipatch

Synonyms Glyceryl Trinitrate; Nitroglycerol; NTG

Therapeutic Category Antianginal Agent; Antihypertensive Agent; Nitrate; Vasodilator; Vasodilator, Coronary

Generic Available Yes

Use Angina pectoris; I.V. for CHF (especially when associated with acute MI); pulmonary hypertension; hypertensive emergencies occurring perioperatively (especially during cardiovascular surgery)

Pregnancy Risk Factor C

Contraindications Hypersensitivity to nitroglycerin, organic nitrates, or any component (including adhesives in transdermal patches); glaucoma; severe anemia; increased ICP; concurrent use with sildenafil (see Drug Interactions); I.V. product is also contraindicated in hypotension, uncontrolled hypokalemia, pericardial tamponade, or constrictive pericarditis

Warnings May cause severe hypotension; use with caution in hypovolemia, hypotension, and right ventricular infarctions; do not chew or swallow sublingual dosage form

Adverse Reactions
Cardiovascular: Flushing, hypotension, pallor, reflex tachycardia, cardiovascular collapse; severe hypotension, bradycardia, and acute coronary vascular insufficiency with abrupt withdrawal
Central nervous system: Dizziness, restlessness, headache
Dermatologic: Allergic contact dermatitis, exfoliative dermatitis
Endocrine & metabolic: Alcohol intoxication from one I.V. formulation
Gastrointestinal: Nausea, vomiting
Miscellaneous: Perspiration

Drug Interactions I.V. nitroglycerin may antagonize the anticoagulant effect of heparin, monitor closely, may need to decrease heparin dosage when nitroglycerin is discontinued; alcohol, beta-blockers, calcium channel blockers may enhance nitroglycerin's hypotensive effect; sildenafil may increase vasodilatory effects and result in severe hypotension

Stability Nitroglycerin adsorbs to plastics; I.V. must be prepared in glass bottles and special administration sets intended for nitroglycerin (nonpolyvinyl chloride) must be used; do not mix with other drugs; store sublingual tablets and ointment in tightly closed container; store at 15°C to 30°C

Mechanism of Action Reduces cardiac oxygen demand by decreasing left ventricular end diastolic pressure and systemic vascular resistance; dilates coronary arteries and improves collateral flow to ischemic regions; vasodilates veins more than arteries

Pharmacodynamics Onset and duration of action is dependent upon dosage form administered; see table on next page.
(Continued)

Nitroglycerin *(Continued)*

Nitroglycerin*

Dosage Form	Onset (min)	Duration
I.V.	1-2	3-5 min
Sublingual	1-3	30-60 min
Translingual spray	2	30-60 min
Buccal, extended release	2-3	3-5 h
Oral, sustained release	40	4-8 h
Topical ointment	20-60	2-12 h
Transdermal	40-60	18-24 h

*Hemodynamic and antianginal tolerance often develops within 24-48 h of continuous nitrate administration.

Adapted from Corwin S and Reiffel, JA, "Nitrate Therapy for Angina Pectoris," *Arch Intern Med*, 1985, 145:538-43 and Franciosa JA, "Nitroglycerin and Nitrates in Congestive Heart Failure," *Heart and Lung*, 1980, 9(5):873-82.

Pharmacokinetics
Protein binding: 60%
Metabolism: Extensive first-pass
Half-life: 1-4 minutes
Elimination: Excretion of inactive metabolites in urine

Usual Dosage Tolerance to the hemodynamic and antianginal effects can develop within 24-48 hours of continuous use

Children: I.V. continuous infusion: Initial: 0.25-0.5 mcg/kg/minute; titrate by 0.5-1 mcg/kg/minute every 3-5 minutes as needed; usual dose: 1-3 mcg/kg/minute; usual maximum dose: 5 mcg/kg/minute; doses up to 20 mcg/kg/minute may be used

Adults:
Oral: 2.5-9 mg every 8-12 hours
I.V. continuous infusion: Initial: 5 mcg/minute, increase by 5 mcg/minute every 3-5 minutes to 20 mcg/minute, then increase as needed by 10 mcg/minute every 3-5 minutes, up to 200 mcg/minute
Sublingual: 0.2-0.6 mg every 5 minutes for maximum of 3 doses in 15 minutes
Ointment: 1" to 2" every 8 hours
Patch, transdermal: Initial: 0.2-0.4 mg/hour, titrate to 0.4-0.8 mg/hour; use a "patch-on" period of 12-14 hours per day and a "patch-off" period of 10-12 hours per day to minimize tolerance
Lingual: 1-2 sprays into mouth onto or under tongue every 3-5 minutes for maximum of 3 sprays in 15 minutes; may administer 5-10 minutes before activities that may precipitate angina
Buccal: Initial: 1 mg every 5 hours while awake (3 times/day); titrate dosage upward if angina occurs with tablet in place

Administration
Oral:
Buccal tablet: Place in buccal pouch and allow to dissolve; do not swallow, chew, or crush
Lingual spray: Do not shake container; spray onto or under tongue with container as close to mouth as possible; do not inhale spray; avoid swallowing immediately after spray; do not expectorate or rinse mouth for 5-10 minutes after use
Sublingual tablet: Place under tongue and allow to dissolve, do not swallow, chew, or crush; do not eat or drink while tablet dissolves
Regular or sustained release capsule/tablet: Administer with a full glass of water on an empty stomach; swallow sustained release capsules/tablets whole, do not crush or chew
Parenteral: I.V. continuous infusion: Dilute in D_5W or NS to 50-100 mcg/mL; maximum concentration not to exceed 400 mcg/mL; rate of infusion (mL/hour) = dose (mcg/kg/minute) x weight (kg) x 60 minutes/hour divided by the concentration (mcg/mL); administer via controlled infusion device
Transdermal: Place on hair-free area of skin; rotate patch sites; **Note:** Some products are a membrane-controlled system (eg, Transderm-Nitro®); do **not** cut these patches to deliver partial doses; rate of drug delivery, reservoir contents, and adhesion may be affected; if partial dose is needed, surface area of patch can be blocked proportionally using adhesive bandage (see Lee, 1997 and see specific product labeling)

Monitoring Parameters Blood pressure, heart rate (continuously with I.V. use)

Patient Information Avoid alcohol; may cause dizziness, headache; if no relief of chest pains after 3 sublingual doses, seek emergency care immediately

Nursing Implications Transdermal patches are now labeled as mg/hour (rates of release used to be described as mg/24 hours)

Additional Information I.V. preparations contain alcohol and/or propylene glycol; may need to use nitrate-free interval (10-12 hours/day) to avoid tolerance development; tolerance may possibly be reversed with acetylcysteine; gradually decrease dose in patients receiving NTG for prolonged period to avoid withdrawal reaction; lingual spray contains 20% alcohol, do not spray toward flames

Dosage Forms

Capsule, sustained release (Nitroglyn® ER, Nitro-Time®): 2.5 mg, 6.5 mg, 9 mg

Infusion, premixed in D_5W: 0.1 mg/mL (250 mL, 500 mL); 0.2 mg/mL (250 mL); 0.4 mg/mL (250 mL, 500 mL)

Injection: 5 mg/mL [contains alcohol and propylene glycol] (5 mL, 10 mL)

Ointment, topical (Nitro-Bid®): 2% [20 mg/g] (1 g, 30 g, 60 g)

Patch, transdermal, topical: Systems designed to deliver 0.1 mg/hour (2.5 mg/24 hours); 0.2 mg/hour (5 mg/24 hours); 0.4 mg/hour (10 mg/24 hours); 0.6 mg/hour (15 mg/24 hours); 0.8 mg/hour (20 mg/24 hours)

Deponit®: 0.1 mg/hour, 0.2 mg/hour, 0.4 mg/hour

Minitran™: 0.1 mg/hour, 0.2 mg/hour, 0.4 mg/hour, 0.6 mg/hour

Nitrek®: 0.2 mg/hour, 0.4 mg/hour, 0.6 mg/hour

Nitro-Dur®: 0.1 mg/hour, 0.2 mg/hour, 0.3 mg/hour, 0.4 mg/hour, 0.6 mg/hour, 0.8 mg/hour

Transderm-Nitro®: 0.1 mg/hour, 0.4 mg/hour

Spray, translingual (Nitrolingual®): 0.4 mg/metered spray [200 metered sprays] (12 g)

Tablet:

Buccal, controlled release (Nitrogard®): 2 mg, 3 mg

Sublingual (NitroQuick®, Nitrostat®, Nitro-Tab®): 0.3 mg, 0.4 mg, 0.6 mg

References

Elkayam U, "Tolerance to Organic Nitrates: Evidence, Mechanisms, Clinical Relevance, and Strategies for Prevention," *Ann Intern Med*, 1991, 114(8):667-77.

Lee HA and Anderson PO, "Giving Partial Doses of Transdermal Patches," *Am J Health Syst Pharm*, 1997, 54(15):1759-60.

♦ **Nitroglycerol** see Nitroglycerin on page 717

♦ **Nitroglyn® ER** see Nitroglycerin on page 717

♦ **Nitroject (Can)** see Nitroglycerin on page 717

♦ **Nitrol (Can)** see Nitroglycerin on page 717

♦ **Nitrolingual®** see Nitroglycerin on page 717

♦ **Nitrong (Can)** see Nitroglycerin on page 717

♦ **Nitropress®** see Nitroprusside on page 719

Nitroprusside (nye troe PRUS ide)

U.S. Brand Names Nitropress®

Canadian Brand Names Nipride

Synonyms Nitroferricyanide

Therapeutic Category Antihypertensive Agent; Vasodilator

Generic Available Yes

Use Management of hypertensive crises; CHF; used for controlled hypotension during anesthesia

Pregnancy Risk Factor C

Contraindications Hypersensitivity to nitroprusside or any component; decreased cerebral perfusion; arteriovenous shunt or coarctation of the aorta (ie, compensatory hypertension)

Warnings Use only as an infusion with D_5W; continuously monitor patient's blood pressure; excessive amounts of nitroprusside can cause cyanide toxicity (usually in patients with decreased liver function) or thiocyanate toxicity (usually in patients with decreased renal function, or in patients with normal renal function but prolonged nitroprusside use)

Precautions Use with caution in patients with severe renal impairment, hepatic failure, hypothyroidism, hyponatremia, increased intracranial pressure

Adverse Reactions

Cardiovascular: Excessive hypotensive response, palpitations, substernal distress

Central nervous system: Restlessness, disorientation, psychosis, headache, increased intracranial pressure

Endocrine & metabolic: Thyroid suppression

Gastrointestinal: Nausea, vomiting

Hematologic: Thiocyanate toxicity

(Continued)

Nitroprusside *(Continued)*

Neuromuscular & skeletal: Weakness

Miscellaneous: Diaphoresis, cyanide toxicity

Stability Discard solution 24 hours after reconstitution and dilution; discard highly colored solutions

Mechanism of Action Causes peripheral vasodilation by direct action on venous and arteriolar smooth muscle, thus reducing peripheral resistance; will increase cardiac output by decreasing afterload; reduces aortal and left ventricular impedance

Pharmacodynamics Hypotensive effects:

Onset of action: Within 2 minutes

Duration: 1-10 minutes

Pharmacokinetics

Half-life: <10 minutes

Thiocyanate: 2.7-7 days

Metabolism: Converted to cyanide by erythrocyte and tissue sulfhydryl group interactions; cyanide is converted in the liver by the enzyme rhodanase to thiocyanate

Elimination: Thiocyanate is excreted in the urine

Usual Dosage Children and Adults: I.V. continuous infusion: Start 0.3-0.5 mcg/kg/minute, titrate to effect; usual dose: 3 mcg/kg/minute; rarely need >4 mcg/kg/minute; maximum dose: 8-10 mcg/kg/minute

Rate (mL/hour) = dose (mcg/kg/minute) x weight (kg) x 60 minutes/hour divided by concentration (mcg/mL)

Administration Parenteral: I.V. continuous infusion only via controlled infusion device; not for direct injection; dilute in plain dextrose solutions only (eg, D_5W); solution should be protected from light, but not necessary to wrap administration set or I.V. tubing. Final concentration for administration: Usual maximum: 200 mcg/mL; in fluid restricted patients a final maximum concentration of 1000 mcg/mL in D_5W has been used. Do not add other medications to nitroprusside solutions.

Monitoring Parameters Blood pressure, heart rate; monitor for cyanide and thiocyanate toxicity; monitor acid-base status as acidosis can be the earliest sign of cyanide toxicity; monitor thiocyanate levels if requiring prolonged infusion (>3 days) or dose ≥4 mcg/kg/minute or patient has renal dysfunction; monitor cyanide blood levels in patients with decreased hepatic function

Reference Range

Thiocyanate:

Toxic: 35-100 µg/mL

Fatal: >200 µg/mL

Cyanide:

Normal <0.2 µg/mL

Normal (smoker): <0.4 µg/mL

Toxic: >2 µg/mL

Potentially lethal: >3 µg/mL

Additional Information Thiocyanate toxicity includes psychoses, blurred vision, confusion, weakness, tinnitus, seizures; cyanide toxicity includes metabolic acidosis, tachycardia, pink skin, decreased pulse, decreased reflexes, altered consciousness, coma, almond smell on breath, methemoglobinemia, dilated pupils

Dosage Forms

Injection, as sodium: 25 mg/mL (2 mL)

Powder for injection, as sodium (Nitropress®): 50 mg

- **NitroQuick®** *see Nitroglycerin on page 717*
- **Nitrostat®** *see Nitroglycerin on page 717*
- **Nitro-Tab®** *see Nitroglycerin on page 717*
- **Nitro-Time®** *see Nitroglycerin on page 717*
- **Nix™ Creme Rinse** *see Permethrin on page 783*
- **Nix Dermal Cream (Can)** *see Permethrin on page 783*

Nizatidine *(ni ZA ti deen)*

U.S. Brand Names Axid®; Axid® AR [OTC]

Canadian Brand Names Apo-Nizatidine; Novo-Nizatidine

Therapeutic Category Gastrointestinal Agent, Gastric or Duodenal Ulcer Treatment; Histamine H_2 Antagonist

Generic Available Yes

Use Treatment and maintenance therapy of duodenal ulcer; treatment of active benign gastric ulcer; esophagitis; gastroesophageal reflux disease (GERD); over-the-counter (OTC) formulation for use in the relief of heartburn, acid indigestion, and sour stomach; adjunctive therapy in the treatment of *Helicobacter pylori*-associated duodenal ulcer

Pregnancy Risk Factor B

Contraindications Hypersensitivity to nizatidine, H_2 antagonists or any component

Warnings Use with caution and modify dosage in patients with impaired renal function

Adverse Reactions

Cardiovascular: Chest pain, ventricular tachycardia (short, asymptomatic episodes)

Central nervous system: Headache, fever, dizziness, insomnia, somnolence, anxiety, nervousness

Dermatologic: Rash, pruritus

Endocrine & metabolic: Hyperuricemia

Gastrointestinal: Nausea, vomiting, diarrhea, flatulence, dyspepsia, constipation, dry mouth, anorexia, abdominal pain

Genitourinary: Impotence

Hematologic: Anemia, thrombocytopenia, eosinophilia, leukopenia

Hepatic: Elevated liver enzymes, jaundice, hepatitis

Neuromuscular & skeletal: Back pain, asthenia, myalgia

Ocular: Amblyopia

Respiratory: Rhinitis, pharyngitis, sinusitis, cough

Miscellaneous: Hypersensitivity reactions, serum sickness

Drug Interactions May increase salicylate serum concentration (high-dose salicylate therapy); decreases absorption of itraconazole, delavirdine, and ketoconazole

Food Interactions Limit xanthine-containing foods and beverages

Stability Nizatidine is stable for 48 hours at room temperature when the contents of a capsule are mixed in Gatorade® lemon-lime, Cran-Grape® grape-cranberry drink, V8®, apple juice, or aluminum- and magnesium hydroxide suspension (approximate concentration 2.5 mg/mL)

Mechanism of Action Competitive inhibition of histamine at H_2-receptors of the gastric parietal cells, which inhibits gastric acid secretion

Pharmacodynamics Peak response: Duodenal ulcer: 4 weeks

Pharmacokinetics

Distribution: V_d: 0.8-1.5 L/kg (adults)

Protein binding: 35%

Bioavailability: Oral: 70%

Half-life, elimination: 2.1 hours; anuric: 3.5-11 hours

Time to peak concentration: 0.5-3 hours

Elimination: 60% excreted unchanged in urine

Usual Dosage Oral:

Infants 6 months to Children 11 years: Limited information available: 6-10 mg/kg/day divided twice daily (see References)

Adults:

Active duodenal and gastric ulcers: 300 mg once daily at bedtime or 150 mg twice daily for 6-8 weeks

Maintenance of healed duodenal ulcer: 150 mg once daily at bedtime for up to 1 year

GERD, esophagitis: 150 mg twice daily for up to 12 weeks

Relief of heartburn, acid indigestion, sour stomach (OTC use): 75 mg 30-60 minutes before meals; no more than 2 tablets/day

Helicobacter pylori-associated duodenal ulcer (limited information): 300 mg twice daily for 4 weeks (combined with clarithromycin and bismuth formulation; followed by 300 mg/day)

Dosage adjustment in renal impairment: Adults:

Active duodenal or gastric ulcer:

Cl_{cr} 20-50 mL/min: 150 mg/day

Cl_{cr} <20 mL/min: 150 mg every other day

Maintenance therapy:

Cl_{cr} 20-50 mL/min: 150 mg every other day

Cl_{cr} <20 mL/min: 150 mg every 3 days

Administration Oral: May administer with or without food; see Stability

Test Interactions False-positive urobilinogen with Multistix®

Patient Information Avoid excessive amounts of caffeinated beverages and aspirin; with self medication, if the symptoms of heartburn, acid indigestion, or sour stomach persist after 2 weeks of continuous use of the drug, consult clinician

Dosage Forms

Capsule (Axid®): 150 mg, 300 mg

Tablet (Axid® AR): 75 mg

(Continued)

Nizatidine *(Continued)*

References
Mikawa K, Nishina K, Maekawa N, et al, "Effects of Oral Nizatidine on Preoperative Gastric Fluid pH and Volume in Children," *Br J Anaesth*, 1994, 73(5):600-4.

Simeone D, Caria MC, Miele E, et al, "Treatment of Childhood Peptic Esophagitis: A Double-Blind Placebo-Controlled Trial of Nizatidine," *J Pediatr Gastroenterol Nur*, 1997, 25(1):51-5.

- ◆ **Nizoral®** *see* Ketoconazole *on page 564*
- ◆ **Noradrenaline Acid Tartrate** *see* Norepinephrine *on page 722*
- ◆ **Norco®** *see* Hydrocodone and Acetaminophen *on page 505*
- ◆ **Norcuron®** *see* Vecuronium *on page 1005*
- ◆ **Nordeoxyguanosine** *see* Ganciclovir *on page 466*
- ◆ **Norditropin® Injection** *see* Human Growth Hormone *on page 498*

Norepinephrine *(nor ep i NEF rin)*

Related Information
Extravasation Treatment *on page 1085*

U.S. Brand Names Levophed®

Synonyms Levarterenol; Noradrenaline Acid Tartrate

Therapeutic Category Adrenergic Agonist Agent; Alpha-Adrenergic Agonist; Sympathomimetic

Generic Available No

Use Treatment of shock which persists after adequate fluid volume replacement; severe hypotension; cardiogenic shock

Pregnancy Risk Factor C

Contraindications Hypersensitivity to norepinephrine, any component, or sulfites

Warnings Potent drug; must be diluted prior to use; monitor hemodynamic status

Precautions Blood/volume depletion should be corrected, if possible, before norepinephrine therapy; extravasation may cause severe tissue necrosis; do **not** give to patients with peripheral or mesenteric vascular thrombosis because ischemia may be increased and the area of infarct extended; use with caution during cyclopropane or halothane anesthesia and in patients with occlusive vascular disease

Adverse Reactions
Cardiovascular: Cardiac arrhythmias, palpitations, bradycardia, tachycardia, hypertension, chest pain, pallor
Central nervous system: Anxiety, headache
Endocrine & metabolic: Uterine contractions
Gastrointestinal: Vomiting
Local: Organ ischemia (due to vasoconstriction of renal and mesenteric arteries), ischemic necrosis and sloughing of superficial tissue after extravasation
Ocular: Photophobia
Respiratory: Respiratory distress
Miscellaneous: Diaphoresis

Drug Interactions Atropine sulfate may block the reflex bradycardia caused by norepinephrine and enhance the pressor response; tricyclic antidepressants, MAO inhibitors, antihistamines (diphenhydramine, tripelennamine), guanethidine, ergot alkaloids, and methyldopa may potentiate the effect of norepinephrine

Stability Readily oxidized, do not use if brown coloration; dilute with D_5W or D_5W/NS; not recommended for dilution in NS; not stable with alkaline solutions

Mechanism of Action Stimulates $beta_1$-adrenergic receptors and alpha-adrenergic receptors causing increased contractility and heart rate as well as vasoconstriction, thereby increasing systemic blood pressure and coronary blood flow; clinically alpha effects (vasoconstriction) are greater than beta effects (inotropic and chronotropic effects)

Pharmacodynamics
Onset of action: Very rapid
Duration: Limited duration following I.V. injection

Pharmacokinetics
Metabolism: By catechol-o-methyltransferase (COMT) and monoamine oxidase (MAO)
Elimination: In urine (84% to 96% as inactive metabolites)

Usual Dosage I.V. (dose stated in terms of **norepinephrine base**):
Children: Initial: 0.05-0.1 mcg/kg/minute, titrate to desired effect; maximum dose: 1-2 mcg/kg/minute
Rate (mL/hour) = dose (mcg/kg/minute) x weight (kg) x 60 minutes/hour divided by concentration (mcg/mL)
Adults: Initial: 4 mcg/minute; titrate to desired response; usual dose: 8-12 mcg/minute as an infusion

ACLS Guidelines 2000: Initial 0.5-1 mcg/minute; titrate to effect
Refractory shock: 8-30 mcg/minute may be required

Administration Parenteral: Administer into large vein to avoid potential extravasation; standard concentration: 4 mcg/mL but 16 mcg/mL has been used safely and with efficacy in situations of extreme fluid restriction

Monitoring Parameters Blood pressure, heart rate, urine output, peripheral perfusion

Additional Information Treat extravasations with local injections of phentolamine (see Extravasation Treatment *on page 1085*)

Dosage Forms Injection, as bitartrate: 1 mg/mL norepinephrine base (4 mL)

Norethindrone (nor eth IN drone)

Related Information
Oral Contraceptives *on page 1087*

U.S. Brand Names Aygestin®; Micronor®; Nor-QD®

Canadian Brand Names Norlutate

Synonyms Norethisterone

Therapeutic Category Contraceptive, Oral; Contraceptive, Progestin Only; Progestin

Generic Available No

Use Treatment of amenorrhea, abnormal uterine bleeding, endometriosis, oral contraceptive

Pregnancy Risk Factor X

Contraindications Hypersensitivity to norethindrone or any component; thromboembolic disorders, severe hepatic disease, breast cancer, cerebral hemorrhage, undiagnosed vaginal bleeding

Warnings Use of any progestin during the first 4 months of pregnancy is not recommended; discontinue if sudden partial or complete loss of vision, proptosis, diplopia, or migraine occur; **there is a higher rate of failure with progestin only contraceptives**; progestin-induced withdrawal bleeding occurs within 3-7 days after discontinuation of drug

Precautions Use with caution in patients with asthma, diabetes mellitus, seizure disorder, migraine, cardiac or renal dysfunction, psychic depression; may affect lipid and carbohydrate metabolism; women with diabetes mellitus or hyperlipidemias should be monitored closely

Adverse Reactions
Cardiovascular: Edema, thromboembolic disorders, hypertension
Central nervous system: Mental depression, nervousness, dizziness, fatigue, headache
Dermatologic: Hirsutism, rash, melasma or chloasma, photosensitivity
Endocrine & metabolic: Breakthrough bleeding, spotting, changes in menstrual flow
Gastrointestinal: Weight gain or loss
Hepatic: Cholestatic jaundice

Drug Interactions Rifampin decreases pharmacologic effect of norethindrone

Food Interactions High-dose vitamin C (1 g/day) may increase adverse effects; increase dietary intake of folate and pyridoxine

Mechanism of Action Inhibits secretion of pituitary gonadotropin (LH) which prevents follicular maturation and ovulation; in the presence of adequate endogenous estrogen, transforms a proliferative endometrium to a secretory one

Pharmacokinetics
Protein binding: 80%
Metabolism: In the liver
Half-life: 5-14 hours
Time to peak serum concentration: 0.5-4 hours

Usual Dosage Adolescents and Adults: Oral:
Amenorrhea and abnormal uterine bleeding: Norethindrone acetate 2.5-10 mg/day for 5-10 days beginning during the latter half of the menstrual cycle
Endometriosis: Norethindrone acetate 5 mg/day for 14 days; increase at increments of 2.5 mg/day every 2 weeks up to 15 mg/day
Contraception: Progesterone only: Norethindrone 0.35 mg every day of the year starting on first day of menstruation

Administration Oral: Administer with food

Test Interactions Thyroid function test, metyrapone test, liver function tests, coagulation tests (prothrombin time, factors VII, VIII, IX, X)

Patient Information Progestin-induced withdrawal bleeding occurs within 3-7 days after discontinuation of the drug; limit caffeine; when used for contraception, if one dose is missed take as soon as remembered, then take the next tablet at the regular
(Continued)

Norethindrone *(Continued)*

time; if two doses are missed, take one of the missed doses, discard the other, and take daily dose at usual time; if three doses are missed, use another form of birth control until menses appear or pregnancy is ruled out

Dosage Forms
Tablet (Micronor®, Nor-QD®): 0.35 mg
Tablet, as acetate (Aygestin®): 5 mg

♦ **Norethisterone** *see* Norethindrone *on page 723*

♦ **Noritate (Can)** *see* Metronidazole *on page 662*

♦ **Norlutate (Can)** *see* Norethindrone *on page 723*

♦ **Normal Human Serum Albumin** *see* Albumin *on page 44*

♦ **Normal Laboratory Values for Children** *see page 1187*

♦ **Normal Saline** *see* Sodium Chloride *on page 906*

♦ **Normal Serum Albumin (Human)** *see* Albumin *on page 44*

♦ **Normodyne®** *see* Labetalol *on page 568*

♦ **Norpace®** *see* Disopyramide *on page 347*

♦ **Norpace® CR** *see* Disopyramide *on page 347*

♦ **Norpramin®** *see* Desipramine *on page 303*

♦ **Nor-QD®** *see* Norethindrone *on page 723*

♦ **North and South American Antisnake-bite Serum** *see* Antivenin (*Crotalidae*) Polyvalent *on page 99*

Nortriptyline *(nor TRIP ti leen)*

Related Information
Comparison of Adverse Effects of Antidepressants *on page 1066*
Comparison of Usual Adult Dosage and Mechanism of Action of Antidepressants *on page 1065*

U.S. Brand Names Aventyl® Hydrochloride; Pamelor®

Canadian Brand Names Alti-Nortriptyline; Apo-Nortriptyline; Gen-Nortriptyline; Norventyl; Novo-Nortriptyline; Nu-Nortriptyline; PMS-Nortriptyline

Therapeutic Category Antidepressant, Tricyclic

Generic Available Yes

Use Treatment of various forms of depression, often in conjunction with psychotherapy; nocturnal enuresis

Pregnancy Risk Factor D

Contraindications Hypersensitivity to nortriptyline or amitriptyline (cross-sensitivity with other tricyclics may occur) or any component; angle-closure glaucoma, use of MAO inhibitors within 14 days (potentially fatal reactions may occur, see Drug Interactions)

Warnings Do not discontinue abruptly in patients receiving high doses chronically; use with extreme caution with renal or hepatic impairment

Precautions Use with caution in patients with cardiac conduction disturbances, cardiovascular disease, seizure disorder, history of urinary retention, hyperthyroidism, or those receiving thyroid hormone replacement

Adverse Reactions Nortriptyline has lower anticholinergic and sedative effects compared to amitriptyline
Cardiovascular: Postural hypotension, arrhythmias, tachycardia, sudden death
Central nervous system: Sedation, fatigue, anxiety, impaired cognitive function, seizures
Dermatologic: Photosensitivity
Endocrine & metabolic: Rarely SIADH
Gastrointestinal: Xerostomia, constipation, increased appetite, weight gain
Genitourinary: Urinary retention
Hematologic: Rarely agranulocytosis, leukopenia, eosinophilia
Hepatic: Cholestatic jaundice, elevated liver enzymes
Neuromuscular & skeletal: Tremor, weakness
Ocular: Blurred vision, increased intraocular pressure
Miscellaneous: Allergic reactions

Drug Interactions Cytochrome P-450 isoenzyme CYP1A2 and CYP2D6 substrate
Nortriptyline may decrease the effects of guanethidine and clonidine (use with clonidine may result in possible hypertensive crisis); nortriptyline may increase the effects of other CNS depressants (including alcohol), adrenergic agents (epinephrine, isoproterenol), anticholinergic agents and warfarin
With MAO inhibitors, hyperpyrexia, hypertension, tachycardia, confusion, seizures, and death have been reported (see Contraindications); the herbal medicine St

John's wort (*Hypericum perforatum*) may increase serious side effects, its use is **not** recommended

Cimetidine, fluoxetine, and methylphenidate may decrease the metabolism and phenobarbital may increase the metabolism of nortriptyline

Food Interactions Riboflavin dietary requirements may be increased

Stability Protect from light

Mechanism of Action Increases the synaptic concentration of serotonin and/or norepinephrine in the central nervous system by inhibition of their reuptake by the presynaptic neuronal membrane

Pharmacodynamics Onset of action: Therapeutic antidepressant effects begin in 7-21 days; maximum effects may not occur for ≥2-3 weeks

Pharmacokinetics

Absorption: Oral: Rapid; well absorbed

Distribution: V_d: 14-22 L/kg; crosses placenta; enters breast milk

Protein binding: 93% to 95%

Metabolism: Undergoes significant first-pass metabolism; primarily detoxified in the liver via hydroxylation followed by glucuronide conjugation

Half-life:

Children (mean ± SD): 18 ± 4 hours

Adults (mean ± SD): 46 ± 24 hours

Time to peak serum concentration: Oral: Within 7-8.5 hours

Elimination: Metabolites and small amounts of unchanged drug excreted in urine; small amounts of biliary elimination occur

Dialysis: Not Dialyzable

Usual Dosage Oral:

Nocturnal enuresis: Children (give dose 30 minutes before bedtime):

6-7 years (20-25 kg): 10 mg/day

8-11 years (25-35 kg): 10-20 mg/day

>11 years (35-54 kg): 25-35 mg/day

Depression:

Children 6-12 years: 1-3 mg/kg/day or 10-20 mg/day in 3-4 divided doses

Adolescents: 1-3 mg/kg/day or 30-50 mg/day in 3-4 divided doses; usual maximum dose: 150 mg/day

Adults: 25 mg 3-4 times/day up to 150 mg/day

Dosing adjustment in hepatic impairment: Use lower doses and slower titration; individualization of dosage is recommended

Administration Oral: May administer with food to decrease GI upset; dilute oral solution in water, milk, or fruit juice immediately before use; do not dilute in grape juice or carbonated beverages

Monitoring Parameters Heart rate, blood pressure, mental status, weight, plasma concentrations

Reference Range Therapeutic: 50-150 ng/mL (SI: 190-570 nmol/L)

Patient Information Avoid alcohol and the herbal medicine St John's wort; limit caffeine; do not discontinue medication abruptly; may cause drowsiness and impair ability to perform activities requiring mental alertness or physical coordination; may cause dry mouth; avoid undo exposure to sun, wear sunscreen

Nursing Implications Treatment duration of nocturnal enuresis is usually ≤3 months

Dosage Forms

Capsule, as hydrochloride: 10 mg, 25 mg, 50 mg, 75 mg

Solution, as hydrochloride: 10 mg/5 mL [contains 4% alcohol] (473 mL)

References

Levy HB, Harper CR, and Weinberg WA, "A Practical Approach to Children Failing in School," *Pediatr Clin North Am*, 1992, 39(4):895-928

- **Novo-Amiodarone (Can)** *see* Amiodarone *on page 72*
- **Novo-Ampicillin (Can)** *see* Ampicillin *on page 88*
- **Novo-Atenol (Can)** *see* Atenolol *on page 111*
- **Novo-AZT (Can)** *see* Zidovudine *on page 1022*
- **Novo-Baclofen (Can)** *see* Baclofen *on page 129*
- **Novo-Buspirone (Can)** *see* Buspirone *on page 159*
- **Novo-Captopril (Can)** *see* Captopril *on page 173*
- **Novo-Carbamaz (Can)** *see* Carbamazepine *on page 175*
- **Novo-Cefaclor (Can)** *see* Cefaclor *on page 186*
- **Novo-Cefadroxil (Can)** *see* Cefadroxil Monohydrate *on page 188*
- **Novo-Chlorhydrate (Can)** *see* Chloral Hydrate *on page 215*
- **Novo-Chlorocap (Can)** *see* Chloramphenicol *on page 218*
- **Novo-Chlorpromazine (Can)** *see* Chlorpromazine *on page 226*
- **Novo-Cholamine (Can)** *see* Cholestyramine Resin *on page 229*
- **Novo-Cimetine (Can)** *see* Cimetidine *on page 234*
- **Novo-Clonazepam (Can)** *see* Clonazepam *on page 254*
- **Novo-Clonidine (Can)** *see* Clonidine *on page 255*
- **Novo-Clopate (Can)** *see* Clorazepate *on page 257*
- **Novo-Cloxin (Can)** *see* Cloxacillin *on page 260*
- **Novo-Cromolyn (Can)** *see* Cromolyn *on page 273*
- **Novo-Cycloprine (Can)** *see* Cyclobenzaprine *on page 278*
- **Novo-Desipramine (Can)** *see* Desipramine *on page 303*
- **Novo-Difenac (Can)** *see* Diclofenac *on page 324*
- **Novo-Difenac-SR (Can)** *see* Diclofenac *on page 324*
- **Novo-Digoxin (Can)** *see* Digoxin *on page 330*
- **Novo-Diltazem (Can)** *see* Diltiazem *on page 337*
- **Novo-Dimenate (Can)** *see* Dimenhydrinate *on page 339*
- **Novo-Dipam (Can)** *see* Diazepam *on page 320*
- **Novo-Dipiradol (Can)** *see* Dipyridamole *on page 346*
- **Novo-Divalproex (Can)** *see* Valproic Acid and Derivatives *on page 998*
- **Novo-Doxepin (Can)** *see* Doxepin *on page 358*
- **Novo-Doxylin (Can)** *see* Doxycycline *on page 362*
- **Novo E (Can)** *see* Vitamin E *on page 1014*
- **Novo-Famotidine (Can)** *see* Famotidine *on page 417*
- **Novo-Fluoxetine (Can)** *see* Fluoxetine *on page 445*
- **Novo-Flupam (Can)** *see* Flurazepam *on page 449*
- **Novo-Flurprofen (Can)** *see* Flurbiprofen *on page 450*
- **Novo-Folacid (Can)** *see* Folic Acid *on page 454*
- **Novo-Furan (Can)** *see* Nitrofurantoin *on page 716*
- **Novo-Furantoin (Can)** *see* Nitrofurantoin *on page 716*
- **Novo-Gesic (Can)** *see* Acetaminophen *on page 29*
- **Novo-Glyburide (Can)** *see* Glyburide *on page 476*
- **Novo-Hexidyl (Can)** *see* Trihexyphenidyl *on page 984*
- **Novo-Hydrazide (Can)** *see* Hydrochlorothiazide *on page 503*
- **Novo-Hydrocort (Can)** *see* Hydrocortisone *on page 506*
- **Novo-Hydroxyzin (Can)** *see* Hydroxyzine *on page 516*
- **Novo-Hylazin (Can)** *see* Hydralazine *on page 501*
- **Novo-Ipramide (Can)** *see* Ipratropium *on page 547*
- **Novo-Ketorolac (Can)** *see* Ketorolac *on page 565*
- **Novo-Levobunolol (Can)** *see* Levobunolol *on page 584*
- **Novo-Lexin (Can)** *see* Cephalexin *on page 207*
- **Novolin 10/90, 20/80, 30/70, 40/60, 50/50 (Can)** *see* Insulin Preparations *on page 538*
- **Novolin® 70/30** *see* Insulin Preparations *on page 538*
- **Novolin® L** *see* Insulin Preparations *on page 538*
- **Novolin Lente (Can)** *see* Insulin Preparations *on page 538*
- **Novolin® N** *see* Insulin Preparations *on page 538*
- **Novolin NPH (Can)** *see* Insulin Preparations *on page 538*
- **Novolin® R** *see* Insulin Preparations *on page 538*
- **Novolin Toronto (Can)** *see* Insulin Preparations *on page 538*
- **Novolin Ultralente (Can)** *see* Insulin Preparations *on page 538*

+ **NovoLog**™ *see* Insulin Preparations *on page 538*
+ **Novo-Loperamide (Can)** *see* Loperamide *on page 603*
+ **Novo-Lorazem (Can)** *see* Lorazepam *on page 609*
+ **Novo-Medopa (Can)** *see* Methyldopa *on page 651*
+ **Novo-Medrone (Can)** *see* Medroxyprogesterone *on page 624*
+ **Novo-Metformin (Can)** *see* Metformin *on page 639*
+ **Novo-Methacin (Can)** *see* Indomethacin *on page 536*
+ **Novo-Mexiletine (Can)** *see* Mexiletine *on page 665*
+ **Novo-Mucilax (Can)** *see* Psyllium *on page 853*
+ **Novo-Naprox (Can)** *see* Naproxen *on page 699*
+ **Novo-Nidazol (Can)** *see* Metronidazole *on page 662*
+ **Novo-Nifedin (Can)** *see* Nifedipine *on page 714*
+ **Novo-Nizatidine (Can)** *see* Nizatidine *on page 720*
+ **Novo-Nortriptyline (Can)** *see* Nortriptyline *on page 724*
+ **Novo-Oxybutynin (Can)** *see* Oxybutynin *on page 744*
+ **Novo-Pen-VK (Can)** *see* Penicillin V Potassium *on page 774*
+ **Novo-Peridol (Can)** *see* Haloperidol *on page 488*
+ **Novo-Pheniram (Can)** *see* Chlorpheniramine *on page 225*
+ **Novo-Pramine (Can)** *see* Imipramine *on page 528*
+ **Novo-Pranol (Can)** *see* Propranolol *on page 847*
+ **Novo-Prazin (Can)** *see* Prazosin *on page 820*
+ **Novo-Prednisolone (Can)** *see* Prednisolone *on page 821*
+ **Novo-Prednisone (Can)** *see* Prednisone *on page 824*
+ **Novo-Profen (Can)** *see* Ibuprofen *on page 520*
+ **Novo-Propoxyn (Can)** *see* Propoxyphene *on page 845*
+ **Novo-Purol (Can)** *see* Allopurinol *on page 53*
+ **Novo-Ranidine (Can)** *see* Ranitidine *on page 865*
+ **Novo-Ridazine (Can)** *see* Thioridazine *on page 953*
+ **Novo-Rythro Encap (Can)** *see* Erythromycin *on page 394*
+ **Novo-Salmol (Can)** *see* Albuterol *on page 45*
+ **Novo-Secobarb (Can)** *see* Secobarbital *on page 893*
+ **Novo-Semide (Can)** *see* Furosemide *on page 462*
+ **Novo-Sertraline (Can)** *see* Sertraline *on page 898*
+ **Novo-Soxazole (Can)** *see* Sulfisoxazole *on page 928*
+ **Novo-Spiroton (Can)** *see* Spironolactone *on page 911*
+ **Novo-Spirozine (Can)** *see* Hydrochlorothiazide and Spironolactone *on page 504*
+ **Novo-Sucralate (Can)** *see* Sucralfate *on page 919*
+ **Novo-Sundac (Can)** *see* Sulindac *on page 930*
+ **Novo-Tetra (Can)** *see* Tetracycline *on page 941*
+ **Novo-Theophyl (Can)** *see* Theophylline *on page 943*
+ **Novo-Timol (Can)** *see* Timolol *on page 962*
+ **Novo-Tolmetin (Can)** *see* Tolmetin *on page 968*
+ **Novo-Trazodone (Can)** *see* Trazodone *on page 977*
+ **Novo-Trimel (Can)** *see* Co-Trimoxazole *on page 270*
+ **Novo-Triolam (Can)** *see* Triazolam *on page 982*
+ **Novo-Triptyn (Can)** *see* Amitriptyline *on page 77*
+ **Novo-Valproic (Can)** *see* Valproic Acid and Derivatives *on page 998*
+ **Novo-Veramil (Can)** *see* Verapamil *on page 1007*
+ **Novo-Zolamide (Can)** *see* Acetazolamide *on page 32*
+ **NP-27**® **[OTC]** *see* Tolnaftate *on page 969*
+ **NPH Iletin**® **II** *see* Insulin Preparations *on page 538*
+ **NS** *see* Sodium Chloride *on page 906*
+ **NSC-373364** *see* Aldesleukin *on page 47*
+ **NTG** *see* Nitroglycerin *on page 717*
+ **Nu-Acyclovir (Can)** *see* Acyclovir *on page 37*
+ **Nu-Alpraz (Can)** *see* Alprazolam *on page 55*
+ **Nu-Amoxi (Can)** *see* Amoxicillin *on page 80*
+ **Nu-Ampi (Can)** *see* Ampicillin *on page 88*
+ **Nu-Atenol (Can)** *see* Atenolol *on page 111*
+ **Nu-Baclo (Can)** *see* Baclofen *on page 129*
+ **Nubain**® *see* Nalbuphine *on page 694*

- ♦ **Nu-Beclomethasone (Can)** *see* Beclomethasone *on page 131*
- ♦ **Nu-Buspirone (Can)** *see* Buspirone *on page 159*
- ♦ **Nu-Capto (Can)** *see* Captopril *on page 173*
- ♦ **Nu-Carbamazepine (Can)** *see* Carbamazepine *on page 175*
- ♦ **Nu-Cefaclor (Can)** *see* Cefaclor *on page 186*
- ♦ **Nu-Cephalex (Can)** *see* Cephalexin *on page 207*
- ♦ **Nu-Cimet (Can)** *see* Cimetidine *on page 234*
- ♦ **Nu-Clonazepam (Can)** *see* Clonazepam *on page 254*
- ♦ **Nu-Clonidine (Can)** *see* Clonidine *on page 255*
- ♦ **Nu-Cloxi (Can)** *see* Cloxacillin *on page 260*
- ♦ **Nu-Cotrimox (Can)** *see* Co-Trimoxazole *on page 270*
- ♦ **Nu-Cyclobenzaprine (Can)** *see* Cyclobenzaprine *on page 278*
- ♦ **Nu-Desipramine (Can)** *see* Desipramine *on page 303*
- ♦ **Nu-Diclo (Can)** *see* Diclofenac *on page 324*
- ♦ **Nu-Diltiaz (Can)** *see* Diltiazem *on page 337*
- ♦ **Nu-Divalproex (Can)** *see* Valproic Acid and Derivatives *on page 998*
- ♦ **Nu-Doxycycline (Can)** *see* Doxycycline *on page 362*
- ♦ **Nu-Erythromycin (Can)** *see* Erythromycin *on page 394*
- ♦ **Nu-Famotidine (Can)** *see* Famotidine *on page 417*
- ♦ **Nu-Fluoxetine (Can)** *see* Fluoxetine *on page 445*
- ♦ **Nu-Flurprofen (Can)** *see* Flurbiprofen *on page 450*
- ♦ **Nu-Glyburide (Can)** *see* Glyburide *on page 476*
- ♦ **Nu-Hydral (Can)** *see* Hydralazine *on page 501*
- ♦ **Nu-Ibuprofen (Can)** *see* Ibuprofen *on page 520*
- ♦ **Nu-Indo (Can)** *see* Indomethacin *on page 536*
- ♦ **Nu-Ipratropium (Can)** *see* Ipratropium *on page 547*
- ♦ **Nu-Iron® [OTC]** *see* Iron Supplements (Oral/Enteral) *on page 548*
- ♦ **Nu-Iron® 150 [OTC]** *see* Iron Supplements (Oral/Enteral) *on page 548*
- ♦ **NuLev™** *see* Hyoscyamine *on page 517*
- ♦ **Nu-Loraz (Can)** *see* Lorazepam *on page 609*
- ♦ **NuLYTELY®** *see* Polyethylene Glycol-Electrolyte Solution *on page 811*
- ♦ **Nu-Medopa (Can)** *see* Methyldopa *on page 651*
- ♦ **Nu-Metformin (Can)** *see* Metformin *on page 639*
- ♦ **Nu-Metoclopramide (Can)** *see* Metoclopramide *on page 657*
- ♦ **Nu-Metop (Can)** *see* Metoprolol *on page 660*
- ♦ **Numzit Teething® [OTC]** *see* Benzocaine *on page 135*
- ♦ **Nu-Naprox (Can)** *see* Naproxen *on page 699*
- ♦ **Nu-Nifed (Can)** *see* Nifedipine *on page 714*
- ♦ **Nu-Nortriptyline (Can)** *see* Nortriptyline *on page 724*
- ♦ **Nu-Oxybutyn (Can)** *see* Oxybutynin *on page 744*
- ♦ **Nu-Pentoxifylline (Can)** *see* Pentoxifylline *on page 781*
- ♦ **Nu-Pen-VK (Can)** *see* Penicillin V Potassium *on page 774*
- ♦ **Nupercainal® [OTC]** *see* Dibucaine *on page 324*
- ♦ **Nupercainal®** *see* Hemorrhoidal Preparations *on page 490*
- ♦ **Nupercainal® Hydrocortisone Cream [OTC]** *see* Hydrocortisone *on page 506*
- ♦ **Nu-Pirox (Can)** *see* Piroxicam *on page 806*
- ♦ **Nu-Prazo (Can)** *see* Prazosin *on page 820*
- ♦ **Nuprin® [OTC]** *see* Ibuprofen *on page 520*
- ♦ **Nu-Prochlor (Can)** *see* Prochlorperazine *on page 834*
- ♦ **Nu-Propranolol (Can)** *see* Propranolol *on page 847*
- ♦ **Nu-Ranit (Can)** *see* Ranitidine *on page 865*
- ♦ **Nuromax®** *see* Doxacurium *on page 356*
- ♦ **Nu-Salbutamol (Can)** *see* Albuterol *on page 45*
- ♦ **Nu-Sulindac (Can)** *see* Sulindac *on page 930*
- ♦ **Nu-Tetra (Can)** *see* Tetracycline *on page 941*
- ♦ **Nu-Timolol (Can)** *see* Timolol *on page 962*
- ♦ **Nutracort®** *see* Hydrocortisone *on page 506*
- ♦ **Nu-Trazodone (Can)** *see* Trazodone *on page 977*
- ♦ **Nutrol C (Can)** *see* Ascorbic Acid *on page 106*
- ♦ **Nutrol E (Can)** *see* Vitamin E *on page 1014*
- ♦ **Nutropin® AQ Injection** *see* Human Growth Hormone *on page 498*

- ♦ **Nutropin® Depot™** *see* Human Growth Hormone *on page 498*
- ♦ **Nutropin® Injection** *see* Human Growth Hormone *on page 498*
- ♦ **Nu-Valproic (Can)** *see* Valproic Acid and Derivatives *on page 998*
- ♦ **Nu-Verap (Can)** *see* Verapamil *on page 1007*
- ♦ **Nyaderm (Can)** *see* Nystatin *on page 729*
- ♦ **Nydrazid® Injection** *see* Isoniazid *on page 554*

Nystatin (nye STAT in)

Related Information
Carbohydrate and Alcohol Content of Liquid Medications for Use in Patients Receiving Ketogenic Diets *on page 1258*

U.S. Brand Names Mycostatin®; Nilstat®; Nystat-Rx®; Nystex®; O-V Staticin®

Canadian Brand Names Candistatin; Nadostine; Nyaderm; PMS-Nystatin

Therapeutic Category Antifungal Agent, Oral Nonabsorbed; Antifungal Agent, Topical; Antifungal Agent, Vaginal

Generic Available Yes

Use Treatment of susceptible cutaneous, mucocutaneous, oral cavity and vaginal fungal infections normally caused by the *Candida* species

Pregnancy Risk Factor B

Contraindications Hypersensitivity to nystatin or any component

Adverse Reactions
Dermatologic: Contact dermatitis, Stevens-Johnson syndrome
Gastrointestinal: Nausea, vomiting, diarrhea
Local: Irritation

Stability Store vaginal inserts in refrigerator; protect from moisture and light

Mechanism of Action Binds to sterols in fungal cell membrane, changing the cell wall permeability allowing for leakage of cellular contents

Pharmacodynamics Onset of symptomatic relief from candidiasis: Within 24-72 hours

Pharmacokinetics
Absorption: Not absorbed through mucous membranes or intact skin; poorly absorbed from the GI tract
Elimination: In feces as unchanged drug

Usual Dosage
Oral candidiasis:
Neonates: 100,000 units 4 times/day or 50,000 units to each side of mouth 4 times/day
Infants: 200,000 units 4 times/day or 100,000 units to each side of mouth 4 times/day
Children and Adults: 400,000-600,000 units 4 times/day; troche: 200,000-400,000 units 4-5 times/day
Cutaneous candidal infections: Children and Adults: Topical: Apply 2-4 times/day
Intestinal infections: Adults: Oral: 500,000-1,000,000 units every 8 hours
Vaginal infections: Adolescents and Adults: Vaginal tablets: Insert 1 tablet/day at bedtime for 2 weeks

Administration
Oral: Shake suspension well before use; suspension should be swished about the mouth and retained in the mouth for as long as possible (several minutes) before swallowing. For neonates and infants, paint nystatin suspension into recesses of the mouth. Troches must be allowed to dissolve slowly and should not be chewed or swallowed whole.
Topical:
Cream or ointment: Gently massage formulation into the skin
Intravaginal: Insert vaginal tablet high in the vagina
Powder: Dust in shoes, in stockings, and on feet for treatment of candidal infection of the feet; also used on very moist lesions

Patient Information Inform physician if irritation or sensitization occur during therapy

Dosage Forms
Cream: 100,000 units/g (15 g, 30 g)
Ointment, topical: 100,000 units/g (15 g, 30 g)
Powder, for preparation of oral suspension: 50 million units, 1 billion units, 2 billion units, 5 billion units
Powder, topical: 100,000 units/g (15 g)
Suspension, oral: 100,000 units/mL (5 mL, 60 mL, 480 mL)
Tablet:
Oral: 500,000 units
(Continued)

Nystatin *(Continued)*

Vaginal: 100,000 units (15 and 30/box with applicator)

Troche: 200,000 units

References

Dismukes WE, Wade JS, Lee JY, et al, "A Randomized, Double-Blind Trial of Nystatin Therapy for the Candidiasis Hypersensitivity Syndrome," *N Engl J Med*, 1990, 323(25):1717-23.

- ◆ **Nystat-Rx**® *see Nystatin on page 729*
- ◆ **Nystex**® *see Nystatin on page 729*
- ◆ **Nytol**® **[OTC]** *see Diphenhydramine on page 342*
- ◆ **Nytol Extra Strength (Can)** *see Diphenhydramine on page 342*
- ◆ **Occlusal**®**-HP [OTC]** *see Salicylic Acid on page 886*
- ◆ **Ocean [OTC]** *see Sodium Chloride on page 906*
- ◆ **OCL**® *see Polyethylene Glycol-Electrolyte Solution on page 811*
- ◆ **Octicair**® **Otic** *see Neomycin, (Bacitracin) Polymyxin B, and Hydrocortisone on page 705*
- ◆ **Octostim (Can)** *see Desmopressin on page 305*

Octreotide Acetate *(ok TREE oh tide AS e tate)*

U.S. Brand Names Sandostatin®; Sandostatin LAR® Depot

Therapeutic Category Antidiarrheal; Antisecretory Agent; Somatostatin Analog

Generic Available No

Use Control of symptoms in patients with metastatic carcinoid, vasoactive intestinal peptide-secreting tumors (VIPomas), and secretory diarrhea; acromegaly

Unlabeled use: AIDS-associated secretory diarrhea, control of bleeding of esophageal varices, breast cancer, cryptosporidiosis, Cushing's syndrome, insulinomas, small bowel fistulas, postgastrectomy dumping syndrome, chemotherapy-induced diarrhea, GVHD-induced diarrhea, Zollinger-Ellison syndrome

Pregnancy Risk Factor B

Contraindications Hypersensitivity to octreotide or any component

Warnings Dosage adjustment may be required to maintain symptomatic control; insulin requirements may be reduced as well as sulfonylurea requirements

Precautions Patients must be monitored closely for biliary tract abnormalities (including biliary obstruction, cholecystitis, and cholelithiasis), hypothyroidism, and glucose tolerance; use with caution in patients with renal impairment

Adverse Reactions

Cardiovascular: Flushing, edema, chest pain, hypertension, palpitations, CHF, orthostatic hypotension, syncope, bradycardia

Central nervous system: Dizziness, fatigue, anxiety, headache, depression, insomnia, fever, chills, seizures, vertigo, hyperesthesia, Bell's palsy

Dermatologic: Erythema, alopecia, bruising, pruritus, rash

Endocrine & metabolic: Hypoglycemia, hyperglycemia, galactorrhea, hypothyroidism

Gastrointestinal: Nausea, diarrhea, abdominal pain, vomiting, constipation, flatulence, fat malabsorption, GI bleeding (rare), xerostomia, dyspepsia, steatorrhea, cholelithiasis, biliary sludge, pancreatitis

Genitourinary: Prostatitis

Hepatic: Hepatitis, jaundice, elevated liver enzymes

Local: Injection site pain, thrombophlebitis

Neuromuscular & skeletal: Weakness, increased CPK, backache, muscle spasm, muscle cramps, arthralgia, tremor, numbness

Ocular: Visual disturbance, ocular burning

Renal: Oliguria, urinary hyperosmolarity

Respiratory: Shortness of breath, rhinorrhea

Drug Interactions Cytochrome P-450 isoenzyme CYP2D6 (high dose) and CYP3A inhibitor

May decrease cyclosporine levels (case report of a transplant rejection) possibly due to decreased cyclosporine bioavailability

Food Interactions Schedule injections between meals to decrease GI effects; may decrease vitamin B_{12} levels and decrease absorption of dietary fats

Stability Store in refrigerator; Sandostatin® injection is stable 14 days at room temperature if protected from light; stable in D_5W or NS for 4 days at room temperature; not compatible in TPN solutions due to glycosyl octreotide conjugate which may have decreased activity; Sandostatin LAR® Depot must be used immediately after reconstitution

Mechanism of Action A synthetic polypeptide which mimics natural somatostatin by inhibiting serotonin release, and the secretion of gastrin, vasoactive intestinal peptide (VIP), insulin, glucagon, secretin, motilin, and pancreatic polypeptide; in animals, also a potent inhibitor of growth hormone

Pharmacodynamics Duration of action: 6-12 hours

Pharmacokinetics

Absorption:

S.C.: Rapid

I.M.(Sandostatin LAR® Depot): 60% to 63% when compared with S.C. immediate release formulation

Distribution: V_d: 13.6 L/kg (adults)

Metabolism: Extensive by the liver

Half-life: 60-110 minutes

Elimination: 32% excreted unchanged in urine

Note: When using Sandostatin LAR® Depot formulation, steady state levels are achieved after 3 injections (3 months of therapy)

Usual Dosage Dosage should be individualized according to the patient's response

Sandostatin®:

Diarrhea:

Infants and Children: I.V., S.C.: Doses of 1-10 mcg/kg every 12 hours have been used in children beginning at the low end of the range and increasing by 0.3 mcg/kg/dose at 3-day intervals; suppression of growth hormone (animal data) is of concern when used as long-term therapy

Adults:

S.C.: Initial: 50 mcg 1-2 times/day

I.V.: Initial: 50-100 mcg every 8 hours; increase by 100 mcg/dose at 48-hour intervals; maximum dose: 500 mcg every 8 hours

The following are effective dosing ranges for specific therapies: Adults: S.C., I.V.:

Carcinoid: 100-600 mcg/day in 2-4 divided doses

VIPomas: 200-300 mcg/day in 2-4 divided doses

Esophageal varices bleeding: I.V. bolus: 25-50 mcg followed by continuous I.V. infusion of 25-50 mcg/hour

Acromegaly: 50 mcg 3 times/day; increase as needed (usual requirement: 100 mcg 3 times/day); maximum dose: 500 mcg 3 times/day; hold dose for 4 weeks per year in patients who have been irradiated, to assess disease activity; resume therapy if growth hormone or somatomedin C (IGF-I) levels increase and signs and symptoms recur

Sandostatin LAR® Depot: May be used in patients who have responded to the immediate release formulation; Adults: I.M.:

Acromegaly: Initial: 20 mg at 4-week intervals for 3 months; dosage may be adjusted based upon the following:

Maintain same dosage **IF**: Growth hormone level <2.5 ng/mL, IGF-I normal, and clinical symptoms controlled

Increase dosage to 30 mg **IF**: Growth hormone level >2.5 ng/mL, IGF-I elevated, and clinical symptoms uncontrolled

Reduce dosage to 10 mg **IF**: Growth hormone level ≤1 ng/mL, IGF-I normal, and clinical symptoms controlled

[May increase dosage to maximum 40 mg every 4 weeks if 30 mg dosage ineffective; it is not recommended to administer dosage at intervals >4 weeks; hold dose for 8 weeks per year in patients who have been irradiated, to assess disease activity; resume therapy if growth hormone or somatomedin C (IGF-I) levels increase and signs and symptoms recur.]

VIPomas, carcinoid: Initial: 20 mg at 4-week intervals; due to the need for serum octreotide to reach therapeutically effective levels following initial injection for Sandostatin LAR® Depot, subcutaneous Sandostatin® injection should be continued at the current dosage **at the same time** for at least the first 2 weeks of therapy (some patients may require 3 or 4 weeks of such therapy). Adjust Sandostatin LAR® Depot dosage after 2 months of therapy depending upon patient response; doses >30 mg are not recommended

Administration Parenteral: Only Sandostatin® injection may be administered I.V., I.M., and S.C.; Sandostatin LAR® Depot may only be administered I.M.

I.V. infusion: Dilute Sandostatin® injection in 50-200 mL NS or D_5W and infuse over 15-30 minutes; in emergency situations, may be administered undiluted by direct I.V. push over 3 minutes; see Stability for compatibility information; allow solution to come to room temperature before administration

I.M. administration: Reconstitute with provided diluent; use immediately after reconstitution; administer into gluteal area only (avoid deltoid injections due to significant pain and discomfort at injection site)

Monitoring Parameters Baseline and periodic ultrasound evaluations for cholelithiasis, blood sugar, baseline and periodic thyroid function tests, fluid and electrolyte

(Continued)

Octreotide Acetate *(Continued)*

balance, fecal fat, and serum carotene determinations; for carcinoid, monitor urinary 5-hydroxyindole acetic acid (5-HIAA), plasma serotonin, plasma substance P; for VIPoma, monitor VIP; vitamin B_{12} levels (chronic therapy); for acromegaly: growth hormone levels, IGF-I (somatomedin C)

Reference Range Vasoactive intestinal peptide (VIP): <75 ng/L; levels vary considerably between laboratories; growth hormone level: <5 ng/mL; IGF-I (somatomedin C): males: <1.9 units/mL, females: <2.2 units/mL

Dosage Forms

Injection: 0.05 mg/mL (1 mL); 0.1 mg/mL (1 mL); 0.2 mg/mL (5 mL); 0.5 mg/mL (1 mL); 1 mg/mL (5 mL)

Injection, microspheres for suspension (Sandostatin LAR® Depot): 10 mg, 20 mg, 30 mg

References

Couper RT, Berzen A, Berall G, et al, "Clinical Response to the Long-Acting Somatostatin Analogue SMS 201-995 in a Child With Congenital Microvillus Atrophy," *Gut,* 1989, 30(7):1020-4.

Jaros W, Biller J, Greer S, et al, "Successful Treatment of Idiopathic Secretory Diarrhea of Infancy With the Somatostatin Analogue SMS 201-995," *Gastroenterology,* 1988, 94(1):189-93.

Katz MD and Erstad BL, "Octreotide, A New Somatostatin Analogue," *Clin Pharm,* 1989, 8(4):255-73.

♦ **Ocu-Carpine®** *see* Pilocarpine *on page 800*
♦ **OcuClear® [OTC]** *see* Oxymetazoline *on page 749*
♦ **Ocufen®** *see* Flurbiprofen *on page 450*

Ocular Lubricant *(OK yoo lar LOO bri kant)*

U.S. Brand Names Duratears® [OTC]; Lacri-Lube® SOP [OTC]

Therapeutic Category Lubricant, Ocular; Ophthalmic Agent, Miscellaneous

Generic Available Yes

Use Ocular lubricant

Contraindications Hypersensitivity to any component

Warnings Discontinue if eye pain, vision change, redness or eye irritation occurs or if condition worsens or persists >72 hours

Adverse Reactions Ocular: Temporary blurring of vision, irritation

Stability Store away from heat

Mechanism of Action Forms an occlusive film on the surface of the eye to lubricate and protect the eye from drying

Usual Dosage Children and Adults: Ophthalmic: Apply $^1/_4$" of ointment to the inside of the lower lid as needed

Administration Ophthalmic: Do not use with contact lenses; to avoid contamination, do not touch tip of container to any surface

Additional Information Contains petrolatum, mineral oil, chlorobutanol and lanolin alcohols

Dosage Forms Ointment, ophthalmic: 3.5 g

♦ **Oculinum®** *see* Botulinum Toxin Type A *on page 149*
♦ **Ocu-Pentolate®** *see* Cyclopentolate *on page 279*
♦ **Ocu-Phrin®** *see* Phenylephrine *on page 789*
♦ **Ocusert Pilo-20®** *see* Pilocarpine *on page 800*
♦ **Ocusert Pilo-40®** *see* Pilocarpine *on page 800*
♦ **Ocutricin® HC Otic** *see* Neomycin, (Bacitracin) Polymyxin B, and Hydrocortisone *on page 705*
♦ **Ocutricin® Ointment** *see* Neomycin, Polymyxin B, and Bacitracin *on page 707*
♦ **Ocu-Trol®** *see* Dexamethasone, Neomycin, and Polymyxin B *on page 309*
♦ **Ocu-Trpoine®** *see* Atropine *on page 116*
♦ **Oesclim (Can)** *see* Estradiol *on page 400*
♦ **Off-Ezy® [OTC]** *see* Salicylic Acid *on page 886*
♦ **OKT3** *see* Muromonab-CD3 *on page 688*
♦ **Oleovitamin A** *see* Vitamin A *on page 1013*
♦ **Oleum Ricini** *see* Castor Oil *on page 186*

Olsalazine *(ole SAL a zeen)*

U.S. Brand Names Dipentum®

Therapeutic Category 5-Aminosalicylic Acid Derivative; Anti-inflammatory Agent

Generic Available No

Use Maintenance of remission of ulcerative colitis in patients intolerant to sulfasalazine

Pregnancy Risk Factor C

Contraindications Hypersensitivity to olsalazine, salicylates, or any component

Warnings Diarrhea is a common adverse effect of olsalazine

Precautions Use with caution in patients with hypersensitivity to sulfasalazine, salicylates, or mesalamine

Adverse Reactions

Cardiovascular: Pericarditis, heart block, hypertension, orthostatic hypotension, edema, chest pain, tachycardia

Central nervous system: Headache, fatigue, drowsiness, depression, insomnia, vertigo, fever

Dermatologic: Erythema nodosum, photosensitivity

Gastrointestinal: Diarrhea, cramps, nausea, dyspepsia, bloating, vomiting, pancreatitis, rectal bleeding, xerostomia

Genitourinary: Urinary frequency, dysuria

Hematologic: Leukopenia, neutropenia, lymphopenia, eosinophilia, thrombocytopenia

Hepatic: Mild cholestatic hepatitis, elevated AST and ALT

Neuromuscular & skeletal: Arthralgia, tremor, paresthesia

Ocular: Blurred vision, dry eyes

Renal: Hematuria, proteinuria

Respiratory: Bronchospasm, respiratory infection

Mechanism of Action Olsalazine is a sodium salt of a salicylate compound that is effectively bioconverted to 5-aminosalicylic acid (5-ASA). The exact mechanism of action appears to be topical rather than systemic. It may diminish colonic inflammation by blocking cyclo-oxygenase and inhibiting colon prostaglandin production in the bowel mucosa.

Pharmacokinetics

Absorption: <3%; very little intact olsalazine is systemically absorbed

Protein binding: High

Metabolism: Mostly by colonic bacteria to the active drug, 5-aminosalicylic acid

Bioavailability: 2.4%

Half-life, elimination: 56 minutes (in serum)

Elimination: Primarily in feces

Usual Dosage Adults: Oral: 1 g/day in 2 divided doses

Administration Oral: Administer with food in evenly divided doses

Patient Information Contact physician if diarrhea occurs; avoid unnecessary exposure to sunlight

Dosage Forms Capsule, as sodium: 250 mg

Omeprazole (oh ME pray zol)

U.S. Brand Names Prilosec™

Canadian Brand Names Losec

Therapeutic Category Gastric Acid Secretion Inhibitor; Gastrointestinal Agent, Gastric or Duodenal Ulcer Treatment; Proton Pump Inhibitor

Generic Available No

Use Treatment and maintenance of healing of severe erosive esophagitis (grade 2 or above) diagnosed by endoscopy; short-term treatment (4-8 weeks) of active duodenal ulcer; short-term treatment of active benign gastric ulcers; short-term treatment of symptomatic gastroesophageal reflux disease (GERD) poorly responsive to customary medical treatment; pathological hypersecretory conditions; peptic ulcer disease; adjunctive treatment of duodenal ulcers associated with *Helicobacter pylori*

Pregnancy Risk Factor C

Contraindications Hypersensitivity to omeprazole or any component

Warnings In long-term (2-year) studies in rats, omeprazole produced a dose-related increase in gastric carcinoid tumors. While available endoscopic evaluations and histologic examinations of biopsy specimens from human stomachs have not detected a risk from short-term exposure to omeprazole, further human data on the effect of sustained hypochlorhydria and hypergastrinemia are needed to rule out the possibility of an increased risk for the development of tumors in humans receiving long-term therapy.

Adverse Reactions

Cardiovascular: Chest pain, tachycardia, bradycardia, palpitations

Central nervous system: Headache, dizziness, vertigo, insomnia, anxiety, hemifacial dysesthesia, nervousness, fever

Dermatologic: Rash, dry skin

Endocrine & metabolic: Hypoglycemia

(Continued)

Omeprazole *(Continued)*

Gastrointestinal: Diarrhea, nausea, abdominal pain, vomiting, constipation, flatulence, discoloration of feces, irritable colon, xerostomia, anorexia, dysgeusia, abdominal pain

Genitourinary: Urinary frequency

Hematologic: Agranulocytosis, pancytopenia, thrombocytopenia, anemia, leukocytosis

Hepatic: Hepatitis, elevated liver function tests, jaundice

Neuromuscular & skeletal: Muscle cramps, myalgia, arthralgia, leg pain, paresthesia, back pain

Otic: Tinnitus

Renal: Hematuria, pyuria, proteinuria, glycosuria

Respiratory: Pharyngeal pain, cough, epistaxis

Drug Interactions Cytochrome P-450 isoenzyme CYP1A2 inducer; isoenzyme CYP2C8, CYP2C18, CYP2C19, and CYP3A3/4 substrate; isoenzyme CYP2C9, CYP3A3/4, CYP2C8, and CYP2C19 inhibitor

Omeprazole inhibits oxidative metabolism; the full potential related to specific drugs remains to be determined; decreases absorption of ketoconazole, itraconazole, iron salts, ampicillin esters; increases half-life (decreased clearance) of diazepam, phenytoin, and warfarin; may increase absorption of digoxin and didanosine; may decrease elimination of methotrexate

Stability Omeprazole stability is a function of pH; it is rapidly degraded in acidic media, but has acceptable stability under alkaline conditions. Prilosec™ is supplied as capsules for oral administration; each capsule of omeprazole contains enteric coated granules to prevent omeprazole degradation by gastric acidity.

Mechanism of Action Suppresses gastric acid secretion by inhibiting the parietal cell membrane enzyme (H^+/K^+)-ATPase or proton pump; demonstrates antimicrobial activity against *Helicobacter pylori*

Pharmacodynamics

Onset of action: 1 hour

Peak effect: 2 hours

Duration: 72 hours

Maximum secretory inhibition: 4 days

Pharmacokinetics

Protein binding: 95%

Metabolism: Extensive first-pass metabolism in the liver

Bioavailability: 30% to 40%; improves slightly with repeated administration

Half-life: 0.5-1 hour

Usual Dosage Oral:

Children: Dosage not established, but a starting dose of 0.6-0.7 mg/kg/day in the morning is recommended; a second dose 12 hours later may be given if necessary; range of effective dosages in the literature: 0.7-3.5 mg/kg/day (Hassall, 2000)

Adults:

Active duodenal ulcer: 20 mg/day for 4-8 weeks

GERD or severe erosive esophagitis: 20 mg/day for 4-8 weeks

Pathological hypersecretory conditions: 60 mg/day to start; doses up to 120 mg 3 times/day have been administered; administer daily doses >80 mg in divided doses

Adjunctive therapy of duodenal ulcers associated with *Helicobacter pylori*: 20 mg twice daily, or 40 mg/day (in combination with antibiotic therapy)

Gastric ulcers: 40 mg/day for 4-8 weeks

Administration Oral: Administer before food or meals; capsule should be swallowed whole, do not chew or crush; because the enteric coating of granules will dissolve in alkaline pH, administration via NG tube should be in acidic juice (eg, apple juice or cranberry juice); stable 30 minutes after mixing; to administer via jejunostomy tube, crush the granules and dissolve in a mixture of water to which a crushed 650 mg sodium bicarbonate tablet has been added

Dosage Forms Capsule, delayed release: 10 mg, 20 mg, 40 mg

Extemporaneous Preparations Omeprazole 2 mg/mL suspension may be made by adding 100 mL 8.4% sodium bicarbonate solution to the contents of ten 20 mg omeprazole capsules; stir for 30 minutes; protect from light; stable 14 days at room temperature and 45 days refrigerated

DiGiacinto JL, Olsen KM, Bergman KL, et al, "Stability of Suspension Formulations of Lansoprazole and Omeprazole Stored in Amber-colored Plastic Oral Syringes," *Ann Pharmacother*, 2000, 34(5):600-4.

References

Gunasekaran TS and Hassall EG, "Efficacy and Safety of Omeprazole for Severe Gastroesophageal Reflux in Children," *J Pediatr*, 1993, 123(1):148-54.

Hassall E, Israel D, Shepherd R, "Omeprazole for Treatment of Chronic Erosive Esophagitis in Children: A Multicenter Study of Efficacy, Safety, Tolerability and Dose Requirements. International Pediatric Omeprazole Study Group," *J Pediatr*, 2000, 137(6):800-7.

Kane DL, "Administration of Omeprazole (Prilosec™) in the Atypical Patient," *Int J Pharm Compounding*, 1997, 1(1):13.

Kato S, Ebina K, Fujii K, et al, "Effect of Omeprazole in the Treatment of Refractory Acid-Related Diseases in Childhood: Endoscopic Healing and Twenty-Four Hour Intragastric Acidity," *J Pediatr*, 1996, 128(3):415-21.

♦ **Omnicef**® *see* Cefdinir *on page 190*

♦ **Omnipen**® *see* Ampicillin *on page 88*

♦ **Omnipen**®-**N** *see* Ampicillin *on page 88*

♦ **Oncaspar**® *see* Pegaspargase *on page 766*

♦ **Oncovin**® *see* Vincristine *on page 1011*

Ondansetron (on DAN se tron)

U.S. Brand Names Zofran®; Zofran® ODT

Therapeutic Category Antiemetic

Generic Available No

Use Prevention of nausea and vomiting associated with highly emetogenic cancer chemotherapy and prevention of postoperative nausea and vomiting

Pregnancy Risk Factor B

Contraindications Hypersensitivity to ondansetron or any component

Warnings Zofran® ODT tablets contain aspartame; avoid use in phenylketonuric patients

Adverse Reactions

Cardiovascular: Tachycardia, bradycardia, angina, syncope

Central nervous system: Lightheadedness, seizures, headache, dizziness, drowsiness, sedation, fatigue, fever, shivers

Dermatologic: Rash, local injection site reaction

Endocrine & metabolic: Hypokalemia

Gastrointestinal: Constipation, diarrhea, abdominal pain, xerostomia

Hepatic: Transient elevations in liver enzymes

Neuromuscular & skeletal: Weakness, musculoskeletal pain, tremor, twitching, ataxia

Ocular: Blurred vision

Respiratory: Bronchospasm

Miscellaneous: Hypersensitivity reactions

Drug Interactions Cytochrome P-450 isoenzyme CYP1A2, CYP2D6, CYP2E1, and CYP3A3/4 substrate

No documented drug interactions; however, ondansetron does contain the same imidazole nucleus as cimetidine and omeprazole; patients receiving concurrent theophylline, phenytoin, or warfarin should be followed closely

Stability

Compatible for 7 days at room temperature when diluted in saline or dextrose solutions; Y-site injection compatibility with bleomycin, carboplatin, carmustine, chlorpromazine, cisplatin, cyclophosphamide, cytarabine, dacarbazine, dactinomycin, daunorubicin, dexamethasone, diphenhydramine, doxorubicin, droperidol, etoposide, fludarabine, ifosfamide, mechlorethamine, methotrexate, mesna, metoclopramide, mitoxantrone, prochlorperazine, promethazine, teniposide, vinblastine, and vincristine

Incompatible with acyclovir, ampicillin, aminophylline, furosemide, ganciclovir, lorazepam, methylprednisolone, and piperacillin

Mechanism of Action Selective 5-HT$_3$ receptor antagonist, blocking serotonin, both peripherally on vagal nerve terminals and centrally in the chemoreceptor trigger zone

Pharmacokinetics

Absorption: Oral: 100%; nonlinear absorption occurs with increasing oral doses; Zofran® ODT tablets are bioequivalent to Zofran® tablets; absorption does not occur via oral mucosa

Distribution: V$_d$: Children: 1.6-1.7 L/kg; Adults: 1.9 L/kg

Protein binding, plasma: 70% to 76%

Metabolism: Extensive first-pass metabolism; primarily by hydroxylation, followed by glucuronidation and sulfate conjugation

Bioavailability: Oral: 50% to 70% due to significant first-pass metabolism; in cancer patients (adult) 85% to 87% bioavailability possibly related to changes in metabolism

(Continued)

Ondansetron *(Continued)*

Half-life:
  Children: 3-7 years: 2.6 hours; 7-12 years: 3.1 hours
  Adults: 4-5 hours
Elimination: In urine and feces; <5% of the parent drug is recovered unchanged in urine
Clearance:
  Children: 3-7 years: 0.5 L/hour/kg; 7-12 years: 0.39 L/hour/kg
  Adults: 25-50.7 L/hour (normal); 16-32 L/hour (cancer)

Usual Dosage

Prevention of chemotherapy-induced nausea and vomiting:
  Oral (all doses given 30 minutes before chemotherapy and repeated at 8-hour intervals):
    Children <4 years: No FDA-approved oral dosage; however, the following dosages based upon body surface area have been used:
      <0.3 m^2: 1 mg 3 times/day
      0.3-0.6 m^2: 2 mg 3 times/day
      0.6-1 m^2: 3 mg 3 times/day
      >1 m^2: 4 mg 3 times/day
      or
    Children 4-11 years: 4 mg 3 times/day
    Children >11 years and Adults: 8 mg 3 times/day or 24 mg once daily
    Adults: Total body irradiation: 8 mg 1-2 hours before each fraction of radiotherapy administered each day
      Single high-dose fraction radiotherapy to abdomen: 8 mg 1-2 hours before irradiation, then 8 mg every 8 hours after first dose for 1-2 days after completion of radiotherapy
      Daily fractionated radiotherapy to abdomen: 8 mg 1-2 hours before irradiation, then 8 mg every 8 hours after first dose for each day of radiotherapy
  I.V.:
    Children >3 years: 0.15 mg/kg/dose infused 30 minutes before the start of emetogenic chemotherapy, with subsequent doses administered 4 and 8 hours after the first dose; decreased effectiveness has been reported when administered for prolonged therapy (eg, more than 3 doses)
    Adults: 0.15 mg/kg/dose infused 30 minutes before the start of emetogenic chemotherapy with subsequent doses administered 4 and 8 hours after the first dose **or as an alternative,** a single dose as follows: 45-80 kg: 8 mg, >80 kg: 12 mg; a few studies have evaluated a single 8 mg loading dose followed by a continuous 1 mg/hour infusion
Prevention of postoperative nausea and vomiting: I.V.: Give immediately before induction of anesthesia, or postoperatively if the patient is symptomatic:
  Children ≥2 years <40 kg: 0.1 mg/kg
  Children >40 kg and Adults: 4 mg
  Note: Repeating a second ondansetron dose in patients who did not achieve adequate control of postoperative nausea and vomiting after a single dose will not provide additional control.
Dosing adjustment in severe hepatic impairment: Adults: Once daily dosage; maximum 8 mg per dose

Administration

Oral: May administer without regard to meals; Zofran® ODT tablet: Place tablet on tongue, it will disintegrate immediately; may also swallow with fluids as whole tablet
Parenteral: I.V.: Dilute in 50 mL I.V. fluid (maximum concentration: 1 mg/mL) and infuse over 15 minutes; single doses for prevention of postoperative nausea/vomiting may be administered I.V. undiluted over 2-5 minutes or I.M.

Dosage Forms

Injection, as hydrochloride: 2 mg/mL (2 mL, 20 mL)
Injection, premixed, as hydrochloride: 32 mg/50 mL
Solution, as hydrochloride: 4 mg/5 mL [strawberry flavor] (50 mL)
Tablet, as hydrochloride: 4 mg, 8 mg, 24 mg
Tablet, orally disintegrating, as ondansetron base (Zofran® ODT): 4 mg, 8 mg

References

"ASHP Therapeutic Guidelines on the Pharmacologic Management of Nausea and Vomiting in Adult and Pediatric Patients Receiving Chemotherapy or Radiation Therapy or Undergoing Surgery," *Am J Health Syst Pharm*, 1999, 56(8):729-64.

Carden PA, Mitchell SL, Waters KD, et al, "Prevention of Cyclophosphamide/Cytarabine-Induced Emesis With Ondansetron in Children With Leukemia," *J Clin Oncol*, 1990, 8(9):1531-5.

Marty M, Pouillart P, Scholl S, et al, "Comparison of the 5-hydroxytryptamine 3 (Serotonin) Antagonist Ondansetron (GR 38032F) With High-Dose Metoclopramide in the Control of Cisplatin-Induced Emesis," *N Engl J Med*, 1990, 322(12):816-21.

Pinkerton CR, Williams D, Wootton C, et al, "5-HT$_3$ Antagonist Ondansetron - An Effective Outpatient Antiemetic in Cancer Treatment," *Arch Dis Child*, 1990, 65(8):822-5.

Roila F and Del Favero A, "Ondansetron Clinical Pharmacokinetics," *Clin Pharmacokinet*, 1995, 29(2):95-109.

Seynaeve C, Schuller J, Buser K, et al, "Comparison of the Anti-emetic Efficacy of Different Doses of Ondansetron, Given as Either a Continuous Infusion or a Single Intravenous Dose, in Acute Cisplatin-Induced Emesis," *Br J Cancer* 1992, 66(1):192-7.

Spahr-Schopfer IA, Lerman J, Sikich N, et al, "Pharmacokinetics of Intravenous Ondansetron in Healthy Children Undergoing Ear, Nose, and Throat Surgery," *Clin Pharmacol Ther*, 1995, 58(3):316-21.

Spector JI, Lester EP, Chevlen EM, et al, "A Comparison of Oral Ondansetron and Intravenous Granisetron for the Prevention of Nausea and Emesis Associated With Cisplatin-Based Chemotherapy," *Oncologist*, 1998, 3(6):432-438.

♦ **Ophthacet**® *see* Sulfacetamide *on page 922*

♦ **Ophthalgan**® *see* Glycerin *on page 478*

♦ **Ophthetic**® *see* Proparacaine *on page 841*

♦ **Ophtho-Bunolol (Can)** *see* Levobunolol *on page 584*

♦ **Ophtho-Tate (Can)** *see* Prednisolone *on page 821*

Opium Tincture (OH pee um TING chur)

Related Information
Overdose and Toxicology *on page 1222*

Synonyms Deodorized Opium Tincture; DTO; Tincture of Opium

Therapeutic Category Analgesic, Narcotic; Antidiarrheal

Generic Available Yes

Use Treatment of diarrhea or relief of pain; **a 25-fold dilution with water** (final concentration 0.4 mg/mL morphine) can be used to treat neonatal abstinence syndrome (opiate withdrawal)

Restrictions C-II

Pregnancy Risk Factor B (D if used for prolonged periods or in high doses at term)

Contraindications Hypersensitivity to opium, morphine, or any component; diarrhea caused by poisoning until the toxic material has been removed; increased intracranial pressure, severe respiratory depression, severe liver or renal insufficiency

Warnings Do not confuse opium tincture with paregoric; opium tincture is 25 times as potent as paregoric; opium shares the toxic potential of opiate agonists, usual precautions of opiate agonist therapy should be observed; some preparations contain sulfites which may cause allergic reactions; opium may mask dehydration by producing fluid retention in the bowel; monitor patients with prolonged or severe diarrhea carefully

Precautions Use with caution in patients with respiratory, hepatic, or renal dysfunction, severe prostatic hypertrophy, or history of narcotic abuse; infants <3 months of age are more susceptible to respiratory depression, use with caution and in reduced doses in this age group

Adverse Reactions
Cardiovascular: Hypotension, bradycardia, peripheral vasodilation
Central nervous system: CNS depression, increased intracranial pressure, drowsiness, dizziness, sedation
Dermatologic: Pruritus
Endocrine & metabolic: Antidiuretic hormone release
Gastrointestinal: Nausea, vomiting, constipation
Genitourinary: Urinary tract spasm, urinary retention
Hepatic: Biliary tract spasm
Ocular: Miosis
Respiratory: Respiratory depression
Miscellaneous: Physical and psychological dependence, histamine release

Drug Interactions CNS depressants (eg, alcohol, narcotics, benzodiazepines, tricyclic antidepressants, MAO inhibitors, phenothiazines) may increase effects/toxicity

Stability Protect from light and excessive heat; do not refrigerate, decreased solubility and precipitation may occur

Mechanism of Action Contains many narcotic alkaloids including morphine; gastric motility inhibition is primarily due to morphine content; decreases digestive secretions, increases GI muscle tone, and reduces GI propulsion

Pharmacodynamics Duration of effect: 4-5 hours

Pharmacokinetics
Absorption: Variable from GI tract
Metabolism: In the liver
Elimination: In urine and bile
(Continued)

Opium Tincture *(Continued)*

Usual Dosage Oral:

Neonates (full-term): Neonatal abstinence syndrome (opiate withdrawal): **Use a 25-fold dilution of opium tincture** (final concentration: 0.4 mg/mL morphine); Initial: Give 0.1 mL/kg or 2 drops/kg of the 25-fold dilution per dose with feedings every 3-4 hours; increase as needed by 0.1 mL/kg or 2 drops/kg of the 25-fold dilution every 3-4 hours until withdrawal symptoms are controlled; usual dose: 0.2-0.5 mL of the 25-fold dilution per dose given every 3-4 hours; it is rare to exceed 0.7 mL of the 25-fold dilution per dose; stabilize withdrawal symptoms for 3-5 days, then gradually decrease the dosage (keeping the same dosage interval) over a 2- to 4-week period

Children:

Diarrhea: 0.005-0.01 mL/kg/dose every 3-4 hours for a maximum of 6 doses/24 hours

Analgesia: 0.01-0.02 mL/kg/dose every 3-4 hours

Adults:

Diarrhea: Usual: 0.6 mL/dose; range: 0.3-1 mL/dose every 3-6 hours to maximum of 6 mL/24 hours

Analgesia: 0.6-1.5 mL/dose every 3-4 hours; usual maximum dose: 6 mL/24 hours

Administration Oral: May administer with food to decrease GI upset; for neonatal abstinence syndrome (opiate withdrawal), use a 25-fold dilution of opium tincture

Monitoring Parameters Respiratory rate, blood pressure, heart rate, resolution of diarrhea or pain, mental status; if using a 25-fold dilution to treat neonatal abstinence syndrome, monitor for resolution of withdrawal symptoms (such as irritability, high-pitched cry, stuffy nose, rhinorrhea, vomiting, poor feeding, diarrhea, sneezing, yawning etc), and signs of overtreatment (such as bradycardia, lethargy, hypotonia, irregular respirations, respiratory depression etc). An abstinence scoring system (eg, Finnegan abstinence scoring system) can be used to more objectively assess neonatal opiate withdrawal symptoms and the need for dosage adjustment. Monitor fluid and electrolyte balance in young children being treated for prolonged or severe diarrhea.

Patient Information Avoid alcohol; may cause drowsiness and impair ability to perform activities requiring mental alertness or physical coordination; may be habit-forming

Nursing Implications Observe patient for excessive sedation, respiratory depression; implement safety measures; assist with ambulation; do not abruptly discontinue after prolonged use

Additional Information Opium tincture contains 10 mg/mL morphine and 17% to 21% alcohol; for treatment of neonatal abstinence syndrome, a 25-fold dilution of opium tincture (final concentration: 0.4 mg/mL morphine) is preferred over paregoric; the 25-fold dilution of opium tincture contains the same morphine concentration as paregoric, but without the high amount of alcohol or additives of paregoric

Dosage Forms Liquid: 10% [0.6 mL equivalent to morphine 6 mg] (120 mL, 480 mL)

References

Kraus DM and Pham JT, "Neonatal Therapy," *Applied Therapeutics: The Clinical Use of Drugs*, 7th ed, Koda-Kimble MA, Young LY, eds, Baltimore, MD: Lippincott Williams & Wilkins, 2001.

Levy M and Spino M, "Neonatal Withdrawal Syndrome: Associated Drugs and Pharmacologic Management," *Pharmacotherapy*, 1993, 13(3):202-11.

"Neonatal Drug Withdrawal. American Academy of Pediatrics Committee on Drugs," *Pediatrics*, 1998, 101(6):1079-88.

- **Opticrom**® *see* Cromolyn *on page 273*
- **Optimyxin (Can)** *see* Bacitracin and Polymyxin B *on page 129*
- **Optivar**™ *see* Azelastine *on page 123*
- **Orabase**®-B [OTC] *see* Benzocaine *on page 135*
- **Oracit**® *see* Citrate and Citric Acid *on page 244*
- **Oracort (Can)** *see* Triamcinolone *on page 979*
- **Orajel**® Maximum Strength [OTC] *see* Benzocaine *on page 135*
- **Orajel**® Mouth-Aid [OTC] *see* Benzocaine *on page 135*
- **Orajel**® Perioseptic [OTC] *see* Carbamide Peroxide *on page 178*
- **Oral Contraceptives** *see page 1087*
- **Oramorph SR**® *see* Morphine Sulfate *on page 683*
- **Oiaprad**® *see* Prednisolone *on page 821*
- **Orasept**® [OTC] *see* Benzocaine *on page 135*
- **Orasol**® [OTC] *see* Benzocaine *on page 135*
- **Orazinc**® [OTC] *see* Zinc Supplements *on page 1026*
- **Orbenin (Can)** *see* Cloxacillin *on page 260*

♦ **Orciprenaline** *see* Metaproterenol *on page 637*
♦ **Oretic**® *see* Hydrochlorothiazide *on page 503*
♦ **ORF17070** *see* Histrelin *on page 496*
♦ **Organex E (Can)** *see* Vitamin E *on page 1014*
♦ **Organidin NR**® *see* Guaifenesin *on page 485*
♦ **ORG NC 45** *see* Vecuronium *on page 1005*
♦ **Oro-Clense (Can)** *see* Chlorhexidine Gluconate *on page 220*
♦ **Orthoclone OKT**®3 *see* Muromonab-CD3 *on page 688*
♦ **Orti C (Can)** *see* Ascorbic Acid *on page 106*
♦ **Os-Cal**® **500 [OTC]** *see* Calcium Supplements *on page 167*

Oseltamivir (o sel TAM e veer)

U.S. Brand Names Tamiflu™
Therapeutic Category Antiviral Agent, Oral; Neuraminidase Inhibitor
Generic Available No
Use Treatment of uncomplicated acute illness due to influenza A and B infection in patients who have been symptomatic for **no more than 2 days**; prophylaxis of influenza A and B (oseltamivir is not a substitute for annual flu vaccination)
Pregnancy Risk Factor C
Contraindications Hypersensitivity to oseltamivir, any component, or other sialic acid-based neuraminidase inhibitors
Precautions Use with caution and modify dosage in patients with renal impairment; oseltamivir does not prevent complication of serious bacterial infection which may begin with or coexist with influenza
Adverse Reactions
  Cardiovascular: Unstable angina, arrhythmia
  Central nervous system: Dizziness, headache, fatigue, insomnia, vertigo, seizure, confusion
  Dermatologic: Rash
  Endocrine & metabolic: Aggravation of diabetes mellitus
  Gastrointestinal: Nausea, vomiting, diarrhea, abdominal pain, pseudomembranous colitis
  Hematologic: Anemia
  Ocular: Conjunctivitis
  Respiratory: Bronchitis, epistaxis
  Miscellaneous: Swelling of face or tongue
Drug Interactions Probenecid (increases serum oseltamivir carboxylate concentration due to decreased tubular secretion in the kidney)
Food Interactions Food has no significant effect on peak oseltamivir plasma concentration or AUC
Stability Store capsule and powder for oral suspension at room temperature. Store reconstituted suspension at room temperature or under refrigeration; stable for 10 days; do not freeze.
Mechanism of Action Inhibits influenza virus neuraminidase which is responsible for detachment of virions from the infected cell's membrane and for viral penetration through respiratory secretions resulting in the inability of the virus to spread within the respiratory tract
Pharmacodynamics Reduction in the median time to improvement: 1.3 days
Pharmacokinetics
  Absorption: Well absorbed from the GI tract
  Distribution: Adults: V_{dss}: 23-26 L
  Protein binding: 3% (oseltamivir carboxylate); 42% (oseltamivir phosphate)
  Metabolism: Prodrug oseltamivir phosphate is metabolized by hepatic esterases to oseltamivir carboxylate (active); neither oseltamivir phosphate or oseltamivir carboxylate are a substrate, inducer, or inhibitor of cytochrome P-450 isoenzymes
  Half-life:
    Oseltamivir phosphate: 1-3 hours
    Oseltamivir carboxylate: 6-10 hours
  Elimination: >99% of oseltamivir carboxylate is eliminated by renal excretion via glomerular filtration and tubular secretion
Usual Dosage Oral:
  Treatment of influenza (treatment should begin within 2 days of onset of flu symptoms):
    Children ≥1-12 years:
      ≤15 kg: 2 mg/kg/dose (maximum dose: 30 mg) twice daily for 5 days
      >15 kg to 23 kg: 45 mg/dose twice daily for 5 days
      >23 kg to 40 kg: 60 mg/dose twice daily for 5 days
(Continued)

Oseltamivir *(Continued)*

>40 kg: 75 mg/dose twice daily for 5 days
Children >12 years and Adults: 75 mg/dose twice daily for 5 days
Prophylaxis of influenza: Adults: 75 mg/dose once daily for at least 7 days or for up to 6 weeks; therapy should begin within 2 days of exposure.
Dosing adjustment in renal impairment: Adults:
Cl$_{cr}$ 10-30 mL/minute:
Treatment of influenza: 75 mg/dose once daily
Prophylaxis of influenza: 75 mg/dose every other day
Cl$_{cr}$ <10 mL/minute: No recommended dosage regimens are available for patients with end-stage renal disease

Administration May administer with or without food; may decrease stomach upset if administered with food; shake suspension well before use

Monitoring Parameters Renal function, serum glucose in patients with diabetes mellitus

Patient Information Oseltamivir is not a substitute for the annual flu vaccination.

Dosage Forms
Capsule, as phosphate: 75 mg (blister package 10)
Powder for oral suspension, as phosphate: 12 mg/mL [tutti-frutti flavor] (100 mL)

References
Hayden FG, Atmar RL, Schilling M, et al, "Use of the Selective Oral Neuraminidase Inhibitor Oseltamivir to Prevent Influenza," *N Engl J Med*, 1999, 341(18):1336-43.
Treanor JJ, Hayden FG, Vrooman PS, et al, "Efficacy and Safety of the Oral Neuraminidase Inhibitor Oseltamivir in Treating Acute Influenza: A Randomized Controlled Trial. US Oral Neuraminidase Study Group," *JAMA*, 2000, 283(8):1016-24.

Oxacillin *(oks a SIL in)*

U.S. Brand Names Bactocill®; Prostaphlin®
Synonyms Isoxazolyl Penicillin; Methylphenyl
Therapeutic Category Antibiotic, Penicillin (Antistaphylococcal)
Generic Available Yes
Use Treatment of bacterial infections such as osteomyelitis, septicemia, endocarditis, and CNS infections due to susceptible penicillinase-producing strains of *Staphylococcus*
Pregnancy Risk Factor B
Contraindications Hypersensitivity to oxacillin, other penicillins, or any component
Warnings Elimination rate will be decreased in neonates
Precautions Use with caution in patients with hypersensitivity to cephalosporins, severe renal impairment; dosage modification required in patients with renal impairment
Adverse Reactions
Central nervous system: Fever
Dermatologic: Rash
Gastrointestinal: Diarrhea, nausea, vomiting, *C. difficile* colitis
Hematologic: Mild leukopenia, agranulocytosis, thrombocytopenia, eosinophilia
Hepatic: Elevated AST, hepatotoxicity
Local: Thrombophlebitis
Renal: Acute interstitial nephritis; hematuria and azotemia have occurred in neonates and infants receiving high-dose oxacillin; albuminuria
Miscellaneous: Hypersensitivity reactions, serum sickness-like reactions
Drug Interactions Probenecid (decreases oxacillin elimination rate)

Food Interactions Food decreases GI absorption

Stability Reconstituted oxacillin 250 mg/1.5 mL solution for injection is stable for 3 days at room temperature or 7 days when refrigerated; reconstituted oxacillin oral solution is stable for 3 days at room temperature or 14 days when refrigerated; injection is incompatible with aminoglycosides and tetracyclines

Mechanism of Action Interferes with bacterial cell wall synthesis during active multiplication by binding to one or more of the penicillin-binding proteins; inhibits the final transpeptidation step of peptidoglycan synthesis causing cell wall death and resultant bactericidal activity against susceptible bacteria

Pharmacokinetics

Absorption: Oral: ~35% to 67%

Distribution: Distributes into bile, pleural, synovial, and pericardial fluids and into lungs and bone; penetrates the blood-brain barrier only when meninges are inflamed; crosses the placenta; appears in breast milk

Protein binding: 90% to 95%

Metabolism: In the liver to active and inactive metabolites

Half-life (prolonged with reduced renal function):

Neonates 8-15 days: 1.6 hours

Children 1 week to 2 years: 0.9-1.8 hours

Adults: 0.3-0.8 hours

Time to peak serum concentration:

Oral: Within 30-120 minutes

I.M.: Within 30-60 minutes

Elimination: By the kidneys and to small degree via bile as parent drug and metabolites

Dialysis: Not dialyzable (0% to 5%)

Usual Dosage

Neonates: I.M., I.V.:

Postnatal age ≤7 days:

≤2000 g: 50 mg/kg/day in divided doses every 12 hours

>2000 g: 75 mg/kg/day in divided doses every 8 hours

Postnatal age >7 days:

<1200 g: 50 mg/kg/day in divided doses every 12 hours

1200-2000 g: 75 mg/kg/day in divided doses every 8 hours

>2000 g: 100 mg/kg/day in divided doses every 6 hours

Infants and Children: I.M., I.V.:

Mild to moderate infections: 100-150 mg/kg/day in divided doses every 6 hours

Severe infections: 150-200 mg/kg/day in divided doses every 4-6 hours; maximum dose: 12 g/day

Children: Oral: 50-100 mg/kg/day divided every 6 hours

Adults:

Oral: 500-1000 mg every 4-6 hours

I.M., I.V.: 250 mg to 2 g/dose every 4-6 hours

Dosing interval in renal impairment: Cl_{cr} <10 mL/minute: Use lower range of the usual dosage

Administration

Oral: Administer on an empty stomach with water 1 hour before or 2 hours after meals

Parenteral:

I.V. push: Administer over 10 minutes at a maximum concentration of 100 mg/mL

I.V. intermittent infusion: Administer over 15-30 minutes at a final concentration ≤40 mg/mL

Monitoring Parameters Periodic CBC with differential, urinalysis, BUN, serum creatinine, AST and ALT

Test Interactions False-positive urinary and serum proteins

Additional Information Sodium content:

1 g injection: 2.8-3.1 mEq

250 mg capsule: 0.7 mEq

250 mg/5 mL oral solution: 0.8 mEq/5 mL

Dosage Forms

Capsule, as sodium: 250 mg, 500 mg

Powder for injection, as sodium: 250 mg, 500 mg, 1 g, 2 g, 4 g, 10 g

Powder for oral solution, as sodium: 250 mg/5 mL (100 mL)

References

Olans RN and Weiner LB, "Reversible Oxacillin Hepatotoxicity," *J Pediatr*, 1976, 89(5):835-8.

Prober CG, Stevenson DK, and Benitz WE, "The Use of Antibiotics in Neonates Weighing Less Than 1200 Grams," *Pediatr Infect Dis J*, 1990, 9(2):111-21.

Oxcarbazepine (ox car BAZ e peen)

U.S. Brand Names Trileptal®

Therapeutic Category Anticonvulsant, Miscellaneous

Generic Available No

Use Adjunctive treatment of partial seizures in pediatric and adult patients; monotherapy of partial seizures in adults

Pregnancy Risk Factor C

Contraindications Hypersensitivity to oxcarbazepine or any component

Warnings Significant hyponatremia may occur; a serum sodium <125 mEq/L has been reported in 2.5% of patients; consider monitoring serum sodium especially in patients who receive other drugs that may cause hyponatremia and in patients with symptoms of hyponatremia (eg, nausea, headache, malaise, confusion, lethargy, or obtundation). Do not abruptly discontinue therapy, withdraw gradually to lessen chance for increased seizure frequency (unless a more rapid withdrawal is required due to safety concerns). Cross-hypersensitivity reactions with carbamazepine may occur (incidence: 25% to 30%); discontinue oxcarbazepine immediately if signs or symptoms of hypersensitivity develop

Precautions CNS adverse effects may occur including somnolence, fatigue, coordination abnormalities (ataxia and gait disturbances), and cognitive symptoms (difficulty concentrating, speech or language problems, and psychomotor slowing); these effects may be more common when oxcarbazepine is used as add-on therapy versus monotherapy. Use with caution and modify dose in patients with renal impairment. Multiple drug interactions may occur (see Drug Interactions).

Adverse Reactions

Central nervous system: Headache, dizziness, somnolence, fatigue, ataxia, tremor, insomnia, cognitive symptoms (psychomotor slowing, difficulty concentrating, speech or language problems), vertigo, anxiety, nervousness, emotional lability

Dermatologic: Rash; rare: Stevens-Johnson syndrome, erythema multiforme, toxic epidermal necrolysis

Endocrine and Metabolic: Hyponatremia (incidence: 2.5%; usually occurs within the first 3 months of therapy, but has been reported in patients more than 1 year after starting medication; serum sodium returns towards normal after discontinuation, reduction of dose, or with conservative treatment such as fluid restriction); reduction in T_4 levels

Gastrointestinal: Nausea, vomiting, abdominal pain, dyspepsia

Neuromuscular & skeletal: Abnormal gait

Ocular: Diplopia, abnormal vision, nystagmus

Miscellaneous: Hypersensitivity reactions; a rare, multi-organ hypersensitivity reaction with rash, lymphadenopathy, fever, eosinophilia, abnormal liver function tests, and arthralgia has also been reported

Drug Interactions Cytochrome P-450 isoenzyme CYP2C19 inhibitor; CYP3A4 and CYP3A5 inducer

Oxcarbazepine may inhibit hepatic metabolism and increase the serum concentrations of phenobarbital (by 14%) and phenytoin (by 40% with high-dose oxcarbazepine; dosage reduction of phenytoin may be needed); may induce hepatic metabolism and decrease serum concentrations of felodipine, lamotrigine, and oral contraceptives such as ethinyl estradiol and levonorgestrel (alternative methods of contraception are recommended)

P-450 enzyme inducers such as carbamazepine, phenobarbital, and phenytoin, may significantly decrease MHD concentrations by 25% to 40%; valproic acid decreases MHD concentrations by 18% and verapamil decreases MHD concentrations by 20%

Food Interactions Food does not affect rate or extent of absorption

Stability Store at controlled room temperature (25°C); dispense in tight container

Mechanism of Action Active 10-monohydroxy metabolite (MHD) is primarily responsible for anticonvulsant activity; exact mechanism unknown; both MHD and oxcarbazepine are thought to decrease the spread of seizure activity by blockade of sodium channels; also increases conductance of potassium and modulates activity of high-voltage activated calcium channels

Pharmacokinetics

Absorption: Oral: Complete

Distribution: MHD: V_d (apparent): Adults: 49 L

Protein binding: Oxcarbazepine: 67%; MHD: 40%, primarily to albumin; parent drug and metabolite do not bind to alpha-1-acid glycoprotein

Metabolism: Oxcarbazepine is extensively metabolized in the liver to its active 10-monohydroxy metabolite (MHD); MHD undergoes further metabolism via glucuronide conjugation; 4% of dose is oxidized to the 10,11-dihydroxy metabolite (DHD) (inactive); 70% of serum concentration appears as MHD, 2% as unchanged oxcarbazepine, and the rest as minor metabolites; **Note:** Unlike carbamazepine, autoinduction of metabolism has not been observed and biotransformation of oxcarbazepine does not result in an epoxide metabolite

Half-life:

Adults:

Oxcarbazepine: 2 hours

MHD: 9 hours

Adults with renal impairment (Cl$_{cr}$ <30 mL/minute): MHD: 19 hours

Time to peak serum concentration: Adults: 3-13 hours (median: 4.5 hours)

Elimination: >95% of dose is excreted in the urine with <1% as unchanged parent drug, 27% as unchanged MHD, 49% as MHD glucuronides, 3% as DHD (inactive), and 13% as conjugate of oxcarbazepine and MHD; <4% excreted in feces

Clearance:

Children <8 years: Increased by 30% to 40% compared to children >8 years and adults

Children >8 years: Values approach adult clearance

Hepatic impairment: Mild to moderate: No effect on pharmacokinetics; Severe: Not studied

Usual Dosage Oral:

Neonates, Infants, and Children <4 years: Not approved for use; controlled trials in children <2 years have not been conducted

Children 4-16 years: Adjunctive therapy: Initial: 8-10 mg/kg/day given in 2 divided doses (usual maximum: 600 mg/day); increase dose slowly over 2 weeks to weight-dependent target maintenance dose:

20-29 kg: 900 mg/day in 2 divided doses

29.1-39 kg: 1200 mg/day in 2 divided doses

>39 kg: 1800 mg/day in 2 divided doses

Note: Use of these pediatric target maintenance doses in one clinical trial resulted in doses ranging from 6-51 mg/kg/day (median dose: 31 mg/kg/day)

Adults:

Adjunctive therapy: Initial: 300 mg twice daily; increase if needed by no more than 600 mg/day at approximately weekly intervals; recommended maintenance dose: 600 mg twice daily; **Note:** Doses >1200 mg/day may have greater efficacy, but most patients are not able to tolerate 2400 mg/day (mostly due to CNS effects); monitor patient closely and measure concentrations of concomitant antiepileptic agents during dosage titration and especially with oxcarbazepine doses >1200 mg/day

Conversion to monotherapy: Initial: 300 mg twice daily with a simultaneous initial reduction of the dose of concomitant antiepileptic drugs (AEDs); withdraw concomitant AEDs completely over 3-6 weeks, while increasing oxcarbazepine dose as needed by no more than 600 mg/day at approximately weekly intervals; recommended oxcarbazepine dose (1200 mg twice daily) should be reached in about 2-4 weeks; **Note:** A lower dose (1200 mg/day) was effective in one study in patients who initiated oxcarbazepine monotherapy

Initiation of monotherapy: Initial: 300 mg twice daily; increase by 300 mg/day every third day to 1200 mg/day; a higher dose (2400 mg/day) was effective in patients who were converted from other AEDs to oxcarbazepine monotherapy.

Dosing adjustment in renal impairment: Cl$_{cr}$ <30 mL/minute: Initial dose: Administer 50% of the normal starting dose; slowly increase the dose if needed, using a slower dosage titration than normal

Dosing adjustment in hepatic impairment:

Mild to moderate hepatic impairment: No dosage adjustment recommended

Severe hepatic impairment: Not evaluated

Administration Oral: May be taken without regard to meals

Monitoring Parameters Seizure frequency, duration and severity; symptoms of CNS depression (dizziness, headache, somnolence) and allergic reaction; consider monitoring serum sodium (particularly during first three months of therapy) especially in patients who receive other drugs that may cause hyponatremia and in patients with symptoms of hyponatremia (eg, nausea, headache, malaise, confusion, lethargy, or obtundation)

Patient Information Inform prescriber if allergic to carbamazepine; do not abruptly discontinue, an increase in seizure activity may result; report excessive somnolence or allergic reactions to physician immediately; report unusual symptoms such as nausea, headache, malaise, confusion, lethargy, or obtundation to physician immediately, blood test for serum sodium may be needed; avoid alcohol; may cause drowsiness and impair ability to perform activities that require mental alertness or physical coordination

Additional Information Symptoms of overdose may include CNS depression (somnolence, ataxia, obtundation); treatment is symptomatic and supportive; (Continued)

Oxcarbazepine *(Continued)*

consider general poisoning management (eg, gastric lavage, activated charcoal); largest reported overdose is 24 g; oxcarbazepine is a keto analogue of carbamazepine

Dosage Forms Tablet: 150 mg, 300 mg, 600 mg

References

Tecoma ES, "Oxcarbazepine," *Epilepsia*, 1999, 40(Suppl 5): S37-46.

♦ **Oxpentifylline** *see* Pentoxifylline *on page 781*

♦ **Oxy (Can)** *see* Salicylic Acid *on page 886*

♦ **Oxy-5® Advanced Formula for Sensitive Skin [OTC]** *see* Benzoyl Peroxide *on page 136*

♦ **Oxy-5® Tinted [OTC]** *see* Benzoyl Peroxide *on page 136*

♦ **Oxy-10® Advanced Formula for Sensitive Skin [OTC]** *see* Benzoyl Peroxide *on page 136*

♦ **Oxy 10® Wash [OTC]** *see* Benzoyl Peroxide *on page 136*

♦ **Oxy® Balance Deep Pore [OTC]** *see* Salicylic Acid *on page 886*

♦ **Oxybutyn (Can)** *see* Oxybutynin *on page 744*

Oxybutynin (oks i BYOO ti nin)

Related Information

Carbohydrate and Alcohol Content of Liquid Medications for Use in Patients Receiving Ketogenic Diets *on page 1258*

U.S. Brand Names Ditropan®; Ditropan® XL

Canadian Brand Names Albert Oxybutynin; Apo-Oxybutynin; Gen-Oxybutynin; Novo-Oxybutynin; Nu-Oxybutyn; Oxybutyn; PMS-Oxybutynin

Therapeutic Category Antispasmodic Agent, Urinary

Generic Available Yes

Use Relief of bladder spasms associated with voiding in patients with uninhibited and reflex neurogenic bladder

Pregnancy Risk Factor B

Contraindications Glaucoma (angle-closure), myasthenia gravis, partial or complete GI obstruction, GU obstruction, ulcerative colitis; hypersensitivity to oxybutynin or any component; intestinal atony, megacolon, toxic megacolon

Precautions Use with caution in patients with hepatic or renal disease, heart disease, hyperthyroidism, reflux esophagitis, hypertension, prostatic hypertrophy, autonomic neuropathy

Adverse Reactions

Cardiovascular: Tachycardia, palpitations, vasodilation

Central nervous system: Drowsiness, dizziness, insomnia, fever, hallucinations

Dermatologic: Rash

Endocrine & metabolic: Hot flashes

Gastrointestinal: Xerostomia, nausea, vomiting, constipation, decreased GI motility

Genitourinary: Impotence, urinary hesitancy or retention

Neuromuscular & skeletal: Weakness

Ocular: Blurred vision, mydriasis, decreased lacrimation, amblyopia, cycloplegia

Miscellaneous: Hypersensitivity reactions, decreased diaphoresis

Drug Interactions Additive sedation with CNS depressants and alcohol; additive anticholinergic effects with antihistamines and anticholinergic agents; decreased haloperidol serum concentrations; may increase digoxin serum levels

Mechanism of Action Direct antispasmodic effect on smooth muscle, also inhibits the action of acetylcholine on smooth muscle; does not block effects at skeletal muscle or at autonomic ganglia

Pharmacodynamics

Immediate release formulation:

Onset of action: Oral: Within 30-60 minutes

Peak effect: 3-6 hours

Duration: 6-10 hours

Extended release formulation: Maximum effects: 3 days

Pharmacokinetics

Absorption: Oral: Rapid and well absorbed

Metabolism: In the liver

Half-life: 1-2.3 hours

Time to peak serum concentration:

Immediate release: Within 60 minutes

Extended release: 12-13 hours

Elimination: In urine

Usual Dosage Oral:
Children:
1-5 years: 0.2 mg/kg/dose 2-4 times/day
>5 years: 5 mg twice daily, up to 5 mg 4 times/day
Adults: 5 mg 2-3 times/day up to 5 mg 4 times/day maximum **or** extended release tablet (Ditropan® XL) 5-10 mg once daily; maximum 30 mg once daily
Note: Should be discontinued periodically to determine whether the patient can manage without the drug and to minimize tolerance to the drug
Administration Oral: May administer with food or milk to decrease GI distress; extended release formulation may be administered with or without food; swallow extended release tablets whole; do not chew or crush
Patient Information Causes drowsiness and may impair ability to perform hazardous activities requiring mental alertness or physical coordination; avoid alcohol; nonabsorbable tablet shell may be seen in stool, but active drug has been released
Dosage Forms
Syrup, as chloride: 5 mg/5 mL (473 mL)
Tablet, as chloride: 5 mg
Tablet, extended release, as chloride (Ditropan® XL): 5 mg, 10 mg, 15 mg

♦ **Oxycocet (Can)** see Oxycodone and Acetaminophen on page 747
♦ **Oxycodan (Can)** see Oxycodone and Aspirin on page 748

Oxycodone (oks i KOE done)

U.S. Brand Names OxyContin®; OxyFast®; OxyIR™; Percolone®; Roxicodone™; Roxicodone™ Intensol™
Canadian Brand Names Supeudol
Therapeutic Category Analgesic, Narcotic
Generic Available Yes
Use Relief of moderate to moderately severe pain
Restrictions C-II
Pregnancy Risk Factor B (D if used for prolonged periods or in high doses at term)
Contraindications Hypersensitivity to oxycodone or any component; significant respiratory depression (in settings without resuscitative equipment or without adequate respiratory monitoring); patients with hypercarbia, severe or acute asthma, paralytic ileus (known or suspected)
Warnings Respiratory depression may occur; use with extreme caution in patients with pre-existing respiratory depression, decreased respiratory reserve, hypoxia, hypercapnia, significant COPD, or cor pulmonale. Hypotension may occur, especially in hypovolemic patients or those receiving medications that compromise vasomotor tone; use with extreme caution in patients with circulatory shock. Orthostatic hypotension may occur in ambulatory patients; physical and psychological dependence may occur; warn patient of possible impairment of alertness or physical coordination (see Patient Information); interactions with other CNS drugs may occur (see Drug Interactions)
Precautions Use with caution in patients with hypersensitivity to other phenanthrene derivative opioid agonists (morphine, codeine, hydrocodone, hydromorphone, oxymorphone, levorphanol). Use with caution in patients with head injury; increased intracranial pressure; CNS depression; respiratory depression; coma; toxic psychosis; seizures; acute abdominal conditions; biliary tract disease; pancreatitis; severe renal, respiratory, or hepatic insufficiency; hypothyroidism; Addison's disease; urethral stricture and in debilitated patients. Use care in prescribing, dispensing, and administering the oral concentrated solution, inappropriate use may cause overdose. Controlled release 80 mg and 160 mg tablets should only be used in patients who are opioid tolerant and who require daily doses of ≥160 mg and ≥320 mg, respectively.
Adverse Reactions
Cardiovascular system: Hypotension, bradycardia, peripheral vasodilation
Central nervous system: CNS depression, increased intracranial pressure, dizziness, drowsiness, sedation, lightheadedness, dysphoria, headache, fatigue
Dermatologic: Pruritus, skin rash
Endocrine & metabolic: Antidiuretic hormone release
Gastrointestinal: Nausea, vomiting, constipation, biliary tract spasm, xerostomia
Genitourinary: Urinary tract spasm, urinary retention
Ocular: Miosis
Respiratory: Respiratory depression
Miscellaneous: Physical and psychological dependence, histamine release, diaphoresis
Drug Interactions Cytochrome P-450 isoenzyme CYP2D6 substrate
(Continued)

Oxycodone *(Continued)*

CNS depressants, phenothiazines, tricyclic antidepressants may potentiate the CNS adverse effects of oxycodone (dosage reduction of one or both agents is recommended; some recommend starting opioid analgesics at $1/3$ to $1/2$ of the normal dose in patients receiving other CNS depressants)

Food Interactions Food does not significantly affect absorption of controlled release tablets; high fat meal may increase peak concentrations of OxyContin® 160 mg tablet by 25%

Stability Store at room temperature; protect from light and moisture

OxyFast® oral concentrate: Stable for 90 days after opening

Mechanism of Action Binds to opiate receptors in the CNS, causing inhibition of ascending pain pathways, altering the perception of and response to pain; produces generalized CNS depression

Pharmacodynamics Duration of pain relief: Oral:

Immediate release: 4-5 hours

Controlled release: 12 hours

Pharmacokinetics

Distribution: Distributes into breast milk; V_{dss}:

Children 2-10 years: Mean: 2.1 L/kg; range: 1.2-3.7 L/kg

Adults: 2.6 L/kg

Protein binding: 38% to 45%

Metabolism: In the liver primarily to noroxycodone (via demethylation) and oxymorphone (via CYP2D6); noroxycodone is the major circulating metabolite, but has much weaker activity than oxycodone; oxymorphone is active, but present in low concentrations; <15% of the dose is metabolized to oxymorphone via CYP2D6; drug and metabolites undergo glucuronide conjugation

Bioavailability: Adults: 60% to 87%

Half-life, apparent: Adults:

Immediate release: 3.2 hours

Controlled release (OxyContin®): 4.5 hours

Half-life, elimination:

Children 2-10 years: 1.8 hours; range: 1.2-3 hours

Adults: 3.7 hours

Adults with renal dysfunction (Cl_{cr} <60 mL/minute): Half-life increases by 1 hour, but peak oxycodone concentrations increase by 50% and AUC increases by 60%

Adults with mild to moderate hepatic dysfunction: Half-life increases by 2.3 hours, peak oxycodone concentrations increase by 50%, and AUC increases by 95%

Elimination: In the urine as unchanged drug (≤19%) and metabolites: Conjugated oxycodone (≤50%), conjugated oxymorphone (≤14%), noroxycodone, and conjugated noroxycodone

Usual Dosage Oral: Doses should be titrated to appropriate effect:

Immediate release products:

Children: 0.05-0.15 mg/kg/dose every 4-6 hours as needed

Adults: Initial: 5 mg every 6 hours as needed; usual: 10-30 mg every 4 hours as needed; more severe pain: ≥30 mg every 4 hours

AHCPR dosing guidelines: Opioid naive patients: (See Carr, 1992 and Jacox, 1994)

Children and Adults <50 kg: Moderate to severe pain: Usual initial dose: 0.2 mg/kg every 3-4 hours

Children and Adults ≥50 kg: Moderate to severe pain: Usual initial dose: 10 mg every 3-4 hours

Controlled release product: Adults: Initial: 10 mg every 12 hours; use immediate-release analgesics as needed for rescue from breakthrough pain or prior to predictable pain from procedures or activities; rescue analgesic should be $1/4$ to $1/3$ of the 12-hour controlled release oxycodone dose; increase the dose of controlled release oxycodone if >2 doses of rescue analgesic are required within 24 hours; dose of controlled release oxycodone may be adjusted every 1-2 days by 25% to 50% (initial increase may be from 10 mg to 20 mg every 12 hours). Mean doses used in open-label trials: Opioid naive patients: 40 mg/day; cancer patients: 105 mg/day (range: 20-720 mg/day)

Note: To convert patients from other opioid or nonopioid analgesics to oxycodone controlled release tablets: See OxyContin® package insert

Dosing adjustment in renal impairment: Cl_{cr} <60 mL/minute: Initiate doses conservatively and carefully titrate dose to appropriate effect

Dosing adjustment in hepatic impairment: Initial: $1/3$ to $1/2$ of the usual dose; carefully titrate dose to appropriate effect

Administration May administer with food to decrease GI upset; swallow sustained release tablets whole, do not crush, chew, or break; avoid high fat meals when initiating controlled (sustained) release 160 mg tablets

Monitoring Parameters Pain relief, respiratory rate, mental status, blood pressure

Patient Information Avoid alcohol; may cause drowsiness and impair ability to perform hazardous activities requiring mental alertness or physical coordination; report the use of other prescription and nonprescription medications to your physician and pharmacist. May be habit-forming; do not abruptly discontinue if therapy lasts more than a few weeks; dose should be tapered to prevent withdrawal. Do not crush, chew, or break controlled release tablets (OxyContin®), as risk of overdose may occur. Empty controlled release tablets may appear in stool after medication is absorbed (this is normal).

Additional Information OxyContin® tablets deliver medication over 12 hours; equianalgesic doses: oral oxycodone 30 mg = morphine 10 mg I.M. = single oral dose morphine 60 mg **or** chronic dosing oral morphine 30 mg

Dosage Forms
Capsule, as hydrochloride, immediate release (OxyIR™): 5 mg
Concentrate, oral, as hydrochloride (OxyFast®, Roxicodone™ Intensol™): 20 mg/mL (30 mL) [contains sodium benzoate]
Solution, oral, as hydrochloride (Roxicodone™): 5 mg/mL (500 mL)
Tablet, as hydrochloride, immediate release:
 Percolone®: 5 mg
 Roxicodone™: 5 mg, 15 mg, 30 mg
Tablet, controlled release, as hydrochloride (OxyContin®): 10 mg, 20 mg, 40 mg, 80 mg, 160 mg

References
Carr D, Jacox A, Chapman CR, et al, "Clinical Practice Guideline Number 1: Acute Pain Management: Operative or Medical Procedures and Trauma," Rockville, Maryland: U.S. Department of Health and Human Services, Public Health Service, Agency for Health Care Policy and Research, AHCPR Publication No 92-0032, 1992.
Jacox A, Carr D, Payne R, et al, "Clinical Practice Guideline Number 9: Management of Cancer Pain," Rockville, Maryland: U.S. Department of Health and Human Services, Public Health Service, Agency for Health Care Policy and Research, AHCPR Publication No. 94-0592, 1994.
Olkkola KT, Hamunen K, and Maunuksela EL, "Clinical Pharmacokinetics and Pharmacodynamics of Opioid Analgesics in Infants and Children," *Clin Pharmacokinet*, 1995, 28(5):385-404.
Olkkola KT, Hamunen K, Seppala T, et al, "Pharmacokinetics and Ventilatory Effects of Intravenous Oxycodone in Postoperative Children," *Br J Clin Pharmacol*, 1994, 38(1):71-6.

Oxycodone and Acetaminophen
(oks i KOE done & a seet a MIN oh fen)

Related Information
Narcotic Analgesics Comparison *on page 1070*
Overdose and Toxicology *on page 1222*

U.S. Brand Names Percocet 2.5/325®; Percocet 5/325®; Percocet 7.5/500®; Percocet 10/650®; Roxicet®; Roxicet® 5/500; Roxilox®; Tylox®

Canadian Brand Names Endocet; Oxycocet; Percocet-Demi

Synonyms Acetaminophen and Oxycodone

Therapeutic Category Analgesic, Narcotic

Generic Available Yes

Use Relief of moderate to severe pain

Restrictions C-II

Pregnancy Risk Factor C

Contraindications Hypersensitivity to oxycodone, acetaminophen, or any component; severe respiratory depression, severe liver or renal insufficiency

Warnings Some preparations contain bisulfites which may cause allergies

Precautions Use with caution in patients with hypersensitivity to other phenanthrene derivative opioid agonists (morphine, codeine, hydrocodone, hydromorphone, oxymorphone, levorphanol)

Adverse Reactions
Cardiovascular: Hypotension, bradycardia, peripheral vasodilation
Central nervous system: CNS depression, increased intracranial pressure, drowsiness, sedation
Dermatologic: Pruritus
Endocrine & metabolic: Antidiuretic hormone release
Gastrointestinal: Nausea, vomiting, constipation, biliary tract spasm
Genitourinary: Urinary tract spasm
Ocular: Miosis
Respiratory: Respiratory depression
Miscellaneous: Physical and psychological dependence, histamine release
(Continued)

Oxycodone and Acetaminophen *(Continued)*

Drug Interactions See Acetaminophen *on page 29* and Oxycodone *on page 745*

Food Interactions Rate of absorption of acetaminophen may be decreased when given with food high in carbohydrates

Mechanism of Action See Acetaminophen *on page 29* and Oxycodone *on page 745*

Pharmacodynamics
Onset of action: Within 10-15 minutes
Peak effect: Within 1 hour
Duration: 3-6 hours

Pharmacokinetics See Acetaminophen *on page 29* and Oxycodone *on page 745*

Usual Dosage Oral (titrate dose to appropriate analgesic effects):
Children: Based on **oxycodone component**: 0.05-0.15 mg/kg/dose up to 5 mg/dose every 4-6 hours as needed
Adults: 1-2 tablets every 4-6 hours as needed for pain; maximum daily dose of acetaminophen: 4 g/day

Administration Oral: May administer with food or milk to decrease GI upset

Monitoring Parameters Pain relief, respiratory rate, mental status, blood pressure

Patient Information Avoid alcohol; may be habit-forming; may cause drowsiness and impair ability to perform hazardous activities requiring mental alertness or physical coordination

Dosage Forms
Caplet (Roxicet® 5/500): Oxycodone hydrochloride 5 mg and acetaminophen 500 mg
Capsule (Roxilox®, Tylox®): Oxycodone hydrochloride 5 mg and acetaminophen 500 mg
Solution, oral (Roxicet®): Oxycodone hydrochloride 5 mg and acetaminophen 325 mg per 5 mL (5 mL, 500 mL)
Tablet:
Percocet 2.5/325®: Oxycodone hydrochloride 2.5 mg and acetaminophen 325 mg
Endocet®, Percocet 5/325®, Roxicet®: Oxycodone hydrochloride 5 mg and acetaminophen 325 mg
Percocet 7.5/500®: Oxycodone hydrochloride 7.5 mg and acetaminophen 500 mg
Percocet 10/650®: Oxycodone hydrochloride 10 mg and acetaminophen 650 mg

References
Olkkola KT, Hamunen K, and Maunuksela EL, "Clinical Pharmacokinetics and Pharmacodynamics of Opioid Analgesics in Infants and Children," *Clin Pharmacokinet*, 1995, 28(5):385-404.

Oxycodone and Aspirin (oks i KOE done & AS pir in)

Related Information
Overdose and Toxicology *on page 1222*

U.S. Brand Names Percodan®; Percodan®-Demi

Canadian Brand Names Endodan; Oxycodan

Synonyms Aspirin and Oxycodone

Therapeutic Category Analgesic, Narcotic

Generic Available Yes

Use Relief of moderate to moderately severe pain

Restrictions C-II

Pregnancy Risk Factor D

Contraindications Hypersensitivity to oxycodone, aspirin, or any component; severe respiratory depression, severe liver, or renal insufficiency

Warnings Contains aspirin, do not use aspirin-containing products in children <16 years of age for chickenpox or flu symptoms due to the association with Reye's syndrome

Precautions Use with caution in patients with hypersensitivity to other phenanthrene derivative opioid agonists (morphine, codeine, hydrocodone, hydromorphone, oxymorphone, levorphanol); contains aspirin, use with caution in patients with impaired renal function, erosive gastritis, peptic ulcer, gout

Adverse Reactions
Cardiovascular: Hypotension, bradycardia, peripheral vasodilation
Central nervous system: CNS depression, increased intracranial pressure, drowsiness, sedation
Dermatologic: Pruritus, rash
Endocrine & metabolic: Antidiuretic hormone release
Gastrointestinal: Nausea, vomiting, constipation, biliary tract spasm, GI distress

Genitourinary: Urinary tract spasm
Hematologic: Inhibition of platelet aggregation (due to aspirin)
Hepatic: Hepatotoxicity (due to aspirin)
Ocular: Miosis
Respiratory: Respiratory depression
Miscellaneous: Histamine release, physical and psychological dependence

Drug Interactions See Aspirin *on page 109* and Oxycodone *on page 745*

Food Interactions Aspirin may increase renal excretion of vitamin C and may decrease serum folate levels

Mechanism of Action See Aspirin *on page 109* and Oxycodone *on page 745*

Pharmacokinetics See Aspirin *on page 109* and Oxycodone *on page 745*

Usual Dosage Oral: Based on **oxycodone-combined salt component**:
Children: 0.05-0.15 mg/kg/dose every 4-6 hours as needed; maximum dose: 5 mg/dose (1 tablet Percodan® or 2 tablets Percodan®-Demi/dose)
  or alternatively:
Percodan®-Demi:
    6-12 years: $^1/_4$ tablet every 6 hours as needed for pain
    >12 years: $^1/_2$ tablet every 6 hours as needed for pain
Adults: Percodan®: 1 tablet every 6 hours as needed for pain or Percodan®-Demi: 1-2 tablets every 6 hours as needed for pain

Administration Oral: May administer with food or milk to decrease GI upset

Monitoring Parameters Pain relief, respiratory rate, mental status, blood pressure

Patient Information Avoid alcohol; may cause drowsiness and impair ability to perform activities requiring mental alertness or physical coordination; may be habit-forming

Additional Information One tablet (Percodan®) contains ~5 mg oxycodone as combined salt

Dosage Forms Tablet:
Percodan®: Oxycodone hydrochloride 4.5 mg, oxycodone terephthalate 0.38 mg, and aspirin 325 mg
Percodan®-Demi: Oxycodone hydrochloride 2.25 mg, oxycodone terephthalate 0.19 mg, and aspirin 325 mg

♦ **OxyContin®** *see* Oxycodone *on page 745*

♦ **Oxyderm (Can)** *see* Benzoyl Peroxide *on page 136*

♦ **OxyFast®** *see* Oxycodone *on page 745*

♦ **OxyIR™** *see* Oxycodone *on page 745*

Oxymetazoline (oks i met AZ oh leen)

Related Information
OTC Cough & Cold Preparations, Pediatric *on page 1072*

U.S. Brand Names Afrin® [OTC]; Afrin® Extra Moisturizing [OTC]; Afrin® Sinus [OTC]; Afrin® with Menthol [OTC]; Duramist Plus® [OTC]; Duration® [OTC]; Genasal® [OTC]; 12-Hour Nasal® [OTC]; Nasal Relief® [OTC]; Neo-Synephrine® 12 Hour [OTC]; Nõstrilla® [OTC]; OcuClear® [OTC]; Sinarest® 12 Hour [OTC]; Twice-A-Day® [OTC]; Vicks Sinex® 12 Hour [OTC]; Visine® L.R. [OTC]; 4-Way® Long Acting [OTC]

Canadian Brand Names Decongestant Nasal Mist; Dristan Long-Lasting Nasal; Drixoral Decongestant Nasal; Nafrine; Ocuclear; Vicks Sinex; Visine Workplace

Therapeutic Category Adrenergic Agonist Agent; Decongestant, Nasal; Nasal Agent, Vasoconstrictor; Vasoconstrictor, Nasal; Vasoconstrictor, Ophthalmic

Generic Available Yes

Use Symptomatic relief of nasal mucosal congestion associated with acute or chronic rhinitis, the common cold, sinusitis, hay fever, or other allergies

Pregnancy Risk Factor C

Contraindications Hypersensitivity to oxymetazoline or any component; patients on MAO inhibitor therapy

Warnings Use for periods exceeding 3 days may result in severe rebound nasal congestion; excessive dosage in children may cause profound CNS depression

Precautions Use with caution in patients with hyperthyroidism, heart disease, hypertension, diabetes mellitus, increased intraocular pressure, or prostatic hypertrophy

Adverse Reactions
Cardiovascular: Hypertension, palpitations, reflex bradycardia, pallor
Central nervous system: Nervousness, dizziness, insomnia, headache, anxiety, tenseness, drowsiness, CNS depression, convulsions, hallucinations
Gastrointestinal: Nausea, vomiting
Ocular: Stinging to eye, mydriasis, increased intraocular pressure, blurred vision
(Continued)

Oxymetazoline *(Continued)*

Respiratory: Sneezing, respiratory difficulty, rebound congestion with prolonged use, dryness of nasal mucosa

Miscellaneous: Diaphoresis

Drug Interactions Anesthetics (discontinue oxymetazoline prior to use of anesthetics that sensitize the myocardium to sympathomimetics, ie, cyclopropane, halothane); MAO inhibitors, methyldopa, tricyclic antidepressants increase hypertensive response

Mechanism of Action Stimulates alpha-adrenergic receptors in the arterioles of the nasal mucosa and arterioles of the conjunctiva to produce vasoconstriction

Pharmacodynamics

Intranasal: Onset of action: Within 5-10 minutes

Duration: 5-6 hours

Pharmacokinetics Metabolic fate is unknown

Usual Dosage

Nasal: Therapy should not exceed 3-5 days; avoid use of 0.05% solution in children <6 years of age

Children 2-5 years: 0.025% solution: 2-3 drops in each nostril twice daily

Children ≥6 years and Adults: 0.05% solution: 2-3 drops or 2-3 sprays or 1-2 metered sprays (Nōstrilla®) into each nostril twice daily

Ophthalmic: Children ≥6 years and Adults: Instill 1-2 drops into the affected eye(s) 2-4 times/day (≥6 hours apart)

Administration

Nasal: Spray or apply drops into each nostril while gently occluding the other

Ophthalmic: Instill drops into conjunctival sac of affected eye(s); avoid contact of bottle tip with skin or eye; finger pressure should be applied to lacrimal sac during and for 1-2 minutes after instillation to decrease the risk of absorption and systemic reactions

Dosage Forms

Nasal, solution, as hydrochloride:

Drops (Afrin®): 0.05% (15 mL, 20 mL)

Spray (Afrin®, Afrin® Extra Moisturizing, Afrin® Sinus, Afrin® With Menthol, Duramist Plus®, Duration®, Genasal®, 4-Way® Long Acting, Nasal Relief®, Neo-Synephrine® 12 Hour, Nōstrilla®, Sinarest® 12 Hour, Vicks Sinex® 12 Hour, Twice-A-Day®, 12-Hour Nasal®): 0.05% (15 mL, 30 mL)

Ophthalmic solution, as hydrochloride (OcuClear®, Visine® L.R.): 0.025% (15 mL, 30 mL)

♦ **Oysco®** *see* Calcium Supplements *on page 167*

♦ **Oyst-Cal 500 [OTC]** *see* Calcium Supplements *on page 167*

♦ **Oystercal® 500** *see* Calcium Supplements *on page 167*

♦ **P-071** *see* Cetirizine *on page 212*

♦ **Pacerone®** *see* Amiodarone *on page 72*

Paclitaxel *(PAK li taks el)*

U.S. Brand Names Taxol®

Therapeutic Category Antineoplastic Agent, Antimicrotubular

Generic Available No

Use Treatment of advanced metastatic breast cancer, metastatic ovarian cancer, and AIDS-related Kaposi's sarcoma that is refractory to conventional therapy; active in lung cancer, head and neck cancer, bladder cancer, malignant melanoma, and other refractory solid tumors, and leukemias

Pregnancy Risk Factor D

Contraindications Hypersensitivity to paclitaxel, Cremophor® EL (polyoxyethylated castor oil) or any component

Warnings The FDA currently recommends that procedures for proper handling and disposal of antineoplastic agents be considered. Anaphylaxis and severe hypersensitivity reactions have occurred in 2% of patients receiving paclitaxel in clinical trials during first or subsequent infusions. **All patients should be premedicated with a corticosteroid, diphenhydramine, and an H_2-receptor antagonist to prevent hypersensitivity reactions.** Patients who experience severe hypersensitivity reactions to paclitaxel should not be rechallenged with the drug. Be prepared to treat a severe hypersensitivity reaction with epinephrine, I.V. fluids, diphenhydramine and a corticosteroid.

CNS toxicity has been reported in pediatric patients receiving high doses of paclitaxel (350-420 mg/m^2 as a 3-hour infusion) which may have resulted from the ethanol contained in the formulation. Severe bone marrow suppression (primarily neutropenia) with resulting infection may occur. In general, do not administer paclitaxel to patients with baseline neutrophil counts <1500/mm³.

Precautions Use with caution in patients with moderate or severe hepatic impairment; dosage adjustment may be necessary in patients with hepatic impairment, severe neutropenia, or peripheral neuropathy

Adverse Reactions

Cardiovascular: Hypotension or hypertension, bradycardia, arrhythmias, flushing, syncope, edema

Central nervous system: Seizures, ataxia, fatigue, headache, fever, confusion

Dermatologic: Alopecia, rash, changes in nail pigmentation

Endocrine & metabolic: Elevations in serum triglyceride levels

Gastrointestinal: Mild to moderate nausea/vomiting, diarrhea, mucositis

Hematologic: Severe neutropenia (dose-limiting toxicity), leukopenia, thrombocytopenia, anemia

Hepatic: Elevated AST, alkaline phosphatase, bilirubin

Local: Erythema, tenderness, swelling at the injection site

Neuromuscular & skeletal: Peripheral neuropathy (dose-dependent, characterized by paresthesia with numbness and tingling in a stocking-and-glove distribution), myalgia, muscle weakness, motor dysfunction, arthralgia

Ocular: Loss of visual acuity, diplopia

Renal: Elevated serum creatinine

Respiratory: Dyspnea

Miscellaneous: Anaphylactoid reactions (dyspnea, bronchospasm, hypotension, generalized urticaria), ethanol intoxication

Drug Interactions Cytochrome P-450 isoenzyme CYP2C8 and CYP3A3/4 substrate Paclitaxel clearance decreases approximately 33% when administered following cisplatin. Since paclitaxel is metabolized by cytochrome P-450 3A4 and 2C8 isozymes, potential drug interactions can occur with agents that are isoenzyme inducers which reduce plasma paclitaxel concentration (ie, phenytoin) or inhibitors (ie, ketoconazole, verapamil, diazepam, cyclosporine, vincristine, etoposide, dexamethasone) which may increase plasma paclitaxel concentration; opiates, antihistamines, or other CNS depressants may potentiate CNS depression caused by ethanol in the paclitaxel formulation

Stability Refrigerate intact vials or store at room temperature; undiluted vials of paclitaxel may precipitate upon refrigeration, but will redissolve at room temperature with no loss in potency; dilution of paclitaxel from 0.3 mg/mL to 1.2 mg/mL in NS or D_5W is stable for up to 48 hours at room temperature; incompatible with amphotericin B, chlorpromazine, hydroxyzine, methylprednisolone, and mitoxantrone

Mechanism of Action An antimicrotubule agent that promotes the assembly of microtubules from tubulin dimers and stabilizes microtubules by preventing depolymerization; results in the inhibition of mitotic cellular functions and cell replication by blocking cells in the late G2 phase and M phase of the cell cycle

Pharmacokinetics

Distribution: Biphasic with initial rapid distribution to the peripheral compartment; later phase is a slow efflux of paclitaxel from the peripheral compartment

V_d: 227-688 L/m²

Protein binding: 89% to 98%

Metabolism: Cytochrome P-450 hepatic isoenzymes metabolize paclitaxel to 6 alpha-hydroxypaclitaxel

Half-life (varies with dose and infusion duration):

Children: 4.6-17 hours

Adults: 1.5-8.4 hours

Elimination: Urinary recovery of unchanged drug: 1.3% to 12.6%

Dialysis: No significant drug removal by hemodialysis

Usual Dosage I.V. infusion (refer to individual protocols):

Children:

Treatment for refractory leukemia is still undergoing investigation: 250-360 mg/m²/dose infused over 24 hours every 14 days

Recurrent Wilms' tumor: 250-350 mg/m²/dose infused over 24 hours every 3 weeks

Adults:

Ovarian carcinoma: 135-175 mg/m²/dose infused over 1-24 hours every 3 weeks

Metastatic breast cancer: 175 mg/m²/dose infused over 3 hours every 3 weeks (protocols have used dosages ranging between 135-250 mg/m²/dose over 1-24 hours every 3 weeks)

Kaposi's sarcoma: 135 mg/m²/dose infused over 3 hours every 3 weeks, or 100 mg/m²/dose infused over 3 hours every 2 weeks

Dosage adjustment in renal impairment: None

(Continued)

Paclitaxel *(Continued)*

Dosage adjustment in hepatic impairment:
Total bilirubin ≤1.5 mg/dL and AST >2x normal limits: Total dose <135 mg/m^2
Total bilirubin 1.6-3.0 mg/dL: Total dose ≤75 mg/m^2
Total bilirubin ≥3.1 mg/dL: Total dose ≤50 mg/m^2

Administration Parenteral: I.V.: Patients should be premedicated with a corticosteroid, diphenhydramine and an H$_2$-receptor antagonist 30-60 minutes prior to paclitaxel administration. To minimize patient exposure to the plasticizer diethylhexylphthalate (DEHP) from polyoxyl 35 castor oil-induced leaching of polyvinyl chloride-containing I.V. infusion bags and administration sets, prepare paclitaxel infusions in glass or in polypropylene or polyolefin bags and administer through polyethylene lined administration sets with a 0.22 micron in-line filter. Paclitaxel can be further diluted in D$_5$W, NS, D$_5$/NS or D$_5$ in Ringer's injection to a final concentration of 0.3-1.2 mg/mL. Paclitaxel has been infused over short (1-3 hours) and long periods (24, 72, and 96 hours to 14 days continuous infusion)

Monitoring Parameters CBC with differential, platelet count, vital signs, ECG, liver function test; observe I.V. injection site for extravasation

Patient Information Avoid alcohol; may cause drowsiness and impair ability to perform hazardous activities requiring mental alertness

Dosage Forms Injection: 30 mg/5 mL vial [vehicle contains polyoxyethylated castor oil and dehydrated alcohol]

References
Woo MH, Gregornik D, Shearer PD, et al, "Pharmacokinetics of Paclitaxel in an Anephric Patient," *Cancer Chemother Pharmacol*, 1999, 43(1):92-6.

♦ **Pain Aid Free (Can)** *see* Acetaminophen *on page 29*
♦ **Palgic® D** *see* Carbinoxamine and Pseudoephedrine *on page 179*
♦ **Palgic® DS** *see* Carbinoxamine and Pseudoephedrine *on page 179*

Palivizumab *(pah li VIZ u mab)*

U.S. Brand Names Synagis®

Therapeutic Category Monoclonal Antibody

Use Prevention of serious lower respiratory tract disease caused by respiratory syncytial virus (RSV) in infants and children <2 years of age with chronic lung disease who have required medical therapy for their chronic lung disease within 6 months before the anticipated RSV season; prevention of serious RSV disease in patients with a history of prematurity (≤28 weeks gestation) up to 12 months of age or infants born at 29-32 weeks of gestation up to 6 months of age; prophylaxis of infants with severe immune deficiency exposed to RSV

Pregnancy Risk Factor C

Contraindications History of severe prior reaction to palivizumab or any component; not recommended for children with cyanotic congenital heart disease

Warnings Anaphylactoid reactions have not been observed following palivizumab administration, but can occur following the administration of proteins. If anaphylaxis or severe allergic reaction occurs, administer epinephrine (1:1000) and provide supportive care as required.

Precautions Use with caution in patients with thrombocytopenia or any coagulation disorder. Safety and efficacy have not been demonstrated for treatment of established RSV disease.

Adverse Reactions
Dermatologic: Rash
Gastrointestinal: Diarrhea, vomiting
Hepatic: Elevated SGOT
Local: Injection site reaction, erythema, induration
Respiratory: Upper respiratory infection, otitis media, rhinitis, pharyngitis, cough

Drug Interactions No formal drug interaction studies have been conducted. Note: No interference with measles, mumps, and rubella vaccines (combined) and varicella vaccine occurs

Stability Store in refrigerator at a temperature between 2°C to 8°C (35.6°F to 46.4°F) in original container; do not freeze; the single-use vial does not contain a preservative

Reconstitute single-use vial with 1 mL of SWI; swirl vial gently for 30 seconds to avoid foaming. Do not shake vial. Allow solution to stand at room temperature for 20 minutes until it clears; solution should be administered within 6 hours of reconstitution.

Mechanism of Action Humanized monoclonal antibody directed to an epitope in the A antigenic site of the respiratory syncytial virus F protein resulting in neutralizing and fusion-inhibitory activity against RSV

Pharmacokinetics
Half-life:
Children <24 months: 20 days
Adults: 18 days
Time to achieve adequate serum antibody titers: 48 hours
Usual Dosage Children: I.M.: 15 mg/kg once monthly during RSV season
Administration Parenteral: Administer I.M., preferably in the anterolateral aspect of the thigh; gluteal muscle should not be used routinely as an injection site because of the risk of damage to the sciatic nerve; injection volume over 1 mL should be given as a divided dose
Monitoring Parameters Observe for anaphylactic or severe allergic reactions
Additional Information RSV prophylaxis should be initiated at the onset of the RSV season. In most areas of the United States, onset of RSV outbreaks is October to December, and termination is March to May, but regional differences occur.
Dosage Forms Injection, lyophilized: 100 mg
References
"Palivizumab, a Humanized Respiratory Syncytial Virus Monoclonal Antibody, Reduces Hospitalization From Respiratory Syncytial Virus Infection in High-Risk Infants. The IMpact-RSV Study Group, ," *Pediatrics*, 1998, 102(3 Pt 1):531-7.
"Prevention of Respiratory Syncytial Virus Infections: Indications for the Use of Palivizumab and Update on the Use of RSV-IGIV. American Academy of Pediatrics Committee on Infectious Diseases and Committee on Fetus and Newborn," *Pediatrics*, 1998, 102(5):1211-6.

♦ **Palmitate-A® [OTC]** *see* Vitamin A *on page 1013*
♦ **2-PAM** *see* Pralidoxime *on page 818*
♦ **Pamelor®** *see* Nortriptyline *on page 724*

Pamidronate (pa mi DROE nate)

U.S. Brand Names Aredia™
Synonyms Aminohydroxypropylidene Diphosphonate; APD
Therapeutic Category Antidote, Hypercalcemia; Bisphosphonate Derivative
Generic Available No
Use Symptomatic treatment of moderate to severe Paget's disease; hypercalcemia associated with malignancy; treatment of osteolytic bone lesions associated with multiple myeloma or metastatic breast cancer
Investigation use: Inhibit bone resorption in severe osteogenesis imperfecta
Pregnancy Risk Factor C
Contraindications Hypersensitivity to pamidronate or any component
Warnings Leukopenia has been observed with oral pamidronate; monitoring of white blood cell counts is suggested; vein irritation and thrombophlebitis may occur with I.V. infusions
Precautions Use with caution in patients with renal impairment; maintain adequate hydration and urinary output during treatment
Adverse Reactions
Cardiovascular: Tachycardia, hypertension, syncope
Central nervous system: Malaise, fever, fatigue, somnolence, insomnia, seizures
Dermatologic: Rash
Endocrine & metabolic: Hypocalcemia, hypophosphatemia, hypothyroidism, hypokalemia, hypomagnesemia, fluid overload
Gastrointestinal: Nausea, anorexia, constipation, GI hemorrhage, abdominal pain, occult blood in stools, abnormal taste
Hematologic: Leukopenia, anemia
Local: Vein irritation, thrombophlebitis
Neuromuscular & skeletal: Bone pain
Ocular: Scleritis, uveitis, conjunctivitis
Respiratory: Rales, rhinitis
Miscellaneous: Moniliasis (associated with 90 mg dosage)
Stability Reconstituted solution stable for 24 hours at room temperature or refrigerated; incompatible with calcium-containing I.V. fluids (ie, Ringer's solution)
Mechanism of Action Pamidronate, a biphosphonate, lowers serum calcium concentrations by binding to bone and inhibiting osteoclast-mediated calcium resorption; this agent does not appear to produce any significant effect on renal tubular calcium handling
Pharmacodynamics
Onset of hypocalcemic effect: 24-48 hours
Maximum effect: 5-7 days
Pharmacokinetics
Absorption: Poorly from the GI tract; pharmacokinetic studies are lacking
Distribution half-life: 1.6 hours
(Continued)

Pamidronate *(Continued)*

Bone half-life: 300 days

Half-life, unmetabolized: 2.5 hours

Elimination: Biphasic; ~50% excreted unchanged in urine within 72 hours

Usual Dosage

Hypercalcemia: I.V.:

Children (limited experience): 0.5-1 mg/kg

Adults: Dosage based upon serum calcium measurement:

Serum calcium 12-13.5 mg/dL: 60-90 mg

Serum calcium >13.5 mg/dL: 90 mg

Consider retreatment if the serum calcium becomes elevated again; allow a minimum of 7 days between each treatment to allow for a full response to the initial treatment

Osteogenesis imperfecta:

Children (limited experience): 0.5-1 mg/kg/day for 3 days; may repeat in 4- to 6-month intervals

Osteolytic bone lesions of breast cancer or multiple myeloma: Adults: 90 mg/month

Paget's disease: Adults: 30 mg for 3 consecutive days

Administration Dilute in 250-500 mL D_5W, $\frac{1}{2}NS$, or NS; infuse over 2-4 hours; in treatment of hypercalcemia, 90 mg doses should be infused over 24 hours

Monitoring Parameters Serum calcium, phosphate, potassium, magnesium, creatinine, hemoglobin, hematocrit, CBC with differential; in addition (Paget's disease) serum alkaline phosphatase, urinary hydroxyproline excretion

Dosage Forms Powder for injection, lyophilized, as disodium: 30 mg, 90 mg

References

Glorieux FH, Bishop NH, Plotkin H, et al, "Cyclic Administration of Pamidronate in Children With Severe Osteogenesis Imperfecta," *N Engl J Med*, 1998, 339(14):947-52.

Lteif AN and Zimmerman D, "Biphosphonates for Treatment of Childhood Hypercalcemia," *Pediatrics*, 1998, 102(4 Pt 1):990-3.

♦ **Panadol (Can)** *see* Acetaminophen *on page 29*

♦ **Pancrease®** *see* Pancrelipase *on page 755*

♦ **Pancrease® MT** *see* Pancrelipase *on page 755*

Pancreatin *(PAN kree a tin)*

U.S. Brand Names Pancreatin 4X 600 mg [OTC]; Pancreatin 8X 900 mg [OTC]; Veg-Pancreatin 4X [OTC]

Therapeutic Category Enzyme, Pancreatic; Pancreatic Enzyme

Generic Available No

Use Replacement therapy in symptomatic treatment of malabsorption syndrome caused by pancreatic enzyme insufficiency

Pregnancy Risk Factor C

Contraindications Hypersensitivity to pancreatin, any component, or to bovine or pork protein; acute pancreatitis; acute exacerbations of chronic pancreatic diseases

Warnings Pancreatin is inactivated by acids; use microencapsulated products whenever possible, since these products permit better dissolution of enzymes in the duodenum and protect the enzyme preparations from acid degradation in the stomach; these products are not bioequivalent, do not substitute without consulting a physician or pharmacist; do not substitute generic pancreatic enzymes for brand name products

Precautions Do not spill powder on hands as is a skin irritant; inhalation of powder may produce an asthmatic attack

Adverse Reactions

Dermatologic: Rash

Endocrine & metabolic: Hyperuricemia

Gastrointestinal: Nausea, abdominal cramps, constipation, diarrhea, colonic strictures, mouth irritation

Ocular: Lacrimation

Renal: Hyperuricosuria

Respiratory: Sneezing, bronchospasm

Miscellaneous: Hypersensitivity reactions

Drug Interactions Calcium carbonate, magnesium hydroxide may decrease effectiveness of enzymes; pancreatin may decrease the response to oral iron therapy; H_2 antagonists (eg, ranitidine, cimetidine) increase effectiveness of pancreatic enzymes

Mechanism of Action Replaces endogenous pancreatic enzymes to assist in digestion of protein, starch and fats

Pharmacokinetics
Absorption: Not absorbed, acts locally in the GI tract
Elimination: In feces

Usual Dosage Oral: The following dosage recommendations are only an approximation for initial dosages; the actual dosage will depend on the digestive requirements of the individual patient

Infants: 2000-4000 lipase units/120 mL (4 ounce) formula
Children ≤4 years: 1000 lipase units/kg/meal (maximum: 2500 lipase units/kg), with $\frac{1}{2}$ dose with each snack
Children >4 years and Adults: 400-500 lipase units/kg/meal (maximum: 2500 lipase units/kg), with $\frac{1}{2}$ dose with each snack

Administration Oral: Swallow capsules/tablets whole; retention in the mouth before swallowing may cause mucosal irritation and stomatitis; administer before or with meals; when administering to infants, may open capsule and spread over acidic foods (applesauce, mashed fruits, rice cereal) in a rubber-tipped teaspoon (use mixture immediately, do not make ahead of time). Place mixture onto the middle of the infant's tongue and then give bottle or breast. As an alternative, the parent may dip a clean finger into the food/enzyme mixture and then place finger into the infant's mouth and allow infant to suck on. Check infant's mouth after eating for lodged enzyme beads and remove.

Monitoring Parameters Stool fat content

Additional Information Concomitant administration of conventional pancreatin enzymes with an H_2-receptor antagonist has been used to decrease acid inactivation of enzyme activity. Colonic strictures have been reported in several pediatric patients. There is a possible association between the development of strictures and a high lipase intake (mean >16,000 units/kg/meal). Patients receiving doses >2500 lipase units/kg/meal or 4000 lipase units/g fat/day should be re-evaluated or titrated downward to lowest effective dose

Dosage Forms See table.

Pancreatin

Product	Dosage Form	Lipase USP Units	Amylase USP Units	Protease USP Units	Pancreatin mg
Pancreatin 4X 600 mg; Veg-Pancreatin	Tablet	1200	60,000	60,000	2400
Pancreatin 8X 900 mg	Tablet	22,500	180,000	180,000	7200

References
Pettei MJ, Leonidas JC, Levinne JJ, et al, "Pancolonic Disease in Cystic Fibrosis and High-Dose Pancreatic Enzyme Therapy," *J Pediatr*, 1994, 125(4):587-9.
Taylor CJ, "Colonic Strictures in Cystic Fibrosis," *Lancet*, 1994, 343(8898):615-6.

♦ **Pancreatin 4X 600 mg [OTC]** *see* Pancreatin *on page 754*
♦ **Pancreatin 8X 900 mg [OTC]** *see* Pancreatin *on page 754*
♦ **Pancrecarb®** *see* Pancrelipase *on page 755*

Pancrelipase *(pan kre LI pase)*

Related Information
Pancreatin *on page 754*

U.S. Brand Names Cotazym®; Cotazym-S®; Creon® 5; Creon® 10; Creon® 20; Digestive Enzymes [OTC]; Hi-Vegi-LIP [OTC]; Kutrase®; Ku-Zyme®; Ku-Zyme® HP; Lipram®; Pancrease®; Pancrease® MT; Pancrecarb®; Ultrase®; Ultrase® MT; Viokase®; Zymase®

Synonyms Lipancreatin

Therapeutic Category Enzyme, Pancreatic; Pancreatic Enzyme

Generic Available Yes

Use Replacement therapy in symptomatic treatment of malabsorption syndrome caused by pancreatic enzyme insufficiency

Pregnancy Risk Factor C

Contraindications Hypersensitivity to pancrelipase, any component, or to pork protein; acute pancreatitis; acute exacerbations of chronic pancreatic diseases

Warnings Pancrelipase is inactivated by acids; use microencapsulated products whenever possible, since these products permit better dissolution of enzymes in the duodenum and protect the enzyme preparations from acid degradation in the stomach; products are not bioequivalent, do not substitute without consulting a
(Continued)

Pancrelipase *(Continued)*

physician or pharmacist; do not substitute generic enzymes for brand name products

Precautions Do not spill powder on hands as is skin irritant; inhalation of powder may produce an asthmatic attack

Adverse Reactions

Dermatologic: Rash

Endocrine & metabolic: Hyperuricemia

Gastrointestinal: Nausea, abdominal cramps, constipation, diarrhea, colonic strictures, mouth irritation

Ocular: Lacrimation

Renal: Hyperuricosuria

Respiratory: Sneezing, bronchospasm

Miscellaneous: Hypersensitivity reactions

Drug Interactions Calcium carbonate, magnesium hydroxide may decrease effectiveness of enzymes; may decrease the response to oral iron therapy; H_2 antagonists (eg, ranitidine, cimetidine) may increase effectiveness of pancreatic enzymes

Mechanism of Action Replaces endogenous pancreatic enzymes to assist in digestion of protein, starch and fats

Pancrelipase

Product	Dosage Form	Lipase USP Units	Amylase USP Units	Protease USP Units
Cotazym® Ku-Zyme® HP	Capsule	8000	30,000	30,000
Cotazym®-S	Capsule, enteric coated spheres	5000	20,000	20,000
Creon® 5	Capsule, delayed release	5000	16,600	18,750
Creon® 10	Capsule, delayed release	10,000	33,200	37,500
Creon® 20	Capsule, delayed release	20,000	66,400	75,000
Digestive Enzymes	Tablet	27.5	19	5
Hi-Vegi-LIP	Tablet	4800	60,000	60,000
Kutrase®	Capsule	2400	30,000	30,000
Ku-Zyme®	Capsule	1200	15,000	15,000
Lipram™ 4500	Capsule	4500	20,000	25,000
Lipram™-PN 16	Capsule	16,000	48,000	48,000
Lipram™-PN 10	Capsule	10,000	30,000	30,000
Lipram™-CR 10	Capsule	10,000	33,200	37,500
Lipram™-CR 20	Capsule	20,000	66,400	75,000
Lipram™-UL 12	Capsule	12,000	39,000	39,000
Lipram™-UL 18	Capsule	18,000	58,500	58,500
Lipram™-UL 20	Capsule	20,000	65,000	65,000
Pancrease®	Capsule, enteric coated microspheres	4500	20,000	25,000
Pancrease® MT 4	Capsule, enteric coated microtablets	4000	12,000	12,000
MT 10		10,000	30,000	30,000
MT 16		16,000	48,000	48,000
MT 20		20,000	56,000	44,000
Pancrecarb® MS-8	Buffered, enteric-coated microspheres	8000	40,000	45,000
Ultrase®	Capsule, enteric coated microspheres	4500	20,000	25,000
MT 12		12,000	39,000	39,000
MT 18		18,000	58,500	58,500
MT 20		20,000	65,000	65,000
Viokase®	Powder	16,800 (per 0.7 g)	70,000 (per 0.7 g)	70,000 (per 0.7 g)
	Tablet	8000	30,000	30,000
Zymase®	Capsule, enteric coated spheres	12,000	24,000	24,000

Pharmacokinetics

Absorption: Not absorbed, acts locally in the GI tract

Elimination: In feces

Usual Dosage The following dosage recommendations are only an approximation for initial dosages. The actual dosage will depend on the digestive requirements of the individual patient. Oral:

Infants: 2000-4000 lipase units/120 mL (4 ounce) formula

Children ≤4 years: 1000 lipase units/kg/meal (maximum: 2500 lipase units/kg), with ¹/₂ dose with each snack

Children >4 years and Adults: 400-500 lipase units/kg/meal (maximum: 2500 lipase units/kg), with ¹/₂ dose with each snack

Occluded feeding tubes: Children and Adults: One tablet of Viokase® crushed with one 325 mg tablet of sodium bicarbonate (to activate the Viokase®) in 5 mL of water can be instilled into the nasogastric tube and clamped for 5 minutes; then flushed with 50 mL of water

Administration Oral: Swallow tablets and capsules whole; do not chew the microspheres or microtablets; retention in the mouth before swallowing may cause mucosal irritation and stomatitis; administer before or with meals; when administering to infants, may open capsule and spread over acidic foods (applesauce, mashed fruits, rice cereal) in a rubber-tipped teaspoon (use mixture immediately, do not make ahead of time). Place mixture onto the middle of the infant's tongue and then give bottle or breast. As an alternative, the parent may dip a clean finger into the food/enzyme mixture and then place finger into the infant's mouth and allow infant to suck on. Check infant's mouth after eating for lodged enzyme beads and remove.

Monitoring Parameters Stool fat content

Additional Information Concomitant administration of conventional pancreatin enzymes with an H_2-receptor antagonist has been used to decrease acid inactivation of enzyme activity. Colonic strictures have been reported in several pediatric patients. There is a possible association between the development of strictures and a high lipase intake (mean >16,000 units/kg/meal). Patients receiving doses >2500 lipase units/kg/meal or 4000 lipase units/g fat/day should be re-evaluated or titrated downward to lowest effective dose

Dosage Forms See table on previous page.

References

Pettei MJ, Leonidas JC, Levinne JJ, et al, "Pancolonic Disease in Cystic Fibrosis and High-Dose Pancreatic Enzyme Therapy," *J Pediatr*, 1994, 125(4):587-9.

Taylor CG, "Colonic Strictures in Cystic Fibrosis," *Lancet*, 1994, 343(8898):615-6.

Pancuronium (pan kyoo ROE nee um)

Therapeutic Category Neuromuscular Blocker Agent, Nondepolarizing; Skeletal Muscle Relaxant, Paralytic

Generic Available Yes

Use Produces skeletal muscle relaxation during surgery after induction of general anesthesia, increases pulmonary compliance during assisted mechanical respiration, facilitates endotracheal intubation

Pregnancy Risk Factor C

Contraindications Hypersensitivity to pancuronium, bromide, or any component

Warnings Ventilation must be supported during neuromuscular blockade; electrolyte imbalance alters blockade

Precautions Use with caution and decrease dose in patients with decreased renal function; many clinical conditions may affect the response to neuromuscular blockade, see table.

Clinical Conditions Affecting Neuromuscular Blockade

Potentiation	Antagonism
Electrolyte abnormalities	Alkalosis
Severe hyponatremia	Hypercalcemia
Severe hypocalcemia	Demyelinating lesions
Severe hypokalemia	Peripheral neuropathies
Hypermagnesemia	Diabetes mellitus
Neuromuscular diseases	
Acidosis	
Acute intermittent porphyria	
Renal failure	
Hepatic failure	

(Continued)

Pancuronium *(Continued)*

Adverse Reactions Most frequent adverse reactions are related to prolongation of pharmacologic actions

Cardiovascular: Tachycardia, hypertension
Dermatologic: Rash, erythema
Gastrointestinal: Excessive salivation
Local: Burning sensation along the vein
Neuromuscular & skeletal: Muscle weakness
Respiratory: Wheezes, bronchospasm
Miscellaneous: Hypersensitivity reactions

Drug Interactions See table.

Potential Drug Interactions

Potentiation	Antagonism
Inhalation anesthetics	Calcium
Desflurane, sevoflurane, enflurane and isoflurane > halothane > nitrous oxide	Carbamazepine
	Phenytoin
	Steroids (chronic administration)
Antibiotics	Theophylline
Aminoglycosides, polymyxins, clindamycin, vancomycin	Anticholinesterases*
Magnesium	Neostigmine, pyridostigmine, edrophonium, echothiophate ophthalmic solution
Antiarrhythmics	Caffeine
Quinidine, procainamide, bretylium, and possibly lidocaine	Azathioprine
Diuretics	
Furosemide, mannitol, thiazides	
Amphotericin B (secondary to hypokalemia)	
Local anesthetics	
Dantrolene (directly depresses skeletal muscle)	
Beta blockers	
Calcium channel blockers	
Ketamine	
Lithium	
Succinylcholine (when administered prior to nondepolarizing neuromuscular-blocking agent)	
Cyclosporine	

*Can prolong the effects of acetylcholine

Stability Refrigerate; however, stable for up to 6 months at room temperature; compatible with D_5W, NS, D_5NS, and LR injections

Mechanism of Action Nondepolarizing neuromuscular blocker which blocks acetylcholine from binding to receptors on motor endplate thus inhibiting depolarization

Pharmacodynamics
Peak effect: I.V. injection: Within 2-3 minutes
Duration: 40-60 minutes (dose dependent)

Pharmacokinetics
Distribution: V_d: Adult: 0.23 L/kg
Protein binding: 87%
Metabolism: 30% to 40% metabolized in liver
Half-life: 110 minutes
Elimination: Primarily in urine (60%) as unchanged drug and bile (40%)
Clearance: Adult: 1.9 mL/kg/minute

Usual Dosage I.V.:
Neonates and Infants: 0.1 mg/kg every 30-60 minutes as needed or as continuous infusion of 0.02-0.04 mg/kg/hour or 0.4-0.6 mcg/kg/minute
Children: 0.15 mg/kg every 30-60 minutes as needed or as continuous infusion 0.03-0.06 mg/kg/hour or 0.5-1 mcg/kg/minute
Adolescents and Adults: 0.15 mg/kg every 30-60 minutes as needed or as a continuous infusion 0.02-0.04 mg/kg/hour or 0.4-0.6 mcg/kg/minute

Dosing adjustment in renal impairment:
Cl$_{cr}$ 10-50 mL/minute: Administer 50% of normal dose
Cl$_{cr}$ <10 mL/minute: Do not use

Administration Parenteral: May be administered undiluted by rapid I.V. injection; for continuous infusion, dilute to 0.01-0.8 mg/mL in D$_5$NS, D$_5$W, LR, or NS.

Monitoring Parameters Heart rate, blood pressure, assisted ventilation status, peripheral nerve stimulator measuring twitch response

Nursing Implications Does not alter the patient's state of consciousness; addition of sedation and analgesia are recommended

Additional Information Patients with hepatic and biliary disease have a larger V$_d$ which may result in a higher total initial dose and possibly a slower onset of effect; the duration of neuromuscular blocking effects may be prolonged in patients with hepatic, biliary, or renal dysfunction

Dosage Forms Injection, as bromide: 1 mg/mL (10 mL); 2 mg/mL (2 mL, 5 mL)

References
Martin LD, Bratton SL, and O'Rourke PP, "Clinical Uses and Controversies of Neuromuscular Blocking Agents in Infants and Children," *Crit Care Med*, 1999, 27(7):1358-68.

♦ **Pandel**® *see* Hydrocortisone *on page 506*
♦ **Panglobulin**™ *see* Immune Globulin (Intravenous) *on page 529*
♦ **PanOxyl**®-AQ *see* Benzoyl Peroxide *on page 136*
♦ **PanOxyl**® Bar [OTC] *see* Benzoyl Peroxide *on page 136*

Papaverine (pa PAV er een)

Therapeutic Category Antimigraine Agent; Vasodilator

Generic Available Yes

Use Relief of peripheral and cerebral ischemia associated with arterial spasm; investigationally for prophylaxis of migraine headache; intracavernosal injection for impotence

Pregnancy Risk Factor C

Contraindications Complete atrioventricular block; Parkinson's disease

Precautions Use with caution in patients with glaucoma; administer I.V. slowly and with caution since arrhythmias and apnea may occur with rapid I.V. use

Adverse Reactions
Cardiovascular: Flushing of the face, tachycardia, hypotension, arrhythmias with rapid I.V. use
Central nervous system: Depression, dizziness, vertigo, drowsiness, sedation, lethargy, headache
Dermatologic: Pruritus
Gastrointestinal: Xerostomia, nausea, constipation
Hepatic: Hepatic hypersensitivity
Local: Thrombosis at the I.V. administration site
Respiratory: Apnea with rapid I.V. use
Miscellaneous: Diaphoresis

Drug Interactions Cytochrome P-450 isoenzyme CYP2D6 substrate
Additive effects with CNS depressants or morphine; papaverine decreases the effects of levodopa

Stability Protect from heat or freezing; do not refrigerate injection; solutions should be clear to pale yellow; precipitates with LR

Mechanism of Action Smooth muscle spasmolytic producing a generalized smooth muscle relaxation including vasodilatation, gastrointestinal sphincter relaxation, bronchiolar muscle relaxation, and potentially a depressed myocardium

Pharmacodynamics Onset of action: Oral: Rapid

Pharmacokinetics
Protein binding: 90%
Metabolism: Rapid in the liver
Bioavailability: Oral: ~54%
Half-life: 30-120 minutes
Elimination: Primarily as metabolites in urine

Usual Dosage
Children: I.M., I.V.: 1.5 mg/kg 4 times/day
Migraine prophylaxis: 6-15 years: Oral: Initial: 5 mg/kg/day given once daily; range: 5-10 mg/kg/day divided into 2-3 doses/day
Adults:
Oral: 75-300 mg 3-5 times/day
Oral, sustained release: 150-300 mg every 12 hours
I.M., I.V.: 30-120 mg every 3 hours as needed
(Continued)

Papaverine (Continued)

Administration

Oral: Administer after or with meals, milk or antacids to decrease nausea; swallow sustained release capsule whole, do not crush or chew

Parenteral: Rapid I.V. administration may result in arrhythmias and fatal apnea; administer slow I.V. over 1-2 minutes

Monitoring Parameters Liver enzymes; intraocular pressure in glaucoma patients

Patient Information May cause dizziness, flushing, headache; may cause drowsiness and impair ability to perform hazardous activities requiring mental alertness or physical coordination

Additional Information Evidence of therapeutic value of systemic use for relief of peripheral and cerebral ischemia related to arterial spasm is lacking

Note: The manufacturer (Eli Lilly) is limiting the distribution of the injectable form to hospitals and similar settings to discourage its use for the treatment of impotence

Further studies are needed to determine the benefit of adding papaverine (60 mg/500 mL) to arterial catheter infusions containing NS or ½NS and heparin 1 unit/mL. One investigation showed a lower risk of arterial catheter failure and longer duration of arterial catheter function in patients 7 months to 5.5 years of age who received papaverine in their arterial catheter solutions; these results should be verified by additional studies before the addition of papaverine to arterial catheter solutions can be recommended; also, papaverine should **not** be used in neonates due to the increased risk of drug-induced cerebral vasodilation and possibility of an intracranial bleed.

Dosage Forms

Capsule, sustained release, as hydrochloride: 150 mg

Injection, as hydrochloride: 30 mg/mL (2 mL, 10 mL)

References

Heulitt MJ, Farrington EA, O'Shea TM, et al, "Double-Blind, Randomized, Controlled Trial of Papaverine-Containing Infusions to Prevent Failure of Arterial Catheters in Pediatric Patients," *Crit Care Med*, 1993, 21(6):825-9.

Sillanpää M and Koponen M, "Papaverine in the Prophylaxis of Migraine and Other Vascular Headache in Children," *Acta Paediatr Scand*, 1978, 67(2):209-12.

♦ **Parabromdylamine** see Brompheniramine on page 152

♦ **Paracetaldehyde** see Paraldehyde on page 760

♦ **Paracetamol** see Acetaminophen on page 29

♦ **Parafon Forte™ DSC** see Chlorzoxazone on page 229

Paraldehyde (par AL de hyde)

Synonyms Paracetaldehyde

Therapeutic Category Anticonvulsant, Miscellaneous; Hypnotic; Sedative

Generic Available Yes

Use Treatment of status epilepticus and tetanus-induced seizures; has been used as a sedative/hypnotic and in the treatment of alcohol withdrawal symptoms

Restrictions C-IV

Pregnancy Risk Factor C

Contraindications Severe hepatic insufficiency, respiratory disease, GI inflammation or ulceration

Warnings Do not abruptly discontinue in patients receiving chronic therapy

Precautions May need to decrease dose in patients with liver disease

Adverse Reactions

Dermatologic: Erythematous rash

Endocrine & metabolic: Metabolic acidosis

Gastrointestinal: Gastric irritation, corrosion of the stomach or rectum

Hepatic: Hepatitis

Respiratory: Coughing, strong and unpleasant breath, pulmonary edema

Miscellaneous: Psychological and physical dependence with prolonged use

Drug Interactions Barbiturates and alcohol may enhance CNS depression

Stability Decomposes with exposure to air and light to acetaldehyde which then oxidizes to acetic acid; store in tightly closed containers; protect from light

Mechanism of Action Unknown mechanism of action; causes depression of CNS, including the ascending reticular activating system to provide sedation/hypnosis and anticonvulsant activity

Pharmacodynamics Hypnosis: Oral:

Onset of action: Within 10-15 minutes

Duration: 6-8 hours

Pharmacokinetics
Distribution: Crosses the placenta
Metabolism: ~70% to 80% in the liver
Half-life:
Neonates: 10 hours
Adults: 3.5-10 hours
Elimination: 30% excreted as unchanged drug in expired air via the lungs; trace amounts are excreted in urine unchanged
Usual Dosage See table.

Paraldehyde

	Sedative	Hypnotic	Seizures
Neonates Rectal			0.3 mL/kg; may repeat once if needed in 4-6 h
Children Oral, rectal	0.15 mL/kg	0.3 mL/kg	0.3 mL/kg every 2-4 h; maximum dose is 5 mL
Adults Oral, rectal	5-10 mL	10-30 mL	

Administration
Oral: Dilute in milk or iced fruit juice
Rectal: Mix paraldehyde 2:1 with oil (cottonseed, olive, or mineral oil)

Do **not** use any plastic equipment for administration, use glass syringes and rubber tubing (paraldehyde will dissolve plastic)

Patient Information Avoid alcohol; causes sedation and impairs ability to perform hazardous activities requiring mental alertness or physical coordination

Nursing Implications Discard unused contents of any container which has been opened for more than 24 hours; do **not** use discolored solution or solutions with strong smell of acetic acid (vinegar); outdated preparations can be toxic

Additional Information Parenteral dosage form is no longer available in the United States

Dosage Forms Liquid, oral or rectal: 1 g/mL (30 mL)

♦ **Paraplatin®** see Carboplatin on page 181

Paregoric (par e GOR ik)
Related Information
Carbohydrate and Alcohol Content of Liquid Medications for Use in Patients Receiving Ketogenic Diets on page 1258
Overdose and Toxicology on page 1222
Synonyms Camphorated Tincture of Opium
Therapeutic Category Analgesic, Narcotic; Antidiarrheal
Generic Available Yes
Use Treatment of diarrhea or relief of pain; neonatal abstinence syndrome (neonatal opiate withdrawal)
Restrictions C-III
Pregnancy Risk Factor B (D when used for long-term or in high-doses)
Contraindications Hypersensitivity to opium or any component (see Additional Information); diarrhea caused by poisoning until the toxic material has been removed
Warnings Some commercial preparations contain sulfites which may cause allergic reactions
Precautions Use with caution in patients with respiratory, hepatic or renal dysfunction, severe prostatic hypertrophy, or history of narcotic abuse; opium shares the toxic potential of opiate agonists, usual precautions of opiate agonist therapy should be observed; infants <3 months of age are more susceptible to respiratory depression, use with caution and in reduced doses in this age group
Adverse Reactions
Cardiovascular: Hypotension, bradycardia, vasodilation
Central nervous system: CNS depression, increased intracranial pressure, drowsiness, dizziness, sedation
Endocrine & metabolic: Antidiuretic hormone release
Gastrointestinal: Nausea, vomiting, constipation, biliary tract spasm
Genitourinary: Urinary tract spasm, urinary retention
Ocular: Miosis
Respiratory: Respiratory depression
(Continued)

Paregoric *(Continued)*

Miscellaneous: Physical and psychological dependence, histamine release

Drug Interactions CNS depressants (eg, alcohol, narcotics, benzodiazepines, tricyclic antidepressants, MAO inhibitors, phenothiazines) may increase effects/ toxicity

Stability Store in light-resistant, tightly closed container; protect from freezing

Mechanism of Action Increases smooth muscle tone in GI tract, decreases motility and peristalsis, diminishes digestive secretions

Pharmacokinetics

Metabolism: Opium is metabolized in the liver

Elimination: In urine, primarily as morphine glucuronide conjugates and as parent compound (morphine, codeine, papaverine, etc)

Usual Dosage Oral:

Neonates (full term): Neonatal abstinence syndrome (opiate withdrawal): Initial: 0.1 mL/kg or 2 drops/kg with feedings every 3-4 hours; increase dosage by 0.1 mL/kg or 2 drops/kg every 3-4 hours until withdrawal symptoms are controlled; it is rare to exceed 0.7 mL/dose. Stabilize withdrawal symptoms for 3-5 days, then gradually decrease the dosage (keeping the same dosing interval) over a 2- to 4-week period.

Children: 0.25-0.5 mL/kg 1-4 times/day

Adults: 5-10 mL 1-4 times/day

Administration Oral: May administer with food to decrease GI upset; shake well before use

Monitoring Parameters Respiratory rate, blood pressure, heart rate, level of sedation; neonatal abstinence syndrome (opiate withdrawal): Monitor for resolution of withdrawal symptoms (such as irritability, high-pitched cry, stuffy nose, rhinorrhea, vomiting, poor feeding, diarrhea, sneezing, yawning, etc) and signs of over treatment (such as bradycardia, lethargy, hypotonia, irregular respirations, respiratory depression, etc); an abstinence scoring system (eg, Finnegan abstinence scoring system) can be used to more objectively assess neonatal opiate withdrawal symptoms and the need for dosage adjustment

Patient Information Avoid alcohol; may cause drowsiness and impair ability to perform hazardous tasks requiring mental alertness; may be habit-forming

Additional Information Do **not** confuse this product with opium tincture which is 25 times **more** potent; each 5 mL of paregoric contains 2 mg morphine equivalent, 0.02 mL anise oil, 20 mg benzoic acid, 20 mg camphor, 0.2 mL glycerin and alcohol; final alcohol content 45%; paregoric also contains papaverine and noscapine; because all of these additives may be harmful to neonates, **a 25-fold dilution of opium tincture** is often preferred for treatment of neonatal abstinence syndrome (opiate withdrawal); see Opium Tincture *on page 737*

Dosage Forms Liquid: 2 mg morphine equivalent/5 mL [equivalent to 20 mg opium powder] (473 mL)

References

Kraus DM and Pham JT, "Neonatal Therapy," *Applied Therapeutics: The Clinical Use of Drugs*, 7th ed, Koda-Kimble MA, Young LY, eds, Baltimore, MD: Lippincott Williams & Wilkins, 2001.

Levy M and Spino M, "Neonatal Withdrawal Syndrome: Associated Drugs and Pharmacologic Management," *Pharmacotherapy*, 1993, 13(3):202-11.

"Neonatal Drug Withdrawal. American Academy of Pediatrics Committee on Drugs," *Pediatrics*, 1998, 101(6):1079-88.

♦ **Parenteral Nutrition (PN)** *see page 1106*

Paromomycin *(par oh moe MYE sin)*

U.S. Brand Names Humatin®

Therapeutic Category Amebicide

Generic Available No

Use Treatment of acute and chronic intestinal amebiasis due to susceptible *Entamoeba histolytica* (not effective in the treatment of extraintestinal amebiasis); tapeworm infestations; adjunctive management of hepatic coma; treatment of cryptosporidial diarrhea

Pregnancy Risk Factor C

Contraindications Hypersensitivity to paromomycin or any component; intestinal obstruction

Warnings May result in overgrowth of nonsusceptible organisms

Precautions Use with caution in patients with impaired GI motility or possible or proven ulcerative bowel lesions; use with caution in patients with impaired renal function

Adverse Reactions

Central nervous system: Headache, vertigo

Dermatologic: Exanthema, rash, pruritus ani

Endocrine & metabolic: Hypocholesterolemia

Gastrointestinal: Diarrhea, abdominal cramps, nausea, vomiting, anorexia, steatorrhea, secondary enterocolitis, pancreatitis

Hematologic: Eosinophilia

Otic: Ototoxicity

Renal: Hematuria

Drug Interactions May decrease digoxin level; increased effect of oral anticoagulants

Food Interactions Paromomycin may cause malabsorption of xylose, sucrose, and fats

Mechanism of Action Acts directly on ameba in the intestinal lumen; interferes with bacterial protein synthesis by binding to 30S ribosomal subunit of susceptible bacteria

Pharmacokinetics

Absorption: Poor from the GI tract

Elimination: Excreted unchanged in feces; portion of oral dose that may be absorbed is excreted in urine

Usual Dosage Oral:

Children:

Intestinal amebiasis (*Entamoeba histolytica*): 25-35 mg/kg/day divided every 8 hours for 7 days

Dientamoeba fragilis infection: 25-30 mg/kg/day divided every 8 hours for 7 days

Tapeworm:

T. saginata, T. solium, D. latum: 11 mg/kg/dose every 15 minutes for 4 doses

H. nana: 45 mg/kg/day once daily for 5-7 days

Adults:

Intestinal amebiasis (*Entamoeba histolytica*): 25-35 mg/kg/day divided every 8 hours for 7 days

Dientamoeba fragilis infection: 25-30 mg/kg/day divided every 8 hours for 7 days

Tapeworm:

T. saginata, T. solium, D. latum: 1 g every 15 minutes for 4 doses

H. nana: 45 mg/kg/day once daily for 5-7 days

Hepatic coma: 4 g/day in 2-4 divided doses for 5-6 days

Cryptosporidial diarrhea: 1.5-2 g/day in 3-4 divided doses for 10-14 days

Administration Oral: Administer with or after meals

Monitoring Parameters Periodic urinalysis and renal function tests; be alert to ototoxicity

Patient Information Notify physician if ringing in ears, hearing loss, or dizziness occurs

Additional Information With the treatment of cestodiasis caused by *T. solium*, paromomycin may cause disintegration of worm segments and release of viable eggs resulting in an increased risk for the development of cysticercosis

Dosage Forms Capsule, as sulfate: 250 mg

References

Danziger LH, Kanyok TP, and Novak RM, "Treatment of Cryptosporidial Diarrhea in an AIDS Patient With Paromomycin," *Ann Pharmacother*, 1993, 27(12):1460-2.

Liu LX and Weller PF, "Antiparasitic Drugs," *N Engl J Med*, 1996, 334(18):1178-84.

Paroxetine (pa ROKS e teen)

Related Information

Comparison of Adverse Effects of Antidepressants *on page 1066*

Comparison of Usual Adult Dosage and Mechanism of Action of Antidepressants *on page 1065*

Serotonin Syndrome *on page 1247*

U.S. Brand Names Paxil®

Therapeutic Category Antidepressant, Selective Serotonin Reuptake Inhibitor (SSRI)

Generic Available No

Use Treatment of depression, obsessive compulsive disorder, panic disorder, social anxiety disorder, and generalized anxiety disorder

Pregnancy Risk Factor C

Contraindications Hypersensitivity to paroxetine or any component; use of MAO inhibitors within 14 days (potentially fatal reactions may occur, see Drug Interactions); concurrent use of thioridazine

Warnings Avoid abrupt discontinuation; taper dosage gradually in patients receiving >20 mg/day as withdrawal symptoms (sweating, dizziness, confusion, and tremor) have been reported following abrupt discontinuation

(Continued)

Paroxetine *(Continued)*

Precautions Use with caution in patients with a history of seizures, mania, renal disease, cardiac disease, or hepatic disease and in suicidal patients, children, or during breast-feeding in lactating women; modify dosage in patients with renal or hepatic impairment; may cause hyponatremia, use with caution in patients with volume depletion or diuretic use; may cause abnormal bleeding (eg, ecchymosis, purpura); use with caution in patients with impaired platelet aggregation; no clinical studies have assessed the combined use of paroxetine and electroconvulsive therapy

Adverse Reactions

Cardiovascular: Palpitations, tachycardia, vasodilation, postural hypotension, bradycardia, hypotension

Central nervous system: Headache, somnolence, dizziness, insomnia, nervousness, agitation, anxiety, migraine

Dermatologic: Alopecia, purpura, ecchymosis

Endocrine & metabolic: Hyponatremia (elderly or volume-depleted patients), SIADH, sexual dysfunction

Gastrointestinal: Nausea, xerostomia, constipation, vomiting, diarrhea, anorexia, flatulence, gastritis

Hematologic: Anemia, leukopenia

Neuromuscular & skeletal: Weakness, tremor, arthritis, paresthesia, asthenia

Ocular: Eye pain

Otic: Ear pain

Respiratory: Asthma

Miscellaneous: Diaphoresis, thirst, bruxism, akinesia

Drug Interactions Cytochrome P-450 isoenzyme CYP2D6 substrate (minor); CYP2D6 and CYP1A2 (high dose) (weak) isoenzyme inhibitor; CYP3A3/4 isoenzyme inhibitor (weak)

Decreased effect with phenobarbital, phenytoin (may also decrease phenytoin levels)

Increased effect/toxicity with alcohol, cimetidine, ritonavir, MAO inhibitors (potential fatal serotonin syndrome: hypertension, hyperthermia, mental status change, myoclonus, hyperpyrexic crisis), dextromethorphan (serotonin syndrome); phenothiazines, type 1C antiarrhythmics; the herbal medicine St John's wort (*Hypericum perforatum*) may increase serious side effects, it use is **not** recommended

Increased effect/toxicity of tricyclic antidepressants, fluoxetine, sertraline, theophylline, warfarin, thioridazine (paroxetine may inhibit the metabolism of thioridazine and increase the risk of serious cardiac effects such as prolongation of the QT_c interval, ventricular arrhythmias, torsade de pointes, and sudden death; concurrent use of thioridazine and paroxetine is contraindicated)

Cyproheptadine may decrease or antagonize effects of paroxetine; use with sumatriptan may cause weakness, incoordination, and hyper-reflexia; paroxetine may decrease the AUC of digoxin by 15%; tryptophan, which can be metabolized to serotonin, may increase serious serotonin side effects and its use is **not** recommended; the combination of paroxetine and pimozide resulted in an oculogyric crisis in a 9-year old boy (Horrigan, 1994); paroxetine may increase or worsen lysergic acid diethylamide (LSD) flashbacks

Food Interactions Food or milk does not significantly affect extent of absorption; food may slightly increase AUC (by 6%), increase peak concentration by 29%, and decrease time to peak from 6.4 hours to 4.9 hours postdose; tryptophan supplements may increase serious side effects

Stability

Oral suspension: Store ≤77°F (25°C)

Tablet: Store between 59°F to 86°F (15°C to 30°C)

Mechanism of Action Paroxetine is a selective serotonin reuptake inhibitor (SSRI), chemically unrelated to tricyclic, tetracyclic, or other antidepressants; the inhibition of serotonin reuptake from CNS neuronal synapses potentiates serotonin activity in the brain

Pharmacodynamics

Onset of action: Antidepressant effects: Within 1-4 weeks

Anti-obsessional and antipanic effects: Up to several weeks

Pharmacokinetics

Absorption: Oral: Well absorbed

Distribution: V_d (adults): Mean: 8.7 L/kg; range: 3-28 L/kg

Protein binding: 95%

Metabolism: Extensive by cytochrome P-450 enzymes via oxidation and methylation followed by glucuronide and sulfate conjugation; nonlinear kinetics may be seen with higher doses and longer duration of therapy due to saturation of P-450 2D6 (CYP2D6), an enzyme partially responsible for metabolism

Bioavailability: Tablet and oral suspension have equal bioavailability

Half-life: Adults: Mean: 21 hours; range: 3-65 hours

Elimination: Metabolites are excreted in urine and bile; 2% of drug excreted unchanged in urine

Usual Dosage Oral:

Children: Limited information is available

Depression: Paroxetine was shown to be effective and well tolerated in an open label clinical trial in 45 children <14 years of age (mean age: 10.7 ± 2 years) with major depression (Rey-Sanchoz, 1997). Doses were initiated at 10 mg/day and adjusted upward on an individual basis with a mean dose of 16.2 mg/day used for an average of 8.4 months. Further studies are needed.

Self-injurious behavior: A 15-year old autistic male with self-injurious behavior was successfully treated with paroxetine 20 mg/day (Snead, 1994). Further studies are needed.

Social phobia: A small case series reported the effective use of paroxetine in 5 pediatric patients with social phobia [2 children (7 and 11 years of age) and 3 adolescents (16, 17, and 18 years of age)]; comorbid diagnoses (obsessive compulsive disorder and/or dysthymia) existed in 3 patients; doses were adjusted on an individual basis; the 7-year old was started on 2.5 mg/day and increased to 5 mg/day after 4 weeks; the 11-year old was started on 5 mg/day and the dose was titrated upwards by 5 mg/day increments every 3-4 weeks to 15 mg/day; adolescents were started on ≤20 mg/day (see Mancini, 1999); further studies are needed

Adults:

Depression: Initial: 20 mg/day given once daily preferably in the morning; increase if needed by 10 mg/day increments at intervals of at least 1 week; maximum dose: 50 mg/day

Obsessive compulsive disorder: Initial: 20 mg/day given once daily preferably in the morning; increase by 10 mg/day increments at intervals of at least 1 week; recommended dose: 40 mg/day; range: 20-60 mg/day; maximum dose: 60 mg/day

Panic disorder: Initial: 10 mg/day given once daily preferably in the morning; increase by 10 mg/day increments at intervals of at least 1 week; recommended dose: 40 mg/day; range: 10-60 mg/day; maximum dose: 60 mg/day

Social anxiety disorder: Initial: 20 mg/day given once daily preferably in the morning; recommended dose: 20 mg/day; range: 20-60 mg/day; doses >20 mg may not have additional benefit

Generalized anxiety disorder: Initial: 20 mg/day given once daily preferably in the morning; recommended dose: 20 mg/day; range: 20-50 mg/day; doses >20 mg may not have additional benefit

Severe hepatic or renal impairment: Adults: Initial: 10 mg/day; increase if needed by 10 mg/day increments at intervals of at least 1 week; maximum dose: 40 mg/day

Administration May be administered without regard to meals; administration with food may decrease GI side effects; shake suspension well before use

Monitoring Parameters Blood pressure, heart rate, liver and renal function

Patient Information Avoid alcohol, tryptophan supplements, and the herbal medicine St John's wort; may cause drowsiness or dizziness and impair ability to perform activities requiring mental alertness or physical coordination; may cause dry mouth; avoid abrupt discontinuation; inform physician if taking or planning to take other medications, supplements, or herbal products

Additional Information Paroxetine is more potent and more selective than other SSRIs (eg, fluoxetine, fluvoxamine, sertraline, and clomipramine) in the inhibition of serotonin reuptake; a recent report describes 5 children (age: 8-15 years) who developed epistaxis (n=4) or bruising (n=1) while receiving SSRI therapy (sertraline) (Lake, 2000)

Dosage Forms Available as paroxetine hydrochloride; mg strength refers to paroxetine

Suspension, oral: 10 mg/5 mL [orange flavor] (250 mL)

Tablet: 10 mg, 20 mg, 30 mg, 40 mg

References

Findling RL, Reed MD, and Blumer JL, "Pharmacological Treatment of Depression in Children and Adolescents," *Paediatr Drugs,* 1999, 1(3):161-82.

Horrigan JP and Barnhill LJ, "Paroxetine-Pimozide Drug Interactions," *J Am Acad Child Adolesc Psychiatry,* 1994, 33(7):1060-1.

Lake MB, Birmaher B, Wassick S, et al, "Bleeding and Selective Serotonin Reuptake Inhibitors in Childhood and Adolescence," *J Child Adolesc Psychopharmacol,* 2000, 10(1):35-8.

(Continued)

Paroxetine *(Continued)*

Mancini C, Van Ameringen M, Oakman JM, et al, "Serotonergic Agents in the Treatment of Social Phobia in Children and Adolescents: A Case Series," *Depress Anxiety*, 1999, 10(1):33-9.

Markel H, Lee A, Holmes RD, et al, "LSD Flashback Syndrome Exacerbated by Selective Serotonin Reuptake Inhibitor Antidepressants in Adolescents," *J Pediatr*, 1994, 125(5 Pt 1):817-9.

Rey-Sanchez F and Guitierrez-Cassares JR, "Paroxetine in Children With Major Depressive Disorder: An Open Trial," *J Am Acad Child Adolesc Psychiatry*, 1997, 36(10):1443-7.

Snead RW, Boon F, and Presberg J, "Paroxetine for Self-Injurious Behavior," *J Am Acad Child Adolesc Psychiatry*, 1994, 33(6):909-10.

◆ **Parvolex (Can)** *see* Acetylcysteine *on page 35*
◆ **Pathocil®** *see* Dicloxacillin *on page 326*
◆ **Paxil®** *see* Paroxetine *on page 763*
◆ **Pazo® Hemorrhoid [OTC]** *see* Hemorrhoidal Preparations *on page 490*
◆ **PCA** *see* Procainamide *on page 829*
◆ **PCE®** *see* Erythromycin *on page 394*
◆ **Pectin and Kaolin** *see* Kaolin and Pectin *on page 561*
◆ **PediaCare® Decongestant Infants [OTC]** *see* Pseudoephedrine *on page 852*
◆ **Pediaflor®** *see* Fluoride *on page 441*
◆ **Pediamist® Pediatric [OTC]** *see* Sodium Chloride *on page 906*
◆ **Pediapred®** *see* Prednisolone *on page 821*
◆ **Pediatric ALS Algorithm, Bradycardia** *see page 1035*
◆ **Pediatric ALS Algorithm, Pulseless Arrest** *see page 1036*
◆ **Pediatric ALS Algorithm, Tachycardia - Rapid Rhythm and Adequate Perfusion** *see page 1037*
◆ **Pediatric ALS Algorithm, Tachycardia - Rapid Rhythm and Evidence of Poor Perfusion** *see page 1038*
◆ **Pediatric HIV** *see page 1162*
◆ **Pediatrix (Can)** *see* Acetaminophen *on page 29*
◆ **Pediazole®** *see* Erythromycin and Sulfisoxazole *on page 397*
◆ **Pedi-Boro® [OTC]** *see* Aluminum Acetate *on page 62*
◆ **Pedi-Dri Topical** *see* Undecylenic Acid and Derivatives *on page 994*
◆ **PediOtic® Otic** *see* Neomycin, (Bacitracin) Polymyxin B, and Hydrocortisone *on page 705*
◆ **Pedi-Pro Topical [OTC]** *see* Undecylenic Acid and Derivatives *on page 994*
◆ **Pedte-Pak-5®** *see* Trace Metals *on page 972*
◆ **Pedtrace-4®** *see* Trace Metals *on page 972*

Pegaspargase *(peg AS par jase)*

Related Information
Emetogenic Potential of Single Chemotherapeutic Agents *on page 1129*

U.S. Brand Names Oncaspar®

Synonyms PEG-L-Asparaginase

Therapeutic Category Antineoplastic Agent, Miscellaneous

Generic Available No

Use Induction treatment of acute lymphoblastic leukemia in combination with other chemotherapeutic agents in patients who have developed hypersensitivity to native forms of L-asparaginase derived from *E. coli* and/or *Erwinia chrysanthemia*; treatment of lymphoma

Pregnancy Risk Factor C

Contraindications Pancreatitis; patients who have had significant hemorrhagic events associated with prior L-asparaginase therapy; patients who have had previous serious allergic reactions to pegaspargase

Warnings The FDA currently recommends that procedures for proper handling and disposal of antineoplastic agents be considered; inhalation of vapors and contact with skin, eyes, or mucous membranes must be avoided; be prepared to treat anaphylaxis at each administration

Precautions Use with caution in patients receiving anticoagulation therapy, aspirin, or NSAIDs; use with caution in patients with hepatic dysfunction or in patients receiving hepatotoxic agents

Adverse Reactions
Cardiovascular: Hypotension, chest pain, tachycardia
Central nervous system: Somnolence, confusion, seizures, fever, chills, headache, dizziness, malaise, coma, mental status changes
Dermatologic: Rash, pruritus, urticaria
Endocrine & metabolic: Hyperglycemia, transient diabetes mellitus, hyperammonemia, hyperuricemia

Gastrointestinal: Protracted nausea and vomiting, abdominal pain, diarrhea, anorexia, pancreatitis

Genitourinary: Hemorrhagic cystitis

Hematologic: Leukopenia; prolonged prothrombin, thrombin and partial thromboplastin times; decreased fibrinogen; thrombosis; hemorrhage

Hepatic: Hepatotoxicity

Neuromuscular & skeletal: Paresthesia, weakness

Renal: Elevated BUN, elevated serum creatinine, renal failure

Respiratory: Cough, bronchospasm, epistaxis

Miscellaneous: Anaphylaxis

Drug Interactions Methotrexate (decreases antineoplastic effect if given immediately prior to MTX); vincristine (increases toxicity if given concomitantly); prednisone (increases hyperglycemic effect); may increase toxicity of highly protein bound drugs; may increase bleeding in patients receiving warfarin, heparin, aspirin, NSAID, or dipyridamole

Stability Store vials in refrigerator; do not freeze; do not administer if there is any indication that the drug has been frozen; avoid excessive agitation, do not shake; do not use if cloudy or if precipitate is present; use of a 0.2 micron filter may result in some loss of potency

Mechanism of Action Hydrolyzes asparagine to aspartic acid and ammonia depleting the exogenous asparagine supply needed by leukemic cells for protein synthesis

Pharmacokinetics

Absorption: Not absorbed from the GI tract; therefore, requires parenteral administration

Distribution: Apparent V_d: Plasma volume

Half-life: 5.73 days; patients who have had a hypersensitivity reaction to asparaginase have a decreased half-life

Elimination: Clearance is unaffected by age, renal function, or hepatic function; not detected in urine

Usual Dosage Refer to individual protocols; Children and Adults:

I.M., I.V.: 2500 units/m²/dose every 14 days; for children with BSA <0.6 m²: 82.5 units/kg every 14 days

Administration

I.M.: Preferred route of administration due to the lower incidence of hepatotoxicity, coagulopathy, and GI and renal disorders compared to the I.V. route; for I.M. administration, limit the volume at a single injection site to 2 mL; if the volume to be administered is >2 mL, use multiple injection sites

I.V.: Infusion in 100 mL of D_5W or NS over a period of 1-2 hours

Monitoring Parameters Vital signs during administration, CBC, urinalysis, serum amylase, liver enzymes, bilirubin, prothrombin time, renal function tests, urine glucose, blood glucose

Patient Information Notify physician if fever, sore throat, painful/burning urination, bruising, bleeding, or shortness of breath occurs

Nursing Implications Patients should be observed for 1 hour following injection; appropriate agents for maintenance of an adequate airway and treatment of a hypersensitivity reaction (antihistamine, epinephrine, oxygen, I.V. corticosteroids) should be readily available

Dosage Forms Injection, preservative free: 750 units/mL

References

Asselin BL, Whitin JC, Cappola DJ, et al, "Comparative Pharmacokinetic Studies of Three Asparaginase Preparations," *J Clin Oncol*, 1993, 11(9):1780-6.

Capizzi RL, "Asparaginase Revisited," *Leuk Lymphoma*, 1993, 10(Suppl):147-50.

♦ **PEG-L-Asparaginase** *see Pegaspargase on page 766*

♦ **Peglyte (Can)** *see Polyethylene Glycol-Electrolyte Solution on page 811*

♦ **PemADD™** *see Pemoline on page 767*

♦ **PemADD™ CT** *see Pemoline on page 767*

Pemoline (PEM oh leen)

Related Information

Carbohydrate and Alcohol Content of Liquid Medications for Use in Patients Receiving Ketogenic Diets *on page 1258*

U.S. Brand Names Cylert®; PemADD™; PemADD™ CT

Synonyms Phenylisohydantoin

Therapeutic Category Central Nervous System Stimulant, Nonamphetamine

Generic Available Yes

Use Attention-deficit/hyperactivity disorder (ADHD) (not first-line therapy, see Warnings); narcolepsy

(Continued)

Pemoline *(Continued)*

Restrictions C-IV

Pregnancy Risk Factor B

Contraindications Liver disease; hypersensitivity to pemoline or any component; children <6 years of age; Tourette's syndrome

Warnings Life-threatening acute hepatic failure may occur; 15 cases of acute hepatic failure were reported to the FDA since 1975; this is 4 to 17 times the expected rate; 12 of the 15 cases resulted in death or liver transplantation; therefore, pemoline is not considered as first-line drug therapy for ADHD. Initiate pemoline only in patients without liver dysfunction/disease and only with normal baseline liver function tests; monitor serum ALT (SGPT) at baseline and every 2 weeks; discontinue drug if serum ALT increases ≥2 times the upper limit of normal, or to a clinically significant level, or if patient develops signs and symptoms of liver failure. Written informed consent (consent form provided by manufacturer; 847-937-7302) should be obtained prior to starting therapy; therapy should be withdrawn if no significant clinical benefit is seen within 3 weeks after completion of dose titration

Precautions Use with caution in patients with renal dysfunction, hypertension, or history of drug abuse; may cause growth suppression in children (monitor carefully); may decrease seizure threshold; may exacerbate thought disorder and behavior disturbance in psychotic children

Adverse Reactions

Central nervous system: Insomnia, seizures, precipitation of Tourette's syndrome, dizziness, hallucinations, headache

Dermatologic: Skin rashes

Endocrine & metabolic: Suppression of linear growth

Gastrointestinal: Stomach ache, nausea, diarrhea, anorexia, weight loss

Hematologic: Aplastic anemia (rare)

Hepatic: Elevated liver enzymes (usually reversible upon discontinuation), jaundice, fatal hepatic failure

Neuromuscular & skeletal: Movement disorders

Miscellaneous: Physical and psychological dependence

Drug Interactions CNS stimulants, CNS depressants, sympathomimetics; may alter insulin requirements in diabetics

Mechanism of Action Blocks the reuptake mechanism of dopaminergic neurons, appears to act at the cerebral cortex and subcortical structures; CNS and respiratory stimulant with weak sympathomimetic effects

Pharmacodynamics

Peak effect: 4 hours; significant benefit on hyperactivity may not be evident until 3rd or 4th week of administration

Duration: 8 hours

Pharmacokinetics

Protein binding: 50%

Metabolism: In the liver

Half-life:

Children: 7-8.6 hours

Adults: 12 hours

Elimination: 43% to 50% excreted unchanged in the urine

Usual Dosage Children ≥6 years: Oral: Initial: 37.5 mg given once daily in the morning, increase by 18.75 mg/day at weekly intervals; effective dose range: 56.25-75 mg/day; maximum dose: 112.5 mg/day; dosage range: 0.5-3 mg/kg/24 hours

Administration Oral: Administer medication in the morning

Monitoring Parameters Liver enzymes; for ADHD: Height, weight

Patient Information Avoid alcohol; avoid caffeine; chewable tablet should be chewed; may cause dizziness; may be habit-forming; do not abruptly discontinue; drug may cause liver failure; inform physician immediately of any signs of liver dysfunction such as dark urine, yellow skin, lack of appetite, GI complaints, general feeling of weakness; comply with blood testing of liver function

Additional Information Treatment of ADHD should include "Drug Holidays" or periodic discontinuation of stimulant medication in order to assess the patient's requirements, to decrease tolerance, and limit suppression of linear growth and weight

Dosage Forms

Tablet: 18.75 mg, 37.5 mg, 75 mg

Tablet, chewable: 37.5 mg

References

Adcock KG, MacElroy DE, Wolford ET, et al, "Pemoline Therapy Resulting in Liver Transplantation," *Ann Pharmacother*, 1998, 32(4):422-5.

Marotta PJ and Roberts EA, "Pemoline Hepatotoxicity in Children," *J Pediatr*, 1998, 132(5):894-7.

Rosh JR, Dellert SF, Narkewicz M, et al, "Four Cases of Severe Hepatotoxicity Associated With Pemoline: Possible Autoimmune Pathogenesis," *Pediatrics*, 1998, 101(5):921-3.

♦ **Pen G** *see* Penicillin G (Parenteral/Aqueous) *on page 772*

Penicillamine (pen i SIL a meen)

Related Information
Overdose and Toxicology *on page 1222*

U.S. Brand Names Cuprimine®; Depen®

Synonyms D-3-Mercaptovaline; β,β-Dimethylcysteine; D-Penicillamine

Therapeutic Category Antidote, Copper Toxicity; Antidote, Lead Toxicity; Chelating Agent, Oral

Generic Available No

Use Treatment of Wilson's disease, cystinuria, adjunct in the treatment of severe rheumatoid arthritis; lead poisoning, primary biliary cirrhosis (as adjunctive therapy following initial treatment with calcium EDTA or BAL)

Pregnancy Risk Factor D

Contraindications Hypersensitivity to penicillamine, any component, and possibly penicillin; patients with renal insufficiency; patients with previous penicillamine-related aplastic anemia or agranulocytosis; concomitant administration with other hematopoietic-depressant drugs (eg, gold, immunosuppressants, antimalarials, phenylbutazone), pregnancy, breast-feeding

Warnings Penicillamine has been associated with fatalities due to agranulocytosis, aplastic anemia, thrombocytopenia, Goodpasture's syndrome, and myasthenia gravis; patients should be warned to promptly report any symptoms suggesting toxicity; interruption of continuous therapy for Wilson's disease or cystinuria even for a few days has been associated with sensitivity reactions upon reinstitution of therapy; approximately 33% of patients will experience an allergic reaction

Precautions Patients on penicillamine for Wilson's disease or cystinuria should receive pyridoxine supplementation 25-50 mg/day; when treating rheumatoid arthritis, daily pyridoxine supplementation is also recommended

Adverse Reactions
Cardiovascular: Edema of the face, feet, or lower legs

Central nervous system: Fever, chills, myasthenic syndrome, fatigue

Dermatologic: Rash, pruritus, pemphigus, increased friability of the skin, exfoliative dermatitis, alopecia, angioedema

Endocrine & metabolic: Iron deficiency, hypoglycemia, thyroiditis

Gastrointestinal: Oral lesions, nausea, vomiting (in children with doses >60 mg/kg/day), epigastric pain, colitis, dysgeusia, ageusia, pancreatitis, sore throat, weight gain

Genitourinary: Urinary incontinence, bloody or cloudy urine

Hematologic: Leukopenia, thrombocytopenia, eosinophilia, aplastic anemia, agranulocytosis, hemolytic anemia

Hepatic: Hepatic dysfunction

Neuromuscular & skeletal: Arthralgia, dermatomyositis, polymyositis, peripheral neuropathy

Ocular: Optic neuritis

Otic: Tinnitus

Renal: Nephrotic syndrome, renal vasculitis, Goodpasture's syndrome, proteinuria, hematuria

Respiratory: Obliterative bronchiolitis, pulmonary fibrosis, interstitial pneumonitis, coughing, wheezing

Miscellaneous: Lymphadenopathy, allergic reactions, SLE-like syndrome, white spots on lips or mouth

Drug Interactions Gold, antimalarials, immunosuppressants, phenylbutazone are associated with similar serious hematologic reactions; iron salts, zinc salts, and antacids decrease penicillamine absorption; decreases serum digoxin levels

Food Interactions Do not administer with milk or food; iron and zinc may decrease drug action; increase dietary intake of pyridoxine; for Wilson's disease, decrease copper in diet and omit chocolate, nuts, shellfish, mushrooms, liver, raisins, broccoli, and molasses; for lead poisoning, decrease calcium in diet

Mechanism of Action Chelates with lead, copper, mercury, iron, and other heavy metals to form stable, soluble complexes that are excreted in the urine; depresses circulating IgM rheumatoid factor levels and *in vitro*, depresses T-cell but not B-cell activity; combines with cystine to form a more soluble compound which prevents the formation of cystine calculi

Pharmacokinetics
Absorption: 40% to 70%

Protein binding: 80% bound to albumin

(Continued)

Penicillamine *(Continued)*

Metabolism: In the liver

Half-life: 1.7-3.2 hours

Time to peak serum concentration: Within 1-2 hours

Elimination: Primarily (30% to 60%) in urine as unchanged drug

Usual Dosage Oral:

Rheumatoid arthritis:

Children: Initial: 3 mg/kg/day (≤250 mg/day) for 3 months, then 6 mg/kg/day (≤500 mg/day) in 2 divided doses for 3 months to a maximum of 10 mg/kg/day (≤1-1.5 g/day) in 3-4 divided doses

Adults: 125-250 mg/day, may increase dose at 1- to 3-month intervals up to 1-1.5 g/day; doses >500 mg/day should be given in divided doses

Wilson's disease (doses titrated to maintain urinary copper excretion >1 mg/day):

Infants and Children: 20 mg/kg/day in 2-4 doses; maximum dose: 1 g/day

Adults: 1 g/day in 4 divided doses; maximum dose: 2 g/day

Cystinuria (doses titrated to maintain urinary cystine excretion at <100-200 mg/day):

Children: 30 mg/kg/day in 4 divided doses; maximum dose: 4 g/day

Adults: Initial: 2 g/day divided every 6 hours (range: 1-4 g/day)

Lead poisoning (continue until blood lead level is <15 μg/dL; treatment duration varies from 4-12 weeks):

Children: 20-30 mg/kg/day in 3-4 divided doses; initiating treatment at 25% of this dose and gradually increasing to the full dose over 2-3 weeks may minimize adverse reactions; maximum dose: 1.5 g/day; a reduced dosage of 15 mg/kg/day in 2 divided doses has been shown to be effective in the treatment of mild to moderate lead poisoning (blood lead concentration 20-40 mcg/dL) with a reduction in adverse effects (Shannon, 2000)

Adults: 1-1.5 g/day in 3-4 divided doses; initiating treatment at 25% of this dose and gradually increasing to the full dose over 2-3 weeks may minimize adverse reactions

Primary biliary cirrhosis: Adults: 250 mg/day to start, increase by 250 mg every 2 weeks up to a maintenance dose of 1 g/day, as 250 mg 4 times/day

Dosing adjustment in renal impairment: Cl_{cr} <50 mL/minute: Avoid use

Administration Oral: Administer on an empty stomach 1 hour before or 2 hours after meals; patients unable to swallow capsules may mix contents of capsule with fruit juice or chilled pureed fruit; patients with cystinuria should drink copious amounts of water

Monitoring Parameters Urinalysis, CBC with differential, hemoglobin, platelet count, liver function tests; weekly measurements of urinary and blood concentrations of the intoxicating metal is indicated (3 months has been tolerated); annual x-ray for renal stones; Wilson's disease: 24-hour urinary copper excretion; quantitative 24-hour urine protein at 1- to 2-week intervals initially (first 2-3 months); urinalysis

Patient Information Possible severe allergic reaction if patient allergic to penicillin; notify physician if unusual bleeding or bruising, or persistent fever, sore throat, or fatigue occur. Report any unexplained cough, shortness of breath, or rash; loss of taste may occur; do not skip or miss doses or discontinue without notifying physician.

Dosage Forms

Capsule (Cuprimine®): 125 mg, 250 mg

Tablet (Depen®): 250 mg

Extemporaneous Preparations A 50 mg/mL suspension may be made by mixing sixty 250 mg capsules with 3 g carboxymethylcellulose, 150 g sucrose, 300 mg citric acid, parabens (methylparaben 120 mg, propylparaben 12 mg, propylene glycol qsad to 100 mL), and purified water to a total volume of 300 mL; cherry flavor may be added. Stability is 30 days refrigerated.

DeCastro FJ, Jaeger RQ, and Rolfe UT, "An Extemporaneously Prepared Penicillamine Suspension Used to Treat Lead Intoxication," *Hosp Pharm*, 1977, 2:446-8.

References

Shannon MW and Townsend MK, "Adverse Effects of Reduced-Dose d-Penicillamine in Children With Mild-to-Moderate Lead Poisoning," *Ann Pharmacother*, 2000, 34(1):15-8.

Penicillin G Benzathine *(pen i SIL in jee BENZ a theen)*

U.S. Brand Names Bicillin® L-A; Permapen®

Synonyms Benzathine Benzylpenicillin; Benzathine Penicillin G; Benzylpenicillin Benzathine

Therapeutic Category Antibiotic, Penicillin

Generic Available No

Use Active against most gram-positive organisms and some spirochetes; used only for the treatment of mild to moderately severe infections (ie, *Streptococcus* pharyngitis) caused by organisms susceptible to low concentrations of penicillin G, or for prophylaxis of infections caused by these organisms such as rheumatic fever prophylaxis

Pregnancy Risk Factor B

Contraindications Hypersensitivity to penicillin or any component

Precautions Use with caution in patients with impaired renal function, impaired cardiac function, pre-existing seizure disorder, or hypersensitivity to cephalosporins

Adverse Reactions
Central nervous system: Convulsions, confusion, lethargy, fever, dizziness
Dermatologic: Rash
Hematologic: Hemolytic anemia
Local: Pain at injection site
Neuromuscular & skeletal: Myoclonus
Renal: Interstitial nephritis
Miscellaneous: Jarisch-Herxheimer reaction, hypersensitivity reactions, anaphylaxis

Drug Interactions Probenecid increases serum concentration of penicillin; antibacterial activity with aminoglycosides is synergistic; tetracyclines, chloramphenicol, and erythromycin may antagonize the activity of penicillin

Stability Store in the refrigerator; avoid freezing

Mechanism of Action Inhibits bacterial cell wall synthesis by binding to one or more of the penicillin-binding proteins; inhibits the final transpeptidation step of peptidoglycan synthesis in bacterial cell wall

Pharmacokinetics
Absorption: I.M.: Slow
Distribution: Minimal concentrations attained in CSF with inflamed or uninflamed meninges
Time to peak serum concentration: Within 12-24 hours; serum levels are usually detectable for 1-4 weeks depending on the dose; larger doses result in more sustained levels rather than higher levels
Elimination: Penicillin G is detected in urine for up to 12 weeks after a single I.M. injection; renal clearance is delayed in neonates, young infants, and patients with impaired renal function

Usual Dosage I.M. (dosage frequency depends on infection being treated):
Neonates >1200 g: Asymptomatic congenital syphilis: 50,000 units/kg for 1 dose
Infants and Children:
Group A streptococcal upper respiratory infection: 25,000-50,000 units/kg as a single dose; maximum dose: 1.2 million units/dose **or**
Children <27 kg: 300,000-600,000 units as a single dose
Children ≥27 kg: 900,000 units as a single dose
Prophylaxis of recurrent rheumatic fever: 25,000-50,000 units/kg every 3-4 weeks; maximum dose: 1.2 million units/dose
Congenital syphilis: 50,000 units/kg every week for 3 weeks; maximum dose: 2.4 million units/dose
Syphilis of more than 1-year duration: 50,000 units/kg every week for 3 successive weeks; maximum dose: 2.4 million units/dose
Adults:
Group A streptococcal upper respiratory infection: 1.2 million units as a single dose
Prophylaxis of recurrent rheumatic fever: 1.2 million units every 3-4 weeks or 600,000 units twice monthly
Early syphilis: 2.4 million units as a single dose in 2 injection sites
Syphilis of more than 1-year duration: 2.4 million units (in 2 injection sites) once weekly for 3 doses

Administration Parenteral: I.M.: Give undiluted injection; administer by deep I.M. injection in the upper outer quadrant of the buttock (adolescents and adults) or into the midlateral muscle of the thigh (infants and children); do **not** give I.V., intra-arterially or S.C.; inadvertent I.V. administration has resulted in thrombosis, severe neurovascular damage, cardiac arrest, and death

Monitoring Parameters CBC, urinalysis, renal function tests

Test Interactions Positive Coombs' [direct], false-positive urinary and/or serum proteins

Nursing Implications S.C. administration may cause pain and induration; avoid repeated I.M. injections into the anterolateral thigh in neonates and infants since quadriceps femoris fibrosis and atrophy may occur

Additional Information Use a penicillin G benzathine/penicillin G procaine combination (ie, Bicillin® C-R) to achieve early peak levels in acute infections

(Continued)

Penicillin G Benzathine *(Continued)*

Dosage Forms Injection: 300,000 units/mL (10 mL); 600,000 units/mL (1 mL, 2 mL, 4 mL)

References

Kaplan EL, Berrios X, Speth J, et al, "Pharmacokinetics of Benzathine Penicillin G: Serum Levels During the 28 Days After Intramuscular Injection of 1,200,000 Units," *J Pediatr*, 1989, 115(1):146-50.

Paryani SG, Vaughn AJ, Crosby M, et al, "Treatment of Asymptomatic Congenital Syphilis: Benzathine Versus Procaine Penicillin G Therapy," *J Pediatr*, 1994, 125(3):471-5.

WHO Study Group, "Rheumatic Fever and Rheumatic Heart Disease," *World Health Organ Tech Rep Ser*, 1988, 764:1-58.

Penicillin G (Parenteral/Aqueous)

(pen i SIL in jee, pa REN ter al, AYE kwee us)

U.S. Brand Names Pfizerpen®

Synonyms Crystalline Penicillin; Pen G

Therapeutic Category Antibiotic, Penicillin

Generic Available Yes

Use Treatment of sepsis, meningitis, pericarditis, endocarditis, pneumonia, and other infections due to susceptible gram-positive organisms (except *Staphylococcus aureus*), some gram-negative organisms such as *Neisseria gonorrhoeae*, or *N. meningitidis* and some anaerobes and spirochetes

Pregnancy Risk Factor B

Contraindications Hypersensitivity to penicillin or any component

Precautions Use with caution in patients with renal impairment, hypersensitivity to cephalosporins, or pre-existing seizure disorder; dosage modification required in patients with renal impairment; further dosage reduction recommended in patients with impaired hepatic and renal function

Adverse Reactions

Central nervous system: Convulsions, confusion, lethargy, fever, dizziness

Dermatologic: Rash, urticaria

Endocrine & metabolic: Electrolyte imbalance

Gastrointestinal: Diarrhea

Hematologic: Hemolytic anemia, neutropenia

Local: Thrombophlebitis

Neuromuscular & skeletal: Myoclonus

Renal: Acute interstitial nephritis

Miscellaneous: Jarisch-Herxheimer reaction, hypersensitivity reactions, anaphylaxis

Drug Interactions Probenecid increases serum concentration of penicillin; antibacterial activity with aminoglycosides is synergistic; tetracyclines, chloramphenicol, and erythromycin may antagonize the activity of penicillin

Food Interactions Food or milk decreases absorption

Stability Reconstituted parenteral solution is stable for 7 days when refrigerated; incompatible with aminoglycosides; inactivated in acidic or alkaline solutions

Mechanism of Action Inhibits bacterial cell wall synthesis by binding to one or more of the penicillin-binding proteins; inhibits the final transpeptidation step of peptidoglycan synthesis in bacterial cell wall

Pharmacokinetics

Absorption: Oral: <30%

Distribution: Penetration across the blood-brain barrier is poor with uninflamed meninges; crosses the placenta; appears in breast milk

Protein binding: 65%

Metabolism: In the liver (10% to 30%) to penicilloic acid

Half-life:

Neonates:

<6 days: 3.2-3.4 hours

7-13 days: 1.2-2.2 hours

>14 days: 0.9-1.9 hours

Infants and Children: 0.5-1.2 hours

Adults: 0.5-0.75 hours with normal renal function

Time to peak serum concentration:

Oral: Within 30-60 minutes

I.M.: Within 30 minutes

Elimination: Penicillin G and its metabolites are excreted in urine mainly by tubular secretion

Dialysis: Moderately dialyzable (20% to 50%)

Usual Dosage
Neonates: I.M., I.V.:
Postnatal age ≤7 days:
≤2000 g: 50,000 units/kg/day in divided doses every 12 hours
Meningitis: 100,000 units/kg/day in divided doses every 12 hours
>2000 g: 75,000 units/kg/day in divided doses every 8 hours
Meningitis: 150,000 units/kg/day in divided doses every 8 hours
Congenital syphilis: 100,000 units/kg/day in divided doses every 12 hours
Group B streptococcal meningitis: 250,000-450,000 units/kg/day in divided doses every 8 hours
Postnatal age >7 days:
<1200 g: 50,000 units/kg/day in divided doses every 12 hours
Meningitis: 100,000 units/kg/day in divided doses every 12 hours
1200-2000 g: 75,000 units/kg/day in divided doses every 8 hours
Meningitis: 150,000 units/kg/day in divided doses every 8 hours
>2000 g: 100,000 units/kg/day in divided doses every 6 hours
Meningitis: 200,000 units/kg/day in divided doses every 6 hours
Congenital syphilis: 150,000 units/kg/day in divided doses every 8 hours
Group B streptococcal meningitis: I.V.: 450,000 units/kg/day in divided doses every 6 hours
Infants and Children:
I.M., I.V.: 100,000 to 250,000 units/kg/day in divided doses every 4-6 hours
Severe infections: 250,000-400,000 units/kg/day in divided doses every 4-6 hours; maximum dose: 24 million units/day
Adults: I.M., I.V.: 2-24 million units/day in divided doses every 4-6 hours
Dosing interval in renal impairment:
Cl_{cr} 10-30 mL/minute: Administer normal dose every 8-12 hours
Cl_{cr} <10 mL/minute: Administer normal dose every 12-18 hours
Administration Parenteral: Administer by I.V. intermittent infusion over 15-60 minutes at a final concentration for administration of 100,000-500,000 units/mL. A final concentration of 50,000 units/mL infused over 15-30 minutes is recommended for neonates and infants. The potassium or sodium content of the dose should be considered when determining the infusion rate.
Monitoring Parameters Periodic serum electrolytes, renal and hematologic function tests
Test Interactions False-positive or negative urinary glucose determination using Clinitest®; positive Coombs' [direct]; false-positive urinary and/or serum proteins
Additional Information
Penicillin G potassium: 1.7 mEq of potassium and 0.3 mEq of sodium per 1 million units of penicillin G
Penicillin G sodium: 2 mEq of sodium per 1 million units of penicillin G
Dosage Forms
Injection, as sodium: 5 million units
Injection:
Frozen premixed, as potassium: 1 million units, 2 million units, 3 million units
Powder, as potassium: 1 million units, 5 million units, 10 million units, 20 million units
References
American Academy of Pediatrics Committee on Infectious Diseases, "Treatment of Bacterial Meningitis," *Pediatrics*, 1988, 81(6):904-7.
Prober CG, Stevenson DK, and Benitz WE, "The Use of Antibiotics in Neonates Weighing Less Than 1200 Grams," *Pediatr Infect Dis J*, 1990, 9(2):111-21.

Penicillin G Procaine (pen i SIL in jee PROE kane)

U.S. Brand Names Crysticillin® A.S.; Pfizerpen®-AS; Wycillin®
Synonyms APPG; Aqueous Procaine Penicillin G; Procaine Benzylpenicillin; Procaine Penicillin G
Therapeutic Category Antibiotic, Penicillin
Generic Available Yes
Use Moderately severe infections due to *Treponema pallidum* and other penicillin G-sensitive microorganisms that are susceptible to low but prolonged serum penicillin concentrations
Pregnancy Risk Factor B
Contraindications Hypersensitivity to penicillin, procaine, or any component
Warnings Some formulations contain a sulfite that may cause allergic-type reactions
Precautions Use with caution in patients with renal impairment, hypersensitivity to cephalosporins, or history of seizures; modify dosage in patients with severe renal impairment
(Continued)

Penicillin G Procaine *(Continued)*

Adverse Reactions
Cardiovascular: Myocardial depression, vasodilation, conduction disturbances

Central nervous system: Seizures, confusion, lethargy, dizziness, disorientation, agitation, hallucinations

Hematologic: Hemolytic anemia

Local: Sterile abscess and pain at injection site

Neuromuscular & skeletal: Myoclonus

Renal: Interstitial nephritis

Miscellaneous: Pseudoanaphylactic reactions, Jarisch-Herxheimer reaction, hypersensitivity reactions

Drug Interactions Probenecid increases serum concentration of penicillin; antibacterial activity with aminoglycosides is synergistic; tetracyclines, chloramphenicol, and erythromycin may antagonize the activity of penicillin

Stability Store in refrigerator

Mechanism of Action Inhibits bacterial cell wall synthesis by binding to one or more of the penicillin-binding proteins; inhibits the final transpeptidation step of peptidoglycan synthesis in bacterial cell wall

Pharmacokinetics
Absorption: I.M.: Slow

Distribution: Penetration across the blood-brain barrier is poor, despite inflamed meninges; appears in breast milk

Time to peak serum concentration: Within 1-4 hours and can persist within the therapeutic range for 15-24 hours

Elimination: Renal clearance is delayed in neonates, young infants, and patients with impaired renal function

Dialysis: Moderately dialyzable (20% to 50%)

Usual Dosage I.M.:
Neonates ≥1200 g: Avoid using in this age group since sterile abscesses and procaine toxicity occur more frequently with neonates than older patients

Congenital syphilis: 50,000 units/kg/day once daily for 10 days; if more than 1 day of therapy is missed, the entire course should be restarted

Infants and Children: 25,000-50,000 units/kg/day in divided doses every 12-24 hours; not to exceed 4.8 million units/24 hours

Congenital syphilis: 50,000 units/kg/day once daily for 10 days; if more than 1 day of therapy is missed, the entire course should be restarted

Adults: 0.6-4.8 million units/day in divided doses every 12-24 hours

When used in conjunction with an aminoglycoside for the treatment of endocarditis caused by susceptible *S. viridans*: 1.2 million units every 6 hours for 2-4 weeks

Neurosyphilis: 2.4 million units once daily for 10 days with probenecid 500 mg every 6 hours

Administration Parenteral: **Do not give I.V., intra-arterially, or S.C.**; procaine suspension for deep I.M. injection only; inadvertent I.V. administration has resulted in neurovascular damage; in infants and children it is preferable to administer I.M. into the midlateral muscles of the thigh; in adults, administer into the gluteus maximus or into the midlateral muscles of the thigh

Monitoring Parameters Periodic renal and hematologic function tests with prolonged therapy

Test Interactions Positive Coombs' [direct], false-positive urinary and/or serum proteins

Nursing Implications Avoid repeated I.M. injections into the anterolateral thigh in neonates and infants since quadriceps femoris fibrosis and atrophy may occur

Dosage Forms Injection, suspension: 300,000 units/mL (10 mL); 500,000 units/mL (1.2 mL); 600,000 units/mL (1 mL, 2 mL, 4 mL)

References
Paryani SG, Vaughn AJ, Crosby M, et al, "Treatment of Asymptomatic Congenital Syphilis: Benzathine Versus Procaine Penicillin G Therapy," *J Pediatr*, 1994, 125(3):471-5.

Penicillin V Potassium *(pen i SIL in vee poe TASS ee um)*

Related Information
Carbohydrate and Alcohol Content of Liquid Medications for Use in Patients Receiving Ketogenic Diets *on page 1258*

U.S. Brand Names Beepen-VK®; Betapen®-VK; Ledercillin® VK; Pen.Vee® K; Robicillin® VK; V-Cillin K®; Veetids®

Canadian Brand Names Apo-Pen-VK; Nadopen-V; Novo-Pen-VK; Nu-Pen-VK; PVF K

Synonyms Phenoxymethyl Penicillin

Therapeutic Category Antibiotic, Penicillin

Generic Available Yes

Use Treatment of mild to moderately severe susceptible bacterial infections involving the upper respiratory tract, skin, and urinary tract; prophylaxis of pneumococcal infections and rheumatic fever

Pregnancy Risk Factor B

Contraindications Hypersensitivity to penicillin or any component

Precautions Use with caution in patients with renal impairment, hypersensitivity to cephalosporins, or history of seizures; dosage adjustment may be necessary in patients with renal impairment

Adverse Reactions

Central nervous system: Convulsions, fever

Dermatologic: Rash

Gastrointestinal: Nausea, diarrhea, vomiting, black hairy tongue, pseudomembranous colitis

Hematologic: Hemolytic anemia

Renal: Acute interstitial nephritis

Miscellaneous: Hypersensitivity reactions, anaphylaxis

Drug Interactions Probenecid (higher, prolonged penicillin serum concentration)

Food Interactions Food or milk may decrease absorption

Stability Refrigerate suspension after reconstitution; discard after 14 days

Mechanism of Action Interferes with bacterial cell wall synthesis during active multiplication by binding to one or more of the penicillin-binding proteins; inhibits the final transpeptidation step of peptidoglycan synthesis causing cell wall death and resultant bactericidal activity against susceptible bacteria

Pharmacokinetics

Absorption: Oral: 60% to 73% from the GI tract

Distribution: Widely distributed to kidneys, liver, skin, tonsils, and into synovial, pleural, and pericardial fluids; appears in breast milk

Protein binding: 80%

Metabolism: 10% to 30%

Half-life: 30 minutes and is prolonged in patients with renal impairment

Time to peak serum concentration: Within 30-60 minutes

Elimination: Penicillin V and its metabolites are excreted in urine mainly by tubular secretion

Usual Dosage Oral:

Systemic infections:

Children <12 years: 25-50 mg/kg/day in divided doses every 6-8 hours; maximum dose: 3 g/day

Children ≥12 years and Adults: 125-500 mg every 6-8 hours

Primary prevention of rheumatic fever (treatment of streptococcal tonsillopharyngitis):

Children: 250 mg 2-3 times/day for 10 days

Adolescents and Adults: 500 mg 2-3 times/day for 10 days

Prophylaxis of pneumococcal infections in children with sickle cell disease and functional or anatomic asplenia: Children:

<2 months to 3 years: 125 mg twice daily

>3-5 years: 250 mg twice daily; may discontinue penicillin prophylaxis after 5 years of age in children who have not experienced invasive pneumococcal infection and have received recommended pneumococcal immunizations

Recurrent rheumatic fever, prophylaxis: Children and Adults: 250 mg twice daily

Administration Oral: Administer with water on an empty stomach 1 hour before or 2 hours after meals; may be administered with food to decrease GI upset

Monitoring Parameters Periodic renal and hematologic function tests during prolonged therapy

Test Interactions False-positive or negative urinary glucose determination using Clinitest®; positive Coombs' [direct]; false-positive urinary and/or serum proteins

Additional Information 0.7 mEq of potassium/250 mg penicillin V; 250 mg = 400,000 units of penicillin

Dosage Forms

Powder for oral solution: 125 mg/5 mL (3 mL, 100 mL, 150 mL, 200 mL); 250 mg/5 mL (100 mL, 150 mL, 200 mL)

Tablet: 125 mg, 250 mg, 500 mg

References

"American Academy of Pediatrics. Committee on Infectious Diseases. Policy Statement: Recommendations for the Prevention of Pneumococcal Infections, Including the Use of Pneumococcal Conjugate

(Continued)

Penicillin V Potassium *(Continued)*

Vaccine (Prevnar™), Pneumococcal Polysaccharide Vaccine, and Antibiotic Prophylaxis," *Pediatrics*, 2000, 106(2 Pt 1):362-6.

Dajani A, Taubert K, Ferrieri P, et al, "Treatment of Acute Streptococcal Pharyngitis and Prevention of Rheumatic Fever: A Statement for Health Professionals. Committee on Rheumatic Fever, Endocarditis, and Kawasaki Disease of the Council on Cardiovascular Disease in the Young, the American Heart Association," *Pediatrics*, 1995, 96(4 Pt 1):758-64.

♦ **Penicilloyl-polylysine** *see* Benzylpenicilloyl-polylysine *on page 138*

♦ **Pentacarinat (Can)** *see* Pentamidine *on page 776*

♦ **Pentam-300® Injection** *see* Pentamidine *on page 776*

Pentamidine *(pen TAM i deen)*

U.S. Brand Names NebuPent™ Inhalation; Pentam-300® Injection

Canadian Brand Names Pentacarinat

Therapeutic Category Antibiotic, Miscellaneous; Antiprotozoal

Generic Available No

Use Treatment and prevention of pneumonia caused by *Pneumocystis carinii* in patients who cannot tolerate or who fail to respond to co-trimoxazole; treatment of African trypanosomiasis; treatment of visceral leishmaniasis caused by *L. donovani*

Pregnancy Risk Factor C

Contraindications Hypersensitivity to pentamidine isethionate or any component (inhalation and injection); do not use concomitantly with didanosine since both drugs can cause pancreatitis

Warnings Healthcare personnel who administer aerosolized pentamidine inhalation therapy, a cough-producing procedure, should be aware of the possibility of secondary exposure to tuberculosis or other infections from patients with undiagnosed pulmonary disease

Precautions Use with caution in patients with diabetes mellitus, renal or hepatic dysfunction, hypertension or hypotension; adjust dose in renal impairment

Adverse Reactions

Cardiovascular: Hypotension, tachycardia, cardiac arrhythmias

Central nervous system: Dizziness, fever, fatigue, delirium

Dermatologic: Rash, itching

Endocrine & metabolic: Hypoglycemia, hyperglycemia, hypocalcemia, hyperkalemia

Gastrointestinal: Nausea, vomiting, metallic taste, pancreatitis

Hematologic: Megaloblastic anemia, neutropenia, leukopenia, thrombocytopenia

Hepatic: Mild hepatic injury

Local: Pain at injection site, thrombophlebitis, sterile abscess, erythema

Renal: Nephrotoxicity, elevated BUN, elevated serum creatinine

With aerosolized pentamidine: Irritation of the airway, cough, transient arterial desaturation, bronchospasm, fatigue, conjunctivitis

Miscellaneous: Jarisch-Herxheimer-like reaction

Drug Interactions Cytochrome P-450 isoenzyme CYP2C19 substrate

Aminoglycosides, amphotericin B, cisplatin and vancomycin (additive nephrotoxicity); didanosine (additive toxicity)

Stability Reconstituted solution is stable for 48 hours at room temperature when protected from light; do not refrigerate due to the possibility of crystallization

Mechanism of Action Interferes with RNA/DNA, phospholipids and protein synthesis through inhibition of oxidative phosphorylation and/or interference with incorporation of nucleotides and nucleic acids into RNA and DNA, in protozoa

Pharmacokinetics

Absorption: I.M.: Well absorbed; limited systemic absorption following pentamidine inhalation therapy

Distribution: Binds to tissues and plasma protein; high concentrations are found in the liver, kidney, adrenals, spleen, lungs and pancreas; poor penetration into CNS; following oral inhalation, high concentrations are found in bronchoalveolar fluid

Half-life, terminal: 6.4-9.4 hours; half-life may be prolonged in patients with severe renal impairment

Elimination: 33% to 66% in urine as unchanged drug

Dialysis: Not appreciably removed by hemodialysis or peritoneal dialysis

Usual Dosage

Children:

Treatment of *Pneumocystis carinii* pneumonia: I.M., I.V. (I.V. preferred): 4 mg/kg/day once daily for 14-21 days

Prophylaxis for *Pneumocystis carinii* pneumonia (See "Note" in Additional Information):

I.M., I.V.: 4 mg/kg/dose every 2-4 weeks **or**

Inhalation: Every month via Respirgard® II nebulizer
  Infants <1 year: Aerosolized pentamidine is administered at doses adjusted for minute ventilation and weight
  Infant dose = 2.27 mg/kg x nebulizer output (L/minute) x wt (kg) divided by alveolar ventilation (L/minute)
  Children <5 years: Some institutions have used a dose of 8 mg/kg
  Children ≥5 years: 300 mg/dose
Treatment of trypanosomiasis: I.M.: 4 mg/kg/day once daily for 10 days
Treatment of visceral leishmaniasis: I.M.: 2-4 mg/kg/day once daily or every 2 days for up to 15 doses
Adults:
  Treatment: I.M., I.V. (I.V. preferred): 4 mg/kg/day once daily for 14 days
  Prevention: Inhalation: 300 mg every 4 weeks via Respirgard® II nebulizer
Dosing adjustment in renal impairment:
  Cl_{cr} 10-30 mL/min: Administer normal dose once every 36 hours
  Cl_{cr} <10 mL/min: Administer normal dose once every 48 hours
Administration
  Oral inhalation: Safe and effective administration via nebulization in children is dependent on patients wearing an appropriately sized pediatric face mask
  Parenteral: May administer deep I.M. or by slow I.V. infusion; rapid I.V. administration can cause severe hypotension; infuse I.V. slowly over a period of at least 60 minutes at a final concentration for administration not to exceed 6 mg/mL
Monitoring Parameters Liver function tests, renal function tests, blood glucose, serum potassium and calcium, CBC with differential and platelet count, EKG, blood pressure
Patient Information Maintain adequate fluid intake; notify physician if fever, cough, or shortness of breath occurs; avoid alcohol
Nursing Implications Patients should receive parenteral pentamidine while lying down and blood pressure should be monitored closely during administration and after completion of the infusion until blood pressure is stabilized; if hypotension occurs due to rapid I.V. administration, slow infusion rate to administer dose over 1-2 hours
Additional Information
  Note: Guidelines for prophylaxis of *Pneumocystis carinii* pneumonia: Initiate PCP prophylaxis for the following patients: All HIV-exposed children at 4-6 weeks of age and continue through the first year of life or until HIV infection has been reasonably excluded; children 1-5 years of age with CD4+ count <500 or CD4+ percentage <15%; children 6-12 years of age with CD4+ count <200 or CD4+ percentage <15%; for children who had a CD4+ count <750 or a CD4+ percentage <15% in the first year of life, prophylaxis should be continued until 2 years of age
  1 mg pentamidine: 1.74 mg pentamidine isethionate
Dosage Forms
  Inhalation, as isethionate: 300 mg
  Powder for injection, as isethionate, lyophilized: 300 mg
References

Hand IL, Wiznia AA, Porricolo M, et al, "Aerosolized Pentamidine for Prophylaxis of *Pneumocystis carinii* Pneumonia in Infants With Human Immunodeficiency Virus Infection," *Pediatr Infect Dis J*, 1994, 13(2):100-4.
Hughes WT, "*Pneumocystis carinii* Pneumonia: New Approaches to Diagnosis, Treatment, and Prevention," *Pediatr Infect Dis J*, 1991, 10(5):391-9.
"1999 USPHS/IDSA Guidelines for the Prevention of Opportunistic Infections in Persons Infected With Human Immunodeficiency Virus," *MMWR Morb Mortal Wkly Rep*, 1999, 48(RR-10):1-66.

♦ **Pentamycetin (Can)** see Chloramphenicol on page 218
♦ **Pentasa®** see Mesalamine on page 634

Pentazocine (pen TAZ oh seen)
Related Information
  Compatibility of Medications Mixed in a Syringe on page 1238
  Narcotic Analgesics Comparison on page 1070
U.S. Brand Names Talwin®; Talwin® NX
Synonyms Pentazocine and Naloxone
Therapeutic Category Analgesic, Narcotic; Opiate Partial Agonist; Sedative
Generic Available No
Use Relief of moderate to severe pain; a sedative prior to surgery; supplement to surgical anesthesia
Restrictions C-IV
Pregnancy Risk Factor B (D if used for prolonged periods or in high doses at term)
Contraindications Hypersensitivity to pentazocine or any component
(Continued)

Pentazocine *(Continued)*

Warnings Pentazocine may precipitate opiate withdrawal symptoms in patients who have been receiving opiates regularly; injection contains sulfites which may cause allergic reaction

Precautions Use with caution in seizure-prone patients, acute MI, patients undergoing biliary tract surgery, patients with renal and hepatic dysfunction, and patients with a history of prior opioid dependence or abuse; decrease dosage in patients with decreased hepatic or renal function

Adverse Reactions

Cardiovascular: Palpitations, hypotension, tachycardia, peripheral vasodilation

Central nervous system: CNS depression, drowsiness, sedation, dizziness, euphoria, lightheadedness (more frequently than morphine), hallucinations, confusion, disorientation, increased intracranial pressure; seizures may occur in seizure-prone patients especially with large I.V. doses

Dermatologic: Pruritus, rash

Endocrine & metabolic: Antidiuretic hormone release

Gastrointestinal: Nausea (more frequently than morphine), vomiting, constipation, biliary tract spasm

Genitourinary: Urinary tract spasm

Local: Tissue damage and irritation with I.M./S.C. use

Ocular: Miosis

Respiratory: Respiratory depression, laryngospasm

Miscellaneous: Physical and psychological dependence, histamine release

Drug Interactions Cytochrome P-450 isoenzyme CYP2D6 substrate

May potentiate or reduce analgesic effect of opiate agonist (ie, morphine), depending on patient's tolerance to opiates; additive effects seen with other CNS depressants; tripelennamine potentiates pentazocine effects and lethality and the two have been abused in combination (Ts and blues) I.V. to provide effects similar to heroin

Stability Store injection at room temperature; do not mix injection with barbiturates, precipitation will occur

Mechanism of Action Binds to opiate receptors in the CNS, causing inhibition of ascending pain pathways, altering the perception of and response to pain; produces generalized CNS depression

Pharmacodynamics

Onset:

Oral, I.M., S.C.: Within 15-30 minutes

I.V.: Within 2-3 minutes

Duration:

Oral: 4-5 hours

Parenteral: 2-3 hours

Pharmacokinetics

Protein binding: 60%

Metabolism: In the liver via oxidative and glucuronide conjugation pathways

Bioavailability: Oral: ~20% due to large first-pass effect; increased oral bioavailability to 60% to 70% in patients with cirrhosis

Half-life: Increased half-life with decreased hepatic function

Children 4-8 years (mean ± SD): 3 ± 1.5 hours

Adults: 2-3 hours

Elimination: Small amounts excreted unchanged in urine

Usual Dosage

Children <14 years: Limited information available:

I.M. doses of 15 mg for children 5-8 years of age and 30 mg for children 9-14 years of age to treat postoperative pain have been used (n=30) (Waterworth, 1974)

In 300 children (1-14 years) I.M. doses ranging from approximately 0.45-1.5 mg/kg in children <27 kg to 0.65-1.9 mg/kg in children >27 kg were used preoperatively (Rita, 1970)

I.V.: Intraoperative: Titrating doses of 0.5 mg/kg every 30-45 minutes as needed for analgesia have been given in 50 children 5-9 years of age; total dose required: 1-1.5 mg/kg (Ray, 1993)

Children >14 years and Adults: Oral: 50 mg every 3-4 hours; may increase to 100 mg/dose if needed; maximum dose: 600 mg/day

Adults:

I.M., S.C.: 30-60 mg every 3-4 hours; maximum: 360 mg/day

I.V.: 30 mg every 3-4 hours; maximum: 360 mg/day

Dosing adjustment in renal impairment: Children and Adults:
Cl$_{cr}$ 10-50 mL/minute: Administer 75% of normal dose
Cl$_{cr}$ <10 mL/minute: Administer 50% of normal dose

Administration
Oral: May be administered with food or milk to decrease GI upset
Parenteral: S.C. route not advised due to tissue damage; rotate injection site for I.M., S.C. use; avoid intra-arterial injection

Monitoring Parameters Respiratory and cardiovascular status; level of pain relief and sedation; blood pressure

Patient Information Avoid alcohol; may cause drowsiness and impair ability to perform hazardous activities requiring mental alertness or physical coordination; may be habit-forming; will cause narcotic withdrawal symptoms in patients currently dependent on narcotics

Additional Information Use only in patients who are not tolerant to or physically dependent upon narcotics

Talwin® NX tablet (pentazocine hydrochloride with naloxone) was formulated to decrease abuse potential of dissolving tablets in water and using as injection

Dosage Forms
Injection, as lactate (Talwin®): 30 mg/mL (1 mL, 1.5 mL, 2 mL, 10 mL)
Tablet, scored (Talwin® NX): Pentazocine hydrochloride 50 mg and naloxone hydrochloride 0.5 mg

References
Hanunen K, Olkkola KT, Seppala T, et al, "Pharmacokinetics and Pharmacodynamics of Pentazocine in Children," *Pharmacol Toxicol*, 1993, 73(2):120-3.
Ray AD and Gupta M, "Clinical Trial of Pentazocine as Analgesic in Pediatric Cases," *J Indian Med Assoc*, 1994, 92(3):77-9.
Rita L, Seleny FL, and Levin RM, "A Comparison of Pentazocine and Morphine for Pediatric Premedication," *Anesth Analg*, 1970, 49(3):377-82.
Waterworth TA, "Pentazocine (Fortal) as Postoperative Analgesic in Children," *Arch Dis Child*, 1974, 49(6):488-90.

♦ **Pentazocine and Naloxone** *see* Pentazocine *on page 777*

Pentobarbital (pen toe BAR bi tal)

Related Information
Compatibility of Medications Mixed in a Syringe *on page 1238*
Laboratory Detection of Drugs in Urine *on page 1234*
Overdose and Toxicology *on page 1222*
Preprocedure Sedatives in Children *on page 1201*

U.S. Brand Names Nembutal®
Canadian Brand Names Nova-Pentobarb; Nova Rectal
Therapeutic Category Anticonvulsant, Barbiturate; Barbiturate; General Anesthetic; Hypnotic; Sedative
Generic Available Yes
Use Short-term treatment of insomnia; preoperative sedation; high-dose barbiturate coma for treatment of increased intracranial pressure or status epilepticus unresponsive to other therapy
Restrictions C-II; C-III (suppositories)
Pregnancy Risk Factor D
Contraindications Marked liver function impairment or latent porphyria; chronic or acute pain; hypersensitivity to barbiturates or any component
Warnings Capsules may contain tartrazine which may cause allergic reactions; commercially available injection contains propylene glycol
Precautions Use with caution in patients with hypovolemic shock, CHF, or hepatic impairment
Adverse Reactions
Cardiovascular: Arrhythmias, bradycardia, hypotension
Central nervous system: Drowsiness, lethargy, CNS excitation or depression, impaired judgment, hypothermia
Dermatologic: Rash
Gastrointestinal: Nausea, vomiting
Local: Arterial spasm, gangrene with inadvertent intra-arterial injection, thrombophlebitis
Renal: Oliguria
Respiratory: Laryngospasm, respiratory depression, apnea (especially with rapid I.V. use)
Miscellaneous: Physical and psychological dependency with chronic use
Drug Interactions Barbiturates are enzyme inducers (monitor patient closely for decreased effect of concomitantly administered medications or increased effect
(Continued)

Pentobarbital *(Continued)*

when barbiturates are discontinued); carbamazepine, chloramphenicol, cimetidine, corticosteroids, CNS depressants, alcohol, doxycycline, warfarin, valproic acid

Food Interactions Food may decrease the rate but not the extent of oral absorption; high doses of pyridoxine may decrease drug effect; barbiturates may increase the metabolism of vitamins D and K; dietary requirements of vitamins D, K, C, B_{12}, folate, and calcium may be increased with long-term use

Stability Protect from light; aqueous solutions are not stable; low pH may cause precipitate; use only clear solution

Mechanism of Action Short-acting barbiturate with sedative, hypnotic, and anticonvulsant properties; depresses CNS activity by binding to barbiturate site at GABA-receptor complex enhancing GABA activity; depresses reticular activating system; higher doses may be gabamimetic

Pharmacodynamics

Onset:
Oral or rectal: 15-60 minutes
I.M.: Within 10-15 minutes
I.V.: Within 1 minute
Duration:
Oral, rectal: 1-4 hours
I.V.: 15 minutes

Pharmacokinetics

Absorption: Oral: ~95%
Distribution: V_d:
Children: 0.8 L/kg
Adults: 1 L/kg
Protein binding: 35% to 55%
Metabolism: Extensive in the liver via hydroxylation and oxidation pathways
Half-life, terminal:
Children: 25 hours
Normal adults: 22 hours; range: 35-50 hours
Elimination: <1% excreted unchanged renally

Usual Dosage

Children:
Sedative: Oral: 2-6 mg/kg/day divided in 3 doses; maximum dose: 100 mg/day
Hypnotic: I.M.: 2-6 mg/kg; maximum dose: 100 mg/dose
Rectal:
2 months to 1 year (10-20 lb): 30 mg
1-4 years (20-40 lb): 30-60 mg
5-12 years (40-80 lb): 60 mg
12-14 years (80-110 lb): 60-120 mg **or**
<4 years: 3-6 mg/kg/dose
>4 years: 1.5-3 mg/kg/dose
Preoperative/preprocedure sedation: ≥6 months:
Oral, I.M., rectal: 2-6 mg/kg; maximum dose: 100 mg/dose
I.V.: 1-3 mg/kg to a maximum of 100 mg until asleep
Conscious sedation prior to a procedure: Children >18 months: I.V.: Initial: 2 mg/kg, additional doses of 1-2 mg/kg may be given every 5-10 minutes until adequate sedation is achieved; maximum total dose: 6 mg/kg or 150-200 mg; mean total dose required (for CT scan sedation): 3.3-4.5 mg/kg
Adolescents: Conscious sedation: Oral, I.V.: 100 mg prior to a procedure
Children and Adults: Pentobarbital coma: I.V.:
Loading dose: 10-15 mg/kg given slowly over 1-2 hours; monitor blood pressure and respiratory rate
Maintenance infusion: Initial: 1 mg/kg/hour; may increase to 2-3 mg/kg/hour; maintain burst suppression on EEG
Adults:
Hypnotic:
Oral: 100-200 mg at bedtime
I.M.: 150-200 mg
I.V.: Initial: 100 mg, may repeat every 1-3 minutes up to 200-500 mg total
Rectal: 120-200 mg at bedtime
Preoperative sedation: I.M.: 150-200 mg

Administration

Oral: May administer with food to decrease GI upset
Parenteral: I.V.: Do not inject >50 mg/minute; rapid I.V. injection may cause respiratory depression, apnea, laryngospasm, bronchospasm, and hypotension; administer over 10-30 minutes; maximum concentration: 50 mg/mL for slow I.V. push;

may dilute in D_5W, $D_{10}W$, NS, ½NS, LR, Ringer's injection, D_5LR, and dextrose/saline combinations for continuous infusion

Monitoring Parameters Vital signs, respiratory status (includes pulse oximetry for conscious sedation), cardiovascular status, CNS status; monitor ICP and cerebral perfusion pressure (CPP) (CPP = MAP - ICP) when using pentobarbital coma to reduce ICP

Reference Range Therapeutic:

Sedation: 1-5 µg/mL (SI: 4-22 µmol/L)

Sleep: 5-15 µg/mL (SI: 22-66 µmol/L)

Coma: 20-40 µg/mL (SI: 88-177 µmol/L)

Patient Information Avoid alcohol; limit caffeine; may be habit-forming; do not abruptly discontinue; may cause drowsiness and impair ability to perform activities requiring mental alertness or physical coordination

Nursing Implications Suppositories should not be divided; parenteral solutions are very alkaline; avoid extravasation; avoid intra-arterial injection

Additional Information Tolerance to hypnotic effect can occur; do not use for >2 weeks to treat insomnia; taper dose to prevent withdrawal; **Note**: Loading doses of 15-35 mg/kg (given over 1-2 hours) have been utilized in pediatric patients for pentobarbital coma but these higher loading doses often cause hypotension requiring vasopressor therapy

I.V. continuous infusions of pentobarbital using initial bolus doses of 1-2 mg/kg followed by initial continuous infusions of 1-2 mg/kg/hour have been used for PICU sedation in six intubated, mechanically ventilated infants (age: 2-17 months) who "failed" sedation with fentanyl and midazolam infusions; doses were titrated to effect and supplemental boluses were administered as needed; further studies are needed (see Tobias, 1995)

Dosage Forms

Capsule, as sodium: 50 mg, 100 mg

Elixir: 18.2 mg/5 mL (473 mL, 4000 mL)

Injection, as sodium: 50 mg/mL (20 mL, 50 mL)

Suppository, rectal, as sodium (C-III): 60 mg, 200 mg

References

Fischer JH and Raineri DL, "Pentobarbital Anesthesia for Status Epilepticus," *Clin Pharm*, 1987, 6(8):601-2.

Hubbard AM, Markowitz RI, Kimmel B, et al, "Sedation for Pediatric Patients Undergoing CT and MRI," *J Comput Assist Tomogr*, 1992, 16(1):3-6.

Pereira JK, Burrows PE, Richards HM, et al, "Comparison of Sedation Regimens for Pediatric Outpatient CT," *Pediatr Radiol*, 1993, 23(5):341-4.

Schaible DH, Cupit GC, Swedlow DB, et al, "High-Dose Pentobarbital Pharmacokinetics in Hypothermic Brain-Injured Children," *J Pediatr*, 1982, 100(4):655-60.

Tobias JD, Deshpande JK, Pietsch JB, et al, "Pentobarbital Sedation for Patients in the Pediatric Intensive Care Unit," *South Med J*, 1995, 88(3):290-4.

♦ **Pentothal®** see Thiopental on page 951

Pentoxifylline (pen toks I fi leen)

U.S. Brand Names Trental®

Canadian Brand Names Albert Pentoxifylline; Apo-Pentoxifylline SR; Nu-Pentoxifylline

Synonyms Oxpentifylline

Therapeutic Category Blood Viscosity Reducer Agent

Generic Available Yes

Use Symptomatic management of peripheral vascular disease, mainly intermittent claudication

Investigational use: AIDS patients with increased tumor necrosis factor, cerebrovascular accidents, cerebrovascular diseases, new onset type I diabetes mellitus, diabetic atherosclerosis, diabetic neuropathy, gangrene, cutaneous polyarteritis nodosa, hemodialysis shunt thrombosis, cerebral malaria, septic shock, sepsis in premature neonates, sickle cell syndromes, vasculitis, Kawasaki disease, Raynaud's syndrome, cystic fibrosis, and persistent pulmonary hypertension of the newborn (case report)

Pregnancy Risk Factor C

Contraindications Hypersensitivity to pentoxifylline, any component, or other xanthine derivatives (eg, caffeine, theophylline, theobromine); recent cerebral or retinal hemorrhage

Warnings Use with caution in patients with renal or hepatic impairment, insulin-treated diabetics, chronic occlusive arterial disease of the limbs, recent surgery, or peptic ulcerations

Adverse Reactions

Cardiovascular: Mild hypotension, angina

(Continued)

781

Pentoxifylline *(Continued)*

Central nervous system: Headache, dizziness, agitation

Gastrointestinal: Dyspepsia, nausea, vomiting

Ocular: Blurred vision

Drug Interactions Cimetidine may increase plasma concentrations of pentoxifylline; pentoxifylline may increase the effect of antihypertensive agents, warfarin, heparin; pentoxifylline may increase serum theophylline levels and toxicity (monitor closely, dosage adjustment of theophylline may be needed)

Food Interactions Food may decrease rate but not extent of absorption

Mechanism of Action Mechanism of action remains unclear; is thought to reduce blood viscosity and improve blood flow by altering the rheology of red blood cells; inhibits production of tumor necrosis factor-alpha; inhibits neutrophil activation and adhesion; increases tissue oxygen levels in patients with peripheral arterial disease; inhibits platelet aggregation

Pharmacodynamics Onset of action: 2-4 weeks with multiple doses

Pharmacokinetics

Absorption: Oral: Well absorbed

Metabolism: Undergoes first-pass in the liver, dose-related (nonlinear) pharmacokinetics

Half-life, apparent:

Parent drug: 24-48 minutes

Metabolites: 60-96 minutes

Time to peak serum concentration: Within 2-4 hours

Elimination: Metabolites excreted in urine; 0% eliminated unchanged in the urine

Usual Dosage Oral:

Children: Minimal information available; one investigation (Furukawa, 1994) found a lower incidence of coronary artery lesions in 22 children (mean age 2 years) treated for acute Kawasaki disease with versus without pentoxifylline 20 mg/kg/day (given in 3 divided doses); all patients received aspirin and I.V. gamma globulin therapy; a lower dose (10 mg/kg/day) was not effective; higher doses have been used investigationally for the treatment of cystic fibrosis (Aronoff 1994)

Adults: 400 mg 3 times/day with meals; decrease to 400 mg twice daily if CNS or GI side effects occur

Administration Oral: Administer with food or antacids to decrease GI upset; swallow extended release tablet whole, do not crush, break, or chew

Test Interactions False positive theophylline level

Patient Information Limit caffeine; if GI or CNS side effects continue, contact physician; while beneficial effects may be seen in 2-4 weeks, continue treatment for at least 8 weeks

Dosage Forms Tablet, extended release: 400 mg

References

Aronoff SC, Quinn FJ, Carpenter LS, et al, "Effects of Pentoxifylline on Sputum Neutrophil Elastase and Pulmonary Function in Patients With Cystic Fibrosis: Preliminary Observations," *J Pediatr*, 1994, 125(6 Pt 1):992-7.

Berman W Jr, Berman N, Pathak D, et al, "Effects of Pentoxifylline (Trental®) on Blood Flow, Viscosity, and Oxygen Transport in Young Adults With Inoperable Cyanotic Congenital Heart Disease," *Pediatr Cardiol*, 1994, 15(2):66-70.

Furukawa S, Matsubara T, Umezawa Y, et al, "Pentoxifylline and Intravenous Gamma Globulin Combination Therapy for Acute Kawasaki Disease," *Eur J Pediatr*, 1994, 153(9):663-7.

Lauterbach R, "Pentoxifylline Treatment of Persistent Pulmonary Hypertension of Newborn," *Eur J Pediatr*, 1993, 152(5):460. (I.V. use)

Lauterbach R, Pawlik D, Tomaszczyk B, et al, "Pentoxifylline Treatment of Sepsis of Premature Infants; Preliminary Clinical Observations," *Eur J Pediatr*, 1994, 153(9):672-4. (I.V. use)

MacDonald MJ, Shahidi NT, Allen DB, et al, "Pentoxifylline in the Treatment of Children With New-Onset Type I Diabetes Mellitus," *JAMA*, 1994, 271(1):27-8.

- ◆ **Percodan®**   *see Oxycodone and Aspirin on page 748*
- ◆ **Percodan®-Demi**   *see Oxycodone and Aspirin on page 748*
- ◆ **Percolone®**   *see Oxycodone on page 745*
- ◆ **Perdium Fiber®** [OTC]   *see Psyllium on page 853*
- ◆ **Perfectoderm® Gel** [OTC]   *see Benzoyl Peroxide on page 136*
- ◆ **Periactin®**   *see Cyproheptadine on page 287*
- ◆ **Peri-Colace®** [OTC]   *see Docusate and Casanthranol on page 351*
- ◆ **Peridex®**   *see Chlorhexidine Gluconate on page 220*
- ◆ **Peridol (Can)** *see Haloperidol on page 488*
- ◆ **Perifoam®** [OTC]   *see Hemorrhoidal Preparations on page 490*
- ◆ **PerioGard®**   *see Chlorhexidine Gluconate on page 220*
- ◆ **Permapen®**   *see Penicillin G Benzathine on page 770*

Permethrin (per METH rin)

U.S. Brand Names Elimite™ Cream; Nix™ Creme Rinse

Canadian Brand Names Kwellada-P; Nix Dermal Cream

Therapeutic Category Antiparasitic Agent, Topical; Pediculocide; Scabicidal Agent

Generic Available No

Use Single application treatment of infestation with *Pediculus humanus capitis* (head louse) and its nits; treatment of *Sarcoptes scabiei* (scabies)

Pregnancy Risk Factor B

Contraindications Hypersensitivity to pyrethroid, pyrethrin, any component, or to chrysanthemums

Precautions For external use only; do not use near the eyes or on mucous membranes such as inside the nose, mouth, or vagina

Adverse Reactions

Dermatologic: Pruritus, erythema, rash of the scalp

Local: Burning, stinging, pain, edema, tingling, numbness, scalp discomfort

Mechanism of Action Inhibits sodium ion influx through nerve cell membrane channels in parasites resulting in delayed repolarization, paralysis, and death of organism

Pharmacokinetics

Absorption: Topical: Minimal (<2%)

Metabolism: By ester hydrolysis to inactive metabolites

Usual Dosage Topical: Children >2 months and Adults:

Head lice: After hair has been washed with shampoo, rinsed with water and towel dried, apply a sufficient volume of creme rinse to saturate the hair and scalp; also apply behind the ears and at the base of the neck; leave on hair for 10 minutes before rinsing off with water; remove remaining nits. May repeat in 1 week if lice or nits still present; in areas of head lice resistance to 1% permethrin, 5% permethrin has been applied to clean, dry hair and left on overnight (8-14 hours) under a shower cap.

Scabies: Apply cream from head to toe; leave on for 8-14 hours before washing off with water; for infants, also apply on the hairline, neck, scalp, temple, and forehead; may reapply in 1 week if live mites appear. Permethrin 5% cream was shown to be safe and effective when applied to an infant <1 month of age with neonatal scabies; time of application was limited to 6 hours before rinsing with soap and water.

Administration Topical: Avoid contact with eyes during application; shake creme rinse well before using

Patient Information Clothing and bedding should be washed in hot water or by dry cleaning to kill the scabies mite

Nursing Implications

To remove nits: Comb hair with a fine-toothed nit comb and apply a damp towel to the scalp for 30-60 minutes

For infestation of eyelashes: Apply petroleum ointment to eyelashes 3-4 times/day for 8-10 days; remove nits mechanically from the eyelashes

For scabies: Itching may continue for several weeks despite successful treatment; oral antihistamines and/or topical corticosteroids may be helpful in relieving symptoms

Additional Information Topical cream formulation contains formaldehyde which is a contact allergen

Dosage Forms

Cream: 5% (60 g)

Creme rinse: 1% (60 mL with comb)

(Continued)

Permethrin *(Continued)*

References

"Drugs for Head Lice," *Med Lett Drugs Ther,* 1997, 39(992):6-7.

Hogan DJ, Schachner L, Tanglertsampan C, "Diagnosis and Treatment of Childhood Scabies and Pediculosis," *Pediatr Clin North Am,* 1991, 38(4):941-57.

Krowchuk DP, Tunnessen WW Jr, and Hurwitz S, "Pediatric Dermatology Update," *Pediatrics,* 1992, 90(2 Pt 1):259-64.

Quarterman MJ and Lesher JL, "Neonatal Scabies Treated With Permethrin 5% Cream," *Pediatr Dermatol,* 1994, 11(3):264-6.

- ◆ **Pernox® [OTC]** *see* Sulfur and Salicylic Acid *on page 929*
- ◆ **Peroxide** *see* Hydrogen Peroxide *on page 509*
- ◆ **Peroxin A5®** *see* Benzoyl Peroxide *on page 136*
- ◆ **Peroxin A10®** *see* Benzoyl Peroxide *on page 136*
- ◆ **Peroxyl®** *see* Hydrogen Peroxide *on page 509*
- ◆ **Persa-Gel®** *see* Benzoyl Peroxide *on page 136*
- ◆ **Persantine®** *see* Dipyridamole *on page 346*
- ◆ **Pertussin® CS [OTC]** *see* Dextromethorphan *on page 316*
- ◆ **Pertussin® DM [OTC]** *see* Dextromethorphan *on page 316*
- ◆ **Pethidine** *see* Meperidine *on page 628*
- ◆ **PFA** *see* Foscarnet *on page 456*
- ◆ **Pfizerpen®** *see* Penicillin G (Parenteral/Aqueous) *on page 772*
- ◆ **Pfizerpen®-AS** *see* Penicillin G Procaine *on page 773*
- ◆ **PGE$_1$** *see* Alprostadil *on page 56*
- ◆ **Phanatuss® [OTC]** *see* Guaifenesin and Dextromethorphan *on page 487*
- ◆ **Pharmaflur®** *see* Fluoride *on page 441*
- ◆ **Pharmilin-DM (Can)** *see* Dextromethorphan *on page 316*
- ◆ **Pharminil DM (Can)** *see* Dextromethorphan *on page 316*
- ◆ **Phazyme® [OTC]** *see* Simethicone *on page 902*
- ◆ **Phazyme® Extra Strength [OTC]** *see* Simethicone *on page 902*
- ◆ **Phazyme® Maximum Strength [OTC]** *see* Simethicone *on page 902*
- ◆ **Phenantoin** *see* Mephenytoin *on page 630*
- ◆ **Phenaphen® With Codeine** *see* Acetaminophen and Codeine *on page 31*
- ◆ **Phenazine®** *see* Promethazine *on page 836*
- ◆ **Phenazo (Can)** *see* Phenazopyridine *on page 784*

Phenazopyridine (fen az oh PEER i deen)

U.S. Brand Names Azo-Standard® [OTC]; Baridium® [OTC]; Prodium™ [OTC]; Pyridiate®; Pyridium®; UTI Relief® [OTC]

Canadian Brand Names Phenazo; Pyronium

Synonyms Phenylazo Diamino Pyridine

Therapeutic Category Analgesic, Urinary; Local Anesthetic, Urinary

Generic Available Yes

Use Symptomatic relief of urinary burning, itching, frequency and urgency in association with urinary tract infection, or following urologic procedures

Pregnancy Risk Factor B

Contraindications Hypersensitivity to phenazopyridine or any component; liver or kidney disease (do not use in patients with Cl$_{cr}$ <50 mL/minute)

Warnings Does not treat infection, acts only as an analgesic; drug should be discontinued if skin or sclera develop a yellow color

Precautions Use with caution in patients with renal impairment

Adverse Reactions

Central nervous system: Vertigo, headache

Dermatologic: Skin pigmentation, rash, pruritus

Gastrointestinal: Stomach cramps

Genitourinary: Discoloration of urine (orange or red)

Hematologic: Methemoglobinemia, hemolytic anemia

Hepatic: Hepatitis

Renal: Transient acute renal failure

Mechanism of Action Exerts local topical anesthetic or analgesic action on urinary tract mucosa through an unknown mechanism

Pharmacokinetics

Metabolism: In the liver and other tissues

Elimination: In urine (where it exerts its action); renal excretion (as unchanged drug) is rapid and accounts for 65% of the drug's elimination

Usual Dosage Oral:

Children: 12 mg/kg/day in 3 divided doses for 2 days if used concomitantly with an antibacterial agent for UTI

Adults: 100-200 mg 3-4 times/day for 2 days if used concomitantly with an antibacterial agent for UTI

Dosing interval in renal impairment:

Cl_{cr} 50-80 mL/minute: Administer every 8-16 hours

Cl_{cr} <50 mL/minute: Avoid use

Administration Oral: Administer with food to decrease GI distress

Test Interactions False-negative Clinistix®, Tes-Tape®, Ictotest®, Acetest®, Ketostix®, urinalysis based upon spectrometry or color reactions

Patient Information May discolor urine orange or red; may stain contact lenses and fabric

Dosage Forms Tablet, as hydrochloride:

Azo-Standard®, Prodium™ [OTC]: 95 mg

Baridium®, UTI Relief®: 97.2 mg

Pyridiate®, Pyridium®: 100 mg

Pyridiate®, Pyridium®: 200 mg

Extemporaneous Preparations A 10 mg/mL suspension may be made by crushing three 200 mg tablets. Mix with a small amount of distilled water or glycerin. Add 20 mL Cologel® and levigate until a uniform mixture is obtained. Add sufficient 2:1 simple syrup/cherry syrup mixture to make a final volume of 60 mL. Store in an amber container. Label "shake well". Stability is 60 days refrigerated.

Handbook on Extemporaneous Formulations, Bethesda MD: American Society of Hospital Pharmacists, 1987.

♦ **Phenergan®** *see* Promethazine *on page 836*

♦ **Phenergan® VC** *see* Promethazine and Phenylephrine *on page 839*

♦ **Phenergan® VC With Codeine** *see* Promethazine, Phenylephrine, and Codeine *on page 840*

♦ **Phenergan® With Codeine** *see* Promethazine and Codeine *on page 838*

Phenobarbital (fee noe BAR bi tal)

Related Information

Antiepileptic Drugs *on page 1208*

Blood Level Sampling Time Guidelines *on page 1220*

Carbohydrate and Alcohol Content of Liquid Medications for Use in Patients Receiving Ketogenic Diets *on page 1258*

Drugs and Breast-Feeding *on page 1243*

Laboratory Detection of Drugs in Urine *on page 1234*

Overdose and Toxicology *on page 1222*

U.S. Brand Names Luminal®

Canadian Brand Names Barbilixir

Synonyms Phenobarbitone; Phenylethylmalonylurea

Therapeutic Category Anticonvulsant, Barbiturate; Barbiturate; Hypnotic; Sedative

Generic Available Yes

Use Management of generalized tonic-clonic (grand mal) and partial seizures; neonatal seizures; febrile seizures in children; sedation; may also be used for prevention and treatment of neonatal hyperbilirubinemia and lowering of bilirubin in chronic cholestasis

Restrictions C-IV

Pregnancy Risk Factor D

Contraindications Hypersensitivity to phenobarbital or any component; pre-existing CNS depression, severe uncontrolled pain, porphyria, severe respiratory disease with dyspnea or obstruction

Warnings Abrupt withdrawal may precipitate status epilepticus

Precautions Use with caution in patients with renal or hepatic impairment

Adverse Reactions

Cardiovascular: Hypotension, circulatory collapse

Central nervous system: Drowsiness, paradoxical excitement, hyperkinetic activity, cognitive impairment, defects in general comprehension, short-term memory deficits, decreased attention span, ataxia

Dermatologic: Skin eruptions, skin rash, exfoliative dermatitis

Hematologic: Megaloblastic anemia

Hepatic: Hepatitis

Respiratory: Respiratory depression, apnea (especially with rapid I.V. use)

Miscellaneous: Psychological and physical dependence

(Continued)

Phenobarbital *(Continued)*

Drug Interactions Cytochrome P-450 isoenzyme CYP1A2, CYP2B6, CYP2C8, CYP3A3/4, and CYP3A5-7 inducer

Phenobarbital may decrease the serum concentration or effect of lamotrigine, ritonavir, saquinavir, delavirdine, ethosuximide, warfarin, oral contraceptives, chloramphenicol, griseofulvin, doxycycline, beta-blockers, theophylline, corticosteroids, teniposide, etoposide, doxorubicin, vincristine, methotrexate, tricyclic antidepressants, cyclosporin, quinidine, haloperidol, and phenothiazines

Valproic acid, methylphenidate, chloramphenicol, felbamate, and propoxyphene may inhibit the metabolism of phenobarbital with resultant increase in phenobarbital serum concentration; ritonavir may affect the metabolism of phenobarbital; phenobarbital and benzodiazepines or other CNS depressants may increase CNS and respiratory depression (especially with I.V. loading doses of phenobarbital)

Food Interactions High doses of pyridoxine may decrease drug effect; barbiturates may increase the metabolism of vitamins D and K; dietary requirements of vitamins D, K, C, B_{12}, folate, and calcium may be increased with long-term use

Stability Protect elixir from light; not stable in aqueous solutions; use only clear solutions; do not add to acidic solutions, precipitation may occur

Mechanism of Action Depresses CNS activity by binding to barbiturate site at GABA-receptor complex enhancing GABA activity; depresses reticular activating system; higher doses may be gabamimetic

Pharmacodynamics Hypnosis:

Onset of action:

Oral: Within 20-60 minutes

I.V.: Within 5 minutes

Peak effect: I.V.: Within 30 minutes

Duration:

Oral: 6-10 hours

I.V.: 4-10 hours

Pharmacokinetics

Absorption: Oral: 70% to 90%

Distribution: V_d:

Neonates: 0.8-1 L/kg

Infants: 0.7-0.8 L/kg

Children: 0.6-0.7 L/kg

Protein binding: 35% to 50%, decreased protein binding in neonates

Metabolism: In the liver via hydroxylation and glucuronide conjugation

Half-life:

Neonates: 45-200 hours

Infants: 20-133 hours

Children: 37-73 hours

Adults: 53-140 hours

Time to peak serum concentration: Oral: Within 1-6 hours

Elimination: 20% to 50% excreted unchanged in urine; clearance can be increased with alkalinization of urine or with oral multiple-dose activated charcoal

Dialysis: Moderately dializable (20% to 50%)

Usual Dosage

Anticonvulsant: Status epilepticus: **Loading dose:** I.V.:

Neonates: 15-20 mg/kg in a single or divided dose

Infants, Children, and Adults: 15-18 mg/kg in a single or divided dose; usual maximum loading dose: 20 mg/kg

Note: In select patients, may give additional 5 mg/kg/dose every 15-30 minutes until seizure is controlled or a total dose of 30 mg/kg is reached; be prepared to support respirations

Anticonvulsant **maintenance dose**: Oral, I.V. (**Note:** Maintenance dose usually starts 12 hours after loading dose):

Neonates: 3-4 mg/kg/day given once daily; assess serum concentrations; increase to 5 mg/kg/day if needed (usually by second week of therapy)

Infants: 5-6 mg/kg/day in 1-2 divided doses

Children:

1-5 years: 6-8 mg/kg/day in 1-2 divided doses

5-12 years: 4-6 mg/kg/day in 1-2 divided doses

>12 years and adults: 1-3 mg/kg/day in 1-2 divided doses

Children:

Sedation: Oral: 2 mg/kg 3 times/day

Hypnotic: I.M., I.V., S.C.: 3-5 mg/kg at bedtime

Hyperbilirubinemia: <12 years: Oral: 3-8 mg/kg/day in 2-3 divided doses; doses up to 12 mg/kg/day have been used

Preoperative sedation: Oral, I.M., I.V.: 1-3 mg/kg 1-1.5 hours before procedure

Adults:

Sedation: Oral, I.M.: 30-120 mg/day in 2-3 divided doses

Hypnotic: Oral, I.M., I.V., S.C.: 100-320 mg at bedtime

Hyperbilirubinemia: Oral: 90-180 mg/day in 2-3 divided doses

Preoperative sedation: I.M.: 100-200 mg 1-1.5 hours before procedure

Administration

Oral: Administer elixir with water, milk, or juice

Parenteral: Do not inject I.V. faster than 1 mg/kg/minute with a maximum of 30 mg/minute for infants and children and 60 mg/minute for adults >60kg; do not administer intra-arterially; avoid extravasation; use only powder for injection for S.C. use, not solutions for injection

Monitoring Parameters CNS status, seizure activity, liver enzymes, CBC with differential, renal function, serum concentrations; I.V. use: Respiratory rate, heart rate, blood pressure; hyperbilirubinemia: bilirubin (total and direct)

Reference Range

Therapeutic: 15-40 µg/mL (SI: 65-172 µmol/L)

Potentially toxic: >40 µg/mL (SI: >172 µmol/L)

Coma: >50 µg/mL (SI: >215 µmol/L)

Potentially lethal: >80 µg/mL (SI: >344 µmol/L)

Patient Information Avoid alcohol; limit caffeine; may be habit-forming; may cause dizziness or drowsiness and impair ability to perform activities requiring mental alertness or physical coordination; do not abruptly discontinue

Nursing Implications Parenteral solutions are very alkaline

Additional Information Injectable solutions contain propylene glycol

A recent study (Relling, 2000) demonstrated that enzyme-inducing antiepileptic drugs (AEDs) (carbamazepine, phenobarbital, and phenytoin) increased systemic clearance of antileukemic drugs (teniposide and methotrexate) and were associated with a worse event-free survival, CNS relapse, and hematologic relapse (ie, lower efficacy), in B-lineage ALL children receiving chemotherapy; the authors recommend using nonenzyme-inducing AEDs in patients receiving chemotherapy for ALL.

Dosage Forms

Elixir: **20 mg/5 mL** (5 mL, 7.5 mL, 15 mL, 120 mL, 473 mL, 946 mL, 4000 mL)

Injection, as sodium: 30 mg/mL (1 mL); 60 mg/mL (1 mL); 65 mg/mL (1 mL); 130 mg/mL (1 mL)

Luminal®: 60 mg/mL (1 mL); 130 mg/mL (1 mL)

Tablet: 15 mg, 16 mg, 30 mg, 32 mg, 60 mg, 65 mg, 100 mg

References

Relling MV, Pui CH, Sandlund JT, et al, "Adverse Effect of Anticonvulsants on Efficacy of Chemotherapy for Acute Lymphoblastic Leukaemia," Lancet, 2000, 356(9226):285-90.

♦ **Phenobarbital, Hyoscyamine, Atropine, and Scopolamine** see Hyoscyamine, Atropine, Scopolamine, and Phenobarbital on page 519

♦ **Phenobarbitone** see Phenobarbital on page 785

♦ **Phenoptic®** see Phenylephrine on page 789

Phenoxybenzamine (fen oks ee BEN za meen)

Related Information

Overdose and Toxicology on page 1222

U.S. Brand Names Dibenzyline®

Therapeutic Category Alpha-Adrenergic Blocking Agent, Oral; Antihypertensive Agent; Vasodilator

Generic Available No

Use Symptomatic management of hypertension and sweating in patients with pheochromocytoma

Pregnancy Risk Factor C

Contraindications Shock

Precautions Use with caution in patients with renal dysfunction, cerebral or coronary arteriosclerosis

Adverse Reactions

Cardiovascular: Postural hypotension, tachycardia, syncope, shock

Central nervous system: Lethargy, headache, dizziness

Gastrointestinal: Vomiting, nausea, diarrhea

Neuromuscular & skeletal: Weakness

Ocular: Miosis

Respiratory: Nasal congestion

Drug Interactions Antagonizes effects of alpha-adrenergic stimulating sympathomimetic agents

(Continued)

Phenoxybenzamine *(Continued)*

Mechanism of Action Produces long-lasting noncompetitive alpha-adrenergic blockade of postganglionic synapses in exocrine glands and smooth muscle

Pharmacodynamics Oral:
Onset of action: Within 2 hours
Peak effect: Within 4-6 hours
Duration: Effects can continue for up to 4 days

Pharmacokinetics
Absorption: Oral: ~20% to 30%
Distribution: Distributes to and may accumulate in adipose tissues
Half-life: Adults: 24 hours
Elimination: Primarily in urine and bile

Usual Dosage Oral:
Children: Initial: 0.2 mg/kg once daily; maximum dose: 10 mg/dose; increase every 4 days by 0.2 mg/kg/day increments; usual maintenance dose: 0.4-1.2 mg/kg/day every 6-8 hours; maximum doses of up to 2-4 mg/kg/day have been recommended

Adults: Initial: 10 mg twice daily; increase dose every other day to usual dose of 10-40 mg every 8-12 hours; higher doses may be needed

Administration Oral: May administer with milk to decrease GI upset

Monitoring Parameters Blood pressure, orthostasis, heart rate

Patient Information Avoid alcohol; may cause dizziness; avoid sudden changes in posture; may cause nasal congestion and constricted pupils; avoid cough, cold, or allergy medications containing sympathomimetics

Dosage Forms Capsule, as hydrochloride: 10 mg

Extemporaneous Preparations
A 2 mg/mL oral liquid preparation made from capsules and with 1% propylene glycol and 0.15% citric acid in distilled water was stable for 7 days when stored in amber glass prescription bottles under refrigeration (4°C). The vehicle is made by dissolving 150 mg of citric acid in a minimal amount of distilled water; then 1 mL of propylene glycol is added and the solution is mixed well; qsad to 100 mL with distilled water. Grind the contents of two 10 mg capsules in a mortar into a fine powder; add a small amount of the vehicle and mix well; transfer to a graduated cylinder and qsad with vehicle to 10 mL; transfer to an amber glass prescription bottle with tight-fitting cap; label "shake well" and "refrigerate" (Lim, 1997).

A stock solution of 10 mg/mL in propylene glycol was stable for 30 days when stored under refrigeration (4°C); when this stock solution was diluted 1:4 (v/v) with syrup (66.7% sucrose) to 2 mg/mL, the preparation was stable for 1 hour at 4°C (see Lim, 1997). **Note**: Although the stock solution is stable for 30 days, it **must be diluted** before administration to decrease the amount of propylene glycol delivered to the patient.

Lim LY, Tan LL, Chan EW, et al "Stability of Phenoxybenzamine Hydrochloride in Various Vehicles," *Am J Health Syst Pharm*, 1997, 54(18):2073-8.

♦ **Phenoxymethyl Penicillin** *see* Penicillin V Potassium *on page 774*

Phentolamine *(fen TOLE a meen)*

Related Information
Extravasation Treatment *on page 1085*
Overdose and Toxicology *on page 1222*

Canadian Brand Names Rogitine

Therapeutic Category Alpha-Adrenergic Blocking Agent, Parenteral; Antidote, Extravasation; Antihypertensive Agent; Diagnostic Agent, Pheochromocytoma; Vasodilator

Generic Available Yes

Use Diagnosis of pheochromocytoma; treatment of hypertension associated with pheochromocytoma or other causes of excess sympathomimetic amines; local treatment of dermal necrosis after extravasation of drugs with alpha-adrenergic effects (dobutamine, dopamine, epinephrine, metaraminol, norepinephrine, phenylephrine)

Pregnancy Risk Factor C

Contraindications Hypersensitivity to phentolamine or any component; renal impairment; coronary or cerebral arteriosclerosis; MI

Precautions Use with caution in patients with gastritis, peptic ulcer; history of cardiac arrhythmias; MI, cerebrovascular spasm, and cerebrovascular occlusion may occur

Adverse Reactions
Cardiovascular: Hypotension, tachycardia, angina, arrhythmias
Central nervous system: Dizziness, headache
Gastrointestinal: Nausea, vomiting, diarrhea, exacerbation of peptic ulcer

Neuromuscular & skeletal: Weakness
Respiratory: Nasal congestion

Stability Reconstituted solution is stable for 48 hours at room temperature and 1 week when refrigerated

Mechanism of Action Competitively blocks alpha-adrenergic receptors to produce brief antagonism of circulating epinephrine and norepinephrine; reduces hypertension caused by alpha effects of catecholamines; also has positive inotropic and chronotropic effects on the heart

Pharmacodynamics
Onset of action:
I.M.: Within 15-20 minutes
I.V.: Immediate
Peak effect:
I.M.: Within 20 minutes
I.V.: Within 2 minutes
Duration:
I.M.: 30-45 minutes
I.V.: Within 15-30 minutes

Pharmacokinetics
Metabolism: In the liver
Half-life: Adults: 19 minutes
Elimination: 10% to 13% excreted in urine as unchanged drug

Usual Dosage
Treatment of alpha-adrenergic drug extravasation: S.C.:
Neonates: Infiltrate area with a small amount (eg, 1 mL) of solution (made by diluting 2.5-5 mg in 10 mL of preservative free NS) within 12 hours of extravasation; do not exceed 0.1 mg/kg or 2.5 mg total
Infants, Children, and Adults: Infiltrate area with a small amount (eg, 1 mL) of solution (made by diluting 5-10 mg in 10 mL of NS) within 12 hours of extravasation; do not exceed 0.1-0.2 mg/kg or 5 mg total
Diagnosis of pheochromocytoma: I.M., I.V.:
Children: 0.05-0.1 mg/kg/dose, maximum single dose: 5 mg
Adults: 5 mg
Hypertension (prior to surgery for pheochromocytoma): I.M., I.V.:
Children: 0.05-0.1 mg/kg/dose given 1-2 hours before pheochromocytomectomy; repeat as needed to control blood pressure; maximum single dose: 5 mg
Adults: 5 mg given 1-2 hours before pheochromocytomectomy; repeat as needed to control blood pressure
Hypertensive crisis due to MAO inhibitor/sympathomimetic amine interaction: I.M., I.V.: Adults: 5-20 mg

Administration Parenteral: Treatment of extravasation: Infiltrate area of extravasation with multiple small injections of a diluted solution (see Usual Dosage); use 27- or 30-gauge needles and change needle between each skin entry; do not inject a volume such that swelling of the extremity or digit with resultant compartment syndrome occurs

Monitoring Parameters Blood pressure, heart rate, orthostasis; treatment of extravasation: site of extravasation, skin color, local perfusion

Nursing Implications When drugs with alpha-adrenergic effects extravasate, they cause local vasoconstriction which causes blanching of the skin and a pale, cold, hard appearance; S.C. phentolamine blocks the alpha-adrenergic receptors and reverses the vasoconstriction; the extravasation area should "pink up" and return to normal skin color; monitor the site of extravasation closely, as repeat doses of S.C. phentolamine may be needed

Additional Information Injection contains mannitol 25 mg/vial

Dosage Forms Powder for injection, as mesylate: 5 mg

♦ **Phenylalanine Mustard** *see* Melphalan *on page 626*
♦ **Phenylazo Diamino Pyridine** *see* Phenazopyridine *on page 784*
♦ **4-Phenylbutyric Acid Sodium** *see* Sodium Phenylbutyrate *on page 907*

Phenylephrine (fen il EF rin)

Related Information
Extravasation Treatment *on page 1085*
OTC Cough & Cold Preparations, Pediatric *on page 1072*
Promethazine and Phenylephrine *on page 839*

U.S. Brand Names AK-Dilate®; AK-Nefrin®; Medicone® [OTC]; Mydfrin®; Neo-Synephrine® Injectable; Neo-Synephrine® Nasal [OTC]; Neo-Synephrine® Ophthalmic; Nostril® [OTC]; Ocu-Phrin®; Phenoptic®; Prefrin™ Liquifilm®; Relief®; Rhinall® [OTC]; Vicks® Sinex® [OTC]

(Continued)

Phenylephrine *(Continued)*

Canadian Brand Names Dionephrine; Minims-Phenylephrine; Prefrin

Therapeutic Category Adrenergic Agonist Agent; Adrenergic Agonist Agent, Ophthalmic; Alpha-Adrenergic Agonist; Nasal Agent, Vasoconstrictor; Ophthalmic Agent, Mydriatic; Sympathomimetic

Generic Available Yes

Use Treatment of hypotension and vascular failure in shock; supraventricular tachycardia; as a vasoconstrictor in regional analgesia; symptomatic relief of nasal and nasopharyngeal mucosal congestion; as a mydriatic in ophthalmic procedures and treatment of wide-angle glaucoma

Pregnancy Risk Factor C

Contraindications Pheochromocytoma, severe hypertension, ventricular tachycardia; hypersensitivity to phenylephrine or any component; acute pancreatitis, hepatitis; peripheral or mesenteric vascular thrombosis, myocardial disease, severe coronary disease, narrow-angle glaucoma (ophthalmic preparation)

Warnings Injection may contain sulfites which may cause allergic reactions in some patients; do not use if solution turns brown or contains a precipitate

Precautions Pressor therapy is **not** a substitute for replacement of blood, plasma, and body fluids in shock; use with caution in patients with hyperthyroidism, bradycardia, partial heart block, myocardial disease, or severe arteriosclerosis; infuse into large veins to prevent extravasation which may cause severe necrosis

Adverse Reactions

Cardiovascular: Hypertension, angina, reflex severe bradycardia, arrhythmias, peripheral vasoconstriction

Central nervous system: Restlessness, excitability, headache, anxiety, nervousness, dizziness

Dermatologic: Pilomotor response, skin blanching

Local: Necrosis if extravasation occurs

Neuromuscular & skeletal: Tremor

Ocular: (Ophthalmic preparation): Transient stinging, browache, blurred vision, photophobia, lacrimation

Respiratory: Respiratory distress, rebound nasal congestion, sneezing, burning, stinging, dryness

Drug Interactions With alpha- and beta-adrenergic blocking agents, may see decreased actions; with oxytocic drugs, may see increased actions; with sympathomimetics and halogenated hydrocarbon anesthetics, tachycardia or arrhythmias may occur; with MAO inhibitors, guanethidine, and bretylium, actions may be potentiated

Stability Compatible when admixed with dextrose, dextrose-saline, Ringer's, LR, NS, and 1/6 M sodium lactate injection

Mechanism of Action Potent, direct-acting alpha-adrenergic stimulator with weak beta-adrenergic activity; causes vasoconstriction of the arterioles of the nasal mucosa and conjunctiva; activates the dilator muscle of the pupil to cause contraction; produces systemic arterial vasoconstriction

Pharmacodynamics

Onset of action:

I.M.: Within 10-15 minutes

I.V.: Following parenteral injection, effects occur immediately

S.C.: 10-15 minutes

Duration:

I.M.: 30 minutes to 2 hours

I.V.: 15-20 minutes

S.C.: 1 hour

Pharmacokinetics

Metabolism: In the liver and intestine by the enzyme monoamine oxidase

Half-life: 2.5 hours

Elimination: Metabolites, routes, and rates of excretion have not been identified

Usual Dosage

Ophthalmic procedures:

Infants <1 year: Instill 1 drop of 2.5% 15-30 minutes before procedures

Children and Adults: Instill 1 drop of 2.5% or 10% solution, may repeat in 10-60 minutes as needed

Nasal decongestant (therapy should not exceed 3-5 days):

Infants >6 months: 1-2 drops of 0.16% every 3 hours

Children:

1-6 years: 2-3 drops every 4 hours of 0.125% solution as needed

6-12 years: 2-3 drops every 4 hours of 0.25% solution as needed

Children >12 years and Adults: 2-3 drops or 1-2 sprays every 4 hours of 0.25% to 0.5% solution as needed; 1% solution may be used in adults in cases of extreme nasal congestion

Hypotension/shock:

Children:

I.M., S.C.: 0.1 mg/kg/dose every 1-2 hours as needed (maximum dose: 5 mg)

I.V. bolus: 5-20 mcg/kg/dose every 10-15 minutes as needed

I.V. infusion: 0.1-0.5 mcg/kg/minute, titrate to desired effect

Adults:

I.M., S.C.: 2-5 mg/dose every 1-2 hours as needed (initial dose should not exceed 5 mg)

I.V. bolus: 0.1-0.5 mg/dose every 10-15 minutes as needed (initial dose should not exceed 0.5 mg)

I.V. infusion: 100-180 mcg/minute, titrate to desired effect; once stabilized, a maintenance rate of 40-60 mcg/minute is usually effective

Paroxysmal supraventricular tachycardia: I.V.:

Children: 5-10 mcg/kg over 20-30 seconds

Adults: 0.25-0.5 mg over 20-30 seconds

Administration

Intranasal: Spray or apply drops into each nostril while gently occluding the other

Ophthalmic: Instill drops into conjunctival sac of affected eye(s); avoid contact of bottle tip with skin or eye; finger pressure should be applied to the lacrimal sac during and for 1-2 minutes after instillation to decrease risk of absorption and systemic reactions

Parenteral: For direct I.V. administration, dilute to 1 mg/mL by adding 1 mL to 9 mL of sterile water, then administer dose over 20-30 seconds; continuous infusion concentrations are usually 20-60 mcg/mL by adding 5 mg to 250 mL I.V. solution (20 mcg/mL) or 15 mg to 250 mL (60 mcg/mL); rate of infusion (mL/hour) = dose (mcg/kg/minute) x weight (kg) x 60 minutes/hour divided by concentration (mcg/mL); administer into a large vein to prevent the possibility of extravasation; use infusion device to control rate of flow; administration into an umbilical arterial catheter is **not** recommended

Monitoring Parameters Heart rate, blood pressure, central venous pressure, arterial blood gases

Nursing Implications Extravasant; avoid I.V. infiltration; extravasation may be treated with local infiltration of phentolamine 5-10 mg diluted in 10-15 mL saline solution

Dosage Forms

Injection, as hydrochloride: 1% [10 mg/mL] (1 mL, 5 mL, 10 mL)

Neo-Synephrine®: 1% [10 mg/mL] (1 mL)

Nasal solution, as hydrochloride:

Drops:

Neo-Synephrine®, Rhinall®: 0.25% (15 mL, 30 mL)

Neo-Synephrine®: 0.5% (15 mL, 30 mL); 1% (15 mL)

Spray:

Neo-Synephrine®, Nostril®, Rhinall®: 0.25% (15 mL, 40 mL)

Neo-Synephrine®, Nostril®, Vicks® Sinex®: 0.5% (15 mL, 30 mL)

Neo-Synephrine®: 1% (15 mL)

Solution, ophthalmic, as hydrochloride:

AK-Nefrin®, Prefrin™ Liquifilm®, Relief®: 0.12% (0.3 mL, 15 mL, 20 mL)

AK-Dilate®, Mydfrin®, Neo-Synephrine®, Ocu-Phrin®, Phenoptic®: 2.5% (2 mL, 3 mL, 5 mL, 15 mL)

AK-Dilate®, Neo-Synephrine®, Neo-Synephrine® Viscous, Ocu-Phrin®: 10% (5 mL, 15 mL)

♦ **Phenylephrine and Cyclopentolate** see Cyclopentolate and Phenylephrine on page 280

♦ **Phenylephrine and Promethazine** see Promethazine and Phenylephrine on page 839

♦ **Phenylephrine, Promethazine, and Codeine** see Promethazine, Phenylephrine, and Codeine on page 840

♦ **Phenylethylmalonylurea** see Phenobarbital on page 785

♦ **Phenylisohydantoin** see Pemoline on page 767

Phenytoin (FEN i toyn)

Related Information

Adult ACLS Algorithm, Stable Ventricular Tachycardia on page 1047

Antiepileptic Drugs on page 1208

Blood Level Sampling Time Guidelines on page 1220

(Continued)

Phenytoin *(Continued)*

Carbohydrate and Alcohol Content of Liquid Medications for Use in Patients Receiving Ketogenic Diets *on page 1258*
Fosphenytoin *on page 458*
Overdose and Toxicology *on page 1222*

U.S. Brand Names Dilantin®

Canadian Brand Names Tremytoine

Synonyms Diphenylhydantoin; DPH

Therapeutic Category Antiarrhythmic Agent, Class I-B; Anticonvulsant, Hydantoin

Generic Available Yes

Use Management of generalized tonic-clonic (grand mal), simple partial and complex partial seizures; prevention of seizures following head trauma/neurosurgery; ventricular arrhythmias, including those associated with digitalis intoxication, prolonged QT interval and surgical repair of congenital heart diseases in children; epidermolysis bullosa

Pregnancy Risk Factor D

Contraindications Hypersensitivity to phenytoin or any component; heart block, sinus bradycardia

Precautions Use with caution in patients with porphyria; discontinue if rash or lymphadenopathy occurs; modify dosage in patients with hepatic or renal dysfunction

Adverse Reactions

Dose-related:

Central nervous system: Slurred speech, dizziness, drowsiness, lethargy, coma, ataxia, dyskinesias

Ocular: Nystagmus, blurred vision, diplopia

Cardiovascular: I.V.: Hypotension, bradycardia, arrhythmias, cardiovascular collapse (especially with rapid I.V. use)

Central nervous system: Fever, mood changes

Dermatologic: Hirsutism, coarsening of facial features, Stevens-Johnson syndrome, rash, exfoliative dermatitis

Endocrine & metabolic: Folic acid depletion, hyperglycemia

Gastrointestinal: Nausea, vomiting, gingival hyperplasia, gum tenderness

Hematologic: Blood dyscrasias, pseudolymphoma, lymphoma

Hepatic: Hepatitis

Local: Venous irritation and pain, thrombophlebitis

Neuromuscular & skeletal: Peripheral neuropathy, osteomalacia

Miscellaneous: Lymphadenopathy, SLE-like syndrome

Drug Interactions Cytochrome P-450 isoenzyme CYP2C9 and CYP2C19 substrate; CYP2Cs, CYP3A3/4, and CYP3A5-7 isoenzyme inducer

Phenytoin may decrease the serum concentration or effectiveness of lamotrigine, ritonavir, saquinavir, delavirdine, felbamate, valproic acid, ethosuximide, primidone, warfarin, oral contraceptives, corticosteroids, teniposide, etoposide, doxorubicin, vincristine, methotrexate, cyclosporine, theophylline, chloramphenicol, rifampin, doxycycline, quinidine, mexiletine, disopyramide, dopamine, or nondepolarizing skeletal muscle relaxants; protein binding of phenytoin can be affected by valproic acid or salicylates; serum phenytoin concentrations may be increased by cimetidine, chloramphenicol, felbamate, zidovudine, isoniazid, trimethoprim, or sulfonamides and decreased by rifampin, zidovudine, cisplatin, vinblastine, bleomycin, antacids (concurrent administration), folic acid, or continuous NG feeds; suspected interaction with nevirapine (monitor closely); ritonavir may affect the metabolism of phenytoin

Food Interactions Tube feedings decrease phenytoin bioavailability; to avoid decreased serum levels with continuous NG feeds, hold feedings for 2 hours prior to and 2 hours after phenytoin administration, if possible; phenytoin may increase the metabolism of vitamins D and K; dietary requirements of vitamins D, K, B_{12}, folate, and calcium may be increased with long-term use; high doses of folate may decrease bioavailability of phenytoin; avoid giving calcium or magnesium supplements at the same time as phenytoin, space administration by ≥2 hours

Stability Parenteral solution may be used as long as there is no precipitate and it is not hazy; slightly yellowed solution may be used; refrigeration may cause precipitate, sometimes the precipitate is resolved by allowing the solution to reach room temperature again; drug may precipitate with pH ≤11.5; do not mix with other medications; may dilute with NS for I.V. infusion, but must be diluted to a concentration <6 mg/mL

Mechanism of Action Stabilizes neuronal membranes and decreases seizure activity by increasing efflux or decreasing influx of sodium ions across cell membranes in the motor cortex during generation of nerve impulses; prolongs effective refractory period and suppresses ventricular pacemaker automaticity, shortens action potential in the heart

Pharmacokinetics

Absorption: Oral: Slow, variable; decreased in neonates

Distribution: V_d:

Neonates:

Premature: 1-1.2 L/kg

Full-term: 0.8-0.9 L/kg

Infants: 0.7-0.8 L/kg

Children: 0.7 L/kg

Adults: 0.6-0.7 L/kg

Protein binding: Adults: 90% to 95%; increased free fraction (decreased protein binding) in neonates (up to 20% free), infants (up to 15% free), and patients with hyperbilirubinemia, hypoalbuminemia, renal dysfunction, or uremia

Metabolism: Follows dose-dependent (Michaelis-Menten) pharmacokinetics; "apparent" or calculated half-life is dependent upon serum concentration, therefore, metabolism is best described in terms of K_m and V_{max}; V_{max} is increased in infants >6 months and children compared to adults; major metabolite (via oxidation) HPPA undergoes enterohepatic recycling and elimination in urine as glucuronides

Bioavailability: Formulation dependent

Time to peak serum concentration: Oral: Dependent upon formulation

Extended release capsule: Within 4-12 hours

Immediate release preparation: Within 2-3 hours

Elimination: <5% excreted unchanged in urine; increased clearance and decreased serum concentrations with febrile illness; highly variable clearance, dependent upon intrinsic hepatic function and dose administered

Usual Dosage

Status epilepticus: I.V.:

Loading dose:

Neonates: 15-20 mg/kg in a single or divided dose;

Infants, Children, and Adults: 15-18 mg/kg in a single or divided dose

Maintenance dose, anticonvulsant (**Note:** Maintenance dose usually starts 12 hours after the loading dose):

Neonates: Initial: 5 mg/kg/day in 2 divided doses; usual: 5-8 mg/kg/day in 2 divided doses; some patients may require dosing every 8 hours

Infants and Children: Initial: 5 mg/kg/day in 2-3 divided doses; usual doses:

0.5-3 years: 8-10 mg/kg/day

4-6 years: 7.5-9 mg/kg/day

7-9 years: 7-8 mg/kg/day

10-16 years: 6-7 mg/kg/day

Some patients require every 8 hours dosing due to fast apparent half-life

Adults: Usual: 300 mg/day or 4-6 mg/kg/day in 2-3 divided doses

Anticonvulsant: Infants, Children and Adults: Oral:

Loading dose: 15-20 mg/kg; based on phenytoin serum concentrations and recent dosing history; administer oral loading dose in 3 divided doses given every 2-4 hours to decrease GI adverse effects and to ensure complete oral absorption

Maintenance dose: Same as I.V. maintenance dose/day listed above. Divide daily dose into 3 doses/day when using suspension, chewable tablets or nonextended release preparations. Extended release preparations may be dosed in adults every 12 or 24 hours if patient is not receiving concomitant enzyme-inducing drugs and apparent half-life is sufficiently long.

Arrhythmias:

Children and Adults: Loading dose: I.V.: 1.25 mg/kg every 5 minutes, may repeat up to total loading dose: 15 mg/kg

Children: Maintenance dose: Oral, I.V.: 5-10 mg/kg/day in 2-3 divided doses

Adults: Loading dose: Oral: 250 mg 4 times/day for 1 day, 250 mg twice daily for 2 days, then maintenance at 300-400 mg/day in divided doses 1-4 times/day

Administration

Oral: May administer with food or milk to decrease GI upset; but to ensure consistent absorption, phenytoin should be administered at the same time with regards to meals; shake oral suspension well prior to each dose; separate administration of antacids or tube feedings and oral phenytoin by 2 hours

Parenteral: I.V.: Neonates: Do not exceed I.V. infusion rate of 0.5 mg/kg/minute; Infants, Children, Adults: Do not exceed I.V. infusion rate of 1-3 mg/kg/minute, maximum rate: 50 mg/minute; I.V. injections should be followed by NS flushes through the same needle or I.V. catheter to avoid local irritation of the vein; I.V. intermittent infusion: Dilute with NS to a concentration <6 mg/mL, use an in-line

(Continued)

Phenytoin *(Continued)*

0.22 micron filter; avoid extravasation; avoid I.M. use due to erratic absorption, pain on injection, and precipitation of drug at injection site

Monitoring Parameters Serum concentrations, CBC with differential, liver enzymes; blood pressure with I.V. use; free and total serum concentrations in patients with hyperbilirubinemia, hypoalbuminemia, renal dysfunction, or uremia

Reference Range

Neonates: Therapeutic: 8-15 μg/mL

Children and Adults:

Therapeutic: 10-20 μg/mL (SI: 40-79 μmol/L); toxicity is measured clinically, some patients require levels outside the suggested therapeutic range

Toxic: >20 μg/mL (SI: >79 μmol/L)

Lethal: >100 μg/mL (SI: >400 μmol/L)

Commonly accepted therapeutic free (unbound) concentration: 1-2 μg/mL

Patient Information Avoid alcohol; do not change brand or dosage without consulting physician; maintain good oral hygiene

Additional Information The 30 mg/5 mL oral suspension is no longer made; injection contains propylene glycol and benzyl alcohol; possible permanent cerebellum damage may occur with chronic toxic serum concentrations

A recent study (Relling, 2000) demonstrated that enzyme-inducing antiepileptic drugs (AEDs) (carbamazepine, phenobarbital, and phenytoin) increased systemic clearance of antileukemic drugs (teniposide and methotrexate) and were associated with a worse event-free survival, CNS relapse, and hematologic relapse, (ie, lower efficacy), in B-lineage ALL children receiving chemotherapy; the authors recommend using nonenzyme-inducing AEDs in patients receiving chemotherapy for ALL.

Dosage Forms

Capsule, as sodium:

Extended: 30 mg, 100 mg

Prompt: 100 mg

Injection, as sodium: 50 mg/mL (2 mL, 5 mL)

Suspension, oral: 125 mg/5 mL (240 mL)

Tablet, chewable: 50 mg

References

Bauer LA and Blouin RA, "Phenytoin Michaelis-Menten Pharmacokinetics in Caucasian Pediatric Patients," *Clin Pharmacokinet,* 1983, 8(6):545-9.

Chiba K, Ishizaki T, Miura H, et al, "Michaelis-Menten Pharmacokinetics of Diphenylhydantoin and Application in the Pediatric Age Patient," *J Pediatr,* 1980, 96(3 Pt 1):479-84.

Relling MV, Pui CH, Sandlund JT, et al, "Adverse Effect of Anticonvulsants on Efficacy of Chemotherapy for Acute Lymphoblastic Leukaemia," *Lancet,* 2000, 356(9226):285-90.

Suzuki Y, Mimaki T, Cox S, et al, "Phenytoin Age-Dose-Concentration Relationship in Children," *Ther Drug Monit,* 1994, 16(2):145-50.

- ◆ **Phillips'**® **Milk of Magnesia [OTC]** *see* Magnesium Supplements *on page 614*
- ◆ **Phillips'**® **M-O [OTC]** *see* Magnesium Supplements *on page 614*
- ◆ **pHisoHex**® *see* Hexachlorophene *on page 495*
- ◆ **Phos-Flur**® *see* Fluoride *on page 441*
- ◆ **Phos-Flur**® **Rinse [OTC]** *see* Fluoride *on page 441*
- ◆ **PhosLo**® **Posture**® **[OTC]** *see* Calcium Supplements *on page 167*

Phosphate Supplements *(FOS fate SUP la ments)*

U.S. Brand Names Fleet® Enema [OTC]; Fleet® Phospho®-Soda [OTC]; K-Phos® M.F.; K-Phos® Neutral; K-Phos® No. 2; K-Phos® Original; Neutra-Phos® [OTC]; Neutra-Phos®-K [OTC]; Uro-KP-Neutral®

Available Salts Potassium Acid Phosphate; Potassium Phosphate; Potassium Phosphate and Sodium Phosphate; Sodium Phosphate

Therapeutic Category Electrolyte Supplement, Oral; Electrolyte Supplement, Parenteral; Laxative, Saline; Phosphate Salt; Potassium Salt; Sodium Salt; Urinary Acidifying Agent

Generic Available Yes

Use Treatment and prevention of hypophosphatemia; short-term treatment of constipation (oral/rectal); evacuation of the colon for rectal and bowel exams; source of phosphate in large volume I.V. fluids; urinary acidifier (potassium acid phosphate) for reduction in formation of calcium stones

Pregnancy Risk Factor C

Contraindications Hyperphosphatemia, hyperkalemia (potassium salt form), hypocalcemia, hypomagnesemia, hypernatremia (sodium salt form), severe renal impairment, severe tissue trauma, heat cramps, CHF, abdominal pain (rectal forms), fecal impaction (rectal forms); patients with infected phosphate kidney stones

Warnings Parenteral **potassium** salt forms: should be administered only in patients with adequate urine flow; must be diluted before I.V. use and infused slowly (see Administration), and patients must be on a cardiac monitor during intermittent infusions

Precautions Use with caution in patients with renal impairment, patients receiving potassium-sparing drugs (potassium salt forms), patients with adrenal insufficiency, cirrhosis

Adverse Reactions

Cardiovascular: Hypotension, edema; **potassium salt form:** arrhythmias, heart block, cardiac arrest

Central nervous system: Tetany, mental confusion, seizures, dizziness, headache

Endocrine & metabolic: Hyperphosphatemia, hyperkalemia **(potassium salt form)**, hypocalcemia, hypernatremia **(sodium salt form)**

Gastrointestinal: Nausea, vomiting, diarrhea, flatulence (oral use)

Local: Phlebitis (parenteral forms)

Neuromuscular & skeletal: Paresthesia, bone and joint pain, arthralgia, weakness, muscle cramps

Renal: Acute renal failure

Drug Interactions Do not give orally at the same time as aluminum- and magnesium-containing antacids or sucralfate which can act as phosphate binders; use of potassium phosphate with potassium-sparing diuretics, ACE inhibitors, or salt substitutes may result in hyperkalemia

Food Interactions Avoid giving with oxalate (ie, berries, nuts, chocolate, beans, celery, tomatoes) or phytate-containing foods (ie, bran, whole wheat)

Stability Phosphate salts may precipitate when mixed with calcium salts; solubility is improved in amino acid parenteral nutrition solutions; check with a pharmacist to determine compatibility

Mechanism of Action Phosphorus participates in bone deposition, calcium metabolism, utilization of B complex vitamins, and as a buffer in acid-base equilibrium; as a laxative, exerts osmotic effect in the small intestine by drawing water into the lumen of the gut, producing distension, promoting peristalsis, and evacuation of the bowel

Pharmacodynamics Onset of action (catharsis):

Oral: 3-6 hours

Rectal: 2-5 minutes

Pharmacokinetics

Absorption: Oral: 1% to 20%

Elimination: Oral forms excreted in feces; I.V. forms are excreted in the urine with over 80% of dose reabsorbed by the kidney

Usual Dosage Note: Phosphate supplements are either sodium or potassium salt forms. Consider the contribution of these electrolytes also when determining appropriate phosphate replacement.

Phosphorus: See table.

Phosphorus - Recommended Daily Allowance (RDA) and Estimated Average Requirement (EAR)

Age	RDA (mmol/day)	EAR (mmol/day)
0-6 mo	–	3.2*
7-12 mo	–	8.9*
1-3 y	14.8	12.3
4-8 y	16.1	13.1
9-18 y	40.3	34
19-30 y	22.6	18.7

*Adequate intake (AI)

I.V. doses should be incorporated into the patient's maintenance I.V. fluids; intermittent I.V. infusion should be reserved for severe depletion situations; requires continuous cardiac monitoring (for potassium salts). **Note:** Doses listed as mmol of **phosphate:**

Hypophosphatemia: Intermittent I.V. infusion: Treatment: It is difficult to provide concrete guidelines for the treatment of severe hypophosphatemia because the extent of total body deficits and response to therapy are difficult to predict. Aggressive doses of phosphate may result in a transient serum elevation followed by redistribution into intracellular compartments or bone tissue. It is recommended (Continued)

Phosphate Supplements *(Continued)*

that repletion of severe hypophosphatemia be done I.V. because large doses of oral phosphate may cause diarrhea and intestinal absorption may be unreliable

Children:

Low dose: 0.08 mmol/kg over 6 hours; use if losses are recent and uncomplicated

Intermediate dose: 0.16-0.24 mmol/kg over 4-6 hours; use if serum phosphorus level 0.5-1 mg/dL

High dose: 0.36 mmol/kg over 6 hours; use if serum phosphorus <0.5 mg/dL

Adults: Varying dosages: 0.15-0.3 mmol/kg/dose over 12 hours; may repeat as needed to achieve desired serum level **or**

15 mmol/dose over 2 hours; use if serum phosphorus <2 mg/dL **or**

Low dose: 0.16 mmol/kg over 4-6 hours; use if serum phosphorus level 2.3-3 mg/dL

Intermediate dose: 0.32 mmol/kg over 4-6 hours; use if serum phosphorus level 1.6-2.2 mg/dL

High dose: 0.64 mmol/kg over 8-12 hours; use if serum phosphorus <1.5 mg/dL

Maintenance:

Children:

I.V.: 0.5-1.5 mmol/kg/day

Oral: 2-3 mmol/kg/day in divided doses

Adults:

I.V.: 50-70 mmol/day

Oral: 50-150 mmol/day in divided doses

Laxative: Oral

Neutra-Phos®, Neutra-Phos®-K, or Uro-KP-Neutral®:

Children <4 years: 1 capsule or packet (250 mg phosphorus/8 mmol) 4 times/day; dilute as instructed

Children >4 years and Adults: 1-2 capsules or packets (250-500 mg phosphorus/8-16 mmol) 4 times/day; dilute as instructed

Fleet® Phospho®-Soda:® Oral:

Children 5-9 years: 5 mL as a single dose

Children 10-12 years: 10 mL as a single dose

Children ≥12 years and Adults: 20-30 mL as a single dose

Laxative: Rectal:

Fleet® Enema:

Children 2-11 years: Contents of one 2.25 oz pediatric enema as a single dose, may repeat

Children ≥12 years and Adults: Contents of one 4.5 oz enema as a single dose, may repeat

Urinary acidification: Adults: Oral (K-Phos® Original): 2 tablets 4 times/day

Administration

Oral: Administer with food to reduce the risk of diarrhea; do not swallow the capsule; contents of 1 capsule or packet should be diluted in 75 mL water before administration; administer tablets with a full glass of water; maintain adequate fluid intake; dilute oral solution with an equal volume of cool water; K-Phos® Original tablets (urinary acidifier) should be dissolved in 6-8 ounces of water before administration

Parenteral: For intermittent I.V. infusion: Peripheral line: Dilute to a maximum concentration of 0.05 mmol/mL; Central line: Dilute to a maximum concentration of 0.12 mmol/mL; maximum rate of infusion: 0.06 mmol/kg/hour; do **not** infuse with calcium containing I.V. fluids

Monitoring Parameters Serum potassium (potassium salt forms), sodium (sodium salt forms), calcium, phosphorus, renal function, reflexes; cardiac monitor (when intermittent infusion or high-dose I.V. replacement of potassium salts needed), stool output (laxative use)

Reference Range Phosphorus:

Newborns: 4.2-9 mg/dL

6 weeks to 18 months: 3.8-6.7 mg/dL

18 months to 3 years: 2.9-5.9 mg/dL

3-15 years: 3.6-5.6 mg/dL

>15 years: 2.5-5 mg/dL

Dosage Forms

Enema

Fleet® Enema: Monobasic **sodium** phosphate 19 g and dibasic sodium phosphate 7 g per 118 mL delivered dose (133 mL)

Fleet® Enema for Children: Monobasic **sodium** phosphate 9.5 g and dibasic sodium phosphate 3.5 g per 59 mL delivered dose (66 mL)

Injection:

Phosphate **(as potassium phosphate)** 3 mmol and **potassium** 4.4 mEq per mL (5 mL, 15 mL, 30 mL)

Phosphate **(as sodium phosphate)** 3 mmol and **sodium** 4 mEq per mL (5 mL, 15 mL, 30 mL, 50 mL)

Powder:

Neutra-Phos®-K: Phosphorus 250 mg [8 mmol] and **potassium** 556 mg [14.25 mEq] per packet

Neutra-Phos®: Phosphorus 250 mg [8 mmol], **potassium** 278 mg [7.125 mEq], and **sodium** 164 mg [7.125 mEq] per packet

Solution, oral (Fleet® Phospho®-Soda): Phosphate 4 mmol/mL; **sodium** phosphate 18 g and sodium biphosphate 48 g per 100 mL (45 mL, 90 mL) (96.4 mEq sodium/ 20 mL)

Tablet:

K-Phos® M.F.: Phosphorus 125.6 mg [4 mmol], **potassium** 44.5 mg [1.1 mEq], and **sodium** 67 mg [2.9 mEq]

K-Phos® Neutral: Phosphorus 250 mg [8 mmol], **potassium** 45 mg [1.1 mEq], and **sodium** 298 mg [13 mEq] per tablet

K-Phos® No. 2: Phosphorus 250 mg [8 mmol], **potassium** 88 mg [2.3 mEq], and **sodium** 134 mg [5.8 mEq]

K-Phos® Original: Phosphorus 114 mg [3.7 mmol] and **potassium** 144 mg [3.7 mEq] per tablet

Uro-KP-Neutral®: Phosphorus 250 mg [8 mmol], **potassium** 49.4 mg [1.27 mEq], and **sodium** 250.5 mg [10.9 mEq]

References

Clark CL, Sacks GS, Dickerson RN, et al, "Treatment of Hypophosphatemia in Patients Receiving Specialized Nutrition Support Using a Graduated Dosing Scheme: Results From a Prospective Clinical Trial," *Crit Care Med*, 1995, 23(9):1504-11.

"Dietary Reference Intakes for Calcium, Phosphorus, Magnesium, Vitamin D, and Fluoride. Standing Committee on the Scientific Evaluation of Dietary Reference Intakes, Food and Nutrition Board, Institute of Medicine," National Academy of Sciences, Washington, DC: National Academy Press, 1997.

Lentz RD, Brown BM, and Kjellstrand CM, "Treatment of Severe Hypophosphatemia," *Ann Intern Med*, 1978, 89(6):941-4.

Lloyd CW and Johnson CE, "Management of Hypophosphatemia," *Clin Pharm*, 1988, 7(2):123-8.

Rosen GH, Boullata JI, O'Rangers EA, et al, "Intravenous Phosphate Repletion Regimen for Critically Ill Patients With Moderate Hypophosphatemia," *Crit Care Med*, 1995, 23(7):1204-10.

◆ **Phosphonoformate** *see* Foscarnet *on page 456*

◆ **3-Phosphoryloxymethyl Phenytoin Disodium** *see* Fosphenytoin *on page 458*

◆ *p*-**Hydroxyampicillin** *see* Amoxicillin *on page 80*

◆ **Phyllocontin (Can)** *see* Aminophylline *on page 69*

◆ **Phylloquinone** *see* Phytonadione *on page 798*

Physostigmine (fye zoe STIG meen)

Related Information

Overdose and Toxicology *on page 1222*

Synonyms Eserine

Therapeutic Category Antidote, Anticholinergic Agent; Cholinergic Agent; Cholinergic Agent, Ophthalmic

Generic Available Yes: Ophthalmic

Use Reverse toxic CNS and cardiac effects caused by anticholinergics and tricyclic antidepressants; ophthalmic solution is used as a miotic in the treatment of open-angle glaucoma

Pregnancy Risk Factor C

Contraindications Hypersensitivity to physostigmine or any component; GI or GU obstruction, asthma, diabetes mellitus, gangrene, severe cardiovascular disease, active uveal inflammation or any inflammatory disease of the iris or ciliary body, glaucoma associated with iridocyclitis; patients receiving depolarizing neuromuscular blockers (eg, succinylcholine)

Warnings Because physostigmine has the potential for producing severe adverse effects, (ie, seizures, bradycardia), routine use as an antidote is controversial; atropine should be readily available to treat severe adverse effects; ophthalmic ointment may delay corneal healing, may cause loss of dark adaptation

Precautions Use with caution in patients with epilepsy, narrow-angle glaucoma, marked vagotonia, parkinsonism, bradycardia; injectable contains benzyl alcohol and bisulfites, avoid in sensitive individuals and neonates

Adverse Reactions

Cardiovascular: Palpitations, bradycardia

Central nervous system: Restlessness, hallucinations, seizures, nervousness

Dermatologic: Burning, redness

(Continued)

Physostigmine (Continued)

Gastrointestinal: Nausea, vomiting, epigastric pain, salivation, diarrhea

Neuromuscular & skeletal: Weakness, muscle twitching

Ocular: Miosis, lacrimation, stinging, burning, eye pain, browache

Respiratory: Dyspnea, bronchospasm, respiratory paralysis, pulmonary edema

Miscellaneous: Diaphoresis

Drug Interactions Additive cholinergic activity with bethanechol and methacholine; succinylcholine

Mechanism of Action Inhibits destruction of acetylcholine by acetylcholinesterase which prolongs the central and peripheral effects of acetylcholine

Pharmacodynamics

Onset of action:

Ophthalmic: Within 20-30 minutes

Parenteral: Within 3-8 minutes

Duration:

Ophthalmic: 12-36 hours

Parenteral: 30 minutes to 1 hour

Pharmacokinetics

Distribution: Widely distributed throughout the body; crosses into the CNS

Half-life: 1-2 hours

Elimination: Via hydrolysis by cholinesterases

Usual Dosage

Reversal of toxic anticholinergic effects:

Children: Reserve for life-threatening situations only: I.V.: 0.01-0.03 mg/kg/dose; may repeat after 15-20 minutes to a maximum total dose of 2 mg

Adults: I.M., I.V., S.C.: 0.5-2 mg initially, repeat every 20 minutes until response or adverse effect occurs; repeat 1-4 mg every 30-60 minutes as life-threatening signs (arrhythmias, seizures, deep come) recur

Preanesthetic reversal: Children and Adults:

I.M., I.V.: Give twice the dose, on a weight basis, of the anticholinergic drug (atropine, scopolamine)

Ophthalmic: Children and Adults: Ointment: Apply small quantity at night or up to 3 times/day

Administration

Ophthalmic: Apply ointment strip to affected eye(s); avoid contact of tube tip with skin or eye; finger pressure should be applied to lacrimal sac during and for 1-2 minutes after instillation to decrease risk of absorption and systemic reaction

Parenteral: Infuse slowly I.V. without additional dilution at a maximum rate of 0.5 mg/minute in children or 1 mg/minute in adults

Monitoring Parameters Heart rate, respiratory rate

Patient Information Burning or stinging may occur with ophthalmic application; may cause loss of dark adaptation; use with caution while driving at night or performing hazardous tasks in poor light

Dosage Forms

Injection, as salicylate: 1 mg/mL (2 mL)

Ointment, ophthalmic, as sulfate: 0.25% (3.5 g)

♦ **Phytomenadione** see Phytonadione on page 798

Phytonadione (fye toe na DYE one)

U.S. Brand Names AquaMEPHYTON®; Mephyton®

Synonyms Methylphytyl Napthoquinone; Phylloquinone; Phytomenadione; Vitamin K_1

Therapeutic Category Nutritional Supplement; Vitamin, Fat Soluble

Generic Available No

Use Prevention and treatment of hypoprothrombinemia caused by vitamin K deficiency or anticoagulant-induced hypoprothrombinemia; hemorrhagic disease of the newborn

Pregnancy Risk Factor C

Contraindications Hypersensitivity to phytonadione or any component

Warnings Ineffective in hereditary hypoprothrombinemia and hypoprothrombinemia caused by severe liver disease; severe hemolytic anemia and hyperbilirubinemia has been reported rarely in neonates following large doses (10-20 mg) of phytonadione

Precautions Severe reactions resembling anaphylaxis or hypersensitivity have occurred rarely during or immediately after I.V. administration (even with proper dilution and rate of administration); restrict I.V. administration for emergency use only; injection contains benzyl alcohol 0.9% as preservative; safe in neonates when used in appropriate doses

Adverse Reactions See Warnings and Precautions

Cardiovascular: Flushing, hypotension, cyanosis

Central nervous system: Dizziness

Gastrointestinal: GI upset, dysgeusia, hyperbilirubinemia (neonates)

Hematologic: Hemolysis

Local: Pain, edema, tenderness at injection site

Miscellaneous: Anaphylactoid reactions, diaphoresis

Respiratory: Dyspnea

Drug Interactions Antagonizes action of warfarin; mineral oil decreases phytonadione absorption

Mechanism of Action Cofactor in the liver synthesis of clotting factors (II, VII, IX, X)

Pharmacodynamics Onset of action: Blood coagulation factors increase within 6-12 hours after oral doses and within 1-2 hours following parenteral administration; after parenteral administration prothrombin time may become normal after 12-14 hours

Pharmacokinetics

Absorption: Oral: From the intestines in the presence of bile

Metabolism: Rapidly in the liver

Elimination: In bile and urine

Usual Dosage I.V. route should be restricted for emergency use only

Hemorrhagic disease of the newborn: Neonates: I.M., S.C.:

Prophylaxis: 0.5-1 mg within 1 hour of birth; may repeat if necessary 6-8 hours later

Treatment: 1-2 mg/dose/day

Oral anticoagulant overdose:

Infants and Children:

No bleeding, rapid reversal needed, patient will require further oral anticoagulant therapy: I.V., S.C.: 0.5-2 mg

No bleeding, rapid reversal needed, patient will **not** require further oral anticoagulant therapy: I.V., S.C.: 2-5 mg

Significant bleeding, not life-threatening: I.V., S.C.: 0.5-2 mg

Significant bleeding, life-threatening: I.V.: 5 mg

Adults: I.V., S.C.: 2.5-10 mg/dose (rarely up to 25-50 mg has been used); may repeat in 6-8 hours if given by I.V., S.C. route; may repeat 12-48 hours after oral route

Vitamin K deficiency due to drugs, malabsorption, or decreased synthesis of vitamin K:

Infants and Children:

Oral: 2.5-5 mg/24 hours

I.M., I.V., S.C.: 1-2 mg/dose as a single dose

Adults:

Oral: 2.5-25 mg/24 hours

I.M., I.V., S.C.: 10 mg

Minimum daily requirement: Not well established

Infants: 1-5 mcg/kg/day

Adults: 0.03 mcg/kg/day

Administration

Oral: May be administered with or without food

Parenteral: Dilute in 5-10 mL I.V. fluid (D_5W or NS) (maximum concentration: 10 mg/mL); infuse over 15-30 minutes; maximum rate of infusion: 1 mg/minute

Monitoring Parameters PT

Additional Information Phytonadione is more effective and is preferred to other vitamin K preparations in the presence of impending hemorrhage; oral absorption depends on the presence of bile salts

Dosage Forms

Injection, aqueous colloidal (AquaMEPHYTON®): 2 mg/mL (0.5 mL); 10 mg/mL (1 mL, 2.5 mL, 5 mL)

Tablet (Mephyton®): 5 mg

Extemporaneous Preparations A 1 mg/mL suspension may be made by crushing six 5 mg tablets, add 5 mL purified water and 5 mL 1% methylcellulose, mix well, add 70% sorbitol to a total volume of 30 mL; shake well, refrigerate, expected stability: 3 days.

Nahata MC and Hipple TF, *Pediatric Drug Formulations*, 4th ed, Cincinnati, OH: Harvey Whitney Books Co, 2000.

References
Michelson AD, Bovill E, Monagle P, et al, "Antithrombic Therapy in Children," *Chest*, 1998, 114(5 Suppl):748S-69S.

♦ **Pilocar**® *see Pilocarpine on page 800*

Pilocarpine (pye loe KAR peen)

U.S. Brand Names Isopto® Carpine; Ocu-Carpine®; Ocusert Pilo-20®; Ocusert Pilo-40®; Pilocar®; Pilopine HS®; Piloptic®; Pilostat®; Salagen®

Canadian Brand Names Diocarpine; Minims-Pilocarpine; Miocarpine

Therapeutic Category Cholinergic Agent; Cholinergic Agent, Ophthalmic; Ophthalmic Agent, Miotic

Generic Available Yes: Hydrochloride Solution

Use

Ophthalmic: Management of chronic simple glaucoma, chronic and acute angle-closure glaucoma; counter effects of cycloplegics

Oral: Symptomatic treatment of xerostomia caused by salivary gland hypofunction resulting from radiotherapy for cancer of the head and neck; and in Sjögren's syndrome

Pregnancy Risk Factor C

Contraindications Hypersensitivity to pilocarpine or any component; when cholinergic effects such as constriction are undesirable, eg, acute inflammatory disease of anterior chamber, acute iritis

Precautions Use with caution in patients with pre-existing retinal disease, CHF, asthma, peptic ulcer, urinary tract obstruction, Parkinson's disease, corneal abrasion, or those predisposed to retinal tears; may occasionally precipitate angle closure by increased resistance to aqueous flow from the posterior to anterior eye chamber

Adverse Reactions

Cardiovascular: Rare hypertension, tachycardia

Central nervous system: Headache

Gastrointestinal (rare): Nausea, vomiting, diarrhea, salivation

Genitourinary: Polyuria

Local: Stinging, burning

Ocular: Miosis, ciliary spasm, blurred vision, retinal detachment, photophobia, acute iritis, keratitis, corneal opacities, lacrimation, browache, conjunctival and ciliary congestion early in therapy

Miscellaneous: Hypersensitivity reactions, diaphoresis

Drug Interactions Topical NSAIDs may decrease pilocarpine effect; increased toxicities when combined with other parasympathomimetics; decreased effectiveness with anticholinergics

Mechanism of Action Directly stimulates cholinergic receptors in the eye causing miosis (by contraction of the iris sphincter), loss of accommodation (by constriction of ciliary muscle), and lowering of intraocular pressure (with decreased resistance to aqueous humor outflow)

Pharmacodynamics

Ophthalmic solution instillation: Miosis:
Onset of action: Within 10-30 minutes
Duration: 4-8 hours

Intraocular pressure reduction:
Onset of action: 1 hour
Duration: 4-12 hours

Ocusert® Pilo application: Miosis:
Onset of effect: 10-30 minutes
Maximal effects: 1.5-2 hours
Duration: 7 days

Oral: Increased salivary flow
Onset of action: 20 minutes
Peak effect: 1 hour
Duration: 3-5 hours

Usual Dosage

Ophthalmic: Children and Adults:
Gel: 0.5" (1.3 cm) ribbon applied to lower conjunctival sac once daily at bedtime; adjust dosage as required to control elevated intraocular pressure
Nitrate solution: Instill 1-2 drops 2-4 times/day
Hydrochloride solution: Instill 1-2 drops up to 6 times/day; adjust the concentration and frequency as required to control elevated intraocular pressure
To counteract the mydriatic effects of sympathomimetic agents: Instill 1 drop of a 1% solution in the affected eye
Ocular systems: Systems are labeled in terms of the mean rate of release of pilocarpine over 7 days; begin with 20 mcg/hour at night; adjust based upon response

Oral: Adults: 5 mg 3 times/day, titration up to 10 mg 3 times/day may be considered for patients who have not responded adequately

Administration

Ophthalmic gel: Instill gel into affected eye(s); close the eye for 1-2 minutes and instruct patient to roll the eyeball in all directions; avoid contact of bottle tip with eye or skin

Ophthalmic solution: Shake well before use; instill into affected eye(s); apply finger pressure to lacrimal sac during and for 1-2 minutes after instillation to decrease drainage into the nose and throat and minimize possible systemic absorption

Oral: May be administered with or without food

Monitoring Parameters Intraocular pressure, funduscopic exam, visual field testing

Patient Information May sting on instillation; notify physician of sweating, urinary retention; usually causes difficulty in dark adaptation; use caution when driving at night or doing hazardous activities in poor light

Additional Information

Ocusert® 20 mcg is approximately equivalent to 0.5% or 1% drops

Ocusert® 40 mcg is approximately equivalent to 2% or 3% drops

Dosage Forms

Gel, ophthalmic, as hydrochloride (Pilopine HS®): 4% (3.5 g)

Ocular therapeutic system

Ocusert® Pilo-20: Releases 20 mcg per hour for 1 week (8s)

Ocusert® Pilo-40: Releases 40 mcg per hour for 1 week (8s)

Solution, ophthalmic, as hydrochloride

Isopto® Carpine: 0.25% (15 mL); 8% (2 mL, 15 mL)

Isopto® Carpine, Ocu-Carpine®, Pilocar®, Piloptic®: 1% (1 mL, 2 mL, 15 mL, 30 mL); 2% (1 mL, 2 mL, 15 mL, 30 mL); 4% (1 mL, 2 mL, 15 mL, 30 mL); 6% (15 mL, 30 mL)

Ocu-Carpine®: 5% (15 mL)

Ocu-Carpine®, Pilocar®, Piloptic®: 0.5% (15 mL, 30 mL)

Ocu-Carpine®, Pilocar®: 3% (15 mL, 30 mL)

Tablet, as hydrochloride (Salagen®): 5 mg

♦ **Pilopine HS®** *see* Pilocarpine *on page 800*
♦ **Piloptic®** *see* Pilocarpine *on page 800*
♦ **Pilostat®** *see* Pilocarpine *on page 800*
♦ **Pima®** *see* Potassium Iodide *on page 815*
♦ **Pin-Rid® [OTC]** *see* Pyrantel Pamoate *on page 855*
♦ **Pin-X® [OTC]** *see* Pyrantel Pamoate *on page 855*

Piperacillin (pi PER a sil in)

U.S. Brand Names Pipracil®

Therapeutic Category Antibiotic, Penicillin (Antipseudomonal)

Generic Available No

Use Treatment of serious infections caused by susceptible strains of gram-positive, gram-negative, and anaerobic bacilli; mixed aerobic-anaerobic bacterial infections or empiric antibiotic therapy in granulocytopenic patients. Primary use is in the treatment of serious carbenicillin-resistant or ticarcillin-resistant *Pseudomonas aeruginosa* infections susceptible to piperacillin.

Pregnancy Risk Factor B

Contraindications Hypersensitivity to piperacillin, penicillins, or any component

Warnings Superinfection has been reported in up to 6% to 8% of patients receiving an extended spectrum penicillin; piperacillin therapy has been associated with an increased incidence of fever and rash in cystic fibrosis patients

Precautions Use with caution in patients with hypersensitivity to cephalosporins; dosage modification required in patients with impaired renal function

Adverse Reactions

Central nervous system: Seizures, fever, headache, dizziness, confusion, drowsiness

Dermatologic: Rash, exfoliative dermatitis

Endocrine & metabolic: Hypokalemia

Gastrointestinal: Diarrhea, vomiting

Hematologic: Hemolytic anemia, eosinophilia, neutropenia, prolonged bleeding time, thrombocytopenia

Hepatic: Elevated liver enzymes, cholestatic hepatitis

Local: Thrombophlebitis

Neuromuscular & skeletal: Myoclonus

Renal: Acute interstitial nephritis

Miscellaneous: Hypersensitivity reactions, anaphylaxis, serum sickness-like reaction

(Continued)

Piperacillin *(Continued)*

Drug Interactions Aminoglycosides (antibacterial activity is synergistic), probenecid (increases serum concentration of piperacillin), vecuronium (prolongs neuromuscular blockade)

Stability Reconstituted piperacillin solution is stable for 24 hours at room temperature and 7 days when refrigerated; incompatible with aminoglycosides

Mechanism of Action Inhibits bacterial cell wall synthesis by binding to one or more of the penicillin-binding proteins; inhibits the final transpeptidation step of peptidoglycan synthesis in bacterial cell walls

Pharmacokinetics

Absorption: I.M.: 70% to 80%

Distribution: Crosses the placenta; distributes into breast milk at low concentrations; penetration across the blood-brain barrier is poor when meninges are uninflamed; good biliary concentration (30-60 times higher than serum concentration)

Protein binding: 22%

Metabolism: 5% to 10%

Half-life: Prolonged with moderately severe renal or hepatic impairment

Neonates:

1-5 days: 3.6 hours

>6 days: 2.1-2.7 hours

Children:

1-6 months: 0.5-1 hours

6 months to 12 years: 0.39-0.5 hours

Adults: 36-80 minutes (dose-dependent)

Time to peak serum concentration: I.M.: Within 30-50 minutes

Elimination: Principally in urine and partially in feces (via bile)

Dialysis: Dialyzable (20% to 50%)

Usual Dosage Safety and efficacy in children <12 years of age has not been established

I.M., I.V.:

Neonates:

≤7 days: 150 mg/kg/day divided every 8 hours

>7 days: 200 mg/kg/day divided every 6 hours

Infants and Children: 200-300 mg/kg/day in divided doses every 4-6 hours; maximum dose: 24 g/day

Higher doses have been used in cystic fibrosis: 350-500 mg/kg/day in divided doses every 4 hours

Adults: 2-4 g/dose every 4-8 hours; maximum dose: 24 g/day

Dosing interval in renal impairment:

Cl_{cr} 20-40 mL/minute: Administer every 8 hours

Cl_{cr} <20 mL/minute: Administer every 12 hours

Administration Parenteral:

I.M.: Reconstitute each gram of piperacillin with at least 2 mL of sterile water, NS, or 0.5% or 1% lidocaine hydrochloride (without epinephrine) to make a 400 mg/mL solution; administer by deep I.M. injection into the gluteus maximus

I.V. push: Administer over 3-5 minutes at a maximum concentration of 200 mg/mL

I.V. intermittent infusion: Administer over 30-60 minutes at a final concentration ≤20 mg/mL

Monitoring Parameters Serum electrolytes, bleeding time especially in patients with renal impairment; periodic tests of renal, hepatic and hematologic function

Test Interactions False-positive urinary and serum proteins, positive Coombs' [direct]

Nursing Implications If the patient is on concurrent aminoglycoside therapy, separate piperacillin administration from the aminoglycoside by at least 30-60 minutes

Additional Information Sodium content of 1 g: 1.85 mEq

Dosage Forms Powder for injection, as sodium: 2 g, 3 g, 4 g, 40 g

References

Placzek M, Whitelaw A, Want S, et al, "Piperacillin in Early Neonatal Infection," *Arch Dis Child*, 1983, 58(12):1006-9.

Prince AS and Neu HC, "Use of Piperacillin, A Semisynthetic Penicillin, in the Therapy of Acute Exacerbations of Pulmonary Disease in Patients With Cystic Fibrosis," *J Pediatr*, 1980, 97(1):148-51.

Thirumoorthi MC, Asmar BI, Buckley JA, et al, "Pharmacokinetics of Intravenously Administered Piperacillin in Preadolescent Children," *J Pediatr*, 1983, 102(6):941-6.

Piperacillin and Tazobactam *(pi PER a sil in & ta zoe BAK tam)*

U.S. Brand Names Zosyn™

Canadian Brand Names Tazocin

Synonyms Tazobactam and Piperacillin

Therapeutic Category Antibiotic, Beta-lactam and Beta-lactamase Combination; Antibiotic, Penicillin (Antipseudomonal)

Generic Available No

Use Treatment of sepsis, gynecologic, intra-abdominal infections, and infections involving skin and skin structures, the lower respiratory tract, and urinary tract caused by piperacillin-resistant, beta-lactamase producing strains that are piperacillin/tazobactam susceptible. Tazobactam expands activity of piperacillin to include beta-lactamase producing strains of *S. aureus, H. influenzae, B. fragilis, Klebsiella, E. coli*, and *Acinetobacter*.

Pregnancy Risk Factor B

Contraindications Hypersensitivity to piperacillin, tazobactam, penicillins, or any component

Warnings Prolonged use may result in superinfection; abnormal platelet aggregation and prolonged bleeding have been reported in patients with renal failure; piperacillin therapy has been associated with an increased incidence of fever and rash in cystic fibrosis patients

Precautions Use with caution in patients with hypersensitivity to cephalosporins or other beta-lactamase inhibitors; use with caution in patients with renal impairment or pre-existing seizure disorder; dosage modification required in patients with impaired renal function

Adverse Reactions

Cardiovascular: Hypertension, hypotension, edema

Central nervous system: Insomnia, headache, dizziness, agitation, confusion, fever, convulsions

Dermatologic: Rash, pruritus, erythema multiforme

Endocrine & metabolism: Hypokalemia

Gastrointestinal: Diarrhea, constipation, nausea, vomiting, dyspepsia, melena, pseudomembranous colitis

Hematologic: Leukopenia, decrease in hemoglobin/hematocrit, eosinophilia, prolonged prothrombin time

Hepatic: Elevated AST, ALT, bilirubin; cholestatic hepatitis

Local: Phlebitis, pain

Renal: Elevated BUN, elevated serum creatinine, interstitial nephritis

Miscellaneous: Hypersensitivity reactions, anaphylaxis

Drug Interactions Probenecid prolongs half-life of piperacillin/tazobactam; vecuronium (prolongs neuromuscular blockade); aminoglycosides (antibacterial activity is synergistic)

Stability Reconstituted piperacillin/tazobactam solution is stable for 24 hours at room temperature and 2 days when refrigerated; incompatible with LR solution and aminoglycosides

Mechanism of Action Inhibits bacterial cell wall synthesis by binding to one or more of the penicillin-binding proteins; inhibits the final transpeptidation step of peptidoglycan synthesis in bacterial cell walls; tazobactam prevents degradation of piperacillin by binding to beta-lactamases

Pharmacokinetics Both AUC and peak concentrations are dose proportional

Distribution: Widely distributed into tissues and body fluids including lungs, intestinal mucosa, female reproductive tissues, interstitial fluid, gallbladder, and bile; penetration into CSF is poor when meninges are uninflamed; piperacillin is excreted into breast milk

Protein binding:

Piperacillin: ~26% to 33%

Tazobactam: 31% to 32%

Metabolism:

Piperacillin: 6% to 9%

Tazobactam: ~22%

Bioavailability: I.M.:

Piperacillin: 71%

Tazobactam: 84%

Half-life:

Piperacillin:

Infants 2-5 months: 1.4 hours

Children 6-23 months: 0.9 hour

Children 2-12 years: 0.7 hour

Adults: 0.7-1.2 hours

Metabolite: 1-1.5 hours

Tazobactam:

Infants 2-5 months: 1.6 hours

Children 6-23 months: 1 hour

(Continued)

Piperacillin and Tazobactam *(Continued)*

Children 2-12 years: 0.8-0.9 hour

Adults: 0.7-0.9 hour

Elimination: Piperacillin and tazobactam are both eliminated by renal tubular secretion and glomerular filtration

Piperacillin: 50% to 70% eliminated unchanged in urine

Tazobactam: Found in urine at 24 hours, with 22% as the inactive metabolite

Dialysis: Hemodialysis removes 30% to 40% of a piperacillin/tazobactam dose; peritoneal dialysis removes 21% of tazobactam and 6% of piperacillin; hepatic impairment does not affect the kinetics of piperacillin or tazobactam significantly

Usual Dosage Safety and efficacy in children <12 years of age has not been established

Infants <6 months of age: I.V.: 150-300 mg of piperacillin component/kg/day in divided doses every 6-8 hours

Infants and Children ≥6 months: I.V.: 240 mg of piperacillin component/kg/day in divided doses every 8 hours; higher doses have been used for serious pseudomonal infections: 300-400 mg of piperacillin component/kg/day in divided doses every 6 hours

Adults: I.V.: 3.375 g (3 g piperacillin/0.375 g tazobactam) every 6 hours

Dosing interval in renal impairment:

Cl_{cr} 20-40 mL/minute: Decrease dose by 30% and administer every 6 hours

Cl_{cr} <20 mL/minute: Decrease dose by 30% and administer every 8 hours

Hemodialysis: Adults: Administer 2.25 g every 8 hours with an additional dose of 0.75 g after each dialysis

Administration Parenteral: I.V. intermittent infusion: May administer over 30 minutes at a maximum concentration of 200 mg/mL (piperacillin component); however, concentrations ≤20 mg/mL are preferred. If the patient is on concurrent aminoglycoside therapy, separate piperacillin and tazobactam administration from the aminoglycoside by at least 30-60 minutes.

Monitoring Parameters Serum electrolytes, bleeding time especially in patients with renal impairment; periodic tests of renal, hepatic, and hematologic function

Test Interactions Positive Coombs' [direct], false-positive urinary and serum proteins; false-positive urine glucose using Clinitest®

Additional Information Sodium content of 1 g piperacillin component: 2.35 mEq

Dosage Forms Injection: Piperacillin sodium 2 g and tazobactam sodium 0.25 g; piperacillin sodium 3 g and tazobactam sodium 0.375 g; piperacillin sodium 4 g and tazobactam sodium 0.5 g (vials at an 8:1 ratio of piperacillin sodium to tazobactam sodium)

References

Bryson HM and Brogden RN, "Piperacillin/Tazobactam. A Review of its Antibacterial Activity, Pharmacokinetic Properties, and Therapeutic Potential," *Drugs*, 1994, 47(3):506-35.

Reed MD, Goldfarb J, Yamashita T, et al, "Single-Dose Pharmacokinetics of Piperacillin and Tazobactam in Infants and Children," *Antimicrob Agents Chemother*, 1994, 38(12):2817-26.

Piperazine *(PI per a zeen)*

U.S. Brand Names Vermizine®

Canadian Brand Names Entacyl; Veriga; Verimex; Versol

Therapeutic Category Anthelmintic

Generic Available Yes

Use Treatment of pinworm (*Enterobius vermicularis*) and roundworm (*Ascaris lumbricoides*) infections; used as an alternative to first-line agents mebendazole or pyrantel pamoate for the treatment of these infections

Pregnancy Risk Factor B

Contraindications Seizure disorders, liver or kidney impairment; hypersensitivity to piperazine or any component

Precautions Use with caution in patients with anemia or malnutrition or patients receiving chlorpromazine; avoid prolonged or repeated piperazine use in children due to potential neurotoxicity

Adverse Reactions

Central nervous system: Dizziness, vertigo, seizures, EEG changes, headache

Gastrointestinal: Nausea, vomiting, diarrhea, abdominal cramps

Hematologic: Hemolytic anemia

Neuromuscular & skeletal: Tremor, weakness

Ocular: Visual impairment, nystagmus

Respiratory: Cough

Miscellaneous: Hypersensitivity reactions (urticaria, erythema multiforme, photodermatitis, fever, arthralgia, bronchospasm)

Drug Interactions Pyrantel pamoate (antagonistic mode of action)

Mechanism of Action Causes muscle paralysis of the roundworm by blocking the effects of acetylcholine at the neuromuscular junction

Pharmacokinetics

Absorption: Well absorbed from the GI tract

Time to peak serum concentration: 1 hour

Elimination: In urine as metabolites and unchanged drug

Usual Dosage Oral:

Pinworms: Children and Adults: 65 mg/kg/day as a single daily dose for 7 days; in severe infections, repeat course after a 1-week interval; not to exceed 2.5 g/day

Roundworms:

Children: 75 mg/kg/day as a single daily dose for 2 days; maximum dose: 3.5 g/day; in severe infections, repeat course after a 1-week interval

Adults: 3.5 g/day for 2 days (in severe infections, repeat course, after a 1-week interval)

Administration Oral: In the case of partial or complete intestinal obstruction due to a heavy roundworm load, administer dose as a solution through a gastrointestinal tube

Monitoring Parameters Stool exam for worms and ova

Nursing Implications Cure rates may be decreased with massive infections or in patients with hypermotility of the GI tract

Dosage Forms

Tablet, as citrate: 250 mg

♦ **Pipracil**® see Piperacillin on page 801

Pirbuterol (peer BYOO ter ole)

U.S. Brand Names Maxair™; Maxair™ Autohaler™

Therapeutic Category Adrenergic Agonist Agent; Antiasthmatic; Beta$_2$-Adrenergic Agonist Agent; Bronchodilator; Sympathomimetic

Generic Available No

Use Prevention and treatment of bronchospasm in patients with reversible airway obstruction due to asthma or COPD

Pregnancy Risk Factor C

Contraindications Hypersensitivity to pirbuterol or or any component

Warnings Paradoxical bronchospasm may occur, especially with the first use of a new cannister

Precautions Use with caution in patients with hyperthyroidism, diabetes mellitus, cardiovascular disorders (including coronary insufficiency or hypertension); excessive or prolonged use can lead to tolerance

Adverse Reactions

Cardiovascular: Tachycardia, palpitations, hypertension, chest pain

Central nervous system: Nervousness, CNS stimulation, anxiety, syncope, hyperactivity, insomnia, dizziness, depression, lightheadedness, drowsiness, headache

Dermatologic: Rash, pruritus, alopecia

Endocrine & metabolic: Hypokalemia

Gastrointestinal: GI upset, xerostomia, glossitis, abdominal pain, vomiting, nausea, unusual taste, hoarseness

Neuromuscular & skeletal: Tremor, weakness, muscle cramping

Respiratory: Irritation of oropharynx, cough, paradoxical bronchospasm

Miscellaneous: Diaphoresis

Drug Interactions Action of pirbuterol is antagonized by beta-adrenergic blocking agents such as propranolol; cardiovascular effects are potentiated in patients also receiving MAO inhibitors or tricyclic antidepressants; concomitant administration of sympathomimetics may result in enhanced cardiovascular effects

Stability Store at room temperature

Mechanism of Action Relaxes bronchial smooth muscle by action on beta$_2$-adrenergic receptors with little effect on heart rate

Pharmacodynamics

Onset: 5 minutes

Peak action: 30-60 minutes

Duration: 5 hours

Pharmacokinetics

Metabolism: Liver (by sulfate conjugation)

Half-life: 2-3 hours

Elimination: 51% excreted in the urine as pirbuterol plus its sulfate conjugate

Usual Dosage Oral inhalation:

Children ≥12 years and Adults: 1-2 inhalations (0.2-0.4 mg) every 4-6 hours; do not exceed 12 inhalations/day

(Continued)

Pirbuterol *(Continued)*

Administration Oral inhalation: Shake well before administration; use spacer for children <8 years of age (Maxair™ Inhaler only); Maxair™ Autohaler™ is breath activated; after sealing lips around mouthpiece, inhale deeply with steady, moderate force; inhalation triggers the release "puff" of medication; do not stop inhalation when puff occurs, but continue to take a deep, full breath; hold breath for 10 seconds, then exhale slowly

Monitoring Parameters Serum potassium, heart rate, pulmonary function tests, respiratory rate; arterial or capillary blood gases (if patient's condition warrants)

Patient Information Do not exceed recommended dosage; rinse mouth with water following each inhalation to help with dry throat and mouth; if more than one inhalation is necessary, wait at least 1 full minute between inhalations; notify physician if palpitations, tachycardia, chest pain, muscle tremors, dizziness, headache, flushing occur, or if breathing difficulty persists

Dosage Forms Aerosol, oral, as acetate:
Maxair™ Inhaler: 0.2 mg/actuation [300 metered doses] (25.6 g)
Maxair™ Autohaler™: 0.2 mg/actuation [80 metered doses] (2.8 g); [400 metered doses] (14 g)

Piroxicam *(peer OKS i kam)*

Related Information
Overdose and Toxicology *on page 1222*

U.S. Brand Names Feldene®

Canadian Brand Names Alti-Piroxicam; Apo-Piroxicam; Brexidol; Fexicam; Gen-Piroxicam; Nu-Pirox; Pro-Piroxicam

Therapeutic Category Analgesic, Non-narcotic; Anti-inflammatory Agent; Nonsteroidal Anti-inflammatory Drug (NSAID), Oral

Generic Available Yes

Use Management of inflammatory diseases and rheumatoid disorders; dysmenorrhea

Pregnancy Risk Factor B (D if used in 3rd trimester)

Contraindications Hypersensitivity to piroxicam, any component, aspirin, or other NSAIDs; active GI bleeding

Precautions Use with caution in patients with impaired cardiac function, hypertension, impaired renal function, GI disease and patients receiving anticoagulants

Adverse Reactions
Cardiovascular: Edema
Central nervous system: Dizziness, headache
Dermatologic: Rash, phototoxic skin eruptions
Gastrointestinal: Nausea, epigastric distress, anorexia, abdominal discomfort, vomiting, GI bleeding, ulcers, perforation
Hematologic: Reduction in hemoglobin and hematocrit, inhibition of platelet aggregation
Hepatic: Hepatitis
Renal: Acute renal failure, elevated BUN, elevated serum creatinine

Drug Interactions Cytochrome P-450 isoenzyme CYP2C9 and CYP2C18 substrate
May increase serum concentrations of lithium; aspirin may decrease piroxicam serum concentrations; GI irritants (eg, potassium supplements) may increase GI adverse effects; piroxicam may decrease antihypertensive effects of ACE inhibitors or angiotensin II antagonists; drug interactions similar to other NSAIDs may also occur; concurrent use of piroxicam with ritonavir is not recommended

Food Interactions Food may decrease the rate but not the extent of absorption

Mechanism of Action Inhibits prostaglandin synthesis by decreasing the activity of the enzyme, cyclo-oxygenase, which results in decreased formation of prostaglandin precursors

Pharmacodynamics Analgesia:
Onset of action: Oral: Within 1 hour
Peak effect: 3-5 hours

Pharmacokinetics
Protein binding: 99%
Metabolism: In the liver
Half-life: 45-50 hours
Elimination: Excreted as metabolites and unchanged drug (~5% to 10%) in the urine; small amount excreted in feces

Usual Dosage Oral:
Children: 0.2-0.3 mg/kg/day once daily; maximum dose: 15 mg/day
Adults: 10-20 mg/day once daily; although associated with increase in GI adverse effects, doses >20 mg/day have been used (ie, 30-40 mg/day)

Administration Oral: May administer with food or milk to decrease GI upset

Monitoring Parameters CBC, BUN, serum creatinine, liver enzymes; periodic ophthalmologic exams with chronic use

Patient Information Avoid alcohol; avoid undo exposure to the sun, use sunscreen

Dosage Forms Capsule: 10 mg, 20 mg

Plicamycin (plye kay MYE sin)

U.S. Brand Names Mithracin®

Synonyms Mithramycin

Therapeutic Category Antidote, Hypercalcemia; Antineoplastic Agent, Antibiotic

Generic Available No

Use Malignant testicular tumors; treatment of hypercalcemia and hypercalciuria of malignancy not responsive to conventional treatment; chronic myelogenous leukemia in blast phase; Paget's disease

Pregnancy Risk Factor D

Contraindications Thrombocytopenia, bleeding diatheses, coagulation disorders, bone marrow function impairment, or hypocalcemia

Warnings The FDA currently recommends that procedures for proper handling and disposal of antineoplastic agents be considered. Discontinue therapy if bleeding or epistaxis occurs; plicamycin may cause permanent sterility and may cause birth defects.

Precautions Use with caution in patients with hepatic or renal impairment; reduce dosage in patients with renal impairment

Adverse Reactions
Cardiovascular: Facial flushing
Central nervous system: Fever, headache, malaise, dizziness, drowsiness
Dermatologic: Rash
Endocrine & metabolic: Hypocalcemia, hypophosphatemia, hypokalemia
Gastrointestinal: Anorexia, stomatitis, nausea, vomiting, diarrhea
Hematologic: Thrombocytopenia, hemorrhagic diathesis (hematemesis, hemoptysis), leukopenia, increase in fibrinolytic activity, prolonged PT
Hepatic: Hepatotoxicity, elevated AST, ALT, and LDH
Local: Phlebitis
Renal: Nephrotoxicity (elevated BUN and serum creatinine, proteinuria)
Respiratory: Epistaxis

Drug Interactions Calcitonin, etidronate, glucagon, aspirin

Stability Refrigeration is recommended but drug remains stable for up to 3 months unrefrigerated; drug is unstable at a pH <4; reconstituted solution is stable for 24 hours at room temperature and 48 hours when refrigerated; chelates divalent cations (especially iron); incompatible with trace element solution

Mechanism of Action Forms a complex with DNA in the presence of magnesium or other divalent cations inhibiting DNA-directed RNA synthesis; may inhibit parathyroid hormone effect on osteoclasts lowering serum calcium concentrations; inhibits bone resorption

Pharmacodynamics
Onset of action for decreasing serum calcium: Within 24-48 hours
Peak effect on calcium levels: 48-72 hours
Duration: 3-15 days

Pharmacokinetics
Distribution: Crosses the blood-brain barrier
Protein-binding: 0%
Half-life, plasma: 1 hour
Elimination: 90% of dose excreted in urine within the first 24 hours

Usual Dosage Adults (dose based on ideal weight): I.V. (refer to individual protocols):

Testicular cancer: 25-30 mcg/kg/day once daily for 8-10 days
Blastic chronic granulocytic leukemia: 25 mcg/kg over 2-4 hours every other day for 3 weeks
(Continued)

Plicamycin *(Continued)*

Hypercalcemia: 15-25 mcg/kg/day once daily for 3-4 days or 25 mcg/kg every 48-72 hours; additional courses of therapy may be given at intervals of 1 week or more if the initial course is unsuccessful. Reduce dose to 12.5 mcg/kg in patients with pre-existing hepatic or renal impairment

Paget's disease: 15 mcg/kg/day once daily for 10 days

Dosing adjustment in renal impairment:

Cl_{cr} 10-50 mL/minute: Decrease dosage by 25%

Cl_{cr} <10 mL/minute: Decrease dosage by 50%

Administration Parenteral: Dose should be diluted in 1 L of D_5W or NS and administered as an I.V. infusion over 4-6 hours; bolus or short infusion over 30-60 minutes in 100-150 mL D_5W is an alternative method of administration; avoid rapid I.V. push injections

Monitoring Parameters Hepatic and renal function tests, CBC, platelet count, prothrombin time; serum electrolytes, calcium and phosphorus

Patient Information Notify physician if fever, sore throat, bleeding, bruising, shortness of breath, or painful urination occur

Nursing Implications Rapid I.V. infusion has been associated with an increased incidence of nausea and vomiting; an antiemetic given prior to and during plicamycin infusion may be helpful. Avoid extravasation since local irritation and cellulitis at the injection site may result; minimize tissue irritation by applying moderate heat to the extravasation site

Additional Information Treatment of hemorrhagic episodes should include transfusion of fresh whole blood or packed red blood cells and fresh frozen plasma, vitamin K, and corticosteroids

Myelosuppressive effects:

WBC: Moderate
Platelets: Moderate
Nadir (days): 7-12
Recovery (days): 21

Dosage Forms Powder for injection: 2.5 mg

References

Mutch RS, Hutson PR, and Lewinsky DB, "Plicamycin: Bolus or Infusion?" *DICP*, 1990, 24(9):885-6.
Ritch PS, "Treatment of Cancer-Related Hypercalcemia," *Semin Oncol*, 1990, 17(2 Suppl 5):26-33.
Stumpf JL, "Pharmacologic Management of Paget's Disease," *Clin Pharm*, 1989, 8(7):485-95.

- **PMS-Amantadine (Can)** *see* Amantadine *on page 62*
- **PMS-Atenolol (Can)** *see* Atenolol *on page 111*
- **PMS-Baclofen (Can)** *see* Baclofen *on page 129*
- **PMS-Benztropine (Can)** *see* Benztropine *on page 137*
- **PMS-Bethanechol Chloride (Can)** *see* Bethanechol *on page 142*
- **PMS-Buspirone (Can)** *see* Buspirone *on page 159*
- **PMS-Captopril (Can)** *see* Captopril *on page 173*
- **PMS-Carbamazepine (Can)** *see* Carbamazepine *on page 175*
- **PMS-Cefaclor (Can)** *see* Cefaclor *on page 186*
- **PMS-Cephalexin (Can)** *see* Cephalexin *on page 207*
- **PMS-Chloral Hydrate (Can)** *see* Chloral Hydrate *on page 215*
- **PMS-Cholestyramine (Can)** *see* Cholestyramine Resin *on page 229*
- **PMS-Cimetidine (Can)** *see* Cimetidine *on page 234*
- **PMS-Clonazepam (Can)** *see* Clonazepam *on page 254*
- **PMS-Conjugated Estrogens (Can)** *see* Estrogens (Conjugated) *on page 402*
- **PMS-Cyproheptadine (Can)** *see* Cyproheptadine *on page 287*
- **PMS-Desipramine (Can)** *see* Desipramine *on page 303*
- **PMS-Dexamethasone (Can)** *see* Dexamethasone *on page 307*
- **PMS-Diazepam (Can)** *see* Diazepam *on page 320*
- **PMS-Diclofenac (Can)** *see* Diclofenac *on page 324*
- **PMS-Diphenhydramine (Can)** *see* Diphenhydramine *on page 342*
- **PMS-Dipivefrin (Can)** *see* Dipivefrin *on page 345*
- **PMS-Docusate Calcium (Can)** *see* Docusate *on page 350*
- **PMS-Docusate Sodium (Can)** *see* Docusate *on page 350*
- **PMS-Erythromycin (Can)** *see* Erythromycin *on page 394*
- **PMS-Fluoxetine (Can)** *see* Fluoxetine *on page 445*
- **PMS-Flurazepam (Can)** *see* Flurazepam *on page 449*
- **PMS-Glyburide (Can)** *see* Glyburide *on page 476*
- **PMS-Haloperidol (Can)** *see* Haloperidol *on page 488*

- **PMS-Hydromorphone (Can)** *see* Hydromorphone *on page 510*
- **PMS-Hydroxyzine (Can)** *see* Hydroxyzine *on page 516*
- **PMS-Imipramine (Can)** *see* Imipramine *on page 528*
- **PMS-Ipratropium (Can)** *see* Ipratropium *on page 547*
- **PMS-Isoniazid (Can)** *see* Isoniazid *on page 554*
- **PMS-Lactulose (Can)** *see* Lactulose *on page 571*
- **PMS-Levobunolol (Can)** *see* Levobunolol *on page 584*
- **PMS-Lidocaine Viscous (Can)** *see* Lidocaine *on page 590*
- **PMS-Lindane (Can)** *see* Lindane *on page 595*
- **PMS-Lithium Carbonate (Can)** *see* Lithium *on page 600*
- **PMS-Loperamine (Can)** *see* Loperamide *on page 603*
- **PMS-Lorazepam (Can)** *see* Lorazepam *on page 609*
- **PMS-Methylphenidate (Can)** *see* Methylphenidate *on page 653*
- **PMS-Metoprolol (Type B) (Can)** *see* Metoprolol *on page 660*
- **PMS-Metoprolol (Type L) (Can)** *see* Metoprolol *on page 660*
- **PMS-Nortriptyline (Can)** *see* Nortriptyline *on page 724*
- **PMS-Nystatin (Can)** *see* Nystatin *on page 729*
- **PMS-Oxybutynin (Can)** *see* Oxybutynin *on page 744*
- **PMS-Prochlorperazine (Can)** *see* Prochlorperazine *on page 834*
- **PMS-Pseudoephedrine (Can)** *see* Pseudoephedrine *on page 852*
- **PMS-Pyrazinamide (Can)** *see* Pyrazinamide *on page 855*
- **PMS-Salbutamol (Can)** *see* Albuterol *on page 45*
- **PMS-Sennosides (Can)** *see* Senna *on page 896*
- **PMS-Sodium Cromoglycate (Can)** *see* Cromolyn *on page 273*
- **PMS-Sodium Polystyrene Sulfonate (Can)** *see* Sodium Polystyrene Sulfonate *on page 908*
- **PMS-Sucralfate (Can)** *see* Sucralfate *on page 919*
- **PMS-Sulfasalazine (Can)** *see* Sulfasalazine *on page 926*
- **PMS-Thioridazine (Can)** *see* Thioridazine *on page 953*
- **PMS-Tobramycin (Can)** *see* Tobramycin *on page 963*
- **PMS-Trazodone (Can)** *see* Trazodone *on page 977*
- **PMS-Trihexyphenidyl (Can)** *see* Trihexyphenidyl *on page 984*
- **PMS-Valproic (Can)** *see* Valproic Acid and Derivatives *on page 998*
- **Pneumococcal Polysaccharide Vaccine, Polyvalent** *see* Pneumococcal Vaccine *on page 809*
- **Pneumococcal Vaccine** *see page 1172*

Pneumococcal Vaccine (noo moe KOK al vak SEEN)

U.S. Brand Names Pneumovax® 23; Pnu-Imune® 23

Synonyms Pneumococcal Polysaccharide Vaccine, Polyvalent

Therapeutic Category Vaccine, Inactivated Bacteria

Use Immunocompetent patients 2-64 years of age with a chronic illness (CHF, sickle cell disease, cardiomyopathy, COPD, diabetes mellitus, chronic liver disease, or CSF leak) or with functional or anatomic asplenia; immunocompromised patients ≥2 years of age with the following conditions: HIV, leukemia, lymphoma, Hodgkin's disease, generalized malignancy, chronic renal failure, nephrotic syndrome or conditions associated with immunosuppression (ie, organ transplantation or long-term corticosteroid therapy); adults ≥65 years of age

Contraindications Hypersensitivity to the vaccine or thimerosal; acute febrile illness; children <2 years of age (antibody response to the vaccine is poor in this age group); pregnancy

Warnings Epinephrine injection (1:1000) must be immediately available in case of anaphylaxis; may cause relapse in patients with stable idiopathic thrombocytopenia purpura

Adverse Reactions

Central nervous system: Low grade fever, Guillain-Barré syndrome

Dermatologic: Rash, urticaria

Neuromuscular & skeletal: Arthralgia

Local: Soreness at the injection site, erythema

Drug Interactions Decreased effect with immunosuppressive agents, live vaccines, immunoglobulin; initiate vaccine at least 2 weeks prior to immunosuppressive therapy and avoid during chemotherapy or radiation therapy

Stability Refrigerate

(Continued)

Pneumococcal Vaccine *(Continued)*

Usual Dosage I.M., S.C.: Children ≥2 years and Adults: 0.5 mL; if an elective splenectomy is planned, administer dose 2 weeks prior to surgery

Revaccination schedule:

Persons 2-64 years of age with functional or anatomic asplenia or immunocompromised persons:

Patients ≤10 years of age: Single revaccination 3-5 years after the previous dose

Patients >10 years of age: Single revaccination ≥5 years after the previous dose

Patients ≥65 years of age: Single revaccination if first dose was ≥5 years ago and patient was <65 years at the time

Administration Parenteral: I.M., S.C.: Do not inject I.V.; avoid intradermal administration; administer S.C. or I.M. into the deltoid muscle or lateral midthigh; pneumococcal vaccine may be given concurrently with other vaccines including MMR, DTP, poliovirus, *H. influenzae* type b, hepatitis B, or influenza vaccine

Patient Information Vaccination does not guarantee protection from fulminant pneumococcal disease in patient's with functional or anatomic asplenia

Nursing Implications Federal law requires that the date of administration, the vaccine manufacturer, lot number of the vaccine, and the administering person's name, title, and address be entered into the patient's permanent medical record

Dosage Forms Injection: 25 mcg of each type of capsular polysaccharide per 0.5 mL

References

Advisory Committee on Immunization Practices, "Prevention of Pneumococcal Disease," *MMWR Morb Mortal Wkly Rep*, 1997, 46(RR-8):1-31.

♦ **Pneumovax® 23** *see Pneumococcal Vaccine on page 809*

♦ **Pnu-Imune® 23** *see Pneumococcal Vaccine on page 809*

♦ **Pod-Ben-25®** *see Podophyllum Resin on page 810*

♦ **Podocon-25™** *see Podophyllum Resin on page 810*

♦ **Podofilm (Can)** *see Podophyllum Resin on page 810*

♦ **Podofin®** *see Podophyllum Resin on page 810*

Podophyllum Resin *(po DOF fil um REZ in)*

U.S. Brand Names Pod-Ben-25®; Podocon-25™; Podofin®

Canadian Brand Names Podofilm

Therapeutic Category Keratolytic Agent

Generic Available Yes

Use Topical treatment of benign growths including external genital and perianal warts (condylomata acuminata), papillomas, fibroids

Pregnancy Risk Factor X

Contraindications Not to be used on birthmarks, moles, or warts with hair growth; cervical, urethral, oral warts; not to be used by diabetic patients or patients with poor circulation; pregnant women; do not apply to normal tissue

Warnings Avoid contact with the eyes as it can cause severe corneal damage; 25% solution should not be applied to or near mucous membranes; podophyllum resin has caused teratogenic effects (skin tags, polyneuritis, limb malformations, septal heart defects) and fetal death when used during pregnancy

Precautions Topical application to large areas or in excessive amounts for prolonged periods should be avoided

Adverse Reactions

Central nervous system: Confusion, lethargy, hallucinations, ataxia, apnea, agitation, seizures

Dermatologic: Pruritus, erythema, scarring

Gastrointestinal: Nausea, vomiting, abdominal pain, diarrhea

Hematologic: Leukopenia, thrombocytopenia

Hepatic: Hepatotoxicity

Local: Pain, local edema

Neuromuscular & skeletal: Peripheral neuropathy, weakness

Renal: Renal failure

Stability Protect from light; avoid exposure to excessive heat

Mechanism of Action Directly affects epithelial cell metabolism by arresting mitosis through binding to a protein subunit of spindle microtubules (tubulin)

Usual Dosage Children and Adults: Topical: 10% to 25% solution in compound benzoin tincture; use 1 drop at a time allowing drying between drops until area is covered; total volume should be limited to <0.5 mL to an area <10 cm² for genital or perianal warts or <2 cm² for vaginal warts per treatment session; therapy may be repeated once weekly for up to 4 applications for the treatment of genital or perianal warts; use 10% solution when applied to or near mucous membranes

Verrucae: 25% solution is applied directly to the wart; remove drug from area of application within 6 hours

Administration Topical: Shake well before using; use protective occlusive dressing around warts to prevent contact with unaffected skin; apply drug to dry surface of affected area

Patient Information Notify physician if undue skin irritation develops

Nursing Implications Solution should be washed off within 1-4 hours for genital and perianal warts and within 1-2 hours for accessible meatal warts

Dosage Forms Liquid, topical: 25% in benzoin (5 mL, 7.5 mL, 30 mL)

References

Goldfarb MT, Gupta AK, Gupta MA, et al, "Office Therapy for Human Papillomavirus Infection in Nongenital Sites," *Dermatol Clin*, 1991, 9(2):287-96.

"1993 Sexually Transmitted Diseases Treatment Guidelines," *MMWR Morb Mortal Wkly Rep*, 1993, 42(RR-14):1-102.

♦ **Polaramine®** *see* Chlorpheniramine *on page 225*

♦ **Poliovirus Vaccine, Live, Inactivated** *see page 1172*

♦ **Poliovirus Vaccine, Live, Trivalent, Oral** *see page 1172*

♦ **Polycidin (Can)** *see* Bacitracin and Polymyxin B *on page 129*

♦ **Polycillin®** *see* Ampicillin *on page 88*

♦ **Polycillin-N®** *see* Ampicillin *on page 88*

♦ **Polycitra®** *see* Citrate and Citric Acid *on page 244*

♦ **Polycitra K®** *see* Citrate and Citric Acid *on page 244*

♦ **Polycitra-LC®** *see* Citrate and Citric Acid *on page 244*

♦ **Polyderm (Can)** *see* Bacitracin and Polymyxin B *on page 129*

Polyethylene Glycol-Electrolyte Solution

(pol i ETH i leen GLY kol ee LEK troe lite soe LOO shun)

U.S. Brand Names CoLyte®; CoLyte®-Flavored; GoLYTELY®; MiraLax™; NuLYTELY®; OCL®

Canadian Brand Names Klean-Prep; Peglyte

Synonyms Colonic Lavage Solution; Electrolyte Lavage Solution

Therapeutic Category Laxative, Bowel Evacuant; Laxative, Osmotic

Generic Available No

Use Bowel cleansing prior to GI examination; treatment of occasional constipation (MiraLax™)

Pregnancy Risk Factor C

Contraindications GI obstruction, gastric retention, bowel perforation, toxic colitis, megacolon

Warnings Do not add flavorings as additional ingredients before use

Precautions May interfere with barium coating of intestinal wall using the double contrast technique; use with caution in patients with ulcerative colitis; use with caution in patients with impaired gag reflex or those who are otherwise prone to regurgitation or aspiration during administration; treatment duration for occasional constipation should not exceed 2 weeks

Adverse Reactions

Dermatologic: Irritative perineal rashes

Endocrine & metabolic: Mild metabolic acidosis with prolonged irrigation periods, electrolyte disturbances

Gastrointestinal: Nausea, cramps, vomiting, abdominal distention, bloating

Drug Interactions Increased peristalsis may decrease absorption of oral medications given within 1 hour of beginning lavage solution

Mechanism of Action Induces catharsis by strong electrolyte and osmotic effects

Pharmacodynamics Onset of action: Bowel cleansing: Within 1-2 hours; constipation: 2-4 days

Usual Dosage

Bowel cleansing: Patient should fast at least 2 hours (preferably 3-4 hours) prior to ingestion:

Children: Oral, nasogastric: 25-40 mL/kg/hour until rectal effluent is clear (usually in 4-10 hours)

Adults:

Oral: Drink 240 mL (8 oz) every 10 minutes until 4 liters are consumed or the rectal effluent is clear

Nasogastric: 20-30 mL/minute (1.2-1.8 L/hour) until 4 liters are administered

Occasional constipation: Adults: Oral: 17 g (~1 heaping tablespoon) daily

(Continued)

Polyethylene Glycol-Electrolyte Solution *(Continued)*

Administration Oral: Add tap water to "fill-line" for reconstitution of powder for solution; no solid foods for 2 hours prior to initiation of therapy; rapid drinking is preferred to drinking small amounts continuously; chilled solution often more palatable; do not add flavorings as additional ingredients before use; MiraLax™ 17 g (dose may be measured using bottle cap) added to 8 oz of water

Monitoring Parameters Electrolytes, BUN, serum glucose, urine osmolality

Patient Information Chilled solution is often more palatable

Nursing Implications First bowel movement should occur in 1 hour

Dosage Forms Powder, for oral solution:

CoLytely®: PEG 3350 240 g, sodium sulfate 22.72 g, sodium bicarbonate 6.72 g, sodium chloride 5.84 g and potassium chloride 2.98 g [also available in pineapple flavor] (4000 mL)

CoLytely®: PEG 3350 227.1 g, sodium sulfate 21.5 g, sodium bicarbonate 6.36 g, sodium chloride 5.53 g and potassium chloride 2.82 g [also available in pineapple flavor] (18 oz)

CoLytely®-Flavored: PEG 3350 240 g, sodium sulfate 22.72 g, sodium bicarbonate 6.72 g, sodium chloride 5.84 g and potassium chloride 2.98 g [with cherry, citrus berry, lemon lime, and pineapple flavor packets] (4000 mL)

GoLytely®: PEG 3350 236 g, sodium sulfate 22.74 g, sodium bicarbonate 6.74 g, sodium chloride 5.86 g and potassium chloride 2.97 g [also available in pineapple flavor] (4000 mL)

GoLytely®: PEG 3350 227 g, sodium sulfate 21.5 g, sodium bicarbonate 6.36 g, sodium chloride 5.53 g and potassium chloride 2.82 g per packet (to make 4000 mL)

MiraLax™: PEG 3350 14 oz (255 g), 27 oz (527 g)

NuLYTELY®: PEG 3350 420 g, sodium bicarbonate 5.72 g, sodium chloride 11.2 g and potassium chloride 1.48 g [also available in cherry, lemon-lime, or orange flavor] (4000 mL)

OCL®: PEG 3350 6 g/100 mL, sodium sulfate 1.29 g/100 mL, sodium bicarbonate 1.68 g/100 mL, sodium chloride 1.46 g/100 mL, potassium chloride 75 mg, and polysorbate 80 30 mg/100 mL (1500 mL)

References

Sondheimer JM, Sokol RJ, Taylor SF, et al, "Safety, Efficacy and Tolerance of Intestinal Lavage in Pediatric Patients Undergoing Diagnostic Colonoscopy," *J Pediatr*, 1991, 119(1):148-52.

Tuggle DW, Hoelzer DJ, Tunell WP, et al, "The Safety and Cost-Effectiveness of Polyethylene Glycol Electrolyte Solution Bowel: Preparation in Infants and Children," *J Pediatr Surg*, 1987, 22(6):513-5.

♦ **Polygam® S/D** *see* Immune Globulin (Intravenous) *on page 529*

♦ **Polymox®** *see* Amoxicillin *on page 80*

Polymyxin B *(pol i MIKS in bee)*

U.S. Brand Names Aerosporin® Injection

Therapeutic Category Antibiotic, Ophthalmic; Antibiotic, Urinary Irrigation; Antibiotic, Miscellaneous

Generic Available Yes

Use Topically for wound irrigation and bladder irrigation against *Pseudomonas aeruginosa*; used occasionally for gut decontamination. Parenteral use of polymyxin B has mainly been replaced by less toxic antibiotics. Reserved for life-threatening infections caused by organisms resistant to the preferred drugs; used as inhalation therapy for gram-negative respiratory infections resistant to preferred drugs; used intrathecally for meningeal infections due to susceptible organisms which are resistant to less toxic antibiotics

Pregnancy Risk Factor B

Contraindications Hypersensitivity to polymyxin or any component

Warnings Polymyxin B can cause serious nephrotoxicity and or neurotoxicity; neurotoxic reactions may be manifested by irritability, weakness, drowsiness, ataxia, perioral paresthesia, numbness of the extremities and blurring of vision. These reactions are usually associated with high serum levels found in patients with impaired renal function or nephrotoxicity. Avoid concurrent or sequential use of other nephrotoxic and neurotoxic drugs, particularly bacitracin, kanamycin, streptomycin, paromomycin, colistin, tobramycin, neomycin, gentamicin, and amikacin. The drug's neurotoxicity can result in respiratory paralysis from neuromuscular blockade, especially when the drug is given soon after anesthesia or muscle relaxants. Polymyxin B sulfate is toxic when given parenterally; **avoid parenteral use whenever possible**.

Precautions Use with caution in patients with myasthenia gravis, patients receiving neuromuscular blocking agents or anesthetics, and in patients with impaired renal function; modify dosage in patients with renal impairment; **I.M. use is not recommended in infants and children due to severe pain at injection site**

Adverse Reactions

Cardiovascular: Facial flushing

Central nervous system: Drowsiness, ataxia, fever, dizziness

Dermatologic: Rash, urticaria

Endocrine & metabolic: Hypocalcemia, hyponatremia, hypokalemia, hypochloremia

Local: Pain at injection site, thrombophlebitis

Neuromuscular & skeletal: Neuromuscular blockade, paresthesia

Ocular: Diplopia

Renal: Nephrotoxicity (hematuria, proteinuria, azotemia)

Respiratory: Respiratory arrest

Miscellaneous: Hypersensitivity reactions

Drug Interactions Neuromuscular blocking agents, anesthetics (increase skeletal muscle relaxation); aminoglycosides, colistin, sodium citrate, parenteral quinidine

Stability Protect from light; incompatible with calcium, magnesium, cephalothin, chloramphenicol, heparin, penicillins; inactivated by acidic or alkaline solutions

Mechanism of Action Binds to phospholipids, alters permeability and damages the bacterial cytoplasmic membrane permitting leakage of intracellular constituents

Pharmacokinetics

Absorption: Well absorbed from the peritoneum; minimal absorption (<10%) from the GI tract (except in neonates), from mucous membranes or intact skin

Distribution: Widely distributed to body tissues in the liver, kidneys, heart, muscle; does not penetrate into CSF or synovial fluid; does not cross the placenta

Half-life: 4.5-6 hours, increased with reduced renal function

Time to peak serum concentration: I.M.: Within 2 hours

Elimination: Primarily as unchanged drug (>60%) in urine via glomerular filtration

Dialysis: Not removed by hemodialysis

Usual Dosage Note: Avoid parenteral use when possible

Infants <2 years:

I.M.: 25,000-40,000 units/kg/day divided every 6 hours

I.V.: 15,000-45,000 units/kg/day by continuous I.V. infusion or divided every 12 hours

Intrathecal: 20,000 units once daily for 3-4 days or 25,000 units once every other day; continue 25,000 units once every other day for at least 2 weeks after cultures of the CSF are negative

Children ≥2 years and Adults:

I.M.: 25,000-30,000 units/kg/day divided every 6 hours

I.V.: 15,000-25,000 units/kg/day divided every 12 hours or by continuous infusion; total daily dose should not exceed 2,000,000 units/day

Bladder irrigation: Continuous irrigation of the urinary bladder for up to 10 days using 20 mg (equal to 200,000 units) added to 1 L of NS; usually no more than 1 L of irrigant is used per day unless urine flow rate is high; administration rate is adjusted to patient's urine output

Topical irrigation or topical solution: 0.1% to 0.3% solution used to irrigate infected wounds; should not exceed 2 million units/day in adults

Gut sterilization: Oral: 100,000-200,000 units/kg/day divided every 6-8 hours

Ophthalmic: A concentration of 0.1% to 0.25% is administered as 1-3 drops every hour, then increasing the interval as response indicates

Inhalation: 2-2.5 mg/kg/day divided every 6 hours; final concentration for administration should not exceed 10 mg/mL

Intrathecal: 50,000 units once daily for 3-4 days, then reduce to once every other day for at least 2 weeks after cultures of the CSF are negative

Dosing adjustment in renal impairment:

Cl_{cr} 5-20 mL/minute: Administer 50% of usual daily dose divided every 12 hours

Cl_{cr} <5 mL/minute: Administer 15% of the usual daily dose divided every 12 hours

Administration Parenteral (avoid parenteral use whenever possible):

I.M.: Not recommended for routine use in infants and children because of the severe pain which occurs with I.M. injection; administer I.M. injections deep into the upper outer quadrant of the gluteal muscles at a final concentration of 250,000 units/mL

I.V.: Infuse drug slowly over 60-90 minutes or by continuous infusion at a concentration of 1000-1667 units/mL in D_5W

Intrathecal: Reconstitute vial with 10 mL NS without preservatives to provide a final concentration of 50,000 units/mL

Monitoring Parameters WBC, serum electrolytes, renal function tests, serum drug concentration, urine output

Reference Range Serum concentration >5 µg/mL are toxic in adults

(Continued)

Polymyxin B *(Continued)*

Additional Information 1 mg = 10,000 units; neuromuscular blockade may be reversed with calcium chloride

Dosage Forms

Injection, as sulfate: 500,000 units (20 mL)

Powder for solution, ophthalmic, as sulfate: 500,000 units (20-50 mL diluent)

♦ **Polymyxin B and Bacitracin** *see* Bacitracin and Polymyxin B *on page 129*

♦ **Polymyxin B and Neomycin** *see* Neomycin and Polymyxin B *on page 705*

♦ **Polymyxin B, Neomycin, and Bacitracin** *see* Neomycin, Polymyxin B, and Bacitracin *on page 707*

♦ **Polymyxin B, Neomycin, and Prednisolone** *see* Neomycin, Polymyxin B, and Prednisolone *on page 707*

♦ **Polymyxin B, Neomycin, (Bacitracin), and Hydrocortisone** *see* Neomycin, (Bacitracin) Polymyxin B, and Hydrocortisone *on page 705*

♦ **Poly-Pred® Liquifilm®** *see* Neomycin, Polymyxin B, and Prednisolone *on page 707*

♦ **Polysporin® Ophthalmic** *see* Bacitracin and Polymyxin B *on page 129*

♦ **Polysporin® Topical** *see* Bacitracin and Polymyxin B *on page 129*

♦ **Polytar® [OTC]** *see* Coal Tar *on page 260*

♦ **Polytopic Ointment (Can)** *see* Bacitracin and Polymyxin B *on page 129*

♦ **Polytracin (Can)** *see* Bacitracin and Polymyxin B *on page 129*

♦ **Poly-Vi-Sol®** *see page 1069*

♦ **Pontocaine®** *see* Tetracaine *on page 940*

Poractant Alfa *(por AKT ant AL fa)*

U.S. Brand Names Curosurf®

Synonyms Porcine Lung Surfactant

Therapeutic Category Lung Surfactant

Generic Available No

Use Treatment of respiratory distress syndrome (RDS) in premature infants

Warnings Rapidly affects oxygenation and lung compliance and should be restricted to a highly supervised use in a clinical setting with immediate availability of clinicians experienced with intubation and ventilatory management of premature infants; if transient episodes of bradycardia and decreased oxygen saturation occur, discontinue the dosing procedure and initiate measures to alleviate the condition; produces rapid improvements in lung oxygenation and compliance that may require immediate reductions in ventilator settings and FiO$_2$.

Precautions Correction of acidosis, hypotension, anemia, hypoglycemia, and hypothermia is recommended prior to administration

Adverse Reactions

Cardiovascular: Transient bradycardia, hypotension

Local: Endotracheal tube blockage

Respiratory: Oxygen desaturation

Stability Store in refrigerator; protect from light; prior to administration, allow to slowly warm to room temperature; artificial warming methods should **not** be used; unused, unopened vials warmed to room temperature may be returned to the refrigerator within 24 hours of warming only once

Mechanism of Action Poractant alfa, an extract of natural porcine lung surfactant, replaces deficient or ineffective endogenous lung surfactant in neonates with respiratory distress syndrome (RDS); surfactant prevents the alveoli from collapsing during expiration by lowering surface tension between air and alveolar surfaces

Usual Dosage Neonates: Intratracheal: Initial: 2.5 mL/kg/dose (200 mg/kg/dose); may repeat 1.25 mL/kg/dose (100 mg/kg/dose) at 12-hour intervals for up to 2 additional doses; maximum total dose: 5 mL/kg

Administration Intratracheal: For intratracheal administration only; suction infant prior to administration; inspect solution to verify complete mixing of the suspension; do not shake; gently turn vial upside-down to obtain uniform suspension; administer intratracheally by instillation through a 5-French end-hole catheter inserted into the infant's endotracheal tube; each dose should be administered as two aliquots, with each aliquot administered into one of the two main bronchi by positioning the infant with either the right or left side dependent

Monitoring Parameters Continuous heart rate and transcutaneous O$_2$ saturation should be monitored during administration; frequent ABG sampling is necessary to prevent postdosing hyperoxia and hypocarbia

Dosage Forms Suspension: 120 mg (1.5 mL); 240 mg (3 mL)

+ **Porcine Lung Surfactant** *see* Poractant Alfa *on page 814*
+ **Pork Regular Iletin® II** *see* Insulin Preparations *on page 538*
+ **Posterisan® [OTC]** *see* Hemorrhoidal Preparations *on page 490*
+ **Potassium Acetate** *see* Potassium Supplements *on page 816*
+ **Potassium Acid Phosphate** *see* Phosphate Supplements *on page 794*
+ **Potassium Bicarbonate** *see* Potassium Supplements *on page 816*
+ **Potassium Chloride** *see* Potassium Supplements *on page 816*
+ **Potassium Citrate** *see* Potassium Supplements *on page 816*
+ **Potassium Gluconate** *see* Potassium Supplements *on page 816*

Potassium Iodide (poe TASS ee um EYE oh dide)

Related Information
Carbohydrate and Alcohol Content of Liquid Medications for Use in Patients Receiving Ketogenic Diets *on page 1258*

U.S. Brand Names Pima®; SSKI®

Synonyms KI; Lugol's Solution; Strong Iodine Solution

Therapeutic Category Antithyroid Agent; Expectorant

Generic Available Yes

Use Facilitate bronchial drainage and cough; reduce thyroid vascularity prior to thyroidectomy; manage thyrotoxic crisis; block thyroidal uptake of radioactive isotopes of iodine in a radiation emergency; treat cutaneous sporotrichosis

Pregnancy Risk Factor D

Contraindications Hypersensitivity to iodides; hyperkalemia, tuberculosis, acute bronchitis, hypothyroidism, Addison's disease, acute dehydration, heat cramps

Warnings Some commercially available products contain sulfites, avoid use in sensitive patients; prolonged use can lead to hypothyroidism

Precautions Use with caution in patients with cystic fibrosis (may have exaggerated susceptibility to goitrogenic effects); may cause flare-up of acne; use with caution in patients with a history of thyroid disease and in patients with cardiac disease or renal failure

Adverse Reactions
Cardiovascular: Arrhythmia
Central nervous system: Fever, headache, confusion
Dermatologic: Urticaria, acne, angioedema, cutaneous hemorrhage
Endocrine & metabolic: Goiter with hypothyroidism, thyroid adenoma, acute parotitis
Gastrointestinal: Metallic taste, GI upset, GI bleeding, soreness of teeth and gums, cutaneous and mucosal hemorrhage
Hematologic: Eosinophilia
Neuromuscular & skeletal: Arthralgia, numbness, paresthesia
Respiratory: Rhinitis
Miscellaneous: Lymph node enlargement

Drug Interactions Potassium-containing medications, ACE inhibitors, and potassium-sparing diuretics may increase serum potassium; lithium and antithyroid drugs may potentiate hypothyroid and goitrogenic effects

Stability Store at room temperature; cold temperatures result in crystallization; warming with shaking will redissolve crystals

Mechanism of Action Reduces viscosity of mucus by increasing respiratory tract secretions; inhibits the release and synthesis of thyroid hormone

Pharmacodynamics Antithyroid effects:
Onset of action: 24-48 hours
Peak effect: 10-15 days after continuous therapy
Duration: May persist up to 6 weeks

Usual Dosage Oral:
Expectorant:
Children: 60-250 mg 4 times/day; maximum single dose: 500 mg
Adults: 300-650 mg 3-4 times/day
Preoperative thyroidectomy: Children and Adults: Given 10-14 days before surgery: 50-250 mg (1-5 drops, 1 g/mL SSKI®) 3 times/day **or** 0.1-0.3 mL (3-5 drops) strong iodine (Lugol's solution) 3 times/day
Graves' disease in neonates: 1 drop strong iodine (Lugol's solution) 3 times/day
Thyrotoxic crisis:
Infants <1 year: 150-250 mg (3-5 drops, 1 g/mL SSKI®) 3 times/day
Children and Adults: 300-500 mg (6-10 drops 1 g/mL SSKI®) 3 times/day **or** 1 mL strong iodine (Lugol's solution) 3 times/day
Cutaneous Sporotrichosis: Oral:
Children: 250-500 mg (5-10 drops, 1 g/mL SSKI®) 3 times/day; increase gradually to a maximum of 1.25-2 g (25-40 drops SSKI®)
(Continued)

Potassium Iodide *(Continued)*

Adults: 250-500 mg (5-10 drops, 1 g/mL SSKI®) 3 times/day; increase gradually to a maximum of 2-2.5 g (40-50 drops SSKI®)

Note: Therapy is continued at the maximum tolerated dosage until the cutaneous lesions have resolved, usually 6-12 weeks

Administration Oral: Administer after meals with food or milk or dilute with a large quantity of water, fruit juice, milk, or broth

Monitoring Parameters Thyroid function tests

Additional Information 10 drops SSKI® = potassium iodide 500 mg

Dosage Forms

Solution, oral:

SSKI®: 1 g/mL (30 mL, 240 mL)

Lugol's Solution, strong iodine: Potassium iodide 100 mg and iodine 50 mg per mL (120 mL, 473 mL)

Syrup (Pima®): 325 mg/5 mL [black raspberry flavor] (473 mL)

♦ **Potassium Phosphate** *see* Phosphate Supplements *on page 794*

♦ **Potassium Phosphate and Sodium Phosphate** *see* Phosphate Supplements *on page 794*

Potassium Supplements *(poe TASS ee um SUP la ments)*

Related Information

Carbohydrate and Alcohol Content of Liquid Medications for Use in Patients Receiving Ketogenic Diets *on page 1258*

U.S. Brand Names Cena-K®; Effer-K™; K+® 8; K+® 10; Kaochlor®; Kaon-Cl®; Kay Ciel®; K+ Care®; K+ Care® ET; K-Dur™; K-Gen®; K-Lor™; Klor-Con® 8; Klor-Con® 10; Klor-Con/25®; Klor-Con® EF; Klorvess® Effervescent; Klotrix®; K-Lyte®; K-Lyte/Cl®; K-lyte DS; K-Tab®; K-Vescent® Potassium Chloride; Micro-K®; Rum-K®; Slow-K®; Tri-K®; Twin-K®

Synonyms KCl (Potassium Chloride)

Available Salts Potassium Acetate; Potassium Bicarbonate; Potassium Chloride; Potassium Citrate; Potassium Gluconate

Therapeutic Category Electrolyte Supplement, Oral; Electrolyte Supplement, Parenteral; Potassium Salt

Generic Available Yes

Use Potassium deficiency; treatment or prevention of hypokalemia

Pregnancy Risk Factor C

Contraindications Severe renal impairment, untreated Addison's disease, heat cramps, hyperkalemia, severe tissue trauma; solid oral dosage forms are contraindicated in patients in whom there is a structural, pathological, and/or pharmacologic cause for delay or arrest in passage through the GI tract; an oral liquid potassium preparation should be used in patients with esophageal compression or delayed gastric emptying time

Warnings Potassium injections should be administered only in patients with adequate urine flow; injection must be diluted before I.V. use and infused slowly (see Administration); some oral products contain the dye tartrazine (avoid use in sensitive individuals)

Precautions Use with caution in patients with cardiac disease, patients receiving potassium-sparing drugs; patients must be on a cardiac monitor during intermittent infusions

Adverse Reactions

Cardiovascular (with rapid I.V. administration): Arrhythmias and cardiac arrest, heart block, hypotension

Central nervous system: Mental confusion

Endocrine & metabolic: Hyperkalemia, metabolic alkalosis (acetate salt)

Gastrointestinal (with oral administration): Nausea, vomiting, diarrhea, abdominal pain, GI lesions, flatulence

Local: Pain at the site of injection, phlebitis

Neuromuscular & skeletal: Muscle weakness, paresthesia, flaccid paralysis

Drug Interactions Potassium-sparing diuretics, salt substitutes, and ACE inhibitors may result in increased serum potassium

Mechanism of Action Potassium is the major cation of intracellular fluid and is essential for the conduction of nerve impulses in heart, brain, and skeletal muscle; contraction of cardiac, skeletal, and smooth muscles; and maintenance of normal renal function, acid-base balance (acetate form), carbohydrate metabolism, and gastric secretion

Pharmacokinetics

Absorption: Well from upper GI tract; enters cells via active transport from extracellular fluid

Elimination: Largely by the kidneys

Usual Dosage I.V. doses should be incorporated into the patient's maintenance I.V. fluids; intermittent I.V. potassium administration should be reserved for severe depletion situations and requires EKG monitoring. Doses listed as mEq of **potassium**. When using microencapsulated or wax matrix formulations, use no more than 20 mEq as a single dose.

Normal daily requirement: Oral, I.V.:

Neonates and Infants: 2-6 mEq/kg/day

Children: 2-3 mEq/kg/day

Adults: 40-80 mEq/day

Prevention of hypokalemia during diuretic therapy: Oral:

Neonates, Infants, and Children: 1-2 mEq/kg/day in 1-2 divided doses

Adults: 20-40 mEq/day in 1-2 divided doses

Treatment of hypokalemia: Oral, I.V.:

Neonates, Infants, and Children: 2-5 mEq/kg/day in divided doses

Adults: 40-100 mEq/day in divided doses

Treatment of hypokalemia: I.V. intermittent infusion (must be diluted prior to administration):

Neonates, Infants, and Children: 0.5-1 mEq/kg/dose (maximum dose: 30 mEq) to infuse at 0.3-0.5 mEq/kg/hour (maximum dose: 1 mEq/kg/hour)

Adults: 10-20 mEq/dose (maximum dose: 40 mEq/dose) to infuse over 2-3 hours (maximum dose: 40 mEq over 1 hour)

Administration

Oral: Sustained release and wax matrix tablets should be swallowed whole, do not crush or chew; effervescent tablets must be dissolved in water before use; administer with food; granules can be diluted or dissolved in water or juice; do not administer liquid full strength, must be diluted in 2-6 parts of water or juice

Parenteral: Potassium must be diluted prior to parenteral administration; maximum recommended concentration (peripheral line): 80 mEq/L; maximum recommended concentration (central line): 150 mEq/L or 15 mEq/100 mL; in severely fluid-restricted patients (with central lines): 200 mEq/L or 20 mEq/100 mL has been used; maximum rate of infusion, see Usual Dosage, I.V. intermittent infusion

Monitoring Parameters Serum potassium, glucose, chloride, pH, urine output (if indicated), cardiac monitor (if intermittent I.V. infusion or potassium I.V. infusion rates >0.25 mEq/kg/hour)

Dosage Forms

Potassium acetate: Injection: 2 mEq/mL (20 mL, 50 mL, 100 mL); 4 mEq/mL (50 mL)

Potassium chloride:

Capsule, controlled release:

Micro-K®: 600 mg [8 mEq]

Micro-K® 10: 750 mg [10 mEq]

Infusion, premixed:

10 mEq in water for injection (50 mL, 100 mL)

10 mEq in D_5W and 1/4 sodium chloride (500 mL, 1000 mL)

10 mEq in D_5W and 1/2 sodium chloride (500 mL, 1000 mL)

10 mEq in D_5W and 1/3 sodium chloride (500 mL)

20 mEq in water for injection (50 mL, 100 mL)

20 mEq in D_5W (1000 mL)

20 mEq in D_5W and 1/4 sodium chloride (1000 mL)

20 mEq in D_5W and 1/2 sodium chloride (1000 mL)

20 mEq in D_5W and 1/3 sodium chloride (1000 mL)

20 mEq in D_5W and NS (1000 mL)

20 mEq in D_5W and LR (1000 mL)

20 mEq in NS (1000 mL)

30 mEq in water for injection (100 mL)

30 mEq in D_5W (1000 mL)

30 mEq in D_5W and 1/4 sodium chloride (1000 mL)

30 mEq in D_5W and 1/2 sodium chloride (1000 mL)

40 mEq in water for injection (100 mL)

40 mEq in D_5W (1000 mL)

40 mEq in D_5W and 1/4 sodium chloride (1000 mL)

40 mEq in D_5W and 1/2 sodium chloride (1000 mL)

40 mEq in D_5W and NS (1000 mL)

40 mEq in D_5W and LR (1000 mL)

(Continued)

Potassium Supplements (Continued)

    40 mEq in NS (1000 mL)
    Injection, concentrate: 2 mEq/mL (5 mL, 10 mL, 20 mL, 250 mL)
    Liquid:
        Cena-K®, Kaochlor®, Kay Ciel®: 20 mEq/15 mL 10% (118 mL, 480 mL, 3840 mL)
        Kaon-Cl®: 40 mEq/15 mL 20% (480 mL, 3840 mL)
        Rum-K®: 30 mEq/15 mL 15% [butter rum flavor] (480 mL)
    Powder:
        Kay Ciel®, K + Care®, K-Lor™, K-Vescent® Potassium Chloride: 20 mEq per packet
        Klor-Con/25®, K-Lyte/Cl®: 25 mEq per packet
    Tablet, controlled release:
        K+® 10, Kaon-Cl® 10, K-Dur® 10, Klor-Con® 10, Klotrix®, K-Tab®: 750 mg [10 mEq]
        K-Dur® 20: 1500 mg [20 mEq]
        Klor-Con® 8, Slow-K®: 600 mg [8 mEq]
    Tablet, extended release: 750 mg [10 mEq]
        K+® 8: 600 mg [8 mEq]
Potassium gluconate:
    Elixir (Kaon®): 20 mEq/15 mL (5 mL, 10 mL, 118 mL, 480 mL, 4000 mL)
    Tablet: 595 mg
Potassium bicarbonate: Tablet for oral solution (K+Care ET): 25 mEq potassium
Potassium bicarbonate and potassium chloride:
    Granules for solution (Klorvess® Effervescent): 20 mEq potassium per packet
    Tablets for solution:
        K-Lyte/CL: 25 mEq potassium
        K-Lyte/CL 50: 50 mEq potassium
Potassium bicarbonate and potassium citrate: Tablet for solution:
    Effer-K™, Klor-Con® EF, K-Lyte®: 25 mEq
    K-Lyte® DS: 50 mEq potassium
Potassium citrate and potassium gluconate: Solution (Twin-K®): 6.7 mEq potassium per 5 mL (480 mL)
Potassium acetate, potassium bicarbonate, and potassium citrate: Solution (Tri-K®): 15 mEq/5 mL (480 mL)
References
Hamill RJ, Robinson LM, Wexler HR, et al, "Efficacy and Safety of Potassium Infusion Therapy in Hypokalemic Critically Ill Patients," *Crit Care Med*, 1991, 19(5):694-9.
Khilnani P, "Electrolyte Abnormalities in Critically Ill Children," *Crit Care Med*, 1992, 20(2):241-50.

♦ **PPL** *see* Benzylpenicilloyl-polylysine *on page 138*

Pralidoxime (pra li DOKS eem)

U.S. Brand Names Protopam®
Synonyms 2-PAM; 2-Pyridine Aldoxime Methochloride
Therapeutic Category Antidote, Anticholinesterase; Antidote, Organophosphate Poisoning
Generic Available No
Use Reverse muscle paralysis associated with toxic exposure to organophosphate anticholinesterase pesticides and chemicals; control of overdosage by anticholinesterase drugs used to treat myasthenia gravis (neostigmine, pyridostigmine)
Pregnancy Risk Factor C
Contraindications Hypersensitivity to pralidoxime or any component; poisonings due to phosphorus, inorganic phosphates, or organic phosphates without anticholinesterase activity
Warnings Not indicated as an antidote for carbamate classes of pesticides and may increase toxicity of carbaryl
Precautions Use with caution in patients with myasthenia gravis; dosage modification required in patients with impaired renal function; use with caution in patients receiving theophylline, succinylcholine, phenothiazines, respiratory depressants (eg, narcotic, barbiturates)
Adverse Reactions
    Cardiovascular: Tachycardia (after rapid I.V. infusion), hypertension
    Central nervous system: Dizziness, headache, drowsiness
    Dermatologic: Rash
    Gastrointestinal: Nausea
    Local: Pain at injection site after I.M. use
    Neuromuscular & skeletal: Muscular weakness, muscle rigidity (after rapid I.V. infusion), transient elevated CPK

Ocular: Blurred vision, diplopia

Respiratory: Hyperventilation, laryngospasm (after rapid I.V. administration)

Drug Interactions Barbiturates potentiated by anticholinesterases

Mechanism of Action Reactivates cholinesterase that had been inactivated by phosphorylation as a result of exposure to organophosphate pesticides; removes the phosphoryl group from the active site of the inactivated enzyme

Pharmacokinetics

Half-life: 0.8-2.7 hours

Time to peak concentration: I.V.: Within 5-15 minutes

Elimination: 80% to 90% excreted unchanged in urine 12 hours after administration

Usual Dosage

Organophosphate poisoning:

Children: I.M., I.V. (use in conjunction with atropine): 20-50 mg/kg/dose; repeat in 1-2 hours if muscle weakness has not been relieved, then at 10- to 12-hour intervals if cholinergic signs recur

Adults: I.M., I.V. (use in conjunction with atropine): 1-2 g; repeat in 1-2 hours if muscle weakness has not been relieved, then at 10- to 12-hour intervals if cholinergic signs recur

Treatment of toxicity from medications used to treat myasthenia gravis: Adults: I.V.: 1-2 g followed by increments of 250 mg every 5 minutes

Administration Parenteral: Reconstitute with 20 mL sterile water (preservative free) resulting in 50 mg/mL solution; dilute in NS to 20 mg/mL and infuse over 15-30 minutes; if a more rapid onset of effect is desired or in a fluid-restricted situation, the maximum concentration is 50 mg/mL; the maximum rate of infusion is over 5 minutes and not exceeding 200 mg/minute

Monitoring Parameters Heart rate, respiratory rate, blood pressure, continuous EKG

Dosage Forms Powder for injection, as chloride: 1 g

♦ **Prandase (Can)** see Acarbose on page 28

Praziquantel (pray zi KWON tel)

U.S. Brand Names Biltricide®

Therapeutic Category Anthelmintic

Generic Available No

Use Treatment of all stages of schistosomiasis caused by *Schistosoma* species pathogenic to humans; also active in the treatment of clonorchiasis, opisthorchiasis, cysticercosis, and many intestinal tapeworm and trematode infections

Pregnancy Risk Factor B

Contraindications Ocular cysticercosis, spinal cysticercosis; hypersensitivity to praziquantel or any component

Precautions Use with caution in patients with severe hepatic disease and in patients with a history of seizures

Adverse Reactions

Central nervous system: Dizziness, drowsiness, fever, headache, vertigo, malaise, CSF reaction syndrome in patients being treated for neurocysticercosis (syndrome includes headache, seizures, intracranial hypertension, increased CSF protein concentrations, hyperthermia)

Dermatologic: Urticarial rash, itching

Gastrointestinal: Abdominal pain, nausea, vomiting, anorexia, diarrhea

Hematologic: Eosinophilia

Miscellaneous: Diaphoresis

Drug Interactions Alcohol may increase CNS depression; phenytoin and carbamazepine may induce metabolism of praziquantel and decrease its activity; cimetidine increases praziquantel serum concentrations

Mechanism of Action Increases the cell permeability to calcium in schistosomes; causes strong contractions and paralysis of worm musculature leading to detachment of suckers from the blood vessel walls and to dislodgment

Pharmacokinetics

Absorption: Oral: ~80%

Distribution: CSF concentration is 14% to 20% of plasma concentration; excreted in breast milk

Protein binding: ~80%

Metabolism: Extensive first-pass effect; metabolized by the liver to hydroxylated and conjugated metabolites

Half-life: 0.8-1.5 hours

Metabolites: 4.5 hours

Time to peak serum concentration: Within 1-3 hours

(Continued)

Praziquantel (Continued)

Elimination: Praziquantel and metabolites excreted mainly in urine (99% as metabolites)

Usual Dosage Children and Adults: Oral:

Schistosomiasis:

S. mansoni, S. haematobium: 20 mg/kg/dose twice daily for 1 day

S. japonicum, S. mekongi: 20 mg/kg/dose 3 times/day for 1 day at 4- to 6-hour intervals

Flukes:

Liver, intestine: 75 mg/kg/day divided every 8 hours for 1 day

Lung: 75 mg/kg/day divided every 8 hours for 2 days

Nanophyetus salmincola: 60 mg/kg/day divided every 8 hours for 1 day

Cysticercosis: 50 mg/kg/day divided every 8 hours for 15 days (adjunctive therapy with dexamethasone is recommended for patients with numerous cysts and for those in whom neurologic symptoms or intracranial hypertension develops); for neurocysticercosis, steroids should be administered **prior** to starting praziquantel

Tapeworms: 5-10 mg/kg as a single dose (25 mg/kg for H. nana)

Administration Oral: Administer with food; tablets can be halved or quartered; do not chew tablets due to bitter taste

Patient Information Avoid alcohol (increased CNS depression); may cause drowsiness and impair ability to perform activities requiring mental alertness or physical coordination

Dosage Forms Tablet, tri-scored: 600 mg

References

King CH and Mahmoud AA, "Drug Five Years Later: Praziquantel," Ann Intern Med, 1989, 110(4):290-6.
Liu LX and Weller PF, "Antiparasitic Drug," N Engl J Med, 1996, 334(18):1178-84.

Prazosin (PRA zoe sin)

Related Information

Overdose and Toxicology on page 1222

U.S. Brand Names Minipress®

Canadian Brand Names Alti-Prazosin; Apo-Prazo; Novo-Prazin; Nu-Prazo

Synonyms Furazosin

Therapeutic Category Alpha-Adrenergic Blocking Agent, Oral; Antihypertensive Agent; Vasodilator

Generic Available Yes

Use Hypertension, severe CHF (in conjunction with diuretics and cardiac glycosides)

Pregnancy Risk Factor C

Contraindications Hypersensitivity to prazosin or any component

Precautions Marked orthostatic hypotension, syncope, and loss of consciousness may occur with first dose ("first dose phenomenon"). This reaction is more likely to occur in patients receiving beta-blockers, diuretics, low sodium diets or larger first doses (ie, >1 mg/dose in adults); avoid rapid increase in dose; use with caution in patients with renal impairment.

Adverse Reactions

Cardiovascular: Orthostatic hypotension, syncope, palpitations, tachycardia, edema

Central nervous system: Dizziness, lightheadedness, nightmares, drowsiness, headache, hypothermia

Dermatologic: Rash

Endocrine & metabolic: Fluid retention, sexual dysfunction

Gastrointestinal: Nausea, xerostomia

Genitourinary: Urinary frequency

Neuromuscular & skeletal: Weakness

Respiratory: Nasal congestion

Drug Interactions Diuretics and antihypertensive medications (especially beta-blockers) may increase prazosin's hypotensive effect

Food Interactions Avoid natural licorice (causes sodium and water retention and increases potassium loss); food has variable effects on absorption

Mechanism of Action Competitively inhibits postsynaptic alpha-adrenergic receptors which results in vasodilation of veins and arterioles and a decrease in total peripheral resistance and blood pressure

Pharmacodynamics Hypotensive effect:

Onset of action: Within 2 hours

Maximum decrease: 2-4 hours

Duration: 10-24 hours

Pharmacokinetics

Distribution: V_d: 0.5 L/kg (hypertensive adults)

Protein-binding: 92% to 97%

Metabolism: Extensive in the liver, metabolites may be active

Bioavailability, oral: 43% to 82%

Half-life, adults: 2-4 hours, increased half-life with CHF

Elimination: 6% to 10% excreted renally as unchanged drug

Usual Dosage Oral:

Children: Initial: 5 mcg/kg/dose (to assess hypotensive effects); usual dosing interval every 6 hours; increase dosage gradually up to 25 mcg/kg/dose every 6 hours; maximum daily dose: 15 mg or 0.4 mg/kg/day (400 mcg/kg/day); may be divided in 2 or 3 doses/day for treatment of hypertension

Adults: Initial: 1 mg/dose 2-3 times/day; usual maintenance dose: 3-15 mg/day in divided doses 2-4 times/day; maximum daily dose: 20 mg

Administration Oral: Administer in a consistent manner with respect to meals

Monitoring Parameters Blood pressure (standing and sitting or supine)

Patient Information Avoid alcohol; rise slowly from sitting or lying position; may cause dizziness; may cause dry mouth

Nursing Implications Be aware of "first-dose phenomenon" (see Precautions); syncope may occur usually within 90 minutes of initial dose

Dosage Forms Capsule, as hydrochloride: 1 mg, 2 mg, 5 mg

References

Friedman WF and George BL, "New Concepts and Drugs in the Treatment of Congestive Heart Failure," *Pediatr Clin North Am*, 1984, 31(6):1197-227.

Sinaiko AR, "Pharmacologic Management of Childhood Hypertension," *Pediatr Clin North Am*, 1993, 40(1):195-212.

♦ **Precose**® *see* Acarbose *on page 28*

♦ **Pred Forte**® *see* Prednisolone *on page 821*

♦ **Pred-G**® *see* Prednisolone and Gentamicin *on page 823*

♦ **Pred Mild**® *see* Prednisolone *on page 821*

♦ **Prednisol**® *see* Prednisolone *on page 821*

Prednisolone (pred NIS oh lone)

Related Information

Asthma Guidelines *on page 1210*

Carbohydrate and Alcohol Content of Liquid Medications for Use in Patients Receiving Ketogenic Diets *on page 1258*

Corticosteroids Comparison, Systemic *on page 1067*

U.S. Brand Names AK-Pred®; Econopred®; Econopred® Plus; Inflamase® Forte; Inflamase® Mild; Orapred®; Pediapred®; Pred Forte®; Pred Mild®; Prednisol®; Prelone®

Canadian Brand Names Ak-Tate; Diopred; Minims-Prednisolone; Novo-Prednisolone; Ophtho-Tate

Synonyms Deltahydrocortisone; Metacortandralone

Therapeutic Category Adrenal Corticosteroid; Antiasthmatic; Anti-inflammatory Agent; Anti-inflammatory Agent, Ophthalmic; Corticosteroid, Ophthalmic; Corticosteroid, Systemic; Glucocorticoid

Generic Available Yes

Use Treatment of endocrine disorders, rheumatic disorders, collagen diseases, dermatologic diseases, allergic states, ophthalmic diseases, respiratory diseases, hematologic disorders, neoplastic diseases, edematous states, and gastrointestinal diseases

Ophthalmic: Treatment of palpebral and bulbar conjunctivitis; corneal injury from chemical, radiation, thermal burns, or foreign body penetration

Pregnancy Risk Factor C

Contraindications Acute superficial herpes simplex keratitis; systemic fungal infections; varicella; hypersensitivity to prednisolone or any component

Warnings Hypothalamic pituitary adrenal (HPA) suppression may occur; acute adrenal insufficiency may occur with abrupt withdrawal after long term use or with stress; withdrawal or discontinuation of corticosteroids should be done carefully; immunosuppression may occur; corticosteroids may mask signs of infection

Precautions Avoid using higher than recommended doses; suppression of HPA axis, suppression of linear growth, or hypercorticism (Cushing's syndrome) may occur; use with caution in patients with hypothyroidism, cirrhosis, ocular herpes simplex, peptic ulcer disease, osteoporosis, myasthenia gravis, hypertension, CHF, nonspecific ulcerative colitis, thromboembolic disorders, and renal dysfunction; Prelone® syrup contains benzoic acid and Orapred® oral solution contains sodium (Continued)

Prednisolone *(Continued)*

benzoate; use with caution in neonates, as these preservatives may displace bilirubin from protein binding sites and at larger doses can cause the gasping syndrome

Adverse Reactions

Cardiovascular: Edema, hypertension, CHF

Central nervous system: Vertigo, seizures, psychoses, pseudotumor cerebri, headache

Dermatologic: Acne, skin atrophy, impaired wound healing, petechiae, bruising

Endocrine & metabolic: Cushing's syndrome, pituitary-adrenal axis suppression, growth suppression, glucose intolerance, hypokalemia, alkalosis, sodium and water retention

Gastrointestinal: Peptic ulcer, nausea, vomiting

Genitourinary: Menstrual irregularities

Neuromuscular & skeletal: Muscle weakness, osteoporosis, fractures

Ocular: Cataracts, increased IOP, glaucoma

Drug Interactions Cytochrome P-450 isoenzyme CYP3A3/4 substrate and inducer

Barbiturates, phenytoin, rifampin, salicylates, toxoids, NSAIDs, diuretics (potassium depleting); caffeine and alcohol may increase risk for GI ulcer; live virus vaccines (increase risk of viral infection); vaccines may have decreased effects

Food Interactions Systemic use of corticosteroids may require a diet with increased potassium, vitamins A, B_6, C, D, folate, calcium, zinc, and phosphorus and decreased sodium

Stability May dilute sodium phosphate salt in dextrose or saline solutions for I.V. administration; dispense oral liquid formulations in tight, light-resistant containers; storage: Prelone® syrup: Store at room temperature, do not refrigerate; Pediapred® oral solution: Store at 4°C to 24°C (39°F to 77°F), may be refrigerated; Orapred® oral solution: Store in refrigerator [2°C to 8°C (36°F to 46°F)]

Mechanism of Action Decreases inflammation by suppression of migration of polymorphonuclear leukocytes and reversal of increased capillary permeability; suppresses the immune system by reducing activity and volume of the lymphatic system

Pharmacokinetics

Absorption: Oral: Well absorbed

Protein binding: 70% to 90% (concentration dependent)

Metabolism: Primarily in the liver, but also metabolized in most tissues, to inactive compounds

Half-life: Adults (serum): 2-4 hours

Elimination: In urine, principally as glucuronide and sulfate-conjugated metabolites

Usual Dosage Dose depends upon condition being treated and response of patient; dosage for infants and children should be based on disease severity and patient response rather than by rigid adherence to dosage guidelines by age, weight, or body surface area. Consider alternate day therapy for long-term therapy. Discontinuation of long-term therapy requires gradual withdrawal by tapering the dose.

Children:

Acute asthma:

Oral: 1-2 mg/kg/day in divided doses 1-2 times/day for 3-10 days; longer treatment may be required; usually given for 5 days

I.V.: 2-4 mg/kg/day divided 3-4 times/day

Anti-inflammatory or immunosuppressive dose: Oral, I.V.: 0.1-2 mg/kg/day in divided doses 1-4 times/day

Nephrotic syndrome: Oral:

Pediatric Nephology Panel recommendations (Hogg, 2000):

Initial: 2 mg/kg/day or 60 mg/m²/day given every day in 1-3 divided doses (maximum dose: 80 mg/day) until urine is protein free for 4-6 weeks; followed by maintenance dose: 2 mg/kg/dose or 40 mg/m²/dose given every other day in the morning; gradually taper and discontinue after 4-6 weeks; **Note:** 6-week daily therapy followed by 6-week alternate day therapy may induce a higher rate of long remission compared to the standard of 4 weeks of daily therapy followed by 4 weeks of alternate day therapy; however, a higher incidence of adverse effects may be seen with the longer regimen and the clinical benefit may be variable

Relapse: Use high-dose daily steroid regimen (listed above) until urine is protein free for 3 days; follow with maintenance-tapering course of alternative therapy (maintenance dose listed above) for 4-6 weeks; subsequent therapy is determined by individual's response and number of relapses (see Hogg, 2000)

British Pediatric Nephrology Consensus Statement (Report of a Workshop by the British Association for Paediatric Nephrology and Research Unit, 1994):

First 3 episodes: Initial: 2 mg/kg/day or 60 mg/m²/day given every day (maximum dose: 80 mg/day) until urine is protein free for 3 consecutive days (maximum dose: 28 days); followed by 1-1.5 mg/kg/dose or 40 mg/m²/dose (maximum: 60 mg/dose) given every other day for 4 weeks

Frequent relapses (long-term maintenance dose): 0.5-1 mg/kg/dose given every other day for 3-6 months

Children and Adults: Ophthalmic suspension: Instill 1-2 drops into conjunctival sac every hour during day, every 2 hours at night until favorable response is obtained, then use 1 drop every 4 hours

Adults: Oral, I.V.: 5-60 mg/day

Administration

Oral: Administer after meals or with food or milk to decrease GI upset

Ophthalmic: Shake suspension well before use; instill drops into affected eye(s); avoid contact of container tip with skin or eye; apply finger pressure to lacrimal sac during and for 1-2 minutes after instillation to decrease risk of absorption and systemic effects

Parenteral: I.V. (**sodium phosphate salt only**): Administer via I.V. infusion; sodium phosphate salt may also be administered I.M., intra-articular, intralesional, or into soft tissue; **do not give acetate salt I.V.**; acetate salt is for I.M., intralesional, intra-articular, or soft tissue administration only

Monitoring Parameters Blood pressure, weight, electrolytes, serum glucose; children's height and growth

Test Interactions Skin tests

Patient Information Avoid alcohol; limit caffeine; do not decrease dose or discontinue without physician's approval; avoid exposure to chicken pox or measles, if exposed, seek medical advice without delay

Dosage Forms

Prednisolone acetate:

Suspension, injection: 25 mg/mL (10 mL, 30 mL); 50 mg/mL (10 mL, 30 mL)

Suspension, ophthalmic:

Pred Mild®: 0.12% (5 mL, 10 mL)

Econopred®: 0.125% (5 mL, 10 mL)

Econopred® Plus, Pred Forte®: 1% (1 mL, 5 mL, 10 mL, 15 mL)

Prednisolone base:

Syrup (Prelone®): 5 mg/5 mL [cherry flavor; contains <0.4% alcohol; dye free; sugar free] (120 mL); 15 mg/5 mL [cherry flavor; contains 5% alcohol] (240 mL, 480 mL)

Tablet: 5 mg

Prednisolone sodium phosphate:

Injection (Key-Pred-SP®): 20 mg/mL (2 mL, 5 mL, 10 mL)

Solution, ophthalmic: 1% (5 mL, 15 mL)

AK-Pred®, Inflamase® Mild: 0.125% (5 mL, 10 mL)

AK-Pred®, Inflamase® Forte: 1% (5 mL, 10 mL, 15 mL)

Solution, oral:

Orapred®: 20 mg/5 mL [**equivalent to 15 mg/5 mL prednisolone base**; dye free; grape flavor; contains 2% alcohol] (240 mL)

Pediapred®: 6.7 mg/5 mL [**equivalent to 5 mg/5 mL prednisolone base**; raspberry flavor] (120 mL)

References

Hogg RJ, Portman RJ, Milliner D, et al, "Evaluation and Management of Proteinuria and Nephrotic Syndrome in Children: Recommendations From a Pediatric Nephrology Panel Established at the National Kidney Foundation Conference on Proteinuria, Albuminuria, Risk, Assessment, Detection, and Elimination (PARADE)," *Pediatrics*, 2000, 105(6):1242-9.

Report of a Workshop by the British Association for Paediatric Nephrology and Research Unit, Royal College of Physicians, "Consensus Statement on Management and Audit Potential for Steroid Responsive Nephrotic Syndrome," *Arch Dis Child*, 1994, 70(2):151-7.

Prednisolone and Gentamicin (pred NIS oh lone & jen ta MYE sin)

U.S. Brand Names Pred-G®

Synonyms Gentamicin and Prednisolone

Therapeutic Category Antibiotic, Ophthalmic; Corticosteroid, Ophthalmic

Generic Available Yes

Use Treatment of steroid responsive inflammatory conditions and superficial ocular infections due to strains of microorganisms susceptible to gentamicin such as *Staphylococcus*, *E. coli*, *H. influenzae*, *Klebsiella*, *Neisseria*, *Pseudomonas*, *Proteus*, and *Serratia* species

Pregnancy Risk Factor C

(Continued)

Prednisolone and Gentamicin *(Continued)*

Contraindications Hypersensitivity to prednisolone, gentamicin, or any component; dendritic keratitis, fungal diseases, vaccinia, varicella, most other viral infections, and mycobacterial infection of the eye. Contraindicated after uncomplicated removal of a corneal foreign body.

Warnings Prolonged use may result in glaucoma, damage to the optic nerve, defects in visual acuity, posterior subcapsular cataract formation, and secondary ocular infections

Adverse Reactions

Local: Burning, stinging, redness

Ocular: Elevation of intraocular pressure, glaucoma, infrequent optic nerve damage, posterior subcapsular cataract formation, superficial punctate keratitis, increased lacrimation

Miscellaneous: Development of secondary infection, allergic sensitization, delayed wound healing

Mechanism of Action See individual monographs for Prednisolone *on page 821* and Gentamicin *on page 469*

Usual Dosage Children and Adults: Ophthalmic: Instill 1 drop 2-4 times/day; during the initial 24-48 hours, the dosing frequency may be increased if necessary, up to 1 drop every hour; or small amount ($\frac{1}{2}$" ribbon) of ointment can be applied into the conjunctival sac 1-3 times/day

Administration Suspension: Shake well before using; instill drop into affected eye; avoid contacting bottle tip with skin or eye; apply finger pressure to lacrimal sac during and for 1-2 minutes after instillation to decrease risk of absorption and systemic effects

Monitoring Parameters With use >10 days, monitor intraocular pressure

Dosage Forms

Ointment, ophthalmic: Prednisolone acetate 0.6% and gentamicin sulfate 0.3% (3.5 g)

Suspension, ophthalmic: Prednisolone acetate 1% and gentamicin sulfate 0.3% (2 mL, 5 mL, 10 mL)

♦ **Prednisolone, Neomycin, and Polymyxin B** *see Neomycin, Polymyxin B, and Prednisolone on page 707*

Prednisone *(PRED ni sone)*

Related Information

Antiepileptic Drugs *on page 1208*

Asthma Guidelines *on page 1210*

Carbohydrate and Alcohol Content of Liquid Medications for Use in Patients Receiving Ketogenic Diets *on page 1258*

Corticosteroids Comparison, Systemic *on page 1067*

U.S. Brand Names Deltasone®; Meticorten®; Sterapred®

Canadian Brand Names Apo-Prednisone; Jaa-Prednisone; Novo-Prednisone; Winpred

Synonyms Deltacortisone; Deltadehydrocortisone

Therapeutic Category Adrenal Corticosteroid; Antiasthmatic; Anti-inflammatory Agent; Corticosteroid, Systemic; Glucocorticoid

Generic Available Yes

Use Management of adrenocortical insufficiency; used for its anti-inflammatory or immunosuppressant effects

Pregnancy Risk Factor C

Contraindications Serious infections, except septic shock or tuberculous meningitis; systemic fungal infections; hypersensitivity to prednisone or any component; varicella

Warnings Hypothalamic pituitary adrenal (HPA) suppression may occur; acute adrenal insufficiency may occur with abrupt withdrawal after long term use or with stress; withdrawal or discontinuation of corticosteroids should be done carefully; immunosuppression may occur; corticosteroids may mask signs of infection

Precautions Avoid using higher than recommended doses; suppression of HPA axis, suppression of linear growth, or hypercorticism (Cushing's syndrome) may occur; use with caution in patients with hypothyroidism, cirrhosis, ocular herpes simplex, peptic ulcer disease, osteoporosis, myasthenia gravis, hypertension, CHF, nonspecific ulcerative colitis, thromboembolic disorders, and renal dysfunction

Adverse Reactions

Cardiovascular: Edema, hypertension, CHF

Central nervous system: Vertigo, seizures, psychoses, pseudotumor cerebri, headache

Dermatologic: Acne, skin atrophy, impaired wound healing, petechiae, bruising

Endocrine & metabolic: Cushing's syndrome, pituitary-adrenal axis suppression, growth suppression, glucose intolerance, hypokalemia, alkalosis, sodium and water retention

Gastrointestinal: Peptic ulcer, nausea, vomiting

Genitourinary: Menstrual irregularities

Neuromuscular & skeletal: Muscle weakness, osteoporosis, fractures

Ocular: Cataracts, increased IOP, glaucoma

Drug Interactions Cytochrome P-450 isoenzyme CYP3A3/4 substrate and inducer
Barbiturates, phenytoin, rifampin, salicylates, toxoids, NSAIDs, diuretics (potassium depleting); caffeine and alcohol may increase risk for GI ulcer; live virus vaccines (increase risk of viral infection); vaccines may have decreased effects

Food Interactions Systemic use of corticosteroids may require a diet with increased potassium, vitamins A, B_6, C, D, folate, calcium, zinc, and phosphorus and decreased sodium

Mechanism of Action Decreases inflammation by suppression of migration of polymorphonuclear leukocytes and reversal of increased capillary permeability; suppresses the immune system by reducing activity and volume of the lymphatic system

Pharmacokinetics Converted rapidly in the liver to prednisolone (active)

Usual Dosage Dose depends upon condition being treated and response of patient; dosage for infants and children should be based on disease severity and patient response rather than by rigid adherence to dosage guidelines by age, weight, or body surface area. Consider alternate day therapy for long-term therapy. Discontinuation of long-term therapy requires gradual withdrawal by tapering the dose. Oral:

Children:

Anti-inflammatory or immunosuppressive: 0.05-2 mg/kg/day divided 1-4 times/day

Acute asthma: 1-2 mg/kg/day in divided doses 1-2 times/day for 3-10 days; longer treatment may be required; usually given for 5 days

Alternative dosing by age for "burst":

<1 year: 10 mg every 12 hours

1-4 years: 20 mg every 12 hours

5-13 years: 30 mg every 12 hours

>13 years: 40 mg every 12 hours

Asthma long-term therapy (alternative dosing by age):

<1 year: 10 mg every other day

1-4 years: 20 mg every other day

5-13 years: 30 mg every other day

>13 years: 40 mg every other day

Nephrotic syndrome:

Pediatric Nephology Panel recommendations (Hogg, 2000):

Initial: 2 mg/kg/day or 60 mg/m²/day given every day in 1-3 divided doses (maximum dose: 80 mg/day) until urine is protein free for 4-6 weeks; followed by maintenance dose: 2 mg/kg/dose or 40 mg/m²/dose given every other day in the morning; gradually taper and discontinue after 4-6 weeks; **Note:** 6-week daily therapy followed by 6-week alternative day therapy may induce a higher rate of long remission compared to the standard of 4 weeks of daily therapy followed by 4 weeks of alternative day therapy; however, a higher incidence of adverse effects may be seen with the longer regimen and the clinical benefit may be variable

Relapse: Use high-dose daily steroid regimen (listed above) until urine is protein free for 3 days; follow with maintenance-tapering course of alternative therapy (maintenance dose listed above) for 4-6 weeks; subsequent therapy is determined by individual's response and number of relapses (see Hogg, 2000)

British Pediatric Nephrology Consensus Statement (Report of a Workshop by the British Association for Paediatric Nephrology and Research Unit, 1994):

First 3 episodes: Initial: 2 mg/kg/day or 60 mg/m²/day given every day (maximum dose: 80 mg/day) until urine is protein free for 3 consecutive days (maximum dose: 28 days); followed by 1-1.5 mg/kg/dose or 40 mg/m²/dose (maximum: 60 mg/dose) given every other day for 4 weeks

Frequent relapses (long-term maintenance dose): 0.5-1 mg/kg/dose given every other day for 3-6 months

Children and Adults: Physiologic replacement: 4-5 mg/m²/day

Adults: 5-60 mg/day in divided doses 1-4 times/day

Administration Oral: Administer after meals or with food or milk to decrease GI upset

(Continued)

Prednisone *(Continued)*

Monitoring Parameters Blood pressure, weight, serum electrolytes, glucose; children's height and growth

Test Interactions Skin tests

Patient Information Avoid alcohol; limit caffeine; do not decrease dose or discontinue without physician's approval

Dosage Forms

Solution:

Concentrate: 5 mg/mL (30 mL)

Oral: 5 mg/5 mL (5 mL, 60 mL, 120 mL, 500 mL)

Tablet: 1 mg, 2.5 mg, 5 mg, 10 mg, 20 mg, 50 mg

Deltasone®: 2.5 mg, 5 mg, 10 mg, 20 mg, 50 mg

Meticorten®: 1 mg

Sterapred®: 5 mg

Sterapred® DS: 10 mg

References

Hogg RJ, Portman RJ, Milliner D, et al, "Evaluation and Management of Proteinuria and Nephrotic Syndrome in Children: Recommendations From a Pediatric Nephrology Panel Established at the National Kidney Foundation Conference on Proteinuria, Albuminuria, Risk, Assessment, Detection, and Elimination (PARADE)," *Pediatrics,* 2000, 105(6):1242-9.

Murphy CM, Coonce SL, and Simon PA, "Treatment of Asthma in Children," *Clin Pharm,* 1991, 10(9):685-703.

Report of a Workshop by the British Association for Paediatric Nephrology and Research Unit, Royal College of Physicians, "Consensus Statement on Management and Audit Potential for Steroid Responsive Nephrotic Syndrome," *Arch Dis Child,* 1994, 70(2):151-7.

- **Prefrin (Can)** *see* Phenylephrine *on page 789*
- **Prefrin™ Liquifilm®** *see* Phenylephrine *on page 789*
- **Pregnyl®** *see* Chorionic Gonadotropin *on page 232*
- **Prelone®** *see* Prednisolone *on page 821*
- **Premarin®** *see* Estrogens (Conjugated) *on page 402*
- **Preparation H® [OTC]** *see* Hemorrhoidal Preparations *on page 490*
- **Preparation H® Hydrocortisone [OTC]** *see* Hydrocortisone *on page 506*
- **Pre-Pen®** *see* Benzylpenicilloyl-polylysine *on page 138*
- **Preprocedure Sedatives in Children** *see page 1201*
- **Pretz-D® [OTC]** *see* Ephedrine *on page 384*
- **Pretz® Irrigation [OTC]** *see* Sodium Chloride *on page 906*
- **Prevacid®** *see* Lansoprazole *on page 578*
- **Prevalite®** *see* Cholestyramine Resin *on page 229*
- **Prevex B (Can)** *see* Betamethasone *on page 140*
- **Prevex HC (Can)** *see* Hydrocortisone *on page 506*
- **PreviDent®** *see* Fluoride *on page 441*
- **PreviDent® 5000 Plus™** *see* Fluoride *on page 441*
- **Prilocaine and Lidocaine** *see* Lidocaine and Prilocaine *on page 594*
- **Prilosec™** *see* Omeprazole *on page 733*
- **Primacor®** *see* Milrinone *on page 672*

Primaquine *(PRIM a kween)*

Therapeutic Category Antimalarial Agent

Generic Available No

Use In conjunction with a blood schizonticidal agent to provide radical cure of *P. vivax* or *P. ovale* malaria after a clinical attack has been confirmed by blood smear or serologic titer; prevention of relapse of *P. ovale* or *P. vivax* malaria; malaria postexposure prophylaxis

Pregnancy Risk Factor C

Contraindications Acutely ill patients who have a tendency to develop granulocytopenia (rheumatoid arthritis, SLE); patients receiving other drugs capable of depressing the bone marrow; patients receiving quinacrine

Precautions Use with caution in patients with G-6-PD deficiency or NADH methemoglobin reductase deficiency

Adverse Reactions

Cardiovascular: Arrhythmias, hypertension

Central nervous system: Headache

Dermatologic: Pruritus

Gastrointestinal: Nausea, vomiting, abdominal cramps

Hematologic: Hemolytic anemia, methemoglobinemia, leukocytosis, leukopenia, agranulocytosis

Ocular: Interference with visual accommodation

Drug Interactions Quinacrine (increased toxicity of primaquine)

Stability Protect from light

Mechanism of Action Eliminates the primary tissue exoerythrocytic forms of *P. falciparum*, *P. malariae*, *P. ovale*, and *P. vivax*; interferes with plasmodial DNA

Pharmacokinetics

Absorption: Oral: Well absorbed

Metabolism: Liver metabolism to carboxyprimaquine, an active metabolite

Half-life: 3.7-9.6 hours

Time to peak serum concentration: Within 6 hours

Elimination: Small amount of unchanged drug excreted in urine

Usual Dosage Oral:

Children: 0.3 mg base/kg/day once daily for 14 days not to exceed 15 mg base/day, or 0.9 mg base/kg once weekly for 8 weeks not to exceed 45 mg base/week

Adults: 15 mg/day (base) once daily for 14 days or 45 mg base once weekly for 8 weeks

Administration Oral: Administer with meals to decrease adverse GI effects; drug has a bitter taste

Monitoring Parameters Periodic CBC, visual color check of urine, hemoglobin

Patient Information Notify physician if a darkening of the urine occurs

Dosage Forms Tablet, as phosphate: 26.3 mg [15 mg base]

References

Lynk A and Gold R, "Review of 40 Children With Imported Malaria," *Pediatr Infect Dis J*, 1989, 8(11):745-50.

Wyler DJ, "Malaria Chemoprophylaxis for the Traveler," *N Engl J Med*, 1993, 329(1):31-7.

♦ **Primatene® Mist [OTC]** *see* Epinephrine *on page 385*
♦ **Primaxin®** *see* Imipenem and Cilastatin *on page 526*

Primidone (PRI mi done)

Related Information

Antiepileptic Drugs *on page 1208*
Carbohydrate and Alcohol Content of Liquid Medications for Use in Patients Receiving Ketogenic Diets *on page 1258*
Drugs and Breast-Feeding *on page 1243*

U.S. Brand Names Mysoline®

Canadian Brand Names Apo-Primidone; Sertan

Therapeutic Category Anticonvulsant, Barbiturate; Barbiturate

Generic Available Yes: Tablet

Use Management of generalized tonic-clonic (grand mal), complex partial and simple partial (focal) seizures

Pregnancy Risk Factor D

Contraindications Hypersensitivity to primidone or any component; porphyria

Precautions Use with caution in patients with renal or hepatic impairment; abrupt discontinuation may precipitate status epilepticus

Adverse Reactions

Central nervous system: Drowsiness, vertigo, lethargy, behavior change, ataxia

Dermatologic: Rash

Gastrointestinal: Nausea, vomiting

Hematologic: Leukopenia, malignant lymphoma-like syndrome, megaloblastic anemia

Ocular: Diplopia, nystagmus

Miscellaneous: Systemic lupus-like syndrome

Drug Interactions Cytochrome P-450 isoenzyme CYP1A2, CYP2B6, CYP2C, CYP2C8, CYP3A3/4, and CYP3A5-7 inducer

Primidone may decrease serum concentrations of ethosuximide, valproic acid, griseofulvin; methylphenidate may increase primidone serum concentrations; phenytoin may decrease primidone serum concentrations; valproic acid may increase phenobarbital concentrations derived from primidone

Food Interactions May increase the metabolism of vitamins D and K; dietary requirements of vitamins D, K, B_{12}, folate, and calcium may be increased with long-term use

Mechanism of Action Decreases neuron excitability, raises seizure threshold similar to phenobarbital

Pharmacokinetics

Distribution: V_d: Adults: 2-3 L/kg

Protein-binding: 99%

(Continued)

Primidone (Continued)

Metabolism: In the liver to phenobarbital (active) and phenylethylmalonamide (PEMA)

Bioavailability: 60% to 80%

Half-life:

Primidone: 10-12 hours

PEMA: 16 hours

Phenobarbital: 52-118 hours (age-dependent)

Time to peak serum concentration: Oral: Within 4 hours

Elimination: Urinary excretion of both active metabolites and unchanged primidone (15% to 25%)

Usual Dosage Oral:

Neonates: 12-20 mg/kg/day in divided doses 2-4 times/day; start with lower dosage and titrate upward

Children <8 years: Initial: 50-125 mg/day given at bedtime; increase by 50-125 mg/day increments every 3-7 days; usual dose: 10-25 mg/kg/day in divided doses 3-4 times/day

Children >8 years and Adults: Initial: 125-250 mg/day at bedtime; increase by 125-250 mg/day every 3-7 days; usual dose: 750-1500 mg/day in divided doses 3-4 times/day with maximum dosage of 2 g/day

Administration Oral: Administer with food to decrease GI upset

Monitoring Parameters Serum primidone and phenobarbital concentrations; CBC with differential; neurological status, seizure frequency, duration, severity

Reference Range

Therapeutic: 5-12 µg/mL (SI: 23-55 µmol/L)

Toxic effects rarely present with levels <10 µg/mL (SI: 46 µmol/L) if phenobarbital concentrations are low

Toxic: >15 µg/mL (SI: >69 µmol/L); monitor both primidone and phenobarbital concentrations

Patient Information Avoid alcohol; limit caffeine; may cause drowsiness and impair ability to perform activities requiring mental alertness or physical coordination; do not abruptly discontinue or change dose without physician approval

Dosage Forms

Suspension, oral: 250 mg/5 mL (240 mL)

Tablet: 50 mg, 250 mg

◆ **Primsol**® see Trimethoprim on page 987

◆ **Principen**® see Ampicillin on page 88

◆ **Prinivil**® see Lisinopril on page 598

◆ **Priscoline**® see Tolazoline on page 967

◆ **Pristinamycin** see Quinupristin/Dalfopristin on page 863

◆ **Privine**® [OTC] see Naphazoline on page 698

◆ **Pro-Amox (Can)** see Amoxicillin on page 80

◆ **Pro-Ampi (Can)** see Ampicillin on page 88

◆ **Pro-Banthine (Can)** see Propantheline on page 840

Probenecid (proe BEN e sid)

Canadian Brand Names Benuryl

Therapeutic Category Adjuvant Therapy, Penicillin Level Prolongation; Antigout Agent; Uric Acid Lowering Agent; Uricosuric Agent

Generic Available Yes

Use Prevention of gouty arthritis; hyperuricemia; prolong serum levels of penicillin/cephalosporin

Pregnancy Risk Factor B

Contraindications Hypersensitivity to probenecid or any component; high dose aspirin therapy; moderate to severe renal impairment (Cl$_{cr}$ <10 mL/minute); children <2 years of age, blood dyscrasias, uric acid kidney stones

Precautions Use with caution in patients with peptic ulcer; hematuria, renal colic; formation of uric acid stones associated with the use of probenecid may be prevented by liberal fluid intake and alkalinization of urine; may not be effective when Cl$_{cr}$ 10-30 mL/minute

Adverse Reactions

Cardiovascular: Flushing

Central nervous system: Dizziness, headache

Dermatologic: Rash

Gastrointestinal: Anorexia, nausea, vomiting, sore gums

Genitourinary: Urinary frequency

Hematologic: Anemia, leukopenia, aplastic anemia, hemolytic anemia (possibly related to G-6-PD deficiency)

Hepatic: Hepatic necrosis

Renal: Nephrotic syndrome, renal colic, uric acid stones

Miscellaneous: Hypersensitivity reactions

Drug Interactions Salicylates and probenecid inhibit the uricosuric actions of each other; probenecid may increase the plasma levels of acyclovir, penicillins, ciprofloxacin, ganciclovir, cephalosporins, methotrexate, dapsone, NSAIDs, and zidovudine; benzodiazepines and thiopental may have prolonged effects; sulfonylureas may have an increase in half-life; clofibrate may have an increased accumulation of its active metabolite; avoid concomitant use with ketorolac since its half-life is increased twofold and levels and toxicity are significantly increased; niacin may inhibit uricosuric effects of probenecid

Mechanism of Action Competitively inhibits the reabsorption of uric acid at the proximal convoluted tubule, thereby promoting its excretion and reducing serum uric acid levels; increases plasma levels of weak organic acids (penicillins, cephalosporins, or other beta-lactam antibiotics) by competitively inhibiting their renal tubular secretion

Pharmacodynamics Exerts maximal effects on penicillin levels after 2 hours; produces maximal renal clearance of uric acid in 30 minutes

Pharmacokinetics

Absorption: Rapid and complete from GI tract

Protein binding: 85% to 95%

Metabolism: In the liver

Half-life: 4-17 hours

Time to peak serum concentration: Within 2-4 hours

Usual Dosage Oral:

Prolongation of penicillin serum levels:

Children 2-14 years: Initial: 25 mg/kg/dose or 0.7 g/m^2/dose as a single dose; maintenance: 40 mg/kg/day or 1.2 g/m^2/day in 4 divided doses (maximum single dose: 500 mg)

Adults: 500 mg 4 times/day

Hyperuricemia: Adults: Initial: 250 mg twice daily for 1 week; increase to 500 mg twice daily; may increase in 500 mg increments every 4 weeks if needed to a maximum of 2-3 g/day; begin therapy 2-3 weeks after an acute gouty attack

Gonorrhea: Adults: 1 g 30 minutes before penicillin, ampicillin, or amoxicillin

Dosing adjustment in renal impairment: Cl_{cr} <50 mL/minute: Avoid use

Administration Oral: Administer with food or antacids to minimize GI effects

Monitoring Parameters Uric acid, renal function, CBC

Test Interactions False-positive glucosuria with Clinitest®; falsely elevated serum theophylline level (Schack & Waxler technique); inhibits renal excretion of phenosulfonphythalein (PSP), 17-ketosteroids, and sulfobromophthalein (BSP)

Patient Information Drink plenty of fluids to reduce the risk of uric acid stones; the frequency of acute gouty attacks may increase during the first 6-12 months of therapy; avoid taking large doses of aspirin or other salicylates; avoid alcohol

Dosage Forms Tablet: 500 mg

Procainamide (proe kane A mide)

Related Information

Adult ACLS Algorithm, Narrow-Complex Supraventricular Tachycardia on page 1046

Adult ACLS Algorithm, Stable Ventricular Tachycardia on page 1047

Adult ACLS Algorithm, V. Fib and Pulseless VT on page 1041

CPR Pediatric Drug Dosages on page 1031

Pediatric ALS Algorithm, Tachycardia - Rapid Rhythm and Adequate Perfusion on page 1037

Pediatric ALS Algorithm, Tachycardia - Rapid Rhythm and Evidence of Poor Perfusion on page 1038

U.S. Brand Names Procanbid®; Pronestyl®; Pronestyl-SR®

Canadian Brand Names Apo-Procainamide; Procan SR

Synonyms PCA; Procaine Amide

Therapeutic Category Antiarrhythmic Agent, Class I-A

Generic Available Yes

Use Ventricular tachycardia, premature ventricular contractions, paroxysmal atrial tachycardia, and atrial fibrillation; to prevent recurrence of ventricular tachycardia, paroxysmal supraventricular tachycardia, atrial fibrillation or flutter; **Note:** Due to proarrhythmic effects, use should be reserved for life-threatening arrhythmias

Pregnancy Risk Factor C

(Continued)

Procainamide *(Continued)*

Contraindications Complete heart block; second or third degree heart block without pacemaker; "torsade de pointes" (twisting of the points), an unusual ventricular tachycardia; pre-existing QT prolongation; hypersensitivity to the procainamide, procaine, related drugs, or any component; myasthenia gravis; SLE

Warnings Serious blood dyscrasias may occur (see Adverse Reactions); long-term administration leads to the development of a positive antinuclear antibody (ANA) test in 50% of patients which may lead to a lupus erythematosus-like syndrome (in 20% to 30% of patients); assess relative benefits and risks if ANA titer becomes positive and consider alternative agent; discontinue procainamide if SLE symptoms develop and change to alternative agent; do not use sustained release preparation for initial therapy; some tablets contain tartrazine; injection may contain bisulfite; 100 mg/mL injection contains benzyl alcohol (use with caution in neonates)

Precautions Use with caution in patients with marked A-V conduction disturbances, bundle-branch block or severe cardiac glycoside intoxication, ventricular arrhythmias in patients with organic heart disease or coronary occlusion, CHF, supraventricular tachyarrhythmias unless digitalis glycoside levels are adequate to prevent marked increases in ventricular rates; drug may accumulate in patients with renal or hepatic dysfunction, dosage adjustment required

Adverse Reactions

Cardiovascular: Hypotension, tachycardia, arrhythmias, A-V block, QT prolongation, widening QRS complex

Central nervous system: Confusion, disorientation, drug fever

Gastrointestinal: Nausea, vomiting, GI complaints

Hematologic: Agranulocytosis, neutropenia, thrombocytopenia, hypoplastic anemia

Hepatic: Hepatomegaly, increased liver enzymes

Miscellaneous: Lupus-like syndrome (arthralgia, positive Coombs' test, thrombocytopenia, rash, myalgia, fever, pericarditis, pleural effusion)

Drug Interactions Cimetidine, ranitidine, amiodarone, beta-blocking agents, trimethoprim may increase plasma procainamide and NAPA concentrations, procainamide dosage adjustment may be required; procainamide may potentiate skeletal muscle relaxants; anticholinergic drugs may have enhanced effects

Food Interactions Procanbid® extended release tablets: A high fat meal may increase extent of absorption by ~20%

Stability Use only clear or slightly yellow solutions; stability of parenteral admixture with D_5W at room temperature (25°C) is 24 hours but 7 days at refrigerated temperature (2°C to 8°C)

Mechanism of Action Class IA antiarrhythmic with anticholinergic and local anesthetic effects; decreases myocardial excitability and conduction velocity and depresses myocardial contractility, by increasing the electrical stimulation threshold of ventricle, His-Purkinje system and through direct cardiac effects

Pharmacodynamics Onset of action: I.M. 10-30 minutes

Pharmacokinetics

Absorption: Oral: Well absorbed; ProcanBid®: Absorption is sustained over 12 hours

Distribution: V_d (decreased with CHF or shock):
  Children: 2.2 L/kg
  Adults: 2 L/kg

Protein binding: 15% to 20%

Metabolism: By acetylation in the liver to produce N-acetyl procainamide (NAPA) (active metabolite)

Bioavailability, oral: 75% to 95%

Half-life:
  Procainamide (dependent upon hepatic acetylator phenotype, cardiac function, and renal function):
    Children: 1.7 hours
    Adults with normal renal function: 2.5-4.7 hours
  NAPA (dependent upon renal function):
    Children: 6 hours
    Adults with normal renal function: 6-8 hours

Time to peak serum concentration:
  Oral (capsule): Within 45 minutes to 2.5 hours
  I.M.: 15-60 minutes

Elimination: Urinary excretion (25% as NAPA)

Dialysis: Moderately dialyzable by hemodialysis (20% to 50%), but not dialyzable by peritoneal dialysis

Usual Dosage Must be titrated to patient's response
Children:
  Oral: 15-50 mg/kg/day divided every 3-6 hours; maximum 4 g/day

I.M.: 20-30 mg/kg/day divided every 4-6 hours; maximum 4 g/day

I.V.:

Loading dose: 3-6 mg/kg/dose over 5 minutes, not to exceed 100 mg/dose; may repeat every 5-10 minutes to maximum total loading dose of 15 mg/kg; do not exceed 500 mg in 30 minutes

Maintenance: Continuous I.V. infusion: 20-80 mcg/kg/minute; maximum dose: 2 g/day

PALS Guidelines 2000 (for perfusing tachycardias): **Note:** Do not routinely administer together with amiodarone:

I.V., I.O.: Loading dose: 15 mg/kg infused over 30-60 minutes; monitor EKG continuously and blood pressure frequently; stop the infusion if hypotension occurs or QRS complex widens by >50% of baseline

Adults:

Oral: Immediate release products: 250-500 mg/dose every 3-6 hours; sustained release: 500 mg to 1 g every 6 hours; extended release (Procanbid®): 1-2 g every 12 hours; usual dose: 50 mg/kg/day or 2-4 g/day

I.V.:

Loading dose: 50-100 mg/dose, repeated every 5-10 minutes until patient controlled; or load with 15-18 mg/kg; maximum loading dose: 1-1.5 g

Maintenance: Continuous I.V. infusion: 3-4 mg/minute; range: 1-6 mg/minute; monitor levels and do not exceed 3 mg/minute for >24 hours in patients with renal failure

Refractory ventricular fibrillation:

Loading dose: 30 mg/minute up to a total of 17 mg/kg

I.V. maintenance infusion: 1-4 mg/minute; monitor levels and do not exceed 3 mg/minute for >24 hours in adults with renal failure

ACLS guidelines 2000:

I.V.: Loading dose: Infuse 20 mg/minute until arrhythmia is controlled, hypotension occurs, QRS complex widens by 50% of its original width, or total of 17 mg/kg is given

I.V. maintenance infusion: 1-4 mg/minute

Dosing interval in renal dysfunction:

Cl_{cr} 10-50 mL/minute: Administer normal dose every 6-12 hours

Cl_{cr} <10 mL/minute: Administer normal dose every 8-24 hours

Administration

Oral: Administer with water on an empty stomach; if GI distress occurs may administer with food or milk to decrease GI upset; swallow extended and sustained release tablets whole, do not chew, break, or crush

Parenteral: I.V.: Do not administer faster than 20-30 mg/minute; severe hypotension can occur with rapid I.V. administration; administer I.V. push over at least 5 minutes; administer I.V. loading doses and intermittent infusions over 25-30 minutes; use concentration of 20-30 mg/mL for loading dose and 2-4 mg/mL for maintenance infusions; rate of infusion (mL/hour) = dose (mcg/kg/minute) x weight (kg) x 60 minutes/hour divided by the concentration

Monitoring Parameters EKG, blood pressure, CBC with differential, platelet count, antinuclear antibody test (ANA); serum drug concentrations, procainamide and NAPA, especially in patients with renal failure or those receiving higher maintenance doses (eg, adults: >3 mg/minute) for >24 hours

Reference Range

Therapeutic:

Procainamide: 4-10 µg/mL (SI: 15-37 µmol/L)

Sum of procainamide and N-acetyl procainamide: 10-30 µg/mL (SI: <110 µmol/L)

Optimal ranges must be ascertained for individual patients, with EKG monitoring

Toxic (procainamide): >10-12 µg/mL (SI: >37-44 µmol/L)

Patient Information Limit alcohol; some sustained release tablets have a wax core that slowly releases the drug, this wax core is not absorbed and will be eliminated in the stool; inform physician if symptoms such as fever, sore throat, chills, bruising, or bleeding occur

Dosage Forms

Capsule, as hydrochloride (Pronestyl®): 250 mg, 375 mg, 500 mg

Injection, as hydrochloride (Pronestyl®): 100 mg/mL (10 mL); 500 mg/mL (2 mL)

Tablet, as hydrochloride (Pronestyl®): 250 mg, 375 mg, 500 mg

Tablet, extended release, as hydrochloride (Procanbid®): 500 mg, 1000 mg

Tablet, sustained release, as hydrochloride: 250 mg, 500 mg, 750 mg, 1000 mg

Pronestyl® SR: 500 mg, 1000 mg

Extemporaneous Preparations Note: Several formulations have been described, some being more complex; for all formulations, the pH must be 4-6 to prevent degradation; some preparations require adjustment of pH; **label all preparations "shake well before use"**

(Continued)

Procainamide (Continued)

A 50 mg/mL oral liquid preparation made from the contents of capsules and 3 different vehicles (cherry syrup, a 1:1 mixture of Ora-Sweet® and Ora-Plus®, or a 1:1 mixture of Ora-Sweet® SF and Ora-Plus®) was stable for 60 days when stored in amber plastic prescription bottles in the dark at room temperature (25°C) or under refrigeration (5°C); empty the contents of twenty-four 250 mg capsules into a mortar; break up the powder and pulverize it; add 20 mL of the vehicle and mix well to form a uniform paste; mix while adding the vehicle in geometric proportions to **almost** 120 mL; transfer to a calibrated bottle and qsad with vehicle to 120 mL; label "protect from light" (Allen, 1996)

A suspension of 50 mg/mL can be made with the capsules, distilled water, and a 2:1 simple syrup/cherry syrup mixture; stability 2 weeks under refrigeration (ASHP, 1987)

Concentrations of 5, 50, and 100 mg/mL oral liquid preparations, (made with the capsules, sterile water for irrigation and cherry syrup) stored at 4°C to 6°C (pH 6) were stable for at least 6 months (Metras, 1992)

A sucrose-based syrup (procainamide 50 mg/mL) made with capsules, distilled water, simple syrup, parabens, and cherry flavoring had a calculated stability of 456 days at 25°C and measured stability of 42 days at 40°C (pH ~5) while a maltitol-based syrup (procainamide 50 mg/mL) made with capsules, distilled water, Lycasin® (a syrup vehicle with 75% w/w maltitol), parabens, sodium bisulfate, saccharin, sodium acetate, pineapple and apricot flavoring, FD & C yellow number 6, (pH adjusted to 5 with glacial acetic acid) had a calculated stability of 97 days at 25°C and a measured stability of 94 days at 40°C. The maltitol-based syrup was more stable than the sucrose-based syrup when temperature was >37°C, but the sucrose-based syrup was more stable at temperatures <37°C (Alexander, 1993)

Alexander KS, Pudipeddi M, and Parker GA, "Stability of Procainamide Hydrochloride Syrups Compounded From Capsules," *Am J Hosp Pharm*, 1993, 50(4):693-8.

Allen LV and Erickson MA, "Stability of Ketoconazole, Metolazone, Metronidazole, Procainamide Hydrochloride, and Spironolactone in Extemporaneously Compounded Oral Liquids," *Am J Health Syst Pharm*, 1996, 53(17):2073-8.

Handbook in Extemporaneous Formulations, Bethesda, MD: American Society of Hospital Pharmacists, 1987.

Metras JI, Swenson CF, and MacDermott MP, "Stability of Procainamide Hydrochloride in an Extemporaneously Compounded Oral Liquid," *Am J Hosp Pharm*, 1992, 49(7):1720-4.

Swenson CF, "Importance of Following Instructions When Compounding," *Am J Hosp Pharm*, 1993, 50(2):261.

References

"Guidelines 2000 for Cardiopulmonary Resuscitation and Emergency Cardiovascular Care, Part 6: Advanced Cardiovascular Life Support, The American Heart Association in Collaboration With the International Liaison Committee on Resuscitation," *Circulation*, 2000, 102(8 Suppl):I86-171.

"Guidelines 2000 for Cardiopulmonary Resuscitation and Emergency Cardiovascular Care, Part 10: Pediatric Advanced Life Support, The American Heart Association in Collaboration With the International Liason Committee on Resuscitation," *Circulation*, 2000, 102(8 Suppl): I291-342.

Singh S, Gelband H, Mehta AV, et al, "Procainamide Elimination Kinetics in Pediatric Patients," *Clin Pharmacol Ther*, 1982, 32(5):607-11.

♦ **Procaine Amide** *see* Procainamide *on page 829*

♦ **Procaine Benzylpenicillin** *see* Penicillin G Procaine *on page 773*

♦ **Procaine Penicillin G** *see* Penicillin G Procaine *on page 773*

♦ **Pro-Cal-Sof® [OTC]** *see* Docusate *on page 350*

♦ **Procanbid®** *see* Procainamide *on page 829*

♦ **Procan SR (Can)** *see* Procainamide *on page 829*

Procarbazine (proe KAR ba zeen)

Related Information
Emetogenic Potential of Single Chemotherapeutic Agents *on page 1129*

U.S. Brand Names Matulane®

Canadian Brand Names Natulan

Synonyms Ibenzmethyzin

Therapeutic Category Antineoplastic Agent, Miscellaneous

Generic Available No

Use Treatment of Hodgkin's disease, non-Hodgkin's lymphoma, brain tumor, bronchogenic carcinoma

Pregnancy Risk Factor D

Contraindications Hypersensitivity to procarbazine or any component; pre-existing bone marrow aplasia

Warnings The FDA currently recommends that procedures for proper handling and disposal of antineoplastic agents be considered; procarbazine is a carcinogen which may cause a secondary acute nonlymphocytic leukemia; procarbazine may cause infertility and is potentially teratogenic

Precautions May potentiate CNS depression when used with phenothiazine derivatives, barbiturates, narcotics, alcohol, tricyclic antidepressants, methyldopa; use with caution in patients with pre-existing renal or hepatic impairment; reduce dosage in patients with marrow disorders, renal impairment (serum creatinine >2 mg/dL and/or a blood urea nitrogen >40 mg/dL), or decreased hepatic function (total bilirubin >3 mg/dL)

Adverse Reactions

Central nervous system: CNS depression, somnolence, confusion, nervousness, irritability, cerebellar ataxia, hallucinations, seizures, nightmares, headache, chills, fever, dizziness

Dermatologic: Dermatitis, alopecia, hypersensitivity rash, pruritus

Endocrine & metabolic: Disulfiram-like reaction, amenorrhea

Gastrointestinal: Nausea, vomiting, diarrhea, stomatitis, anorexia

Genitourinary: Azoospermia, ovarian failure

Hematologic: Myelosuppression, thrombocytopenia, pancytopenia, hemolysis

Neuromuscular & skeletal: Arthralgia, myalgia, tremor, neuropathy, weakness

Ocular: Nystagmus, diplopia, photophobia

Miscellaneous: Flu-like syndrome

Drug Interactions Alcohol (disulfiram-like reaction with nausea, vomiting, headache, sedation, and visual disturbances); MAO inhibitors, tricyclic antidepressants, ephedrine, epinephrine, isoproterenol (hypertensive crisis, tremor, excitation, cardiac palpitations, angina); narcotics, phenothiazines, barbiturates, methyldopa (additive CNS depression); phenytoin, phenobarbital (increases cytotoxic activity of procarbazine)

Food Interactions Avoid food with high tyramine content (cheese, tea, dark beer, coffee, cola drinks, wine, bananas) as hypertensive crisis, tremor, excitation, cardiac palpitations, and angina may occur

Stability Unstable in water or aqueous solution; avoid contact of the drug with moisture

Mechanism of Action Inhibits DNA, RNA, and protein synthesis; may damage DNA directly via free-radical formation and suppress mitosis

Pharmacokinetics

Absorption: Oral: Well absorbed

Distribution: Crosses the blood-brain barrier and distributes into CSF, liver, kidney, intestine, and skin

Metabolism: In the liver; first-pass conversion to cytotoxic metabolites

Half-life: 10 minutes

Time to peak serum concentration: Within 1 hour

Elimination: In urine (<5% as unchanged drug) and 70% as metabolites

Usual Dosage Oral (refer to individual protocols; base dosage on ideal body weight):

Children:

Hodgkin's disease: 50-100 mg/m^2/day once daily for 10-14 days of a 28-day cycle

BMT aplastic anemia conditioning regimen: 12.5 mg/kg/dose every other day for 4 doses

Brain tumor: 75 mg/m^2 at hour 1 on day 1; repeat cycle every 2-4 weeks if tolerated; **or** 100 mg/m^2 on days 1-14 of a treatment course

Neuroblastoma and medulloblastoma: Doses as high as 100-200 mg/m^2/day once daily have been used

Adults: Initial: 2-4 mg/kg/day in single or divided doses for 7 days then increase dose to 4-6 mg/kg/day until response is obtained or leukocyte count decreases to <4000/mm^3 or the platelet count decreases to <100,000/mm^3; maintenance: 1-2 mg/kg/day

Administration Oral: Administer with food or after meals; total daily dose may be administered at a single time or in divided doses throughout the day to minimize GI toxicity

Monitoring Parameters CBC with differential, platelet count, and reticulocyte count; urinalysis, liver function test, renal function test

Patient Information Notify physician of fever, sore throat, bleeding, or bruising; avoid alcohol (disulfiram-like reaction with nausea, vomiting, headache, sedation, and visual disturbances)

Additional Information Myelosuppressive effects:

WBC: Moderate

(Continued)

Procarbazine *(Continued)*

Platelets: Moderate
Onset (days): 14
Nadir (days): 21
Recovery (days): 28

Dosage Forms Capsule, as hydrochloride: 50 mg

References

Longo DL, Young RC, Wesley M, et al, "Twenty Years of MOPP Therapy for Hodgkin's Disease," *J Clin Oncol*, 1986, 4(9):1295-306.

Rodriguez LA, Prados M, Silver P, et al, "Re-evaluation of Procarbazine for the Treatment of Recurrent Malignant Central Nervous System Tumors," *Cancer*, 1989, 64(12):2420-3.

♦ **Procardia**® *see* Nifedipine *on page 714*

♦ **Procardia XL**® *see* Nifedipine *on page 714*

Prochlorperazine *(proe klor PER a zeen)*

Related Information

Carbohydrate and Alcohol Content of Liquid Medications for Use in Patients Receiving Ketogenic Diets *on page 1258*

Compatibility of Medications Mixed in a Syringe *on page 1238*

Overdose and Toxicology *on page 1222*

U.S. Brand Names Compazine®

Canadian Brand Names Nu-Prochlor; PMS-Prochlorperazine; Stemetil

Therapeutic Category Antiemetic; Antipsychotic Agent; Phenothiazine Derivative

Generic Available Yes

Use Management of nausea and vomiting; acute and chronic psychosis; treatment of intractable migraine headaches

Pregnancy Risk Factor C

Contraindications Hypersensitivity to prochlorperazine or any component; cross-sensitivity with other phenothiazines may exist; avoid use in patients with narrow-angle glaucoma; bone marrow suppression; severe liver or cardiac disease; severe toxic CNS depression or coma

Warnings High incidence of extrapyramidal reactions especially in children, reserve use in children <5 years of age to those who are unresponsive to other antiemetics; incidence of extrapyramidal reactions is increased with acute illnesses such as chicken pox, measles, CNS infections, gastroenteritis, and dehydration; injection contains sulfites which may cause allergic reactions; lowers seizure threshold, use cautiously in patients with seizure history; some products contain tartrazine dye, avoid use in sensitive individuals; discontinue use at least 48 hours before myelography and do not resume until 24 hours post myelography

Precautions Safety and efficacy have not been established in children <9 kg or <2 years of age

Adverse Reactions Incidence of extrapyramidal reactions are higher with prochlorperazine than chlorpromazine

Cardiovascular: Hypotension (especially with I.V. use); orthostatic hypotension; tachycardia, arrhythmias, sudden death

Central nervous system: Sedation, drowsiness, restlessness, anxiety; extrapyramidal reactions which include dystonic reactions such as spasm of neck muscles, torticollis, extensor rigidity of back muscles, opisthotonos, trismus, and mandibular tics; pseudoparkinsonian signs and symptoms, tardive dyskinesia, neuroleptic malignant syndrome, seizures, altered central temperature regulation

Dermatologic: Hyperpigmentation, pruritus, rash, photosensitivity

Endocrine & metabolic: Amenorrhea, galactorrhea, gynecomastia, abnormal glucose tolerance

Gastrointestinal: GI upset, xerostomia, constipation, weight gain

Genitourinary: Impotence, urinary retention

Hematologic: Agranulocytosis, leukopenia (usually in patients with large doses for prolonged periods), thrombocytopenia, hemolytic anemia, eosinophilia

Hepatic: Cholestatic jaundice

Ocular: Retinal pigmentation, blurred vision

Miscellaneous: Anaphylactoid reactions

Drug Interactions Phenothiazines inhibit the ability of bromocriptine to lower serum prolactin concentrations; benztropine (and other anticholinergics) may inhibit the therapeutic response to prochlorperazine; sulfadoxine-pyamthamine, propranolol, and chloroquine may increase prochlorperazine concentrations; cigarette smoking may enhance the hepatic metabolism of prochlorperazine; concurrent use of prochlorperazine and antihypertensives may produce additive hypotensive effects; antihypertensive effects of guanethidine and guanadrel may be inhibited by prochlorperazine; concurrent use with TCAs may produce increased toxicity or altered therapeutic response; prochlorperazine may inhibit the antiparkinsonian effect of levodopa; prochlorperazine plus lithium may rarely produce neurotoxicity; barbiturates may reduce prochlorperazine concentrations; prochlorperazine and CNS depressants (ethanol, narcotics) may produce additive CNS depressant effects; prochlorperazine and trazodone may produce additive hypotensive effects; use with cisapride may increase the risk of malignant arrhythmias

Food Interactions Increase dietary intake of riboflavin

Stability Protect from light; clear or slightly yellow solutions may be used; incompatible with aminophylline, amphotericin B, ampicillin, calcium salts, cephalothin, foscarnet (Y-site), furosemide, hydrocortisone, hydromorphone, methohexital, midazolam, penicillin G, pentobarbital, phenobarbital, thiopental

Mechanism of Action Blocks postsynaptic mesolimbic dopaminergic receptors in the brain, including the medullary chemoreceptor trigger zone; exhibits a strong alpha-adrenergic blocking effect and depresses the release of hypothalamic and hypophyseal hormones

Pharmacodynamics
Onset of action:
Oral: 30-40 minutes
I.M.: Within 10-20 minutes
Rectal: Within 60 minutes
Duration:
I.M., oral extended release: 12 hours
Rectal, oral immediate release: 3-4 hours

Usual Dosage
Antiemetic:
Children >10 kg:
Oral, rectal: 0.4 mg/kg/day in 3-4 divided doses; **or** as an alternative:
10-14 kg: 2.5 mg every 12-24 hours as needed; maximum dose: 7.5 mg/day
15-18 kg: 2.5 mg every 8-12 hours as needed; maximum dose: 10 mg/day
19-39 kg: 2.5 mg every 8 hours or 5 mg every 12 hours as needed; maximum dose: 15 mg/day
I.M.: 0.1-0.15 mg/kg/dose; usual: 0.13 mg/kg/dose; change to oral as soon as possible
I.V.: Not recommended
Adults:
Oral: 5-10 mg 3-4 times/day; usual maximum dose: 40 mg/day
Oral, extended release: 10 mg twice daily or 15 mg once daily
I.M.: 5-10 mg every 3-4 hours; usual maximum dose: 40 mg/day
I.V.: 2.5-10 mg; maximum 10 mg/dose or 40 mg/day; may repeat dose every 3-4 hours as needed
Rectal: 25 mg twice daily
Treatment of intractable migraine headaches (limited information available): I.V.: Children: 0.15 mg/kg as a single dose in 20 children between the ages of 8-17 years combined with I.V. hydration has been used (Kabbouche, 2001)
Treatment of psychoses:
Children 2-12 years:
Oral, rectal: 2.5 mg 2-3 times/day, increase dosage as needed to a maximum daily dose of 20 mg for 2-5 years and 25 mg for 6-12 years
I.M.: 0.13 mg/kg/dose, change to oral as soon as possible
Adults:
Oral: 5-10 mg 3-4 times/day, increase as needed to a daily maximum dose of 150 mg
I.M.: 10-20 mg every 4 hours as needed, change to oral as soon as possible

Administration
Oral: Administer with food or water
Parenteral: I.M. is preferred; avoid I.V. administration; if necessary, may be administered by direct I.V. injection at a maximum rate of 5 mg/minute; do not administer by S.C. route (tissue damage may occur)

Monitoring Parameters CBC with differential and periodic ophthalmic exams (if chronically used)

Test Interactions False-positives for phenylketonuria, urinary amylase, uroporphyrins, urobilinogen

Patient Information Limit caffeine; causes drowsiness and may impair ability to perform hazardous tasks requiring mental alertness or physical coordination; may cause dry mouth; avoid unnecessary exposure to sunlight

Nursing Implications Avoid skin contact with oral solution or injection, contact dermatitis has occurred
(Continued)

Prochlorperazine *(Continued)*

Additional Information Use lowest possible dose in pediatric patients to try to decrease incidence of extrapyramidal reactions

Dosage Forms

Injection, as edisylate: 5 mg/mL (2 mL, 10 mL)

Suppository, rectal: 2.5 mg, 5 mg, 25 mg (12/box)

Syrup, as edisylate: 5 mg/5 mL (120 mL)

Tablet, as maleate: 5 mg, 10 mg

References

Kabbouche MA, Vockell AL, LeCates SL, et al, "Tolerability and Effectiveness of Prochlorperazine for Intractable Migraine in Children," *Pediatrics*, 2001, 107(4):E62, www.pediatrics.org/cgi/content/full/107/4/e62.

- ◆ **Procrit**® *see* Epoetin Alfa *on page 388*
- ◆ **Proctocort**™ *see* Hydrocortisone *on page 506*
- ◆ **ProctoCream**® **HC** *see* Hydrocortisone *on page 506*
- ◆ **ProctoFoam**® **[OTC]** *see* Hemorrhoidal Preparations *on page 490*
- ◆ **Procytox (Can)** *see* Cyclophosphamide *on page 281*
- ◆ **Prodiem Plain (Can)** *see* Psyllium *on page 853*
- ◆ **Prodium**™ **[OTC]** *see* Phenazopyridine *on page 784*
- ◆ **Profasi**® *see* Chorionic Gonadotropin *on page 232*
- ◆ **Profilnine**® **SD** *see* Factor IX Complex (Human) *on page 414*
- ◆ **Proglycem**® *see* Diazoxide *on page 323*
- ◆ **Prograf**® *see* Tacrolimus *on page 934*
- ◆ **Pro-Indo (Can)** *see* Indomethacin *on page 536*
- ◆ **Proleukin**® *see* Aldesleukin *on page 47*
- ◆ **Proloprim**® *see* Trimethoprim *on page 987*
- ◆ **Pro-Lorazepam (Can)** *see* Lorazepam *on page 609*

Promethazine *(proe METH a zeen)*

Related Information

Compatibility of Medications Mixed in a Syringe *on page 1238*

Overdose and Toxicology *on page 1222*

Promethazine and Phenylephrine *on page 839*

U.S. Brand Names Phenazine®; Phenergan®

Canadian Brand Names Histantil

Therapeutic Category Antiemetic; Phenothiazine Derivative; Sedative

Generic Available Yes

Use Symptomatic treatment of various allergic conditions and motion sickness; sedative and an antiemetic

Pregnancy Risk Factor C

Contraindications Hypersensitivity to promethazine or any component; narrow-angle glaucoma, severe toxic CNS depression or coma, prostatic hypertrophy, GI or GU obstruction

Warnings Do not give S.C. or intra-arterially, necrotic lesions may occur; injection may contain sulfites which may cause allergic reactions in some patients; rapid I.V. administration may produce a transient fall in blood pressure; slow I.V. administration may produce a slightly elevated blood pressure

Precautions Use with caution in patients with cardiovascular disease, impaired liver function, asthma, peptic ulcer, sleep apnea, seizures, hypertensive crisis; avoid in patients with suspected Reye's syndrome

Adverse Reactions

Cardiovascular: Tachycardia, bradycardia, hypotension (rapid I.V. administration), hypertension (slow I.V. administration), palpitations

Central nervous system: Sedation (pronounced), drowsiness, confusion, fatigue, excitation, extrapyramidal reactions, dystonia, tardive dyskinesia

Dermatologic: Photosensitivity, rash, angioedema

Gastrointestinal: Xerostomia, GI upset, increased appetite, weight gain, abdominal pain, diarrhea, nausea

Genitourinary: Urinary retention

Hematologic: Thrombocytopenia, leukopenia, agranulocytosis (rare)

Hepatic: Cholestatic jaundice, hepatitis

Ocular: Blurred vision

Neuromuscular & skeletal: Arthralgia, tremor, paresthesia, myalgia

Respiratory: Thickening of bronchial secretions, pharyngitis

Miscellaneous: Allergic reactions

Drug Interactions CYP2D6 enzyme substrate

Phenothiazines inhibit the ability of bromocriptine to lower serum prolactin concentrations; benztropine (and other anticholinergics) may inhibit the therapeutic response to promethazine; sulfadoxine-pyrimethamine, propranolol, and chloroquine may increase promethazine concentrations; cigarette smoking may enhance the hepatic metabolism of promethazine; concurrent use of promethazine with an antihypertensive may produce additive hypotensive effects; antihypertensive effects of guanethidine and guanadrel may be inhibited by promethazine; concurrent use with TCA may produce increased toxicity or altered therapeutic response; promethazine may inhibit the antiparkinsonian effect of levodopa; promethazine plus lithium may rarely produce neurotoxicity; barbiturates may reduce promethazine concentrations; promethazine may reverse the pressor effects of epinephrine; promethazine and CNS depressants (ethanol, narcotics) may produce additive CNS depressant effects; promethazine and trazodone may produce additive hypotensive effects; use with cisapride may increase the risk of malignant arrhythmias

Food Interactions Increase dietary intake of riboflavin

Stability Protect from light; **compatible** (when comixed in the same syringe) with atropine, chlorpromazine, diphenhydramine, droperidol, fentanyl, glycopyrrolate, hydromorphone, hydroxyzine hydrochloride, meperidine, midazolam, nalbuphine, pentazocine, prochlorperazine, scopolamine; **incompatible** when mixed with aminophylline, cefoperazone (Y-site), chloramphenicol, dimenhydrinate (same syringe), foscarnet (Y-site), furosemide, heparin, hydrocortisone, methohexital, penicillin G, pentobarbital, phenobarbital, thiopental

Mechanism of Action Blocks postsynaptic mesolimbic dopaminergic receptors in the brain; exhibits a strong alpha-adrenergic blocking effect and depresses the release of hypothalamic and hypophyseal hormones; competes with histamine for the H_1-receptor

Pharmacodynamics

Onset of action:

Oral, I.M.: Within 20 minutes

I.V.: 3-5 minutes

Duration: 2-8 hours

Pharmacokinetics

Absorption: 88%

Bioavailability: 25% (due to first pass metabolism)

Half-life: 16-19 hours

Metabolism: In the liver

Elimination: Principally as inactive metabolites in the urine and in the feces

Usual Dosage

Children:

Antihistamine: Oral: 0.1 mg/kg/dose every 6 hours during the day and 0.5 mg/kg/dose at bedtime as needed

Antiemetic: Oral, I.M., I.V., rectal: 0.25-1 mg/kg 4-6 times/day as needed

Motion sickness: Oral: 0.5 mg/kg 30 minutes to 1 hour before departure, then every 12 hours as needed

Sedation: Oral, I.M., I.V., rectal: 0.5-1 mg/kg/dose every 6 hours as needed

Adults:

Antihistamine:

Oral, rectal: 12.5 mg 3 times/day and 25 mg at bedtime

I.M., I.V.: 25 mg, may repeat in 2 hours when necessary; switch to oral route as soon as feasible

Antiemetic: Oral, I.M., I.V., rectal: 12.5-25 mg every 4 hours as needed

Motion sickness: Oral: 25 mg 30 minutes to 1 hour before departure, then every 12 hours as needed

Sedation: Oral, I.M., I.V., rectal: 25-50 mg/dose; repeat every 4-6 hours if needed

Administration

Oral: Administer with food, water, or milk to decrease GI distress

Parenteral: I.M. administration is preferred; avoid I.V. use (see Warnings); in selected patients, promethazine has been administered I.V. diluted to a maximum concentration of 25 mg/mL and infused at a maximum rate of 25 mg/minute; avoid S.C. administration, promethazine is a chemical irritant which may produce necrosis

Test Interactions Alters the flare response in intradermal allergen tests; false negative and positive reactions with pregnancy tests relying on immunological reactions between hCG and anti-hCG

Patient Information Causes drowsiness and may impair ability to perform hazardous tasks which require mental alertness or physical coordination; may cause (Continued)

Promethazine *(Continued)*

photosensitivity; avoid excessive sunlight; notify physician of involuntary movements or feelings of restlessness; may cause dry mouth

Additional Information Although promethazine has been used in combination with meperidine and chlorpromazine as a premedication (lytic cocktail), this combination may have a higher rate of adverse effects compared to alternative sedative/analgesics

Dosage Forms

Injection, as hydrochloride: 25 mg/mL (1 mL, 10 mL); 50 mg/mL (1 mL, 10 mL)
Phenazine®: 50 mg/mL (10 mL)
Phenergan®: 25 mg/mL (1 mL); 50 mg/mL (1 mL)
Suppository, rectal, as hydrochloride (Phenergan®): 12.5 mg, 25 mg, 50 mg
Syrup, as hydrochloride: 6.25 mg/5 mL (120 mL, 240 mL, 480 mL, 4000 mL)
Phenergan®: 6.25 mg/5 mL (120 mL, 480 mL)
Tablet, as hydrochloride (Phenergan®): 12.5 mg, 25 mg, 50 mg

References
Strenkoski-Nix LC, Ermer J, DeCleene S, et al, "Pharmacokinetics of Promethazine Hydrochloride After Administration of Rectal Suppositories and Oral Syrup to Healthy Subjects," *Am J Health Syst Pharm*, 2000, 57(16):1499-505.

Promethazine and Codeine (proe METH a zeen & KOE deen)

U.S. Brand Names Phenergan® With Codeine
Synonyms Codeine and Promethazine
Therapeutic Category Antitussive; Cough Preparation; Phenothiazine Derivative
Generic Available Yes
Use Temporary relief of coughs and upper respiratory symptoms associated with allergy or the common cold
Restrictions C-V
Pregnancy Risk Factor C
Contraindications Hypersensitivity to promethazine, codeine, or any component; lower respiratory tract symptoms, including asthma; concurrent use of MAO inhibitors, narrow-angle glaucoma
Precautions Use with caution in patients with cardiovascular disease, impaired liver function, impaired renal function, sleep apnea, seizures, hypertensive crisis, suspected Reye's syndrome; hypersensitivity reactions to morphine, hydrocodone, hydromorphone, levorphanol, oxycodone, oxymorphone

Adverse Reactions

Promethazine:
Cardiovascular: Tachycardia, bradycardia, palpitations
Central nervous system: Sedation (pronounced), confusion, drowsiness, restlessness, anxiety, extrapyramidal reactions, tardive dyskinesia, seizures
Dermatologic: Rash, photosensitivity
Endocrine & metabolic: Antidiuretic hormone release
Gastrointestinal: GI upset, xerostomia, constipation
Genitourinary: Urinary retention
Hematologic: Agranulocytosis, leukopenia (rare), thrombocytopenia
Hepatic: Cholestatic jaundice, hepatitis
Neuromuscular & skeletal: Arthralgia, tremor, paresthesia, myalgia
Ocular: Blurred vision
Respiratory: Thickening of bronchial secretions, pharyngitis
Miscellaneous: Allergic reactions

Codeine:
Cardiovascular: Palpitations, orthostatic hypotension, tachycardia or bradycardia, peripheral vasodilation
Central nervous system: CNS depression, dizziness, sedation, euphoria, hallucination, seizures
Dermatologic: Pruritus
Gastrointestinal: Nausea, vomiting, constipation, biliary tract spasm
Genitourinary: Urinary tract spasm
Ocular: Miosis
Respiratory: Respiratory depression
Miscellaneous: Physical and psychological dependence, histamine release, allergic reactions

Drug Interactions See Promethazine *on page 836* and Codeine *on page 262*
Food Interactions Increase fluids, fiber intake, and riboflavin in diet
Mechanism of Action See individual monographs for Codeine *on page 262* and Promethazine *on page 836*

Usual Dosage Oral (**in terms of codeine**):

Children: 1-1.5 mg/kg/day divided every 4 hours as needed; maximum dose: 30 mg/day **or**

2-6 years: 1.25-2.5 mL every 4-6 hours as needed or 2.5-5 mg/dose every 4-6 hours as needed; maximum dose: 30 mg codeine/day

6-12 years: 2.5-5 mL every 4-6 hours as needed or 5-10 mg/dose every 4-6 hours as needed; maximum dose: 60 mg codeine/day

Adults: 10-20 mg/dose every 4-6 hours as needed; maximum dose: 120 mg codeine/day; or 5-10 mL every 4-6 hours as needed

Administration Oral: Administer with food or water to decrease GI upset

Test Interactions Alters the flare response in intradermal allergen tests; false negative and positive reactions with pregnancy tests relying on immunological reactions between hCG and anti-hCG

Patient Information Causes drowsiness and may impair ability to perform hazardous activities which require mental alertness or physical coordination; may cause dry mouth; avoid unnecessary exposure to sunlight

Dosage Forms Syrup: Promethazine hydrochloride 6.25 mg and codeine phosphate 10 mg per 5 mL (5 mL, 120 mL, 240 mL, 473 mL)

Promethazine and Phenylephrine

(proe METH a zeen & fen il EF rin)

U.S. Brand Names Phenergan® VC; Promethazine VC Plain Syrup; Promethazine VC Syrup

Synonyms Phenylephrine and Promethazine

Therapeutic Category Antihistamine/Decongestant Combination

Generic Available Yes

Use Temporary relief of upper respiratory symptoms associated with allergy or the common cold

Pregnancy Risk Factor C

Contraindications Hypersensitivity to promethazine, phenylephrine, or any component; asthma, peripheral vascular disease, narrow-angle glaucoma, severe hypertension, cardiovascular disease, liver disease, patients receiving MAO inhibitors

Precautions Use with caution in patients with cardiovascular disease, impaired liver function, asthma, peptic ulcer, sleep apnea, seizures, hypertensive crisis; avoid in patients with suspected Reye's syndrome

Adverse Reactions

Promethazine:

Cardiovascular: Hypertension, hypotension, tachycardia

Central nervous system: Sedation (pronounced), drowsiness, confusion, fatigue, excitation, extrapyramidal reactions, dystonia, tardive dyskinesia

Dermatologic: Photosensitivity, rash, angioedema

Gastrointestinal: Xerostomia, GI upset, increased appetite, weight gain, abdominal pain, diarrhea, nausea

Genitourinary: Urinary retention

Hematologic: Thrombocytopenia, leukopenia, agranulocytosis (rare)

Hepatic: Cholestatic jaundice, hepatitis

Ocular: Blurred vision

Neuromuscular & skeletal: Arthralgia, tremor, paresthesia, myalgia

Respiratory: Thickening of bronchial secretions, pharyngitis

Miscellaneous: Allergic reactions

Phenylephrine:

Cardiovascular: Hypertension, angina, reflex severe bradycardia, arrhythmias, peripheral vasoconstriction

Central nervous system: Restlessness, excitability, headache, anxiety, nervousness, dizziness

Dermatologic: Pilomotor response, skin blanching

Neuromuscular & skeletal: Tremor

Respiratory: Respiratory distress, rebound nasal congestion, sneezing, burning, stinging, dryness

Drug Interactions See Promethazine *on page 836* and Phenylephrine *on page 789*

Food Interactions Increase dietary intake of riboflavin

Usual Dosage Oral:

Children:

2-6 years: 1.25 mL every 4-6 hours, not to exceed 7.5 mL in 24 hours

6-12 years: 2.5 mL every 4-6 hours, not to exceed 15 mL in 24 hours

Children >12 years and Adults: 5 mL every 4-6 hours, not to exceed 30 mL in 24 hours

(Continued)

Promethazine and Phenylephrine *(Continued)*

Administration Oral: Administer with food, water, or milk to decrease GI distress

Test Interactions Alters the flare response in intradermal allergen tests; false negative and positive reactions with pregnancy tests relying on immunological reactions between hCG and anti-hCG

Patient Information Causes drowsiness and may impair ability to perform hazardous activities requiring mental alertness or physical coordination; may cause dry mouth; avoid unnecessary exposure to sunlight

Dosage Forms Liquid: Promethazine hydrochloride 6.25 mg and phenylephrine hydrochloride 5 mg per 5 mL (120 mL, 240 mL, 480 mL, 4000 mL)

Promethazine, Phenylephrine, and Codeine

(proe METH a zeen, fen il EF rin, & KOE deen)

U.S. Brand Names Mallergan-VC® With Codeine; Phenergan® VC With Codeine

Synonyms Codeine, Promethazine, and Phenylephrine; Phenylephrine, Promethazine, and Codeine

Therapeutic Category Antihistamine/Decongestant Combination; Antitussive; Cough Preparation

Generic Available Yes

Use Temporary relief of coughs and upper respiratory symptoms including nasal congestion

Restrictions C-V

Pregnancy Risk Factor C

Contraindications Hypersensitivity to promethazine, codeine, phenylephrine, or any component; asthma, peripheral vascular disease; patients receiving MAO inhibitors

Warnings See individual monographs for Promethazine *on page 836*, Phenylephrine *on page 789*, and Codeine *on page 262*

Precautions See individual monographs for Promethazine *on page 836*, Phenylephrine *on page 789*, and Codeine *on page 262*

Adverse Reactions See individual monographs for Promethazine *on page 836*, Phenylephrine *on page 789*, and Codeine *on page 262*

Drug Interactions See individual monographs for Promethazine *on page 836*, Phenylephrine *on page 789*, and Codeine *on page 262*

Food Interactions Increase fluids, fiber intake, and riboflavin in diet

Usual Dosage Oral: Not recommended for children <2 years of age

Children (**dose expressed in terms of codeine**): 1-1.5 mg/kg/day divided every 4-6 hours, maximum dose: 30 mg/day **or**

<6 years:

Weight 25 lb: 1.25-2.5 mL every 4-6 hours, not to exceed 6 mL/24 hours

Weight 30 lb: 1.25-2.5 mL every 4-6 hours, not to exceed 7 mL/24 hours

Weight 35 lb: 1.25-2.5 mL every 4-6 hours, not to exceed 8 mL/24 hours

Weight 40 lb: 1.25-2.5 mL every 4-6 hours, not to exceed 9 mL/24 hours

6-11 years: 2.5-5 mL every 4-6 hours, not to exceed 15 mL/24 hours

Children ≥12 years and Adults: 5 mL every 4-6 hours, not to exceed 30 mL/24 hours

Administration Oral: Administer with food or water to decrease GI upset

Patient Information May cause dry mouth; avoid unnecessary exposure to sunlight

Dosage Forms Liquid: Promethazine hydrochloride 6.25 mg, phenylephrine hydrochloride 5 mg, and codeine phosphate 10 mg per 5 mL with alcohol 7% (120 mL, 240 mL, 480 mL, 4000 mL)

♦ **Promethazine VC Plain Syrup** *see* Promethazine and Phenylephrine *on page 839*

♦ **Promethazine VC Syrup** *see* Promethazine and Phenylephrine *on page 839*

♦ **Pronestyl®** *see* Procainamide *on page 829*

♦ **Pronestyl-SR®** *see* Procainamide *on page 829*

♦ **Propaderm (Can)** *see* Beclomethasone *on page 131*

♦ **Propanthel (Can)** *see* Propantheline *on page 840*

Propantheline (proe PAN the leen)

Canadian Brand Names Pro-Banthine; Propanthel

Therapeutic Category Anticholinergic Agent; Antispasmodic Agent, Gastrointestinal; Antispasmodic Agent, Urinary

Generic Available Yes: 15 mg tablet

Use Adjunctive treatment of peptic ulcer, irritable bowel syndrome, pancreatitis, ureteral and urinary bladder spasm; to reduce duodenal motility during diagnostic radiologic procedures

Pregnancy Risk Factor C

Contraindications Narrow-angle glaucoma; hypersensitivity to propantheline or any component; ulcerative colitis; toxic megacolon; obstructive disease of the GI or urinary tract

Warnings Infants, patients with Down's syndrome, and children with spastic paralysis or brain damage may be hypersensitive to antimuscarinic effects

Precautions Use with caution in febrile patients, patients with hyperthyroidism, hepatic, cardiac, or renal disease, hypertension, GI infections, diarrhea, reflux esophagitis

Adverse Reactions
Cardiovascular: Tachycardia, palpitations, flushing
Central nervous system: Insomnia, drowsiness, dizziness, nervousness, headache
Dermatologic: Rash, dry skin
Endocrine & metabolic: Suppression of lactation
Gastrointestinal: Xerostomia, nausea, vomiting, constipation, dry throat, dysphagia
Genitourinary: Impotence, urinary retention
Ocular: Mydriasis, blurred vision
Neuromuscular & skeletal: Weakness
Respiratory: Dry nose
Miscellaneous: Allergic reactions, diaphoresis (decreased)

Drug Interactions May increase potential of potassium chloride wax-matrix preparations to cause intestinal lesions due to decreased peristalsis; increased effect/toxicity with anticholinergics, disopyramide, narcotic analgesics, bretylium, type I antiarrhythmics, antihistamines, phenothiazines, tricyclic antidepressants, corticosteroids (increased IOP), CNS depressants (sedation), adenosine, amiodarone, beta-blockers, amoxapine

Mechanism of Action Competitively blocks the action of acetylcholine at postganglionic parasympathetic receptor sites

Pharmacodynamics
Onset of action: Within 30-45 minutes
Duration: 4-6 hours

Pharmacokinetics
Metabolism: In the liver and GI tract
Elimination: In urine, bile, and other body fluids

Usual Dosage Oral:
Antisecretory:
Children: 1-2 mg/kg/day in 3-4 divided doses
Adults: 15 mg 3 times/day before meals or food and 30 mg at bedtime; for mild manifestations: 7.5 mg 3 times/day
Antispasmodic:
Children: 2-3 mg/kg/day in divided doses every 4-6 hours and at bedtime
Adults: 15 mg 3 times/day before meals or food and 30 mg at bedtime

Administration Oral: Administer 30 minutes before meals and at bedtime

Patient Information Causes drowsiness and may impair ability to perform hazardous tasks requiring mental alertness or physical coordination; notify physician if skin rash, flushing, or eye pain occurs; or if difficulty in urinating, constipation, or sensitivity to light becomes severe or persists; maintain good oral hygiene habits, because lack of saliva may increase chance of cavities

Dosage Forms Tablet, as bromide: 15 mg

♦ **Propa Ph [OTC]** see Salicylic Acid on page 886

Proparacaine (proe PAR a kane)

U.S. Brand Names Alcaine®; Ophthetic®
Canadian Brand Names Diocaine
Synonyms Proxymetacaine
Therapeutic Category Local Anesthetic, Ophthalmic
Generic Available Yes
Use Local anesthesia for tonometry, gonioscopy; suture removal from cornea; removal of corneal foreign body; cataract extraction, glaucoma surgery; short operative procedure involving the cornea and conjunctiva
Pregnancy Risk Factor C
Contraindications Hypersensitivity to proparacaine or any component
Precautions Use with caution in patients with cardiac disease, hyperthyroidism
Adverse Reactions
Dermatologic: Allergic contact dermatitis
Local: Irritation, stinging, sensitization
Ocular: Keratitis, iritis, erosion of the corneal epithelium, conjunctival congestion and hemorrhage, corneal opacification
(Continued)

Proparacaine *(Continued)*

Mechanism of Action Local anesthetic; prevents initiation and transmission of impulse at the nerve cell membrane by decreasing ion permeability

Pharmacodynamics
Onset of action: Within 20 seconds of instillation
Duration: 15-20 minutes

Usual Dosage Children and Adults:
Ophthalmic surgery: Instill 1 drop of 0.5% solution in eye every 5-10 minutes for 5-7 doses
Tonometry, gonioscopy, suture removal: Instill 1-2 drops of 0.5% solution in eye just prior to procedure

Administration Ophthalmic: Instill drops into affected eye(s); avoid contact of bottle tip with skin or eye

Patient Information Do not rub eye until anesthesia has worn off

Dosage Forms Ophthalmic, solution, as hydrochloride: 0.5% (15 mL)

♦ **Propine**® *see Dipivefrin on page 345*

♦ **Pro-Piroxicam (Can)** *see Piroxicam on page 806*

♦ **Proplex**® **T** *see Factor IX Complex (Human) on page 414*

Propofol *(PROE po fole)*

U.S. Brand Names Diprivan®

Therapeutic Category General Anesthetic

Generic Available Yes

Use Induction of anesthesia in children ≥3 years and adults; maintenance of anesthesia in children ≥2 months and adults; initiation and maintenance of monitored anesthesia care sedation in adults; continuous sedation of adult intensive care unit patients

Pregnancy Risk Factor B

Contraindications Hypersensitivity to propofol, sulfites (generic product contains sodium metabisulfite), disodium edetate (Diprivan® contains disodium edetate), or any component (eg, soybean oil, egg yolk phospholipid, or egg lecithin); patients who are not intubated or mechanically ventilated; other contraindications to general anesthesia or sedation apply

Warnings Not recommended for induction of anesthesia in children <3 years or for maintenance of anesthesia in infants <2 months of age; not recommended for monitored anesthesia care sedation in children; **not recommended for sedation of PICU patients. Note: The FDA is very concerned about the safety of propofol in PICU patients.** The results of a manufacturer's randomized controlled clinical trial (n=327) revealed an increase in the number of deaths in PICU patients treated with Diprivan® versus other standard sedative agents. Diprivan® was administered at initial infusion rates of 5.5 mg/kg/hour and titrated to maintain a standardized level of sedation. Twenty-one of the 25 deaths occurred in patients who received propofol. The FDA's review of the data did not find a correlation of the deaths with an underlying disease state, nor did the review identify a definite pattern to the causes of death. A new clinical trial will be conducted to address this issue (see http://www.FDA.gov/medwatch/safety/2001/dipvivan_deardoc.pdf). The use of propofol in PICU patients, especially at high doses for prolonged periods of time may be associated with certain toxicities; metabolic acidosis with fatal cardiac failure has occurred in several children (4 weeks to 11 years of age) who received propofol infusions at average rates of infusion of 4.5-10 mg/kg/hour for 66-115 hours (maximum rates of infusion 6.2-11.5 mg/kg/hour); see Parke, 1992; Strickland, 1995; and Bray, 1995.

Patients require continuous monitoring and airway management; cardiovascular and respiratory resuscitation equipment should be available; decrease the dose in ASA III or IV, elderly, debilitated, or hypovolemic patients; not recommended for use in obstetrics, cesarean deliveries, lactating women, patients with increased ICP or impaired cerebral circulation. Abrupt discontinuation may result in rapid awakening, anxiety, agitation, and resistance to mechanical ventilation. Although products contain preservatives, rapid growth of micro-organisms can occur; failure to use aseptic technique can result in microbial contamination and fever, sepsis, infection, life-threatening illnesses, or death; discard I.V. tubing and unused portions after 12 hours; **do not use if microbial contamination is suspected.**

Propofol should be administered by qualified healthcare professionals trained in advanced cardiac life support and anesthetic drug use (when used for general anesthesia and monitored anesthesia care sedation) or management of critically ill patients (when used for sedation in intensive care patient).

Precautions Use with caution in patients with seizures or history of epilepsy, or severe cardiac or respiratory disease; I.V. injection may produce transient local pain; perioperative myoclonia may occur; decrease dose and rate of infusion for elderly, debilitated, or ASA III/IV patients. Abrupt discontinuation in pediatric patients may cause agitation, hyperirritability, tremulousness, and flushing of hands and feet. Increased frequency of bradycardia, jitteriness, and agitation have also been observed.

Diprivan® contains disodium edetate which can chelate trace metals, including zinc; as much as 10 mg of elemented zinc may be lost per day when calcium disodium edetate is used in gram doses to treat heavy metal poisonings; no reports of zinc deficiency or low zinc levels have been reported with Diprivan®, however, the manufacturer recommends that Diprivan® not be infused for >5 days without giving a "drug holiday"; during this time off of Diprivan®, replacement of estimated or measured urine zinc losses is recommended. **Note:** The generic product does not contain disodium edetate, but contains metabisulfite as the preservative; sulfites may cause hypersensitivity reactions

Adverse Reactions
Cardiovascular: Hypotension (dose related), bradycardia, myocardial depression, flushing
Central nervous system: Fever, headache, dizziness
Dermatologic: Rash, pruritus
Endocrine & metabolic: Hyperlipidemia; fatal metabolic acidosis has been reported
Gastrointestinal: Nausea, vomiting, abdominal cramping
Genitourinary: Discoloration of urine (green)
Local: Pain at injection site (especially when administered via small vein); **Note:** Dilution with D_5W or administration of lidocaine pretreatment may decrease local pain
Neuromuscular & skeletal: Myalgia, twitching, clonic/myoclonic movement
Respiratory: Respiratory acidosis, respiratory depression, apnea
Miscellaneous: Anaphylaxis, anaphylactoid reactions

Drug Interactions Theophylline may antagonize the CNS effects of propofol; propofol may increase serum concentrations of alfentanil; increased toxicity may occur with acetazolamide (cardiorespiratory instability), CNS depressants, atracurium (anaphylaxis), phenothiazines, fentanyl (increased concentration of propofol), guanabenz, MAO inhibitors, narcotic analgesics, vecuronium (increased neuromuscular blockade); in pediatric patients, concurrent use of propofol with fentanyl may cause serious bradycardia

Stability Does not require refrigeration; protect from light; do not use if there is evidence of separation of phases of emulsion, particulate matter, or discoloration; discard unused portions at end of surgical procedure; ICU use: Discard tubing and unused portions after 12 hours; dilute with D_5W only; do not dilute to <2 mg/mL; diluted emulsion is more stable in glass; stability in plastic: 95% potency after 2 hours; may administer with D_5W, LR, D_5LR, $D_5/^1/_2NS$, $D_5/^1/_4NS$; do not administer with blood or blood products through the same I.V. catheter; do not mix with other drugs

Mechanism of Action Propofol is a hindered phenolic compound with intravenous general anesthetic properties. The drug is unrelated to any of the currently used barbiturate, opioid, benzodiazepine, arylcyclohexylamine, or imidazole intravenous anesthetic agents.

Pharmacodynamics
Onset of anesthesia: Within 30 seconds after bolus infusion
Duration: ~3-10 minutes depending on the dose, rate and duration of administration; with prolonged use (eg, 10 days ICU sedation), propofol accumulates in tissues and redistributes into plasma when the drug is discontinued, so that the time to awakening (duration of action) is increased; however, if dose is titrated on a daily basis, so that the minimum effective dose is utilized, time to awakening may be within 10-15 minutes even after prolonged use

Pharmacokinetics
Distribution: Large volume of distribution; highly lipophilic
V_d (apparent): Children 4-12 years: 5-10 L/kg
V_{dss}:
Adults: 170-350 L
Adults (10-day infusion): 60 L/kg
Protein binding: 97% to 99%
Metabolism: In the liver via glucuronide and sulfate conjugation
Half-life (three-compartment model):
Alpha: 2-8 minutes
Beta (second distribution): ~40 minutes
(Continued)

Propofol *(Continued)*

Terminal: ~200 minutes; range: 300-700 minutes

Terminal (after 10-day infusion): 1-3 days

Elimination: ~90% excreted in urine as metabolites and <1% as unchanged drug

Usual Dosage Dosage must be individualized based on total body weight and titrated to the desired clinical effect; wait at least 3-5 minutes between dosage adjustments to clinically assess drug effects; smaller doses are required when used with narcotics; the following are general dosing guidelines:

General anesthesia:

I.V. induction: (See "Symbols and Abbreviations Used in This Handbook" in front section of this book for explanation of ASA classes):

Children ≥3 years, ASA I or II: 2.5-3.5 mg/kg; use a lower dose for children ASA III or IV

Adults, ASA I or II, <55 years: 2-2.5 mg/kg (~40 mg every 10 seconds until onset of induction)

Elderly, debilitated, hypovolemic, or ASA III or IV: 1-1.5 mg/kg (~20 mg every 10 seconds until onset of induction)

Cardiac anesthesia: 0.5-1.5 mg/kg (~20 mg every 10 seconds until onset of induction)

Neurosurgical patients: 1-2 mg/kg (~20 mg every 10 seconds until onset of induction)

Maintenance: I.V. infusion:

Infants ≥2 months to Children 16 years, ASA I or II: Initial: 200-300 mcg/kg/minute; decrease dose after 30 minutes if clinical signs of light anesthesia are absent; usual infusion rate: 125-150 mcg/kg/minute; younger pediatric patients may require larger infusion rates compared to older children

Adults, ASA I or II, <55 years: Initial: 150-200 mcg/kg/minute for 10-15 minutes; decrease by 30% to 50% during first 30 minutes of maintenance; usual infusion rate: 100-200 mcg/kg/minute

Elderly, debilitated, hypovolemic, ASA III or IV: 50-100 mcg/kg/minute

Cardiac anesthesia:

Low dose propofol with primary opioid: 50-100 mcg/kg/minute (see manufacturer's labeling)

Primary propofol with secondary opioid: 100-150 mcg/kg/minute

Neurosurgical patients: 100-200 mcg/kg/minute

Maintenance: I.V. intermittent bolus: Adults, ASA I or II, <55 years: 20-50 mg increments as needed

Monitored Anesthesia Care sedation:

Initiation:

Adults, ASA I or II, <55 years: Slow I.V. infusion: 100-150 mcg/kg/minute for 3-5 minutes; slow injection: 0.5 mg/kg over 3-5 minutes

Elderly, debilitated, neurosurgical, or ASA III or IV patients: Use similar doses to healthy adults; avoid rapid I.V. boluses

Maintenance:

Adults, ASA I or II, <55 years: I.V. infusion using variable rates (preferred over intermittent boluses): 25-75 mcg/kg/minute; incremental bolus doses: 10 mg or 20 mg

Elderly, debilitated, neurosurgical, or ASA III or IV patients: Use 80% of healthy adult dose; **do not** use rapid bolus doses (single or repeated)

ICU sedation in intubated mechanically ventilated patients: Avoid rapid bolus injection; individualize dose and titrate to response

Adults: Continuous infusion: Initial: 0.3 mg/kg/hour; increase by 0.3-0.6 mg/kg/hour every 5-10 minutes until desired sedation level is achieved; usual maintenance: 0.3-3 mg/kg/hour or higher; reduce dose by 80% in elderly, debilitated, and ASA III or IV patients; reduce dose after adequate sedation established and adjust to response (ie, evaluate frequently to use minimum dose for sedation)

Administration Parenteral: I.V.: Shake injection well before use; administer pediatric induction doses over 20-30 seconds; do not administer via filter with <5-micron pore size

Monitoring Parameters Respiratory rate, blood pressure, heart rate, oxygen saturation, ABGs, depth of sedation; serum lipids or triglycerides with use >24 hours

Nursing Implications May change urine color to green

Additional Information Due to poor water solubility, the I.V. formulation is an isotonic oil-in-water emulsion and contains soybean oil, glycerol, egg lecithin, and sodium hydroxide (for pH adjustment); the brand name and generic product differ in the preservative used; Diprivan® contains 0.005% disodium edetate, while the generic product contains sodium metabisulfite (0.25 mg/mL); propofol injection contains ~0.1 g of fat/mL (1.1 kcal/mL)

Dosage Forms Injection: 10 mg/mL (20 mL, 50 mL, 100 mL)

References

Bray RJ, "Fatal Myocardial Failure Associated With a Propofol Infusion in a Child," *Anaesthesia*, 1995, 50(1):94.

Parke TJ, Stevens JE, Rice ASC, et al, "Metabolic Acidosis and Fatal Myocardial Failure After Propofol Infusion in Children: Five Case Reports," *BMJ*, 1992, 305(6854):613-6.

Strickland RA and Murray MJ, "Fatal Metabolic Acidosis in a Pediatric Patient Receiving an Infusion of Propofol in the Intensive Care Unit: Is There a Relationship?" *Crit Care Med*, 1995, 23(2):405-9.

Propoxyphene (proe POKS i feen)

Related Information

Overdose and Toxicology *on page 1222*

U.S. Brand Names Darvon®; Darvon-N®

Canadian Brand Names Novo-Propoxyn; 624 Tablets

Synonyms Dextropropoxyphene

Therapeutic Category Analgesic, Narcotic

Generic Available Yes: Capsule

Use Management of mild to moderate pain

Restrictions C-IV

Pregnancy Risk Factor C (D if used for prolonged periods)

Contraindications Hypersensitivity to propoxyphene or any component

Warnings Do not exceed recommended dosage

Precautions Use with caution in patients with renal or hepatic dysfunction, or when substituting propoxyphene for opiates in narcotic dependent patients; reduce dose in patients with hepatic dysfunction; avoid use in patients with Cl_{cr} <10 mL/minute

Adverse Reactions

Central nervous system: Dizziness, lightheadedness, sedation, paradoxical excitement and insomnia, headache

Dermatologic: Rashes

Gastrointestinal: GI upset, nausea, vomiting, constipation

Hepatic: Elevated liver enzymes

Neuromuscular & skeletal: Weakness

Miscellaneous: Psychologic and physical dependence

Drug Interactions Cytochrome P-450 isoenzyme CYP3A3/4 inhibitor

CNS depressants, alcohol, MAO inhibitors, may potentiate adverse effects; propoxyphene may inhibit the metabolism and increase the serum concentrations of carbamazepine, phenobarbital, tricyclic antidepressants, and warfarin; concurrent use of propoxyphene with ritonavir is not recommended

Food Interactions Food may decrease rate of absorption, but may slightly increase bioavailability

Mechanism of Action Binds to opiate receptors in the CNS, causing inhibition of ascending pain pathways, altering the perception of and response to pain; produces generalized CNS depression

Pharmacodynamics

Onset of effects: Oral: Within 30-60 minutes

Duration: 4-6 hours

Pharmacokinetics

Metabolism: In the liver to an active metabolite (norpropoxyphene) and inactive metabolites

Bioavailability: Oral: 30% to 70% due to first-pass effect

Half-life, adults: 8-24 hours (mean: ~15 hours)

Norpropoxyphene, adults: 34 hours

Dialysis: Not dialyzable (0% to 5%)

Usual Dosage Oral:

Children: Dose not well established; doses of propoxyphene hydrochloride of 2-3 mg/kg/day divided every 6 hours have been used

Adults:

Hydrochloride: 65 mg every 3-4 hours as needed for pain; maximum dose: 390 mg/day

Napsylate: 100 mg every 4 hours as needed for pain; maximum dose: 600 mg/day

Dosing adjustment in renal impairment: Cl_{cr} <10 mL/minute: Avoid use

Dosing adjustment in hepatic impairment: Reduced doses should be used

Administration Oral: May administer with food to decrease GI upset

Monitoring Parameters Pain relief, respiratory rate, blood pressure, mental status; liver enzymes with long-term use

Test Interactions False-positive methadone test

(Continued)

Propoxyphene *(Continued)*

Patient Information Avoid alcohol; may be habit-forming; may cause dizziness or drowsiness and impair ability to perform activities requiring mental alertness or physical coordination

Additional Information Propoxyphene does not possess any anti-inflammatory or antipyretic actions; it possesses little, if any, antitussive effects; propoxyphene napsylate 100 mg is equivalent to 65 mg of propoxyphene hydrochloride; several cases utilizing propoxyphene in children for opioid detoxification have been reported (see References)

Dosage Forms
Capsule, as hydrochloride (Darvon®): 65 mg
Tablet, as napsylate (Darvon-N®): 100 mg

References
Hasday JD and Weintraub M, "Propoxyphene in Children With Iatrogenic Morphine Dependence," *Am J Dis Child*, 1983, 137(8):745-8.

Propoxyphene and Acetaminophen
(proe POKS i feen & a seet a MIN oh fen)

Related Information
Narcotic Analgesics Comparison *on page 1070*
Overdose and Toxicology *on page 1222*

U.S. Brand Names Darvocet-N® 50; Darvocet-N® 100; Wygesic®

Synonyms Acetaminophen and Propoxyphene

Therapeutic Category Analgesic, Narcotic

Generic Available Yes

Use Management of mild to moderate pain

Restrictions C-IV

Pregnancy Risk Factor C

Contraindications Hypersensitivity to propoxyphene, acetaminophen, or any component

Warnings Do not exceed recommended dosage

Precautions Use with caution in patients with renal or hepatic dysfunction or when substituting propoxyphene for opiates in narcotic dependent patients

Adverse Reactions
Propoxyphene:
Central nervous system: Dizziness, lightheadedness, sedation, paradoxical excitement, insomnia, headache
Dermatologic: Rashes
Gastrointestinal: GI upset, nausea, vomiting, constipation
Hepatic: Elevated liver enzymes
Neuromuscular & skeletal: Weakness
Miscellaneous: Psychologic and physical dependence
Acetaminophen:
Dermatologic: Rash
Hematologic: Blood dyscrasias (neutropenia, pancytopenia, leukopenia)
Hepatic: Hepatic necrosis with overdose
Renal: Renal injury with chronic use
Miscellaneous: Hypersensitivity reactions (rare)

Drug Interactions See Propoxyphene *on page 845* and Acetaminophen *on page 29*

Food Interactions Food may decrease rate of absorption of propoxyphene, but may slightly increase bioavailability; the rate of absorption of acetaminophen may be decreased when given with food high in carbohydrates

Pharmacodynamics See individual monographs for Propoxyphene *on page 845* and Acetaminophen *on page 29*

Pharmacokinetics See individual monographs for Propoxyphene *on page 845* and Acetaminophen *on page 29*

Usual Dosage Adults: Oral:
Darvocet-N® 50: 1-2 tablets every 4 hours as needed; maximum dose: 600 mg propoxyphene napsylate/day
Darvocet-N® 100 or Wygesic®: 1 tablet every 4 hours as needed; maximum dose: 600 mg propoxyphene napsylate/day

Administration Oral: Administer with water on an empty stomach; may administer with food to decrease GI upset

Monitoring Parameters Pain relief, respiratory rate, blood pressure, mental status; liver enzymes with long-term use

Test Interactions False-positive methadone test

Patient Information Avoid alcohol; may be habit-forming; may cause dizziness, drowsiness and impair ability to perform hazardous tasks requiring mental alertness

Additional Information Propoxyphene napsylate 100 mg is equivalent to 65 mg of propoxyphene hydrochloride

Dosage Forms Tablet:

Darvocet-N® 50: Propoxyphene napsylate 50 mg and acetaminophen 325 mg

Darvocet-N® 100: Propoxyphene napsylate 100 mg and acetaminophen 650 mg

Wygesic®: Propoxyphene hydrochloride 65 mg and acetaminophen 650 mg

Propranolol (proe PRAN oh lole)

Related Information

Carbohydrate and Alcohol Content of Liquid Medications for Use in Patients Receiving Ketogenic Diets *on page 1258*

Overdose and Toxicology *on page 1222*

U.S. Brand Names Inderal®; Inderal® LA

Canadian Brand Names Apo-Propranolol; Novo-Pranol; Nu-Propranolol

Therapeutic Category Antianginal Agent; Antiarrhythmic Agent, Class II; Antihypertensive Agent; Antimigraine Agent; Beta-Adrenergic Blocker

Generic Available Yes

Use Management of hypertension, angina pectoris, pheochromocytoma, essential tremor, tetralogy of Fallot cyanotic spells, and arrhythmias (such as atrial fibrillation and flutter, A-V nodal re-entrant tachycardias, and catecholamine-induced arrhythmias); prevention of MI, migraine headache; symptomatic treatment of hypertrophic subaortic stenosis; short-term adjunctive therapy of thyrotoxicosis

Pregnancy Risk Factor C

Contraindications Hypersensitivity to propranolol or any component; uncompensated CHF, cardiogenic shock, bradycardia or heart block, asthma, hyperactive airway disease, chronic obstructive lung disease, Raynaud's syndrome

Warnings In patients with angina pectoris, exacerbation of angina and, in some cases, MI occurred following abrupt discontinuance of therapy; hypoglycemia may occur, particularly in infants and children (whether the patient has diabetes mellitus or not), especially during fasting before surgery; hypoglycemia may also occur after prolonged physical exertion and in patients with renal dysfunction

Precautions Propranolol may block hypoglycemia-induced tachycardia and blood pressure changes, use with caution in patients with diabetes mellitus; use with caution in patients with renal or hepatic dysfunction; avoid I.V. use in patients receiving calcium channel blockers (eg, verapamil) (effects may be potentiated); patients receiving beta blockers who have a history of anaphylactic reactions, may be more reactive to a repeated allergen challenge and may not be responsive to the usual epinephrine doses used to treat an allergic reaction

Adverse Reactions

Cardiovascular: Hypotension, impaired myocardial contractility, CHF, bradycardia, worsening of A-V conduction disturbances

Central nervous system: Lightheadedness, insomnia, vivid dreams, lethargy, depression

Endocrine & metabolic: Hypoglycemia [also blunts warning signs of hypoglycemia (eg, tachycardia)], hyperglycemia

Gastrointestinal: Nausea, vomiting, diarrhea, GI distress

Hematologic: Agranulocytosis

Neuromuscular & skeletal: Weakness

Respiratory: Bronchospasm

Miscellaneous: Cold extremities

Drug Interactions Cytochrome P-450 isoenzyme, CYP1A2, CYP2C18, CYP2C19, and CYP2D6 substrate

Phenobarbital, rifampin may increase propranolol clearance and may decrease its activity; cimetidine may reduce propranolol clearance and may increase its effects; aluminum-containing antacid may reduce GI absorption of propranolol; flecainide, hydralazine, quinidine, verapamil may increase cardiovascular adverse effects

Food Interactions Avoid natural licorice (causes sodium and water retention and increases potassium loss); protein-rich foods may increase bioavailability; a change in diet from high carbohydrate/low protein to low carbohydrate/high protein may result in increased oral clearance

Stability Injection is compatible in saline, incompatible with bicarbonate; protect injection from light

Mechanism of Action Nonselective beta-adrenergic blocker (class II antiarrhythmic); competitively blocks response to beta$_1$ and beta$_2$-adrenergic stimulation (Continued)

Propranolol *(Continued)*

which results in decrease in heart rate, myocardial contractility, blood pressure, and myocardial oxygen demand

Pharmacodynamics Beta blockade: Oral:

Onset of action: Within 1-2 hours

Duration: ~6 hours

Pharmacokinetics

Distribution: V_d: Adults: 3.9 L/kg; crosses the placenta; small amounts appear in breast milk

Protein-binding (Alpha$_1$-acid glycoprotein and albumin):

Newborns: 60% to 68%

Adults: 93%

Metabolism: Extensive first-pass effect, metabolized in the liver to active and inactive compounds

Bioavailability: 30% to 40%; oral bioavailability may be increased in Down syndrome children

Half-life (prolonged with hepatic dysfunction):

Neonates and Infants: Possible increased half-life

Children: 3.9-6.4 hours

Adults: 4-6 hours

Elimination: Metabolites are excreted primarily in urine (96% to 99%); <1% excreted in urine as unchanged drug

Dialysis: Not dialyzable: (0% to 5%)

Usual Dosage

Neonates:

Oral: Initial: 0.25 mg/kg/dose every 6-8 hours; increase slowly as needed to maximum of 5 mg/kg/day

I.V.: Initial: 0.01 mg/kg slow I.V. push over 10 minutes; may repeat every 6-8 hours as needed; increase slowly to maximum of 0.15 mg/kg/dose every 6-8 hours

Arrhythmias:

Oral:

Children: Initial: 0.5-1 mg/kg/day in divided doses every 6-8 hours; titrate dosage upward every 3-5 days; usual dose: 2-4 mg/kg/day; higher doses may be needed; do not exceed 16 mg/kg/day or 60 mg/day

Adults: Initial: 10-20 mg/dose every 6-8 hours, increase gradually; usual range: 40-320 mg/day

I.V.:

Children: 0.01-0.1 mg/kg slow I.V. over 10 minutes; maximum dose: 1 mg (infants); 3 mg (children)

Adults: 1 mg/dose slow I.V.; repeat every 5 minutes up to a total of 5 mg

Hypertension: Oral:

Children: Initial: 0.5-1 mg/kg/day in divided doses every 6-12 hours; increase gradually every 3-5 days; usual dose: 1-5 mg/kg/day; maximum dose: 8 mg/kg/day

Adults: Initial: 40 mg twice daily or 60-80 mg once daily as sustained release capsules; increase dosage every 3-5 days; usual dose: ≤320 mg divided in 2-3 doses/day or once daily as sustained release; maximum daily dose: 640 mg

Migraine headache prophylaxis: Oral:

Children: 0.6-1.5 mg/kg/day divided every 8 hours; maximum dose: 4 mg/kg/day

or

≤35 kg: 10-20 mg 3 times/day

>35 kg: 20-40 mg 3 times/day

Adults: Initial: 80 mg/day divided every 6-8 hours (or once daily as sustained release capsule); increase by 20-40 mg/dose every 3-4 weeks to a maximum of 160-240 mg/day given in divided doses every 6-8 hours (or once daily as sustained release capsules)

Tetralogy spells: Infants and Children:

Oral: Usual: 1-2 mg/kg/dose every 6 hours, may initiate at 1/2 the usual dose; may increase by 1 mg/kg/day every 24 hours to maximum of 5 mg/kg/day; if refractory may increase slowly to a maximum of 10-15 mg/kg/day but must carefully monitor heart rate, heart size, and cardiac contractility (Garson, 1981).

I.V.: 0.15-0.25 mg/kg/dose slow I.V.; may repeat in 15 minutes

Thyrotoxicosis:

Neonates: Oral: 2 mg/kg/day in divided doses every 6-12 hours; occasionally higher doses may be required

Adolescents and Adults: Oral: 10-40 mg/dose every 6 hours

Adults: I.V.: 1-3 mg/dose slow I.V. as a single dose

Administration
    Oral: Administer with food; do not chew or crush sustained action capsules, swallow whole; mix concentrated oral solution with water, fruit juice, liquid, or semisolid food before administration
    Parenteral: I.V. administration should not exceed 1 mg/minute; administer slow I.V. over 10 minutes in children; maximum concentration for injection: 1 mg/mL
Monitoring Parameters EKG, blood pressure
Reference Range Therapeutic: 50-100 ng/mL (SI: 190-390 nmol/L) at end of dosing interval
Patient Information Avoid alcohol; do not discontinue abruptly; may mask fast heart rate of hypoglycemia, but sweating will still occur
Nursing Implications The I.V. dose is much smaller than oral dose
Additional Information Not indicated for hypertensive emergencies; do not abruptly discontinue therapy, taper dosage gradually over 2 weeks
Dosage Forms
    Capsule, sustained action, as hydrochloride (Inderal® LA): 60 mg, 80 mg, 120 mg, 160 mg
    Injection, as hydrochloride (Inderal®): 1 mg/mL (1 mL)
    Solution, oral, as hydrochloride: 4 mg/mL [strawberry-mint flavor; alcohol free] (5 mL, 500 mL); 8 mg/mL [strawberry-mint flavor; alcohol free] (500 mL)
    Solution, oral, concentrate, as hydrochloride: 80 mg/mL (30 mL)
    Tablet, as hydrochloride (Inderal®): 10 mg, 20 mg, 40 mg, 60 mg, 80 mg

References
Garson A Jr, Gillette PC, and McNamara DG, "Propranolol: The Preferred Palliation for Tetralogy of Fallot," *Am J Cardiol*, 1981, 47(5):1098-104.
Lai CW, Ziegler DK, Lansky LL, et al, "Hemiplegic Migraine in Childhood: Diagnostic and Therapeutic Aspects," *J Pediatr*, 1982, 101(5):696-9.
Pickoff AS, Zies L, Ferrer PL, et al, "High-Dose Propranolol Therapy in the Management of Supraventricular Tachycardia," *J Pediatr*, 1979, 94(1):144-6.
Rasoulpour M and Marinelli KA, "Systemic Hypertension," *Clin Perinatol*, 1992, 19(1):121-37.
Sinaiko AR, "Pharmacologic Management of Childhood Hypertension," *Pediatr Clin North Am*, 1993, 40(1):195-212.

♦ **Propulsid®** *see* Cisapride *U.S. - Available Via Limited-Access Protocol Only on page 239*
♦ **2-Propylpentanoic Acid** *see* Valproic Acid and Derivatives *on page 998*

Propylthiouracil (proe pil thye oh YOOR a sil)
Canadian Brand Names Propyl-Thyracil
Synonyms PTU
Therapeutic Category Antithyroid Agent
Generic Available Yes
Use Palliative treatment of hyperthyroidism; adjunct to ameliorate hyperthyroidism in preparation for surgical treatment or radioactive iodine therapy; management of thyrotoxic crisis
Pregnancy Risk Factor D
Contraindications Hypersensitivity to propylthiouracil or any component
Warnings May cause agranulocytosis, thyroid hyperplasia, thyroid carcinoma (usage >1 year)
Precautions Use with caution in patients receiving other drugs known to cause agranulocytosis
Adverse Reactions
    Cardiovascular: Edema, cutaneous vasculitis
    Central nervous system: Drowsiness, vertigo, dizziness, headache, drug fever
    Dermatologic: Rash, urticaria, pruritus, exfoliative dermatitis, alopecia, skin pigmentation
    Gastrointestinal: Nausea, vomiting, ageusia, sialadenopathy, constipation
    Hematologic: Agranulocytosis, leukopenia, thrombocytopenia, bleeding, hypoprothrombinemia
    Hepatic: Jaundice, hepatitis
    Neuromuscular & skeletal: Arthralgia, paresthesia, neuritis
    Renal: Nephritis
    Respiratory: Interstitial pneumonitis
    Miscellaneous: Lymphadenopathy
Drug Interactions Anticoagulants (enhanced anticoagulant activity)
Mechanism of Action Inhibits the synthesis of thyroid hormones by blocking the oxidation of iodine in the thyroid gland; blocks synthesis of thyroxine and triiodothyronine
    (Continued)

Propylthiouracil *(Continued)*

Pharmacodynamics For significant therapeutic effects 24-36 hours are required; remission of hyperthyroidism usually does not occur before 4 months of continued therapy

Pharmacokinetics
Distribution: Breast milk to plasma ratio: 0.1
Protein binding: 75% to 80%
Metabolism: Hepatic
Bioavailability: 80% to 95%
Half-life: 1.5-5 hours
  End-stage renal disease: 8.5 hours
Time to peak serum concentration: Oral: Within 1 hour; persists for 2-3 hours
Elimination: 35% excreted in urine

Usual Dosage Oral:
Neonates: 5-10 mg/kg/day in divided doses every 8 hours
Children: 5-7 mg/kg/day in divided doses every 8 hours **or**
  6-10 years: 50-150 mg/day divided every 8 hours
  ≥10 years: 150-300 mg/day divided every 8 hours
  Maintenance: $^{1}/_{3}$-$^{2}/_{3}$ of the initial dose in divided doses every 8-12 hours; this begins usually after 2 months on an effective initial dosage
Adults: Initial: 300-450 mg/day in divided doses every 8 hours (doses of 600-1200 mg/day are sometimes needed); maintenance: 100-150 mg/day in divided doses every 8-12 hours

Dosing adjustment in renal impairment: Adjustment is not necessary

Administration Oral: Administer with food

Monitoring Parameters CBC with differential, liver function tests, platelets, thyroid function tests (TSH, T_3, T_4), prothrombin time

Reference Range See normal values for thyroid function in Normal Laboratory Values for Children *on page 1187*

Dosage Forms Tablet: 50 mg

Extemporaneous Preparations A 5 mg/mL oral suspension may be made by crushing twenty 50 mg propylthiouracil tablets; add by geometric proportions 1:1 mixture of Ora-Plus® and Ora-Sweet® to a final volume of 200 mL; stable 91 days at 4°C and 70 days at 25°C
  Nahata MC, Morosco RS, and Trowbridge JM, "Stability of Propylthiouracil in Extemporaneously Prepared Oral Suspensions at 4 and 25 Degrees C," *Am J Health Syst Pharm*, 2000, 57(12):1141-3.

References
Raby C, Lagorce JF, Jambut-Absil AC, et al, "The Mechanism of Action of Synthetic Antithyroid Drugs: Iodine Complexation During Oxidation of Iodide," *Endocrinology*, 1990, 126(3):1683-91.

♦ **Propyl-Thyracil (Can)** *see* Propylthiouracil *on page 849*
♦ **2-Propylvaleric Acid** *see* Valproic Acid and Derivatives *on page 998*
♦ **Prosedyl (Can)** *see* Quinidine *on page 860*
♦ **Pro-Sof® Plus [OTC]** *see* Docusate and Casanthranol *on page 351*
♦ **Prostaglandin E₁** *see* Alprostadil *on page 56*
♦ **Prostaphlin®** *see* Oxacillin *on page 740*
♦ **Prostigmin®** *see* Neostigmine *on page 708*
♦ **Prostin VR Pediatric® Injection** *see* Alprostadil *on page 56*

Protamine *(PROE ta meen)*

Therapeutic Category Antidote, Heparin
Generic Available Yes
Use Treatment of heparin overdosage; neutralize heparin during surgery or dialysis procedures
Pregnancy Risk Factor C
Contraindications Hypersensitivity to protamine or any component
Warnings Heparin rebound associated with anticoagulation and bleeding has been reported to occur occasionally; symptoms typically occur 8-9 hours after protamine administration, but may occur as long as 18 hours later
Precautions Use with caution in patients allergic to fish, with prior history of vasectomy, patients receiving protamine-containing insulin or previous protamine therapy
Adverse Reactions
Cardiovascular: Hypotension, bradycardia, flushing, pulmonary hypertension
Central nervous system: Lassitude
Gastrointestinal: Nausea, vomiting
Neuromuscular & skeletal: Back pain

Respiratory: Dyspnea

Miscellaneous: Hypersensitivity reactions

Stability Refrigerate; stable for at least 2 weeks at room temperature

Mechanism of Action Combines with strongly acidic heparin to form a stable complex (salt) neutralizing the anticoagulant activity of both drugs

Pharmacodynamics Onset of action: Heparin neutralization occurs within 5 minutes following I.V. injection

Pharmacokinetics Elimination: Unknown

Usual Dosage I.V.: Protamine dosage is determined by the most recent dosage of heparin or low molecular weight heparin (LMWH); 1 mg of protamine neutralizes 90 USP units of heparin (lung), 115 USP units of heparin (intestinal), and 1 mg (100 units) LMWH; maximum dose: 50 mg

Heparin overdosage: Since blood heparin concentrations decrease rapidly **after** heparin administration, adjust the protamine dosage depending upon the duration of time since heparin administration as follows (see table):

Time Since Last Heparin Dose (min)	Dose of Protamine (mg) to Neutralize 100 units of Heparin
<30	1
30-60	0.5-0.75
60-120	0.375-0.5
>120	0.25-0.375

If heparin is administered by deep S.C. injection, use 1-1.5 mg protamine per 100 units heparin; this may be done by administering a portion of the dose (eg, 25-50 mg) slowly I.V. followed by the remaining portion as a continuous infusion over 8-16 hours (the expected absorption time of the S.C. heparin dose)

LMWH overdosage: If most recent LMWH dose has been administered within the last 4 hours, use 1 mg protamine per 1 mg (100 units) LMWH; a second dose of 0.5 mg protamine per 1 mg (100 units) LMWH may be given if APTT remains prolonged 2-4 hours after the first dose

Administration Parenteral: Reconstitute vial with 5 mL SWI; if using protamine in neonates, reconstitute with preservative free SWI; resulting solution equals 10 mg/mL; inject without further dilution over 10 minutes not to exceed 5 mg/minute; maximum of 50 mg in any 10-minute period

Monitoring Parameters Coagulation tests, APTT or ACT, cardiac monitor, and blood pressure monitor required during administration

Dosage Forms Injection, as sulfate: 10 mg/mL (5 mL, 25 mL)

References

Monagle P, Michelson AD, Bovill E, et al, "Antithrombic Therapy in Children," *Chest*, 2001, 119:344S-70S.

Protirelin (proe TYE re lin)

U.S. Brand Names Thyrel® TRH

Canadian Brand Names Relefact TRH

Synonyms Lopremone

Therapeutic Category Diagnostic Agent, Thyroid Function

Generic Available No

Use Adjunct in the diagnostic assessment of thyroid function, and an adjunct to other diagnostic procedures in assessment of patients with pituitary or hypothalamic dysfunction; also causes release of prolactin from the pituitary and is used to detect defective control of prolactin secretion.

Pregnancy Risk Factor C

Contraindications Hypersensitivity to protirelin or any component

Warnings Due to transient changes in blood pressure (both increases and decreases), monitor blood pressure frequently during and at frequent intervals during first 15 minutes after administration; patient should be supine before, during, and immediately after administration

Adverse Reactions

Cardiovascular: Marked changes in blood pressure (hypotension or hypertension), flushing, chest tightness

Central nervous system: Lightheadedness, anxiety, seizures (rare), drowsiness

Endocrine & metabolic: Breast enlargement

Gastrointestinal: Nausea, dysgeusia, abdominal discomfort, xerostomia

Genitourinary: Urinary frequency

Miscellaneous: Diaphoresis

Drug Interactions Aspirin in therapeutic doses, pharmacologic doses of steroids, levodopa, and thyroid hormones reduce TSH response to protirelin

(Continued)

Protirelin *(Continued)*

Mechanism of Action Increases release of thyroid stimulating hormone (TSH) from the anterior pituitary

Pharmacodynamics Peak TSH levels occur in 20-30 minutes; TSH returns to baseline after about 3 hours

Pharmacokinetics Mean plasma half-life: 5 minutes

Usual Dosage I.V.:
Infants and Children: 7 mcg/kg to a maximum dose of 500 mcg
Adults: 500 mcg (range 200-500 mcg)

Administration Parenteral: Administer undiluted direct I.V. over 15-30 seconds with the patient remaining supine for an additional 15 minutes (see Warnings)

Monitoring Parameters Blood pressure, prolactin, TSH, T_4, and T_3

Nursing Implications Keep patient supine during drug administration

Dosage Forms Injection: 500 mcg/mL (1 mL)

- ♦ **Protopam**® *see* Pralidoxime *on page 818*
- ♦ **Protopic**® *see* Tacrolimus *on page 934*
- ♦ **Protostat**® **Oral** *see* Metronidazole *on page 662*
- ♦ **Protrin (Can)** *see* Co-Trimoxazole *on page 270*
- ♦ **Protropin**® **Injection** *see* Human Growth Hormone *on page 498*
- ♦ **Protylol (Can)** *see* Dicyclomine *on page 326*
- ♦ **Proventil**® *see* Albuterol *on page 45*
- ♦ **Proventil**® **HFA** *see* Albuterol *on page 45*
- ♦ **Provera**® *see* Medroxyprogesterone *on page 624*
- ♦ **Proxigel**® **[OTC]** *see* Carbamide Peroxide *on page 178*
- ♦ **Proxymetacaine** *see* Proparacaine *on page 841*
- ♦ **Prozac**® *see* Fluoxetine *on page 445*
- ♦ **Prozac**® **Weekly**™ *see* Fluoxetine *on page 445*
- ♦ **Prudoxin**™ *see* Doxepin *on page 358*
- ♦ **P & S (Can)** *see* Salicylic Acid *on page 886*

Pseudoephedrine *(soo doe e FED rin)*

Related Information
OTC Cough & Cold Preparations, Pediatric *on page 1072*

U.S. Brand Names Cenafed® [OTC]; Children's Silfedrine® [OTC]; Decofed® Syrup [OTC]; Dimetapp® Decongestant [OTC]; Efidac/24® [OTC]; Genaphed® [OTC]; PediaCare® Decongestant Infants [OTC]; Sudafed® [OTC]; Sudafed® 12 Hour [OTC]; Triaminic® AM Decongestant Formula [OTC]; Triaminic® Infant Decongestant [OTC]

Canadian Brand Names Balminil Decongestant; Congest Aid; Congest-Eze; Contac Cold Nondrowsy; Decongestant Tablets; Drixoral ND; Eltor 120; Maxenal; Nasal Sinus Relief; PMS-Pseudoephedrine; Pseudofrin; Tantafed

Synonyms *d*-Isoephedrine

Therapeutic Category Adrenergic Agonist Agent; Decongestant; Sympathomimetic

Generic Available Yes

Use Temporary symptomatic relief of nasal congestion due to common cold, upper respiratory allergies, and sinusitis; also promotes nasal or sinus drainage

Pregnancy Risk Factor C

Contraindications Hypersensitivity to pseudoephedrine or any component; MAO inhibitor therapy, severe hypertension, severe coronary artery disease

Precautions Use with caution in patients with hyperthyroidism, diabetes mellitus, prostatic hypertrophy, mild-moderate hypertension, arrhythmias

Adverse Reactions
Cardiovascular: Tachycardia, palpitations, arrhythmias
Central nervous system: Nervousness, excitability, dizziness, insomnia, drowsiness, headache, seizures, hallucinations
Gastrointestinal: Nausea, vomiting
Neuromuscular & skeletal: Tremor, weakness
Miscellaneous: Diaphoresis

Drug Interactions Additive effects with other sympathomimetics; hypertensive crisis with MAO inhibitors; phenothiazines and tricyclic antidepressants potentiate pressor effects; propranolol (beta-blockers)

Mechanism of Action Directly stimulates alpha-adrenergic receptors of respiratory mucosa causing vasoconstriction; directly stimulates beta-adrenergic receptors causing bronchial relaxation, increased heart rate and contractility

Pharmacodynamics
Onset of action: Oral: Decongestant effects occur within 15-30 minutes
Duration: 4-6 hours (up to 12 hours with extended release formulation administration)

Pharmacokinetics
Distribution: Children: V_d: 2.4-2.6 L/kg; breast milk to plasma ratio: 2.6-3.3
Metabolism: Incomplete in the liver to inactive metabolite
Half-life:
  Children 3.1 hours
  Adults: 9-16 hours
Elimination: 55% to 75% of dose excreted unchanged in urine
  Clearance:
    Children: 9.2-10.3 mL/minute/kg
    Adults: 7.3-7.6 mL/minute/kg

Usual Dosage Oral:
Children:
  <2 years: 4 mg/kg/day in divided doses every 6 hours
  2-5 years: 15 mg every 6 hours; maximum dose: 60 mg/24 hours
  6-12 years: 30 mg every 6 hours; maximum dose: 120 mg/24 hours
  Children >12 years and Adults: 60 mg every 6 hours; maximum dose: 240 mg/24 hours or extended release product: 120 mg every 12 hours

Administration Oral: Administer with water or milk to decrease GI distress; swallow timed release tablets or capsules whole, do not chew or crush

Test Interactions False-positive test for amphetamines by EMIT assay

Dosage Forms
Drops, oral, as hydrochloride (Dimetapp® Decongestant Pediatric, PediaCare® Decongestant Infants, Triaminic® Infant Decongestant): 7.5 mg/0.8 mL (15 mL)
Liquid, as hydrochloride: 15 mg/5 mL (120 mL)
  Decofed®, Children's Silfedrine®: 30 mg/5 mL (120 mL, 240 mL, 473 mL)
Liquigels (Dimetapp® Decongestant): 30 mg
Syrup, as hydrochloride:
  Cenafed®: 30 mg/5 mL (480 mL, 4000 mL)
  Triamine® AM Decongestant Formula: 15 mg/5 mL (118 mL)
Tablet, as hydrochloride:
  Cenaphed®, Sudafed®: 60 mg
  Genaphed®, Sudafed®: 30 mg
Tablet, extended release, as hydrochloride:
  Efidac® 24: 240 mg
  Sudafed® 12 Hour: 120 mg

References
Simons FE, Gu X, Watson WT, et al, "Pharmacokinetics of the Orally Administered Decongestants Pseudoephedrine and Phenylpropanolamine in Children," *J Pediatr*, 1996, 129(5):729-34.

♦ **Pseudoephedrine and Brompheniramine** *see* Brompheniramine and Pseudoephedrine *on page 153*
♦ **Pseudoephedrine and Carbinoxamine** *see* Carbinoxamine and Pseudoephedrine *on page 179*
♦ **Pseudoephedrine and Triprolidine** *see* Triprolidine and Pseudoephedrine *on page 989*
♦ **Pseudofrin (Can)** *see* Pseudoephedrine *on page 852*
♦ **Pseudomonic Acid A** *see* Mupirocin *on page 687*
♦ **psoriGel® [OTC]** *see* Coal Tar *on page 260*

Psyllium (SIL i yum)
U.S. Brand Names Fiberall®; Genfiber® [OTC]; Hydrocil® [OTC]; Konsyl® [OTC]; Konsyl-D® [OTC]; Metamucil® [OTC]; Modane® Bulk [OTC]; Natural Fiber Laxative® [OTC]; Perdium Fiber® [OTC]; Reguloid® [OTC]; Serutan® [OTC]; Syllact® [OTC]
Canadian Brand Names Novo-Mucilax; Prodiem Plain
Synonyms Plantago Seed; Plantain Seed; Psyllium Hydrophilic Mucilloid
Therapeutic Category Laxative, Bulk-Producing
Generic Available Yes
Use Treatment of chronic atonic or spastic constipation and in constipation associated with rectal disorders; management of irritable bowel syndrome; adjunctive treatment with low cholesterol and saturated fat diet to reduce risk of coronary artery disease
Pregnancy Risk Factor B
Contraindications Fecal impaction, GI obstruction; hypersensitivity to psyllium or any component
Warnings Products may contain aspartame; avoid use in phenylketonurics; inhalation of psyllium powder may produce allergic reactions in susceptible individuals
(Continued)

Psyllium *(Continued)*

Precautions Use with caution in patients with esophageal strictures, ulcers, stenosis, or intestinal adhesions

Adverse Reactions

Gastrointestinal: Esophageal or bowel obstruction, diarrhea, constipation, abdominal cramps

Respiratory: Bronchospasm

Miscellaneous: Rhinoconjunctivitis, anaphylaxis upon inhalation in susceptible individuals

Drug Interactions Decreased effect of warfarin, digitalis, potassium-sparing diuretics, salicylates, tetracyclines, nitrofurantoin

Mechanism of Action Adsorbs water in the intestine to form a viscous liquid which promotes peristalsis and reduces transit time

Pharmacodynamics

Onset of action: 12-24 hours

Peak effect: May take 2-3 days

Pharmacokinetics Absorption: Oral: Generally not absorbed; small amounts of grain extract present in the preparation have been reportedly absorbed following colonic hydrolysis

Usual Dosage Oral:

Children 6-11 years: $^{1}/_{2}$-1 rounded teaspoonful in 4 oz glass of liquid 1-3 times/day

Adults: 1-2 rounded teaspoonfuls or 1-2 packets or 1-2 wafers in 8 oz glass of liquid 1-4 times/day

Administration Oral: Granules and powder must be mixed in a glass of water or juice; drink a full glass of liquid with each dose

Patient Information Each dose must be taken with full glass of water; inadequate fluid intake may result in throat swelling and choking

Nursing Implications Inhalation of psyllium dust may cause sensitivity to psyllium (runny nose, watery eyes, wheezing)

Additional Information 3.4 g psyllium hydrophilic mucilloid/7 g powder is equivalent to a rounded teaspoonful or 1 packet

Dosage Forms

Granules:

Perdiem Fiber®: 82% (250 g)

Serutan®: 3.4 g/dose (540 g)

Powder: 2 g/dose; 3.4 g/dose; 3.5 g/dose; 6 g/dose

Fiberall®: 3.4 g/dose [regular, orange, tropical fruit flavors] (300 g, 450 g)

Genfiber®: 3.4 g/dose [regular and orange flavors] (397 g, 595 g)

Hydrocil® Instant: 3.5 g/dose (3.7 g unit dose packets, 300 g)

Konsyl®: 6 g/dose (6 g unit dose packets, 300 g, 450 g)

Konsyl-D®: 3.4 g/dose [with dextrose] (6.5 unit dose packets, 325 g, 500 g)

Konsyl® Easy Mix Formula: 6 g/dose [sugar free] (250 g)

Konsyl® for Kids: 2 g/dose [bubblegum flavor] (280 g)

Konsyl® Orange: 3.4 g/dose [with sucrose] (12 g unit dose packets, 425 g, 538 g)

Metamucil®: 3.4 g/dose [regular or orange flavor] (390 g, 570 g, 870 g, 1254 g)

Metamucil® Smooth Texture: 3.4 g/dose [regular or orange flavor; also available sugar free] (unit dose packets, 300 g, 450 g, 609 g, 660 g, 699 g, 912 g, 1368 g)

Modane® Bulk: 3.4 g/dose (390 g)

Natural Fiber Laxative®: 3.4 g/dose [smooth texture] (370 g, 420 g, 570 g)

Reguloid®: 3.4 g/dose [regular and orange flavor; also available sugar free] (300 g, 390 g, 450 g, 570 g)

Wafers: 3.4 g/dose

Fiberall®: 3.4 g/dose [oatmeal raisin or fruit-nut flavor] (14s)

Metamucil®: 3.4 g/dose [apple crisp or cinnamon spice flavor] (24s)

- **Psyllium Hydrophilic Mucilloid** *see* Psyllium *on page 853*
- **P.T.E.-4®** *see* Trace Metals *on page 972*
- **P.T.E.-5®** *see* Trace Metals *on page 972*
- **Pteroylglutamic Acid** *see* Folic Acid *on page 454*
- **PTU** *see* Propylthiouracil *on page 849*
- **Pulmicort® Respules™** *see* Budesonide *on page 154*
- **Pulmicort® Turbuhaler®** *see* Budesonide *on page 154*
- **Pulmophylline (Can)** *see* Theophylline *on page 943*
- **Pulmozyme®** *see* Dornase Alfa *on page 355*
- **Purge® [OTC]** *see* Castor Oil *on page 186*
- **Purinethol®** *see* Mercaptopurine *on page 631*
- **PVF K (Can)** *see* Penicillin V Potassium *on page 774*

Pyrantel Pamoate (pi RAN tel PAM oh ate)

U.S. Brand Names Antiminth® [OTC]; Pin-Rid® [OTC]; Pin-X® [OTC]; Reese's® Pinworm Medicine [OTC]

Canadian Brand Names Combantrin; Jaa Pyral

Therapeutic Category Anthelmintic

Generic Available No

Use Roundworm (*Ascaris lumbricoides*), pinworm (*Enterobius vermicularis*), and hookworm (*Ancylostoma duodenale* and *Necator americanus*) infestations, and trichostrongyliasis

Pregnancy Risk Factor C

Contraindications Hypersensitivity to pyrantel pamoate or any component

Precautions Use with caution in patients with liver impairment, anemia, malnutrition

Adverse Reactions

Central nervous system: Dizziness, drowsiness, insomnia, headache, fever

Dermatologic: Rash

Gastrointestinal: Nausea, vomiting, anorexia, diarrhea, abdominal cramps, tenesmus

Hepatic: Elevated liver enzymes

Neuromuscular & skeletal: Weakness

Drug Interactions Piperazine (antagonist)

Stability Protect from light

Mechanism of Action Promotes release of acetylcholine and inhibits cholinesterase causing neuromuscular paralysis of susceptible helminths

Pharmacokinetics

Absorption: Oral: Poor

Metabolism: Undergoes partial hepatic metabolism

Time to peak serum concentration: Within 1-3 hours

Elimination: In feces (50% as unchanged drug) and urine (7% as unchanged drug)

Usual Dosage Children and Adults: Oral:

Roundworm, pinworm, or trichostrongyliasis: 11 mg/kg administered as a single dose; maximum dose: 1 g; dosage should be repeated after 2 weeks for pinworm infection

Hookworm: 11 mg/kg/day once daily for 3 days

Maximum daily dose: 1 g

Administration Oral: May mix drug with milk or fruit juice; may administer with or without food

Monitoring Parameters Stool for presence of eggs, worms, and occult blood; serum AST and ALT

Patient Information Hygienic precaution is essential to prevent reinfection

Nursing Implications Shake suspension well before pouring to assure accurate dosage; fasting or purgation is not required prior to administration

Dosage Forms

Capsule, as pamoate: 180 mg

Liquid, as pamoate: 50 mg/mL (30 mL); 144 mg/mL (30 mL)

Suspension, oral, as pamoate: 50 mg/mL [caramel-currant flavor] (60 mL)

Pyrazinamide (peer a ZIN a mide)

Canadian Brand Names PMS-Pyrazinamide; Tebrazid

Synonyms Pyrazinoic Acid Amide

Therapeutic Category Antitubercular Agent

Generic Available No

Use In combination with other antituberculosis agents in the treatment of *Mycobacterium* tuberculosis infection (especially useful in disseminated and meningeal tuberculosis); CDC currently recommends a 3 or 4 multidrug regimen which includes pyrazinamide, rifampin, INH, and at times ethambutol or streptomycin for the treatment of tuberculosis

Pregnancy Risk Factor C

Contraindications Severe hepatic damage; hypersensitivity to pyrazinamide or any component

Precautions Use with caution in patients with renal failure, gout, or diabetes mellitus

Adverse Reactions

Central nervous system: Malaise, fever

Dermatologic: Urticaria, rash, photosensitivity

Endocrine & metabolic: Gout, hyperuricemia

Gastrointestinal: Nausea, vomiting, anorexia

Hepatic: Hepatotoxicity (increased incidence with doses >30 mg/kg/day), jaundice

Neuromuscular & skeletal: Arthralgia

(Continued)

Pyrazinamide *(Continued)*

Drug Interactions Isoniazid (decreased INH serum levels)

Mechanism of Action Converted to pyrazinoic acid in susceptible strains of *Mycobacterium* which lowers the pH of the environment

Pharmacokinetics

Absorption: Oral: Well absorbed

Distribution: Widely distributed into body tissues and fluids including the liver, lung, and CSF

Protein binding: 50%

Metabolism: In the liver

Half-life: 9-10 hours, prolonged with reduced renal or hepatic function

Time to peak serum concentration: Within 2 hours

Elimination: In urine (4% as unchanged drug)

Usual Dosage Oral:

Infants, Children, and Adolescents: 20-40 mg/kg/day in divided doses every 12-24 hours for the first 2 months of active treatment; daily dose not to exceed 2 g; **or** daily pyrazinamide for 2 weeks followed by directly observed therapy of 50 mg/kg/dose twice weekly to a maximum of 2 g/dose for 6 weeks

Adults: 15-30 mg/kg/day in 1-4 divided doses for the first 2 months of active treatment; maximum daily dose: 3 g/day; or daily pyrazinamide for 2 weeks followed by directly observed therapy of 50-70 mg/kg/dose twice weekly to a maximum of 4 g/dose for 6 weeks

Monitoring Parameters Periodic liver function tests, serum uric acid

Patient Information Notify physician if fatigue, weakness, nausea, vomiting, or joint pain and swelling occur; avoid excessive sunlight

Dosage Forms Tablet: 500 mg

Extemporaneous Preparations

Pyrazinamide suspension can be compounded with simple syrup or 0.5% methylcellulose with simple syrup at a concentration of 100 mg/mL; the suspension is stable for 2 months at 4°C or 25°C when stored in glass or plastic bottles

To prepare pyrazinamide suspension in 0.5% methylcellulose with simple syrup: Crush 200 pyrazinamide 500 mg tablets and mix with a suspension containing 500 mL of 1% methylcellulose and 500 mL simple syrup. Add to this a suspension containing 140 crushed pyrazinamide tablets in 350 mL of 1% methylcellulose and 350 mL of simple syrup to make 1.7 L of suspension containing pyrazinamide 100 mg/mL in 0.5% methylcellulose with simple syrup.

Nahata MC, Morosco RS, and Peritre SP, "Stability of Pyrazinamide in Two Suspensions," *Am J Health-Syst Pharm*, 1995, 52:1558-60.

References

Ad Hoc Committee of the Scientific Assembly on Microbiology, Tuberculosis and Pulmonary Infections, "Treatment of Tuberculosis and Tuberculosis Infection in Adults and Children," *Clin Infect Dis*, 1995, 21:9-27.

American Academy of Pediatrics, Committee on Infectious Diseases, "Chemotherapy for Tuberculosis in Infants and Children," *Pediatrics*, 1992, 89(1):161-5.

Starke JR, "Multidrug Therapy for Tuberculosis in Children," *Pediatr Infect Dis J*, 1990, 9(11):785-93.

Starke JR and Correa AG, "Management of Mycobacterial Infection and Disease in Children," *Pediatr Infect Dis J*, 1995, 14(6):455-70.

♦ **Pyrazinoic Acid Amide** *see* Pyrazinamide *on page 855*

♦ **Pyridiate®** *see* Phenazopyridine *on page 784*

♦ **2-Pyridine Aldoxime Methochloride** *see* Pralidoxime *on page 818*

♦ **Pyridium®** *see* Phenazopyridine *on page 784*

Pyridostigmine *(peer id oh STIG meen)*

Related Information

Overdose and Toxicology *on page 1222*

U.S. Brand Names Mestinon®; Regonol®

Therapeutic Category Antidote; Neuromuscular Blocking Agent; Cholinergic Agent

Generic Available No

Use Symptomatic treatment of myasthenia gravis by improving muscle strength; reversal of effects of nondepolarizing neuromuscular blocking agents

Pregnancy Risk Factor C

Contraindications Hypersensitivity to pyridostigmine, bromides, or any component; GI or GU obstruction

Warnings Overdosage may result in cholinergic crisis, this must be distinguished from myasthenic crisis; adequate facilities should be available for cardiopulmonary resuscitation when testing and adjusting dose for myasthenia gravis; have atropine and epinephrine ready to treat hypersensitivity reactions; injection contains benzyl alcohol; avoid use in neonates

Precautions Use with caution in patients with epilepsy, asthma, bradycardia, hyperthyroidism, arrhythmias, recent coronary occlusion, vagotonia, or peptic ulcer

Adverse Reactions

Cardiovascular: Bradycardia, hypotension, arrhythmias, A-V block, syncope

Central nervous system: Headache, convulsions, drowsiness, dizziness

Dermatologic: Rash

Gastrointestinal: Nausea, vomiting, diarrhea, increased peristalsis, abdominal cramps, dysphagia, salivation

Genitourinary: Urinary frequency

Local: Thrombophlebitis (after I.V. administration)

Neuromuscular & skeletal: Muscle cramps, weakness

Ocular: Miosis, lacrimation, diplopia, conjunctival hyperemia

Respiratory: Increased bronchial secretions, bronchospasm, laryngospasm, dyspnea

Miscellaneous: Diaphoresis

Drug Interactions Corticosteroids and magnesium may decrease effect of pyridostigmine; increases neuromuscular blocking effects of succinylcholine; atropine is direct antagonist

Stability Protect oral solution from light

Mechanism of Action Competitively inhibits destruction of acetylcholine by acetylcholinesterase which facilitates transmission of impulses across myoneural junction producing generalized cholinergic responses such as miosis, increased tonus of skeletal and intestinal musculature, bronchial and ureteral constriction, bradycardia, and increased salivary and sweat gland production

Pharmacodynamics

Onset of action:

Oral: 30-45 minutes

I.M.: <15 minutes

I.V.: Within 2-5 minutes

Duration:

Oral: 3-6 hours

I.M., I.V.: 2-3 hours

Pharmacokinetics

Absorption: Oral: Very poor (10% to 20%) from the GI tract

Metabolism: In the liver and at tissue site by cholinesterases

Usual Dosage Myasthenia gravis (dosage should be adjusted so patient takes larger doses prior to time of greatest fatigue)

Oral:

Neonates: 5 mg every 4-6 hours

Children: 7 mg/kg/day in 5-6 divided doses

Adults: Initial: 60 mg 3 times/day with maintenance dose ranging from 60 mg to 1.5 g/day (incremental increases every 48 hours or more if needed)

I.M., I.V.:

Neonates and Children: 0.05-0.15 mg/kg/dose (maximum single dose: 10 mg)

Adults: 2 mg every 2-3 hours (or 1/30th of oral dose)

Reversal of nondepolarizing neuromuscular blocker: I.V.:

Children: 0.1-0.25 mg/kg/dose preceded by atropine or glycopyrrolate

Adults: 10-20 mg preceded by atropine or glycopyrrolate

Administration

Parenteral: Administer direct I.V. slowly over 2-4 minutes; patients receiving large parenteral doses should be pretreated with atropine

Oral: Swallow sustained release tablets whole, do not chew or crush

Monitoring Parameters Muscle strength, heart rate, vital capacity

Dosage Forms

Injection, as bromide (with benzyl alcohol) (Mestinon®, Regonol®): 5 mg/mL (2 mL, 5 mL)

Syrup, as bromide (Mestinon®): 60 mg/5 mL [raspberry flavor] (480 mL)

Tablet, as bromide (Mestinon®): 60 mg

Pyridoxine (peer i DOKS een)

Related Information

Antiepileptic Drugs on page 1208

Synonyms Vitamin B$_6$

Therapeutic Category Antidote, Cycloserine Toxicity; Antidote, Hydrazine Toxicity; Antidote, Mushroom Toxicity; Drug-induced Neuritis, Treatment Agent; Nutritional Supplement; Vitamin, Water Soluble

(Continued)

Pyridoxine *(Continued)*

Generic Available Yes

Use Prevention and treatment of vitamin B_6 deficiency, pyridoxine-dependent seizures in infants; treatment of drug-induced deficiency (eg, isoniazid or hydralazine); treatment of acute intoxication of isoniazid, cycloserine, hydrazine, mushroom (genus *Gyromitra*)

Pregnancy Risk Factor A (C if dose exceeds RDA recommendation)

Contraindications Hypersensitivity to pyridoxine or any component

Adverse Reactions

Central nervous system: Sensory neuropathy (after chronic administration of large doses), seizures (following I.V. administration of very large doses), headache

Gastrointestinal: Nausea

Hematologic: Decreased serum folic acid concentration

Hepatic: Elevated AST

Local: Burning or stinging at injection site

Neuromuscular & skeletal: Paresthesia

Respiratory: Respiratory distress

Miscellaneous: Allergic reactions have been reported

Drug Interactions Decreases levodopa effectiveness when used without carbidopa; decreases serum levels of phenobarbital and phenytoin

Mechanism of Action Precursor to pyridoxal and pyridoxamine which function as cofactors in the metabolism of proteins, carbohydrates, and fats; also aids in the release of liver and muscle stored glycogen and in the synthesis of GABA (within the CNS) and heme

Pharmacokinetics

Absorption: Readily from the GI tract; primarily in jejunum

Metabolism: Converted to pyridoxal (active form in liver)

Half-life, biologic: 15-20 days

Elimination: By liver metabolism

Usual Dosage

Adequate intake: Infants:

<6 months: 0.1 mg (0.01 mg/kg)

6-12 months: 0.3 mg (0.03 mg/kg)

Recommended daily allowance:

1-3 years: 0.5 mg

4-8 years: 0.6 mg

9-13 years: 1 mg

14-19 years:

Male: 1.3 mg

Female: 1.2 mg

20-50 years: 1.3 mg

>50 years:

Male: 1.7 mg

Female: 1.5 mg

Pyridoxine-dependent seizures: Oral, I.M., I.V.:

Neonates and Infants: Initial: 10-100 mg; maintenance: Oral: 50-100 mg/day

Dietary deficiency: Oral:

Children: 5-25 mg/day for 3 weeks, then 1.5-2.5 mg/day in multivitamin product

Adults: 2.5-10 mg/day until clinical signs are corrected, then 2-5 mg/day (dosage found in multivitamin products)

Drug-induced neuritis (eg, isoniazid, hydralazine, penicillamine, cycloserine): Oral:

Children:

Treatment: 10-50 mg/day

Prophylaxis: 1-2 mg/kg/day

Adults:

Cycloserine: Treatment 100-300 mg/day in divided doses

Isoniazid or penicillamine: Treatment: 100-200 mg/day for 3 weeks; prophylaxis: 25-100 mg/day

Acute intoxication: Children and Adults:

Hydrazine: 25 mg/kg: $^1/_3$ dose I.M. and $^2/_3$ dose I.V. infusion over 3 hours

Isoniazid: Dose equal to isoniazid ingested given as a first dose of 1-4 g I.V., followed by 1 g I.M. every 30 minutes until total dosage completed

Mushroom ingestion (genus *Gyromitra*): I.V.: 25 mg/kg; repeat as necessary to a maximum total dose of 15-20 g

Administration Parenteral: Administer slow I.V.

Monitoring Parameters When administering large I.V. doses, monitor respiratory rate, heart rate, and blood pressure

Reference Range 30-80 ng/mL

Test Interactions False positive urobilinogen spot test using Ehrlich's reagent

Dosage Forms

Injection, as hydrochloride: 100 mg/mL (10 mL, 30 mL)

Tablet, as hydrochloride: 25 mg, 50 mg, 100 mg, 250 mg, 500 mg

Tablet, extended release, as hydrochloride: 200 mg

Extemporaneous Preparations A 1 mg/mL oral solution has an expected stability of 30 days when refrigerated when compounded as follows: Withdraw 100 mg (1 mL of a 100 mg/mL injection) from a vial with a needle and syringe, add to 99 mL of simple syrup in an amber bottle; keep in refrigerator

Nahata MC and Hipple TF, *Pediatric Drug Formulations*, 4th ed, Cincinnati, OH: Harvey Whitney Books Co, 2000.

Pyrimethamine (peer i METH a meen)

U.S. Brand Names Daraprim®

Therapeutic Category Antimalarial Agent

Generic Available No

Use Used in combination with sulfadiazine for treatment of toxoplasmosis; used in combination with dapsone as primary or secondary prophylaxis for *Pneumocystis carinii* in HIV-infected patients; pyrimethamine has been used for chemoprophylaxis of malaria, however, due to severe adverse reactions and reports of resistance to pyrimethamine, other antimalarial agents are now generally preferred

Pregnancy Risk Factor C

Contraindications Megaloblastic anemia; hypersensitivity to pyrimethamine, chloroguanide, or any component; resistant malaria and patients with seizure disorders

Precautions Use with caution in patients with impaired renal or hepatic function and in patients with possible folate deficiency

Adverse Reactions

Cardiovascular: Shock

Central nervous system: Seizures, fever, fatigue, ataxia, headache

Dermatologic: Rash, photosensitivity

Endocrine & metabolic: Folic acid deficiency

Gastrointestinal: Anorexia, abdominal cramps, vomiting, atrophic glossitis, diarrhea

Hematologic: Megaloblastic anemia, leukopenia, thrombocytopenia, agranulocytosis, pancytopenia, pulmonary eosinophilia

Neuromuscular & skeletal: Tremor

Renal: Hematuria

Respiratory: Respiratory failure

Drug Interactions Para-aminobenzoic acid, sulfonamides

Mechanism of Action Inhibits parasitic dihydrofolate reductase resulting in inhibition of tetrahydrofolic acid synthesis

Pharmacokinetics

Absorption: Oral: Well absorbed

Distribution: V_d: Adults: 2.9 L/kg; appears in breast milk; distributed to the kidneys, lung, liver, and spleen

Protein binding: 80% to 87%

Half-life: 111 hours (range: 54-148 hours)

Time to peak serum concentration: Within 2-6 hours

Elimination: Pyrimethamine and metabolites are excreted in urine

Usual Dosage Oral:

Toxoplasmosis (with sulfadiazine):

Newborns and Infants: Initial: 2 mg/kg/day divided every 12 hours for 2 days, then 1 mg/kg/day once daily given with sulfadiazine for the first 6 months; next 6 months: 1 mg/kg/day 3 times/week with sulfadiazine; oral folinic acid 5-10 mg 3 times/week should be administered to prevent hematologic toxicity

Children: 2 mg/kg/day divided every 12 hours for 3 days followed by 1 mg/kg/day (maximum: 25 mg/day) once daily or divided twice daily for 4 weeks given with sulfadiazine; oral folinic acid 5-10 mg 3 times/week should be administered to prevent hematologic toxicity

Adults: 50-75 mg/day together with 1-4 g of a sulfonamide plus oral folinic acid 5-10 mg 3 times/week for 1-3 weeks depending on patient's tolerance and response, then reduce dose by 50% and continue for 4-5 weeks **or** 25-50 mg/day for 3-4 weeks

Prophylaxis for first episode of *Toxoplasma gondii*:

Children ≥1 month of age: 1 mg/kg/day once daily with dapsone plus oral folinic acid 5 mg every 3 days

Adolescents and Adults: 50 mg once weekly with dapsone plus oral folinic acid 25 mg once weekly

(Continued)

859

Pyrimethamine *(Continued)*

Prophylaxis for recurrence of *Toxoplasma gondii*:

Children ≥1 month of age: 1 mg/kg/day once daily given with sulfadiazine or clindamycin, plus oral folinic acid 5 mg every 3 days

Adolescents and Adults: 25-75 mg once daily in combination with sulfadiazine or clindamycin, plus oral folinic acid 10-25 mg daily

Prophylaxis for first episode or recurrence of *Pneumocystis carinii*:

Adolescents and Adults: 50-75 mg once weekly in combination with dapsone plus oral folinic acid 25 mg once weekly

Administration Oral: Administer with meals to minimize vomiting

Monitoring Parameters CBC including platelet counts

Patient Information Notify physician if rash, sore throat, pallor, or glossitis occurs

Additional Information Folinic acid may be given in a dosage of 3-9 mg/day for 3 days, or 5 mg every 3 days, or as required to reverse symptoms or to prevent hematologic problems due to pyrimethamine-induced folic acid deficiency

Dosage Forms Tablet: 25 mg

Extemporaneous Preparations Pyrimethamine tablets may be crushed to prepare oral suspensions of the drug in a 1:1 mixture of simple syrup and 1% methylcellulose to yield a suspension with a pyrimethamine concentration of 2 mg/mL; stable for at least 91 days when stored in plastic or glass prescription bottles at 4°C or 25°C

Nahata MC, Morosco RS, and Hipple TF, "Stability of Pyrimethamine in a Liquid Dosage Formulation Stored for Three Months," *Am J Health-Syst Pharm*, 1997, 54:2714-6.

References

"1997 USPHS/IDSA Guidelines for the Prevention of Opportunistic Infections in Persons Infected With Human Immunodeficiency Virus," *MMWR Morb Mortal Wkly Rep*, 1997, 46(RR-12):1-46.

Van Voorhis WC, "Therapy and Prophylaxis of Systemic Protozoan Infections," *Drugs*, 1990, 40(2):176-202.

Quinidine *(KWIN i deen)*

U.S. Brand Names Quinaglute® Dura-Tabs®; Quinidex® Extentabs®

Canadian Brand Names Apo-Quinidine; Biquin; Prosedyl; Quinate; Quinobarb

Therapeutic Category Antiarrhythmic Agent, Class I-A

Generic Available Yes

Use Prophylaxis after cardioversion of atrial fibrillation and/or flutter to maintain normal sinus rhythm; also used to prevent reoccurrence of paroxysmal supraventricular tachycardia, paroxysmal A-V junctional rhythm, paroxysmal ventricular tachycardia, paroxysmal atrial fibrillation, and atrial or ventricular premature contractions; also has activity against *Plasmodium falciparum* malaria

Pregnancy Risk Factor C

Contraindications Patients with complete A-V block with an A-V junctional or idioventricular pacemaker; patients with intraventricular conduction defects (marked widening of QRS complex); patients with cardiac glycoside-induced A-V conduction disorders; hypersensitivity to quinidine, any component, or cinchona derivatives

Warnings May cause syncope, most likely due to ventricular tachycardia or fibrillation; syncope may subside spontaneously, but occasionally may be fatal; discontinue quinidine if syncope occurs

Precautions Use with caution in patients with myocardial depression, sick sinus syndrome, incomplete A-V block, cardiac glycoside intoxication, hepatic and/or renal insufficiency, myasthenia gravis; hemolysis may occur in patients with G-6-PD deficiency; quinidine-induced hepatotoxicity, including granulomatous hepatitis, increased serum AST and alkaline phosphatase concentrations, and jaundice may occur; use with caution in nursing women; adjust dose with severe renal impairment

Adverse Reactions

Cardiovascular: Syncope, hypotension, tachycardia, heart block, ventricular fibrillation, vascular collapse, severe hypotension with rapid I.V. administration

Central nervous system: Fever, headache

Dermatologic: Angioedema, rash

Gastrointestinal: GI disturbances, nausea, vomiting, cramps

Hematologic: Blood dyscrasias, thrombotic thrombocytopenic purpura

Hepatic: Elevated AST; elevated alkaline phosphatase, jaundice, granulomatous hepatitis

Respiratory: Respiratory depression

Miscellaneous: Cinchonism (nausea, tinnitus, headache, impaired hearing or vision, vomiting, abdominal pain, vertigo, confusion, delirium, syncope)

Drug Interactions Cytochrome P-450 isoenzyme CYP3A3/4 and CYP3A5-7 substrate; CYP2D6 and CYP3A3/4 isoenzyme inhibitor

Quinidine potentiates nondepolarizing and depolarizing muscle relaxants; diltiazem, verapamil, delavirdine, saquinavir, amiodarone, alkalinizing agents, and cimetidine may increase quinidine serum concentrations; phenobarbital, phenytoin, and rifampin may decrease quinidine serum concentrations. Quinidine may increase plasma concentration of digoxin; closely monitor digoxin concentrations; digoxin dosage may need to be reduced (by one-half) when quinidine is initiated; new steady-state digoxin plasma concentrations occur in 5-7 days. Beta-blockers plus quinidine may increase bradycardia; quinidine may enhance coumarin anticoagulants; potential interaction with ritonavir, concurrent use is not recommended

Food Interactions Excessive intake of fruit juices or vitamin C may decrease urine pH and result in increased clearance of quinidine with decreased serum concentration; alkaline foods may result in increased quinidine serum concentrations; food has a variable effect on absorption of sustained release formulation; grapefruit juice significantly increases the AUC of 3-hydroxyquinidine (a metabolite of quinidine)

Stability Do not use discolored parenteral solution

Mechanism of Action Class IA antiarrhythmic with anticholinergic, local anesthetic, and mild negative inotropic effects; depresses phase 0 of the action potential; decreases myocardial excitability, conduction velocity, and myocardial contractility by decreasing sodium influx during depolarization and potassium efflux in repolarization; also reduces calcium transport across cell membrane

Pharmacokinetics

Distribution: V_d: Adults: 2-3.5 L/kg, decreased V_d with CHF, malaria; increased V_d with cirrhosis; crosses the placenta; appears in breast milk

Protein-binding:

Newborns: 60% to 70%

Adults: 80% to 90%

Decreased protein binding with cyanotic congenital heart disease, cirrhosis, or acute MI

Metabolism: Extensive in the liver (50% to 90%) to inactive compounds

Bioavailability:

Sulfate: 80%

Gluconate: 70%

Half-life, plasma (increased half-life with elderly, cirrhosis, and CHF):

Children: 2.5-6.7 hours

Adults: 6-8 hours

Elimination: In urine (15% to 25% as unchanged drug)

Dialysis: Slightly dialyzable (5% to 20%) by hemodialysis; not removed by peritoneal dialysis

Usual Dosage Note: Dose expressed in terms of the salt: 267 mg of quinidine gluconate = 200 mg of quinidine sulfate

Children: Test dose (for idiosyncratic reaction, intolerance, syncope, thrombocytopenia) (sulfate, oral or gluconate, I.M.): 2 mg/kg or 60 mg/m^2

Oral (quinidine sulfate): Usual: 30 mg/kg/day or 900 mg/m^2/day given in 5 daily doses or 6 mg/kg every 4-6 hours; range: 15-60 mg/kg/day in 4-5 divided doses

I.V. (quinidine gluconate): 2-10 mg/kg/dose every 3-6 hours as needed (I.V. route **not** recommended)

Adults: Test dose (for idiosyncratic reaction, intolerance, syncope, thrombocytopenia): 200 mg administered several hours before full dosage

Oral (sulfate): 100-600 mg/dose every 4-6 hours; begin at 200 mg/dose and titrate to desired effect

Oral (gluconate): 324-972 mg every 8-12 hours

I.M.: 400 mg/dose every 4-6 hours

(Continued)

Quinidine *(Continued)*

I.V.: 200-400 mg/dose diluted and given at a rate ≤10 mg/minute

Dosing adjustment in renal impairment: Children and Adults: Cl_{cr} <10 mL/minute: Administer 75% of normal dose

Administration

Oral: Administer with water on an empty stomach, but may administer with food or milk to decrease GI upset; best to administer in a consistent manner with regards to meals; swallow sustained-release tablets whole, do not chew or crush

Parenteral: I.V.: Maximum rate of infusion: 10 mg/minute; maximum concentration: 16 mg/mL; I.V. tubing length should be minimized (quinidine may be significantly adsorbed to polyvinyl chloride tubing)

Monitoring Parameters CBC with differential, platelet count, liver and renal function tests, and serum concentrations should be routinely performed during long-term administration

Reference Range Optimal therapeutic level is method dependent

Therapeutic: 2-7 µg/mL (SI: 6.2-15.4 µmol/L)

Toxic: >8 µg/mL (SI: >18 µmol/L)

Patient Information Notify physician if fever, rash, unusual bruising or bleeding, visual disturbances, or ringing in the ears occurs; avoid excessive intake of fruit juices or vitamin C

Additional Information Use of sustained release products is not recommended in children

Dosage Forms

Injection, as gluconate: 80 mg/mL (10 mL)

Tablet, as sulfate: 200 mg, 300 mg

Tablet:

Sustained action, as sulfate (Quinidex® Extentabs®): 300 mg

Sustained release, as gluconate (Quinaglute® Dura-Tabs®): 324 mg

Extemporaneous Preparations

A 10 mg/mL oral liquid preparation made from tablets and 3 different vehicles (cherry syrup, a 1:1 mixture of Ora-Sweet® and Ora-Plus®, or a 1:1 mixture of Ora-Sweet® SF and Ora-Plus®) was stable for 60 days when stored in amber plastic prescription bottles in the dark at room temperature (25°C) or under refrigeration (5°C); Grind six 200 mg tablets in a mortar into a fine powder; add 15 mL of the vehicle and mix well to form a uniform paste; mix while adding the vehicle in geometric proportions to **almost** 120 mL; transfer to a calibrated bottle and qsad to 120 mL; label "shake well" and "protect from light" (Allen 1998).

Allen LV and Erickson MA, "Stability of Bethanechol Chloride, Pyrazinamide, Quinidine Sulfate, Rifampin, and Tetracycline in Extemporaneously Compounded Oral Liquids," *Am J Health Syst Pharm*, 1998, 55(17):1804-9.

References

Pickoff AS, Singh S, and Gelband H, *The Medical Management of Cardiac Arrhythmias in Cardiac Arrhythmias in the Neonate, Infant and Child*, Roberts NK and Gelband H, ed, Norwalk, CT: Appleton-Century-Crofts, 1983.

Szefler SJ, Pieroni DR, Gingell RL, et al, "Rapid Elimination of Quinidine in Pediatric Patients," *Pediatrics*, 1982, 70(3):370-5.

Quinine *(KWYE nine)*

U.S. Brand Names Legatrin® [OTC]; Quinamm®; Quiphile®; Q-vel®

Therapeutic Category Antimalarial Agent; Skeletal Muscle Relaxant, Miscellaneous

Generic Available Yes

Use Suppression or treatment of chloroquine-resistant *P. falciparum* malaria (inactive against sporozoites, pre-erythrocytic or exoerythrocytic forms of plasmodia); treatment of *Babesia microti* infection; prevention and treatment of nocturnal recumbency leg muscle cramps

Pregnancy Risk Factor D

Contraindications Tinnitus, optic neuritis, G-6-PD deficiency; hypersensitivity to quinine or any component; history of black water fever; pregnancy

Precautions Use with caution in patients with cardiac arrhythmias (quinine has quinidine-like activity), in patients with myasthenia gravis, and in patients with impaired liver function

Adverse Reactions

Cardiovascular: Flushing of the skin, anginal symptoms, conduction disturbances, ventricular tachycardia

Central nervous system: Fever, headache, confusion

Dermatologic: Rash, pruritus

Endocrine & metabolic: Hypoglycemia

Gastrointestinal: Nausea, vomiting, epigastric pain

Hematologic: Hemolysis, thrombocytopenia

Hepatic: Hepatitis

Ocular: Visual disturbances

Otic: Tinnitus, impaired hearing

Miscellaneous: Hypersensitivity reactions, cinchonism (nausea, tinnitus, headache, impaired hearing or vision, vomiting, abdominal pain, vertigo, confusion, delirium, syncope)

Drug Interactions Quinine may decrease the clearance of digoxin or digitoxin leading to increased plasma concentrations of these cardiac glycosides; cimetidine (prolongs half-life of quinine), aluminum-containing antacids (decreases quinine absorption); quinine may potentiate the effects of neuromuscular blocking agents; oral anticoagulants, urinary alkalinizers (may increase quinine toxicity); mefloquine (additive cardiotoxicity)

Stability Protect from light

Mechanism of Action Depresses oxygen uptake and carbohydrate metabolism; intercalates into DNA, disrupting the parasite's replication and transcription; affects calcium distribution within muscle fibers and decreases the excitability of the motor end-plate region

Pharmacokinetics

Absorption: Oral: Readily absorbed, mainly from the upper small intestine

Distribution: Widely distributed to body tissues and fluids including small amounts into bile and CSF; crosses the placenta; excreted into breast milk

V_d (children): 0.8 L/kg

V_d (adults): 1.9 L/kg

Protein binding: 70% to 90%

Metabolism: Primarily in the liver via hydroxylation pathways

Half-life:

Children: 6-12 hours

Adults: 8-14 hours

Time to peak serum concentration: Within 1-3 hours

Elimination: In bile and saliva with <5% excreted unchanged in urine

Not effectively removed by peritoneal dialysis, removed by hemodialysis

Usual Dosage Oral:

Children:

Treatment of chloroquine-resistant malaria: 30 mg/kg/day in divided doses every 8 hours for 3-7 days in conjunction with another agent; maximum dose: 2 g/day

Babesiosis: 25 mg/kg/day, divided every 8 hours for 7 days; maximum dose: 650 mg/dose

Adults:

Treatment of chloroquine-resistant malaria: 650 mg every 8 hours for 3-7 days in conjunction with another agent

Suppression of malaria: 325 mg twice daily and continued for 6 weeks after exposure

Babesiosis: 650 mg every 6-8 hours for 7 days

Leg cramps: 200-300 mg at bedtime

Administration Oral: Do not crush tablets or capsule to avoid bitter taste

Monitoring Parameters CBC with platelet count, liver function tests, blood glucose, ophthalmologic examination

Patient Information Report to physician if tinnitus, hearing loss, rash, or visual disturbances occur during therapy

Additional Information Parenteral form of quinine (dihydrochloride) is no longer available from the CDC; quinidine gluconate should be used instead; the FDA has banned over-the-counter (OTC) drug products containing quinine sold for treatment and/or prevention of malaria, as well as, products labeled for treatment or prevention of nocturnal leg cramps

Dosage Forms

Capsule, as sulfate: 64.8 mg, 65 mg, 200 mg, 300 mg, 325 mg

Tablet, as sulfate: 162.5 mg, 260 mg

References

Schulbe DE, "Quinine Ban Signals Change for Pharmacists, APhA," *Pharmacy Today*, 1995, 1(12):6.

♦ **Quinobarb (Can)** see Quinidine on page 860

♦ **Quinsana® Plus Topical [OTC]** see Undecylenic Acid and Derivatives on page 994

Quinupristin/Dalfopristin (kwi NYOO pris tin/dal FOE pris tin)

U.S. Brand Names Synercid®

Synonyms Pristinamycin; RP59500

(Continued)

Quinupristin/Dalfopristin *(Continued)*

Therapeutic Category Antibiotic, Streptogramin

Use Treatment of serious or life-threatening infections caused by vancomycin-resistant *Enterococcus faecium*; treatment of complicated skin and skin structure infections caused by *Staphylococcus aureus* (methicillin-susceptible and methicillin-resistant strains) or *Streptococcus pyogenes*

Pregnancy Risk Factor B

Contraindications Hypersensitivity to quinupristin, dalfopristin, other streptogramins (pristinamycin or virginiamycin), or to any component

Warnings Quinupristin/dalfopristin inhibit cytochrome P-450 3A4 metabolism of cyclosporine, midazolam, nifedipine, and terfenadine. There was a 77% increase in cyclosporine's half-life with a 63% increase in the AUC. Cyclosporine levels should be closely monitored in patients who are receiving quinupristin/dalfopristin therapy concomitantly. Coadministration of quinupristin/dalfopristin with cytochrome P-450 3A4 substrates with narrow therapeutic ranges require serum concentration monitoring of these drugs. Concurrent use with astemizole, terfenadine, and cisapride is not recommended. Superinfections and pseudomembranous colitis have been reported with the use of quinupristin/dalfopristin. Resistance to quinupristin/dalfopristin has been reported in a few cases of *Enterococcus faecium* infections.

Precautions Use with caution in patients with hepatic or renal dysfunction; dosage reduction may be necessary in patients with hepatic cirrhosis; may cause pain and phlebitis when infused through a peripheral line; episodes of severe arthralgia and myalgia have been reported which improve with a dose frequency reduction to "q12h" or discontinuation of quinupristin/dalfopristin

Adverse Reactions

Central nervous system: Headache

Dermatologic: Rash, pruritus, urticaria

Hepatic: Elevated AST, ALT, bilirubin

Local: Pain, edema, inflammation at infusion site; thrombophlebitis

Neuromuscular & skeletal: Arthralgia, myalgia

Miscellaneous: Superinfection

Drug Interactions Cytochrome P-450 isoenzyme CYP3A4 inhibitor

Quinupristin/dalfopristin may increase plasma concentration of cyclosporine, tacrolimus, astemizole, terfenadine, delavirdine, nevirapine, indinavir, ritonavir, vinca alkaloids, docetaxel, paclitaxel, midazolam, diazepam, dihydropyridines, verapamil, diltiazem, HMG-CoA reductase inhibitors, cisapride, methylprednisolone, carbamazepine, quinidine, lidocaine, disopyramide (see Warnings)

Stability Unopened vials should be stored in a refrigerator at 2°C to 8°C; reconstituted drug is stable for 1 hour at room temperature; infusion bag is stable for 5 hours at room temperature and for 54 hours if refrigerated at 2°C to 8°C; incompatible with NS and heparin; compatible with aztreonam, ciprofloxacin, fluconazole, haloperidol, metoclopramide, morphine, and potassium chloride during Y-site administration

Mechanism of Action Inhibits bacterial protein synthesis by binding to the 50S bacterial ribosomal subunit resulting in peptide chain elongation inhibition and peptidyl transferase inhibition

Pharmacokinetics

Distribution:

V_d: Quinupristin: 0.45 L/kg

V_d: Dalfopristin: 0.24 L/kg

Protein binding:

Quinupristin: 23% to 32%

Dalfopristin: 50% to 56%

Metabolism: Quinupristin is conjugated with glutathione and cysteine to active metabolites; dalfopristin is hydrolyzed to an active metabolite

Half-life:

Quinupristin: 0.85 hour

Dalfopristin: 0.7 hour

Elimination: 75% to 77% excreted in the bile and feces

Usual Dosage Dosage is expressed in terms of combined "mg" of quinupristin plus dalfopristin: I.V.:

Children: Limited information is available; quinupristin/dalfopristin has been used in a limited number of pediatric patients under a compassionate use protocol

Treatment of vancomycin-resistant *Enterococcus faecium* infection: 7.5 mg/kg/dose every 8 hours

Treatment of vancomycin-resistant *Enterococcus faecium* CNS shunt infection: 7.5 mg/kg/dose every 8 hours (plus 1 mg intrathecal dose daily at the time of shunt tap was used in an 8-month old infant for 68 days in one case report; 1 or

2 mg doses every day for 5-33 days have been administered intrathecally in 6 patients)

Treatment of complicated skin and skin structure infection: 7.5 mg/kg/dose every 12 hours for at least 7 days

Adolescents ≥16 years and Adults:

Treatment of vancomycin-resistant *Enterococcus faecium* infection: 7.5 mg/kg/dose every 8 hours

Treatment of complicated skin and skin structure infection: 7.5 mg/kg/dose every 12 hours

Dosage adjustment in hepatic impairment: Dosage adjustment may be necessary, but exact recommendations cannot be made at this time

Administration Parenteral: Reconstitute vial by slowly adding 5 mL D_5W or sterile water for injection to make a 100 mg/mL solution; gently swirl the vial contents without shaking to minimize foam formation; further dilute the reconstituted solution with D_5W to a final maximum concentration for administration via peripheral line of 2 mg/mL; maximum concentration for administration via a central line is 5 mg/mL; if an injection site reaction occurs, the dose can be further diluted to a final concentration of <1 mg/mL; administer infusion over 60 minutes; following infusion of quinupristin/dalfopristin, the infusion line should be flushed with D_5W to minimize venous irritation; **DO NOT FLUSH** with saline or heparin solutions due to incompatibility

Monitoring Parameters CBC, liver function test; monitor infusion site closely

Nursing Implications If moderate to severe venous irritation occurs following peripheral quinupristin/dalfopristin administration, consider increasing the infusion volume, changing infusion sites, or establishing central venous access; administration of hydrocortisone or diphenhydramine did not decrease infusion site reactions

Dosage Forms Powder for injection: 500 mg vial (150 mg quinupristin and 350 mg dalfopristin)

References

Gransden WR, King A, Marossy D, et al, "Quinupristin/Dalfopristin in Neonatal *Enterococcus faecium* Meningitis," *Arch Dis Child Fetal Neonatal Ed*, 1998, 78(3):F235-6.

Gray JW, Darbyshire PJ, Beath SV, et al, "Experience With Quinupristin/Dalfopristin in Treating Infections With Vancomycin-Resistant *Enterococcus faecium* in Children," *Pediatr Infect Dis J*, 2000, 19(3):234-8.

Nachman SA, Verma R, and Egnor M, "Vancomycin-Resistant *Enterococcus faecium* Shunt Infection in an Infant: An Antibiotic Cure," *Microb Drug Resist*, 1995, 1(1):95-6

♦ **Quiphile**® *see* Quinine *on page 862*

♦ **Quixin**™ **Ophthalmic** *see* Levofloxacin *on page 586*

♦ **QVAR**™ **40 mcg** *see* Beclomethasone *on page 131*

♦ **QVAR**™ **80 mcg** *see* Beclomethasone *on page 131*

♦ **Q-vel**® *see* Quinine *on page 862*

♦ **Rabies Immune Globulin, Human** *see page 1172*

♦ **Rabies Virus Vaccine, Human Diploid** *see page 1172*

♦ **Racemic Epinephrine** *see* Epinephrine *on page 385*

♦ **Radiostol (Can)** *see* Ergocalciferol *on page 392*

♦ **R-albuterol** *see* Levalbuterol *on page 583*

Ranitidine (ra NI ti deen)

Related Information

Carbohydrate and Alcohol Content of Liquid Medications for Use in Patients Receiving Ketogenic Diets *on page 1258*

U.S. Brand Names Zantac®; Zantac® 75 [OTC]

Canadian Brand Names Alti-Ranitidine; Apo-Ranitidine; Gen-Ranitidine; Novo-Ranidine; Nu-Ranit

Therapeutic Category Gastrointestinal Agent, Gastric or Duodenal Ulcer Treatment; Histamine H_2 Antagonist

Generic Available Yes (except gel capsules, effervescent granules and tablets)

Use Short-term treatment of active duodenal ulcers and benign gastric ulcers; long-term prophylaxis of duodenal ulcer and gastric hypersecretory states; gastroesophageal reflux disease (GERD); recurrent postoperative ulcer; treatment and prophylaxis of erosive esophagitis; upper GI bleeding, prevention of acid-aspiration pneumonitis during surgery, and prevention of stress-induced ulcers; over-the-counter (OTC) formulation for use in the relief of heartburn, acid indigestion, and sour stomach

Pregnancy Risk Factor B

Contraindications Hypersensitivity to ranitidine or any component or other H_2 antagonists; patients with history of acute porphyria

Warnings Zantac® 150 EFFERdose® tablets and Zantac® 150 EFFERdose® granules contain phenylalamine and should be avoided in phenylketonurics

(Continued)

Ranitidine *(Continued)*

Precautions Use with caution in patients with liver and renal impairment; dosage modification required in patients with renal impairment

Adverse Reactions

Cardiovascular: Bradycardia, tachycardia

Central nervous system: Dizziness, sedation, malaise, mental confusion, headache, hallucinations, anxiety

Dermatologic: Rash, alopecia, erythema multiforme

Endocrine & metabolic: Gynecomastia

Gastrointestinal: Constipation, nausea, vomiting, abdominal discomfort, pancreatitis (rare)

Hematologic: Thrombocytopenia, aplastic anemia (rare), granulocytopenia, leukopenia

Hepatic: Hepatitis

Local: Transient pain at injection site

Neuromuscular & skeletal: Arthralgias

Renal: Elevated serum creatinine

Drug Interactions CYP2D6 and 3A3/4 enzyme inhibitor

Variable effects on warfarin; antacids may decrease absorption of ranitidine; ranitidine decreases the absorption of ketoconazole and itraconazole

Stability Protect injection from light; stable for 48 hours at room temperature or 30 days when frozen in D_5W or NS; stable for 24 hours in TPN solutions; stable for 24 hours in TPN with lipids

Mechanism of Action Competitive inhibition of histamine at H_2-receptors of the gastric parietal cells, which inhibits gastric acid secretion

Pharmacokinetics

Distribution: V_d: 1.4 L/kg; minimally penetrates the blood-brain barrier; breast milk to plasma ratio: 1.9-6.7

Protein binding: 15%

Metabolism: In the liver

Bioavailability: Oral: ~50%

Half-life:

Infants: 3.5 hours

Children 3.5-16 years: 1.8-2 hours

Adults:

Normal renal and hepatic function: 2-3 hours

Decreased renal function: 8.7 hours

Time to peak serum concentration: Oral: 1-3 hours

Elimination: 30% (oral) or 70% (I.V.) eliminated as unchanged drug in the urine and in feces

Hemodialysis: Slightly dialyzable (5% to 20%)

Usual Dosage

Premature and Term Infants <2 weeks:

Oral: 2 mg/kg/day divided every 12 hours

I.V.: 1.5 mg/kg/dose as loading dose, then 12 hours later maintenance dose of 1.5-2 mg/kg/day divided every 12 hours

Continuous infusion: 1.5 mg/kg/dose as loading dose followed by 0.04-0.08 mg/kg/hour infusion (or 1-2 mg/kg/day)

Children ≥1 month to 16 years:

Gastric/duodenal ulcer:

Oral:

Treatment: 2-4 mg/kg/day divided twice daily; maximum: 300 mg/day

Maintenance: 2-4 mg/kg/day divided twice daily; maximum: 150 mg/day

I.V.: 2-4 mg/kg/day divided every 6-8 hours; maximum: 150 mg/day

GERD and erosive esophagitis:

Oral: 4-10 mg/kg/day divided twice daily; maximum: GERD: 300 mg/day; erosive esophagitis: 600 mg/day

I.V.: 2-4 mg/kg/day divided every 6-8 hours; maximum: 150 mg/day **or as an alternative**

Continuous infusion: Initial: 1 mg/kg/dose for one dose followed by infusion of 0.08-0.17 mg/kg/hour or 2-4 mg/kg/day

Children ≥16 years and Adults:

Treatment of duodenal or gastric ulcers, GERD, maintenance of erosive esophagitis: Oral: 150 mg/dose twice daily or 300 mg at bedtime

Prophylaxis of recurrent duodenal ulcer: Oral: 150 mg at bedtime

Gastric hypersecretory conditions:

Oral: 150 mg twice daily; maximum: 600 mg/day

I.M., I.V.: 50 mg/dose every 6-8 hours (dose not to exceed 400 mg/day)

Continuous I.V. infusion: Initial 50 mg I.V. followed by 6.25 mg/hour titrated to gastric pH >4.0 for prophylaxis or >7.0 for treatment; **continuous I.V. infusion is preferred in patients with active bleeding**

Erosive esophagitis: Oral: 150 mg 4 times/day

Pathologic hypersecretory conditions (eg, Zollinger-Ellison syndrome):

Continuous I.V. infusion: Initial 50 mg I.V. followed by 1 mg/kg/hour infusion; titrate dosage in 0.5 mg/kg/hour increments to maintain gastric acid output at <10 mEq/hour; doses up to 2.5 mg/kg/hour (220 mg/hour) have been used

Oral: 150 mg twice daily; more frequent administration may be indicated depending upon response; doses up to 6.3 g/day have been used in severe cases

Relief of heartburn, acid indigestion, sour stomach (OTC use): Oral: 75 mg 30-60 minutes before eating; no more than 2 tablets/day

Dosing interval in renal impairment:

Cl_{cr} 10-50 mL/minute: Administer at 75% of normal dose or administer every 18-24 hours

Cl_{cr} <10 mL/minute: Administer at 50% of normal dose or administer every 18-24 hours

Administration

Oral: Administer with meals and at bedtime; EFFERdose® tablets and granules must be dissolved in 6-8 ounces of water before use

Parenteral: Intermittent I.V. infusion preferred over direct injection to decrease risk of bradycardia; for intermittent infusion, infuse over 15-30 minutes, at a usual concentration of 0.5 mg/mL; for direct I.V. injection, administer over a period not less than 5 minutes at a final concentration not to exceed 2.5 mg/mL

Monitoring Parameters AST, ALT, serum creatinine; when used to prevent stress-related GI bleeding, measure the intragastric pH and try to maintain pH >4; gastric acid secretion (<10 mEq/hour)

Test Interactions False-positive urine protein using Multistix®; gastric acid secretion test, skin test allergen extracts

Patient Information Avoid excessive amounts of coffee and aspirin; when self-medicating, if symptoms of heartburn, acid indigestion, or sour stomach persist after 2 weeks of continuous use of the drug, consult a clinician.

Additional Information Causes fewer CNS adverse reactions and drug interactions compared to cimetidine; safety and efficacy of full-dose therapy extending beyond 8 weeks have not been determined

Dosage Forms

Granules, effervescent, as hydrochloride (EFFERdose®): 150 mg

Infusion, preservative free, as hydrochloride, in NaCl 0.45%: 1 mg/mL (50 mL)

Injection, as hydrochloride: 25 mg/mL (2 mL, 6 mL, 40 mL)

Syrup, as hydrochloride: 15 mg/mL [peppermint flavor] (10 mL, 473 mL)

Tablet, as hydrochloride

Zantac®: 150 mg, 300 mg

Zantac® 75: 75 mg

Tablet, effervescent, as hydrochloride (EFFERdose®): 150 mg

References

Blumer JL, Rothstein FC, Kaplan BS, et al, "Pharmacokinetic Determination of Ranitidine Pharmacodynamics in Pediatric Ulcer Disease," *J Pediatr*, 1985, 107(2):301-6.

Eddleston JM, Booker PD, and Green JR, "Use of Ranitidine in Children Undergoing Cardiopulmonary Bypass," *Crit Care Med*, 1989, 17(1):26-9.

Fontana M, Massironi E, Rossi A, et al, "Ranitidine Pharmacokinetics in Newborn Infants," *Arch Dis Child*, 1993, 68(5 Spec No):602-3.

Lopez-Herce J, Albajara L, Codoceo R, et al, "Ranitidine Prophylaxis in Acute Gastric Mucosal Damage in Critically Ill Pediatric Patients," *Crit Care Med*, 1988, 16(6):591-93.

Morris DL, Markham SJ, Beechey A, et al, "Ranitidine-Bolus or Infusion Prophylaxis for Stress Ulcer," *Crit Care Med*, 1988, 16(3):229-32.

Roberts CJ, "Clinical Pharmacokinetics of Ranitidine," *Clin Pharmacokinet*, 1984, 9(3):211-21.

- **Regutol® [OTC]** *see Docusate on page 350*
- **Rejuva (Can)** *see Tretinoin on page 978*
- **Relefact TRH (Can)** *see Protirelin on page 851*
- **Relief®** *see Phenylephrine on page 789*
- **Relisorm (Can)** *see Gonadorelin on page 482*
- **Remular® S** *see Chlorzoxazone on page 229*
- **Renova®** *see Tretinoin on page 978*
- **Resectisol®** *see Mannitol on page 619*
- **Respa-DM®** *see Guaifenesin and Dextromethorphan on page 487*
- **Respa-GF** *see Guaifenesin on page 485*
- **RespiGam™** *see Respiratory Syncytial Virus Immune Globulin (Intravenous) on page 868*

Respiratory Syncytial Virus Immune Globulin (Intravenous)

(RES peer rah tor ee sin SISH al VYE rus i MYUN GLOB yoo lin in tra VEE nus)

U.S. Brand Names RespiGam™

Synonyms RSV-IGIV; RSV-IVIG

Therapeutic Category Immune Globulin

Generic Available No

Use Prevention of serious lower respiratory tract infection caused by RSV in children <24 months of age with BPD who are receiving supplemental oxygen; history of prematurity (≤32 weeks gestation); prophylaxis of infants with severe immune deficiency exposed to RSV; prophylaxis of infants and children with severe immunosuppression (eg, BMT patient exposed to RSV)

Pregnancy Risk Factor C

Contraindications History of a severe reaction associated with the administration of RSV-IGIV or other human immunoglobulin preparations; patients with IgA deficiency; hypersensitivity to any component

Warnings Adverse reactions may be related to the rate of administration; loop diuretics should be available for the management of patients who are at risk for fluid overload; epinephrine and diphenhydramine should be available for treatment of acute hypersensitivity reactions. Aseptic meningitis syndrome (onset of several hours to 2 days following RSV-IGIV administration: Symptoms of severe headache, drowsiness, fever, photophobia, painful eye movements, muscle rigidity, nausea and vomiting with pleocytosis and elevated protein levels in CSF have occurred in 3 patients in the PREVENT trial); (see Additional Information)

Precautions Use with caution in patients with underlying pulmonary disease since these patients are sensitive to extra fluid volume; immunization with MMR and varicella vaccines should be deferred for 9 months after the last RSV-IGIV dose

Adverse Reactions

Cardiovascular: Tachycardia, hypertension, edema, hypotension, heart murmur, cyanosis

Central nervous system: Fever/pyrexia (6%), dizziness, anxiety, aseptic meningitis syndrome

Dermatologic: Rash, eczema, pruritus

Gastrointestinal: Vomiting (6%), diarrhea, gastroenteritis

Local: Injection site inflammation

Respiratory: Respiratory distress, wheezing, rales, hypoxia, tachypnea, cyanosis, cough, rhinorrhea, dyspnea

Drug Interactions Live virus vaccine (ie, MMR, measles, varicella) when given during or within 10 months after RSV-IGIV administration; antibody response to DPT, DTaP, OPV, and *H. influenzae* b vaccine may be lower

Stability Refrigerate; do not freeze; do not shake vials; compatible with dextrose 5% through dextrose 20% with or without sodium chloride

Pharmacokinetics Half-life: 22-28 days

Usual Dosage I.V. infusion: Infants and Young Children: 750 mg/kg once monthly during RSV season (starting November with the last infusion in April).

Administration Infusion should start within 6 hours and be completed by 12 hours after vial entry; an in-line filter is not necessary, but if one is used, the pore size should be larger than 15 µM; if dilution is needed, a dilution of no greater than 1:2 should be used.

The infusion schedule is as follows:

Initial infusion rate for the first 15 minutes: 1.5 mL/kg/hour, then increase infusion rate for the next 15 minutes to 3 mL/kg/hour

30 minutes to end of infusion: 6 mL/kg/hour

Maximum infusion rate: 6 mL/kg/hour

Monitoring Parameters Heart rate, blood pressure, temperature, respiratory rate; observe for retractions and rales

Additional Information PREVENT (Prophylaxis of RSV in elevated-risk neonates trial) was a multicenter, randomized, double-blind, placebo-controlled trial (n=250 RSV-IGIV, n=260 placebo) among infants ≤24 months, born prematurely (≤35 weeks gestation), or children with BPD and a requirement for supplemental oxygen within the past 6 months. Each patient received a monthly infusion from November through April. The trial showed that children treated with RSV-IGIV had less RSV hospitalizations (20 days vs. 35 days, p=0.047); fewer RSV hospital days per 100 days (60 days vs. 129 days, p=0.045); fewer RSV hospital days with supplemental oxygen (34 days vs. 85 days, p=0.007). There was no difference between the two groups for ICU admissions, RSV ICU days per 100 children, RSV mechanical ventilation or days of ventilation per 100 children. (Groothius, 1993)

RSV-IGIV is a sterile liquid without preservatives purified using Cohn-Oncley cold ethanol fractionation and further treatment with a solvent-detergent partitioning method; contains trace amounts of IgA and IgM, sucrose and albumin; sodium content: 20-30 mEq/L

Dosage Forms Injection, preservative free: 1000 mg, 2500 mg (50 mL)

References

American Academy of Pediatrics Committee on Infectious Diseases, Committee on Fetus and Newborn, "Respiratory Syncytial Virus Immune Globulin Intravenous: Indications for Use," *Pediatrics*, 1997, 99(4):645-50.

Ellenberg SS, Epstein JS, Fratantoni JC, et al, "A Trial of RSV Immune Globulin in Infants and Young Children: The FDA's View," *N Engl J Med*, 1994, 331(3):203-5.

Groothius JR, Simoes EA, Levin MJ, et al, "Prophylactic Administration of Respiratory Syncytial Virus Immune Globulin to High-Risk Infants and Young Children. The Respiratory Syncytial Virus Immune Globulin Study Group," *N Engl J Med*, 1993, 329(21):1524-30.

♦ **Retin-A**® *see Tretinoin on page 978*

♦ **Retina-A**® **Micro** *see Tretinoin on page 978*

♦ **Retinoic Acid** *see Tretinoin on page 978*

♦ **Retisol-A (Can)** *see Tretinoin on page 978*

♦ **Retrovir**® *see Zidovudine on page 1022*

♦ **Reversol**® *see Edrophonium on page 373*

♦ **Revitalose-C-1000 (Can)** *see Ascorbic Acid on page 106*

♦ **R-Gene**® *see Arginine on page 104*

♦ **rGM-CSF** *see Sargramostim on page 890*

♦ **Rheomacrodex**® *see Dextran on page 311*

♦ **Rhesonativ**® *see Rh₀(D) Immune Globulin (Intramuscular) on page 869*

♦ **Rheumatrex**® **Oral** *see Methotrexate on page 648*

♦ **Rhinalar (Can)** *see Flunisolide on page 438*

♦ **Rhinall**® **[OTC]** *see Phenylephrine on page 789*

♦ **Rhinocort**® *see Budesonide on page 154*

♦ **Rhinocort**® **Aqua**™ *see Budesonide on page 154*

♦ **Rhinosyn-DMX**® **[OTC]** *see Guaifenesin and Dextromethorphan on page 487*

♦ **Rho-Clonazepam (Can)** *see Clonazepam on page 254*

♦ **Rhodacine (Can)** *see Indomethacin on page 536*

Rh₀(D) Immune Globulin (Intramuscular)
(ar aych oh (dee) i MYUN GLOB yoo lin)

U.S. Brand Names HypRho®-D; HypRho®-D Mini-Dose; MICRhoGAM™; Mini-Gamulin® Rh; Rhesonativ®; RhoGAM™

Therapeutic Category Immune Globulin

Generic Available No

Use Prevention of isoimmunization in Rh-negative individuals exposed to Rh-positive blood during delivery of an Rh-positive infant, as a result of an abortion, following amniocentesis or abdominal trauma, or following a transfusion accident; prevention of hemolytic disease of the newborn if there is a subsequent pregnancy with an Rh-positive fetus

Pregnancy Risk Factor C

Contraindications Rh₀(D)-positive patient; hypersensitivity to immune globulins or to thimerosal; transfusion of Rh₀(D)-positive blood in previous 3 months; prior sensitization to Rh₀(D)

Warnings Do not inject I.V.; do not administer to the neonate

Precautions Use with caution in patients with thrombocytopenia or bleeding disorders, patients with IgA deficiency
(Continued)

Rh_o(D) Immune Globulin (Intramuscular) *(Continued)*

Adverse Reactions
Central nervous system: Lethargy, fever
Gastrointestinal: Splenomegaly
Hepatic: Elevated bilirubin
Local: Pain at the injection site
Neuromuscular & skeletal: Myalgia

Drug Interactions Live virus vaccines (Rh_o(D) may interfere with immune response to measles, mumps, rubella)

Stability Refrigerate; may be stable for up to 30 days at room temperature; avoid freezing

Mechanism of Action Suppresses the immune response and antibody formation of Rh-negative individuals to Rh-positive red blood cells

Pharmacokinetics
Distribution: Appears in breast milk, however not absorbed by the nursing infant
Half-life: 23-26 days

Usual Dosage Adults: Administer to mother **NOT** to infant; I.M.:
Obstetrical usage: 1 vial (300 mcg) prevents maternal sensitization if fetal packed red blood cell volume that has entered the maternal circulation is <15 mL; if it is more, give additional vials. The number of vials = RBC volume of the calculated fetomaternal hemorrhage divided by 15 mL
Postpartum prophylaxis: 300 mcg within 72 hours of delivery
Antepartum prophylaxis: 300 mcg at approximately 26-28 weeks gestation; followed by 300 mcg within 72 hours of delivery if infant is Rh-positive
Following miscarriage, abortion, or termination of ectopic pregnancy at up to 13 weeks of gestation: 50 mcg ideally within 3 hours, but may be given up to 72 hours after; if pregnancy has been terminated at 13 or more weeks of gestation, administer 300 mcg within 72 hours

Administration Parenteral: Administer I.M. preferably in the anterolateral aspects of the upper thigh or the deltoid muscle of the upper arm. The total volume can be given in divided doses at different sites at one time or may be divided and given at intervals, provided the total dosage is given within 72 hours of the fetomaternal hemorrhage or transfusion.

Dosage Forms
Injection: Each vial contains one single dose 300 mcg of Rh_o(D) immune globulin
Injection, microdose: Each vial contains one single dose of microdose, 50 mcg of Rh_o(D) immune globulin

Rh_o(D) Immune Globulin (Intravenous)
(ar aych oh (dee) i MYUN GLOB yoo lin, in tra VEE nus)

U.S. Brand Names WinRho SDF®

Synonyms Rh_o(D) Immune Human Globulin; Rh_oIGIV

Therapeutic Category Immune Globulin

Use Treatment of nonsplenectomized, Rh_o(D) positive children and adults with chronic idiopathic thrombocytopenic purpura (ITP), children with acute ITP, or children and adults with ITP secondary to HIV infection; prevention of isoimmunization in Rh-negative individuals exposed to Rh-positive blood during delivery of an Rh-positive infant, within 72 hours of an abortion, following amniocentesis or abdominal trauma, or following a transfusion accident; prevention of hemolytic disease of the newborn if there is a subsequent pregnancy with an Rh-positive infant

Pregnancy Risk Factor C

Contraindications Hypersensitivity to immune globulin, thimerosal, or any component; IgA deficiency

Warnings When used for ITP in a patient who is Rh_o(D)-positive, a decrease in hemoglobin concentration as a result of destruction of Rh_o(D)-positive red blood cells can be expected; reduce WinRho SDF® dosage in these patients to minimize risk of increasing the severity of anemia; these patients should be monitored for signs and/or symptoms of intravascular hemolysis, clinically compromising anemia, and renal insufficiency; when used for suppression of Rh isoimmunization, the drug is administered to the mother **not** the infant; use only the I.V. route when treating ITP; anaphylactic hypersensitivity reactions can occur; studies indicate that there is no discernible risk of transmitting HIV or hepatitis B

Precautions Use with caution in patients with thrombocytopenia or bleeding disorders or individuals with hemoglobin concentrations <8 g/dL

Adverse Reactions
Cardiovascular: Hypotension, vasodilation
Central nervous system: Fever, headache, chills, dizziness, somnolence

Dermatologic: Rash, pruritus
Local: Discomfort and swelling at injection site
Gastrointestinal: Abdominal pain, diarrhea
Genitourinary: Hemoglobinuria
Hematologic: Hemolysis (hemoglobin decrease of >2 g/dL in 5% to 10% of ITP patients)
Neuromuscular & skeletal: Back pain, myalgia, hyperkinesia
Miscellaneous: Hypersensitivity reactions

Drug Interactions May interfere with the immune response to live virus vaccines (allow 3 months after administration of vaccine)

Stability Refrigerate do not freeze; reconstituted powder is stable 12 hours at room temperature

Mechanism of Action The $Rh_o(D)$ antigen is responsible for most cases of Rh sensitization, which occurs when Rh-positive fetal RBCs enter the maternal circulation of an Rh-negative woman. Injection of anti-D globulin results in opsonization of the fetal RBCs, which are then phagocytized in the spleen, preventing immunization of the mother. Injection of anti-D into an Rh-positive patient with ITP coats the patient's own D-positive RBCs with antibody and, as they are cleared by the spleen, they saturate the capacity of the spleen to clear antibody-coated cells, sparing antibody-coated platelets. Other proposed mechanisms involve the generation of cytokines following the interaction between antibody-coated RBCs and macrophages.

Pharmacodynamics
Onset of effect:
Rh isoimmunization: I.V.: 8 hours; ITP: I.V.: 1-2 days
Peak response: ITP: 7-14 days
Duration of effect: ITP: (single dose) 30 days

Pharmacokinetics
Half-life, elimination:
I.M.: 5-10 days
I.V.: 24 days
Time to peak concentration:
I.M.: 5-10 days
I.V.: 2 hours

Usual Dosage
ITP: **I.V. only:** Children and Adults:
Initial:
Hemoglobin ≥10 g/dL: 50 mcg/kg (250 international units/kg) as single dose or divided into 2 doses given on separate days
Hemoglobin <10 g/dL: 25-40 mcg/kg (125-200 international units/kg) as single dose or divided into 2 doses given on separate days
Hemoglobin <8 g/dL: Use with caution (see Precautions and Warnings)
Maintenance (usage dependent upon clinical response, platelet count, hemoglobin, red blood cell counts, and reticulocyte levels)
Response to initial dose: 25-60 mcg/kg (125-300 international units/kg) as single dose
Nonresponse to initial therapy:
Hemoglobin >10 g/dL: 50-60 mcg/kg (250-300 international units/kg) as single dose
Hemoglobin 8-10 g/dL: 25-40 mcg/kg (125-200 international units/kg) as single dose
Hemoglobin <8 g/dL: Use with caution (see Precautions and Warnings)
Suppression of Rh isoimmunization: **Adult female:** I.V. or I.M.: see table

I.V. Rh$_o$D Immune Globulin Dosage in Pregnancy and Obstetrical Conditions

Condition	Dosage
28 weeks gestation	300 mcg (1500 international units); repeat every 12 weeks throughout pregnancy
Postpartum (if newborn Rh-positive)	120 mcg (600 international units) **as soon as possible**, preferably <72 hours, after delivery; if baby's Rh status is not known by 72 hours, administer as soon as possible up to 28 days after delivery
Threatened abortion at any time	300 mcg (1500 international units) as soon as possible within 72 hours
Amniocentesis and chronic villus sampling before 34 weeks gestation	300 mcg (1500 international units) within 72 hours; repeat every 12 weeks throughout pregnancy
Abortion, amniocentesis, or any other manipulation after 34 weeks gestation	120 mcg (600 international units) within 72 hours

(Continued)

Rh$_o$(D) Immune Globulin (Intravenous) *(Continued)*

Treatment of exposure to incompatible blood transfusion or massive fetal hemorrhage; within 72 hours of event: **Adult female:**

Exposed to Rh$_o$(D) positive whole blood:

I.M.: 12 mcg (60 international units)/mL blood; administer in 1200 mcg (6000 international units) aliquots every 12 hours until the total calculated dose is administered

I.V.: 9 mcg (45 international units)/mL blood; administer in 600 mcg (3000 international units) aliquots every 8 hours until the total calculated dose is administered

Exposed to Rh$_o$(D) positive red blood cells:

I.M.: 24 mcg (120 international units)/mL cells administer in 1200 mcg (6000 international units) aliquots every 12 hours until the total calculated dose is administered

I.V.: 18 mcg (90 international units)/mL cells; administer in 600 mcg (3000 international units) aliquots every 8 hours until the total calculated dose is administered

Administration Parenteral: WinRho SDF® is the only immune globulin product available that can be administered **both** I.M. and I.V.; however, **for the treatment of ITP, it must be administered I.V.**

I.M.: Reconstitute 120 mcg and 300 mcg vials with 1.25 mL NS and the 100 mcg vial with 8.5 mL NS; gently swirl vial; do not shake; administer into the deltoid muscle of upper arm or the anterolateral aspect of the upper thigh; the gluteal region is not recommended for routine administration due to the potential risk of sciatic nerve injury; if gluteal area is used, administer only in the upper, outer quadrant

I.V.: Reconstitute 120 mcg and 300 mcg vials with 2.5 mL NS and 8.5 mL NS for the 1000 mcg vial; gently swirl vial; do not shake; infuse over 3-5 minutes

Monitoring Parameters ITP: CBC, reticulocytes, UA, renal function

Additional Information WinRho SDF® 1 mcg = 5 international units

Dosage Forms Injection, freeze dried: 120 mcg (600 international units); 300 mcg (1500 international units); 1000 mcg (5000 international units) [each vial is accompanied with NS diluent]

References

Gaines AR, "Acute Onset Hemoglobinemia and/or Hemoglobinuria and Sequela Following Rh(o)(D) Immune Globulin Intravenous Administration in Immune Thrombocytopenic Purpura Patients," *Blood*, 2000, 95(8):2523-9.

♦ **Rh$_o$(D) Immune Human Globulin** *see* Rh$_o$(D) Immune Globulin (Intravenous) *on page 870*

♦ **RhoGAM™** *see* Rh$_o$(D) Immune Globulin (Intramuscular) *on page 869*

♦ **Rho-Haloperidol (Can)** *see* Haloperidol *on page 488*

♦ **Rh$_o$IGIV** *see* Rh$_o$(D) Immune Globulin (Intravenous) *on page 870*

♦ **Rhoxal-Atenolol (Can)** *see* Atenolol *on page 111*

♦ **Rhoxal-Famotidine (Can)** *see* Famotidine *on page 417*

♦ **Rhoxal-Salbutamol (Can)** *see* Albuterol *on page 45*

♦ **Rhoxal-Valproic (Can)** *see* Valproic Acid and Derivatives *on page 998*

♦ **rHuEPO** *see* Epoetin Alfa *on page 388*

♦ **rHuEPO-α** *see* Epoetin Alfa *on page 388*

Ribavirin *(rye ba VYE rin)*

U.S. Brand Names Virazole®

Synonyms ICN-1299; RTCA; Tribavirin

Therapeutic Category Antiviral Agent, Inhalation Therapy

Generic Available No

Use Treatment of patients with RSV infections; specially indicated for treatment of severe lower respiratory tract RSV infections in patients with an underlying compromising condition (prematurity, BPD and other chronic lung conditions, congenital heart disease, immunodeficiency, immunosuppression), and recent transplant recipients; may also be used in other viral infections including influenza A and B and adenovirus

Pregnancy Risk Factor X

Contraindications Females of childbearing age

Warnings Ribavirin is potentially mutagenic, tumor-promoting, and gonadotoxic; there is evidence that ribavirin is teratogenic in small animals

Precautions Use with caution in patients requiring assisted ventilation because precipitation of the drug in the respiratory equipment may interfere with safe and effective patient ventilation; carefully monitor patients with COPD and asthma for deterioration of respiratory function

Adverse Reactions
Cardiovascular: Hypotension, cardiac arrest
Central nervous system: Headache
Dermatologic: Rash, skin irritation
Hematologic: Anemia
Ocular: Conjunctivitis
Respiratory: Mild bronchospasm, worsening of respiratory function, nasal and throat irritation

Drug Interactions Ribavirin antagonizes the antiviral activity of zidovudine and zalcitabine against HIV

Stability Reconstituted solution is stable for 24 hours at room temperature

Mechanism of Action Inhibits replication of RNA and DNA viruses; inhibits influenza virus RNA polymerase activity and interferes with the expression of messenger RNA resulting in inhibition of viral protein synthesis

Pharmacokinetics
Absorption: Systemically absorbed from the respiratory tract following nasal and oral inhalation; absorption is dependent upon respiratory factors and method of drug delivery; maximal absorption occurs with the use of the aerosol generator via an endotracheal tube
Distribution: Highest concentrations are found in the respiratory tract and erythrocytes
Metabolism: Occurs intracellularly and may be necessary for drug action; metabolized by the liver to deribosylated ribavirin (active metabolite)
Half-life:
Respiratory tract secretions: ~2 hours
Plasma:
Children: 6.5-11 hours
Adults: 24 hours; half-life is much longer in the erythrocyte (16-40 days), which can be used as a marker for intracellular metabolism
Time to peak serum concentration: Aerosol inhalation: At the end of the inhalation period
Elimination: Hepatic metabolism is the major route of elimination with 40% of the drug cleared renally as unchanged drug and metabolites

Usual Dosage Infants, Children, and Adults: Aerosol inhalation:
Use with Viratek® small particle aerosol generator (SPAG-2) at a concentration of 20 mg/mL (6 g reconstituted with 300 mL of sterile water without preservatives); 6 g ribavirin vial has also been diluted with 300 mL of sterile NS solution rather than sterile water to achieve a near isotonic solution.
Note: Dose actually delivered to the patient will depend on patient's minute ventilation
Continuous aerosolization: 12-18 hours/day for 3 days, or up to 7 days in length
Intermittent aerosolization: (high-dose, short-duration aerosol): 2 g over 2 hours 3 times/day at a concentration of 60 mg/mL (6 g reconstituted with 100 mL of sterile water without preservatives) in **non-mechanically ventilated** patients for 3-7 days has been used to permit easier accessibility for patient care and limit environmental exposure of healthcare worker. Due to apparent increased potential for crystallization of the high-dose 60 mg/mL solution around areas of turbulent flow such as bends in tubing or connector pieces, use of high-dose therapy in individuals with an endotracheal tube in place is **not** recommended.

Administration Ribavirin should be administered in well-ventilated rooms (at least 6 air changes/hour)

Mechanically ventilated patients: Ribavirin can potentially be deposited in the ventilator delivery system depending on temperature, humidity, and electrostatic forces; this deposition can lead to malfunction or obstruction of the expiratory valve, resulting in inadvertently high positive end-expiratory pressures. The use of one-way valves in the inspiratory lines, a breathing circuit filter in the expiratory line, and frequent monitoring and filter replacement have been effective in preventing these problems.

Monitoring Parameters Respiratory function, hemoglobin, reticulocyte count, CBC, I & O

Nursing Implications Healthcare workers who are pregnant or who may become pregnant should be advised of the potential risks of exposure and counseled about risk reduction strategies including alternate job responsibilities; limit contact by visitors with patients receiving ribavirin; ribavirin may adsorb to contact lenses
(Continued)

Ribavirin (Continued)

Additional Information RSV season is usually December to April; viral shedding period for RSV is usually 3-8 days

Dosage Forms Powder for aerosol: 6 g (100 mL)

References

American Academy of Pediatrics Committee on Infectious Diseases, "Reassessment of the Indications for Ribavirin Therapy in Respiratory Syncytial Virus Infections," *Pediatrics*, 1996, 97(1):137-40.

Englund JA, Piedra PA, Ahn Y-M, et al, "High-Dose, Short-Duration Ribavirin Aerosol Therapy Compared With Standard Ribavirin Therapy in Children With Suspected Respiratory Syncytial Virus Infection," *J Pediatr*, 1994, 125:635-41.

Janai HK, Marks MI, Zaleska M, et al, "Ribavirin: Adverse Drug Reactions 1986 to 1988," *Pediatr Infect Dis J*, 1990, 9(3):209-11.

Meert KL, Sarnaik AP, Gelmini MJ, et al, "Aerosolized Ribavirin in Mechanically Ventilated Children With Respiratory Syncytial Virus Lower Respiratory Tract Disease: A Prospective, Double-Blind, Randomized Trial," *Crit Care Med*, 1994, 22(4):566-72.

Smith DW, Frankel LR, Mathers LH, et al, "A Controlled Trial of Aerosolized Ribavirin in Infants Receiving Mechanical Ventilation for Severe Respiratory Syncytial Virus Infection," *N Engl J Med*, 1991, 325(1):24-9.

Riboflavin (RYE boe flay vin)

Synonyms Lactoflavin; Vitamin B_2; Vitamin G

Therapeutic Category Nutritional Supplement; Vitamin, Water Soluble

Generic Available Yes

Use Prevention of riboflavin deficiency and treatment of ariboflavinosis; microcytic anemia associated with glutathione reductase deficiency

Pregnancy Risk Factor A (C if dose exceeds RDA recommendation)

Contraindications Hypersensitivity to riboflavin or any component

Adverse Reactions Genitourinary: Discoloration of urine (bright yellow) with large doses

Drug Interactions Probenecid

Food Interactions Food increases the extent of GI absorption

Stability Protect from light

Mechanism of Action Converted to coenzymes which act as hydrogen-carrier molecules, which are necessary for normal tissue respiration; also needed for activation of pyridoxine and conversion of tryptophan to niacin

Pharmacokinetics

Absorption: Readily via GI tract; GI absorption is decreased in patients with hepatitis, cirrhosis, or biliary obstruction

Metabolism: Metabolic fate unknown

Half-life, biologic: 66-84 minutes

Elimination: 9% eliminated unchanged in urine

Usual Dosage Oral:

Riboflavin deficiency:

Children: 3-10 mg/day in divided doses

Adults: 5-30 mg/day in divided doses

Adequate intake: Infants:

<6 months: 0.3 mg (0.04 mg/kg)

6-12 months: 0.4 mg (0.04 mg/kg)

Recommended daily allowance (RDA):

Children:

1-3 years: 0.5 mg

4-8 years: 0.6 mg

9-13 years: 0.9 mg

14-18 years:

Male: 1.3 mg

Female: 1 mg

19-70 years:

Male: 1.3 mg

Female: 1.1 mg

Microcytic anemia associated with glutathione reductase deficiency: Adults: 10 mg daily for 10 days

Administration Oral: Administer with food

Monitoring Parameters CBC and reticulocyte counts (if anemic when treating deficiency)

Test Interactions Large doses may interfere with urinalysis based on spectrometry; may cause false elevations in fluorometric determinations of catecholamines and urobilinogen

Patient Information Large doses may cause bright yellow urine

Dosage Forms
Capsule: 100 mg
Tablet: 10 mg, 25 mg, 50 mg, 100 mg

♦ **Rid-a-Pain-HP**® **[OTC]** *see* Capsaicin *on page 172*

♦ **Ridaura**® *see* Auranofin *on page 119*

♦ **Ridenol**® **[OTC]** *see* Acetaminophen *on page 29*

Rifabutin (rif a BYOO tin)

U.S. Brand Names Mycobutin®

Synonyms Ansamycin

Therapeutic Category Antibiotic, Miscellaneous; Antitubercular Agent

Generic Available No

Use Prevention of disseminated *Mycobacterium avium* complex (MAC) in patients with advanced HIV infection; utilized in multiple drug regimens for treatment of MAC

Pregnancy Risk Factor B

Contraindications Hypersensitivity to rifabutin, any component, or other rifamycin; rifabutin is contraindicated in patients with a WBC <1000/mm^3 or a platelet count <50,000 mm^3

Warnings Rifabutin as a single agent must not be administered to patients with active tuberculosis since its use may lead to the development of tuberculosis that is resistant to both rifabutin and rifampin; rifabutin should be discontinued in patients with AST >500 international units/L or if total bilirubin is >3 mg/dL

Precautions Use with caution in patients with liver impairment

Adverse Reactions
Central nervous system: Fever, headache, seizures, confusion, insomnia
Dermatologic: Rash, staining of skin (brown-orange)
Gastrointestinal: Abdominal pain, diarrhea, dyspepsia, nausea, vomiting, dysgeusia, flatulence
Genitourinary: Discoloration of urine (brown-orange)
Hematologic: Thrombocytopenia, anemia, leukopenia, neutropenia
Hepatic: Elevated liver enzymes
Neuromuscular & skeletal: Arthralgia, myositis
Ocular: Uveitis
Miscellaneous: Discoloration of body fluids (brown-orange)

Drug Interactions Cytochrome P-450 isoenzyme CYP3A3/4 inducer
May decrease the serum concentration or effect of dapsone, verapamil, methadone, ketoconazole, digoxin, theophylline, barbiturates, protease inhibitors, non-nucleoside reverse transcriptase inhibitors, anticoagulants, corticosteroids, zidovudine, cyclosporine, quinidine, and oral contraceptives (alternative form of contraception should be considered); indinavir and ritonavir increase rifabutin concentrations (decrease daily rifabutin dose by 50% if given with indinavir or decrease rifabutin adult dose to 150 mg 2-3 times per week if given with ritonavir); protease inhibitors, erythromycin, clarithromycin, ketoconazole, fluconazole, and itraconazole may increase serum concentration of rifabutin

Food Interactions High-fat meal may decrease the rate but not the extent of absorption

Mechanism of Action Inhibits DNA-dependent RNA polymerase at the beta subunit which prevents chain initiation

Pharmacokinetics
Absorption: Oral: Readily absorbed
Distribution: To body tissues including the lungs, liver, spleen, eyes, and kidneys
Protein binding: 85%
Metabolism: To active and inactive metabolites
Half life, terminal: 45 hours (range: 16-69 hours)
Time to peak serum concentration: 2-4 hours
Elimination: Renal and biliary clearance of unchanged drug is 10%; 30% excreted in feces

Usual Dosage Oral:
Children: Efficacy and safety of rifabutin have not been established in children; a limited number of HIV-positive children with MAC (n=22) have been given rifabutin for MAC prophylaxis; dosages of up to 75 mg/day have been given to children <4 years of age (~5-6 mg/kg/day)
Infants and Children: Prophylaxis for first episode of MAC in HIV-infected patients:
Children <6 years: 5 mg/kg once daily
Children ≥6 years: 300 mg once daily
Infants and Children: Prophylaxis for recurrence of MAC in HIV-infected patients:
5 mg/kg (maximum dose: 300 mg) once daily in combination with clarithromycin
(Continued)

Rifabutin *(Continued)*

Adolescents and Adults:

Prophylaxis for first episode of MAC in HIV-infected patient: 300 mg once daily; for patients who experience gastrointestinal upset, rifabutin can be administered 150 mg twice daily with food

Prophylaxis for recurrence of MAC in HIV-infected patient: 300 mg once daily as a component of a multiple drug regimen

Administration Oral: May administer with or without food or mix with applesauce; administer with food to decrease GI upset

Monitoring Parameters Periodic liver function tests, CBC with differential, platelet count, hemoglobin, hematocrit

Patient Information May discolor skin, urine, tears, perspiration, or other body fluids to a brown-orange color; soft contact lenses may be permanently stained

Dosage Forms Capsule: 150 mg

Extemporaneous Preparations A 20 mg/mL rifabutin suspension is made by placing the powder from eight 150 mg rifabutin capsules into a glass mortar, levigating with 20 mL of a 1:1 vehicle of Ora-Sweet® and Ora-Plus® and triturating the mixture to make a paste. Additional vehicle is added in geometric proportion levigating until a uniform mixture is obtained; qsad to 60 mL with vehicle. Stable for 12 weeks at 4°C, 25°C, 30°C, and 40°C. Label "shake well before using."

Haslam JL, Egodage KL, Chen Y, et al, "Stability of Rifabutin in Two Extemporaneously Compounded Oral Liquids," *Am J Health Syst Pharm*, 1999, 56(4):333-6.

References

1999 USPHS/IDSA Guidelines for the Prevention of Opportunistic Infections in Persons Infected With Human Immunodeficiency Virus, *MMWR Morb Mortal Wkly Rep*, 1999, 48(RR-10): 1-6 6.

Krause PJ, Hight DW, Schwartz AN, et al, "Successful Management of *Mycobacterium intracellulare* Pneumonia in a Child," *Pediatr Infect Dis*, 1986, 5(2):269-71.

Levin RH and Bolinger AM, "Treatment of Nontuberculous Mycobacterial Infections in Pediatric Patients," *Clin Pharm*, 1988, 7(7):545-51.

Starke JR and Correa AG, "Management of Mycobacterial Infection and Disease in Children," *Pediatr Infect Dis J*, 1995, 14(6):455-70.

♦ **Rifadin**® *see* Rifampin *on page 876*

♦ **Rifampicin** *see* Rifampin *on page 876*

Rifampin *(RIF am pin)*

U.S. Brand Names Rifadin®; Rimactane®

Canadian Brand Names Rofact

Synonyms Rifampicin

Therapeutic Category Antibiotic, Miscellaneous; Antitubercular Agent

Generic Available No

Use Used in combination with other antitubercular drugs for the treatment of active tuberculosis; elimination of meningococci from asymptomatic carriers; prophylaxis in contacts of patients with *Haemophilus influenzae* type B infection; used in combination with other anti-infectives in the treatment of staphylococcal infections

Pregnancy Risk Factor C

Contraindications Hypersensitivity to rifampin or any component

Precautions Use with caution in patients with liver impairment; modification of dosage should be considered in patients with severe liver impairment

Adverse Reactions

Central nervous system: Drowsiness, fatigue, confusion, ataxia, fever, headache

Dermatologic: Rash, pruritus

Gastrointestinal: Nausea, vomiting, diarrhea, stomatitis, anorexia

Hematologic: Eosinophilia, blood dyscrasias (leukopenia, thrombocytopenia), hemolytic anemia

Hepatic: Hepatitis, cholestatic jaundice

Local: Irritation at the I.V. site

Neuromuscular & skeletal: Myalgias, arthralgia

Renal: Renal failure, interstitial nephritis

Miscellaneous: Flu-like syndrome; discoloration of body fluids (red-orange)

Drug Interactions Cytochrome P-450 isoenzyme CYP3A3/4 substrate; isoenzyme CYP1A2, CYP2C9, CYP2C18, CYP2C19, CYP3A3/4, and CYP3A5-7 inducer

Rifampin induces liver enzymes which may decrease the plasma concentration of the following drugs: verapamil, diltiazem, nifedipine, methadone, digoxin, cyclosporine, corticosteroids, oral anticoagulants, theophylline, barbiturates, chloramphenicol, ketoconazole, oral contraceptives (alternate form of contraception should be considered), protease inhibitors, non-nucleoside reverse transcriptase inhibitors, and quinidine; halothane or isoniazid (additive hepatotoxic effects)

Food Interactions Food may delay and reduce the amount of rifampin absorbed

Stability Reconstituted I.V. solution is stable for 24 hours at room temperature; once the reconstituted I.V. solution is further diluted in D_5W (preferably) or NS, the I.V. infusion solution should be administered within 4 hours of preparation to avoid precipitation

Mechanism of Action Inhibits bacterial RNA synthesis by binding to the beta subunit of DNA-dependent RNA polymerase, blocking RNA transcription

Pharmacokinetics

Absorption: Oral: Well absorbed

Distribution: Highly lipophilic; crosses the blood-brain barrier and is widely distributed into body tissues and fluids such as the liver, lungs, gallbladder, bile, tears, and breast milk; distributes into CSF when meninges are inflamed

Protein binding: 80%

Metabolism: Undergoes enterohepatic recycling; metabolized in the liver to a deacetylated metabolite (active)

Half-life: 3-4 hours, prolonged with hepatic impairment

Time to peak serum concentration: Oral: Within 2-4 hours

Elimination: Principally in feces (60% to 65%) and urine (~30%)

Dialysis: Plasma rifampin concentrations are not significantly affected by hemodialysis or peritoneal dialysis

Usual Dosage Oral (I.V. infusion dose is the same as for the oral route):

Tuberculosis:

Children: 10-20 mg/kg/day in divided doses every 12-24 hours

Adults: 10 mg/kg/day administered once daily; maximum dose: 600 mg/day

American Thoracic Society and CDC currently recommend twice weekly therapy as part of a short-course regimen which follows 1-2 months of daily treatment of uncomplicated pulmonary tuberculosis in the compliant patient

Children: 10-20 mg/kg/dose (up to 600 mg) twice weekly under supervision to ensure compliance

Adults: 10 mg/kg (up to 600 mg) twice weekly

H. influenzae prophylaxis:

Neonates <1 month: 10 mg/kg/day every 24 hours for 4 days

Infants and Children: 20 mg/kg/day every 24 hours for 4 days, not to exceed 600 mg/dose

Adults: 600 mg every 24 hours for 4 days

Meningococcal prophylaxis:

<1 month: 10 mg/kg/day in divided doses every 12 hours for 2 days

Infants and Children: 20 mg/kg/day in divided doses every 12 hours for 2 days, not to exceed 600 mg/dose

Adults: 600 mg every 12 hours for 2 days

Nasal carriers of Staphylococcus aureus:

Children: 15 mg/kg/day divided every 12 hours for 5-10 days in combination with other antibiotics

Adults: 600 mg once daily for 5-10 days in combination with other antibiotics

Administration

Oral: Administer 1 hour before or 2 hours after a meal on an empty stomach; may administer with food to decrease GI distress; may mix contents of capsule with applesauce or jelly

Parenteral: Do not administer I.M. or S.C.; administer I.V. preparation once daily by slow I.V. infusion over 30 minutes to 3 hours at a final concentration not to exceed 6 mg/mL

Monitoring Parameters Periodic monitoring of liver function (AST, ALT); bilirubin, CBC

Patient Information May discolor urine, tears, sweat, or other body fluids to a red-orange color; soft contact lenses may be permanently stained

Nursing Implications The compounded oral suspension must be shaken well before using

Dosage Forms

Capsule: 150 mg, 300 mg

Powder for injection: 600 mg (contains a sulfite)

Extemporaneous Preparations Rifampin oral suspension can be compounded with simple syrup or wild cherry syrup at a concentration of 10 mg/mL; the suspension is stable for 4 weeks at room temperature or in a refrigerator when stored in a glass amber prescription bottle. However, there are some experts who do not recommend using rifampin syrup formulated from capsules due to conflicting reports indicating that the product is unstable (14.5% to 68% of labeled potency after preparation). It may be preferable to perform trituration, rather than simple mixing in syrup when preparing rifampin oral suspension.

(Continued)

Rifampin *(Continued)*

Nahata MC, Morosco RS, and Hipple TF, "Effect of Preparation Method and Storage on Rifampin Concentration in Suspensions," *Ann Pharmacother*, 1994, 28(2):182-5.

References

American Academy of Pediatrics Committee on Infectious Diseases, "Chemotherapy for Tuberculosis in Infants and Children," *Pediatrics*, 1992, 89(1):161-5.

Starke JR, "Modern Approach to the Diagnosis and Treatment of Tuberculosis in Children," *Pediatr Clin North Am*, 1988, 35(3):441-64.

Starke JR, "Multidrug Therapy for Tuberculosis in Children," *Pediatr Infect Dis J*, 1990, 9(11):785-93.

♦ **rIFN-α** *see* Interferon Alfa-2a *on page 542*

♦ **rIFN-α2** *see* Interferon Alfa-2b *on page 544*

♦ **Rimactane®** *see* Rifampin *on page 876*

Rimantadine (ri MAN ta deen)

U.S. Brand Names Flumadine®

Therapeutic Category Antiviral Agent, Oral

Generic Available No

Use Prophylaxis (adults and children) and treatment (adults) of influenza A viral infection

Pregnancy Risk Factor C

Contraindications Hypersensitivity to rimantadine, amantadine, or any component

Precautions Use with caution in patients with liver disease, epilepsy, history of recurrent eczematoid dermatitis, uncontrolled psychosis, severe psychoneurosis, and in patients receiving CNS stimulant drugs; modify dosage in patients with renal impairment, severe hepatic dysfunction, or active seizure disorder

Adverse Reactions

Cardiovascular: Orthostatic hypotension, edema

Central nervous system: Dizziness, confusion, headache, insomnia, difficulty in concentrating, anxiety, restlessness, irritability, hallucinations; CNS adverse effects are less than with amantadine

Gastrointestinal: Nausea, vomiting, xerostomia

Genitourinary: Urinary retention

Drug Interactions Anticholinergic agents, CNS stimulants may possibly increase adverse effects

Food Interactions Food does not affect rate or extent of absorption

Mechanism of Action Blocks the uncoating of influenza A viral RNA and prevents penetration of the virus into host cell; inhibits M_2 protein in the assembly of progeny virions

Pharmacokinetics

Absorption: Oral: Well absorbed

Distribution: Adults: 17-25 L/kg

Protein binding: ~40%

Metabolism: Extensively in the liver via hydroxylation and glucuronidation

Half-life:

Children 4-8 years: 13-38 hours

Adults: 24-36 hours

Elimination: <25% excreted unchanged in the urine

Dialysis: Hemodialysis: Negligible effect

Usual Dosage Oral: (See Additional Information for duration of therapy)

Prophylaxis:

Children <10 years: 5 mg/kg once daily; maximum dose: 150 mg/day

Children >10 years and Adults: 100 mg twice daily (see Note)

Treatment: Adults: 100 mg twice daily (see Note)

Note: Patients with severe hepatic or renal dysfunction or elderly nursing home patients: 100 mg/day

Administration Oral: May administer with food

Patient Information May cause dizziness or confusion and may impair ability to perform activities requiring mental alertness or physical coordination; may cause dry mouth

Additional Information Not active against influenza B; treatment or prophylaxis in immunosuppressed patients has not been fully evaluated

Duration of treatment: 5-7 days; optimal duration not established

Duration of prophylactic therapy: For at least 10 days after known exposure; usually for 6-8 weeks during influenza A season or local outbreak (or until vaccine produces sufficient antibody titers)

Duration of fever and other symptoms can be reduced if rimantadine therapy is started within the first 48 hours of influenza A illness

During an outbreak of influenza, administer rimantadine prophylaxis for 2-3 weeks after influenza vaccination until vaccine antibody titers are sufficient to provide protection

Dosage Forms
Syrup, as hydrochloride: 50 mg/5 mL (240 mL)
Tablet, as hydrochloride: 100 mg

♦ **Riopan® [OTC]** see Antacid Preparations on page 95
♦ **Riphenidate (Can)** see Methylphenidate on page 653
♦ **Ritalin®** see Methylphenidate on page 653
♦ **Ritalin-SR®** see Methylphenidate on page 653

Ritonavir (rit ON uh veer)
Related Information
Adult and Adolescent HIV on page 1166
Pediatric HIV on page 1162
U.S. Brand Names Norvir®
Therapeutic Category Antiretroviral Agent; HIV Agents (Anti-HIV Agents); Protease Inhibitor
Use Treatment of HIV infection in combination with other antiretroviral agents. (**Note:** HIV regimens consisting of **three** antiretroviral agents are strongly recommended)
Pregnancy Risk Factor B
Contraindications Hypersensitivity to ritonavir or any component
Warnings Ritonavir is a potent CYP3A enzyme inhibitor which interacts with numerous drugs. Due to potential serious and/or life-threatening drug interactions, the following drugs should not be coadministered with ritonavir: amiodarone, astemizole, bepridil, bupropion, cisapride, clozapine, dihydroergotamine, ergotamine, flecainide, encainide, meperidine, pimozide, piroxicam, propafenone, propoxyphene, quinidine, rifabutin, terfenadine, alprazolam, clorazepate, diazepam, estazolam, flurazepam, midazolam, triazolam, and zolpidem (see Drug Interactions); avoid concurrent use of St John's wort (may lead to loss of virologic response and/or resistance). Spontaneous bleeding episodes have been reported in patients with hemophilia type A and B. New onset diabetes mellitus, exacerbation of diabetes, and hyperglycemia have been reported in HIV-infected patients receiving protease inhibitors.
Precautions Use caution in patients with hepatic insufficiency
Adverse Reactions
Central nervous system: Headache, confusion
Endocrine & metabolic: Elevated triglycerides and cholesterol, increased creatine phosphokinase; rare: hyperglycemia, diabetes, ketoacidosis
Gastrointestinal: Nausea, vomiting, diarrhea, taste perversion, abdominal pain, anorexia, pancreatitis
Hematologic: Rare: Spontaneous bleeding episodes in hemophiliacs
Hepatic: Elevated liver enzymes, hepatitis
Neuromuscular & skeletal: Circumoral and peripheral paresthesias, weakness
Miscellaneous: Allergic reaction (urticaria, rash, bronchospasm, angioedema)
Drug Interactions Cytochrome P-450 isoenzyme CYP1A2, CYP2A6, CYP2C9, CYP2C19, CYP2E1, and CYP3A3/4 substrate; isoenzyme CYP2D6 substrate (minor); isoenzyme CYP1A2 inducer; isoenzyme CYP2A6, CYP2C9, CYP1A2, CYP2C19, CYP2D6, CYP2E1, and CYP3A3/4 inhibitor
Increases plasma concentration of amiodarone, astemizole, warfarin (monitor anticoagulant effect), bepridil, bupropion, cisapride, clozapine, dihydroergotamine, encainide, ergotamine, flecainide, meperidine, pimozide, piroxicam, propafenone, propoxyphene, quinidine, rifabutin, and terfenadine; inhibits metabolism of alprazolam, clorazepate, diazepam, estazolam, flurazepam, midazolam, triazolam, and zolpidem resulting in profound and prolonged sedation; 77% increase in clarithromycin AUC (decrease clarithromycin dose in patients with renal impairment); 145% increase in desipramine AUC (consider dosage reduction); 13% decrease in didanosine AUC (if patient is on concurrent ritonavir and didanosine therapy, doses should be spaced 2.5 hours apart); 40% decrease in ethinyl estradiol AUC (consider alternative contraceptive measures); 43% decrease in theophylline AUC (monitor theophylline levels); metronidazole (disulfiram-like reaction); inhibits indinavir and saquinavir metabolism; coadministration with nelfinavir increases concentration of nelfinavir; ritonavir decreases methadone serum concentrations; the herbal medicine, St John's wort (*Hypericum perforatum*) may significantly decrease concentrations of ritonavir and is **not** recommended for concurrent use
(Continued)

Ritonavir *(Continued)*

Stability Refrigerate capsules; liquid formulation is stable for 30 days at room temperature; liquid formulation should be stored in the original container; protect from light

Mechanism of Action A protease inhibitor which acts on an enzyme late in the HIV replication process after the virus has entered into the cell's nucleus preventing cleavage of protein precursors essential for HIV infection of new cells and viral replication. Saquinavir- and zidovudine-resistant HIV isolates are generally susceptible to ritonavir but strains resistant to ritonavir are usually cross-resistant to indinavir and saquinavir.

Pharmacokinetics

Absorption: Well absorbed

Distribution: High concentrations in serum and lymph nodes

Protein binding: 98% to 99%

Time to peak serum concentration: 2-4 hours

Metabolism: In the liver by the cytochrome P-450 enzyme 3A (CYP3A) to an active and inactive metabolite

Half-life: 3-5 hours

Elimination: Renal clearance is negligible

Usual Dosage Oral:

Neonates: Under investigation in PACTG 354

Children ≤12 years: Initial: 250 mg/m²/dose twice daily; titrate upward by 50 mg/m²/dose twice daily increments over 5 days, up to 400 mg/m²/dose twice daily; dosage range: 350-400 mg/m²/dose twice daily (every 12 hours); maximum dose: 600 mg/dose twice daily

Adolescents and Adults: 600 mg twice daily; may use a dose titration schedule to reduce adverse events (nausea/vomiting) by initiating therapy at 300 mg twice daily; increase dose by 100 mg twice daily increments over 5 days up to a maximum dose of 600 mg twice daily

Administration Administer with food to increase absorption; consider reserving liquid formulation for use in patients receiving tube feeding due to its bad taste. May mix liquid formulation with milk, chocolate milk, vanilla or chocolate pudding or ice cream, or a liquid nutritional supplement. Other techniques used to increase tolerance in children include dulling the taste buds by chewing ice, giving popsicles or spoonfuls or partially frozen orange or grape juice concentrates before administration of ritonavir; coating the mouth with peanut butter to eat before the dose; administration of strong-tasting foods such as maple syrup, cheese, or strong-flavored chewing gum immediately after a dose.

Monitoring Parameters Liver function tests, blood glucose levels, CD4 cell count, plasma levels of HIV RNA

Patient Information If dose is missed, take the next dose as soon as possible; however, if a dose is skipped, do not double the next dose

Dosage Forms

Capsule: 100 mg (contains ethanol and polyoxyl 35 castor oil)

Solution: 80 mg/mL (240 mL) (contains ethanol and polyoxyl 35 castor oil)

References

Danner SA, Carr A, Leonard JM, et al, "A Short-Term Study of the Safety, Pharmacokinetics, and Efficacy of Ritonavir, an Inhibitor of HIV-1 Protease. European-Australian Collaborative Ritonavir Study Group," *N Engl J Med*, 1995, 333(23):1528-33.

Mueller BU, Zuckerman J, Nelson J, et al, "A Phase I/II Study of the Protease Inhibitor Ritonavir (ABT-538) in Children With HIV Infection," *Eleventh International Conference on AIDS*, Vancouver, Canada, 1996.

Working Group on Antiretroviral Therapy and Medical Management of HIV-Infected Children, "Guidelines for the Use of Antiretroviral Agents in Pediatric HIV Infection," January 7, 2000, http://www.hivatis.org.

+ **Robinul®** *see* Glycopyrrolate *on page 479*
+ **Robinul® Forte** *see* Glycopyrrolate *on page 479*
+ **Robitussin® [OTC]** *see* Guaifenesin *on page 485*
+ **Robitussin® A-C** *see* Guaifenesin and Codeine *on page 486*
+ **Robitussin Children's (Can)** *see* Dextromethorphan *on page 316*
+ **Robitussin® Cough Calmers [OTC]** *see* Dextromethorphan *on page 316*
+ **Robitussin®-DM [OTC]** *see* Guaifenesin and Dextromethorphan *on page 487*
+ **Robitussin® Pediatric [OTC]** *see* Dextromethorphan *on page 316*
+ **Rocaltrol®** *see* Calcitriol *on page 166*
+ **Rocephin®** *see* Ceftriaxone *on page 204*

Rocuronium (roe kyoor OH nee um)

U.S. Brand Names Zemuron®

Therapeutic Category Neuromuscular Blocker Agent, Nondepolarizing; Skeletal Muscle Relaxant, Paralytic

Generic Available No

Use Produces skeletal muscle relaxation during surgery after induction of general anesthesia, increases pulmonary compliance during assisted mechanical respiration, facilitates endotracheal intubation

Pregnancy Risk Factor B

Contraindications Hypersensitivity to rocuronium or any component

Warnings Dosage adjustment needed in patients with severe hepatic disease; ventilation must be supported during neuromuscular blockade

Precautions Many clinical conditions may potentiate or antagonize neuromuscular blockade, see table.

Clinical Conditions Affecting Neuromuscular Blockade

Potentiation	Antagonism
Electrolyte abnormalities	Alkalosis
Severe hyponatremia	Hypercalcemia
Severe hypocalcemia	Demyelinating lesions
Severe hypokalemia	Peripheral neuropathies
Hypermagnesemia	Diabetes mellitus
Neuromuscular diseases	
Acidosis	
Acute intermittent porphyria	
Renal failure	
Hepatic failure	

Increased sensitivity in patients with myasthenia gravis, Eaton-Lambert syndrome; resistance to neuromuscular blockade in burn patients (>30% of body) for period of 5-70 days postinjury; resistance to neuromuscular blockade in patients with muscle trauma, denervation, immobilization, infection

Adverse Reactions Most frequent adverse reactions are associated with prolongation of its pharmacologic actions
Cardiovascular: Hypotension, hypertension, arrhythmias, tachycardia
Dermatologic: Rash, pruritus
Gastrointestinal: Vomiting
Local: Injection site edema
Neuromuscular & skeletal: Muscle weakness
Respiratory: Bronchospasm
Miscellaneous: Hiccups

Drug Interactions See table on next page.

Stability Refrigerate; unopened vials are stable 60 days at room temperature; open vials are stable for 30 days at room temperature; compatible with NS and D$_5$W; do not mix with alkaline solutions

Mechanism of Action Nondepolarizing neuromuscular blocking agent which blocks neural transmission at the myoneural junction by binding with cholinergic receptor sites

Pharmacodynamics
Peak effect:
  Children: 30 seconds to 1 minute
  Adults: 1-3.7 minutes

(Continued)

Rocuronium *(Continued)*

Duration:
Children:
3-12 months: 40 minutes
1-12 years: 27 minutes
Adults: 20-94 minutes (dose-related) (most prolonged in elderly ≥65 years of age)

Potential Drug Interactions

Potentiation	Antagonism
Inhalation anesthetics	Calcium
Desflurane, sevoflurane, enflurane and	Carbamazepine
isoflurane > halothane > nitrous	Phenytoin
oxide	Steroids (chronic administration)
Antibiotics	Theophylline
Aminoglycosides, polymyxins,	Anticholinesterases*
clindamycin, vancomycin	Neostigmine, pyridostigmine,
Magnesium	edrophonium, echothiophate
Antiarrhythmics	ophthalmic solution
Quinidine, procainamide, bretylium, and	Caffeine
possibly lidocaine	Azathioprine
Diuretics	
Furosemide, mannitol, thiazides	
Amphotericin B (secondary to hypokalemia)	
Local anesthetics	
Dantrolene (directly depresses skeletal muscle)	
Beta blockers	
Calcium channel blockers	
Ketamine	
Lithium	
Succinylcholine (when administered prior to nondepolarizing neuromuscular-blocking agent)	
Cyclosporine	

*Can prolong the effects of acetylcholine

Pharmacokinetics

Distribution: V_d:
Children: 0.21-0.36 L/kg
Adults: 0.22-0.26 L/kg
Hepatic dysfunction: 0.53 L/kg
Renal dysfunction: 0.34 L/kg
Protein binding: ~30%
Half-life:
Alpha elimination: 1-2 minutes
Beta elimination:
Children:
3-12 months: 1.3 ± 0.5 hours
3-8 years: 0.8 ± 0.3 hours
Adults: 1.4-2.4 hours
Hepatic dysfunction: 4.3 hours
Renal dysfunction: 2.4 hours
Elimination: Primarily biliary excretion (70%); up to 30% of dose excreted unchanged in urine

Usual Dosage I.V.:

Infants: 0.5 mg/kg/dose repeat every 20-30 minutes as needed
Children and Adults: Initial: 0.6-1.2 mg/kg/dose with repeat doses of 0.2 mg/kg every 20-30 minutes
Continuous infusion: 10-12 mcg/kg/minute
Note: While I.V. administration is preferred, I.M. administration in single doses of 1 mg/kg (infants) and 1.8 mg/kg (children) has been used successfully (Kaplan, 1999).

Administration Parenteral: May be administered undiluted by rapid I.V. injection; for continuous infusion, dilute with NS, D_5W, or LR to a concentration of 0.5-1 mg/mL

Monitoring Parameters Peripheral nerve stimulator measuring twitch response, heart rate, blood pressure, assisted ventilation status

Nursing Implications Does not alter the patient's state of consciousness; addition of sedation and analgesia are recommended

Dosage Forms Injection, as bromide: 10 mg/mL (5 mL, 10 mL)

References

Kaplan RF, Uejima T, Lobel G, et al, "Intramuscular Rocuronium in Infants and Children: A Multicenter Study to Evaluate Tracheal Intubating Conditions, Onset, and Duration of Action," *Anesthesiology*, 1999, 91(3):633-8.

Martin LD, Bratton SL, and O'Rourke PP, "Clinical Uses and Controversies of Neuromuscular Blocking Agents in Infants and Children," *Crit Care Med*, 1999, 27(7):1358-68.

Reynolds LM, Lau M, Brown R, et al, "Bioavailability of Intramuscular Rocuronium in Infants and Children," *Anesthesiology*, 1997, 87(5):1096-105.

Willets LS, "Rocuronium for Tracheal Intubation," *Ped Pharmacotherapy*, 2000, 6(10):1-6.

♦ **Rofact (Can)** *see* Rifampin *on page 876*

♦ **Roferon-A**® *see* Interferon Alfa-2a *on page 542*

♦ **Rogaine**® **[OTC]** *see* Minoxidil *on page 676*

♦ **Rogaine**® **Extra Strength [OTC]** *see* Minoxidil *on page 676*

♦ **Rogitine (Can)** *see* Phentolamine *on page 788*

♦ **Rolaids**® **[OTC]** *see* Calcium Supplements *on page 167*

♦ **Rolene (Can)** *see* Betamethasone *on page 140*

♦ **Romazicon**® *see* Flumazenil *on page 436*

♦ **Romilar**® **AC** *see* Guaifenesin and Codeine *on page 486*

♦ **Rondec**® *see* Carbinoxamine and Pseudoephedrine *on page 179*

♦ **Rondec-TR**® *see* Carbinoxamine and Pseudoephedrine *on page 179*

Rosiglitazone (ROSE i gli ta zone)

U.S. Brand Names Avandia®

Therapeutic Category Antidiabetic Agent, Oral; Antidiabetic Agent, Thiazolidinedione

Generic Available No

Use Type 2 diabetes mellitus (noninsulin-dependent, NIDDM) when diet and exercise alone do not result in adequate glycemic control; may be used in combination with metformin or a sulfonylurea

Pregnancy Risk Factor C

Contraindications Hypersensitivity to rosiglitazone or any component; moderate to severe liver disease (transaminases >2.5 times the upper limit of normal at baseline); patients who experienced jaundice during troglitazone therapy; type 1 diabetes mellitus; diabetic ketoacidosis

Warnings Avoid use in patients with NYHA class 3 or 4 heart failure; idiosyncratic hepatotoxicity has been reported with another thiazolidinedione agent (troglitazone); two cases of hepatocellular injury (Forman, et al and Al-Salman, 2000) have been reported occurring within 2-3 weeks after initiation of rosiglitazone therapy; LFTs in these patients revealed severe hepatocellular injury which responded with rapid improvement of liver function and resolution of symptoms upon discontinuation of rosiglitazone; monitoring should include periodic determinations of liver function

Precautions Use with caution in patients with heart failure or edema; may increase plasma volume and/or increase cardiac hypertrophy; use with caution in patients with elevated transaminases (AST or ALT) and in patients with anemia or depressed leukocyte counts (may reduce hemoglobin, hematocrit, and/or WBC)

Adverse Reactions

Cardiovascular: Edema

Central nervous system: Headache, fatigue

Endocrine & metabolic: Weight gain, elevated total LDL and HDL cholesterol, hyperglycemia, hypoglycemia

Gastrointestinal: Diarrhea

Hematologic: Anemia

Hepatic: Elevated transaminases, elevated bilirubin

Neuromuscular & skeletal: Back pain

Respiratory: Upper respiratory tract infection, sinusitis

Miscellaneous: Injury

Drug Interactions Cytochrome P-450 isoenzyme CYP2C8 substrate; isoenzyme CYP2C9 (minor)

Food Interactions Peak concentrations are lower by 28% and delayed when administered with food; these effects are not believed to be clinically significant

Mechanism of Action Thiazolidinedione antidiabetic agent that lowers blood glucose by improving target cell response to insulin, without increasing pancreatic

(Continued)

883

Rosiglitazone *(Continued)*

insulin secretion; this mechanism of action is dependent on the presence of insulin for activity

Pharmacodynamics Maximum effect: Up to 12 weeks

Pharmacokinetics

Distribution: V_{dss} (apparent): 17.6 L

Protein binding: 99.8%

Metabolism: Hepatic (99%), metabolism by cytochrome P-450 isoenzyme CYP2C8, minor metabolism via CYP2C9

Bioavailability: 99%

Half-life: 3-4 hours

Time to peak serum concentration: 1 hour

Elimination: As metabolites, in urine (64%) and feces (23%)

Usual Dosage Adults: Oral: Initial: 4 mg in single or divided doses twice daily; after 8-12 weeks of treatment the dosage may be increased to 8 mg daily in single or divided doses twice daily. **Note:** When changing patients from troglitazone to rosiglitazone, a 1-week washout is recommended before initiating therapy with rosiglitazone

Dosage adjustment in renal impairment: No dosage adjustment is required

Dosage comment in hepatic impairment: Clearance is significantly lower in hepatic impairment. Therapy should not be initiated if the patient exhibits active liver disease with increased transaminases (>2.5 times the upper limit of normal) at baseline (see Contraindications and Warnings)

Administration Oral: May be taken without regard to meals

Monitoring Parameters Signs and symptoms of hypoglycemia, fasting blood glucose, hemoglobin A_{1c}; liver enzymes: baseline, every 2 months for the first 12 months of therapy, and periodically thereafter; patients with an elevation in ALT >3 times the upper limit of normal should be rechecked as soon as possible; if the ALT levels remain >3 times the upper limit of normal, therapy with rosiglitazone should be discontinued

Reference Range Target range:

Blood glucose: Fasting and preprandial: 80-120 mg/dL; bedtime: 100-140 mg/dL

Glycosylated hemoglobin (hemoglobin A_{1c}): <7%

Patient Information Follow directions of prescriber; if dose is missed at the usual meal, take it with next meal; do not double dose if daily dose is missed completely; more frequent monitoring is required during periods of stress, trauma, surgery, pregnancy, increased activity, or exercise; avoid alcohol; report chest pain, rapid heartbeat or palpitations, abdominal pain, fever, rash, hypoglycemic reactions, yellowing of skin or eyes, dark urine or light stool, or unusual fatigue or nausea/vomiting.

Dosage Forms Tablet: 2 mg, 4 mg, 8 mg

References

Al-Salman J, Arjomand H, Kemp DG, et al, "Hepatocellular Injury in a Patient Receiving Rosiglitazone. A Case Report," *Ann Intern Med*, 2000, 132(2):121-4.

DeFronzo RA, "Pharmacologic Therapy for Type 2 Diabetes Mellitus," *Ann Intern Med*, 1999, 131(4):281-303.

Forman LM, Simmons DA, and Diamond RH, "Hepatic Failure in a Patient Taking Rosiglitazone," *Ann Intern Med*, 2000, 132(2):118-21.

+ **Rubidomycin** *see* Daunorubicin *on page 298*
+ **Rubion (Can)** *see* Cyanocobalamin *on page 277*
+ **Rum-K®** *see* Potassium Supplements *on page 816*
+ **RWJ17070** *see* Histrelin *on page 496*
+ **Rythmodan (Can)** *see* Disopyramide *on page 347*
+ **S₂® [OTC]** *see* Epinephrine *on page 385*
+ **Sabulin (Can)** *see* Albuterol *on page 45*

Sacrosidase (sak RO se dase)

U.S. Brand Names Sucraid®
Therapeutic Category Sucrase Deficiency, Treatment Agent
Generic Available No
Use Oral replacement therapy in congenital sucrase-isomaltase deficiency (CSID)
Pregnancy Risk Factor C
Contraindications Hypersensitivity to sacrosidase or any component, yeast and yeast products and glycerol
Warnings Hypersensitivity reactions to sacrosidase, including bronchospasm, have been reported; administer initial doses in a setting where acute hypersensitivity reactions may be treated within a few minutes; skin testing may be performed prior to administration to potentially identify patients at risk for hypersensitivity reactions.
Precautions Use with caution in CSID patients with diabetes mellitus, as Sucraid® will improve absorption of the products of sucrose hydrolysis (glucose and fructose); diet and/or insulin dosage may need to be adjusted
Adverse Reactions
  Central nervous system: Insomnia, headache, nervousness
  Endocrine & metabolic: Dehydration
  Gastrointestinal: Abdominal pain, vomiting, nausea, diarrhea, constipation
  Respiratory: Bronchospasm
  Miscellaneous: Hypersensitivity reactions (see Warnings)
Drug Interactions None as yet have been identified
Food Interactions May be inactivated or denatured if administered with fruit juice, warm or hot food or liquids; since isomaltase deficiency is not affected by sacrosidase, adherence to a low-starch diet may be required to decrease symptomatology
Stability Refrigerate at 4°C to 8°C (36°F to 46°F); protect from light; discard 4 weeks after opening
Mechanism of Action Sacrosidase is a naturally occurring GI enzyme which breaks down the disaccharide sucrose into its monosaccharide components; this hydrolysis is necessary to allow absorption of these nutrients
Pharmacokinetics Metabolism: Sacrosidase is metabolized in the GI tract to individual amino acids which are systemically absorbed
Usual Dosage Oral:
  Infants and Children ≤15 kg: 8500 international units (1 mL) per meal or snack
  Children >15 kg and Adults: 17,000 international units (2 mL) per meal or snack
Administration Oral: Dilute in 2-4 ounces of water, milk, or formula; approximately ¹/₂ of the dose may be taken before, and the remainder of the dose at the completion of, each meal or snack; do not administer with fruit juices, warm or hot food or liquids (see Food Interactions)
Monitoring Parameters Breath hydrogen test, oral sucrose tolerance test, urinary disaccharides, intestinal disaccharidases (measured from small bowel biopsy)
  CSID symptomatology: Diarrhea, abdominal pain, gas and bloating
Additional Information 1 mL = 22 drops from sacrosidase container tip
Dosage Forms Solution, oral: 8500 international units/mL (118 mL)
References
  Treem WR, McAdams L, Stanford L, et al, "Sacrosidase Therapy for Congenital Sucrose-Isomaltase Deficiency," *J Pediatr Gastroenterol Nutr*, 1999, 28(2):137-42.

+ **Safe Tussin® 30 [OTC]** *see* Guaifenesin and Dextromethorphan *on page 487*
+ **Safeway Nasal (Can)** *see* Sodium Chloride *on page 906*
+ **Saizen® Injection** *see* Human Growth Hormone *on page 498*
+ **Salac® [OTC]** *see* Salicylic Acid *on page 886*
+ **Sal-Acid®** *see* Salicylic Acid *on page 886*
+ **Salactic® [OTC]** *see* Salicylic Acid *on page 886*
+ **Salagen®** *see* Pilocarpine *on page 800*
+ **Salazopyrin (Can)** *see* Sulfasalazine *on page 926*
+ **Salazopyrin EN-Tabs (Can)** *see* Sulfasalazine *on page 926*
+ **Salbutamol** *see* Albuterol *on page 45*

♦ **Salicylazosulfapyridine** *see* Sulfasalazine *on page 926*

Salicylic Acid (sal i SIL ik AS id)

U.S. Brand Names Compound W® [OTC]; Compound W® One Step Wart Remover [OTC]; DHS Sal®; Dr. Scholl's® Callus Remover [OTC]; Dr. Scholl's® Clear Away [OTC]; Dr. Scholl's® Corn Remover [OTC]; Duofilm® [OTC]; Duoplant® [OTC]; Fostex® Medicated Cleansing [OTC] Freezone® [OTC]; Fung-O® [OTC]; Gordofilm® [OTC]; Hydrisalic™ [OTC]; Ionil® [OTC]; Ionil® Plus [OTC]; Keralyt® [OTC]; Lupi-care™ Dandruff [OTC]; Lupicare™ Psoriasis [OTC]; Maxi-Strength Wart Remover [OTC]; Mediplast® [OTC]; MG217Sal-Acid® [OTC]; Mosco® Corn and Callus Remover [OTC]; Neutrogena® Acne Wash [OTC]; Neutrogena® Body Clear™ [OTC]; Neutrogena® Clear Pore [OTC]; Neutrogena® Healthy Scalp [OTC]; Neutrogena® Maximum Strength T/Sal® [OTC]; Neutrogena® On The Spot® Acne Patch [OTC]; Occlusal®-HP [OTC]; Off-Ezy® [OTC]; Oxy® Balance Deep Pore [OTC]; Propa Ph [OTC]; Salac® [OTC]; Sal-Acid®; Salactic® [OTC]; Sal Plant® [OTC]; Stri-dex® Body Focus [OTC]; Stri-dex® Maximum Strength [OTC]; Stri-dex® Regular Strength [OTC]; Trans-Ver-Sal® [OTC]; Wart-Off® Maximum Strength [OTC]; Wart Remover [OTC]

Canadian Brand Names Acnex; Anti-Acne Control Formula; Anti-Acne Spot Treatment; Blemish Control; Carnation; Clean & Clear Deep Cleaning Astringent; Clean & Clear Invisible Blemish; Clearasil Cleanser; Clearasil Clearstick; Clearasil Pads; Clear Pore Treatment; Clearskin Medicated Wash; Clearskin Overnight Acne Treatment; Duoforte; Neostrata Astringent Acne; Off-Ezy; Oxy; P & S; Salseb; Scholl One Step; Scholl Zino; Sebcur; Soluver; Trans-Plantar; Trans-Ver-Sal; X-Seb

Therapeutic Category Keratolytic Agent

Generic Available Yes

Use Topically for its keratolytic effect in controlling seborrheic dermatitis or psoriasis of body and scalp, dandruff, and other scaling dermatoses; to remove warts, corns, calluses; also used in the treatment of acne

Pregnancy Risk Factor C

Contraindications Hypersensitivity to salicylic acid or any component; children <2 years of age

Warnings Should not be used systemically due to severe irritating effect on GI mucosa; prolonged use over large areas, especially in children, may result in salicylate toxicity; do not apply on irritated, reddened, or infected skin; do not use on moles, birthmarks, warts with hair growing from them, or genital warts

Precautions For external use only; avoid contact with eyes, face, and other mucous membranes

Adverse Reactions
Dermatologic: Facial scarring, erythema, scaling
Local: Irritation, burning

Mechanism of Action Produces desquamation of hyperkeratotic epithelium; increases hydration of the stratum corneum causing the skin to swell, soften, and desquamate

Pharmacokinetics
Absorption: Topical: Readily absorbed
Time to peak serum concentration: Within 5 hours when applied with an occlusive dressing
Elimination: Salicyluric acid (52%), salicylate glucuronides (42%), and salicylic acid (6%) are the major metabolites identified in urine after percutaneous absorption

Usual Dosage Children ≥2 years and Adults: Topical:
Lotion, cream, gel: Apply a thin layer to the affected area once or twice daily
Plaster: Cut to size that covers the corn or callus, apply and leave in place for 48 hours; do not exceed 5 applications over a 14-day period
Shampoo: Initial: Use daily or every other day; apply to wet hair and massage vigorously into the scalp; rinse hair thoroughly after shampooing; 1-2 treatments/week will usually maintain control
Solution: Apply a thin layer directly to wart using brush applicator once daily as directed for 1 week or until the wart is removed

Administration Topical: For external use only; when applying in concentrations >10%, protect surrounding normal tissue with petrolatum

Monitoring Parameters Signs and symptoms of salicylate toxicity: Nausea, vomiting, dizziness, tinnitus, loss of hearing, lethargy, diarrhea, psychic disturbances

Nursing Implications For warts: Before applying product, soak area in warm water for 5 minutes; dry area thoroughly, then apply medication

Dosage Forms

Cream:

Fostex® Medicated Cleansing Cream, Neutrogena® Oil Free Acne Cream: 2% (120 g, 200 g)

Lupicare® Dandruff, Lupicare® II Psoriasis Skin, Lupicare® Psoriasis Scalp: 2.5% (56 g, 113 g, 227 g)

Foam (Salac®): 2% (100 g)

Gel:

DuoPlant® Exact Pore Treatment, Neutrogena® Clear Pore Treatment, Oxy® Balance Deep Cleansing Shower Gel, Stri-Dex® Body Focus: 2% (60 g, 240 g, 296 mL)

Hydrisalic™, Keralyt®: 6% (30 g)

Compound W®, Dr. Scholl's® Clear Away Gel, DuoPlant®, Sal-Plant® Gel: 17% (7.5 g, 14 g, 15 g)

Liquid, topical:

Propa® PH: 0.5% (180 mL)

Neutrogena® Acne Wash, Neutrogena® Body Clear™ Body Wash, Neutrogena® Body Clear™ Body Scrub, Salac®: 2% (180 mL, 250 mL)

Compound W®, Dr. Scholl's® Clear Away, Duofilm®, Fung-O®, Maxi-Strength Wart Remover, Occlusal®-HP, Off-Ezy®, Salactic® Film, Wart Remover, Wart Off® Maximum Strength: 17% (9.3 mL, 10 mL, 13.5 mL, 15 mL)

Gordofilm®: 16.7% (15 mL)

Freezone® Maximum Strength, Mosco® Corn and Callus Remover: 17.7% (9.3 mL, 10 mL)

Lotion (Neutrogena® Body Clear™ Body Lotion, Oxy® Balance All Night Deep Pore): 2% (177 mL, 250 mL)

Ointment (MG217 Sal-Acid): 3% (56 g)

Patch, transdermal:

Neutrogena® On the Spot® Acne Patch: 2% (27s)

Trans-Ver-Sal®: 15% [6 mm PediaPatch, 12 mm AdultPatch, 20 mm PlantarPatch] (10s, 12s, 15s, 25s, 40s)

Duofilm®: 17% (18s)

Compund W® One Step Wart Remover, Dr. Scholl's® Callus Remover Pad, Dr. Scholl's® Clear Away One Step Pad, Dr. Scholl's® Corn Remover Pad: 40% (6s, 9s, 12s, 14s)

Plaster (Mediplast®, Sal-Acid®): 40% (14s, 25s)

Pledgets:

Oxy® Balance Deep Pore Cleansing, Stri-Dex® Regular Strength: 0.5% (55s, 90s)

Oxy® Balance Deep Pore Cleansing Maximum Strength, Stri-Dex® Maximum Strength: 2% (32s, 55s, 90s)

Shampoo:

Neutrogena® Healthy Scalp: 1.8% (90 mL, 180 mL)

Ionil®, Ionil® Plus, Lupicare® Psoriasis Shampoo: 2% (120 mL, 240 mL, 480 mL, 960 mL)

DHS Sal®, Neutrogena® Maximum Strength T/Sal®: 3% (120 mL, 135 mL)

Soap: 2% (114 g)

♦ **Salicylic Acid and Sulfur** *see* Sulfur and Salicylic Acid *on page 929*

♦ **SalineX® [OTC]** *see* Sodium Chloride *on page 906*

Salmeterol (sal ME te role)

Related Information

Asthma Guidelines *on page 1210*

U.S. Brand Names Serevent®; Serevent® Diskus®

Therapeutic Category Adrenergic Agonist Agent; Antiasthmatic; Beta$_2$-Adrenergic Agonist Agent; Bronchodilator

Generic Available No

Use Maintenance treatment of asthma and COPD; prevention of bronchospasm in patients >4 years of age with reversible obstructive airway disease; prevention of exercise-induced bronchospasm in children >4 years of age and adults

Pregnancy Risk Factor C

Contraindications Hypersensitivity to salmeterol, adrenergic amines, or any component

Warnings Cardiovascular effects are not common with salmeterol when used in recommended doses. Salmeterol is not meant to relieve acute asthmatic symptoms. Acute episodes should be treated with short-acting beta$_2$ agonist. Do not increase the frequency of salmeterol use. Paroxysmal bronchospasm (which can be fatal) has been reported with this and other inhaled agents. If this occurs, discontinue treatment; most commonly occurs with first use of a new canister or vial

(Continued)

Salmeterol *(Continued)*

Precautions Use with caution in patients with cardiovascular disorders, convulsive disorders, thyrotoxicosis, or others who are sensitive to the effects of sympathomimetic amines

Adverse Reactions

Cardiovascular: Prolonged QT_c interval (large doses), tachycardia, palpitations, arrhythmias

Central nervous system: Dizziness, headache, nervousness, hyperactivity, insomnia, malaise

Dermatologic: Rash, pruritus

Endocrine & metabolic: Hypokalemia

Gastrointestinal: GI upset, diarrhea, nausea

Neuromuscular & skeletal: Joint and back pain, tremors, muscle cramps

Respiratory: Respiratory arrest, cough, pharyngitis, paradoxical bronchospasm (see Warnings)

Miscellaneous: Hypersensitivity reactions, tachyphylaxis

Drug Interactions Cytochrome P-450 isoenzyme CYP3A3/4 substrate

Additive effects with beta-adrenergic agents; MAO inhibitors and tricyclic antidepressants potentiate cardiovascular effects; beta-blocking agents antagonize effects; increased potassium losses with diuretics

Stability The therapeutic effect may decrease when the cannister is cold, therefore, the canister should remain at room temperature. Do not store at temperatures >120°F. Serevent® Diskus® is stable for 6 weeks after protective foil is removed.

Mechanism of Action Relaxes bronchial smooth muscle by selective action on beta$_2$-receptors with little effect on heart rate

Pharmacodynamics

Onset of effect: 10-20 minutes

Peak effect: 3 hours

Duration: Up to 12 hours

Pharmacokinetics

Protein binding: 94% to 95%

Metabolism: Extensive via hydroxylation

Half-life: 3-4 hours

Usual Dosage Children >4 years and Adults:

Maintenance and prevention of asthma, COPD

Inhalation, oral:

Serevent®: 42 mcg (2 actuations/puffs) twice daily, 12 hours apart

Serevent® Diskus®: 50 mcg (1 actuation/puff) twice daily, 12 hours apart

Prevention of exercise-induced asthma: Inhalation: Serevent® 42 mcg (2 actuations/puffs) 30-60 minutes prior to exercise; additional doses should not be used for 12 hours; patients who are using salmeterol twice daily should **not** use an additional salmeterol dose prior to exercise; if twice daily use is not effective during exercise, consider other appropriate therapy

Administration Inhalation:

Serevent®: Shake well before use; before using inhaler for first time or if unused for more than 4 weeks, "test spray" 4 times into the air; use Serevent® with spacer device in children <8 years of age

Serevent® Diskus®: May not be used with a spacer

Monitoring Parameters Pulmonary function tests

Patient Information Do not use to treat acute symptoms; do not exceed the prescribed dose of salmeterol; do not stop using inhaled or oral corticosteroids without medical advice even if feeling better; avoid spraying in eyes; remove the cannister and rinse the plastic case and cap under warm water and dry daily. Store cannister with nozzle end down.

Additional Information When salmeterol is initiated in patients previously receiving a short-acting beta agonist, instruct the patient to discontinue the regular use of the short-acting beta agonist and to utilize the shorter-acting agent for symptomatic or acute episodes only. Although each puff delivers 25 mcg the amount delivered through the mouthpiece is actually 21 mcg per puff.

Dosage Forms

Aerosol, oral, as xinafoate (Serevent®): 21 mcg/actuation [60 inhalations] (6.5 g), [120 inhalations] (13 g)

Inhalation, powder, oral, as xinafoate (Serevent® Diskus®): 50 mcg/actuation (28 blisters, 60 blisters)

References

Meyer JM, Wenzel CL, and Kradjan WA, "Salmeterol: A Novel, Long-Acting Beta$_2$-Agonist," *Ann Pharmacother*, 1993, 27(12):1478-87.

♦ **Salofalk (Can)** *see* Mesalamine *on page 634*

♦ **Sal Plant® [OTC]** *see* Salicylic Acid *on page 886*

♦ **Salseb (Can)** *see* Salicylic Acid *on page 886*

♦ **Salt Poor Albumin** *see* Albumin *on page 44*

♦ **Sal-Tropine™** *see* Atropine *on page 116*

♦ **Sandimmune®** *see* Cyclosporine *on page 284*

♦ **Sandoglobulin®** *see* Immune Globulin (Intravenous) *on page 529*

♦ **Sandostatin®** *see* Octreotide Acetate *on page 730*

♦ **Sandostatin LAR® Depot** *see* Octreotide Acetate *on page 730*

♦ **SangCya™** *see* Cyclosporine *on page 284*

♦ **Sani-Supp® Suppository [OTC]** *see* Glycerin *on page 478*

Saquinavir (sa KWIN a veer)

Related Information
Adult and Adolescent HIV *on page 1166*

U.S. Brand Names Fortovase®; Invirase®

Therapeutic Category Antiretroviral Agent; HIV Agents (Anti-HIV Agents); Protease Inhibitor

Generic Available No

Use Treatment of HIV infection in combination with other antiretroviral agents; **(Note:** HIV regimens consisting of **three** antiretroviral agents are strongly recommended); in a randomized, double-blind study of 297 patients, a triple drug combination of saquinavir, zalcitabine, and zidovudine reduced HIV-1 replication, increased CD4+ cell counts, and decreased levels of activation markers in serum more than did treatment with zidovudine and either saquinavir or zalcitabine; postexposure chemoprophylaxis following occupational exposure to HIV

Pregnancy Risk Factor B

Contraindications Hypersensitivity to saquinavir or any component; concurrent therapy with astemizole, terfenadine, cisapride, midazolam, triazolam, ergot derivatives, simvastatin, or lovastatin

Warnings Spontaneous bleeding episodes have been reported in patients with hemophilia receiving an HIV protease inhibitor; new onset diabetes mellitus, exacerbation of diabetes and hyperglycemia have been reported in HIV-infected patients receiving protease inhibitors. Due to potential serious and/or life-threatening drug interactions, certain drugs are contraindicated (see Contraindications and Drug Interactions).

Precautions Use with caution in patients with diabetes mellitus, hepatic impairment or in patients receiving drugs which induce or are substrates of cytochrome P-450 3A; interaction studies with saquinavir (metabolized by cytochrome P-450 3A) and terfenadine, astemizole, or cisapride have not been conducted; concurrent use with terfenadine, astemizole, or cisapride is not recommended

Adverse Reactions
Cardiovascular: Cyanosis, heart murmur, hypotension, hypertension, syncope

Central nervous system: Confusion, ataxia, headache, dizziness, seizures, fever, hallucinations, asthenia, agitation, fatigue

Dermatologic: Rash, photosensitivity reaction, acne

Endocrine & metabolic: Hypoglycemia, increased creatine phosphokinase; rare: hyperglycemia, diabetes, ketoacidosis; buffalo hump

Gastrointestinal: Diarrhea, abdominal discomfort, nausea, vomiting, stomatitis

Hematologic: Hemolytic anemia, pancytopenia, thrombocytopenia, microhemorrhages; rare: spontaneous bleeding episodes in hemophiliacs

Hepatic: Elevated ALT, AST, bilirubin, and amylase

Neuromuscular & skeletal: Parethesias, peripheral neuropathy, tremor, arthralgia

Respiratory: Cough

Drug Interactions Cytochrome P-450 isoenzyme CYP3A3/4 substrate and inhibitor Rifampin decreases saquinavir concentrations by 80%; rifabutin, nevirapine, phenobarbital, phenytoin, dexamethasone, carbamazepine may decrease saquinavir concentrations; saquinavir may increase concentrations of calcium channel blockers, clindamycin, dapsone, quinidine, astemizole, terfenadine, cisapride, ergot alkaloid derivatives, midazolam, triazolam, lovastatin, simvastatin, and atorvastatin; ketoconazole, delavirdine, clarithromycin, indinavir, nelfinavir, ritonavir may increase saquinavir levels; saquinavir decreases delavirdine levels; the herbal medicine St John's wort (*Hypericum perforatum*) decreases AUC and plasma concentration of saquinavir

Food Interactions Presence of a high fat meal maximizes bioavailability of saquinavir; grapefruit juice may increase saquinavir levels

(Continued)

Saquinavir *(Continued)*

Stability

Fortovase®: Store capsules in refrigerator; stable for 3 months if stored at room temperature

Invirase®: Store at room temperature in tightly closed bottles

Mechanism of Action Saquinavir is an HIV protease inhibitor which acts late in the life cycle of the virus inside the cell by blocking the cleavage of a polyprotein precursor into structural proteins required for the assembly of infectious virions in lymphocytes and monocytes

Pharmacokinetics

Distribution: CSF concentration is negligible when compared to concentrations from matched plasma samples; partitions into tissues

Protein binding: 98%

Metabolism: Extensive first-pass effect; hepatic metabolism by cytochrome P-450 3A system to inactive metabolites

Bioavailability:

Invirase®: 4% (increased in the presence of food)

Fortovase®: Relative to Invirase® is ~331%

Half-life: Adults: 13 hours

Elimination: 88% of dose eliminated in feces; 1% excreted in urine

Usual Dosage Oral:

Children: Safety and efficacy in children and adolescents <16 years of age have not been established; Fortovase®: 50 mg/kg/dose 3 times/day is under study in Pediatric AIDS Clinical Trials Group protocol 397

Adults:

Invirase®: 600 mg 3 times/day; lower doses (<1800 mg/day) have not shown effective antiviral activity

Fortovase®: 1200 mg 3 times/day

Administration Oral: Administer within 2 hours after a full meal to increase absorption; avoid taking saquinavir with grapefruit juice

Monitoring Parameters Liver function tests, triglyceride levels, blood glucose levels, CD4 cell count, plasma levels of HIV RNA

Patient Information Saquinavir is not a cure for HIV infection; if a dose is missed, take the next dose as soon as possible; however, if a dose is skipped, do not double the next dose; notify physician if numbness, tingling, persistent severe abdominal pain, nausea, or vomiting occurs. Report the use of other medications, nonprescription medications, and herbal or natural products to your physician and pharmacist; since sun exposure can cause photosensitivity reactions, use of sunscreen or protective clothing is recommended.

Dosage Forms

Capsule, as mesylate (Invirase®): 200 mg

Capsule, soft gelatin, as base (Fortovase®): 200 mg

References

Collier AC, Coombs RW, Schoenfeld DA, et al, "Treatment of Human Immunodeficiency Virus Infection With Saquinavir, Zidovudine, and Zalcitabine," *N Engl J Med*, 1996, 334(16):1011-7.

Mueller BU, "Antiviral Chemotherapy," *Curr Opin Pediatr*, 1997, 9(2):178-83.

Working Group on Antiretroviral Therapy and Medical Management of HIV-Infected Children, "Guidelines for the Use of Antiretroviral Agents in Pediatric HIV Infection," January 7, 2000, http://www.hivatis.org.

♦ **Sarafem**™ *see* Fluoxetine *on page 445*

Sargramostim *(sar GRAM oh stim)*

U.S. Brand Names Leukine®

Synonyms GM-CSF; Granulocyte Macrophage Colony Stimulating Factor; rGM-CSF

Therapeutic Category Colony-Stimulating Factor

Generic Available No

Use Accelerates myeloid recovery in patients undergoing autologous or allogeneic BMT; mobilize hematopoietic progenitor cells into peripheral blood for collection by leukapheresis; accelerate myeloid engraftment following autologous peripheral blood progenitor cell transplantation; increase neutrophil counts in patients with malignancies receiving myelosuppressive chemotherapy; increase leukocyte counts in patients with severe aplastic anemia

Pregnancy Risk Factor C

Contraindications Excessive leukemic myeloid blasts in bone marrow or peripheral blood ≥10%; history of idiopathic thrombocytopenic purpura; hypersensitivity to GM-CSF, yeast-derived products, or any component

Precautions Use with caution in patients with autoimmune or chronic inflammatory disease, hypertension, cardiovascular disease, pulmonary disease, or renal or hepatic impairment

Rapid increase in peripheral blood counts: If ANC is >20,000/mm³ or platelets >500,000/mm³, decrease dose by 50% or discontinue drug (counts will fall to normal within 3-7 days after discontinuing drug)

Growth factor potential: Caution with myeloid malignancies; do **not** administer within 24 hours prior to or after chemotherapy or 12 hours prior to or after radiation therapy

Adverse Reactions
Cardiovascular: Hypotension, tachycardia, flushing, pericardial effusion, fluid retention, venous thrombosis

Central nervous system: Malaise, fever, headache, chills

Dermatologic: Rash

Endocrine & metabolic: Polydipsia

Gastrointestinal: Nausea, vomiting, diarrhea, stomatitis, GI hemorrhage

Hepatic: Elevated liver function tests

Neuromuscular & skeletal: Bone pain, myalgia, rigors, weakness

Respiratory: Dyspnea

Miscellaneous: "First dose" reaction (fever, hypotension, tachycardia, rigors, flushing, nausea, vomiting, dyspnea)

Drug Interactions Lithium and corticosteroids may potentiate myeloproliferative effects of sargramostim

Stability Store vial in the refrigerator; stable after reconstitution for 6 hours at room temperature; use only NS to prepare I.V. infusion solution; GM-CSF at a concentration ≥10 mcg/mL is compatible with TPN during Y-site administration

Mechanism of Action Stimulates proliferation, differentiation and functional activity of neutrophils, eosinophils, monocytes and macrophages

Pharmacodynamics
Onset of action: Increase in WBC in 7-14 days

Duration: WBC will return to baseline within 1 week after discontinuing drug

Pharmacokinetics
Half-life: 2 hours

Time to peak serum concentration: S.C.: Within 3 hours

Usual Dosage I.V., S.C.:
Children (no dosing for children has been FDA approved): 250 mcg/m²/day once daily for 21 days to begin 2-4 hours after the marrow infusion on day 0 of BMT or not less than 24 hours after chemotherapy. If significant adverse effects or "first dose" reaction is seen at this dose, discontinue the drug until toxicity resolves, then restart at a reduced dose of 125 mcg/m²/day

Aplastic anemia: 8-32 mcg/kg/day once daily

Cancer chemotherapy recovery: 3-15 mcg/kg/day once daily for 14-21 days; maximum dose: 30 mcg/kg/day or 1500 mcg/m²/day

Adults: 250 mcg/m²/day once daily for 21 days to begin 2-4 hours after BMT, or not less than 24 hours after chemotherapy (to minimize first dose reaction, start with low doses and increase gradually)

Aplastic anemia: 15-480 mcg/m² once daily

Cancer chemotherapy recovery: 3-15 mcg/kg/day once daily for 10 days

Administration Parenteral:
I.V.: Administer as a 30-minute, 2-hour, or 6-hour I.V. infusion or by continuous I.V. infusion. Do not shake solution to avoid foaming. Dilute in NS; if the final concentration of GM-CSF in NS is <10 mcg/mL, then add 1 mg albumin per mL of I.V. fluid. Albumin acts as a carrier molecule to prevent drug adsorption to the I.V. tubing. Albumin should be added to the saline prior to addition of GM-CSF.

S.C.: Reconstituted 250 mcg/mL or 500 mcg/mL solution may be administered without further dilution; rotate injection sites

Monitoring Parameters CBC with differential, platelets; renal/liver function tests, especially with previous dysfunction; vital signs, weight; pulmonary function

Reference Range Excessive leukocytosis (WBC >50,000 cells/mm³, ANC >20,000 cells/mm³)

Patient Information Possible bone pain may occur

Nursing Implications Can premedicate with analgesics and antipyretics; control bone pain with non-narcotic analgesics

Additional Information Produced by recombinant DNA technology using a yeast-derived expression system

Dosage Forms
Injection: 500 mcg (1 mL)

Powder for injection (lyopholized): 250 mcg

References
Lieschke GJ and Burgess AW, "Granulocyte Colony-Stimulating Factor and Granulocyte-Macrophage Colony-Stimulating Factor," (1) N Engl J Med, 1992, 327(1):28-35.

(Continued)

Sargramostim *(Continued)*

Lieschke GJ and Burgess AW, "Granulocyte Colony-Stimulating Factor and Granulocyte-Macrophage Colony-Stimulating Factor," (2) *N Engl J Med*, 1992, 327(2):99-106.

Stute N, Furman WL, Schell M, et al, "Pharmacokinetics of Recombinant Human Granulocyte - Macrophage Colony - Stimulating Factor in Children After Intravenous and Subcutaneous Administration," *J Pharm Sci*, 1995, 84(7):824-8.

Trissel LA, Bready BB, Kwan JW, et al, "Visual Compatibility of Sargramostim With Selected Antineoplastic Agents, Anti-infectives, or Other Drugs During Simulated Y-Site Injection," *Am J Hosp Pharm*, 1992, 49(2):402-6.

♦ **Sarna HC (Can)** *see* Hydrocortisone *on page 506*

♦ **S.A.S (Can)** *see* Sulfasalazine *on page 926*

♦ **Scabene®** *see* Lindane *on page 595*

♦ **Scheinpharm Testone-Cyp (Can)** *see* Testosterone *on page 938*

♦ **Scheinpharm Triamcine-A (Can)** *see* Triamcinolone *on page 979*

♦ **Scholl Athlete's Foot (Can)** *see* Tolnaftate *on page 969*

♦ **Scholl One Step (Can)** *see* Salicylic Acid *on page 886*

♦ **Scholl Zino (Can)** *see* Salicylic Acid *on page 886*

♦ **Scopace™** *see* Scopolamine *on page 892*

Scopolamine *(skoe POL a meen)*

Related Information
Overdose and Toxicology *on page 1222*

U.S. Brand Names Isopto® Hyoscine; Scopace™; Transderm Scop®

Canadian Brand Names Buscopan; Transderm-V

Synonyms Hyoscine

Therapeutic Category Anticholinergic Agent; Anticholinergic Agent, Ophthalmic; Anticholinergic Agent, Transdermal; Ophthalmic Agent, Mydriatic

Generic Available Yes

Use Preoperative medication to produce amnesia and decrease salivary and respiratory secretions; to produce cycloplegia and mydriasis (ophthalmic formulation); treatment of iridocyclitis (ophthalmic formulation); prevention of motion sickness (transdermal formulation)

Pregnancy Risk Factor C

Contraindications Hypersensitivity to scopolamine or any component; patients hypersensitive to belladonna or barbiturates may be hypersensitive to scopolamine; narrow-angle glaucoma, GI or GU obstruction, thyrotoxicosis, tachycardia secondary to cardiac insufficiency, paralytic ileus, myasthenia gravis

Warnings Drug withdrawal symptoms such as nausea, vomiting, headache, dizziness, and equilibrium disturbance have been reported following removal of transdermal system, primarily in patients using the system for more than 3 days

Precautions Use with caution with hepatic or renal dysfunction since adverse CNS effects occur more often in these patients; use with caution in infants and children since they may be more susceptible to adverse effects of scopolamine

Adverse Reactions
Cardiovascular: Tachycardia, palpitations
Central nervous system: Disorientation, drowsiness, hallucinations, confusion, psychosis, delirium, excitement, restlessness
Gastrointestinal: Xerostomia, constipation, nausea, vomiting, dysphagia, dysgeusia
Genitourinary: Urinary retention
Ocular: Blurred vision, cycloplegia, mydriasis, photophobia, increased intraocular pressure
Miscellaneous: Anaphylaxis, allergic reactions
Note: Systemic adverse effects have been reported with both the topical and ophthalmic preparations

Drug Interactions Additive adverse effects with other anticholinergic agents and amantadine; GI absorption of the following drugs may be affected: acetaminophen, levodopa, ketoconazole, digoxin (tablets only), riboflavin, KCl wax-matrix preparations; additive CNS effects with other CNS depressants, alcohol

Stability Physically compatible when mixed in the same syringe with atropine, butorphanol, chlorpromazine, dimenhydrinate, diphenhydramine, droperidol, fentanyl, glycopyrrolate, hydromorphone, hydroxyzine, meperidine, metoclopramide, morphine, pentazocine, pentobarbital, perphenazine, prochlorperazine, promazine, promethazine, or thiopental

Mechanism of Action Blocks the action of acetylcholine at parasympathetic sites in smooth muscle, secretory glands and the CNS; antagonizes histamine and serotonin

Pharmacodynamics
Onset of effect:
Oral, I.M.: 30 minutes to 1 hour
I.V.: 10 minutes
Transdermal: 4 hours
Duration of effect:
Oral, I.M.: 4-6 hours
I.V.: 2 hours
Transdermal: 72 hours

Pharmacokinetics
Absorption: Well absorbed by all routes of administration
Metabolism: In the liver

Usual Dosage
Preoperatively and antiemetic: I.M., I.V., S.C.:
Children: 6 mcg/kg/dose (maximum dose: 0.3 mg/dose); may be repeated every 6-8 hours
Adults: 0.3-0.65 mg; may be repeated 3-4 times/day
Motion sickness: Transdermal:
Children >12 years and Adults: Apply 1 disc behind the ear at least 4 hours prior to exposure every 3 days as needed
Ophthalmic:
Refraction:
Children: Instill 1 drop of 0.25% to eye(s) twice daily for 2 days before procedure
Adults: Instill 1-2 drops of 0.25% to eye(s) 1 hour before procedure
Iridocyclitis:
Children: Instill 1 drop of 0.25% to eye(s) up to 3 times/day
Adults: Instill 1-2 drops of 0.25% to eye(s) up to 3 times/day

Administration
Oral: May be administered without regard to food
Parenteral: I.V.: Dilute with an equal volume of SWI and administer by direct I.V. injection over 2-3 minutes
Transdermal: Apply patch to hairless area behind one ear; wash hands before and after application; if becomes dislodged, replace with fresh patch
Ophthalmic: Instill drops to conjunctival sac of affected eye(s); avoid contact of bottle tip with skin or eye; finger pressure should be applied to lacrimal sac during and for 1-2 minutes after instillation to decrease risk of absorption and systemic reactions

Patient Information Causes drowsiness and may impair ability to perform hazardous activities requiring mental alertness or physical coordination; may cause blurred vision if contacts eye; may cause dry mouth; avoid alcohol

Additional Information Transdermal disc is programmed to deliver *in vivo* 0.5 mg over 3 days

Dosage Forms
Disc, transdermal (Transderm Scop®): 1.5 mg/disc (4s)
Injection, as hydrobromide: 0.4 mg/mL (1 mL)
Solution, ophthalmic, as hydrobromide (Isopto® Hyoscine): 0.25% (5 mL, 15 mL)
Tablet, soluble, as hydrobromide (Scopace™): 0.4 mg

- Scopolamine, Hyoscyamine, Atropine, and Phenobarbital *see* Hyoscyamine, Atropine, Scopolamine, and Phenobarbital *on page 519*
- Scot-Tussin® [OTC] *see* Guaifenesin *on page 485*
- Scot-Tussin® Allergy Relief [OTC] *see* Diphenhydramine *on page 342*
- Scot-Tussin® Diabetes Cough Formula [OTC] *see* Dextromethorphan *on page 316*
- Scot-Tussin® Senior Clear [OTC] *see* Guaifenesin and Dextromethorphan *on page 487*
- SeaMist® [OTC] *see* Sodium Chloride *on page 906*
- Sebcur (Can) *see* Salicylic Acid *on page 886*
- Sebex® [OTC] *see* Sulfur and Salicylic Acid *on page 929*
- Sebulex® [OTC] *see* Sulfur and Salicylic Acid *on page 929*

Secobarbital (see koe BAR bi tal)

Related Information
Laboratory Detection of Drugs in Urine *on page 1234*

U.S. Brand Names Seconal™
Canadian Brand Names Novo-Secobarb
Synonyms Quinalbarbitone
Therapeutic Category Barbiturate; Hypnotic; Sedative
(Continued)

Secobarbital *(Continued)*

Generic Available Yes

Use Short-term treatment of insomnia; preanesthetic agent

Restrictions C-II

Pregnancy Risk Factor D

Contraindications Hypersensitivity to secobarbital or any component, pre-existing CNS depression, severe uncontrolled pain, porphyria, severe respiratory disease with dyspnea or obstruction

Precautions Use with caution in patients with hypovolemic shock, CHF, hepatic impairment, respiratory dysfunction or depression, previous addiction to the sedative/hypnotic group, chronic or acute pain, renal dysfunction; tolerance or psychological and physical dependence may occur with prolonged use

Adverse Reactions

Cardiovascular: Hypotension, cardiac arrhythmias, bradycardia

Central nervous system: Dizziness, lightheadedness, drowsiness, "hangover" effect, lethargy, impaired judgment, CNS depression or paradoxical excitation, hypothermia, nightmares, hallucinations

Dermatologic: Rash, exfoliative dermatitis, Stevens-Johnson syndrome

Gastrointestinal: Nausea, vomiting, constipation

Hematologic: Megaloblastic anemia, thrombocytopenia, agranulocytosis

Respiratory: Respiratory depression, apnea

Miscellaneous: Psychological and physical dependence with prolonged use

Drug Interactions Cytochrome P-450 isoenzyme CYP2C9, CYP3A3/4, and CYP3A5-7 inducer

Barbiturates are enzyme inducers (monitor patients closely for decreased effect of concomitantly administered medications or increased effect when barbiturates are discontinued)

Secobarbital may decrease the serum concentration or effect of ethosuximide, warfarin, oral contraceptives, chloramphenicol, griseofulvin, doxycycline, beta-blockers, cyclophosphamide, theophylline, corticosteroids, tricyclic antidepressants, quinidine, haloperidol, and phenothiazines. Secobarbital given with other CNS depressants may increase CNS and respiratory depression. Chloramphenicol, valproic acid, and chlorpropamide may inhibit the metabolism of secobarbital with a resultant increase in secobarbital serum concentration.

Food Interactions High doses of pyridoxine may decrease drug effect; barbiturates may increase the metabolism of vitamins D and K

Mechanism of Action Depresses CNS activity by binding to barbiturate site at GABA-receptor complex enhancing GABA activity; depresses reticular activating system; higher doses may be gabamimetic

Pharmacodynamics

Onset: Hypnosis: Oral: 15-30 minutes

Duration: Hypnosis: Oral: 3-4 hours with 100 mg dose

Pharmacokinetics

Absorption: Oral: Well absorbed (90%)

Distribution: V_d: Adult: 1.5 L/kg; crosses the placenta; appears in breast milk

Protein binding: 45% to 60%

Metabolism: In the liver by the microsomal enzyme system

Half-life:

Children: 2-13 years: 2.7-13.5 hours

Adults: 15-40 hours; mean 28 hours

Time to peak serum concentration: Oral: Within 2-4 hours

Elimination: Renally as inactive metabolites and small amounts as unchanged drug

Dialysis: Hemodialysis: Slightly dialyzable (5% to 20%)

Usual Dosage Oral:

Children:

Preoperative sedation: 2-6 mg/kg (maximum dose: 100 mg/dose) 1-2 hours before procedure

Sedation: 6 mg/kg/day divided every 8 hours

Adults:

Hypnotic: Usual: 100 mg/dose at bedtime; range 100-200 mg/dose

Preoperative sedation: 100-300 mg 1-2 hours before procedure

Monitoring Parameters Blood pressure, heart rate, respiratory rate, pulse oximetry, CNS status

Patient Information Avoid alcohol and other CNS depressants; may be habit-forming; may cause dizziness or drowsiness and impair ability to perform activities requiring mental alertness or physical coordination; do not abruptly discontinue

Additional Information Effectiveness for insomnia decreases greatly after 2 weeks of use; alkalinization of urine does not significantly increase excretion; withdraw slowly over 5-6 days after prolonged use to avoid sleep disturbances and rapid eye movement (REM) rebound

Dosage Forms Capsule: 100 mg

References

Levine HL, Cohen ME, Duffner PK, et al, "Rectal Absorption and Disposition of Secobarbital in Epileptic Children," *Pediatr Pharmacol (New York)*, 1982, 2(1):33-8.

Nahata MC, Starling S, and Edwards RC, "Prolonged Sedation Associated With Secobarbital in Newborn Infants Receiving Ventilatory Support," *Am J Perinatol*, 1991, 8(1):35-6.

Wolfert RR and Cox RM, "Room Temperature Stability of Drug Products Labeled for Refrigerated Storage," *Am J Hosp Pharm*, 1975, 32(6):585-7.

♦ **Seconal**™ *see Secobarbital on page 893*

Secretin (Synthetic Porcine) (SEE kre tin)

Therapeutic Category Diagnostic Agent, Pancreatic Exocrine Insufficiency; Diagnostic Agent, Gastrinoma (Zollinger-Ellison Syndrome)

Generic Available No

Use Diagnosis of gastrinoma (Zollinger-Ellison syndrome) and diagnosis of pancreatic exocrine dysfunction (Chronic pancreatitis)

Pregnancy Risk Factor C

Contraindications Do not give to patients with acute pancreatitis until attack has subsided

Precautions Patients with a history of hypersensitivity, allergy or asthma should receive an I.V. test dose of 0.2 mcg; use with caution in patients who are highly nervous or have an excessive gag reflex; patients receiving anticholinergics, patients who have had a vagotomy, or patients with inflammatory bowel disease may have a reduced response to secretin; patients with alcoholic or other liver diseases may have an increased response to secretin

Adverse Reactions

Cardiovascular: Hypotension

Central nervous system: Headache, fever

Gastrointestinal: Abdominal discomfort and cramps, diarrhea, nausea

Miscellaneous: Hypersensitivity reactions, diaphoresis

Drug Interactions Anticholinergics may reduce response to secretin

Stability Store in freezer (-20°C); should be used immediately after reconstitution

Mechanism of Action Secretin is a naturally-occurring hormone secreted by cells in the duodenal and upper jejunal mucosa which increases the volume and bicarbonate content of pancreatic juice; when used as a diagnostic agent, synthetic porcine secretin stimulates an increase in gastrin release in patients with Zollinger-Ellison syndrome when compared with normal patients; gastrin bicarbonate concentration is reduced in patients with chronic pancreatitis when compared with a normal patient's response to secretin

Pharmacodynamics

Peak output of pancreatic secretions: Within 30 minutes

Duration: At least 2 hours

Pharmacokinetics

Protein binding: 40%

Inactivated by proteolytic enzymes if administered orally

Metabolism: Metabolic fate is thought to be hydrolysis to smaller peptides

Half-life: 2.84 ±0.62 minutes

Elimination: Clearance: 14.8 ±0.7 mL/minute

Usual Dosage Children and Adults: I.V.:

Pancreatic function: 0.2 mcg/kg as single dose

Gastrinoma (Zollinger-Ellison): 0.4 mcg/kg as single dose

Administration Parenteral: Reconstitute with 8 mL of NS resulting in a 2 mcg/mL solution; **do not shake**; use immediately by direct I.V. injection slowly over 1 minute

Monitoring Parameters Peak bicarbonate concentration of duodenal fluid aspirate (chronic pancreatitis); serum gastrin (gastrinoma)

Reference Range

Peak gastric bicarbonate concentration:

Normal: 94-134 mEq/L

Chronic pancreatitis: <80 mEq/L

Severe pancreatitis: <50 mEq/L

Serum gastrin:

Normal: ≤110 pg/mL

Gastrinoma: >110 pg/mL

(Continued)

Secretin (Synthetic Porcine) *(Continued)*

Nursing Implications Patients should fast at least 12 hours before testing for Zollinger-Ellison syndrome

Additional Information Available currently as an orphan drug by contacting the manufacturer ChiRhoClin, Inc.

Dosage Forms Powder for injection: 16 mcg (10 mL)

- ◆ **Sedatuss DM (Can)** *see* Dextromethorphan *on page 316*
- ◆ **Selax (Can)** *see* Docusate *on page 350*
- ◆ **Selenium** *see* Trace Metals *on page 972*

Selenium Sulfide (se LEE nee um SUL fide)

U.S. Brand Names Exsel®; Selsun®; Selsun Blue® [OTC]

Canadian Brand Names Versel

Therapeutic Category Antiseborrheic Agent, Topical; Shampoos

Generic Available Yes

Use To treat itching and flaking of the scalp associated with dandruff; to control scalp seborrheic dermatitis; treatment of tinea versicolor

Pregnancy Risk Factor C

Contraindications Hypersensitivity to selenium or any component

Warnings Safety in infants has not been established; avoid use in children <2 years of age

Precautions Do not use on damaged skin to avoid any systemic toxicity

Adverse Reactions

Central nervous system: Lethargy

Dermatologic: Alopecia, discoloration of hair

Gastrointestinal: Vomiting following long-term use on damaged skin, abdominal pain, garlic breath

Local: Local irritation

Neuromuscular & skeletal: Tremor

Miscellaneous: Perspiration

Mechanism of Action May block the enzymes involved in growth of epithelial tissue

Pharmacokinetics Absorption: Not absorbed topically through intact skin, but can be absorbed topically through damaged skin

Usual Dosage Children ≥ 2 years and Adults: Topical:

Dandruff, seborrhea: Massage 5-10 mL into wet scalp, leave on scalp 2-3 minutes, rinse thoroughly and repeat application; alternatively, 5-10 mL of shampoo is applied and allowed to remain on scalp for 5-10 minutes before being rinsed off thoroughly without a repeat application; shampoo twice weekly for 2 weeks initially, then use once every 1-4 weeks as indicated depending upon control

Tinea versicolor: Apply the 2.5% lotion in a thin layer covering the body surface from the face to the knees; leave on skin for 30 minutes, then rinse thoroughly; apply every day for 7 days; then follow with monthly applications for 3 months to prevent recurrences

Administration Topical: For external use only; avoid contact with eyes or acutely inflamed skin

Patient Information Remove all jewelry before using the lotion; wash hands thoroughly following application of the lotion; may discolor hair

Dosage Forms Lotion, shampoo:

Selsun Blue®: 1% (120 mL, 210 mL, 240 mL, 330 mL)

Exsel®, Selsun®: 2.5% (120 mL)

References

Lester RS, "Topical Formulary for the Pediatrician," *Pediatr Clin North Am*, 1983, 30(4):749-65.

- ◆ **Sele-Pak®** *see* Trace Metals *on page 972*
- ◆ **Selepen®** *see* Trace Metals *on page 972*
- ◆ **Selsun®** *see* Selenium Sulfide *on page 896*
- ◆ **Selsun Blue® [OTC]** *see* Selenium Sulfide *on page 896*

Senna (SEN na)

Related Information

Carbohydrate and Alcohol Content of Liquid Medications for Use in Patients Receiving Ketogenic Diets *on page 1258*

U.S. Brand Names Black Draught® [OTC]; Senna-Gen® [OTC]; Senokot® [OTC]; Senolax® [OTC]; X-Prep® Liquid [OTC]

Canadian Brand Names Ex-Lax Chocolated; Ex-Lax Extra Strength; Ex-Lax Sugar Coated; Laxative Pills; PMS-Sennosides; Riva-Senna

Therapeutic Category Laxative, Stimulant

Generic Available Yes

Use Short-term treatment of constipation; evacuate the colon for bowel or rectal examinations

Pregnancy Risk Factor C

Contraindications Hypersensitivity to senna or any component; nausea and vomiting; undiagnosed abdominal pain, appendicitis, intestinal obstruction or perforation

Precautions Avoid prolonged use (>1 week); chronic use may lead to dependency, fluid and electrolyte imbalance, vitamin and mineral deficiencies

Adverse Reactions

Endocrine & metabolic: Electrolyte and fluid imbalance

Gastrointestinal: Nausea, vomiting, diarrhea, abdominal cramps, perianal irritation, discoloration of feces

Genitourinary: Discoloration of urine

Drug Interactions Docusate may enhance the absorption of senna

Mechanism of Action Active metabolite (aglycone) acts as a local irritant on the colon, stimulates Auerbach's plexus to produce peristalsis

Pharmacodynamics Onset of action:

Oral: Within 6-24 hours

Rectal: Evacuation occurs in 30 minutes to 2 hours

Pharmacokinetics

Metabolism: In the liver

Elimination: In the feces (via bile) and in urine

Usual Dosage

Children: Oral: 10-20 mg/kg/dose at bedtime; maximum daily dose: 872 mg

- Granules: >27 kg: $1/2$ teaspoon at bedtime to a maximum of 1 teaspoon twice daily
- Tablet: >27 kg: 1 tablet at bedtime to a maximum of 2 tablets twice daily
- Syrup:
  - 1 month to 1 year: 1.25-2.5 mL at bedtime up to a maximum of 5 mL/day
  - 1-5 years: 2.5-5 mL at bedtime to a maximum of 10 mL/day
  - 5-15 years: 5-10 mL at bedtime to a maximum of 20 mL/day

Adults: Oral:

- Granules: 1 teaspoonful at bedtime, not to exceed 2 teaspoonfuls twice daily
- Syrup: 2-3 teaspoonfuls at bedtime, not to exceed 3 teaspoonfuls twice daily
- Tablet: 2 tablets at bedtime, not to exceed 4 tablets twice daily

Rectal:

- Children >27 kg: $1/2$ suppository at bedtime
- Adults: 1 suppository at bedtime; repeat in 2 hours if necessary

Administration Oral: Administer with water; syrup can be taken with juice or milk to mask taste

Monitoring Parameters I & O, frequency of bowel movements, serum electrolytes if severe diarrhea occurs

Patient Information May discolor urine or feces; drink plenty of fluids

Dosage Forms

Granules: 326 mg/teaspoonful

Suppository, rectal: 652 mg

Syrup: 218 mg/5 mL (60 mL, 240 mL)

Tablet: 187 mg, 217 mg, 600 mg

References

Perkin JM, "Constipation in Childhood: A Controlled Comparison Between Lactulose and Standardized Senna," *Curr Med Res Opin*, 1977, 4(8):540-3.

- **Senna-Gen® [OTC]** *see* Senna *on page 896*
- **Senokot® [OTC]** *see* Senna *on page 896*
- **Senolax® [OTC]** *see* Senna *on page 896*
- **Sensorcaine®** *see* Bupivacaine *on page 158*
- **Sensorcaine-MPF®** *see* Bupivacaine *on page 158*
- **Septa® Ointment [OTC]** *see* Neomycin, Polymyxin B, and Bacitracin *on page 707*
- **Septisol®** *see* Hexachlorophene *on page 495*
- **Septra®** *see* Co-Trimoxazole *on page 270*
- **Septra® DS** *see* Co-Trimoxazole *on page 270*
- **Serevent®** *see* Salmeterol *on page 887*
- **Serevent® Diskus®** *see* Salmeterol *on page 887*
- **Seromycin® Pulvules®** *see* Cycloserine *on page 283*
- **Serostim® Injection** *see* Human Growth Hormone *on page 498*
- **Serotonin Syndrome** *see page 1247*

♦ **Sertan (Can)** *see* Primidone *on page 827*

Sertraline (SER tra leen)
U.S. Brand Names Zoloft®
Canadian Brand Names Apo-Sertraline; Novo-Sertraline
Therapeutic Category Antidepressant, Selective Serotonin Reuptake Inhibitor (SSRI)
Generic Available No
Use Treatment of depression, obsessive-compulsive disorder, panic disorder (with or without agoraphobia), post-traumatic stress disorder
Pregnancy Risk Factor C
Contraindications Hypersensitivity to sertraline or any component; use of MAO inhibitors within 14 days (potentially fatal reactions may occur, see Drug Interactions); oral concentrate in patients receiving disulfiram (contains 12% alcohol)
Precautions Use with caution in patients with seizure disorders, concomitant illnesses that may effect hepatic metabolism or hemodynamic responses (eg, unstable cardiac disease, recent MI), and in suicidal patients; use with caution and decrease dose in patients with hepatic dysfunction; may result in hyponatremia, SIADH, significant weight loss, decrease in serum uric acid (mild uricosuric effect, use with caution in patient at risk of uric acid nephropathy), activation of mania/ hypomania, or abnormal platelet function; dropper for oral concentrate contains dry natural rubber, use with caution in patients with latex allergy
Adverse Reactions
  Central nervous system: Agitation, dizziness, headache, insomnia, nervousness, fatigue, somnolence, fever, impaired concentration, activation of mania or hypomania, emotional lability, abnormal thinking, seizures (0.2%)
  Dermatologic: Rash
  Endocrine & metabolic: Weight loss; SIADH, hyponatremia (elderly or volume-depleted patients); decreased serum uric acid, sexual dysfunction, decreased libido
  Gastrointestinal: Nausea, vomiting, diarrhea, loose stools, xerostomia, constipation, anorexia, dyspepsia
  Hematologic: Altered platelet function, purpura
  Neuromuscular & skeletal: Tremor, paresthesia, hyperkinesia, twitching, malaise
  Ocular: Abnormal vision
  Respiratory: Epistaxis
  Miscellaneous: Diaphoresis
Drug Interactions Cytochrome P-450 isoenzyme CYP3A3/4 and CYP2D6 (minor) substrate; CYP2C9, CYP2C19, and CYP3A3/4 isoenzyme inhibitor; weak inhibitor of CYP1A2 and CYP2D6

  Use within 2 weeks of MAO inhibitors may result in fever, tremors, rigidity, myoclonus, autonomic instability, rapid fluctuations in vital signs, irritability, confusion, extreme agitation, delirium, and coma; sertraline may displace highly protein bound drugs and cause adverse effects; may increase prothrombin time in patients receiving warfarin; use with sumatriptan may cause weakness, incoordination, and hyper-reflexia; although lithium levels were not significantly affected in one study, monitoring of lithium levels and appropriate dosage adjustments is recommended in patients initiating sertraline therapy. Tryptophan (which can be metabolized to serotonin) and the herbal medicine St John's wort (*Hypericum perforatum*), may increase serious side effects; use of these agents is **not recommended**.

  Sertraline may decrease the metabolism of tricyclic antidepressants, tolbutamide, diazepam, flecainide, propafenone, and other drugs metabolized by CYP enzymes (monitoring of serum drug concentrations and dosage reduction of these agents may be required); cimetidine may increase sertraline concentrations; the following drugs may increase the risk of serotonin syndrome if given with selective serotonin reuptake inhibitors: Amitriptyline, amphetamines, buspirone, dihydroergotamine, erythromycin, fentanyl, meperidine, nefazodone, sumatriptan, sympathomimetics, tramadol
Food Interactions Tryptophan supplements may increase serious side effects
  Tablets: Food may slightly increase AUC, increase peak concentrations by 25% and shorten the time to peak plasma concentrations
  Oral concentrate: Food may prolong the rate, but does not effect the extent of absorption
Stability Store at room temperature
Mechanism of Action Selective inhibitor of CNS neuronal serotonin uptake; minimal effects on reuptake of norepinephrine or dopamine; does not significantly bind to alpha-adrenergic, benzodiazepine, cholinergic, dopamine, GABA, histamine,

or serotonin receptors; may therefore be useful in patients at risk from sedation, hypotension and anticholinergic effects of tricyclic antidepressants; does not inhibit monoamine oxidase

Pharmacodynamics Maximum effect may take several weeks

Pharmacokinetics

Protein binding: 98%

Metabolism: Significant first pass effect; undergoes N-demethylation to N-desmethylsertraline (significantly less active than sertraline); both parent and metabolite undergo oxidative deamination, followed by reduction, hydroxylation and conjugation with glucuronide (**Note:** Children 6-17 years may metabolize sertraline slightly better than adults, as pediatric AUCs and peak concentrations were 22% lower than adults when adjusted for weight; however, lower doses are recommended for younger pediatric patients to avoid excessive drug levels)

Bioavailability: Tablets approximately equal to oral solution

Half-life: Parent: Mean: 26 hours; metabolite (N-desmethylsertraline): 62-104 hours
    Children: 6-12 years: Mean: 26.2 hours
    Children: 13-17 years: Mean: 27.8 hours
    Adults: 18-45 years: Mean: 27.2 hours

Elimination: 40% to 45% of dose eliminated in urine (none as unchanged drug); 40% to 45% eliminated in feces (12% to 14% as unchanged drug)

Clearance: May be decreased in patients with hepatic impairment

Dialysis: Not likely to remove significant amount of drug due to large V_d

Usual Dosage Oral: (**Note:** See Additional Information)

Children 6-12 years:

Depression: Initial: 25 mg once daily; titrate dose upwards if clinically needed; may increase by 25-50 mg/day increments at intervals of at least 1 week; mean final dose in 21 children (8-18 years of age) was 100 ± 53 mg or 1.6 mg/kg/day (n=11); range: 25-200 mg/day; maximum dose: 200 mg/day (see Tierney, 1995); avoid excessive dosing

Obsessive-compulsive disorder: Initial: 25 mg once daily; titrate dose upwards if clinically needed; increase by 25-50 mg/day increments at intervals of at least 1 week; range: 25-200 mg/day; maximum dose: 200 mg/day; avoid excessive dosing

Adolescents 13-17 years:

Depression: Initial 50 mg once daily; titrate dose upwards if clinically needed; may increase by 50 mg/day increments at intervals of at least 1 week; mean final dose in 13 adolescents was 110 ± 50 mg or about 2 mg/kg/day (see McConville, 1996); in another study using a slower titration, the mean dose at week 6 was 93 mg (n=41) and at week 10 was 127 mg (n=34) (see Ambrosini, 1999)

Obsessive-compulsive disorder: Initial: 50 mg once daily; titrate dose upwards if clinically needed; increase by 50 mg/day increments at intervals of at least 1 week; range: 25-200 mg/day; maximum dose: 200 mg/day

Adults:

Depression and obsessive-compulsive disorder: Initial: 50 mg once daily; titrate dose upwards if clinically needed; increase by 50 mg/day increments at intervals of at least 1 week; range: 50-200 mg/day; maximum dose: 200 mg/day

Panic disorder and post-traumatic stress disorder: Initial: 25 mg once daily; increase dose after 1 week to 50 mg once daily; titrate dose further if clinically needed; increase by 50 mg/day increments at intervals of at least 1 week; range: 50-200 mg/day; maximum dose: 200 mg/day

Dosing adjustment in renal impairment: None needed

Dosing adjustment in hepatic impairment: Use with caution and in reduced doses

Administration Oral: May be administered without regard to food; administer once daily dosage in morning or evening. Must dilute oral concentrate before use; measure dose with dropper provided and mix with 4 ounces of water, orange juice, lemonade, ginger ale, or lemon/lime soda; do not mix with other liquids; take dose immediately after mixing, do not mix ahead of time; sometimes a slight haze may be seen after mixing (this is normal)

Monitoring Parameters Weight and growth in children if long-term therapy; uric acid, CBC, liver function, serum sodium, urine output

Patient Information May cause dizziness or drowsiness and impair ability to perform activities requiring mental alertness or physical coordination; may cause dry mouth; report the use of other medications, nonprescription medications, and herbal or natural products to your physician and pharmacist; avoid alcohol, tryptophan supplements, and the herbal medicine, St John's wort

Nursing Implications If patient experiences somnolence, administer dose at bedtime; if patient experiences insomnia, administer dose in morning

(Continued)

Sertraline *(Continued)*

Additional Information Two larger studies of children and adolescents with depression and obsessive-compulsive disorder utilized a forced upward dosage titration of sertraline to 200 mg/day; these studies conclude that the adult dosage titration regimen can be used in children ≥6 years and adolescents (see Alderman, 1998 and March, 1998); however, other studies in adults (see Fabre, 1995) demonstrate that lower sertraline doses (50 mg/day) are as effective as higher doses with fewer adverse effects and discontinuations of therapy. Further studies are needed in pediatric patients to identify optimal doses; clinically, doses should be individually titrated based on patient response and adverse effects.

A recent report (Lake, 2000) describes 5 children (age 8-15 years) who developed epistaxis (n=4) or bruising (n=1) while receiving sertraline therapy. Due to limited long-term studies, the clinical usefulness of sertraline should be periodically reevaluated in patients receiving the drug for extended intervals; effects of long term use of sertraline on pediatric growth, development, and maturation have not been directly assessed.

Dosage Forms Available as sertraline hydrochloride; mg strength refers to sertraline
Concentrate, oral: 20 mg/mL (60 mL) [contains 12% alcohol]
Tablet: 25 mg, 50 mg, 100 mg

References

Alderman J, Wolkow R, Chung M, et al, "Sertraline Treatment of Children and Adolescents With Obsessive-Compulsive Disorder or Depression: Pharmacokinetics, Tolerability, and Efficacy," *J Am Acad Child Adolesc Psychiatry*, 1998, 37(4):386-94.

Ambrosini PJ, Wagner KD, Biederman J, et al, "Multicenter Open-Label Sertraline Study in Adolescent Outpatients With Major Depression," *J Am Acad Child Adolesc Psychiatry*, 1999, 38(5):566-72.

Fabre LF, Abuzzahab FS, Amin M, et al, "Sertraline Safety and Efficacy in Major Depression: A Double-Blind Fixed-Dose Comparison With Placebo," *Biol Psychiatry*, 1995, 38(9):592-602.

Findling RL, Reed MD, and Blumer JL, "Pharmacological Treatment of Depression in Children and Adolescents," *Paediatr Drugs*, 1999, 1(3):161-82.

Lake MB, Birmaher B, Wassick S, et al, "Bleeding and Selective Serotonin Reuptake Inhibitors in Childhood and Adolescence," *J Child Adolesc Psychopharmacol*, 2000, 10(1):35-8.

March JS, Biederman J, Wolkow R, et al, "Sertraline in Children and Adolescents With Obsessive-Compulsive Disorder: A Multicenter Randomized Controlled Trial," *JAMA*, 1998, 280(20):1752-6.

McConville BJ, Minnery KL, Sorter MT, et al, "An Open Study of the Effects of Sertraline on Adolescent Major Depression," *J Child Adolesc Psychopharmacol*, 1996, 6(1):41-51.

Thomsen PH, "Obsessive-Compulsive Disorder: Pharmacological Treatment," *Eur Child Adolesc Psychiatry*, 2000, 9 Suppl 1:I76-84.

Tierney E, Joshi PT, Llinas JF, et al, "Sertraline for Major Depression in Children and Adolescents: Preliminary Clinical Experience," *J Child Adolesc Psychopharmacol*, 1995; 5(1):13-27.

♦ **Serutan®** [OTC] *see* Psyllium *on page 853*

♦ **Shohl's Solution, Modified** *see* Citrate and Citric Acid *on page 244*

♦ **Silace (Can)** *see* Docusate *on page 350*

♦ **Siladryl®** [OTC] *see* Diphenhydramine *on page 342*

♦ **Silafed®** [OTC] *see* Triprolidine and Pseudoephedrine *on page 989*

♦ **Silapap®** [OTC] *see* Acetaminophen *on page 29*

♦ **Silphen DM®** [OTC] *see* Dextromethorphan *on page 316*

♦ **Siltussin DM®** [OTC] *see* Guaifenesin and Dextromethorphan *on page 487*

♦ **Siltussin® SA** [OTC] *see* Guaifenesin *on page 485*

♦ **Silvadene®** *see* Silver Sulfadiazine *on page 901*

Silver Nitrate *(SIL ver NYE trate)*

U.S. Brand Names Dey-Drop® Ophthalmic Solution

Therapeutic Category Ophthalmic Agent, Miscellaneous; Topical Skin Product

Generic Available Yes

Use Prevention of gonococcal ophthalmia neonatorum; cauterization of wounds and sluggish ulcers, removal of granulation tissue and warts

Pregnancy Risk Factor C

Contraindications Not for use on broken skin or cuts; hypersensitivity to silver nitrate or any component

Warnings Do not use applicator sticks on the eyes; repeated applications of the ophthalmic solution into the eye can cause cauterization of the cornea and blindness; not effective for the prevention of neonatal chlamydial conjunctivitis

Adverse Reactions

Dermatologic: Staining of the skin

Hematologic: Methemoglobinemia

Local: Burning and skin irritation

Ocular: Cauterization of the cornea, blindness, chemical conjunctivitis

Drug Interactions Sulfacetamide eye preparations are incompatible with silver nitrate solutions

Stability Store applicator sticks in a dry place since moisture causes the oxidized film to dissolve; protect from light

Mechanism of Action Free silver ions precipitate bacterial proteins by combining with chloride in tissue forming silver chloride; coagulates cellular protein to form an eschar

Pharmacokinetics Absorption: Not readily absorbed from mucous membranes

Usual Dosage

Neonates: Ophthalmic: Instill 2 drops immediately after birth into conjunctival sac of each eye as a single dose; do not irrigate eyes following instillation of eye drops; silver nitrate prophylaxis should be administered immediately after delivery or no later than 1 hour after delivery

Children and Adults:

Sticks: Apply to mucous membranes and other moist skin surfaces only on area to be treated 2-3 times/week for 2-3 weeks

Topical solution: Apply a cotton applicator dipped in solution on the affected area 2-3 times/week for 2-3 weeks

Monitoring Parameters With prolonged use, monitor methemoglobin levels

Patient Information Discontinue topical preparation if redness or irritation develop; silver nitrate solution may stain skin

Nursing Implications Silver nitrate solutions stain skin and utensils

Dosage Forms

Applicator, topical: 75% with potassium nitrate 25% (6")

Ointment, topical: 10% (30 g)

Solution:

Ophthalmic: 1% (wax ampuls)

Topical: 10% (30 mL); 25% (30 mL); 50% (30 mL)

References

Cushing AH and Smith S, "Methemoglobinemia With Silver Nitrate Therapy of a Burn: Report of a Case," *J Pediatr*, 1969, 74(4):613-5.

Hammerschlag MR, Cummings C, Roblin PM, et al, "Efficacy of Neonatal Ocular Prophylaxis for the Prevention of Chlamydial and Gonococcal Conjunctivitis," *N Engl J Med*, 1989, 320(12):769-72.

Silver Sulfadiazine (SIL ver sul fa DYE a zeen)

U.S. Brand Names Silvadene®; SSD® AF; SSD® Cream; Thermazene®

Canadian Brand Names Dermazin; Flamazine

Therapeutic Category Antibiotic, Topical

Generic Available No

Use Adjunct in the prevention and treatment of infection in second and third degree burns

Pregnancy Risk Factor C

Contraindications Hypersensitivity to silver sulfadiazine or any component; premature infants or neonates <2 months of age since sulfas may displace bilirubin from protein binding sites and cause kernicterus

Precautions Use with caution in patients with G-6-PD deficiency and renal impairment; sulfadiazine may accumulate in patients with impaired hepatic or renal function

Adverse Reactions

Dermatologic: Itching, rash, erythema multiforme, discoloration of skin

Hematologic: Hemolytic anemia, leukopenia, agranulocytosis, aplastic anemia, thrombocytopenia

Hepatic: Hepatitis

Local: Pain, burning

Renal: Interstitial nephritis

Miscellaneous: Serum hyperosmolality (due to propylene glycol component in the cream), hypersensitivity reactions to sulfas

Drug Interactions Topical proteolytic enzymes (silver may inactivate enzymes)

Stability Discard if cream is darkened (reacts with heavy metals resulting in release of silver)

Mechanism of Action Acts upon the bacterial cell wall and cell membrane

Pharmacokinetics

Absorption: Significant percutaneous absorption of sulfadiazine can occur especially when applied to extensive burns

Half-life: 10 hours and is prolonged in patients with renal insufficiency

Time to peak serum concentration: Within 3-11 days of continuous topical therapy

Elimination: ~50% excreted unchanged in urine

Usual Dosage Children and Adults: Topical: Apply once or twice daily with a sterile gloved hand; apply to a thickness of $1/16$"; burned area should be covered with cream at all times

(Continued)

Silver Sulfadiazine *(Continued)*

Administration Topical: Apply to cleansed, debrided burned areas

Monitoring Parameters Serum electrolytes, UA, renal function test, CBC in patients with extensive burns on long-term treatment

Patient Information For external use only; may discolor skin

Additional Information Contains methylparaben and propylene glycol

Dosage Forms Cream, topical: 1% [10 mg/g] (20 g, 50 g, 100 g, 400 g, 1000 g)

References

Kulick MI, Wong R, Okarma TB, et al, "Prospective Study of Side Effects Associated With the Use of Silver Sulfadiazine in Severely Burned Patients," *Ann Plast Surg*, 1985, 14(5):407-18.

Lockhart SP, Rushworth A, Azmy AA, et al, "Topical Silver Sulfadiazine: Side Effects and Urinary Excretion," *Burns Incl Therm Inj*, 1983, 10(1):9-12.

Simethicone (sye METH i kone)

Related Information

Carbohydrate and Alcohol Content of Liquid Medications for Use in Patients Receiving Ketogenic Diets *on page 1258*

U.S. Brand Names Alka-Seltzer® Gas Relief [OTC]; Flatulex® [OTC]; Gas-X® [OTC]; Gas-X® Maximum Strength [OTC]; Genasyme® [OTC]; Maalox Anti-Gas® [OTC]; Maalox Anti-Gas® Extra Strength; Mylanta Gas® [OTC]; Mylanta Gas® Maximum Strength [OTC]; Mylicon® [OTC]; Phazyme® [OTC]; Phazyme® Extra Strength [OTC]; Phazyme® Maximum Strength [OTC]

Canadian Brand Names Ovol

Synonyms Activated Dimethicone; Activated Methylpolysiloxane

Therapeutic Category Antiflatulent

Generic Available Yes: Tablet

Use Relieve flatulence, functional gastric bloating, and postoperative gas pains

Pregnancy Risk Factor C

Food Interactions Avoid gas-forming foods

Mechanism of Action Spreads on surface of aqueous liquids forming a film of low surface tension which collapses foam bubbles; allows mucous-surrounded gas bubbles to coalesce and be expelled

Pharmacokinetics Elimination: In feces

Usual Dosage Oral:

Infants and Children <2 years: 20 mg 4 times/day

Children 2-12 years: 40 mg 4 times/day

Children >12 years and Adults: 40-125 mg after meals and at bedtime as needed, not to exceed 500 mg/day

Administration Oral: Administer after meals or at bedtime; chew tablets thoroughly before swallowing; mix with water, infant formula or other liquids

Patient Information Avoid carbonated beverages

Dosage Forms

Softgels:

Alka-Seltzer® Gas Relief, Gas-X® Extra Strength, Mylanta Gas® Maximum Strength, Phazyme® Extra Strength: 125 mg

Phazyme® Maximum Strength: 166 mg

Suspension (Flatulex®, Genasym®, Mylicon®, Phazyme®): 40 mg/0.6 mL (30 mL)

Tablet, chewable:

Gas-X®, Genasyme®, Maalox Anti-Gas®, Mylanta Gas®: 80 mg

Gas-X® Extra Strength, Mylanta Gas® Maximum Strength: 125 mg

Maalox Anti-Gas® Extra Strength: 150 mg

Phazyme® Maximum Strength: 166 mg

◆ **Simply Allergy®** [OTC] *see* Diphenhydramine *on page 342*

◆ **Simply Sleep®** [OTC] *see* Diphenhydramine *on page 342*

◆ **Sinarest® 12 Hour** [OTC] *see* Oxymetazoline *on page 749*

◆ **Sinequan®** *see* Doxepin *on page 358*

◆ **Singulair®** *see* Montelukast *on page 682*

◆ **Sirop Dentition (Can)** *see* Benzocaine *on page 135*

◆ **Sirop Expectorant (Can)** *see* Guaifenesin *on page 485*

◆ **Sleep Aid (Can)** *see* Diphenhydramine *on page 342*

◆ **Sleep-Eze D (Can)** *see* Diphenhydramine *on page 342*

◆ **Sleepinal®** [OTC] *see* Diphenhydramine *on page 342*

◆ **Slo-bid™** *see* Theophylline *on page 943*

◆ **Slo-Niacin®** [OTC] *see* Niacin *on page 711*

◆ **Slo-Phyllin®** *see* Theophylline *on page 943*

◆ **Slow FE®** [OTC] *see* Iron Supplements (Oral/Enteral) *on page 548*

- **Slow-K®** *see* Potassium Supplements *on page 816*
- **Slow-Mag® [OTC]** *see* Magnesium Supplements *on page 614*
- **SM-7338** *see* Meropenem *on page 633*
- **SMX-TMP** *see* Co-Trimoxazole *on page 270*
- **Snake (Pit Vipers) Antivenin** *see* Antivenin (*Crotalidae*) Polyvalent *on page 99*
- **Sodium 2-Mercaptoethane Sulfonate** *see* Mesna *on page 636*
- **Sodium 4-Phenylbutyrate** *see* Sodium Phenylbutyrate *on page 907*

Sodium Acetate (SOW dee um AS e tate)

Therapeutic Category Alkalinizing Agent, Parenteral; Electrolyte Supplement, Parenteral; Sodium Salt

Generic Available Yes

Use Sodium salt replacement; correction of acidosis through conversion of acetate to bicarbonate

Pregnancy Risk Factor C

Contraindications Alkalosis, hypocalcemia, edema, cirrhosis, excessive chloride losses, hypernatremia

Warnings Avoid extravasation

Precautions Use with caution in patients with hepatic failure, CHF or other sodium-retaining conditions

Adverse Reactions

Cardiovascular: Thrombosis, hypervolemia, edema, cerebral hemorrhage

Endocrine & metabolic: Hypernatremia, hypokalemic metabolic alkalosis, hypocalcemia

Local: Extravasant, local cellulitis

Respiratory: Pulmonary edema

Stability Protect from light, heat, and from freezing; **incompatible** with acids, acidic salts, catecholamines, atropine

Mechanism of Action Sodium is the principal extracellular cation; functions in fluid and electrolyte balance, osmotic pressure control, and water distribution; acetate is metabolized to bicarbonate which neutralizes hydrogen ion concentration and raises blood and urinary pH

Usual Dosage Sodium acetate is metabolized to bicarbonate on an equimolar basis outside the liver; administer in large volume I.V. fluids as a sodium source. Dosage is dependent upon the clinical condition, fluid, electrolytes and acid-base balance of the patient.

Maintenance sodium requirements: I.V.:
Neonates, Infants, and Children: 3-4 mEq/kg/day; maximum dose: 100-150 mEq/day
Adults: 154 mEq/day

Metabolic acidosis: If sodium acetate is desired over sodium bicarbonate, the amount of acetate may be dosed utilizing the equation found in the sodium bicarbonate monograph as each mEq acetate is converted to a mEq of HCO_3; see Sodium Bicarbonate *on page 904*

Administration Parenteral: Must be diluted prior to I.V. administration; infuse hypertonic solutions (>154 mEq/L) via a central line; maximum rate of administration: 1 mEq/kg/hour

Monitoring Parameters Serum electrolytes including calcium, arterial blood gases (if indicated)

Additional Information Sodium and acetate content of 1 g: 7.3 mEq

Dosage Forms Injection: 2 mEq/mL (20 mL, 50 mL, 100 mL); 4 mEq/mL (50 mL, 100 mL)

- **Sodium Acid Carbonate** *see* Sodium Bicarbonate *on page 904*

Sodium Benzoate (SOW dee um BENZ oh ate)

Therapeutic Category Ammonium Detoxicant; Hyperammonemia Agent; Urea Cycle Disorder (UCD) Treatment Agent

Generic Available Yes

Use Adjunctive therapy for the prevention and treatment of hyperammonemia due to suspected or proven urea cycle disorders

Precautions Use with caution in patients with Reye's syndrome, propionic or methylmalonic acidemia; use with caution in neonates with hyperbilirubinemia due to potential displacement of bilirubin from albumin binding sites

Adverse Reactions

Endocrine & metabolic: Metabolic acidosis

Gastrointestinal: Nausea, vomiting

(Continued)

Sodium Benzoate *(Continued)*

Mechanism of Action Assists in lowering serum ammonia levels by activation of a nonurea cycle pathway (the benzoate-hippurate pathway); ammonia in the presence of benzoate will conjugate with glycine to form hippurate which is excreted by the kidney

Pharmacokinetics

Half-life: 0.75-7.4 hours

Elimination: Clearance is largely attributable to metabolism with urinary excretion of hippurate, the major metabolite

Usual Dosage Investigational use (not FDA approved): Oral, I.V.:

Infants and Children: 0.25 g/kg bolus followed by 0.25 g/kg/day as continuous infusion or divided every 6-8 hours

Adolescents and Adults: Initial 5.5 g/m^2 bolus followed by 5.5 g/m^2/day as continuous I.V. infusion or divided every 6-8 hours

Administration Not available commercially

Oral: Must be compounded using chemical powder

I.V.: I.V. solutions must also be compounded and tested for sterility and pyrogenicity prior to use; infuse bolus (with sodium phenylacetate) over 90 minutes in 25-35 mL/kg $D_{10}W$

Monitoring Parameters Plasma ammonia and amino acids

Additional Information Used to treat urea cycle enzyme deficiency in combination with arginine; a maximum of 1 mole nitrogen is removed for every 1 mole of benzoate administered

Dosage Forms Powder: 454 g

References

Batshaw ML, "Hyperammonemia," *Curr Probl Pediatr,* 1984, 14(11):1-69.

Batshaw ML and Brusilow SW, "Treatment of Hyperammonemic Coma Caused by Inborn Errors of Urea Synthesis," *J Pediatr,* 1980, 97(6):893-900.

Batshaw ML, MacArthur RB, and Tuchman M, "Alternative Pathway Therapy for Urea Cycle Disorders: Twenty Years Later," *J Pediatr,* 2001, 138(1 Suppl):S46-54.

Green TP, Marchessault RP, and Freese DK, "Disposition of Sodium Benzoate in Newborn Infants With Hyperammonemia," *J Pediatr,* 1983, 102(5):785-90.

Maestri NE, Hauser ER, Bartholomew D, et al, "Prospective Treatment of Urea Cycle Disorders," *J Pediatr,* 1991, 119(6):923-8.

Summar M, "Current Strategies for the Management of Neonatal Urea Cycle Disorders," *J Pediatr,* 2001, 138(1 Suppl):S30-9.

Sodium Bicarbonate *(SOW dee um bye KAR bun ate)*

Related Information

Adult ACLS Algorithm, Asystole *on page 1043*

Adult ACLS Algorithm, Pulseless Electrical Activity *on page 1042*

Antacid Preparations *on page 95*

CPR Pediatric Drug Dosages *on page 1031*

U.S. Brand Names Neut®

Canadian Brand Names Brioschi

Synonyms Baking Soda; $NaHCO_3$; Sodium Acid Carbonate; Sodium Hydrogen Carbonate

Therapeutic Category Alkalinizing Agent, Oral; Alkalinizing Agent, Parenteral; Antacid; Electrolyte Supplement, Oral; Electrolyte Supplement, Parenteral; Sodium Salt

Generic Available Yes

Use Management of metabolic acidosis; antacid; alkalinization of urine; stabilization of acid base status in cardiac arrest (see Warnings) and treatment of life-threatening hyperkalemia

Pregnancy Risk Factor C

Contraindications Alkalosis, hypocalcemia, hypernatremia; unknown abdominal pain, inadequate ventilation during cardiopulmonary resuscitation; excessive chloride losses

Warnings Avoid extravasation, tissue necrosis can occur due to the hypertonicity of $NaHCO_3$; use of I.V. $NaHCO_3$ should be reserved for documented metabolic acidosis and for life-threatening hyperkalemia; routine use in cardiac arrest is not recommended; patient should be adequately ventilated before administering in cardiac arrest

Precautions Use with caution in patients with CHF or other sodium-retaining conditions, renal insufficiency

Adverse Reactions

Cardiovascular: Edema, cerebral hemorrhage (especially with rapid injection of the hyperosmotic $NaHCO_3$ solution in infants)

Central nervous system: Tetany, intracranial acidosis

Endocrine & metabolic: Metabolic alkalosis, hypernatremia, hypokalemia, hypocalcemia, hyperosmolality

Gastrointestinal: Gastric distention, flatulence may occur with oral administration

Local: Tissue necrosis, ulceration after I.V. extravasation

Respiratory: Pulmonary edema

Drug Interactions Chlorpropamide, lithium, methotrexate, salicylates, and tetracycline have increased renal clearance with alkaline urine; anorexiants, flecainide, mecamylamine, quinidine, and sympathomimetics have decreased renal clearance with alkaline urine; concurrent doses with iron may decrease iron absorption

Stability Do not mix $NaHCO_3$ with calcium salts, catecholamines, atropine

Mechanism of Action Dissociates to provide bicarbonate ion which neutralizes hydrogen ion concentration and raises blood and urinary pH

Pharmacodynamics

Onset of action:

Oral, as antacid: 15 minutes

I.V.: Rapid

Duration:

Oral: 1-3 hours

I.V.: 8-10 minutes

Pharmacokinetics

Absorption: Oral: Well absorbed

Elimination: Reabsorbed by kidney and <1% is excreted in urine

Usual Dosage

Cardiac arrest: See Warnings; patient should be adequately ventilated before administering $NaHCO_3$

Infants: 1 mEq/kg slow IVP initially; may repeat with 0.5 mEq/kg in 10 minutes one time, or as indicated by the patient's acid-base status

Children and Adults: 1 mEq/kg IVP initially; may repeat with 0.5 mEq/kg in 10 minutes one time, or as indicated by the patient's acid-base status

Metabolic acidosis: Dosage should be based on the following formula if blood gases and pH measurements are available:

Neonates, Infants and Children: HCO_3^-(mEq) = 0.3 x weight (kg) x base deficit (mEq/L) **or** HCO_3^-(mEq) = 0.5 x weight (kg) x [24 - serum HCO_3^-(mEq/L)]

Adults: HCO_3^-(mEq) = 0.2 x weight (kg) x base deficit (mEq/L) **or** HCO_3^-(mEq) = 0.5 x weight (kg) x [24 - serum HCO_3^-(mEq/L)]

If acid-base status is not available: Dose for older Children and Adults: 2-5 mEq/kg I.V. infusion over 4-8 hours; subsequent doses should be based on patient's acid-base status

Prevention of hyperuricemia secondary to tumor lysis syndrome (urinary alkalinization) (refer to individual protocols):

Infants and Children:

I.V.: 120-200 mEq/m²/day diluted in maintenance I.V. fluids of 3000 mL/m²/day; titrate to maintain urine pH between 6-7

Oral: 12 g/m²/day divided into 4 doses; titrate to maintain urine pH between 6-7

Chronic renal failure: Oral: Initiate when plasma HCO_3^- <15 mEq/L:

Children: 1-3 mEq/kg/day in divided doses

Adults: 20-36 mEq/day in divided doses

Renal tubular acidosis: Oral:

Distal:

Children: 2-3 mEq/kg/day in divided doses

Adults: 0.5-2 mEq/kg/day given in 4-5 divided doses

Proximal: Children and Adults: Initial: 5-10 mEq/kg/day in divided doses; maintenance: Increase as required to maintain serum bicarbonate in the normal range

Urine alkalinization: Oral:

Children: 1-10 mEq (84-840 mg)/kg/day in divided doses; dose should be titrated to desired urinary pH

Adults: 48 mEq (4 g) initially, then 12-24 mEq (1-2 g) every 4 hours; dose should be titrated to desired urinary pH; doses up to 16 g/day have been used

Antacid: Oral: Adults: 325 mg to 2 grams 1-4 times/day

Administration

Oral: Administer 1-3 hours after meals

Parenteral: For direct I.V. administration: in neonates and infants, use the 0.5 mEq/mL solution or dilute the 1 mEq/mL solution 1:1 with **sterile water**; in children and adults, the 1 mEq/mL solution may be used; administer slowly (maximum rate in neonates and infants: 10 mEq/minute); for infusion, dilute to a maximum concentration of 0.5 mEq/mL in dextrose solution and infuse over 2 hours (maximum rate of administration: 1 mEq/kg/hour)

Monitoring Parameters Serum electrolytes including calcium, urinary pH, arterial blood gases (if indicated)

(Continued)

Sodium Bicarbonate *(Continued)*

Additional Information 1 mEq NaHCO$_3$ is equivalent to 84 mg; each g of NaHCO$_3$ provides 12 mEq each of sodium and bicarbonate ions

Dosage Forms

Injection (Neut®): 4% [40 mg/mL = 2.4 mEq/5 mL] (5 mL); 4.2% [42 mg/mL = 5 mEq/ 10 mL] (10 mL); 5% (500 mL); 7.5% [75 mg/mL = 8.92 mEq/10 mL] (50 mL); 8.4% [84 mg/mL = 10 mEq/10 mL] (10 mL, 50 mL)

Injection, premixed: 5% (500 mL)

Powder: 120 g, 480 g

Tablet: 325 mg [3.8 mEq]; 650 mg [7.6 mEq]

Sodium Chloride (SOW dee um KLOR ide)

U.S. Brand Names Adsorbonac® [OTC]; Afrin® Saline Mist [OTC]; AK-NaCl® [OTC]; Ayr® [OTC]; Ayr® Baby Saline [OTC]; Ayr® Saline Mist [OTC]; Breathe Free® [OTC]; Broncho® Saline [OTC]; Entsol™ [OTC]; HuMIST® [OTC]; Muro 128® [OTC]; NaSal™ [OTC]; Nasal Moist® [OTC]; Ocean [OTC]; Pediamist® Pediatric [OTC]; Pretz® Irrigation [OTC]; SalineX® [OTC]; SeaMist® [OTC]

Canadian Brand Names Certified Nasal; EFA Steri; Minims-Sodium Chloride; Safeway Nasal; Salinex; Thalaris

Synonyms NaCl; Normal Saline; NS; 1/2NS

Therapeutic Category Electrolyte Supplement, Oral; Electrolyte Supplement, Parenteral; Lubricant, Ocular; Sodium Salt

Generic Available Yes

Use Prevention of muscle cramps and heat prostration; restoration of sodium ion in hyponatremia; restores moisture to nasal membranes; reduction of corneal edema; source of electrolytes and water for expansion of the extracellular fluid compartment

Pregnancy Risk Factor C

Contraindications Hypersensitivity to sodium chloride or any component; hypertonic uterus, hypernatremia, fluid retention

Warnings Sodium toxicity is almost exclusively related to how fast a sodium deficit is corrected; both rate and magnitude of correction are extremely important

Precautions Use with caution in patients with CHF, renal insufficiency, cirrhosis, hypertension

Adverse Reactions

Cardiovascular: Edema, thrombosis, hypervolemia

Endocrine & metabolic: Hypernatremia, dilution of serum electrolytes, overhydration

Gastrointestinal: Nausea, vomiting (oral use)

Local: Phlebitis (with concentrations >0.9%)

Respiratory: Pulmonary edema

Mechanism of Action Principal extracellular cation; functions in fluid and electrolyte balance, osmotic pressure control and water distribution

Pharmacokinetics

Absorption: Oral, I.V.: Rapid

Distribution: Widely distributed

Elimination: Mainly in urine but also in sweat, tears, and saliva

Usual Dosage Dosage depends upon clinical condition, fluid, electrolyte and acid-base balance of patient; hypertonic solution (>0.9%) should only be used for the initial treatment of acute serious symptomatic hyponatremia; see Fluid and Electrolyte Requirements in Children *on page 1102*

Maintenance sodium requirements: Oral, I.V.:

Premature neonates: 2-8 mEq/kg/day

Term neonates: 1-4 mEq/kg/day

Infants and Children: 3-4 mEq/kg/day; maximum dose: 100-150 mEq/day

Adults: 154 mEq/day

Nasal: Children and Adults: Use as often as needed

Heat cramps: Adults: Oral: 0.5-1 g, up to 5-10 times/day (5 g/day maximum)

Ophthalmic, ointment: Children and Adults: Apply once daily or more often as needed

To correct acute, serious hyponatremia: mEq sodium = [desired sodium (mEq/L) - actual sodium (mEq/L)] x 0.6 x wt (kg); for acute correction use 125 mEq/L as the desired serum sodium; acutely correct serum sodium in 5 mEq/L/dose increments; more gradual correction in increments of 10 mEq/L/day is indicated in the asymptomatic patient

Administration

Nasal: Spray into 1 nostril while gently occluding other

Ophthalmic: Apply to affected eye(s); avoid contact of bottle tip with eye or skin

Oral: Administer with full glass of water

Parenteral: Infuse hypertonic solutions (>0.9% saline) via central line only; maximum rate of administration: 1 mEq/kg/hour

Monitoring Parameters Serum sodium, chloride, I & O, weight

Reference Range Serum/plasma sodium levels:
Premature neonates: 132-140 mEq/L
Full-term neonates: 133-142 mEq/L
Infants ≥2 months to Adults: 135-145 mEq/L

Nursing Implications Bacteriostatic NS should not be used for diluting or reconstituting drugs for administration in neonates

Additional Information Normal saline (0.9%) = 154 mEq/L; 3% NaCl = 513 mEq/L; 5% NaCl = 855 mEq/L

Dosage Forms
Gel, nasal (Nasal Moist®): 0.65% (30 g)
Injection: 0.45% (25 mL, 50 mL, 100 mL, 500 mL, 1000 mL, 2000 mL); 0.9% (1 mL, 2 mL, 3 mL, 5 mL, 10 mL, 20 mL, 25 mL, 30 mL, 50 mL, 100 mL, 150 mL, 250 mL, 500 mL, 1000 mL, 1500 mL, 2000 mL, 3000 mL); 3% (500 mL); 5% (500 mL)
Injection:
Bacteriostatic: 0.9% (10 mL, 20 mL, 30 mL)
Concentrated: 14.6% (2.5 mEq/mL) (20 mL, 40 mL); 23.4% (4 mEq/mL) (30 mL, 50 mL, 100 mL, 250 mL)
Ointment, ophthalmic (AK-NaCl®, Muro 128®): 5% (3.5 g)
Solution:
Inhalation: 0.45% (3 mL, 5 mL); 0.9% (3 mL, 5 mL)
Broncho® Saline: 0.9% (90 mL, 240 mL)
Irrigation: 0.45% (1500 mL, 2000 mL); 0.9% (250 mL, 500 mL, 1000 mL, 1500 mL, 2000 mL, 3000 mL, 4000 mL, 5000 mL)
Nasal:
Afrin®, Saline Mist, Ayr®, Ayr® Baby Saline, Ayr® Saline Mist, Breather Free®, HuMIST®, NaSal™, Nasal Moist®, Ocean, SeaMist®: 0.65% (15 mL, 30 mL, 45 mL, 50 mL)
Entosol™: 3% (30 mL, 100 mL, 240 mL)
Pediamist® Pediatric: 0.5% (15 mL); 0.6% (15 mL)
Pretz® Irrigation: 0.75% (240 mL)
Salinex®: 0.4% (15 mL, 50 mL)
Ophthalmic (Adsorbonac®, Muro 128®): 2% (15 mL) 5% (15 mL, 30 mL)
Tablet: 1 g (17 mEq)

♦ **Sodium Edetate** see Edetate Disodium on page 372
♦ **Sodium Etidronate** see Etidronate Disodium on page 411
♦ **Sodium Ferric Gluconate** see Iron Supplements (Parenteral) on page 551
♦ **Sodium Hydrogen Carbonate** see Sodium Bicarbonate on page 904
♦ **Sodium Hyposulfate** see Sodium Thiosulfate on page 909

Sodium Phenylbutyrate (SOW dee um fen il BYOO ti rate)

U.S. Brand Names Buphenyl®

Synonyms Ammonapse; 4-Phenylbutyric Acid Sodium; Sodium 4-Phenylbutyrate

Therapeutic Category Ammonium Detoxicant; Hyperammonemia Agent; Urea Cycle Disorder (UCD) Treatment Agent

Use Adjunctive therapy in the chronic management of patients with urea cycle disorder involving deficiencies of carbamoylphosphate synthetase, ornithine transcarbamylase, or argininosuccinic acid synthetase; provides an alternative pathway for waste nitrogen excretion

Pregnancy Risk Factor C

Contraindications Hypersensitivity to phenylbutyrate, or any component; patients with severe hypertension, heart failure or renal dysfunction; **phenylbutyrate is not indicated in the treatment of acute hyperammonemia**

Precautions Use cautiously in patients with renal or hepatic dysfunction and in patients who must maintain a low sodium diet as each gram of drug contains 125 mg sodium

Adverse Reactions
Cardiovascular: Edema, arrhythmias, syncope
Central nervous system: Headache, depression
Dermatologic: Rash
Endocrine & metabolic: Amenorrhea, menstrual dysfunction, acidosis, alkalosis, hyperchloremia, hyperuricemia, hypokalemia, hypernatremia, hyperphosphatemia
Gastrointestinal: Anorexia, abnormal taste, abdominal pain, nausea, vomiting, weight gain, gastritis; rare: peptic ulcer, rectal bleeding, pancreatitis
Hematologic: Anemia, leukopenia, leukocytosis, thrombocytopenia, aplastic anemia
(Continued)

Sodium Phenylbutyrate *(Continued)*

Hepatic: Hypoalbuminemia, elevated liver enzymes, elevated bilirubin

Renal: Renal tubular acidosis

Miscellaneous: Offensive body odor

Drug Interactions Haloperidol, valproic acid and corticosteroids increase ammonia concentrations and may decrease effectiveness of sodium phenylbutyrate; probenecid may decrease urinary excretion

Food Interactions Avoid mixing with acidic-type beverages (eg, colas, lemonade, grape juice) since drug may precipitate

Stability Store at room temperature (59°F to 86°F); after opening, containers should be kept tightly closed

Mechanism of Action Sodium phenylbutyrate is a prodrug that, when given orally, is rapidly converted to phenylacetate. Phenylacetate is conjugated with glutamine to form the active compound phenylacetylglutamine. Phenylacetylglutamine serves as a substitute for urea and is excreted in the urine carrying with it 2 moles nitrogen (equivalent to urea) per mole of phenylacetylglutamine thus assisting in the clearance of nitrogenous waste in patients with urea cycle disorders.

Pharmacokinetics

Distribution: V_d: 0.2 L/kg

Metabolism: conjugation to phenylacetylglutamine (active form); undergoes nonlinear Michaelis-Menten elimination kinetics

Half-life: 0.8 hours (parent compound); 1.2 hours (phenylacetate)

Time to peak serum concentration:

Powder: 1 hour

Tablet: 1.35 hours

Elimination: 80% of metabolite excreted in urine in 24 hours

Usual Dosage Oral:

Neonates, Infants, and Children <20 kg: 450-600 mg/kg/day divided four to six times daily; maximum daily dose 20 g/day

Children >20 kg and Adults: 9.9-13 g/m^2/day, divided four to six times daily; maximum daily dose 20 g/day

Administration Oral: Administer with meals or feedings; mix powder with food or drink; avoid mixing with acidic beverages (eg, most fruit juices or colas)

Monitoring Parameters Plasma ammonia and glutamine concentrations, serum electrolytes, proteins, hepatic and renal function tests, physical signs/symptoms of hyperammonemia (ie, lethargy, ataxia, confusion, vomiting, seizures, and memory impairment)

Patient Information It is important to follow the dietary restrictions required when treating this disorder, the medication must be taken in strict accordance with the prescribed regimen; avoid altering the dosage without the prescriber's knowledge; the powder formulation has a very salty taste

Additional Information Teaspoon and tablespoon measuring devices are provided with the powder; each 1 g powder contains 0.94 g sodium phenylbutyrate = 125 mg sodium; each tablet contains 0.5 g sodium phenylbutyrate = 62 mg sodium

Dosage Forms

Powder: 3.2 g [sodium phenylbutyrate 3 g] per **teaspoon or** 9.1 g [sodium phenylbutyrate 8.6 g] per **tablespoon**

Tablet: 500 mg

References

Batshaw ML, MacArthur RB, and Tuchman M, "Alternative Pathway Therapy for Urea Cycle Disorders: Twenty Years Later," *J Pediatr*, 2001, 138(1 Suppl):S46-S55.

Berry GT and Steiner RD, "Long-Term Management of Patients With Urea Cycle Disorders," *J Pediatr*, 2001, 138(1 Suppl):S56-60.

Brusilow SW, "Phenylacetylglutamine May Replace Urea as a Vehicle for Waste Nitrogen Excretion," *Pediatr Res*, 1991, 29(2):147-50.

Maestri NE, Brusilow SW, Clissold DB, et al, "Long-Term Treatment of Girls With Ornithine Transcarbamylase Deficiency," *N Engl J Med*, 1996, 335(12):855-9.

♦ **Sodium Phosphate** *see* Phosphate Supplements *on page 794*

Sodium Polystyrene Sulfonate

(SOW dee um pol ee STYE reen SUL fon ate)

Related Information

Carbohydrate and Alcohol Content of Liquid Medications for Use in Patients Receiving Ketogenic Diets *on page 1258*

U.S. Brand Names Kayexalate®; Kionex™; SPS®

Canadian Brand Names K-Exit; PMS-Sodium Polystyrene Sulfonate

Therapeutic Category Antidote, Hyperkalemia

Generic Available Yes

Use Treatment of hyperkalemia

Pregnancy Risk Factor C

Contraindications Hypersensitivity to sodium polystyrene sulfonate or any component; hypernatremia; intestinal obstruction or perforation (oral use)

Warnings Avoid using the commercially available liquid product in neonates due to the preservative content. Enema may be prepared with powder and diluted with sorbitol 10% solution or oral solution may be made by dilution with 25% sorbitol solution. Treatment with this drug alone may be insufficient to rapidly correct severe hyperkalemia; other more rapidly effective appropriate measures should be used; enema will reduce the serum potassium faster than oral administration, but the oral route will result in a greater reduction over several hours.

Precautions Use with caution in patients with severe CHF, hypertension, or edema; small amounts of magnesium and calcium may also be lost in binding

Adverse Reactions

Endocrine & metabolic: Hypokalemia, hypocalcemia, hypomagnesemia, hypernatremia

Gastrointestinal: Anorexia, nausea, vomiting, constipation, intestinal necrosis

Drug Interactions Cation-donating antacids (such as magnesium hydroxide or calcium carbonate)

Food Interactions Never mix in orange juice

Mechanism of Action Removes potassium by exchanging sodium ions for potassium ions in the intestine before the resin is passed from the body

Pharmacodynamics Onset of action: Within 2-24 hours

Pharmacokinetics Elimination: Remains in the GI tract to be completely excreted in the feces (primarily as potassium polystyrene sulfonate)

Usual Dosage

Children:

Oral: 1 g/kg/dose every 6 hours

Rectal: 1 g/kg/dose every 2-6 hours

Adults:

Oral: 15 g 1-4 times/day

Rectal: 30-50 g every 6 hours

Administration

Oral or NG: Administer as ~25% sorbitol solution; shake suspension well before use

Enema: Shake suspension well before use; see Warnings; retain enema in colon for at least 30-60 minutes or several hours, if possible

Monitoring Parameters Serum sodium, potassium, calcium, magnesium, EKG (if applicable)

Additional Information 1 g of resin binds ~1 mEq of potassium; 4.1 mEq sodium per g of powder

Dosage Forms Oral or rectal:

Powder for suspension:

Kionex™: 454 g

Kayexalate®: 480 g

Suspension (SPS®): 15 g/60 mL [with sorbitol and alcohol] (60 mL, 120 mL, 200 mL, 500 mL)

♦ **Sodium Sulamyd®** *see Sulfacetamide on page 922*

Sodium Thiosulfate (SOW dee um thye oh SUL fate)

U.S. Brand Names Versiclear™

Synonyms Disodium Thiosulfate Pentahydrate; Sodium Hyposulfate; Thiosulfuric Acid

Therapeutic Category Antidote, Cisplatin; Antidote, Cyanide; Antidote, Extravasation; Antifungal Agent, Topical

Generic Available Yes

Use

Parenteral: Used alone or with sodium nitrite or amyl nitrite in cyanide poisoning or arsenic poisoning; reduce the risk of nephrotoxicity associated with cisplatin therapy; local infiltration (in diluted form) of selected chemotherapy extravasation

Topical: Treatment of tinea versicolor, acne

Pregnancy Risk Factor C

Contraindications Hypersensitivity to sodium thiosulfate or any component

Precautions Discontinue if irritation or sensitivity occurs; rapid I.V. infusion has caused transient hypotension and EKG changes in dogs

Adverse Reactions

Cardiovascular: Hypotension

(Continued)

909

Sodium Thiosulfate *(Continued)*

Central nervous system: Coma, CNS depression secondary to thiocyanate intoxication, psychosis, confusion
Dermatologic: Contact dermatitis
Local: Local irritation
Neuromuscular & skeletal: Weakness
Otic: Tinnitus

Stability Stable diluted in NS or D_5W at concentrations of 1.5% and 9.76% sodium thiosulfate for 24 hours

Mechanism of Action
Prevention of cyanide toxicity: By providing an extra sulfur group to the enzyme rhodanase, it increases the rate of detoxification of cyanide
Prevention of cisplatin nephrotoxicity: Complexes with cisplatin to form a compound that is nontoxic to either normal or cancerous cells

Pharmacokinetics
Half-life, elimination: 0.65 hours
Elimination: 28.5% excreted unchanged in the urine

Usual Dosage
Cyanide and nitroprusside antidote: I.V.: See Usual Dosage in Cyanide Antidote Kit on page 275
Prevention of cisplatin nephrotoxicity: Adults: I.V.: 12 g over 6 hours in association with cisplatin **or** 9 g/m^2 I.V. bolus then 1.2 g/m^2/hour for 6 hours; should be administered before or during cisplatin administration
Chemotherapy infiltration: Children and Adults: Dilute 10% sodium thiosulfate 4-8 mL with 6 mL sterile water to make $1/6$ to $1/3$ molar solution; as local infiltration for the following chemotherapy agents:
Mechlorethamine: Use 2 mL for each mg infiltrated
Cis-platinum: 2 mL for each 100 mg infiltrated; use only for large infiltrates (>20 mL) and concentrations >0.5 mg/mL of cis-platinum
Topical use (antifungal, acne): Children and Adults: 25% solution: Apply thin film twice daily to affected areas for several weeks to months

Administration
Parenteral: I.V.: Inject slowly, over at least 10 minutes; rapid administration may cause hypotension
Topical: Do not apply topically to or near eyes; thoroughly cleanse and dry affects areas prior to application

Dosage Forms
Injection: 100 mg/mL (10 mL); 250 mg/mL (50 mL)
Lotion (Vesiclear™): 25% with salicylic acid 1% and isopropyl alcohol 10% (120 mL)

References
Hall AH and Rumack BH, "Hydroxocobalamin/Sodium Thiosulfate as a Cyanide Antidote," *J Emerg Med*, 1987, 5(2):115-21.
Naughton M, "Acute Cyanide Poisoning," *Anaesth Intensive Care*, 1974, 2(4):351-6.

♦ **SoFlax (Can)** *see* Docusate *on page 350*
♦ **Soflax EX (Can)** *see* Bisacodyl *on page 143*
♦ **Solarcaine® [OTC]** *see* Benzocaine *on page 135*
♦ **Solarcaine® Aloe Extra Burn Relief [OTC]** *see* Lidocaine *on page 590*
♦ **Solarcaine Lidocaine (Can)** *see* Lidocaine *on page 590*
♦ **Solganal®** *see* Aurothioglucose *on page 120*
♦ **Solu-Cortef®** *see* Hydrocortisone *on page 506*
♦ **Solu-Crom (Can)** *see* Cromolyn *on page 273*
♦ **Solugel (Can)** *see* Benzoyl Peroxide *on page 136*
♦ **Solu-Medrol®** *see* Methylprednisolone *on page 655*
♦ **Solurex®** *see* Dexamethasone *on page 307*
♦ **Solurex L.A.®** *see* Dexamethasone *on page 307*
♦ **Soluver (Can)** *see* Salicylic Acid *on page 886*
♦ **Somatrem** *see* Human Growth Hormone *on page 498*
♦ **Somatropin** *see* Human Growth Hormone *on page 498*
♦ **Sominex® [OTC]** *see* Diphenhydramine *on page 342*
♦ **Somnol (Can)** *see* Flurazepam *on page 449*
♦ **Som Pam (Can)** *see* Flurazepam *on page 449*

Sorbitol *(SOR bi tole)*
Therapeutic Category Laxative, Hyperosmolar; Laxative, Osmotic
Generic Available Yes

Use Humectant; sweetening agent; hyperosmotic laxative; facilitates the passage of sodium polystyrene sulfonate or a charcoal-toxin complex through the intestinal tract

Contraindications Anuria

Adverse Reactions

Endocrine & metabolic: Fluid and electrolyte losses, lactic acidosis

Gastrointestinal: Diarrhea, abdominal distress, nausea, vomiting

Mechanism of Action A polyalcoholic sugar with osmotic cathartic actions

Pharmacodynamics

Onset of action: Oral: Mean time to first stool in patients receiving a charcoal-sorbitol slurry:

Children (ingestions):

6.4 hours (dose: 1.5 g/kg in 4 patients)

8.48 hours (dose: 2 g/kg in 33 patients)

Adults:

Nonpoisoned volunteers: 1.6 hours (dose: 2 g/kg)

Ingestion: 7.2 hours (14 adults; dose not specified)

Pharmacokinetics

Absorption: Oral, rectal: Poor

Metabolism: Mainly in the liver to fructose

Usual Dosage Hyperosmotic laxative (as single dose, at infrequent intervals):

Children 2-11 years:

Oral: 2 mL/kg (as 70% solution)

Rectal enema: 30-60 mL as 25% to 30% solution

Children ≥12 years and Adults:

Oral: 30-150 mL (as 70% solution)

Rectal enema: 120 mL as 25% to 30% solution

Adjunct to sodium polystyrene sulfonate: 15 mL as 70% solution orally until diarrhea occurs (10-20 mL/2 hours) or 20-100 mL as an oral vehicle for the sodium polystyrene sulfonate resin

When administered with charcoal: Oral:

Children: 4.3 mL/kg of 35% sorbitol with 1 g/kg of activated charcoal or maximum dose: 2 g/kg sorbitol with activated charcoal

Adults: 4.3 mL/kg of 70% sorbitol with 1 g/kg of activated charcoal

Monitoring Parameters Serum electrolytes, I & O

Dosage Forms

Solution, oral: 70% (480 mL)

Solution, irrigation: 3% (3000 mL, 5000 mL); 3.3% (2000 mL, 4000 mL)

References

Charney EB and Bodurtha JN, "Intractable Diarrhea Associated With the Use of Sorbitol," *J Pediatr*, 1981, 98:157-8.

James LP, Nichols MH, and King WD, "A Comparison of Cathartics in Pediatric Ingestions," *Pediatrics*, 1995, 96(2 Pt 1):235-8.

Kumar A, Weatherly MR, and Beaman DC, "Sweeteners, Flavorings, and Dyes in Antibiotic Preparations," *Pediatrics*, 1991, 87(3):352-60.

♦ **Spectazole**™ *see* Econazole *on page 370*

♦ **Spectro Gram (Can)** *see* Chlorhexidine Gluconate *on page 220*

♦ **Spectro Tar (Can)** *see* Coal Tar *on page 260*

Spironolactone (speer on oh LAK tone)

U.S. Brand Names Aldactone®

Canadian Brand Names Novo-Spiroton

Therapeutic Category Antihypertensive Agent; Diuretic, Potassium Sparing

Generic Available Yes

Use Management of edema associated with excessive aldosterone excretion; hypertension; primary hyperaldosteronism; hypokalemia; treatment of hirsutism; cirrhosis of liver accompanied by edema or ascites

Pregnancy Risk Factor C

Contraindications Hypersensitivity to spironolactone or any component; renal failure, anuria, hyperkalemia

Warnings Spironolactone has been shown to be tumorigenic in toxicity studies using 25-250 times the usual human dose in rats

Precautions Use with caution in patients with dehydration, hyponatremia, impaired renal clearance (Cl_{cr} <50 mL/minute) or hepatic dysfunction; patients receiving other potassium-sparing diuretics or potassium supplements

Adverse Reactions

Cardiovascular: Arrhythmia

Central nervous system: Lethargy, headache, mental confusion, fever, ataxia

Dermatologic: Rash, urticaria

(Continued)

Spironolactone *(Continued)*

Endocrine & metabolic: Hyperkalemia, dehydration, hyponatremia, hyperchloremic metabolic acidosis, postmenopausal bleeding, amenorrhea, gynecomastia (in males); breast tenderness, deepening of voice, and increased hair growth (in females)

Gastrointestinal: Anorexia, nausea, vomiting, diarrhea, gastritis, cramping, gastric bleeding

Genitourinary: Dysuria

Hematologic: Agranulocytosis

Neuromuscular & skeletal: Weakness, numbness or paresthesia in hands, feet or lips, lower back or side pain

Renal: Decreased renal function (including renal failure)

Respiratory: Cough, shortness of breath, dyspnea, hoarseness

Drug Interactions Potassium, other potassium-sparing diuretics, and ACE inhibitors (eg, captopril) may additively increase the serum potassium; may decrease digoxin clearance and attenuate its inotropic effect; decreased hypoprothrombinemic effect of oral anticoagulants; salicylates may interfere with natriuretic action of spironolactone

Food Interactions Avoid natural licorice (causes sodium and water retention and increases potassium loss) and salt substitutes

Mechanism of Action Competes with aldosterone for receptor sites in the distal renal tubules, increasing sodium chloride and water excretion while conserving potassium and hydrogen ions; may block the effect of aldosterone on arteriolar smooth muscle as well

Pharmacokinetics

Distribution: V_d: Breast milk to plasma ratio: 0.51-0.72

Protein binding: 91% to 98%

Metabolism: In the liver to multiple metabolites, including canrenone (active)

Half-life:

Spironolactone: 78-84 minutes

Canrenone: 13-24 hours

Time to peak serum concentration: Within 1-3 hours (primarily as the active metabolite)

Elimination: Urinary and biliary

Usual Dosage Oral:

Neonates: Diuretic: 1-3 mg/kg/day every 12-24 hours

Children:

Diuretic, hypertension: 1.5-3.3 mg/kg/day or 60 mg/m²/day in divided doses every 6-24 hours

Diagnosis of primary aldosteronism: 100-400 mg/m²/day in divided doses

Adults:

Edema, hypertension, hypokalemia: 25-200 mg/day in 1-2 divided doses

Diagnosis of primary aldosteronism: 100-400 mg/day in 1-2 divided doses

Hirsutism in women: 50-200 mg/day in 1-2 divided doses

CHF: Patients with severe heart failure already using an ACE inhibitor and a loop diuretic ± digoxin: 25 mg/day, increase or reduce depending on individual response and evidence of hyperkalemia

Dosing interval in renal impairment:

Cl_{cr} 10-50 mL/minute: Administer every 12-24 hours

Cl_{cr} <10 mL/minute: Avoid use

Administration Oral: Administer with food

Monitoring Parameters Serum potassium, sodium, and renal function

Test Interactions May cause false elevation in serum digoxin concentrations measured by RIA

Patient Information May cause drowsiness and impair ability to perform hazardous tasks which require mental alertness or physical coordination

Dosage Forms Tablet: 25 mg, 50 mg, 100 mg

Extemporaneous Preparations

A 5 mg/mL suspension may be made by crushing tablets, levigating with a small amount of distilled water or glycerin; dilute with 1 part Cologel® and 2 parts simple syrup and/or cherry syrup to make the final concentration; stable 60 days when refrigerated (ASHP, 1987)

A 1 mg/mL suspension may be compounded by crushing ten 25 mg tablets, add a small amount of water and soak for 5 minutes; add 50 mL 1.5% carboxymethylcellulose, 100 mL syrup NF, and mix; use a sufficient quantity of purified water to a total volume of 250 mL; stable at room temperature or refrigerated for 3 months (Nahata, 1993)

A 25 mg/mL suspension may be made by crushing one-hundred twenty-five 25 mg tablets, add in geometric proportions a 1:1 mixture of Ora-Sweet® and Ora-Plus® or Ora-Sweet® SF and Ora-Plus® to a total volume of 120 mL; stable 60 days refrigerated stored in amber bottles; shake well (Allen, 1996)

Allen LV and Erickson MA, "Stability of Labetalol Hydrochloride, Metoprolol Tartrate, Verapamil Hydrochloride, and Spironolactone With Hydrochlorothiazide in Extemporaneously Compounded Oral Liquids," *Am J Health Syst Pharm*, 1996, 53(19):2304-9.

Handbook on Extemporaneous Formulations, Bethesda, MD: American Society of Hospital Pharmacists, 1987.

Nahata MC, Morosco RS, and Hipple TF, "Stability of Spironolactone in an Extemporaneously Prepared Suspension at Two Temperatures," *Ann Pharmacother*, 1993, 27:1198-9.

♦ **Spironolactone and Hydrochlorothiazide** *see* Hydrochlorothiazide and Spironolactone *on page 504*

♦ **Sporanox®** *see* Itraconazole *on page 559*

♦ **SPS®** *see* Sodium Polystyrene Sulfonate *on page 908*

♦ **SSD® AF** *see* Silver Sulfadiazine *on page 901*

♦ **SSD® Cream** *see* Silver Sulfadiazine *on page 901*

♦ **SSKI®** *see* Potassium Iodide *on page 815*

♦ **Stagesic®** *see* Hydrocodone and Acetaminophen *on page 505*

♦ **Statex (Can)** *see* Morphine Sulfate *on page 683*

♦ **Staticin®** *see* Erythromycin *on page 394*

♦ **Stat Touch 2® [OTC]** *see* Chlorhexidine Gluconate *on page 220*

Stavudine (STAV yoo deen)

Related Information
Adult and Adolescent HIV *on page 1166*
Pediatric HIV *on page 1162*

U.S. Brand Names Zerit®

Synonyms d4T; 2',3'-didehydro-3'-deoxythymidine

Therapeutic Category Antiretroviral Agent; HIV Agents (Anti-HIV Agents); Nucleoside Reverse Transcriptase Inhibitor (NRTI)

Generic Available No

Use Treatment of HIV infection in combination with other antiretroviral agents. (**Note:** HIV regimens consisting of **three** antiretroviral agents are strongly recommended)

Pregnancy Risk Factor C

Contraindications Hypersensitivity to stavudine or any component

Warnings The major clinical toxicity of stavudine is peripheral neuropathy which has occurred in 15% to 21% of patients in controlled trials; lactic acidosis and severe hepatomegaly with steatosis is a rare but potentially life-threatening toxicity associated with the use of NRTIs

Precautions Use with caution in patients with a history of peripheral neuropathy, or hepatic or renal impairment; dosage adjustment required in patients with impaired renal function

Adverse Reactions
Central nervous system: Headache, fever, insomnia, malaise, dizziness, nervousness, increased energy, mania

Dermatologic: Rash, pruritus

Gastrointestinal: Abdominal pain, diarrhea, nausea, vomiting, anorexia, pancreatitis

Hepatic: Elevated AST and ALT

Neuromuscular & skeletal: Peripheral neuropathy (tingling, burning, pain, numbness of hands or feet), weakness

Otic: Ear pain

Respiratory: Rhinitis, cough

Drug Interactions Drugs associated with peripheral neuropathy (chloramphenicol, cisplatin, dapsone, ethionamide, gold, hydralazine, iodoquinol, isoniazid, lithium, metronidazole, nitrofurantoin, pentamidine, phenytoin, ribavirin, vincristine) may increase risk for stavudine peripheral neuropathy; drugs that decrease renal function could decrease clearance of stavudine; stavudine should not be administered in combination with zidovudine (poor antiretroviral effect); concurrent use with didanosine and hydroxyurea may increase risk of pancreatitis, lactic acidosis, and severe hepatomegaly; methadone may decrease stavudine levels by 27% (no dosage adjustment needed)

Stability
Capsules: Store in tightly closed containers at room temperature

(Continued)

Stavudine *(Continued)*

Oral solution: Reconstitute powder for oral solution according to manufacturer's instructions; keep refrigerated; solution is stable for 30 days

Mechanism of Action Antiviral activity is dependent on intracellular conversion of stavudine to the active metabolite d4-triphosphate; Inhibits replication of retroviruses by competing with thymidine triphosphate for viral RNA-directed DNA polymerase and incorporation into DNA

Pharmacokinetics

Distribution: Penetrates into the CSF achieving 16% to 97% of concomitant plasma concentrations; distributes into extravascular spaces

Metabolism: Converted intracellularly to active triphosphate form

Bioavailability: Children: 61% to 78%; adults: 80%

Half-life, elimination: Children: 1.1 hours; adults: 1.2-1.45 hours

Time to peak serum concentration: 0.5-0.75 hours

Elimination: 24% to 57% is excreted unchanged in the urine

Usual Dosage Oral:

Neonates: Under investigation in PACTG 332

Children <30 kg: 1 mg/kg/dose every 12 hours; do not exceed adult doses

Adolescent and Adults:

30-59 kg: 30 mg every 12 hours

≥60 kg: 40 mg every 12 hours

Dosing adjustment in renal impairment:

Cl_{cr} 26-50 mL/minute: Decrease dose by 50% (eg, ≥60 kg: administer 20 mg every 12 hours)

Cl_{cr} <10-25 mL/minute: Decrease dose by 75% (eg, ≥60 kg: administer 20 mg every 24 hours)

Dosing adjustment in hepatic impairment: no data

Administration Oral: Administer with or without food; shake solution well before using

Monitoring Parameters Periodic CBC with differential, hemoglobin, renal function, liver enzymes, serum amylase, CD4 cell count, HIV RNA plasma levels, signs/symptoms of peripheral neuropathy

Patient Information Avoid alcohol. Stavudine is not a cure; notify physician if tingling, burning, pain, or numbness of hands or feet occurs

Dosage Forms

Capsule: 15 mg, 20 mg, 30 mg, 40 mg

Powder for oral solution: 1 mg/mL (200 mL)

References

Kline MW, Dunkle LM, Church JA, et al, "A Phase I/II Evaluation of Stavudine (d4T) in Children With Human Immunodeficiency Virus Infection," *Pediatrics*, 1995, 96(2 Pt 1):247-52.

Working Group on Antiretroviral Therapy and Medical Management of HIV-Infected Children, "Guidelines for the Use of Antiretroviral Agents in Pediatric HIV Infection," April 15, 1999, http://www.hivatis.org.

♦ **Stemetil (Can)** *see* Prochlorperazine *on page 834*

♦ **Sterapred®** *see* Prednisone *on page 824*

♦ **Stie VAA (Can)** *see* Tretinoin *on page 978*

♦ **Stimate®** *see* Desmopressin *on page 305*

♦ **St. Joseph® Cough Suppressant [OTC]** *see* Dextromethorphan *on page 316*

♦ **Streptase®** *see* Streptokinase *on page 914*

Streptokinase *(strep toe KYE nase)*

U.S. Brand Names Streptase®

Therapeutic Category Thrombolytic Agent

Generic Available No

Use Thrombolytic agent used in treatment of recent severe or massive deep vein thrombosis, pulmonary emboli, MI, arterial thrombosis or embolism, and occluded arteriovenous cannulas

Pregnancy Risk Factor C

Contraindications Hypersensitivity to streptokinase or any component; recent streptococcal infection; any internal bleeding; CVA or intracranial or intraspinal surgery (within 2 months); severe uncontrolled hypertension; brain carcinoma

Warnings Bleeding may occur; avoid I.M. injections

Precautions Relative contraindications: major surgery within the last 10 days, GI bleeding, recent trauma, severe hypertension

Adverse Reactions

Cardiovascular: Hypotension, arrhythmias, flushing

Central nervous system: Fever

Dermatologic: Itching, urticaria, angioneurotic edema

Hematologic: Surface bleeding, internal bleeding, cerebral hemorrhage

Neuromuscular & skeletal: Musculoskeletal pain

Respiratory: Bronchospasm

Drug Interactions Anticoagulants, antiplatelet agents, antifibrinolytic agents

Stability Store unopened vials at room temperature; store reconstituted solutions in refrigerator and use within 24 hours

Mechanism of Action Promotes thrombolysis; activates the conversion of plasminogen to plasmin by forming a complex, exposing plasminogen-activating site, and cleaving a peptide bond that converts plasminogen to plasmin; plasmin degrades fibrin, fibrinogen and other procoagulant proteins into soluble fragments; effective both outside and within the formed thrombus/embolus

Pharmacodynamics

Onset of action: Activation of plasminogen: Almost immediate

Duration:

Fibrinolytic effects: Only a few hours

Anticoagulant effects: 12-24 hours

Pharmacokinetics

Half-life, biologic: 83 minutes

Elimination: By circulating antibodies and via the reticuloendothelial system

Usual Dosage

Children: Safety and efficacy not established

Thromboses: I.V.: *Chest*, 2001 recommendations: Initial (loading dose): 2000 units/kg followed by 2000 units/kg/hour for 6-12 hours; some patients may require longer or shorter courses of treatment; dose should be individualized based on response

Clotted catheter: **Note: Not recommended** due to possibility of allergic reactions with repeated doses: 10,000-25,000 units diluted in NS to a final volume equivalent to catheter volume; instill into catheter and leave in place for 1 hour, then aspirate contents out of catheter and flush catheter with NS

Adults:

Thromboses: I.V.: 250,000 units to start, then 100,000 units/hour for 24-72 hours depending on location

Cannula occlusion: **Note:** Not recommended due to possibility of allergic reactions with repeated doses: 250,000 units into cannula, clamp for 2 hours, then aspirate contents out of catheter and flush with NS; **Note:** Serious adverse effects (hypersensitivity reactions, hypotension, apnea, and bleeding), some of which were life-threatening, have been reported with this use and dose; lower doses of 3000 units/hour for 12-24 hours infused into each lumen have been successfully used (see Phelps, 2001)

Administration Parenteral: I.V.: Dilute in NS (preferred) or D$_5$W; maximum concentration: 1.5 million units/50 mL

Monitoring Parameters For systemic therapy: Blood pressure, thrombin clotting time, PTT, APTT, fibrinogen level, fibrin/fibrinogen degradation products, D-dimers, platelet count, hemoglobin, hematocrit, signs of bleeding

Nursing Implications For intravenous or intracoronary use only; avoid I.M. injections

Additional Information Best results are realized if used within 5-6 hours of MI; antibodies to streptokinase remain for 3-6 months after initial dose, use another thrombolytic enzyme (ie, urokinase) if repeat thrombolytic therapy is indicated

Failure of thrombolytic agents in newborns/neonates may occur due to the low plasminogen concentrations (~50% to 70% of adult levels); streptokinase- induced clot lysis may be more impaired than urokinase or TPA in these patients; supplementing plasminogen (via administration of fresh frozen plasma) may possibly help

Dosage Forms Powder for injection: 250,000 units (6.5 mL); 750,000 units (6.5 mL); 1,500,000 units (50 mL)

References

Andrew M, Brooker L, Leaker M, et al, "Fibrin Clot Lysis by Thrombolytic Agents Is Impaired in Newborns Due to a Low Plasminogen Concentration," *Thromb Haemost*, 1992, 68(3):325-30.

Kothari SS, Varma S, and Wasir HS, "Thrombolytic Therapy in Infants and Children," *Am Heart J*, 1994, 127(3):651-7.

Monagle P, Michelson AD, Bovill E, et al, "Antithrombotic Therapy in Children," *Chest*, 2001, 119:344S-70S.

Nowak-Göttl U, Auberger K, Halimeh S, et al, "Thrombolysis in Newborns and Infants," *Thromb Haemost*, 1999, 82(Suppl 1):112-6.

Phelps KC and Verazino KC, "Alternatives to Urokinase for the Management of Central Venous Catheter Occlusion," *Hospital Pharmacy*, 2001, 36(3): 265-74.

Streptomycin (strep toe MYE sin)

Related Information

Overdose and Toxicology *on page 1222*

(Continued)

Streptomycin *(Continued)*

Therapeutic Category Antibiotic, Aminoglycoside; Antitubercular Agent

Generic Available Yes

Use Combination therapy of active tuberculosis; used in combination with other agents for treatment of streptococcal or enterococcal endocarditis, mycobacterial infections, plague, tularemia, and brucellosis

Pregnancy Risk Factor D

Contraindications Hypersensitivity to streptomycin or any component

Warnings Aminoglycosides are associated with significant nephrotoxicity or ototoxicity; the ototoxicity is directly proportional to the amount of drug given and the duration of treatment; tinnitus or vertigo are indications of vestibular injury and impending bilateral irreversible deafness; renal damage is usually reversible

Precautions Use with caution in patients with pre-existing vertigo, tinnitus, hearing loss, neuromuscular disorders, or renal impairment; modify dosage in patients with renal impairment

Adverse Reactions

Cardiovascular: Myocarditis, cardiovascular collapse

Central nervous system: Dizziness, vertigo, headache, ataxia

Dermatologic: Toxic epidermal necrolysis

Gastrointestinal: Vomiting

Hematologic: Bone marrow suppression

Neuromuscular & skeletal: Neuromuscular blockade

Otic: Ototoxicity, hearing loss

Renal: Nephrotoxicity

Miscellaneous: Hypersensitivity reactions, serum sickness

Drug Interactions Additive nephrotoxicity with acyclovir, amphotericin B, cisplatin, vancomycin; additive ototoxicity with ethacrynic acid, furosemide, urea, mannitol; potentiates neuromuscular blocking action of succinylcholine, tubocurarine

Stability Streptomycin injection should be stored in the refrigerator

Mechanism of Action Inhibits bacterial protein synthesis by binding directly to the 30S ribosomal subunits causing faulty peptide sequence to form in the protein chain

Pharmacokinetics

Distribution: Distributes into most body tissues and fluids except the brain; small amounts enter the CSF only with inflamed meninges; crosses the placenta; small amounts appear in breast milk

Protein binding: 34%

Half-life (prolonged with renal impairment):

Newborns: 4-10 hours

Adults: 2-4.7 hours

Time to peak serum concentration: I.M.: Within 1-2 hours

Elimination: 30% to 90% of dose excreted as unchanged drug in urine, with small amount (1%) excreted in bile, saliva, sweat, and tears

Usual Dosage I.M. (I.V. in patients who cannot tolerate I.M. injections):

Newborns: 10-20 mg/kg/day once daily

Infants: 20-30 mg/kg/day in divided doses every 12 hours

Children:

Tuberculosis: 20-40 mg/kg/day once daily, not to exceed 1 g/day; **or** 20-40 mg/kg/ dose twice weekly under direct observation, not to exceed 1.5 g/dose; usually discontinued after 2-3 months of therapy or as soon as isoniazid and rifampin susceptibility is established

Other infections: 20-40 mg/kg/day in combination with other antibiotics divided every 6-12 hours

Plague: 30 mg/kg/day divided every 8-12 hours

Adults:

Tuberculosis: 15 mg/kg/day once daily, not to exceed 1 g/day; **or** 25-30 mg/kg/ dose twice weekly under direct observation, not to exceed 1.5 g/dose

Enterococcal endocarditis: 1 g every 12 hours for 2 weeks, then 500 mg every 12 hours for 4 weeks in combination with penicillin

Streptococcal endocarditis: 1 g every 12 hours for 1 week, then 500 mg every 12 hours for 1 week

Tularemia: 1-2 g/day in divided doses for 7-10 days or until patient is afebrile for 5-7 days

Plague: 2 g/day in divided doses until the patient is afebrile for at least 3 days

Dosing adjustment in renal impairment:

Cl_{cr} 50-80 mL/minute: Administer 7.5 mg/kg/dose every 24 hours

Cl_{cr} 10-50 mL/minute: Administer 7.5 mg/kg/dose every 24-72 hours

Cl_{cr} <10 mL/minute: Administer 7.5 mg/kg/dose every 72-96 hours

Administration Parenteral:

I.M.: Inject deep I.M. into a large muscle mass; administer at a concentration not to exceed 500 mg/mL; rotate injection sites

I.V.: I.V. infusion through a peripheral or central line; 12-15 mg/kg/dose is diluted in 100 mL of NS; infuse over 30-60 minutes

Monitoring Parameters Hearing (audiogram), BUN, creatinine; serum concentration of the drug should be monitored in patients with renal impairment; eighth cranial nerve damage is usually preceded by high-pitched tinnitus, roaring noises, sense of fullness in ears, or impaired hearing and may persist for weeks after drug is discontinued

Reference Range Therapeutic serum concentrations: Peak: 15-40 µg/mL; trough: <5 µg/mL

Test Interactions False-positive urine glucose with Benedict's solution

Additional Information For use by patients with active tuberculosis that is resistant to isoniazid and rifampin or patients with active tuberculosis in areas where resistance is common and whose drug susceptibility is not yet known. Pfizer will distribute streptomycin directly to physicians and health clinics at no charge. Call Pfizer at 1-800-254-4445.

Dosage Forms Powder for injection, as sulfate: 1 g

References

Ad Hoc Committee of the Scientific Assembly on Microbiology, Tuberculosis, and Pulmonary Infections, "Treatment of Tuberculosis and Tuberculosis Infection in Adults and Children," *Clin Infect Dis*, 1995, 21:9-27.

American Academy of Pediatrics Committee on Infectious Diseases, "Chemotherapy for Tuberculosis in Infants and Children," *Pediatrics* 1992, 89(1):161-5.

Arguedas AG and Wehrle PP, "New Concepts for Antimicrobial Use in Central Nervous System Infections," *Semin Pediatr Infect Dis*, 1991, 2(1):36-42.

Lorin MI, Hsu KH, and Jacob SC, "Treatment of Tuberculosis in Children," *Pediatr Clin North Am*, 1983, 30(2):333-48.

♦ **Stri-dex® Body Focus [OTC]** *see* Salicylic Acid *on page 886*
♦ **Stri-dex® Maximum Strength [OTC]** *see* Salicylic Acid *on page 886*
♦ **Stri-dex® Regular Strength [OTC]** *see* Salicylic Acid *on page 886*
♦ **Strong Iodine Solution** *see* Potassium Iodide *on page 815*
♦ **Sublimaze®** *see* Fentanyl *on page 422*

Succimer (SUKS i mer)

U.S. Brand Names Chemet®

Synonyms DMSA

Therapeutic Category Antidote, Lead Toxicity; Chelating Agent, Oral

Generic Available No

Use Treatment of lead poisoning in children with blood levels >45 mcg/dL; not indicated for prophylaxis of lead poisoning in a lead-containing environment

Pregnancy Risk Factor C

Contraindications Hypersensitivity to succimer or any component

Warnings Elevated blood lead levels and associated symptoms may return rapidly after discontinuation due to redistribution of lead from bone stores to soft tissues and blood; monitor blood lead levels for "rebound" after therapy

Precautions Use with caution in patients with renal or hepatic impairment; adequate hydration should be maintained during therapy

Adverse Reactions The most common events attributable to succimer have been observed in about 10% of patients treated

Central nervous system: Headache, fatigue, dizziness

Dermatologic: Rash, pruritus

Gastrointestinal: Nausea, vomiting, diarrhea, appetite loss, metallic taste, hemorrhoidal symptoms, sulfurous odor to breath, sore throat

Hematologic: Thrombocytosis, eosinophilia, reversible neutropenia

Hepatic: Transiently elevated AST, ALT, alkaline phosphatase, and serum cholesterol

Neuromuscular & skeletal: Paresthesia, sensorimotor neuropathy, back, rib, kneecap, and leg pains

Ocular: Watery eyes, cloudy film in eye

Renal: Sulfurous odor to urine, decreased urination, proteinuria

Respiratory: Rhinorrhea, nasal congestion

Miscellaneous: Flu-like symptoms

Drug Interactions Not recommended to be used concomitantly with edetate calcium disodium or penicillamine

Mechanism of Action Forms stable water-soluble complexes with lead resulting in increased urinary excretion; also chelates other toxic heavy metals such as arsenic and mercury

(Continued)

917

Succimer *(Continued)*

Pharmacokinetics
Absorption: Oral: Rapid, variable
Metabolism: Extensive to mixed succimer-cysteine disulfides
Half-life, elimination: 2 days
Time to peak serum concentration: ~1-2 hours
Elimination: ~25% in urine with peak urinary excretion occurring between 2-4 hours after dosing; of the total amount of succimer eliminated in urine, 90% is eliminated as mixed succimer-cysteine disulfide conjugates; 10% is excreted unchanged; fecal excretion of succimer probably represents unabsorbed drug

Usual Dosage Children and Adults: Oral: 10 mg/kg/dose (or 350 mg/m²/dose) every 8 hours for 5 days followed by 10 mg/kg/dose (or 350 mg/m²/dose) every 12 hours for 14 days

Note: Concomitant iron therapy has been reported in a small number of children without the formation of a toxic complex with iron (as seen with dimercaprol); courses of therapy may be repeated if indicated by weekly monitoring of blood lead levels; lead levels should be stabilized to <15 mcg/dL; 2 weeks between courses is recommended unless more timely treatment is indicated by lead levels

Dosing adjustment in renal/hepatic impairment: Administer with caution and monitor closely

Administration Oral: Ensure adequate patient hydration; for patients who cannot swallow the capsule, sprinkle the medicated beads on a small amount of soft food or administer with a fruit juice to mask the odor

Monitoring Parameters Blood lead levels, serum aminotransferases

Test Interactions Falsely elevated serum creatine phosphokinase (CPK); false-positive urine ketones with Ketostix®, falsely decreased uric acid measurements

Dosage Forms Capsule: 100 mg

References
Mann KV and Travers JD, "Succimer, An Oral Lead Chelator," *Clin Pharm*, 1991, 10(12):914-22.

Succinylcholine *(suks in il KOE leen)*

U.S. Brand Names Anectine®; Quelicin®

Synonyms Suxamethonium

Therapeutic Category Neuromuscular Blocker Agent, Depolarizing; Skeletal Muscle Relaxant, Paralytic

Generic Available Yes

Use Used to produce skeletal muscle relaxation in procedures of short duration such as endotracheal intubation or endoscopic exams

Pregnancy Risk Factor C

Contraindications Hypersensitivity to succinylcholine chloride or any component; history of decreased concentrations and/or decreased activity of plasma pseudo-cholinesterase; malignant hyperthermia; myopathies associated with elevated serum creatinine values; narrow-angle glaucoma; penetrating eye injuries

Warnings Malignant hyperthermia may be triggered by succinylcholine use; monitor closely for signs/symptoms; some products contain benzyl alcohol; avoid use in neonates

Precautions As rare reports of acute rhabdomyolysis with hyperkalemia followed by ventricular dysrhythmias, cardiac arrest, and death have been reported in children with undiagnosed skeletal muscle myopathy, use with caution in patients recovering from severe trauma; use with caution in patients with pre-existing hyperkalemia, paraplegia, extensive or severe burns, extensive denervation of skeletal muscle because of disease or injury to the CNS or with degenerative or dystrophic neuromuscular disease

Adverse Reactions
Cardiovascular: Bradycardia, hypotension, cardiac arrhythmias, flushing, cardiac arrest, hypertension, tachycardia
Central nervous system: Malignant hyperthermia
Dermatologic: Rash
Endocrine & metabolic: Hyperkalemia, myoglobinemia
Gastrointestinal: Increased intragastric pressure, salivation
Neuromuscular & skeletal: Myalgia due to muscle fasciculations, muscle weakness
Ocular: Increased intraocular pressure
Renal: Myoglobinuria
Respiratory: Apnea, bronchospasm, respiratory depression

Drug Interactions Decreased neuromuscular blockade with diazepam; increased neuromuscular blockade with promazine, cyclophosphamide, oral contraceptives, glucocorticoids, MAO inhibitors, oxytocin, phenothiazines, quinidine, beta-blocking agents, procainamide, lidocaine, lithium, trimethaphan, furosemide, magnesium, chloroquine, acetylcholine, anticholinesterases, amphotericin B, and thiazide diuretics (due to electrolyte imbalances); cyclophosphamide, aminoglycosides, clindamycin may increase bradycardia; narcotic analgesics and inhalation anesthetics may increase the risk of sinus arrest; increased arrhythmias with digoxin (due to potassium changes)

Stability Injection is incompatible with alkaline solutions; store in refrigerator; stability at room temperature is product specific; check with each manufacturer

Mechanism of Action Acts similarly to acetylcholine, produces depolarization of the motor endplate at the myoneural junction which causes sustained flaccid skeletal muscle paralysis

Pharmacodynamics
I.M.:
Onset of effect: 2-3 minutes
Duration: 10-30 minutes
I.V.:
Onset of action: Within 30-60 seconds
Duration: ~4-6 minutes

Pharmacokinetics
Metabolism: Succinylcholine is rapidly hydrolyzed by plasma pseudocholinesterase
Elimination: 10% excreted unchanged in urine

Usual Dosage
Children:
I.M.: 2.5-4 mg/kg (maximum dose: 150 mg)
I.V.: Initial: 1-2 mg/kg; maintenance: 0.3-0.6 mg/kg every 5-10 minutes as needed; because of the risk of malignant hyperthermia, use of continuous infusions is **not** recommended in infants and children
Adults: I.M., I.V.: 0.6 mg/kg (range: 0.3-1.1 mg/kg), up to 150 mg total dose; maintenance: 0.04-0.07 mg/kg every 5-10 minutes as needed
Continuous infusion: 2.5 mg/minute (range: 0.5-10 mg/minute)
Note: Pretreatment with atropine may reduce occurrence of bradycardia
Dosing adjustment in hepatic impairment: Dose should be decreased in patients with severe liver disease

Administration Parenteral: I.V.: May be administered by rapid I.V. injection without further dilution; I.M.: Injection should be made deeply

Monitoring Parameters Heart rate, serum potassium, assisted ventilator status, peripheral nerve stimulator measuring twitch response

Dosage Forms Injection, as chloride:
Anectine®: 20 mg/mL (10 mL)
Quelicin®: 20 mg/mL (5 mL, 10 mL); 50 mg/mL (10 mL); 100 mg/mL (10 mL)

♦ **Sucraid**® *see* Sacrosidase *on page 885*

Sucralfate (soo KRAL fate)
Related Information
Carbohydrate and Alcohol Content of Liquid Medications for Use in Patients Receiving Ketogenic Diets *on page 1258*
U.S. Brand Names Carafate®
Canadian Brand Names Apo-Sucralfate; Novo-Sucralate; PMS-Sucralfate; Sulcrate; Sulcrate Suspension Plus
Synonyms Aluminum Sucrose Sulfate, Basic
Therapeutic Category Gastrointestinal Agent, Gastric or Duodenal Ulcer Treatment
Generic Available No
Use Short-term management of duodenal ulcers
Unlabeled use: Gastric ulcers; suspension may be used topically for treatment of stomatitis due to cancer chemotherapy or other causes of esophageal, gastric, and rectal erosions; treatment of NSAID mucosal damage; prevention of stress ulcers
Pregnancy Risk Factor B
Contraindications Hypersensitivity to sucralfate or any component
Warnings Because of the potential for sucralfate to alter the absorption of some drugs, separate administration times (administer other medications 2 hours before or after sucralfate) should be considered when alterations in bioavailability are believed to be critical
Precautions Use with caution in renal failure due to accumulation of aluminum
Adverse Reactions
Cardiovascular: Facial edema
(Continued)

Sucralfate *(Continued)*

Central nervous system: Dizziness, sleepiness, vertigo, headache

Dermatologic: Rash, pruritus, angioedema

Gastrointestinal: Constipation, diarrhea, nausea, gastric discomfort, indigestion, xerostomia, flatulence

Neuromuscular & skeletal: Back pain

Respiratory: Laryngospasm, rhinitis, respiratory difficulty

Drug Interactions Absorption of orally administered tetracycline, phenytoin, keto-conazole, quinidine, ranitidine, colistin, gentamicin, amphotericin B, sodium and potassium phosphate salts, digoxin, sustained release theophylline, quinolones, and cimetidine may be decreased (separate administration by 2 hours); aluminum-containing antacids may increase total body burden of aluminum; antacids, cimetidine, and ranitidine when administered concomitantly may decrease sucralfate's activity (gastric acidity is required for sucralfate to form its protective barrier)

Food Interactions Interferes with absorption of vitamin A, vitamin D, vitamin E, and vitamin K

Mechanism of Action Aluminum salt of sulfated sucrose which in the presence of acid pH (gastric acid) forms a complex, paste-like substance that adheres to the damaged mucosal area. This selectively forms a protective coating that protects the lining against peptic acid, pepsin, and bile salts.

Pharmacodynamics GI protection effect:

Onset of action: 1-2 hours

Duration: Up to 6 hours

Pharmacokinetics

Absorption: Oral: <5%

Metabolism: Not metabolized

Elimination: 90% excreted in stool; small amounts that are absorbed are excreted in the urine as unchanged compounds

Usual Dosage Oral:

Children: Dose not established; doses of 40-80 mg/kg/day divided every 6 hours have been used

Stomatitis: 5-10 mL (1 g/10 mL); swish and spit or swish and swallow 4 times/day

Adults:

Stress ulcer prophylaxis: 1 g 4 times/day

Stress ulcer treatment: 1 g every 4 hours

Duodenal ulcer:

Treatment: 1 g 4 times/day for 4-8 weeks, or alternatively 2 g twice daily; treatment is recommended for 4-8 weeks in adults

Maintenance: Prophylaxis: 1 g twice daily

Stomatitis: 1 g/10 mL suspension, swish and spit or swish and swallow 4 times/day

Proctitis: Rectal enema: 2 g/20 mL daily

Dosage comment in renal impairment: Aluminum salt is minimally absorbed (<5%), however, may accumulate in renal failure

Administration

Oral: Administer on an empty stomach 1 hour before meals and at bedtime (see Warnings); tablet may be broken or dissolved in water before ingestion; do not administer antacids within 30 minutes of administration; shake suspension well before use

Rectal: May administer oral suspension as rectal enema; shake suspension well before use

Additional Information There is approximately 14-16 mEq acid neutralizing capacity per 1g sucralfate

Dosage Forms

Suspension, oral: 1 g/10 mL (420 mL)

Tablet: 1 g

References

Melko GP, Turco TF, Phelan TF, et al, "Treatment of Radiation-Induced Proctitis With Sucralfate Enemas," *Ann Pharmacother*, 1999, 33(12):1274-6.

Sufentanil (soo FEN ta nil)

Related Information
Overdose and Toxicology *on page 1222*

U.S. Brand Names Sufenta®

Therapeutic Category Analgesic, Narcotic; General Anesthetic

Generic Available No

Use Analgesia; analgesia adjunct; anesthetic agent

Restrictions C-II

Pregnancy Risk Factor C

Contraindications Hypersensitivity to sufentanil or any component; increased intracranial pressure; severe respiratory depression

Warnings May cause severe respiratory depression; rapid I.V. infusion may result in skeletal muscle and chest wall rigidity → impaired ventilation → respiratory distress, apnea, bronchoconstriction, laryngospasm, arrest; inject slowly over 3-5 minutes; nondepolarizing skeletal muscle relaxant may be required

Precautions Use with caution in patients with head injuries, hepatic impairment, pulmonary disease, or with use of MAO inhibitors within past 14 days; sufentanil shares the toxic potential of opiate agonists, precautions of opiate agonist therapy should be observed

Adverse Reactions
Cardiovascular: Bradycardia, hypotension, peripheral vasodilation
Central nervous system: CNS depression, drowsiness, dizziness, sedation
Dermatologic: Erythema, pruritus, rash
Endocrine & metabolic: ADH release
Gastrointestinal: Nausea, vomiting, constipation, biliary tract spasm
Genitourinary: Urinary tract spasm
Neuromuscular & skeletal: Skeletal and thoracic muscle rigidity, especially after rapid I.V. administration
Ocular: Miosis, blurred vision
Respiratory: Respiratory depression, apnea
Miscellaneous: Physical and psychological dependence with prolonged use

Drug Interactions Cytochrome P-450 isoenzyme CYP3A3/4 substrate
CNS depressants, phenothiazines, MAO inhibitors, tricyclic antidepressants may potentiate adverse effects of opiates; beta-blocker therapy may potentiate sufentanil bradycardia

Mechanism of Action Binds with stereospecific receptors at many sites within the CNS, increases pain threshold, alters pain reception, inhibits ascending pain pathways; ultra short-acting narcotic

Pharmacodynamics
Onset of action: 1-3 minutes
Duration: Dose dependent; anesthesia adjunct doses: 5 minutes

Pharmacokinetics
Distribution: V_{dss}:
Children 2-8 years: 2.9 ± 0.6 L/kg
Adults: 1.7 ± 0.2 L/kg
Protein binding (alpha$_1$.acid glycoprotein):
Neonates: 79%
Adults:
Male: 93%
Postpartum women: 91%
Metabolism: Primarily by the liver via demethylation and dealkylation
Half-life, elimination:
Neonates: 382-1162 minutes
Children 2-8 years: 97 ± 42 minutes
Adolescents 10-15 years: 76 ± 33 minutes
Adults: 164 ± 22 minutes
Elimination: ~2% excreted unchanged in the urine; 80% of dose excreted in urine (mostly as metabolites) within 24 hours
Clearance:
Children 2-8 years: 30.5 ± 8.8 mL/minute/kg
Adolescents: 12.8 ± 12 mL/minute/kg
Adults: 12.7 ± 0.8 mL/minute/kg

Usual Dosage Doses should be titrated to appropriate effects; wide range of doses, dependent upon desired degree of analgesia or anesthesia; use lean body weight to dose patients who are >20% above ideal body weight

Children <12 years: Anesthesia: I.V.: Initial: 10-25 mcg/kg; maintenance: Up to 25-50 mcg as needed
(Continued)

921

Sufentanil *(Continued)*

Adults: I.V.:
    Adjunct to general anesthesia:
        Low dose: Initial: 0.5-1 mcg/kg; maintenance: 10-25 mcg as needed
        Moderate dose: Initial: 2-8 mcg/kg; maintenance: 10-50 mcg as needed
        Anesthesia: Initial: 8-30 mcg/kg; maintenance: 10-50 mcg as needed

Administration Parenteral: I.V.: Slow I.V. injection or by infusion

Monitoring Parameters Respiratory rate, blood pressure, heart rate, oxygen saturation, neurological status (for degree of analgesia/anesthesia)

Nursing Implications Patient may develop rebound respiratory depression postoperatively

Dosage Forms Injection, as citrate: 50 mcg/mL (1 mL, 2 mL, 5 mL)

References

Guay J, Gaudreault P, Tang A, et al, "Pharmacokinetics of Sufentanil in Normal Children," *Can J Anaesth*, 1992, 39(1):14-20.

Seguin JH, Erenberg A, and Leff RD, "Safety and Efficacy of Sufentanil Therapy in the Ventilated Infant," *Neonatal Netw*, 1994, 13(4):37-40.

♦ **Sulbactam and Ampicillin** *see* Ampicillin and Sulbactam *on page 90*

♦ **Sulcrate (Can)** *see* Sucralfate *on page 919*

♦ **Sulcrate Suspension Plus (Can)** *see* Sucralfate *on page 919*

♦ **Sulf-10®** *see* Sulfacetamide *on page 922*

Sulfacetamide *(sul fa SEE ta mide)*

U.S. Brand Names AK-Sulf®; Bleph®-10; Cetamide®; I-Sulfacet®; Ophthacet®; Sodium Sulamyd®; Sulf-10®; Sulfair®

Canadian Brand Names Diosulf

Therapeutic Category Antibiotic, Ophthalmic; Antibiotic, Sulfonamide Derivative

Generic Available Yes

Use Treatment and prophylaxis of conjunctivitis, corneal ulcers, and other superficial ocular infections due to susceptible organisms; adjunctive treatment with systemic sulfonamides for therapy of trachoma

Pregnancy Risk Factor C

Contraindications Hypersensitivity to sulfacetamide, any component, or sulfonamides; infants <2 months of age; epithelial herpes simplex keratitis, vaccinia, varicella, and other viral diseases of the cornea and conjunctiva; fungal diseases of the ocular structures

Warnings Antibacterial activity may be decreased in the presence of purulent exudates containing para-aminobenzoic acid (PABA); nonsusceptible organisms such as fungi may proliferate with prolonged or repeated use of sulfonamide preparations; hemolysis may occur in patients with G-6-PD deficiency

Precautions Use with caution in patients with severe dry eye or G-6-PD deficiency

Adverse Reactions

Central nervous system: Headache, fever

Dermatologic: Stevens-Johnson syndrome, exfoliative dermatitis, toxic epidermal necrolysis, rash, photosensitivity

Hematologic: Bone marrow suppression

Local: Irritation, stinging and burning (especially with 30% solution), itching

Ocular: Blurred vision, transient epithelial keratitis, reactive hyperemia, conjunctival edema

Miscellaneous: Hypersensitivity reactions, syndrome resembling systemic lupus erythematosus

Drug Interactions Silver, gentamicin (antagonism)

Stability Protect from light; discolored or cloudy solutions should not be used; incompatible with silver and zinc sulfate; sulfacetamide is inactivated by blood or purulent exudates

Mechanism of Action Interferes with bacterial growth by inhibiting bacterial folic acid synthesis through competitive antagonism of PABA

Pharmacodynamics Onset of action: Improvement of conjunctivitis is usually seen within 3-6 days

Pharmacokinetics

Distribution: Excreted in breast milk

Half-life: 7-13 hours

Elimination: When absorbed, excreted primarily in urine as unchanged drug

Usual Dosage Children >2 months and Adults: Ophthalmic:

Ointment: Apply to lower conjunctival sac 1-4 times/day and at bedtime or apply ½" to 1" into the conjunctival sac at night in conjunction with the use of drops during the day

Solution: Instill 1-2 drops into the lower conjunctival sac every 1-3 hours according to severity of infection during the waking hours and less frequently at night; **Note:** 30% solution is used for more severe infections

Trachoma (30% solution): 2 drops every 2 hours (concomitant use of systemic sulfonamide therapy is recommended)

Administration Ophthalmic: Avoid contact of tube or bottle tip with skin or eye; solution: Apply finger pressure to lacrimal sac during and for 1-2 minutes after instillation to decrease risk of absorption and systemic effects

Monitoring Parameters Response to therapy

Patient Information Eye drops may burn and sting when first instilled; may cause sensitivity to bright light

Dosage Forms Ophthalmic, as sodium:

Ointment: 10% (3.5 g, 3.75 g)

Solution: 10% (1 mL, 2 mL, 2.5 mL, 3.75 mL, 5 mL, 15 mL); 15% (2 mL, 5 mL, 15 mL); 30% (5 mL, 15 mL)

References

Lohr JA, Austin RD, Grossman M, et al, "Comparison of Three Topical Antimicrobials for Acute Bacterial Conjunctivitis," *Pediatr Infect Dis J,* 1988, 7(9):626-9.

Sulfadiazine (sul fa DYE a zeen)

Therapeutic Category Antibiotic, Sulfonamide Derivative

Generic Available Yes

Use Adjunctive treatment in toxoplasmosis; treatment of urinary tract infections and nocardiosis; rheumatic fever prophylaxis in penicillin-allergic patient; uncomplicated attack of malaria

Pregnancy Risk Factor B (D at term)

Contraindications Porphyria; hypersensitivity to any sulfa drug or any component; infants <2 months of age due to competition with bilirubin for protein-binding sites (unless indicated for the treatment of congenital toxoplasmosis); pregnant women during third trimester

Precautions Use with caution in patients with impaired hepatic function or impaired renal function, urinary obstruction, blood dyscrasia, G-6-PD deficiency; dosage modification required in patients with renal impairment

Adverse Reactions

Cardiovascular: Vasculitis

Central nervous system: Dizziness, fever, headache

Dermatologic: Rash, exfoliative dermatitis, Stevens-Johnson syndrome, photosensitivity, urticaria

Gastrointestinal: Nausea, vomiting, abdominal pain

Genitourinary: Crystalluria

Hematologic: Granulocytopenia, leukopenia, thrombocytopenia, aplastic anemia, hemolytic anemia

Hepatic: Jaundice, hepatitis

Renal: Acute nephropathy, hematuria

Miscellaneous: Serum sickness-like reactions

Drug Interactions PABA, procaine; tetracaine antagonizes antibacterial action of sulfonamides; paraldehyde increases potential for crystalluria; displaces agents from protein binding sites: coumarin anticoagulants increase bleeding, MTX increases toxicity, sulfonylurea antidiabetic agents (hypoglycemia)

Food Interactions Supplemental folinic acid should be administered to reverse symptoms or prevent problems due to folic acid deficiency; avoid large quantities of vitamin C or acidifying agents (cranberry juice) to prevent crystalluria

Stability Protect from light

Mechanism of Action Interferes with bacterial growth by inhibiting bacterial folic acid synthesis through competitive antagonism of PABA

Pharmacokinetics

Absorption: Oral: Well absorbed

Distribution: Excreted in breast milk; diffuses into CSF with higher concentrations reached when meninges are inflamed; distributed into most body tissues

Protein binding: 32% to 56%

Metabolism: Metabolized by N-acetylation

Half-life: 10 hours

Time to peak serum concentration: Within 4 hours

Elimination: In urine as metabolites (15% to 40%) and as unchanged drug (43% to 60%)

(Continued)

Sulfadiazine *(Continued)*

Usual Dosage Oral:

Congenital toxoplasmosis: Newborns: 100 mg/kg/day divided every 12 hours for 12 months in conjunction with pyrimethamine 1 mg/kg/day once daily and supplemental folinic acid 5 mg every 3 days for first 6 months, then pyrimethamine 1 mg/kg/day 3 times/week and folinic acid 10 mg 3 times/week for the next 6 months

Toxoplasmosis:

Children: 120-200 mg/kg/day divided every 6 hours in conjunction with pyrimethamine 2 mg/kg/day divided every 12 hours for 3 days followed by 1 mg/kg/day once daily (maximum dose: 25 mg/day) with supplemental folinic acid 5-10 mg every 3 days

Adults: 2-8 g/day divided every 6 hours in conjunction with pyrimethamine 25 mg/day and with supplemental folinic acid 5-10 mg every 3 days

Prophylaxis of recurrent rheumatic fever:

≤30 kg: 500 mg once daily

>30 kg: 1 g once daily

Administration Oral: Administer with water on an empty stomach

Monitoring Parameters CBC, renal function tests, urinalysis

Patient Information Drink plenty of fluids; avoid prolonged exposure to sunlight; limit alcohol; notify physician if rash, sore throat, fever, arthralgia, shortness of breath, or jaundice occurs

Dosage Forms Tablet: 500 mg

Extemporaneous Preparations Tablets may be crushed to prepare oral suspension of the drug in water or with a sucrose-containing solution; aqueous suspension with concentrations of 100 mg/mL should be stored in the refrigerator and used within 7 days

References

Frenkel JK, "Toxoplasmosis," *Pediatr Clin North Am*, 1985, 32(4):917-32.

Sulfadoxine and Pyrimethamine

(sul fa DOKS een & peer i METH a meen)

U.S. Brand Names Fansidar®

Synonyms Pyrimethamine and Sulfadoxine

Therapeutic Category Antimalarial Agent

Generic Available No

Use Treatment of *Plasmodium falciparum* malaria in patients in whom chloroquine resistance is suspected; malaria prophylaxis for travelers to areas where chloroquine-resistant malaria is endemic

Pregnancy Risk Factor C

Contraindications Hypersensitivity to any sulfa drug, pyrimethamine, or any component; porphyria, megaloblastic anemia, severe renal insufficiency; children <2 months of age due to competition with bilirubin for protein binding sites; pregnant women at term; do not use for treatment of malaria acquired in Southeast Asia or the Amazon Basin since resistance to sulfadoxine and pyrimethamine has been reported

Warnings Fatalities associated with sulfonamides, although rare, have occurred due to severe reactions including Stevens-Johnson syndrome, toxic epidermal necrolysis, hepatic necrosis, agranulocytosis, aplastic anemia and other blood dyscrasias; discontinue use at first sign of rash or any sign of adverse reaction; hemolysis may occur in patients with G-6-PD deficiency

Precautions Use with caution in patients with renal or hepatic impairment, patients with possible folate deficiency, patients with bronchial asthma, and patients with seizure disorders

Adverse Reactions

Cardiovascular: Vasculitis

Central nervous system: Seizures, headache, insomnia, ataxia, fatigue, hyperesthesia

Dermatologic: Erythema multiforme, Stevens-Johnson syndrome, toxic epidermal necrolysis, rash, photosensitivity, urticaria, pruritus

Endocrine & metabolic: Folic acid deficiency

Gastrointestinal: Anorexia, vomiting, gastritis, glossitis, diarrhea, abdominal cramps

Hematologic: Megaloblastic anemia, leukopenia, thrombocytopenia, pancytopenia, agranulocytosis, pulmonary eosinophilia

Hepatic: Hepatic necrosis; jaundice; elevated ALT, AST

Neuromuscular & skeletal: Tremor

Respiratory: Respiratory failure

Drug Interactions Para-aminobenzoic acid, folic acid

Stability Protect from light

Mechanism of Action Sulfadoxine interferes with bacterial folic acid synthesis and growth via competitive inhibition of para-aminobenzoic acid; pyrimethamine inhibits microbial dihydrofolate reductase, resulting in inhibition of tetrahydrofolic acid synthesis

Pharmacokinetics

Absorption: Oral: Well absorbed

Distribution: Excreted in breast milk; pyrimethamine is distributed to kidneys, lungs, liver, and spleen; sulfadoxine is widely distributed in the body

Protein binding:

Pyrimethamine: 80% to 87%

Sulfadoxine: 90% to 95%

Half-life:

Pyrimethamine: 111 hours

Sulfadoxine: 169 hours

Time to peak serum concentration: Within 2-8 hours

Elimination: In urine as parent compounds and several unidentified metabolites

Usual Dosage Children ≥ 2 months and Adults: Oral:

Treatment of acute attack of malaria: A single dose of the following number of Fansidar® tablets is used in sequence with quinine on last day of quinine therapy:

2-11 months: 1/4 tablet

1-3 years: 1/2 tablet

4-8 years: 1 tablet

9-14 years: 2 tablets

>14 years: 3 tablets

Adults: 3 tablets on last day of quinine therapy

Malaria prophylaxis (for areas where chloroquine-resistant *P. falciparum* exists):

Short-term travel (≤3 weeks): Travelers should carry pyrimethamine-sulfadoxine for use as presumptive self-treatment if a febrile illness develops while taking chloroquine for prophylaxis. Take single dose in the event of febrile illness when medical attention is not immediately available:

2-11 months: 1/4 tablet

1-3 years: 1/2 tablet

4-8 years: 1 tablet

9-14 years: 2 tablets

>14 years and Adults: 3 tablets

Administration Oral: Administer with meals

Monitoring Parameters Liver function tests, CBC including platelet counts, renal function tests and urinalysis should be performed periodically

Patient Information Drink plenty of fluids; avoid prolonged exposure to the sun; notify physician if rash, sore throat, pallor, glossitis, fever, arthralgia, cough, shortness of breath, or jaundice occurs; limit alcohol

Additional Information Leucovorin should be administered to reverse signs and symptoms of folic acid deficiency

Dosage Forms Tablet: Sulfadoxine 500 mg and pyrimethamine 25 mg

References

Lynk A and Gold R, "Review of 40 Children With Imported Malaria," *Pediatr Infect Dis J*, 1989, 8(11):745-50.

Randall G and Seidel JS, "Malaria," *Pediatr Clin North Am*, 1985, 32(4):893-916.

♦ **Sulfair®** *see* Sulfacetamide *on page 922*

♦ **Sulfalax® [OTC]** *see* Docusate *on page 350*

♦ **Sulfamethoprim®** *see* Co-Trimoxazole *on page 270*

Sulfamethoxazole (sul fa meth OKS a zole)

U.S. Brand Names Gantanol®

Canadian Brand Names Apo-Sulfamethoxazole

Therapeutic Category Antibiotic, Sulfonamide Derivative

Generic Available Yes: Tablet

Use Treatment of urinary tract infections, nocardiosis, chlamydial infections, toxoplasmosis, acute otitis media, and acute exacerbations of chronic bronchitis due to susceptible organisms

Pregnancy Risk Factor B (D at term)

Contraindications Porphyria; hypersensitivity to sulfa drug or any component; infants <2 months of age (sulfas compete with bilirubin for protein binding sites which may result in kernicterus in newborns); pregnant women during third trimester

Warnings Should not be used for group A beta-hemolytic streptococcal infections

(Continued)

Sulfamethoxazole *(Continued)*

Precautions Maintain adequate fluid intake to prevent crystalluria; use with caution in patients with renal or hepatic impairment, patients with G-6-PD deficiency, and in patients with urinary obstruction

Adverse Reactions
Cardiovascular: Vasculitis
Central nervous system: Dizziness, fever, headache, vertigo, disorientation
Dermatologic: Rash, exfoliative dermatitis, Stevens-Johnson syndrome, photosensitivity
Gastrointestinal: Nausea, vomiting, anorexia, stomatitis, pseudomembranous colitis
Genitourinary: Crystalluria
Hematologic: Granulocytopenia, leukopenia, thrombocytopenia, aplastic anemia, hemolytic anemia, neutropenia
Hepatic: Jaundice, hepatitis
Renal: Acute nephropathy
Miscellaneous: Serum sickness-like reactions

Drug Interactions Warfarin, sulfonylurea antidiabetic agents, methotrexate, (displaces sulfonylureas, warfarin, and methotrexate from protein binding sites)

Food Interactions Avoid large quantities of vitamin C or acidifying agents (cranberry juice) to prevent crystalluria; food decreases the rate but does not reduce the extent of absorption

Stability Protect from light

Mechanism of Action Interferes with bacterial growth by inhibiting bacterial folic acid synthesis through competitive antagonism of PABA

Pharmacokinetics
Absorption: Oral: 70% to 90%
Distribution: Crosses the placenta; widely distributed into most body tissues
Protein binding: 50% to 70%
Metabolism: Primarily in the liver to a N-acetylated metabolite (inactive but contributes to nephrotoxicity) and a N-glucuronide conjugate
Half-life: 7-12 hours, prolonged with renal impairment
Time to peak serum concentration: Within 3-4 hours
Elimination: Unchanged drug (20%) and its metabolites are excreted in urine
Dialysis: Moderately dialyzable (20% to 50%)

Usual Dosage Oral:
Children ≥2 months: Initial: 50-60 mg/kg/dose one time, followed by 50-60 mg/kg/day divided every 12 hours, not to exceed 75 mg/kg/day or a maximum dose: 3 g/24 hours
Adults: 2 g stat, followed by 1 g 2-3 times/day; maximum dose: 3 g/24 hours
Dosing adjustment in renal impairment:
Cl_{cr} 10-30 mL/minute: Decrease usual dose by 50%
Cl_{cr} <10 mL/minute: Decrease usual dose by 75%

Administration Oral: Administer with a glass of water on an empty stomach; shake suspension well before use

Monitoring Parameters CBC, UA, renal function test

Patient Information Report to physician any sore throat, mouth sores, rash, jaundice, unusual bleeding or fever; drink plenty of fluids; avoid vitamin C products; avoid prolonged exposure to sunlight

Dosage Forms Tablet: 500 mg

♦ **Sulfamethoxazole and Trimethoprim** *see* Co-Trimoxazole *on page 270*
♦ **Sulfamylon**® *see* Mafenide *on page 613*

Sulfasalazine *(sul fa SAL a zeen)*

Related Information
Drugs and Breast-Feeding *on page 1243*

U.S. Brand Names Azulfidine®; Azulfidine® EN-tabs®

Canadian Brand Names Alti-Sulfasalazine; Apo-Sulfasalazine; PMS-Sulfasalazine; Salazopyrin; Salazopyrin EN-Tabs; S.A.S

Synonyms Salicylazosulfapyridine

Therapeutic Category 5-Aminosalicylic Acid Derivative; Anti-inflammatory Agent

Generic Available Yes

Use Management of ulcerative colitis; treatment of active Crohn's disease and juvenile rheumatoid arthritis

Pregnancy Risk Factor B (D at term)

Contraindications Hypersensitivity to sulfasalazine, sulfa drugs, or any component; porphyria, GI or GU obstruction; hypersensitivity to salicylates; children <2 years of age

Precautions Use with caution in patients with renal impairment, G-6-PD deficiency, blood dyscrasias, or bronchial asthma

Adverse Reactions Incidence of adverse effects increase with dosage >4 g/day and in slow acetylators of sulfapyridine

Cardiovascular: Vasculitis

Central nervous system: Headache, fever, convulsions, vertigo, malaise, mood changes

Dermatologic: Rash, toxic epidermal necrolysis, urticaria, Stevens-Johnson syndrome, photosensitivity, staining of skin (orange-yellow)

Gastrointestinal: Nausea, vomiting, diarrhea, pancreatitis, anorexia

Genitourinary: Crystalluria, infertility (oligospermia), discoloration of urine (orange-yellow)

Hematologic: Hemolytic anemia, agranulocytosis, neutropenia, leukopenia

Hepatic: Elevated liver enzymes, jaundice, cholestatic jaundice, cirrhosis, liver necrosis/failure

Otic: Tinnitus

Renal: Nephrotoxicity

Respiratory: Fibrosing alveolitis, pulmonary eosinophilia

Miscellaneous: Serum sickness-like reaction

Drug Interactions

Decreased effect of iron, digoxin, folic acid, and PABA or PABA metabolites of drugs (ie, procaine, proparacaine, tetracaine)

Increased effect of oral anticoagulants, methotrexate, and oral hypoglycemic agents (as with other sulfa drugs)

Food Interactions Need to increase dietary intake of iron; since sulfasalazine impairs folate absorption, consider providing 1 mg/day folate supplement

Mechanism of Action Acts locally in the colon to decrease the inflammatory response and interfere with secretion by inhibiting prostaglandin synthesis; therapeutic effect may result from antibacterial action with change in intestinal flora

Pharmacodynamics

Onset for JRA: minimum trial of 3 months is necessary;

Onset for ulcerative colitis: >3-4 weeks

Pharmacokinetics

Absorption: Oral: 10% to 15% as unchanged drug from the small intestine; upon administration, the drug is split into sulfapyridine and 5-aminosalicylic acid (5-ASA) in the colon

Distribution: Breast milk to plasma ratio: 0.09-0.17

Metabolism: Both components are metabolized in the liver; slow acetylators have higher plasma sulfapyridine concentrations

Half-life:

Sulfasalazine:

Single dose: 5.7 hours

Multiple doses: 7.6 hours

Sulfapyridine:

Single dose: 8.4 hours

Multiple doses: 10.4 hours

Time to peak serum concentration:

Serum sulfasalazine: Within 1.5-6 hours

Serum sulfapyridine (active metabolite): Within 6-24 hours

Elimination: Primarily in urine (as unchanged drug, components, and acetylated metabolites); small amounts appear in feces

Usual Dosage Oral:

Children ≥2 years:

Ulcerative colitis:

Mild exacerbation: 40-50 mg/kg/day divided every 6 hours

Moderate-severe exacerbation: 50-75 mg/kg/day divided every 4-6 hours, not to exceed 6 g/day

Maintenance dose: 30-50 mg/kg/day divided every 4-8 hours; not to exceed 2 g/day

Juvenile rheumatoid arthritis (JRA): Initial: 10 mg/kg/day; increase weekly by 10 mg/kg/day; usual dose: 30-50 mg/kg/day in 2 divided doses; maximum dose: 2 g/day

Adults: 1 g 3-4 times/day divided every 4-6 hours, not to exceed 6 g/day; maintenance: 2 g/day divided every 6-12 hours

Administration Oral: Administer after meals or with food; do not administer with antacids

Monitoring Parameters Stool frequency, hematocrit, reticulocyte count, CBC, urinalysis, renal function tests, liver function tests

(Continued)

Sulfasalazine *(Continued)*

Patient Information Maintain adequate fluid intake; may cause orange-yellow discoloration of urine and skin; may stain soft contact lenses yellow; avoid prolonged exposure to sunlight

Additional Information Good response to sulfasalazine for JRA is most likely to occur in HLA B27-positive boys who are older than 9 years of age at onset of arthritis

Dosage Forms

Tablet (Azulfidine®): 500 mg

Tablet, enteric coated (Azulfidine® EN-tabs®): 500 mg

References

American College of Rheumatology Ad Hoc Committee on Clinical Guidelines, "Guidelines for the Management of Rheumatoid Arthritis," *Arthritis Rheum*, 1996, 39(5):713-22.

Giannini EH and Cawkwell GD, "Drug Treatment in Children With Juvenile Rheumatoid Arthritis," *Pediatr Clin North Am*, 1995, 42(5):1099-125.

Kirschner BS, "Inflammatory Bowel Disease in Children," *Pediatr Clin North Am*, 1988, 35(1):189-208.

♦ **Sulfatrim®** *see Co-Trimoxazole on page 270*

♦ **Sulfatrim® DS** *see Co-Trimoxazole on page 270*

♦ **Sulfimycin®** *see Erythromycin and Sulfisoxazole on page 397*

Sulfisoxazole *(sul fi SOKS a zole)*

Related Information

Carbohydrate and Alcohol Content of Liquid Medications for Use in Patients Receiving Ketogenic Diets *on page 1258*

U.S. Brand Names Gantrisin®

Canadian Brand Names Novo-Soxazole; Sulfizole

Synonyms Sulphafurazole

Therapeutic Category Antibiotic, Sulfonamide Derivative

Generic Available Yes

Use Treatment of uncomplicated urinary tract infections, otitis media, *Chlamydia*; nocardiosis; treatment of acute pelvic inflammatory disease in prepubertal children

Pregnancy Risk Factor B (D at term)

Contraindications Hypersensitivity to any sulfa drug or any component; porphyria; infants <2 months of age (sulfas compete with bilirubin for protein binding sites which may result in kernicterus in newborns); patients with urinary obstruction; pregnant women during third trimester; nursing mothers

Precautions Use with caution in patients with G-6-PD deficiency (hemolysis may occur), hepatic or renal impairment; dosage modification required in patients with renal impairment; risk of crystalluria should be considered in patients with impaired renal function

Adverse Reactions

Cardiovascular: Vasculitis

Central nervous system: Dizziness, headache, fever, vertigo, disorientation

Dermatologic: Rash, Stevens-Johnson syndrome, photosensitivity, exfoliative dermatitis

Gastrointestinal: Nausea, vomiting, anorexia, stomatitis, pseudomembranous colitis

Genitourinary: Crystalluria (rare)

Hematologic: Thrombocytopenia, leukopenia, agranulocytosis, aplastic anemia, hemolytic anemia, neutropenia

Hepatic: Jaundice, hepatitis

Renal: Nephrotoxicity

Miscellaneous: Hypersensitivity reactions

Drug Interactions Methotrexate, tolbutamide, chlorpropamide, oral anticoagulants (displaced from protein binding sites); PABA (antagonizes the antibacterial activity of sulfas); thiopental (competes for plasma protein binding)

Food Interactions Interferes with folate absorption

Stability Protect from light

Mechanism of Action Interferes with bacterial growth by inhibiting bacterial folic acid synthesis through competitive antagonism of PABA

Pharmacokinetics

Absorption: Sulfisoxazole acetyl is hydrolyzed in the GI tract to sulfisoxazole which is readily absorbed

Distribution: Crosses the placenta; excreted into breast milk; distributes into extra-cellular space; CSF concentration ranges from 8% to 57% of blood concentration in patients with normal meninges

Protein binding: 85% to 88%

Metabolism: In the liver by acetylation and glucuronide conjugation to inactive compounds

Half-life: 4-8 hours, prolonged with renal impairment

Time to peak serum concentration: Within 2-4 hours

Elimination: Primarily in urine (95% within 24 hours), 40% to 60% as unchanged drug

Dialysis: >50% removed by hemodialysis

Usual Dosage

Infants ≥2 months and Children: Oral: Initial: 75 mg/kg for 1 dose, followed by 120-150 mg/kg/day in divided doses every 4-6 hours; not to exceed 6 g/day

Pelvic inflammatory disease: 100 mg/kg/day in divided doses every 6 hours; used in combination with ceftriaxone

Chlamydia trachomatis: 100 mg/kg/day divided every 6 hours; maximum dose: 2 g/day

Prophylaxis of UTI: 10-20 mg/kg/day divided every 12 hours

Adults: Oral: 2-4 g stat, followed by 4-8 g/day in divided doses every 4-6 hours

Children and Adults: Ophthalmic: Solution: Instill 1-2 drops to conjunctiva of affected eye every 2-3 hours

Dosing interval in renal impairment:

Cl_{cr} 10-50 mL/minutes: Administer every 8-12 hours

Cl_{cr} <10 mL/minute: Administer every 12-24 hours

Administration

Ophthalmic: Avoid contact of bottle tip with skin or eye; apply finger pressure to lacrimal sac during and for 1-2 minutes after instillation of drops to decrease risk of absorption and systemic effects

Oral: Administer with a glass of water on an empty stomach; shake suspension well before use

Monitoring Parameters CBC, urinalysis, renal function tests

Test Interactions False-positive protein in urine; false-positive urine glucose with Clinitest®

Patient Information Avoid prolonged exposure to sunlight; report to physician any sore throat, mouth sores, rash, unusual bleeding, or fever; limit alcohol

Nursing Implications Maintain adequate patient fluid intake

Dosage Forms

Suspension, oral, pediatric, as acetyl: 500 mg/5 mL [raspberry flavor] (480 mL)

Tablet: 500 mg

References

"Practice Parameter: The Diagnosis, Treatment, and Evaluation of the Initial Urinary Tract Infection in Febrile Infants and Young Children. American Academy of Pediatrics. Committee on Quality Improvement. Subcommittee on Urinary Tract Infection," *Pediatrics*, 1999, 103(4 Pt 1):843-52.

Thoene DE and Johnson CE, "Pharmacotherapy of Otitis Media," *Pharmacotherapy*, 1991, 11(3):212-21.

♦ **Sulfisoxazole and Erythromycin** *see* Erythromycin and Sulfisoxazole *on page 397*

♦ **Sulfizole (Can)** *see* Sulfisoxazole *on page 928*

Sulfur and Salicylic Acid (SUL fur & sal i SIL ik AS id)

U.S. Brand Names MG217 Medicated Tar-Free [OTC]; Pernox® [OTC]; Sebex® [OTC]; Sebulex® [OTC]

Canadian Brand Names Meted; Sebex

Synonyms Salicylic Acid and Sulfur

Therapeutic Category Antiseborrheic Agent, Topical

Generic Available Yes

Use Therapeutic shampoo for dandruff and seborrheal dermatitis; acne skin cleanser

Contraindications Hypersensitivity to sulfur, salicylic acid, or any component

Warnings For external use only; avoid contact with eyes; discontinue use if skin irritation develops

Precautions Infants are more sensitive to sulfur than adults; do not use in children <2 years of age

Adverse Reactions Topical preparations containing 2% to 5% sulfur generally are well tolerated; concentration >15% is very irritating to the skin; higher concentrations (eg, 10% or higher) may cause systemic toxicity

Cardiovascular: Collapse (with sulfur concentration >10%)

Central nervous system: Dizziness, headache

Gastrointestinal: Vomiting

Local: Irritation

Neuromuscular & skeletal: Muscle cramps

Stability Preparations containing sulfur may react with metals including silver and copper, resulting in discoloration of the metal

(Continued)

Sulfur and Salicylic Acid *(Continued)*

Mechanism of Action Salicylic acid works synergistically with sulfur in its keratolytic action to break down keratin and promote skin peeling

Pharmacokinetics Absorption: 1% of topically applied sulfur is absorbed; sulfur is reduced to hydrogen sulfide

Usual Dosage Children ≥2 years and Adults: Topical:

Shampoo: Initial: Massage onto wet scalp; leave lather on scalp for 5 minutes, rinse, repeat application, then rinse thoroughly; use daily or every other day; 1-2 treatments/week will usually maintain control

Soap: Use daily or every other day

Administration Topical: Avoid contact with the eyes; for external use only

Patient Information Contact physician if condition worsens or rash or irritation develops

Dosage Forms

Cleanser (Pernox® Scrub Cleanser): Sulfur 2% and salicylic acid 1.5% (60 mL, 120 mL)

Shampoo

Sebex®, Sebulex®: Sulfur 2% and salicylic acid 2% (120 mL, 240 mL)

MG217 Medicated Tar-Free: Colloidal sulfur 5% and salicylic acid 3% (120 mL, 240 mL)

Soap: Precipitated sulfur 5% and salicylic acid 3% (116 g)

Sulindac *(sul IN dak)*

Related Information

Overdose and Toxicology *on page 1222*

U.S. Brand Names Clinoril®

Canadian Brand Names Apo-Sulin; Novo-Sundac; Nu-Sulindac

Therapeutic Category Analgesic, Non-narcotic; Anti-inflammatory Agent; Nonsteroidal Anti-inflammatory Drug (NSAID), Oral

Generic Available Yes

Use Management of inflammatory disease, rheumatoid disorders; acute gouty arthritis

Pregnancy Risk Factor B (D in 3rd trimester or near delivery)

Contraindications Hypersensitivity to sulindac, any component, aspirin, or other NSAIDs

Precautions Use with caution in patients with peptic ulcer disease, GI bleeding, bleeding abnormalities, impaired renal or hepatic function, CHF, hypertension, and patients receiving anticoagulants

Adverse Reactions

Cardiovascular: Edema

Central nervous system: Dizziness, nervousness, headache

Dermatologic: Rash, pruritus

Gastrointestinal: Abdominal pain; GI bleeding, ulcer, perforation; nausea; vomiting; diarrhea; constipation

Hematologic: Thrombocytopenia, agranulocytosis, inhibition of platelet aggregation, bone marrow suppression

Hepatic: Hepatitis

Otic: Tinnitus

Renal: Renal impairment

Respiratory: Bronchospasm

Drug Interactions Sulindac may potentiate effects of warfarin; probenecid may increase serum concentration of sulindac; dimethyl sulfoxide or ASA may decrease sulindac serum concentration; sulindac may increase methotrexate serum concentrations and may increase cyclosporin nephrotoxicity; potassium supplements and other GI irritants may increase GI adverse effects; effects of antihypertensive agents, furosemide, thiazides may be decreased; drug interactions similar to other NSAIDs may also occur

Food Interactions Food may decrease rate and extent of absorption

Mechanism of Action Inhibits prostaglandin synthesis by decreasing the activity of the enzyme, cyclo-oxygenase, which results in decreased formation of prostaglandin precursors

Usual Dosage Oral:

Children: Dose not established; doses of 4 mg/kg/day divided in 2 doses have been used

Adults: 150-200 mg twice daily; not to exceed 400 mg/day

Administration Oral: Administer with food or milk to decrease GI upset

Monitoring Parameters Liver enzymes, BUN, serum creatinine, CBC with differential, platelet count; periodic ophthalmologic exams with chronic use

Patient Information Avoid alcohol; may cause dizziness; do not take with aspirin
Dosage Forms Tablet: 150 mg, 200 mg

♦ **Sulphafurazole** *see* Sulfisoxazole *on page 928*

Sumatriptan (SOO ma trip tan)
Related Information
Serotonin Syndrome *on page 1247*
U.S. Brand Names Imitrex®
Therapeutic Category Antimigraine Agent
Generic Available No
Use
Injection, intranasal, and tablets: Acute treatment of migraine with or without aura
Injection: Acute treatment of cluster headaches
Pregnancy Risk Factor C
Contraindications I.V. administration (coronary vasospasm may occur); ischemic heart disease, Prinzmetal angina, cerebrovascular or peripheral vascular syndromes (eg, stroke, TIA, ischemic bowel disease), severe hepatic impairment, patients with signs or symptoms of ischemic heart disease, MI, silent MI, uncontrolled hypertension; concomitant use of ergotamine derivatives (within last 24 hours), vasoconstrictive drugs, methysergide, or MAO inhibitors; use of MAO inhibitors within past 2 weeks; hypersensitivity to sumatriptan or any component; management of hemiplegic or basilar migraine
Warnings Life-threatening or fatal hypersensitivity reactions may occur; rarely, serious coronary events including acute MI, life-threatening arrhythmias, and death, may occur; avoid use in patients with risk factors for coronary artery disease, unless cardiovascular disease can be ruled out; consider administering first dose under close supervision to patients at high risk for coronary disease; EKG should be performed if angina-like symptoms occur; periodically evaluate cardiovascular system in patients with risk factors for coronary artery disease
Precautions Temporary increases in peripheral vascular resistance and blood pressure may occur; use with caution in patients with impaired hepatic or renal function, epilepsy; cross-hypersensitivity to sulfonamides is possible; other potentially serious neurological conditions should be ruled out prior to acute migraine therapy; sumatriptan (given at five times the maximum oral single dose) has caused corneal opacities in dogs; other animal studies suggest it may bind to the melanin of the eye; human studies are not available
Adverse Reactions
Cardiovascular: Hypertension; flushing; chest tightness, pressure, pain; coronary artery vasospasm; vascular ischemia; colonic ischemia; rarely: acute MI, life-threatening arrhythmias
Central nervous system: Dizziness, drowsiness, headache
Gastrointestinal: Nausea, vomiting, abdominal discomfort; bad or unusual taste (with intranasal use)
Local: Injection site reaction (59%), pain, redness at injection site
Neuromuscular & skeletal: Weakness, myalgia, neck pain with stiffness
Miscellaneous: Atypical sensations of tingling, heat, flushing, burning, heaviness, pressure, tightness, numbness; jaw, mouth, tongue discomfort; diaphoresis; rarely: hypersensitivity reactions (potentially fatal anaphylaxis or anaphylactoid reactions)
Drug Interactions Use with ergot-containing drugs may result in prolonged vasospasm reactions; vasoconstrictive drugs; methysergide; MAO inhibitors (MAO inhibitors may significantly increase sumatriptan serum concentrations; use of MAO inhibitors is contraindicated); selective serotonin reuptake inhibitors (may cause weakness, incoordination, hyper-reflexia; monitor patients carefully)
Food Interactions Food slightly delays the rate but not the extent of oral absorption
Stability Store at 2°C to 20°C (36°F to 86°F); protect from light
Mechanism of Action Selective agonist for serotonin (5-HT$_1$) receptor in cranial arteries; causes vasoconstriction and reduces sterile inflammation associated with antidromic neuronal transmission correlating with relief of migraine
Pharmacodynamics Migraine pain relief:
Onset:
Oral: 1-1.5 hours
S.C.: 10 minutes to 2 hours
Maximum effect: Oral: 2-4 hours
Pharmacokinetics
Distribution: Adults:
V_d (central): 50 L;
V_d (apparent): 2.4 L/kg
(Continued)

Sumatriptan *(Continued)*

Protein binding: 14% to 21%

Metabolism: In the liver to an indole acetic acid metabolite (inactive) which then undergoes ester glucuronide conjugation; may be metabolized by monoamine oxidase (MAO)

Bioavailability:

Oral: ~15%; may be significantly increased with liver disease

Intranasal: 17% (compared to S.C.)

S.C.: 97%

Half-life:

Distribution: 15 minutes

Terminal: 2 hours; range: 1-4 hours

Time to peak serum concentration:

Oral: Healthy adults: 2 hours; during migraine attacks: 2.5 hours

S.C.: Range: 5-20 minutes; mean: 12 minutes

Elimination: 60% of an oral dose is renally excreted (primarily as metabolites), 40% is eliminated via the feces, and only 3% as unchanged drug; 42% of an intranasal dose is excreted as the indole acetic acid metabolite with 3% excreted in the urine unchanged; 22% of a S.C. dose is excreted in urine unchanged and 38% as the indole acetic acid metabolite

Usual Dosage

Children and Adolescents <18 years: Use not recommended:

Intranasal: A randomized, double-blind, placebo-controlled, single-attack study in adolescent migraine patients (12-17 years of age) used sumatriptan nasal spray in doses of 5 mg (n=128), 10 mg (n=133), and 20 mg (n=118). Compared to placebo, the percent of patients with headache relief (reduction in headache pain) at 1 hour postdose was significantly greater for the 10 mg and 20 mg group and at 2 hours postdose was significantly greater for the 5 mg group. The percent of patients with **complete** headache relief at 2 hours was significantly greater for the 20 mg group. Younger patients (12-14 years of age) had higher efficacy rates at lower doses, but patients 15-17 years of age had the highest efficacy with the 20 mg doses (Winner, 2000); additional studies are needed

Oral: Efficacy of oral sumatriptan was **not** established in placebo-controlled trials in patients 12-17 years of age (n=701) with doses of 25-100 mg; adverse events were similar to adults; frequency of adverse events was dose- and age-dependent (increased frequency of adverse events in younger patients); postmarketing reports include the occurrence of MI in a 14-year-old male after oral sumatriptan with symptoms occurring within 1 day of drug use

S.C.: An open-labeled prospective trial in 17 children 6-16 years of age with juvenile migraine used S.C. doses of 6 mg in 15 children 30-70 kg, and 3 mg/dose in two children who weighed 22 kg and 30 kg (MacDonald, 1994); additional studies are needed

Adults:

Intranasal: Initial single dose: 5 mg, 10 mg, or 20 mg administered in one nostril, given as soon as possible after the onset of migraine; 10 mg dose may be administered as 5 mg in each nostril; may repeat after 2 hours; maximum: 40 mg/day

Oral: Initial single dose: 25 mg given as soon as possible after the onset of a migraine; range: 25-100 mg/dose; maximum single dose: 100 mg; may repeat after 2 hours; maximum: 200 mg/day

S.C.: 6 mg given as soon as possible after the onset of a migraine; a second injection (≤6 mg) may be administered at least 1 hour after the initial dose; maximum dose: 12 mg/24 hours

Dosing adjustment in hepatic dysfunction: Adults: Oral: Maximum single dose: 50 mg

Administration

Intranasal: Each nasal spray unit is preloaded with 1 dose; **do not** test the spray unit before use; remove unit from plastic pack when ready to use; while sitting down, gently blow nose to clear nasal passages; keep head upright and close one nostril gently with index finger; hold container with other hand, with thumb supporting bottom and index and middle fingers on either side of nozzle; insert nozzle into nostril about $1/2$ inch; close mouth; take a breath through nose while releasing spray into nostril by pressing firmly on blue plunger; remove nozzle from nostril; keep head level for 10-20 seconds and gently breathe in through nose and out through mouth; **do not breathe deeply**

Oral: Administer with fluids

Parenteral: S.C. use only; do **not** administer I.M.; do **not** administer I.V. (may cause coronary vasospasm)

Patient Information If pain or tightness in chest or throat occurs, notify physician; females should avoid pregnancy; pain at injection site lasts <1 hour

Additional Information Safety of treating >4 headaches per month is not established; sumatriptan is **not** indicated for migraine prophylaxis

Dosage Forms

Injection, as succinate: 12 mg/mL (base) (0.5 mL, 2 mL)

Spray, intranasal: 5 mg (100 μL unit dose spray device); 20 mg (100 μL unit dose spray device)

Tablet, as succinate: 25 mg, 50 mg, 100 mg (base)

Extemporaneous Preparations A 5 mg/mL oral liquid preparation made from tablets and 3 different vehicles (Ora-Sweet®, Ora-Sweet® SF, or Syrpalta® syrups) was stable for 21 days when stored in amber glass bottles in the dark under refrigeration (4°C); **Note:** Preparations with Ora-Sweet® and Ora-Sweet® SF used Ora-Plus® as a suspending vehicle; grind nine 100 mg tablets in a mortar into a fine powder; add 40 mL of Ora-Plus® Suspending Vehicle, 5 mL at a time, and mix thoroughly between each addition; **Note:** The suspending vehicle helps to facilitate dispersion of the tablets and is used only if Ora-Sweet® or Ora-Sweet® SF is the vehicle to be used (ie, suspending vehicle is not used if preparation uses Syrpalta® syrup as the vehicle); transfer to a calibrated amber glass bottle; rinse mortar and pestle 5 times with 10 mL of Ora-Plus® suspension vehicle pouring into bottle each time; qsad with appropriate syrup (Ora-Sweet® or Ora-Sweet® SF) to 180 mL; label "shake well," "refrigerate," and "protect from light"; (**Note:** This study also tested microbial growth on days 0 and 28; no growth of bacteria or fungus occurred) (Fish, 1997)

Fish DN, Beall HD, Goodwin SD, et al, "Stability of Sumatriptan Succinate in Extemporaneously Prepared Oral Liquids," *Am J Health Syst Pharm*, 1997, 54(14):1619-22.

References

MacDonald JT, "Treatment of Juvenile Migraine With Subcutaneous Sumatriptan," *Headache*, 1994, 34(10):581-2.

Scott AK, "Sumatriptan Clinical Pharmacokinetics," *Clin Pharmacokinet*, 1994, 27(5):337-44.

Winner P, Rothner AD, Saper J, et al, "A Randomized, Double-Blind, Placebo-Controlled Study of Sumatriptan Nasal Spray in the Treatment of Acute Migraine in Adolescents," *Pediatrics*, 2000, 106(5):989-97.

- **Sumycin®** *see* Tetracycline *on page 941*
- **Super C (Can)** *see* Ascorbic Acid *on page 106*
- **Superdophilus® [OTC]** *see Lactobacillus acidophilus* and *Lactobacillus bulgaricus on page 571*
- **Supeudol (Can)** *see* Oxycodone *on page 745*
- **Supprelin™** *see* Histrelin *on page 496*
- **Suprax®** *see* Cefixime *on page 193*
- **Surfak® [OTC]** *see* Docusate *on page 350*
- **Survanta®** *see* Beractant *on page 138*
- **Sustiva™** *see* Efavirenz *on page 374*
- **Suxamethonium** *see* Succinylcholine *on page 918*
- **Syllact® [OTC]** *see* Psyllium *on page 853*
- **Symadine®** *see* Amantadine *on page 62*
- **Symmetrel®** *see* Amantadine *on page 62*
- **Synacthen** *see* Cosyntropin *on page 269*
- **Synacthen Depot (Can)** *see* Cosyntropin *on page 269*
- **Synagis®** *see* Palivizumab *on page 752*
- **Synalar®** *see* Fluocinolone *on page 439*
- **Synemol®** *see* Fluocinolone *on page 439*
- **Synercid®** *see* Quinupristin/Dalfopristin *on page 863*
- **Synflex (Can)** *see* Naproxen *on page 699*
- **Synthetic Lung Surfactant** *see* Colfosceril *on page 265*
- **Synthroid®** *see* Levothyroxine *on page 588*
- **Syracol-CF® [OTC]** *see* Guaifenesin and Dextromethorphan *on page 487*
- **Syrup DM (Can)** *see* Dextromethorphan *on page 316*
- **Syrup DM-E (Can)** *see* Guaifenesin and Dextromethorphan *on page 487*
- **T₃** *see* Liothyronine *on page 597*

- **T₄ Thyroxine** *see* Levothyroxine *on page 588*
- **624 Tablets (Can)** *see* Propoxyphene *on page 845*
- **Tac™-3** *see* Triamcinolone *on page 979*

Tacrolimus (ta KROE li mus)

U.S. Brand Names Prograf®; Protopic®

Synonyms FK506

Therapeutic Category Immunosuppressant Agent

Generic Available No

Use

Oral/injection: Immunosuppressant used with corticosteroids to prevent graft versus host disease in patients who have received organ transplants and are not responding to cyclosporine

Topical: Moderate to severe atopic dermatitis in patients not responsive to conventional therapy or when conventional therapy is not appropriate

Pregnancy Risk Factor C

Contraindications Hypersensitivity to tacrolimus, polyoxyl 60 hydrogenated castor oil, or any component

Warnings Avoid use with other immunosuppressants; immunosuppression with tacrolimus may result in increased susceptibility to infection and the possible development of lymphoma; adequate airway, supportive measures, and agents for treating anaphylaxis should be available when tacrolimus is administered I.V.

Precautions Use with caution and modify dosage in patients with hepatic or renal impairment

Adverse Reactions

Cardiovascular: Hypertension, hypotension, peripheral edema, chest pain, myocardial hypertrophy, angina pectoris, palpitations, CHF, hypertrophic obstructive cardiomyopathy

Central nervous system: Encephalopathy, headache, hallucinations, pain, fever, seizures, altered mental status, insomnia, dizziness

Dermatologic: Pruritus, rash

Endocrine & metabolic: Hyperkalemia, hyperglycemia, hypomagnesemia, hypophosphatemia

Gastrointestinal: Diarrhea, nausea, vomiting, constipation, dyspepsia

Hematologic: Anemia, thrombocytopenia, leukocytosis, eosinophilia

Hepatic: Hepatotoxicity; elevated AST, ALT, and LDH

Neuromuscular & skeletal: Tremor, paresthesia, back pain, arthralgia

Ocular: Abnormal vision

Otic: Tinnitus

Renal: Nephrotoxicity, elevated BUN and serum creatinine

Respiratory: Pleural effusion, respiratory distress

Miscellaneous: Increased susceptibility to infections, lymphoproliferative disorders, anaphylaxis (may be due to polyoxyl 60 hydrogenated castor oil injectable vehicle)

Topical:

Cardiovascular: Peripheral edema

Central nervous system: Headache, fever, hyperesthesia, pain

Dermatologic: Skin burning, pruritus, erythema, acne, urticaria, rash

Endocrine & metabolic: Dysmenorrhea

Gastrointestinal: Diarrhea, abdominal pain, nausea

Respiratory: Cough, rhinitis

Drug Interactions Cytochrome P-450 isoenzyme CYP3A3/4 substrate

Diltiazem, verapamil, nifedipine, fluconazole, itraconazole, ketoconazole, cimetidine, clarithromycin, erythromycin, methylprednisolone, protease inhibitors, metoclopramide, cyclosporine, and oral clotrimazole increase tacrolimus serum concentrations; antacids, cholestyramine, sodium polystyrene sulfonate, carbamazepine, phenobarbital, primidone, phenytoin, rifabutin, and rifampin decrease tacrolimus serum concentrations; additive nephrotoxicity when used with NSAIDs, nephrotoxic antibiotics, amphotericin B, or cyclosporine

Food Interactions Food reduces the rate and extent of absorption by ~27%; grapefruit juice may increase tacrolimus blood concentration

Stability Reconstitution: Stable for 24 hours when mixed in D_5W or NS in glass or polyolefin containers; 24-hour stability in plastic syringes stored at 24°C; no need to protect from light; do not store in polyvinyl chloride containers since the polyoxyl 60 hydrogenated castor oil injectable vehicle may leach phthalates from polyvinyl chloride containers; polyvinyl-containing administration sets adsorb drug and may lead to a lower dose being delivered to the patient; tacrolimus is unstable in alkaline media; do not mix with acyclovir or ganciclovir

Mechanism of Action Binds to an intracellular protein forming a complex which inhibits phosphatase activity of calcineurin resulting in the inhibition of T-cell activation

Pharmacokinetics

Absorption: Erratic and incomplete oral absorption (5% to 67%)

Distribution: Distributes to erythrocytes, breast milk, lung, kidneys, pancreas, liver, placenta, heart, and spleen; V_d: 5-65 L/kg (V_d is increased in pediatric patients versus adults)

Protein binding: 75% to 97% to alpha-acid glycoprotein (some binding to albumin)

Metabolism: Hepatic metabolism through the cytochrome P-450 system

Bioavailability:

Oral:

Children: 10% to 52%

Adults: 7% to 28%

Topical: <0.5%

Half-life, elimination: 3.5-40.5 hours (mean: 8.7 hours)

Time to peak serum concentration: Oral: 1-4 hours

Elimination: Primarily in bile; <1% excreted unchanged in urine

Clearance: 7-103 mL/minute/kg (average: 30 mL/minute/kg); clearance may be higher in children

Usual Dosage

Children:

Oral: 0.3 mg/kg/day divided every 12 hours; children generally require higher maintenance dosages on a mg/kg basis than adults

I.V. continuous infusion: 0.05-0.15 mg/kg/day

Children ≥2 years: Topical: Moderate to severe atopic dermatitis: Apply 0.03% ointment to affected area twice daily; continue applications for 1 week after symptoms have cleared

Adults:

Oral: 0.15-0.3 mg/kg/day divided every 12 hours

I.V. continuous infusion: 0.05-0.1 mg/kg/day

Dosing adjustment in renal or hepatic impairment: Patients with renal or hepatic impairment should receive the lowest dose in the dosage range

Administration

Oral: Administer on an empty stomach; use oral syringe or glass container (not plastic or foam cup) when administering this medication; do not administer with grapefruit juice; do not administer within 2 hours before or after antacids

Parenteral: May administer by I.V. continuous infusion; I.V. concentrate for injection must be diluted to 0.004-0.02 mg/mL in NS or D_5W prior to administration; PVC-free administration tubing should be used to minimize the potential for significant drug absorption onto the tubing; begin no sooner than 6-hours post-transplant; continue only until oral medication can be tolerated

Topical: For external use only; do not cover with occlusive dressings; rub ointment in gently and completely onto clean, dry skin

Monitoring Parameters Liver enzymes, BUN, serum creatinine, glucose, potassium, magnesium, phosphorus, blood tacrolimus concentrations, CBC with differential; blood pressure, neurologic status, EKG

Reference Range Limited data correlating serum level to therapeutic efficacy/toxicity:

Trough (whole blood ELISA): 9.8-19.4 ng/mL

Trough (HPLC): 0.5-1.5 ng/mL

Patient Information Administer dose at the same time each day; you will be susceptible to infection (avoid crowds and people with infections); notify physician if you develop increased urination, thirst, chest pain, acute headache or dizziness, symptoms of respiratory infection, rash, unusual bruising or bleeding

Nursing Implications Patients receiving I.V. tacrolimus should be under continuous observation for at least the first 30 minutes following dosage initiation; adequate airway, supportive measures, and agents for treating anaphylaxis should be available when tacrolimus is administered I.V.

Additional Information Tacrolimus should be initiated no sooner than 6 hours after transplant; convert I.V. tacrolimus to oral form as soon as possible or within 2-3 days (the oral formulation should be started 8-12 hours after stopping the I.V. infusion); when switching a patient from cyclosporine to tacrolimus, allow at least 24 hours after discontinuing cyclosporine before initiating tacrolimus therapy to minimize the risk of nephrotoxicity

Dosage Forms

Capsule (Prograf®): 0.5 mg, 1 mg, 5 mg

Injection (Prograf®): 5 mg/mL [with alcohol and polyoxyl 60 hydrogenated castor oil] (1 mL)

Ointment, topical (Protopic®): 0.03% (30 g, 60g); 0.1% (30 g, 60 g)

(Continued)

Tacrolimus *(Continued)*

Extemporaneous Preparations A 0.5 mg/mL suspension has been prepared by mixing the contents of six 5 mg tacrolimus capsules with equal amounts of Ora-Plus® and Simple Syrup, NF to make a final volume of 60 mL. When compounding tacrolimus oral suspension, protect hands with latex gloves. The suspension is stable for 56 days when stored at room temperature in either glass or plastic amber prescription bottles. Label "shake well before using."

Jacobson PA, Johnson CE, West NJ, et al, "Stability of Tacrolimus in an Extemporaneously Compounded Oral Liquid," *Am J Health Sys Pharm* , 1997, 54(2):178-80.

References
Asante-Korang A, Boyle GJ, Webber SA, et al, "Experience of FK506 Immune Suppression in Pediatric Heart Transplantation: A Study of Long-Term Adverse Effects," *J Heart Lung Transplant*, 1996, 15(4):415-22.

McDiarmid SV, Colonna JO, Shaked A, et al, "Differences in Oral FK506 Dose Requirements Between Adults and Pediatric Liver Transplant Patients," *Transplantation*, 1993, 55(6):1328-32.

Menegaux F, Keeffe EB, Andrews BT, et al, "Neurological Complications of Liver Transplantation in Adult Versus Pediatric Patients," *Transplantation*, 1994, 58(4):447-50.

♦ **Tagamet®** *see* Cimetidine *on page 234*

♦ **Tagamet-HB® [OTC]** *see* Cimetidine *on page 234*

♦ **Talwin®** *see* Pentazocine *on page 777*

♦ **Talwin® NX** *see* Pentazocine *on page 777*

♦ **Tambocor®** *see* Flecainide *on page 427*

♦ **Tamiflu™** *see* Oseltamivir *on page 739*

♦ **Tantafed (Can)** *see* Pseudoephedrine *on page 852*

♦ **Tantaphen (Can)** *see* Acetaminophen *on page 29*

♦ **TAO®** *see* Troleandomycin *on page 989*

♦ **Tapanol® [OTC]** *see* Acetaminophen *on page 29*

♦ **Tapazole®** *see* Methimazole *on page 644*

♦ **Tarabine® PFS** *see* Cytarabine *on page 290*

♦ **Tar Distillate (Can)** *see* Coal Tar *on page 260*

♦ **Targel (Can)** *see* Coal Tar *on page 260*

♦ **Taro-Carbamazepine (Can)** *see* Carbamazepine *on page 175*

♦ **Taro-Sone (Can)** *see* Betamethasone *on page 140*

♦ **Tavist®** *see* Clemastine *on page 249*

♦ **Tavist®-1 [OTC]** *see* Clemastine *on page 249*

♦ **Taxol®** *see* Paclitaxel *on page 750*

♦ **Tazicef®** *see* Ceftazidime *on page 201*

♦ **Tazidime®** *see* Ceftazidime *on page 201*

♦ **Tazobactam and Piperacillin** *see* Piperacillin and Tazobactam *on page 802*

♦ **Tazocin (Can)** *see* Piperacillin and Tazobactam *on page 802*

♦ **3TC** *see* Lamivudine *on page 572*

♦ **3TC, Abacavir, and AZT** *see* Abacavir, Lamivudine, and Zidovudine *on page 26*

♦ **3TC, Abacavir, and ZDV** *see* Abacavir, Lamivudine, and Zidovudine *on page 26*

♦ **3TC, Abacavir, and Zidovudine** *see* Abacavir, Lamivudine, and Zidovudine *on page 26*

♦ **3TC, ABC, and AZT** *see* Abacavir, Lamivudine, and Zidovudine *on page 26*

♦ **3TC, ABC, and ZDV** *see* Abacavir, Lamivudine, and Zidovudine *on page 26*

♦ **3TC and AZT** *see* Lamivudine and Zidovudine *on page 574*

♦ **3TC and ZDV** *see* Lamivudine and Zidovudine *on page 574*

♦ **T-Cell Growth Factor** *see* Aldesleukin *on page 47*

♦ **TCGF** *see* Aldesleukin *on page 47*

♦ **TCN** *see* Tetracycline *on page 941*

♦ **Tebrazid (Can)** *see* Pyrazinamide *on page 855*

♦ **Tegopen®** *see* Cloxacillin *on page 260*

♦ **Tegretol®** *see* Carbamazepine *on page 175*

♦ **Tegretol®-XR** *see* Carbamazepine *on page 175*

♦ **Tempra® [OTC]** *see* Acetaminophen *on page 29*

♦ **Tenolin (Can)** *see* Atenolol *on page 111*

♦ **Tenormin®** *see* Atenolol *on page 111*

♦ **Tensilon®** *see* Edrophonium *on page 373*

Terbutaline (ter BYOO ta leen)

Related Information
Asthma Guidelines *on page 1210*

U.S. Brand Names Brethine®

Canadian Brand Names Bricanyl

Therapeutic Category Adrenergic Agonist Agent; Antiasthmatic; Beta$_2$-Adrenergic Agonist Agent; Bronchodilator; Sympathomimetic; Tocolytic Agent

Generic Available No

Use Bronchodilator for relief of reversible bronchospasm in patients with asthma, bronchitis, and emphysema

Pregnancy Risk Factor B

Contraindications Hypersensitivity to terbutaline or any component

Warnings Paradoxical bronchoconstriction may occur with excessive use; if it occurs, discontinue terbutaline immediately

Precautions Use with caution in patients with diabetes mellitus, hypertension, hyperthyroidism, history of seizures, or cardiac disease; excessive or prolonged use may lead to tolerance

Adverse Reactions
Cardiovascular: Tachycardia, hypertension, arrhythmias, flushing
Central nervous system: Drowsiness, headache, nervousness, seizures, dizziness
Gastrointestinal: Nausea, vomiting, dysgeusia
Neuromuscular & skeletal: Tremor
Otic: Tinnitus
Respiratory: Dyspnea, bronchospasm (with excessive use), pharyngitis, dry throat, chest tightness
Miscellaneous: Diaphoresis

Drug Interactions Additive effects with other sympathomimetics; increased pressor response with methyldopa, MAO inhibitors, oxytocic drugs, and tricyclic antidepressants

Mechanism of Action Relaxes bronchial smooth muscle and muscles of peripheral vasculature by action on beta$_2$-receptors with less effect on heart rate

Pharmacodynamics
Onset of action:
Oral: 30 minutes
Oral inhalation: 5-30 minutes
S.C.: 6-15 minutes
Duration:
Oral: 4-8 hours
Oral inhalation: 3-6 hours
S.C.: 1.5-4 hours

Pharmacokinetics
Absorption: 33% to 50%
Distribution: Breast milk to plasma ratio: <2.9
Metabolism: Possible first-pass metabolism after oral use
Half-life: 11-16 hours
Elimination: Primarily (60%) unchanged in urine after parenteral use

Usual Dosage
Children <12 years:
Oral: Initial: 0.05 mg/kg/dose every 8 hours, increase gradually, up to 0.15 mg/kg/dose; maximum daily dose: 5 mg
S.C.: 0.005-0.01 mg/kg/dose to a maximum of 0.4 mg/dose every 15-20 minutes for 2 doses
Children ≥12 years and Adults:
Oral: 2.5-5 mg/dose every 6-8 hours; maximum daily dose:
12-15 years: 7.5 mg
>15 years: 15 mg
S.C.: 0.25 mg/dose repeated in 15-30 minutes for one time only; a total dose of 0.5 mg should not be exceeded within a 4-hour period
Note: Continuous I.V. infusion has been used successfully in children with asthma; a 2-10 mcg/kg loading dose followed by an 0.08-0.4 mcg/kg/minute continuous infusion; depending upon the clinical response, the dosage may require titration in increments of 0.1-0.2 mcg/kg/minute every 30 minutes; doses as high as 6 mcg/kg/minute have been used.
Nebulization: Children and Adults: 0.01-0.03 mL/kg (1 mg = 1 mL using injection); minimum dose: 0.1 mL; maximum dose: 2.5 mL diluted with 1-2 mL NS, every 4-6 hours

Administration
Oral: May administer with or without food
(Continued)

Terbutaline *(Continued)*

Parenteral: May administer undiluted, direct I.V. over 5-10 minutes; for continuous infusion, dilute to a maximum concentration of 1 mg/mL

Monitoring Parameters Heart rate, blood pressure, respiratory rate, arterial or capillary blood gases (if applicable)

Dosage Forms

Injection, as sulfate: 1 mg/mL (1 mL)

Tablet, as sulfate: 2.5 mg, 5 mg

Extemporaneous Preparations A 1 mg/mL suspension made from terbutaline tablets in simple syrup NF is stable 30 days when refrigerated

Horner RK and Johnson CE, "Stability of An Extemporaneously Compounded Terbutaline Sulfate Oral Liquid," *Am J Hosp Pharm*, 1991, 48(2):293-5.

References

Bohn D, Kalloghlian A, Jenkins J, et al, "Intravenous Salbutamol in the Treatment of Status Asthmaticus in Children," *Crit Care Med*, 1984, 12(10):892-6.

Canny GJ and Levison H, "Aerosols - Therapeutic Use and Delivery in Childhood Asthma," *Ann Allergy*, 1988, 60(1):11-9.

Fuglsang G, Pedersen S, and Borgstrom L, "Dose-Response Relationships of I.V. Administered Terbutaline in Children With Asthma," *J Pediatr*, 1989, 114(2):315-20.

Goldenhersh N and Rachelefsky GS, "Childhood Asthma: Management," *Pediatr Rev*, 1989, 10(9):259-67.

Expert Panel Report 2, "Guidelines for the Diagnosis and Management of Asthma," *Clinical Practice Guidelines*, National Institutes of Health, National Heart, Lung, and Blood Institute, NIH Publication No. 94-4051, April, 1997.

Rachelefsky GS and Siegel SC, "Asthma in Infants and Children - Treatment of Childhood Asthma: Part II," *J Allergy Clin Immunol*, 1985, 76(3):409-25.

Tipton WR and Nelson HS, "Frequent Parenteral Terbutaline in the Treatment of Status Asthmaticus in Children," *Ann Allergy*, 1987, 58(4):252-6.

♦ **Tersa-Tar (Can)** *see* Coal Tar *on page 260*

♦ **TESPA** *see* Thiotepa *on page 954*

♦ **Testoderm®** *see* Testosterone *on page 938*

♦ **Testoderm® TTS** *see* Testosterone *on page 938*

♦ **Testoderm® with Adhesive** *see* Testosterone *on page 938*

♦ **Testopel®** *see* Testosterone *on page 938*

Testosterone *(tes TOS ter one)*

U.S. Brand Names Androderm®; AndroGel®; Delatestryl®; Depo®-Testosterone; Testoderm®; Testoderm® TTS; Testoderm® with Adhesive; Testopel®

Canadian Brand Names Andriol; Scheinpharm Testone-Cyp

Synonyms Aqueous Testosterone

Therapeutic Category Androgen

Generic Available Yes

Use Androgen replacement therapy in the treatment of delayed male puberty; male hypogonadism

Restrictions C-III

Pregnancy Risk Factor X

Contraindications Severe renal, hepatic, or cardiac disease; male patients with prostatic or breast cancer, hypercalcemia, pregnancy; hypersensitivity to testosterone or any component

Warnings May accelerate bone maturation without producing compensating gain in linear growth; perform radiographic examination of the hand and wrist every 6 months to determine the rate of bone maturation (when using in prepubertal children)

Precautions Use with caution in patients with hepatic, cardiac, or renal dysfunction

Adverse Reactions

Cardiovascular: Flushing, edema, hypertension, tachycardia

Central nervous system: Excitation, aggressive behavior, sleeplessness, anxiety, mental depression, headache, nervousness

Dermatologic: Acne, hirsutism, urticaria

Endocrine & metabolic: Gynecomastia, hypercalcemia, hypoglycemia, increased serum cholesterol, hyperlipemia, hyponatremia, increased or decreased libido

Gastrointestinal: Nausea, abdominal pain, diarrhea

Genitourinary: Epididymitis, priapism, bladder irritability

Hematologic: Leukopenia, suppression of clotting factors, polycythemia

Hepatic: Cholestatic hepatitis, peliosis hepatitis, hepatocellular carcinoma (high doses), elevated liver function tests

Local: Inflammation and itching at injection site

Neuromuscular & skeletal: Myalgia

Drug Interactions Cytochrome P-450 isoenzyme CYP3A3/4 and CYP3A5-7 substrate

Potentiates effects of oral anticoagulants; increases propranolol clearance

Mechanism of Action Principal endogenous androgen responsible for promoting the growth and development of the male sex organs and maintaining secondary sex characteristics in androgen-deficient males

Pharmacodynamics Duration of effect: Based upon the route of administration and the specific testosterone ester used; the cypionate and enanthate esters have the longest duration, up to 2-4 weeks after I.M. administration; pellets 3-4 months

Pharmacokinetics

Protein binding: 98%

Metabolism: Inactivation in liver

Half-life: 10-100 minutes

Elimination: 90% excreted in urine as metabolites

Usual Dosage

Children: I.M.:

Male hypogonadism:

Initiation of pubertal growth: 40-50 mg/m^2/dose (cypionate or enanthate ester) monthly until the growth rate falls to prepubertal levels

Terminal growth phase: 100 mg/m^2/dose (cypionate or enanthate ester) monthly until growth ceases

Maintenance virilizing dose: 100 mg/m^2/dose (cypionate or enanthate ester) twice monthly

Delayed puberty: 40-50 mg/m^2/dose monthly (cypionate or enanthate ester) for 6 months

Adults: Hypogonadism:

Testosterone or testosterone propionate: I.M.: 10-25 mg 2-3 times/week

Testosterone cypionate or enanthate:

I.M.: 50-400 mg every 2-4 weeks

Transdermal: 5-6 mg/day initially (use 4 mg/day if scrotal area cannot accommodate 6 mg/day system); adjust dosage in 3-4 weeks depending upon testosterone level

Testosterone pellets: S.C.: Dosage depends on the minimum daily requirements of testosterone propionate [each 25 mg testosterone propionate weekly equals 150 mg (2 pellets)]; usual dose (testosterone pellets): 150-450 mg (2-6 pellets) every 3 months

AndroGel®: Transdermal gel: Males >18 years: Initial: 5 g applied once daily (preferably in the morning); may increase as needed to a maximum of 10 g once daily

Adults: Postpubertal cryptorchism: Testosterone or testosterone propionate: I.M.: 10-25 mg 2-3 times/week

Administration

Parenteral: Administer deep I.M.; not for I.V. administration; pellets only are for S.C. administration

Topical: Apply Testoderm® or Testoderm® with Adhesive transdermal system to scrotum; apply Testoderm® TTS or Androderm® to skin on the arm back or upper buttocks; **do not** apply these two formulations (Testoderm® TTS and Androderm®) to the scrotum; skin should be clean and dry, scrotal hair should be dry-shaved; do not use chemical depilatories; apply transdermal system firmly for 10 seconds. If system should fall off <12 hours from initial application, it may be reapplied; if >12 hours, apply new system at the next scheduled time. Apply AndroGel® to clean, dry, intact skin of the shoulder and upper arms and/or abdomen. Upon opening the packet(s), the entire contents should be squeezed into the palm of the hand and immediately applied to the application site(s). Application sites should be allowed to dry for a few minutes prior to dressing. Hands should be washed with soap and water after application. **Do not apply AndroGel® to the genitals**

Monitoring Parameters Periodic liver function tests, radiologic examination of wrist and hand every 6 months (when using in prepubertal children); hemoglobin, hematocrit, testosterone level, serum electrolytes

Reference Range Testosterone, Urine:

Male: 100-1500 ng/24 hours

Female: 100-500 ng/24 hours

Nursing Implications 0.1% triamcinolone cream may be applied to skin under Androderm® to decrease irritation

Additional Information Testosterone 5% cream, not available commercially (must be compounded), has been effective in the treatment of microphallus when applied topically for 21 days

(Continued)

Testosterone *(Continued)*

Dosage Forms

Injection:

Aqueous suspension: 50 mg/mL (10 mL); 100 mg/mL (10 mL)

In oil, as cypionate (Depo®-Testosterone): 100 mg/mL (10 mL); 200 mg/mL (1 mL, 10 mL)

In oil, as enanthate (Delatestryl®): 200 mg/mL (1 mL, 5 mL, 10 mL)

In oil, as propionate: 100 mg/mL (10 mL)

Pellets, for subcutaneous implantation (Testopel®): 75 mg

Transdermal gel (AndroGel® 1%): 25 mg [2.5 g gel/packet] (30s); 50 mg (5 g gel/packet) (30s)

Transdermal system:

Androderm®: 2.5 mg/day (60s), 5 mg/day (60s)

Testoderm®: 4 mg/day (30s), 6 mg/day (30s)

Tesoderm® TTS: 5 mg/day (30s)

Testoderm® with Adhesive: 6 mg/day (30s)

♦ **Tetanus Immune Globulin, Human** *see page 1172*

♦ **Tetanus Toxoid, Adsorbed** *see page 1172*

♦ **Tetanus Toxoid, Fluid** *see page 1172*

Tetracaine (TET ra kane)

U.S. Brand Names AK-T-Caine™; Cepacol Viractin® [OTC]; Pontocaine®

Canadian Brand Names Ametop; Minims-Tetracaine

Synonyms Amethocaine

Therapeutic Category Analgesic, Topical; Local Anesthetic, Injectable; Local Anesthetic, Ophthalmic; Local Anesthetic, Oral; Local Anesthetic, Topical

Generic Available Yes

Use Local anesthesia in the eye for various diagnostic and examination purposes; spinal anesthesia; topical anesthesia for local skin disorders; local anesthesia for mucous membranes

Pregnancy Risk Factor C

Contraindications Hypersensitivity to tetracaine or any component; ophthalmic secondary bacterial infection, patients with liver disease; CNS disease, meningitis (if used for epidural or spinal anesthesia); myasthenia gravis, impaired cardiac conduction

Warnings Parenteral form may contain sulfites which may cause severe hypersensitivity reactions in sensitive individuals

Precautions Use with caution in patients with cardiac disease and hyperthyroidism

Adverse Reactions

Cardiovascular: Cardiac arrest, bradycardia, myocardial depression, cardiac arrhythmias, hypotension

Central nervous system: Anxiety, apprehension, nervousness, disorientation, seizures, drowsiness, unconsciousness

Dermatologic: Urticaria, contact dermatitis with topical form

Gastrointestinal: Nausea, vomiting

Local: Stinging, burning at injection site

Ocular: Lacrimation, photophobia, corneal epithelial erosion, keratitis, corneal opacification, miosis

Otic: Tinnitus

Respiratory: Respiratory arrest

Drug Interactions Inhibits sulfonamide activity; enhances CNS depression of other CNS depressants

Mechanism of Action Blocks both the generation and conduction of sensory, motor, and autonomic nerve fibers by decreasing the neuronal membrane's permeability to sodium ions, which results in decreasing the rate of depolarization of the nerve membrane

Pharmacodynamics

Onset of action:

Ophthalmic instillation: Anesthetic effects occur within 60 seconds

Topical: Within 3 minutes when applied to mucous membranes

Duration: 1.5-3 hours

Pharmacokinetics

Metabolism: By the liver

Elimination: Metabolites are renally excreted

Usual Dosage

Children: Safety and efficacy have not been established

Adults:

Cream: Apply to affected area as needed

Injection: Dosage varies with the anesthetic procedure, the degree of anesthesia required, and the individual patient response; it is administered by subarachnoid injection for spinal anesthesia:

Perineal anesthesia: 5 mg

Perineal and lower extremities: 10 mg

Anesthesia extending up to the costal margin: 15-20 mg

Low spinal anesthesia (saddle block): 2-5 mg

Ophthalmic: Solution: Instill 1-2 drops

Administration

Ophthalmic: Apply drops to conjunctiva of affected eye(s); avoid contact of bottle tip with skin or eye; finger pressure should be applied to lacrimal sac during and for 1-2 minutes after instillation to decrease risk of absorption and systemic reactions

Parenteral: Subarachnoid administration by experienced individuals only

Patient Information Do not touch or rub eye until anesthesia (if ophthalmic) has worn off

Nursing Implications Not for prolonged use topically

Dosage Forms

Gel, as hydrochloride (Cepacol Viractin®): 2% (7.1 g)

Injection, as hydrochloride (Pontocaine®): 1% [10 mg/mL] (2 mL)

Injection, as hydrochloride, with dextrose 6% (Pontocaine®): 0.3% [3 mg/mL] (5 mL)

Ointment, topical, as hydrochloride (Pontocaine®): 0.5% [5 mg/mL] (28 g)

Powder for injection, as hydrochloride (Pontocaine®): 20 mg

Solution, as hydrochloride:

Ophthalmic: 0.5% [5 mg/mL] (1 mL, 2 mL, 15 mL)

AK-T-Caine™: 0.5% (15 mL)

Pontocaine®: 0.5% (15 mL, 59 mL)

Topical (Pontocaine®): 2% [20 mg/mL] (30 mL, 118 mL)

♦ **Tetracap**® *see* Tetracycline *on page 941*

♦ **Tetracosactide** *see* Cosyntropin *on page 269*

Tetracycline (tet ra SYE kleen)

Related Information

Carbohydrate and Alcohol Content of Liquid Medications for Use in Patients Receiving Ketogenic Diets *on page 1258*

U.S. Brand Names Sumycin®; Tetracap®

Canadian Brand Names Apo-Tetra; Novo-Tetra; Nu-Tetra

Synonyms TCN

Therapeutic Category Acne Products; Antibiotic, Ophthalmic; Antibiotic, Tetracycline Derivative; Antibiotic, Topical

Generic Available Yes

Use

Children, Adolescents and Adults: Treatment of Rocky Mountain spotted fever caused by susceptible *Rickettsia* or brucellosis

Adolescents and Adults: Presumptive treatment of chlamydial infection in patients with gonorrhea

Children >8 years, Adolescents and Adults: Treatment of moderate to severe inflammatory acne vulgaris, Lyme disease, mycoplasmal disease or *Legionella*

Pregnancy Risk Factor D; B (topical)

Contraindications Hypersensitivity to tetracycline or any component; pregnancy; children ≤8 years; use of tetracyclines during tooth development may cause permanent discoloration of the teeth, enamel hypoplasia and retardation of skeletal development and bone growth with risk being greatest for children <4 years and in those receiving high doses

Warnings Photosensitivity reaction may occur with this drug; avoid prolonged exposure to sunlight or tanning equipment; prolonged use may result in superinfection

Precautions Use with caution in patients with renal and liver impairment; dosage modification required in patients with renal impairment

Adverse Reactions

Central nervous system: Pseudotumor cerebri, fever

Dermatologic: Rash, exfoliative dermatitis, photosensitivity, angioedema, discoloration of nails

Gastrointestinal: Nausea, vomiting, diarrhea, stomatitis, glossitis, antibiotic-associated pseudomembranous colitis, esophagitis, oral candidiasis

Hematologic: Hemolytic anemia

Hepatic: Hepatotoxicity

(Continued)

Tetracycline *(Continued)*

Neuromuscular & skeletal: Injury to growing bones and teeth
Renal: Renal damage, Fanconi-like syndrome
Respiratory: Pulmonary infiltrates with eosinophilia
Miscellaneous: Hypersensitivity reactions, candidal superinfection

Drug Interactions Calcium-, magnesium- or aluminum-containing antacids; iron, zinc; kaolin-, pectin-, or bismuth-containing antidiarrheals decrease tetracycline absorption. Tetracycline enhances the hypoprothrombinemic effect of warfarin; methoxyflurane increases chance of nephrotoxicity; concomitant use with isotretinoin has been associated with cases of pseudotumor cerebri

Food Interactions Tetracyclines decrease absorption of magnesium, zinc, calcium, dairy products, iron, and amino acids; calcium, dairy products, iron supplements decrease tetracycline absorption

Stability Protect from light; outdated tetracyclines have caused a Fanconi-like syndrome

Mechanism of Action Inhibits bacterial protein synthesis by binding to the 30S and possibly the 50S ribosomal subunit(s) of susceptible bacteria preventing additions of amino acids to the growing peptide chain; may also cause alterations in the cytoplasmic membrane

Pharmacokinetics

Distribution: Widely distributed to most body fluids and tissues including ascitic, synovial and pleural fluids; bronchial secretions; appears in breast milk; poor penetration into CSF

Absorption:
Oral: 75%
I.M.: Poor, with less than 60% of dose absorbed
Protein binding: 30% to 60%
Half-life: 6-12 hours with normal renal function and is prolonged with renal impairment
Time to peak serum concentration: Within 2-4 hours
Elimination: Primary route is the kidney, with 60% of a dose excreted as unchanged drug in urine, small amounts appear in bile
Dialysis: Slightly dialyzable (5% to 20%)

Usual Dosage

Children >8 years:
Oral: 25-50 mg/kg/day in divided doses every 6 hours; not to exceed 3 g/day
Ophthalmic:
Ointment: Apply every 2-12 hours
Suspension: Instill 1-2 drops 2-4 times/day
Adolescents and Adults:
Oral: 250-500 mg/dose every 6-12 hours
Ophthalmic:
Ointment: Apply every 2-12 hours
Suspension: Instill 1-2 drops 2-4 times/day
Topical:
Ointment: Apply small amount of ointment to cleansed area 2-3 times daily
Solution: Acne: Apply each morning and evening

Dosing adjustment in renal impairment:
Cl_{cr} 50-80 mL/minute: Administer every 8-12 hours
Cl_{cr} 10-50 mL/minute: Administer every 12-24 hours
Cl_{cr} <10 mL/minute: Administer every 24 hours

Administration

Oral: Administer 1 hour before or 2 hours after meals with adequate amounts of fluid; avoid taking antacids, calcium, iron, dairy products, or milk formulas within 3 hours of tetracyclines; shake suspension well before use

Ophthalmic: Avoid contact of tube or bottle tip with skin or eye; instill ointment or drops in the lower conjunctival sac; apply finger pressure to lacrimal sac during and for 1-2 minutes after instillation of drops to decrease risk of absorption and systemic effects; shake suspension well before use

Topical: Acne: Topical solution should be applied to cleansed affected area; reconstitute topical solution by inserting the plastic applicator unit containing the powder into the bottle containing the diluent; apply solution by tilting the bottle and rubbing applicator tip over the skin while gently applying pressure

Monitoring Parameters Renal, hepatic, and hematologic function tests

Test Interactions False-negative urine glucose with Clinistix®

Patient Information Avoid prolonged exposure to sunlight or sunlamps; may discolor nails

Dosage Forms
Capsule, as hydrochloride (Sumycin®, Tetracap®): 250 mg, 500 mg
Suspension, oral, as hydrochloride (Sumycin®): 125 mg/5 mL (480 mL)
Tablet, as hydrochloride (Sumycin®): 250 mg, 500 mg

References
American Academy of Pediatrics. Committee on Drugs. "Requiem for Tetracyclines," *Pediatrics*, 1975, 55(1):142-3.

- **Tetrahydrocannabinol** *see* Dronabinol *on page 364*
- **Texacort®** *see* Hydrocortisone *on page 506*
- **TG** *see* Thioguanine *on page 950*
- **6-TG** *see* Thioguanine *on page 950*
- **T/Gel® [OTC]** *see* Coal Tar *on page 260*
- **T-Gesic®** *see* Hydrocodone and Acetaminophen *on page 505*
- **Thalaris (Can)** *see* Sodium Chloride *on page 906*
- **THAM®** *see* Tromethamine *on page 990*
- **THC** *see* Dronabinol *on page 364*
- **Theo-24®** *see* Theophylline *on page 943*
- **Theochron®** *see* Theophylline *on page 943*
- **Theo-Dur®** *see* Theophylline *on page 943*
- **Theolair™** *see* Theophylline *on page 943*

Theophylline (thee OF i lin)

Related Information
Asthma Guidelines *on page 1210*
Blood Level Sampling Time Guidelines *on page 1220*
Carbohydrate and Alcohol Content of Liquid Medications for Use in Patients Receiving Ketogenic Diets *on page 1258*
Overdose and Toxicology *on page 1222*

U.S. Brand Names Aerolate III®; Aerolate® JR; Aerolate® SR; Elixophyllin®; Quibron®-T; Quibron®-T/SR; Slo-bid™; Slo-Phyllin®; Theo-24®; Theochron®; Theo-Dur®; Theolair™; T-Phyl®; Uni-Dur®; Uniphyl®

Canadian Brand Names Apo-Theo LA; Novo-Theophyl; Pulmophylline

Therapeutic Category Antiasthmatic; Bronchodilator; Respiratory Stimulant; Theophylline Derivative

Generic Available Yes

Use Treatment of symptoms and reversible airway obstruction due to chronic asthma, chronic bronchitis, or COPD; treatment of idiopathic apnea of prematurity in neonates

Pregnancy Risk Factor C

Contraindications Hypersensitivity to theophylline or any component

Warnings If a patient develops signs and symptoms of theophylline toxicity (eg, persistent, repetitive vomiting), a serum theophylline level should be measured and subsequent doses held; due to potential saturation of theophylline clearance at serum levels within or (in some patients) less than the therapeutic range, dosage adjustments should be made in small increments (maximum dosage adjustment: 25%); due to wide interpatient variability, theophylline serum level measurements must be used to optimize therapy and prevent serious toxicity

Precautions Use with caution in patients with peptic ulcer, hyperthyroidism, seizure disorders, hypertension, and patients with cardiac arrhythmias (excluding bradyarrhythmias)

Adverse Reactions See table.

Theophylline Serum Levels (μg/mL)*	Adverse Reactions
15-25	GI upset, GE reflux, diarrhea, nausea, vomiting, abdominal pain, nervousness, headache, insomnia, agitation, dizziness, muscle cramp, tremor
25-35	Tachycardia, occasional PVC
>35	Ventricular tachycardia, frequent PVC, seizure

*Adverse effects do not necessarily occur according to serum levels. Arrhythmia and seizure can occur without seeing the other adverse effects.

Drug Interactions Cytochrome P-450 isoenzyme CYP1A2, CYP2E1, and CYP3A3/4 substrate
(Continued)

Theophylline *(Continued)*

Decreases adenosine, esmolol, benzodiazepine, and pancuronium effects; increases lithium clearance; increases CNS side effects with ephedrine; increases risk of cardiac arrhythmias with halothane; decreases zafirlukast serum levels; for medications which alter theophylline clearance, see tables.

Clinical Factors Reported to Affect Theophylline Clearance

Decreased Theophylline Level	Increased Theophylline Level
Smoking (cigarettes, marijuana)	Acute pulmonary edema
High protein/low carbohydrate diet	Cessation of smoking (after chronic use)
Charcoal broiled beef	Cor pulmonale
	Congestive heart failure
	Hypothyroidism
	Fever (≥102° for 24 hours or more, or lesser temperature elevations for longer periods)
	Hepatic cirrhosis/acute hepatitis
	Renal failure in infants <3 mo of age
	Sepsis with multisystem organ failure
	Shock
	Viral illness

Medications Affecting Theophylline Clearance Resulting in Either Increased or Decreased Serum Levels

Decreased Theophylline Level	Increased Theophylline Level
Aminoglutethimide	Alcohol
Carbamazepine	Allopurinol (>600 mg/day)
Isoproterenol (I.V.)	Beta-blockers
Isoniazid*	Calcium channel blockers
Ketoconazole	Cimetidine
Loop diuretics*	Ciprofloxacin
Nevirapine	Clarithromycin
Phenobarbital	Corticosteroids
Phenytoin	Disulfiram
Rifampin	Ephedrine
Ritonavir	Erythromycin
Sulfinpyrazone	Esmolol
Sympathomimetics	Influenza virus vaccine
	Interferon, human recombinant alpha 2-a and 2-b
	Isoniazid*
	Loop diuretics*
	Methotrexate
	Mexiletine
	Oral contraceptives
	Propafenone
	Propranolol
	Tacrine
	Thiabendazole
	Thyroid hormones
	Troleandomycin (TAO®)
	Verapamil
	Zileuton

*Both increased and decreased theophylline levels have been reported.

Food Interactions Food does not appreciably affect the absorption of liquid, fast-release products and most sustained release products; however, food may induce a sudden release (dose-dumping) of once-daily sustained release products resulting in an increase in serum drug levels and potential toxicity; avoid excessive amounts of caffeine; avoid extremes of dietary protein and carbohydrate intake; limit char-coal-broiled foods and caffeinated beverages

Mechanism of Action Competitively inhibits two isoenzymes of the enzyme phosphodiesterase resulting in increased levels of cyclic adenine monophosphate (cAMP) which may be responsible for most of theophylline's effects; effects on the myocardium and neuromuscular transmission may be due to the intracellular translocation of ionized calcium; overall, theophylline produces the following effects:

relaxation of the smooth muscle of the respiratory tract, suppression of the response of airways to stimuli, increases the force of contraction of diaphragmatic muscles; pulmonary, coronary, and renal artery dilation; CNS stimulation, diuresis, stimulation of catecholamine release, gastric acid secretion, and relaxation of biliary and GI smooth muscle

Pharmacokinetics

Absorption: Oral: Rapid and complete with up to 100% absorption depending upon the formulation used

Distribution: V_d: 0.45 L/kg; distributes into breast milk; breast milk to plasma ratio: 0.67; crosses the placenta and into the CSF

Protein binding: 40%; decreased protein binding in neonates (due to a greater percentage of fetal albumin), hepatic cirrhosis, uncorrected acidemia, women in third trimester of pregnancy, and geriatric patients

Metabolism: In the liver by demethylation and oxidation; theophylline is metabolized to caffeine (active); in neonates this theophylline-derived caffeine accumulates (due to decreased hepatic metabolism) and significant concentrations of caffeine may occur; a substantial decrease in serum caffeine concentrations occurs after 40 weeks postconceptional age

Half-life: See table.

Theophylline Clearance and Half-Life With Respect to Age and Altered Physiological States*

Patient Group	Mean Clearance (mL/kg/min)	Mean Half-life (h)
Premature infants		
postnatal age 3-15 d	0.29	30
postnatal age 25-57 d	0.64	20
Term infants		
postnatal age 1-2 d	Not reported†	25
postnatal age 3-30 wk‡	Not reported†	11
Children		
1-4 y	1.7	3.4
4-12 y	1.6	Not reported†
13-15 y	0.9	Not reported†
16-17 y	1.4	3.7 (range: 1.5-5.9)
Adults		
16-60 (nonsmoking)	0.65	8.2
>60 y (nonsmoking, healthy)	0.41	9.8
Acute pulmonary edema	0.33	19
Cystic fibrosis (14-28 y)	1.25	6
Liver disease		
acute hepatitis	0.35	19.2
cholestasis	0.65	14.4
cirrhosis	0.31	32
Sepsis with multiorgan failure	0.46	18.8
Hypothyroid	0.38	11.6
Hyperthyroid	0.8	4.5
COPD >60 y, nonsmoking >1 y	0.54	11

*From Hendeles L, 1995

†Either not reported or not reported in a comparable format

‡Maturation of clearance in premature infants and term infants is most closely related to postconceptional age (PCA); adult clearance values are reached at approximately 55 weeks PCA and higher pediatric values at approximately 60 weeks PCA (Kraus, 1993).

Elimination: In urine; children >3 months and adults excrete 10% in urine as unchanged drug; neonates excrete approximately 50% of the dose unchanged in urine

Usual Dosage Oral (see Aminophylline *on page 69* for I.V. doses):

Loading dose:

Neonates: Apnea of prematurity: 4 mg/kg/dose
(Continued)

945

Theophylline *(Continued)*

Infants and Children: Treatment of acute bronchospasm: (to achieve a serum level of about 10 mcg/mL; loading doses should be given using a rapidly absorbed oral product **not** a sustained release product):

If no theophylline has been administered in the previous 24 hours: 5 mg/kg theophylline

If theophylline has been administered in the previous 24 hours: 2.5 mg/kg theophylline may be given in emergencies when serum levels are not available

A modified loading dose (mg/kg) may be calculated (when the serum level is known) by: [Blood level desired - blood level measured] divided by 2 (for every 1 mg/kg theophylline given, the blood level will rise by approximately 2 mcg/mL)

Maintenance dose: See table.

Maintenance Dose for Acute Symptoms

Population Group	Oral Theophylline (mg/kg/day)
Premature infant or newborn to 6 wk (for apnea/bradycardia)	4*
6 wk to 6 mo	10*
Infants 6 mo to 1 y	12-18*
Children 1-9 y	20-24
Children 9-12 y, adolescent daily smokers of cigarettes or marijuana, and otherwise healthy adult smokers <50 y	16
Adolescents 12-16 y (nonsmokers)	13
Otherwise healthy nonsmoking adults (including elderly patients)	10 (not to exceed 900 mg/day)
Cardiac decompensation, cor pulmonale, and/ or liver dysfunction	5 (not to exceed 400 mg/day)
*Alternative dosing regimen for full-term infants <1 year of age: Total daily dose (mg) = [(0.2 x age in weeks) + 5] x weight (kg) Postnatal Age <26 weeks: Total daily dose divided every 8 hours Postnatal Age >26 weeks: Total daily dose divided every 6 hours	

These recommendations, based on mean clearance rates for age or risk factors, were calculated to achieve a serum level of 10 mcg/mL (5 mcg/mL for newborns with apnea/bradycardia). In newborns and infants, a fast-release oral product can be used. The total daily dose can be divided every 12 hours in newborns and every 6-8 hours in infants. In children and healthy adults, a slow-release product can be used. The total daily dose can be divided every 8-12 hours.

Use ideal body weight for obese patients

Dose should be further adjusted based on serum levels. Guidelines for drawing theophylline serum levels are shown in the table.

Guidelines for Drawing Theophylline Serum Levels

Dosage Form	Time to Draw Level*
I.V. bolus	30 min after end of 30-min infusion
I.V. continuous infusion	12-24 h after initiation of infusion
P.O. liquid, fast-release formulation	Peak: 1 h postdose after at least 1 day of therapy Trough: Just before a dose after at least 1 day of therapy

*The time to achieve steady-state serum levels is prolonged in patients with longer half-lives (eg, premature neonates, infants, and adults with cardiac or liver failure (see theophylline half-life table). In these patients, serum theophylline levels should be drawn after 48-72 hours of therapy; serum levels may need to be done prior to steady-state to assess the patient's current progress or evaluate potential toxicity.

Administration

Oral: Sustained release preparations should be administered with a full glass of water, whole or cut by half only; do not crush; sustained release capsule forms may be opened and sprinkled on soft foods; do not chew or crush beads

Parenteral: Premade I.V. infusion bags for continuous infusion usage; rate of infusion dependent upon dosage; loading doses using I.V. infusion should be administered over 20-30 minutes

Monitoring Parameters Respiratory rate, heart rate, serum theophylline level, arterial or capillary blood gases (if applicable); number and severity of apnea spells (apnea of prematurity)

Reference Range
Therapeutic levels:
Asthma: 10-15 µg/mL (peak level)
Apnea of prematurity: 6-14 µg/mL
Toxic concentration: >20 µg/mL

Test Interactions May elevate uric acid levels

Patient Information Contact physician whenever nausea, vomiting, persistent headache, or irregular heartbeats occur; notify physician if a new illness develops (especially if high fevers); do not alter time, dose, or frequency of administration without physician knowledge; avoid drinking or eating of large quantities of caffeine-containing beverages or food

Additional Information Due to improved theophylline clearance during the first year of life, serum concentration determinations and dosage adjustments may be needed to optimize therapy

Dosage Forms
Capsule:
Timed release: 100 mg, 125 mg, 200 mg, 300 mg **[12 hours]**
Aerolate®: 65 mg [III]; 130 mg [JR], 260 mg [SR] **[8-12 hours]**
Slo-bid™: 50 mg, 75 mg, 100 mg, 125 mg, 200 mg, 300 mg **[8-12 hours]**
Theo-24®: 100 mg, 200 mg, 300 mg, 400 mg **[24 hours]**
Elixir (Elixophyllin®): 80 mg/15 mL (480 mL, 4000 mL)
Infusion, in D_5W:
200 mg [4 mg/mL] (50 mL), [2 mg/mL] (100 mL)
400 mg [4 mg/mL] (100 mL), [1.6 mg/mL] (250 mL), [0.8 mg/mL] (500 mL)
800 mg [3.2 mg/mL] (250 mL), [1.6 mg/mL] (500 mL), [0.8 mg/mL] (1000 mL)
Solution, oral: 80 mg/15 mL (15 mL, 18.75 mL)
Syrup (Slo-Phyllin®) [alcohol free, sugar free]: 80 mg/15 mL (500 mL)
Tablet, immediate release:
Quibron®-T: 300 mg
Slo-Phyllin®: 200 mg
Theolair™: 125 mg, 250 mg
Tablet, timed release: 100 mg, 200 mg, 300 mg, 450 mg **[12-24 hours]**
Quibron®-T/SR: 300 mg **[8-12 hours]**
Theochron®: 100 mg, 200 mg, 300 mg **[12-24 hours]**
Theo-Dur®: 100 mg, 200 mg, 300 mg, 450 mg **[8-24 hours]**
Theolair-SR®: 300 mg, 500 mg **[8-24 hours]**
T-Phyl®: 200 mg **[8-12 hours]**
Uni-Dur®: 400 mg, 600 mg **[24 hours]**
Uniphyl®: 400 mg, 600 mg **[24 hours]**

References
Hendeles L, Jenkins J, and Temple R, "Revised FDA Labeling Guideline for Theophylline Oral Dosage Forms," *Pharmacotherapy*, 1995, 15(4):409-427.
Kearney TE, Manoguerra AS, Curtis GP, et al, "Theophylline Toxicity and the Beta-Adrenergic System," *Ann Intern Med*, 1985, 102(6):766-9.
Kraus DM, Fischer JH, Reitz SJ, et al, "Alterations in Theophylline Metabolism During the First Year of Life," *Clin Pharmacol Ther*, 1993, 54(4):351-9.
Upton RA, "Pharmacokinetic Interactions Between Theophylline and Other Medication (Part I)," *Clin Pharmacokinet*, 1991, 20(1):66-80.

♦ **Theophylline Ethylenediamine** *see Aminophylline on page 69*

♦ **Thera-Flur®** *see Fluoride on page 441*

♦ **Thera-Flur-N®** *see Fluoride on page 441*

♦ **Thermazene®** *see Silver Sulfadiazine on page 901*

♦ **Theroxide® Wash [OTC]** *see Benzoyl Peroxide on page 136*

Thiabendazole (thye a BEN da zole)

U.S. Brand Names Mintezol®

Synonyms Tiabendazole

Therapeutic Category Anthelmintic

Generic Available No

Use Treatment of strongyloidiasis, cutaneous larva migrans, visceral larva migrans, dracunculosis, trichinosis, and mixed helminthic infections

Pregnancy Risk Factor C

Contraindications Hypersensitivity to thiabendazole or any component; pregnancy
(Continued)

Thiabendazole (Continued)

Precautions Use with caution in patients with renal or hepatic impairment, malnutrition, anemia, or dehydration

Adverse Reactions

Cardiovascular: Flushing, hypotension, bradycardia

Central nervous system: Dizziness, drowsiness, vertigo, seizures, fever, malaise, headache, chills, hallucinations

Dermatologic: Rash, Stevens-Johnson syndrome, erythema multiforme, pruritus

Endocrine & metabolic: Hyperglycemia

Gastrointestinal: Nausea, vomiting, diarrhea, anorexia

Genitourinary: Malodor of the urine

Hematologic: Leukopenia

Hepatic: Hepatotoxicity, jaundice, cholestasis

Neuromuscular & skeletal: Paresthesia, numbness

Ocular: Blurred vision

Otic: Tinnitus

Renal: Nephrotoxicity, hematuria

Miscellaneous: Hypersensitivity reactions, lymphadenopathy

Drug Interactions Increases serum theophylline concentrations (monitor serum theophylline level in patients receiving both drugs concomitantly)

Mechanism of Action Inhibits helminth-specific mitochondrial fumarate reductase

Pharmacokinetics

Absorption: From the GI tract and through the skin

Metabolism: Extensive in the liver via hydroxylation and conjugation with sulfuric and/or glucuronic acid

Time to peak serum concentration: Within 1-2 hours

Elimination: In feces (5%) and urine (87%), primarily as conjugated metabolites

Usual Dosage

Oral:

Children and Adults: 50 mg/kg/day divided every 12 hours (maximum dose: 3 g/day)

Strongyloidiasis: For 2 consecutive days (5 days or longer for disseminated disease)

Cutaneous larva migrans: For 2-5 consecutive days

Visceral larva migrans: For 5-7 consecutive days

Trichinosis: For 2-4 consecutive days

Angiostrongylosis: 50-75 mg/kg/day divided every 8-12 hours for 3 days

Dracunculosis: 50-75 mg/kg/day divided every 12 hours for 3 days

Topical: Cutaneous larva migrans: Instead of oral therapy, thiabendazole 10% to 15% suspension or a 10% ointment in white petrolatum has been applied topically to lesions 4-6 times/day

Administration Oral: Administer after meals; chew tablet well before swallowing; shake suspension well before use

Monitoring Parameters Periodic renal and hepatic function tests, serum glucose

Patient Information May cause drowsiness and impair ability to perform activities requiring mental alertness or physical coordination; avoid driving or operating machinery

Nursing Implications Purgation is not required prior to use

Dosage Forms

Suspension, oral: 500 mg/5 mL (120 mL)

Tablet, chewable: 500 mg [orange flavor]

References

Walden J, "Parasitic Diseases. Other Roundworms. *Trichuris*, Hookworm, and *Strongyloides*," *Prim Care*, 1991, 18(1):53-74.

Zygmunt DJ, "*Strongyloides stearcoralis*," *Infect Control Hosp Epidemiol*, 1990, 11(9):495-7.

♦ **Thiamazole** *see* Methimazole *on page 644*

♦ **Thiamilate® [OTC]** *see* Thiamine *on page 948*

Thiamine (THYE a min)

U.S. Brand Names Thiamilate® [OTC]

Canadian Brand Names Betaxin

Synonyms Aneurine; Thiaminium; Vitamin B_1

Therapeutic Category Nutritional Supplement; Vitamin, Water Soluble

Generic Available Yes

Use Treatment of thiamine deficiency including beriberi, Wernicke's encephalopathy syndrome, and peripheral neuritis associated with pellagra; alcoholic patients with altered sensorium; various genetic metabolic disorders

Pregnancy Risk Factor A (C if dose exceeds RDA recommendation)
Contraindications Hypersensitivity to thiamine or any component
Warnings Large doses should be given in divided doses for better oral absorption
Precautions Use parenteral route cautiously, see Adverse Reactions
Adverse Reactions
  Cardiovascular: Cardiovascular collapse and death (primarily following repeated I.V. administration), warmth
  Dermatologic: Rash, angioedema
  Genitourinary: Discoloration of urine (bright yellow) with large doses
  Neuromuscular & skeletal: Paresthesia
Drug Interactions I.V. dextrose solutions increase thiamine requirement; thiamine may enhance the effects of neuromuscular blocking agents
Food Interactions High carbohydrate diets may increase thiamine requirement
Stability Unstable with alkaline or neutral solutions
Mechanism of Action An essential coenzyme in carbohydrate metabolism; combines with adenosine triphosphate to form thiamine pyrophosphate
Pharmacokinetics
  Absorption:
    Oral: Poor
    I.M.: Rapid and complete
  Metabolism: In the liver
  Elimination: Renally as unchanged drug only after body storage sites become saturated
Usual Dosage
  Adequate intake: Infants:
    <6 months: 0.2 mg (0.03 mg/kg)
    6-12 months: 0.3 mg (0.03 mg/kg)
  Recommended daily allowance (RDA):
    1-3 years: 0.5 mg
    4-8 years: 0.6 mg
    9-13 years: 0.9 mg
    14-18 years:
      Male: 1.2 mg
      Female: 1 mg
    ≥19 years:
      Male: 1.2 mg
      Female: 1.1 mg
  Dietary supplement (depends on caloric or carbohydrate content of the diet)
    Oral:
      Infants: 0.3-0.5 mg/day
      Children: 0.5-1 mg/day
      Adults: 1-2 mg/day
    Note: The above doses can be found in multivitamin preparations
  Thiamine deficiency (beriberi):
    Children: 10-25 mg/dose I.M. or I.V. daily (if critically ill), or 10-50 mg/dose orally every day for 2 weeks, then 5-10 mg/dose orally daily for 1 month
    Adults: 5-30 mg/dose I.M. or I.V. 3 times/day (if critically ill); then orally 5-30 mg/day in single or divided doses 3 times/day for 1 month
  Wernicke's encephalopathy: Adults: Initial: 100 mg I.V., then 50-100 mg/day I.M. or I.V. until consuming a regular, balanced diet
  Metabolic disorders: Oral: Adults: 10-20 mg/day (dosages up to 4 g/day in divided doses have been used)
Administration
  Oral: May administer with or without food
  Parenteral: Administer by slow I.V. injection or I.M.
Reference Range Normal values: 1.6-4 mg/dL
Test Interactions False-positive for uric acid using the phosphotungstate method and for urobilinogen using the Ehrlich's reagent; large doses may interfere with the spectrophotometric determination of serum theophylline concentration
Patient Information May color urine bright yellow
Additional Information Dietary sources include legumes, pork, beef, whole grains, yeast, fresh vegetables; a deficiency state can occur in as little as 3 weeks following total dietary absence
Dosage Forms
  Injection, as hydrochloride: 100 mg/mL (1 mL, 2 mL, 30 mL)
  Tablet, as hydrochloride: 25 mg, 50 mg, 100 mg, 250 mg, 500 mg
  Tablet, enteric coated, as hydrochloride (Thiamilate®): 20 mg

♦ **Thiaminium** see Thiamine on page 948

Thiethylperazine (thye eth il PER a zeen)

Related Information

Overdose and Toxicology *on page 1222*

U.S. Brand Names Torecan®

Therapeutic Category Antiemetic; Phenothiazine Derivative

Generic Available No

Use Relief of nausea and vomiting

Pregnancy Risk Factor X

Contraindications Severe CNS depression, comatose states; hypersensitivity to thiethylperazine or any component; pregnancy

Warnings Safety and efficacy in children <12 years of age have not been established; postural hypotension may occur after I.M. injection; the injectable form contains sulfite which may cause allergic reactions in sensitive individuals; tablet contains yellow No.5 (tartrazine) which may cause allergic reactions in sensitive individuals; avoid use in children and adolescents whose signs and symptoms are suggestive of Reye's syndrome

Adverse Reactions

Cardiovascular: Hypotension, peripheral edema

Central nervous system: Drowsiness, extrapyramidal effects, seizures, fever, headache, neuroleptic malignant syndrome

Gastrointestinal: Xerostomia

Hepatic: Cholestatic jaundice (occasional)

Neuromuscular & skeletal: Trigeminal neuralgia

Ocular: Blurred vision

Respiratory: Dryness of mucous membranes

Drug Interactions Additive effects with anticholinergic agents and other phenothiazines; additive CNS depression with sedatives and antihistamines

Mechanism of Action Blocks postsynaptic mesolimbic dopaminergic receptors in the brain including the medullary chemoreceptor trigger zone; exhibits a strong alpha-adrenergic blocking effect and depresses the release of hypothalamic and hypophyseal hormones

Pharmacodynamics

Onset of action: Oral, I.M.: Antiemetic effects occur within 30 minutes

Duration: ~4 hours

Usual Dosage Children >12 years and Adults: Oral, I.M.: 10 mg 1-3 times/day as needed

Administration Parenteral: Inject I.M. deeply into large muscle mass, patient should be lying down and remain so for at least 1 hour; I.V. and S.C. routes of administration are not recommended

Patient Information Causes drowsiness and may impair ability to perform hazardous tasks requiring mental alertness or physical coordination; may cause photosensitivity; avoid excessive sunlight

Dosage Forms

Injection, as maleate: 5 mg/mL (2 mL)

Tablet, as maleate: 10 mg

Thioguanine (thye oh GWAH neen)

Related Information

Emetogenic Potential of Single Chemotherapeutic Agents *on page 1129*

Canadian Brand Names Lanvis

Synonyms 2-Amino-6-mercaptopurine; TG; 6-TG; 6-Thioguanine; Tioguanine

Therapeutic Category Antineoplastic Agent, Antimetabolite

Generic Available No

Use Remission induction in acute myelogenous (nonlymphocytic) leukemia; treatment of chronic myelogenous leukemia and acute lymphocytic leukemia

Pregnancy Risk Factor D

Contraindications History of previous therapy resistance with thioguanine and in patients resistant to mercaptopurine; hypersensitivity to thioguanine or any component

Warnings The FDA currently recommends that procedures for proper handling and disposal of antineoplastic agents be considered; thioguanine is potentially carcinogenic and teratogenic

Precautions Use with caution and reduce dose of thioguanine in patients with renal or hepatic impairment

Adverse Reactions

Central nervous system: Neurotoxicity

Dermatologic: Skin rash, photosensitivity, staining of skin or eyes (yellow)

Endocrine & metabolic: Hyperuricemia

Gastrointestinal: Mild nausea or vomiting, anorexia, stomatitis, diarrhea

Hematologic: Myelosuppression (leukopenia, thrombocytopenia, anemia)

Hepatic: Hepatitis, jaundice, veno-occlusive hepatic disease

Neuromuscular & skeletal: Unsteady gait

Drug Interactions Busulfan (increases busulfan toxicity)

Food Interactions Enhanced absorption if administered between meals

Mechanism of Action Purine analog that is incorporated into DNA and RNA resulting in the inhibition of synthesis and utilization of purine nucleotides

Pharmacokinetics

Absorption: Oral: 30% (variable and incomplete)

Distribution: Crosses the placenta; does not appear to cross into CSF

Metabolism: Rapid and extensive hepatic metabolism by methylation of thioguanine to 2-amino-6-methylthioguanine (active) and inactive compounds

Half-life, terminal: 11 hours

Time to peak serum concentration: Within 8-12 hours

Elimination: Metabolites excreted in urine

Usual Dosage Oral (refer to individual protocols):

Infants <3 years: Combination drug therapy for ANLL: 3.3 mg/kg/day in divided doses twice daily for 4 days

Children and Adults:

Single agent chemotherapy for ANLL: 2-3 mg/kg/day once daily calculated to nearest 20 mg

Induction of remission in patients with acute leukemia (combination therapy): 75-200 mg/m^2/day in 1-2 divided doses for 5-7 days or until remission is attained

Administration Oral: Administer between meals on an empty stomach

Monitoring Parameters CBC with (differential, platelet count), liver function tests, hemoglobin, hematocrit, serum uric acid

Patient Information Notify physician if fever, sore throat, bleeding, bruising, yellow discoloration of skin or eyes, or leg swelling occurs; avoid prolonged exposure to sunlight

Nursing Implications Ensure adequate patient hydration, alkalinization of the urine, and/or administration of allopurinol to prevent hyperuricemia

Additional Information Myelosuppressive effects:

WBC: Moderate

Platelets: Moderate

Onset (days): 7-10

Nadir (days): 14

Recovery (days): 21

Dosage Forms Tablet, scored: 40 mg

Extemporaneous Preparations A 40 mg/mL oral suspension compounded from tablets which were crushed, mixed with a volume of Cologel® suspending agent equal to 1/3 the final volume, and brought to the final volume with a 2:1 mixture of simple syrup and cherry syrup was stable for 84 days when stored in an amber bottle at room temperature

Dressman JB and Poust RI, "Stability of Allopurinol and Five Antineoplastics in Suspension," *Am J Hosp Pharm*, 1983, 40:616-8.

References

Culbert SJ, Shuster JJ, Land VJ, et al, "Remission Induction and Continuation Therapy in Children With Their First Relapse of Acute Lymphoid Leukemia: A Pediatric Oncology Group Study," *Cancer*, 1991, 67(1):37-42.

Steuber CP, Civin C, Krischer J, et al, "A Comparison of Induction and Maintenance Therapy for Acute Nonlymphocytic Leukemia in Childhood: Results of a Pediatric Oncology Group Study," *J Clin Oncol*, 1991, 9(2):247-58.

♦ **6-Thioguanine** *see* Thioguanine *on page 950*

Thiopental (thye oh PEN tal)

Related Information

Preprocedure Sedatives in Children *on page 1201*

U.S. Brand Names Pentothal®

Therapeutic Category Anticonvulsant, Barbiturate; Barbiturate; General Anesthetic; Hypnotic; Sedative

Generic Available Yes

Use Induction of anesthesia; adjunct for intubation in head injury patients; control of convulsive states; treatment of elevated intracranial pressure

Restrictions C-III

Pregnancy Risk Factor C

(Continued)

Thiopental *(Continued)*

Contraindications Porphyria (variegate or acute intermittent); hypersensitivity to thiopental, pentobarbital, any component, or other barbiturates

Precautions Use with caution in patients with asthma or pharyngeal infections because cough, laryngospasm, or bronchospasms may occur; use with caution in patients with hypotension, severe cardiovascular disease, hepatic or renal dysfunction; avoid extravasation or intra-arterial injection which may cause necrosis due to pH of 10.6; ensure patient has intravenous access

Adverse Reactions
Cardiovascular: Decreased cardiac output, hypotension
Local: Necrosis with I.V. extravasation
Renal: Decreased urine output
Respiratory: Cough, laryngospasm, bronchospasm, respiratory depression, apnea
Miscellaneous: Anaphylaxis

Drug Interactions Barbiturates are enzyme inducers (monitor patients closely for decreased effect of concomitantly administered medications or increased effect when barbiturates are discontinued); CNS depressants

Stability Solutions are alkaline and incompatible with drugs with acidic pH, such as succinylcholine, atropine sulfate

Mechanism of Action Ultra-short-acting barbiturate; depresses CNS activity by binding to barbiturate site at GABA-receptor complex enhancing GABA activity; depresses reticular activating system; higher doses may be gabamimetic

Pharmacodynamics Anesthesia effects:
Onset of action: I.V.: 30-60 seconds
Duration: 5-30 minutes

Pharmacokinetics
Distribution: V_d: Adults: 1.4 L/kg
Protein binding: 72% to 86%
Metabolism: In the liver primarily to inactive metabolites but pentobarbital is also formed
Half-life, adults: 3-11.5 hours (shorter half-life in children)

Usual Dosage
Induction anesthesia: I.V.:
Neonates: 3-4 mg/kg
Infants: 5-8 mg/kg
Children 1-12 years: 5-6 mg/kg
Children >12 years and Adults: 3-5 mg/kg
Maintenance anesthesia: I.V.:
Children: 1 mg/kg as needed
Adults: 25-100 mg as needed
Increased intracranial pressure: Children: I.V.: 1.5-5 mg/kg/dose; repeat as needed to control intracranial pressure; larger doses (30 mg/kg) to induce coma after hypoxic-ischemic injury do not appear to improve neurologic outcome
Seizures: I.V.:
Children: 2-3 mg/kg/dose, repeat as needed
Adults: 75-250 mg/dose, repeat as needed
Sedation: Rectal:
Children: 5-10 mg/kg/dose
Adults: 3-4 g/dose

Administration Parenteral: Avoid rapid I.V. injection (may cause hypotension or decreased cardiac output); may administer by intermittent infusion over 10-60 minutes at a maximum concentration of 50 mg/mL

Monitoring Parameters Respiratory rate, heart rate, blood pressure

Reference Range
Therapeutic:
Hypnotic: 1-5 µg/mL (SI: 4.1-20.7 µmol/L)
Coma: 30-100 µg/mL (SI: 124-413 µmol/L)
Anesthesia: 7-130 µg/mL (SI: 29-536 µmol/L)

Nursing Implications Avoid extravasation, necrosis may occur

Additional Information Accumulation may occur with chronic dosing due to lipid solubility; prolonged recovery occurs due to redistribution of thiopental from fat stores; therefore, thiopental is usually not used for procedures lasting >15-20 minutes; sodium content, injection: 4.9 mEq/g

Dosage Forms Powder for injection, as sodium: 250 mg, 400 mg, 500 mg, 1 g, 2.5 g, 5 g

♦ **Thioplex®** *see Thiotepa on page 954*

Thioridazine (thye oh RID a zeen)

Related Information

Overdose and Toxicology *on page 1222*

U.S. Brand Names Mellaril®; Mellaril-S®

Canadian Brand Names Apo-Thioridazine; Novo-Ridazine; PMS-Thioridazine

Therapeutic Category Antipsychotic Agent; Phenothiazine Derivative

Generic Available Yes

Use Due to prolongation of the QT_c interval (see Warnings), thioridazine is currently indicated only for the treatment of refractory schizophrenic patients; in the past, the drug had been used for management of psychotic disorders; depressive neurosis; dementia in elderly; severe behavioral problems in children

Pregnancy Risk Factor C

Contraindications Concurrent therapy with propranolol, pindolol, fluvoxamine, fluoxetine, paroxetine, drugs that inhibit cytochrome P-450 isoenzyme CYP2D6, drugs that prolong the QT_c interval, and patients with reduced levels of CYP2D6, a history of cardiac arrhythmias, congenital long QT syndrome, or a $Q-T_c$ interval >450 msec (adults); severe CNS depression; hypersensitivity to thioridazine or any component; cross-sensitivity to other phenothiazines may exist; avoid use in patients with narrow-angle glaucoma, blood dyscrasias, severe liver or cardiac disease

Warnings Prolongation of the QT_c interval may occur and may be associated with torsade de pointes arrhythmias and sudden death

Precautions Use with caution in patients with severe cardiovascular disorder or seizures

Adverse Reactions Sedation and anticholinergic effects are more pronounced than extrapyramidal effects; EKG changes and retinal pigmentation are more common than with chlorpromazine

Cardiovascular: Hypotension, orthostatic hypotension, tachycardia, arrhythmias

Central nervous system: Sedation, drowsiness, restlessness, anxiety, extrapyramidal reactions, pseudoparkinsonian signs and symptoms, tardive dyskinesia, neuroleptic malignant syndrome, seizures, altered central temperature regulation

Dermatologic: Hyperpigmentation, pruritus, rash, contact dermatitis, photosensitivity (rare)

Endocrine & metabolic: Amenorrhea, galactorrhea, gynecomastia

Gastrointestinal: GI upset, xerostomia, constipation, weight gain

Genitourinary: Urinary retention

Hematologic: Agranulocytosis, leukopenia (usually in patients with large doses for prolonged periods)

Hepatic: Cholestatic jaundice

Ocular: Retinal pigmentation (usually in patients receiving larger than recommended doses), blurred vision, brownish coloring of vision, decreased night vision, decreased visual acuity (may be irreversible)

Miscellaneous: Anaphylactoid reactions

Drug Interactions Cytochrome P-450 isoenzyme CYP1A2 and CYP2D6 substrate; CYP2D6 isoenzyme inhibitor

Additive effects with alcohol and other CNS depressants; concurrent use with lithium has caused acute encephalopathy-like syndrome (rare); increased cardiac arrhythmias with tricyclic antidepressants; epinephrine may cause hypotension; drugs that inhibit the metabolism of thioridazone (eg, fluoxetine, paroxetine) or drugs that prolong the QT_c interval may increase the risk of serious adverse effects, such as QT_c prolongation, serious ventricular arrhythmias (eg, torsade de pointes) and sudden death (such drugs are contraindicated; see Contraindications); mixing liquid thioridazine with carbamazepine suspension will result in precipitation of an orange rubbery mass (see also Contraindications)

Food Interactions May increase dietary requirements for riboflavin; liquid thioridazine formulations may precipitate with enteral formulas

Mechanism of Action Blocks postsynaptic mesolimbic dopaminergic receptors in the brain; exhibits a strong alpha-adrenergic blocking effect and depresses the release of hypothalamic and hypophyseal hormones

Pharmacokinetics

Protein binding: 99%

Metabolism: In the liver to active and inactive metabolites

Bioavailability: 25% to 33%

Half-life: Adults: 9-30 hours

Dialyzable: Not dialyzable: (0% to 5%)

Usual Dosage Oral:

Children >2 years: Initial: 0.5 mg/kg/day in 2-3 divided doses; range: 0.5-3 mg/kg/day; usual: 1 mg/kg/day in 2-3 divided doses; maximum dose: 3 mg/kg/day

(Continued)

Thioridazine *(Continued)*

Behavior problems: Initial: 10 mg 2-3 times/day, increase gradually

Severe psychoses: Initial: 25 mg 2-3 times/day, increase gradually

Children >12 years and Adults:

Psychoses: Initial: 25-100 mg 3 times/day with gradual increments as needed and tolerated; maximum daily dose: 800 mg/day in 2-4 divided doses; maintenance: 10-200 mg/dose 2-4 times/day

Depressive disorders, dementia: Initial: 25 mg 3 times/day; maintenance dose: 20-200 mg/day

Administration Oral: Administer with water, food, or milk to decrease GI upset; dilute the oral concentrate with water or juice before administration; do not administer liquid thioridazine simultaneously with carbamazepine suspension (see Drug Interactions); do not mix liquid thioridazine with enteric formulas (see Food Interactions)

Monitoring Parameters Baseline and periodic EKG and serum potassium; periodic eye exam, CBC with differential, blood pressure, liver enzyme tests

Test Interactions False-positives for phenylketonuria, urinary amylase, uroporphyrins, urobilinogen

Patient Information Avoid alcohol; may cause drowsiness and impair ability to perform activities requiring mental alertness or physical coordination; may cause dry mouth; avoid skin contact with oral suspension or solution, may cause contact dermatitis; rarely causes photosensitivity, avoid excess sun exposure, use sunscreen; do not discontinue or alter dose without physician approval

Additional Information In cases of overdoses, cardiovascular monitoring and continuous EKG monitoring should be performed; avoid drugs (such as quinidine, disopyramide, and procainamide) that may further prolong the QT interval

Dosage Forms

Concentrate, oral, as hydrochloride (Mellaril®): 30 mg/mL [contains 3% alcohol] (120 mL); 100 mg/mL [contains 4.2% alcohol] (3.4 mL, 120 mL)

Suspension, oral, as hydrochloride (Mellaril-S®): 5 mg/mL [buttermint flavor] (480 mL); 20 mg/mL [buttermint flavor] (480 mL)

Tablet, as hydrochloride (Mellaril®): 10 mg, 15 mg, 25 mg, 50 mg, 100 mg, 150 mg, 200 mg

References

Aman MG, Marks RE, Turbott SH, et al, "Clinical Effects of Methylphenidate and Thioridazine in Intellectually Subaverage Children," *J Am Acad Child Adolesc Psychiatry*, 1991, 30(2):246-56.

♦ **Thiosulfuric Acid** *see* Sodium Thiosulfate *on page 909*

Thiotepa *(thye oh TEP a)*

Related Information

Emetogenic Potential of Single Chemotherapeutic Agents *on page 1129*

U.S. Brand Names Thioplex®

Synonyms TESPA; Triethylenethiophosphoramide; TSPA

Therapeutic Category Antineoplastic Agent, Alkylating Agent

Generic Available No

Use Treatment of superficial tumors of the bladder; palliative treatment of adenocarcinoma of breast or ovary; lymphomas and sarcomas; meningeal neoplasms; control of pleural, pericardial or peritoneal effusions caused by metastatic tumors; high-dose regimens with autologous bone marrow transplantation

Pregnancy Risk Factor D

Contraindications Hypersensitivity to thiotepa or any component; severe myelosuppression with leukocyte count <3000/mm^3 or platelet count <150,000 mm^3; pregnancy

Warnings The FDA currently recommends that procedures for proper handling and disposal of antineoplastic agents be considered. The drug is potentially mutagenic, carcinogenic, teratogenic, and may cause fertility impairment.

Precautions Reduce dosage in patients with hepatic, renal, or bone marrow dysfunction

Adverse Reactions

Central nervous system: Dizziness, fever, headache, confusion, somnolence

Dermatologic: Alopecia, rash, pruritus, hyperpigmentation of skin with high-dose therapy

Endocrine & metabolic: Amenorrhea, hyperuricemia, azoospermia

Gastrointestinal: Nausea, vomiting, stomatitis, esophagitis, anorexia, mucositis

Genitourinary: Rarely hemorrhagic cystitis

Hematologic: Leukopenia (nadir: 7-10 days), anemia, thrombocytopenia (nadir: 3 weeks), granulocytopenia

Hepatic: Elevated liver transaminase and bilirubin (high-dose therapy)

Local: Pain at injection site

Renal: Hematuria

Miscellaneous: Anaphylaxis

Drug Interactions Succinylcholine (thiotepa inhibits pseudocholinesterase activity; prolongs muscular paralysis); other alkylating agents (intensifies toxicity)

Stability Refrigerate, protect from light; the reconstituted 10 mg/mL solution is chemically stable for 5 days when stored in the refrigerator; since it contains no preservatives use within 8 hours; unstable in acid medium. Thiotepa is stable for 24 hours at a concentration of 1-5 mg/mL in NS when stored at room temperature; at 0.5 mg/mL, thiotepa is stable for 8 hours at room temperature; stability decreases significantly at concentrations <0.5 mg/mL (1 hour).

Mechanism of Action Polyfunctional alkylating agent that reacts with DNA phosphate groups to produce cross-linking of DNA strands leading to inhibition of DNA, RNA, and protein synthesis

Pharmacokinetics

Absorption: Variable absorption through serous membranes and from I.M. injection sites; bladder mucosa: 10% to 100% and is increased with mucosal inflammation or tumor infiltration

Distribution: V_{dss}: 0.7-1.6 L/kg; distributes into CSF

Protein binding: 8% to 13%

Metabolism: In the liver via oxidative desulfuration (cytochrome P-450 microsomal enzyme system) primarily to TEPA (active metabolite)

Half-life, terminal:

Thiotepa: 109 minutes (51.6-212 minutes) with dose-dependent clearance

TEPA: 10-21 hours

Elimination: Very little thiotepa or active metabolite are excreted unchanged in urine (1.5% of thiotepa dose)

Usual Dosage Refer to individual protocols

Children: I.V.: Sarcomas: 25-65 mg/m^2 as a single dose every 3-4 weeks

High-dose thiotepa with ABMT: One regimen uses 300 mg/m^2/dose over 3 hours; repeat every 24 hours for a total of 3 doses; maximum tolerated dose over 3 days: 900-1125 mg/m^2

Adults:

I.V.: 0.3-0.4 mg/kg at 1- to 4-week intervals or 0.2 mg/kg (6 mg/m^2)/day for 4-5 days, repeat at 2- to 4-week intervals; continuous infusion: 15-35 mg/m^2 over 48 hours

Intracavitary: 0.6-0.8 mg/kg; dose should not be repeated more frequently than at a 1 week interval

Administration

Bladder instillation: Prepare with 30-60 mg diluted in 30-60 mL sterile water and instill by catheter and retain for 2 hours

Intrapleural or pericardial: Dose is further diluted to a volume of 10-20 mL in NS or D$_5$W;

Intraperitoneal: Administration requires dilution in larger volumes (up to 2 L)

I.V.: Filter through a 0.22 micron filter (Millex-GS) prior to administration; administer direct I.V. over 5 minutes at a final concentration of 10 mg/mL; administer I.V. intermittent or continuous infusion at a final concentration for administration of 1 mg/mL (thiotepa may be further diluted in D$_5$W, NS, or LR)

Monitoring Parameters CBC with differential and platelet count, uric acid, urinalysis

Patient Information Notify physician if fever, sore throat, bleeding, or bruising occurs

Nursing Implications If thiotepa solution comes in contact with skin or mucosa, the affected area should be washed with soap and water immediately or affected mucosa should be rinsed thoroughly with water.

Additional Information Myelosuppressive effects:

WBC: Moderate

Platelets: Severe

Onset (days): 7-10

Nadir (days): 14-20

Recovery (days): 28

Dosage Forms Powder for injection: 15 mg

References

Grovas AC, Boyett JM, Lindsley K, et al, "Regimen-Related Toxicity of Myeloablative Chemotherapy With BCNU, Thiotepa, and Etoposide Followed by Autologous Stem Cell Rescue for Children With Newly Diagnosed Glioblastoma Multiforme: Report From the Children's Cancer Group," *Med Pediatr Oncol*, 1999, 33(2):83-7.

(Continued)

Thiotepa *(Continued)*

Heideman R, Cole D, Balis F, et al, "Phase I and Pharmacokinetic Evaluation of Thiotepa in the Cerebro-spinal Fluid and Plasma of Pediatric Patients: Evidence for Dose-Dependent Plasma Clearance of Thiotepa," *Cancer Res*, 1989, 49(3):736-41.

Herzig GP, "Phase I-II Studies of High-Dose Thiotepa and Autologous BMT in Patients With Refractory Malignancies," *Adv Cancer Chemotherapy*, 1987, 17-29 (proceedings of a symposium, Oct 1986)

Saarinen UM, Hovi L, and Makipern CA, "High Dose Thiotepa With Autologous Bone Marrow Rescue in Pediatric Solid Tumors," *Proc Am Soc Clin Oncol*, 1989, 8:303.

Thiothixene (thye oh THIKS een)

Related Information
Overdose and Toxicology *on page 1222*

U.S. Brand Names Navane®

Therapeutic Category Antipsychotic Agent; Phenothiazine Derivative

Generic Available Yes

Use Management of psychotic disorders

Pregnancy Risk Factor C

Contraindications Hypersensitivity to thiothixene or any component; cross-sensitivity with other phenothiazines may exist; avoid use in patients with narrow-angle glaucoma, bone marrow suppression, severe liver or cardiac disease

Precautions Use with caution in patients with cardiovascular disease or seizures

Adverse Reactions Sedation and extrapyramidal effects occur more often
Cardiovascular: Hypotension (especially with parenteral use), orthostatic hypotension, tachycardia, arrhythmias
Central nervous system: Sedation, drowsiness, restlessness, anxiety, insomnia, extrapyramidal reactions, tardive dyskinesia, neuroleptic malignant syndrome, seizures, altered central temperature regulation
Dermatologic: Rash, photosensitivity
Endocrine & metabolic: Amenorrhea, galactorrhea, gynecomastia
Gastrointestinal: GI upset, xerostomia, constipation, weight gain
Genitourinary: Urinary retention
Hematologic: Agranulocytosis, leukopenia
Ocular: Retinal pigmentation, blurred vision

Drug Interactions Cytochrome P-450 isoenzyme CYP1A2 substrate
Alcohol and other CNS depressants, anticholinergics, or hypotensive agents may increase adverse effects

Food Interactions May cause increase in dietary riboflavin requirements

Mechanism of Action Elicits antipsychotic activity by postsynaptic blockade of CNS dopamine receptors resulting in inhibition of dopamine-mediated effects; also has alpha-adrenergic blocking activity

Usual Dosage Oral:
Children ≤12 years: Not well established; 0.25 mg/kg/day in divided doses
Children >12 years and Adults: Initial: 2 mg 3 times/day, up to 20-30 mg/day; maximum dose: 60 mg/day

Administration Oral: Administer with food or water

Monitoring Parameters Periodic eye exam, CBC with differential, blood pressure, liver enzyme tests

Patient Information Avoid alcohol; limit caffeine; may cause drowsiness and impair ability to perform activities requiring mental alertness or physical coordination; may cause dry mouth; avoid excessive sunlight, use sunscreen

Dosage Forms
Capsule: 1 mg, 2 mg, 5 mg, 10 mg, 20 mg
Concentrate, oral, as hydrochloride: 5 mg/mL (30 mL, 120 mL)

References
Wiener JM, "Psychopharmacology in Childhood Disorders," *Psychiatr Clin North Am*, 1984, 7(4):831-43.

♦ **Thorazine®** *see* Chlorpromazine *on page 226*
♦ **Thrombin-JMI®** *see* Thrombin (Topical) *on page 956*

Thrombin (Topical) (THROM bin, TOP i kal)

U.S. Brand Names Thrombin-JMI®; Thrombogen®

Therapeutic Category Hemostatic Agent

Generic Available No

Use Hemostasis whenever minor bleeding from capillaries and small venules is accessible

Pregnancy Risk Factor C

Contraindications Hypersensitivity to thrombin, any component, or material of bovine origin

Warnings Do not inject - for topical use only

Adverse Reactions
Central nervous system: Fever
Miscellaneous: Allergic reactions

Stability Following reconstitution, use immediately; stable 3 hours refrigerated; stable frozen (reconstituted) for 48 hours

Mechanism of Action Catalyzes the conversion of fibrinogen to fibrin

Usual Dosage Topical: Apply powder directly to the site of bleeding or on oozing surfaces or use 1000-2000 units/mL of solution where bleeding is profuse; use 100 units/mL for bleeding from skin or mucosal surfaces

Administration Topical: May be applied directly as a powder or as reconstituted solution; the most effective hemostasis results when the thrombin mixes freely with blood as it appears; use sterile water or NS to reconstitute thrombin powder to desired concentration; **not for injection**

Additional Information One unit is amount required to clot 1 mL of standardized fibrinogen solution in 15 seconds

Dosage Forms Powder:
Thrombin-JMI®: 1000 units, 5000 units, 10,000 units, 20,000 units, 50,000 units
Thrombin-JMI® Spray Kit: 5000 unit, 10,000 units, 20,000 units
Thrombin-JMI® Syringe Spray Kit: 10,000 units, 20,000 units
Thrombogen®: 5000 units, 10,000 units, 20,000 units
Thrombogen® Spray Kit: 10,000 units, 20,000 units

- **Thrombogen®** *see* Thrombin (Topical) *on page 956*
- **Thymocyte Stimulating Factor** *see* Aldesleukin *on page 47*
- **Thyrel® TRH** *see* Protirelin *on page 851*
- **Tiabendazole** *see* Thiabendazole *on page 947*

Tiagabine (tye AG a bene)

U.S. Brand Names Gabitril®

Therapeutic Category Anticonvulsant, Miscellaneous

Generic Available No

Use Adjunctive therapy of partial epilepsy

Pregnancy Risk Factor C

Contraindications Hypersensitivity to tiagabine or any component

Warnings Do not abruptly discontinue therapy, withdraw gradually to lessen chance for increased seizure frequency (unless a more rapid withdrawal is required due to safety concerns); exacerbation of EEG abnormalities associated with CNS adverse events (cognitive and neuropsychiatric) may occur in patients with an EEG history of spike and wave discharges and may require dosage adjustment; nonconvulsant status epilepticus has also been reported and may respond to dosage reduction or discontinuation

Precautions Use with caution in patients with hepatic impairment; possible long-term ophthalmologic effects exist (more studies are needed); use with caution with alcohol or other CNS depressants

Adverse Reactions
Central nervous system: Impaired concentration, speech/language problems, confusion, somnolence, fatigue, dizziness, nervousness, depression, ataxia, insomnia, emotional lability, headache
Gastrointestinal: Nausea, abdominal pain, diarrhea
Neuromuscular & skeletal: Asthenia, tremor

Drug Interactions Cytochrome P-450 isoenzyme CYP3A substrate, may also be metabolized by CYP1A2, 2D6, or 2C19
Tiagabine may decrease valproic acid concentrations by ~10%; carbamazepine, phenytoin, primidone, and phenobarbital may increase tiagabine clearance by 60%; naproxen, salicylates, and valproic acid may decrease tiagabine protein binding and increase the free concentration

Food Interactions Food may decrease the rate but not the extent of absorption

Stability Protect from moisture and light; store at room temperature

Mechanism of Action Exact mechanism unknown; thought to potentiate the action of GABA (an inhibitory neurotransmitter) by selectively binding to the GABA uptake carrier and blocking GABA uptake into presynaptic neurons. This allows more GABA to be available at its site of action to bind to postsynaptic neuronal receptors.

Pharmacokinetics
Absorption: Rapid and nearly complete (>95%)
Distribution: Mean V_d:
Children 3-10 years: 2.4 L/kg
Adults: 1.3-1.6 L/kg
(Continued)

Tiagabine *(Continued)*

V_d values are more similar between children and adults when expressed as L/m^2

Protein binding: 96%, mainly to albumin and alpha$_1$-acid glycoprotein

Metabolism: Extensive in the liver via oxidation and glucuronidation; undergoes enterohepatic recirculation

Bioavailability: 90%

Diurnal effect: Trough concentrations and AUC are lower in the evening versus morning

Half-life:
Children 3-10 years: Mean: 5.7 hours (range: 2-10 hours)
Children 3-10 years receiving enzyme-inducing AEDs: Mean: 3.2 hours (range: 2-7.8 hours)
Adults (normal volunteers): 7-9 hours
Adults receiving enzyme-inducing AEDs: 4-7 hours

Time to peak serum concentration: Fasting state: ~45 minutes

Elimination: ~2% excreted unchanged in urine; 25% excreted in urine and 63% excreted in feces as metabolites

Clearance:
Children 3-10 years: 4.2 ± 1.6 mL/minute/kg
Children 3-10 years receiving enzyme-inducing AEDs: 8.6 ± 3.3 mL/minute/kg
Adults (normal volunteers): 109 mL/minute
Adult patients: 1.9 ± 0.5 mL/minute/kg
Adults receiving enzyme-inducing AEDs: 6.3 ± 3.5 mL/minute/kg

Clearance values are more similar between children and adults when expressed as mL/minute/m^2

Hepatic impairment: Clearance of unbound drug is decreased by 60%

Usual Dosage Oral: **Note:** Doses were determined in patients receiving enzyme-inducing AEDs; lower doses or slower titration may be required in patients not receiving enzyme-inducing agents

Children <12 years: Only limited preliminary information is available; dosing guidelines are not established (see Adkins, 1998 and Pellock, 1999)

Children 12-18 years: Initial: 4 mg once daily for 1 week, then 8 mg/day given in 2 divided doses for 1 week, then increase weekly by 4-8 mg/day; administer in 2-4 divided doses per day; titrate dose to response; maximum dose: 32 mg/day (doses >32 mg/day have been used in select adolescent patients for short periods of time)

Adults: Initial: 4 mg once daily for 1 week, then increase weekly by 4-8 mg/day; administer in 2-4 divided doses per day; titrate dose to response; maximum dose: 56 mg/day. **Note:** Twice daily dosing may not be well tolerated and dosing 3 times/day is the currently favored dosing frequency (see Kalviainen, 1998).

Dosing adjustment in renal impairment: None needed

Dosing adjustment in hepatic impairment: Reduced doses and longer dosing intervals may be required

Administration Oral: Administer with food (to avoid rapid increase in plasma concentrations and adverse CNS effects)

Monitoring Parameters Seizure frequency, duration, and severity

Reference Range Not established

Patient Information May cause dizziness or drowsiness and impair ability to perform activities requiring mental alertness or physical coordination

Additional Information Population pharmacokinetic analysis suggests that tiagabine may be administered at similar doses without adjustment for age, gender, or body weight in epilepsy patients ≥ 11 years of age (see Samara, 1998)

Dosage Forms Tablet, as hydrochloride: 2 mg, 4 mg, 12 mg, 16 mg, 20 mg

References
Adkins JC and Noble S, "Tiagabine. A Review of Its Pharmacodynamic and Pharmacokinetic Properties and Therapeutic Potential in the Management of Epilepsy," *Drugs*, 1998, 55(3):437-60.

Gustavson LE, Boellner SW, Granneman GR, et al, "A Single-Dose Study to Define Tiagabine Pharmacokinetics in Pediatric Patients With Complex Partial Seizures," *Neurology*, 1997, 48(4):1032-7.

Kalviainen R, Brodie MJ, Duncan J, et al, "A Double-Blind, Placebo-Controlled Trial of Tiagabine Given Three-Times Daily as Add-On Therapy for Refractory Partial Seizures. Northern European Tiagabine Study Group," *Epilepsy Res*, 1998, 30(1):31-40.

Leach JP and Brodie MJ, "Tiagabine," *Lancet*, 1998, 351(9097):203-7.

Pellock JM, "Managing Pediatric Epilepsy Syndromes With New Antiepileptic Drugs," *Pediatrics*, 1999, 104(5 Pt 1):1106-16.

Samara EE, Gustavson LE, El-Shourbagy T, et al, "Population Analysis of the Pharmacokinetics of Tiagabine in Patients With Epilepsy," *Epilepsy*, 1998, 39(8):868-73.

♦ **Tiamol (Can)** *see* Fluocinonide *on page 440*

♦ **Tiazac®** *see* Diltiazem *on page 337*

♦ **Ticar**® *see* Ticarcillin *on page 959*

Ticarcillin (tye kar SIL in)

U.S. Brand Names Ticar®

Therapeutic Category Antibiotic, Penicillin (Antipseudomonal)

Generic Available No

Use Treatment of infections such as septicemia, acute and chronic respiratory tract infections, skin and soft tissue infections, and urinary tract infections due to susceptible strains of *Pseudomonas*, *Proteus*, *Escherichia coli*, and *Enterobacter*

Pregnancy Risk Factor B

Contraindications Hypersensitivity to ticarcillin, any component, or penicillins

Warnings Prolonged use may result in superinfection

Precautions Use with caution in patients with CHF due to ticarcillin's high sodium content; dosage modification required in patients with impaired renal and/or hepatic function

Adverse Reactions

Central nervous system: Seizures, headache, fever

Dermatologic: Rash

Endocrine & metabolic: Hypernatremia, hypokalemia, metabolic alkalosis

Gastrointestinal: Diarrhea, pseudomembranous colitis, stomatitis, nausea

Genitourinary: Cystitis, hematuria

Hematologic: Inhibition of platelet aggregation, leukopenia, neutropenia, eosinophilia, prolonged prothrombin time, bleeding diathesis, hemolytic anemia, decreased hemoglobin and hematocrit

Hepatic: Elevated AST and ALT, hepatitis

Local: Phlebitis

Renal: Elevated BUN, elevated serum creatinine

Miscellaneous: Hypersensitivity reactions including anaphylaxis; superinfection

Drug Interactions Aminoglycosides (antibacterial activity is synergistic), probenecid (increases serum concentration of ticarcillin); may alter renal elimination of lithium

Stability Reconstituted ticarcillin solution 200-300 mg/mL is stable for 24 hours at room temperature or 72 hours when refrigerated; incompatible with aminoglycosides

Mechanism of Action Inhibits bacterial cell wall synthesis by binding to one or more of the penicillin-binding proteins; inhibits the final transpeptidation step of peptidoglycan synthesis in bacterial cell walls

Pharmacokinetics

Absorption: I.M.: 86%

Distribution: V_d: Neonates: 0.42-0.76 L/kg; distributed into breast milk at low concentrations; attains high concentrations in bile; minimal concentrations attained in CSF with uninflamed meninges

Protein binding: 45% to 65%

Metabolism: 10%

Half-life, adults: 1-1.3 hours, prolonged with renal impairment and/or hepatic impairment

Neonates:

<1 week: 3.5-5.6 hours

1-8 weeks: 1.3-2.2 hours

Children 5-13 years: 0.9 hours

Time to peak serum concentration: I.M.: Within 30-75 minutes

Elimination: Almost entirely in urine as unchanged drug and its metabolites with small amounts excreted in feces (3.5%)

Dialysis: Moderately dialyzable (20% to 50%)

Usual Dosage Ticarcillin is generally only given I.M. for the treatment of uncomplicated urinary tract infections

Neonates: I.V.:

Postnatal age ≤7 days:

≤2000 g: 150 mg/kg/day in divided doses every 12 hours

>2000 g: 225 mg/kg/day in divided doses every 8 hours

Postnatal age >7 days:

<1200 g: 150 mg/kg/day in divided doses every 12 hours

1200-2000 g: 225 mg/kg/day in divided doses every 8 hours

>2000 g: 300 mg/kg/day in divided doses every 6-8 hours

Infants and Children:

I.M.: 50-100 mg/kg/day in divided doses every 6-8 hours

I.V.: 200-300 mg/kg/day in divided doses every 4-6 hours; doses as high as 400 mg/kg/day divided every 4-6 hours have been used in acute pulmonary exacerbations of cystic fibrosis

Maximum dose: 24 g/day

(Continued)

Ticarcillin *(Continued)*

Adults:
  I.M.: 1 g every 6 hours
  I.V.: 1-4 g every 4-6 hours; maximum dose: 24 g/day
  Dosing interval in renal impairment:
    Cl_{cr} 10-30 mL/minute: Administer every 8 hours
    Cl_{cr} <10 mL/minute: Administer every 12 hours

Administration Parenteral:
  I.M.: Reconstitute each gram of ticarcillin with 2 mL SWI or 1% lidocaine hydrochloride injection (without epinephrine) to make a 385 mg/mL solution; administer by deep I.M. injection into a large muscle mass
  I.V.: Ticarcillin may be administered I.V. push over 10-20 minutes or by I.V. intermittent infusion over 30-120 minutes at a final concentration not to exceed 100 mg/mL; concentrations ≤50 mg/mL are preferred for peripheral intermittent infusions to avoid vein irritation; if the patient is on concurrent aminoglycoside therapy, separate ticarcillin administration from the aminoglycoside by at least 30-60 minutes

Monitoring Parameters Serum electrolytes, bleeding time, and periodic tests of renal, hepatic, and hematologic function

Test Interactions False-positive urinary or serum protein, positive Coombs' [direct]

Additional Information Sodium content of 1 g: 5.2-6.5 mEq

Dosage Forms Powder for injection, as disodium: 1 g, 3 g, 20 g, 30 g

References
Brogden RN, Heel RC, Speight TM, et al, "Ticarcillin: A Review of Its Pharmacological Properties and Therapeutic Efficacy," *Drugs*, 1980, 20(5):325-52.

Nelson JD, Kusmiesz H, Shelton S, et al, "Clinical Pharmacology and Efficacy of Ticarcillin in Infants and Children," *Pediatrics*, 1978, 61(6):858-63.

Ticarcillin and Clavulanate Potassium

(tye kar SIL in & klav yoo LAN ate poe TASS ee um)

U.S. Brand Names Timentin®

Synonyms Clavulanate Potassium and Ticarcillin

Therapeutic Category Antibiotic, Beta-lactam and Beta-lactamase Combination; Antibiotic, Penicillin (Antipseudomonal)

Generic Available No

Use Treatment of infections caused by susceptible organisms involving the lower respiratory tract, urinary tract, skin and skin structures, bone and joint, and septicemia. Clavulanate expands activity of ticarcillin to include beta-lactamase producing strains of *S. aureus*, *H. influenzae*, *Moraxella catarrhalis*, *B. fragilis*, *Klebsiella*, and *Proteus* species

Pregnancy Risk Factor B

Contraindications Hypersensitivity to ticarcillin, clavulanate, or penicillin

Warnings Abnormal platelet aggregation and prolonged bleeding have been reported in patients with renal impairment receiving high doses; prolonged use may result in superinfection

Precautions Use with caution and modify dosage in patients with renal impairment; use with caution in patients with CHF due to high sodium content of the formulation

Adverse Reactions
  Central nervous system: Seizures, headache, fever
  Dermatologic: Rash
  Endocrine & metabolic: Hypernatremia, hypokalemia, metabolic alkalosis
  Gastrointestinal: Diarrhea, stomatitis, nausea, pseudomembranous colitis
  Genitourinary: Cystitis, hematuria
  Hematologic: Eosinophilia, leukopenia, decreased hemoglobin and hematocrit, inhibition of platelet aggregation, prolongation of bleeding time, neutropenia, hemolytic anemia
  Hepatic: Elevated ALT and AST, hepatitis
  Local: Thrombophlebitis
  Renal: Elevated BUN, elevated serum creatinine
  Miscellaneous: Hypersensitivity reactions including anaphylaxis; superinfection

Drug Interactions Aminoglycosides (antibacterial activity is synergistic), probenecid (increases serum concentration of ticarcillin)

Stability Reconstituted 200 mg/mL solution is stable for 6 hours at room temperature and 72 hours when refrigerated; darkening of drug indicates loss of potency of clavulanate potassium; incompatible with sodium bicarbonate and aminoglycosides

Mechanism of Action Ticarcillin inhibits bacterial cell wall synthesis by binding to one or more of the penicillin-binding proteins; inhibits the final transpeptidation step of peptidoglycan synthesis in bacterial cell walls; clavulanic acid inhibits degradation of ticarcillin by binding to beta-lactamases

Pharmacokinetics

Distribution: Ticarcillin is distributed into tissue, interstitial fluid, pleural fluid, bile, and breast milk; low concentrations of ticarcillin distribute into the CSF but increase when meninges are inflamed

V_{dss} ticarcillin: 0.22 L/kg

V_{dss} clavulanic acid: 0.4 L/kg

Protein binding:

Ticarcillin: 45% to 65%

Clavulanic acid: 9% to 30%

Metabolism: Clavulanic acid is metabolized in the liver

Half-life: In patients with normal renal function

Neonates:

Clavulanic acid: 1.9 hours

Ticarcillin: 4.4 hours

Children (1 month to 9.3 years):

Clavulanic acid: 54 minutes

Ticarcillin: 66 minutes

Adults:

Clavulanic acid: 66-90 minutes

Ticarcillin: 66-72 minutes

Clavulanic acid does not affect the clearance of ticarcillin

Elimination:

Children: 71% of the ticarcillin and 50% of the clavulanic acid dose are excreted unchanged in the urine over 4 hours

Adults: 45% of clavulanate is excreted unchanged in urine, whereas 60% to 90% of ticarcillin is excreted unchanged in urine

Dialysis: Removed by hemodialysis

Usual Dosage I.V.:

Term neonates and Infants <3 months: 200-300 mg ticarcillin component/kg/day divided every 6-8 hours

Infants ≥3 months and Children:

Mild to moderate infection: 200 mg ticarcillin component/kg/day divided every 6 hours

Severe infections that occur outside the CNS: 300 mg ticarcillin component/kg/day in divided doses every 4-6 hours; maximum dose: 18-24 g/day

Adults: 3.1 g (ticarcillin 3 g plus clavulanic acid 0.1 g) every 4-6 hours; maximum dose: 18-24 g/day

Urinary tract infections: 3.1 g every 6-8 hours

Dosing interval in renal impairment:

Cl_{cr} 10-30 mL/minute: Administer every 8 hours

Cl_{cr} <10 mL/minute: Administer every 12 hours

Dosing interval in hepatic impairment and a Cl_{cr} <10 mL/minute: Administer every 24 hours

Administration

Parenteral: Administer by I.V. intermittent infusion over 30 minutes; final concentration for administration should not exceed 100 mg/mL of ticarcillin; however, concentrations ≤50 mg/mL are preferred; if the patient is on concurrent aminoglycoside therapy, separate ticarcillin and clavulanate potassium administration from the aminoglycoside by at least 30-60 minutes

Monitoring Parameters

Serum electrolytes, periodic renal, hepatic and hematologic function tests

Test Interactions

Positive Coombs' [direct], false-positive urinary and serum proteins

Additional Information

Sodium content of 1 g: 4.75 mEq

Potassium content of 1 g: 0.15 mEq

Dosage Forms

Infusion, premixed (frozen): Ticarcillin disodium 3 g and clavulanic acid 0.1 (100 mL)

Powder for injection: Ticarcillin disodium 3 g and clavulanic acid 0.1 g (3.1 g, 31 g)

References

Begue P, Quiniou F, Quinet B, "Efficacy and Pharmacokinetics of Timentin® in Paediatric Infections," *J Antimicrob Chemother*, 1986, 17(Suppl C):81-91.

Reed MD, Yamashita TS, and Blumer JL, "Pharmacokinetic-Based Ticarcillin/Clavulanic Acid Dose Recommendations for Infants and Children," *J Clin Pharmacol*, 1995, 35(7):658-65.

Stutman HR and Marks MI, "Review of Pediatric Antimicrobial Therapies," *Semin Pediatr Infect Dis*, 1991, 2:3-17.

◆ **Tigan®** *see* Trimethobenzamide *on page 986*

◆ **Tilade®** *see* Nedocromil *on page 701*

TIMOLOL

♦ **Tim-Ak (Can)** *see* Timolol *on page 962*
♦ **Timentin®** *see* Ticarcillin and Clavulanate Potassium *on page 960*

Timolol (TYE moe lole)

Related Information
Overdose and Toxicology *on page 1222*

U.S. Brand Names Betimol®; Blocadren®; Timoptic®; Timoptic® OcuDose®; Timoptic-XE®

Canadian Brand Names Apo-Timol; Apo-Timop; Beta-Tim; Gen-Timolol; Novo-Timol; Nu-Timolol; Tim-Ak

Therapeutic Category Antihypertensive Agent; Antimigraine Agent; Beta-Adrenergic Blocker; Beta-Adrenergic Blocker, Ophthalmic

Generic Available Yes

Use Ophthalmic dosage form used to treat elevated intraocular pressure such as glaucoma or ocular hypertension; orally for treatment of hypertension and angina and for prevention of MI and migraine headaches

Pregnancy Risk Factor C

Contraindications Uncompensated CHF, cardiogenic shock, bradycardia or heart block, bronchial asthma, severe chronic obstructive pulmonary disease or history of asthma, CHF or bradycardia

Warnings Severe CNS, cardiovascular and respiratory adverse effects have been seen following ophthalmic use; some products may contain sulfites which can cause allergic reactions

Precautions Similar to other beta-blockers; use with caution in patients with decreased renal or hepatic function (dosage adjustment required); use with a miotic in angle-closure or narrow-angle glaucoma; use with caution in patients with diabetes mellitus, may block hypoglycemia-induced tachycardia and blood pressure changes

Adverse Reactions
Cardiovascular: Bradycardia, arrhythmia, hypotension, syncope
Central nervous system: Dizziness, headache
Dermatologic: Rash
Gastrointestinal: Diarrhea, nausea
Local (ocular): Irritation, conjunctivitis, keratitis, visual disturbances; transient (30 seconds to 5 minutes) blurred vision after instillation of ophthalmic gel
Respiratory: Bronchospasm

Drug Interactions Cytochrome P-450 isoenzyme CYP2D6 substrate
Verapamil, nifedipine, diltiazem, digitalis, quinidine may increase adverse cardiac effects; NSAIDs may decrease antihypertensive effects of timolol; patients receiving beta blockers, who have a history of anaphylactic reactions, may be more reactive to a repeated allergen challenge and may not be responsive to the usual epinephrine doses used to treat an allergic reaction; use of timolol with clonidine may increase the rebound hypertension seen with clonidine withdrawal; drug interactions similar to other beta-blockers may occur

Stability Ophthalmic: Store at room temperature; do not freeze; protect from light

Mechanism of Action Blocks both beta₁- and beta₂-adrenergic receptors; reduces intraocular pressure by reducing aqueous humor production or possibly outflow; reduces blood pressure by blocking adrenergic receptors and decreasing sympathetic outflow; produces negative chronotropic and negative inotropic activity

Pharmacodynamics Hypotensive effects:
Onset of action: Oral: Within 15-45 minutes
Peak effect: 30-150 minutes
Duration:
Oral: 4 hours
Ophthalmic (intraocular effects): 24 hours

Pharmacokinetics
Protein binding: <10%
Metabolism: Extensively in the liver, extensive first-pass effect
Bioavailability: Oral: ~60%
Half-life: Adults: 2-4 hours; prolonged with reduced renal function
Elimination: Urinary excretion (15% to 20% as unchanged drug)
Dialysis: Not readily dialyzable

Usual Dosage
Ophthalmic:
Gel (Timoptic-XE®): Adults: 0.25% or 0.5% gel, instill 1 drop once daily; do not exceed 1 drop once daily of 0.5% gel
Solution (Timoptic®): Children and Adults: Initial: 0.25% solution, instill 1 drop twice daily; increase to 0.5% solution if response not adequate; decrease to 1

962

drop/day if controlled; do not exceed 1 drop twice daily of 0.5% solution (see Additional Information)

Oral:

Children: No information regarding pediatric dose is currently available in literature

Adults:

Hypertension: Initial: 10 mg twice daily, increase gradually every 7 days, usual dosage: 20-40 mg/day in 2 divided doses; maximum dose: 60 mg/day

Prevention of MI: 10 mg twice daily initiated within 1-4 weeks after infarction

Migraine headache: Initial: 10 mg twice daily, increase to maximum of 30 mg/day

Administration

Ophthalmic: Apply gentle pressure to lacrimal sac during and immediately following instillation (1 minute) or instruct patient to gently close eyelid after administration, to decrease systemic absorption of ophthalmic drops; avoid contact of bottle tip with skin or eye; remove contact lenses prior to administration (Timoptic® contains benzalkonium chloride which may adsorb to soft contact lenses); lenses may be inserted 15 minutes after Timoptic® administration. Gel: Invert container, shake once before use; administer other topical ophthalmic medications at least 10 minutes before Timoptic-XE®

Oral: May be administered without regard to food

Monitoring Parameters Heart rate, blood pressure; liver enzymes, BUN, serum creatinine with long-term oral use; monitor respiratory rate, CNS status, and cardiovascular status with ophthalmic use in patients at risk for adverse effects (eg, asthmatics, CHF patients, etc)

Patient Information Potential visual disturbances from ophthalmic use may impair ability to perform hazardous duties such as driving or operating machinery

Nursing Implications Discontinue medication if breathing difficulty occurs

Additional Information Ophthalmic: Use lowest effective dose in pediatric patients. Children had higher plasma concentrations vs adults following ophthalmic use; some achieved therapeutic levels; this may result in increased adverse systemic effects. The concurrent use of 2 ophthalmic beta blockers is not recommended.

Dosage Forms

Gel, ophthalmic, as maleate (Timoptic-XE®): 0.25% (2.5 mL, 5 mL); 0.5% (2.5 mL, 5 mL)

Solution, ophthalmic, as hemihydrate (Betimol®): 0.25% (5 mL, 10 mL, 15 mL); 0.5% (5 mL, 10 mL, 15 mL)

Solution, ophthalmic, as maleate (Timoptic®): 0.25% (2.5 mL, 5 mL, 10 mL, 15 mL); 0.5% (2.5 mL, 5 mL, 10 mL, 15 mL)

Solution, ophthalmic, preservative free, as maleate, single use (Timoptic® OcuDose®): 0.25% (0.2 mL); 0.5% (0.2 mL)

Tablet, as maleate (Blocadren®): 5 mg, 10 mg, 20 mg

References

Hoskins HD, Hetherington J Jr, Magee SD, et al, "Clinical Experience With Timolol in Childhood Glaucoma," *Arch Ophthalmol*, 1985, 103(8):1163-5.

Passo MS, Palmer EA, and Van Buskirk EM, "Plasma Timolol in Glaucoma Patients," *Ophthalmology*, 1984, 91(11):1361-3.

Tobramycin (toe bra MYE sin)

Related Information

Blood Level Sampling Time Guidelines *on page 1220*

Overdose and Toxicology *on page 1222*

U.S. Brand Names AKTob®; Nebcin®; TOBI™; Tobrex®; Tomycine™

Canadian Brand Names PMS-Tobramycin; Tomycine

Therapeutic Category Antibiotic, Aminoglycoside; Antibiotic, Ophthalmic

(Continued)

Tobramycin *(Continued)*

Generic Available Yes

Use Treatment of documented or suspected infections caused by susceptible gram-negative bacilli including *Pseudomonas aeruginosa*; nonpseudomonal enteric bacillus infection which is more sensitive to tobramycin than gentamicin based on susceptibility tests; susceptible organisms in lower respiratory tract infections, septicemia; intra-abdominal, skin, bone, and urinary tract infections; empiric therapy in cystic fibrosis and immunocompromised patients; used topically to treat superficial ophthalmic infections caused by susceptible bacteria; inhalation therapy management of cystic fibrosis patients with *P. aeruginosa*

Pregnancy Risk Factor D

Contraindications Hypersensitivity to tobramycin, any component, or aminoglycosides

Warnings I.M., I.V.: Aminoglycosides are associated with significant nephrotoxicity or ototoxicity; the ototoxicity is directly proportional to the amount of drug given and the duration of treatment; tinnitus or vertigo are indications of vestibular injury and impending irreversible bilateral deafness; renal damage is usually reversible. Some formulations contain sulfites which may cause allergic reactions; transient tinnitus has been reported in tobramycin inhalation-treated patients; bronchospasm can occur with inhalation of tobramycin. Aminoglycosides can cause fetal harm when administered to a pregnant woman; aminoglycosides have been associated with several reports of total, irreversible, bilateral congenital deafness in pediatric patients exposed *in utero*

Precautions Use with caution in patients with renal impairment, pre-existing auditory or vestibular impairment, patients receiving anesthetics or neuromuscular blocking agents, and in patients with neuromuscular disorders; dosage modification required in patients with impaired renal function

Adverse Reactions

Central nervous system: Vertigo, gait instability, fever, ataxia, dizziness, headache

Dermatologic: Allergic contact dermatitis, rash

Endocrine & metabolic: Hypomagnesemia

Gastrointestinal: Nausea, vomiting

Hematologic: Granulocytopenia, thrombocytopenia, eosinophilia

Hepatic: Elevated AST and ALT

Local: Thrombophlebitis

Neuromuscular & skeletal: Neuromuscular blockade, paresthesia, tremor, weakness

Ocular: Ophthalmic use: Lacrimation, itching, edema of the eyelid, keratitis

Otic: Ototoxicity (may be associated with high serum aminoglycoside concentrations persisting for prolonged periods) with tinnitus, hearing loss; early toxicity usually affects high-pitched sound

Renal: Nephrotoxicity (high trough levels) with proteinuria, reduction in glomerular filtration rate, elevated serum creatinine, decrease in urine specific gravity, casts in urine and possible electrolyte wasting

Respiratory: With inhalation therapy: Voice alteration, bronchospasm, dyspnea, increased cough, pharyngitis, hoarseness

Drug Interactions Increased toxicity: Concurrent use of amphotericin B, cephalosporins, penicillins, loop diuretics, urea, mannitol, vancomycin, cisplatin, indomethacin; potentiates effect of neuromuscular blocking agents and botulinum toxin

Stability Incompatible with penicillins, cephalosporins, heparin

Inhalation solution: Store in refrigerator; upon removal from the refrigerator, the solution may be stored at room temperature for up to 28 days; do not use solution if it is cloudy or contains particles; a darkened yellow solution does not indicate loss of potency; protect from intense light; incompatible with dornase alfa (may precipitate)

Mechanism of Action Inhibits cellular initiation of bacterial protein synthesis by binding to 30S and 50S ribosomal subunits resulting in a defective bacterial cell membrane

Pharmacokinetics

Absorption:

Oral: Poor

I.M.: Rapid and complete

Inhalation: Low systemic bioavailability although peak tobramycin serum concentration 1 hour after inhalation ranges between 0.95-1.05 mg/mL

Distribution: Crosses the placenta; distributes primarily in the extracellular fluid volume; poor penetration into the CSF and into bronchial secretions; drug accumulates in the renal cortex; small amounts distribute into bile, sputum, saliva, tears, and breast milk

V_d: Increased by fever, edema, ascites, fluid overload, and in neonates; V_d is decreased in patients with dehydration

Neonates: 0.45 ± 0.1 L/kg
Infants: 0.4 ± 0.1 L/kg
Children: 0.35 ± 0.15 L/kg
Adolescents: 0.3 ± 0.1 L/kg
Adults: 0.2-0.3 L/kg

Protein binding: <30%

Half-life:
Neonates:
≤1200 g: 11 hours
>1200 g: 2-9 hours
Infants: 4 ± 1 hour
Children: 2 ± 1 hour
Adolescents: 1.5 ± 1 hour
Adults with normal renal function: 2-3 hours, directly dependent upon glomerular filtration rate; impaired renal function: 5-70 hours

Time to peak serum concentration:
I.M.: Within 30-60 minutes
I.V.: 30 minutes after a 30-minute infusion

Elimination: With normal renal function, ~90% to 95% of dose excreted in urine within 24 hours

Dialysis: Dialyzable (50% to 100%)

Usual Dosage Dosage should be based on an estimate of ideal body weight except in neonates (neonatal dosage should be based on actual weight unless the patient has hydrocephalus or hydrops fetalis)

Neonates: I.M., I.V.:
Preterm neonates <1000 g: 3.5 mg/kg/dose every 24 hours
0-4 weeks, <1200 g: 2.5 mg/kg/dose every 18 hours
Postnatal age ≤7 days:
1200-2000 g: 2.5 mg/kg/dose every 12 hours
>2000 g: 2.5 mg/kg/dose every 12 hours
Postnatal age >7 days:
1200-2000 g: 2.5 mg/kg/dose every 8-12 hours
>2000 g: 2.5 mg/kg/dose every 8 hours

Infants and Children <5 years: I.M., I.V.: 2.5 mg/kg/dose every 8 hours*
Pulmonary infection in cystic fibrosis: 2.5-3.3 mg/kg/dose every 6-8 hours
Patients on hemodialysis: 1.25-1.75 mg/kg/dose postdialysis

Children ≥5 years: I.M., I.V.: 2-2.5 mg/kg/dose every 8 hours*
Pulmonary infection in cystic fibrosis: 2.5-3.3 mg/kg/dose every 6-8 hours
Patients on hemodialysis: 1.25-1.75 mg/kg/dose postdialysis

*Note: Some patients may require larger or more frequent doses if serum levels document the need (ie, cystic fibrosis, patients undergoing continuous hemofiltration, patients with major burns, or febrile granulocytopenic patients); modify dose based on individual patient requirements as determined by renal function, serum drug concentrations, and patient-specific clinical parameters.

Children and Adults: Ophthalmic:
Ointment: Apply 0.5" ribbon into the affected eye 2-3 times/day; for severe infections, apply ointment every 3-4 hours
Solution:
Mild to moderate infections: Instill 1-2 drops every 4 hours
Severe infections: instill 2 drops every 30-60 minutes initially, then reduce to less frequent intervals

Inhalation:
Standard aerosolized tobramycin:
Children: 40-80 mg 2-3 times/day
Adults: 60-80 mg 3 times/day
High dose regimen: Children ≥6 years and Adults: 300 mg every 12 hours (do not administer doses less than 6 hours apart); administer in repeated cycles of 28 days on drug followed by 28 days off drug

Adults: I.M., I.V.: 3-6 mg/kg/day in 3 divided doses; studies of once daily dosing have used I.V. doses of 4-6.6 mg/kg once daily
Patients on hemodialysis: 0.5-0.7 mg/kg/dose postdialysis

Dosing in Renal Impairment:
Children and Adults: 2.5 mg/kg (2-3 serum level measurements should be obtained after the initial dose to measure the half-life in order to determine the frequency of subsequent doses)

(Continued)

Tobramycin *(Continued)*

Administration

Inhalation (high-dose regimen): Use a PARI LC Plus™ reusable nebulizer and a DeVilbiss Pulmo-Aide® air compressor for administration of tobramycin by inhalation; patient should be sitting or standing upright and breathing normally through the mouthpiece of the nebulizer

Ophthalmic: Avoid contact of tube or bottle tip with skin or eye; apply finger pressure to lacrimal sac during and for 1-2 minutes after instillation of drops to decrease risk of absorption and systemic effects

Parenteral: Administer by I.M., I.V. slow intermittent infusion over 30-60 minutes or by direct injection over 15 minutes; final I.V. concentration for administration should not exceed 10 mg/mL; administer other antibiotics such as penicillins and cephalosporins at least 1 hour before or after tobramycin

Monitoring Parameters Urinalysis, urine output, BUN, serum creatinine, peak and trough serum tobramycin levels; be alert to ototoxicity, audiograms

Not all pediatric patients who receive aminoglycosides require monitoring of serum aminoglycoside concentrations. Indications for use of aminoglycoside serum concentration monitoring include:

Treatment course >5 days

Patients with decreased or changing renal function

Patients with a poor therapeutic response

Infants <3 months of age

Atypical body constituency (obesity, expanded extracellular fluid volume)

Clinical need for higher doses or shorter intervals (cystic fibrosis, burns, endocarditis, meningitis, relatively resistant organism)

Patients on hemodialysis or chronic ambulatory peritoneal dialysis

Signs of nephrotoxicity or ototoxicity

Concomitant use of other nephrotoxic agents

Patients on high-dose aerosolized tobramycin: Peak tobramycin level obtained 1 hour following inhalation to identify patients who are significant absorbers

Reference Range

Peak: 4-12 µg/mL; peak values are 2-3 times greater with once daily dosing regimens

Trough: 0.5-2 µg/mL

Test Interactions Aminoglycoside serum levels measured in blood taken from Silastic® central line catheters can sometimes give falsely high readings

Patient Information Report any dizziness or sensation of ringing or fullness in ears to the physician

Nursing Implications Obtain serum concentration after the third dose except in neonates or patients with rapidly changing renal function in whom levels need to be measured sooner; peak tobramycin serum concentrations are drawn 30 minutes after the end of a 30-minute infusion, immediately on completion of a 1-hour I.V. infusion or 1 hour after an intramuscular injection; the trough is drawn just before the next dose; provide optimal patient hydration and perfusion

Dosage Forms

Injection, as sulfate

Nebcin® Pediatric: 10 mg/mL (2 mL)

Nebcin®: 40 mg/mL (2 mL)

Ointment, ophthalmic (Tobrex®): 0.3% [3 mg/g] (3.5 g)

Powder for injection (Nebcin®): 40 mg/mL (1.2 g vials)

Solution for inhalation, ampul, preservative free (TOBI™): 60 mg/mL (5 mL)

Solution, ophthalmic (AKTob®, Tobrex®, Tomycine™): 0.3% [3 mg/mL] (5 mL)

References

Gilbert DN, "Once-Daily Aminoglycoside Therapy," *Antimicrob Agents Chemother*, 1991, 35(3):399-405.

Green TP, Mirkin BL, Peterson PK, et al, "Tobramycin Serum Level Monitoring in Young Patients With Normal Renal Function," *Clin Pharmacokinet*, 1984, 9(5):457-68.

Nahata MC, Powell DA, Durrell DE, et al, "Effect of Gestational Age and Birth Weight on Tobramycin Kinetics in Newborn Infants," *J Antimicrob Chemother*, 1984, 14(1):59-65.

Ramsey BW, Burns J, Smith A, et al, "Safety and Efficacy of Tobramycin for Inhalation in Patients With Cystic Fibrosis: The Results of Two Phase III Placebo Controlled Clinical Trials," *Pediatr Pulmonol*, 1997, (Suppl 14):137-8, S10.3.

Ramsey BW, Dorkin HL, Eisenberg JD, et al, "Efficacy of Aerosolized Tobramycin in Patients With Cystic Fibrosis," *N Engl J Med*, 1993, 328(24):1740-6.

Shaw PK, Braun TL, Liebergen A, et al, "Aerosolized Tobramycin Pharmacokinetics in Cystic Fibrosis Patients," *J Pediatr Pharm Pract*, 1997, 2(1):23-6.

♦ **Tobrex®** *see* Tobramycin *on page 963*

♦ **Tofranil®** *see* Imipramine *on page 528*

♦ **Tofranil-PM®** *see* Imipramine *on page 528*

Tolazoline (tole AZ oh leen)

Related Information
Overdose and Toxicology *on page 1222*

U.S. Brand Names Priscoline®

Synonyms Benzazoline

Therapeutic Category Alpha-Adrenergic Blocking Agent, Parenteral; Antihypertensive Agent; Vasodilator

Generic Available No

Use Persistent pulmonary hypertension of the newborn (PPHN), also known as persistent fetal circulation (PFC); peripheral vasospastic disorders

Pregnancy Risk Factor C

Contraindications Hypersensitivity to tolazoline or any component; known or suspected coronary artery disease

Warnings May activate stress ulcers via stimulation of gastric secretions

Precautions Use with caution in patients with mitral stenosis, gastritis, peptic ulcers; use with caution and decrease dose in patients with renal dysfunction

Adverse Reactions
Cardiovascular: Hypotension, flushing, tachycardia, arrhythmias
Endocrine & metabolic: Hypochloremic alkalosis
Gastrointestinal: Increased secretions, nausea, vomiting, diarrhea, epigastric discomfort, GI bleeding
Hematology: Agranulocytosis, thrombocytopenia, pancytopenia
Ocular: Mydriasis
Renal: Oliguria
Respiratory: Pulmonary hemorrhage
Miscellaneous: Increased pilomotor activity

Drug Interactions A paradoxical decrease in blood pressure followed by a significant rebound increase in blood pressure can be seen when epinephrine or norepinephrine is administered with tolazoline; a disulfiram reaction may possibly be seen with concomitant ethanol use

Stability Compatible in D_5W, $D_{10}W$ and saline solutions; do not mix with other drugs

Mechanism of Action Competitively blocks alpha-adrenergic receptors to produce brief antagonism of circulating epinephrine and norepinephrine; reduces hypertension caused by catecholamines and causes vascular smooth muscle relaxation (direct action); results in peripheral vasodilation and decreased peripheral resistance; GI adverse effects and peripheral vasodilation mediated via histamine-like action

Pharmacodynamics Peak effects: Within 30 minutes

Pharmacokinetics
Distribution: V_d: Neonates: 1.6 L/kg
Half-life, neonates: 3-10 hours; increased half-life with decreased renal function, oliguria
Elimination: Rapid in urine primarily as unchanged drug

Usual Dosage
Neonates: I.V.:
Initial: 1-2 mg/kg over 10-15 minutes via scalp vein or upper extremity
Maintenance: I.V. continuous infusion: 1-2 mg/kg/hour; **Note:** Some neonatal centers use lower maintenance doses (eg, 0.15-0.3 mg/kg/hour or 0.5-1 mg/kg/hour)
Acute vasospasm "cath toes": 0.25 mg/kg/hour (no load)
Adults: Peripheral vasospastic disorder: I.M., I.V., S.C.: 10-50 mg 4 times/day
Dosing adjustment in renal dysfunction: Neonates: Urine output <0.9 mL/kg/hour: Decrease dose by 50%

Administration Parenteral: I.V.: Usual maximum concentration: 0.1 mg/mL

Monitoring Parameters Heart rate, blood pressure, respiratory rate, blood gases, serum chloride and bicarbonate

Additional Information Little experience with infusions >48 hours; acidosis may decrease tolazoline's effects

Dosage Forms Injection, as hydrochloride: 25 mg/mL (4 mL)

References
Ward RM, Daniel CH, Kendig JW, et al, "Oliguria and Tolazoline Pharmacokinetics in the Newborn," *Pediatrics*, 1986, 77(3):307-15.

♦ **Tolectin**® *see* Tolmetin *on page 968*

♦ **Tolectin**® **DS** *see* Tolmetin *on page 968*

Tolmetin (TOLE met in)

Related Information
Overdose and Toxicology *on page 1222*

U.S. Brand Names Tolectin®; Tolectin® DS

Canadian Brand Names Novo-Tolmetin

Therapeutic Category Analgesic, Non-narcotic; Nonsteroidal Anti-inflammatory Drug (NSAID), Oral

Generic Available Yes

Use Treatment of inflammatory and rheumatoid disorders, including juvenile rheumatoid arthritis

Pregnancy Risk Factor C (D in 3rd trimester or near delivery)

Contraindications Hypersensitivity to tolmetin, any component, aspirin, or other NSAIDs

Precautions Use with caution in patients with upper GI disease, impaired renal function, CHF, hypertension, and patients receiving anticoagulants; although rare, anaphylactoid reactions occur more commonly with tolmetin than other NSAIDs

Adverse Reactions

Cardiovascular: Edema

Central nervous system: Dizziness, nervousness, drowsiness, headache

Dermatologic: Rash, urticaria

Gastrointestinal: Nausea, abdominal pain, dyspepsia, diarrhea, constipation; GI bleeding, ulcer, perforation

Hematologic: Anemia, leukopenia, prolongation of bleeding time

Hepatic: Hepatitis

Otic: Tinnitus

Renal: Acute renal failure, renal dysfunction

Drug Interactions Tolmetin may potentiate the effects of warfarin and may increase prothrombin time and bleeding; aspirin may decrease tolmetin serum concentration; tolmetin may increase serum concentrations of methotrexate; tolmetin may decrease antihypertensive effects of ACE inhibitors or angiotensin II antagonists; drug interactions similar to other NSAIDs may also occur

Food Interactions Food or milk may decrease the extent of oral absorption

Mechanism of Action Inhibits prostaglandin synthesis by decreasing the activity of the enzyme, cyclo-oxygenase, which results in decreased formation of prostaglandin precursors

Pharmacokinetics

Absorption: Oral: Well absorbed

Protein binding: 99%

Metabolism: In the liver via oxidation and conjugation

Half-life, elimination: 5 hours

Time to peak serum concentration: Within 30-60 minutes

Elimination: Excreted in the urine as metabolites or conjugates

Usual Dosage Oral:

Children ≥2 years:

Anti-inflammatory: Initial: 20 mg/kg/day in 3-4 divided doses, then 15-30 mg/kg/day in 3-4 divided doses; maximum dose: 30 mg/kg/day

Analgesic: 5-7 mg/kg/dose every 6-8 hours

Adults: 400 mg 3 times/day; usual dose: 600 mg to 1.8 g/day; maximum dose: 2 g/day

Administration Oral: May administer with food, milk, or antacids to decrease GI adverse effects

Monitoring Parameters CBC with differential, liver enzymes, occult blood loss, BUN, serum creatinine; periodic ophthalmologic exams

Patient Information Avoid alcohol; may cause dizziness or drowsiness and impair ability to perform activities requiring mental alertness or physical coordination

Dosage Forms

Capsule, as sodium (Tolectin® DS): 400 mg

Tablet, as sodium (Tolectin®): 200 mg, 600 mg

References

Berde C, Ablin A, Glazer J, et al, "American Academy of Pediatrics Report of the Subcommittee on Disease-Related Pain in Childhood Cancer," *Pediatrics*, 1990, 86(5 Pt 2):818-25.

Hollingworth P, "The Use of Non-Steroidal Anti-inflammatory Drugs in Paediatric Rheumatic Diseases," *Br J Rheumatol*, 1993, 32(1):73-7.

Rose CD and Doughty RA, "Pharmacological Management of Juvenile Rheumatoid Arthritis," *Drugs*, 1992, 43(6):849-63.

Tolnaftate (tole NAF tate)

U.S. Brand Names Absorbine Jr.® Antifungal [OTC]; Aftate® [OTC]; NP-27® [OTC]; Tinactin® [OTC]; Tinactin® Jock Itch [OTC]; Ting® [OTC]

Canadian Brand Names Avon Footworks; Pitrex; Scholl Athlete's Foot

Therapeutic Category Antifungal Agent, Topical

Generic Available Yes

Use Treatment of tinea pedis, tinea cruris, tinea corporis, tinea manuum caused by *Trichophyton rubrum*, *T. mentagrophytes*, *T. tonsurans*, *M. canis*, *M. audouinii*, and *E. floccosum*; also effective in the treatment of tinea versicolor infections due to *Malassezia furfur*

Pregnancy Risk Factor C

Contraindications Hypersensitivity to tolnaftate or any component; nail and scalp infections

Adverse Reactions
Dermatologic: Pruritus, contact dermatitis
Local: Irritation, stinging
Miscellaneous: Hypersensitivity reaction, sensitization to butylated hydroxytoluene component of cream, solution, and aerosol powder

Mechanism of Action Distorts the hyphae and stunts mycelial growth in susceptible fungi

Pharmacodynamics Onset of action: Response may be seen 24-72 hours after initiation of therapy

Usual Dosage Children and Adults: Topical: Apply 1-3 drops of solution or a small amount of cream or powder and rub into the affected areas 2-3 times/day for 2-4 weeks

Administration Topical: Wash and dry affected area before drug application; avoid contact with eyes

Monitoring Parameters Resolution of skin infection

Patient Information Avoid contact with the eyes; apply to clean dry area; consult the physician if a skin irritation develops or if the skin infection worsens or does not improve after 10 days of therapy

Additional Information Usually not effective alone for the treatment of infections involving hair follicles or nails

Dosage Forms
Aerosol, topical:
Liquid (Aftate®, Tinactin®, Ting®): 1% (59.2 mL, 90 mL, 113 mL, 120 mL)
Powder (Aftate®, NP-27®, Tinactin®, Tinactin® Jock Itch): 1% (100 g, 105 g)
Cream (NP-27®, Tinactin®, Tinactin® Jock Itch, Ting®): 1% (15 g, 30 g, 96 g)
Gel, topical (Absorbine Jr.® Antifungal): 1% (21 g)
Powder, topical (Tinactin®, Ting®): 1% (45 g, 90 g)
Solution, topical (Absorbine Jr.® Antifungal, Tinactin®): 1% (10 mL, 30 mL, 60 mL)

♦ **Tolu-Sed® DM [OTC]** *see* Guaifenesin and Dextromethorphan *on page 487*
♦ **Tomycine™** *see* Tobramycin *on page 963*
♦ **Topactin (Can)** *see* Fluocinonide *on page 440*
♦ **Topamax®** *see* Topiramate *on page 969*
♦ **Topilene (Can)** *see* Betamethasone *on page 140*

Topiramate (toe PYE ra mate)

U.S. Brand Names Topamax®

Therapeutic Category Anticonvulsant, Miscellaneous

Generic Available No

Use Adjunctive treatment of primary generalized tonic-clonic seizures or partial epilepsy in children 2-16 years of age and adults; also used for treatment of Lennox-Gastaut syndrome; may potentially be useful in infantile spasms

Pregnancy Risk Factor C

Contraindications Hypersensitivity to topiramate or any component

Warnings Do not abruptly discontinue therapy, withdraw gradually to lessen chance for increased seizure frequency; CNS adverse effects are common (see Adverse Reactions); avoid use with alcohol, CNS depressants, or carbonic anhydrase inhibitors (see Drug Interactions)

Precautions Use with caution and decrease the dose in patients with renal dysfunction; use with caution in patients allergic to sulfa drugs and in patients with hepatic impairment

Adverse Reactions
Central nervous system: Ataxia, difficulty in concentrating, dizziness, memory difficulties, fatigue, nervousness, somnolence, psychomotor slowing, speech/
(Continued)

Topiramate *(Continued)*

language problems, confusion, depression, anxiety, cognitive problems; irritability and sleep disturbances (reported in children); **Note:** Somnolence and fatigue are the most common CNS adverse effects in children

Gastrointestinal: Weight loss, anorexia, nausea

Hematologic: Purpura

Neuromuscular & skeletal: Paresthesia, tremor

Ocular: Nystagmus, diplopia, abnormal vision

Renal: Nephrolithiasis

Respiratory: Epistaxis

Drug Interactions Cytochrome P-450 isoenzyme CYP2C19 substrate and inhibitor Phenytoin and carbamazepine may significantly decrease topiramate serum concentrations (topiramate dosage increase may be needed); valproic acid may decrease topiramate concentrations; topiramate may decrease serum concentrations of valproic acid, digoxin, and ethinyl estradiol (may decrease the efficacy of oral contraceptives); alcohol or other CNS depressants may increase adverse CNS effects; carbonic anhydrase inhibitors may increase the risk of nephrolithiasis or paresthesia; topiramate may increase phenytoin serum concentrations by 25% in some patients

Food Interactions Food may decrease the rate but not the extent of absorption

Stability Protect from moisture; store at room temperature

Mechanism of Action Exact mechanism unknown; thought to decrease the spread of seizure activity by blockade of sodium channels, potentiation of GABA (an inhibitory neurotransmitter) and antagonism of kainate activation of glutamate (an excitatory amino acid) subtype receptors; also inhibits carbonic anhydrase (minor effect)

Pharmacokinetics Note: Sprinkle capsule is bioequivalent to tablet

Absorption: Rapid

Distribution: V_d: Adults: 0.6-0.8 L/kg

Protein binding: 13% to 17%

Metabolism: Minor amounts metabolized in liver via hydroxylation, hydrolysis, and glucuronidation; percentage of dose metabolized in liver and clearance are increased in patients receiving enzyme inducers

Bioavailability: Tablet: 80% (relative to a prepared solution)

Half-life:

Adults: 19-23 hours (mean 21 hours)

Adults with renal impairment: 59 ± 11 hours (n=7)

Time to peak serum concentration: 2 hours; range: 1.4-4.3 hours

Elimination: 70% of dose excreted unchanged in urine; may undergo renal tubular reabsorption

Clearance:

Children 4-17 years: ~50% higher than adults (per kg)

Adults: 20-30 mL/minute

Renal impairment: Reduced

Hepatic impairment: May be reduced

Dialysis: Significantly hemodialyzed; dialysis clearance: 120 mL/minute (4-6 times higher than in adults with normal renal function); supplemental doses may be required

Usual Dosage Oral:

Children 2-16 years:

Partial onset seizures: Initial: 1-3 mg/kg/day (maximum: 25 mg) given nightly for 1 week; increase at 1- to 2-week intervals by 1-3 mg/kg/day given in 2 divided doses; titrate dose to response; usual maintenance: 5-9 mg/kg/day given in 2 divided doses

Primary generalized tonic-clonic seizures: Use slower initial titration rate; titrate to 6 mg/kg/day by the end of 8 weeks

Adolescents ≥17 years and Adults:

Partial onset seizures: Initial: 25-50 mg/day given daily for 1 week; increase at weekly intervals by 25-50 mg/day; titrate dose to response; usual maintenance: 200 mg twice daily; maximum dose: 1600 mg/day

Primary generalized tonic-clonic seizures: Use slower initial titration rate; titrate upwards to recommended dose by the end of 8 weeks

Dosing adjustment in renal impairment: Cl_{cr} <70 mL/minute/1.73 m²: Administer 50% of the usual dose; titrate more slowly due to prolonged half-life

Dosing adjustment in hepatic impairment: Carefully adjust dose as plasma concentrations may be increased if normal dosing is used

Administration May be administered without regard to food; broken tablets have a bitter taste; tablets may be crushed, mixed with water, and administered immediately. Swallow sprinkle capsules whole or open and sprinkle contents on small amount of soft food (eg, 1 teaspoonful of applesauce); swallow sprinkle/food mixture immediately; do not chew; do not store for later use; drink fluids after dose to make sure mixture is completely swallowed

Monitoring Parameters Seizure frequency, duration, and severity; renal function

Reference Range Not applicable; plasma topiramate concentrations have not been shown to correlate with clinical efficacy

Patient Information Ensure adequate fluid intake to avoid kidney stone formation; may cause dizziness or drowsiness and impair ability to perform activities requiring mental alertness or physical coordination; avoid alcohol

Dosage Forms
Capsule: 15 mg, 25 mg
Tablet: 25 mg, 100 mg, 200 mg

References

Doose DR, Walker SA, Gisclon LG, et al, "Single-Dose Pharmacokinetics and Effect of Food on the Bioavailability of Topiramate, a Novel Antiepileptic Drug," *J Clin Pharmacol*, 1996, 36(10):884-91.

Glauser TA, "Preliminary Observations on Topiramate in Pediatric Epilepsies," *Epilepsia*, 1997, 38(Suppl 1):S37-41.

Glauser TA, "Topiramate Use in Pediatric Patients," *Can J Neurol Sci*, 1998, 25(3):S8-12.

Glauser TA, Clark PO, and Strawsburg R, "A Pilot Study of Topiramate in the Treatment of Infantile Spasms," *Epilepsia*, 1998, 39(12):1324-8.

Pellock JM, "Managing Pediatric Epilepsy Syndromes With New Antiepileptic Drugs," *Pediatrics*, 1999, 104(5 Pt 1):1106-16.

Sachdeo RC, "Topiramate. Clinical Profile in Epilepsy," *Clin Pharmacokinet*, 1998, 34(5):335-46.

♦ **Topisone (Can)** *see* Betamethasone *on page 140*

♦ **Toprol XL®** *see* Metoprolol *on page 660*

♦ **Topsyn (Can)** *see* Fluocinonide *on page 440*

♦ **Toradol®** *see* Ketorolac *on page 565*

♦ **Torecan®** *see* Thiethylperazine *on page 950*

♦ **Tornalate®** *see* Bitolterol *on page 146*

Torsemide (TOR se mide)

U.S. Brand Names Demadex®

Therapeutic Category Antihypertensive Agent; Diuretic, Loop

Generic Available No

Use Management of edema associated with CHF and hepatic or renal disease; used alone or in combination with antihypertensives in treatment of hypertension

Pregnancy Risk Factor B

Contraindications Hypersensitivity to torsemide, any component, or other sulfonylureas; anuria

Warnings Loop diuretics are potent diuretics, excess amounts can lead to profound diuresis with fluid and electrolyte loss; close medical supervision and dose evaluation is required

Adverse Reactions
Cardiovascular: Orthostatic hypotension, EKG abnormality, chest pain, atrial fibrillation, ventricular tachycardia, syncope
Central nervous system: Headache, dizziness, insomnia, nervousness
Dermatologic: Rash, photosensitivity
Endocrine & metabolic: Hyponatremia, hypokalemia, hypochloremia, alkalosis, hypocalcemia, dehydration, hyperuricemia, gout
Gastrointestinal: Diarrhea, nausea, constipation, dyspepsia, GI hemorrhage, stomach cramps, pancreatitis
Genitourinary: Excessive urination
Hematologic: Agranulocytosis, anemia
Neuromuscular & skeletal: Myalgia, arthralgia, weakness
Otic: Ototoxicity
Renal: Prerenal azotemia, interstitial nephritis, nephrocalcinosis

Drug Interactions Cytochrome P-450 isoenzyme CYP2C9 substrate
Increased risk of ototoxicity with aminoglycosides and cis-platinum; increased anticoagulant effects of warfarin; increased risk of digoxin toxicity when used alone or combined with other medications which cause increased potassium losses (eg, corticosteroids, amphotericin B); decreased glucose tolerance which may result in increased requirements of sulfonylureas and other antidiabetic agents; decreased diuretic effects of torsemide when combined with NSAIDs; increased lithium serum levels; increased salicylate levels with potential toxicity (with high dose salicylates)

Stability Stable for 24 hours at room temperature when mixed with D_5W or NS

Mechanism of Action Inhibits reabsorption of sodium and chloride in the ascending loop of Henle and distal renal tubule, interfering with the chloride-binding cotransport (Continued)

Torsemide *(Continued)*

system, thus causing increased excretion of water, sodium, chloride, magnesium, and calcium

Pharmacodynamics
Onset of effect:
Oral: 60 minutes
I.V.: 10 minutes
Peak effect:
Oral: 60-120 minutes
I.V.: Within 60 minutes
Duration: Oral, I.V.: 6-8 hours

Pharmacokinetics
Absorption: Oral: Rapid
Distribution: V_d: 12-15 L (adults)
Protein binding: Plasma: ~97% to 99%
Metabolism: Hepatic by cytochrome P-450, 80%
Bioavailability: 80% to 90%
Half-life: 3.5 hours (range 2-4 hours); 7-8 hours in cirrhosis (dose modification appears unnecessary)
Elimination: 20% eliminated unchanged in urine

Usual Dosage Adults: Oral, I.V.:
Edema: 10-20 mg once daily; titrate upward as needed (maximum dose: 200 mg/day)
Hepatic cirrhosis: 5-10 mg once daily
Hypertension: Initial: 5 mg once daily; increase to 10 mg if ineffective after 4-6 weeks of therapy

Administration
Oral: May be administered with food or milk
Parenteral: May be administered undiluted direct I.V. over 3-5 minutes

Monitoring Parameters Renal function, serum electrolytes, and fluid intake and output, blood pressure

Patient Information Rise slowly from a lying or sitting position to minimize dizziness, lightheadedness or fainting; also use extra care when exercising, standing for long periods of time; take last dose of day early in the evening to prevent nocturia

Additional Information 10-20 mg torsemide is approximately equivalent to:
Furosemide 40 mg
Bumetanide 1 mg

Dosage Forms
Injection: 10 mg/mL (2 mL, 5 mL)
Tablet: 5 mg, 10 mg, 20 mg, 100 mg

- ◆ **Totacillin®** *see* Ampicillin *on page 88*
- ◆ **Totacillin®-N** *see* Ampicillin *on page 88*
- ◆ **Touro® DM** *see* Guaifenesin and Dextromethorphan *on page 487*
- ◆ **Touro Ex®** *see* Guaifenesin *on page 485*
- ◆ **t-PA** *see* Alteplase *on page 58*
- ◆ **T-Phyl®** *see* Theophylline *on page 943*
- ◆ **Trace Elements** *see* Trace Metals *on page 972*

Trace Metals *(trase MET als)*

Related Information
Parenteral Nutrition (PN) *on page 1106*

U.S. Brand Names Iodopen®; Molypen®; M.T.E.-4®; M.T.E.-5®; M.T.E.-6®; M.T.E.-7®; Multe-Pak-4®; Neotrace-4®; Pedte-Pak-5®; Pedtrace-4®; P.T.E.-4®; P.T.E.-5®; Sele-Pak®; Selepen®

Synonyms Multiple Trace Metals; Neonatal Trace Metals; Selenium; Trace Elements

Available Salts Ammonium Molybdate; Chromium Chloride; Copper Sulfate; Cupric Chloride; Iodine Sodium; Manganese Chloride; Manganese Sulfate; Zinc Chloride; Zinc Sulfate

Therapeutic Category Mineral, Parenteral; Trace Element, Parenteral; Trace Element, Multiple, Neonatal

Generic Available Yes

Use Prevent and correct trace metal deficiencies

Pregnancy Risk Factor C

Contraindications Do not give by direct injection because of potential for phlebitis, tissue irritation, and potential to increase renal loss of minerals from a bolus injection

Warnings Some products may contain benzyl alcohol which has been associated with fatal "gasping" syndrome in premature infants. Metals may accumulate in conditions of renal failure or biliary obstruction; consider reduction in dosage or deletion of copper and manganese in patients with biliary obstruction; avoid copper use in patients with Wilson's disease; administration of copper in the absence of zinc or zinc in the absence of copper may cause decreases in their respective plasma levels; molybdenum promotes the utilization of copper and increases its excretion; excessive amounts of molybdenum may produce copper deficiency; multiple trace metal solutions present a risk of overdosage when the need for one trace element is appreciably higher than for others in the formulation; utilization of individual trace metal solutions may be needed. Consider reduction in dosage or deletion of selenium and chromium in patients with renal dysfunction.

Adverse Reactions The following describe the symptomatology associated with excess trace metals

Chromium: Nausea, vomiting, GI ulcers, renal and hepatic dysfunction, convulsions, coma

Copper: Prostration, behavioral changes, diarrhea, progressive marasmus, hypotonia, photophobia, hepatic dysfunction, peripheral edema

Manganese: Irritability, speech disturbances, abnormal gait, headache, anorexia, apathy, impotence, cholestatic jaundice, movement disorders

Molybdenum: Gout-like syndrome with increased blood levels of uric acid and xanthine oxidase

Selenium: Alopecia, weak nails, dermatitis, dental defects, GI disorders, nervousness, mental depression, metallic taste, garlic odor of breath and sweat

Zinc: Profuse diaphoresis, decreased consciousness, blurred vision, tachycardia, hypothermia

Drug Interactions Oral zinc decreases quinolone and tetracycline absorption

Food Interactions Decreased absorption of oral zinc when given with bran products, protein, and phytates

Mechanism of Action

Chromium: Part of glucose tolerance factor, an essential activator of insulin-mediated reactions; helps maintain normal glucose metabolism and peripheral nerve function

Copper: Cofactor for serum ceruloplasmin, helps maintain normal rates of red and white cell formation

Manganese: Activator for several enzymes including manganese-dependent superoxide dismutase and pyruvate carboxylase; activates glycosyl transferases involved in mucopolysaccharide synthesis

Molybdenum: Constituent of the enzymes xanthine oxidase, sulfite oxidase, and aldehyde oxidase

Selenium: Part of glutathione peroxidase which protects cell components from oxidative damage due to peroxides produced in cellular metabolism

Zinc: A cofactor for >70 different enzymes; facilitates wound healing, helps maintain normal growth rates, normal skin hydration, and the senses of taste and smell

Pharmacokinetics

Chromium: 10% to 20% oral absorption; excretion primarily via kidneys and bile

Copper: 30% oral absorption; 80% elimination via bile; intestinal wall 16% and urine 4%

Manganese: 10% oral absorption; excretion primarily via bile; ancillary routes via pancreatic secretions or reabsorption into the intestinal lumen occur during periods of biliary obstruction

Molybdenum: 30% to 70% oral absorption; primarily renal excretion; some biliary excretion associated with an enterohepatic cycle

Selenium: Very poor oral absorption; 75% excretion via kidneys, remainder via feces, lung, and skin

Zinc: 20% to 30% oral absorption; 90% excretion in stools, remainder via urine and perspiration

Usual Dosage See table on next page.

Administration Parenteral: Must be diluted prior to use and infused as component of parenteral nutrition or parenteral solutions

Reference Range

Chromium: 0.18-0.47 ng/mL (SI: 35-90 nmol/L); some laboratories report much higher

*Copper: ~0.7-1.5 µg/mL (SI: 11-24 µmol/L); levels are higher in pregnant women and children

Manganese: 18-30 µg/dL (SI: 2.3-3.8 µmol/L)

(Continued)

Trace Metals *(Continued)*

Selenium: 95-165 ng/mL (SI: 120-209 nmol/L)
Zinc: 70-120 µg/dL (SI: 10-18.4 µmol/L)

*May not be a meaningful measurement of body stores

Trace Mineral Daily Requirements*

	Infants	Children (≥3 mo to ≤5 y)	Older Children, Adolescents, and Adults
Chromium†	0.2 mcg/kg	0.14-0.2 mcg/kg (max: 5 mcg)	5-15 mcg
Copper‡	20 mcg/kg	20 mcg/kg (max: 300 mcg)	0.2-0.5 mg
Iodide§	1 mcg/kg	1 mcg/kg	1 mcg/kg
Manganese‡	1 mcg/kg	2-10 mcg/kg (max: 50 mcg)	50-150 mcg
Selenium†¶	2-3 mcg/kg	2-3 mcg/kg (max: 30 mcg)	30-40 mcg
Zinc	400 mcg/kg (preterm) 300 mcg/kg (term <3 mo)	100 mcg/kg (max: 5 mg)	2-5 mg

*Recommended intakes of trace elements cannot be achieved through the use of a commercially available combination trace element product. Only through the use of individualized trace element products can recommended intakes be achieved.

†Omit in patients with renal dysfunction.

‡Omit in patients with obstructive jaundice.

§Percutaneous absorption from protein-bound iodine may be adequate.

¶Indicated for use in long-term parenteral nutrition patients.

Multiple Trace Metal Parenteral Solutions

	Content per mL					
	Chromium (mcg)	Copper (mg)	Iodide (mcg)	Manganese (mg)	Selenium (mcg)	Zinc (mg)
Pedtrace-4®	0.85	0.1	—	0.025	—	0.5
Multiple trace element neonatal	0.85	0.1	—	0.025	—	1.5
Neotrace-4®	0.85	0.1	—	0.025	—	1.5
PedTE-PAK-4®	1	0.1	—	0.025	—	1
P.T.E.-4®	1	0.1	—	0.025	—	1
Multiple trace element pediatric	1	0.1	—	0.03	—	0.5
Trace metals additive in NS	2	0.2	—	0.16	—	0.8
M.T.E.-4®	4	0.4	—	0.1	—	1
MulTE-PAK-4®	4	0.4	—	0.1	—	1
Multiple trace element	4	0.4	—	0.1	—	1
Multiple trace element conc	10	1	—	0.5	—	5
M.T.E.-4® conc	10	1	—	0.5	—	5
PTE-5®	1	0.1	—	0.025	15	1
M.T.E.-5®	4	0.4	—	0.1	20	1
MulTE-PAK-5®	4	0.4	—	0.1	20	1
Multiple trace element w/ selenium	4	0.4	—	0.1	20	1
M.T.E.-5® conc	10	1	—	0.5	60	5
Multiple trace element w/ selenium concentrated	10	1	—	0.5	60	5
M.T.E.-6®	4	0.4	25	0.1	20	1
M.T.E.-7®*	4	0.4	25	0.1	20	1
M.T.E.-6® conc	10	1	75	0.5	60	5

*With 25 mcg molybdenum.

Additional Information Persistent diarrhea or excessive GI fluid losses from ostomy sites may grossly increase zinc losses

Dosage Forms See table on previous page.

Injection [elemental equivalence]:

Chromium, as chromic chloride (hexahydrate): 0.0205 mg/mL [0.004 mg/mL] (10 mL)

Copper:

As cupric chloride: 1.07 mg/mL [0.4 mg/mL] (10 mL)

As sulfate: 1.57 mg/mL [0.4 mg/mL] (10 mL)

Iodine, as iodine sodium (Iodopen®): 0.118 mg/mL [0.1 mg/mL] (10 mL)

Manganese:

As chloride: 0.36 mg/mL [0.1 mg/mL] (10 mL)

As sulfate: 0.31 mg/mL [0.1 mg/mL] (10 mL)

Molybdenum, as ammonium molybdate (tetrahydrate) (Molypen®): 46 mcg/mL [25 mcg/mL] (10 mL)

Selenium, as selenious acid (Selepen®): 0.0654 mg/mL [0.04 mg/mL] (10 mL, 30 mL)

Zinc:

As chloride: 2.09 mg/mL [1 mg/mL] (10 mL, 50 mL)

As sulfate: 21.95 mg/mL [5 mg/mL] (5 mL)

Anhydrous: 2.46 mg/mL [1 mg/mL] (10 mL)

Heptahydrate: 4.39 mg/mL [1 mg/mL] (10 mL)

References

Dahlstrom KA, Ament ME, Medhin MG, et al, "Serum Trace Elements in Children Receiving Long-Term Parenteral Nutrition," *J Pediatr*, 1986, 109(4):625-30.

Fell JM, Reynolds AP, Meadows N, et al, "Manganese Toxicity in Children Receiving Long-Term Parenteral Nutrition," *Lancet*, 1996, 347(9010):1218-21.

Greene HL, Hambridge KM, Schanler R, et al, "Guidelines for the Use of Vitamins, Trace Elements, Calcium, Magnesium and Phosphorus in Infants and Children Receiving Total Parenteral Nutrition: Report of the Subcommittee on Pediatric Nutrient Requirements From the Committee on Clinical Practice Issues of The American Society for Clinical Nutrition," *Am J Clin Nutr*, 1988, 48(5):1324-42.

Litov RE, and Combs GF Jr, "Selenium in Pediatric Nutrition," *Pediatrics*, 1991, 87(3):339-51.

♦ **Tracrium**® *see Atracurium on page 114*

♦ **Trandate**® *see Labetalol on page 568*

Tranexamic Acid (tran eks AM ik AS id)

U.S. Brand Names Cyklokapron®

Synonyms AMCA; CL-65336; transAMCA

Therapeutic Category Antihemophilic Agent

Generic Available No

Use Prevention of excessive bleeding after tonsillectomy; short-term use (2-8 days) in hemophilia patients during and following tooth extraction; primary menorrhagia; prevention of GI hemorrhage and hemorrhage following ocular trauma; recurrent epistaxis; hereditary angioneurotic edema

Pregnancy Risk Factor B

Contraindications Hypersensitivity to tranexamic acid or any component; subarachnoid hemorrhage; acquired defective color vision, active intravascular clotting process

Warnings Patients receiving therapy for a long duration should have baseline and frequent ophthalmologic exams; do not administer concomitantly with factor IX complex concentrates or anti-inhibitor coagulant concentrates due to increased risk of thrombosis

Precautions Dosage modification required in patients with renal impairment; use with caution in patients with cardiovascular, renal, cerebrovascular disease, or transurethral prostatectomy

Adverse Reactions

Cardiovascular: Hypotension (with rapid I.V. administration), thromboembolic complications

Central nervous system: Cerebral ischemia and infarction (when used in the treatment of subarachnoid hemorrhage), headache, hydrocephalus, giddiness

Gastrointestinal: Nausea, diarrhea, vomiting

Hematologic: Thrombocytopenia, coagulation defects, abnormal bleeding times

Ocular: Visual abnormalities (focal areas of retinal degeneration have been seen in animals), central venous stasis retinopathy

Drug Interactions Chlorpromazine

Stability Incompatible with solutions containing penicillin; compatible with dextrose, saline, and electrolyte solutions

(Continued)

Tranexamic Acid *(Continued)*

Mechanism of Action Forms a reversible complex that displaces plasminogen from fibrin resulting in inhibition of fibrinolysis; it also inhibits the proteolytic activity of plasmin

Pharmacokinetics

Distribution: Breast milk levels are 1% of serum; CSF levels are 10% of plasma

Protein binding: 3%

Bioavailability:

Oral: 33% to 35%

I.M.: 100%

Half-life: 2 hours

Time to peak serum concentration:

Oral: 3 hours

I.M.: 1 hour

I.V.: 5 minutes

Elimination: Elimination characteristics differ by route of administration: after I.V. administration 95% excreted as unchanged drug in urine vs 39% after oral administration

Usual Dosage Dental extraction in hemophiliacs: Children and Adults: 10 mg/kg I.V. immediately before surgery, then 25 mg/kg/dose orally 3-4 times/day for 2-8 days

Alternatives:

10 mg/kg/dose I.V. 3-4 times/day if unable to take orally

25 mg/kg/dose orally 3-4 times/day beginning 1 day prior to surgery

Menorrhagia: Oral: Adolescents and Adults: 1-1.5 g (12-25 mg/kg/dose) 3-4 times daily for 3-4 days

Adults: Oral:

Epistaxis: 1.5 g 3 times/day

Ocular trauma: 1 g 3 times/day

Dosing adjustment in renal impairment: Adults: See table.

Tranxemic Acid Dosage Adjustments in Renal Impairment (Adult Data)

Serum Creatinine (mg/dL)	I.V. dose	Oral dose
1.36-2.83	10 mg/kg twice daily	15 mg/kg twice daily
>2.83-5.66	10 mg/kg once daily	15 mg/kg once daily
>5.66	10 mg/kg every 48 h or 5 mg/kg every 24 h	15 mg/kg every 48 h or 7.5 mg/kg every 24 h

Administration

Parenteral: May be administered by direct I.V. injection at a maximum rate of 100 mg/minute (1 mL/minute)

Oral: May be administered with food

Monitoring Parameters Ophthalmologic exams (baseline and at regular intervals) of chronic therapy

Reference Range 5-10 µg/mL is required to decrease fibrinolysis

Dosage Forms

Injection: 100 mg/mL (10 mL)

Tablet: 500 mg

Trazodone (TRAZ oh done)

Related Information
Comparison of Adverse Effects of Antidepressants *on page 1066*
Comparison of Usual Adult Dosage and Mechanism of Action of Antidepressants *on page 1065*
Drugs and Breast-Feeding *on page 1243*
Serotonin Syndrome *on page 1247*

U.S. Brand Names Desyrel®

Canadian Brand Names Alti-Trazodone; Apo-Trazodone; Gen-Trazodone; Novo-Trazodone; Nu-Trazodone; PMS-Trazodone; Trazorel

Therapeutic Category Antidepressant

Generic Available Yes

Use Treatment of depression

Pregnancy Risk Factor C

Contraindications Hypersensitivity to trazodone or any component

Warnings Monitor closely and use with extreme caution in patients with cardiac disease or arrhythmias

Adverse Reactions Possesses fewer anticholinergic and cardiac adverse effects than tricyclic antidepressants
Cardiovascular: Postural hypotension (5%), arrhythmias
Central nervous system: Drowsiness (20% to 50%), sedation, dizziness, insomnia, confusion, agitation, seizures, extrapyramidal reactions, headache
Gastrointestinal: Xerostomia, constipation, nausea, vomiting
Genitourinary: Prolonged priapism (1:6000), urinary retention (rare)
Hepatic: Hepatitis
Neuromuscular & skeletal: Weakness
Ocular: Blurred vision (15% to 30%)

Drug Interactions Cytochrome P-450 isoenzyme CYP2D6 and CYP3A3/4 substrate
May antagonize the antihypertensive effects of clonidine and methyldopa; may increase the serum concentrations of phenytoin or digoxin; effects may be additive with other CNS depressants, alcohol; fluoxetine may increase trazodone serum concentration

Food Interactions Food may decrease the rate but not the extent of absorption

Mechanism of Action Inhibits reuptake of serotonin; minimal or no effect on reuptake of norepinephrine or dopamine; possesses little if any anticholinergic effects; alpha-adrenergic blockade thought to be responsible for orthostatic hypotension and dry mouth

Pharmacodynamics Maximum antidepressant effect: ~2-6 weeks

Pharmacokinetics
Protein binding: 85% to 95%
Metabolism: In the liver via hydroxylation and oxidation
Half-life, elimination: 5-9 hours, prolonged in elderly and obese patients
Elimination: Primarily in urine (74%) with ~21% excreted in feces

Usual Dosage Oral:
Children 6-18 years: Initial: 1.5-2 mg/kg/day in divided doses; increase gradually every 3-4 days as needed; maximum dose: 6 mg/kg/day in 3 divided doses
Adolescents: Initial: 25-50 mg/day; increase to 100-150 mg/day in divided doses
Adults: Initial: 150 mg/day in 3 divided doses (may increase by 50 mg/day every 3-7 days); maximum dose: 600 mg/day

Administration Oral: Administer after meals or a snack to decrease lightheadedness, sedation, and postural hypotension

Monitoring Parameters Blood pressure, mental status, liver enzymes

Reference Range
Therapeutic: 0.5-2.5 µg/mL (SI: 1-6 µmol/L)
Potentially toxic: >2.5 µg/mL (SI: >6 µmol/L)
Toxic: >4 µg/mL (SI: >10 µmol/L)

Patient Information Avoid alcohol; may cause drowsiness and impair ability to perform hazardous tasks that require mental alertness or physical coordination; may cause dry mouth

Additional Information Mean doses of ~5 mg/kg/day were used in 22 children 5-12 years of age to treat severe behavioral disorders (Zubieta, 1992). Doses of 1 mg/kg/day given in 3 divided doses were used for migraine prophylaxis in 40 patients 7-18 years of age (Battistella, 1993). Further studies are needed before trazodone can be recommended in children for these indications.

Dosage Forms Tablet: 50 mg, 100 mg, 150 mg, 300 mg

References
Battistella PA, Ruffilli R, Cernetti R, et al, "A Placebo-Controlled Crossover Trial Using Trazodone in Pediatric Migraine," *Headache*, 1993, 33(1):36-9.

(Continued)

TRETINOIN

Trazodone *(Continued)*

Zubieta JK and Alessi NE, "Acute and Chronic Administration of Trazodone in the Treatment of Disruptive Behavior Disorders in Children," *J Clin Psychopharmacol*, 1992, 12(5):346-51.

♦ **Trazorel (Can)** *see* Trazodone *on page 977*
♦ **Trecator®-SC** *see* Ethionamide *on page 407*
♦ **Tremytoine (Can)** *see* Phenytoin *on page 791*
♦ **Trental®** *see* Pentoxifylline *on page 781*

Tretinoin (TRET i noyn)

U.S. Brand Names Altinac™; Avita®; Renova®; Retin-A®; Retina-A® Micro
Canadian Brand Names Rejuva; Retisol-A; Stie VAA; Vesanoid
Synonyms Retinoic Acid; *trans*-Retinoic Acid; Vitamin A Acid
Therapeutic Category Acne Products; Retinoic Acid Derivative; Vitamin, Topical
Generic Available No
Use Treatment of acne vulgaris, photodamaged skin, and some skin cancers
Pregnancy Risk Factor C
Contraindications Hypersensitivity to tretinoin or any component; sunburn
Warnings Avoid contact with abraded skin, mucous membranes, eyes, mouth, angles of the nose; avoid excessive exposure to sunlight or sunlamps
Precautions Use with caution in patients with eczema
Adverse Reactions
Cardiovascular: Edema
Dermatologic: Excessive dryness, erythema, scaling of the skin, hyperpigmentation or hypopigmentation, photosensitivity, initial acne flare-up
Local: Stinging, blistering
Drug Interactions Sulfur, benzoyl peroxide, salicylic acid, and resorcinol potentiate adverse reactions seen with tretinoin
Food Interactions Avoid excessive intake of vitamin A
Mechanism of Action Keratinocytes in the sebaceous follicle become less adherent which allows for easy removal; inhibits microcomedone formation and eliminates lesions already present
Pharmacodynamics
Onset of therapeutic effects: 2-3 weeks
Optimal effects: May require 6 weeks or longer
Pharmacokinetics
Absorption: Topical: Minimum absorption
Metabolism: In the liver
Elimination: In bile and urine
Usual Dosage Children >12 years and Adults: Topical: Begin therapy with a weaker formulation of tretinoin (0.025% cream or 0.01% gel) and increase the concentration as tolerated; apply once daily before retiring or on alternate days; if stinging or irritation develop, decrease frequency of application
Administration Topical: Apply to dry skin (wait at least 15-30 minutes to apply after cleansing); avoid contact with eyes, mucous membranes, mouth, or open wounds
Patient Information Minimize exposure to sunlight; use of a sunscreen is recommended; avoid washing face more frequently than 2-3 times/day; avoid using topical preparations with high alcoholic content during treatment period
Additional Information Liquid preparation generally is more irritating
Dosage Forms
Cream:
Renova®: 0.02% (20 g, 40 g)
Avita®: 0.025% (20 g, 45 g)
Altinac™, Retin-A®: 0.025% (20 g, 45 g); 0.05% (20 g, 45 g); 0.1% (20 g, 45 g)
Renova®: 0.05% (20 g, 40 g, 60 g)
Retin-A® Micro: 0.1% (20 g, 45 g)
Gel, topical
Retin-A®: 0.01% (15 g, 45 g); 0.025% (15 g, 45 g)
Avita®: 0.025% (15 g, 45 g)
Liquid, topical (Retin-A®): 0.05% (28 mL)
References

Winston MH, Shalita AR, "Acne Vulgaris, Pathogenesis and Treatment," *Pediatr Clin North Am*, 1991, 38(4):889-903.

♦ **Triacet™** *see* Triamcinolone *on page 979*
♦ **Triacetyloleandomycin** *see* Troleandomycin *on page 989*
♦ **Triadapin (Can)** *see* Doxepin *on page 358*
♦ **Triaderm (Can)** *see* Triamcinolone *on page 979*

♦ **Triam-A**® *see* Triamcinolone *on page 979*

Triamcinolone (trye am SIN oh lone)
Related Information
Asthma Guidelines *on page 1210*
Corticosteroids Comparison, Topical *on page 1068*
Estimated Comparative Daily Dosages for Inhaled Corticosteroids *on page 1216*
U.S. Brand Names Amcort®; Aristocort®; Aristocort® A; Aristocort® Forte; Aristospan®; Azmacort®; Clinacort®; Kenalog®; Kenalog-10®; Kenalog-40®; Kenalog® in Orabase®; Ken-Jec 40®; Nasacort®; Nasacort® AQ; Tac™-3; Triacet™; Triam-A®; Triam Forte®; Triderm®; Tri-Nasal®
Canadian Brand Names Oracort; Scheinpharm Triamcine-A; Triaderm
Therapeutic Category Adrenal Corticosteroid; Antiasthmatic; Anti-inflammatory Agent; Corticosteroid, Inhalant (Oral); Corticosteroid, Intranasal; Corticosteroid, Systemic; Corticosteroid, Topical; Glucocorticoid
Generic Available Yes
Use
Oral inhalation: Long-term (chronic) control of persistent bronchial asthma; **NOT** indicated for the relief of acute bronchospasm. Also used to help reduce or discontinue oral corticosteroid therapy for asthma.
Intranasal: Management of seasonal and perennial allergic rhinitis
Systemic: Immunosuppression; relief of severe inflammation
Topical: Relief of inflammation and pruritus associated with corticosteroid-responsive dermatoses
Pregnancy Risk Factor C
Contraindications Hypersensitivity to triamcinolone or any component; primary treatment of status asthmaticus; systemic fungal infections; serious infections, except septic shock or tuberculous meningitis
Warnings Fatalities have occurred due to adrenal insufficiency in asthmatic patients during and after switching from systemic corticosteroids to aerosol steroids; several months may be required for full recovery of the adrenal glands; patients receiving higher doses of systemic corticosteroids (eg, adults receiving ≥20 mg of prednisone per day) may be at greater risk; during this period of adrenal suppression, aerosol steroids do **not** provide the systemic corticosteroid needed to treat patients requiring stress doses (ie, patients with major stress such as trauma, surgery, or infections); when used at high doses hypothalamic - pituitary - adrenal (HPA) suppression may occur; use with inhaled or systemic corticosteroids (even alternate-day dosing) may increase risk of HPA suppression; withdrawal and discontinuation of corticosteroids should be done carefully; immunosuppression may occur
Precautions Avoid using higher than recommended doses; suppression of HPA function, suppression of linear growth, or hypercorticism (Cushing's syndrome) may occur; use with extreme caution in patients with respiratory tuberculosis, untreated systemic infections, or ocular herpes simplex
Adverse Reactions
Cardiovascular: Facial edema, hypertension
Central nervous system: Fatigue
Dermatologic: Itching, hypertrichosis, skin atrophy, hyperpigmentation, hypopigmentation, acne
Endocrine & metabolic: Cushingoid state, sodium retention, pituitary-adrenal axis suppression, potential growth suppression, glucose intolerance, hypokalemia
Gastrointestinal: Oral candidiasis, dry throat, xerostomia, peptic ulcer
Local: Burning, sterile abscesses
Neuromuscular & skeletal: Osteoporosis
Ocular: Cataracts
Respiratory: Hoarseness, wheezing, cough
Drug Interactions Cytochrome P-450 isoenzyme CYP3A3/4 inducer
Barbiturates, phenytoin, rifampin increase the metabolism of triamcinolone; salicylates; NSAIDs, caffeine and alcohol may increase risk of GI ulcer; live virus vaccines (increase risk of viral infection); vaccines may have decreased effects
Food Interactions Systemic use of corticosteroids may require a diet with increased potassium, vitamins A, B_6, C, D, folate, calcium, zinc, and phosphorus and decreased sodium
Mechanism of Action Controls the rate of protein synthesis, depresses the migration of polymorphonuclear leukocytes and fibroblasts, reverses capillary permeability, and stabilizes lysosomal membranes at the cellular level to prevent or control inflammation
Pharmacokinetics
Time to peak serum concentration: I.M.: Within 8-10 hours
(Continued)

Triamcinolone *(Continued)*

Half-life: 88 minutes

Usual Dosage

I.M. (as acetonide or hexacetonide): Children: 6-12 years: 0.03-0.2 mg/kg at 1- to 7-day intervals

Intra-articular (as hexacetonide): Children >12 years and Adults: 2-20 mg every 3-4 weeks

Intra-articular, intrabursal, or tendon-sheath injection: Children: 6-12 years: 2.5-15 mg, repeat as needed

Intra-articular, intrasynovial, intralesional (as diacetate or acetonide): Children >12 years and Adults: 2.5-40 mg, repeat as needed when signs and symptoms recur

Intralesional, sublesional (as diacetate or acetonide): Children >12 years and Adults: Up to 1 mg per injection site and may be repeated 1 or more times weekly; multiple sites may be injected if they are 1 cm or more apart, not to exceed 30 mg

Intranasal:

Nasacort®:

Children 6-11 years: Initial: 2 sprays in each nostril once daily; titrate to lowest effective dose once symptoms are controlled

Children >12 years and Adults: Initial: 2 sprays in each nostril once daily; may increase after 4-7 days up to 4 sprays in each nostril once daily, 2 sprays in each nostril twice daily, or 1 spray in each nostril 4 times/day

Nasacort AQ®: Children >12 years and Adults: Initial: 2 sprays in each nostril once daily; titrate to lowest effective dose once symptoms are controlled; usual maintenance dose: 1 spray in each nostril once daily

Tri-Nasal®: Children >12 years and Adults: Initial: 2 sprays in each nostril once daily; may increase to maximum dose of 4 sprays in each nostril once daily or 2 sprays in each nostril twice daily; may initiate at maximum doses if faster relief of symptoms is required; titrate to lowest effective dose once symptoms are controlled

Oral: Children >12 years and Adults: 4-100 mg/day in 1-4 divided doses

Oral inhalation: Doses should be titrated to the lowest effective dose once asthma is controlled; maintenance doses may be given twice daily. Manufacturer recommendation:

Children: 6-12 years: 1-2 puffs given 3-4 times/day; maximum dose: 12 puffs/day

Children >12 years and Adults: 2 puffs given 3-4 times/day; for severe asthma: 12-16 puffs/day divided into 3-4 doses/day; maximum dose: 16 puffs/day

NIH Guidelines (NIH, 1997) [give in divided doses 3-4 times/day]:

Children:

"Low" dose: 400-800 mcg/day (4-8 puffs/day)

"Medium" dose: 800-1200 mcg/day (8-12 puffs/day)

"High" dose: >1200 mcg/day (>12 puffs/day)

Adults:

"Low" dose: 400-1000 mcg/day (4-10 puffs/day)

"Medium" dose: 1000-2000 mcg/day (10-20 puffs/day)

"High" dose: >2000 mcg/day (>20 puffs/day)

Topical: Children and Adults: Apply a thin film 2-3 times/day

Administration

Oral: May administer with meals to decrease GI upset

Oral inhalant: Shake canister well before use; use a spacer device for children <8 years of age; do not spray in eyes

Intranasal: Shake container well before use; clear nasal passages by blowing nose prior to use; do not spray in eyes

Parenteral: Avoid S.C. use; do not inject I.V.; acetonide or hexacetonide may be administered I.M.; see Usual Dosage for other parenteral routes of administration

Topical: Apply sparingly to affected area, gently rub in until disappears; avoid application on face; do not occlude area unless directed; do not use on open skin; avoid contact with eyes

Monitoring Parameters Oral inhalation: Check mucus membranes for signs of fungal infection; monitor growth in pediatric patients

Patient Information Notify physician if condition being treated persists or worsens; do not decrease dose or discontinue without physicians approval; avoid exposure to chicken pox or measles, if exposed seek medical advice without delay

Oral inhalant: Rinse mouth with water without swallowing to decrease chance of oral candidiasis; report sore mouth or mouth lesions to physician

Nursing Implications Once daily oral doses should be given in the morning

Additional Information Oral inhalation: If bronchospasm with wheezing occurs after use, a fast-acting bronchodilator may be used

Dosage Forms
Triamcinolone acetonide
Aerosol:
  Nasal inhaler (Nasacort®): 55 mcg per actuation [100 activations] (10 g)
  Nasal spray
    Nasacort® AQ: 55 mcg per actuation [120 activations] (16.5 g)
    Tri-Nasal®: 50 mcg per actuation [120 actuations] (15 mL)
  Oral inhaler (Azmacort®): 100 mcg per actuation (20 g)
  Topical (Kenalog®): 0.2 mg/2-second spray (63 g)
Cream:
  Aristocort® A, Kenalog®: 0.025% (15 g, 60 g, 80 g, 454 g)
  Aristocort®, Aristocort® A, Kenalog®, Triacet™, Triderm®: 0.1% (15 g, 60 g, 80 g, 90 g, 240 g, 454 g)
  Aristocort® A, Kenalog®: 0.5% (15 g, 20 g, 80 g)
Injection:
  Tac™-3: 3 mg/mL (5 mL)
  Kenalog-10®: 10 mg/mL (5 mL)
  Ken-Jec 40®, Kenalog-40®, Triam-A®: 40 mg/mL (1 mL, 5 mL, 10 mL)
Lotion (Kenalog®): 0.025% (60 mL); 0.1% (60 mL)
Ointment, topical: 0.025% (15 g, 80 g, 454 g); 0.5% (15 g)
  Aristocort® A, Kenalog®, Triderm®: 0.1% (15 g, 28 g, 30 g, 60 g, 80 g, 90 g, 454 g)
Paste, dental (Kenalog® in Orabase®): 0.1% (5 g)
Triamcinolone diacetate
Injection:
  Aristocort®: 25 mg/mL [for intralesional use only] (5 mL)
  Amcort®, Aristocort® Forte, Clinacort®, Triam Forte®: 40 mg/mL (1 mL, 5 mL)
Triamcinolone hexacetonide
Injection:
  Aristospan®: 5 mg/mL [for intralesional use only] (5 mL)
  Aristospan®: 20 mg/mL [for intra-articular use only] (1 mL, 5 mL)
Triamcinolone oral
Tablet (Aristocort®): 4 mg

References
Expert Panel Report 2, "Guidelines for the Diagnosis and Management of Asthma," *Clinical Practice Guidelines*, National Institutes of Health, National Heart, Lung, and Blood Institute, NIH Publication No. 94-4051, April, 1997.

♦ **Triam Forte®** *see* Triamcinolone *on page 979*
♦ **Triaminic® AM Decongestant Formula [OTC]** *see* Pseudoephedrine *on page 852*
♦ **Triaminic® Infant Decongestant [OTC]** *see* Pseudoephedrine *on page 852*

Triamterene (trye AM ter een)
U.S. Brand Names Dyrenium®
Therapeutic Category Antihypertensive Agent; Diuretic, Potassium Sparing
Generic Available No
Use Used alone or in combination with other diuretics to treat edema and hypertension; decreases potassium excretion caused by kaliuretic diuretics
Pregnancy Risk Factor B
Contraindications Hypersensitivity to triamterene or any component; severe renal or hepatic impairment, hyperkalemia
Precautions Use with caution in patients with impaired hepatic or renal function, history of renal calculi, diabetes mellitus; patients receiving other potassium-sparing diuretics or potassium supplements
Adverse Reactions
Cardiovascular: Hypotension
Central nervous system: Dizziness, headache
Endocrine & metabolic: Hyperkalemia, hyponatremia, hypomagnesemia, hyperchloremia, hyperuricemia, metabolic acidosis
Dermatologic: Photosensitivity
Gastrointestinal: Nausea, vomiting, diarrhea, xerostomia
Genitourinary: Slight alkalinization of urine
Hematologic: Blood dyscrasias, thrombocytopenia, megaloblastic anemia
Hepatic: Abnormal liver function
Neuromuscular & skeletal: Muscle cramps, weakness
Renal: Prerenal azotemia, nephrolithiasis (rare), reversible acute renal failure
Miscellaneous: Allergic reactions have been reported
(Continued)

Triamterene (Continued)

Drug Interactions Increased risk of hyperkalemia if given together with other potassium-sparing diuretics (ie, spironolactone); may increase risk of hyperkalemia with ACE inhibitors, (ie, captopril, enalapril); concomitant administration of triamterene and indomethacin may increase nephrotoxicity; increased risk of hyperkalemia with potassium-containing preparations; may increase lithium toxicity by decreasing lithium clearance; may increase amantadine toxicity possibly by decreasing its renal excretion

Food Interactions Avoid salt substitutes and diets with increased potassium

Mechanism of Action Interferes with potassium/sodium exchange (active transport) in the distal tubule, cortical collecting tubule and collecting duct by inhibiting sodium, potassium-ATPase; decreases calcium excretion; increases magnesium loss

Pharmacodynamics
Onset of action: Diuresis occurs within 2-4 hours
Duration: 7-9 hours
Note: Maximum therapeutic effect may not occur until after several days of therapy

Pharmacokinetics
Absorption: Oral: Unreliably absorbed
Metabolism: Hepatic conjugation
Half-life: 100-150 minutes
Elimination: 21% excreted unchanged in urine

Usual Dosage Oral:
Children: 2-4 mg/kg/day in 1-2 divided doses; maximum dose: 6 mg/kg/day and not to exceed 300 mg/day
Adults: 25-100 mg/day in 1-2 divided doses; maximum dose: 300 mg/day

Administration Oral: Administer with food to avoid GI upset

Monitoring Parameters Electrolytes (sodium, potassium, magnesium, HCO_3, chloride), CBC, BUN, creatinine, platelets

Test Interactions Interferes with fluorometric assay of quinidine

Patient Information Avoid unnecessary sun exposure; may cause dry mouth

Additional Information Abrupt discontinuation of therapy may result in rebound kaliuresis; taper off gradually

Dosage Forms Capsule: 50 mg, 100 mg

♦ **Triatec-30 (Can)** see Acetaminophen and Codeine on page 31

Triazolam (trye AY zoe lam)

Related Information
Overdose and Toxicology on page 1222

U.S. Brand Names Halcion®

Canadian Brand Names Apo-Triazo; Gen-Triazolam; Novo-Triolam

Therapeutic Category Benzodiazepine; Hypnotic; Sedative

Generic Available Yes

Use Short-term treatment of insomnia

Restrictions C-IV

Pregnancy Risk Factor X

Contraindications Hypersensitivity to triazolam or any component, cross-sensitivity with other benzodiazepines may occur; severe uncontrolled pain; pre-existing CNS depression; narrow-angle glaucoma; not to be used in pregnancy or lactation

Warnings Abrupt discontinuance may precipitate withdrawal or rebound insomnia

Adverse Reactions
Central nervous system: Drowsiness, anterograde amnesia, confusion, bizarre behavior, agitation, dizziness, hallucinations, nightmares, headache, ataxia
Gastrointestinal: Xerostomia, nausea, vomiting
Hepatic: Cholestatic jaundice
Miscellaneous: Physical and psychological dependence

Drug Interactions Cytochrome P-450 isoenzyme CYP3A3/4 and CYP3A5-7 substrate
CNS depressants, alcohol may increase CNS adverse effects; cimetidine, erythromycin may decrease and enzyme inducers may increase the metabolism of triazolam; protease inhibitors (indinavir, nelfinavir, lopinavir, ritonavir, saquinavir) and delavirdine may potentially decrease triazolam's metabolism and increase triazolam serum concentrations; concurrent use of triazolam with protease inhibitors or delavirdine is not recommended; ketoconazole, itraconazole may increase intensity and duration of triazolam effects

Food Interactions Food may decrease the rate of absorption; grapefruit juice significantly increases the bioavailability of oral triazolam

Mechanism of Action Depresses all levels of the CNS, including the limbic and reticular formation, by binding to the benzodiazepine site on the gamma-aminobutyric acid (GABA) receptor complex and modulating GABA, which is a major inhibitory neurotransmitter in the brain

Pharmacodynamics Hypnotic effects:
Onset: Within 15-30 minutes
Duration: 6-7 hours

Pharmacokinetics
Distribution: V_d: 0.8-1.8 L/kg
Protein binding: 89%
Metabolism: Extensive in the liver
Half-life: 1.7-5 hours
Elimination: In urine as unchanged drug and metabolites

Usual Dosage Oral:
Children <18 years: Dosage not established; investigational doses of 0.02 mg/kg given as an elixir have been used in children (n=20) for sedation prior to dental procedures; further studies are needed before this dose can be recommended
Adults: 0.125-0.25 mg at bedtime

Administration Oral: Administer dose in bed, since onset of hypnotic effect is rapid; do not administer with grapefruit juice

Monitoring Parameters Liver enzymes with prolonged use

Patient Information Avoid alcohol; may be habit-forming with long-term use; do not discontinue abruptly; may cause drowsiness and impair ability to perform activities requiring mental alertness or physical coordination; take dose in bed at bedtime; may also cause daytime drowsiness; may cause dry mouth

Additional Information Onset of action is rapid, patient should be in bed when taking medication

Dosage Forms Tablet: 0.125 mg, 0.25 mg

References
Meyer ML, Mourino AP, and Farrington FH, "Comparison of Triazolam to a Chloral Hydrate/Hydroxyzine Combination in the Sedation of Pediatric Dental Patients," *Pediatr Dent*, 1990, 12(5):283-7.

♦ **Tribavirin** *see Ribavirin on page 872*
♦ **Trichloroacetaldehyde Monohydrate** *see Chloral Hydrate on page 215*
♦ **Tricosal®** *see Choline Magnesium Trisalicylate on page 231*
♦ **Triderm®** *see Triamcinolone on page 979*

Triethanolamine Polypeptide Oleate-Condensate
(trye eth a NOLE a meen pol i PEP tide OH lee ate-KON den sate)

U.S. Brand Names Cerumenex® Otic

Therapeutic Category Otic Agent, Cerumenolytic

Generic Available No

Use Removal of ear wax (cerumen)

Pregnancy Risk Factor C

Contraindications Perforated tympanic membrane or otitis media; hypersensitivity to triethanolamine polypeptide oleate-condensate or any component

Warnings Discontinue if sensitization or irritation occurs

Precautions Avoid undue exposure to skin during administration and the flushing out of ear canal; exposure of ear canal to otic solution should be limited to 15-30 minutes

Adverse Reactions Local: Localized dermatitis, mild erythema and pruritus, severe eczematoid reactions involving the external ear and periauricular tissue

Mechanism of Action Emulsifies and disperses accumulated cerumen for easier removal

Pharmacodynamics Onset of effect: Produces slight disintegration of very hard ear wax by 24 hours

Usual Dosage Children and Adults: Otic: Fill ear canal, insert cotton plug; allow to remain 15-30 minutes; flush ear with lukewarm water as a single treatment; if a second application is needed for unusually hard impactions, repeat the procedure

Monitoring Parameters Evaluate hearing before and after instillation of medication

Patient Information For external use in the ear only; warm to body temperature before using to improve effect

Nursing Implications Avoid undue exposure of the drug to the periaural skin

Dosage Forms Solution, otic: 10% (6 mL, 12 mL)

References
Mehta AK, "An *In Vitro* Comparison of the Disintegration of Human Ear Wax by Five Cerumenolytics Commonly Used in General Practice," *Br J Clin Pract*, 1985, 39(5):200-3.

♦ **Triethylenethiophosphoramide** *see Thiotepa on page 954*

♦ **Trifluorothymidine** *see* Trifluridine *on page 984*

Trifluridine (trye FLURE i deen)
U.S. Brand Names Viroptic®
Synonyms F_3T; Trifluorothymidine
Therapeutic Category Antiviral Agent, Ophthalmic
Generic Available No
Use Treatment of primary keratoconjunctivitis and recurrent epithelial keratitis caused by herpes simplex virus types I and II
Pregnancy Risk Factor C
Contraindications Hypersensitivity to trifluridine or any component
Adverse Reactions
   Cardiovascular: Hyperemia
   Local: Burning, stinging
   Ocular: Palpebral edema, epithelial keratopathy, keratitis, stromal edema, increased intraocular pressure
   Miscellaneous: Hypersensitivity reactions
Stability Store in refrigerator; storage at room temperature may result in a solution with altered pH which could result in ocular discomfort upon administration and/or decreased potency
Mechanism of Action Interferes with viral replication by incorporating into viral DNA in place of thymidine, inhibiting thymidylate synthetase resulting in the formation of defective proteins
Pharmacodynamics Onset of action: Response to treatment occurs within 2-7 days; epithelial healing is complete in 1-2 weeks
Pharmacokinetics Absorption: Ophthalmic: Systemic absorption is negligible, while corneal penetration is adequate
Usual Dosage Children and Adults: Ophthalmic: Instill 1 drop into affected eye every 2 hours while awake, to a maximum of 9 drops/day, until re-epithelialization of corneal ulcer occurs; then use 1 drop every 4 hours for another 7 days; do **not** exceed 21 days of treatment
Administration Ophthalmic: Avoid contact of bottle tip with skin or eye; instill drops onto the cornea of the affected eye(s); apply finger pressure to lacrimal sac during and for 1-2 minutes after instillation to decrease risk of absorption and systemic effects
Monitoring Parameters Ophthalmologic exam (test for corneal staining with fluorescein or rose Bengal)
Additional Information Found to be effective in 138 of 150 patients unresponsive or intolerant to idoxuridine or vidarabine
Dosage Forms Solution, ophthalmic: 1% (7.5 mL)

♦ **Triglycerides, Medium Chain** *see* Medium Chain Triglycerides *on page 623*
♦ **Trihexyphen (Can)** *see* Trihexyphenidyl *on page 984*

Trihexyphenidyl (trye heks ee FEN i dil)
Related Information
   Overdose and Toxicology *on page 1222*
U.S. Brand Names Artane®
Canadian Brand Names Apo-Trihex; Novo-Hexidyl; PMS-Trihexyphenidyl; Trihexyphen
Synonyms Benzhexol
Therapeutic Category Anticholinergic Agent; Antidote, Drug-induced Dystonic Reactions; Anti-Parkinson's Agent
Generic Available Yes: Tablet
Use Adjunctive treatment of Parkinson's disease; also used in treatment of drug-induced extrapyramidal effects and acute dystonic reactions
Pregnancy Risk Factor C
Contraindications Hypersensitivity to trihexyphenidyl or any component; children younger than 3 years of age; patients with narrow-angle glaucoma, GI or GU obstruction; myasthenia gravis, achalasia
Precautions Use with caution in patients with hyperthyroidism, renal or hepatic dysfunction, hypertension, hiatal hernia, tachycardia, cardiac arrhythmias, peptic ulcer, esophageal reflux; use with caution in hot weather or during exercise
Adverse Reactions
   Cardiovascular: Tachycardia
   Central nervous system: Dizziness, nervousness, drowsiness, agitation, delirium, headache
   Dermatologic: Rash

Gastrointestinal: Xerostomia, nausea, constipation
Genitourinary: Urinary hesitancy or retention
Neuromuscular & skeletal: Weakness
Ocular: Blurred vision, mydriasis, increased intraocular tension

Drug Interactions May increase gastric degradation of levodopa and decrease the amount of levodopa absorbed by delaying gastric emptying; antagonizes the therapeutic effects of cholinergic agents (tacrine, donepezil) and neuroleptics; increases central and/or peripheral anticholinergic effects when administered with amantadine, rimantadine, narcotic analgesics, phenothiazines and other antipsychotics (especially with high anticholinergic activity), tricyclic antidepressants, quinidine and some other antiarrhythmics, and antihistamines

Mechanism of Action Presumed to act by blocking excess acetylcholine at cerebral synapses; many of its effects are due to its pharmacologic similarities with atropine

Pharmacodynamics
Onset of effect: 1 hour
Peak effect: 2-3 hours
Duration: 6-12 hours

Pharmacokinetics
Metabolism: Metabolic fate undetermined
Bioavailability: 100%
Half-life: 5.6-10.2 hours
Elimination: Some urinary excretion

Usual Dosage Adults: Oral:
Extrapyramidal: 5-15 mg/day in 3-4 divided doses
Parkinsonism: 1 mg daily; increase by 2 mg increments every 3-5 days to 6-10 mg/day (maximum daily dosage: 12-15 mg); doses >10 mg/day should be divided into 3-4 doses

Administration Oral: Administer with food or water to decrease GI irritation

Monitoring Parameters Intraocular pressure monitoring (baseline and at regular intervals)

Patient Information Causes drowsiness and may impair ability to perform hazardous duties requiring mental alertness or physical coordination

Dosage Forms
Elixir, as hydrochloride: 2 mg/5 mL (480 mL)
Tablet, as hydrochloride: 2 mg, 5 mg

♦ **Tri-K®** *see* Potassium Supplements *on page 816*
♦ **Trikacide (Can)** *see* Metronidazole *on page 662*
♦ **Trileptal®** *see* Oxcarbazepine *on page 742*
♦ **Trilisate®** *see* Choline Magnesium Trisalicylate *on page 231*
♦ **Trimethaphan Camphorsulfonate** *see* Trimethaphan Camsylate *on page 985*

Trimethaphan Camsylate (trye METH a fan KAM si late)

U.S. Brand Names Arfonad® Injection

Synonyms Trimethaphan Camphorsulfonate

Therapeutic Category Alpha-Adrenergic Blocking Agent, Parenteral; Anticholinergic Agent; Antihypertensive Agent; Ganglionic Blocking Agent

Generic Available No

Use Hypertensive emergencies; controlled hypotension during surgery

Pregnancy Risk Factor D

Contraindications Hypersensitivity to trimethaphan camsylate or any component; hypovolemia or shock; anemia; respiratory insufficiency

Precautions Use with caution in patients with allergies; cardiac, hepatic, or renal dysfunction; diabetes mellitus, Addison's disease, or glaucoma

Adverse Reactions
Cardiovascular: Hypotension (especially orthostatic), tachycardia (especially in children and young adults)
Central nervous system: Restlessness
Dermatologic: Itching, urticaria
Endocrine & metabolic: With prolonged use (>48-72 hours) sodium and water retention
Gastrointestinal: Anorexia, nausea, vomiting, xerostomia, adynamic ileus
Genitourinary: Urinary retention
Ocular: Mydriasis, cycloplegia
Neuromuscular & skeletal: Weakness
Respiratory: Apnea, respiratory arrest (especially with doses >6 mg/minute)
(Continued)

Trimethaphan Camsylate *(Continued)*

Drug Interactions Anesthetics, procainamide, diuretics and other hypotensive agents may increase hypotensive effects of trimethaphan; effects of tubocurarine and succinylcholine may be prolonged by trimethaphan

Stability Solution should be freshly prepared and any unused portion discarded

Mechanism of Action Blocks transmission in both adrenergic and cholinergic ganglia by blocking stimulation from presynaptic receptors to postsynaptic receptors mediated by acetylcholine; possesses direct peripheral vasodilatory activity and is a weak histamine releaser

Pharmacodynamics
Onset of action: I.V.: Immediate
Peak effects: 5 minutes
Duration: 10-30 minutes

Pharmacokinetics
Metabolism: Primarily by postganglionic pseudocholinesterase
Elimination: Urinary excretion

Usual Dosage I.V.:
Children: 50-150 mcg/kg/minute
Adults: Initial: 0.5-2 mg/minute; titrate to effect; usual dose: 0.3-6 mg/minute

Administration Parenteral: Must be diluted; usually administered by I.V. continuous infusion at a final concentration of 1 mg/mL in D_5W

Monitoring Parameters Blood pressure and heart rate continuously

Dosage Forms Injection: 50 mg/mL (10 mL)

Trimethobenzamide *(trye meth oh BEN za mide)*

Related Information
Compatibility of Medications Mixed in a Syringe *on page 1238*

U.S. Brand Names Tigan®

Therapeutic Category Antiemetic

Generic Available No

Use Control of nausea and vomiting (especially for long-term antiemetic therapy)

Pregnancy Risk Factor C

Contraindications Hypersensitivity to trimethobenzamide, any component, or benzocaine (contained in suppository); suppositories are contraindicated in premature infants or neonates

Precautions Use cautiously in infants and children; may mask emesis due to Reye's syndrome or mimic CNS effects of Reye's syndrome in patients with emesis of other etiologies

Adverse Reactions
Cardiovascular: Hypotension (especially after I.M. use)
Central nervous system: Drowsiness, sedation, extrapyramidal symptoms, dizziness, seizures, coma, depression, opisthotonos
Dermatologic: Hypersensitivity skin reactions
Gastrointestinal: Diarrhea
Hematologic: Blood dyscrasias
Hepatic: Jaundice
Local: Pain, stinging, burning at I.M. injection site
Ocular: Blurred vision

Mechanism of Action Acts centrally to inhibit stimulation of the medullary chemoreceptor trigger zone

Pharmacodynamics
Onset of action:
Oral: 10-40 minutes
I.M.: 15-35 minutes
Duration:
Oral: 3-4 hours
I.M.: 2-3 hours

Pharmacokinetics
Metabolism: Not well determined
Bioavailability: Oral dose is ~60% of I.M. dose
Elimination: 20% excreted unchanged in urine in 24 hours

Usual Dosage Do not use rectally in neonates and infants
Children:
Oral, rectal: 15-20 mg/kg/day (400-500 mg/m²/day) divided into 3-4 doses; **or as an alternative**
<13.6 kg (30 lbs): 100 mg 3-4 times/day
13.6-41 kg (30-90 lbs): 100-200 mg 3-4 times/day

I.M.: Not recommended

Adults:

Oral: 250 mg 3-4 times/day

I.M., rectal: 200 mg 3-4 times/day

Administration

Oral: May administer with or without food

Parenteral: I.M. use only, **not** for I.V. use

Patient Information Causes drowsiness and may impair ability to perform activities requiring mental alertness or physical coordination

Additional Information Note: Less effective than phenothiazines but may be associated with fewer side effects

Dosage Forms

Capsule, as hydrochloride: 100 mg, 250 mg

Injection, as hydrochloride: 100 mg/mL (2 mL, 20 mL)

Suppository, rectal, as hydrochloride: 100 mg, 200 mg

Trimethoprim (trye METH oh prim)

Related Information

Blood Level Sampling Time Guidelines *on page 1220*

U.S. Brand Names Primsol®; Proloprim®; Trimpex®

Synonyms TMP

Therapeutic Category Antibiotic, Miscellaneous

Generic Available Yes: Tablets

Use Treatment of urinary tract infections caused by susceptible *Escherichia coli*, *Proteus mirabilis*, *Klebsiella pneumoniae*, *Enterobacter* species, and coagulase-negative *Staphylococcus* (including *S. saprophyticus*); prophylaxis of urinary tract infections; in combination with other agents for treatment of *Pneumocystis carinii* pneumonia; treatment of otitis media caused by susceptible *Streptococcus pneumoniae* and *Haemophilus influenzae* (not indicated for *Moraxella catarrhalis* due to consistent resistance); not indicated for prolonged administration or prophylaxis of otitis media

Pregnancy Risk Factor C

Contraindications Hypersensitivity to trimethoprim or any component; megaloblastic anemia due to folate deficiency

Warnings May cause folate deficiencies with subsequent bone marrow suppression and blood dyscrasias; monitor patients for fever, sore throat, purpura, or pallor; discontinue trimethoprim if bone marrow depression occurs; leucovorin (folinic acid) may be needed to restore normal hematopoiesis

Precautions Use with caution in patients with impaired renal or hepatic function or with possible folate deficiency; decrease dose in patients with renal dysfunction; safety is not established in infants <2 months of age; effectiveness for treatment of acute otitis media is not established in infants <6 months of age; oral solution contains propylene glycol and sodium benzoate (avoid use in neonates)

Adverse Reactions

Central nervous system: Fever, headache, aseptic meningitis

Dermatologic: Rash, pruritus, exfoliative dermatitis

Hematologic: Megaloblastic anemia, neutropenia, leukopenia, thrombocytopenia, methemoglobinemia

Hepatic: Elevated liver enzymes, cholestatic jaundice

Gastrointestinal: Nausea, vomiting, epigastric distress

Renal: Elevated BUN and serum creatinine

Drug Interactions Use with other folate antagonists (methotrexate, pyrimethamine) may increase risk of megaloblastic anemia; trimethoprim may decrease the metabolism of phenytoin resulting in increased phenytoin serum concentrations; cyclosporine, dapsone, procainamide, rifampin, warfarin

Food Interactions May cause folic acid deficiency, supplements may be needed

Stability Store tablets and solution at 15°C to 25°C (59°F to 77°F); protect from light

Mechanism of Action Binds to the enzyme dihydrofolate reductase in bacteria and inhibits conversion of dihydrofolic acid to tetrahydrofolate (functional form of folic acid). This results in depletion of folic acid, interference with bacterial biosynthesis of nucleic acids and protein production, and inhibition of microbial growth.

Pharmacokinetics

Absorption: Oral: Readily and extensively absorbed (90% to 100%)

Distribution: Penetrates into middle ear fluid with a mean peak middle ear fluid concentration in children 1-12 years of 2 mcg/mL after a single 4 mg/kg dose; crosses the placenta; excreted in breast milk

V_d:

Newborns: ~2.7 L/kg

(Continued)

Trimethoprim *(Continued)*

Infants: 1.5 L/kg
Children 1-10 years: ~1 L/kg
Adults: 1.3-1.8 L/kg
Protein binding: 42% to 46%
Metabolism: Partially (10% to 20%) metabolized in the liver via demethylation, oxidation, and hydroxylation
Bioavailability: Similar for tablets and solution
Half-life (prolonged in renal dysfunction):
Newborns: ~19 hours
Infants 2 months to 1 year: 3-6 hours; mean: 4.6 hours
Children 1-10 years: 3-5.5 hours
Adults, normal renal function: 8-11 hours
Adults, anuric: 20-50 hours
Time to peak serum concentration: Within 1-4 hours
Elimination: Significantly excreted in urine (60% to 80%) as unchanged drug via glomerular filtration and tubular secretion; increased renal excretion with acidic urine
Dialysis: Moderately dialyzable (20% to 50%)

Usual Dosage Oral:
Infants ≥6 months and Children: Acute otitis media: 10 mg/kg/day in divided doses every 12 hours for 10 days
Infants and Children <12 years: Urinary tract infection: Treatment: 4-6 mg/kg/day in divided doses every 12 hours for 10 days
Children ≥12 years and Adults:
Urinary tract infection: Treatment: 100 mg every 12 hours or 200 mg every 24 hours for 10 days
Prophylaxis: 100 mg once daily
Pneumocystis carinii pneumonia treatment (given with dapsone): 15-20 mg/kg/day in 4 divided doses for 21 days
Dosing adjustment in renal impairment:
Cl$_{cr}$ 15-30 mL/minute: Administer 50% of normal dose
Cl$_{cr}$ <15 mL/minute: Avoid use

Administration Oral: Administer on an empty stomach; may administer with milk or food if GI upset occurs

Monitoring Parameters CBC with differential, platelet count, liver enzyme tests, bilirubin, serum creatinine and BUN

Reference Range Therapeutic:
Peak: 5-15 mg/L
Trough: 2-8 mg/L

Test Interactions May falsely increase creatinine determination measured by the Jaffé alkaline picrate assay; may interfere with determination of serum methotrexate when measured by methods that use a bacterial dihydrofolate reductase as the binding protein (eg, the competitive binding protein technique); does **not** interfere with RIA for methotrexate

Patient Information Report any skin rash, persistent or severe fatigue, fever, sore throat, or unusual bleeding or bruising; complete full course of therapy

Additional Information Not effective versus *Pseudomonas* or *B. fragilis*; discontinue if bone marrow suppression occurs

Dosage Forms
Solution, oral, as hydrochloride (Primsol®): 50 mg/5 mL [as base] [bubblegum flavor, dye free, alcohol free] (473 mL)
Tablet:
Proloprim®: 100 mg, 200 mg
Trimpex®: 100 mg

References
Hoppu K, "Age Differences in Trimethoprim Pharmacokinetics: Need for Revised Dosing in Children?" *Clin Pharmacol Ther*, 1987, 41(3):336-43.
Hoppu K, Koskimies O, and Vilska J, "Trimethoprim in the Treatment of Acute Urinary Tract Infections in Children," *Int J Clin Pharmacol Ther Toxicol*, 1988, 26(2):65-8.
Leff RD, Cho CT, and Reed MD, "Safety and Efficacy of Trimethoprim Hydrochloride Solution for the Treatment of Children With Otitis Media," *Journal of Pediatric Pharmacy Practice*, 1998, 3(1): 33-9.

♦ **Trimethoprim and Sulfamethoxazole** *see* Co-Trimoxazole *on page 270*

♦ **Trimox**® *see* Amoxicillin *on page 80*

♦ **Trimpex**® *see* Trimethoprim *on page 987*

♦ **Tri-Nasal**® *see* Triamcinolone *on page 979*

♦ **Trinipatch (Can)** *see* Nitroglycerin *on page 717*

♦ **Triostat**™ *see* Liothyronine *on page 597*

♦ **Triple Antibiotic®** *see* Neomycin, Polymyxin B, and Bacitracin *on page 707*
♦ **Triple Care Cream (Can)** *see* Zinc Oxide *on page 1026*
♦ **Triposed® [OTC]** *see* Triprolidine and Pseudoephedrine *on page 989*

Triprolidine and Pseudoephedrine
(trye PROE li deen & soo doe e FED rin)

Related Information
OTC Cough & Cold Preparations, Pediatric *on page 1072*
Overdose and Toxicology *on page 1222*

U.S. Brand Names Actifed® Cold and Allergy [OTC]; Allerfrin® [OTC]; Allerphed® [OTC]; Aprodine® [OTC]; Genac® [OTC]; Silafed® [OTC]; Triposed® [OTC]

Synonyms Pseudoephedrine and Triprolidine

Therapeutic Category Antihistamine/Decongestant Combination; Sympathomimetic

Generic Available Yes

Use Temporary relief of nasal congestion, running nose, sneezing, itching of nose or throat and itchy, watery eyes due to common cold, hay fever or other upper respiratory allergies

Pregnancy Risk Factor C

Contraindications Hypersensitivity to triprolidine, any component, or pseudoephedrine; severe hypertension or coronary artery disease; MAO inhibitor therapy, GI or GU obstruction, narrow-angle glaucoma

Warnings Not recommended for use in children <4 months of age

Precautions Use with caution in patients with mild to moderate high blood pressure, heart disease, diabetes mellitus, asthma, thyroid disease, or prostatic hypertrophy

Adverse Reactions
Cardiovascular: Hypertension, tachycardia
Central nervous system: Sedation, CNS stimulation, headache
Gastrointestinal: Nausea, vomiting, xerostomia, anorexia

Drug Interactions MAO inhibitors, beta-blocking agents, other sympathomimetics, methyldopa, reserpine, alpha-blocking agents, CNS depressants

Usual Dosage Oral:
Children: May dose according to **pseudoephedrine** component: 4 mg/kg/day in divided doses 3-4 times/day **or**
4 months to 2 years: 1.25 mL 3-4 times/day
2-4 years: 2.5 mL 3-4 times/day
4-6 years: 3.75 mL 3-4 times/day
6-12 years: 5 mL or ½ tablet 3-4 times/day
Children >12 years and Adults: 10 mL or 1 tablet 3-4 times/day

Administration Oral: Administer with food or milk to decrease GI irritation

Patient Information May cause drowsiness and may impair ability to perform activities requiring mental alertness or physical coordination

Dosage Forms
Syrup (Allerfrin®, Allerphed®, Aprodine®, Silafed®, Triposed®): Triprolidine hydrochloride 1.25 mg and pseudoephedrine hydrochloride 30 mg per 5 mL (120 mL, 240 mL, 480 mL, 3840 mL)
Tablet (Actifed® Cold and Allergy, Allerfrim®, Aprodine®, Genac®): Triprolidine hydrochloride 2.5 mg and pseudoephedrine hydrochloride 60 mg

♦ **Tris Buffer** *see* Tromethamine *on page 990*
♦ **Tris(hydroxymethyl)aminomethane** *see* Tromethamine *on page 990*
♦ **Trisulfa (Can)** *see* Co-Trimoxazole *on page 270*
♦ **Trisulfa-S (Can)** *see* Co-Trimoxazole *on page 270*
♦ **Tri-Vi-Flor®** *see page 1069*
♦ **Tri-Vi-Sol®** *see page 1069*
♦ **Tri-Vit** *see page 1069*
♦ **Tri-Vit With Fluoride** *see page 1069*
♦ **Trizivir™** *see* Abacavir, Lamivudine, and Zidovudine *on page 26*

Troleandomycin (troe lee an doe MYE sin)
U.S. Brand Names TAO®

Synonyms Triacetyloleandomycin

Therapeutic Category Antibiotic, Macrolide

Generic Available No

Use Adjunct in the treatment of severe corticosteroid-dependent asthma due to its steroid-sparing properties; obsolete antibiotic with spectrum of activity similar to erythromycin
(Continued)

Troleandomycin *(Continued)*

Pregnancy Risk Factor C

Contraindications Hypersensitivity to troleandomycin or any component; concomitant administration of terfenadine, astemizole, pimozide, or cisapride with troleandomycin may result in QT interval prolongation, ventricular tachycardia, and torsade de pointes

Warnings Cholestatic hepatitis has been reported in patients who have received troleandomycin for 2 weeks or longer and in cases where repeated courses were administered

Precautions Use with caution in patients with impaired hepatic function.

Adverse Reactions

Central nervous system: Fever

Dermatologic: Urticaria, rash

Gastrointestinal: Abdominal cramping, nausea, vomiting, diarrhea, rectal burning, esophagitis

Hepatic: Cholestatic hepatitis, jaundice

Drug Interactions Cytochrome P-450 isoenzyme CYP3A3/4 substrate; isoenzyme CYP3A3/4 and CYP3A5-7 inhibitor

Troleandomycin inhibits the cytochrome P-450 microsomal enzyme system decreasing clearance of theophylline (see Additional Information), cisapride, triazolam, pimozide, astemizole, and terfenadine; interferes with metabolism of ergotamine and carbamazepine potentiating their action; decreases methylprednisolone clearance from a linear first order decline to a nonlinear decline in plasma concentration

Food Interactions Food delays the rate, but not the extent of absorption

Mechanism of Action Troleandomycin has an undefined action independent of its effects on steroid elimination

Pharmacokinetics

Time to peak serum concentration: Oral: Within 2 hours

Elimination: 10% to 25% excreted in urine as active drug; excreted in feces via bile

Usual Dosage Oral:

Children: 25-40 mg/kg/day divided every 6 hours

Adjunct in corticosteroid-dependent asthma: 14 mg/kg/day in divided doses every 6-12 hours not to exceed 250 mg every 6 hours; dose is tapered to once daily then alternate day dosing

Adults: 250-500 mg 4 times/day

Monitoring Parameters Hepatic function tests

Patient Information Report any prodromal symptoms of hepatitis (fatigue, weakness, nausea, vomiting, dark urine, or yellowing of eyes)

Additional Information For patients on both troleandomycin and theophylline: Troleandomycin can significantly reduce theophylline clearance resulting in higher serum theophylline concentrations; empiric reduction in theophylline dosage appears to be indicated with the initiation of troleandomycin

Dosage Forms Capsule: 250 mg

References

Brenner AM and Szefler SJ, "Troleandomycin in the Treatment of Severe Asthma," *Immunol Allergy Clin North Am*, 1991, 11(1):91-102.

Kamada AK, Hill MR, Brenner AM, et al, "Effect of Low-Dose Troleandomycin on Theophylline Clearance: Implications for Therapeutic Drug Monitoring," *Pharmacotherapy*, 1992, 12(2):98-102.

Spector SL, Katz FH, and Farr RS, "Troleandomycin: Effectiveness in Steroid-Dependent Asthma and Bronchitis," *J Allergy Clin Immunol*, 1974, 54(6):367-79.

Tromethamine *(troe METH a meen)*

U.S. Brand Names THAM®

Synonyms Tris Buffer; Tris(hydroxymethyl)aminomethane

Therapeutic Category Alkalinizing Agent, Parenteral

Generic Available No

Use Correction of metabolic acidosis associated with cardiac bypass surgery or cardiac arrest; to correct excess acidity of stored blood that is preserved with acid citrate dextrose (ACD); to prime the pump-oxygenator during cardiac bypass surgery; indicated in severe metabolic acidosis in patients in whom sodium or carbon dioxide elimination is restricted [eg, infants needing alkalinization after receiving maximum sodium bicarbonate (8-10 mEq/kg/24 hours)]

Pregnancy Risk Factor C

Contraindications Uremia or anuria; chronic respiratory acidosis; salicylate intoxication; hypersensitivity to tromethamine or any component

Warnings Avoid infusion via low-lying umbilical venous catheters due to associated risk of hepatocellular necrosis; due to osmotic effects, use of sodium bicarbonate for the treatment of acidotic neonates and infants with RDS may be preferred

Precautions Reduce dose and monitor pH carefully in renal impairment

Adverse Reactions

Cardiovascular: Venospasm

Endocrine & metabolic: Hyperosmolality of serum, hyperkalemia, hypoglycemia

Hepatic: Liver cell destruction from direct contact with tromethamine, hemorrhagic hepatic necrosis (when administered through umbilical vein at concentrations ≥1.2 M)

Local: Tissue irritation, necrosis with extravasation

Respiratory: Respiratory depression, apnea

Mechanism of Action Proton acceptor, which combines with hydrogen ions to form bicarbonate and buffer

Pharmacokinetics 30% of dose is not ionized; rapidly eliminated by kidneys

Usual Dosage I.V.: Dose depends on severity and progression of acidosis:

Neonates: Manufacturer's recommendation: 1 mL/kg for each pH unit below 7.4

Infants, Children, and Adults:

Empiric dosage based upon base deficit: Tromethamine mL of 0.3 M solution = body weight (kg) x base deficit (mEq/L); maximum: 500 mg/kg/dose = 13.9 mL/kg/dose using 0.3 M solution

Metabolic acidosis with cardiac arrest: Tromethamine mL of 0.3 M solution: 3.5-6 mL/kg/dose (126-216 mg/kg/dose); maximum: 500 mg/kg/dose = 13.9 mL/kg/dose using 0.3 M solution

Excess acidity of acid citrate dextrose priming blood: Tromethamine mL of 0.3 M solution: 14-70 mL added added to each 500 mL of blood

Acidosis during cardiac bypass surgery: Tromethamine mL of 0.3 M solution: 9 mL/kg (324 mg/kg/dose); maximum dose: 1000 mL (36 g) as single dose

Administration Parenteral: Maximum concentration: 0.3 molar; infuse slowly over at least 1 hour; administer into a central venous line

Monitoring Parameters Serum electrolytes, arterial blood gases, serum pH, blood sugar, EKG monitoring, renal function tests

Additional Information 1 mM = 120 mg = 3.3 mL = 1 mEq of THAM®

Dosage Forms Injection (THAM®): 18 g [0.3 molar] (500 mL)

♦ **Tronolane®** *see* Hemorrhoidal Preparations *on page 490*

♦ **Tropicacyl®** *see* Tropicamide *on page 991*

Tropicamide (troe PIK a mide)

U.S. Brand Names Mydriacyl®; Tropicacyl®

Canadian Brand Names Diotrope; Minims-Tropicamide

Synonyms Bistropamide

Therapeutic Category Ophthalmic Agent, Mydriatic

Generic Available Yes

Use Short-acting mydriatic used in diagnostic procedures; as well as preoperatively and postoperatively; treatment of some cases of acute iritis, iridocyclitis, and keratitis

Pregnancy Risk Factor C

Contraindications Glaucoma, adhesions between the iris and the lens; hypersensitivity to tropicamide or any component

Warnings Tropicamide may cause an increase in intraocular pressure

Precautions Use with caution in infants and children since tropicamide may cause potentially dangerous CNS disturbances and psychotic reactions

Adverse Reactions

Cardiovascular: Tachycardia, flushing

Central nervous system: Parasympathetic stimulation, drowsiness, headache, behavioral disturbances, psychotic reactions

Gastrointestinal: Xerostomia

Local: Transient stinging

Ocular: Blurred vision, photophobia, increased intraocular pressure, follicular conjunctivitis

Miscellaneous: Allergic reactions

Stability Store at room temperature; do not refrigerate

Mechanism of Action Prevents the sphincter muscle of the iris and the muscle of the ciliary body from responding to cholinergic stimulation producing pupillary dilation and paralysis of accommodation

Pharmacodynamics

Maximum mydriatic effect: ~20-40 minutes

(Continued)

Tropicamide *(Continued)*

Duration: ~6-7 hours
Maximum cycloplegic effect:
Peak: 20-35 minutes
Duration: <6 hours

Usual Dosage Children and Adults: Ophthalmic:

Cycloplegia: Instill 1-2 drops (1%); may repeat in 5 minutes. The exam must be performed within 30 minutes after the repeat dose; if the patient is not examined within 20-30 minutes, instill an additional drop. Concentrations <1% are inadequate for producing satisfactory cycloplegia.

Mydriasis: Instill 1-2 drops (0.5%) 15-20 minutes before exam; may repeat every 30 minutes as needed

Administration Ophthalmic: To minimize systemic absorption, apply finger pressure on the lacrimal sac for 1-2 minutes following instillation of the ophthalmic solution; avoid contact of bottle tip with skin or eye

Patient Information May cause blurred vision; do not drive or engage in hazardous activities while the pupils are dilated; may cause sensitivity to light

Dosage Forms Solution, ophthalmic: 0.5% (2 mL, 15 mL); 1% (2 mL, 3 mL, 15 mL)

References

Caputo AR and Schnitzer RE, "Systemic Response to Mydriatic Eyedrops in Neonates: Mydriatics in Neonates," *J Pediatr Ophthalmol Strabismus*, 1978, 15(2):109-22.

♦ **T/Scalp**® **[OTC]** *see Hydrocortisone on page 506*
♦ **TSPA** *see Thiotepa on page 954*
♦ **T-Stat**® *see Erythromycin on page 394*

Tubocurarine *(too boe kyoor AR een)*

Synonyms *d*-Tubocurarine

Therapeutic Category Neuromuscular Blocker Agent, Nondepolarizing; Skeletal Muscle Relaxant, Paralytic

Generic Available No

Use Adjunct to anesthesia to induce skeletal muscle relaxation

Pregnancy Risk Factor C

Potential Drug Interactions

Potentiation	Antagonism
Inhalation anesthetics	Calcium
Desflurane, sevoflurane, enflurane and	Carbamazepine
isoflurane > halothane > nitrous	Phenytoin
oxide	Steroids (chronic administration)
Antibiotics	Theophylline
Aminoglycosides, polymyxins,	Anticholinesterases*
clindamycin, vancomycin	Neostigmine, pyridostigmine,
Magnesium	edrophonium, echothiophate
Antiarrhythmics	ophthalmic solution
Quinidine, procainamide, bretylium, and	Caffeine
possibly lidocaine	Azathioprine
Diuretics	
Furosemide, mannitol, thiazides	
Amphotericin B (secondary to hypokalemia)	
Local anesthetics	
Dantrolene (directly depresses skeletal muscle)	
Beta blockers	
Calcium channel blockers	
Ketamine	
Lithium	
Succinylcholine (when administered prior to nondepolarizing neuromuscular-blocking agent)	
Cyclosporine	

*Can prolong the effects of acetylcholine

Contraindications Hypersensitivity to tubocurarine or any component

Warnings Ventilation must be supported during neuromuscular blockade; some commercially available products may contain sulfites and benzyl alcohol; avoid products with benzyl alcohol in neonates

Precautions Use with caution in patients with renal impairment, respiratory depression, impaired hepatic or endocrine function, myasthenia gravis; several clinical conditions may antagonize or potentiate neuromuscular blockade, see table.

Clinical Conditions Affecting Neuromuscular Blockade

Potentiation	Antagonism
Electrolyte abnormalities	Alkalosis
Severe hyponatremia	Hypercalcemia
Severe hypocalcemia	Demyelinating lesions
Severe hypokalemia	Peripheral neuropathies
Hypermagnesemia	Diabetes mellitus
Neuromuscular diseases	
Acidosis	
Acute intermittent porphyria	
Renal failure	
Hepatic failure	

Adverse Reactions Most frequent adverse reactions are related to prolongation of its pharmacologic actions
Cardiovascular: Cardiac arrhythmias, hypotension, tachycardia or bradycardia
Gastrointestinal: Decreased GI motility, increased salivation
Neuromuscular & skeletal: Muscle weakness
Respiratory: Bronchospasm
Miscellaneous: Allergic reactions, hypersensitivity reactions

Drug Interactions See table on previous page.

Stability Refrigerate; incompatible with barbiturates

Mechanism of Action Nondepolarizing neuromuscular blocking agent which blocks acetylcholine from binding to receptors on motor endplate thus inhibiting depolarization; also has histamine-releasing and ganglionic blocking properties

Pharmacodynamics
Onset of effect:
I.M.: Unpredictable, 10-25 minutes
I.V.: 2-5 minutes
Duration: 20-30 minutes

Pharmacokinetics Elimination: ~33% to 75% of parenteral dose excreted unchanged in urine in 24 hours; about 11% excreted in bile through a specific organic cation secretion mechanism

Usual Dosage I.V.:
Neonates <1 month: 0.3 mg/kg as a single dose; maintenance: 0.1 mg/kg/dose as needed to maintain paralysis
Children: 0.2-0.5 mg/kg as a single dose; maintenance: 0.04-0.1 mg/kg/dose as needed to maintain paralysis
Adults: 0.5-0.6 mg/kg or 0.3 mg/kg after initial dose of succinylcholine for intubation; administer maintenance doses every 40-60 minutes as needed
Dosing adjustment in renal impairment: May accumulate with multiple doses and, therefore, reduction in subsequent doses is recommended
Cl_{cr} 50-80 mL/minute: Administer 75% of normal dose
Cl_{cr} 10-50 mL/minute: Administer 50% of normal dose
Cl_{cr} <10 mL/minute: Avoid use
Dosing in hepatic impairment: Larger doses may be necessary

Administration Parenteral: May infuse direct I.V. without further dilution over a period of 1-1½ minutes

Monitoring Parameters Respiratory status, heart rate, blood pressure, mechanical ventilator status, peripheral nerve stimulator measuring twitch response

Nursing Implications Does **not** alter the patient's state of consciousness; addition of sedation and analgesia is recommended

Dosage Forms Injection, as chloride: 3 mg/mL [3 units/mL] (5 mL, 10 mL, 20 mL)

♦ **Tumor Lysis Syndrome, Management** *see page 1158*
♦ **Tums**® **[OTC]** *see* Antacid Preparations *on page 95*
♦ **Tums**® **[OTC]** *see* Calcium Supplements *on page 167*
♦ **Tums**® **E-X [OTC]** *see* Calcium Supplements *on page 167*

- **Tums® Ultra® [OTC]** *see* Calcium Supplements *on page 167*
- **Tuss-DM® [OTC]** *see* Guaifenesin and Dextromethorphan *on page 487*
- **Tussin® [OTC]** *see* Guaifenesin *on page 485*
- **Tussin® DM [OTC]** *see* Guaifenesin and Dextromethorphan *on page 487*
- **Tussin DM Antitussive (Can)** *see* Dextromethorphan *on page 316*
- **Tussin GF Expectorant (Can)** *see* Guaifenesin *on page 485*
- **Tussi-Organidin® DM NR** *see* Guaifenesin and Dextromethorphan *on page 487*
- **Tussi-Organidin® NR** *see* Guaifenesin and Codeine *on page 486*
- **Tussi-Organidin® S-NR** *see* Guaifenesin and Codeine *on page 486*
- **Tusstat®** *see* Diphenhydramine *on page 342*
- **Twice-A-Day® [OTC]** *see* Oxymetazoline *on page 749*
- **Twin-K®** *see* Potassium Supplements *on page 816*
- **Tylenol® [OTC]** *see* Acetaminophen *on page 29*
- **Tylenol No. 3 with Codeine without Caffeine (Can)** *see* Acetaminophen and Codeine *on page 31*
- **Tylenol® With Codeine** *see* Acetaminophen and Codeine *on page 31*
- **Tylenol with Codeine No 4 (Can)** *see* Acetaminophen and Codeine *on page 31*
- **Tylox®** *see* Oxycodone and Acetaminophen *on page 747*
- **UCB-P071** *see* Cetirizine *on page 212*
- **UDCA** *see* Ursodiol *on page 996*
- **Ulcidine (Can)** *see* Famotidine *on page 417*
- **Ultrase®** *see* Pancrelipase *on page 755*
- **Ultrase® MT** *see* Pancrelipase *on page 755*
- **Unasyn®** *see* Ampicillin and Sulbactam *on page 90*

Undecylenic Acid and Derivatives
(un de sil EN ik AS id & dah RIV ah tivs)

U.S. Brand Names Caldesene® Topical [OTC]; Cruex® Topical [OTC]; Fungoid® Topical Solution; Merlenate® Topical [OTC]; Pedi-Dri Topical; Pedi-Pro Topical [OTC]; Quinsana® Plus Topical [OTC]; Undoguent® Topical [OTC]

Canadian Brand Names Desenex

Synonyms Zincundecate

Therapeutic Category Antifungal Agent, Topical

Generic Available Yes

Use Treatment of athlete's foot (tinea pedis), ringworm (except nails and scalp), prickly heat, jock itch (tinea cruris), diaper rash, and other minor skin irritations due to superficial dermatophytes

Contraindications Hypersensitivity to undecylenic acid and derivatives or any component; fungal infections of the scalp or nails

Warnings Do not apply to blistered, raw, or oozing areas of skin or over deep wounds or puncture wounds

Adverse Reactions
Dermatologic: Rash
Local: Skin irritation, stinging, sensitization

Mechanism of Action Undecylenic acid is a fatty acid with fungistatic activity that retards proliferation of the fungus by altering the conditions of growth; zinc undecylenate provides an astringent action that aids in the reduction of inflammation and irritation

Pharmacodynamics Onset of action: Improvement in erythema and pruritus may be seen within 1 week after initiation of therapy

Usual Dosage Children and Adults: Topical: Apply as needed twice daily for 2-4 weeks

Administration Topical: Clean and dry the affected area before topical application; if the solution is sprayed or applied onto the affected area, allow area to air dry; ointment or cream should be applied at night, the powder may be applied during the day or used alone when a drying effect is needed

Monitoring Parameters Resolution of skin infection

Patient Information For external use only; avoid contact with the eye; do not inhale the powder

Dosage Forms
Cream: Total undecylenate 20% (15 g, 82.5 g)
Foam, topical: Undecylenic acid 10% (42.5 g)
Liquid, topical: Undecylenic acid 10% (42.5 g)
Ointment, topical: Total undecylenate 22% (30 g, 60 g, 454 g); total undecylenate 25% (60 g, 454 g)

Powder, topical: Calcium undecylenate 10% (45 g, 60 g, 120 g); total undecylenate 22% (45 g, 54 g, 81 g, 90 g, 105 g, 165 g, 454 g)

Solution, topical: Undecylenic acid 25% (29.57 mL)

♦ **Undoguent**® **Topical [OTC]** *see* Undecylenic Acid and Derivatives *on page 994*
♦ **Uni-Dur**® *see* Theophylline *on page 943*
♦ **Unipen**® **Injection** *see* Nafcillin *on page 693*
♦ **Unipen**® **Oral** *see* Nafcillin *on page 693*
♦ **Uniphyl**® *see* Theophylline *on page 943*
♦ **Uni-Pro**® **[OTC]** *see* Ibuprofen *on page 520*
♦ **Unisom**® **Maximum Strength [OTC]** *see* Diphenhydramine *on page 342*
♦ **Unithroid**® *see* Levothyroxine *on page 588*
♦ **Urasal (Can)** *see* Methenamine *on page 643*
♦ **Urea Peroxide** *see* Carbamide Peroxide *on page 178*
♦ **Urecholine**® *see* Bethanechol *on page 142*
♦ **Urex**® *see* Methenamine *on page 643*
♦ **Urocit**®**-K** *see* Citrate and Citric Acid *on page 244*

Urokinase (yoor oh KIN ase)

U.S. Brand Names Abbokinase®
Therapeutic Category Thrombolytic Agent
Generic Available No
Use Thrombolytic agent used in treatment of recent severe or massive deep vein or arterial thrombosis, pulmonary emboli, and occluded arteriovenous cannulas
Pregnancy Risk Factor B
Contraindications Hypersensitivity to urokinase or any component; internal bleeding; CVA (within 2 months); brain carcinoma, bacterial endocarditis, anticoagulant therapy, surgery or trauma within past 10 days
Warnings Stop urokinase administration if any signs of bleeding occur. Due to problems in the manufacturing process, the FDA recommended on January 25, 1999, that Abbokinase® be reserved for critical use in specific patients after consideration has been given to alternative agents; Abbokinase® is made from kidney cell cultures that come from human neonates (postmortem harvesting); deficiencies in the harvesting and manufacturing process may have increased the risk of transmission of an infectious agent; the FDA does not know of any cases of infectious diseases that were transmitted by the use of Abbokinase®; the manufacturer is in the process of correcting the problems and has added additional tests (but the new processes and tests have not been fully validated). For further information, see http://www.fda.gov/medwatch/safety/1999/safety99.htm
Precautions Systemic use: Use with caution in patients with severe hypertension, recent lumbar puncture, patient receiving I.M. administration of medications. If indicated, febrile patients should receive antibiotics for at least 24 hours prior to urokinase therapy; obtain an echocardiogram in febrile patients prior to therapy to rule out intracardiac vegetations; pretreatment lab studies should include platelet count, PT/PTT, fibrinogen, fibrin degradation products, plasminogen, antithrombin III, protein S, protein C.
Adverse Reactions
Central nervous system: Fever
Dermatologic: Rash
Hematologic: Internal bleeding
Local: Bleeding, hematoma at I.M. or L.P. sites
Respiratory: Bronchospasm
Miscellaneous: Allergic reactions
Drug Interactions Anticoagulants, aspirin
Stability Store 250,000 unit vials in refrigerator; powder for 5000 unit/mL ("open-cath") should be stored below 77°F; avoid freezing; reconstitute by gently rolling and tilting, **do not shake**; does not contain preservative; the 5000 unit vial should be reconstituted just prior to use; discard unused portion; a reconstituted 250,000 unit vial is stable for 24 hours under refrigeration
Mechanism of Action Promotes thrombolysis by directly activating plasminogen to plasmin, which degrades fibrin, fibrinogen, and other procoagulant plasma proteins
Pharmacodynamics
Onset of action: I.V.: Fibrinolysis occurs rapidly
Duration: 4 or more hours
Pharmacokinetics
Half-life: 10-20 minutes
(Continued)

Urokinase *(Continued)*

Elimination: Cleared by the liver with a small amount excreted in the urine and the bile

Usual Dosage

Infants, Children, and Adults:

Arterial or venous thrombosis or pulmonary emboli: I.V.: Loading dose: 4400 units/kg over 10 minutes, followed by 4400 units/kg/hour for 6-12 hours; some patients may require longer (12-72 hours) or shorter courses of treatment; dose should be individualized based on response; continuous infusion doses of 4000-10,000 units/kg/hour have been used; reassess clot size every 12-24 hours

Occluded I.V. catheters:

5000 units/mL concentration; (use only Abbokinase® Open Cath), the volume to instill into the catheter is equal to the internal volume of the catheter; administer in each lumen over 1-2 minutes, leave in lumen for 1-4 hours, then **aspirate out of catheter**, flush catheter with NS; may repeat with 10,000 units in each lumen if 5000 units fails to clear the catheter; **do not infuse into the patient**

Continuous I.V. infusion: 150-200 units/kg/hour in each lumen for 8-48 hours; infuse at a rate of at least 20 mL/hour in children and adults

Dialysis patients: 5000 units is administered in each lumen over 1-2 minutes; leave urokinase in lumen for 1-2 days, then aspirate out of lumen

Adults: MI: Intracoronary: 6000 units/minute up to 2 hours

Administration Parenteral: I.V. infusion: Usual concentration: 1250-1500 units/mL; maximum concentration not yet defined

Abbokinase® Open Cath 5000 unit product is **not** for systemic administration, it must be aspirated out of the catheter; do **not** dilute Abbokinase® Open Cath for I.V. infusion

Monitoring Parameters CBC, reticulocyte, platelet count; fibrinogen level, plasminogen, fibrin/fibrinogen degradation products, D-dimer, PT, APTT, thrombin clotting time, ATIII, protein C, ACT, urinalysis

Reference Range Systemic thrombolysis: Usual desired pediatric lower limit for fibrinogen level is 100 mg/dL

Nursing Implications Use 0.22 or 0.45 micron filter during I.V. systemic therapy

Additional Information Failure of thrombolytic agents in newborns/neonates may occur due to the low plasminogen concentrations (~50% to 70% of adult levels); higher doses of urokinase may be needed, supplementing plasminogen (via administration of fresh frozen plasma) may possibly help

Dosage Forms

Powder for injection, preservative free: 250,000 units

Powder for injection, catheter clear, preservative free: 5000 units, 9000 units

References

Andrew M, Brooker L, Leaker M, et al, "Fibrin Clot Lysis by Thrombolytic Agents Is Impaired in Newborns Due to a Low Plasminogen Concentration," *Thromb Haemost*, 1992, 68(3):325-30.

Bagnall HA, Gomperts E, and Atkinson JB, "Continuous Infusion of Low-Dose Urokinase in the Treatment of Central Venous Catheter Thrombosis in Infants and Children," *Pediatrics*, 1989, 83(6):963-6.

Kothari SS, Varma S, and Wasir HS, "Thrombolytic Therapy in Infants and Children," *Am Heart J*, 1994, 127(3):651-7.

Manco-Johnson MJ, Nuss R, Hays T, et al, "Combined Thrombolytic and Anticoagulant Therapy for Venous Thrombosis in Children," *J Pediatr*, 2000, 136(4):446-53.

Monagle P, Michelson AD, Bovill E, et al, "Antithrombotic Therapy in Children," *Chest*, 2001, 119:334S-70S.

Nowak-Gottl U, Auberger K, Halimeh S, et al, "Thrombolysis in Newborns and Infants," *Thromb Haemost*, 1999, 82 (Suppl 1):112-6.

Phelps KC and Verazino KC, "Alternatives to Urokinase for the Management of Central Venous Catheter Occlusion," *Hospital Pharmacy*, 2001, 36(3): 265-74.

♦ **Uro-KP-Neutral**® *see* Phosphate Supplements *on page 794*

♦ **Urolene Blue**® *see* Methylene Blue *on page 653*

♦ **Uro-Mag**® **[OTC]** *see* Magnesium Supplements *on page 614*

♦ **Uromitexan (Can)** *see* Mesna *on page 636*

♦ **Uroplus**® **DS** *see* Co-Trimoxazole *on page 270*

♦ **Uroplus**® **SS** *see* Co-Trimoxazole *on page 270*

♦ **Urozide (Can)** *see* Hydrochlorothiazide *on page 503*

♦ **Ursacol** *see* Ursodiol *on page 996*

♦ **Urso**® *see* Ursodiol *on page 996*

♦ **Ursodeoxycholic Acid** *see* Ursodiol *on page 996*

Ursodiol *(ER soe dye ole)*

U.S. Brand Names Actigall™; Urso®

Synonyms UDCA; Ursacol; Ursodeoxycholic Acid

Therapeutic Category Gallstone Dissolution Agent

Generic Available No

Use Gallbladder stone dissolution; prevention of gallstone formation (obese patients experiencing rapid weight loss); primary biliary cirrhosis (Urso®)

   Unlabeled use: facilitate bile excretion in infants with biliary atresia; cholestasis secondary to PN; improve the hepatic metabolism of essential fatty acids in patients with cystic fibrosis

Pregnancy Risk Factor B

Contraindications Hypersensitivity to ursodiol or any component; not to be used with calcified cholesterol stones, radiopaque stones, bile pigment stones, or stones larger than 20 mm in diameter; allergy to bile acids; patients with compelling reasons for cholecystectomy (eg, unremitting acute cholecystitis, cholangitis, biliary obstruction)

Warnings Gallbladder stone dissolution may take several months of therapy; complete dissolution may not occur and recurrence of stones within 5 years has been observed in 50% of patients

Precautions Use with caution in patients with a nonvisualizing gallbladder and those with chronic liver disease

Adverse Reactions

   Central nervous system: Headache, fatigue, anxiety, depression, sleep disorder

   Dermatologic: Rash, pruritus, hair thinning

   Gastrointestinal: Diarrhea, biliary pain, constipation, stomatitis, flatulence, nausea, vomiting, abdominal pain

   Hepatic: Elevated liver enzymes

   Neuromuscular & skeletal: Arthralgias, myalgia, back pain

   Respiratory: Cough, rhinitis

Drug Interactions Decreased effect with aluminum-containing antacids, cholestyramine, colestipol, clofibrate, oral contraceptives (estrogens), activated charcoal

Stability Do not store above 30°C (86°F)

Mechanism of Action Decreases the cholesterol content of bile and bile stones by reducing the secretion of cholesterol from the liver and the fractional reabsorption of cholesterol by the intestines

Pharmacokinetics

   Absorption: 90%

   Metabolism: Undergoes extensive enterohepatic recycling; following hepatic conjugation and biliary secretion, the drug is hydrolyzed to active ursodiol, where it is recycled or transformed to lithocholic acid by colonic microbial flora

   Half-life: 100 hours

   Elimination: In feces via bile

Usual Dosage Oral:

   Biliary atresia: Infants: 10-15 mg/kg/day once daily

   Improvement in the hepatic metabolism of essential fatty acids in cystic fibrosis: Children: 30 mg/kg/day

   TPN-induced cholestasis: Infants and Children: 30 mg/kg/day in 3 divided doses

   Gallstone dissolution: Adults: 8-10 mg/kg/day in 2-3 divided doses; maintenance therapy: 250 mg/day at bedtime for 6 months to 1 year; use beyond 24 months is not established

   Gallstone prevention: Adults: 300 mg twice daily

   Primary biliary cirrhosis: Adults: 13-15 mg/kg/day in 4 divided doses

Administration Oral: Administer with food or, if a single dosage, at bedtime

Monitoring Parameters ALT, AST, sonogram, oral cholecystogram before therapy and every 6 months during therapy; obtain ultrasound images of gallbladder at 6-month intervals for the first year of therapy

Patient Information Frequent blood work necessary to follow drug effects; report any persistent nausea, vomiting, abdominal pain

Additional Information 30% to 50% of patients have stone recurrence after dissolution

Dosage Forms

   Capsule (Actigall™): 300 mg

   Tablet, film-coated (Urso®): 250 mg

Extemporaneous Preparations

   A 20 mg/mL ursodiol suspension may be made by opening seventeen 300 mg capsules; add in geometric proportions a 1:1 mixture of Ora-Sweet®:Ora-Plus® or 1% methylcellulose:syrup NF to a total volume of 255 mL; stable 91 days refrigerated. (Nahata, 1999)

   A 25 mg/mL ursodiol suspension may be made by opening ten 300 mg capsules; mix with 10 mL Glycerin, USP until smooth mixture is obtained. Add 60 mL Ora-Plus® and continue to levigate until a smooth mixture is achieved. Transfer (Continued)

Ursodiol *(Continued)*

mixture to a light-resistent bottle; add a small amount of Orange Syrup, NF to wash remaining drug from the mortar to bottle. Add additional syrup to make final volume of 120 mL. Label "shake well"; stable 60 days at room temperature or refrigerated. (Johnson, 1995)

A 60 mg/mL ursodiol suspension may be made in a similar method by opening twelve 300 mg capsules and wetting with sufficient glycerin and triturating to make a fine paste; gradually add simple syrup to make a final volume of 60 mL. Label "shake well"; stable 35 days in refrigerator. (Mallett, 1997)

Johnson CE and Nesbitt J, "Stability of Ursodiol in an Extemporaneously Compounded Oral Liquid," *Am J Health Syst Pharm*, 1995, 52(16):1798-800.

Mallett MS, Hagan RL, and Peters DA, "Stability of Ursodiol 25 mg/mL in an Extemporaneously Prepared Oral Liquid," *Am J Health-Syst Pharm*, 1997, 54(12):1401-4.

Nahata MC, Morosco RS, and Hipple TF, "Stability of Ursodiol in Two Extemporaneously Prepared Oral Suspensions," *J Appl Ther Res*, 1999, 3:221-4.

References

Colombo C, Setchell KD, Podda M, et al, "Effect of Ursodeoxycholic Acid Therapy for Liver Disease Associated With Cystic Fibrosis," *J Pediatr*, 1990, 117(3):482-9.

Lepage G, Paradis K, Lacaille F, et al, "Ursodeoxycholic Acid Improves the Hepatic Metabolism of Essential Fatty Acids and Retinol in Children With Cystic Fibrosis," *J Pediatr*, 1997, 130(1)52-8.

Spagnuolo MI, Iorio R, Vegnente A, et al, "Ursodeoxycholic Acid for Treatment of Cholestasis in Children on Long-Term Total Parenteral Nutrition - A Pilot Study," *Gastroenterology*, 1996, 111(3):716-9.

Ullrich D, Rating D, Schroter W, et al, "Treatment With Ursodeoxycholic Acid Renders Children With Biliary Atresia Suitable for Liver Transplantation," *Lancet*, 1987, 2(8571):1324.

♦ **UTI Relief**® **[OTC]** *see* Phenazopyridine *on page 784*

♦ **Vagifem**® *see* Estradiol *on page 400*

♦ **Valergen**® *see* Estradiol *on page 400*

♦ **Valium**® *see* Diazepam *on page 320*

Valproic Acid and Derivatives (val PROE ik AS id & dah RIV ah tivs)

Related Information

Antiepileptic Drugs *on page 1208*

Blood Level Sampling Time Guidelines *on page 1220*

Carbohydrate and Alcohol Content of Liquid Medications for Use in Patients Receiving Ketogenic Diets *on page 1258*

Serotonin Syndrome *on page 1247*

U.S. Brand Names Depacon™; Depakene®; Depakote®; Depakote®-ER

Canadian Brand Names Alti-Valproic; Apo-Divalproex; Apo-Valproic; Deproic; Epiject; Epival; Gen-Valproic; Novo-Divalproex; Novo-Valproic; Nu-Divalproex; Nu-Valproic; PMS-Valproic; Rhoxal-Valproic

Synonyms Dipropylacetic Acid; DPA; 2-Propylpentanoic Acid; 2-Propylvaleric Acid; VPA

Therapeutic Category Anticonvulsant, Miscellaneous; Infantile Spasms, Treatment

Generic Available Yes

Use Management of simple and complex partial seizures, simple and complex absence seizures, mixed seizure types, myoclonic and generalized tonic-clonic (grand mal) seizures; may be effective in infantile spasms; divalproex sodium is also indicated for the treatment of manic episodes of bipolar disorders (manic-depressive illness) in adults and the prevention of migraine headaches

Pregnancy Risk Factor D

Contraindications Hypersensitivity to valproic acid or derivatives or any component; hepatic dysfunction

Warnings Hepatic failure resulting in death may occur; children <2 years of age (especially those on polytherapy, with congenital metabolic disorders, with seizure disorders and mental retardation, or with organic brain disease) are at considerable risk; monitor patients closely for appearance of malaise, loss of seizure control, weakness, facial edema, anorexia, jaundice and vomiting; hepatotoxicity has been reported after 3 days to 6 months of therapy. Pancreatitis resulting in death may occur; pancreatitis may be hemorrhagic and rapidly progress to death; onset has occurred shortly after starting therapy and after several years of treatment; monitor patients closely for nausea, vomiting, anorexia, and abdominal pain and evaluate promptly; discontinue valproate if pancreatitis occurs. Dose-related thrombocytopenia may occur. I.V. valproate is not recommended for the prophylaxis of post-traumatic seizures in patients with acute head trauma

Precautions Valproate may stimulate the replication of HIV and CMV *in vitro*; clinical effects are unknown

Adverse Reactions

Central nervous system: Drowsiness, irritability, confusion, restlessness, hyperactivity, malaise, headache, ataxia, dizziness, asthenia

Dermatologic: Alopecia, erythema multiforme

Endocrine & metabolic: Hyperammonemia, impaired fatty-acid oxidation, carnitine deficiency

Gastrointestinal: Nausea, vomiting, diarrhea, dyspepsia, constipation, pancreatitis (potentially fatal), weight gain, taste perversion (I.V.)

Hematologic: Thrombocytopenia (risk increases significantly with serum levels ≥110 mcg/mL (females) or ≥135 mcg/mL (males)), prolongation of bleeding time

Hepatic: Transiently elevated liver enzymes, liver failure (can be fatal)

Local: I.V.: Pain and local reaction at injection site

Neuromuscular & skeletal: Tremor

Ocular: Diplopia, blurred vision

Drug Interactions
Cytochrome P-450 isoenzyme CYP2C19 substrate; CYP2C9 and CYP2D6 isoenzyme inhibitor, CYP3A3/4 isoenzyme inhibitor (weak)

Valproic acid may displace phenytoin and diazepam from protein binding sites. Aspirin may displace valproic acid from protein binding sites which may result in toxicity. Valproic acid may significantly increase phenobarbital serum concentrations in patients receiving phenobarbital or primidone. Valproic acid may increase zidovudine, amitriptyline, or nortriptyline concentrations; valproic acid may inhibit the metabolism of lamotrigine and phenytoin. Phenobarbital, primidone, phenytoin, and carbamazepine may decrease serum levels of valproic acid; felbamate may increase plasma concentrations of valproic acid; antacids may increase the oral absorption of valproic acid.

Food Interactions
Dietary carnitine requirements may be increased; food may decrease the rate but not the extent of absorption

Stability
Injection: Stable for 24 hours at room temperature when diluted in D$_5$W, NS, or LR; discard unused portion of vial (does not contain preservative)

Mechanism of Action
Causes increased availability of gamma-aminobutyric acid (GABA), an inhibitory neurotransmitter, to brain neurons or may enhance the action of GABA or mimic its action at postsynaptic receptor sites

Pharmacokinetics

Protein binding: 80% to 90% (dose dependent); decreased protein binding in neonates, elderly, and patients with renal impairment or chronic hepatic disease

Distribution: Distributes into CSF at concentrations similar to unbound concentration in plasma (ie, ~10% of total plasma concentration)

Metabolism: Extensive in liver via glucuronide conjugation and oxidation

Bioavailability: Oral: Equivalent to I.V.; **Depakote®-ER tablets are not bioequivalent to Depakote® delayed release tablets**; mean bioavailability of Depakote®-ER tablets is 81% to 89%, relative to Depakote® delayed release tablets

Half-life: Increased with liver disease

Newborns (exposed to VPA *in utero*): 30-60 hours

Newborns 1st week of life: 40-45 hours

Newborns <10 days: 10-67 hours

Children >2 months: 7-13 hours

Children 2-14 years: Mean: 9 hours; range: 3.5-20 hours

Adults: 8-17 hours

Time to peak serum concentration:

Oral: 1-4 hours; divalproex (enteric coated): 3-5 hours

I.V.: At the end of the infusion

Elimination: 2% to 3% excreted unchanged in urine; faster clearance in children who receive other antiepileptic drugs and those who are younger; age and polytherapy explain 80% of interpatient variability in total clearance; children >10 years of age have pharmacokinetic parameters similar to adults

Usual Dosage
Note: Depakote®-ER is only approved for prophylaxis of migraine headaches; use of Depakote®-ER in pediatric patients is not recommended; do not confuse Depakote®-ER with Depakote®. **Erroneous substitution of Depakote® (delayed release tablets) for Depakote®-ER has resulted in toxicities; only Depakote®-ER is intended for once daily administration.**

Seizures: Children and Adults:

Oral: Initial: 10-15 mg/kg/day in 1-3 divided doses; increase by 5-10 mg/kg/day at weekly intervals until therapeutic levels are achieved; maintenance: 30-60 mg/kg/day in 2-3 divided doses; Depakote® and Depakote® Sprinkle® can be given twice daily

Note: Children receiving more than 1 anticonvulsant (ie, polytherapy) may require doses up to 100 mg/kg/day in 3-4 divided doses

(Continued)

Valproic Acid and Derivatives *(Continued)*

I.V.: Total daily I.V. dose is equivalent to the total daily oral dose, however, I.V. dose should be divided with a frequency of every 6 hours; if I.V. form is administered 2-3 times/day, close monitoring of trough levels is recommended; switch patients to oral product as soon as clinically possible (I.V. use has not been studied for >14 days)

Rectal: Dilute syrup 1:1 with water for use as a retention enema; loading dose: 17-20 mg/kg one time; maintenance: 10-15 mg/kg/dose every 8 hours

Prophylaxis of migraine headaches: Adults: Oral:

Depakote®: Initial: 250 mg twice daily; increase dose based on patient response; maximum dose: 1000 mg/day

Depakote®-ER: Initial: 500 mg once daily for 7 days; may increase if needed to 1000 mg once daily; range: 500-1000 mg/day; dose should be individualized; if smaller dosage adjustments are needed, use Depakote® delayed release tablets; may initiate treatment with lower dose of Depakote® delayed release tablet in patients who have GI upset

Mania: Adults: Oral: Initial: 750 mg/day in divided doses; adjust dose as rapidly as possible to desired clinical effect or plasma concentration; maximum recommended dose: 60 mg/kg/day

Dosing adjustment in renal impairment: Cl_{cr} <10 mL/minute: No dosage adjustment is needed for patients on hemodialysis (unbound clearance of valproate is reduced (27%) in these patients, but hemodialysis reduces valproate concentrations by ~20%)

Administration

Oral: May administer with food to decrease adverse GI effects; do not administer with carbonated drinks; do not administer tablet with milk; may mix contents of Depakote® Sprinkle® capsule with semisolid food (eg, applesauce, pudding, mashed potatoes) and swallow immediately, but do not crush or chew sprinkle beads; swallow delayed release and extended release tablets whole, do not crush, break, or chew

I.V.: Dilute dose with at least 50 mL of D_5W, NS, or LR; infuse over 60 minutes; maximum infusion rate: 20 mg/minute

Monitoring Parameters Liver enzymes, bilirubin, serum ammonia, CBC with platelets, serum concentrations

Reference Range

Therapeutic: 50-100 µg/mL (SI: 350-690 µmol/L)

Toxic: >100-150 µg/mL (SI: >690-1040 µmol/L)

Seizure control may improve at levels >100 µg/mL (SI: >690 µmol/L), but toxicity may occur

Test Interactions False-positive result for urine ketones; altered thyroid function tests

Patient Information Avoid alcohol; may cause drowsiness and impair ability to perform activities requiring mental alertness and physical coordination; notify physician if nausea, vomiting, loss of appetite, abdominal pain, yellow skin, general feeling of weakness, or bleeding or easy bruising occurs

Nursing Implications Instruct patients/parents to report signs or symptoms of hepatotoxicity and pancreatitis (see Warnings); GI side effects of divalproex may be less than valproic acid

Additional Information A valproic acid associated Reye's-like syndrome has been reported (see Hilmas, 2000). Acute intoxications: Naloxone may reverse the CNS depressant effects but may also block the action of other anticonvulsants; carnitine may reduce the ammonia level; multiple dosing of activated charcoal can enhance elimination.

Routine prophylactic use of carnitine in children receiving valproic acid to avoid carnitine deficiency and hepatotoxicity is probably not indicated (Freeman, 1994); a case of fatal hepatotoxic reaction has been reported in a child receiving valproic acid despite carnitine supplementation (Murphy, 1993)

Sodium content of valproate sodium syrup: 5 mL = 23 mg (1 mEq of sodium); safety of I.V. form has not been well studied in children <2 years of age

Dosage Forms

Capsule, sprinkle, as divalproex sodium (Depakote® Sprinkle®): 125 mg

Capsule, as valproic acid (Depakene®): 250 mg

Injection, as sodium valproate (Depacon™): 100 mg/mL (5 mL)

Syrup, as sodium valproate (Depakene®): 250 mg/5 mL (50 mL, 480 mL)

Tablet, delayed release, as divalproex sodium (Depakote®): 125 mg, 250 mg, 500 mg

Tablet, extended release, as divalproex sodium (Depakote®-ER): 500 mg

References

Cloyd JC, Fischer JH, Kriel RL, et al, "Valproic Acid Pharmacokinetics in Children. IV. Effects of Age and Antiepileptic Drugs on Protein Binding and Intrinsic Clearance," *Clin Pharmacol Ther*, 1993, 53(1):22-9.

Cloyd JC, Kriel RL, Fischer JH, et al, "Pharmacokinetics of Valproic Acid in Children: I. Multiple Antiepileptic Drug Therapy," *Neurology*, 1983, 33(2):185-91.

Dreifuss FE, Santilli N, Langer DH, et al, "Valproic Acid Hepatic Fatalities: A Retrospective Review," *Neurology*, 1987, 37(3):379-85.

Freeman JM, Vining EP, Cost S, et al, "Does Carnitine Administration Improve the Symptoms Attributed to Anticonvulsant Medications?: A Double-Blinded, Crossover Study," *Pediatrics*, 1994, 93(6 Pt 1):893-5.

Hilmas E and Lee CK, "Valproic Acid-Related Reye's-Like Syndrome," *The Journal of Pediatric Pharmacy Practice*, 2000, 5(3):149-55.

Murphy JV, Groover RV and Hodge C, "Hepatotoxic Effects in a Child Receiving Valproate and Carnitine," *J Pediatr*, 1993, 123(2):318-20.

♦ **Vancenase®** *see* Beclomethasone *on page 131*

♦ **Vancenase® AQ** *see* Beclomethasone *on page 131*

♦ **Vancenase® AQ 84 mcg** *see* Beclomethasone *on page 131*

♦ **Vanceril®** *see* Beclomethasone *on page 131*

♦ **Vanceril® 84 mcg Double Strength** *see* Beclomethasone *on page 131*

♦ **Vancocin®** *see* Vancomycin *on page 1001*

♦ **Vancocin CP (Can)** *see* Vancomycin *on page 1001*

♦ **Vancoled®** *see* Vancomycin *on page 1001*

Vancomycin (van koe MYE sin)

Related Information

Blood Level Sampling Time Guidelines *on page 1220*

Carbohydrate and Alcohol Content of Liquid Medications for Use in Patients Receiving Ketogenic Diets *on page 1258*

Endocarditis Prophylaxis *on page 1160*

U.S. Brand Names Lyphocin®; Vancocin®; Vancoled®

Canadian Brand Names Vancocin CP

Therapeutic Category Antibiotic, Miscellaneous

Generic Available Yes

Use Treatment of patients with the following infections or conditions: Infections due to documented or suspected methicillin-resistant *S. aureus* or beta-lactam resistant coagulase negative *Staphylococcus*; serious or life-threatening infections (ie, endocarditis, meningitis, osteomyelitis) due to documented or suspected staphylococcal or streptococcal infections in patients who are allergic to penicillins and/or cephalosporins; empiric therapy of infections associated with central lines, VP shunts, hemodialysis shunts, vascular grafts, prosthetic heart valves; used orally for staphylococcal enterocolitis or for antibiotic-associated pseudomembranous colitis produced by *C. difficile*

Pregnancy Risk Factor C

Contraindications Hypersensitivity to vancomycin or any component; avoid in patients with previous hearing loss

Precautions Use with caution in patients with renal impairment or those receiving other nephrotoxic or ototoxic drugs; dosage modification required in patients with impaired renal function

Adverse Reactions Rapid infusion associated with red neck or red man syndrome: Erythema multiforme-like reaction with intense pruritus, tachycardia, hypotension, rash involving face, neck, upper trunk, back and upper arms; red man or red neck syndrome usually develops during a rapid infusion of vancomycin or with doses ≥15-20 mg/kg/hour; reaction usually dissipates in 30-60 minutes

Cardiovascular: Cardiac arrest

Central nervous system: Fever, chills

Dermatologic: Red neck or red man syndrome, urticaria, macular skin rash

Gastrointestinal: Nausea

Hematologic: Neutropenia, eosinophilia

Local: Phlebitis

Neuromuscular & skeletal: Lower back pain

Otic: Ototoxicity associated with prolonged serum concentration >40 µg/mL

Renal: Nephrotoxicity (higher incidence with trough concentrations >10 µg/mL)

Miscellaneous: Hypersensitivity reactions

Drug Interactions Anesthetic agents (erythema, hypotension, hypothermia, and facial flushing); concurrent ototoxic or nephrotoxic drugs including loop diuretics, cisplatin, and aminoglycosides

Stability After the oral or parenteral solution is reconstituted, refrigerate and use within 2 weeks; incompatible with heparin, phenobarbital, and ceftazidime

(Continued)

Vancomycin *(Continued)*

Mechanism of Action Inhibits bacterial cell wall synthesis; blocks glycopeptide polymerization of the phosphodisaccharide-pentapeptide complex in the second stage of cell wall synthesis by binding tightly to D-alanyl-D-alanine portion of cell wall precursor

Pharmacokinetics

Absorption:

Oral: Poor

I.M.: Erratic

Intraperitoneal administration can result in 38% systemic absorption

Distribution: Widely distributed in body tissues and fluids including pericardial, pleural, ascites, and synovial fluids; low concentration in CSF if meninges are inflamed

Protein binding: 55%

Metabolism: <3%

Half-life, biphasic: Prolonged significantly with reduced renal function

Terminal:

Newborns: 6-10 hours

3 months to 4 years: 4 hours

>3 years: 2.2-3 hours

Adults: 5-8 hours

Elimination: Primarily via glomerular filtration; excreted as unchanged drug in the urine (80% to 90%); oral doses are excreted primarily in the feces; presence of malignancy in children is associated with an increase in vancomycin clearance

Dialysis: Not dialyzable (0% to 5%)

Usual Dosage Initial dosage recommendation:

Neonates: I.V.:

Postnatal age ≤7 days:

<1200 g: 15 mg/kg/day given every 24 hours

1200-2000 g: 10-15 mg/kg/dose given every 12-18 hours

>2000 g: 10-15 mg/kg/dose given every 8-12 hours

Postnatal age >7 days:

<1200 g: 15 mg/kg/day given every 24 hours

1200-2000 g: 10-15 mg/kg/dose given every 8-12 hours

>2000 g: 15-20 mg/kg/dose given every 8 hours

Infants >1 month and Children: I.V.: 40 mg/kg/day in divided doses every 6-8 hours

Nonobese pediatric cancer patients with normal renal function (n=28, age range: 9 months to 13 years): initial dosage regimen of 60 mg/kg/day divided every 6 hours has been recommended

Staphylococcal central nervous system infection: I.V.: 60 mg/kg/day in divided doses every 6 hours; maximum dose: 1 g/dose

Adults (with normal renal function): I.V.: 0.5 g every 6 hours or 1 g every 12 hours; maximum dose: 4 g/day

Dosing interval in renal impairment:

Cl_{cr} >90 mL/minute: Administer normal dose every 6 hours

Cl_{cr} 70-89 mL/minute: Administer normal dose every 8 hours

Cl_{cr} 46-69 mL/minute: Administer normal dose every 12 hours

Cl_{cr} 30-45 mL/minute: Administer normal dose every 18 hours

Cl_{cr} 15-29 mL/minute: Administer normal dose every 24 hours

Renal dysfunction, end stage renal disease, or on dialysis: 10-20 mg/kg; subsequent dosages and frequency of administration are best determined by measurement of serum levels and assessment of renal insufficiency

Intrathecal/intraventricular:

Neonates: 5-10 mg/day

Children: 5-20 mg/day

Adults: 20 mg/day

Oral (antibiotic-associated pseudomembraneous colitis: Metronidazole is the drug of initial choice per 2000 Red Book recommendations):

Children: 40 mg/kg/day in divided doses every 6 hours for 7-10 days; not to exceed 2 g/day

Adults: 0.5-2 g/day in divided doses every 6-8 hours

Prophylaxis of endocarditis in penicillin allergic patients: I.V.:

GI or genitourinary procedures:

Children: 20 mg/kg 1 hour prior to the procedure **plus** gentamicin 1.5 mg/kg 30 minutes prior to the procedure

Adults: 1 g 1 hour prior to the procedure **plus** gentamicin 1.5 mg/kg (maximum dose: 120 mg) 30 minutes prior to the procedure

Administration

Parenteral: Administer vancomycin by I.V. intermittent infusion over 60 minutes at a final concentration not to exceed 5 mg/mL; if a maculopapular rash appears on face, neck, trunk, and upper extremities, slow the infusion rate to administer dose over 1½ to 2 hours and increase the dilution volume; the reaction usually dissipates in 30-60 minutes; administration of antihistamines just before the infusion may also prevent or minimize this reaction

Intrathecal/Intraventricular: Dilute in NS without preservatives to a final concentration between 2-5 mg/mL

Monitoring Parameters Periodic renal function tests, urinalysis, serum vancomycin concentrations, WBC; audiogram (in patients who concurrently receive ototoxic chemotherapy)

Reference Range

Peak: 25-40 µg/mL
Trough: 5-10 µg/mL

Patient Information Report pain at infusion site; dizziness, fullness or ringing in ears with I.V. use

Nursing Implications Do not administer I.M.; peak levels are drawn 30 minutes to 1 hour after the completion of a 1-hour infusion; troughs are obtained just before the next dose

Dosage Forms

Capsule, as hydrochloride (Vancocin®): 125 mg, 250 mg

Powder for oral solution, as hydrochloride (Vancocin®): 1 g [provides 250 mg/5 mL when mixed]; 10 g [provides 500 mg/6 mL when mixed]

Powder for injection, as hydrochloride (Lyphocin®, Vancocin®, Vancoled®): 500 mg, 1 g, 5 g, 10 g

References

American Academy of Pediatrics Committee on Infectious Diseases, "Treatment of Bacterial Meningitis," *Pediatrics*, 1988, 81(6):904-7.

Chang D, "Influence of Malignancy on the Pharmacokinetics of Vancomycin in Infants and Children," *Pediatr Infect Dis J*, 1995, 14(8):667-73.

Chang D, Liem L, and Malogolowkin M, "A Prospective Study of Vancomycin Pharmacokinetics and Dosage Requirements in Pediatric Cancer Patients," *Pediatr Infect Dis J*, 1994, 13(11):969-74.

Leonard MB, Koren G, Stevenson DK, et al, "Vancomycin Pharmacokinetics in Very Low Birth Weight Neonates," *Pediatr Infect Dis J*, 1989, 8(5):282-6.

Matzke GR, Zhanel GG, and Guay DRP, "Clinical Pharmacokinetics of Vancomycin," *Clin Pharmacokinet*, 1986, 11(4):257-82.

Rodvold KA, Everett JA, Pryka RD, and Kraus DM, "Pharmacokinetics and Administration Regimens of Vancomycin in Neonates, Infants and Children," *Clin Pharmacokinet*, 1997, 33(1):32-51.

Rybak MJ, Albrecht LM, Boike SC, et al, "Nephrotoxicity of Vancomycin, Alone and With an Aminoglycoside," *J Antimicrob Chemother*, 1990, 25(4):679-87.

♦ **Vanoxide® [OTC]** *see* Benzoyl Peroxide *on page 136*
♦ **Vantin®** *see* Cefpodoxime *on page 199*
♦ **Varicella-Zoster Immune Globulin (Human)** *see page 1172*
♦ **VasoClear® [OTC]** *see* Naphazoline *on page 698*
♦ **Vasocon®** *see* Naphazoline *on page 698*

Vasopressin (vay soe PRES in)

Related Information

Adult ACLS Algorithm, Cardiac Arrest *on page 1039*
Adult ACLS Algorithm, Comprehensive ECC *on page 1040*
Adult ACLS Algorithm, V. Fib and Pulseless VT *on page 1041*

U.S. Brand Names Pitressin®
Synonyms ADH; Antidiuretic Hormone; 8-Arginine Vasopressin
Therapeutic Category Antidiuretic Hormone Analog; Hormone, Posterior Pituitary
Generic Available No

Use Treatment of diabetes insipidus; prevention and treatment of postoperative abdominal distention; differential diagnosis of diabetes insipidus; adjunct in the treatment of acute massive hemorrhage of GI tract or esophageal varices; treatment of ventricular fibrillation or tachycardia refractory to initial defibrillation (see Adult ACLS Algorithms *on page 1039*)

Pregnancy Risk Factor B
Contraindications Hypersensitivity to vasopressin or any component
Warnings I.V. infiltration may lead to severe vasoconstriction and localized tissue necrosis
Precautions Use with caution in patients with seizure disorders, migraine, asthma, vascular disease, renal disease, cardiac disease, goiter with cardiac complications, arteriosclerosis, chronic nephritis with nitrogen retention
(Continued)

Vasopressin *(Continued)*

Adverse Reactions

Cardiovascular: Circumoral pallor; with high doses: hypertension, bradycardia, arrhythmias, venous thrombosis, vasoconstriction, angina, heart block, cardiac arrest

Central nervous system: Vertigo, fever, headache

Dermatologic: Urticaria

Endocrine & metabolic: Water intoxication, hyponatremia

Gastrointestinal: Abdominal cramps, nausea, vomiting, flatus, diarrhea

Neuromuscular & skeletal: Tremor

Respiratory: Wheezing, bronchoconstriction

Miscellaneous: Diaphoresis

Drug Interactions

Decreased antidiuretic activity: Lithium, demeclocycline, large doses of epinephrine, heparin (therapeutic doses), alcohol

Increased antidiuretic activity: Chlorpropamide, carbamazepine, phenformin, tricyclic antidepressants, clofibrate, fludrocortisone

Mechanism of Action Increases cyclic adenosine monophosphate (cAMP) which increases water permeability at the distal convoluted tubule and collecting duct resulting in decreased urine volume and increased urine osmolality; causes peristalsis by directly stimulating the smooth muscle in the GI tract (in doses greater than those required for its antidiuretic action); causes vasoconstriction (primarily of capillaries and small arterioles)

Pharmacodynamics I.M., S.C.:

Onset of action: 1 hour

Duration of action: 2-8 hours

Pharmacokinetics Destroyed by trypsin in GI tract, must be administered parenterally

Half-life: 10-20 minutes

Metabolism: Most of dose is rapidly metabolized in liver and kidney

Usual Dosage

Diabetes insipidus:

I.M., S.C.: (Highly variable dosage; titrate dosage based upon serum and urine sodium and osmolality in addition to fluid balance and urine output)

Children: 2.5-10 units 2-4 times/day

Adults: 5-10 units 2-4 times/day as needed (range: 5-60 units/day)

Continuous infusion: Children and Adults: Initial: 0.5 milliunit/kg/hour (0.0005 unit/kg/hour); double dosage as needed every 30 minutes to a maximum of 10 milliunit/kg/hour

Abdominal distention: Adults: I.M.: 5 units initially, then repeated every 3-4 hours; dosage may be increased to 10 units if necessary

Ventricular fibrillation or tachycardia unresponsive to initial defibrillation: Adults: I.V.: 40 units as a single dose only (see Adult ACLS Algorithms *on page 1039*)

GI hemorrhage: I.V. continuous infusion (may also be infused directly into the superior mesenteric artery):

Children: Initial: 0.002-0.005 units/kg/minute; titrate dose as needed; maximum dose: 0.01 units/kg/minute; if bleeding stops for 12 hours, then taper off over 24-48 hours

Adults: Initial: I.V.: 0.2-0.4 unit/minute, then titrate dose as needed; if bleeding stops, continue at same dose for 12 hours, taper off over 24-48 hours

Dosing adjustment in hepatic impairment: Some patients with cirrhosis respond to much lower doses

Administration Parenteral: Continuous infusion: Dilute in NS or D_5W to a final concentration of 0.1-1 unit/mL; see Usual Dosage for rate of infusion

Monitoring Parameters Fluid intake and output, urine specific gravity, urine and serum osmolality, serum and urine sodium

Dosage Forms Injection, aqueous: 20 pressor units/mL (0.5 mL, 1 mL)

References

Tuggle DW, Bennett KG, Scott J, et al, "Intravenous Vasopressin and Gastrointestinal Hemorrhage in Children," *J Pediatr Surg*, 1988, 23(7):627-9.

Vecuronium (ve KYOO roe nee um)

U.S. Brand Names Norcuron®

Synonyms ORG NC 45

Therapeutic Category Neuromuscular Blocker Agent, Nondepolarizing; Skeletal Muscle Relaxant, Paralytic

Generic Available No

Use Adjunct to anesthesia, to facilitate endotracheal intubation, and provide skeletal muscle relaxation during surgery or mechanical ventilation

Pregnancy Risk Factor C

Contraindications Hypersensitivity to vecuronium or any component

Warnings Ventilation must be supported during neuromuscular blockade; use only by individuals who are experienced in the maintenance of an adequate airway and respiratory support

Precautions Use with caution in patients with hepatic impairment, neuromuscular disease, myasthenia gravis; many clinical conditions may potentiate or antagonize neuromuscular blockade, see table.

Clinical Conditions Affecting Neuromuscular Blockade

Potentiation	Antagonism
Electrolyte abnormalities	Alkalosis
Severe hyponatremia	Hypercalcemia
Severe hypocalcemia	Demyelinating lesions
Severe hypokalemia	Peripheral neuropathies
Hypermagnesemia	Diabetes mellitus
Neuromuscular diseases	
Acidosis	
Acute intermittent porphyria	
Renal failure	
Hepatic failure	

Potential Drug Interactions

Potentiation	Antagonism
Inhalation anesthetics	Calcium
Desflurane, sevoflurane, enflurane and	Carbamazepine
isoflurane > halothane > nitrous	Phenytoin
oxide	Steroids (chronic administration)
Antibiotics	Theophylline
Aminoglycosides, polymyxins,	Anticholinesterases*
clindamycin, vancomycin	Neostigmine, pyridostigmine,
Magnesium	edrophonium, echothiophate
Antiarrhythmics	ophthalmic solution
Quinidine, procainamide, bretylium, and	Caffeine
possibly lidocaine	Azathioprine
Diuretics	
Furosemide, mannitol, thiazides	
Amphotericin B (secondary to hypokalemia)	
Local anesthetics	
Dantrolene (directly depresses skeletal muscle)	
Beta blockers	
Calcium channel blockers	
Ketamine	
Lithium	
Succinylcholine (when administered prior to nondepolarizing neuromuscular-blocking agent)	
Cyclosporine	

*Can prolong the effects of acetylcholine

(Continued)

1005

Vecuronium *(Continued)*

Adverse Reactions Most frequent reactions are associated with prolongation of its pharmacologic effect

Cardiovascular: Arrhythmias, tachycardia, hypotension, hypertension

Dermatologic: Urticaria, rash

Neuromuscular & skeletal: Muscle weakness

Respiratory: Respiratory insufficiency, bronchospasm, apnea

Drug Interactions See table on previous page.

Stability Stable for 5 days at room temperature when reconstituted with bacteriostatic water; stable for 24 hours at room temperature when reconstituted with preservative free sterile water (avoid preservatives in neonates); do not mix with alkaline drugs; compatible with dextrose, NS, or LR

Mechanism of Action Nondepolarizing neuromuscular blocker which blocks acetylcholine from binding to receptors on motor endplate thus inhibiting depolarization

Pharmacodynamics

Onset of effects: Within 1-3 minutes

Duration of effect (dose dependent): 30-40 minutes

Pharmacokinetics

Distribution: V_d:

Infants: 0.36 L/kg

Children: 0.2 L/kg

Adults: 0.27 L/kg

Protein binding: 60% to 80%

Half-life, distribution: Adults: 4 minutes

Half-life, elimination:

Infants: 65 minutes

Children: 41 minutes

Adults: 65-75 minutes

Elimination: Vecuronium bromide and its metabolite(s) appear to be excreted principally in feces via biliary elimination (50%); the drug and its metabolite(s) are also excreted in urine (25%); the rate of elimination is appreciably reduced with hepatic dysfunction but not with renal dysfunction

Usual Dosage I.V.:

Neonates: 0.1 mg/kg/dose; maintenance: 0.03-0.15 mg/kg/dose every 1-2 hours as needed

Infants >7 weeks to 1 year: 0.1 mg/kg/dose; repeat every hour as needed; may be administered as a continuous infusion at 1-1.5 mcg/kg/minute (0.06-0.09 mg/kg/hour)

Children >1 year: 0.1 mg/kg/dose; repeat every hour as needed; may be administered as a continuous infusion at 1.5-2.5 mcg/kg/minute (0.09-0.15 mg/kg/hour)

Adults: 0.1 mg/kg/dose; repeat every hour as needed; may be administered as a continuous infusion at 1.5-2 mcg/kg/minute (0.09-0.12 mg/kg/hour)

Dosing adjustment in hepatic impairment: Dose reductions are necessary in patients with cirrhosis or cholestasis

Administration Parenteral: I.V.: Dilute vial to a maximum concentration of 2 mg/mL and administer by rapid direct injection; for continuous infusion, dilute to a maximum concentration of 1 mg/mL

Monitoring Parameters Assisted ventilation status, heart rate, blood pressure, peripheral nerve stimulator measuring twitch response

Nursing Implications Does not alter the patient's state of consciousness; addition of sedation and analgesia is recommended

Additional Information Produces minimal, if any, histamine release

Dosage Forms Powder for injection, as bromide: 10 mg, 20 mg

References

Martin LD, Bratton SL, and O'Rourke PP, "Clinical Uses and Controversies of Neuromuscular Blocking Agents in Infants and Children," *Crit Care Med*, 1999, 27(7):1358-68.

♦ **Ventolin® Rotocaps®** *see* Albuterol *on page 45*
♦ **VePesid®** *see* Etoposide *on page 412*

Verapamil (ver AP a mil)

U.S. Brand Names Calan®; Calan® SR; Covera-HS®; Isoptin®; Isoptin® SR; Verelan®; Verelan® PM
Canadian Brand Names Alti-Verapamil; Apo-Verap; Chronovera; Gen-Verapamil; Novo-Veramil; Nu-Verap
Synonyms Iproveratril
Therapeutic Category Antianginal Agent; Antiarrhythmic Agent, Class IV; Antihypertensive Agent; Calcium Channel Blocker
Generic Available Yes
Use Angina, hypertension; I.V. for supraventricular tachyarrhythmias (PSVT, atrial fibrillation, atrial flutter)
Pregnancy Risk Factor C
Contraindications Sinus bradycardia; advanced heart block; ventricular tachycardia; cardiogenic shock; hypersensitivity to verapamil or any component; atrial fibrillation or flutter associated with accessory conduction pathways
Warnings Avoid I.V. use in neonates and young infants due to severe apnea, bradycardia, hypotensive reactions, and cardiac arrest; I.V. use is discouraged in children due to hypotension and myocardial depression; monitor EKG and blood pressure closely in patients receiving I.V. therapy; have I.V. calcium chloride 10 mg/kg available at bedside to treat hypotension. I.V. administration, hypertrophic cardiomyopathy, sick sinus syndrome, moderate to severe CHF, concomitant therapy with beta-blockers or digoxin can all increase the incidence of adverse effects.
Precautions Use with caution in patients with sick sinus syndrome, severe left ventricular dysfunction, hepatic or renal impairment, hypertrophic cardiomyopathy (especially obstructive), concomitant therapy with beta-blockers or digoxin; reduce dose in patients with severe renal dysfunction
Adverse Reactions
  Cardiovascular: Hypotension, bradycardia; first, second, or third degree A-V block, worsening heart failure
  Central nervous system: Dizziness, fatigue, seizures (occasionally with I.V. use), headache
  Gastrointestinal: Constipation, nausea, abdominal discomfort
  Hepatic: Elevated hepatic enzymes
  Respiratory: May precipitate insufficiency of respiratory muscle function in Duchenne muscular dystrophy
Drug Interactions Cytochrome P-450 isoenzyme CYP1A2 and CYP3A3/4 substrate; CYP3A3/4 isoenzyme inhibitor
  Increased cardiovascular adverse effects with beta-adrenergic blocking agents, digoxin, quinidine, and disopyramide. Verapamil may increase serum concentrations of caffeine, ethanol, digoxin, quinidine, carbamazepine, and cyclosporine necessitating a decrease in dosage. Phenobarbital and rifampin may decrease verapamil serum concentrations by increasing hepatic metabolism. Avoid combination with disopyramide, discontinue disopyramide 48 hours before starting therapy, do not restart until 24 hours after verapamil has been discontinued.
Food Interactions Sprinkling contents of capsule onto food does not affect oral absorption
Stability Store injection at room temperature; protect from heat and from freezing; use only clear solutions; compatible in solutions of pH of 3-6, but may precipitate in solutions having a pH ≥6
Mechanism of Action Inhibits calcium ion from entering the "slow channels" or select voltage-sensitive areas of vascular smooth muscle and myocardium during depolarization; produces a relaxation of coronary vascular smooth muscle and coronary vasodilation; increases myocardial oxygen delivery in patients with vasospastic angina
Pharmacodynamics
  Peak effects:
    Oral (nonsustained tablets): 2 hours
    I.V.: 1-5 minutes
  Duration:
    Oral: 6-8 hours
    I.V.: 10-20 minutes
Pharmacokinetics
  Protein binding:
    Neonates: ~60%
    Adults: 90%
  (Continued)

Verapamil (Continued)

Metabolism: Extensive first-pass effect, metabolized in the liver to several inactive dealkylated metabolites; major metabolite is norverapamil which possesses weak hemodynamic effects

Bioavailability: Oral: 20% to 30%

Half-life:

Infants: 4.4-6.9 hours

Adults (single dose): 2-8 hours, increased up to 12 hours with multiple dosing

Increased half-life with hepatic cirrhosis

Elimination: 70% of dose excreted in urine (3% to 4% as unchanged drug), and 16% in feces

Usual Dosage

Infants <1 year: I.V.: **Not recommended** (see Warnings); administer with continuous EKG monitoring, have I.V. calcium available at bedside: 0.1-0.2 mg/kg (usual: 0.75-2 mg/dose) may repeat dose in 30 minutes if adequate response not achieved

Children 1-16 years: I.V.: 0.1-0.3 mg/kg/dose (**Note:** PALS 2000 guidelines recommend 0.1 mg/kg); maximum dose: 5 mg/dose; may repeat dose in 30 minutes if adequate response not achieved; maximum for second dose: 10 mg/dose

Children: Oral (dose not well established):

4-8 mg/kg/day in 3 divided doses

or

1-5 years: 40-80 mg every 8 hours

>5 years: 80 mg every 6-8 hours

Note: A mean daily dose of ~5 mg/kg/day (range: 2.3-8.1 mg/kg/day) was used in 22 children 15 days to 17 years of age receiving chronic oral therapy for SVT (n=20) or hypertrophic cardiomyopathy (n=2) (Piovan, 1995)

Adults:

Oral: 240-480 mg/24 hours divided 3-4 times/day or divided 1-2 times/day for extended release products

I.V. (ACLS 2000 guidelines): PSVT (narrow complex, unresponsive to vagal maneuvers and adenosine, in patients with preserved cardiac function): Initial: 2.5-5 mg; if no response in 15-30 minutes and no adverse effects seen, give 5-10 mg every 15-30 minutes to a maximum total dose of 20 mg

I.V.: 5-10 mg (0.075-0.15 mg/kg); may repeat 10 mg (0.15 mg/kg) 15-30 minutes after the initial dose if needed and if patient tolerated initial dose

I.V. continuous infusion: Loading dose: 5-10 mg; may repeat in 30 minutes if adequate response is not achieved; follow with continuous infusion: 5 mg/hour; titrate dose to ventricular rate; usual: 5-10 mg/hour; range: 4-24 mg/hour. **Note:** Previously recommended doses of 0.005 mg/kg/minute (5 mcg/kg/minute) will result in doses of ~20 mg/hour and may produce adverse effects such as hypotension; lower infusion rates (5-10 mg/hour) are effective in most adult patients.

Dosing adjustment in renal impairment: Children and Adults: Cl_{cr} <10 mL/minute: Administer 50% to 75% of normal dose

Administration

Oral: Nonsustained-release tablets can be administered with or without food; administer sustained release tablet with food or milk; swallow sustained released preparations whole, do not chew or crush

Parenteral:

I.V.: Infuse I.V. dose over 2-3 minutes; infuse I.V. over 3-4 minutes if blood pressure is in the lower range of normal; Maximum concentration: 2.5 mg/mL

I.V. continuous infusion: Final concentration for administration: 0.5-2.5 mg/mL

Monitoring Parameters EKG, blood pressure, heart rate; hepatic enzymes with long-term use

Patient Information Avoid alcohol; limit caffeine

Dosage Forms

Capsule, extended release, as hydrochloride (Verelan® PM): 100 mg, 200 mg, 300 mg

Capsule, sustained release, as hydrochloride: 120 mg, 180 mg, 240 mg

Verelan®: 120 mg, 180 mg, 240 mg, 360 mg

Injection, as hydrochloride: 2.5 mg/mL (2 mL, 4 mL)

Isoptin®: 2.5 mg/mL (2 mL, 4 mL)

Tablet, as hydrochloride: 40 mg, 80 mg, 120 mg

Calan®: 40 mg, 80 mg, 120 mg

Tablet, sustained release, as hydrochloride: 120 mg, 180 mg, 240 mg

Calan® SR, Isoptin® SR: 120 mg, 180 mg, 240 mg

Covera-HS®: 180 mg, 240 mg

Extemporaneous Preparations

A 50 mg/mL oral suspension may be made using twenty 80 mg verapamil tablets (regular, not sustained release), 3 mL of purified water USP, 8 mL of methylcellulose 1% and simple syrup qs ad to 32 mL; stability is 91 days under refrigeration; shake well before use (Nahata, 2000)

A 50 mg/mL oral liquid preparation made from tablets (regular, not sustained release) and 3 different vehicles (cherry syrup, a 1:1 mixture of Ora-Sweet® and Ora-Plus®, or a 1:1 mixture of Ora-Sweet® SF and Ora-Plus®) was stable for 60 days when stored in amber plastic prescription bottles in the dark at room temperature (25°C) or under refrigeration (5°C); grind seventy-five 80 mg tablets in a mortar into a fine powder; add 40 mL of the vehicle and mix well to form a uniform paste; mix while adding the vehicle in geometric proportions to **almost** 120 mL; transfer to a calibrated bottle and qsad with vehicle to make 120 mL; label "shake well" and "protect from light" (Allen, 1996).

Allen LV and Erickson MA, "Stability of Labetalol Hydrochloride, Metoprolol Tartrate, Verapamil Hydrochloride, and Spironolactone With Hydrochlorothiazide in Extemporaneously Compounded Oral Liquids," *Am J Health Syst Pharm,* 1996, 53(19):2304-9.

Nahata MC and Hipple TF, *Pediatric Drug Formulations,* 4th ed, Cincinnati, OH: Harvey Whitney Books Co, 2000.

References
Barbarash RA, Bauman JL, Lukazewski AA, et al, "Verapamil Infusions in the Treatment of Atrial Tachyarrhythmias," *Crit Care Med,* 1986, 14(10):886-8.

"Guidelines 2000 for Cardiopulmonary Resuscitation and Emergency Cardiovascular Care, Part 6: Advanced Cardiovascular Life Support, The American Heart Association in Collaboration With the International Liaison Committee on Resuscitation," *Circulation,* 2000, 102(8 Suppl):I86-171.

"Guidelines 2000 for Cardiopulmonary Resuscitation and Emergency Cardiovascular Care, Part 10: Pediatric Advanced Life Support, The American Heart Association in Collaboration With the International Liaison Committee on Resuscitation," *Circulation,* 2000, 102(8 Suppl): I291-342.

Piovan D, Padrini R, Svalato Moreolo G, et al, "Verapamil and Norverapamil Plasma Levels in Infants and Children During Chronic Oral Treatment," *Ther Drug Monit,* 1995, 17(1):60-7.

Sapire DW, O'Riordan AC, and Black IF, "Safety and Efficacy of Short- and Long-Term Verapamil Therapy in Children With Tachycardia," *Am J Cardiol,* 1981, 48(6):1091-7.

Shakibi JG, "Arrhythmias in Infants and Children," *Pediatrician,* 1981, 10(1-3):117-22.

- ◆ **Verelan®** *see* Verapamil *on page 1007*
- ◆ **Verelan® PM** *see* Verapamil *on page 1007*
- ◆ **Veriga (Can)** *see* Piperazine *on page 804*
- ◆ **Verimex (Can)** *see* Piperazine *on page 804*
- ◆ **Vermizine®** *see* Piperazine *on page 804*
- ◆ **Vermox®** *see* Mebendazole *on page 620*
- ◆ **Versed®** *see* Midazolam *on page 669*
- ◆ **Versel (Can)** *see* Selenium Sulfide *on page 896*
- ◆ **Versiclear™** *see* Sodium Thiosulfate *on page 909*
- ◆ **Versol (Can)** *see* Piperazine *on page 804*
- ◆ **Vesanoid (Can)** *see* Tretinoin *on page 978*
- ◆ **Vibramycin®** *see* Doxycycline *on page 362*
- ◆ **Vibra-Tabs®** *see* Doxycycline *on page 362*
- ◆ **Vicks® 44E [OTC]** *see* Guaifenesin and Dextromethorphan *on page 487*
- ◆ **Vicks Formula 44® Cough Relief [OTC]** *see* Dextromethorphan *on page 316*
- ◆ **Vicks® Pediatric Formula 44E [OTC]** *see* Guaifenesin and Dextromethorphan *on page 487*
- ◆ **Vicks Sinex (Can)** *see* Oxymetazoline *on page 749*
- ◆ **Vicks® Sinex® [OTC]** *see* Phenylephrine *on page 789*
- ◆ **Vicks Sinex® 12 Hour [OTC]** *see* Oxymetazoline *on page 749*
- ◆ **Vicodin®** *see* Hydrocodone and Acetaminophen *on page 505*
- ◆ **Vicodin® ES** *see* Hydrocodone and Acetaminophen *on page 505*

Vidarabine (vye DARE a been)

U.S. Brand Names Vira-A®

Synonyms Adenine Arabinoside; Ara-A; Arabinofuranosyladenine

Therapeutic Category Antiviral Agent, Ophthalmic

Generic Available No

Use Treatment of acute keratoconjunctivitis and epithelial keratitis due to herpes simplex virus

Pregnancy Risk Factor C

Contraindications Hypersensitivity to vidarabine or any component; concurrent application of a corticosteroid in the treatment of herpes simplex keratitis

Warnings Vidarabine is potentially mutagenic, teratogenic, and oncogenic
(Continued)

Vidarabine *(Continued)*

Adverse Reactions Ocular: Keratitis, photophobia, lacrimation, foreign body sensation, uveitis, stromal edema, blurred vision, burning

Stability Store at room temperature; avoid freezing

Mechanism of Action Inhibits viral DNA synthesis by blocking DNA polymerase or virus-induced ribonucleotide reductase

Pharmacokinetics

Absorption: Systemic absorption is not expected to occur following ophthalmic use

Distribution: Trace amounts detected in the aqueous humor if there is an epithelial defect in the cornea

Protein binding:

Vidarabine: 20% to 30%

Ara-hypoxanthine: 0% to 3%

Elimination: Following administration, rapidly deaminated by red cell adenosine deaminase to ara-hypoxanthine (active); excreted in urine as vidarabine (1% to 3%) and the active metabolite (40% to 53%)

Usual Dosage Children and Adults: Ophthalmic: Keratoconjunctivitis: Apply ½" of ointment in lower conjunctival sac 5 times/day every 3 hours while awake until complete re-epithelialization has occurred, then twice daily for an additional 7 days

Administration Ophthalmic: Instill 1 cm of ointment in lower conjunctival sac of the affected eye; avoid contact of tube tip with skin or eye

Patient Information Ophthalmic ointment may cause sensitivity to bright light; minimize light sensitivity by wearing sunglasses

Dosage Forms Ointment, ophthalmic, as monohydrate: 3% [30 mg/mL = 28 mg/mL base] (3.5 g)

♦ **Videx® Oral** *see Didanosine on page 327*

Vinblastine *(vin BLAS teen)*

Related Information

Emetogenic Potential of Single Chemotherapeutic Agents *on page 1129*

Extravasation Treatment *on page 1085*

U.S. Brand Names Velban®

Synonyms Vincaleukoblastine; VLB

Therapeutic Category Antineoplastic Agent, Mitotic Inhibitor

Generic Available Yes

Use Palliative treatment of Hodgkin's disease; advanced testicular germinal-cell cancers; non-Hodgkin's lymphoma, histiocytosis, and choriocarcinoma

Pregnancy Risk Factor D

Contraindications Hypersensitivity to vinblastine or any component; severe leukopenia

Warnings The FDA currently recommends that procedures for proper handling and disposal of antineoplastic agents be considered; vinblastine may cause fetal toxicity when administered to pregnant women; for I.V. use only; **intrathecal administration may result in death**

Precautions Avoid extravasation; dosage modification required in patients with impaired liver function or neurotoxicity; dosage should be reduced in patients with recent exposure to radiation therapy or chemotherapy

Adverse Reactions

Cardiovascular: Tachycardia, orthostatic hypotension

Central nervous system: Depression, malaise, seizures, headache

Dermatologic: Rashes, mild alopecia, photosensitivity

Endocrine & metabolic: Hyperuricemia

Gastrointestinal: Nausea, hemorrhagic enterocolitis, vomiting, constipation, abdominal pain, paralytic ileus, stomatitis

Genitourinary: Urinary retention

Hematologic: Myelosuppression: Leukopenia (nadir: 4-10 days), thrombocytopenia

Local: Severe tissue burn if infiltrated

Neuromuscular & skeletal: Jaw pain, myalgia, peripheral neuropathy, paresthesia

Drug Interactions Cytochrome P-450 isoenzyme CYP3A3/4 and CYP3A5-7 substrate; isoenzyme CYP2D6 inhibitor

Concomitant administration with mitomycin has resulted in severe bronchospasm and shortness of breath; may decrease serum phenytoin concentrations

Stability Store in refrigerator; 1 mg/mL solutions prepared with preserved NS injection is stable for 30 days when refrigerated and protected from light. **Note:** Vinblastine must be dispensed in overwrap which bears the statement "Do not remove covering until the moment of injection. Fatal if given intrathecally. For I.V. use only."

Mechanism of Action Binds to microtubular protein of the mitotic spindle causing metaphase arrest

Pharmacokinetics

Distribution: Poor penetration into CSF; rapidly distributed into body tissues; V_{dss}: 27.3 L/kg

Protein binding: 75%

Metabolism: Extensive in the liver to a more active metabolite

Half-life, terminal: 24 hours

Elimination: Biliary excretion (95%)

Usual Dosage Vinblastine may be administered at intervals of every 7 days or greater and only after leukocyte count has returned to at least 4000/mm³; maintenance therapy should be titrated according to leukocyte count

I.V. (refer to individual protocols):

Children:

Hodgkin's disease: 2.5-6 mg/m²/day once every 1-2 weeks for 3-6 weeks; maximum weekly dose: 12.5 mg/m²

Histiocytosis: 0.4 mg/kg once ever 7-10 days

Germ cell tumor: 0.2 mg/kg on days 1 and 2 of cycle every 3 weeks times 4 cycles

Adults: 3.7-18.5 mg/m²/day every 7-10 days or 0.1-0.5 mg/kg/day once weekly or 1.4-1.8 mg/m²/day for 5 days given as an I.V. continuous infusion

Dosing adjustment in hepatic impairment: Children and Adults: Direct serum bilirubin concentration >3 mg/dL: Reduce dose 50%

Administration Parenteral: **Do not administer intrathecally, death may occur**; do not administer I.M. or S.C. since the drug is very irritating; may be administered IVP directly into the vein or through a Y-site of a freely running I.V. over a 1-minute period at a concentration for administration of 1 mg/mL; I.V. continuous infusion: Each day's dose may be diluted in 1000 mL of D₅W or NS; administer over 24 hours

Monitoring Parameters CBC with differential and platelet count, serum uric acid, hepatic function tests

Patient Information Report to physician any fever, sore throat, bleeding, or bruising; avoid contact with the eyes since the drug is very irritating and corneal ulceration may result; avoid direct exposure to sunlight

Nursing Implications Maintain adequate hydration. Allopurinol may be given to prevent uric acid nephropathy; stool softeners may be helpful in preventing constipation; vinblastine is a tissue irritant and can cause sloughing upon extravasation; check vein patency before drug administration; care should be taken to avoid extravasation. If extravasation occurs, local injection of hyaluronidase into the leading edge of the extravasation site and a warm compress can be used for treatment; apply warm pack immediately for 30-60 minutes, then alternate off/on every 15 minutes for 1 day. Refer to Extravasation Treatment *on page 1085.*

Additional Information Myelosuppressive effects:

Nadir (days): 4-10

Recovery (days): 7-14

Dosage Forms

Injection, as sulfate: 1 mg/mL (10 mL)

Powder for injection, as sulfate (Velban®): 10 mg

References

Balis FM, Holcenberg JS and Bleyer WA, "Clinical Pharmacokinetics of Commonly Used Anticancer Drugs," *Clin Pharmacokinet*, 1983, 8(3):202-32.

Crom WR, Glynn-Barnhart AM, Rodman JH, et al, "Pharmacokinetics of Anticancer Drugs in Children," *Clin Pharmacokinet*, 1987, 12(3):168-213.

Tannock I, Ehrlichman C, Perrault D, et al, "Failure of 5-Day Vinblastine Infusion in the Treatment of Patients With Advanced Refractory Breast Cancer," *Cancer Treat Rep*, 1982, 66(9):1783-4.

Yap HY, Blumenschein GR, Keating MJ, et al, "Vinblastine Given as a Continuous 5-Day Infusion in the Treatment of Refractory Breast Cancer," *Cancer Treat Rep*, 1980, 64(2-3):279-83.

♦ **Vincaleukoblastine** *see* Vinblastine *on page 1010*

♦ **Vincasar® PFS** *see* Vincristine *on page 1011*

Vincristine (vin KRIS teen)

Related Information

Emetogenic Potential of Single Chemotherapeutic Agents *on page 1129*

Extravasation Treatment *on page 1085*

U.S. Brand Names Oncovin®; Vincasar® PFS

Synonyms LCR; Leurocristine; VCR

Therapeutic Category Antineoplastic Agent, Mitotic Inhibitor

Generic Available Yes

Use Treatment of leukemias, Hodgkin's disease, neuroblastoma, malignant lymphomas, Wilms' tumor, and rhabdomyosarcoma

(Continued)

Vincristine *(Continued)*

Pregnancy Risk Factor D

Contraindications Hypersensitivity to vincristine or any component; patients with demyelinating form of Charcot-Marie-Tooth syndrome

Warnings The FDA currently recommends that procedures for proper handling and disposal of antineoplastic agents be considered; vincristine may cause fetal toxicity when administered to pregnant women; for I.V. use only; **intrathecal administration may result in death.**

Precautions Dosage modification required in patients with impaired hepatic function, patients receiving other neurotoxic drugs, or patients with pre-existing neuromuscular disease; avoid extravasation

Adverse Reactions

Cardiovascular: Orthostatic hypotension

Central nervous system: Neurotoxicity, seizures, CNS depression, cranial nerve paralysis

Dermatologic: Alopecia, rash

Endocrine & metabolic: Hyperuricemia, SIADH

Gastrointestinal: Constipation, paralytic ileus, nausea, vomiting, diarrhea, stomatitis

Local: Pain, cellulitis and tissue necrosis if infiltrated, phlebitis

Neuromuscular & skeletal: Jaw pain, leg pain, myalgia, numbness, motor difficulties, cramping, weakness

Ocular: Extraocular muscle paresis, photophobia

Respiratory: Dyspnea

Drug Interactions Cytochrome P-450 isoenzyme CYP3A3/4 and CYP3A5-7 substrate; isoenzyme CYP2D6 inhibitor

Asparaginase may decrease vincristine clearance; acute pulmonary reactions may occur with concomitant use of mitomycin C; concurrent administration with itraconazole may result in an increased severity of neuromuscular side effects

Stability Store in refrigerator; injectable solution is stable for 1 month at room temperature. **Note:** Vincristine must be dispensed in overwrap which bears the statement "Do not remove covering until the moment of injection. Fatal if given intrathecally. For I.V. use only."

Mechanism of Action Binds to microtubular protein of the mitotic spindle causing metaphase arrest

Pharmacokinetics

Distribution: Poor penetration into the CSF; V_{dss}: 120 L/m^2

Protein binding: 75%

Metabolism: Extensive in the liver

Half-life, terminal: 24 hours

Elimination: Primarily in bile (~80%)

Clearance:

Infants: Vincristine clearance is more closely related to body weight than to body surface area

Children 2-18 years: 482 mL/minute/m^2 (faster clearance in children <10 years of age than in adolescents)

Usual Dosage I.V. (refer to individual protocols):

Children ≤10 kg or BSA <1 m^2: Initial therapy: 0.05 mg/kg once weekly then titrate dose; maximum single dose: 2 mg

Children >10 kg or BSA ≥1 m^2: 1-2 mg/m^2, may repeat once weekly for 3-6 weeks; maximum single dose: 2 mg

Neuroblastoma: I.V. continuous infusion with doxorubicin: 1 mg/m^2/day for 72 hours

Adults: 0.4-1.4 mg/m^2 up to 2 mg; may repeat every week

Dosing adjustment in hepatic impairment: Children and Adults: Direct serum bilirubin concentration >3 mg/dL: Dosage reduction of 50% is recommended

Administration Parenteral: **Do not administer intrathecally, death may occur;** do not administer I.M. or S.C. since the drug is very irritating; I.V.: Vincristine is administered IVP or through a Y-site of a freely running I.V. over a period of 1 minute at a concentration for administration of 1 mg/mL; may administer as a dilute I.V. infusion

Monitoring Parameters Serum electrolytes (sodium), hepatic function tests, neurologic examination, CBC, hemoglobin, serum uric acid

Patient Information Stool softener should be used for constipation prophylaxis; report to physician any fever, sore throat, bleeding, bruising, or shortness of breath

Nursing Implications Maintain adequate hydration. Allopurinol may be given to prevent uric acid nephropathy; vincristine is a tissue irritant; care should be taken to avoid extravasation. If extravasation occurs, local injection of hyaluronidase into the leading edge of the extravasation site and a warm compress can be used for treatment; apply warm pack immediately for 30-60 minutes, then alternate off/on every 15 minutes for 1 day; refer to Extravasation Treatment *on page 1085.* Avoid contact with the eye since vincristine is very irritating.

Dosage Forms Injection, as sulfate: 1 mg/mL (1 mL, 2 mL, 5 mL)

References
Crom WR, deGraaf SS, Synold T, et al, "Pharmacokinetics of Vincristine in Children and Adolescents With Acute Lymphocytic Leukemia," *J Pediatr*, 1994, 125(4):642-9.

Woods WG, O'Leary M, and Nesbit ME, "Life-Threatening Neuropathy and Hepatotoxicity in Infants During Induction Therapy for Acute Lymphoblastic Leukemia," *J Pediatr*, 1981, 98(4):642-5.

♦ **Vioform® [OTC]** *see* Clioquinol *on page 252*

♦ **Viokase®** *see* Pancrelipase *on page 755*

♦ **Viosterol** *see* Ergocalciferol *on page 392*

♦ **Vira-A®** *see* Vidarabine *on page 1009*

♦ **Viracept®** *see* Nelfinavir *on page 702*

♦ **Viramune®** *see* Nevirapine *on page 710*

♦ **Virazole®** *see* Ribavirin *on page 872*

♦ **Viroptic®** *see* Trifluridine *on page 984*

♦ **Visine® L.R. [OTC]** *see* Oxymetazoline *on page 749*

♦ **Visine Workplace (Can)** *see* Oxymetazoline *on page 749*

♦ **Vistaril®** *see* Hydroxyzine *on page 516*

♦ **Vita-C® [OTC]** *see* Ascorbic Acid *on page 106*

♦ **Vitacarn®** *see* Carnitine *on page 184*

Vitamin A (VYE ta min aye)

Related Information
Carbohydrate and Alcohol Content of Liquid Medications for Use in Patients Receiving Ketogenic Diets *on page 1258*

U.S. Brand Names Aquasol A® [OTC]; Palmitate-A® [OTC]

Synonyms Oleovitamin A

Therapeutic Category Nutritional Supplement; Vitamin, Fat Soluble

Generic Available Yes

Use Treatment and prevention of vitamin A deficiency; supplementation in children 6 months to 2 years with measles

Pregnancy Risk Factor A (X if dose exceeds RDA recommendation)

Contraindications Hypervitaminosis A; hypersensitivity to vitamin A or any component

Warnings Patients receiving >25,000 units/day should be closely monitored for toxicity

Adverse Reactions Seen only with doses exceeding physiologic replacement
Central nervous system: Irritability, drowsiness, vertigo, delirium, headache, coma, increased intracranial pressure
Dermatologic: Erythema, peeling skin
Gastrointestinal: Vomiting, diarrhea
Ocular: Visual disturbances, papilledema

Drug Interactions Cholestyramine decreases absorption of vitamin A; neomycin and mineral oil may also interfere with vitamin A absorption; retinoids may have additive adverse effects; enhances hypoprothrombinemic effects of warfarin

Stability Protect injectable preparation from light

Mechanism of Action Needed for bone development, growth, visual adaptation to darkness, testicular and ovarian function, and as a cofactor in many biochemical processes

Pharmacokinetics
Absorption: Vitamin A in dosages **not** exceeding physiologic replacement is well absorbed after oral administration; water miscible preparations are absorbed more rapidly than oil preparations; large oral doses, conditions of fat malabsorption, low protein intake, or hepatic or pancreatic disease reduce oral absorption
Metabolism: Conjugated with glucuronide, undergoes enterohepatic circulation
Elimination: In feces via biliary elimination

Usual Dosage Recommended daily allowance (RDA):
<1 year: 375 mcg* (1250 units)
1-3 years: 400 mcg* (1330 units)
4-6 years: 500 mcg* (1670 units)
7-10 years: 700 mcg* (2330 units)
>10 years: Female: 800 mcg* (2670 units); Male: 1000 mcg* (3330 units)
*mcg retinol equivalent (0.3 mcg retinol = 1 unit vitamin A)
Daily dietary supplement: Oral:
Infants up to 6 months: 1500 units
(Continued)

Vitamin A *(Continued)*

Children:
6 months to 3 years: 1500-2000 units
4-6 years: 2500 units
7-10 years: 3300-3500 units
Children >10 years and Adults: 4000-5000 units

Vitamin A supplementation in measles (recommendation of the World Health Organization): Children: Oral: Give as a single dose; repeat the next day and at 4 weeks for children with ophthalmologic evidence of vitamin A deficiency:
6 months to 1 year: 100,000 units
>1 year: 200,000 units

Note: Use of vitamin A in measles is recommended only for patients 6 months to 2 years of age hospitalized with measles and its complications **or** patients >6 months of age who have any of the following risk factors and who are not already receiving vitamin A: immunodeficiency, ophthalmologic evidence of vitamin A deficiency including night blindness, Bitot's spots or evidence of xerophthalmia, impaired intestinal absorption, moderate to severe malnutrition including that associated with eating disorders, or recent immigration from areas where high mortality rates from measles have been observed

Note: Monitor patients closely; dosages >25,000 units/kg have been associated with toxicity

Vitamin A deficiency (varying recommendations available):
Severe deficiency with xerophthalmia:
Children 1-8 years: Oral: 5000 units/kg/day for 5 days or until recovery occurs; I.M.: 5000-15,000 units/day for 10 days
Children >8 years and Adults: Oral: 500,000 units/day for 3 days, then 50,000 units/day for 14 days; then 10,000-20,000 units/day for 2 months; I.M.: 50,000-100,000 units/day for 3 days; then 50,000 units/day for 14 days

Prophylactic therapy for children at risk for developing deficiency: Oral: Given every 4-6 months:
Infants ≤1 year: 100,000 units
Children >1 year: 200,000 units

Malabsorption syndrome (prophylaxis): Children >8 years and Adults: Oral: 10,000-50,000 units/day of water miscible product

Administration

Oral: Administer with food or milk
Parenteral: I.M. only

Additional Information 1 USP vitamin A unit = 0.3 mcg of all-*trans* isomer of retinol; 1 RE (retinol equivalent) = 1 mcg of all-*trans*-retinol

Dosage Forms

Capsule: 8000 units, 10,000 units, 25,000 units, 50,000 units
Injection (Aquasol-A®): 50,000 units/mL (2 mL)
Tablet: 5000 units, 10,000 units, 15,000 units
Palmitate-A®: 5000 units, 15,000 units

References

Committee on Infectious Diseases, "Vitamin A in the Treatment of Measles," *Pediatrics*, 1993, 91(5):1014-5.
DeMaeyer EM, "The WHO Programme of Prevention and Control of Vitamin A Deficiency, Xerophthalmia, and Nutritional Blindness," *Nutr Health*, 1986, 4(2):105-12.
Hussey GD and Klein M, "A Randomized, Controlled Trial of Vitamin A in Children With Severe Measles," *N Engl J Med*, 1990, 323(3):160-4.

- **Vitamin A Acid** *see* Tretinoin *on page 978*
- **Vitamin B$_1$** *see* Thiamine *on page 948*
- **Vitamin B$_2$** *see* Riboflavin *on page 874*
- **Vitamin B$_3$** *see* Niacin *on page 711*
- **Vitamin B$_6$** *see* Pyridoxine *on page 857*
- **Vitamin B$_{12}$** *see* Cyanocobalamin *on page 277*
- **Vitamin B$_{12}$** *see* Hydroxocobalamin *on page 512*
- **Vitamin C** *see* Ascorbic Acid *on page 106*
- **Vitamin D$_2$** *see* Ergocalciferol *on page 392*

Vitamin E *(VYE ta min ee)*

Related Information

Carbohydrate and Alcohol Content of Liquid Medications for Use in Patients Receiving Ketogenic Diets *on page 1258*

U.S. Brand Names Aquasol E® Oral [OTC]; Aquavit-E®; Freeda® Vitamin E; Nature's Bounty® Vitamin E; Vitec® [OTC]

Canadian Brand Names Novo E; Nutrol E; Organex E

Synonyms *d*-Alpha Tocopherol; *dl*-Alpha Tocopherol

Therapeutic Category Nutritional Supplement; Vitamin, Fat Soluble; Vitamin, Topical

Generic Available Yes

Use Prevention and treatment of vitamin E deficiency

Pregnancy Risk Factor A (C if dose exceeds RDA recommendation)

Contraindications Hypersensitivity to vitamin E or any component

Warnings Necrotizing enterocolitis has been associated with oral administration of large dosages (eg, >200 units/day) of a hyperosmolar vitamin E preparation in low birth weight infants

Adverse Reactions

Central nervous system: Headache

Dermatologic: Rash

Endocrine & metabolic: Gonadal dysfunction; decreased serum thyroxine and triiodothyronine; increased cholesterol and triglycerides

Gastrointestinal: Nausea, diarrhea, intestinal cramps, necrotizing enterocolitis (see Warnings)

Neuromuscular & skeletal: Weakness

Ocular: Blurred vision

Renal: Creatinuria and increased serum creatinine kinase; increased urinary estrogens and androgens

Drug Interactions Iron, mineral oil, warfarin

Mechanism of Action Antioxidant which prevents oxidation of vitamin A and C; protects polyunsaturated fatty acids in membranes from attack by free radicals and protects red blood cells against hemolysis by oxidizing agents

Pharmacokinetics

Absorption: Oral: Depends upon the presence of bile; absorption is reduced in conditions of malabsorption, in low birth weight premature infants, and as dosage increases; water miscible preparations are better absorbed than oil preparations

Metabolism: In the liver to glucuronides

Elimination: Primarily in bile

Usual Dosage 1 unit vitamin E = 1 mg *dl*-alpha-tocopherol acetate. Oral:

Vitamin E - Recommended Daily Allowance (RDA) and Estimated Average Requirement (EAR)

Age	RDA (mg/day)	EAR (mg/day)
0-6 mo	–	4 (6 units)
7-12 mo	–	6 (9 units)
1-3 y	6 (9 units)	5 (7.5 units)
4-8 y	7 (10.5 units)	6 (9 units)
9-13 y	11 (16.5 units)	9 (13.5 units)
≥14 y	15 (22.5 units)	12 (18 units)

Vitamin E deficiency:

Neonates, premature, low birth weight: 25-50 units/day results in normal levels within 1 week

Children (with malabsorption syndrome): 1 unit/kg/day of water miscible vitamin E (to raise plasma tocopherol concentrations to the normal range within 2 months and to maintain normal plasma concentrations)

Adults: 60-75 units/day

Prevention of vitamin E deficiency:

Neonates:

Low birth weight: 5 units/day

Full-term: 5 units/L of formula ingested

Adults: 30 units/day

Prevention of retinopathy of prematurity or BPD secondary to O_2 therapy: Neonates and Infants: (American Academy of Pediatrics considers this use investigational and routine use is not recommended): 15-30 units/kg/day to maintain plasma levels between 1.5-2 mcg/mL (may need as high as 100 units/kg/day)

Cystic fibrosis, beta-thalassemia, sickle cell anemia may require higher daily maintenance doses: Infants, Children, and Adolescents:

Cystic fibrosis: 100-400 units/day

Beta-thalassemia: 750 units/day

Sickle cell: 450 units/day

Topical: Apply a thin layer over affected area

(Continued)

Vitamin E *(Continued)*

Administration Oral: May administer with or without food

Monitoring Parameters Plasma tocopherol concentrations

Reference Range Plasma tocopherol: 6-14 µg/mL

Dosage Forms

Capsule: 100 units, 200 units, 400 units, 600 units, 800 units 1000 units

Capsule, water miscible: 400 units

Cream: 50 mg/g (15 g, 60 g, 75 g, 120 g, 454 g)

Nature's Bounty® Vitamin E Cream: 100 units/g (57 g)

Drops, oral (Aquasol E®, Aquavit-E®): 15 units/0.3 mL (12 mL, 30 mL)

Liquid, topical: 30 mL, 60 mL

Freeda® Vitamin E Liquid: 4600 units/5 mL [oral or topical] (30 mL, 60 mL)

Lotion: 120 mL, 480 mL

Vitec®: 90 mL

Oil: 30 mL, 60 mL

Nature's Bounty® Vitamin E Oil: 100 units/0.25 mL [oral or topical] (60 mL)

Tablet: 100 units, 200 units, 400 units, 500 units, 800 units

References

American Academy of Pediatrics Committee on Fetus and Newborn, "Vitamin E and the Prevention of Retinopathy of Prematurity," *Pediatrics*, 1985, 76(2):315-6.

Warfarin *(WAR far in)*

Related Information

Overdose and Toxicology *on page 1222*

U.S. Brand Names Coumadin®

Therapeutic Category Anticoagulant

Generic Available Yes

Use Prophylaxis and treatment of venous thromboembolic disorders; prevention of arterial thromboembolism in patients with prosthetic heart valves or atrial fibrillation; prevention of death, venous thromboembolism, and recurrent MI after acute MI

Pregnancy Risk Factor X

Contraindications Hypersensitivity to warfarin or any component; severe liver or kidney disease; open wounds; uncontrolled bleeding; GI ulcers; neurosurgical procedures; malignant hypertension; pregnancy

Warnings Concomitant use with vitamin K may decrease anticoagulant effect; monitor carefully; concomitant use with ethacrynic acid, indomethacin, NSAIDs, phenylbutazone, or aspirin increases warfarin's anticoagulant effect and may cause severe GI irritation; oral anticoagulant therapy is usually avoided in neonates due to a greater potential risk of bleeding (see Monagle, 2001)

Precautions Do not switch brands once desired therapeutic response has been achieved; use with caution in patients with active tuberculosis, diabetes mellitus, or heparin-induced thrombocytopenia with deep vein thrombosis; use with caution in patients with or at risk for hemorrhage, necrosis, or gangrene

Adverse Reactions

Central nervous system: Fever

Dermatologic: Skin lesions, skin necrosis; hair loss (rare in children)

Gastrointestinal: Anorexia, nausea, vomiting, diarrhea

Hematologic: Hemorrhage

Respiratory: Hemoptysis; tracheal calcification (rare in children)

Drug Interactions Cytochrome P-450 isoenzyme CYP1A2 substrate (minor), CYP2C8, CYP2C9, CYP2C18, CYP2C19, and CYP3A3/4 isoenzyme substrate; CYP2C9 isoenzyme inhibitor

Alcohol, alteplase, amiodarone, anabolic steroids, aspirin, amoxicillin, barbiturates, carbamazepine, cefaclor, chloral hydrate, chloramphenicol, chlordiazepoxide, cholestyramine, cimetidine, clofibrate, cloxacillin, co-trimoxazole, disulfiram, erythromycin, fluconazole, griseofulvin, isoniazid, ketoconazole, metronidazole, miconazole (systemic or intravaginal use), nafcillin, omeprazole, phenylbutazone, phenytoin, phenobarbital, piroxicam, prednisone, propranolol, ranitidine, rifampin, salicylates, streptokinase, sucralfate, sulfonamides, urokinase, vitamin K, zafirlukast, zileuton; ritonavir and delavirdine may decrease warfarin metabolism; concurrent use of delavirdine and warfarin is not recommended; suspected drug interaction with nevirapine (monitor closely)

Food Interactions Vitamin K can reverse the anticoagulation effects of warfarin; large amounts of food high in vitamin K (such as green leafy vegetables) may reverse warfarin, decrease prothrombin time, and lead to therapeutic failure; a balanced diet with a consistent intake of vitamin K is essential; avoid large amounts of alfalfa, asparagus, broccoli, brussel sprouts, cabbage, cauliflower, green teas, kale, lettuce, spinach, turnip greens, watercress; avoid enteral feeds high in vitamin K. **Note:** Breast-fed infants may be more sensitive to warfarin due to low amounts of vitamin K in breast milk.

High doses of vitamin A, E, or C may alter PT; use caution with fish oils or omega 3 fatty acids; avoid fried or boiled onions as they may increase drug effect by increasing fibrinolytic activity; avoid herbal teas and remedies such as tonka beans, melilot, and woodruff as they contain natural coumarins and will increase effect of warfarin; avoid large amounts of liver, avocado, soy protein, soybean oil, papain.

Stability

Tablets and injection: Protect from light

Injection: Use within 4 hours after reconstitution, do not refrigerate, discard unused portion (does not contain preservative)

Mechanism of Action Interferes with hepatic synthesis of vitamin K-dependent coagulation factors (II, VII, IX, X)

Pharmacodynamics Anticoagulation effects:

Onset of action: Within 36-72 hours

Peak effect: Within 5-7 days

Pharmacokinetics

Absorption: Oral: Rapid

Metabolism: In the liver

Half-life: 42 hours, highly variable among individuals

Usual Dosage Oral:

Infants and Children: **To maintain an International Normalized Ratio (INR) between 2-3:**

Initial loading dose on day 1 (if baseline INR is 1-1.3): 0.2 mg/kg (maximum dose: 10 mg); use initial loading dose of 0.1 mg/kg if patient has liver dysfunction

Loading dose for days 2-4: doses are dependent upon patient's INR

if INR is 1.1-1.3, repeat the initial loading dose

if INR is 1.4-1.9, give 50% of the initial loading dose

if INR is 2-3, give 50% of the initial loading dose

if INR is 3.1-3.5, give 25% of the initial loading dose

if INR is >3.5, hold the drug until INR <3.5, then restart at 50% less than the previous dose

Maintenance dose guidelines for day 5 of therapy and beyond: doses are dependent upon patient's INR

if INR is 1.1-1.4, increase dose by 20% of previous dose

if INR is 1.5-1.9, increase dose by 10% of previous dose

if INR is 2-3, do not change the dose

if INR is 3.1-3.5, decrease dose by 10% of previous dose

if INR is >3.5, hold the drug and check INR daily until INR <3.5, then restart at 20% less than the previous dose

Usual maintenance dose: ~0.1 mg/kg/day; range: 0.05-0.34 mg/kg/day; the dose in mg/kg/day is inversely related to age; in one study (Andrew, 1994), to attain an INR of 2-3, children <12 months of age required a mean dose of 0.32 mg/kg/day, but children 11-18 years required a mean dose of 0.09 mg/kg/day; to attain an INR of 1.3-1.8, children <12 months (n=2) required 0.24 and 0.27 mg/kg/day, but children >1 year required a mean of 0.08 mg/kg/day (range: 0.03-0.17 mg/kg/day); consistent anticoagulation may be difficult to maintain in children <5 years of age

(Continued)

Warfarin *(Continued)*

Adults: 5-15 mg/day for 2-5 days, then adjust dose according to results of INR or PT; usual maintenance dose ranges from 2-10 mg/day

I.V.: (For patients who cannot take oral form): I.V. dose is equal to oral dose

Administration

Oral: May administer on an empty or full stomach

Parenteral: I.V. use only; do not administer I.M.; reconstitute 5 mg vial with 2.7 mL SWI to produce 2 mg/mL solution; administer by slow I.V. injection over 1-2 minutes into peripheral vein

Monitoring Parameters INR (preferred) or prothrombin time; hemoglobin, hematocrit, signs and symptoms of bleeding

Reference Range The INR is now the standard test used to monitor warfarin anticoagulation; the desired INR is based upon indication; due to the lack of pediatric clinical trials assessing optimal INR ranges and clinical outcomes, the desired INR ranges for children are extrapolated from adult studies; the optimal therapeutic INR ranges may possibly be lower in children versus adults. Further pediatric studies are needed (see Monagle, 2001)

For pediatric patients, a target INR of 2.5 (range: 2-3) is recommended for the treatment of venous thromboembolisms. A target INR of 3.0 (range: 2.5-3.5) is recommended for children with mechanical prosthetic heart valves. Low-dose warfarin (INR target range: 1.4-1.9) is recommended for the following situations: Children with substantial risks for bleeding or when monitoring is not possible; initial treatment of children with an old thrombus or those who are at a significant risk for thromboembolism; following 3 months of therapeutic doses of warfarin in children with a new thrombus and a long-term predisposing cause for recurrent thromboembolism (see Monagle, 2001) (see Additional Information).

For Adults, an INR of 2-3 is recommended for most venous thrombotic diseases including prevention and treatment of DVT, treatment of PE, prevention of systemic embolism (due to atrial fibrillation, valvulvar heart disease, acute MI, and cardiac valve replacement with tissue valves). An INR of 2.5-3.5 is recommended for cardiac valve replacement with mechanical prosthetic valves (high risk), but for a bileaflet mechanical valve in the aortic position an INR of 2-3 is recommended. An INR of 2.5-3.5 is recommended in adults to prevent recurrent MI (Hirsh, 2001)

Note: If INR is not available, prothrombin time should be $1\frac{1}{2}$ to 2 times the control.

Patient Information Avoid alcohol; limit caffeine; report any signs of bleeding to physician at once (eg, gums bleeding, dark brown urine, black tar-like stools); avoid hazardous activities; use soft toothbrush; carry Medi-Alert® ID identifying drug use; be aware of other drugs and foods to avoid

Nursing Implications Be aware of drug interactions and foods that contain vitamin K which can alter anticoagulant effects; avoid I.M. injections of drugs

Additional Information Usual duration of therapy: **first venous thrombotic event:** treat for at least 3 months; after 3 months, low-dose warfarin (INR 1.5-1.8) or LMWH is recommended as an option in children with first time central venous line-related DVT until the central venous line is removed; **recurrent central venous line related thromboembolic events:** after initial 3 months of warfarin therapy, low-dose warfarin (INR 1.5-1.8) or LMWH is recommended until removal of the central venous line; if thromboembolism recurs during low-dose therapy, increase to a therapeutic dose and continue until central venous line is removed or for at least 3 months; **idiopathic thrombotic event:** treat for at least 6 months; **recurrent noncentral venous line related thrombotic event:** after initial 3 months of warfarin therapy (recommendation: 1-3 months), treat with therapeutic or low-dose warfarin (or LMWH) indefinitely; mechanical prosthetic heart valves: treat for life (see Monagle, 2001)

Overdoses of warfarin may be treated with vitamin K, to reverse warfarin's anticoagulation effect

Dosage Forms

Powder for injection, as sodium, lyophilized: 5 mg

Tablet, as sodium: 1 mg, 2 mg, 2.5 mg, 3 mg, 4 mg, 5 mg, 6 mg, 7.5 mg, 10 mg

References

Andrew M, Marzinotto V, Brooker LA, et al, "Oral Anticoagulation Therapy in Pediatric Patients: A Prospective Study," *Thromb Haemost,* 1994, 71(3):265-9.

David M and Andrew M, "Venous Thromboembolic Complications in Children," *J Pediatr,* 1993, 123(3):337-46.

Fihn SD "Aiming for Safe Anticoagulation," *N Engl J Med,* 1995, 333(1):54-5.

Hirsh J, Dalen JE, Anderson DR, et al, "Oral Anticoagulants. Mechanism of Action, Clinical Effectiveness, and Optimal Therapeutic Range," *Chest,* 2001, 119:8S-21S.

Monagle P, Michelson AD, Bovill E, et al, "Antithrombotic Therapy in Children," *Chest,* 2001, 119:344S-70S.

Wells PS, Holbrook AM, Crowther NR, et al, "Interactions of Warfarin With Drugs and Food," *Ann Intern Med*, 1994, 121(9):676-83.

- **Wart-Off® Maximum Strength [OTC]** *see* Salicylic Acid *on page 886*
- **Wart Remover [OTC]** *see* Salicylic Acid *on page 886*
- **4-Way® Long Acting [OTC]** *see* Oxymetazoline *on page 749*
- **Westcort®** *see* Hydrocortisone *on page 506*
- **White Mineral Oil** *see* Mineral Oil *on page 675*
- **Wigraine®** *see* Ergotamine *on page 393*
- **Winpred (Can)** *see* Prednisone *on page 824*
- **WinRho SDF®** *see* Rh₀(D) Immune Globulin (Intravenous) *on page 870*
- **Wood Sugar** *see* d-Xylose *on page 367*
- **Wyamycin® S** *see* Erythromycin *on page 394*
- **Wycillin®** *see* Penicillin G Procaine *on page 773*
- **Wydase®** *see* Hyaluronidase *on page 500*
- **Wygesic®** *see* Propoxyphene and Acetaminophen *on page 846*
- **Wymox®** *see* Amoxicillin *on page 80*
- **Xanax®** *see* Alprazolam *on page 55*
- **Xopenex™** *see* Levalbuterol *on page 583*
- **X-Prep® Liquid [OTC]** *see* Senna *on page 896*
- **X-Seb (Can)** *see* Salicylic Acid *on page 886*
- **Xylocaine®** *see* Lidocaine *on page 590*
- **Xylocaine® MPF** *see* Lidocaine *on page 590*
- **Xylocaine® MPF With Epinephrine** *see* Lidocaine and Epinephrine *on page 593*
- **Xylocaine® Viscous** *see* Lidocaine *on page 590*
- **Xylocaine® With Epinephrine** *see* Lidocaine and Epinephrine *on page 593*
- **Xylocard (Can)** *see* Lidocaine *on page 590*
- **Xylo-Pfan® [OTC]** *see* d-Xylose *on page 367*
- **Xylose** *see* d-Xylose *on page 367*
- **Yellow Fever Vaccine** *see page 1172*
- **Yodoxin®** *see* Iodoquinol *on page 546*

Zafirlukast (za FIR loo kast)

Related Information

Asthma Guidelines *on page 1210*

U.S. Brand Names Accolate®

Therapeutic Category Antiasthmatic; Leukotriene Receptor Antagonist

Use Prophylaxis and chronic treatment of asthma

Pregnancy Risk Factor B

Contraindications Hypersensitivity to zafirlukast or any component

Warnings Zafirlukast is not indicated for use in the reversal of bronchospasm in acute asthma attacks, including status asthmaticus. Therapy with zafirlukast can be continued during acute exacerbations of asthma. An increased proportion of zafirlukast patients (>55 years of age) reported infections as compared to placebo-treated patients; these infections were mostly mild or moderate in intensity, predominantly affected the respiratory tract, were dose-proportional to the total milligrams of zafirlukast exposure, and associated with coadministration of inhaled corticosteroids.

Precautions Use with caution in patients receiving warfarin (see Drug Interactions) and patients with liver disease; dosage reduction in patients with hepatic impairment may be needed; discontinue therapy if liver dysfunction occurs; where no other attributable cause of liver dysfunction is identified, do not resume zafirlukast therapy

Adverse Reactions

Central nervous system: Headache, dizziness, pain, fever, asthenia

Gastrointestinal: Nausea, diarrhea, abdominal pain, vomiting, dyspepsia, xerostomia

Hepatic: Elevated liver enzymes, hepatitis, hyperbilirubinemia

Neuromuscular & skeletal: Myalgia, weakness, arthralgia

Respiratory: Rhinitis, pharyngitis

Miscellaneous: Infections (primarily respiratory), hypersensitivity reactions

Drug Interactions Cytochrome P-450 isoenzyme CYP2C9 substrate; CYP2C9 and CYP3A3/4 isoenzyme inhibitor

Erythromycin, terfenadine, and theophylline decrease zafirlukast serum levels; aspirin increases plasma levels of zafirlukast; coadministration of zafirlukast with warfarin results in a clinically significant increase in prothrombin time (PT)

Food Interactions Food decreases zafirlukast absorption by 40%

(Continued)

Zafirlukast *(Continued)*

Stability Store tablets at controlled room temperature; protect from light and moisture; dispense in original airtight container

Mechanism of Action Zafirlukast is a selective and competitive leukotriene-receptor antagonist (LTRA) of cysteinyl leukotrienes C_4 (LTC$_4$), D_4 (LTD$_4$), and E_4 (LTE$_4$). This activity produces inhibition of the effects of these leukotrienes on bronchial smooth muscle resulting in the attenuation of bronchoconstriction and decreased vascular permeability, mucosal edema, and mucus production.

Pharmacodynamics Asthma symptom improvement:
Duration of effect: 12 hours
Time to maximal effects: 2-6 weeks

Pharmacokinetics
Absorption: Rapid
Distribution: Extensively excreted into breast milk; breast milk to plasma ratio: 0.15
Protein binding: 99%, predominantly albumin
Metabolism: Extensively metabolized by liver via cytochrome P-450 isoenzyme CYP2C9 pathway
Half-life, elimination: 10 hours
Time to peak serum concentration: 2-4 hours
Elimination: Fecal (90%) and urine (10%)

Usual Dosage Oral:
Children 7-11 years: 10 mg twice daily
Children ≥12 years and Adults: 20 mg twice daily
Dosing adjustment in hepatic impairment: In patients with hepatic impairment (ie, biopsy-proven cirrhosis), there is a 50% to 60% greater C_{max} and AUC compared to normal subjects; these patients should be monitored closely for adverse effects and dosage reductions made if indicated (see Precautions)

Administration Oral: Administer at least 1 hour before or 2 hours after a meal

Monitoring Parameters Pulmonary function tests (FEV-1, PEF), improvement in asthma symptoms, liver function tests

Reference Range Plasma levels not clinically indicated; plasma zafirlukast serum concentrations exceeding 5 ng/mL at 12-14 hours following oral doses have correlated with activity; mean trough serum levels at doses of 20 mg twice daily were 20 ng/mL

Patient Information Take regularly as prescribed, even during symptom-free periods. Do not use to treat acute episodes of asthma. Do not decrease the dose or stop taking any other asthma medications unless instructed by a physician. Nursing women should not take zafirlukast.

Dosage Forms Tablet: 10 mg, 20 mg

Zalcitabine *(zal SITE a been)*

Related Information
Adult and Adolescent HIV *on page 1166*
Pediatric HIV *on page 1162*

U.S. Brand Names Hivid®

Synonyms ddC; Dideoxycytidine

Therapeutic Category Antiretroviral Agent; HIV Agents (Anti-HIV Agents); Nucleoside Reverse Transcriptase Inhibitor (NRTI)

Generic Available No

Use Treatment of HIV infection in combination with other antiretroviral agents. (**Note:** HIV regimens consisting of **three** antiretroviral agents are strongly recommended)

Pregnancy Risk Factor C

Contraindications Hypersensitivity to zalcitabine or any component

Warnings An accumulative dose-related, clinically disabling peripheral neuropathy (treatment-limiting), or fatal pancreatitis may occur; discontinue therapy in patients with symptoms of pancreatitis until pancreatitis can be ruled out; cases of fatal lactic acidosis and severe hepatomegaly with steatosis may occur; hepatic failure and death (which may be related to underlying hepatitis B) have been reported (rare); discontinue therapy in patients with clinical or laboratory signs suggestive of lactic acidosis or hepatotoxicity (eg, steatosis and hepatomegaly even without marked elevations of liver enzymes) or if liver function tests increase to >5 times the upper limit of normal

Precautions Use with extreme caution in patients with pre-existing peripheral neuropathy; avoid use in patients with moderate or severe peripheral neuropathy; use with caution in patients at risk for developing peripheral neuropathy [patients with low CD4 count (<50 cells/mm^2), diabetes mellitus, weight loss, concurrent therapy with other drugs that cause peripheral neuropathy]; zalcitabine may exacerbate existing liver dysfunction in patients with a previous history of liver disease or alcohol abuse; increased liver function tests were observed in patients on zalcitabine therapy; use with caution in patients with hepatic impairment; obtain CBC and clinical chemistry tests prior to and during therapy; obtain serum amylase and triglyceride levels and use with caution in patients with history of pancreatitis, increased amylase, ethanol abuse or patients receiving hyperalimentation; use with caution and adjust dose in patients with renal dysfunction; multiple potentially serious drug interactions exist (see Drug Interactions)

Adverse Reactions

Cardiovascular: Chest pain, edema, hypertension, palpitations, syncope, atrial fibrillation, tachycardia, CHF, heart racing

Central nervous system: Headache, dizziness, fever, malaise, fatigue, chest pain

Dermatologic: Pruritus, rash (may be erythematous, maculopapular, follicular or other)

Endocrine & metabolic: Lactic acidosis (rare, but potentially fatal), hyperglycemia, hypocalcemia

Gastrointestinal: Oral ulcers, nausea, esophageal ulcers, dysphagia, anorexia, abdominal pain, vomiting, diarrhea, constipation, pancreatitis (1.1%; can be fatal), weight loss

Hematologic: Leukopenia, absolute neutrophil count alteration, anemia, granulocytosis, neutrophilia, thrombocytopenia

Hepatic: Jaundice, hepatitis; severe hepatomegaly with steatosis (can be fatal)

Neuromuscular & skeletal: Peripheral neuropathy (22% to 35%), myalgia, arthralgia, weakness, foot pain, myositis

Respiratory: Pharyngitis, epistaxis

Miscellaneous: Anaphylactoid reactions, hypersensitivity reactions, night sweats

Drug Interactions Magnesium- and aluminum-containing antacids and metoclopramide may decrease the bioavailability of zalcitabine; amphotericin, foscarnet, probenecid, cimetidine, and aminoglycosides may interfere with the renal elimination of zalcitabine and potentiate the risk of peripheral neuropathy or other zalcitabine toxicities; drugs associated with peripheral neuropathy (chloramphenicol, cisplatin, dapsone, disulfiram, ethionamide, glutethimide, gold, hydralazine, iodoquinol, isoniazid, lithium, metronidazole, nitrofurantoin, pentamidine, phenytoin, ribavirin, and vincristine) may increase the risk for zalcitabine peripheral neuropathy; concomitant use of zalcitabine with didanosine is not recommended (increased risk of peripheral neuropathy); one case of fulminant pancreatitis associated with concomitant zalcitabine and pentamidine use has been reported; if I.V. pentamidine is required to treat *Pneumocystis carinii* pneumonia, treatment with zalcitabine should be interrupted

Food Interactions Food decreases the rate and extent of absorption (AUC decreased by 14%)

Stability Tablets should be stored in tightly closed bottles at 59°F to 86°F

Mechanism of Action A nucleoside (pyrimidine) analogue that is converted within cells to the active metabolite dideoxycytidine triphosphate (ddCTP) which serves as an alternative substrate to deoxycytidine triphosphate (dCTP), a natural substrate for cellular DNA polymerase and reverse transcriptase; inhibits HIV viral enzyme reverse transcriptase and DNA synthesis causing chain termination

Pharmacokinetics

Distribution: V_{dss}:

Children: 9.3 L/m^2

Adults: 0.53 L/kg

CSF levels are 9% to 37% of serum levels (mean 20%)

Protein binding: Minimal, <4%

Metabolism: Converted intracellularly to active triphosphate form; minimal hepatic metabolism; primary identified metabolite is dideoxyuridine

Bioavailability:

Children: 29% to 100% (mean: 54%)

Adults: >80%

Half-life:

Children: Mean: 1.4 hours

Adults: 1-3 hours (mean: 2 hours)

Adults with Cl_{cr} <55 mL/minute: up to 8.5 hours

Elimination: Primarily renal with 60% of dose excreted unchanged in urine within 24 hours; elimination is prolonged in patients with renal dysfunction

Dialysis: Hemodialysis reduces plasma levels by 50%

Usual Dosage Oral: (Use in combination with other antiretroviral agents)

Neonates: Dose unknown

(Continued)

Zalcitabine *(Continued)*

Infants and Children <13 years: Usual dose: 0.01 mg/kg every 8 hours; range: 0.005-0.01 mg/kg every 8 hours

Adolescents and Adults: 0.75 mg 3 times/day

Dosing adjustment in severe renal impairment: Adults:

Cl_{cr} 10-40 mL/minute: 0.75 mg every 12 hours

Cl_{cr} <10 mL/minute: 0.75 mg every 24 hours

Administration Oral: Administer on an empty stomach 1 hour before or 2 hours after a meal; do not administer concurrently with antacids

Monitoring Parameters Renal function, CD4 counts, viral load, CBC with differential, liver enzymes, serum chemistries, serum amylase, triglyceride, signs/symptoms of peripheral neuropathy

Patient Information Avoid alcohol; zalcitabine is not a cure; notify physician if numbness, tingling, persistent severe abdominal pain, nausea, or vomiting occurs; take zalcitabine every day as prescribed; do not change dose or discontinue without physician's advice; if a dose is missed, take it as soon as possible, then return to normal dosing schedule; if a dose is skipped, do **not** double the next dose

Additional Information Adverse events may be increased in patients with decreased CD4 cell counts; an oral 0.1 mg/mL zalcitabine raspberry syrup formulation is available on an investigational basis from Roche Pharmaceuticals as part of a U.S. pediatric compassionate use study (NV14610)

Dosage Forms Tablet: 0.375 mg, 0.75 mg

References

Adkins JC, Peters DH, and Faulds D, "Zalcitabine. An Update of Its Pharmacodynamic and Pharmacokinetic Properties and Clinical Efficacy in the Management of HIV Infection," *Drugs*, 1997, 53(6):1054-80.

Bakshi SS, Britto P, Capparelli E, et al, "Evaluation of Pharmacokinetics, Safety, Tolerance, and Activity of Combination of Zalcitabine and Zidovudine in Stable, Zidovudine-Treated Pediatric Patients With Human Immunodeficiency Virus Infection. AIDS Clinical Trials Group Protocol 190 Team," *J Infect Dis*, 1997, 175(5):1039-50.

Chadwick EG, Nazareno LA, Nieuwenhuis TJ, et al, "Phase I Evaluation of Zalcitabine Administered to Human Immunodeficiency Virus-Infected Children," *J Infect Dis*, 1995, 172(6):1475-9.

Pizzo PA, Butler K, Balis F, et al, "Dideoxycytidine Alone and in an Alternating Schedule With Zidovudine in Children With Symptomatic Human Immunodeficiency Virus Infection," *J Pediatr*, 1990, 117(5):799-808.

Spector SA, "HIV Therapy Advances. Pediatric Antiretroviral Choices," *AIDS*, 1994, 8(Suppl 3):S15-8.

Spector SA, Blanchard S, Wara DW, et al, "Comparative Trial of Two Dosages of Zalcitabine in Zidovudine-Experienced Children With Advanced Human Immunodeficiency Virus Disease. Pediatric AIDS Clinical Trials Group," *Pediatr Infect Dis J*, 1997, 16(6):623-6.

Working Group on Antiretroviral Therapy and Medical Management of HIV-Infected Children, "Guidelines for the Use of Antiretroviral Agents in Pediatric HIV Infection," January 7, 2000, http://www.hivatis.org.

Zidovudine *(zye DOE vyoo deen)*

Related Information

Adult and Adolescent HIV *on page 1166*

Carbohydrate and Alcohol Content of Liquid Medications for Use in Patients Receiving Ketogenic Diets *on page 1258*

Pediatric HIV *on page 1162*

U.S. Brand Names Retrovir®

Canadian Brand Names Apo-Zidovudine; Novo-AZT

Synonyms Azidothymidine; AZT; Compound S; ZDV

Therapeutic Category Antiretroviral Agent; HIV Agents (Anti-HIV Agents); Nucleoside Reverse Transcriptase Inhibitor (NRTI)

Generic Available No

Use Treatment of HIV infection in combination with other antiretroviral agents; **(Note:** HIV regimens consisting of **three** antiretroviral agents are strongly recommended); chemoprophylaxis after occupational exposure to HIV; chemoprophylaxis to reduce perinatal HIV transmission

Pregnancy Risk Factor C

Contraindications Life-threatening hypersensitivity to zidovudine or any component

Warnings Associated with hematologic toxicity including granulocytopenia and severe anemia requiring transfusions; zidovudine treatment should be stopped in children with an absolute neutrophil count <500 cells/mm^3 until marrow recovery is observed; use of erythropoietin, filgrastim, or reduced zidovudine dosage may be necessary in some patients; use has been associated with potentially fatal lactic acidosis and severe hepatomegaly with steatosis; zidovudine has been shown to be carcinogenic in rats and mice

Precautions Use with caution in patients with bone marrow compromise or in patients with impaired renal or hepatic function; reduce dosage or interrupt therapy in patients with anemia and/or granulocytopenia, myopathy, renal or hepatic impairment

Adverse Reactions

Central nervous system: Malaise, dizziness, manic syndrome, seizures, confusion, fever, severe headache, insomnia, asthenia

Dermatologic: Rash, pigmentation of nails (blue)

Endocrine & metabolic: Lactic acidosis

Gastrointestinal: Nausea, diarrhea, vomiting, anorexia

Hematologic: Granulocytopenia, thrombocytopenia, leukopenia, anemia

Hepatic: Cholestatic hepatitis, hepatomegaly; elevated serum AST, LDH, and alkaline phosphatase

Neuromuscular & skeletal: Myalgia, tremor, weakness; unusual: myopathy, myositis

Drug Interactions Acyclovir; coadministration with drugs that increase zidovudine concentration (acetaminophen, atovaquone, methadone, valproic acid, cimetidine, indomethacin, lorazepam, fluconazole, probenecid, aspirin) may increase toxicity of zidovudine; flucytosine, pentamidine, co-trimoxazole may increase hematologic side effects; didanosine, foscarnet, ganciclovir, zalcitabine (synergistic antiretroviral activity); ribavirin (antagonistic); coadministration with rifampin or rifabutin may increase metabolism of zidovudine; clarithromycin decreases zidovudine concentration by interfering with its absorption (administer doses 4 hours apart); do not administer in combination with stavudine (poor antiretroviral effect)

Food Interactions Folate or vitamin B$_{12}$ deficiency increases zidovudine-associated myelosuppression

Stability Diluted I.V. zidovudine solution is stable for 24 hours when refrigerated

Mechanism of Action Zidovudine is a thymidine analog that enters the cell and is phosphorylated by cellular kinases to the active metabolite zidovudine triphosphate which serves as an alternative substrate to deoxythymidine triphosphate for incorporation by reverse transcriptase; inhibits HIV viral polymerases and DNA synthesis

Pharmacokinetics

Absorption: Oral: Well absorbed (66% to 70%)

Distribution: Significant penetration into the CSF; crosses the placenta

Protein binding: 25% to 38%

Metabolism: Extensive first-pass effect; metabolized in the liver via glucuronidation to inactive metabolites

Bioavailability:

Neonates <14 days: 89%

Infants: 60%

Half-life, terminal: 60 minutes

Premature neonate: 6.3 hours

Full-term neonates: 3.1 hours

Older infants: 1.9 hours

Time to peak serum concentration: Within 30-90 minutes

Elimination: Urinary excretion (63% to 95%)

Oral: 72% to 74% of drug excreted in urine as metabolites and 14% to 18% as unchanged drug

I.V.: 45% to 60% excreted in urine as metabolites and 18% to 29% as unchanged drug

Usual Dosage

Premature Infants: (Standard neonatal dose may be excessive in premature infants) Under investigation in PACTG 331: Oral: 1.5 mg/kg/dose every 12 hours from birth to 2 weeks of age; then increase to 2 mg/kg/dose every 8 hours after 2 weeks of age

(Continued)

Zidovudine (Continued)

Neonates:
Oral: 2 mg/kg/dose every 6 hours
I.V.: 1.5 mg/kg/dose every 6 hours

Children:
Oral: 160 mg/m^2/dose every 8 hours; dosage range: 90 mg/m^2/dose to 180 mg/m^2/dose every 6-8 hours; some Working Group members use a dose of 180 mg/m^2 every 12 hours when using in drug combinations with other antiretroviral compounds, but data on this dosing in children is limited
I.V. continuous infusion: 20 mg/m^2/hour
I.V. intermittent infusion: 120 mg/m^2/dose every 6 hours

Dosing adjustment in children with zidovudine toxicity:
Hemoglobin <8 g/dL: Reduce zidovudine dose by 30%

Children >12 years and Adults:
Oral: 200 mg 3 times/day or 300 mg twice daily
HIV postexposure prophylaxis: 600 mg/day in divided doses (eg, 300 mg twice daily, 200 mg 3 times/day or 100 mg every 4 hours) in combination with lamivudine 150 mg twice daily and indinavir 800 mg 3 times/day are first-line agents for HIV postexposure prophylaxis
I.V.: 1-2 mg/kg/dose every 4 hours

Administration
Oral: May administer with food (although the manufacturer recommends administration 30 minutes before or 1 hour after a meal with a glass of water); the patient should be in an upright position while taking zidovudine capsules to minimize the risk of esophageal ulceration
Parenteral: Do not administer I.M.; do not administer I.V. push or by rapid infusion; infuse I.V. zidovudine over 1 hour at a final concentration not to exceed 4 mg/mL in D$_5$W

Monitoring Parameters CBC with differential, hemoglobin, MCV, reticulocyte count, serum creatine kinase, CD4 cell count, HIV RNA plasma levels, renal and hepatic function tests

Patient Information Zidovudine is not a cure for AIDS. Take zidovudine as directed. Notify physician if muscle weakness, shortness of breath, headache, insomnia, signs of infection, unusual bleeding, or rash occur.

Additional Information Conversion from oral to I.V. dose: I.V. dose = $^2/_3$ of the oral dose

Dosage Forms
Capsule: 100 mg
Concentration for injection (for I.V. infusion): 10 mg/mL (20 mL)
Syrup: 50 mg/5 mL [strawberry flavor] (240 mL)
Tablet: 300 mg

References
Carpenter CC, Fischel MA, Hammer SM, et al, "Antiretroviral Therapy for HIV Infection in 1997. Updated Recommendations of the International AIDS Society - USA Panel," *JAMA*, 1997, 277(24):1962-9.

CDC and the National Foundation for Infectious Disease, "Public Health Service Guidelines for the Management of Health-Care Worker Exposures to HIV and Recommendations for Postexposure Prophylaxis," *MMWR Morb Mortal Wkly Rep*, May 15, 1998/47 (RR-7):29-30.

Mueller BU, Jacobsen F, Butler KM, et al, "Combination Treatment With Azidothymidine and Granulocyte Colony-Stimulating Factor in Children With Human Immunodeficiency Virus Infection," *J Pediatr*, 1992, 121(5 Pt 1):797-802.

Volberding PA, Lagakos SW, Koch MA, et al, "Zidovudine in Asymptomatic Human Immunodeficiency Virus Infection. A Controlled Trial in Persons With Fewer Than 500 CD4-Positive Cells Per Cubic Millimeter. The AIDS Clinical Trials Group of the National Institute of Allergy and Infectious Diseases," *N Engl J Med*, 1990, 322(14):941-9.

Working Group on Antiretroviral Therapy and Medical Management of HIV-Infected Children, "Guidelines for the Use of Antiretroviral Agents in Pediatric HIV Infection," April 15, 1999, http://www.hivatis.org.

♦ **Zidovudine, Abacavir, and Lamivudine** *see* Abacavir, Lamivudine, and Zidovudine *on page 26*
♦ **Zidovudine and Lamivudine** *see* Lamivudine and Zidovudine *on page 574*
♦ **Zilactin Baby (Can)** *see* Benzocaine *on page 135*
♦ **Zilactin®-B Medicated [OTC]** *see* Benzocaine *on page 135*
♦ **Zilactin®-L [OTC]** *see* Lidocaine *on page 590*

Zileuton (zye LOO ton)

Related Information
Asthma Guidelines *on page 1210*
U.S. Brand Names Zyflo™
Therapeutic Category Antiasthmatic; Leukotriene Receptor Antagonist
Use Prophylaxis and chronic treatment of asthma

Pregnancy Risk Factor C

Contraindications Active liver disease or transaminase elevations greater than or equal to three times the upper limit of normal; hypersensitivity to zileuton or any ingredient

Warnings Coadministration of zileuton with theophylline, propranolol, astemizole, and terfenadine is associated with significant increases in serum levels of these agents which may require reductions in dosage; elevated terfenadine and astemizole levels have been associated with severe cardiovascular effects including QT interval prolongation, ventricular tachycardia, ventricular fibrillation, death, cardiac arrest, hypotension, and palpitations; elevations of one or more liver function tests may occur during therapy; these laboratory abnormalities may progress, remain unchanged, or resolve with continued therapy; zileuton is **not** indicated for use in the reversal of bronchospasm in acute asthma attacks, including status asthmaticus; zileuton can be continued during acute exacerbations of asthma.

Precautions Use with caution in patients who consume substantial quantities of alcohol or have a past history of liver disease

Adverse Reactions

Cardiovascular: Chest pain

Central nervous system: Headache, pain, dizziness, fever, insomnia, fatigue, nervousness, somnolence

Gastrointestinal: Dyspepsia, nausea, abdominal pain, constipation, flatulence

Hematologic: Low white blood cell count

Hepatic: Elevated liver enzymes

Neuromuscular & skeletal: Myalgia, arthralgia, weakness, paresthesias, asthenia

Ocular: Conjunctivitis

Drug Interactions Cytochrome P-450 isoenzyme CYP1A2, CYP2C9, and CYP3A3/4 substrate; CYP1A2 and CYP3A3/4 isoenzyme inhibitor

Increased toxicity: Coadministration of zileuton with propranolol or theophylline results in an approximate doubling of serum concentrations (propranolol or theophylline); coadministration of zileuton with warfarin results in a clinically significant increase in prothrombin time (PT); coadministration of zileuton with terfenadine or astemizole results in a decrease in clearance leading to an increase in terfenadine or astemizole serum levels (elevated serum levels have been associated with severe cardiovascular effects, see Warnings)

Mechanism of Action Specific inhibitor of 5-lipoxygenase and thus inhibits leukotriene (LTB1, LTC1, LTD1, and LTE1) formation. Leukotrienes are substances that induce numerous biological effects including augmentation of neutrophil and eosinophil migration, neutrophil and monocyte aggregation, leukocyte adhesion, increased capillary permeability and smooth muscle contraction.

Pharmacodynamics After discontinuation of zileuton therapy, 5-lipoxygenase activity (eg, return of leukotriene B4 levels to baseline) occurred in approximately 7 days. See table.

Zileuton Pharmacodynamic Parameters

Parameter	Inhibition of Leukotriene B4 Production	Increased FEV-1
Onset of effect	0.5-1 h	30 min
Peak effect	2-4 h	1 h
Maximal effect	5-8 h	4 wk

Pharmacokinetics

Absorption: Rapidly absorbed

Distribution: V_d: 1.2 L/kg

Protein binding: 93%

Metabolism: Several metabolites in plasma and urine; metabolized by the cytochrome P-450 isoenzymes CYP1A2, CYP2C9, and CYP3A4

Half-life: 2.1-2.5 hours

Time to peak serum concentration: 1-3 hours

Elimination: Predominantly via metabolism; <0.5% excreted unchanged in urine

Clearance: 7 mL/minute/kg

Usual Dosage Oral: Children ≥12 years and Adults: 600 mg 4 times daily with meals and at bedtime

Dosing adjustment in hepatic impairment: Contraindicated in patients with active liver disease

Administration May administer without regard to meals

(Continued)

Zileuton *(Continued)*

Monitoring Parameters Monitor serum ALT before treatment begins, once monthly for the first 3 months, every 2-3 months for the remainder of the first year and periodically thereafter for patients receiving long-term zileuton therapy; complete blood count periodically when on long-term therapy; pulmonary function tests, improvement in asthma symptoms

Patient Information Inform patients that zileuton is indicated for the chronic treatment of asthma and to take regularly as prescribed even during symptom-free periods. Zileuton is not a bronchodilator; do not use to treat acute episodes of asthma. When taking zileuton, do not decrease the dose or stop taking any other asthma medications unless instructed by a physician.

If experiencing signs or symptoms of liver dysfunction (right upper quadrant pain, nausea, fatigue, lethargy, pruritus, jaundice, or "flu-like" symptoms), contact a physician immediately.

Zileuton can interact with other drugs. While taking zileuton, consult a physician or pharmacist before starting or stopping any prescription or nonprescription medicines.

Dosage Forms Tablet: 600 mg

♦ **Zinacef®** *see* Cefuroxime *on page 205*

♦ **Zinaderm (Can)** *see* Zinc Oxide *on page 1026*

♦ **Zincate®** *see* Zinc Supplements *on page 1026*

♦ **Zinc Carbonate** *see* Zinc Supplements *on page 1026*

♦ **Zinc Chloride** *see* Trace Metals *on page 972*

♦ **Zinc Chloride** *see* Zinc Supplements *on page 1026*

♦ **Zinc Gluconate** *see* Zinc Supplements *on page 1026*

♦ **Zincoderm (Can)** *see* Zinc Oxide *on page 1026*

♦ **Zincofax (Can)** *see* Zinc Oxide *on page 1026*

Zinc Oxide *(zingk OKS ide)*

U.S. Brand Names Ammens® Medicated Deodorant [OTC]; Balmex® [OTC]; Boudreaux's® Butt Paste [OTC]; Critic-Aid Skin Care® [OTC]; Desitin® [OTC]; Desitin® Creamy [OTC]

Canadian Brand Names Babys Own Ointment; Diaper Rash; Egozinc; Infazinc; Johnson's Diaper Rash; Triple Care Cream; Zinaderm; Zincoderm; Zincofax

Synonyms Lassar's Zinc Paste

Therapeutic Category Topical Skin Product

Generic Available Yes

Use Protective coating for mild skin irritations and abrasions; soothing and protective ointment to promote healing of chapped skin, diaper rash

Contraindications Hypersensitivity to zinc oxide or any component

Stability Avoid prolonged storage at temperatures >30°C

Mechanism of Action Mild astringent, protective and weak antiseptic action

Usual Dosage Infants, Children, and Adults: Topical: Apply several times daily to affected area

Administration Topical: For external use only; do not use in the eyes

Patient Information Paste is easily removed with mineral oil

Dosage Forms
Ointment, topical: 20% (30 g, 60 g, 480 g); 40% (120 g)
    Balmex®: 11.3% (60 g, 120 g, 480 g)
    Desitin®: 40% (30 g, 60 g, 90 g, 120 g, 270 g, 480 g)
    Desitin® Creamy: 10% (60 g, 120 g)
Paste, topical:
    Boudreaux's® Butt Paste: 16% (30 g, 60 g, 120 g, 480 g)
    Critic-Aid Skin Care®: 20% (71 g, 170 g)
Powder, topical (Ammens® Medicated Deodorant): 9.1% (187.5 g, 330 g)

♦ **Zinc Sulfate** *see* Trace Metals *on page 972*

♦ **Zinc Sulfate** *see* Zinc Supplements *on page 1026*

Zinc Supplements *(zink SUP la ments)*

U.S. Brand Names Cold-Eeze® [OTC]; Galzin™; Orazinc® [OTC]; Zincate®

Available Salts Zinc Carbonate; Zinc Chloride; Zinc Gluconate; Zinc Sulfate

Therapeutic Category Mineral, Oral; Mineral, Parenteral

Generic Available Yes

Use Treatment and prevention of zinc deficiency states; may improve wound healing in those who are zinc deficient

Pregnancy Risk Factor C

Contraindications Hypersensitivity to zinc salts or any component

Warnings Do not administer undiluted by direct injection into a peripheral vein due to potential for phlebitis, tissue irritation, and potential increased renal loss of minerals from a bolus injection; administration of zinc in absence of copper may decrease plasma copper levels; excessive intake in healthy persons may be deleterious as decreases in HDL (high-density lipoproteins) and impairment of immune system function have been reported

Adverse Reactions

Cardiovascular: Hypotension, tachycardia (excessive doses)

Central nervous system: Hypothermia (excessive doses)

Gastrointestinal: Indigestion, nausea, vomiting

Hematologic: Neutropenia, leukopenia

Hepatic: Jaundice (excessive doses)

Ophthalmic: Blurred vision (excessive doses)

Respiratory: Pulmonary edema (excessive doses)

Miscellaneous: Profuse diaphoresis

Drug Interactions Zinc may decrease penicillamine, tetracycline, and quinolone absorption; iron decreases zinc absorption; agents which increase gastric pH, such as H_2-blockers, may decrease zinc absorption

Food Interactions Coffee, foods high in phytate (eg, whole grain cereals & legumes), bran, and dairy products reduce zinc absorption; avoid foods high in calcium or phosphorus

Mechanism of Action A cofactor for more than 70 enzymes which are important to carbohydrate and protein metabolism, zinc helps to maintain normal growth and tissue repair, normal skin hydration, and senses of taste and smell

Pharmacokinetics

Absorption: pH dependent; poor from GI tract (20% to 30%); solubilized by conversion to zinc chloride in the presence of gastric acid

Distribution: Storage sites are liver and skeletal muscle; serum levels do not adequately reflect whole-body zinc status

Protein binding: 55% bound to albumin; 40% bound to alpha 1-macroglobulin

Elimination: 90% in feces with only traces appearing in urine and perspiration

Usual Dosage Clinical response may not occur for up to 6-8 weeks

RDA: Oral:

Neonates and Infants <12 months: 5 mg **elemental** zinc/day

Children 1-10 years: 10 mg **elemental** zinc/day

Children ≥11 years and Adults: Male: 15 mg **elemental** zinc/day; Female: 12 mg **elemental** zinc/day

Zinc deficiency: Oral:

Infants and Children: 0.5-1 mg **elemental** zinc/kg/day divided 1-3 times/day; larger doses may be needed if impaired intestinal absorption or an excessive loss of zinc (eg, excessive, prolonged diarrhea)

Adults: 25-50 mg **elemental** zinc/dose (110-220 mg zinc sulfate) 3 times/day

Supplement to parenteral nutrition solutions (clinical response may not occur for up to 6-8 weeks): (See Trace Metals): I.V. (all doses are mcg of **elemental** zinc):

Premature Infants: 400 mcg/kg/day

Term Infants <3 months: 300 mcg/kg/day

Infants ≥3 months and Children ≤5 years: 100 mcg/kg/day (maximum: 5 mg/day)

Children >5 years and Adolescents: 2-5 mg/day

Adults:

Stable metabolically: 2.5-4 mg **elemental** zinc/day; catabolic state: Increase by an additional 2 mg/day (eg, 4.5-6 mg **elemental** zinc/day)

Stable with fluid loss from small bowel: Additional 12.2 mg **elemental** zinc/L parenteral nutrition or 17.1 mg **elemental** zinc/kg of stool or ileostomy output

Wound healing: Oral: Adults: 50 mg **elemental** zinc (220 mg zinc sulfate) 3 times daily in patients with low serum zinc levels (<110 mcg/dL)

Administration

Oral: Administer oral formulation with food if GI upset occurs

Parenteral: Dilute as component of daily parenteral nutrition or maintenance fluids; do not give undiluted by direct injection into a peripheral vein due to potential for phlebitis and tissue irritation, and potential to increase renal losses of minerals from a bolus injection

Monitoring Parameters Patients on parenteral nutrition or chronic therapy should have periodic serum copper and serum zinc levels; alkaline phosphatase, taste

(Continued)

Zinc Supplements *(Continued)*

acuity, mental depression, wound healing (if indicated), growth (if indicated), skin integrity

Reference Range

Serum: 70-130 µg/dL

Patient Information Do not exceed recommended dose

Dosage Forms

Zinc acetate (Galzin™): Capsule: 25 mg, 50 mg

Zinc chloride: Injection: 1 mg elemental zinc/mL (10 mL, 50 mL)

Zinc, elemental:

Lozenges: 10 mg, 15 mg

Cold-Eeze®: 13.3 mg

Tablet: 30 mg, 60 mg

Zinc gluconate (14.3% zinc): Tablet: 15 mg (elemental zinc 2 mg), 50 mg [elemental zinc 7 mg]

Zinc sulfate (23% zinc):

Capsule (Zincate®): 220 mg [elemental zinc 50 mg]

Injection: 1 mg elemental zinc/mL (10 mL); 5 mg elemental zinc/mL (5 mL)

Tablet: 66 mg [elemental zinc 15 mg]

Orazinc®: 110 mg [elemental zinc 25 mg]

Tablet, extended release: 220 mg [elemental zinc 50 mg]

- **Zincundecate** *see* Undecylenic Acid and Derivatives *on page 994*
- **Zinecard**® *see* Dexrazoxane *on page 310*
- **Zithromax**™ *see* Azithromycin *on page 124*
- **Zofran**® *see* Ondansetron *on page 735*
- **Zofran**® **ODT** *see* Ondansetron *on page 735*
- **Zoloft**® *see* Sertraline *on page 898*
- **Zonalon**® *see* Doxepin *on page 358*
- **ZORprin**® *see* Aspirin *on page 109*
- **Zostrix**® **[OTC]** *see* Capsaicin *on page 172*
- **Zostrix**®**-HP [OTC]** *see* Capsaicin *on page 172*
- **Zosyn**™ *see* Piperacillin and Tazobactam *on page 802*
- **Zovirax**® *see* Acyclovir *on page 37*
- **ZVD and 3TC** *see* Lamivudine and Zidovudine *on page 574*
- **Zydone**® *see* Hydrocodone and Acetaminophen *on page 505*
- **Zyflo**™ *see* Zileuton *on page 1024*
- **Zyloprim**® *see* Allopurinol *on page 53*
- **Zymase**® *see* Pancrelipase *on page 755*
- **Zymenol**® **[OTC]** *see* Mineral Oil *on page 675*
- **Zyrtec**® *see* Cetirizine *on page 212*

APPENDIX TABLE OF CONTENTS

APPENDIX TABLE OF CONTENTS

CPR PEDIATRIC DRUG DOSAGES

(PALS Medications for Cardiac Arrest and Symptomatic Arrhythmias)

Drug	Dose	Remarks
Adenosine	0.1 mg/kg	Rapid I.V., I.O. bolus
	Repeat dose: 0.2 mg/kg	Rapid flush to central circulation
	Maximum single dose: 12 mg	Monitor ECG during dose
Amiodarone for pulseless VF/VT	I.V., I.O.: 5 mg/kg	Rapid I.V. bolus
Amiodarone for perfusing tachycardias	Loading dose: I.V., I.O.: 5 mg/kg	I.V. over 20-60 minutes
	Maximum dose: 15 mg/kg/day	Routine use in combination with drugs prolonging QT interval is **not** recommended; hypotension is most frequent side effect
Atropine sulfate*	I.V.: 0.02 mg/kg (minimum dose = 0.1 mg)	May give I.V., I.O., or E.T.
	Maximum single dose (may repeat once): Children: 0.5 mg Adolescents: 1 mg	Tachycardia and pupil dilation may occur but **not** fixed dilated pupils
Calcium chloride 10% = 100 mg/mL (=27.2 mg/mL elemental Ca)	I.V., I.O.: 20 mg/kg (0.2 mL/kg)	Give slow I.V. push for hypocalcemia, hypermagnesemia, calcium channel blocker toxicity, preferably via central vein; monitor heart rate - bradycardia may occur
Calcium gluconate 10% = 100 mg/mL (=9 mg/mL elemental Ca)	I.V., I.O.: 60-100 mg/kg (0.6-1 mL/kg)	Give slow I.V. push for hypocalcemia, hypermagnesemia, calcium channel blocker toxicity, preferably via central vein
Epinephrine for symptomatic bradycardia*	I.V., I.O.: 0.01 mg/kg (1:10,000; 0.1 mL/kg) E.T.: 0.1 mg/kg (1:1000; 0.1 mL/kg)	Tachyarrhythmias, hypertension may occur
Epinephrine for pulseless arrest*	First dose: I.V., I.O.: 0.01 mg/kg (1:10,000; 0.1 mL/kg) E.T.: 0.1 mg/kg (1:1000; 0.1 mL/kg) Subsequent doses: Repeat initial dose or may increase up to 10 times (0.1 mg/kg, 1:1000, 0.1 mL/kg) Administer epinephrine every 3-5 minutes I.V., I.O., E.T. doses as high as 0.2 mg/kg of 1:1000 may be effective	
Epinephrine for **neonatal** resuscitation	I.V., E.T.: 0.01-0.03 mg/kg (1:10,000; 0.1-0.3 mL/kg) Repeat every 3-5 minutes as indicated	Data in neonates is not sufficient to recommend higher doses for E.T. route; I.O. route not commonly used in the newly born (umbilical vein is more accessible, smaller bones are fragile, I.O. space is small in premature infants), but may be used in neonate and older infant.
Glucose (10%, 25%, or 50%)	I.V., I.O.: 0.5-1 g/kg • 1-2 mL/kg 50% • 2-4 mL/kg 25% • 5-10 mL/kg 10%	For suspected hypoglycemia; avoid hyperglycemia
Lidocaine*	I.V., I.O., E.T.: 1 mg/kg	Rapid bolus
Lidocaine infusion	I.V., I.O. (start after a bolus): 20-50 mcg/kg/min	1-2.5 mL/kg/hour of 120 mg/100 mL solution or use "Rule of 6"

CPR PEDIATRIC DRUG DOSAGES (Continued)

Drug	Dose	Remarks
Magnesium sulfate (500 mg/mL)	I.V., I.O.: 25-50 mg/kg Maximum dose: 2 g/dose	Rapid I.V. infusion for torsades or suspected hypomagnesemia; 10- to 20-minute infusion for asthma that responds poorly to beta-adrenergic agonists
Naloxone*	≤5 years or ≤20 kg: 0.1 mg/kg >5 years or >20 kg: 2 mg	For total reversal of narcotic effect. Use small repeated doses (0.01-0.03 mg/kg) titrated to desired effect
Procainamide for perfusing tachycardias (100 mg/mL and 500 mg/mL)	Loading dose: I.V., I.O.: 15 mg/kg	Infusion over 30-60 minutes; routine use in combination with drugs prolonging QT interval is **not** recommended
Sodium bicarbonate (1 mEq/mL and 0.5 mEq/mL)	I.V., I.O.: 1 mEq/kg/dose	Infuse slowly and only if ventilation is adequate

I.V. = intravenous; I.O. = intraosseous; E.T. = endotracheal

*For endotracheal administration, use higher doses (2-10 times the I.V. dose); dilute medication with NS to a volume of 3-5 mL and follow with several positive-pressure ventilations.

Adapted with permission of Lippincott Williams & Wilkins, "Guidelines 2000 for Cardiopulmonary Resuscitation and Emergency Cardiovascular Care. Part 10: Pediatric Advanced Life Support. The American Heart Association in Collaboration With the International Liaison Committee on Resuscitation," *Circulation*, 2000, 102(8 Suppl):I308.

EMERGENCY PEDIATRIC DRIP CALCULATIONS

Drips

Drug	Dose	Calculation*	Rate & Dose
Dobutamine	5-20 mcg/kg/min	6 x body wt (kg) is the mg added to make 100 mL	1 mL/h = 1 mcg/kg/min
Dopamine	2-20 mcg/kg/min	6 x body wt (kg) is the mg added to make 100 mL	1 mL/h = 1 mcg/kg/min
Epinephrine	0.1-1 mcg/kg/min	0.6 x body wt (kg) is the mg added to make 100 mL	1 mL/h = 0.1 mcg/kg/min
Isoproterenol	0.1-1 mcg/kg/min	0.6 x body wt (kg) is the mg added to make 100 mL	1 mL/h = 0.1 mcg/kg/min
Lidocaine	20-50 mcg/kg/min	120 mg in 100 mL of D_5W	1 mL/kg/h = 20 mcg/kg/min

Note: Patients ≥40 kg and those requiring fluid restriction may need more concentrated solutions in order to deliver less fluid per hour. In those cases, or as an alternative to the listed calculations above, use the following equation:

$$\text{Rate (mL/h)} = \frac{\text{dose (mcg/kg/min)} \times \text{weight (kg)} \times 60 \text{ min/h}}{\text{concentration (mcg/mL)}}$$

NEONATAL RESUSCITATION ALGORITHM

Algorithm for Resuscitation of the Newly Born Infant

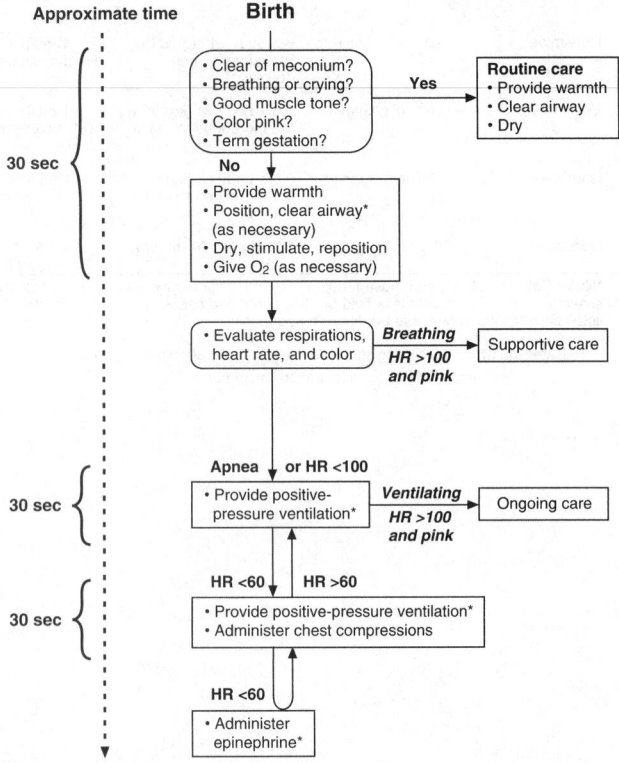

*Endotracheal intubation may be considered at several steps.

Epinephrine dose for neonatal resuscitation: I.V., E.T.: 0.01-0.03 mg/kg (1:10,000; 0.1-0.3 mL/kg). Repeat every 3-5 minutes as indicated. Data in neonates is not sufficient to recommend higher doses for E.T. route; I.O. route not commonly used in the newly born (umbilical vein is more accessible, smaller bones are fragile, I.O. space is small in premature infants), but may be used in neonate and older infant.

Adapted with permission of Lippincott Williams & Wilkins, "Guidelines 2000 for Cardiopulmonary Resuscitation and Emergency Cardiovascular Care, Part 11: Neonatal Resuscitation, the American Heart Association in Collaboration With the International Liaison Comittee in Resuscitation," *Circulation*, 2000, 102(8 Suppl):I349.

PEDIATRIC ALS ALGORITHMS

PALS Bradycardia Algorithm

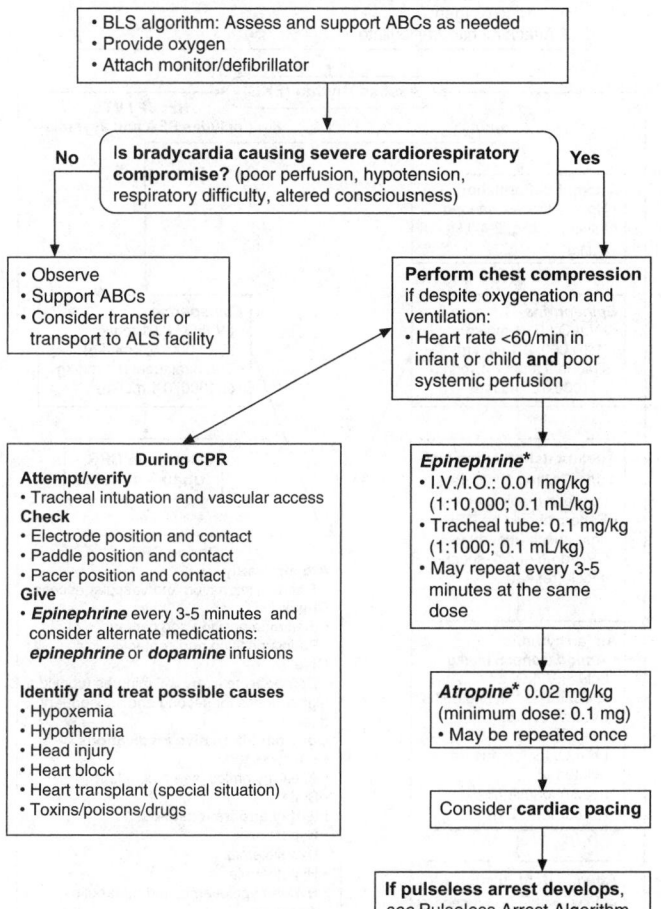

* BLS algorithm: Assess and support ABCs as needed
* Provide oxygen
* Attach monitor/defibrillator

No ⟵ Is bradycardia causing severe cardiorespiratory compromise? (poor perfusion, hypotension, respiratory difficulty, altered consciousness) ⟶ **Yes**

* Observe
* Support ABCs
* Consider transfer or transport to ALS facility

Perform chest compression if despite oxygenation and ventilation:
* Heart rate <60/min in infant or child **and** poor systemic perfusion

During CPR
Attempt/verify
* Tracheal intubation and vascular access
Check
* Electrode position and contact
* Paddle position and contact
* Pacer position and contact
Give
* *Epinephrine* every 3-5 minutes and consider alternate medications: *epinephrine* or *dopamine* infusions

Identify and treat possible causes
* Hypoxemia
* Hypothermia
* Head injury
* Heart block
* Heart transplant (special situation)
* Toxins/poisons/drugs

*Epinephrine**
* I.V./I.O.: 0.01 mg/kg (1:10,000; 0.1 mL/kg)
* Tracheal tube: 0.1 mg/kg (1:1000; 0.1 mL/kg)
* May repeat every 3-5 minutes at the same dose

*Atropine** 0.02 mg/kg (minimum dose: 0.1 mg)
* May be repeated once

Consider **cardiac pacing**

If pulseless arrest develops, *see* Pulseless Arrest Algorithm

*Give atropine first for bradycardia due to suspected increased vagal tone or primary AV block.

Adapted with permission of Lippincott Williams & Wilkins, "Guidelines 2000 for Cardio-pulmonary Resuscitation and Emergency Cardiovascular Care, Part 10: Pediatric Advanced Life Support, The American Heart Association in Collaboration With the International Liaison Committee on Resuscitation," *Circulation*, 2000, 102(8 Suppl):I313.

PEDIATRIC ALS ALGORITHMS *(Continued)*

PALS Pulseless Arrest Algorithm

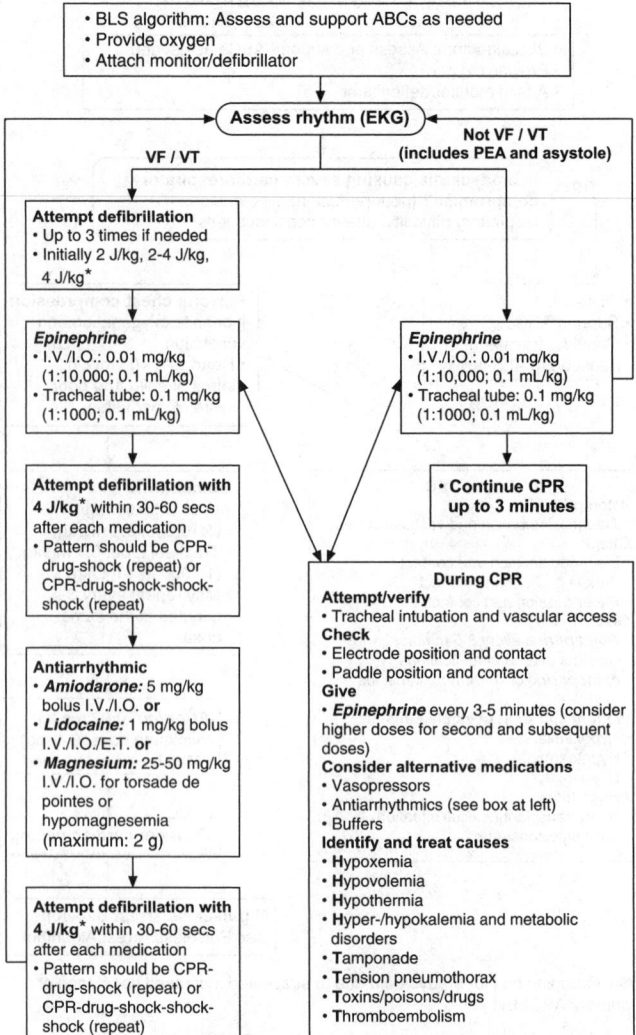

*Alternative waveforms and higher doses are Class Indeterminate for children.

Adapted with permission of Lippincott Williams & Wilkins, "Guidelines 2000 for Cardiopulmonary Resuscitation and Emergency Cardiovascular Care, Part 10: Pediatric Advanced Life Support, The American Heart Association in Collaboration With the International Liaison Committee on Resuscitation," *Circulation*, 2000, 102(8 Suppl):I311.

PALS Tachycardia Algorithm
for Infants and Children With Rapid Rhythm and
Adequate Perfusion

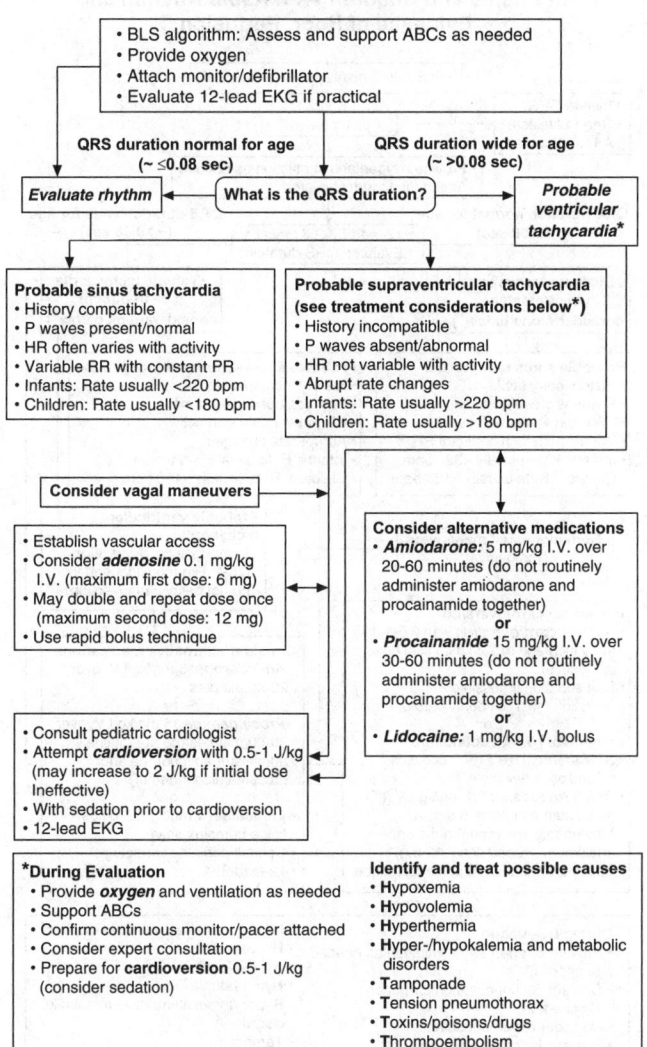

- BLS algorithm: Assess and support ABCs as needed
- Provide oxygen
- Attach monitor/defibrillator
- Evaluate 12-lead EKG if practical

QRS duration normal for age
(~ ≤0.08 sec)

QRS duration wide for age
(~ >0.08 sec)

Evaluate rhythm

What is the QRS duration?

Probable ventricular tachycardia*

Probable sinus tachycardia
- History compatible
- P waves present/normal
- HR often varies with activity
- Variable RR with constant PR
- Infants: Rate usually <220 bpm
- Children: Rate usually <180 bpm

Probable supraventricular tachycardia
(see treatment considerations below*)
- History incompatible
- P waves absent/abnormal
- HR not variable with activity
- Abrupt rate changes
- Infants: Rate usually >220 bpm
- Children: Rate usually >180 bpm

Consider vagal maneuvers

- Establish vascular access
- Consider *adenosine* 0.1 mg/kg I.V. (maximum first dose: 6 mg)
- May double and repeat dose once (maximum second dose: 12 mg)
- Use rapid bolus technique

Consider alternative medications
- *Amiodarone:* 5 mg/kg I.V. over 20-60 minutes (do not routinely administer amiodarone and procainamide together)

  or
- *Procainamide* 15 mg/kg I.V. over 30-60 minutes (do not routinely administer amiodarone and procainamide together)

  or
- *Lidocaine:* 1 mg/kg I.V. bolus

- Consult pediatric cardiologist
- Attempt *cardioversion* with 0.5-1 J/kg (may increase to 2 J/kg if initial dose ineffective)
- With sedation prior to cardioversion
- 12-lead EKG

*During Evaluation
- Provide *oxygen* and ventilation as needed
- Support ABCs
- Confirm continuous monitor/pacer attached
- Consider expert consultation
- Prepare for *cardioversion* 0.5-1 J/kg (consider sedation)

Identify and treat possible causes
- Hypoxemia
- Hypovolemia
- Hyperthermia
- Hyper-/hypokalemia and metabolic disorders
- Tamponade
- Tension pneumothorax
- Toxins/poisons/drugs
- Thromboembolism
- Pain

Adapted with permission of Lippincott Williams & Wilkins, "Guidelines 2000 for Cardiopulmonary Resuscitation and Emergency Cardiovascular Care, Part 10: Pediatric Advanced Life Support, The American Heart Association in Collaboration With the International Liaison Committee on Resuscitation," *Circulation*, 2000, 102(8 Suppl):I315.

PEDIATRIC ALS ALGORITHMS *(Continued)*

PALS Tachycardia Algorithm
for Infants and Children With Rapid Rhythm and
Evidence of Poor Perfusion

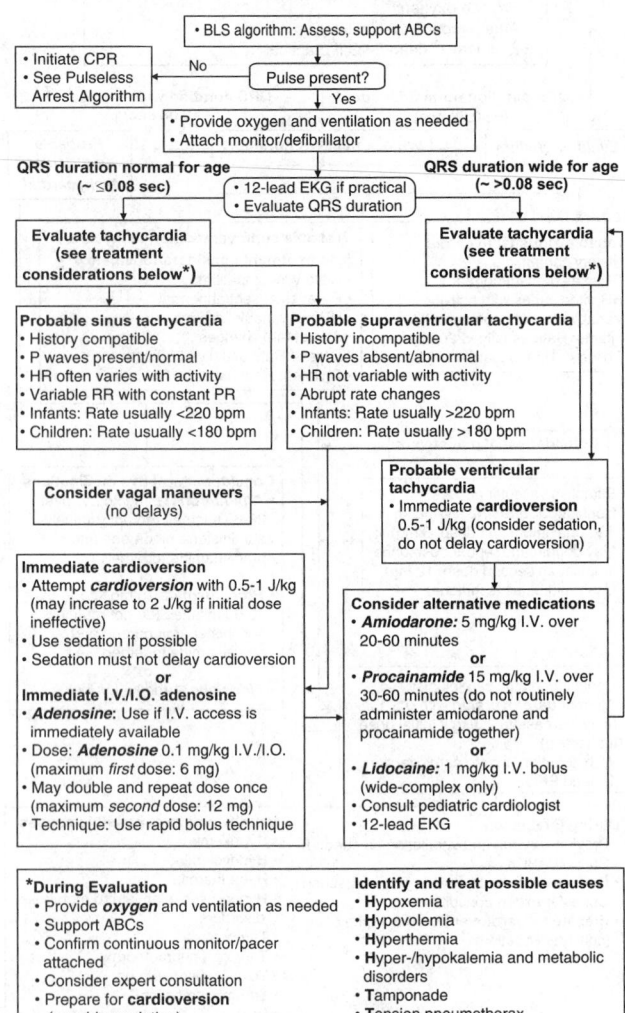

Adapted with permission of Lippincott Williams & Wilkins, "Guidelines 2000 for Cardiopulmonar Resuscitation and Emergency Cardiovascular Care, Part 10: Pediatric Advanced Life Support, The American Heart Association in Collaboration With the International Liaison Committee on Resuscitation," *Circulation*, 2000, 102(8 Suppl):I316.

ADULT ACLS ALGORITHMS

ILCOR Universal / International ACLS Algorithm

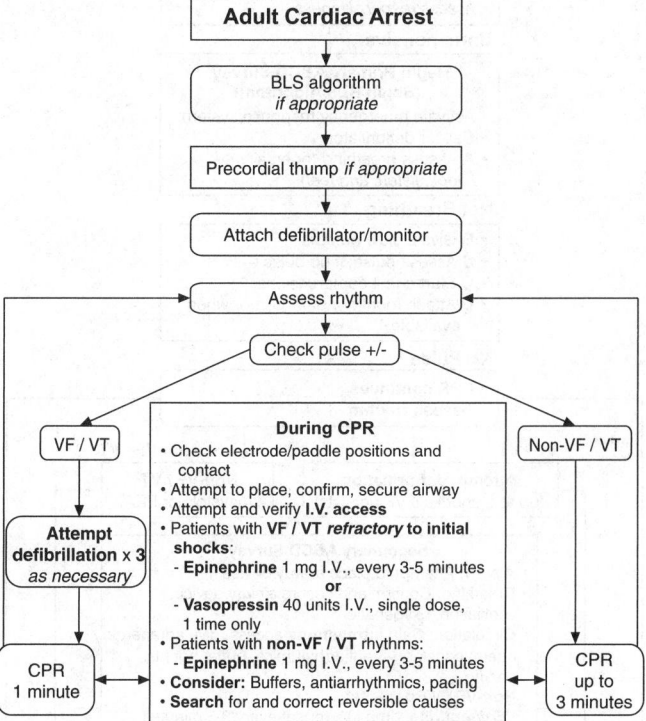

Adult Cardiac Arrest

↓

BLS algorithm
if appropriate

↓

Precordial thump *if appropriate*

↓

Attach defibrillator/monitor

↓

Assess rhythm

↓

Check pulse +/-

VF / VT

↓

Attempt defibrillation × **3**
as necessary

↓

CPR
1 minute

During CPR
- Check electrode/paddle positions and contact
- Attempt to place, confirm, secure airway
- Attempt and verify **I.V.** access
- Patients with **VF / VT** *refractory* to initial **shocks**:
  - **Epinephrine** 1 mg I.V., every 3-5 minutes
    or
  - **Vasopressin** 40 units I.V., single dose, 1 time only
- Patients with **non-VF / VT** rhythms:
  - **Epinephrine** 1 mg I.V., every 3-5 minutes
- **Consider:** Buffers, antiarrhythmics, pacing
- **Search** for and correct reversible causes

Non-VF / VT

↓

CPR
up to
3 minutes

Consider causes that are potentially reversible

- **H**ypovolemia
- **H**ypoxia
- **H**ydrogen ion - acidosis
- **H**yper-/hypokalemia, other metabolic
- **H**ypothermia

- "**T**ablets" (drug OD, accidents)
- **T**amponade, cardiac (pericardiocentesis)
- **T**ension pneumothorax (decompress)
- **T**hrombosis, coronary (ACS); (fibrinolytics)
- **T**hrombosis, pulmonary (embolism, fibrinolytics, surgical evacuation)

Adapted with permission of Lippincott Williams & Wilkins, "Guidelines 2000 for Cardiopulmonary Resuscitation and Emergency Cardiovascular Care, Part 6: Advanced Cardiovascular Life Support, The American Heart Association in Collaboration With the International Liaison Committee on Resuscitation," *Circulation*, 2000, 102(8 Suppl):I143.

ADULT ACLS ALGORITHMS *(Continued)*

Comprehensive ECC Algorithm

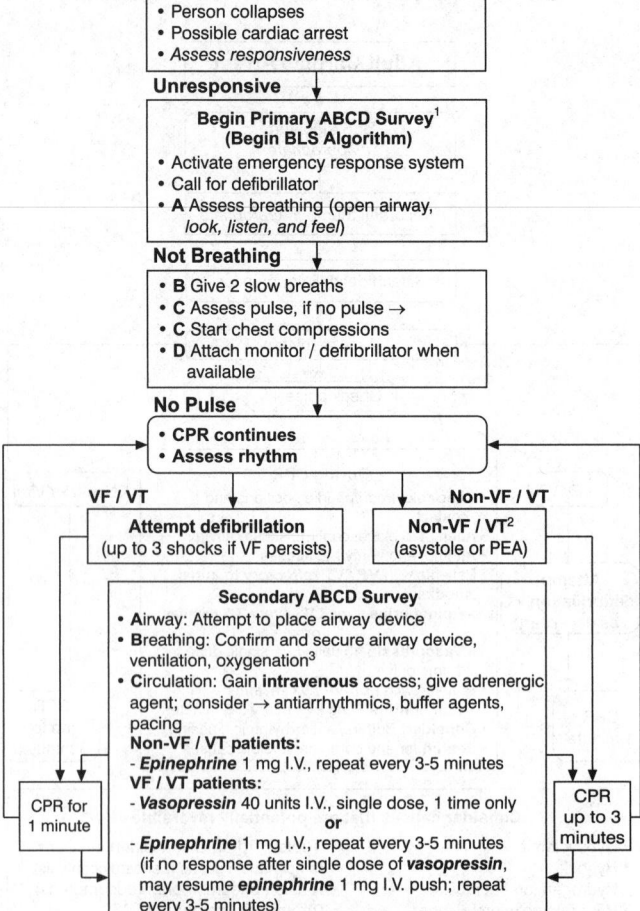

- Person collapses
- Possible cardiac arrest
- *Assess responsiveness*

Unresponsive

Begin Primary ABCD Survey[1]
(Begin BLS Algorithm)
- Activate emergency response system
- Call for defibrillator
- **A** Assess breathing (open airway, *look, listen, and feel*)

Not Breathing

- **B** Give 2 slow breaths
- **C** Assess pulse, if no pulse →
- **C** Start chest compressions
- **D** Attach monitor / defibrillator when available

No Pulse

- CPR continues
- Assess rhythm

VF / VT

Attempt defibrillation
(up to 3 shocks if VF persists)

Non-VF / VT

Non-VF / VT[2]
(asystole or PEA)

Secondary ABCD Survey
- Airway: Attempt to place airway device
- Breathing: Confirm and secure airway device, ventilation, oxygenation[3]
- Circulation: Gain **intravenous** access; give adrenergic agent; consider → antiarrhythmics, buffer agents, pacing
  Non-VF / VT patients:
  - *Epinephrine* 1 mg I.V., repeat every 3-5 minutes
  VF / VT patients:
  - *Vasopressin* 40 units I.V., single dose, 1 time only
    or
  - *Epinephrine* 1 mg I.V., repeat every 3-5 minutes (if no response after single dose of *vasopressin*, may resume *epinephrine* 1 mg I.V. push; repeat every 3-5 minutes)
- **D**ifferential **D**iagnosis: Search for and treat reversible causes[4]

CPR for 1 minute

CPR up to 3 minutes

[1]Do not attempt resuscitation if any objective indicators of DNAR status or clinical indicators that resuscitation attempts are not indicated (eg, signs of death).
[2]Recommendation is to consider non-VF / VT rhythms as one rthythm when the patient is in cardiac arrest.
[3]Use 2 methods to confirm tube placement: Primary physical examination criteria plus a secondary device (qualitative and quantitative measures of end-tidal CO_2).
[4]Reversible causes: See ILCOR Universal / International ACLS Algorithm.

Adapted with permission of Lippincott Williams & Wilkins, "Guidelines 2000 for Cardiopulmonary Resuscitation and Emergency Cardiovascular Care, Part 6: Advanced Cardiovascular Life Support, The American Heart Association in Collaboration With the International Liaison Committee on Resuscitation," *Circulation*, 2000, 102(8 Suppl):I144.

Ventricular Fibrillation / Pulseless VT Algorithm

Primary ABCD Survey[1]
Focus: Basic CPR and defibrillation

- **Check** responsiveness
- **Activate** emergency response system
- **Call** for defibrillator

A Airway: Open the airway
B Breathing: Provide positive-pressure ventilations
C Circulation: Give chest compressions
D Defibrillation: Assess for and shock VF / pulseless VT, up to 3 times
(200 J, 200-300 J, 360 J, or equivalent *biphasic*) if necessary

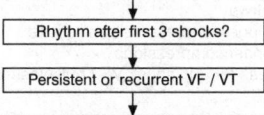

Rhythm after first 3 shocks?

Persistent or recurrent VF / VT

Secondary ABCD Survey
Focus: More advanced assessments and treatments

A Airway: Place airway device as soon as possible
B Breathing: Confirm airway device placement by exam plus confirmation device[2]
B Breathing: Secure airway device; purpose-made tube holders preferred[3]
B Breathing: Confirm effective oxygenation and ventilation[4]
C Circulation: Establish I.V. access
C Circulation: Identify rhythm → monitor
C Circulation: Administer drugs appropriate for rhythm and condition
D Differential Diagnosis: Search for and treat identified reversible causes

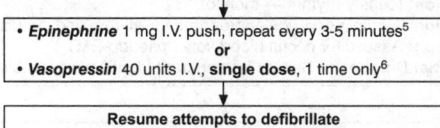

- *Epinephrine* 1 mg I.V. push, repeat every 3-5 minutes[5]
or
- *Vasopressin* 40 units I.V., **single dose**, 1 time only[6]

Resume attempts to defibrillate
1 x 360 J (or equivalent *biphasic*) within 30-60 seconds

Consider antiarrhythmics:[7]
Amiodarone (IIb): 300 mg I.V. push. If VF/pulseless VT recurs, consider a second dose of 150 mg (maximum cumulative dose: 2.2 g over 24 hours)
Lidocaine (indeterminate): 1-1.5 mg/kg I.V. push. Consider repeat in 3-5 minutes to maximum cumulative dose of 3 mg/kg
Magnesium sulfate (IIb if hypomagnesemic state): 1-2 g I.V. in polymorphic VT (torsade de pointes) and suspected hypomagnesemic state
Procainamide (IIb for intermittent/recurrent VF / VT): 30 mg/min in refractory VF (maximum total dose: 17 mg/kg) - acceptable but not recommended due to prolonged administration time
Consider buffers

Resume attempts to defibrillate

[1]Do not attempt resuscitation if any objective indicators of DNAR status or clinical indicators that resuscitation attempts are not indicated (eg, signs of death).
[2]Consider continuous qualitative end-tidal CO_2 monitor (Class IIa - acceptable, probably effective).
[3]Commercial purpose-made tracheal tube holders recommended (Class IIb - acceptable, possibly effective).
[4]End-tidal CO_2 monitor and oxygen saturation monitor.
[5]If this fails, higher doses of epinephrine (up to 0.2 mg/kg) are acceptable (growing evidence of potential harm).
[6]No evidence about value of repeat vasopressin doses.
[7]Numbers in parentheses represent strength of recommendation (Class IIb - acceptable, possibly effective).

Adapted with permission of Lippincott Williams & Wilkins, "Guidelines 2000 for Cardiopulmonary Resuscitation and Emergency Cardiovascular Care, Part 6: Advanced Cardiovascular Life Support, The American Heart Association in Collaboration With the International Liaison Committee on Resuscitation," *Circulation*, 2000, 102(8 Suppl):I147.

ADULT ACLS ALGORITHMS *(Continued)*

Pulseless Electrical Activity Algorithm

(PEA = rhythm on monitor, without detectable pulse)

Primary ABCD Survey[1]
Focus: *Basic CPR and defibrillation*

- **Check** responsiveness
- **Activate** emergency response system
- **Call** for defibrillator

A Airway: Open the airway
B Breathing: Provide positive-pressure ventilations
C Circulation: Give chest compressions
D Defibrillation: Assess for and shock VF / pulseless VT

Secondary ABCD Survey
Focus: *More advanced assessments and treatments*

A Airway: Place airway device as soon as possible
B Breathing: Confirm airway device placement by exam plus confirmation device[2]
B Breathing: Secure airway device; purpose-made tube holders preferred[3]
B Breathing: Confirm effective oxygenation and ventilation[4]
C Circulation: Establish I.V. access
C Circulation: Identify rhythm → monitor
C Circulation: Administer drugs appropriate for rhythm and condition
C Circulation: Assess for occult blood flow ("pseudo-EMT")
D Differential Diagnosis: Search for and treat identified reversible causes

---

Review for most frequent causes[5]

- Hypovolemia
- Hypoxia
- Hydrogen ion - acidosis
- Hyper-/hypokalemia
- Hypothermia

- "Tablets" (drug OD, accidents)
- Tamponade, cardiac
- Tension pneumothorax
- Thrombosis, coronary (ACS)
- Thrombosis, pulmonary (embolism)

- ***Epinephrine*** 1 mg I.V. push, repeat every 3-5 minutes[6]

- ***Atropine*** 1 mg I.V. (if PEA rate is **slow**), repeat every 3-5 minutes as needed, to a total dose of 0.04 mg/kg

---

[1]Do not attempt resuscitation if any objective indicators of DNAR status or clinical indicators that resuscitation attempts are not indicated (eg, signs of death).

[2]Consider continuous qualitative end-tidal CO_2 monitor (Class IIa - acceptable, probably effective).

[3]Commercial purpose-made tracheal tube holders recommended (Class IIb - acceptable, possibly effective).

[4]End-tidal CO_2 monitor and oxygen saturation monitor.

[5]Sodium bicarbonate 1 mEq/kg recommended in the following:

Class I: If patient has known, preexisting hyperkalemia

Class IIa: Known, preexisting bicarbonate-responsive acidosis, in tricyclic antidepressant overdose, or to alkalinize the urine in aspirin or other drug overdoses

Class IIb: In intubated and ventilated patients with long arrest interval, or on return of circulation after a long arrest interval

Note: Ineffective or harmful in hypercarbic acidosis (Class III)

[6]If this fails, higher doses of epinephrine (up to 0.2 mg/kg) are acceptable (growing evidence of potential harm).

Adapted with permission of Lippincott Williams & Wilkins, "Guidelines 2000 for Cardiopulmonary Resuscitation and Emergency Cardiovascular Care, Part 6: Advanced Cardiovascular Life Support, The American Heart Association in Collaboration With the International Liaison Committee on Resuscitation," *Circulation*, 2000, 102(8 Suppl):I151.

Asystole: The Silent Heart Algorithm

Primary ABCD Survey[1]
Focus: *Basic CPR and defibrillation*

- **Check** responsiveness
- **Activate** emergency response system
- **Call** for defibrillator

A Airway: Open the airway
B Breathing: Provide positive-pressure ventilations
C Circulation: Give chest compressions
C Confirm true asystole
D Defibrillation: Assess for VF / pulseless VT; shock if indicated

Rapid scene survey: Any evidence personnel should **not** attempt resuscitation?

Secondary ABCD Survey[2,3]
Focus: *More advanced assessments and treatments*

A Airway: Place airway device as soon as possible
B Breathing: Confirm airway device placement by exam plus confirmation device
B Breathing: Secure airway device; purpose-made tube holders preferred[4]
B Breathing: Confirm effective oxygenation and ventilation[5]
C Circulation: Confirm true asystole
C Circulation: Establish I.V. access
C Circulation: Identify rhythm → monitor
C Circulation: Administer drugs appropriate for rhythm and condition
C Circulation: Give medications appropriate for rhythm and condition
D Differential Diagnosis: Search for and treat identified reversible causes

---

Transcutaneous pacing
If considered, perform immediately

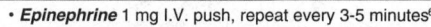

- ***Epinephrine*** 1 mg I.V. push, repeat every 3-5 minutes[6]

- ***Atropine*** 1 mg I.V., repeat every 3-5 minutes up to a total of 0.04 mg/kg

---

Asystole persists
Withhold or cease resuscitation efforts?

- Consider quality of resuscitation?
- Atypical clinical features present?
- Support for cease-efforts protocols in place?

---

[1]Do not attempt resuscitation if any objective indicators of DNAR status or clinical indicators that resuscitation attempts are not indicated (eg, signs of death).
[2]Confirm true asystole.
[3]Sodium bicarbonate 1 mEq/kg indicated for patients with tracheal intubation plus long arrest intervals, on return of spontaneous circulation if long arrest interval, tricyclic antidepressant overdose, to alkalinize urine (eg, ASA overdose). **Note:** Ineffective or harmful in hypercarbic acidosis.
[4]Commercial purpose-made tracheal tube holders recommended (Class IIb - acceptable, possibly effective).
[5]End-tidal CO_2 monitor and oxygen saturation monitor
[6]If this fails, higher doses of epinephrine (up to 0.2 mg/kg) are acceptable (growing evidence of potential harm).

Adapted with permission of Lippincott Williams & Wilkins, "Guidelines 2000 for Cardiopulmonary Resuscitation and Emergency Cardiovascular Care, Part 6: Advanced Cardiovascular Life Support, The American Heart Association in Collaboration With the International Liaison Committee on Resuscitation," *Circulation*, 2000, 102(8 Suppl):I153.

ADULT ACLS ALGORITHMS *(Continued)*

Bradycardia Algorithm

Bradycardia
- **Slow** (absolute bradycardia = rate <60 bpm)
  or
- **Relatively slow** (rate less than expected relative to underlying condition or cause)

Primary ABCD Survey
- Assess ABCs
- Secure airway noninvasively
- Ensure monitor / defibrillator is available

Secondary ABCD Survey
- Assess secondary ABCs (invasive airway management needed?)
- Oxygen - I.V. access - monitor - fluids
- Vital signs, pulse oximeter, monitor BP
- Obtain and review 12-lead EKG
- Obtain and review portable chest x-ray
- Problem-focused history
- Problem-focused physical examination
- Consider causes (differential diagnoses)

Serious signs or symptoms?[1]
Due to the bradycardia?

No → Type II second-degree AV block[2]
or
Third-degree AV block?

Yes → **Intervention sequence[3]**
- *Atropine* 0.5-1 mg[4]
- *Transcutaneous pacing* if available
- *Dopamine* 5-20 mcg/kg/min
- *Epinephrine* 2-10 mcg/min

No → Observe

Yes →
- Prepare for transvenous pacer[5]
- If symptoms develop, use transcutaneous pacemaker until transvenous pacer placed

[1]Signs/symptoms must be attributable to slow rate. Manifestations include chest pain, shortness of breath, decreased LOC, hypotension, shock, CHF, pulmonary congestion.
[2]Never treat combination of third-degree heart block and ventricular escape beats with lidocaine (or any agent which suppresses ventricular escape rhythms).
[3]Do not delay transcutaneous pacing in symptomatic patients while waiting for I.V. access or for atropine to take effect; denervated transplanted hearts will not respond to atropine - go directly to catecholamine infusion or pacing.
[4]Atropine should be repeated every 3-5 minutes up to 0.03-0.04 mg/kg total dose; use every 3 minutes in severe clinical conditions.
[5]Verify patient tolerance and mechanical capture. Use analgesia and sedation as needed.

Adapted with permission of Lippincott Williams & Wilkins, "Guidelines 2000 for Cardiopulmonary Resuscitation and Emergency Cardiovascular Care, Part 6: Advanced Cardiovascular Life Support, The American Heart Association in Collaboration With the International Liaison Committee on Resuscitation," *Circulation*, 2000, 102(8 Suppl):I156.

Tachycardia Overview Algorithm

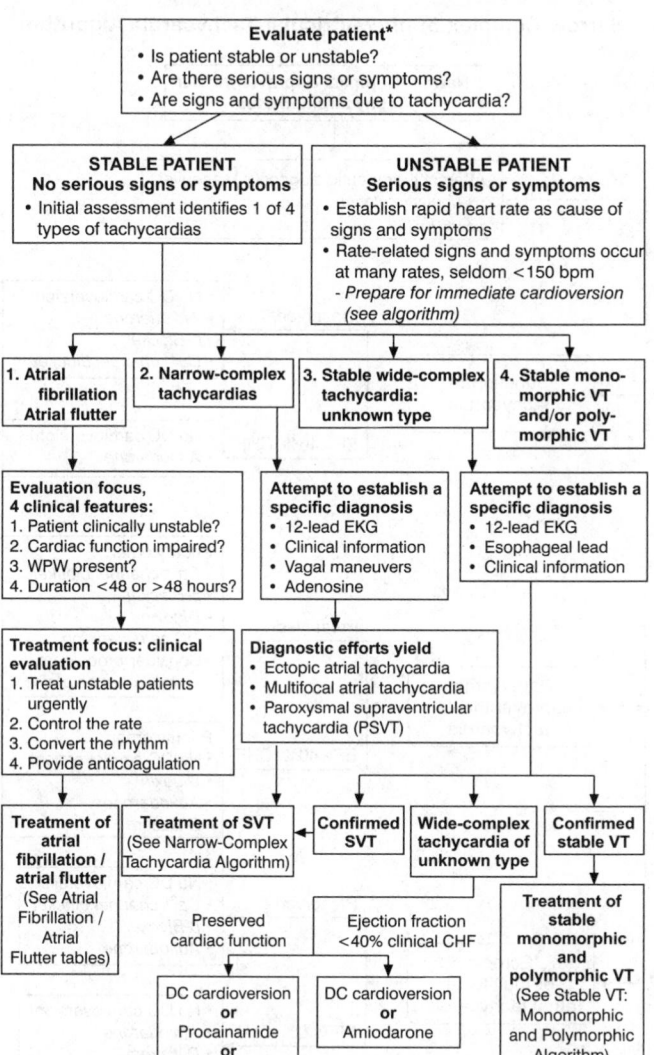

Evaluate patient*
- Is patient stable or unstable?
- Are there serious signs or symptoms?
- Are signs and symptoms due to tachycardia?

STABLE PATIENT
No serious signs or symptoms
- Initial assessment identifies 1 of 4 types of tachycardias

UNSTABLE PATIENT
Serious signs or symptoms
- Establish rapid heart rate as cause of signs and symptoms
- Rate-related signs and symptoms occur at many rates, seldom <150 bpm
  - *Prepare for immediate cardioversion (see algorithm)*

1. Atrial fibrillation Atrial flutter

2. Narrow-complex tachycardias

3. Stable wide-complex tachycardia: unknown type

4. Stable monomorphic VT and/or polymorphic VT

Evaluation focus, 4 clinical features:
1. Patient clinically unstable?
2. Cardiac function impaired?
3. WPW present?
4. Duration <48 or >48 hours?

Attempt to establish a specific diagnosis
- 12-lead EKG
- Clinical information
- Vagal maneuvers
- Adenosine

Attempt to establish a specific diagnosis
- 12-lead EKG
- Esophageal lead
- Clinical information

Treatment focus: clinical evaluation
1. Treat unstable patients urgently
2. Control the rate
3. Convert the rhythm
4. Provide anticoagulation

Diagnostic efforts yield
- Ectopic atrial tachycardia
- Multifocal atrial tachycardia
- Paroxysmal supraventricular tachycardia (PSVT)

Treatment of atrial fibrillation / atrial flutter (See Atrial Fibrillation / Atrial Flutter tables)

Treatment of SVT (See Narrow-Complex Tachycardia Algorithm)

Confirmed SVT

Wide-complex tachycardia of unknown type

Confirmed stable VT

Treatment of stable monomorphic and polymorphic VT (See Stable VT: Monomorphic and Polymorphic Algorithm)

Preserved cardiac function

Ejection fraction <40% clinical CHF

DC cardioversion or Procainamide or Amiodarone

DC cardioversion or Amiodarone

*Unstable condition must be related to the tachycardia. Signs and symptoms may include chest pain, shortness of breath, decreased LOC, hypotension, shock, pulmonary congestion, CHF, and AMI.

Adapted with permission of Lippincott Williams & Wilkins, "Guidelines 2000 for Cardiopulmonary Resuscitation and Emergency Cardiovascular Care, Part 6: Advanced Cardiovascular Life Support, The American Heart Association in Collaboration With the International Liaison Committee on Resuscitation," *Circulation*, 2000, 102(8 Suppl):I159.

ADULT ACLS ALGORITHMS *(Continued)*

Narrow-Complex Supraventricular Tachycardia Algorithm

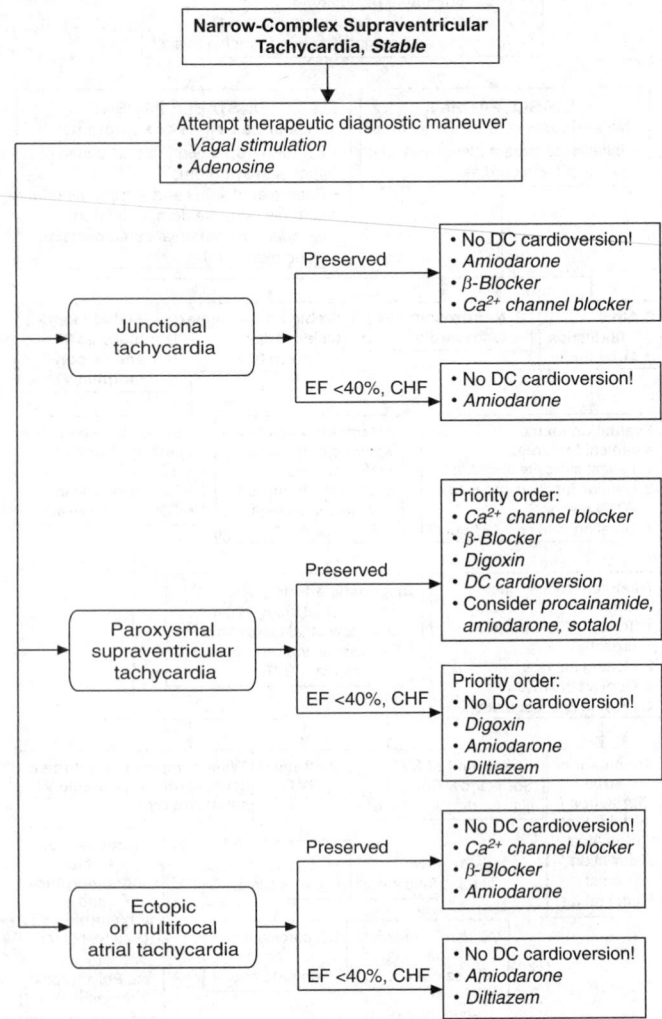

Adapted with permission of Lippincott Williams & Wilkins, "Guidelines 2000 for Cardiopulmonary Resuscitation and Emergency Cardiovascular Care, Part 6: Advanced Cardiovascular Life Support, The American Heart Association in Collaboration With the International Liaison Committee on Resuscitation," *Circulation*, 2000, 102(8 Suppl):I162.

Stable Ventricular Tachycardia
(Monomorphic or Polymorphic) Algorithm

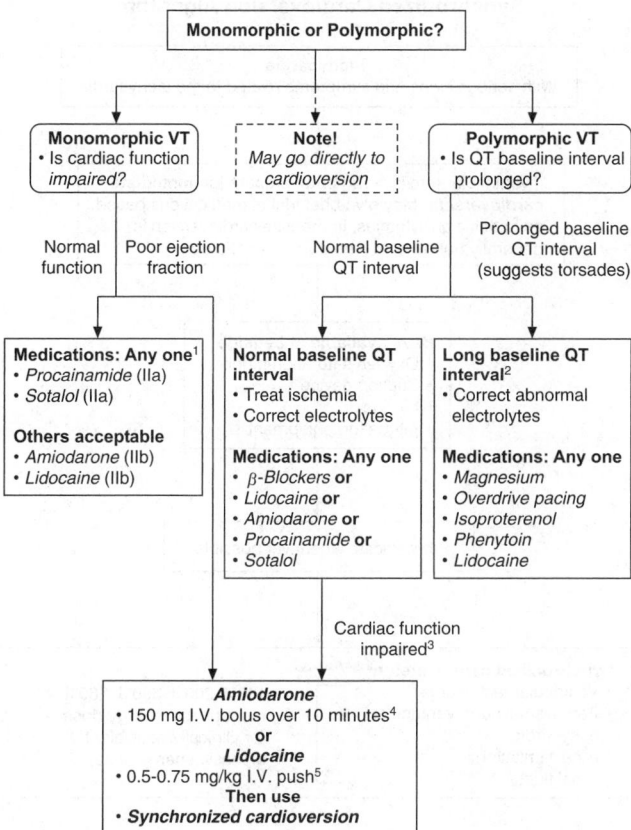

[1]Use just one agent at a time. **Note:** Numbers in parentheses represent strength of recommendation, not antiarrhythmic classification.

[2]Stop/avoid treatments which prolong QT. Identify and treat any electrolyte abnormalities.

[3]Clinical signs suggestive of impaired LV function (EF <40% or CHF).

[4]Repeat 150 mg I.V. over 10 minutes every 10-15 minutes as needed. Alternative infusion: 360 mg over 6 hours, then 540 mg over the remaining 18 hours. Maximum total dose: 2.2 g in 24 hours.

[5]Repeat every 5-10 minutes, then infuse 1-4 mg/min. Maximum total dose: 3 mg/kg (or 300 mg) over 1 hour.

Note: Class IIa recommendation: Acceptable, probably effective;
Class IIb: Acceptable, possibly effective.

Adapted with permission of Lippincott Williams & Wilkins, "Guidelines 2000 for Cardiopulmonary Resuscitation and Emergency Cardiovascular Care, Part 6: Advanced Cardiovascular Life Support, The American Heart Association in Collaboration With the International Liaison Committee on Resuscitation," *Circulation*, 2000, 102(8 Suppl):I163.

ADULT ACLS ALGORITHMS *(Continued)*

Synchronized Cardioversion Algorithm

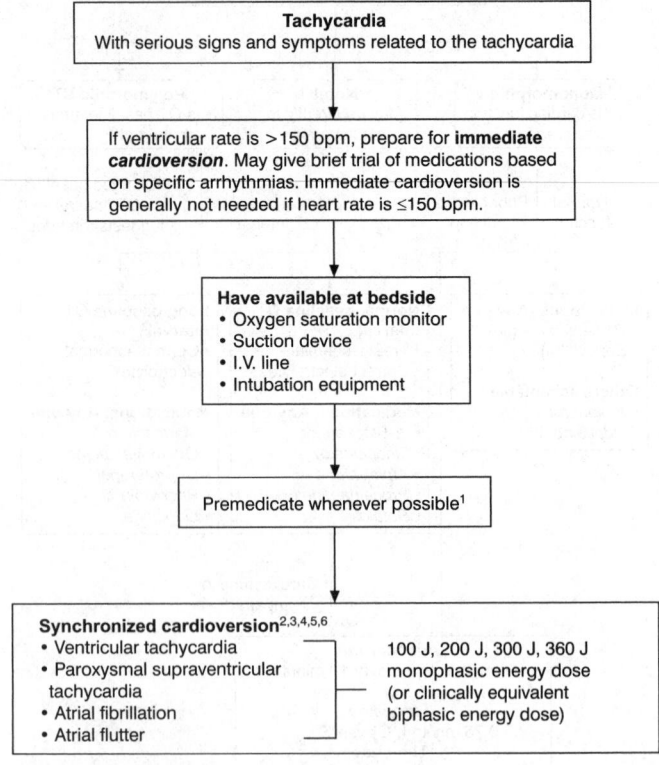

Tachycardia
With serious signs and symptoms related to the tachycardia

If ventricular rate is >150 bpm, prepare for **immediate cardioversion**. May give brief trial of medications based on specific arrhythmias. Immediate cardioversion is generally not needed if heart rate is ≤150 bpm.

Have available at bedside
- Oxygen saturation monitor
- Suction device
- I.V. line
- Intubation equipment

Premedicate whenever possible[1]

Synchronized cardioversion[2,3,4,5,6]
- Ventricular tachycardia
- Paroxysmal supraventricular tachycardia
- Atrial fibrillation
- Atrial flutter

100 J, 200 J, 300 J, 360 J monophasic energy dose (or clinically equivalent biphasic energy dose)

[1]Effective regimens have included a sedative (eg, **diazepam**, **midazolam**, **barbiturates**, **etomidate**, **ketamine**, **methohexital**) with or without an analgesic agent (eg, **fentanyl**, **morphine**, **meperidine**). Many experts recommend anesthesia if service is readily available.

[2]Both monophasic and biphasic waveforms are acceptable if documented as clinically equivalent to reports of monophasic shock success.

[3]Note possible need to resynchronize after each cardioversion.

[4]If delays in synchronization occur and clinical condition is critical, go immediately to unsynchronized shocks.

[5]Treat polymorphic ventricular tachycardia (irregular form and rate) like ventricular fibrillation: see ventricular fibrillation/pulseless ventricular tachycardia algorithm.

[6]Paroxysmal supraventricular tachycardia and atrial flutter often respond to lower energy levels (start with 50 J).

Adapted with permission of Lippincott Williams & Wilkins, "Guidelines 2000 for Cardiopulmonary Resuscitation and Emergency Cardiovascular Care, Part 6: Advanced Cardiovascular Life Support, The American Heart Association in Collaboration With the International Liaison Committee on Resuscitation," *Circulation*, 2000, 102(8 Suppl):I164.

ATRIAL FIBRILLATION / ATRIAL FLUTTER

Atrial Fibrillation / Atrial Flutter in Normal Cardiac Function — Control of Rate and Rhythm

Control Rate		Convert Rhythm	
Heart Function Preserved	Impaired Heart Function EF <40% or CHF	Duration <48 Hours	Duration >48 Hours or Unknown
Note: AF >48-hours duration: Use agents to convert rhythm with extreme caution in patient not receiving adequate anticoagulation because of possible embolic complications Use only one of the following agents:* • Calcium channel blocker (Class I) • Beta blocker (Class I) • Other drugs (class IIb recommendations) eg, digoxin, amiodarone	Not applicable	**Consider:** • DC cardioversion Use only one of the following agents:* • Amiodarone (Class IIa) • Ibutilide (Class IIa) • Flecainide (Class IIa) • Propafenone (Class IIa) • Procainamide (Class IIa) • Other drugs (class IIb recommendations) eg, sotalol, disopyramide	**NO DC CARDIOVERSION!** **Note:** Conversion of AF to NSR with drugs or shock may cause embolization of atrial thrombi unless patient has adequate anticoagulation. Use antiarrhythmic agents with extreme caution (see Note above) if AF is >48-hours duration **OR** *Delayed cardioversion* Anticoagulation for 3 weeks at proper levels • Cardioversion, *then* • Anticoagulation for 4 more weeks **OR** *Early cardioversion* • Begin I.V. heparin at once • TEE to exclude atrial clot, *then* • Cardioversion within 24 hours, *then* • Anticoagulation for 4 more weeks

Legend: AF: Atrial fibrillation; Class I: Acceptable, definitely effective; Class IIa: Acceptable, probably effective; Class IIb: Acceptable, possibly effective; Class III: Not indicated, may be harmful; EF: Ejection fraction; NSR: Normal sinus rhythm; TEE: Transesophageal echocardiogram

*Occasionally, two of the named antiarrhythmic agents may be used, but use of these agents in combination may have proarrhythmic potential; classes listed represent the *Class of Recommendation* rather than the Vaughn-Williams classification of antiarrhythmics.

Adapted with permission from Lippincott Williams & Wilkins, "Guidelines 2000 for Cardiopulmonary Resuscitation and Emergency Cardiovascular Care. Part 6: Advanced Cardiovascular Life Support. The American Heart Association in Collaboration With the International Liaison Committee on Resuscitation," *Circulation*, 2000, 102(8 Suppl), I160-1.

ATRIAL FIBRILLATION / ATRIAL FLUTTER *(Continued)*

Atrial Fibrillation / Atrial Flutter in Impaired Heart Function (EF <40% or CHF) — Control of Rate and Rhythm

	Control Rate		Convert Rhythm	
	Heart Function Preserved	Impaired Heart Function EF <40% or CHF	Duration <48 Hours	Duration >48 Hours or Unknown
	Not applicable	**Note:** AF >48-hours duration: Use agents to convert rhythm with extreme caution in patient not receiving adequate anticoagulation because of possible embolic complications Use only one of the following agents:* • Digoxin (Class IIb) • Diltiazem (Class IIb) • Amiodarone (Class IIb)	**Consider:** • DC cardioversion OR • Amiodarone (Class IIb)	• **Anticoagulation** (as described in "Control of Rate and Rhythm - Normal Cardiac Function"), followed by • **DC Cardioversion**

Legend: AF: Atrial fibrillation; Class I: Acceptable, definitely effective; Class IIa: Acceptable, probably effective; Class IIb: Acceptable, possibly effective; Class III: Not indicated, may be harmful; EF: Ejection fraction; NSR: Normal sinus rhythm; TEE: Transesophageal echocardiogram

*Occasionally, two of the named antiarrhythmic agents may be used, but use of these agents in combination may have proarrhythmic potential; classes listed represent the *Class of Recommendation* rather than the Vaughn-Williams classification of antiarrhythmics.

Adapted with permission from Lippincott Williams & Wilkins, "Guidelines 2000 for Cardiopulmonary Resuscitation and Emergency Cardiovascular Care. Part 6: Advanced Cardiovascular Life Support. The American Heart Association in Collaboration With the International Liaison Committee on Resuscitation." *Circulation*, 2000, 102(8 Suppl), I160-1.

Atrial Fibrillation / Atrial Flutter in
Wolff-Parkinson-White Syndrome — Control of Rate and Rhythm

Control Rate		Convert Rhythm	
Heart Function Preserved	**Impaired Heart Function EF <40% or CHF**	**Duration <48 Hours**	**Duration >48 Hours or Unknown**
Note: AF >48-hours duration: Use agents to convert rhythm with extreme caution in patient not receiving adequate anticoagulation because of possible embolic complications • DC Cardioversion **OR** • **Primary antiarrhythmic agents** Use only one of the following agents:* • Amiodarone (Class IIb) • Flecainide (Class IIb) • Procainamide (Class IIb) • Propafenone (Class IIb) • Sotalol (Class IIb) • **Class III (can be harmful)** • Adenosine • Beta-blockers • Calcium channel blockers • Digoxin	**Note:** AF >48-hours duration: Use agents to convert rhythm with extreme caution in patient not receiving adequate anticoagulation because of possible embolic complications • DC Cardioversion **OR** • Amiodarone (Class IIb)	• DC Cardioversion **OR** • **Primary antiarrhythmic agents** Use only one of the following agents:* • Amiodarone (Class IIb) • Flecainide (Class IIb) • Procainamide (Class IIb) • Propafenone (Class IIb) • Sotalol (Class IIb) • **Class III (can be harmful)** • Adenosine • Beta-blockers • Calcium channel blockers • Digoxin	• **Anticoagulation** (as described in "Control of Rate and Rhythm - Normal Cardiac Function"), followed by • **DC Cardioversion**

Legend: AF: Atrial fibrillation; Class I: Acceptable, definitely effective; Class IIa: Acceptable, probably effective; Class IIb: Acceptable, possibly effective; Class III: Not indicated, may be harmful; EF: Ejection fraction; NSR: Normal sinus rhythm; TEE: Transesophageal echocardiogram

*Occasionally, two of the named antiarrhythmic agents may be used, but use of these agents in combination may have proarrhythmic potential; classes listed represent the *Class of Recommendation* rather than the Vaughn-Williams classification of antiarrhythmics.

Adapted with permission from Lippincott Williams & Wilkins, "Guidelines 2000 for Cardiopulmonary Resuscitation and Emergency Cardiovascular Care, Part 6: Advanced Cardiovascular Life Support. The American Heart Association in Collaboration With the International Liaison Committee on Resuscitation," *Circulation*, 2000, 102(8 Suppl), I160-1..

NORMAL HEART RATES

Age	Mean Heart Rate (beats/minute)	Heart Rate Range (2nd – 98th percentile)
<1 d	123	93-154
1-2 d	123	91-159
3-6 d	129	91-166
1-3 wk	148	107-182
1-2 mo	149	121-179
3-5 mo	141	106-186
6-11 mo	134	109-169
1-2 y	119	89-151
3-4 y	108	73-137
5-7 y	100	65-133
8-11 y	91	62-130
12-15 y	85	60-119

Adapted from *The Harriet Lane Handbook*, 12th ed, Greene MG, ed, St Louis, MO: Mosby Yearbook, 1991.

Normal QRS Axes
(in degrees)

Age	Mean	Range
1 wk – 1 mo	+110	+30 to +180
1–3 mo	+70	+10 to +125
3 mo – 3 y	+60	+10 to +110
>3 y	+60	+20 to +120
Adults	+50	−30 to +105

INTERVALS AND SEGMENTS
OF AN EKG CYCLE

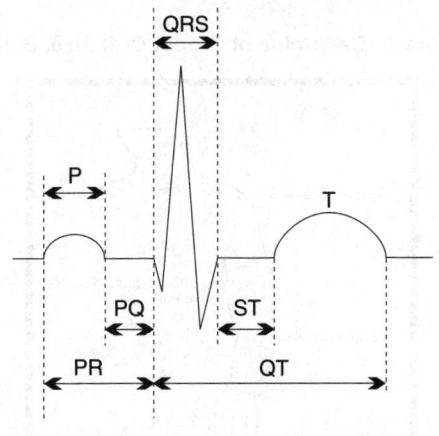

HEXAXIAL REFERENCE
SYSTEM

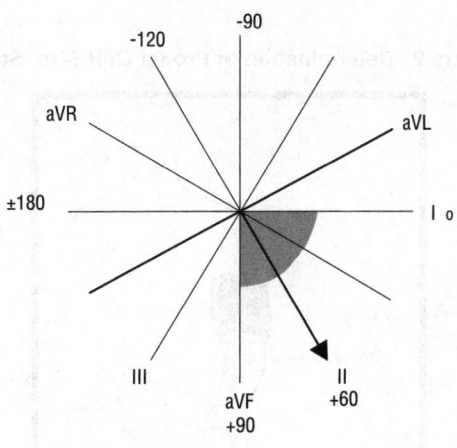

MEASURING PEDIATRIC BLOOD PRESSURE

Figure 1. Determine of Proper Cuff Size, Step 1

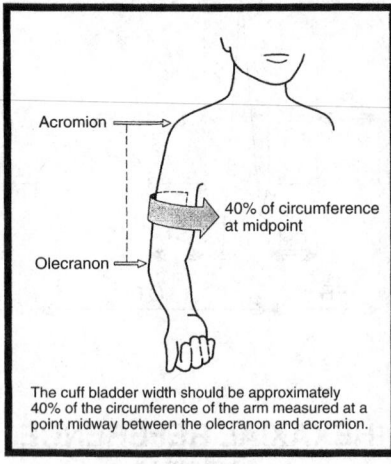

The cuff bladder width should be approximately 40% of the circumference of the arm measured at a point midway between the olecranon and acromion.

Figure 2. Determination of Proper Cuff Size, Step 2

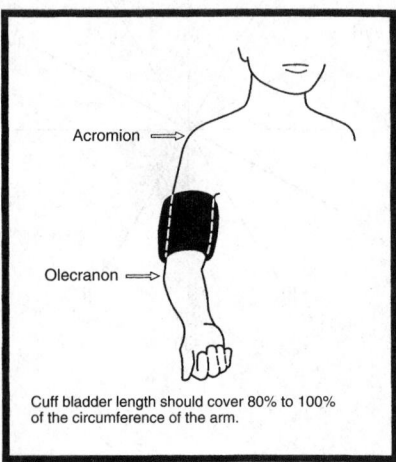

Cuff bladder length should cover 80% to 100% of the circumference of the arm.

Figure 3. Blood Pressure Measurement

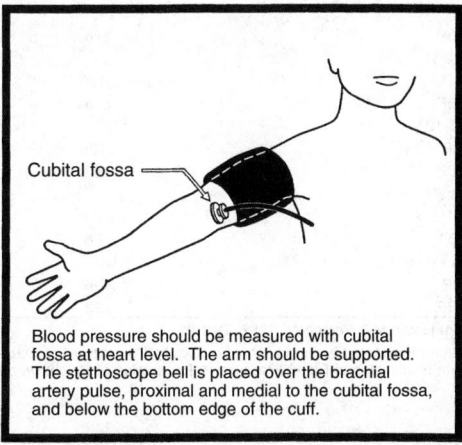

Cubital fossa

Blood pressure should be measured with cubital
fossa at heart level. The arm should be supported.
The stethoscope bell is placed over the brachial
artery pulse, proximal and medial to the cubital fossa,
and below the bottom edge of the cuff.

Used with permission: Perloff D, Grim C, Flack J, et al, "Human Blood Pressure
Determination by Sphygmomanometry," *Circulation*, 1993, 88:2460-7.

HYPERTENSION, CLASSIFICATION BY AGE GROUP*

Age Group	Significant Hypertension (mm Hg)	Severe Hypertension (mm Hg)
Newborn (7 d)		
systolic BP	≥96	≥106
Newborn (8-30 d)		
systolic BP	≥104	≥110
Infant (<2 y)		
systolic BP	≥112	≥118
diastolic BP	≥74	≥82
Children (3-5 y)		
systolic BP	≥116	≥124
diastolic BP	≥76	≥84
Children (6-9 y)		
systolic BP	≥122	≥130
diastolic BP	≥78	≥86
Children (10-12 y)		
systolic BP	≥126	≥134
diastolic BP	≥82	≥90
Adolescents (13-15 y)		
systolic BP	≥136	≥144
diastolic BP	≥86	≥92
Adolescents (16-18 y)		
systolic BP	≥142	≥150
diastolic BP	≥92	≥98

Adapted from Horan MJ, *Pediatrics*, 1987, 79:1-25.

*See also Blood Pressure Measurement, Age Specific Percentiles *on page 9999* and 90th and 95th Percentiles of Blood Pressure by Percentiles of Height *on page 9999*

BLOOD PRESSURE IN PREMATURE INFANTS, NORMAL

(Birth weight 600-1750 g)*

Day	600-999 g		1000-1249 g	
	S (± 2SD)	D (± 2SD)	S (± 2SD)	D (± 2SD)
1	37.9 (17.4)	23.2 (10.3)	44 (22.8)	22.5 (13.5)
3	44.9 (15.7)	30.6 (12.3)	48 (15.4)	36.5 (9.6)
7	50 (14.8)	30.4 (12.4)	57 (14)	42.5 (16.5)
14	50.2 (14.8)	37.4 (12)	53 (30)	
28	61 (23.5)	45.8 (27.4)	57 (30)	

Day	1250-1499 g		1500-1750 g	
	S (± 2SD)	D (± 2SD)	S (± 2SD)	D (± 2SD)
1	48 (18)	27 (12.4)	47 (15.8)	26 (15.6)
3	59 (21.1)	40 (13.7)	51 (18.2)	35 (10)
7	68 (14.8)	40 (11.3)	66 (23)	41 (24)
14	64 (21.2)	36 (24.2)	76 (34.8)	42 (20.3)
28	69 (31.4)	44 (26.2)	73 (5.6)	50 (9.9)

*Blood pressure was obtained by the Dinamap method.

S = systolic; D = diastolic; SD = standard deviation.

Modified from Ingelfinger JR, Powers L, and Epstein MF, "Blood Pressure Norms in Low-Weight Infants: Birth Through Four Weeks", *Pediatr Res*, 1983, 17:319A.

BLOOD PRESSURE MEASUREMENTS, AGE-SPECIFIC PERCENTILES

Blood Pressure Measurements: Ages 0-12 Months, Boys

Korotkoff phase IV (K4) used for diastolic BP. Reproduced with permission from Horan MJ, *Pediatrics*, 1987, 79:11-25.

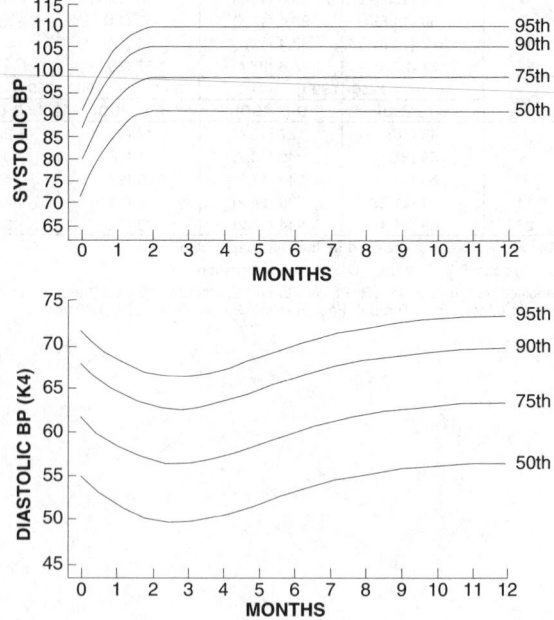

90th PERCENTILE												
SYSTOLIC BP	87	101	106	106	106	105	105	105	105	105	105	105	105
DIASTOLIC BP	68	65	63	63	63	65	66	67	68	68	69	69	69
HEIGHT CM	51	59	63	66	68	70	72	73	74	76	77	78	80
WEIGHT KG	4	4	5	5	6	7	8	9	9	10	10	11	11

Blood Pressure Measurements: Ages 0-12 Months, Girls

Korotkoff phase IV (K4) used for diastolic BP. Reproduced with permission from Horan MJ, *Pediatrics*, 1987, 79:11-25.

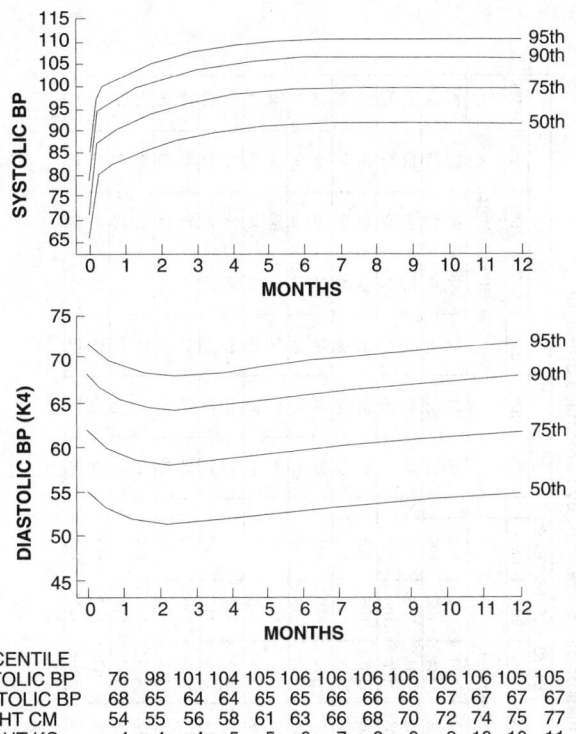

90th PERCENTILE													
SYSTOLIC BP	76	98	101	104	105	106	106	106	106	106	106	105	105
DIASTOLIC BP	68	65	64	64	65	65	66	66	66	67	67	67	67
HEIGHT CM	54	55	56	58	61	63	66	68	70	72	74	75	77
WEIGHT KG	4	4	4	5	5	6	7	8	9	9	10	10	11

BLOOD PRESSURE MEASUREMENTS, AGE-SPECIFIC PERCENTILES *(Continued)*

90th and 95th Percentiles of Blood Pressure by Percentiles of Height

BOYS AGE 1-9 YEARS

Age (y)	BP Percentiles† →	Systolic BP (mm Hg)							Diastolic BP (mm Hg)‡						
	Height Percentiles* →	5%	10%	25%	50%	75%	90%	95%	5%	10%	25%	50%	75%	90%	95%
1	90th	94	95	97	98	100	102	102	50	51	52	53	54	54	55
	95th	98	99	101	102	104	106	106	55	55	56	57	58	59	59
2	90th	98	99	100	102	104	105	106	55	55	56	57	58	59	59
	95th	101	102	104	106	108	109	110	59	59	60	61	62	63	63
3	90th	100	101	103	105	107	108	109	59	59	60	61	62	63	63
	95th	104	105	107	109	111	112	113	63	63	64	65	66	67	67
4	90th	102	103	105	107	109	110	111	62	62	63	64	65	66	66
	95th	106	107	109	111	113	114	115	66	67	67	68	70	71	71
5	90th	104	105	106	108	110	112	112	65	65	66	67	68	69	69
	95th	108	109	110	112	114	115	116	69	70	70	71	72	73	74
6	90th	105	106	108	110	111	113	114	67	68	69	70	70	71	72
	95th	109	110	112	114	115	117	117	72	72	73	74	75	76	76
7	90th	106	107	109	111	113	114	115	69	70	71	72	72	73	74
	95th	110	111	113	115	116	118	119	74	74	75	76	77	78	78
8	90th	107	108	110	112	114	115	116	71	71	72	73	74	75	75
	95th	111	112	114	116	118	119	120	75	76	76	77	78	79	80
9	90th	109	110	112	113	115	117	117	72	73	73	74	75	76	76
	95th	113	114	116	117	119	121	121	76	77	78	79	80	80	81

*Height percentile determined by standard growth curves.

† Blood pressure percentile determined by a single measurement

‡Korotkoff phase V (K5) used for diastolic BP

Source: National Institutes of Health, National Heart, Lung, and Blood Institute, "Update on the Task Force Report (1987) on High Blood Pressure in Children and Adolescents: A Working Group Report from the National High Blood Pressure Education Program," NIH No, 96-3790, 1996.

		Systolic BP (mm Hg)							Diastolic BP (mm Hg)‡						
	Height Percentiles* →	5%	10%	25%	50%	75%	90%	95%	5%	10%	25%	50%	75%	90%	95%
Age (y)	BP Percentiles† ↓														
10	90th	110	112	113	115	117	118	119	73	74	74	75	76	77	78
	95th	114	115	117	119	121	122	123	77	78	79	80	80	81	82
11	90th	112	113	115	117	119	120	121	74	74	75	76	77	78	78
	95th	116	117	119	121	123	124	125	78	79	79	80	81	82	83
12	90th	115	116	117	119	121	123	123	75	75	76	77	78	78	79
	95th	119	120	121	123	125	126	127	79	79	80	81	82	83	83
13	90th	117	118	120	122	124	125	126	75	76	76	77	78	79	80
	95th	121	122	124	126	128	129	130	79	80	81	82	83	83	84
14	90th	120	121	123	125	126	128	128	76	76	77	78	79	80	80
	95th	124	125	127	128	130	132	132	80	81	81	82	83	84	85
15	90th	123	124	125	127	129	131	131	77	77	78	79	80	81	81
	95th	127	128	129	131	133	134	135	81	82	83	83	84	85	86
16	90th	125	126	128	130	132	133	134	79	79	80	81	82	82	83
	95th	129	130	132	134	136	137	138	83	83	84	85	86	87	87
17	90th	128	129	131	133	134	136	136	81	81	82	83	84	85	85
	95th	132	133	135	136	138	140	140	85	85	86	87	88	89	89

*Height percentile determined by standard growth curves.

† Blood pressure percentile determined by a single measurement

‡Korotkoff phase V (K5) used for diastolic BP

Source: National Institutes of Health, National Heart, Lung, and Blood Institute, "Update on the Task Force Report (1987) on High Blood Pressure in Children and Adolescents: A Working Group Report from the National High Blood Pressure Education Program," NIH No, 96-3790, 1996.

BLOOD PRESSURE MEASUREMENTS, AGE-SPECIFIC PERCENTILES (Continued)

GIRLS AGE 1-9 YEARS

Age (y)	BP Percentiles† →	Systolic BP (mm Hg)							Diastolic BP (mm Hg)‡						
	Height Percentiles* →	5%	10%	25%	50%	75%	90%	95%	5%	10%	25%	50%	75%	90%	95%
1	90th	97	98	99	100	102	103	104	53	53	53	54	55	56	56
	95th	101	102	103	104	105	107	107	57	57	57	58	59	60	60
2	90th	99	99	100	102	103	104	105	57	57	58	58	59	60	61
	95th	102	103	104	105	107	108	109	61	61	62	62	63	64	65
3	90th	100	100	102	103	104	105	106	61	61	61	62	63	63	64
	95th	104	104	105	107	108	109	110	65	65	65	66	67	67	68
4	90th	101	102	103	104	106	107	108	63	63	64	65	65	66	67
	95th	105	106	107	108	109	111	111	67	67	68	69	69	70	71
5	90th	103	103	104	106	107	108	109	65	66	66	67	68	68	69
	95th	107	107	108	110	111	112	113	69	70	70	71	72	72	73
6	90th	104	105	106	107	109	110	111	67	67	68	69	69	70	71
	95th	108	109	110	111	112	114	114	71	71	72	73	73	74	75
7	90th	106	107	108	109	110	112	112	69	69	69	70	71	72	72
	95th	110	110	112	113	114	115	116	73	73	73	74	75	76	76
8	90th	108	109	110	111	112	113	114	70	70	71	71	72	73	74
	95th	112	112	113	115	116	117	118	74	74	75	75	76	77	78
9	90th	110	110	112	113	114	115	116	71	72	72	73	74	74	75
	95th	114	114	115	117	118	119	120	75	76	76	77	78	78	79

*Height percentile determined by standard growth curves.

† Blood pressure percentile determined by a single measurement.

‡Korotkoff phase V (K5) used for diastolic BP

Source: National Institutes of Health, National Heart, Lung, and Blood Institute, "Update on the Task Force Report (1987) on High Blood Pressure in Children and Adolescents: A Working Group Report from the National High Blood Pressure Education Program," NIH No, 96-3790, 1996.

GIRLS AGE 10-17 YEARS

Age (y)	BP Percentile†	Systolic BP (mm Hg)							Diastolic BP (mm Hg)‡						
	Height Percentiles* →	5%	10%	25%	50%	75%	90%	95%	5%	10%	25%	50%	75%	90%	95%
10	90th	112	112	114	115	116	117	118	73	73	73	74	75	76	76
	95th	116	116	117	119	120	121	122	77	77	77	78	79	80	80
11	90th	114	114	116	117	118	119	120	74	74	75	75	76	77	77
	95th	118	118	119	121	122	123	124	78	78	79	79	80	81	81
12	90th	116	116	118	119	120	121	122	75	75	76	76	77	78	78
	95th	120	120	121	123	124	125	126	79	79	80	80	81	82	82
13	90th	118	118	119	121	122	123	124	76	76	77	78	78	79	80
	95th	121	122	123	125	126	127	128	80	80	81	82	82	83	84
14	90th	119	120	121	122	124	125	126	77	77	78	79	79	80	81
	95th	123	124	125	126	128	129	130	81	81	82	83	83	84	85
15	90th	121	121	122	124	125	126	127	78	78	79	79	80	81	82
	95th	124	125	126	128	129	130	131	82	82	83	83	84	85	86
16	90th	122	122	123	125	126	127	128	79	79	79	80	81	82	82
	95th	125	126	127	128	130	131	132	83	83	83	84	85	86	86
17	90th	122	123	124	125	126	128	128	79	79	79	80	81	82	82
	95th	126	126	127	129	130	131	132	83	83	83	84	85	86	86

*Height percentile determined by standard growth curves.

† Blood pressure percentile determined by a single measurement

‡Korotkoff phase V (K5) used for diastolic BP

Source: National Institutes of Health, National Heart, Lung, and Blood Institute, "Update on the Task Force Report (1987) on High Blood Pressure in Children and Adolescents: A Working Group Report from the National High Blood Pressure Education Program," NIH No, 96-3790, 1996.

ANTIHYPERTENSIVE AGENTS BY CLASS

Alpha 2 Agonists
Clonidine
Methyldopa

Alpha 1 Antagonists
Prazosin

Beta Antagonists
Atenolol
Esmolol
Nadolol
Propranolol
Timolol

Mixed Alpha/Beta Antagonists
Labetalol

Calcium Channel Blockers
Diltiazem
Nifedipine
Verapamil

Angiotensin Converting Enzyme Inhibitors
Captopril
Enalapril/Enalaprilat
Lisinopril

Nitrates
Isosorbide dinitrate
Nitroglycerin

Ganglionic Blockers
Trimethaphan

Diuretics
Amiloride
Bumetanide
Chlorothiazide
Ethacrynic acid
Furosemide
Hydrochlorothiazide
Mannitol
Metolazone
Spironolactone
Torsemide
Triamterene

Vasodilators (Direct-acting)
Diazoxide
Hydralazine
Minoxidil
Nitroprusside

ANTIDEPRESSANT AGENTS

Comparison of Usual Adult Dosage and Mechanism of Action

Drug	Usual Adult Dosage (mg/d)	Reuptake Inhibition	
		Norepinephrine	Serotonin
First-Generation Antidepressants *Tricyclic Antidepressants*			
Amitriptyline (Elavil®, Endep®)	100-300	Moderate	High
Clomipramine† (Anafranil®)	100-250	Moderate	High
Desipramine (Norpramin®, Pertofrane®)	100-300	High	Low
Doxepin (Adapin®, Sinequan®)	100-300	Low	Moderate
Imipramine (Janimine®, Tofranil®)	100-300	Moderate	Moderate
Nortriptyline (Aventyl®, Pamelor®)	50-200	Moderate	Low
Protriptyline (Vivactil®)	15-60	Moderate	Low
Trimipramine (Surmontil®)	100-300	Low	Low
Monoamine Oxidase Inhibitors			
Phenelzine (Nardil®)	15-90	—	—
Tranylcypromine (Parnate®)	10-40	—	—
Second-Generation Antidepressants *Older Second-Generation Antidepressants*			
Amoxapine (Asendin®)	100-400	Moderate	Low
Maprotiline (Ludiomil®)	100-225	Moderate	Low
Trazodone (Desyrel®)	150-500	Very low	Moderate
Newer Second-Generation Antidepressants			
Bupropion (Wellbutrin®)	300-450‡	Very low§	Very low§
Third-Generation Antidepressants *Selective Serotonin Reuptake Inhibitors*			
Fluoxetine (Prozac®)	10-40	Very low	High
Fluvoxamine (Luvox®)	100-300	Very low	Very high
Paroxetine (Paxil®)	20-50	Very low	Very high
Sertraline (Zoloft®)	50-150	Very low	Very high
Serotonin/Norepinephrine Reuptake Inhibitors			
Venlafaxine (Effexor®)	75-375	Very high	Very high
Atypical Antidepressants with 5HT2 Receptor Antagonist Properties			
Mirtazapine (Remeron®)**	15-45	Very low	Very low
Nefazodone (Serzone®)**	300-600	Very low	High

†Not approved by FDA for depression

‡Not to exceed 150 mg/dose to minimize seizure risk

§Norepinephrine and serotonin reuptake inhibition is minimal, but inhibits dopamine reuptake

**These agents work primarily through antagonizing the postsynaptic 5HT2 receptor.

ANTIDEPRESSANT AGENTS *(Continued)*

Comparison of Adverse Effects

Drug	ACH	Drowsiness	Orthostatic Hypotension	Cardiac Arrhythmias	GI Distress	Weight Gain
Adverse Effects						
First-Generation Antidepressants *Tricyclic Antidepressants*						
Amitriptyline (Elavil®, Endep®)	4+	4+	4+	3+	0	4+
Clomipramine† (Anafranil®)	4+	4+	2+	3+	1+	4+
Desipramine (Norpramin®, Pertofrane®)	1+	2+	2+	2+	0	1+
Doxepin (Adapin®, Sinequan®)	3+	4+	2+	2+	0	4+
Imipramine (Janimine®, Tofranil®)	3+	3+	4+	3+	1+	4+
Nortriptyline (Aventyl®, Pamelor®)	2+	2+	1+	2+	0	1+
Protriptyline (Vivactil®)	2+	1+	2+	3+	0	0
Trimipramine (Surmontil®)	4+	4+	3+	3+	0	4+
Monoamine Oxidase Inhibitors						
Phenelzine (Nardil®)	2+	2+	2+	1+	1+	3+
Tranylcypromine (Parnate®)	2+	1+	2+	1+	1+	2+
Second-Generation Antidepressants *Older Second-Generation Antidepressants*						
Amoxapine (Asendin®)	2+	2+	2+	2+	0	2+
Maprotiline (Ludiomil®)	2+	3+	2+	2+	0	2+
Trazodone (Desyrel®)	0	4+	3+	1+	1+	2+
Newer Second-Generation Antidepressants						
Bupropion (Wellbutrin®)	0	0	0	1+	1+	0
Third-Generation Antidepressants *Selective Serotonin Reuptake Inhibitors*						
Fluoxetine (Prozac®)	0	0	0	0	3+¶	0
Fluvoxamine (Luvox®)	0	0	0	0	3+¶	0
Paroxetine (Paxil®)	1+	1+	0	0	3+¶	1+
Sertraline (Zoloft®)	0	0	0	0	3+¶	0
Serotonin/Norepinephrine Reuptake Inhibitors						
Venlafaxine# (Effexor®)	1+	1+	0	1+	3+¶	0
Atypical Antidepressants with 5HT2 Receptor Antagonist Properties						
Mirtazapine (Remeron®)	1+	2+	0	0	3+	0
Nefazodone (Serzone®)	1+	1+	0	0	1+	0

Key: ACH = anticholinergic effects (dry mouth, blurred vision, urinary retention, constipation); 0 - 4+ = absent or rare - relatively common.

†Not approved by FDA for depression

¶Nausea is usually mild and transient

#Comparative studies evaluating the adverse effects of venlafaxine in relation to other antidepressants have not been performed

CORTICOSTEROIDS, SYSTEMIC

Relative Potencies and Equivalent Doses of Corticosteroids

(Glucocorticoid potency compared to hydrocortisone "mg" for "mg" basis)

Compound	Gluco-corticoid Potency	Mineralo-corticoid Potency	Equivalent Dose (mg)	Duration* of Action
Cortisone (Cortone®)	0.8	++	25	S
Injection: 50 mg/mL suspension				
Tablet: 5 mg				
Dexamethasone (Decadron®, Dexone®, Hexadrol®)	25-30	0	0.75	L
Elixir: 0.5 mg/5 mL				
Injection: 4 mg/mL				
Intensol: 1 mg/mL				
Tablet: 0.25 mg, 0.5 mg, 0.75 mg, 1 mg, 1.5 mg, 2 mg, 4 mg				
Fludrocortisone (Florinef®)	10	+++++		I
Tablet: 0.1 mg				
Hydrocortisone (Cortef®)	1	++	20	S
Injection: 50 mg/mL				
Suspension: 10 mg/5 mL				
Tablet: 5 mg, 10 mg, 20 mg				
Methylprednisolone (Medrol®, Solu-Medrol®, Depo-Medrol®)	5	0	4	I
Injection: 40 mg, 125 mg, 500 mg, 1 g				
Injection, susp: 80 mg/mL				
Tablet: 2 mg, 4 mg, 16 mg, 24 mg				
Prednisolone (Delta-Cortef®, Prelone® Syrup, Pediapred®)	4	+	5	I
Liquid: 5 mg/5 mL				
Syrup: 15 mg/5 mL				
Tablet: 5 mg				
Prednisone (Deltasone®, Liquid Pred®, Orasone®)	4	+	5	I
Liquid: 5 mg/5 mL				
Tablet: 1 mg, 2.5 mg, 5 mg, 10 mg, 20 mg, 50 mg				

*S = Short, 8-12 hours biologic activity

I = Intermediate, 12-36 hours biologic activity

L = Long, 36-54 hours biologic activity

Reference

Knoben JE, and Anderson PO, *Handbook of Clinical Drug Data*, 6th ed, Drug Intelligence Pub, Inc, 1988.

CORTICOSTEROIDS, TOPICAL

The following topical corticosteroid preparations are grouped according to relative anti-inflammatory activity. Preparations in each group are approximately equivalent.

Drug	Dosage Form
Lowest Potency	
Hydrocortisone	0.5% cream, ointment
Hydrocortisone	1% cream, ointment
Hydrocortisone	2.5% cream, ointment
Hydrocortisone	1% solution
Hydrocortisone	1% lotion
Low Potency	
Alclometasone Dipropionate (Aclovate®)	0.05% cream, ointment
Desonide (Tridesilon®)	0.05% cream, ointment
Fluocinolone Acetonide	
(Fluonid®)	0.01% solution
(Synalar®)	0.01% cream
Low Intermediate Potency	
Betamethasone Valerate (Valisone®)	0.01% cream
Flurandrenolide (Cordran®)*	0.025% cream, ointment
Hydrocortisone Valerate (Westcort®)	0.2% cream, ointment
Triamcinolone Acetonide (Kenalog®)	0.025% cream, ointment, lotion
High Intermediate Potency	
Betamethasone Valerate (Valisone®)	0.1% cream, ointment, lotion
Desoximetasone (Topicort®)	0.05% gel
Fluocinolone Acetonide (Synalar®)*	0.025% cream, ointment
Flurandrenolide (Cordran®)*	0.05% cream, ointment, lotion
Halcinonide (Halog®)	0.025% cream
Triamcinolone Acetonide (Aristocort®, Kenalog®)	0.1% cream, ointment, lotion
High Potency	
Amcinonide (Cyclocort®)*	0.1% ointment
Betamethasone Dipropionate (Diprosone®)	0.05% cream, ointment, lotion
Desoximetasone (Topicort®)	0.25% cream, ointment
Diflorasone Diacetate (Florone®)	0.05% cream, ointment
Fluocinolone Acetonide (Synalar®-HP)	0.2% cream
Fluocinonide (Lidex®)	0.05% cream, ointment, solution
Halcinonide (Halog®)	0.1% cream, ointment, solution
Triamcinolone Acetonide (Aristocort®, Kenalog®)	0.5% cream, ointment

*Does not contain propylene glycol.

Reference
Cornell RC and Stoughton RB, "The Use of Topical Steroids in Psoriasis," *Dermatol Clin*, 1984, 2:397-407.

MULTIPLE VITAMIN PRODUCTS

Product	Content Given Per	A IU	D IU	E IU	C mg	FA mg	B$_1$ mg	B$_2$ mg	B$_3$ mg	B$_5$ mg	B$_6$ mg	B$_{12}$ mcg	Elemental Fe mg	Fluoride mg	Other
Drops															
Poly-Vi-Sol®	1 mL	1500	400	5	35		0.5	0.6	8		0.4	2			
Poly-Vi-Sol® with Iron	1 mL	1500	400	5	35		0.5	0.6	8		0.4	2	10		
Tri-Vi-Sol®	1 mL	1500	400		35										
Tri-Vi-Flor® 0.25 mg	1 mL	1500	400		35									0.25	
Adek®	1 mL	1500	400	40	45		0.5	0.6	6	3	0.6	4			Biotin 15 mcg, vitamin K 0.1 mg, zinc 5 mg, beta carotene 1 mg
Liquid															
Theragran®	5 mL	5000	400		200	0.2	10	10	300	21.4	4.1	5			
Vi-Daylin® Multivitamin	5 mL	2500	400	15	60	0.4	1.05	1.2	13.5		1.05	4.5			
B Complex	5 mL						2.3	1	6.7		0.3				
Tablet															
Adek®	1 tablet	4000	400	150	60	0.2	1.2	1.3	10	10	1.5	12			Zinc 1.1 mg, beta carotene 3 mg, vitamin K, biotin 50 mcg
Centrum Jr® with Iron	1 tablet	5000	400	30	60	0.4	1.5	1.7	20	10	2	6	18		Biotin 45 mcg, zinc 15 mg, Ca, Cu 1, Mg, Mn, Mo, P, vitamin K
Nephro-Vite®	1 tablet				100	1	1.5	1.7	20	5	10	6			Biotin 150 mcg
Poly-Vi-Flor® 1 mg	1 tablet	2500	400	15	60	0.3	1.05	1.2	13.5		1.05	4.5		1	
Poly-Vi-Sol®	1 tablet	2500	400	15	60	0.3	1.05	1.2	13.5		1.05	4.5			
Vi-Daylin® with Iron	1 tablet	2500	400	15	60	0.3	1.05	1.2	13.5		1.05	4.5	12		
Capsule															
Nephrocaps®	1 capsule				100	1	1.5	1.7	20	5	10	6			Biotin 150 mcg

NARCOTIC ANALGESICS COMPARISON

Drug	Dosage Form	Onset (min)	Duration (h)	Equi-analgesic I.M. Dose (mg)	Equi-analgesic P.O. Dose (mg)	Parenteral Oral Ratio	Partial Antagonist
Alfentanil hydrochloride	Inj: 500 mcg/mL 5 mL amp	Immediate (I.V.)	ND	ND	—	—	No
Codeine	Inj: 30 mg/mL as phosphate Tab: 15 mg, 30 mg as sulfate, 60 mg as phosphate	10-30 (I.M.)	4-6 (I.M.)	120	200	1/2-2/3	No
Fentanyl citrate (Sublimaze®)	Inj: 50 mcg/mL 2 mL, 10 mL amp	7-8 (I.M.)	1-2 (I.M.); 0.5-1 (I.V.)	0.1-0.2	—	—	No
Hydrocodone and acetaminophen	Tab: 5 mg hydrocodone + 500 mg acetaminophen (Vicodin®)	ND	4-6 (P.O.)	—	ND	ND	No
Hydromorphone hydrochloride (Dilaudid®)	Inj: 2 mg/mL amp Tab: 2 mg	15-30 (I.M.)	4-5 (I.M.)	1.5	7.5	1/5	No
Meperidine hydrochloride (Demerol®)	Inj: 25 mg/0.5 mL, 50 mg/mL, 100 mg/mL amp Syrup: 10 mg/mL Tab: 50 mg	10-45 (I.M.)	2-4 (I.M.)	75-100	300	1/3-1/2	No
Methadone hydrochloride (Dolophine®)	Inj: 10 mg/mL amp Solution: 1 mg/mL Tab: 5 mg, 10 mg	30-60 (I.M.)	4-6 (I.M.); duration increases with repeated use due to cumulative effects	10	20	1/2	No

Drug	Dosage Form	Onset (min)	Duration (h)	Equi-analgesic I.M. Dose (mg)	Equi-analgesic P.O. Dose (mg)	Parenteral Oral Ratio	Partial Antagonist
Morphine sulfate	Inj: 10 mg/mL, 15 mg/mL amp, 2 mg/mL Carboject®, 1 mg/mL 30 mL PCA syringe Inj, preservative free: 1 mg/mL 10 mL vial, 5 mg/10 mL amp (Duramorph® PF) Solution: 10 mg/5 mL, 20 mg/5 mL Tab (soluble): 10 mg, 30 mg Tab (controlled release): 30 mg (MS Contin®)	15-60 (epidural or I.T.) 15-30 (S.C.)	4-5 (I.M.) (S.C.)	10	60	1/6; ratio decreases to 1/1.5-2.5 upon chronic dosing	No
Oxycodone hydrochloride and acetaminophen (P.O.) (Percodan®, Tylox®)	Cap: Oxycodone 5 mg + acetaminophen 500 mg Tab: Oxycodone (~5 mg) + acetaminophen 325 mg	15-30 (P.O.)	4-6 (P.O.)	—	30	—	No
Pentazocine (Talwin® NX)	Inj: 30 mg/mL as lactate, 1 mL, 1.5 mL, 2 mL uni-amp or Carboject®, 10 mL vial Tab: 50 mg with 0.5 mg naloxone (Talwin® NX)	15-30 (I.M.) (P.O.)	2-3 (I.M) 4-5 (P.O.)	50	150	1/3	Yes
Propoxyphene and acetaminophen (P.O.) (Darvocet-N® 50, Darvocet-N® 100, Darvon®)	Cap: Propoxyphene HCl (Darvon®) 32 mg, 65 mg Tab: Propoxyphene napsylate 50 mg + acetaminophen 325 mg (Darvocet-N® 50); Propoxyphene napsylate 100 mg + acetaminophen 650 mg (Darvocet-N® 100)	30-60 (P.O.)	4-6 (P.O.)	—	HCl salt: 130 Napsylate salt: 200	—	No

ND = no data.

*These values are based on adult studies. Duration may be shorter in children due to faster elimination (in general) compared to adults.

OTC COUGH AND COLD PREPARATIONS, PEDIATRIC

Commonly Used Pediatric OTC Cough & Cold Preparations

Brand Name	Type of Preparation
Actifed®	Antihistamine/Decongestant
Benadryl® Allergy Decongestant Elixir	Antihistamine/Decongestant
Children's Dimetapp® Cold & Allergy	Antihistamine/Decongestant
Children's Dimetapp® Cold & Cough	Antihistamine/Antitussive/Decongestant
Chlor-Trimeton® Allergy 4-Hour	Antihistamine
Dimetane®	Antihistamine/Decongestant
Dimetapp® Cold and Congestion	Antitussive/Decongestant/Expectorant
Dimetapp® Elixir Cold and Allergy	Antihistamine/Decongestant
Dimetapp® Infant Drops	Decongestant
Dimetapp® Infant Drops Decongestant and Cough	Antitussive/Decongestant
Dorcol® Children's Cough Syrup	Antitussive/Decongestant/Expectorant
Neosynephrine® 12-Hour Children's Nose Drops	Decongestant
Neosynephrine® Nose Drops/Nasal Spray	Decongestant
Organidin® NR	Expectorant
Pediacare® Infant Oral Drops	Decongestant
Pediacare® Cough-Cold Formula	Antihistamine/Antitussive/Decongestant
Pediacare® "Night Rest"	Antihistamine/Antitussive/Decongestant
Robitussin®	Expectorant
Robitussin-CF®	Antitussive/Decongestant/Expectorant
Robitussin-DM®	Antitussive/Expectorant
Robitussin-PE®	Decongestant/Expectorant
Robitussin® Pediatric Cough Suppressant	Antitussive
Sudafed®	Decongestant
Sudafed Plus	Antihistamine/Decongestant
Triaminic® Cold & Cough Soft Chews	Antihistamine/Antitussive/Decongestant
Triaminic Cold & Allergy Syrup® (orange)	Antihistamine/Decongestant
Triaminic® Cold, Cough, and Fever	Antihistamine/Antitussive/Decongestant
Triaminic-DM® Throat Pain and Cough Syrup (dark red)	Antitussive/Decongestant
Tylenol® Cold, Children's	Antihistamine/Decongestant
Vick's Nyquil®, Children's	Antihistamine/Antitussive/Decongestant
Vick's Pediatric Formula 44® Cough and Cold	Antihistamine/Antitussive/Decongestant
Vick's Pediatric Formula 44® Cough and Congestion	Antitussive/Decongestant

Content of Commonly Used Pediatric Cough & Cold Preparations

The following chart lists the contents of the more common OTC cough and cold preparations. Products are grouped by preparation type. For specific recommendations, see individual drug monographs.

Brand Name	Generic(s)	Strength	Other Information
Decongestants			
Neosynephrine® 12-Hour Children's Nose Drops	Oxymethazoline	0.025%	Benzalkonium chloride, phenylmercuric acetate 0.002% as preservative
Neosynephrine® Nose Drops/Nasal Spray	Phenylephrine	0.16% 0.125% 0.25% 0.25%-0.5%	Infants >6 mo 1-6 y >6-12 y >12 y to adult
Pediacare® Infant Oral Drops	Pseudoephedrine	7.5 mg/0.8 mL	–
Dimetapp® Infant Drops	Pseudoephedrine	7.5 mg/0.8 mL	–
Sudafed®	Pseudoephedrine	15 mg/5 mL 30 mg/5 mL 30 mg/tab 60 mg/tab 120 mg/tab or cap (timed release) 240 mg/tab (timed release)	–
Antihistamines			
Chlor-Trimeton® Allergy 4-Hour	Chlorpheniramine	2 mg/5 mL	5% EtOH
Expectorants			
Organidin® NR Robitussin®	Guaifenesin	100 mg/5 mL	–
Antitussives			
Robitussin® Pediatric Cough Suppressant	Dextromethorphan HBr	7.5 mg/5 mL	–
Antihistamine/Decongestants			
Actifed®	Triprolidine	1.25 mg/5 mL 2.5 mg/tab	–
	Pseudoephedrine	30 mg/5 mL 60 mg/tab	
Benadryl®Allergy Decongestant Liquid	Diphenhydramine Pseudoephedrine	12.5 mg/5 mL 30 mg/5 mL	–
Dimetane®	Phenylephrine Brompheniramine	5 mg/5 mL 2 mg/5 mL	2.3% EtOH
Children's Dimetapp® Elixir Cold & Allergy	Brompheniramine Pseudoephedrine	1 mg/5 mL 15 mg/5 mL	–
Dimetapp® Cold & Allergy	Chlorpheniramine Phenylephrine	2 mg/tab 5 mg/tab	Acetaminophen 325 mg/tab
Sudafed Plus	Chlorpheniramine Pseudoephedrine	2 mg/5 mL 4 mg/tab 30 mg/5 mL 60 mg/tab	–
Triaminic® Cold & Allergy (orange)	Chlorpheniramine Pseudoephedrine	1 mg/5 mL 15 mg/5 mL	–
Tylenol® Cold, Children's	Chlorpheniramine Pseudoephedrine	1 mg/5 mL 0.5 mg/tab 15 mg/5 mL 7.5 mg/tab	Acetaminophen 160 mg/5 mL 80 mg/tab

OTC COUGH AND COLD PREPARATIONS, PEDIATRIC
(Continued)

Brand Name	Generic(s)	Strength	Other Information
Antitussive/Decongestant			
Dimetapp® Infant Drops Decongestant & Cough	Dextromethorphan	2.5 mg/0.8 mL	–
	Pseudoephedrine	7.5 mg/0.8 mL	
Triaminic-DM® Throat Pain & Cough	Dextromethorphan	5 mg/5 mL	Acetaminophen 160 mg
	Pseudoephedrine	15 mg/5 mL	
Vick's® Pediatric Formula 44 Cough & Congestion	Dextromethorphan	5 mg/5 mL	–
	Pseudoephedrine	10 mg/5 mL	
Antitussive/Expectorant			
Robitussin-DM®	Dextromethorphan	10 mg/5 mL	1.4% EtOH
	Guaifenesin	100 mg/5 mL	
Decongestant/Expectorant			
Robitussin-PE®	Pseudoephedrine	30 mg/5 mL	1.4% EtOH
	Guaifenesin	100 mg/5 mL	
Antihistamine/Antitussive/Decongestant			
Children's Dimetapp® DM Cold & Cough	Brompheniramine	1 mg/5 mL	–
	Dextromethorphan	5 mg/5 mL	
	Pseudoephedrine	15 mg/5 mL	
Pediacare® Cough-Cold Formula	Chlorpheniramine	1 mg/5 mL 0.5 mg/tab 1 mg/chew tab	–
	Dextromethorphan	5 mg/5 mL 2.5 mg/tab 5 mg/chew tab	
	Pseudoephedrine	15 mg/5 mL 7.5 mg/tab 15 mg/chew tab	
Pediacare® "Night Rest"	Chlorpheniramine	1 mg/5 mL	–
	Dextromethorphan	7.5 mg/5 mL	
	Pseudoephedrine	15 mg/5 mL	
Triaminic® Cold & Cough Soft Chews	Chlorpheniramine	1 mg/chew tab	–
	Dextromethorphan	5 mg/chew tab	
	Pseudoephedrine	15 mg/chew tab	
Triaminic® Cold, Cough, & Fever	Chlorpheniramine	1 mg/5 mL	Acetaminophen 160 mg
	Dextromethorphan	7.5 mg/5 mL	
	Pseudoephedrine	15 mg/5 mL	
Vick's Nyquil®, Children's	Chlorpheniramine	0.67 mg/5 mL	–
	Dextromethorphan	5 mg/5 mL	
	Pseudoephedrine	10 mg/5 mL	
Vick's Pediatric Formula 44® Cough & Cold	Chlorpheniramine	0.67 mg/5 mL	–
	Dextromethorphan	5 mg/5 mL	
	Pseudoephedrine	10 mg/5 mL	
Antitussive/Decongestant/Expectorant			
Dorcol® Children's Cough Syrup	Dextromethorphan	5 mg/5 mL	
	Pseudoephedrine	15 mg/5 mL	
	Guaifenesin	50 mg/5 mL	
Dimetapp® Cold & Congestion	Dextromethorphan	10 mg/caplet	–
	Pseudoephedrine	30 mg/caplet	
	Guaifenesin	200 mg/caplet	
Robitussin-CF®	Dextromethorphan	10 mg/5 mL	4.75% EtOH
	Pseudoephedrine	30 mg/5 mL	
	Guaifenesin	100 mg/5 mL	

Note: Due to an association with phenylpropanolamine use and hemorrhagic stroke, the FDA has recommended the withdrawal of phenylpropanolamine and phenylpropanolamine-containing products (November, 2000).

CONVERSIONS

Apothecary-Metric Exact Equivalents

1 gram (g)	=	15.43 grains	0.1 mg	=	1/600 gr
1 milliliter (mL)	=	16.23 minims	0.12 mg	=	1/500 gr
1 minim	=	0.06 mL	0.15 mg	=	1/400 gr
1 grain (gr)	=	64.8 milligrams	0.2 mg	=	1/300 gr
1 fluid ounce (fl. oz)	=	29.57 mL	0.3 mg	=	1/200 gr
1 pint (pt)	=	473.2 mL	0.4 mg	=	1/150 gr
1 ounce (oz)	=	28.35 grams	0.5 mg	=	1/120 gr
1 pound (lb)	=	453.6 grams	0.6 mg	=	1/100 gr
1 kilogram (kg)	=	2.2 pounds	0.8 mg	=	1/80 gr
1 quart (qt)	=	946.4 mL	1 mg	=	1/65 gr

Apothecary-Metric Approximate Equivalents*

Liquids			Solids		
1 teaspoonful	=	5 mL	$1/4$ grain	=	15 mg
1 tablespoonful	=	15 mL	$1/2$ grain	=	30 mg
			1 grain	=	60 mg
			$1 1/2$ grain	=	100 mg
			5 grains	=	300 mg
			10 grains	=	600 mg

*Use exact equivalents for compounding and calculations requiring a high degree of accuracy.

Pounds-Kilograms

1 pound = 0.45359 kilograms
1 kilogram = 2.2 pounds

Temperature Conversion

Celsius to Fahrenheit = (°C x 9/5) + 32 = °F
Fahrenheit to Celsius = (°F - 32) x 5/9 = °C

CYTOCHROME P-450 ENZYMES AND DRUG METABOLISM

Background

The cytochrome P-450 enzymes are a "superfamily" of enzymes that catalyze the biotransformation (metabolism) of endogenous and exogenous lipophilic substances. These enzymes are considered to be the most important of the phase I enzymes and account for the majority of drug metabolism in humans. Enzyme "families," known as isoenzymes, are located primarily in the liver. The nomenclature of this system has been standardized. Isoenzyme "families" are identified using a CYP prefix, followed by an Arabic number (eg, CYP1). Subfamilies are designated by a letter following the number (eg, CYP1A) and individual isoenzymes are numbered sequentially within the subfamily (eg, CYP1A2). Cytochrome P-450 isoenzymes that are important in the metabolism of drugs in humans are primarily found in the CYP1, CYP2, and CYP3 families.

Enzymes may be inhibited (slowing metabolism through this pathway) or induced (increased in activity or number). Individual drugs metabolized by a specific enzyme are identified as substrates for the isoenzyme. Considerable effort has been expended in recent years to classify drugs metabolized by this system as either an inhibitor, inducer, or substrate of a specific isoenzyme. It should be noted that a drug may demonstrate complex activity within this scheme, acting as an inhibitor of one isoenzyme while serving as a substrate for another.

By recognizing that a substrate's metabolism may be dramatically altered by concurrent therapy with either an inducer or inhibitor, potential interactions may be identified and addressed. For example, a drug which inhibits CYP1A2 is likely to block metabolism of theophylline (a substrate for this isoenzyme). Because of this interaction, the dose of theophylline required to maintain a consistent level in the patient should be reduced when an inhibitor is added. Failure to make this adjustment may lead to supratherapeutic theophylline concentrations and potential toxicity.

This approach does have limitations. For example, the metabolism of specific drugs may have primary and secondary pathways. The contribution of secondary pathways to the overall metabolism may limit the impact of any given inhibitor. In addition, there may be up to a tenfold variation in the concentration of an isoenzyme across the broad population. In fact, a complete absence of an isoenzyme may occur in some genetic subgroups. Finally, the relative potency of inhibition, relative to the affinity of the enzyme for its substrate, demonstrates a high degree of variability. These issues make it difficult to anticipate whether a theoretical interaction will have a clinically relevant impact in a specific patient.

The details of this enzyme system continue to be investigated, and information is expanding daily. However, to be complete, it should be noted that other enzyme systems also influence a drug's pharmacokinetic profile. For example, a key enzyme system regulating the absorption of drugs is the p-glycoprotein system. Recent evidence suggests that some interactions originally attributed to the cytochrome system may, in fact, have been the result of inhibition of this enzyme.

The following tables represent an attempt to detail the available information with respect to isoenzyme activities. Within certain limits, they may be used to identify potential interactions. Of particular note, an effort has been made in each drug monograph to identify involvement of a particular isoenzyme in the drug's metabolism. These tables are intended to supplement the limited space available to list drug interactions in the monograph. Consequently, they may be used to define a greater range of both actual and potential drug interactions.

CYTOCHROME P-450 ENZYMES AND RESPECTIVE METABOLIZED DRUGS

CYP1A2

Substrates

Acetaminophen
Acetanilid
Albendazole (minor)
Alosetron
Aminophylline
Amitriptyline (demethylation)
Antipyrine
Apomorphine
Betaxolol
Caffeine
Chlorpromazine
Clomipramine (demethylation)
Clozapine
Cyclobenzaprine (demethylation)
Desipramine (demethylation)
Diazepam
Estradiol
Estradiol and medroxyprogesterone
Fluvoxamine
Haloperidol (minor)
Imipramine (demethylation)
Levobupivacaine
Levomepromazine
Maprotiline
Methadone
Metoclopramide

Mirtazapine (hydroxylation)
Nortriptyline
Olanzapine (demethylation, hydroxylation)
Ondansetron
Phenacetin
Phenothiazines
Pimozide (minor)
Propafenone
Propranolol
Riluzole
Ritonavir
Ropinirole
Ropivacaine
Tacrine
Tamoxifen
Testosterone
Theophylline
Thioridazine
Thiothixene
Trifluoperazine
Verapamil
Warfarin (R-warfarin, minor pathway)
Zileuton
Ziprasidone (minor)
Zopiclone

Inducers

Albendazole
Carbamazepine
Charbroiled foods
Cigarette smoke
Cruciferous vegetables (cabbage, brussels
    sprouts, broccoli, cauliflower)
Modafinil (weak)

Nicotine
Omeprazole
Phenobarbital
Phenytoin
Primidone
Rifampin
Ritonavir

Inhibitors

Anastrozole
Cimetidine
Ciprofloxacin
Citalopram (weak)
Clarithromycin
Diethyldithiocarbamate
Diltiazem
Enoxacin
Entacapone (high dose)
Erythromycin
Ethinyl estradiol
Fluvoxamine
Fluoxetine (high dose)

Grapefruit juice
Isoniazid
Ketoconazole
Mexiletine
Mibefradil
Moricizine (possible)
Norfloxacin
Paroxetine (high dose)(weak)
Ritonavir
Sertraline (weak)
Tacrine
Tertiary TCAs
Zileuton

CYTOCHROME P-450 ENZYMES AND DRUG METABOLISM *(Continued)*

CYP2A6

Substrates

Dexmedetomidine	Ritonavir
Letrozole	Tamoxifen
Montelukast	Tolcapone
Nicotine	

Inducers

Barbiturates

Inhibitors

Diethyldithiocarbamate	Methoxsalen
Entacapone (high dose)	Ritonavir
Letrozole	Tranylcypromine

CYP2B6

Substrates

Antipyrine	Nicotine
Bupropion (hydroxylation)	Orphenadrine
Cyclophosphamide	Tamoxifen
Ifosfamide	

Inducers

Modafinil (weak)	Phenytoin
Phenobarbital	Primidone

Inhibitors

Diethyldithiocarbamate	Orphenadrine

CYP2C
(Specific isozyme has not been identified)

Substrates

Antipyrine	Mephobarbital
Carvedilol	Tamoxifen
Clozapine (minor)	Ticrynafen
Mestranol	

Inducers

Carbamazepine	Primidone
Haloperidol	Rifampin
Phenobarbital	Sulfinpyrazone
Phenytoin	

Inhibitors

Isoniazid	Ketoprofen
Ketoconazole	Miconazole

CYP2C8

Substrates

Carbamazepine	Paclitaxel
Diazepam	Pioglitazone
Diclofenac	Retinoic acid
Ibuprofen	Rosiglitazone
Mephobarbital	Tolbutamide
Naproxen (5-hydroxylation)	Warfarin (S-warfarin)
Omeprazole	

Inducers

Carbamazepine	Primidone
Phenobarbital	Rifampin
Phenytoin	Rifapentine

Inhibitors

Anastrozole	Omeprazole

CYP2C9

Substrates

Alosetron
Amitriptyline (demethylation)
Amoxapine
Carvedilol
Celecoxib
Dapsone
Diclofenac
Flurbiprofen
Fluvastatin
Glimepiride
Hexobarbital
Ibuprofen
Imipramine (demethylation)
Indomethacin
Irbesartan
Losartan
Mefenamic acid
Metronidazole
Mirtazapine
Montelukast
Naproxen (5-hydroxylation)
Nateglinide
Omeprazole
Phenytoin
Piroxicam
Quetiapine (minor pathway)
Ritonavir
Rosiglitazone (minor)
Sildenafil citrate (minor pathway)
Tenoxicam
Tetrahydrocannabinol
Tolbutamide
Torsemide
Warfarin (S-warfarin)
Zafirlukast (hydroxylation)
Zileuton

Inducers

Carbamazepine
Fluconazole
Fluoxetine
Phenobarbital
Phenytoin
Rifampin
Rifapentine

Inhibitors

Amiodarone
Anastrozole
Chloramphenicol
Cimetidine
Clopidogrel (high conc - *in vitro*)
Co-trimoxazole
Diclofenac
Disulfiram
Entacapone (high dose)
Flurbiprofen
Fluconazole
Fluoxetine
Fluvastatin
Fluvoxamine (potent)
Isoniazid
Ketoconazole (weak)
Ketoprofen
Leflunomide (*in vitro* only)
Metronidazole
Nateglinide
Omeprazole
Phenylbutazone
Ritonavir
Sertraline
Sulfamethoxazole-trimethoprim
Sulfaphenazole
Sulfinpyrazone
Sulfonamides
Sulindac
Troglitazone
Valproic acid
Warfarin (R-warfarin)
Zafirlukast

CYP2C18

Substrates

Dronabinol
Naproxen
Omeprazole
Piroxicam
Proguanil
Propranolol
Retinoic acid
Tolbutamide
Warfarin

Inducers

Carbamazepine
Phenobarbital
Phenytoin
Rifampin

Inhibitors

Cimetidine
Fluconazole
Fluvastatin
Isoniazid

CYTOCHROME P-450 ENZYMES AND DRUG METABOLISM *(Continued)*

CYP2C19

Substrates

Amitriptyline (demethylation)	Mephobarbital
Amoxapine	Moclobemide
Apomorphine	Olanzapine (minor)
Barbiturates	Omeprazole
Carisoprodol	Pantoprazole
Citalopram	Pentamidine
Clomipramine (demethylation)	Phenytoin
Desmethyldiazepam	Proguanil
Diazepam (N-demethylation, minor pathway)	Propranolol
Divalproex sodium	Ritonavir
Hexobarbital	Tolbutamide
Imipramine (demethylation)	Topiramate
Lansoprazole	Valproic acid
Mephenytoin	Warfarin (R-warfarin)

Inducers

Carbamazepine	Phenytoin
Phenobarbital	Rifampin

Inhibitors

Cimetidine	Omeprazole
Citalopram (weak)	Oxcarbazepine
Disulfiram	Proguanil
Entacapone (high conc)	Ritonavir
Felbamate	Sertraline
Fluconazole	Telmisartan
Fluoxetine	Teniposide
Fluvastatin	Tolbutamide
Fluvoxamine	Topiramate
Isoniazid	Tranylcypromine
Ketoconazole (weak)	Troglitazone
Letrozole	Warfarin (R-warfarin)
Modafinil	

CYP2D6

Substrates

Amitriptyline (hydroxylation)	Encainide
Amoxapine	Ethylmorphine
Amphetamine	Fenfluramine
Betaxolol	Flecainide
Bisoprolol	Fluoxetine (minor pathway)
Brofaromine	Fluphenazine
Bufuronol	Halofantrine
Captopril	Haloperidol (minor pathway)
Carvedilol	Hydrocodone
Cevimeline	Hydrocortisone
Chlorpheniramine	Hydroxyamphetamine
Chlorpromazine	Imipramine (hydroxylation)
Cinnarizine	Labetalol
Clomipramine (hydroxylation)	Lidocaine
Clozapine (minor pathway)	Loratadine
Codeine (hydroxylation, o-demethylation)	Maprotiline
Cyclobenzaprine (hydroxylation)	m-Chlorophenylpiperazine (m-CPP)
Cyclophosphamide	Meperidine
Debrisoquin	Methadone
Delavirdine	Methamphetamine
Desipramine	Metoclopramide
Dexfenfluramine	Metoprolol
Dextromethorphan (o-demethylation)	Mexiletine
Dihydrocodeine	Mianserin
Diphenhydramine	Mirtazapine (hydroxylation)
Dolasetron	Molindone
Donepezil	Morphine
Doxepin	Nortriptyline (hydroxylation)

Olanzapine (minor, hydroxymethylation)
Ondansetron
Orphenadrine
Oxycodone
Papaverine
Paroxetine (minor pathway)
Penbutolol
Pentazocine
Perhexiline
Perphenazine
Phenformin
Pindolol
Promethazine
Propafenone
Propoxyphene
Propranolol
Quetiapine (minor pathway)
Remoxipride

Risperidone
Ritonavir (minor)
Ropivacaine
Selegiline
Sertindole
Sertraline (minor pathway)
Sparteine
Tamoxifen
Thioridazine**
Tiagabine
Timolol
Tolterodine
Tramadol
Trazodone
Trimipramine
Tropisetron
Venlafaxine (o-desmethylation)
Yohimbine

Inhibitors

Amiodarone
Celecoxib
Chloroquine
Chlorpromazine
Cimetidine
Citalopram
Clomipramine
Codeine
Delavirdine
Desipramine
Dextropropoxyphene
Diltiazem
Doxorubicin
Entacapone (high dose)
Fluoxetine
Fluphenazine
Fluvoxamine
Haloperidol
Labetalol
Lobeline
Lomustine
Methadone

Mibefradil
Moclobemide
Norfluoxetine
Paroxetine
Perphenazine
Primaquine
Propafenone
Propoxyphene
Quinacrine
Quinidine
Ranitidine
Risperidone (weak)
Ritonavir
Sertindole
Sertraline (weak)
Thioridazine
Valproic acid
Venlafaxine (weak)
Vinblastine
Vincristine
Vinorelbine
Yohimbine

CYP2E1

Substrates

Acetaminophen
Acetone
Aniline
Benzene
Caffeine
Chloral hydrate
Chlorzoxazone
Clozapine
Dapsone
Dextromethorphan
Enflurane
Ethanol
Halothane

Isoflurane
Isoniazid
Methoxyflurane
Nitrosamine
Ondansetron
Phenol
Ritonavir
Sevoflurane
Styrene
Tamoxifen
Theophylline (minor pathway)
Venlafaxine

Inducers

Ethanol
Isoniazid

Mitoxantrone (weak - *in vitro*)

Inhibitors

Diethyldithiocarbamate (disulfiram metabolite)
Dimethyl sulfoxide
Disulfiram

Entacapone (high dose)
Ritonavir

CYTOCHROME P-450 ENZYMES AND DRUG METABOLISM (Continued)

CYP3A3/4

Substrates

Acetaminophen
Albendazole
Alfentanil
Alosetron
Alprazolam**
Amiodarone
Amitriptyline (minor)
Amlodipine
Amoxapine
Amprenavir
Anastrozole
Androsterone
Antipyrine
Apomorphine
Argatroban (minor)
Astemizole**
Atorvastatin
Benzphetamine
Bepridil
Bexarotene
Bromazepam
Bromocriptine
Budesonide
Bupropion (minor)
Buspirone
Busulfan
Caffeine
Cannabinoids
Carbamazepine
Cevimeline
Cerivastatin
Chlordiazepoxide
Chlorpromazine
Cilostazol
Cimetidine
Cisapride**
Citalopram
Clarithromycin
Clindamycin
Clofibrate
Clomipramine
Clonazepam
Clorazepate
Clozapine
Cocaine
Codeine (demethylation)
Cortisol
Cortisone
Cyclobenzaprine (demethylation)
Cyclophosphamide
Cyclosporine
Dapsone
Dehydroepiandrostendione
Delavirdine
Desmethyldiazepam
Dexamethasone
Dextromethorphan (minor, N-demethylation)
Diazepam (minor; hydroxylation, N-demethylation)
Digitoxin
Diltiazem
Disopyramide
Docetaxel
Dofetilide (minor)
Dolasetron
Donepezil
Doxorubicin
Doxycycline
Dronabinol
Enalapril
Erythromycin
Estradiol
Estradiol and medroxyprogesterone
Ethinyl estradiol
Ethosuximide
Etoposide
Exemestane
Felodipine
Fentanyl
Fexofenadine
Finasteride
Fluoxetine
Flutamide
Fluticasone
Gemfibrozil
Glyburide
Granisetron
Halofantrine
Haloperidol
Hydrocortisone
Hydroxyarginine
Ifosfamide
Imipramine
Indinavir
Isradipine
Itraconazole
Ketoconazole
Lansoprazole (minor)
Letrozole
Levobupivacaine
Lidocaine
Loratadine
Losartan
Lovastatin
Methadone
Mibefradil
Miconazole
Midazolam
Mifepristone
Mirtazapine (N-demethylation)
Modafinil
Montelukast
Nateglinide
Navelbine
Nefazodone
Nelfinavir**
Nevirapine
Nicardipine
Nifedipine
Niludipine
Nimodipine
Nisoldipine
Nitrendipine
Omeprazole (sulfonation)
Ondansetron
Oral contraceptives
Orphenadrine
Paclitaxel
Pantoprazole
Pimozide**
Pioglitazone
Pravastatin
Prednisone
Progesterone

Proguanil
Propafenone
Quercetin
Quetiapine
Quinidine
Quinine
Repaglinide
Retinoic acid
Rifampin
Risperidone
Ritonavir**
Salmeterol
Saquinavir
Sertindole
Sertraline
Sibutramine##
Sildenafil citrate
Simvastatin
Sirolimus
Sufentanil
Tacrolimus
Tamoxifen
Temazepam
Teniposide
Terfenadine**

Testosterone
Tetrahydrocannabinol
Theophylline
Tiagabine
Tolcapone
Tolterodine
Toremifene
Trazodone
Tretinoin
Triazolam**
Troglitazone
Troleandomycin
Venlafaxine (N-demethylation)
Verapamil
Vinblastine
Vincristine
Warfarin (R-warfarin)
Yohimbine
Zaleplon (minor pathway)
Zatosetron
Zidovudine
Zileuton
Ziprasidone
Zolpidem**
Zonisamide

Inducers

Carbamazepine
Dexamethasone
Ethosuximide
Glucocorticoids
Griseofulvin
Nafcillin
Nelfinavir
Nevirapine
Oxcarbazepine
Phenobarbital
Phenylbutazone

Phenytoin
Primidone
Progesterone
Rifabutin
Rifapentine
Rifampin
Rofecoxib (mild)
St John's wort
Sulfadimidine
Sulfinpyrazone
Troglitazone

Inhibitors

Amiodarone
Amprenavir
Anastrozole
Azithromycin
Cannabinoids
Cimetidine
Clarithromycin**
Clotrimazole
Cyclosporine
Danazol
Delavirdine
Dexamethasone
Diethyldithiocarbamate
Diltiazem
Dirithromycin
Disulfiram
Entacapone (high dose)
Erythromycin**
Ethinyl estradiol
Fluconazole (weak)
Fluoxetine
Fluvoxamine**
Gestodene
Grapefruit juice
Haloperidol
Indinavir
Isoniazid
Itraconazole**
Ketoconazole**

Lopinavir and Ritonavir
Metronidazole
Mibefradil**
Miconazole (moderate)
Modafinil (minor)
Nefazodone**
Nelfinavir
Nevirapine
Nicardipine
Norfloxacin
Norfluoxetine
Omeprazole (weak)
Oxiconazole
Paroxetine (weak)
Propoxyphene
Quinidine
Quinine**
Quinupristin and dalfopristin
Ranitidine
Ritonavir**
Saquinavir
Sertindole
Sertraline
Troglitazone
Troleandomycin
Valproic acid (weak)
Verapamil
Zafirlukast
Zileuton

CYTOCHROME P-450 ENZYMES AND DRUG METABOLISM (Continued)

CYP3A4/5

Inducer

Oxcarbazepine

CYP3A5-7

Substrates

Cortisol	Terfenadine
Estradiol and medroxyprogesterone	Testosterone
Ethinyl estradiol	Triazolam
Lovastatin	Vinblastine
Nifedipine	Vincristine
Quinidine	

Inducers

Phenobarbital	Primidone
Phenytoin	Rifampin

Inhibitors

Clotrimazole	Miconazole
Ketoconazole	Troleandomycin
Metronidazole	

**Contraindications:
Terfenadine, astemizole, cisapride, and triazolam contraindicated with nefazodone
Pimozide contraindicated with CYP3A3/4 inhibitors
Alprazolam and triazolam contraindicated with ketoconazole and itraconazole
Terfenadine, astemizole, and cisapride contraindicated with fluvoxamine
Terfenadine contraindicated with mibefradil, ketoconazole, erythromycin, clarithromycin, troleandomycin
Thioridazine contraindicated with CYP2D6 inhibitors
Ritonavir contraindicated with triazolam, zolpidem, astemizole, rifabutin, quinine, clarithromycin, troleandomycin
Mibefradil contraindicated with astemizole
Nelfinavir contraindicated with rifabutin

\#\#Do not use with SSRIs, sumatriptan, lithium, meperidine, fentanyl, dextromethorphan, or pentazocine within 2 weeks of an MAOI.

References

Baker GB, Urichuk CJ, and Coutts RT, "Drug Metabolism and Metabolic Drug-Drug Interactions in Psychiatry," *Child Adolescent Psychopharm News (Suppl).*
DeVane CL, "Pharmacogenetics and Drug Metabolism of Newer Antidepressant Agents," *J Clin Psychiatry,* 1994, 55(Suppl 12):38-45.
Drug Interactions Analysis and Management. Cytochrome (CYP) 450 Isozyme Drug Interactions, Vancouver, WA: Applied Therapeutics, Inc, 523-7.
Ereshefsky L, "Drug-Drug Interactions Involving Antidepressants: Focus on Venlafaxine," *J Clin Psychopharmacol,* 1996, 16(3 Suppl 2):375-535.
Ereshefsky L, *Psychiatr Annal,* 1996, 26:342-50.
Fleishaker JC and Hulst LK, "A Pharmacokinetic and Pharmacodynamic Evaluation of the Combined Administration of Alprazolam and Fluvoxamine," *Eur J Clin Pharmacol,* 1994, 46(1):35-9.
Flockhart DA, et al, *Clin Pharmacol Ther,* 1996, 59:189.
Ketter TA, Flockhart DA, Post RM, et al, "The Emerging Role of Cytochrome P-450 3A in Psychopharmacology," *J Clin Psychopharmacol,* 1995, 15(6):387-98.
Michalets EL, "Update: Clinically Significant Cytochrome P-450 Drug Interactions," *Pharmacotherapy,* 1998, 18(1):84-112.
Nemeroff CB, DeVane CL, and Pollock BG, "Newer Antidepressants and the Cytochrome P450 System," *Am J Psychiatry,* 1996, 153(3):311-20.
Pollock BG, "Recent Developments in Drug Metabolism of Relevance to Psychiatrists," *Harv Rev Psychiatry,* 1994, 2(4):204-13.
Richelson E, "Pharmacokinetic Drug Interactions of New Antidepressants: A Review of the Effects on the Metabolism of Other Drugs," *Mayo Clin Proc,* 1997, 72(9):835-47.
Riesenman C, "Antidepressant Drug Interactions and the Cytochrome P450 System: A Critical Appraisal," *Pharmacotherapy,* 1995, 15(6 Pt 2):84S-99S.
Schmider J, Greenblatt DJ, von Moltke LL, et al, "Relationship of *In Vitro* Data on Drug Metabolism to *In Vivo* Pharmacokinetics and Drug Interactions: Implications for Diazepam Disposition in Humans," *J Clin Psychopharmacol,* 1996, 16(4):267-72.
Slaughter RL, *Pharm Times,* 1996, 7:6-16.
Watkins PB, "Role of Cytochrome P450 in Drug Metabolism and Hepatotoxicity," *Semin Liver Dis,* 1990, 10(4):235-50.

EXTRAVASATION TREATMENT

Medication Extravasated	Cold/Warm Pack	Antidote
Chemotherapeutic agents		
DNA Intercalators		

Amsacrine
  Daunorubicin
  Doxorubicin
	Cold	None

Vinca alkaloids		

Paclitaxel
  Vinblastine
  Vincristine
  Vindesine
  Vinorelbine
	Warm	Hyaluronidase (Wydase®)
		1. Add 1 mL NS to 150 units vial to make 150 units/mL concentration
		2. Administer 0.2 mL injection subcutaneously or intradermally into the extravasation site at the leading edge;
		Note: Some institutions utilize a 1:10 dilution in infants and children; prepare by mixing 0.1 mL of 150 units/mL solution with 0.9 mL NS in 1 mL syringe to make final concentration = 15 units/mL

Alkylating agents		

Cisplatin
  Mechlorethamine
  (Nitrogen mustard)
	Cold	Sodium thiosulfate
		1/6 molar solution: mix 4 mL of 10% sodium thiosulfate with 6 mL of sterile water; inject 2 mL for each mg mechlorethamine or 100 mg cisplatinum (use only for large cisplatinum infiltrates >20 mL and when using cisplatinum concentrations >0.5 mg/mL; no data for use in cisplatinum infusions in children)

Other vesicant chemotherapeutic agents	Cold	None
Vasopressors		
Dobutamine Dopamine Epinephrine Metaraminol Norepinephrine Phenylephrine	None	Phentolamine (Regitine®) Mix 5 mg with 9 mL of NS Inject a small amount of this dilution into extravasated area. Blanching should reverse immediately. Monitor site. If blanching should recur, additional injections of phentolamine may be needed.
I.V. fluids and other medications		
Nafcillin Calcium	Cold	Hyaluronidase (Wydase®) As described above

BURN MANAGEMENT

Modified Lund-Browder Burn Assessment Chart
Estimation of Total Body Surface Area of Burn Involvement*
(% by site and age)

Site†	0-1 years	1-4 years	5-9 years	10-14 years	15 years	Adult
Head	9.5	8.5	6.5	5.5	4.5	3.5
Neck	0.5	0.5	0.5	0.5	0.5	0.5
Trunk	13	13	13	13	13	13
Upper arm	2	2	2	2	2	2
Forearm	1.5	1.5	1.5	1.5	1.5	1.5
Hand	1.5	1.5	1.5	1.5	1.5	1.5
Perineum	1	1	1	1	1	1
Buttock (each)	2.5	2.5	2.5	2.5	2.5	2.5
Thigh	2.75	3.25	4	4.25	4.5	4.75
Leg	2.5	2.5	2.75	3	3.25	3.5
Foot	1.75	1.75	1.75	1.75	1.75	1.75

*Applies only to second- and third-degree burns

†Percentage for each site is only for **a single extremity with** anterior **OR** posterior involvement. Percentage should be **doubled if both anterior and posterior** involvement of a single extremity.

The total body surface area of burn involvement is determined by the sum of the percentages of each site.

Adapted from Coren CV, "Burn Injuries in Children," *Pediatric Annals*, 1987, 16(4):328-39.

Parkland Fluid Replacement Formula

A guideline for replacement of deficits and ongoing losses (**Note:** For infants, maintenance fluids may need to be added to this): Administer 4 mL/kg/% burn of Ringer's lactate (glucose may be added but beware of stress hyperglycemia) over the first 24 hours; half of this total is given over the first 8 hours **calculated from the time of injury**; the remaining half is given over the next 16 hours. The second 24-hour fluid requirements average 50% to 75% of first day's requirement. Concentrations and rates best determined by monitoring weight, serum electrolytes, urine output, NG losses, etc.

Colloid may be added after 18-24 hours (1 g/kg/day of albumin) to maintain serum albumin >2 g/100 mL.

Potassium is generally withheld for the first 48 hours due to the large amount of potassium that is released from damaged tissues. To manage serum electrolytes, monitor urine electrolytes twice weekly and replace calculated urine losses.

ORAL CONTRACEPTIVES

Brand Name	Type	Progestin	Estrogen	Availability
Brevicon® Genora®0.5/35 Modicon® Nelova®0.5/35E	Combo	Norethindrone 0.5 mg	Ethinyl estradiol 35 mcg	21, 28
Demulen®1/35	Combo	Ethynodiol diacetate 1 mg	Ethinyl estradiol 35 mcg	21, 28
Demulen®1/50	Combo	Ethynodiol diacetate 1 mg	Ethinyl estradiol 50 mcg	21, 28
Desogen®	Combo	Desogestrel 0.15 mg	Ethinyl estradiol 30 mcg	28
Jenest™-28	Biphasic			28
	1-7 d	Norethindrone 0.5 mg	Ethinyl estradiol 35 mcg	
	8-21 d	Norethindrone 1 mg	Ethinyl estradiol 35 mcg	
	22-28 d	Inert	—	
Lo/Ovral®	Combo	Norgestrel 0.3 mg	Ethinyl estradiol 30 mcg	21, 28
Loestrin 21®1.5/30	Combo	Norethindrone acetate 1.5 mg	Ethinyl estradiol 30 mcg	21
Loestrin® Fe 1.5/30	Combo/Iron 21-28 d	Norethindrone acetate 1.5 mg	Ethinyl estradiol 30 mcg	28
Loestrin 21® 1/20	Combo	Norethindrone acetate 1 mg	Ethinyl estradiol 20 mcg	21
Loestrin® Fe 1/20	Combo/Iron 21-28 d	Norethindrone acetate 1 mg	Ethinyl estradiol 20 mcg	28
Genora® 1/35 N.E.E.® 1/35 Nelova®1/35 E Norinyl®1+35 Ortho-Novum™1/35	Combo	Norethindrone 1 mg	Ethinyl estradiol 35 mcg	21, 28
Genora® 1/50 Nelova®1/50M Norethin® 1/50M Norinyl®1+50 Ortho-Novum™1/50	Combo	Norethindrone 1 mg	Mestranol 50 mcg	21, 28
Levlen® Levora® Nordette®	Combo	Levonorgestrel 0.15 mg	Ethinyl estradiol 20 mcg	21, 28
Micronor®	Progestin only	Norethindrone 0.35 mg	—	28
Norlestrin® 2.5/50	Combo	Norethindrone acetate 2.5 mg	Ethinyl estradiol 30 mcg	21
Nor-QD®	Progestin only	Norethindrone 0.35 mg	—	42
Ortho-Cept®	Combo	Desogestrel 0.15 mg	Ethinyl estradiol 30 mcg	21, 28
Ortho-Cyclen®	Combo	Norgestimate 0.25 mg	Ethinyl estradiol 35 mcg	21, 28
Nelova™ 10/11	Biphasic			21, 28
	1-10 d	Norethindrone 0.5 mg	Ethinyl estradiol 35 mcg	
	11-21 d	Norethindrone 1 mg	Ethinyl estradiol 35 mcg	
	22-28 d	Inert	—	
Ortho-Novum™10/11	Biphasic			21, 28
	1-10 d	Norethindrone 0.5 mg	Ethinyl estradiol 35 mcg	
	11-21 d	Norethindrone 1 mg	Ethinyl estradiol 35 mcg	
	22-28 d	Inert	—	
Ortho-Novum™ 7/7/7	Triphasic			21, 28
	1-7 d	Norethindrone 0.5 mg	Ethinyl estradiol 35 mcg	
	8-14 d	Norethindrone 0.75 mg	Ethinyl estradiol 35 mcg	
	15-21 d	Norethindrone 1 mg	Ethinyl estradiol 35 mcg	
	22-28 d	Inert	—	

ORAL CONTRACEPTIVES *(Continued)*

Brand Name	Type	Progestin	Estrogen	Availability
Ortho Tri-Cyclen®	Triphasic			
	1-7 d	Norgestimate 0.18 mg	Ethinyl estradiol 35 mcg	21, 28
	8-14 d	Norgestimate 0.215 mg	Ethinyl estradiol 35 mcg	
	15-21 d	Norgestimate 0.25 mg	Ethinyl estradiol 35 mcg	
	22-28 d	Inert	—	
Ovcon® 35	Combo	Norethindrone 0.4 mg	Ethinyl estradiol 35 mcg	21, 28
Ovcon® 50	Combo	Norethindrone 1 mg	Ethinyl estradiol 50 mcg	21, 28
Ovral®	Combo	Norgestrel 0.5 mg	Ethinyl estradiol 50 mcg	21, 28
Ovrette®	Progestin only	Norgestrel 0.075 mg	—	28
Tri-Norinyl®	Triphasic			
	1-7 d	Norethindrone 0.5 mg	Ethinyl estradiol 35 mcg	21, 28
	8-16 d	Norethindrone 1 mg	Ethinyl estradiol 35 mcg	
	17-21 d	Norethindrone 0.5 mg	Ethinyl estradiol 35 mcg	
	22- 28 d	Inert	—	
Tri-Phasil® Tri-Levlen®	Triphasic			
	1-6 d	Levonorgestrel 0.05 mg	Ethinyl estradiol 30 mcg	21, 28
	7-11 d	Levonorgestrel 0.075 mg	Ethinyl estradiol 40 mcg	
	12-21 d	Levonorgestrel 0.125 mg	Ethinyl estradiol 30 mcg	
	22- 28 d	Inert	—	

Combo = Monophasic combination

Monophasic Oral Contraceptives
In Order of Decreasing Estrogen Content

Estrogen	Brand Name (Progestin Content)
Mestranol 50 mcg	Genora®1/50, Nelova®1/50M, Norethin®1/50M, Norinyl®1+50, Ortho-Novum®1/50 **(Norethindrone 1 mg)**
Ethinyl estradiol 50 mcg	Ovcon®-50 **(Norethindrone 1 mg)**
	Demulen ®1/50 **(Ethynodiol diacetate 1 mg)**
	Ovral® **(Norgestrel 0.5 mg)**
Ethinyl estradiol 35 mcg	Genora ®1/35, N.E.E ®1/35, Nelova®1/35E, Norethin®1/35E, Norinyl®1+35, Ortho-Novum®1/35 **(Norethindrone 1 mg)**
	Brevicon ®, Genora ®0.5/35, Modicon®, Nelova ®0.5/35E **(Norethindrone 0.5 mg)**
	Ovcon®-35 **(Norethindrone 0.4 mg)**
	Ortho-Cyclen® **(Norgestimate 0.25 mg)**
	Demulen® 1/35 **(Ethynodiol diacetate 1 mg)**
Ethinyl estradiol 30 mcg	Loestrin 21® 1.5/30, Loestrin®Fe 1.5/30 **(Norethindrone acetate 1.5 mg)**
	Lo/Ovral® **(Norgestrel 0.3 mg)**
	Desogen®, Ortho-Cept® **(Desogestrel 0.15 mg)**
Ethinyl estradiol 20 mcg	Levlen®, Levora®, Nordette® **(Levonorgestrel 0.15 mg)**
	Loestrin 21® 1/20, Loestrin®Fe 1/20 **(Norethindrone acetate 1 mg)**

Hormonal Effects of Progestins

	Progestin Effect	Estrogen Effect	Antiestrogen Effect	Androgen Effect
Norethynodrel	+1	+3	0	0
Norethindrone	+1	+1 (Low dose)	+1 (Higher doses)	+2
Norethindrone acetate	+1	+1	+3	+2
Ethynodiol diacetate	+2	+1 (Low dose)	+1 (Higher doses)	+2
Norgestimate	+3	0	+3	0
Desogestrel	+3	0/+1	+3	0/+1
Norgestrel/ levonorgestrel	+3	0	+2	+3

0=No effect; +1=Slight effect; +2=Moderate effect; +3=Pronounced effect

Adapted from *Facts and Comparisons*, St Louis, MO; Facts and Comparisons, Inc, 1996.

Signs/Symptoms of Hormonal Imbalance With Oral Contraceptives

Estrogen Excess	Fluid retention, edema, cyclic weight gain, "bloating," hypertension, breast fullness/tenderness, nausea, migraine headache, melasma, telangiectasia, cervical mucorrhea, and polyposis
Estrogen Deficiency	Increased spotting, early or midcycle breakthrough bleeding, hypomenorrhea
Progestin Excess	Fatigue, lethargy, depression, decreased libido, increased appetite, weight gain, breast regression, monilial vaginitis, hypomenorrhea, hair loss, hirsutism, acne, oily scalp. **Note:** Hair loss, hirsutism, acne, and oily scalp are effects of the androgenic activity of progestins.
Progestin Deficiency	Amenorrhea, late breakthrough bleeding, hypermenorrhea

FLUIDS, ELECTROLYTES, & NUTRITION

ENTERAL NUTRITIONAL PRODUCT FORMULARY, INFANTS

Milk Based Formulas*
(Indications: Feeding normal term infants or sick infants without special nutritional requirements)

	Human Milk	Enfamil® With Iron	Similac® With Iron
Calories /100 mL	67	67.6	67.6
Protein g/100 mL	1.0	1.42	1.45
Protein source	Mature Term human milk	60% whey 40% casein	Nonfat milk
Carbohydrate g/100 mL	6.8	7.4	7.23
Carbohydrate source	Lactose	Lactose	Lactose
Fat g/100 mL	4.0	3.6	3.65
Fat source	Human milk, fat	45% palm oil† 20% coconut oil 20% soy oil 15% high oleic sunflower oil	Soy and coconut oils§
Osmolality mOsm/kg	300	300	300
Sodium mEq/L (mg/L)	7.8 (180)	8 (183)	8.0 (183)
Potassium mEq/L (mg/L)	13.5 (525)	18.7 (730)	18.2 (710)
Chloride mEq/L (mg/L)	11.9 (420)	12 (426)	12.2 (433)
Calcium mEq/L (mg/L)	14 (280)	26.4 (528)	24.6 (492)
Phosphorus mEq/L (mg/L)	9 (140)	20.5 (358)	25.2 (380)
Iron mg/L	0.3	12.2 (4.7)¶	12.2 (1.49)¶

*Information based on manufacturer's literature as of 1999 and is subject to change.

†Enfamil® with iron powder: 45% corn oil, 55% coconut oil.

§Similac® with iron powder: coconut and corn oil.

¶Low iron formulation in parenthesis.

Hypercaloric Milk Based Formulas – 24*†
(Indications: Fluid restriction, increased caloric demands)

	Enfamil® 24	Similac® 24
Calories /100 mL	81.1	81.2
Protein g/100 mL	1.8	2.2
Protein source	Nonfat milk and whey	Nonfat milk
Carbohydrate g/100 mL	8.3	8.53
Carbohydrate source	Lactose	Lactose
Fat g/100 mL	4.5	4.28
Fat source	45% palm oil 20% coconut oil 20% soy oil 15% high oleic sunflower oil	Soy and coconut oils
Osmolality mOsm/kg	360	380
Sodium mEq/L (mg/L)	9.6 (220)	12.2 (280)
Potassium mEq/L (mg/L)	22.3 (870)	27.4 (1070)
Chloride mEq/L (mg/L)	14.4 (510)	18.6 (660)
Calcium mEq/L (mg/L)	31.4 (628)	36.4 (730)
Phosphorus mEq/L (mg/L)	27.6 (427)	36.8 (570)
Iron mg/L	14.6 (5.7)¶	15 (14.5)¶

*Information based on manufacturer's literature as of 1999 and is subject to change; 24 calories/oz

†To approximate values for the content of a 30 cal/oz formula (made by dilution of a powder formulation) multiply the value desired, found in a 20 cal/oz formula, by 1.5 (20 cal/oz formula contents for Enfamil® and Similac® are listed in preceding Milk Based Formula chart). For example, the fat in a 30 cal/oz Enfamil® formula = 1.5 x 3.6 = 5.4 g/100 mL.

¶Low iron formulation in parentheses

FLUIDS, ELECTROLYTES, & NUTRITION *(Continued)*

Soy Formulas*
(Indications: Lactose deficiency, milk intolerance, or galactosemia)

	Prosobee®	Isomil®
Calories /100 mL	67.6	67.6
Protein g/100 mL	2	1.8
Protein source	Soy protein isolate	Soy protein isolate
Carbohydrate g/100 mL	6.8	6.83
Carbohydrate source	Corn syrup solids	Corn syrup and sucrose
Fat g/100 mL	3.6	3.69
Fat source	45% palm oil† 20% coconut oil 20% soy oil 15% high oleic sunflower oil	Soy and coconut oils
Osmolality mOsm/kg	200	230
Sodium mEq/L (mg/L)	10.6 (243)	13 (300)
Potassium mEq/L (mg/L)	21 (825)	18.7 (730)
Chloride mEq/L (mg/L)	15.3 (561)	11.9 (420)
Calcium mEq (mg/L)	31.8 (636)	35.5 (710)
Phosphorus mEq/L (mg/L)	32.4 (500)	32.9 (510)
Iron mg/L	12.8	12

*Information based on manufacturer's literature as of 1999 and is subject to change.

†Prosobee® powder: 45% corn oil, 55% coconut oil.

Hypercaloric Soy Formulas – 24*†
(Indications: Fluid restriction, increased caloric demands)

	Prosobee® 24
Calories /100 mL	81.1
Protein g/100 mL	2.4
Protein source	Soy protein isolate
Carbohydrate g/100 mL	8.2
Carbohydrate source	Corn syrup solids
Fat g/100 mL	4.3
Fat source	45% palm oil 20% coconut oil 20% soy oil 15% high oleic sunflower oil
Osmolality mOsm/kg	240
Sodium mEq/L (mg/L)	12.7 (292)
Potassium mEq/L (mg/L)	25.2 (990)
Chloride mEq/L (mg/L)	19 (672)
Calcium mEq/L (mg/L)	38 (761)
Phosphorus mEq/L (mg/L)	38.9 (602)
Iron mg/L	15.2

*Information based on manufacturer's literature as of 1999 and is subject to change.

†To approximate values for the content of a 27 or 30 cal/oz formula (made by dilution of a powder based formulation), multiply the value desired, found in the 20 cal/oz formula (20 cal/oz formula contents for Prosobee® are listed in the preceding Soy Formulas chart), by the following factors: 1.35 (27 cal/oz) or 1.5 (30 cal/oz).

FLUIDS, ELECTROLYTES, & NUTRITION *(Continued)*

Casein Hydrolysate Formulas*
(Indications: For infants whose renal or cardiovascular functions would benefit from lowered mineral levels)

	Similac® PM 60/40
Calories /100 mL	67.6
Protein g/100 mL	1.58
Protein source	Whey and caseinate
Carbohydrate g/100 mL	6.9
Carbohydrate source	Lactose
Fat g/100 mL	3.78
Fat source	Soy and coconut oils†
Osmolality mOsm/kg	280
Sodium mEq/L (mg/L)	7 (160)
Potassium mEq/L (mg/L)	14.9 (580)
Chloride mEq/L (mg/L)	11.3 (400)
Calcium mEq/L (mg/L)	19 (380)
Phosphorus mEq/L (mg/L)	12.3 (190)
Iron mg/L	1.5
Special uses	Renal and cardiovascular disease

*Information based on manufacturer's literature as of 1999 and is subject to change.

†Similac® PM 60/40 powder: corn and coconut oil.

Casein Hydrolysate Formulas*
(Indications: For infants requiring low molecular weight peptides or amino acids)

	Nutramigen®	Pregestimil®
Calories /100 mL	67.6	68
Protein g/100 mL	1.9	1.9
Protein source	Casein hydrolysate, L-cystine, L-tyrosine, and L-tryptophan	Casein hydrolysate, L-cystine, L-tyrosine, and L-tryptophan
Carbohydrate g/100 mL	7.4	6.8
Carbohydrate source	Corn syrup solids and modified corn starch	Corn syrup solids, dextrose, and modified corn starch
Fat g/100 mL	3.4	3.8
Fat source	Palm olein, soy, coconut, high-oleic sunflower oils	60% MCT oil 20% corn oil 20% high oleic sunflower oil
Osmolality mOsm/kg	320	320
Sodium mEq/L (mg/L)	13.8 (318)	11.5 (264)
Potassium mEq/L (mg/L)	19 (744)	18.9 (737)
Chloride mEq/L (mg/L)	16.4 (582)	16.4 (581)
Calcium mEq/L (mg/L)	31.8 (636)	31.8 (636)
Phosphorus mEq/L (mg/L)	27.3 (426)	27.3 (423)
Iron mg/L	12.2	12.8
Special uses	Sensitivity to intact proteins, galactosemia	Malabsorption, cystic fibrosis

*Information based on manufacturer's literature as of 1999 and is subject to change.

To approximate values for the content of a 24, 27, or 30 cal/oz formula (made by dilution of a powder based formulation), multiply the value desired, found in the above 20 cal/oz formula, by the following factors: 1.2 (24 cal/oz), 1.35 (27 cal/oz), or 1.5 (30 cal/oz).

Other Infant and Pediatric Formulas* – Special Care
(Indications: Premature infant formulas designed for rapidly growing LBW infants)

	Human Milk Fortifier	Special Care 20 With Fe	Special Care 24 With Fe	Neosure
Calories /100 mL	80.6	67.6	81.2	74.6
Protein g/100 mL	2.2	1.83	2.2	2
Protein source	Nonfat milk and whey protein concentrate	Nonfat milk and whey protein concentrate	Nonfat milk and whey protein concentrate	Nonfat milk and whey protein concentrate
Carbohydrate g/100 mL	8.55	7.17	8.61	7.7
Carbohydrate source	Corn syrup solids and lactose	Hydrolyzed cornstarch and lactose	Hydrolyzed cornstarch and lactose	Corn syrup solids and lactose
Fat g/100 mL	4.37	3.67	4.41	4
Fat source	Medium chain triglycerides and coconut oils	Medium chain triglycerides, soy, and coconut oils	Medium chain triglycerides, soy, and coconut oils	Medium chain triglycerides, soy, and coconut oils
Osmolality mOsm/kg	280	210	252	250
Sodium mEq/L (mg/L)	15.3 (350)	12.6 (290)	15.2 (350)	10.4 (246)
Potassium mEq/L (mg/L)	26.6 (1040)	22.3 (870)	26.9 (1050)	27 (1060)
Chloride mEq/L (mg/L)	18.6 (660)	15.5 (550)	18.6 (660)	15.7 (560)
Calcium mEq/L (mg/L)	84.7 (1694)	60.8 (1220)	72.8 (1460)	39 (784)
Phosphorus mEq/L (mg/L)	60.2 (935)	39.4 (610)	47 (730)	29.6 (460)
Iron mg/L	3	12.2 (2.5)†	14.6 (3.0)†	13.4

*Information based on manufacturer's literature as of 1999 and is subject to change.
†Low iron formulation in parentheses.

ENTERAL FORMULAS – PEDIATRIC

(A selection of the commonly used enteral feedings for children 1-10 years of age)

	Pediasure®	Peptamen Junior®	Vivonex® Pediatric	Boost®	Carnation Instant Breakfast®*	Ensure®	Ensure® HN	Sustacal® Liquid
Calories/oz	30	30	24	30	28	30	30	30
Calories/mL	1.06	1.06	0.8	1.01	0.94	1.06	1.06	1.0
Carbohydrate g/100 mL	11	13.8	12.6	17.4	14.6	14	14	14.0
Carbohydrate source	Corn syrup solids, sucrose	Maltodextrin, corn starch	Maltodextrin, modified starch	Sucrose, corn syrup solids	Maltodextrin, sucrose, lactose	Corn syrup solids, sucrose	Corn syrup solids, sucrose	Corn syrup solids, sucrose
Protein g/100 mL	3.0	3.0	2.4	4.3	4.5	3.7	4.4	6.1
Protein source	Caseinate, whey protein conc	Hydrolyzed whey protein	L-amino acids	Milk protein conc	Nonfat milk	Caseinates, soy protein isolate	Caseinates, soy protein isolate	Casein, soy protein isolate
Fat g/100 mL	5.0	3.8	2.4	1.7	1.9	3.7	3.5	2.3
Fat source	High-oleic safflower, soy, and MCT oils	MCT, soy, and canola oils	MCT and soy solids	Canola, sunflower, and corn oils	Butterfat	Corn oil	Corn oil	Partially hydrogenated soy oil
Osmolality mOsm/kg	310	260 unflavored 360 vanilla	360	590-620	661-747	470	470	650
Sodium mg/100 mL (mEq/100 mL)	38 (1.7)	46 (2)	40 (1.7)	55 (2.4)	90 (3.9)	83 (3.6)	79.1 (3.4)	93 (4.0)
Potassium mg/100 mL (mEq/100 mL)	131 (3.4)	132 (3.4)	120 (3.1)	169 (4.3)	250 (6.4)	154 (3.9)	154 (3.9)	204 (5.2)
Iron (mg/100 mL)	1.4	1.4	1.0	–	–	–	–	–

*Mixed with 2% milk as directed.

FLUIDS, ELECTROLYTES, & NUTRITION *(Continued)*

ENTERAL FORMULAS – ADOLESCENTS, ADULTS

	Isocal®	Osmolite®	Osmolite HN®	Jevity®*
Calories/mL	1.06	1.06 ·	1.06	1.06
Carbohydrate g/100 mL	13.5	15.1	14.4	15.0
Carbohydrate source	Maltodextrin	Corn syrup solids	Corn syrup solids	Corn syrup solids
Protein g/100 mL	3.4	3.7	4.4	4.4
Protein source	Caseinate, soy protein isolate	Caseinate, soy protein isolate	Caseinate, soy protein isolate	Caseinates
Fat g/100 mL	4.4	3.5	3.5	3.5
Fat source	Soy oil, MCT oil	High-oleic safflower, canola, and MCT oils	High-oleic safflower, canola, and MCT oils	High-oleic safflower, canola, and MCT oils
Osmolality mOsm/kg	270	300	300	300
Sodium mg/100 mL (mEq/100 mL)	53 (2.3)	63 (2.7)	92 (4.0)	91.6 (4.0)
Potassium mg/100 mL (mEq/100 mL)	132 (3.4)	100 (2.6)	154 (3.9)	154 (3.9)

*Contains 13.6 g/L soy fiber.

ENTERAL FORMULAS WITH HIGH CALORIC DENSITY

	Ensure Plus®	Ensure Plus HN®	Sustacal Plus®	Sustagen®	TraumaCal®
Calories/mL	1.5	1.5	1.5	1.9	1.5
Carbohydrate g/100 mL	20	20	19	31.6	14.5
Carbohydrate source	Corn syrup solids, sucrose	Corn syrup solids, sucrose	Corn syrup solids, sucrose	Corn syrup solids, lactose, dextrose	Corn syrup solids, sucrose
Protein g/100 mL	5.4	6.2	6.1	11.5	8.3
Protein source	Caseinate, soy protein isolate	Caseinate, soy protein isolate	Caseinates	Cow's milk, caseinates	Caseinates
Fat g/100 mL	5.3	5.0	5.8	1.7	6.8
Fat source	Corn oil	Corn oil	Corn oil	Butterfat	Soy oil, MCT oil
Osmolality mOsm/kg	690	650	630	1130	490
Sodium mg/100 mL (mEq/100 mL)	104 (4.5)	117 (5.1)	85 (3.7)	92 (4.0)	120 (5.2)
Potassium mg/100 mL (mEq/100 mL)	192 (4.9)	179 (4.6)	148 (3.8)	296 (7.6)	140 (3.6)

ENTERAL FORMULAS WITH MODIFIED PROTEIN – "ELEMENTAL"
Adolescents and Adults

	Criticare HN®	Peptamen®	Tolerex®	Vivonex Plus®
Calories/mL	1.06	1.0	1.0	1.0
Carbohydrate g/100 mL	22	12.7	22.6	19.0
Carbohydrate source	Maltodextrin, modified corn starch	Maltodextrin, corn starch	Maltodextrin	Maltodextrin, modified starch
Protein g/100 mL	3.8	4.0	2.1	4.5
Protein source	Hydrolyzed casein, L-amino acids	Hydrolyzed whey	L-amino acids	L-amino acids
Fat g/100 mL	0.53	3.9	0.1	0.7
Fat source	Safflower oil	Sunflower and MCT oils	Safflower oil	Soy oil
Osmolality mOsm/kg	650	270 unflavored 380 vanilla	550 unflavored 617-678 flavored	650
Sodium mg/100 mL (mEq/100 mL)	63 (2.7)	50 (2.2)	46 (2.0)	61 (2.7)
Potassium mg/100 mL (mEq/100 mL)	132 (3.4)	125 (3.2)	117 (3.0)	110 (2.8)

FLUIDS, ELECTROLYTES, & NUTRITION *(Continued)*

Nutritional Modules*

	Polycose® Liquid	Polycose® Powder	Promod® Powder†
Indication	Carbohydrate additive for use as a caloric supplement which is readily mixable in most foods, enteral formulas or beverages without appreciably altering their taste	Carbohydrate additive for use as a caloric supplement which is readily mixable in most foods, enteral formulas or beverages without appreciably altering their taste	Protein supplement which mixes readily in enteral formulas, most foods, or beverages without appreciably altering their taste
Calories	2/mL	3.8/g‡	4.2/g
Protein (g)	—	—	0.76/g
Protein source	—	—	Whey protein concentrate
Carbohydrate (g)	0.5/mL	0.94/g	<0.1/g
Carbohydrate source	Glucose polymers	Glucose polymers	Lactose
Fat (g)	—	—	<0.09/g
Fat source	—	—	Soy lecithin
Osmolality mOsm/kg	900	900 in solution	—
Sodium mEq/L (mg/L)	<0.03/mL (<0.7/mL)	<0.05/g (<1.1/g)	<0.099/g (<2.3/g)
Potassium mEq/L (mg/L)	<0.002/mL (<0.06/mL)	<0.003/g (<0.1/g)	<0.25/g (<9.85/g)
Chloride mEq/L (mg/L)	<0.04/mL (<1.4/mL)	<0.06/g (<2.23/g)	—
Calcium mEq/L (mg/L)	<0.01/mL (<0.2/mL)	<0.02/g (<0.3/g)	<0.33/g (<6.67/g)
Phosphorus mEq/L (mg/L)	(<0.03/mL)	(<0.05/g)	(<5/g)
Iron mg/L	—	—	—

*These products are not complete formulations and should not be used as a sole source of nutrition.

†1 scoop = 6.6 g, 1 tsp = 1.3 g, 1 tbsp = 4 g.

‡1 tsp (2 g) = 8 calories, 1 tbsp (6 g) = 23 calories, ¼ cup (24 g) = 95 calories.

Nutritional Modules*

	Vegetable Oil†	Microlipid®	MCT Oil®‡	Whole Milk
Indications	Inexpensive fat source for calories and essential fatty acids	50% fat emulsion for use as a source of calories or essential fatty acids; it mixes easily and stays in emulsion	Fat supplement for use for patients who cannot efficiently digest and absorb long-chain fats	
Calories	8/mL	4.5/mL	7.67/mL	157/8 oz
Protein (g)	—	—	—	8/8 oz
Protein source	—	—	—	82% casein, 18% whey
Carbohydrate (g)	—	—	—	11/8 oz
Carbohydrate source	—	—	—	Lactose
Fat (g)	0.93/mL	0.5/mL•	0.93/mL	8.9/8 oz
Fat source	Corn, soybean, sunflower or safflower oils♦	Safflower oil, polyglycerol esters, soy lecithin	Lipid fraction of coconut oil (consists primarily of C_8 and C_{10} saturated fatty acids)	Butter fat
Osmolality mOsm/kg	—	60	—	288
Sodium mEq/L (mg/L)	—	—	—	5.3/8 oz (122/8 oz)
Potassium mEq/L (mg/L)	—	—	—	9/8 oz (351/8 oz)
Chloride mEq/L (mg/L)	—	—	—	7/8 oz (247/8 oz)
Calcium mEq/L (mg/L)	—	—	—	14.4/8 oz (288/8 oz)
Phosphorus mEq/L (mg/L)	—	—	—	14.6/8 oz (227/8 oz)
Iron mg/L	—	—	—	0.12/8 oz

*These products are not complete formulations and should not be used as a sole source of nutrition.

†1 tbsp = 14 g.

‡Does not contain essential fatty acids.

•1 tbsp = 5.5 g linoleic.

♦% of linoleic from fat: soybean oil 51%, corn oil 58%, sunflower oil 65%, safflower oil 77%.

FLUID AND ELECTROLYTE REQUIREMENTS IN CHILDREN

Maintenance Fluids (Two methods)

Surface area method (most commonly used in children >10 kg): 1500-2000 mL/m^2/day

Body weight method

<10 kg	100 mL/kg/day
11-20 kg	1000 mL + 50 mL/kg (for each kg >10)
>20 kg	1500 mL + 20 mL/kg (for each kg >20)

Maintenance Electrolytes (See specific electrolyte in Alphabetical Listing of Drugs for more detailed information)

Sodium: 3-4 mEq/kg/day **or** 30-50 mEq/m^2/day
Potassium: 2-3 mEq/kg/day **or** 20-40 mEq/m^2/day

Dehydration Fluid Therapy

Goals of therapy:

- Restore circulatory volume to prevent shock (10% to 15% dehydration)
- Restore combined intracellular and extracellular deficits of water and electrolytes within 24 hours
- Maintain adequate water and electrolytes
- Resolve homeostatic distortions (eg, acidosis)
- Replace ongoing losses

Analysis of the Severity of Dehydration by Physical Signs

Clinical Sign	Mild*	Moderate*	Severe*
Pre-illness body weight	5% loss	10% loss	15% loss
Skin turgor	↓	Tenting	Tenting
Mucous membranes	Dry	Very dry	Parched
Skin color	Pale	Grey	Mottled
Urine output	↓	↓↓	Azotemic
Blood pressure	Normal	Normal, ↓	↓↓
Heart rate	Normal, ↑	↑	↑↑
Fontanelle (<7 mo)	Flat	Soft	Sunken
CNS	Consolable	Irritable	Lethargic/coma

*Postpubertal children and adults experience the same symptoms with mild, moderate, and severe dehydration associated with 3%, 6%, and 9% losses in body weight respectively.

Restoration of Circulatory Volume (10% to 15% dehydration estimate)

Fluid boluses of 20 mL/kg using crystalloid (eg, normal saline) or 10 mL/kg colloid (eg, 5% albumin) administered as rapidly as possible; repeat until improved circulation (eg, warm skin, decreased heart rate (towards normal), improved capillary refill time, urine output restored).

Classification of Dehydration (based upon the serum sodium concentration)

Isotonic	130-150 mEq/L
Hypotonic	<130 mEq/L
Hypertonic	>150 mEq/L

Estimated Water & Electrolyte Deficits in Dehydration
(moderate to severe)

Type of Dehydration	Water (mL/kg)	Na+ (mEq/kg)	K+ (mEq/kg)	Cl⁻ and HCO₃⁻ (mEq/kg)
Isotonic	100-150	8-10	8-10	16-20
Hypotonic	50-100	10-14	10-14	20-28
Hypertonic	120-180	2-5	2-5	4-10

Current Pediatric Diagnosis & Treatment, 10th ed, 1991.

Water deficit may also be calculated (in isotonic dehydration):

$$\text{Water deficit (mL)} = \frac{\% \text{ dehydration x wt (kg) x 1000 g/kg}}{100}$$

Assessment of Water Loss in Relation to Serum Na⁺ Concentrations
Degree of Dehydration as % Body Weight

Serum Na⁺	Mild	Moderate	Severe
Isotonic	5%	10%	15%
Hypotonic (Na⁺< 130)	4%	6%	8%
Hypertonic (Na⁺ >150)	7%	12%	17%

Example of Fluid Replacement
(assume 10 kg infant with 10% isotonic dehydration)

	Water	Sodium (mEq)	Potassium (mEq)
Maintenance	1000 mL	40	20
Deficit*	1000 mL	80	80
Total	2000 mL	120	100

*Reduce this total by any fluid boluses given initially.

First 8 hours: Replace $\frac{1}{3}$ maintenance water   = 330 mL

Replace $\frac{1}{2}$ deficit water = 500 mL

Total   830 mL/8 h = 103 mL/h

Replace $\frac{1}{2}$ of Na⁺ & K⁺ = 60 mEq sodium/803 mL; 50 mEq potassium/803 mL (It is suggested that the maximum potassium initially used is 40 mEq/L and is **not** started until urine output has been established.)

The actual order would appear as: $D_5\frac{1}{2}NS$ at 103 mL/hour for 8 hours; add 40 mEq/L KCl after patient voids.

Second 16 hours: Replace $\frac{2}{3}$ maintenance water = 670 mL

Replace $\frac{1}{2}$ deficit water = 500 mL

Total   1260 mL/16 h = 79 mL/h

Replace remainder of sodium and potassium.

The actual order would appear as: $D_5\frac{1}{3}NS$ with KCl 40 mEq/L at 79 mL/hour for 16 hours. (Use of $\frac{1}{4}NS$ may be more desirable for convenience.)

FLUID AND ELECTROLYTE REQUIREMENTS IN CHILDREN *(Continued)*

Analysis of Ongoing Losses

Electrolyte Composition of Biological Fluids (mEq/L)

Fluid Type	Sodium	Potassium	Chloride	Total HCO_3^-
Stomach	20-120	5-25	90-160	0-5
Duodenal drainage	20-140	3-30	30-120	10-50
Biliary tract	120-160	3-12	70-130	30-50
Small intestine Initial drainage	100-140	4-40	60-100	30-100
Small intestine Established drainage	4-20	4-10	10-100	40-120
Pancreatic	110-160	4-15	30-80	70-130
Diarrheal stool	10-25	10-30	30-120	10-50

Current Pediatric Diagnosis & Treatment, 9th ed, Appleton & Lange, 1987.

Because of the wide range of normal values, specific analyses are suggested in individual cases.

Alterations of Maintenance Fluid Requirements

Fever	Increase maintenance fluids by 12% per degree centigrade above 37°C (eg, do **not** correct for 38°C, but increase fluids by 24% for fever of 39°C)
Hyperventilation	Increase maintenance fluids by 10-60 mL/100 kcal BEE (basal energy expenditure)
Sweating	Increase maintenance fluids by 10-25 mL/100 kcal BEE (basal energy expenditure)
Hyperthyroidism	Variable increase in maintenance fluids: 25%-50%
GI loss and renal disease	Monitor and analyze output; adjust therapy accordingly
Renal failure	Maintenance fluids are equal to insensible losses (300 mL/m^3) + urine replacement (mL for mL)

Oral Rehydration

Due to the high worldwide incidence of dehydration from infantile diarrhea, effective, inexpensive oral rehydration solutions have been developed. In the U.S., a typical effective solution for rehydration contains 50-60 mEq/L sodium, 20-30 mEq/L potassium, 30 mEq/L bicarbonate or its equivalent, and sufficient chloride to provide electroneutrality. Two percent to 3% glucose facilitates electrolyte absorption and short-term calories. The following table describes the electrolyte/sugar content of commonly used oral rehydration solutions.

Composition of Frequently Used Oral Electrolyte Replacement Solutions

Solutions	% CHO	Na$^+$ (mEq/L)	K$^+$ (mEq/L)	Cl$^-$ (mEq/L)	HCO$^-$ (mEq/L)
Normal saline		154		154	
Ringer's lactate		130	4	109	28
Dextrose 5% in 0.25% NaCl	5% glucose	38		38	
WHO solution	2% glucose or 4% sucrose	90	20	80	30 citrate
WHO solution, modified	2% glucose	55	25	30	50
Rehydralyte®	2.5% glucose	75	20	65	30 citrate
Ricelyte®	3% carbohydrate	50	25	45	34 citrate
Resol®	2% glucose	50	20	50	34 citrate
Rice water	2.5% carbohydrate	90	20	30	80
Pedialyte® (Ross)	2.5% glucose	45	20	35	30 citrate
Infalyte® (Penwalt)	3% glucose	50	25	45	34
Gatorade®	2.6% glucose, 2% fructose	23.5	<1	17	
Apple juice	3.2% glucose, 1.3% sucrose, 7.5% fructose	<1	25		
Orange juice 1:3 (dilution with water)	1% glucose, 1.2% fructose	<1	50		50 citrate
Grape juice	1.6% glucose, 2.1% fructose	0.2-0.7	8-11		8
One package cherry gelatin dissolved in 4 cups water		24	Needs added K$^+$		
Coca-Cola®		1.6	<1		13.4 citrate
Pepsi-Coal®		6.5	0.8		
Beef broth		120	10		
Chicken broth		250	8		

Adapted from Aranda-Michel, J and Giannella RA, "Acute Diarrhea" A Practical Review," *Am J of Med,* 1999, 106:670-6.

PARENTERAL NUTRITION (PN)

The following information is intended as a brief overview of the use of parenteral nutrition in infants and children.

General Indications for Use

Parenteral nutrition is the provision of required nutrients by the intravenous route to replenish, optimize, or maintain nutritional status.

Specific Indications

Parenteral nutrition of **all** required nutrients (total parenteral nutrition) is indicated in patients for whom it is expected that it would be impossible or dangerous to enterally administer nutrition. Parenteral nutrition in combination with enteral nutrition is indicated in patients who are expected to be unable to meet their nutritional needs by the enteral route alone within 5 days.

1. Patients with an inability to absorb nutrients via the gastrointestinal tract which may include the following: severe diarrhea, short bowel syndrome, developmental anomalies of the GI tract, inflammatory bowel disease, cystic fibrosis, or anatomic or functional loss of GI integrity.

2. Severe malnutrition.

3. Severe catabolic states such as: burns, trauma, or sepsis.

4. Patients undergoing high dose chemotherapy, radiation, and bone marrow transplantation.

5. Patients whose clinical condition may necessitate complete bowel rest (eg, necrotizing enterocolitis, pancreatitis, GI fistulas, or recent GI surgery).

6. Intensive care low-birth-weight infants.

7. Neonatal asphyxia.

8. Meconium ileus.

9. Respiratory distress syndrome (RDS).

Nutritional Assessment

As many as 33% of hospitalized pediatric patients are malnourished and require nutritional therapy. The type of nutritional support indicated depends on the underlying disease, the degree of gastrointestinal function, and the severity of malnutrition. Acutely malnourished patients have an increased risk for serious infection, postoperative complications, and death. Indicators of acute protein-calorie malnutrition include low weight for height, low serum albumin, lymphopenia, decreased body fat folds, and decreased arm muscle area. Nutritional screening may be done by the dietitian. Those patients who are at nutritional risk should receive a complete nutritional assessment.

Nutritional Requirements

Approximate requirements for energy and protein at various ages for normal subjects are listed in the first table at the end of this section. Patients who are severely malnourished or markedly catabolic may require higher levels to achieve catch-up growth or meet increased requirements. Patients who are well-nourished and/or inactive may require less.

During parenteral nutrition, 10% to 16% of calories should be in the form of amino acids to achieve optimal benefit (approximately 2-3 g/kg/day in infants and 1.5-2.5 g/kg/day ideal body weight in older patients). Exceptions include patients with renal or hepatic failure (where less protein is indicated), or in the treatment of severe trauma, head injury, or sepsis (where more protein may be indicated).

PN ORDERING

Fluid Intake

The patient should be given a total volume of fluid reasonable for his/her age and cardiovascular status. It is generally safe to start with the fluid maintenance level of 1500 mL/m^2/day in children. The fluid requirements in preterm infants are extremely variable due to much greater insensible water losses from radiant warmers and bili-lights. While the standard fluid maintenance of 100 mL/kg/day may be sufficient for term infants, intakes of up to 150 mL/kg/day may be necessary in the very low birth weight infants. Be sure to consider significant fluid intake from medications or other I.V. fluids and enteral diets in planning the fluids available for parenteral nutrition.

Dextrose

For central PN, dextrose is usually begun with a 10% to 12.5% solution or a solution providing dextrose at no more than 5 mg/kg/minute (in neonates and premature infants). The concentration is advanced, if tolerated, by 2.5% to 5% per day (2-2.5 mg/kg/minute increments in neonates and premature infants) to the desired caloric density, usually 20% to 25% dextrose. Fluid restricted patients often need 30% to 35% dextrose to meet their energy needs. For peripheral PN, 5% to 12.5% dextrose is utilized.

Dextrose calculations:

% Dextrose = Dextrose (g)/100 mL

Dextrose calorie value = 3.4 kcal/g

$$\text{Dextrose infusion rate (mg/kg/minute)} = \frac{\text{rate (mL/h) x \% dextrose x 0.166}}{\text{weight (kg)}}$$

$$\text{\% Dextrose desired*} = \frac{\text{desired rate (mg/kg/min) x weight (kg)}}{0.166 \text{ x rate (mL/h)}}$$

*Do not use dextrose concentrations <5% due to hypotonicity.

Amino Acids

Amino acids may be described as either a "standard" mixture of essential and nonessential amino acids or "specialized" mixtures. Specialized mixtures are intended for use in patients whose physiologic or metabolic needs may not be met with the "standard" amino acid compositions. Examples of specialized solutions include:

Trophamine®, Aminosyn® PF	Indicated for use in premature infants and young children due to addition of taurine, L-glutamic acid, L-aspartic acid, increased amounts of histidine, and reduction in amounts of methionine, alanine, phenylalanine, and glycine. Supplementation with a cysteine additive has been recommended.
Hepatamine®	Indicated for treatment in patients with hepatic encephalopathy due to cirrhosis or hepatitis or in patients with liver disease who are intolerant of standard amino acid solutions. Contains higher percentage of branched-chain amino acids and a lower percentage of aromatic amino acids than standard mixtures.
Nephramine®, Aminosyn® RF	Indicated for use in patients with compromised renal function who are intolerant of standard amino acid solutions. Contains a mixture of essential amino acids and histidine.

PARENTERAL NUTRITION (PN) *(Continued)*

Amino acid calculations:

% amino acid	=	amino acid (g)/100mL
Grams of protein	=	grams of nitrogen x 6.25
% amino acid desired	=	$\dfrac{\text{(g amino acid/kg) x weight (kg) x 100}}{\text{total PN fluid volume (mL)}}$

Fat Emulsion (FE)

There are three roles for intravenous fat in parenteral nutrition:

1. to provide nonprotein calories
2. to provide essential fatty acids and a "balanced" calorie source
3. to provide calories in catabolic patients with limited ability to excrete CO_2

The FE dosage is increased as tolerated daily (see General Guidelines for Initiation and Advancement for PN following). The maximum fat intake is 4 g/kg/day and no more than 60% of the total daily caloric intake. It is administered as a continuous infusion over 24 hours or at a rate no greater than 0.15-0.2 g/kg/hour via a Y-connector with the dextrose-amino acid I.V. line. In patients receiving cyclic PN, the FE should be administered over the duration of the PN infusion. The triglyceride concentration should be checked before the first infusion and daily as the dose is increased. Subsequently, it should be monitored at least weekly. Triglyceride concentrations should be maintained at <150 mg/dL in neonates, <350 mg/dL in renal patients, and <250 mg/dL in other patients. FE should be used cautiously in neonates with hyperbilirubinemia due to displacement of bilirubin from albumin by the free fatty acids. An increase in free bilirubin may increase the risk of kernicterus. Significant displacement occurs when the free fatty acid to serum albumin molar ratio (FFA/SA) >6. For example, infants with a total bilirubin >8-10 mg/dL (assuming an albumin concentration of 2.5-3 g/dL) should not receive more parenteral FE than required to meet the essential fatty acid requirement of 0.5-1 g/kg/day.

Note: Avoid use of 10% FE in preterm infants because a greater accumulation of plasma lipids occurs due to the greater phospholipid load of the 10% concentration.

Fat emulsion calculations:

20% FE = 20 g fat/100 mL = 2 kcal/mL

Desired 20% FE (mL)	=	$\dfrac{\text{(\% total kcal as fat) x (total kcal)}}{2\ \text{kcal/mL}}$

or as an alternative

Desired 20% FE (mL)	=	FE (g/kg) x weight (kg) x 5 mL/g

General Guidelines for Initiation and Advancement of PN*

Age	Initiation and Advancement	Dextrose	Protein (g/kg/ day)	Fat (g/kg/ day)
Premature infant	Initial	4-6 mg/kg/min	0.5-1.5	0.5
	Daily Increase	1-2.5 mg/kg/min	0.5-1	0.5
	Maximum	18 mg/kg/min	2.5-3	3
Term infant to 1 year	Initial	7-9 mg/kg/min	1-1.5	0.5-1
	Daily Increase	1-2.5 mg/kg/min	1	0.5-1
	Maximum	21 mg/kg/min	2.5-3	4
Children 1-10 years	Initial Dextrose Concentration	10% to 12.5%	1-1.5	1
	Daily Increase	5% increments	1	1
	Maximum	15 mg/kg/min	2-2.5	3
>10 years	Initial Dextrose Concentration	10% to 15%	1-1.5	1
	Daily Increase	5% increments	1	1
	Maximum	8.5 mg/kg/min *	1.5-2	3

*Rate of advancement may be limited by metabolic tolerance (eg, hyperglycemia, azotemia, hypertriglyceridemia)

Reference

National Advisory Group on Standards and Practice Guidelines for Parenteral Nutrition, "Safe Practices for Parenteral Nutrition Formulation," *JPEN*, 1998, 22(2):49-66.

MINERALS, TRACE ELEMENTS, AND VITAMINS

Guideline for Daily Electrolyte Requirements

	Neonates (mEq/kg)	Infants/Children (mEq/kg)	Adolescents
Sodium	2-5	2-6	60-150 mEq/d
Potassium	2-4	2-4	60-150 mEq/d
Calcium gluconate*	3-4	1-2.5	10-20 mEq/d
Magnesium	0.3-0.5	0.3-0.5	10-30 mEq/d
Phosphate*	1-2 mmol/kg	0.5-1 mmol/kg	10-40 mmol/d

*Calcium-phosphate stability in parenteral nutrition solutions is dependent upon the pH of the solution, temperature, and relative concentration of each ion. The pH of the solution is primarily dependent upon the amino acid concentration. The higher the percentage amino acids the lower the pH, the more soluble the calcium and phosphate. Individual commercially available amino acid solutions vary significantly with respect to pH lowering potential and consequent calcium phosphate compatibility. See the pharmacist for specific calcium phosphate stability information.

Vitamins

A pediatric parenteral multivitamin product is indicated for children <11 years of age. Children >11 years of age may receive adult multivitamin formulations.

Dosage:

Pediatric MVI:
Neonates: 2 mL/kg/d; maximum 5 mL/d
Infants and children ≤11 y: 5 mL
Children >11 y and adults: Use adult formulation 10 mL/d

PARENTERAL NUTRITION (PN) *(Continued)*

Trace Mineral Daily Requirements*

	Infants	Children (≥3 mo to ≤5 y)	Older Children and Adolescents
Chromium†	0.2 mcg/kg	0.14-0.2 mcg/kg (max: 5 mcg)	5-15 mcg
Copper‡	20 mcg/kg	20 mcg/kg (max: 300 mcg)	0.2-0.5 mg
Iodide§	1 mcg/kg	1 mcg/kg	1 mcg/kg
Manganese‡	1 mcg/kg	2-10 mcg/kg (max: 50 mcg)	50-150 mcg
Selenium†¶	2-3 mcg/kg	2-3 mcg/kg (max: 30 mcg)	30-40 mcg
Zinc	400 mcg/kg (preterm) 300 mcg/kg (term <3 mo)	100 mcg/kg (max: 5 mg)	2-5 mg

*Recommended intakes of trace elements cannot be achieved through the use of a single pediatric trace element produce. Only through the use of individualized trace element products can recommended intakes be achieved.

†Omit in patients with renal dysfunction.

‡Omit in patients with obstructive jaundice.

§Percutaneous absorption from protein-bound iodine may be adequate.

¶Indicated for use in long-term parenteral nutrition patients.

These are recommended daily trace mineral requirements. Additional supplementation may be indicated in clinical conditions resulting in excessive losses. For example, additional zinc may be needed in situations of excessive gastrointestinal losses.

Developing the PN Goal Regimen

The purpose of this example is to illustrate the thought process in determining what dextrose and amino acid solution and fat emulsion intake would provide the desired daily fluid calorie and protein goals.

1. Calculate the fluid, protein, and caloric goals. Example:

    Weight = 10 kg
    Fluids = 100 mL/kg/day = 1000 mL
    Calories = 100 kcal/kg/day = 1000 kcal
    Protein = 2.5 g/kg/day = 25 g

2. If fat emulsion (FE) comprises 40% to 60% of the total daily calories, using the above example: 40% of 1000 kcal = 400 kcal.

    400 kcal ÷ 2 kcal/mL (20% FE) = 200 mL

3. To determine the goal dextrose concentration calculate the total daily calories remaining. Example:

1000 kcal	(total daily calories)
- 400 kcal	(daily calories from fats)
600 kcal	(total daily calories remaining)

4. Determine the concentration of dextrose to achieve the total daily calories remaining. Example:

    600 kcal ÷ 3.4 kcal/g x [100 ÷ 800 mL*] = 22%

    *Total daily fluids desired minus that from fats.

5. Calculate percent amino acid solution to achieve goal protein intake. Example:

    [25 g (total protein) ÷ 800 mL (total fluid)] x 100 = 3.1%

    This patient's goal regimen would be: dextrose 22%, amino acid 3.1%, 800 mL/day plus fat emulsion 20% 200 mL/day.

Parenteral Nutrition Monitoring Guidelines

Parameter	Initial	Maintenance
	Frequency	
Body weight	Daily	Daily
Height or length	Weekly	Weekly
Triceps Skin Fold (TSF)/ Midarm Circumference (MAC)	PRN	PRN
Calories/protein intakes	Daily	PRN
Intake/output	Every 8 hours	Every 8 hours
Urine glucose	Every 4 hours	Every 8 hours
Urine specific gravity	Every 8 hours	Every 8 hours
Urine protein	Every 8 hours	Every 8 hours
Electrolytes	Daily	1-2 times weekly
Ca, Mg, PO$_4$	Daily	Weekly
BUN/Cr	Daily	Weekly
Serum glucose	Daily	Weekly
Albumin	Weekly	Weekly
Triglycerides	Daily	Weekly
Transferrin or prealbumin	Weekly	Weekly
Bilirubin, direct	Once	PRN (after 2 weeks minimum PN)
Liver function tests	Once	PRN

Nutritional Guidelines for Pediatric Patients*

Age	kcal/kg/d	Protein g/kg/d
Preterm neonate	120-140	2.5-3
Term infant - 1 y	90-120	2-2.5
1-7 y	75-90	1.5-2
12 y	60-75	1.5-2
12-18 y	30-60	0.8-2

*Kerner JA, Manual of Pediatric Parenteral Nutrition, Wiley & Sons, Inc, 1983.

PN kcal/mL*

Dextrose Concentration						
5%	10%	15%	20%	25%	30%	35%
0.17	0.34	0.51	0.68	0.85	1.02	1.19

Dextrose provides 3.4 kcal/g.

Intralipid 10% provides 1.1 kcal/mL.

Intralipid 20% provides 2 kcal/mL.

*Calories derived from amino acids are not included.

PARENTERAL NUTRITION (PN) *(Continued)*

Y-Site Compatibility of Medications With TPN and Lipid
(Administered in D_5W or NS via Y-connector into PN line)

Medication	PN	Lipid	Comments
Acetazolamide	I	—	
Acyclovir	I	—	Visual precipitate forms
Albumin	C	I	May crack emulsion
Aldesleukin	C	C	
Alprostadil	—	—	
Amikacin	C	I	Causes oiling out of fat emulsion
Aminophylline	C	C	Incompatible with insulin; caution with high concentration of Ca/Phos
Amphotericin B	I	I	Formation of fine yellow particles
Ampicillin	I	I	
Ampicillin/sulbactam	I	—	
Atracurium	C	—	
Azlocillin	C	C	
Aztreonam	C	—	
Bicarbonate	I	I	Incompatible with many electrolytes; precipitate forms
Cefamandole	C	C	
Cefazolin	C	C	
Cefepime	C	—	
Cefonicid	—	—	
Cefoperazone	C	—	
Cefotaxime	C	C	
Cefotetan	—	—	
Cefoxitin	C	C	
Ceftazidime	C	—	
Ceftizoxime	—	—	
Ceftriaxone	C	—	
Cefuroxime	C	—	
Cephalothin	C	C	
Cephapirin	C	C	
Cephradine	I	—	Heavy precipitate of Ca/Phos due to increased pH
Chloramphenicol	C	C	
Cimetidine	C	C	
Ciprofloxacin	C	C	
Chlorothiazide	I	—	Precipitate forms
Clindamycin	C	C	
Co-trimoxazole	I	—	Precipitate forms
Cyanocobalamin	C	C	
Cyclophosphamide	C	—	
Cyclosporine	C	C	
Cytarabine	C	—	
Dexamethasone (sodium phosphate)	C	—	
Digoxin	C	C	
Diphenhydramine	C	C	
Dobutamine	C	—	
Dopamine	C	C	

Y-Site Compatibility of Medications With TPN and Lipid
(continued)

Medication	PN	Lipid	Comments
Doxycycline	C	—	
Droperidol	—	—	
Epinephrine	C	—	
Epoetin alfa	C	—	
Erythromycin	C	C	
Famotidine	C	C	
Fentanyl	C	—	
Filgrastim	I	C	Incompatible with salt solutions
Fluconazole	C	—	
Fluorouracil	C	—	
Folic acid	C	C	
Foscarnet	C	—	
Fosphenytoin	C	—	
Furosemide	C	C	
Ganciclovir	I	—	Precipitate forms
Gentamicin	C	C	
Granisetron	C	—	
Haloperidol (lactate)	C	—	
Heparin	C	C	
Hydralazine	C	—	
Hydrocortisone	C	C	
Hydromorphone	C	—	
Idarubicin	C	—	
IL-2	C	C	
Imipenem/cilastatin	I	—	Significant loss of activity noted after 15 minutes
Indomethacin	I	—	
Insulin, regular	C	C	
Iron dextran	C	I	Causes oiling out of fat emulsion
Isoproterenol	C	C	
Kanamycin	C	C	
Levofloxacin	—	—	
Levorphanol	—	—	
Lidocaine	C	C	
Meperidine	C	—	
Meropenem	—	—	
Metaraminol	—	—	
Methicillin	C	I	Microscopic globule coalescence noted in 24 hours
Methotrexate	C	—	
Methyldopa	C	I	May crack emulsion
Methylprednisolone	C	—	
Metoclopramide	C	—	
Metronidazole	C	—	
Mezlocillin	C	C	
Miconazole	C	—	
Midazolam	I	—	Precipitate forms
Morphine	C	C	
Moxalactam	C	—	

PARENTERAL NUTRITION (PN) *(Continued)*

Y-Site Compatibility of Medications With TPN and Lipid *(continued)*

Medication	PN	Lipid	Comments
Nafcillin	C	C	
Netilmicin	C	—	
Norepinephrine	C	C	
Octreotide	I	C	
Ondansetron	C	—	
Oxacillin	C	C	
Penicillin G Na/K	C	C	
Pentamidine	—	—	
Phenytoin	I	I	Immediate precipitate
Phytonadione	C	C	
Piperacillin	C	C	
Propofol	C	—	
Ranitidine	C	I	Loss of 10% of ranitidine activity after 24 hours
Sargramostim	C	—	
Sodium bicarbonate	I	I	Incompatible with many electrolytes; precipitate forms
Tetracycline	C	I	Highly acidic pH may disrupt emulsion
Thiamine	C	C	
Ticarcillin	C	C	
Ticarcillin/clavulanate	—	—	
Trimethoprim/ sulfamethoxazole	I	—	Precipitate forms
Tobramycin	C	C	
Urokinase	C	—	
Vancomycin	C	—	
Verapamil	—	—	
Vitamin K	C	—	

C = Compatible, may simultaneously infuse drug and TPN/lipid.

I = Incompatible, drug should be given through a **separate** I.V. line or turn off the TPN/liquid during drug administration. Flush I.V. line with normal saline **before** and **after** drug administration.

— = Information on compatibility not available. Give drug through a **separate** I.V. line or turn off TPN infusion during drug administration. Flush line with normal saline **before** and **after** drug administration.

Reference
Trissel LA, "Handbook on Injectable Drugs," 10th ed, Bethesda, MD: American Society of Health-System Pharmacists, Inc, 1998.

Pharmacologic considerations of mixing medications with PN solutions include:

Adsorption — bag, bottle, tubing, filter
Blood levels
Site of injection/administration
Flush
Amino acid-dextrose concentrations

pH factors
Temperature
Additives in solution
Heparin dose

GROWTH CHARTS

CDC Growth Charts: United States

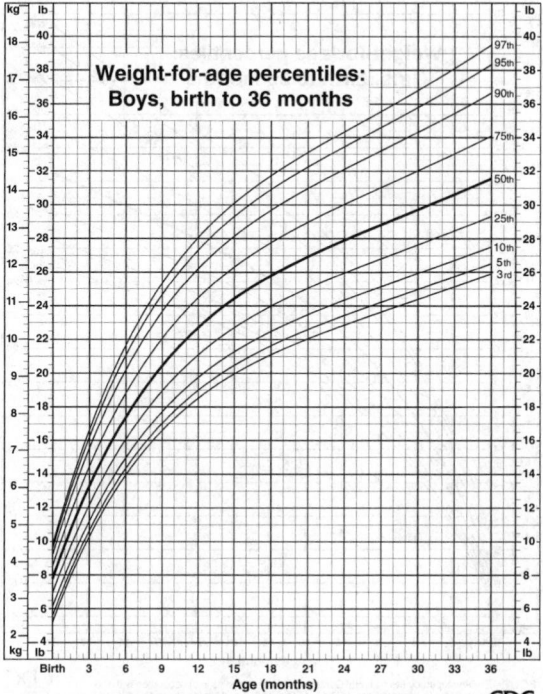

Weight-for-age percentiles:
Boys, birth to 36 months

SOURCE: Developed by the National Center for Health Statistics in collaboration with the National Center for Chronic Disease Prevention and Health Promotion (2000). Available at http://www.cdc.gov/growthcharts

GROWTH CHARTS *(Continued)*

CDC Growth Charts: United States

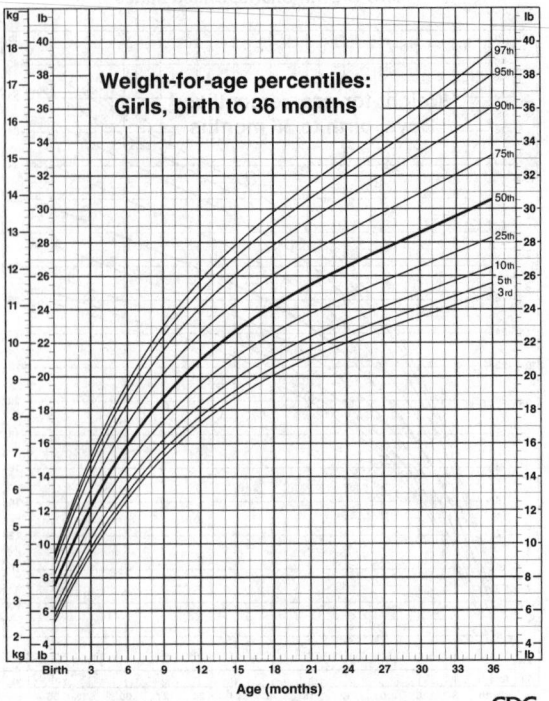

Weight-for-age percentiles:
Girls, birth to 36 months

SOURCE: Developed by the National Center for Health Statistics in collaboration with the National Center for Chronic Disease Prevention and Health Promotion (2000).
Available at http://www.cdc.gov/growthcharts

1116

CDC Growth Charts: United States

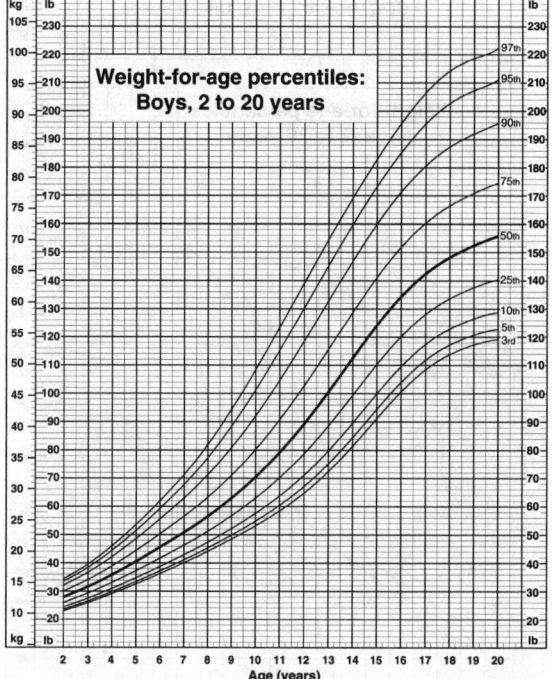

**Weight-for-age percentiles:
Boys, 2 to 20 years**

SOURCE: Developed by the National Center for Health Statistics in collaboration with the
National Center for Chronic Disease Prevention and Health Promotion (2000).
Available at http://www.cdc.gov/growthcharts

CDC

CDC Growth Charts: United States

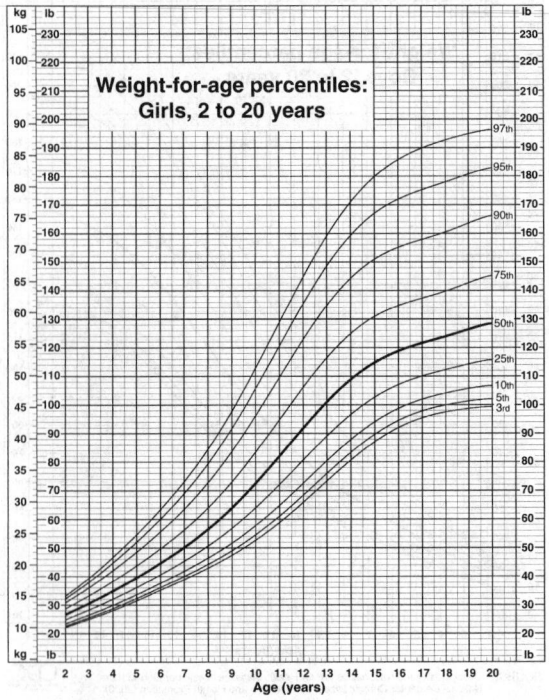

Weight-for-age percentiles:
Girls, 2 to 20 years

SOURCE: Developed by the National Center for Health Statistics in collaboration with the
National Center for Chronic Disease Prevention and Health Promotion (2000).
Available at http://www.cdc.gov/growthcharts

CDC Growth Charts: United States

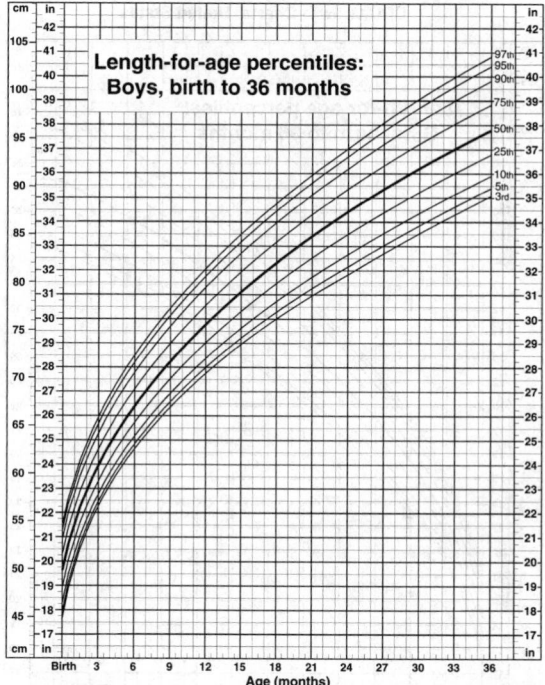

Length-for-age percentiles:
Boys, birth to 36 months

SOURCE: Developed by the National Center for Health Statistics in collaboration with the National Center for Chronic Disease Prevention and Health Promotion (2000).
Available at http://www.cdc.gov/growthcharts

GROWTH CHARTS *(Continued)*

CDC Growth Charts: United States

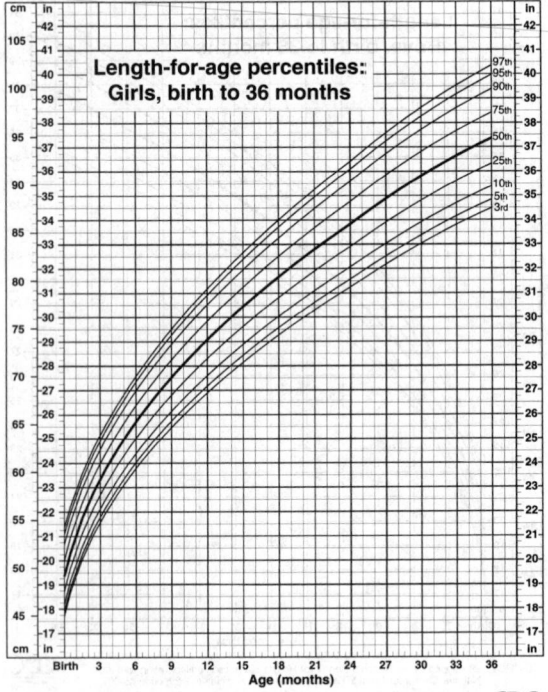

Length-for-age percentiles: Girls, birth to 36 months

SOURCE: Developed by the National Center for Health Statistics in collaboration with the National Center for Chronic Disease Prevention and Health Promotion (2000).
Available at http://www.cdc.gov/growthcharts

CDC Growth Charts: United States

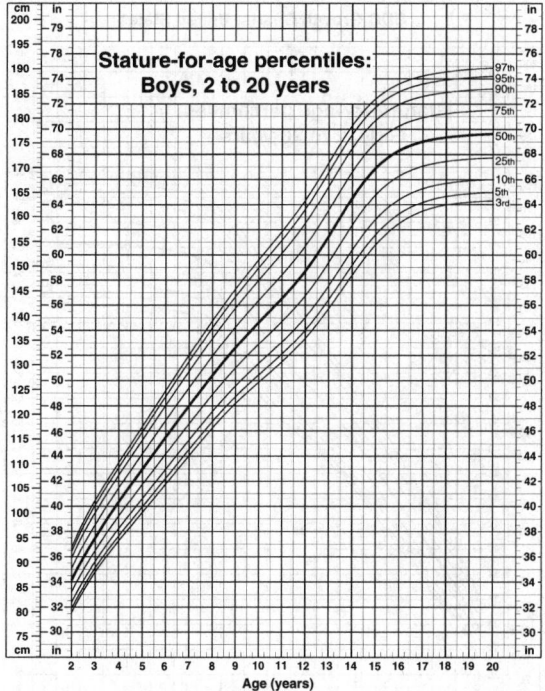

Stature-for-age percentiles:
Boys, 2 to 20 years

Age (years)

SOURCE: Developed by the National Center for Health Statistics in collaboration with the National Center for Chronic Disease Prevention and Health Promotion (2000).

Available at http://www.cdc.gov/growthcharts

GROWTH CHARTS *(Continued)*

CDC Growth Charts: United States

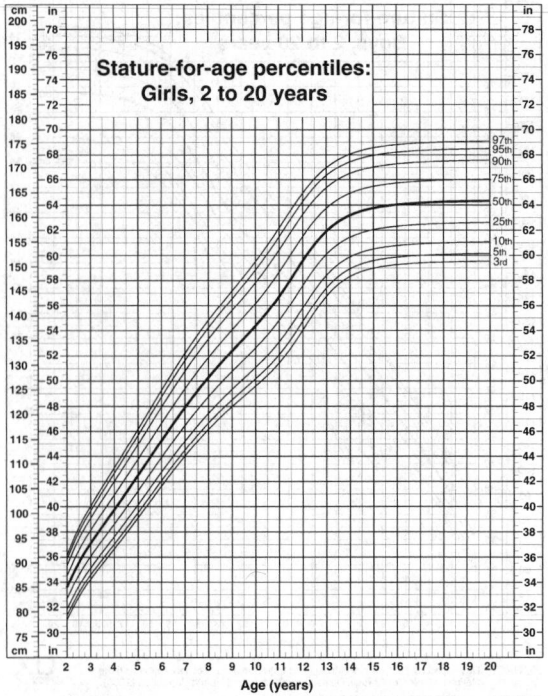

Stature-for-age percentiles:
Girls, 2 to 20 years

SOURCE: Developed by the National Center for Health Statistics in collaboration with the National Center for Chronic Disease Prevention and Health Promotion (2000).

Available at http://www.cdc.gov/growthcharts

CDC Growth Charts: United States

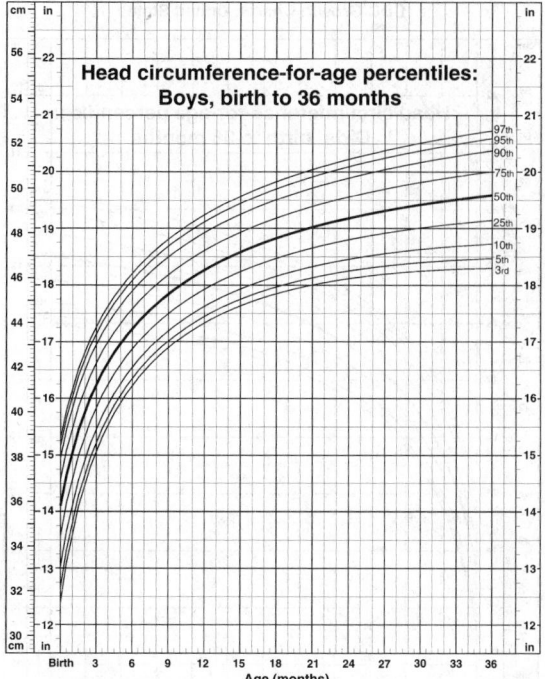

Head circumference-for-age percentiles:
Boys, birth to 36 months

SOURCE: Developed by the National Center for Health Statistics in collaboration with the
National Center for Chronic Disease Prevention and Health Promotion (2000).
Available at http://www.cdc.gov/growthcharts

GROWTH CHARTS *(Continued)*

CDC Growth Charts: United States

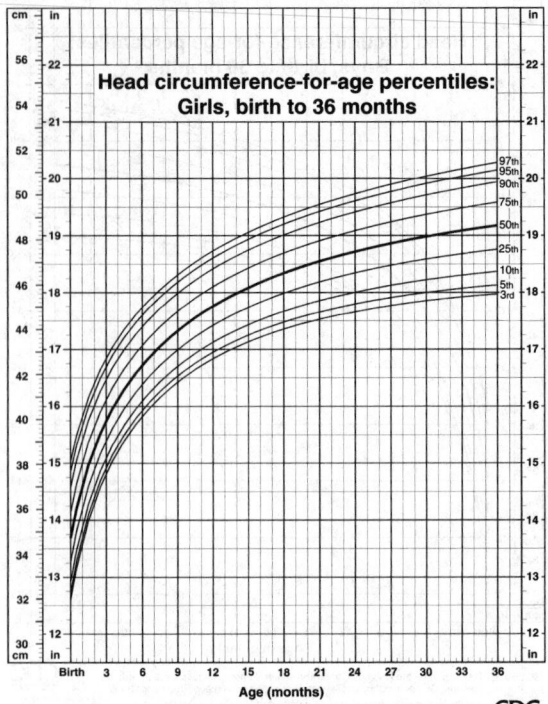

Head circumference-for-age percentiles: Girls, birth to 36 months

Age (months)

SOURCE: Developed by the National Center for Health Statistics in collaboration with the National Center for Chronic Disease Prevention and Health Promotion (2000).
Available at http://www.cdc.gov/growthcharts

IDEAL BODY WEIGHT CALCULATION

Adults (18 years and older)

IBW (male) = 50 + (2.3 x height in inches over 5 feet)
IBW (female) = 45.5 + (2.3 x height in inches over 5 feet)

IBW is in kg.

Children

a. 1-18 years (Traub and Johnson, 1980)

$$IBW = \frac{(height^2 \times 1.65)}{1000}$$

IBW is in kg.
Height is in cm.

b. 5 feet and taller (Traub and Johnson, 1980)

IBW (male) = 39 + (2.27 x height in inches over 5 feet)
IBW (female) = 42.2 + (2.27 x height in inches over 5 feet)

IBW is in kg.

c. 1-17 years (Traub and Kichen, 1983)

$$IBW = 2.396e^{0.01883 \, (height)}$$

IBW is in kg.
Height is in cm.

References

Traub SL and Johnson CE, "Comparison of Methods of Estimating Creatinine Clearance in Children," *Am J Hosp Pharm*, 1980, 37(2):195-201.
Traub SL and Kichen L, "Estimating Ideal Body Mass in Children," *Am J Hosp Pharm*, 1983, 40(1):107-10.

BODY SURFACE AREA OF CHILDREN AND ADULTS

Calculating Body Surface Area in Children

In a child of average size, find weight and corresponding surface area on the boxed scale to the left; or, use the nomogram to the right. Lay a straightedge on the correct height and weight points for the child, then read the intersecting point on the surface area scale.

FOR CHILDREN OF NORMAL HEIGHT AND WEIGHT

NOMOGRAM

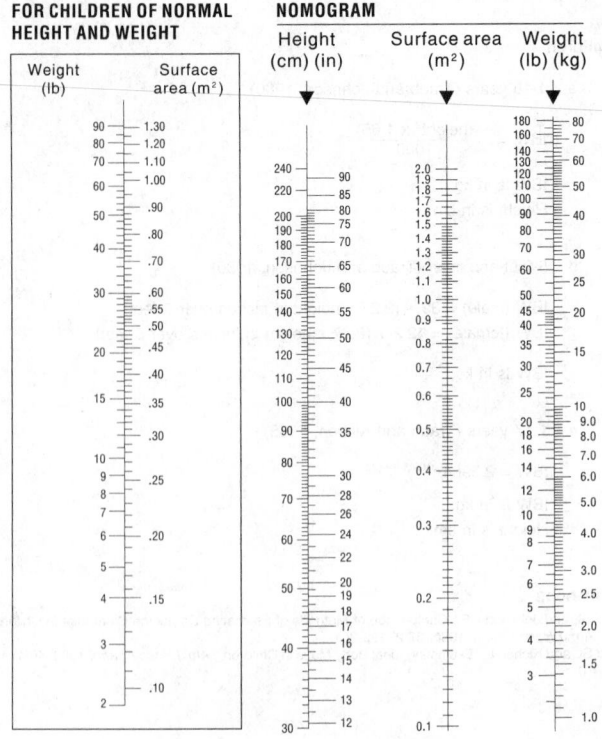

BODY SURFACE AREA FORMULA
(Adult and Pediatric)

$$BSA\ (m^2) = \sqrt{\frac{Ht\ (in)\ x\ Wt\ (lb)}{3131}}\ \ \text{or, in metric: } BSA\ (m^2) = \sqrt{\frac{Ht\ (cm)\ x\ Wt\ (kg)}{3600}}$$

References

Lam TK and Leung DT, "More on Simplified Calculation of Body Surface Area," *N Engl J Med*, 1988, 318(17):1130 (Letter).

Mosteller RD, "Simplified Calculation of Body Surface Area", *N Engl J Med*, 1987, 317(17):1098 (Letter).

AVERAGE WEIGHTS AND SURFACE AREAS

Average Weight and Surface Area of Preterm Infants, Term Infants, and Children

Age	Average Weight (kg)*	Approximate Surface Area (m²)
Weeks Gestation		
26	0.9-1	0.1
30	1.3-1.5	0.12
32	1.6-2	0.15
38	2.9-3	0.2
40 (term infant at birth)	3.1-4	0.25
Months		
3	5	0.29
6	7	0.38
9	8	0.42
Year		
1	10	0.49
2	12	0.55
3	15	0.64
4	17	0.74
5	18	0.76
6	20	0.82
7	23	0.90
8	25	0.95
9	28	1.06
10	33	1.18
11	35	1.23
12	40	1.34
Adults	70	1.73

*Weights from age 3 months and over are rounded off to the nearest kilogram.

PHYSICAL DEVELOPMENT

Weight gain first 6 weeks
20 g/day

Birth weight
regained by day 14
doubles by age 4 mo
triples by age 12 mo
quadruples by age 2 y

Teeth
1st tooth 6-18 mo
teeth = age (mo) − 6
(until 30 mo)

Head circumference
35 cm at birth
44 cm by 6 mo
47 cm by 1 y
1 cm/mo for 1st y
3 cm/mo 2nd y

Length
increases 50% by age 1 y
doubles by age 4 y
triples by age 13 y

Tanner Stages of Sexual Development

Stage	Characteristics	Age at onset (mean ± SD)
Genital stages: Male		
1	Prepubertal	
2	Scrotum and testes enlarge; skin of scrotum reddens and rugations appear	11.4 ± 1.1 y
3	Penis lengthens; testes enlarge further	12.9 ± 1 y
4	Penis growth continues in length and width; glans develops adult form	13.8 ± 1 y
5	Development completed; adult appearance	14.9 ± 1.1 y
Breast development: Female		
1	Prepubertal	
2	Breast buds appear; areolae enlarge	11.2 ± 1.1 y
3	Elevation of breast contour; areolae enlarge	12.2 ± 1.1 y
4	Areolae and papilla form a secondary mound on breast	13.1 ± 1.2 y
5	Adult form	15.3 ± 1.7 y
Menarche		
Pubic hair: Both sexes		13.5 ± 1 y
1	Prepubertal, no coarse hair	
2	Longer, silky hair appears at base of penis or along labia	F: 11.7 ± 1.2 y M: 12 ± 1 y
3	Hair coarse, kinky, spreads over pubic bone	F: 12.4 ± 1.1 y M: 13.9 ± 1 y
4	Hair of adult quality but not spread to junction of medial thigh with perineum	F: 13 ± 1 y M: 14.4 ± 1.1 y
5	Spread to medial thigh	F: 14.4 ± 1.1 y M: 15.2 ± 1.1 y
6	"Male escutcheon"	Variable if occurs
Maximum growth rate		
Male at 14.1±0.9 y		
Female at 12.1±0.9 y		

EMETOGENIC POTENTIAL OF SINGLE CHEMOTHERAPEUTIC AGENTS

Class I — Low (<10%)

Asparaginase/Pegaspargase
Bleomycin
Busulfan
Chlorambucil (oral)
Cladribine
Corticosteroids
Cyclophosphamide (oral)
Fludarabine

Hydroxyurea
Melphalan (oral)
Mercaptopurine
Methotrexate <50 mg/m^2
Thioguanine (oral)
Vinblastine
Vincristine

Class II — Moderately Low (10% to 30%)

Cytarabine <500 mg/m^2
Doxorubicin ≤20 mg/m^2
Etoposide
Fluorouracil <1000 mg/m^2
Gemcitabine
Interferon-beta

Lomustine
Methotrexate ≥50-250 mg/m^2
Mitomycin <8 mg/m^2
Paclitaxel
Raltitrexed
Thiotepa

Class III — Moderate (30% to 60%)

Amsacrine
Azacitidine
Cyclophosphamide <750 mg/m^2
Cytarabine 500-1000 mg/m^2
Daunorubicin
Docetaxel
Doxorubicin >20 mg to <60 mg/m^2
Fluorouracil ≥1000 mg/m^2
Idarubicin
Ifosfamide

Irinotecan
Methotrexate >250 mg/m^2 to ≤1000 mg/m^2
Mitomycin ≥8 mg/m^2
Mitoxantrone
Teniposide
Topotecan
Tretinoin
Vinorelbine

Class IV — Moderately High (60% to 90%)

Actinomycin D
Aldesleukin
Carboplatin 200-400 mg/m^2
Carmustine <250 mg
Cisplatin <50 mg/m^2
Cyclophosphamide 750-1500 mg/m^2

Cytarabine >1000 mg/m^2
Dacarbazine <500 mg/m^2
Doxorubicin ≥60 mg/m^2
Melphalan 20-80 mg/m^2
Methotrexate >1000 mg/m^2
Procarbazine (oral)

Class V — High (>90%)

Busulfan (as part of BMT regimen)
Carboplatin >500 mg/m^2
Carmustine ≥250 mg/m^2
Cisplatin ≥50 mg/m^2
Cyclophosphamide ≥1500 mg/m^2

Dacarbazine ≥500 mg/m^2
Mechlorethamine
Melphalan >80 mg/m^2
Pentostatin

COMPATIBILITY OF CHEMOTHERAPY AND RELATED SUPPORTIVE CARE MEDICATIONS

Compatible: The drugs are physically compatible when mixed in the same container or infused through the same I.V. line simultaneously.

Y-site compatible: The drugs are physically compatible when infused through the same I.V. line simultaneously.

Incompatible: The drugs are physically incompatible when mixed in the same container, or infused through the same I.V. line simultaneously.

Variable compatibility: The compatibility of the drugs varies according to the concentration and/or diluent of the drugs. Please refer to the table at the end of this section for more information on variable compatibility.

Abbreviations

AA	Amino acid solution
BNS	Bacteriostatic normal saline
BWI	Bacteriostatic water for injection
D_5W	5% dextrose in water
D_5/NS	5% dextrose in 0.9% sodium chloride
D_5/$\frac{1}{4}$NS	5% dextrose in 0.225% sodium chloride
D_5/$\frac{1}{2}$NS	5% dextrose in 0.45% sodium chloride
D_5LR	5% dextrose in lactated Ringer's injection
$D_{10}W$	10% dextrose in water
$D_{10}W$/0.01% albumin	10% dextrose in water with 0.01% albumin
$D_{10}W$/0.05% albumin	10% dextrose in water with 0.05% albumin
$D_{10}W$/0.1% albumin	10% dextrose in water with 0.1% albumin
D_{10}/NS	10% dextrose in water in 0.9% sodium chloride
LR	Lactated Ringer's injection
NS	0.9% sodium chloride (normal saline)
SWI	Sterile water for injection
TPN	Total parenteral nutrition solution

Reported Compatibilities and Incompatibilities of Parenteral Dosage Forms

Aldesleukin

Compatible:

D₅W

SWI

Y-Site Compatible:

Amikacin	Fluconazole	Ondansetron
Amphotericin	Foscarnet	Piperacillin
Calcium gluconate	Gentamicin	Potassium chloride
Cotrimoxazole	Heparin	Ranitidine
Diphenhydramine	Magnesium sulfate	Thiethylperazine
Dopamine	Metoclopramide	Ticarcillin
Fat emulsion	Morphine	Tobramycin

Incompatible:

Ganciclovir	Pentamidine	Promethazine
Heparin	Prochlorperazine	

Amifostine

Compatible:

NS

Y-Site Compatible:

Amikacin	Diphenhydramine	Mannitol
Aminophylline	Dobutamine	Mechlorethamine
Ampicillin	Dopamine	Meperidine
Ampicillin/sulbactam	Doxorubicin	Mesna
Aztreonam	Doxycycline	Methotrexate
Bleomycin	Droperidol	Methylprednisolone
Bumetanide	Enalaprilat	Metoclopramide
Buprenophine	Etoposide	Metronidazole
Butorphanol	Famotidine	Mezlocillin
Calcium gluconate	Floxuridine	Mitomycin
Carboplatin	Fluconazole	Mitoxantrone
Carmustine	Fludarabine	Morphine
Cefamandole	Fluorouracil	Nalbuphine
Cefepime	Furosemide	Netilmicin
Cefotaxime	Gallium nitrate	Ondansetron
Cefotetan	Gemcitabine	Piperacillin
Cefoxitin	Gentamicin	Plicamycin
Ceftazidime	Granisetron	Potassium chloride
Ceftizoxime	Haloperidol	Promethazine
Ceftriaxone	Heparin	Ranitidine
Cefuroxime	Hydrocortisone sodium phosphate	Sodium bicarbonate
Cimetidine		Streptozocin
Ciprofloxacin	Hydrocortisone sodium succinate	Teniposide
Clindamycin		Thiotepa
Cotrimoxazole	Hydromorphone	Ticarcillin
Cyclophosphamide	Idarubicin	Ticarcillin/clavulanate
Cytarabine	Ifosfamide	Tobramycin
Dacarbazine	Imipenem/cilastatin	Trimetrexate
Dactinomycin	Leucovorin	Vancomycin
Daunomycin	Lorazepam	Vinblastine
Dexamethasone	Magnesium sulfate	Vincristine

Incompatible:

Acyclovir	Cisplatin	Minocycline
Amphotericin	Ganciclovir	Prochlorperazine
Chlorpromazine	Hydroxyzine	

COMPATIBILITY OF CHEMOTHERAPY AND RELATED SUPPORTIVE CARE MEDICATIONS *(Continued)*

Asparaginase

Compatible:

D$_5$W	NS	SWI

Y-Site Compatible:

Methotrexate	Sodium bicarbonate

Bleomycin

Compatible:

BNS	Dexamethasone	Leucovorin
BWI	Diphenhydramine	Metoclopramide
SWI	Droperidol	Phenytoin
Amikacin	Fluorouracil	Streptomycin
Amsacrine	Furosemide	Tobramycin
Ceftazidime	Gentamicin	Vinblastine
Cephapirin	Heparin	Vincristine
Cimetidine	Hydrocortisone sodium	
Dacarbazine	phosphate	

Y-Site Compatible:

Allopurinol	Doxorubicin, liposomal	Paclitaxel
Amifostine	Filgrastim	Piperacillin
Aztreonam	Fludarabine	Sargramostim
Cefepime	Gemcitabine	Teniposide
Cisplatin	Methotrexate	Thiotepa
Cyclophosphamide	Mitomycin	Vinorelbine
Doxorubicin	Ondansetron	

Incompatible:

Aminophylline	Diazepam	Nafcillin
Ascorbic acid	Doxapram	Penicillin G
Cefazolin	Hydrocortisone sodium	Terbutaline
Cephalothin	succinate	

Variable Compatibility:

D$_5$W	NS

Busulfan

Compatible:

D$_5$W	NS

Carboplatin

Compatible:

D$_5$W	Etoposide	Ifosfamide
SWI	Floxuridine	

Y-Site Compatible:

Allopurinol	Fludarabine	Propofol
Amifostine	Gemcitabine	Sargramostim
Aztreonam	Granisetron	Teniposide
Cefazolin	Ondansetron	Thiotepa
Doxorubicin, liposomal	Piperacillin	TPN
Filgrastim	Piperacillin/tazobactam	Vinorelbine

Incompatible:

Fluorouracil	Mesna	Sodium bicarbonate

Variable Compatibility:

D$_5$/NS	D$_5$/^{1}/$_2$NS	NS
D$_5$/^{1}/$_4$NS		

Carmustine

Compatible:
D_5W	SWI	Dacarbazine
NS		

Y-Site Compatible:
Amifostine	Gemcitabine	Sargramostim
Aztreonam	Ondansetron	Teniposide
Cefepime	Piperacillin	Thiotepa
Filgrastim	Piperacillin/tazobactam	Vinorelbine
Fludarabine		

Incompatible:
Allopurinol	Sodium bicarbonate

Cisplatin

Compatible:
D_5/NS	Cephalothin	Ifosfamide
$D_5/^1/_4NS$	Cyclophosphamide	Leucovorin
$D_5/^1/_2NS$	Floxuridine	Mannitol
NS	Hydroxyzine	Mechlorethamine
Cefazolin	Hydroxyurea	Ondansetron

Y-Site Compatible:
Allopurinol	Filgrastim	Mitomycin
Aztreonam	Fludarabine	Morphine
Bleomycin	Fluorouracil	Paclitaxel
Bumetanide	Furosemide	Potassium chloride
Chlorpromazine	Ganciclovir	Prochlorperazine
Cimetidine	Gemcitabine	Promethazine
Dexamethasone	Granisetron	Propofol
Diphenhydramine	Heparin	Ranitidine
Doxapram	Hydromorphone	Sargramostim
Doxorubicin	Lorazepam	Teniposide
Doxorubicin, liposomal	Methotrexate	Thiotepa
Droperidol	Methylprednisolone	Vinorelbine
Famotidine	Metoclopramide	

Incompatible:
Amifostine	Gallium nitrate	Piperacillin
Amsacrine	Mesna	Piperacillin/tazobactam
Cefepime	Oxacillin	Sodium bicarbonate

Variable Compatibility:
D_5W	SWI	Etoposide

Cladribine

Compatible:
NS

Cyclophosphamide

Compatible:
D_5W	AA 4.25%/$D_{25}W$	Hydroxyzine
D_5/NS	Cisplatin	Mesna
D_5/LR	Dacarbazine	Methotrexate
NS	Etoposide	Mitoxantrone
LR	Fluorouracil	Ondansetron
SWI		

Y-Site Compatible:
Allopurinol	Clindamycin	Heparin
Amifostine	Cotrimoxazole	Hydromorphone
Amikacin	Dexamethasone	Idarubicin
Ampicillin	Diphenhydramine	Kanamycin
Azlocillin	Doxapram	Leucovorin
Aztreonam	Doxorubicin	Lorazepam
Bleomycin	Doxorubicin, liposomal	Methylprednisolone
Cefamandole	Doxycycline	Metoclopramide
Cefazolin	Droperidol	Metronidazole
Cefepime	Erythromycin	Mezlocillin
Cefoperazone	Famotidine	Minocycline
Cefotaxime	Filgrastim	Mitomycin
Cefoxitin	Fludarabine	Morphine
Ceftriaxone	Furosemide	Moxalactam
Cephalothin	Gallium nitrate	Nafcillin
Cephapirin	Ganciclovir	Oxacillin
Chloramphenicol	Gemcitabine	Paclitaxel
Chlorpromazine	Gentamicin	Penicillin G
Cimetidine	Granisetron	Piperacillin

COMPATIBILITY OF CHEMOTHERAPY AND RELATED SUPPORTIVE CARE MEDICATIONS (Continued)

Piperacillin/tazobactam	Sodium bicarbonate	TPN
Prochlorperazine	Teniposide	Vancomycin
Promethazine	Thiotepa	Vinblastine
Propofol	Ticarcillin	Vincristine
Ranitidine	Ticarcillin/clavulanate	Vinorelbine
Sargramostim	Tobramycin	

Cytarabine

Compatible:

BNS	NS	Hydroxyurea
BWI	LR	Lincomycin
D$_5$W	AA 4.25%/D$_{25}$W	Mitoxantrone
D$_5$/NS	Corticotropin	Ondansetron
D$_5$/^{1}/$_4$NS	Dacarbazine	Potassium chloride
D$_5$/^{1}/$_2$NS	Daunomycin	Prednisolone
D$_5$/LR	Etoposide	Sodium bicarbonate
D$_{10}$/NS	Hydroxyzine	Vincristine

Y-Site Compatible:

Amifostine	Filgrastim	Piperacillin
Amsacrine	Fludarabine	Piperacillin/tazobactam
Aztreonam	Furosemide	Prochlorperazine
Cefepime	Gemcitabine	Promethazine
Chlorpromazine	Granisetron	Propofol
Cimetidine	Heparin	Ranitidine
Dexamethasone	Idarubicin	Sargramostim
Diphenhydramine	Lorazepam	Teniposide
Doxorubicin, liposomal	Metoclopramide	Thiotepa
Droperidol	Morphine	TPN
Famotidine	Paclitaxel	Vinorelbine

Incompatible:

Allopurinol	Gallium nitrate	Nafcillin
Ceftazidime	Ganciclovir	Oxacillin
Fluorouracil	Insulin	Penicillin G

Variable Compatibility:

Cephalothin	Hydrocortisone sodium	Methylprednisolone
Gentamicin	phosphate	

Dacarbazine

Compatible:

NS	Cyclophosphamide	Mercaptopurine
SWI	Cytarabine	Methotrexate
Bleomycin	Dactinomycin	Ondansetron
Carmustine	Doxorubicin	Vinblastine
Cimetidine	Fluorouracil	

Y-Site Compatible:

Amifostine	Granisetron	Sargramostim
Aztreonam	Hydrocortisone sodium	Teniposide
Doxorubicin, liposomal	phosphate	Thiotepa
Filgrastim	Lidocaine	Vinorelbine
Fludarabine	Paclitaxel	

Incompatible:

D$_5$W	Hydrocortisone sodium	Piperacillin
Allopurinol	succinate	Piperacillin/tazobactam
Cefepime		

Variable Compatibility:

Heparin

Dactinomycin

Compatible:

D$_5$W	SWI	Dacarbazine
NS		

Y-Site Compatible:

Allopurinol	Fludarabine	Teniposide
Amifostine	Gemcitabine	Thiotepa
Aztreonam	Ondansetron	Vinorelbine
Cefepime	Sargramostim	

Incompatible:

| BNS | BWI | Filgrastim |

Daunomycin

Compatible:

D$_5$W	SWI	Hydrocortisone sodium
NS	Cytarabine	succinate
LR	Etoposide	

Y-Site Compatible:

Amifostine	Methotrexate	Teniposide
Filgrastim	Ondansetron	Thiotepa
Gemcitabine	Sodium bicarbonate	Vinorelbine

Incompatible:

Allopurinol	Dexamethasone	Piperacillin
Aztreonam	Fludarabine	Piperacillin/tazobactam
Cefepime		

Dexrazoxane

Compatible:

D$_5$W

Y-Site Compatible:

Gemcitabine

Diphenhydramine

Compatible:

Amikacin	Glycopyrrolate	Penicillin G (sodium and
Aminophylline	Hydrocortisone sodium	potassium)
Ascorbic acid	succinate	Pentazocine
Atropine	Hydromorphone	Perphenazine
Bleomycin	Hydroxyzine	Prochlorperazine
Butorphanol	Lidocaine	Promazine
Cephapirin	Meperidine	Promethazine
Chlorpromazine	Methicillin	Ranitidine
Cimetidine	Methyldopate	Scopolamine
Colistimethate	Metoclopramide	Sufentanil
Dimenhydrinate	Midazolam	Thiothixene
Droperidol	Morphine	Polymyxin B
Erythromycin	Nalbuphine	Vitamin B complex
Fentanyl	Nafcillin	with C
Fluphenazine	Netilmicin	

Y-Site Compatible:

Acyclovir	Filgrastim	Methotrexate
Aldesleukin	Fluconazole	Ondansetron
Amifostine	Fludarabine	Paclitaxel
Amsacrine	Gallium nitrate	Piperacillin/tazobactam
Aztreonam	Gemcitabine	Potassium chloride
Ciprofloxacin	Granisetron	Sargramostim
Cisplatin	Heparin	Tacrolimus
Cyclophosphamide	Idarubicin	Teniposide
Cytarabine	Melphalan	Thiotepa
Doxorubicin	Meperidine	Vinorelbine

COMPATIBILITY OF CHEMOTHERAPY AND RELATED SUPPORTIVE CARE MEDICATIONS *(Continued)*

Incompatible:

Allopurinol	Cephalothin	Pentobarbital
Amobarbital	Dexamethasone	Secobarbital
Amphotericin	Foscarnet	Thiopental
Cefepime	Haloperidol	

Variable Compatibility:

Diatrizoate	Iodipamide

Docetaxel

Compatible:

D₅W	NS

Y-Site Compatible:
Gemcitabine

Incompatible:
Doxorubicin, liposomal

Doxorubicin

Compatible:

D₅W	LR	Ondansetron
NS	Dacarbazine	Vincristine

Y-Site Compatible:

Amifostine	Fludarabine	Paclitaxel
Aztreonam	Gemcitabine	Prochlorperazine
Bleomycin	Granisetron	Promethazine
Chlorpromazine	Hydromorphone	Propofol
Cimetidine	Leucovorin	Ranitidine
Cisplatin	Lorazepam	Sargramostim
Cyclophosphamide	Methotrexate	Sodium bicarbonate
Dexamethasone	Methylprednisolone	Teniposide
Diphenhydramine	Metoclopramide	Thiotepa
Famotidine	Mitomycin	Vinorelbine
Filgrastim	Morphine	

Incompatible:

Allopurinol	Gallium nitrate	Piperacillin/tazobactam
Aminophylline	Ganciclovir	TPN
Cefepime	Heparin	Paclitaxel
Cephalothin	Hydrocortisone sodium	Tobramycin
Diazepam	succinate	
Furosemide		

Variable Compatibility:

Fluorouracil	Vinblastine

Doxorubicin, Liposomal

Compatible:
D₅W

Y-Site Compatible:

Allopurinol	Dacarbazine	Leucovorin
Aldesleukin	Dexamethasone	Lorazepam
Aminophylline	Diphenhydramine	Magnesium sulfate
Ampicillin	Dobutamine	Mesna
Aztreonam	Dopamine	Methotrexate
Bleomycin	Droperidol	Methylprednisolone
Calcium chloride	Enalaprilat	Metronidazole
Calcium gluconate	Etoposide	Mezlocillin
Cefazolin	Famotidine	Netilmicin
Cefepime	Fluconazole	Ondansetron
Cefoperazone	Fluorouracil	Piperacillin
Cefoxitin	Furosemide	Potassium chloride
Ceftizoxime	Ganciclovir	Prochlorperazine
Ceftriaxone	Gentamicin	Ranitidine
Chlorpromazine	Granisetron	Ticarcillin
Cimetidine	Haloperidol	Ticarcillin/clavulanate
Ciprofloxacin	Heparin	Tobramycin
Cisplatin	Hydrocortisone sodium	Vancomycin
Clindamycin	succinate	Vinblastine
Cotrimoxazole	Hydromorphone	Vincristine
Cyclophosphamide	Ifosfamide	Vinorelbine
Cytarabine		

Incompatible:

Amphotericin
Buprenorphine
Ceftazidime
Docetaxel
Gallium nitrate
Hydroxyzine

Mannitol
Meperidine
Metoclopramide
Miconazole
Mitoxantrone

Morphine
Ofloxacin
Piperacillin/tazobactam
Promethazine
Sodium bicarbonate

Droperidol

Compatible:

Atropine
Bleomycin
Butorphanol
Chlorpromazine
Cimetidine
Cisplatin
Cyclophosphamide
Dimenhydrinate
Diphenhydramine

Doxorubicin
Fentanyl
Glycopyrrolate
Hydroxyzine
Meperidine
Metoclopramide
Midazolam
Mitomycin
Morphine

Nalbuphine
Pentazocine
Perphenazine
Prochlorperazine
Promazine
Promethazine
Scopolamine
Vinblastine
Vincristine

Y-Site Compatible:

Amifostine
Aztreonam
Filgrastim
Fluconazole
Fludarabine
Gemcitabine
Hydrocortisone sodium
    succinate

Idarubicin
Melphalan
Ondansetron
Paclitaxel
Potassium chloride
Sargramostim

Teniposide
Thiotepa
Vinorelbine
Vitamin B complex
    with C

Incompatible:

Allopurinol
Cefepime
Fluorouracil
Foscarnet

Furosemide
Heparin
Leucovorin
Methotrexate

Nafcillin
Pentobarbital
Piperacillin/tazobactam

Erythropoietin

Compatible:

BNS

D_{10}/0.05% albumin

D_{10}/0.1% albumin

Incompatible:

D_{10}W
D_{10}/0.01% albumin

NS

SWI

Etoposide

Compatible:

D_5W
NS
LR
Carboplatin

Cyclophosphamide
Cytarabine
Daunomycin
Floxuridine

Fluorouracil
Hydroxyzine
Ifosfamide
Ondansetron

Y-Site Compatible:

Allopurinol
Amifostine
Aztreonam
Doxorubicin, liposomal
Fludarabine
Gemcitabine

Granisetron
Haloperidol
Methotrexate
Paclitaxel
Piperacillin

Piperacillin/tazobactam
Sargramostim
Sodium bicarbonate
Teniposide
Vinorelbine

Incompatible:

Cefoperazone
Ceftazidime

Cefepime
Filgrastim

Gallium nitrate
Idarubicin

Variable Compatibility:

Cisplatin

Mannitol

Potassium chloride

COMPATIBILITY OF CHEMOTHERAPY AND RELATED SUPPORTIVE CARE MEDICATIONS *(Continued)*

Filgrastim

Compatible:
D$_5$W   SWI

Y-Site Compatible:

Acyclovir	Dexamethasone	Mechlorethamine
Allopurinol	Diphenhydramine	Meperidine
Amikacin	Doxorubicin	Mesna
Aminophylline	Doxycycline	Methotrexate
Ampicillin	Droperidol	Metoclopramide
Ampicillin/sulbactam	Enalaprilat	Miconazole
Aztreonam	Fat emulsion	Minocycline
Bleomycin	Floxuridine	Mitoxantrone
Bumetanide	Fluconazole	Morphine
Buprenorphine	Fludarabine	Nalbuphine
Butorphanol	Gallium nitrate	Netilmicin
Calcium gluconate	Ganciclovir	Ondansetron
Carboplatin	Gentamicin	Plicamycin
Carmustine	Haloperidol	Potassium chloride
Cefazolin	Hydrocortisone sodium	Promethazine
Cefotetan	phosphate	Ranitidine
Ceftazidime	Hydrocortisone sodium	Sodium bicarbonate
Chlorpromazine	succinate	Streptozocin
Cimetidine	Hydromorphone	Ticarcillin
Cisplatin	Hydroxyzine	Ticarcillin/clavulanate
Cotrimoxazole	Idarubicin	Tobramycin
Cyclophosphamide	Ifosfamide	Vancomycin
Cytarabine	Imipenem/cilastatin	Vinblastine
Dacarbazine	Leucovorin	Vincristine
Daunomycin	Lorazepam	Vinorelbine

Incompatible:

NS	Ceftizoxime	Mannitol
Amphotericin	Ceftriaxone	Methylprednisolone
Amsacrine	Cefuroxime	Metronidazole
Cefepime	Dactinomycin	Mezlocillin
Cefonicid	Etoposide	Mitomycin
Cefoperazone	Fluorouracil	Piperacillin
Cefotaxime	Furosemide	Prochlorperazine
Cefoxitin	Heparin	Thiotepa

Floxuridine

Compatible:

D$_5$W	Carboplatin	Fluorouracil
NS	Cisplatin	Heparin
SWI	Etoposide	Leucovorin

Y-Site Compatible:

Amifostine	Gemcitabine	Sargramostim
Aztreonam	Ondansetron	Teniposide
Filgrastim	Paclitaxel	Thiotepa
Fludarabine	Piperacillin/tazobactam	Vinorelbine

Incompatible:
Allopurinol   Cefepime

Fludarabine

Compatible:
D$_5$W   NS   SWI

Y-Site Compatible:

Allopurinol	Cefotaxime	Doxorubicin
Amifostine	Cefotetan	Doxycycline
Amikacin	Ceftazidime	Droperidol
Aminophylline	Ceftizoxime	Etoposide
Ampicillin	Ceftriaxone	Famotidine
Ampicillin/sulbactam	Cefuroxime	Filgrastim
Amsacrine	Cimetidine	Floxuridine
Aztreonam	Cisplatin	Fluconazole
Bleomycin	Cotrimoxazole	Fluorouracil
Butorphanol	Cyclophosphamide	Furosemide
Carboplatin	Cytarabine	Gemcitabine
Carmustine	Dacarbazine	Gentamicin
Cefazolin	Dactinomycin	Haloperidol
Cefepime	Dexamethasone	Heparin
Cefoperazone	Diphenhydramine	

Hydrocortisone sodium
phosphate
Hydrocortisone sodium
succinate
Hydromorphone
Ifosfamide
Imipenem/cilastatin
Lorazepam
Magnesium sulfate
Mannitol
Mechlorethamine
Meperidine
Mesna
Methotrexate

Methylprednisolone
Metoclopramide
Mezlocillin
Minocycline
Mitoxantrone
Morphine
Multivitamins
Nalbuphine
Netilmicin
Ondansetron
Pentostatin
Piperacillin
Piperacillin/tazobactam

Potassium chloride
Promethazine
Ranitidine
Sodium bicarbonate
Teniposide
Tetracycline
Ticarcillin
Ticarcillin/clavulanate
Tobramycin
Vancomycin
Vinblastine
Vincristine
Vinorelbine

Incompatible:

Acyclovir
Amphotericin
Chlorpromazine

Daunomycin
Ganciclovir
Hydroxyzine

Miconazole

Prochlorperazine

Fluorouracil

Compatible:

D$_5$W
D$_5$/LR
NS
Bleomycin
Cephalothin

Cyclophosphamide
Dacarbazine
Etoposide
Floxuridine
Ifosfamide

Magnesium sulfate
Methotrexate
Mitoxantrone
Prednisolone
Vincristine

Y-Site Compatible:

Allopurinol
Amifostine
Aztreonam
Cefepime
Cisplatin
Doxorubicin, liposomal
Fludarabine
Furosemide
Gemcitabine

Granisetron
Heparin
Hydrocortisone sodium
succinate
Mannitol
Metoclopramide
Mitomycin
Paclitaxel
Piperacillin

Piperacillin/tazobactam
Potassium chloride
Propofol
Sargramostim
Teniposide
Thiotepa
Vinblastine
Vitamin B complex

Incompatible:

Carboplatin
Cytarabine
Diazepam
Droperidol

Epirubicin
Filgrastim
Gallium nitrate

Ondansetron
TPN
Vinorelbine

Variable Compatibility:

Doxorubicin

Leucovorin

Gemcitabine

Compatible:

NS

Y-Site Compatible:

Amifostine
Amikacin
Aminophylline
Ampicillin
Ampicillin/sulbactam
Aztreonam
Bleomycin
Bumetanide
Buprenorphine
Butorphanol
Calcium gluconate
Carboplatin
Carmustine
Cefazolin
Cefonicid
Cefotetan
Cefoxitin
Ceftazidime
Ceftizoxime
Ceftriaxone
Cefuroxime
Chlorpromazine
Cimetidine
Ciprofloxacin
Cisplatin
Clindamycin
Cyclophosphamide
Cytarabine

Dactinomycin
Daunomycin
Dexamethasone
Dexrazoxane
Diphenhydramine
Dobutamine
Docetaxel
Dopamine
Doxorubicin
Doxycycline
Droperidol
Enalaprilat
Etoposide
Etoposide phosphate
Famotidine
Floxuridine
Fludarabine
Fluorouracil
Fluconazole
Gallium nitrate
Gentamicin
Granisetron
Haloperidol
Heparin
Hydrocortisone sodium
phosphate
Hydrocortisone sodium
succinate

Hydromorphone
Hydroxyzine
Idarubicin
Ifosfamide
Leucovorin
Lorazepam
Mannitol
Meperidine
Mesna
Metoclopramide
Metronidazole
Miconazole
Minocycline
Mitoxantrone
Morphine
Nalbuphine
Netilmicin
Ofloxacin
Ondansetron
Paclitaxel
Plicamycin
Potassium chloride
Promethazine
Ranitidine
Sodium bicarbonate
Streptozocin
Teniposide
Thiotepa

COMPATIBILITY OF CHEMOTHERAPY AND RELATED SUPPORTIVE CARE MEDICATIONS *(Continued)*

Ticarcillin	Trimethoprim	Vincristine
Ticarcillin/clavulanate	Vancomycin	Vinorelbine
Tobramycin	Vinblastine	Zidovudine
Topotecan		

Incompatible:

Acyclovir	Ganciclovir	Mezlocillin
Amphotericin	Imipenem/cilastatin	Mitomycin
Cefoperazone	Irinotecan	Piperacillin
Cefotaxime	Methotrexate	Piperacillin/tazobactam
Furosemide	Methylprednisolone	Prochlorperazine

Haloperidol

Compatible:

Hydromorphone	Sufentanil

Y-Site Compatible:

Amifostine	Gemcitabine	Paclitaxel
Amsacrine	Lidocaine	Phenylephrine
Aztreonam	Lorazepam	Tacrolimus
Cimetidine	Melphalan	Teniposide
Dobutamine	Midazolam	Theophylline
Dopamine	Nitroglycerin	Thiotepa
Famotidine	Norepinephrine bitar-	TPN
Filgrastim	trate	Vinorelbine
Fludarabine	Ondansetron	

Incompatible:

Allopurinol	Foscarnet	Ketorolac
Cefepime	Gallium nitrate	Piperacillin/tazobactam
Diphenhydramine	Heparin	Sargramostim
Fluconazole	Hydroxyzine	

Variable Compatibility:

Benztropine	Diamorphine	Sodium nitroprusside
Cyclizine		

Heparin

Compatible:

Aminophylline	Dopamine	Metronidazole
Amphotericin	Enalaprilat	Nafcillin
Ascorbic acid	Erythromycin	Norepinephrine
Bleomycin	Esmolol	Octreotide
Calcium gluconate	Floxacillin	Potassium chloride
Cefepime	Fluconazole	Prednisolone
Cephapirin	Flumazenil	Promazine
Chloramphenicol	Furosemide	Ranitidine
Cibenzoline	Isoproterenol	Sodium bicarbonate
Clindamycin	Lidocaine	Verapamil
Cloxacillin	Lincomycin	Vitamin B complex
Colistimethate	Methyldopa	with C
Dimenhydrinate	Methylprednisolone	

Y-Site Compatible:

Acyclovir	Digoxin	Melphalan
Aldesleukin	Diphenhydramine	Menadiol sodium
Allopurinol	Edrophonium	diphosphate
Amifostine	Epinephrine	Methicillin
Ampicillin	Erythromycin	Methotrexate
Ampicillin/sulbactam	Esmolol	Methoxamine
Atracurium	Estrogens, conjugated	Methyldopa
Atropine	Ethacrynate	Metoclopramide
Aztreonam	Famotidine	Metronidazole
Betamethasone sodium	Fentanyl	Midazolam
phosphate	Fludarabine	Minocycline
Cefazolin	Fluorouracil	Mitomycin
Cefotetan	Foscarnet	Morphine
Ceftazidime	Gallium nitrate	Neostigmine
Ceftriaxone	Gemcitabine	Nitroglycerin
Cephalothin	Hydralazine	Ondansetron
Chlordiazepoxide	Hydrocortisone sodium	Oxacillin
Chlorpromazine	succinate	Oxytocin
Cimetidine	Insulin	Paclitaxel
Cisplatin	Kanamycin	Pancuronium
Cyanocobalamin	Leucovorin	Penicillin G potassium
Cyclophosphamide	Lorazepam	Pentazocine
Cytarabine	Magnesium sulfate	Phytonadione

Piperacillin	Streptokinase	TPN
Piperacillin/tazobactam	Succinylcholine	Trimethobenzamide
Procainamide	Tacrolimus	Trimethaphan
Prochlorperazine	Teniposide	Vercuronium
Propranolol	Theophylline	Vinblastine
Pyridostigmine	Thiotepa	Vincristine
Sargramostim	Ticarcillin	Vinorelbine
Scopolamine	Ticarcillin/clavulanate	Zldovudine
Sodium nitroprusside		

Incompatible:

Alteplase	Doxorubicin	Levorphanol
Amikacin	Doxycycline	Methadone
Amiodarone	Ergotamine	Methotrimeprazine
Amsacrine	Filgrastim	Phenytoin
Ciprofloxacin	Gentamicin	Polymyxin B
Codeine phosphate	Haloperidol	Streptomycin
Daunomycin	Hyaluronidase	Tobramycin
Diazepam	Idarubicin	Triflupromazine
Dobutamine	Labetatol	

Variable Compatibility:

Cephalothin	Hydrocortisone sodium	Promethazine
Dacarbazine	succinate	Quinidine gluconate
Diltiazem	Methylprednisolone	Vancomycin
Droperidol	Penicillin G sodium	

Hydroxyzine

Compatible:

Atropine	Etoposide	Pentazocine
Benzquinamide	Fentanyl	Mesna
Bupivacaine	Fluphenazine	Methotrexate
Butorphanol	Glycopyrrolate	Nafcillin
Chlorpromazine	Hydromorphone	Perphenazine
Cimetidine	Lidocaine	Procaine
Cisplatin	Meperidine	Prochlorperazine
Codeine	Methotrimeprazine	Promazine
Cyclophosphamide	Metoclopramide	Promethazine
Cytarabine	Midazolam	Scopolamine
Diphenhydramine	Morphine	Sufentanil
Doxapram	Nalbuphine	Thiothixene
Droperidol	Oxymorphone	

Y-Site Compatible:

Aztreonam	Gemcitabine	Teniposide
Ciprofloxacin	Melphalan	Thiotepa
Filgrastim	Ondansetron	Vinorelbine
Foscarnet	Sufentanil	

Incompatible:

Allopurinol	Fluconazole	Pentobarbital
Amifostine	Fludarabine	Phenobarbital
Aminophylline	Haloperidol	Piperacillin/tazobactam
Amobarbital	Ketorolac	Ranitidine
Cefepime	Paclitaxel	Sargramostim
Chloramphenicol	Penicillin G (sodium and	
Diphenhydramine	potassium)	

Idarubicin

Compatible:

D$_5$W	NS	LR
D$_5$/NS		

Y-Site Compatible:

Amifostine	Droperidol	Metoclopramide
Amikacin	Erythromycin	Potassium chloride
Aztreonam	Filgrastim	Ranitidine
Ciprofloxacin	Gemcitabine	Sargramostim
Cyclophosphamide	Imipenem/cilastatin	Thiotepa
Cytarabine	Magnesium sulfate	Vinorelbine
Diphenhydramine	Mannitol	

Incompatible:

Acyclovir	Furosemide	Methotrexate
Allopurinol	Gentamicin	Mezlocillin
Ampicillin/sulbactam	Heparin	Piperacillin/tazobactam
Cefazolin	Hydrocortisone sodium	Sodium bicarbonate
Cefepime	succinate	Teniposide
Ceftazidime	Lorazepam	Vancomycin
Dexamethasone	Meperidine	Vincristine
Etoposide		

COMPATIBILITY OF CHEMOTHERAPY AND RELATED SUPPORTIVE CARE MEDICATIONS *(Continued)*

Ifosfamide

Compatible:

D₅W	NS	Cisplatin
D₅/NS	LR	Etoposide
D₅/¼NS	SWI	Fluorouracil
D₅/LR	Carboplatin	

Y-Site Compatible:

Allopurinol	Gemcitabine	Sargramostim
Amifostine	Granisetron	Sodium bicarbonate
Aztreonam	Ondansetron	Teniposide
Doxorubicin, liposomal	Paclitaxel	Thiotepa
Filgrastim	Piperacillin	TPN
Fludarabine	Piperacillin/tazobactam	Vinorelbine
Gallium nitrate	Propofol	

Incompatible:

Cefepime	Methotrexate

Variable Compatibility:

Epirubicin	Mesna

Irinotecan

Compatible:
   D₅W

Incompatible:
   Gemcitabine

Leucovorin

Compatible:

BWI	NS	Bleomycin
D₅W	LR	Cisplatin
D₁₀/NS	SWI	Floxuridine

Y-Site Compatible:

Amifostine	Furosemide	Sodium bicarbonate
Aztreonam	Gemcitabine	Tacrolimus
Cefepime	Heparin	Teniposide
Cyclophosphamide	Methotrexate	Thiotepa
Doxorubicin	Metoclopramide	TPN
Doxorubicin, liposomal	Mitomycin	Vinblastine
Filgrastim	Piperacillin	Vincristine
Fluconazole	Piperacillin/tazobactam	

Incompatible:

Droperidol	Foscarnet	Trimetrexate

Variable Compatibility:
   Fluorouracil

Lorazepam

Compatible:

Cimetidine	Hydromorphone

Y-Site Compatible:

Acyclovir	Diltiazem	Melphalan
Albumin	Doxorubicin	Methotrexate
Amifostine	Erythromycin	Metronidazole
Amikacin	Etomidate	Morphine
Amoxicillin	Fentanyl	Paclitaxel
Amoxicillin/clavulanate	Filgrastim	Pancuronium
Amsacrine	Fluconazole	Piperacillin
Atracurium	Fludarabine	Piperacillin/tazobactam
Bumetanide	Furosemide	Potassium chloride
Cefepime	Gemcitabine	Ranitidine
Cefotaxime	Gentamicin	Tacrolimus
Ciprofloxacin	Granisetron	Teniposide
Cisplatin	Haloperidol	Thiotepa
Cotrimoxazole	Heparin	Vancomycin
Cyclophosphamide	Hydrocortisone sodium	Vercuronium
Cytarabine	succinate	Vinorelbine
Dexamethasone	Kantaserin	Zidovudine

Incompatible:

Aldesleukin	Gallium nitrate	Sargramostim
Aztreonam	Idarubicin	Sufentanil
Buprenorphine	Imipenem/cilastatin	
Floxacillin	Ondansetron	Thiopental

Variable Compatibility:

Foscarnet

Mechlorethamine

Compatible:

NS   SWI

Y-Site Compatible:

Amifostine	Fludarabine	Sargramostim
Aztreonam	Granisetron	Teniposide
Filgrastim	Ondansetron	Vinorelbine

Incompatible:

D_5W	Cefepime	Methohexital
Allopurinol		

Melphalan

Compatible:

NS

Y-Site Compatible:

Acyclovir	Doxycycline	Methotrexate
Amikacin	Droperidol	Methylprednisolone
Aminophylline	Enalaprilat	Metoclopramide
Ampicillin	Etoposide	Metronidazole
Aztreonam	Famotidine	Miconazole
Bleomycin	Filgrastim	Minocycline
Bumetanide	Floxuridine	Mitomycin
Buprenorphine	Fluconazole	Mitoxantrone
Butorphanol	Fludarabine	Morphine
Calcium gluconate	Fluorouracil	Nalbuphine
Carboplatin	Furosemide	Netilmicin
Carmustine	Gallium nitrate	Ondansetron
Cefazolin	Ganciclovir	Pentostatin
Cefepime	Gentamicin	Piperacillin
Cefoperazone	Haloperidol	Plicamycin
Cefotaxime	Heparin	Potassium chloride
Cefotetan	Hydrocortisone sodium	Prochlorperazine
Ceftazidime	phosphate	Promethazine
Ceftriaxone	Hydrocortisone sodium	Ranitidine
Cefuroxime	succinate	Sodium bicarbonate
Cimetidine	Hydromorphone	Streptozocin
Cisplatin	Hydroxyzine	Teniposide
Cotrimoxazole	Idarubicin	Thiotepa
Cyclophosphamide	Ifosfamide	Ticarcillin
Cytarabine	Imipenem/cilastatin	Ticarcillin/clavulanate
Dacarbazine	Lorazepam	Tobramycin
Dactinomycin	Mannitol	Vancomycin
Daunomycin	Mechlorethamine	Vinblastine
Diazepam	Meperidine	Vincristine
Doxorubicin	Mesna	Vinorelbine

Incompatible:

D_5W	SWI	Chlorpromazine
LR	Amphotericin	

COMPATIBILITY OF CHEMOTHERAPY AND RELATED SUPPORTIVE CARE MEDICATIONS *(Continued)*

Mesna

Compatible:

BWI	LR	Hydroxyzine
D_5W	Cyclophosphamide	Ifosfamide
NS		

Y-Site Compatible:

Allopurinol	Gallium nitrate	Sargramostim
Amifostine	Gemcitabine	Sodium acetate
Aztreonam	Granisetron	Teniposide
Cefepime	Methotrexate	Thiotepa
Doxorubicin, liposomal	Ondansetron	TPN
Filgrastim	Paclitaxel	Vinorelbine
Fludarabine	Piperacillin/tazobactam	

Incompatible:

Carboplatin	Cisplatin	Chlorpromazine

Methadone

Incompatible:

Aminophylline	Phenytoin	Pentobarbital
Ammonium chloride	Heparin	Sodium bicarbonate
Amobarbital	Methicillin	
Chlorothiazide	Nitrofurantoin	Thiopental

Methotrexate

Compatible:

D_5W	Cyclophosphamide	Imipenem/cilastatin
NS	Cytarabine	Mercaptopurine
LR	Dacarbazine	Ondansetron
SWI	Fluorouracil	Sodium bicarbonate
Amino acid 4.25%/D_{25}W	Hydroxyzine	Vincristine
Cephalothin		

Y-Site Compatible:

Allopurinol	Doxorubicin, liposomal	Methylprednisolone
Amifostine	Etoposide	Mitomycin
Asparaginase	Famotidine	Morphine
Aztreonam	Filgrastim	Oxacillin
Bleomycin	Fludarabine	Paclitaxel
Cefepime	Furosemide	Piperacillin/tazobactam
Ceftriaxone	Gallium nitrate	Prochlorperazine
Cimetidine	Ganciclovir	Ranitidine
Cisplatin	Granisetron	Sargramostim
Daunomycin	Heparin	Teniposide
Dexchlorpheniramine	Hydromorphone	Thiotepa
Diphenhydramine	Leucovorin	Vinblastine
Doxapram	Lorazepam	Vindesine
Doxorubicin	Mesna	Vinorelbine

Incompatible:

Dexamethasone	Midazolam	Promethazine
Gemcitabine		Propofol
Idarubicin	Nalbuphine	
Ifosfamide	Prednisolone	TPN

Variable Compatibility:

Droperidol	Metoclopramide	Vancomycin

Metoclopramide

Compatible:

D_5W	Multivitamins	Potassium phosphate
NS	Potassium acetate	Verapamil
Clindamycin	Potassium chloride	TPN
Mannitol		

Y-Site Compatible:

Acyclovir	Fluconazole	Morphine
Aldesleukin	Fludarabine	Ondansetron
Amifostine	Fluorouracil	Paclitaxel
Aztreonam	Foscarnet	Piperacillin/tazobactam
Bleomycin	Gallium nitrate	Sargramostim
Ciprofloxacin	Gemcitabine	Sufentanil
Cisplatin	Heparin	Tacrolimus
Cyclophosphamide	Idarubicin	Teniposide
Cytarabine	Leucovorin	Thiotepa
Diltiazem	Melphalan	Vinblastine
Doxorubicin	Meperidine	Vincristine
Droperidol	Methotrexate	Vinorelbine
Famotidine	Mitomycin	Zidovudine
Filgrastim		

Incompatible:

Allopurinol	Cephalothin	Floxacillin
Ampicillin	Chloramphenicol	Furosemide
Calcium gluconate	Dexamethasone	Penicillin G potassium
Cefepime	Erythromycin	Sodium bicarbonate

Metronidazole

Compatible:

Amikacin	Cefuroxime	Heparin
Aminophylline	Cephalothin	Hydrocortisone
Cefazolin	Chloramphenicol	Moxalactam
Cefotaxime	Ciprofloxacin	Multielectrolyte concen-
Cefotetan	Clindamycin	trate
Cefoxitin	Disopyramide	Multivitamins
Ceftazidime	Floxacillin	Netilmicin
Ceftizoxime	Fluconazole	Penicillin G potassium
Ceftriaxone	Gentamicin	Tobramycin

Y-Site Compatible:

Acyclovir	Gemcitabine	Perphenazine
Allopurinol	Heparin	Piperacillin/tazobactam
Amifostine	Hydromorphone	Sargramostim
Cefepime	Labetatol	Tacrolimus
Cyclophosphamide	Lorazepam	Teniposide
Diltiazem	Magnesium sulfate	Theophylline
Enalaprilat	Melphalan	Thiotepa
Esmolol	Meperidine	TPN
Fluconazole	Midazolam	Vinorelbine
Foscarnet	Morphine	

Incompatible:

Aztreonam	Dopamine	Filgrastim

Variable Compatibility:

Ampicillin	Cefamandole

COMPATIBILITY OF CHEMOTHERAPY AND RELATED SUPPORTIVE CARE MEDICATIONS *(Continued)*

Mitomycin

Compatible:

NS	Hydrocortisone sodium	
LR	succinate	
Dexamethasone		

Y-Site Compatible:

Allopurinol	Droperidol	Ondansetron
Amifostine	Fluorouracil	Teniposide
Bleomycin	Furosemide	Thiotepa
Cisplatin	Leucovorin	Vinblastine
Cyclophosphamide	Methotrexate	Vincristine
Doxorubicin	Metoclopramide	

Incompatible:

Aztreonam	Gemcitabine	Sargramostim
Cefepime		
Filgrastim	Piperacillin/tazobactam	Vinorelbine

Variable Compatibility:

D_5W	SWI	Heparin

Mitoxantrone

Compatible:

D_5W	Cyclophosphamide	Fluorouracil
D_5/NS		
NS	Cytarabine	Potassium chloride

Y-Site Compatible:

Allopurinol	Gemcitabine	Teniposide
Amifostine	Ondansetron	Thiotepa
Filgrastim	Sargramostim	Vinorelbine
Fludarabine		

Incompatible:

Aztreonam	Heparin	Piperacillin/tazobactam
Cefepime	Paclitaxel	
Doxorubicin, liposomal	Piperacillin	Propofol

Variable Compatibility:

Hydrocortisone sodium	Hydrocortisone sodium	TPN
phosphate	succinate	

Ondansetron

Compatible:

D_5W	Dexamethasone	Mannitol
NS	Doxorubicin	Meperidine
LR	Etoposide	Methotrexate
Cisplatin	Fluconazole	Morphine
Cyclophosphamide	Hydrocortisone sodium	Ranitidine
Cytarabine	succinate	
Dacarbazine		

Y-Site Compatible:

Aldesleukin	Droperidol	Miconazole
Amifostine	Famotidine	Mitomycin
Amikacin	Filgrastim	Mitoxantrone
Aztreonam	Floxuridine	Paclitaxel
Bleomycin	Fludarabine	Pentostatin
Carboplatin	Gallium nitrate	Piperacillin/tazobactam
Carmustine	Gemcitabine	Potassium chloride
Cefazolin	Gentamicin	Prochlorperazine
Cefotaxime	Haloperidol	Promethazine
Cefoxitin	Heparin	Sodium acetate
Ceftazidime	Hydrocortisone sodium	Streptozocin
Ceftizoxime	phosphate	Teniposide
Cefuroxime	Hydromorphone	Thiotepa
Chlorpromazine	Hydroxyzine	Ticarcillin
Cimetidine	Ifosfamide	Ticarcillin/clavulanate
Dactinomycin	Imipenem/cilastatin	TPN
Daunomycin	Magnesium sulfate	Vancomycin
Diphenhydramine	Mechlorethamine	Vinblastine
Doxorubicin, liposomal	Mesna	Vincristine
Doxycycline	Metoclopramide	Vinorelbine

Incompatible:

Acyclovir	Amsacrine	Methylprednisolone
Allopurinol	Cefepime	Mezlocillin
Aminophylline	Cefoperazone	Piperacillin
Amphotericin	Furosemide	Sargramostim
Ampicillin	Ganciclovir	Sargramostim
Ampicillin/sulbactam	Lorazepam	Sodium bicarbonate

Variable Compatibility:

Fluorouracil

Paclitaxel

Compatible:

NS

Y-Site Compatible:

Acyclovir	Etoposide	Mannitol
Amikacin	Famotidine	Meperidine
Aminophylline	Floxuridine	Mesna
Ampicillin/sulbactam	Fluconazole	Methotrexate
Bleomycin	Fluorouracil	Metoclopramide
Butorphanol	Furosemide	Morphine
Calcium chloride	Ganciclovir	Nalbuphine
Carboplatin	Gemcitabine	Ondansetron
Cefepime	Gentamicin	Pentostatin
Cefotetan	Granisetron	Potassium chloride
Ceftazidime	Haloperidol	Prochlorperazine
Cefuroxime	Heparin	Propofol
Cimetidine	Hydrocortisone sodium phosphate	Ranitidine
Cyclophosphamide	Hydrocortisone sodium succinate	Sodium bicarbonate
Cytarabine	Hydromorphone	Thiotepa
Dacarbazine	Ifosfamide	TPN
Dexamethasone	Lorazepam	Vancomycin
Diphenhydramine	Magnesium sulfate	Vinblastine
Doxorubicin		Vincristine
Droperidol		

Incompatible:

Amphotericin	Doxorubicin, liposomal	Methylprednisolone
Chlorpromazine	Hydroxyzine	Mitoxantrone

Variable Compatibility:

D_5W Cisplatin

Pentostatin

Compatible:

NS   LR

Y-Site Compatible:

Fludarabine	Paclitaxel	Sargramostim
Ondansetron		

Variable Compatibility:

D_5W

COMPATIBILITY OF CHEMOTHERAPY AND RELATED SUPPORTIVE CARE MEDICATIONS *(Continued)*

Phytonadione

Compatible:

Amikacin	Chloramphenicol	Doxapram
Calcium gluceptate	Cimetidine	Sodium bicarbonate
Cefapirin	Netilmicin	TPN

Y-Site Compatible:

Ampicillin	Hydrocortisone sodium	Tolazoline
Epinephrine	succinate	Vitamin B complex
Famotidine	Potassium chloride	with C
Heparin		

Incompatible:

Dobutamine	Ranitidine

Plicamycin

Compatible:

D_5W	SWI	Piperacillin
NS		

Y-Site Compatible:

Allopurinol	Filgrastim	Teniposide
Amifostine	Gemcitabine	Vinorelbine
Aztreonam	Piperacillin/tazobactam	

Incompatible:

Cefonicid

Prochlorperazine

Compatible:

Amikacin	Erythromycin	Sodium bicarbonate
Ascorbic acid	Ethacrinate	Vitamin B complex
Dexamethasone	Lidocaine	with C
Dimenhydrinate	Nafcillin	

Y-Site Compatible:

Amsacrine	Hydrocortisone sodium	Potassium chloride
Cisplatin	succinate	Sargramostim
Cyclophosphamide	Melphalan	Sufentanil
Cytarabine	Methotrexate	Teniposide
Doxorubicin	Ondansetron	Thiotepa
Fluconazole	Paclitaxel	Vinorelbine
Heparin		

Incompatible:

Aldesleukin	Cefepime	Gallium nitrate
Allopurinol	Cephalothin	Gemcitabine
Amifostine	Chloramphenicol	Methohexital
Aminophylline	Floxacillin	Penicillin G sodium
Amphotericin	Fludarabine	Piperacillin/tazobactam
Ampicillin	Foscarnet	Phenobarbital
Aztreonam	Filgrastim	Thiopental
Calcium gluceptate	Furosemide	

Variable Compatibility:

Calcium gluconate	Penicillin G potassium

Promethazine

Compatible:

Amikacin	Chloroquine	Vitamin B complex
Ascorbic acid	Netilmicin	with C

Y-Site Compatible:

Amifostine	Cytarabine	Melphalan
Amsacrine	Doxorubicin	Ondansetron
Aztreonam	Filgrastim	Sargramostim
Ciprofloxacin	Fluconazole	Teniposide
Cisplatin	Fludarabine	Thiotepa
Cyclophosphamide	Gemcitabine	Vinorelbine

Incompatible:

Aldesleukin	Chlorothiazide	Methohexital
Allopurinol	Floxacillin	Methotrexate
Aminophylline	Foscarnet	Penicillin G (sodium and
Cefepime	Furosemide	potassium)
Cefoperazone	Heparin	Pentobarbital
Cefotetan	Hydrocortisone sodium	Piperacillin/tazobactam
Ceftizoxime	succinate	Thiopental
Chloramphenicol	Methicillin	

Variable Compatibility:

Potassium chloride

Sargramostim

Compatible:

BWI	NS	SWI
D₅W		

Y-Site Compatible:

Allopurinol	Dacarbazine	Mechlorethamine
Amikacin	Dactinomycin	Meperidine
Aminophylline	Dexamethasone	Mesna
Aztreonam	Diphenhydramine	Methotrexate
Bleomycin	Dobutamine	Metoclopramide
Butorphanol	Doxorubicin	Metronidazole
Calcium gluconate	Doxycycline	Mezlocillin
Carboplatin	Droperidol	Miconazole
Carmustine	Etoposide	Minocycline
Cefazolin	Famotidine	Mitoxantrone
Cefepime	Fentanyl	Netilmicin
Cefotetan	Floxuridine	Pentostatin
Cefoxitin	Fluconazole	Piperacillin/tazobactam
Ceftizoxime	Fluorouracil	Potassium chloride
Ceftriaxone	Furosemide	Prochlorperazine
Cefuroxime	Gentamicin	Promethazine
Cimetidine	Heparin	Ranitidine
Cisplatin	Human immune globulin	Teniposide
Cotrimoxazole	Idarubicin	Ticarcillin
Cyclophosphamide	Ifosfamide	Ticarcillin/clavulanate
Cyclosporine	Magnesium sulfate	Vinblastine
Cytarabine	Mannitol	Vincristine

Incompatible:

Acyclovir	Hydrocortisone sodium	Mitomycin
Ampicillin	phosphate	Morphine
Ampicillin/sulbactam	Hydrocortisone sodium	Nalbuphine
Cefonicid	succinate	Ondansetron
Cefoperazone	Hydromorphone	Piperacillin
Chlorpromazine	Hydroxyzine	Sodium bicarbonate
Ganciclovir	Imipenem/cilastatin	Tobramycin
Haloperidol	Methylprednisolone	

Variable Compatibility:

Amphotericin	Ceftazidime	Vancomycin
Amsacrine		

COMPATIBILITY OF CHEMOTHERAPY AND RELATED SUPPORTIVE CARE MEDICATIONS *(Continued)*

Streptozocin

Compatible:

D_5W	NS	SWI

Y-Site Compatible:

Filgrastim	Ondansetron	Thiotepa
Gemcitabine	Teniposide	Vinorelbine
Granisetron		

Incompatible:

Allopurinol	Cefepime	Piperacillin/tazobactam
Aztreonam	Piperacillin	

Teniposide

Compatible:

D_5W	NS	LR

Y-Site Compatible:

Acyclovir	Dacarbazine	Mechlorethamine
Allopurinol	Dactinomycin	Meperidine
Amifostine	Daunomycin	Mesna
Amikacin	Dexamethasone	Methotrexate
Aminophylline	Diphenhydramine	Methylprednisolone
Amphotericin	Doxorubicin	Metoclopramide
Ampicillin	Doxycycline	Metronidazole
Ampicillin/sulbactam	Droperidol	Mezlocillin
Aztreonam	Enalaprilat	Miconazole
Bleomycin	Etoposide	Midazolam
Bumetanide	Famotidine	Mitomycin
Buprenorphine	Floxuridine	Mitoxantrone
Butorphanol	Fluconazole	Morphine
Calcium gluconate	Fludarabine	Nalbuphine
Carboplatin	Fluorouracil	Netilmicin
Carmustine	Furosemide	Ondansetron
Cefazolin	Gallium nitrate	Piperacillin
Cefonicid	Ganciclovir	Plicamycin
Cefoperazone	Gemcitabine	Potassium chloride
Cefotaxime	Gentamicin	Prochlorperazine
Cefotetan	Haloperidol	Promethazine
Cefoxitin	Heparin	Ranitidine
Ceftazidime	Hydrocortisone sodium phosphate	Sargramostim
Ceftizoxime		Sodium bicarbonate
Ceftriaxone	Hydrocortisone sodium succinate	Streptozocin
Cefuroxime		Thiotepa
Chlorpromazine	Hydromorphone	Ticarcillin
Cimetidine	Hydroxyzine	Ticarcillin/clavulanate
Cisplatin	Ifosfamide	Tobramycin
Corticotropin	Imipenem/cilastatin	Vancomycin
Cotrimoxazole	Leucovorin	Vinblastine
Cyclophosphamide	Lorazepam	Vincristine
Cytarabine	Mannitol	Vinorelbine

Incompatible:

Idarubicin

Thiethylperazine

Compatible:

NS	Hydromorphone	Ranitidine
Butorphanol	Midazolam	

Y-Site Compatible:

Aldesleukin

Incompatible:

Ketorolac	Perphenazine

Variable Compatibility:

Nalbuphine

Thiotepa

Compatible:

NS	SWI

Y-Site Compatible:

Acyclovir	Daunomycin	Mannitol
Allopurinol	Dexamethasone	Meperidine
Amifostine	Diphenhydramine	Mesna
Amikacin	Dobutamine	Methotrexate
Aminophylline	Dopamine	Methylprednisolone
Amphotericin	Doxorubicin	Metoclopramide
Ampicillin	Doxycycline	Metronidazole
Ampicillin/sulbactam	Droperidol	Mezlocillin
Aztreonam	Enalaprilat	Miconazole
Bleomycin	Etoposide	Mitomycin
Bumetanide	Famotidine	Mitoxantrone
Buprenorphine	Floxuridine	Morphine
Butorphanol	Fluconazole	Nalbuphine
Calcium gluconate	Fludarabine	Netilmicin
Carboplatin	Fluorouracil	Ofloxacin
Carmustine	Furosemide	Ondansetron
Cefazolin	Gallium nitrate	Paclitaxel
Cefepime	Ganciclovir	Piperacillin
Cefonicid	Gemcitabine	Piperacillin/tazobactam
Cefoperazone	Gentamicin	Plicamycin
Cefotaxime	Granisetron	Potassium chloride
Cefotetan	Haloperidol	Prochlorperazine
Cefoxitin	Heparin	Promethazine
Ceftazidime	Hydrocortisone sodium phosphate	Ranitidine
Ceftizoxime		Sodium bicarbonate
Ceftriaxone	Hydrocortisone sodium succinate	Streptozocin
Cefuroxime		Teniposide
Chlorpromazine	Hydromorphone	Ticarcillin
Cimetidine	Hydroxyzine	Ticarcillin/clavulanate
Ciprofloxacin	Idarubicin	Tobramycin
Cotrimoxazole	Ifosfamide	TPN
Cyclophosphamide	Imipenem/cilastatin	Vancomycin
Cytarabine	Leucovorin	Vinblastine
Dacarbazine	Lorazepam	Vincristine
Dactinomycin	Magnesium sulfate	

Incompatible:

Cisplatin	Filgrastim	Minocycline

Topotecan

Compatible:

D$_5$W	NS	LR

Y-Site Compatible:

Gemcitabine

COMPATIBILITY OF CHEMOTHERAPY AND RELATED SUPPORTIVE CARE MEDICATIONS *(Continued)*

Trimetrexate

Compatible:

D$_5$W

Y-Site Compatible:

Amifostine

Incompatible:

BNS	D$_5$/LR	Calcium chloride
D$_5$/NS	D$_{10}$/NS	Chloride ion
D$_5$/¼NS	NS	Leucovorin
D$_5$/½NS	LR	Potassium chloride

Vinblastine

Compatible:

BNS	NS	Bleomycin
D$_5$W	LR	Dacarbazine

Y-Site Compatible:

Allopurinol	Fludarabine	Paclitaxel
Amifostine	Fluorouracil	Piperacillin
Aztreonam	Gemcitabine	Piperacillin/tazobactam
Cisplatin	Leucovorin	Sargramostim
Cyclophosphamide	Methotrexate	Teniposide
Doxorubicin, liposomal	Metoclopramide	Vincristine
Droperidol	Mitomycin	Vinorelbine
Filgrastim	Ondansetron	

Incompatible:

Cefazolin   Furosemide

Variable Compatibility:

Doxorubicin   Heparin

Vincristine

Compatible:

D$_5$W	Bleomycin	Fluorouracil
NS	Cytarabine	Methotrexate
LR	Doxorubicin	

Y-Site Compatible:

Allopurinol	Filgrastim	Ondansetron
Amifostine	Fludarabine	Paclitaxel
Aztreonam	Gemcitabine	Piperacillin/tazobactam
Cisplatin	Granisetron	Sargramostim
Cyclophosphamide	Heparin	Teniposide
Doxapram	Leucovorin	Vinblastine
Doxorubicin, liposomal	Metoclopramide	Vinorelbine
Droperidol	Mitomycin	

Incompatible:

Cefepime	Idarubicin	Sodium bicarbonate
Furosemide		

Vinorelbine

Compatible:

D$_5$W   NS   LR

D$_5$/^{1}/$_2$NS

Y-Site Compatible:

Amikacin	Doxycycline	Lorazepam
Aztreonam	Droperidol	Mannitol
Bleomycin	Enalaprilat	Mechlorethamine
Bumetanide	Etoposide	Meperidine
Buprenorphine	Famotidine	Mesna
Butorphanol	Filgrastim	Methotrexate
Calcium gluconate	Fluconazole	Metoclopramide
Carboplatin	Fludarabine	Metronidazole
Carmustine	Fluorouracil	Minocycline
Cefotaxime	Gallium nitrate	Mitoxantrone
Ceftazidime	Gemcitabine	Morphine
Ceftizoxime	Gentamicin	Nalbuphine
Chlorpromazine	Haloperidol	Netilmicin
Cimetidine	Heparin	Ondansetron
Cisplatin	Hydrocortisone sodium	Plicamycin
Cyclophosphamide	phosphate	Streptozocin
Cytarabine	Hydrocortisone sodium	Teniposide
Dacarbazine	succinate	Ticarcillin
Dactinomycin	Hydromorphone	Ticarcillin/clavulanate
Daunomycin	Hydroxyzine	Tobramycin
Dexamethasone	Idarubicin	Vinblastine
Diphenhydramine	Ifosfamide	Vincristine
Doxorubicin	Imipenem/cilastatin	Vindesine
Doxorubicin, liposomal		

Incompatible:

Acyclovir	Cefoperazone	Furosemide
Allopurinol	Cefotetan	Ganciclovir
Aminophylline	Ceftriaxone	Methylprednisolone
Amphotericin	Cefuroxime	Mitomycin
Ampicillin	Cotrimoxazole	Sodium bicarbonate
Cefazolin	Fluorouracil	Thiotepa

COMPATIBILITY OF CHEMOTHERAPY AND RELATED SUPPORTIVE CARE MEDICATIONS *(Continued)*

Drug	Variable Compatibility
Carboplatin	Solutions in saline are less stable than in dextrose.
Carmustine	Solutions should be dispensed in glass and protected from light. Solutions are stable for <8 hours under most circumstances.
Cisplatin	Must have a chloride concentration of at least 0.2% in the final solution. The commercial product has a NS concentration. Etoposide + mannitol + potassium chloride in normal saline precipitates within 24 hours; when in $D_5/^1/_2NS$, it is stable for 24 hours.
Dacarbazine	Heparin 100 units/mL with dacarbazine 25 mg/mL is **incompatible**. Heparin 100 units/mL with dacarbazine 10 mg/mL is **compatible.**
Filgrastim	Gentamicin is reported to be physically **compatible** for Y-site injection, but with a decrease in biologic activity. Imipenem/cilastatin with filgrastim 40 mcg/mL is reported to be physically **compatible** for Y-site injection, but with a decrease in biologic activity.
Fluorouracil	Doxorubicin 2 mg/mL with fluorouracil 50 mg/mL is **compatible** for 13 minutes. Doxorubicin 0.5-1 mg/mL with fluorouracil 50 mg/mL is **incompatible**. Fluorouracil with doxorubicin is **Y-site compatible.** Variable compatibility with leucovorin.
Mesna	**Compatible** with ifosfamide. **Incompatible** with ifosfamide and epinephrine.
Leucovorin	Variable compatibility with fluorouracil.
Mitomycin	Mitomycin 50 mg/L in NS has a color change and 10% loss of drug concentration in 12 hours. Mitomycin 1 g/L in SWI precipitates in 24 hours under refrigeration. Other temperatures and concentrations are reported to be stable. Mitomycin in D_5W is **incompatible** in 20 mg/L; **compatible** in 40 mg/L. Mitomycin 500 mg/L with heparin 33,300 units/L in NS is **compatible**. PVC containers of mitomycin 167 mg/L with heparin 33,300 units/L in NS is **compatible**. Glass containers of mitomycin 167 mg/L with heparin 33,300 units/L in NS are **incompatible**.
Pentostatin	Pentostatin 20 mg/mL in D_5W at room temperature: a 2% loss of drug in 24 hours; 8% to 10% loss in 48 hours; and a 10% loss in 54 hours. Under refrigeration, there is no loss in 96 hours. There is a 10% loss in 23 hours at room temperature of pentostatin 2 mg/mL in D_5W
Sargramostim	Amphotericin B 0.6 mg/mL in D_5W with sargramostim 10 mcg/mL in NS forms immediate precipitate. Amphotericin B 0.6 mg/mL in D_5W with sargramostim 10 mcg/mL in D_5W is **Y-site compatible**. Amsacrine with sargramostim in NS forms immediate precipitate. Amsacrine with sargramostim in D_5W is **Y-site compatible**. Ceftazidime 40 mg/mL in NS with sargramostim 10 mcg/mL in NS is **incompatible**, with particle formation within 4 hours. Ceftazidime 40 mg/mL with sargramostim 6 or 15 mcg/mL is **compatible** for 2 hours (Y-site **compatible**). Vancomycin 20 mg/mL and sargramostim 6 mcg/mL is **incompatible**. Vancomycin 10 mg/mL and sargramostim 10 mcg/mL is **Y-site compatible**. Vancomycin 20 mg/mL and sargramostim 15 mcg/mL is **Y-site compatible**.
Vancomycin	Vancomycin 5 mg/mL with methotrexate 30 mg/mL is **compatible** for 2 hours, precipitates within 4 hours. Other concentrations tested were **compatible** for 1 hour. Vancomycin with methotrexate is **Y-site compatible**.
Vinblastine	In various volumes, doxorubicin 2 mg/mL with vinblastine 1 mg/mL yields erratic assay results. Vinblastine with doxorubicin is **Y-site compatible**. Heparin 200 units/mL with vinblastine 1 mg/mL is **incompatible** in a syringe for 13 minutes. Heparin 500 units/mL with vinblastine 0.5 mg/mL is **compatible** in a syringe for 13 minutes.

Suggested Readings

Hall PD, Yui D, Lyons S, et al, "Compatibility of Filgrastim With Selected Antimicrobial Drugs During Simulated Y-Site Administration," *Am J Health-System Pharm*, 1997, 54:184-9.

McGuire TR, Narducci WA, and Fox JL, "Compatibility and Stability of Ondansetron Hydrochloride, Dexamethasone and Lorazepam in Injectable Solutions," *Am J Health-System Pharm*, 1993, 50:1410-4.

Najari Z and Rucho WJ, "Compatibility of Commonly Used Bone Marrow Drugs During Y-Site Delivery," *Am J Health-System Pharm*, 1997, 54:181-4.

Trissel LA, Chandler SW, and Folstad JT, "Visual Compatibility of Amsacrine With Selected Drugs During Simulated Y-Site Injection," *Am J Hospital Pharm*, 1990, 47:2525-8.

Trissel LA, Bready BB, Kwan JW, et al, "Visual Compatibility of Sargramostim With Selected Antineoplastic Agents, Anti-infectives, or Other Drugs During Simulated Y-Site Injection," *Am J Hospital Pharm*, 1992, 49:402-6.

Trissel LA and Martinez JF, "Physical Compatibility of Melphalan With Selected Drugs During Simulated Y-Site Administration," *Am J Hospital Pharm*, 1993, 50:2359-63.

Trissel LA and Martinez JF, Visual, "Turbidimetric and Particle-Content Assessment of Compatibility of Vinorelbine Tartrate With Selected Drugs During Simulated Y-Site Injection," *Am J Hospital Pharm*, 1994, 51:495-9.

Trissel LA and Martinez JF, "Physical Compatibility of Allopurinol Sodium With Selected Drugs During Simulated Y-Site Administration," *Am J Hospital Pharm*, 1994, 51:1792-9.

Trissel LA and Martinez JF, "Compatibility of Filgrastim With Selected Drugs During Simulated Y-Site Administration," *Am J Hospital Pharm*, 1994, 51:1907-13.

Trissel LA and Martinez JF, "Screening Teniposide For Y-Site Compatibility," *Hospital Pharm*, 1994, 29:1010, 1012-4, 1017.

Trissel LA, *Handbook on Injectable Drugs*, 9th Ed. Bethesda, MD: Am Society Health-Systems Pharmacists, 1996.

Trissel LA, *Supplement to Handbook on Injectable Drugs*, 9th Ed. Bethesda, MD: Am Society of Health-Systems Pharmacists, 1997.

Trissel LA, Gilbert DL, and Martinez JF, "Compatibility of Granisetron Hydrochloride With Selected Drugs During Simulated Y-Site Administration," *Am J Health-System Pharm*, 1997, 54:56-60.

Trissel LA, Gilbert DL, and Martinez JF, "Compatibility of Propofol With Selected Drugs During Simulated Y-Site Administration," *Am J Health-System Pharm*, 1997, 54:1287-92.

Trissel LA, Gilbert DL, Martinez JF, et al, "Compatibility of Parenteral Nutrient Solutions With Selected Drugs During Simulated Y-Site Administration," *Am J Health-System Pharm*, 1997, 54:1295-300.

Trissel LA, Gilbert DL, and Martinez JF, "Compatibility of Doxorubicin Hydrochloride Liposome With Selected Other Drugs During Simulated Y-Site Administration," *Am J Health-System Pharm*, 1997; 54:2708-13.

Trissel LA, Martinez JF, and Gilbert DL, "Compatibility of Gemcitabine Hydrochloride With 107 Selected Drugs During Simulated Y-Site Administration," *J Am Pharmaceutical Association*, 1999, 39 (4):514-18.

Zhang Y, Xu QA, Trissel LA, et al, "Compatibility and Stability of Paclitaxel Combined With Cisplatin and With Carboplatin in Infusion Solutions," *Ann Pharmacother*, 1997, 31 (12):1465-70.

HEMATOLOGIC ADVERSE EFFECTS OF DRUGS

Drug	Red Cell Aplasia	Thrombocy-topenia	Neutrope-nia	Pancytope-nia	Hemolysis
Acetazolamide		+	+	+	
Allopurinol			+		
Amiodarone	+				
Amphotericin B				+	
Amrinone		++			
Asparaginase		+++	+++	+++	++
Barbiturates		+		+	
Benzocaine					++
Captopril			++		+
Carbamazepine		++	+		
Cephalosporins			+		++
Chloramphenicol		+	++	+++	
Chlordiazepoxide			+	+	
Chloroquine		+			
Chlorothiazides		++			
Chlorpropamide	+	++	+	++	+
Chlortetracycline				+	
Chlorthalidone			+		
Cimetidine		+	++	+	
Codeine		+			
Colchicine				+	
Cyclophosphamide		+++	+++	+++	+
Dapsone					+++
Desipramine		++			
Digitalis		+			
Digitoxin		++			
Erythromycin		+			
Estrogen		+		+	
Ethacrynic acid			+		
Fluorouracil		+++	+++	+++	+
Furosemide		+	+		
Gold salts	+	+++	+++	+++	
Heparin		++		+	
Ibuprofen			+		+
Imipramine			++		
Indomethacin		+	++	+	
Isoniazid		+		+	
Isosorbide dinitrate					+
Levodopa					++
Meperidine		+			
Meprobamate		+	+	+	
Methimazole			++		
Methyldopa		++			+++
Methotrexate		+++	+++	+++	++
Methylene blue					+
Metronidazole			+		
Nalidixic acid					+
Naproxen				+	
Nitrofurantoin			++		+
Nitroglycerine		+			
Penicillamine		++	+		
Penicillins		+	++	+	+++
Phenazopyridine				.	+++
Phenothiazines		+	++	+++	+

Drug	Red Cell Aplasia	Thrombocy-topenia	Neutrope-nia	Pancytope-nia	Hemolysis
Phenylbutazone		+	++	+++	+
Phenytoin		++	++	++	+
Potassium iodide		+			
Prednisone		+			
Primaquine					+++
Procainamide			+		
Procarbazine		+	++	++	+
Propylthiouracil		+	++	+	+
Quinidine		+++	+		
Quinine		+++	+		
Reserpine		+			
Rifampicin		++	+		+++
Spironolactone			+		
Streptomycin		+		+	
Sulfamethoxazole with trimethoprim			+		
Sulfonamides	+	++	++	++	++
Sulindac	+	+	+	+	
Tetracyclines		+			+
Thioridazine			++		
Tolbutamide		++	+	++	
Triamterene					+
Valproate	+				
Vancomycin			+		

+ = rare or single reports.

++ = occasional reports.

+++ = substantial number of reports.

Adapted from D'Arcy PF and Griffin JP, eds, *Iatrogenic Diseases*, New York, NY: Oxford University Press, 1986, 128-30.

TUMOR LYSIS SYNDROME, MANAGEMENT

Tumor lysis syndrome (TLS) may be seen with any tumor that is undergoing rapid cell turnover as a result of high growth fraction or high cell death due to therapy. It occurs most often in Burkitt's lymphoma and T-cell ALL, both of which have large tumor burdens and high sensitivity to chemotherapy. Acute lysis of tumor cells results in the rapid release of potassium, phosphates, and nucleic acids into the circulation. Hypocalcemia, hyperuricemia, and renal failure may result. Secondary acute precipitation of calcium and urates in the kidney, tumor infiltration of the kidney, obstructive uropathy, and dehydration may increase the primary metabolic disturbances. The following chart reviews the management of TLS.

Therapy	Infants & Children	Adolescents & Adults
Hydration (patients typically present with dehydration; I.V. fluids should be started immediately)	3000-6000 mL/m^2/day	3000-6000 mL/m^2/day
	D$_5$W $^1/_4$ NS (+ sodium bicarbonate)	D$_5$W $^1/_4$ NS (+ sodium bicarbonate)
	Maintain urine output at ≥1 mL/kg/hour	Maintain urine output at 100-150 mL/hour
	Maintain urine specific gravity at ≤1.010	Maintain urine specific gravity at ≤1.010
	Strict monitoring of I & O	Strict monitoring of I & O
Alkalinization	50-100 mEq/L sodium bicarbonate in I.V. fluid	50-100 mEq/L sodium bicarbonate in I.V. fluid
	Maintain urine pH at 7.0-7.5	Maintain urine pH at 7.0-7.5
	Reduce bicarbonate if serum bicarbonate >30 mEq/L or urine pH >7.5	Reduce bicarbonate if serum bicarbonate >30 mEq/L or urine pH >7.5
Uric acid reduction	Allopurinol: I.V., oral: 200-400 mg/m^2/day in 1-3 divided doses (maximum: 600 mg/day) Urate oxidase: I.V. (investigational, see protocol): 0.2 mg/kg/dose once or twice daily	Allopurinol: I.V.: 200-400 mg/m^2/day in 1-3 divided doses (maximum: 600 mg/day) Oral: 600-800 mg/day in 1-2 doses
Diuretics (avoid if hypovolemic)	Furosemide: I.V.: 1 mg/kg/dose as needed Mannitol: I.V.: 0.25-0.5 g/kg/dose as needed	Furosemide: I.V.: 20-40 mg/dose as needed Mannitol: I.V.: 0.25-0.5 g/kg/dose as needed
Phosphate reduction	Aluminum hydroxide: Oral: 50 mg/kg/dose every 8 hours	Aluminum hydroxide: Oral: 30-40 mL/dose every 6-8 hours
Dialysis indications (peritoneal dialysis is much less efficient for reducing uric acid than other modalities, and is contraindicated in patients with abdominal tumors.)	Potassium level >6 mEq/L	
	Uric acid level >10 mg/dL	
	Creatinine >10 times normal	
	Uremia	
	Phosphorus >10 mg/dL or rapidly rising	
	Symptomatic hypocalcemia	
	Severe, unmanageable hypertension	
	Volume overload	

Kelly KM and Lange B, "Oncologic Emergencies," *Pediatr Clin North Am*, 1997, 44(4):809-30.

HOTLINE PHONE NUMBERS

AIDS Hotline	800-590-2437
AMA Foreign Drug	312-464-4575
AMA Library Answer Center	312-464-4818
American Association of Poison Control Centers (AAPCC) Poison Prevention	202-625-3333
American College of Clinical Pharmacy (ACCP)	816-531-2177
American Dental Association (ADA)	800-621-8099
American Medical Association (AMA)	312-464-5000
American Pharmaceutical Association (APhA)	202-628-4410
American Association of Health-System Pharmacists	301-657-3000
Animal Poison Care Hotline (24-hours)	800-548-2423
Canadian Pharmaceutical Association	613-523-7877
Center for Disease Control	1-800-311-3435

Use this number for the following departments also:

- CDC Disease Information
- CDC Epidemiology Program
- CDC Immunity Division
- CDC Influenza Branch
- CDC International Travelers Information
- CDC Parasitic Division
- CDC STDs
- CDC Tuberculosis Section

FDA (Rare Diseases/Orphan Drugs)	800-300-7469
National Cancer Institute	301-496-1196
Asthma and Allergy Foundation of America	1-800-7-ASTHMA
Cancer Treatment (of NCI)	1-800-4-CANCER
Epilepsy Foundation of America	301-459-3700
National Council on Patient Information & Education	301-656-8565
National Institute of Health	301-496-4000
National Poison Center	202-362-3867
Emergency	202-625-3333
Parental Stress	800-632-8188
Pediatric Pharmacy Advocacy Group (PPAG) Membership and Drug Information	720-981-7356
Pesticides (Mon-Fri, 6:30 AM - 4:30 PM Pacific)	800-858-7378
Rocky Mountain Poison Control Information	800-525-6115

ENDOCARDITIS PROPHYLAXIS*

	Dosage for Adults	Dosage for Children†
DENTAL AND UPPER RESPIRATORY PROCEDURES		
Oral§		
Amoxicillin¶	2 g 1 h before procedure	50 mg/kg 1 h before procedure
Penicillin allergy:		
Clindamycin or	600 mg 1 h before procedure	20 mg/kg 1 h before procedure
Cephalexin or	2 g 1 h before procedure	50 mg/kg 1 h before procedure
Azithromycin or Clarithromycin	500 mg 1 h before procedure	15 mg/kg 1 h before procedure
Parenteral§		
Ampicillin	2 g I.M. or I.V. 30 minutes before procedure	50 mg/kg I.M. or I.V. 30 minutes before procedure
Penicillin allergy:		
Clindamycin or	600 mg I.V. 30 minutes before procedure	20 mg/kg I.V. 30 minutes before procedure
Cefazolin (not to be used in individuals with immediate-type hypersensitivity reaction to penicillins)	1 g I.M. or I.V. 30 minutes before procedure	25 mg/kg I.M. or I.V. 30 minutes before procedure
GASTROINTESTINAL AND GENITOURINARY PROCEDURES‡		
Oral§		
Amoxicillin for moderate risk patients	2 g 1 h before procedure	50 mg/kg 1 h before procedure
Parenteral§		
Ampicillin for moderate risk patients	2 g I.M. or I.V. 30 minutes before procedure	50 mg/kg I.M. or I.V. 30 minutes before procedure
Ampicillin **plus**	2 g I.M. or I.V. 30 minutes before procedure; ampicillin 1 g I.M./I.V. or amoxicillin 1 g P.O. 6 h later	50 mg/kg I.M. or I.V. 30 minutes before procedure and 25 mg/kg I.M./I.V. or amoxicillin 25 mg/kg P.O. 6 h later
Gentamicin for high-risk patients	1.5 mg/kg (max: 120 mg) I.M. or I.V. 30 minutes before procedure	1.5 mg/kg I.M. or I.V. 30 minutes before procedure

	Dosage for Adults	Dosage for Children†
Penicillin allergy:		
Vancomycin for moderate-risk patients	1 g I.V. infused **slowly over 1 h**; complete infusion within 30 minutes before procedure	20 mg/kg I.V. infused **slowly over 1 h**; complete infusion within 30 minutes before procedure
Vancomycin **plus**	1 g I.V. infused slowly over 1 h; complete infusion within 30 minutes before procedure	20 mg/kg I.V. infused slowly over 1 h; complete infusion within 30 minutes before procedure
Gentamicin for high-risk patients	1.5 mg/kg (max: 120 mg) I.M. or I.V. 30 minutes before procedure	1.5 mg/kg I.M. or I.V. 30 minutes before procedure

*Endocarditis prophylaxis recommended

High-risk category:

Prosthetic cardiac valves

Previous bacterial endocarditis

Complex cyanotic congenital heart disease (eg, single ventricle states, transposition of the great arteries, tetralogy of Fallot)

Surgically constructed systemic pulmonary shunts or conduits

Moderate-risk category:

Most other congenital cardiac malformations (other than high-risk category)

Acquired valvar dysfunction (eg, rheumatic heart disease)

Hypertrophic cardiomyopathy

Mitral valve prolapse with valvar regurgitation and/or thickened leaflets

†Children's dose should not exceed adult dosage.

‡For a review of the risk of bacteremia and endocarditis with various procedures, see Mandell GL, Bennett JE, Dolin R, eds, *Principles and Practice of Infectious Diseases*, 4th ed, New York, NY: Churchill Livingstone, 1995, 794.

§Oral regimens are more convenient and safer. Parenteral regimens are more likely to be effective; they are recommended especially for patients with prosthetic heart valves, those who have had endocarditis previously, or those taking continuous oral penicillin for rheumatic fever prophylaxis.

¶Amoxicillin is recommended because of its excellent bioavailability and good activity against streptococci and enterococci.

References
Dajani AS, Taubert KA, Wilson W, et al, "Prevention of Bacterial Endocarditis. Recommendations by the American Heart Association," *JAMA*, 1997, 277(22):1794-1801.

PEDIATRIC HIV

Selected tables from the Centers for Disease Control and Prevention, "Guidelines for the Use of Antiretroviral Agents in Pediatric HIV Infection," first published in *MMWR,* 1998:47(No.RR-4), April 17, 1998, updated as a "Living Document", January 7, 2000, located at (URL) http://www.hivatis.org.

Table 1. 1994 Revised Human Immunodeficiency Virus Pediatric Classification System: Immune Categories Based on Age-specific CD4+ T-lymphocyte and Percentage*

Immune Category	<12 mo		1-5 y		6-12 y	
	No./μL	%	No./μL	%	No./μL	%
Category 1 no suppression	≥1500	≥25	≥1000	≥25	≥500	≥25
Category 2 moderate suppression	750-1499	15-24	500-999	15-24	200-499	15-24
Category 3 severe suppression	<750	<15	<500	<15	<200	<15

*Modified from: "1994 Revised Classification System for Human Immunodeficiency Virus Infection in Children Less Than 13 Years of Age," *MMWR,* 1994, 43(RR-12):1-10.

Table 2. 1994 Revised Human Immunodeficiency Virus Pediatric Classification System: Clinical Categories*

Category N: Not Symptomatic
Children who have no signs or symptoms considered to be the result of HIV infection or who have only **one** of the conditions listed in category A

Category A: Mildly Symptomatic
Children with **two** or more of the following conditions, but none of the conditions listed in categories B and C:

- Lymphadenopathy (≥0.5 cm at more than two sites; bilateral = one site)
- Hepatomegaly
- Splenomegaly
- Dermatitis
- Parotitis
- Recurrent or persistent upper respiratory infection, sinusitis, or otitis media

Category B: Moderately Symptomatic
Children who have symptomatic conditions other than those listed for category A or category C that are attributed to HIV infection. Examples of conditions in clinical category B include, but are not limited to, the following:

- Anemia (<8 g/dL), neutropenia (<1000/mm³), or thrombocytopenia (<100,000/mm³) persisting ≥30 days
- Bacterial meningitis, pneumonia, or sepsis (single episode)
- Candidiasis, oropharyngeal (ie, thrush) persisting for >2 months in children aged >6 months
- Cardiomyopathy
- Cytomegalovirus infection with onset before age 1 month
- Diarrhea, recurrent or chronic
- Hepatitis
- Herpes simplex virus (HSV) stomatitis, recurrent (ie, more than two episodes within 1 year)
- HSV bronchitis, pneumonitis, or esophagitis with onset before age 1 month
- Herpes zoster (ie, shingles) involving at least two distinct episodes or more than one dermatome
- Leiomyosarcoma

INFECTIOUS DISEASES/IMMUNOLOGY

- Lymphoid interstitial pneumonia (LIP) or pulmonary lymphoid hyperplasia complex
- Nephropathy
- Nocardiosis
- Fever lasting >1 month
- Toxoplasmosis with onset before age 1 month
- Varicella, disseminated (ie, complicated chickenpox)

Category C: Severely Symptomatic

Children who have any condition listed in the 1987 surveillance case definition for acquired immunodeficiency syndrome, with the exception of LIP (which is a category B condition).

---

*Modified from: "1994 Revised Classification System for Human Immunodeficiency Virus Infection in Children Less Than 13 Years of Age," *MMWR*, 1994, 43(RR-12):1-10.

Table 3. Indications for Initiation of Antiretroviral Therapy in Children With Human Immunodeficiency Virus (HIV) Infection*

- Clinical symptoms associated with HIV infection (ie, clinical categories A, B, or C [Table 2])
- Evidence of immune suppression, indicated by CD4+ T-lymphocyte absolute number or percentage (ie, immune category 2 or 3 [Table 1])
- Age <12 months - regardless of clinical, immunologic, or virologic status
- For asymptomatic children ≥1 year of age with normal immune status, two options can be considered:
  1. Preferred approach: Initiate therapy regardless of age or symptom status
  2. Alternative approach: Defer treatment in situations in which the risk for clinical disease progression is low and other factors (eg, concern for the durability of response, safety, and adherence) favor postponing treatment. In such cases, the healthcare provider should regularly monitor virologic, immunologic, and clinical status. Factors to be considered in deciding to initiate therapy include the following:
     - High or increasing HIV RNA copy number
     - Rapidly declining CD4+ T-lymphocyte number or percentage to values approaching those indicative of moderate immune suppression (ie, immune category 2 [Table 1])
     - Development of clinical symptoms

***Indications for initiation of antiretroviral therapy in postpubertal HIV-infected adolescents should follow the adult guidelines.** (Office of Public Health and Science, Department of Health and Human Services. Availability of report of NIH panel to define principles of therapy of HIV infection and guidelines for the use of antiretroviral agents in HIV-infected adults. Federal Register, 1997, 62:33417-8 and updated as "Guidelines for the Use of Antiretroviral Agents in HIV-Infected Adults and Adolescents," January 28, 2000, http://www.hivatis.org. See page 1133).

PEDIATRIC HIV *(Continued)*

Table 4. Recommended Antiretroviral Regimens for Initial Therapy for Human Immunodeficiency Virus (HIV) Infection in Children

Strongly Recommended

Clinical trial evidence of clinical benefit and/or sustained suppression of HIV replication in adults and/or children.

- One highly active protease inhibitor plus two nucleoside analogue reverse transcriptase inhibitors (NRTIs)

    – Preferred protease inhibitor for infants and children who cannot swallow pills or capsules: nelfinavir or ritonavir; alternative for children who can swallow pills or capsules: indinavir

    – Recommended dual NRTI combinations: the most data on use in children are available for the combinations of zidovudine (ZDV) and dideoxyinosine (ddl) and for ZDV and lamivudine (3TC); more limited data is available for the combinations of stavudine (d4T) and ddl, d4T and 3TC, and ZDV and zalcitabine (ddC)*

- Alternative for children who can swallow capsules: Efavirenz (Sustiva®)** plus 2 NRTIs (see above) or efavirenz (Sustiva®) plus nelfinavir and 1 NRTI

Recommended as an Alternative

Clinical trial evidence of suppression of HIV replication, but 1) durability may be less in adults and/or children than with strongly recommended regimens; or 2) the durability of suppression is not yet defined; or 3) evidence of efficacy may not outweigh potential adverse consequences (eg, toxicity, drug interactions, cost, etc).

- Nevirapine and two NRTIs
- Abacavir in combination with ZDV and 3TC

Offer Only in Special Circumstances

Clinical trial evidence of 1) limited benefit for patients, or 2) data are inconclusive, but may be reasonably offered in special circumstances.

- Two NRTIs
- Amprenavir in combination with 2 NRTIs or abacavir

Not Recommended

Evidence against use because of 1) overlapping toxicity, and/or 2) because use may be virologically undesirable

- Any monotherapy†
- d4T and ZDV
- ddC and ddl
- ddC and d4T
- ddC and 3TC

---

*ddC is not available in a liquid preparation commercially, although a liquid formulation is available through a compassionate use program of the manufacturer (Hoffman-LaRoche Inc, Nutley, New Jersey). ZDV and ddC is a less preferred choice for use in combination with a protease inhibitor.

Efavirenz is currently available only in capsule form, but liquid preparation is currently being evaluated. There are currently no data on appropriate dosage of efavirenz in children <3 years of age. **Note: A liquid efavirenz preparation is available from the manufacturer (DuPont Pharmaceuticals Company, Wilmington, Delaware) through an expanded access program for HIV-infected children and adolescents 3-16 years of age.

†Except for ZDV chemoprophylaxis administered to HIV-exposed infants during the first 6 weeks of life to prevent perinatal HIV transmission; if an infant is identified as HIV-infected while receiving ZDV prophylaxis, therapy should be changed to a combination antiretroviral drug regimen.

Table 5. Considerations for Changing Antiretroviral Therapy for Human Immunodeficiency Virus (HIV)-Infected Children

Virologic Considerations*

- Less than a minimally acceptable virologic response after 8-12 weeks of therapy; for children receiving antiretroviral therapy with two nucleoside analogue reverse transcriptase inhibitors (NRTIs) and a protease inhibitor, such a response is defined as a <10-fold (1.0 $\log_{10}$) decrease from baseline HIV RNA levels; for children who are receiving less potent antiretroviral therapy (ie, dual NRTI combinations), an insufficient response is defined as a <5-fold (0.7 $\log_{10}$) decrease in HIV RNA levels from baseline

- HIV RNA not suppressed to undetectable levels after 4-6 months of antiretroviral therapy†

- Repeated detection of HIV RNA in children who initially responded to antiretroviral therapy with undetectable levels‡

- A reproducible increase in HIV RNA copy number among children who have had a substantial HIV RNA response, but still have low levels of detectable HIV RNA; such an increase would warrant change in therapy if, after initiation of the therapeutic regimen, a >3-fold (0.5 $\log_{10}$) increase in copy number for children ≥2 years of age and a >5-fold (0.7 $\log_{10}$) increase is observed for children <2 years of age

Immunologic Considerations*

- Change in immunologic classification (Table 1)§

- For children with CD4+ T-lymphocyte percentages of <15% (ie, those in immune category 3), a persistent decline of five percentiles or more in CD4+ cell percentage (eg, from 15% to 10%)

- A rapid and substantial decrease in absolute CD4+ T-lymphocyte count (eg, a >30% decline in <6 months)

Clinical Considerations

- Progressive neurodevelopmental deterioration

- Growth failure defined as persistent decline in weight-growth velocity despite adequate nutritional support and without other explanation

- Disease progression defined as advancement from one pediatric clinical category to another (eg, from clinical category A to clinical category B)**

*At least two measurements (taken 1 week apart) should be performed before considering a change in therapy.

†The initial HIV RNA level of the child at the start of therapy and the level achieved with therapy should be considered when contemplating potential drug changes. For example, an immediate change in therapy may not be warranted if there is a sustained 1.5-2.0 $\log_{10}$ decrease in HIV RNA copy number, even if RNA remains detectable at low levels.

‡More frequent evaluation of HIV RNA levels should be considered if the HIV RNA increase is limited (eg, if when using an HIV RNA assay with a lower limit of detection of 1000 copies/mL, there is a ≤0.7 $\log_{10}$ increase from undetectable to approximately 5000 copies/mL in an infant <2 years of age).

§Minimal changes in CD4+ T-lymphocyte percentile that may result in change in immunologic category (eg, from 26% to 24%, or 16% to 14%) may not be as concerning as a rapid substantial change in CD4+ percentile within the same immunologic category (eg, a drop from 35% to 25%).

**In patients with stable immunologic and virologic parameters, progression from one clinical category to another may not represent an indication to change therapy. Thus, in patients whose disease progression is not associated with neurologic deterioration or growth failure, virologic and immunologic considerations are important in deciding whether to change therapy.

ADULT AND ADOLESCENT HIV

Selected tables from the Centers for Disease Control and Prevention, "Report of the NIH Panel to Define Principles of Therapy of HIV Infection and Guidelines for the Use of Antiretroviral Agents in HIV-Infected Adults and Adolescents," first published in *MMWR,* 1998:47(No. RR-5), April 24, 1998, updated as a "Living Document," April 23, 2001, located at (URL) http://www.hivatis.org.

Indications for Plasma HIV RNA Testing*

Clinical Indication	Information	Use
Syndrome consistent with acute HIV infection	Establishes diagnosis when HIV antibody test is negative or indeterminate	Diagnosis†
Initial evaluation of newly diagnosed HIV infection	Baseline viral load "set point"	Decision to start or defer therapy
Every 3-4 months in patients not on therapy	Changes in viral load	Decision to start therapy
2-8 weeks after initiation of antiretroviral therapy	Initial assessment of drug efficacy	Decision to continue or change therapy
3-4 months after start of therapy	Maximal effect of therapy	Decision to continue or change therapy
Every 3-4 months in patients on therapy	Durability of antiretroviral effect	Decision to continue or change therapy
Clinical event or significant decline in CD4+ T cells	Association with changing or stable viral load	Decision to continue, initiate, or change therapy

*Acute illness (eg, bacterial pneumonia, tuberculosis, HSV, PCP, etc) and immunizations can cause increases in plasma HIV RNA for 2-4 weeks; viral load testing should not be performed during this time. Plasma HIV RNA results should usually be verified with a repeat determination before starting or making changes in therapy.

†Diagnosis of HIV infection determined by HIV RNA testing should be confirmed by standard methods (such as Western blot serology) performed 2-4 months after the initial indeterminate or negative test.

Recommendations for the Use of Drug Resistance Assays

Clinical Setting / Recommendation	Rationale
Recommended	
Virologic failure during HAART*	Determine the role of resistance in drug failure and maximize the number of active drugs in the new regimen, if indicated.
Suboptimal suppression of viral load after initiation of antiretroviral therapy	Determine the role of resistance and maximize the number of active drugs in the new regimen, if indicated.
Consider	
Acute HIV infection	Determine if drug-resistant virus was transmitted and change regimen accordingly.
Not Generally Recommended	
Chronic HIV infection prior to initiation of therapy	Uncertain prevalence of resistant virus. Current assays may not detect minor drug-resistant species.
After discontinuation of drugs	Drug-resistant mutations may become minor species in the absence of selective drug pressure. Current assays may not detect minor drug-resistant species.
Plasma viral load <1000 HIV RNA copies/mL	Resistance assays cannot be reliably performed because of low copy number of HIV RNA.

*HAART: Highly active antiretroviral therapy

Risks and Benefits of Delayed Initiation of Therapy and of Early Therapy in the Asymptomatic HIV-Infected Patient

*Risks and Benefits of Delayed Therapy**

Benefits of Delayed Therapy

- Avoid negative effects on quality of life (ie, inconvenience)
- Avoid drug-related adverse events
- Delay in development of drug resistance
- Preserve maximum number of available and future drug options when HIV disease risk is highest

Risks of Delayed Therapy

- Possible risk of irreversible immune system depletion
- Possible greater difficulty in suppressing viral replication
- Possible increased risk of HIV transmission

*Risks and Benefits of Early Therapy**

Benefits of Early Therapy

- Control of viral replication easier to achieve and maintain
- Delay or prevention of immune system compromise
- Lower risk of resistance with complete viral suppression
- Possible decreased risk of HIV transmission†

Risks of Early Therapy

- Drug-related reduction in quality of life
- Greater cumulative drug-related adverse events
- Earlier development of drug resistance, if viral suppression is suboptimal
- Limitation of future antiretroviral treatment options

*See table, "Indications for the Initiation of Antiretroviral Therapy in the Chronically HIV-1 Infected Patient," for consensus recommendations regarding when to initiate therapy.

†The risk of viral transmission still exists; antiretroviral therapy cannot substitute for primary HIV prevention measures (eg, use of condoms and safer sex practices).

Goals of HIV Therapy and Tools to Achieve Them

Goals of Therapy

Maximal and durable suppression of viral load
Restoration and/or preservation of immunologic function
Improvement of quality of life
Reduction of HIV-related morbidity and mortality

Tools to Achieve Goals of Therapy

Maximize adherence to the antiretroviral regimen
Rational sequencing of drugs
Preservation of future treatment options
Use of resistance testing in selected clinical settings

ADULT AND ADOLESCENT HIV *(Continued)*

Indications for the Initiation of Antiretroviral Therapy in the Chronically HIV-1 Infected Patient

Clinical Category	CD4+ T Cell Count	Plasma HIV RNA	Recommendation
Symptomatic (AIDS, severe symptoms)	Any value	Any value	Treat
Asymptomatic, AIDS	CD4+ T cells <200/mm³	Any value	Treat
Asymptomatic	CD4+ T cells >200/mm³ but <350/mm³	Any value	Treatment should generally be offered, though controversy exists.*
Asymptomatic	CD4+ T cells >350/mm³	>30,000 (bDNA) **or** >55,000 (RT-PCR)	Some experts would recommend initiating therapy, recognizing that the 3-year risk of developing AIDS in untreated patients is >30%. In the absence of very high levels of plasma HIV RNA, some would defer therapy and monitor the CD4+ T cell count and level of plasma HIV RNA more frequently. Clinical outcomes data after initiating therapy are lacking.
Asymptomatic	CD4+ T cells >350/mm³	<30,000 (bDNA) **or** <55,000 (RT-PCR)	Many experts would defer therapy and observe, recognizing that the 3-year risk of developing AIDS in untreated patients is <15%.

*Clinical benefit has been demonstrated in controlled trials only for patients with CD4+ T cells <200/mm³. However, most experts would offer therapy at a CD4+ T cell threshold <350/mm³. All decisions to initiate therapy should be based on prognosis for disease-free survival in the absence of treatment, as determined by the CD4+ T cell count and level of plasma HIV RNA, the potential benefits and risks of therapy, and the willingness of the patient to accept therapy.

Recommended Antiretroviral Agents for Initial Treatment of Established HIV Infection

This table provides a guide to the use of available treatment regimens for individuals with no prior or limited experience on HIV therapy. In accordance with the established goals of HIV therapy, priority is given to regimens in which clinical trials data suggest the following: Sustained suppression of HIV plasma RNA (particularly in patients with high baseline viral load) and sustained increase in CD4+T cell count (in most cases over 48 weeks), and favorable clinical outcome (ie, delayed progression to AIDS and death). Particular emphasis is given to regimens that have been compared directly with other regimens that perform sufficiently well with regard to these parameters to be included in the "Strongly Recommended" category. Additional consideration is given to the regimen's pill burden, dosing frequency, food requirements, convenience, toxicity, and drug interaction profile compared with other regimens.

It is important to note that all antiretroviral agents, including those in the "Strongly Recommended" category, have potentially serious toxic and adverse events associated with their use (see individual drug monographs).

Antiretroviral drug regimens are comprised of one choice each from column A and column B. Drugs are listed in alphabetical, not priority order:

	Column A	Column B
Strongly Recommended	Efavirenz Indinavir Nelfinavir Ritonavir + Indinavir* Ritonavir/Lopinavir† Ritonavir + Saquinavir (SGC‡ or HGC‡)	Stavudine + Didanosine§ Stavudine + Lamivudine Zidovudine + Didanosine Zidovudine + Lamivudine
Recommended as an Alternative	Abacavir Amprenavir Delavirdine Nelfinavir + Saquinavir-SGC Nevirapine Ritonavir Saquinavir-SGC	Didanosine + Lamivudine Zidovudine + Zalcitabine
No Recommendation; Insufficient Data¶	Hydroxyurea in combination with antiretroviral drugs Ritonavir + Amprenavir Ritonavir + Nelfinavir	
Not Recommended; Should Not be Offered (All monotherapies, whether from column A or B#)	Saquinavir-HGC•	Stavudine + Zidovudine Zalcitabine + Didanosine Zalcitabine + Lamivudine Zalcitabine + Stavudine

*Based on expert opinion.

†Co-formulated as Kaletra®.

‡Saquinavir-SGC, soft-gel capsule (Fortovase®); Saquinavir-HGC, hard-gel capsule (Invirase®).

§Pregnant women may be at increased risk for lactic acidosis and liver damage when treated with the combination of stavudine and didanosine. This combination should be used in pregnant women only when the potential benefit clearly outweighs the potential risk.

¶This category includes drugs or combinations for which information is too limited to allow a recommendation for or against use.

#Zidovudine monotherapy may be considered for prophylactic use in pregnant women with low viral load and high CD4+ T cell counts to prevent perinatal transmission.

•Use of saquinavir-HGC (Invirase®) is not recommended, except in combination with ritonavir.

ADULT AND ADOLESCENT HIV *(Continued)*

Guidelines for Changing an Antiretroviral Regimen for Suspected Drug Failure

- Criteria for changing therapy include a suboptimal reduction in plasma viremia after initiation of therapy, reappearance of viremia after suppression to undetectable, significant increases in plasma viremia from the nadir of suppression, and declining CD4⁺ T cell numbers.

- When the decision to change therapy is based on viral load determination, it is preferable to confirm with a second viral load test.

- Distinguish between the need to change a regimen due to drug intolerance or inability to comply with the regimen versus failure to achieve the goal of sustained viral suppression; single agents can be changed in the event of drug intolerance.

- In general, do not change a single drug or add a single drug to a failing regimen; it is important to use at least two new drugs and preferably to use an entirely new regimen with at least three new drugs. If susceptibility testing indicates resistance to only one agent in a combination regimen, it may be possible to replace only that drug; however, this approach requires clinical validation.

- Many patients have limited options for new regimens of desired potency; in some of these cases, it is rational to continue the prior regimen if partial viral suppression was achieved.

- In some cases, regimens identified as suboptimal for initial therapy are rational due to limitations imposed by toxicity, intolerance, or nonadherence. This especially applies in late-stage disease. For patients with no rational alternative options who have virologic failure with return of viral load to baseline (pretreatment levels) and a declining CD4⁺ T cell count, there should be consideration for discontinuation of antiretroviral therapy.

- Experience is limited with regimens using combinations of two protease inhibitors or combinations of protease inhibitors with NNRTIs; for patients with limited options due to drug intolerance or suspected resistance, these regimens provide possible alternative treatment options.

- There is limited information about the value of restarting a drug that the patient has previously received. Susceptibility testing may be useful in this situation if clinical evidence suggestive of the emergence of resistance is observed. However, testing for phenotypic or genotypic resistance in peripheral blood virus may fail to detect minor resistant variants. Thus, the presence of resistance is more useful information in altering treatment strategies than the absence of detectable resistance.

- Avoid changing from ritonavir to indinavir, or vice versa, for drug failure, since high-level cross-resistance is likely.

- Avoid changing among NNRTIs for drug failure, since high-level cross-resistance is likely.

- The decision to change therapy and the choice of a new regimen requires that the clinician have considerable expertise in the care of persons living with HIV. Physicians who are less experienced in the care of persons with HIV infection are strongly encouraged to obtain assistance through consultation with or referral to a clinician with considerable expertise in the care of HIV-infected patients.

Acute Retroviral Syndrome: Associated Signs and Symptoms (Expected Frequency)

- Fever (96%)
- Lymphadenopathy (74%)
- Pharyngitis (70%)
- Rash (70%)
  - Erythematous maculopapular with lesions on face and trunk and sometimes extremities, including palms and soles
  - Mucocutaneous ulceration involving mouth, esophagus, or genitals
- Myalgia or arthralgia (54%)
- Diarrhea (32%)
- Headache (32%)
- Nausea and vomiting (27%)
- Hepatosplenomegaly (14%)
- Weight loss (13%)
- Thrush (12%)
- Neurologic symptoms (12%)
  - Meningoencephalitis or aseptic meningitis
  - Peripheral neuropathy or radiculopathy
  - Facial palsy
  - Guillain-Barré syndrome
  - Brachial neuritis
  - Cognitive impairment or psychosis

Zidovudine (ZDV) Perinatal Transmission Prophylaxis Regimen

Antepartum	Initiation at 14-34 weeks gestation and continued throughout pregnancy: A. PACTG 076 regimen: ZDV 100 mg 5 times daily B. Acceptable alternative regimen: ZDV 200 mg 3 times daily or ZDV 300 mg 2 times daily
Intrapartum	During labor, ZDV 2 mg/kg I.V. over 1 hour, followed by a continuous infusion of 1 mg/kg/hour I.V. until delivery
Postpartum	Oral administration of ZDV to the newborn (ZDV syrup, 2 mg/kg every 6 hours) for the first 6 weeks of life, beginning at 8-12 hours after birth

IMMUNIZATION GUIDELINES

Standards for Pediatric Immunization Practices

Standard 1.   Immunization services are readily available.

Standard 2.   There are no barriers or unnecessary prerequisites to the receipt of vaccines.

Standard 3.   Immunization services are available free or for a minimal fee.

Standard 4.   Providers utilize all clinical encounters to screen and, when indicated, immunize children.

Standard 5.   Providers educate parents and guardians about immunizations in general terms.

Standard 6.   Providers question parents or guardians about contraindications and, before immunizing a child, inform them in specific terms about the risks and benefits of the immunizations their child is to receive.

Standard 7.   Providers follow only true contraindications.

Standard 8.   Providers administer simultaneously all vaccine doses for which a child is eligible at the time of each visit.

Standard 9.   Providers use accurate and complete recording procedures.

Standard 10.   Providers co-schedule immunization appointments in conjunction with appointments for other child health services.

Standard 11.   Providers report adverse events following immunization promptly, accurately, and completely.

Standard 12.   Providers operate a tracking system.

Standard 13.   Providers adhere to appropriate procedures for vaccine management.

Standard 14.   Providers conduct semiannual audits to assess immunization coverage levels and to review immunization records in the patient populations they serve.

Standard 15.   Providers maintain up-to-date, easily retrievable medical protocols at all locations where vaccines are administered.

Standard 16.   Providers operate with patient-oriented and community-based approaches.

Standard 17.   Vaccines are administered by properly trained individuals.

Standard 18.   Providers receive ongoing education and training on current immunization recommendations.

Recommended by the National Vaccine Advisory Committee, April 1992.
Modified by the United States Public Health Service, 1993.
Endorsed by the American Academy of Pediatrics, May 1992.

The Standards represent the consensus of the National Vaccine Advisory Committee (NVAC) and of a broad group of medical and public health experts about what constitutes the most desirable immunization practices. It is recognized by the NVAC that not all of the current immunization practices of public and private providers are in compliance with the Standards. Nevertheless, the Standards are expected to be useful as a means of helping providers to identify needed changes, to obtain resources if necessary, and to actually implement the desirable immunization practices in the future.

Table 1. Dosage and Administration Guidelines for Vaccines Available in the United States

Vaccine	Dosage	Route of Administration	Type
DT*	0.5 mL	I.M.; do not give S.C.	Toxoids
Td*	0.5 mL	I.M.; do not give S.C.	Toxoids
DTP*	0.5 mL	I.M.; do not give S.C.	Diphtheria and tetanus toxoids with killed *B. pertussis* organisms
DTaP (Acel-Imune®, Tripedia®, Infanrix®)†††	0.5 mL	I.M.; do not give S.C.	Diphtheria and tetanus toxoids with inactivated acellular pertussis
DTP-HbOC (Tetramune®)⁺	0.5 mL	I.M.; do not give S.C.	Diphtheria and tetanus toxoids with killed *B. pertussis* organisms and *Haemophilus* b conjugate (diphtheria CRM_{197} protein conjugate)
DTaP-PRP-T (Tripedia®/ActHIB®, TriHIBit®)	0.5 mL	I.M.; do not give S.C.	Polysaccharide-protein conjugate with toxoids and inactivated bacteria
Haemophilus B conjugate vaccine	0.5 mL	I.M. PRP-D, HbOC, or PRP-T can be given S.C. in individuals at risk of hemorrhage	Polysaccharide protein conjugate
ProHIBit® (PRP-D), manufactured by Connaught Laboratories	0.5 mL (for children ≥12 mo)	I.M.	Polysaccharide (diphtheria toxoid conjugate)
HibTITER® (HbOC),† manufactured by Lederle Laboratories	0.5 mL	I.M.	Oligosaccharide (diphtheria CRM_{197} protein conjugate)
PedvaxHIB® (PRP-OMP),‡ manufactured by MSD	0.5 mL	I.M.; do not give S.C.	Polysaccharide (meningococcal protein conjugate)
ActHIB®, OmniHIB® (PRP-T), manufactured by Pasteur Merieux Serums & Vaccines	0.5 mL	I.M.	Tetanus toxoid protein conjugate
Haemophilus B conjugate – PRP-OMP and hepatitis B (recombinant) (Comvax®)	0.5 mL	I.M.; do not give S.C.	Polysaccharide-protein conjugate with inactivated virus
Hepatitis A vaccine, inactivated		I.M.; do not give S.C.	Inactivated virus
Havrix®			
Children 2-18 y:	0.5 mL (720 ELISA units) with 2nd dose given 6-12 mo later		
Children >18 y and adults:	1 mL (1440 ELISA units) with 2nd dose given 6-12 mo later		
Vaqta®			
Children 2-17 y:	0.5 mL (25 units) with 2nd dose given 6-18 mo later		
Children >17 y and adults:	1 mL (50 units) with 2nd dose given 6 mo later		

IMMUNIZATION GUIDELINES *(Continued)*

Table 1. Dosage and Administration Guidelines for Vaccines Available in the United States *(continued)*

Vaccine	Dosage	Route of Administration	Type
Hepatitis B§		I.M. in the anterolateral thigh or in the deltoid muscle[][]	Yeast recombinant-derived inactivated viral antigen
Infants born to HB$_s$Ag-negative mothers, children, and adolescents <20 y[]			
Recombivax HB® (MSD)	5 mcg (0.5 mL)		
Engerix-B® (SKF)	10 mcg (0.5 mL)		

Infants born to HB$_s$Ag-positive mothers (both immunization with hepatitis B and administration of 0.5 mL hepatitis B immune globulin is recommended for **infants** born to HB$_s$Ag-positive mothers using different administration sites) within 12 hours of birth; administer vaccine at birth; repeat vaccine dose at 1 and 6 months following the initial dose

Recombivax HB® (MSD)	5 mcg (0.5 mL)		
Engerix-B® (SKF)	10 mcg (0.5 mL)		
Adults ≥20 y			
Recombivax HB® (MSD)	10 mcg (1 mL)		
Engerix-B® (SKF)	20 mcg (1 mL)		
Dialysis patients and immunosuppressed patients			
Recombivax HB® (MSD)	<20 y: 20 mcg (0.5 mL); ≥20 y, 40 mcg (1 mL) using special dialysis formulation		
Engerix-B® (SKF)¶	<20 y, 20 mcg (1 mL); ≥20 y, 40 mcg (2 mL), give as two 1 mL doses at different sites		
Influenza		I.M. (2 doses 4+ weeks apart in children <9 years of age not previously immunized; only 1 dose needed for annual updates)	Inactivated virus subvirion (split) (contraindicated in patients allergic to chicken eggs)
Split virus only in pediatric patients			
6-35 mo	0.25 mL (1 or 2 doses)		
3-8 y	0.5 mL (1 or 2 doses)		
≥9 y	0.5 mL (1 dose)		
Measles	0.5 mL	S.C.	Live virus (contraindicated in patients with anaphylactic allergy to neomycin)

Most areas: Two doses (1st dose at 15 months with MMR; 2nd dose at 4-6 years or 11-12 years, depending on local school entry requirements)

High-risk area: Two doses (1st dose at 12 months with MMR; 2nd dose as above)

Children 6-15 months in epidemic situations: Dose is given at the time of first contact with a health care provider; children <1 year of age should receive single antigen measles vaccine. If vaccinated before 1 year, revaccinate at 15 months with MMR. A 3rd dose is administered at 4-6 years or 11-12 years, depending on local school entry requirements.

Meningococcal	0.5 mL#	S.C.	Polysaccharide
MMR•	0.5 mL	S.C.	Live virus

Table 1. Dosage and Administration Guidelines for Vaccines Available in the United States *(continued)*

Vaccine	Dosage	Route of Administration	Type
MR	0.5 mL	S.C.	Live virus
Mumps	0.5 mL	S.C.	Live virus
Pneumococcal heptavalent (Prevnar®)♦	0.5 mL	I.M.	Protein-conjugated polysaccharide
Pneumococcal polyvalent♦ ♦	0.5 mL (≥2 y)	I.M. or S.C. (I.M. preferred)	Polysaccharide
Poliovirus (OPV) trivalent	0.5 mL	Oral	Live virus
Poliovirus (IPV)**· trivalent	0.5 mL	S.C. or I.M.	Inactivated virus
Rabies			
Human diploid cell vaccine (Imovax®)	1 mL	I.M.‡‡ or	Inactivated virus
(HDCV)	0.1 mL	I.D.§§	
Rabies vaccine adsorbed (RVA)	1 mL	I.M.‡‡	Inactivated virus
Purified chick embryo cell (PCEC) (RabAvert™)	1 mL	I.M.‡‡	Inactivated virus
Rubella	0.5 mL (≥12 mo)¶¶	S.C.	Live virus
Tetanus (adsorbed)##	0.5 mL	I.M.	Toxoid
Tetanus (fluid)	0.5 mL	I.M., S.C.	Toxoid
Varicella (Varivax®)	0.5 mL	S.C.	Live virus
Children 12 mo - 12 y: Single 0.5 mL dose			
Adolescents ≥13 y and adults: 0.5 mL dose x 2 (second 0.5 mL dose is administered 4 to 8 weeks later)			
Yellow fever	0.5 mL••	S.C.	Live attenuated virus

*DT & DTP for use in children <7 years of age. Td contains same amount of tetanus toxoid as DT & DTP, but a reduced dose of diphtheria toxoid. Td for use in children ≥7 years of age.

†††DTaP is the recommended vaccine for primary vaccination against diphtheria, tetanus, and pertussis; including completion of the series in children who have received 1 or more doses of whole-cell DTP. The occurrence of fever and local reactions is lower with acellular pertussis vaccine than with whole-cell DTP.

⁺DTP-HbOC may be substituted for DTP and *Haemophilus* b conjugate vaccines which are administered separately, whenever recommended schedules for use of these 2 vaccines coincide. Initiate at 2 months of age for 3 doses (2 months, 4 months, and 6 months), followed by a 4th dose at 15-18 months of age. DTaP and *Haemophilus* b conjugate vaccine may be administered separately as an alternative to DTP-HbOC at 15-18 months of age.

†The conjugate (HbCV) vaccine is preferred over the polysaccharide (HbPV) vaccine. In children with a high risk for *Haemophilus influenzae* type b disease and HbCV is unavailable, an acceptable alternate is to give HbPV at 18 months of age with a 2nd dose at 24 months of age. Children <5 years of age who were previously vaccinated with HbPV between 18-23 months of age should be revaccinated with a single dose of HbCV at least 2 months after the initial dose of HbPV. Either HbCV or HbPV can be administered up to the 5th birthday. However, they are generally not recommended for children >5 years of age.

‡PRP-OMP (PedvaxHIB®) manufactured by Merck, Sharp & Dohme is initiated at 2 months of age for 3 doses (2 months, 4 months and 12 months). If initiated at 7-11 months of age, 3 doses are administered (initial 2 doses at 2-month intervals, 3rd dose at 15-18 months of age); if initiated at 12-14 months of age, 2 doses are administered at 2- to 3-month intervals between doses; if initiated at 15-59 months of age, 1 dose is administered.

§Hepatitis B vaccine can be given at the same time with DTP, HbOC, polio, and/or MMR; administer 3 doses at 0, 1, and 6 months).

[]Administer to newborns at 0-2 days of age before hospital discharge; repeat at 1-2 months and 6-18 months following the initial dose. If not vaccinated at birth, administer at 2, 4, and 6-18 months of age.

¶Engerix-B® — an alternate schedule for postexposure prophylaxis or more rapid induction using 4 doses at 0, 1, 2, and 12 months of age is recommended.

#Indicated in children ≥2 years of age at risk (anatomic or functional asplenia, those with terminal complement component or properdin deficiencies), in epidemic or highly endemic

IMMUNIZATION GUIDELINES *(Continued)*

areas. The American College Health Association recommends immunization of college students.

•See measles.

♦Routine administration to all children ≤23 months at 2, 4, 6, and 12-15 months. Initial dose should be given no earlier than at 6 weeks of age. Recommended for children 24-59 months who are at high risk for invasive pneumococcal infection.

♦♦Indicated for children with sickle cell disease; asplenia; nephrotic syndrome or chronic renal failure; conditions associated with immunosuppression; CSF leaks; HIV infection. Advisory Committee on Immunization Practices (ACIP) also recommends that patients ≥2 years of age with chronic cardiovascular disease, chronic pulmonary disease, diabetes mellitus, or chronic liver disease receive pneumococcal immunization. Patients ≥2 years of age living in special environments in which the risk of invasive pneumococcal disease is high (ie, Alaskan native and certain American Indian populations) should receive pneumococcal immunization.

**The primary series consists of 3 doses. The first 2 doses should be administered at an interval of 8 weeks beginning at 2 months of age (minimum age of 6 weeks). The 3rd dose should be given at 6-18 months of age. A booster dose of 0.5 mL should be given to all children who have completed the primary series, before entering school. However, if the 3rd dose of the primary series is given on or after the 4th birthday, a 4th dose is not required before entering school. When polio vaccine is given to persons >18 years of age, IPV should be given.

‡‡In infants and small children, I.M. injection can be given into the midlateral aspect of the thigh; in older children and adults, I.M. injection can be given into the deltoid muscle. For postexposure prophylaxis, repeat doses are given on days 3, 7, 14, and 28 after the first dose. Initiate and complete immunization series with one vaccine product. Intradermal vaccine is not advised for postexposure prophylaxis.

§§For pre-exposure prophylaxis against rabies for high-risk individuals, 1 mL I.M. or 0.1 mL intradermal is administered on days 0, 7, and 21 (or 28). Both I.M. and I.D. dosage forms are available. Preferred site for intradermal administration is the skin in the deltoid area. Patients taking chloroquine or mefloquine should only receive rabies vaccine by the I.M. route. Do **not** administer intradermally to minimize potential for vaccine failure.

[][]Aluminum-absorbed vaccines must be injected deep in the muscle mass and not S.C. because they can cause local irritation, inflammation, granuloma formation, and necrosis. Only patients (ie, hemophiliacs) who are at risk of hemorrhage following I.M. injections should receive hepatitis B vaccine S.C.

¶¶As MMR in a 2-dose schedule.

##Adsorbed preferred to fluid toxoid because of longer lasting immunity.

••≥9 months of age living in or traveling to endemic areas. Contraindicated in infants <4 months of age and in patients who have had an anaphylactic reaction to eggs. Increased risk of encephalitis associated with use of yellow fever vaccine in infants <9 months of age.

Note: For each vaccine, check the manufacturer's package insert for specific product information since preparations may change from time to time.

References

Advisory Committee on Immunization Practices, Measles Prevention, Recommendations of the Immunization Practices Advisory Committee, *MMWR* 1989, 38(5-9):1-18.

American Academy of Pediatrics, Report of the Committee on Infectious Diseases (Red Book), 25th ed, 2000.

American Academy of Pediatrics, Committee on Infectious Diseases, "Acellular Pertussis Vaccines: Recommendations for Use as the Fourth and Fifth Doses," *Pediatrics*, 1992, 90:121-3.

American Academy of Pediatrics, Committee on Infectious Diseases, "Universal Hepatitis B Immunization," *Pediatrics*, 1992, 89:795-800.

American Academy of Pediatrics, Committee on Infectious Diseases, "Recommendations for the Use of Live Attenuated Varicella Vaccine," *Pediatrics*, 1995, 95(5):791-6.

American Academy of Pediatrics, Committee on Infectious Diseases, "Policy Statement: Recommendations for the Prevention of Pneumococcal Infections, Including the Use of Pneumococcal Conjugate Vaccine (Prevnar®), Pneumococcal Polysaccharide Vaccine, and Antibiotic Prophylaxis," *Pediatrics*, 2000, 106(2 Pt 1): 362-6.

American Academy of Pediatrics, Committee on Infectious Diseases, "Recommended Childhood Immunization Schedule – United States, January-December 2001," *Pediatrics*, 2001, 107(1):202-4.

Table 2. Persons Who Should Receive Pre-exposure Hepatitis B Immunization

- All infants

- Children at high risk for early childhood HBV infection

- Adolescents: Hepatitis B vaccination should be given by or before 11-12 years of age. Special efforts should be made to vaccinate all adolescents, not only those at high risk

- Hemophiliac patients and other recipients of certain blood products

- Intravenous drug abusers

- Heterosexual persons who have had more than one sex partner in the previous 6 months and/or those with a recent episode of a sexually transmitted disease

- Sexually active men who have sex with men

- Household and sexual contacts of HB$_s$Ag-positive persons

- Members of households with adoptees who are hepatitis B surface antigen-positive

- Children and other household contacts in populations of high HBV endemicity

- Staff and residents of institutions for the developmentally disabled

- Staff of nonresidential day care and school programs for developmentally disabled if attended by known HB$_s$Ag-positive persons

- Hemodialysis patients

- Healthcare workers and others with occupational risk of exposure to blood or blood-contaminated body fluid

- International travelers to areas of high or intermediate HBV endemicity

- Inmates of long-term correctional facilities

*Adapted from American Academy of Pediatrics, Report of the Committee on Infectious Diseases, *Red Book*, 25th ed, 2000, 296.

See **Table 3** for recommended Hepatitis B immunization schedule.

IMMUNIZATION GUIDELINES *(Continued)*

Table 3. Childhood Immunization Schedule
Recommended Childhood Immunization Schedule
United States, January - December 2001

Vaccines[1] are listed under routinely recommended ages. Bars indicate range of recommended ages for immunization. Any dose not given at the recommended age should be given as a "catch up" immunization at any subsequent visit when indicated and feasible.

Ovals indicate vaccines to be given if previously recommended doses were missed or given earlier than the recommended minimum age.

Age ▶ Vaccine ▼	Birth	1 mo	2 mo	4 mo	6 mo	12 mo	15 mo	18 mo	24 mo	4-6 y	11-12 y	14-18 y
Hepatitis B[2]	Hep B #1											
		Hep B #2			Hep B #3						(Hep B[2])	
Diphtheria, Tetanus, Pertussis[3]			DTaP	DTaP	DTaP		DTaP[3]			DTaP	Td	
H. influenzae type b[4]			Hib	Hib	Hib	Hib						
Inactivated Polio[5]			IPV	IPV		IPV[5]				IPV[5]		
Pneumococcal Conjugate[6]			PCV	PCV	PCV	PCV						
Measles, Mumps, Rubella[7]						MMR				MMR[7]	(MMR[7])	
Varicella[8]						Var					(Var[8])	
Hepatitis A[9]										Hep A-in selected areas[9]		

1 This schedule indicates the recommended ages for routine administration of currently licensed childhood vaccines as of 11/1/00, for children through 18 years of age. Additional vaccines may be licensed and recommended during the year. Licensed combination vaccines may be used whenever any components of the combination are indicated and its other components are not contraindicated. Providers should consult the manufacturers' package inserts for detailed recommendations.

2 Infants born to HBsAg-negative mothers should receive the 1st dose of hepatitis B (Hep B) vaccine by age 2 months. The 2nd dose should be at least one month after the 1st dose. The 3rd dose should be administered at least 4 months after the 1st dose and at least 2 months after the 2nd dose, but not before 6 months of age for infants.

Infants born to HBsAg-positive mothers should receive hepatitis B vaccine and 0.5 mL hepatitis B immune globulin (HBIG) within 12 hours of birth at separate sites. The 2nd dose is recommended at 1-2 months of age and the 3rd dose at 6 months of age.

Infants born to mothers whose HBsAg status is unknown should receive hepatitis B vaccine within 12 hours of birth. Maternal blood should be drawn at the time of delivery to determine the mother's HBsAg status; if the HBsAg test is positive, the infant should receive HBIG as soon as possible (no later than 1 week of age).

All children and adolescents who have not been immunized against hepatitis B should begin the series during any visit. Special efforts should be made to immunize children who were born in or whose parents were born in areas of the world with moderate or high endemicity of hepatitis B virus infection.

3 The 4th dose of DTaP (diphtheria and tetanus toxoids and acellular pertussis vaccine) may be administered as early as 12 months of age, provided 6 months have elapsed since the 3rd dose and the child is unlikely to return at age 15-18 months. Td (tetanus and diphtheria toxoids) is recommended at 11-12 years of age if at least 5 years have elapsed since the last dose of DTP, DTaP, or DT. Subsequent routine Td boosters are recommended every 10 years.

4 Three *Haemophilus influenzae* type b (Hib) conjugate vaccines are licensed for infant use. If PRP-OMP (PedvaxHIB® and ComVax® [Merck]) is administered at 2 and 4 months of age, a dose at 6 months is not required. Because clinical studies in infants have demonstrated that using some combination products may induce a lower immune response to the Hib vaccine component, DTaP/Hib combination products should not be used for primary immunization in infants at 2, 4, or 6 months of age, unless FDA-approved for these ages.

5 An all-IPV schedule is recommended for routine childhood polio vaccination in the United States. All children should receive four doses of IPV at 2 months, 4 months, 6-18 months, and 4-6 years of age. Oral polio vaccine (OPV) should be used only in selected circumstances. (See MMWR *Morb Mortal Wkly Rep* May 19, 2000/49(RR-5);1-22).

6 The heptavalent conjugate pneumococcal vaccine (PCV) is recommended for all children 2-23 months of age. It also is recommended for certain children 24-59 months of age. (See MMWR *Morb Mortal Wkly Rep* Oct. 6, 2000/49(RR-9);1-35).

7 The 2nd dose of measles, mumps, and rubella (MMR) vaccine is recommended routinely at 4-6 years of age but may be administered during any visit, provided at least 4 weeks have elapsed since receipt of the 1st dose and that both doses are administered beginning at or after 12 months of age. Those who have not previously received the second dose should complete the schedule by the 11- to 12-year-old visit.

8 Varicella (Var) vaccine is recommended at any visit on or after the first birthday for susceptible children, ie, those who lack a reliable history of chickenpox (as judged by a healthcare provider) and who have not been immunized. Susceptible persons 13 years of age or older should receive 2 doses, given at least 4 weeks apart.

9 Hepatitis A (Hep A) is shaded to indicate its recommended use in selected states and/or regions, and for certain high risk groups; consult your local public health authority. (See MMWR *Morb Mortal Wkly Rep* Oct. 1, 1999, 48(RR-12): 1-37.

Adapted from the Advisory Committee on Immunization Practices (ACIP), the American Academy of Pediatrics (AAP), and the American Academy of Family Physicians (AAFP).

For additional information about the vaccines listed refer to the National Immunization Program Home Page at *www.cdc.gov/nip*

Table 4. Recommended Immunization Schedules for Children Not Immunized in the First Year of Life

Recommended Time/Age	Immunization(s)*	Comments
Younger Than 7 Years		
First visit	DTaP, Hib, HBV, MMR	If indicated, tuberculin testing may be done at same visit.
		If child is ≥5 y of age, Hib is not indicated in most circumstances.
Interval after first visit		
1 mo (4 wk)	DTaP, IPV, HBV, Var†	The second dose of IPV may be given if accelerated poliomyelitis immunization is necessary, such as for travelers to areas where polio is endemic.
2 mo	DTaP, Hib, IPV	Second dose of Hib is indicated only if the first dose was received when <15 mo.
≥8 mo	DTaP, HBV, IPV	IPV and HBV are not given if the third doses were given earlier.
Age 4-6 y (at or before school entry)	DTaP, IPV, MMR‡	DTaP is not necessary if the fourth dose was given after the fourth birthday; IPV is not necessary if the third dose was given after the fourth birthday.
Age 11-12 y	See Table 3	
7-12 Years		
First visit	HBV, MMR, dT, IPV	
Interval after first visit		
2 mo (8 wk)	HBV, MMR,‡ Var,§ dT, IPV	IPV also may be given 1 mo after the first visit if accelerated poliomyelitis immunization is necessary.
8-14 mo	HBV,§ dT, IPV	IPV is not given if the third dose was given earlier.
Age 11-12 y	See Table 3	

Adapted from American Academy of Pediatrics, Report of the Committee on Infectious Diseases, *Red Book*, 25th ed, 2000.

*If all needed vaccines cannot be administered simultaneously, priority should be given to protecting the child against those diseases that pose the greatest immediate risk. In the United States, these diseases for children <2 years usually are measles and *Haemophilus influenzae* type b infection; for children >7 years, they are measles, mumps, and rubella. Before 13 years of age, immunity against hepatitis B and varicella should be ensured. DTaP, HBV, Hib, MMR, and Var can be given simultaneously at separate sites if failure of the patient to return for future immunizations is a concern.

†Varicella vaccine can be administered to susceptible children any time after 12 months of age. Unimmunized children who lack a reliable history of varicella should be immunized before their 13th birthday.

‡Minimal interval between doses of MMR is 1 month (4 weeks).

§HBV may be given earlier in a 0-, 2-, and 4-month schedule.

IMMUNIZATION GUIDELINES *(Continued)*

Table 5. Spacing Live and Killed Antigen Administration Guidelines

Antigen Combinations	Recommended Minimum Interval Between Doses
≥2 killed antigens	None. May be given simultaneously or at any interval between doses.
Killed and live antigens	None. May be given simultaneously or at any interval between doses. (**Exception:** Concurrent administration of cholera and yellow fever vaccines should be avoided. Separate these vaccines by at least 3 weeks.)
	Vaccines associated with systemic reactions (cholera, plague and parenteral typhoid) should be given on separate occasions.

Table 6. Passive Immunization Agents — Immune Globulins

Immune Globulin	Dosage	Route
Hepatitis B (H-BIG®)		I.M.
percutaneous inoculation	0.06 mL/kg/dose (within 24 hours) (5 mL max)	
perinatal	0.5 mL/dose (within 12 hours of birth)	
sexual exposure	0.06 mL/kg/dose (within 14 days of contact) (5 mL max)	
Immune globulin (IG)		I.M.*
hepatitis A prophylaxis	0.02 mL/kg/dose (as soon as possible or within 2 weeks after exposure) (postexposure prophylaxis)	
<2 y:	0.06 mL/kg/dose (≥3 months or long-term exposure) repeat every 5 months with continuous exposure	
≥2 y:	0.02 mL/kg (3- to 5-month exposure) may be given to travelers whose departure is imminent with hepatitis A vaccine 0.06 mL/kg (long-term exposure) and hepatitis A vaccine	
hepatitis B	0.06 mL/kg/dose (H-BIG® should be used)	
hepatitis C	0.06 mL/kg/dose (percutaneous exposure)	
measles†	0.25 mL/kg/dose (max: 15 mL/dose) (within 6 days of exposure) 0.5 mL/kg/dose (max: 15 mL/dose) (immunocompromised children)	
Rabies‡	20 IU/kg/dose (within 3 days)	
Tetanus (serious, contaminated, wounds; <3 previous tetanus vaccine doses)	250-500 units/dose	I.M.
Varicella-zoster§ (VZIG)	Within 48 hours but not later than 96 hours after exposure	I.M.¶
	0-10 kg 125 units = 1 vial	
	10.1-20 kg 250 units = 2 vials	
	20.1-30 kg 375 units = 3 vials	
	30.1-40 kg 500 units = 4 vials	
	>40 kg 625 units = 5 vials	

*Deep I.M. in the gluteal region for large doses only. Deltoid muscle or the anterolateral aspect of the thigh are preferred sites for injection. No greater than 5 mL/site in adults or large children; 1-3 mL/site in small children and infants. Max: 20 mL at one time. Pregnant women and infants should receive a thimerosol-free preparation.

†IG prophylaxis may not be indicated in a patient who has received IGIV within 3 weeks of exposure.

‡$^1/_2$ of dose used to infiltrate the wound with the remaining $^1/_2$ of dose given I.M. Rabies immune globulin is not recommended in previously HDCV immunized patients.

§Infants born to women who develop varicella within 5 days before or 48 hours after delivery should receive 125 units I.M. as a single dose.

¶No greater than 2.5 mL of VZIG/one injection site. Doses >2.5 mL should be divided and administered at different sites.

Table 7. Suggested Intervals Between Administration of Immune Globulin Preparations for Various Indications and Measles Immunization*

Indication	Dose (including mg IgG/kg)	Time Interval (mo) Before Measles Vaccination
Tetanus (TIG) prophylaxis	I.M.: 250 units (10 mg IgG/kg)	3
Hepatitis A (IG) prophylaxis		
Contact prophylaxis	I.M.: 0.02 mL/kg (3.3 mg IgG/kg)	3
International travel	I.M.: 0.06 mL/kg (10 mg IgG/kg)	3
Hepatitis B prophylaxis (HBIG)	I.M.: 0.06 mL/kg (10 mg IgG/kg)	3
Rabies immune globulin (RIG)	I.M.: 20 IU/kg (22 mg IgG/kg)	4
Varicella prophylaxis (VZIG)	I.M.: 125 units/10 kg (20-40 mg IgG/kg) (max: 625 units)	5
Measles prophylaxis (IG)		
Standard (ie, nonimmunocompromised contact)	I.M.: 0.25 mL/kg (40 mg IgG/kg)	5
Immunocompromised contact	I.M.: 0.50 mL/kg (80 mg IgG/kg)	6
Blood transfusion		
RBCs, washed	I.V.: 10 mL/kg (negligible IgG/kg)	0
RBCs, adenine-saline added	I.V.: 10 mL/kg (10 mg IgG/kg)	3
Packed RBCs	I.V.: 10 mL/kg (20-60 mg IgG/kg)	5
Whole blood cells	I.V.: 10 mL/kg (80-100 mg IgG/kg)	6
Plasma/platelet products	I.V.: 10 mL/kg (160 mg IgG/kg)	7
Replacement therapy for immune deficiencies	I.V.: 300-400 mg/kg (as IGIV)†	8
Immune thrombocytopenic purpura‡	I.V.: 400 mg/kg (as IGIV)	8
	I.V.: 1000 mg/kg (as IGIV)	10
Kawasaki disease	I.V.: 2 g/kg (as IGIV)	11
RSV prophylaxis	I.V.: 750 mg/kg (as RSV-IVIG)	9

*This table is not intended for determining the correct indications and dosage for the use of immune globulin preparations. Unvaccinated persons may not be fully protected against measles during the entire suggested time interval, and additional doses of immune globulin and/or measles vaccine may be indicated after measles exposure. The concentration of measles antibody in a particular immune globulin preparation can vary by lot. The rate of antibody clearance after receipt of an immune globulin preparation also can vary. The recommended time intervals are extrapolated from an estimated half-life of 30 days of passively acquired antibody and an observed interference with the immune response to measles vaccine for 5 months after a dose of 80 mg IgG/kg.

†Measles vaccination is recommended for most HIV-infected children who do not have evidence of severe immunosuppression, but it is contraindicated for patients who have congenital disorders of the immune system.

‡Formerly referred to as idiopathic thrombocytopenic purpura.

Modified from *Red Book 2000: Report of the Committee on Infectious Diseases*, 25th ed, Elk Grove Village, IL: American Academy of Pediatrics, 390.

IMMUNIZATION GUIDELINES *(Continued)*

Table 8. Recommended for Routine Immunization of HIV-Infected Children — United States

Vaccine	Known HIV Infection	
	Asymptomatic	Symptomatic
DTaP	Yes	Yes
OPV	No	No
IPV	Yes	Yes
MMR	Yes	Yes*
Hib	Yes	Yes
Pneumococcal	Yes	Yes
Influenza†	Yes	Yes
Varicella	Consider	Consider
BCG	No	No
Hepatitis A	‡	‡
Hepatitis B	Yes	Yes

*Severely immunocompromised HIV-infected children should not receive MMR.

†Administer influenza vaccine each autumn and repeat annually for HIV-exposed infants ≥6 months of age, HIV-infected children and adolescents, and household contacts of HIV-infected persons.

‡The immune response in immunocompromised persons, including persons with HIV, may be suboptimal.

CONTRAINDICATIONS AND PRECAUTIONS TO IMMUNIZATIONS

Vaccine	Contraindications	Precautions	Vaccine May Be Given
All vaccines (DTaP, IPV, OPV, MMR, Hib, HBV, Var)	Anaphylactic reaction to a vaccine or a vaccine component is a contraindication to further dose of that vaccine	Moderate or severe illnesses with or without a fever	• Mild to moderate local reaction (soreness, redness, swelling) following a dose • Low-grade or moderate fever following a prior dose • Mild acute illness with or without low-grade fever • Current antimicrobial therapy • Convalescent phase of illnesses • Prematurity • Recent exposure to an infectious disease • History of penicillin or fact that relatives have such allergies • Pregnancy of mother or household contact • Unimmunized household contact
DTaP	Encephalopathy within 7 days of administration of previous dose of DTaP	• Temperature of 40.5°C within 48 hours after vaccination with a prior dose of DTaP • Collapse or shock-like state within 48 hours of receiving a prior dose of DTaP • Seizures within 3 days of receiving a prior dose of DTaP • Persistent inconsolable crying lasting 3 hours, within 48 hours of receiving a prior dose of DTaP • GBS within 6 weeks after a dose	• Family history of seizures • Family history of sudden infant death syndrome • Family history of an adverse event after DTaP administration
IPV	Anaphylactic reaction to neomycin or streptomycin	Pregnancy	

CONTRAINDICATIONS AND PRECAUTIONS TO IMMUNIZATIONS *(Continued)*

Vaccine	Contraindications	Precautions	Vaccine May Be Given
OPV	• Infection with HIV or a household contact with HIV • Known altered immunodeficiency (hematologic and solid tumors, congenital immunodeficiency, and long-term immunosuppressive therapy) • Immunodeficient household contact	Pregnancy	• Breast-feeding • Current antimicrobial therapy • Mild diarrhea
MMR	• Pregnancy • Anaphylactic reaction to neomycin or gelatin • Known altered immunodeficiency (hematologic and solid tumors, congenital immunodeficiency, severe HIV infection, and long-term immunosuppressive therapy)	• Recent (within 3-11 months, depending on product and dose) immune globulin administration • Thrombocytopenia or history of thrombocytopenic purpura	• Tuberculosis or positive PPD • Simultaneous tuberculin skin testing • Breast-feeding • Pregnancy of mother of recipient • Immunodeficient family member or household contact • Infection with HIV • Nonanaphylactic reactions to eggs or neomycin
Hib	None		
Hepatitis B	Anaphylactic reaction to baker's yeast		Pregnancy
Varicella	• Pregnancy • Anaphylactic reaction to neomycin or gelatin • Infection with HIV • Known altered immunodeficiency (hematologic and solid tumors, congenital immunodeficiency, and long-term immunosuppressive therapy)	• Recent immune globulin administration • Family history of immunodeficiency	• Pregnancy in the mother of the recipient • Immunodeficiency in a household contact • Household contact with HIV

Adapted from American Academy of Pediatrics, Report of the Committee on Infectious Diseases, *Red Book*, 25th ed, 2000.

SKIN TESTS FOR DELAYED HYPERSENSITIVITY

Skin tests for delayed hypersensitivity are used diagnostically to assess previous infection (ie, PPD, histoplasmin, and coccidioidin) or used to evaluate cellular immune function by testing for anergy (ie, mumps, *Candida*, tetanus toxoid, trichophyton, PPD). Anergy, a defect in cell-mediated immunity, is characterized by a depressed response or lack of response to skin testing with injected antigens. Anergy has been associated with congenital and acquired immunodeficiencies, and malnutrition.

Candida 1:100

Dose = 0.1 mL intradermally (30% of children younger than 18 months of age and 50% older than 18 months of age respond)

Can be used as a control antigen

Coccidioidin 1:100

Dose = 0.1 mL intradermally (apply with PPD **and** a control antigen)
Mercury derivative used as a preservative for spherulin.

Histoplasmin 1:100

Dose = 0.1 mL intradermally (yeast derived)

Multitest CMI (*Candida,* diphtheria toxoid, tetanus toxoid, *Streptococcus,* old tuberculin, *Trichophyton, Proteus* antigen, and negative control)

Press loaded unit into the skin with sufficient pressure to puncture the skin and allow adequate penetration of all points.

Mumps 40 cfu per mL

Dose = 0.1 mL intradermally (contraindicated in patients allergic to eggs, egg products, or thimerosal)

Purified Protein Derivative 5 TU (PPD* Mantoux Tuberculin)

Screening for tuberculosis:

Children who have no risk factors but who reside in high-prevalence regions: skin test at 4-6 years and 11-16 years of age

Children exposed to HIV-infected individuals, homeless, residents of nursing homes, institutionalized adolescents, users of illicit drugs, incarcerated adolescents and migrant farm workers: skin test every 2-3 years

Children at high risk (children infected with HIV, incarcerated adolescents): annual skin testing

Dose = 0.1 mL intradermally

Definition of positive Mantoux skin test (regardless of previous BCG administration):

Reaction ≥5 mm for high-risk group (children in close contact with known or suspected infectious cases of tuberculosis; children suspected to have disease based on clinical and/or roentgenographic evidence; and children with underlying host factors (immunosuppressive conditions, receiving immunosuppressive therapy, and HIV infection).

Reaction ≥10 mm for children <4 years; those with medical diseases who are at increased risk for dissemination or for those at increased risk because of environmental exposure.

Reaction ≥15 mm for children ≥4 years of age including those with no risk factors.

*PPD 1 TU (first strength) is only used in individuals suspected of being highly sensitive. PPD 250 TU (second strength) is used only for individuals

SKIN TESTS FOR DELAYED HYPERSENSITIVITY
(Continued)

who fail to respond to a previous injection of 5 TU, or anergic patients in whom TB is suspected.

Tetanus Toxoid 1:5

Dose = 0.1 mL intradermally (29% of children younger than 2 years of age and 78% older than 2 years of age respond if they have received 3 immunizing doses)

Can be used as a control antigen.

Tine Test

Indication: survey and screen for exposure to tuberculosis (grasp forearm firmly; stretch the skin of the volar surface tightly; apply the tines to the selected site; press for at least one second so that a circular halo impression is left on the skin)

General Information

1. Intradermal skin tests should be injected in the flexor surface of the forearm.

2. A pale wheal 6-10 mm in diameter should form over the needle tip as soon as the injection is administered. If no bleb forms, the injection must be repeated.

3. Space skin tests at least 2 inches apart to prevent reactions from overlapping.

4. Read skin tests for diameter of induration and presence of erythema at 24, 48, and 72 hours. Reactions occurring before 24 hours are indicative of an immediate rather than a delayed hypersensitivity reaction.

5. False-negative results may occur in patients with malnutrition, viral infections, febrile illnesses, immunodeficiency disorders, severe disseminated infections, uremia, patients who have received immunosuppressive therapy (steroids, antineoplastic agents), patients who have received a recent live attenuated virus vaccine (MMR, measles).

6. False-positive results may occur in patients sensitive to ingredients in the skin test solution such as thimerosal; cross-sensitivity between similar antigens; or with improper interpretation of skin test.

7. Side effects are pain, blisters, extensive erythema and necrosis at the injection site.

   *Emergency equipment and epinephrine should be readily available to treat severe allergic reactions that may occur.

Recommended Interpretation of Skin Test Reactions

Reaction	Local Reaction	
	After Intradermal Injections of Antigens	After Dinitrochlorobenzene
1+	Erythema >10 mm and/or induration >1-5 mm	Erythema and/or induration covering <1/2 area of dosing site
2+	Induration 6-10 mm	Induration covering >1/2 area of dose site
3+	Induration 11-20 mm	Vesiculation and induration at dose site or spontaneous flare at days 7-14 at the site
4+	Induration >20 mm	Bulla or ulceration at dose site or spontaneous flare at days 7-14 at the site

References

American Academy of Pediatrics Committee on Infectious Diseases, "Screening for Tuberculosis in Infants and Children," *Pediatrics*, 1994, 93(1):131-4.

American Academy of Pediatrics Committee on Infectious Diseases, "Update on Tuberculosis Skin Testing of Children," *Pediatrics*, 1996, 97(2):282-4.

NORMAL LABORATORY VALUES FOR CHILDREN

		Normal Values
CHEMISTRY		
Albumin	0-1 y	2.0-4.0 g/dL
	1 y to adult	3.5-5.5 g/dL
Ammonia	Newborns	90-150 µg/dL
	Children	40-120 µg/dL
	Adults	18-54 µg/dL
Amylase	Newborns	0-60 units/L
	Adults	30-110 units/L
Bilirubin, conjugated, direct	Newborns	<1.5 mg/dL
	1 mo to adult	0-0.5 mg/dL
Bilirubin, total	0-3 d	2.0-10.0 mg/dL
	1 mo to adult	0-1.5 mg/dL
Bilirubin, unconjugated, indirect		0.6-10.5 mg/dL
Calcium	Newborns	7.0-12.0 mg/dL
	0-2 y	8.8-11.2 mg/dL
	2 y to adult	9.0-11.0 mg/dL
Calcium, ionized, whole blood		4.4-5.4 mg/dL
Carbon dioxide, total		23-33 mEq/L
Chloride		95-105 mEq/L
Cholesterol	Newborns	45-170 mg/dL
	0-1 y	65-175 mg/dL
	1-20 y	120-230 mg/dL
Creatinine	0-1 y	≤0.6 mg/dL
	1 y to adult	0.5-1.5 mg/dL
Glucose	Newborns	30-90 mg/dL
	0-2 y	60-105 mg/dL
	Children to Adults	70-110 mg/dL
Iron		
	Newborns	110-270 µg/dL
	Infants	30-70 µg/dL
	Children	55-120 µg/dL
	Adults	70-180 µg/dL
Iron binding	Newborns	59-175 µg/dL
	Infants	100-400 µg/dL
	Adults	250-400 µg/dL
Lactic acid, lactate		2-20 mg/dL
Lead, whole blood		<10 µg/dL
Lipase		
	Children	20-140 units/L
	Adults	0-190 units/L
Magnesium		1.5-2.5 mEq/L
Osmolality, serum		275-296 mOsm/kg
Osmolality, urine		50-1400 mOsm/kg
Phosphorus	Newborns	4.2-9.0 mg/dL
	6 wk to 19 mo	3.8-6.7 mg/dL
	19 mo to 3 y	2.9-5.9 mg/dL
	3-15 y	3.6-5.6 mg/dL
	>15 y	2.5-5.0 mg/dL

NORMAL LABORATORY VALUES FOR CHILDREN
(Continued)

Normal Values

CHEMISTRY

Potassium, plasma	Newborns	4.5-7.2 mEq/L
	2 d to 3 mo	4.0-6.2 mEq/L
	3 mo to 1 y	3.7-5.6 mEq/L
	1-16 y	3.5-5.0 mEq/L
Protein, total	0-2 y	4.2-7.4 g/dL
	>2 y	6.0-8.0 g/dL
Sodium		136-145 mEq/L
Triglycerides	Infants	0-171 mg/dL
	Children	20-130 mg/dL
	Adults	30-200 mg/dL
Urea nitrogen, blood	0-2 y	4-15 mg/dL
	2 y to Adult	5-20 mg/dL
Uric acid	Male	3.0-7.0 mg/dL
	Female	2.0-6.0 mg/dL

ENZYMES

Alanine aminotransferase (ALT) (SGPT)	0-2 mo	8-78 units/L
	>2 mo	8-36 units/L
Alkaline phosphatase (ALKP)	Newborns	60-130 units/L
	0-16 y	85-400 units/L
	>16 y	30-115 units/L
Aspartate aminotransferase (AST)	Infants	18-74 units/L
(SGOT)	Children	15-46 units/L
	Adults	5-35 units/L
Creatine kinase (CK)	Infants	20-200 units/L
	Children	10-90 units/L
	Adult male	0-206 units/L
	Adult female	0-175 units/L
Lactate dehydrogenase (LDH)	Newborns	290-501 units/L
	1 mo to 2 y	110-144 units/L
	>16 y	60-170 units/L

Blood Gases

	Arterial	Capillary	Venous
pH	7.35-7.45	7.35-7.45	7.32-7.42
pCO_2 (mm Hg)	35-45	35-45	38-52
pO_2 (mm Hg)	70-100	60-80	24-48
HCO_3 (mEq/L)	19-25	19-25	19-25
TCO_2 (mEq/L)	19-29	19-29	23-33
O_2 saturation (%)	90-95	90-95	40-70
Base excess (mEq/L)	-5 to +5	-5 to +5	-5 to +5

Thyroid Function Tests

T₄ (thyroxine)	1-7 d	10.1-20.9 µg/dL
	8-14 d	9.8-16.6 µg/dL
	1 mo to 1 y	5.5-16.0 µg/dL
	>1 y	4.0-12.0 µg/dL
FTI	1-3 d	9.3-26.6
	1-4 wk	7.6-20.8
	1-4 mo	7.4-17.9
	4-12 mo	5.1-14.5
	1-6 y	5.7-13.3
	>6 y	4.8-14.0
T₃	Newborns	100-470 ng/dL
	1-5 y	100-260 ng/dL
	5-10 y	90-240 ng/dL
	10 y to Adult	70-210 ng/dL
T₃ uptake		35%-45%
TSH	Cord	3-22 µIU/mL
	1-3 d	<40 µIU/mL
	3-7 d	<25 µIU/mL
	>7 d	0-10 µIU/mL

NORMAL LABORATORY VALUES FOR CHILDREN
(Continued)

Hematology Values

Age	Hgb (g/dL)	Hct (%)	RBC (mill/mm³)	RDW	MCV (fL)	MCH (pg)	MCHC (%)	PLTS (x 10³/mm³)
0-3 d	15.0-20.0	45-61	4.0-5.9	<18	95-115	31-37	29-37	250-450
1-2 wk	12.5-18.5	39-57	3.6-5.5	<17	86-110	28-36	28-38	250-450
1-6 mo	10.0-13.0	29-42	3.1-4.3	<16.5	74-96	25-35	30-36	300-700
7 mo to 2 y	10.5-13.0	33-38	3.7-4.9	<16	70-84	23-30	31-37	250-600
2-5 y	11.5-13.0	34-39	3.9-5.0	<15	75-87	24-30	31-37	250-550
5-8 y	11.5-14.5	35-42	4.0-4.9	<15	77-95	25-33	31-37	250-550
13-18 y	12.0-15.2	36-47	4.5-5.1	<14.5	78-96	25-35	31-37	150-450
Adult male	13.5-16.5	41-50	4.5-5.5	<14.5	80-100	26-34	31-37	150-450
Adult female	12.0-15.0	36-44	4.0-4.9	<14.5	80-100	26-34	31-37	150-450

WBC and Diff

Age	WBC (x 10^3/mm³)	Segs	Bands	Lymphs	Monos	Eosinophils	Basophils	Atypical Lymphs	No. of NRBCs
0-3 d	9.0-35.0	32-62	10-18	19-29	5-7	0-2	0-1	0-8	0-2
1-2 wk	5.0-20.0	14-34	6-14	36-45	6-10	0-2	0-1	0-8	0
1-6 mo	6.0-17.5	13-33	4-12	41-71	4-7	0-3	0-1	0-8	0
7 mo to 2 y	6.0-17.0	15-35	5-11	45-76	3-6	0-3	0-1	0-8	0
2-5 y	5.5-15.5	23-45	5-11	35-65	3-6	0-3	0-1	0-8	0
5-8 y	5.0-14.5	32-54	5-11	28-48	3-6	0-3	0-1	0-8	0
13-18 y	4.5-13.0	34-64	5-11	25-45	3-6	0-3	0-1	0-8	0
Adults	4.5-11.0	35-66	5-11	24-44	3-6	0-3	0-1	0-8	0

Segs = segmented neutrophils
Bands = band neutrophils
Lymphs = lymphocytes
Monos = monocytes

NORMAL LABORATORY VALUES FOR CHILDREN
(Continued)

Erythrocyte Sedimentation Rates and Reticulocyte Counts

Sedimentation rate, Westergren	Children	0-20 mm/hour
	Adult male	0-15 mm/hour
	Adult female	0-20 mm/hour
Sedimentation rate, Wintrobe	Children	0-13 mm/hour
	Adult male	0-10 mm/hour
	Adult female	0-15 mm/hour
Reticulocyte count	Newborns	2%-6%
	1-6 mo	0%-2.8%
	Adults	0.5%-1.5%

Cerebrospinal Fluid Values, Normal

		% PMNs
Cell count		
Preterm mean	9 (0-25.4 WBC/mm^3)	57%
Term mean	8.2 (0-22.4 WBC/mm^3)	61%
>1 mo	0.7	0
Glucose		
Preterm	24-63 mg/dL	mean 50
Term	34-119 mg/dL	mean 52
Children	40-80 mg/dL	
CSF glucose/blood glucose		
Preterm	55-105%	
Term	44-128%	
Children	50%	
Lactic acid dehydrogenase	5-30 units/mL	mean 20 units/mL
Myelin basic protein	<4 ng/mL	
Pressure: Initial LP (mm H$_2$O)		
Newborns	80-110 (<110)	
Infants/children	<200 (lateral recumbent position)	
Respiratory movements	5-10	
Protein		
Preterm	65-150 mg/dL	mean 115
Term	20-170 mg/dL	mean 90
Children		
Ventricular	5-15 mg/dL	
Cisternal	5-25 mg/dL	
Lumbar	5-40 mg/dL	

APGAR SCORING SYSTEM

Sign	Score		
	0	1	2
Heart rate	Absent	Under 100 beats per minute	Over 100 beats per minute
Respiratory effort	Absent	Slow (irregular)	Good crying
Muscle tone	Limp	Some flexion of extremities	Active motion
Reflex irritability	No response	Grimace	Cough or sneeze
Color	Blue, pale	Pink body, blue extremities	All pink

From Apgar V, "A Proposal for a New Method of Evaluation of the Newborn Infant," *Anesth Analg*, 1953, 32:260.

FETAL HEART RATE MONITORING

Normal Heart Rates

Fetal heart rate (FHR) 120-160 bpm. Isolated accelerations are normal and considered reassuring. Mild (100-120 bpm) and transient bradycardias may be normal. Normal fetal heart rate tracings show beat-to-beat variability of 5-10 bpm (poor beat-to-beat variability suggests fetal hypoxia).

Abnormal Heart Rates

Bradycardia (FHR <120 bpm): Potential causes include fetal distress, drugs, congenital heart block (associated with maternal SLE, congenital cardiac defects).

Tachycardia (FHR >160 bpm): Potential causes include maternal fever, chorioamnionitis, drugs, fetal dysrhythmias, eg, SVT (with or without fetal CHF).

Decreased Beat-to-Beat Variability

Results from fetal CNS depression. Potential causes include fetal hypoxia, fetal sleep, fetal immaturity, and maternal narcotic/sedative administration.

Fetal Heart Rate Decelerations

Type 1 (early decelerations)

- Seen most commonly in late labor
- Mirror uterine contractions in time of onset, duration, and resolution
- Uniform shape
- Usually associated with good beat-to-beat variability
- Heart rate may dip to 60-80 bpm
- Associated with fetal head compression (increases vagal tone)
- Considered benign, and not representative of fetal hypoxia

APGAR SCORING SYSTEM *(Continued)*

Type 2 (late decelerations)

- Deceleration 10-30 seconds after onset of uterine contraction
- Heart rate fails to return to baseline after contraction is completed
- Asymmetrical shape (longer deceleration, shorter acceleration)
- Late decelerations of 10-20 bpm may be significant
- Probably associated with fetal CNS and myocardial depression

Type 3 (variable decelerations)

- Heart rate variations do not correlate with uterine contractions
- Variable shape and duration
- Occur occasionally in many normal labors
- Concerning if severe (HR <60 bpm), prolonged (duration >60 seconds), associated with poor beat-to-beat variability, or combined with late decelerations
- Associated with cord compression (including nuchal cord)

Reference
Manual of Neonatal Care, Joint Program in Neonatology, 1991.

CREATININE CLEARANCE ESTIMATING METHODS IN PATIENTS WITH STABLE RENAL FUNCTION

The following formulas provide an acceptable estimate of the patient's creatinine clearance except when:

a. The patient's serum creatinine is changing rapidly (either up or down).

b. Patients are markedly emaciated.

In these situations (a and b above), certain assumptions have to be made:

a. In patients with rapidly rising serum creatinines (ie, increasing by >0.5-0.7 mg/dL/day), it is best to assume that the patient's creatinine clearance is probably less than 10 mL/minute.

b. In emaciated patients, although their actual creatinine clearance is less than their calculated creatinine clearance (because of decreased creatinine production), it is not possible to predict easily how much less.

Estimation of creatinine clearance using serum creatinine and body length* (to be used when an adequate timed specimen cannot be obtained). **Note:** This formula may not provide an accurate estimation of creatinine clearance for infants <6 months of age or for patients with severe starvation or muscle wasting.

$$CL_{cr} = K \times L/S_{cr}$$

where:

Cl_{cr} = creatinine clearance in mL/minute/1.73 m^2

K = constant of proportionality that is age specific

Age	K
Low birth weight ≤1 y	0.33
Full-term ≤1 y	0.45
2-12 y	0.55
13-21 y female	0.55
13-21 y male	0.70

L = length in cm

S_{cr} = serum creatinine concentration in mg/dL

Reference

Schwartz GJ, Brion LP, and Spitzer A, "The Use of Plasma Creatinine Concentration for Estimating Glomerular Filtration Rate in Infants, Children and Adolescents," *Ped Clin N Amer,* 1987, 34:571-90.

Children 1-18 years

Method 1: (Traub SL, Johnson CE, *Am J Hosp Pharm*, 1980, 37:195-201)

Equation:

$$Cl_{cr} = \frac{0.48 \times (height)}{S_{cr}}$$

where

Cl_{cr} = creatinine clearance in mL/min/1.73 m^2

S_{cr} = serum creatinine in mg/dL

Height = height in cm

Method 2: See nomogram.

CREATININE CLEARANCE ESTIMATING METHODS IN PATIENTS WITH STABLE RENAL FUNCTION *(Continued)*

Children 1-18 Years

The nomogram below is for rapid evaluation of endogenous creatinine clearance (Cl_{cr}) in pediatric patients.

To predict Cl_{cr} connect the child's S_{cr} (serum creatinine) and Ht (height) with a ruler and read the Cl_{cr} where the ruler intersects the center line.

Adults 18 years and older

Method 1: (Cockroft DW and Gault MH, *Nephron*, 1976, 16:31-41)

Estimated creatinine clearance (Cl_{cr}) (mL/min):

$$\text{Male} = \frac{(140 - \text{age})\ \text{IBW (kg)}}{72 \times \text{serum creatinine}}$$

$$\text{Female} = \text{Estimated } Cl_{cr} \text{ male} \times 0.85$$

Note: The use of the patient's ideal body weight (IBW) is recommended for the above formula except when the patient's actual body weight is less than ideal. Use of the IBW is especially important in obese patients. See appendix Growth & Development section for Ideal Body Weight Calculation.

Method 2: (Jelliffe RW, *Ann Intern Med*, 1973, 79:604)

Estimated creatinine clearance (Cl_{cr}) (mL/min/1.73 m^2):

$$\text{Male} = \frac{98 - 0.8\ (\text{age} - 20)}{\text{serum creatinine}}$$

$$\text{Female} = \text{Estimated } Cl_{cr} \text{ male} \times 0.90$$

RENAL FUNCTION TESTS

Endogenous creatinine clearance vs age (timed collection)

Creatinine clearance (mL/min/1.73 m^2) = ($Cr_uV/S_{cr}T$) (1.73/A)

where:

Cr_u	=	Urine creatinine concentration (mg/dL)
V	=	Total urine volume collected during sampling period (mL)
S_{Cr}	=	Serum creatinine concentration (mg/dL)
T	=	Duration of sampling period (min) (24 h = 1440 min)
A	=	Body surface area (m^2)

Age-specific normal values

5-7 d	50.6±5.8 mL/min/1.73 m^2
1-2 mo	64.6±5.8 mL/min/1.73 m^2
5-8 mo	87.7±11.9 mL/min/1.73 m^2
9-12 mo	86.9±8.4 mL/min/1.73 m^2
≥18 mo	
male	124±26 mL/min/1.73 m^2
female	109±13.5 mL/min/1.73 m^2
Adults	
male	105±14 mL/min/1.73 m^2
female	95±18 mL/min/1.73 m^2

Note: In patients with renal failure (creatinine clearance <25 mL/min), creatinine clearance may be elevated over GFR because of tubular secretion of creatinine.

Serum BUN/Serum Creatinine Ratio

Serum BUN (mg/dL):serum creatinine (mg/dL)

Normal BUN:creatinine ratio is 10-15.

BUN:creatinine ratio >20 suggests prerenal azotemia (also seen with high urea-generation states such as GI bleeding).

BUN:creatinine ratio <5 may be seen with disorders affecting urea biosynthesis such as urea cycle enzyme deficiencies and with hepatitis.

Fractional Sodium Excretion

Fractional sodium secretion (FENa) = Na_uS_{cr}/Na_sCr_u x 100%

where:

Na_u	=	Urine sodium (mEq/L)
Na_s	=	Serum sodium (mEq/L)
Cr_u	=	Urine creatinine (mg/dL)
S_{Cr}	=	Serum creatinine (mg/dL)

FENa <1% suggests prerenal failure
FENa >2% suggest intrinsic renal failure
(for newborns, normal FENa is approximately 2.5%)

Note: Disease states associated with a falsely elevated FENa include severe volume depletion (>10%), early acute tubular necrosis and volume depletion in chronic renal disease. Disorders associated with a lowered FENa include acute glomerulonephritis, hemoglobinuric or myoglobinuric renal failure, nonoliguric acute tubular necrosis, and acute urinary tract obstruction. In addition, FENa may be <1% in patients with acute renal failure **and** a second condition predisposing to sodium retention (eg, burns, congestive heart failure, nephrotic syndrome).

RENAL FUNCTION TESTS *(Continued)*

Urine Calcium/Urine Creatinine Ratio (spot sample)

Urine calcium (mg/dL): urine creatinine (mg/dL)

Normal values <0.21 (mean values 0.08 males, 0.06 females)

Premature infants show wide variability of calcium:creatinine ratio, and tend to have lower thresholds for calcium loss than older children. Prematures without nephrolithiasis had mean Ca:Cr ratio of 0.75±0.76. Infants with nephrolithiasis had mean Ca:Cr ratio of 1.32±1.03 (Jacinto, et al, *Pediatrics*, vol 81, p 31).

Urine Protein/Urine Creatinine Ratio (spot sample)

P_u/Cr_u	Total Protein Excretion (mg/m²/day)
0.1	80
1	800
10	8000
where:	
P_u =	Urine protein concentration (mg/dL)
Cr_u =	Urine creatinine concentration (mg/dL)

Serum Osmolality

Predicted serum osmolality =

2 x Na (mEq/L) + BUN (mg/dL) / 2.8 + glucose (mg/dL) / 18

High Anion Gap (see Toxicology section)

ACID/BASE ASSESSMENT

Henderson-Hasselbalch Equation

$$pH = 6.1 + \log (HCO_3^- / (0.03) (pCO_2))$$

Alveolar Gas Equation

P_iO_2 = f_iO_2 x (total atmospheric pressure – vapor pressure of H_2O at 37°C)

= f_iO_2 x (760 mm Hg – 47 mm Hg)

PAO_2 = P_iO_2 – $PACO_2$ / R

Alveolar/arterial oxygen gradient = PAO_2 – PaO_2

Normal ranges:

Children	15-20 mm Hg
Adults	20-25 mm Hg

Where:

P_iO_2	=	Oxygen partial pressure of inspired gas (mm Hg) (150 mm Hg in room air at sea level)
f_iO_2	=	Fractional pressure of oxygen in inspired gas (0.21 in room air)
PAO_2	=	Alveolar oxygen partial pressure
$PACO_2$	=	Alveolar carbon dioxide partial pressure
PaO_2	=	Arterial oxygen partial pressure
R	=	Respiratory exchange quotient (typically 0.8, increases with high carbohydrate diet, decreases with high fat diet)

Acid/Base Disorders

Acute metabolic acidosis (<12 h duration)

$PaCO_2$ expected = 1.5 (HCO_3^-) + 8±2

or

expected change in pCO = (1-1.5) x change in HCO_3^-

Acute metabolic alkalosis (<12 h duration)

expected change in pCO_2 = (0.5-1) x change in HCO_3^-

Acute respiratory acidosis (<6 h duration)

expected change in HCO_3^- = 0.1 x pCO_2

Acute respiratory acidosis (>6 h duration)

expected change in HCO_3^- = 0.4 x change in pCO_2

Acute respiratory alkalosis (<6 h duration)

expected change in HCO_3^- = 0.2 x change in pCO_2

Acute respiratory alkalosis (>6 h duration)

expected change in HCO_3^- = 0.5 x change in pCO_2

ACUTE DYSTONIC REACTIONS, MANAGEMENT

1. **Confirm that patient has stable airway and adequate respiratory activity.**

2. Administer **one** of the following:

   Diphenhydramine 0.7-1 mg/kg/dose I.V./P.O. q4-6h prn **or**

   Hydroxyzine 0.5-1 mg/kg/dose I.M./P.O. q4-6h prn
   (adult dose: 25-100 mg I.M./P.O. q6h) **or**

   Children >3 years: Benztropine 0.02-0.05 mg/kg/dose or maximum of 1-2 mg I.V./P.O. (avoid use in children <3 years of age except in cases of extreme emergency)

Agents which predispose patients to acute dystonic reactions, such as phenothiazine neuroleptics or antiemetics, often have long therapeutic half-lives. Anticholinergic administration should therefore be continued for 6-24 hours after discontinuation of phenothiazine therapy.

PREPROCEDURE SEDATIVES IN CHILDREN

Purpose: The following table is a guide to aid the clinician in the selection of the most appropriate sedative to sedate a child for a procedure. One must also consider:

- Not all patients require sedation. It is dependent on the procedure and age of the child.

- When sedation is desired, one must consider the time of onset, the duration of action, and the route of administration.

- Each of the following drugs is well absorbed when given by the suggested routes and doses.

- Each drug was assigned an "intensity" based upon the class of drug, dose, and route.[1]

  - Conscious sedation: A medically controlled state of depressed consciousness that retains the patient's ability to independently and continuously maintain a patent airway, respond appropriately to physical stimulation and/or verbal commands. The protective reflexes are maintained.

  - Deep sedation: A medically controlled state of depressed consciousness associated with partial or complete loss of protective reflexes and inability to respond appropriately to physical stimulation and/or verbal commands.

- Those drugs classified as producing deep sedation require more frequent monitoring postprocedure.

- For painful procedures, an analgesic agent needs to be administered.

Sedatives Used to Produce Conscious Sedation

Drug	Route	Dose (mg/kg)	Onset (min)	Duration (h)	Comments
Chloral hydrate	P.O./P.R.	25-100	10-20	4-8	May cause hepatic neoplasms in rats; maximum single dose: infants: 1 g; children: 2 g
Diazepam[2,3] (Valium®)	P.O.	0.2-0.3 90 min prior	60-90	6-8	Maximum oral dose: 10 mg
	I.V.	0.1-0.2	1-3	6-8	Maximum dose I.V.: 5 mg; due to poor absorption and tissue irritation, I.M. route **not** recommended
	P.R.	0.2-0.4	2-10	6-8	May use I.V. solution rectally
"DPT" cocktail[4] (Demerol®, Phenergan®, Thorazine®)	I.M.	Demerol® 1-2, Phenergan® 0.5-1, Thorazine® 0.5-1	30	2-14	May be mixed in single syringe; I.M. only. This combination of agents may have a higher rate of adverse effects compared with alternative sedative/analgesics.
Fentanyl	Transmucosal	5-15 mcg/kg	5-15	1-2	Maximum transmucosal dose: 400 mcg
	I.M.	1-3 mcg/kg	7-15	1-2	
	I.V.	1-3 mcg/kg	Immediate	30-60 min	
Lorazepam[5] (Ativan®)	P.O.	0.05; 90-120 min prior	60	8-12	
	Deep I.M.	0.05; 90-120 min prior	30-60	8-12	
	I.V.	0.05; over 5-10 min	15-30	8-12	

PREPROCEDURE SEDATIVES IN CHILDREN *(Continued)*

Sedatives Used to Produce Conscious Sedation *(continued)*

Drug	Route	Dose (mg/kg)	Onset (min)	Duration (h)	Comments
Meperidine (Demerol®)	P.O.	2-4	10-15	2-4	Doses I.M./I.V. >2 mg/kg are considered deep sedation
	I.M.	0.5-2	10-15	2-4	
	I.V.	0.5-2	5	2-3	
Midazolam[6,7] (Versed®)	P.O.	0.2-0.4; 30-45 min prior	20-30	1-2	Maximum oral dose: 15 mg
	Deep I.M.	0.1-0.15; 30-60 min prior	15	1-2	Maximum total dose: 10 mg
	I.V.	**6 mo - 5 y:** 0.05-0.1; **6-12 y:** 0.025-0.05; **>12 y - Adult:** 2.5-5 mg (total dose); give over 10-20 min	1-5	1-2	Maximum concentration: 1 mg/mL; maximum I.M./I.V. dose: 6 mo - 5 y: 6 mg 6 y - Adult: 10 mg
	P.R.	0.3	20-30	1-2	Dilute injection in 5 mL NS; administer rectally
	Intranasal	0.2-0.3	5	30-60 min	Administer nasally: Use a 1 mL needle-less syringe into the nares over 15 seconds; use 5 mg/mL concentration; ½ dose may be administered into each nare
Morphine	P.O.	0.2-0.5	20-30	3-5	
	I.M.	0.05-0.2	20-30	3-5	
	I.V.	0.05-0.2	10-15	2-5	

Note: See individual drug monographs for further information.

Sedatives Used to Produce Deep Sedation

Drug	Route	Dose (mg/kg)	Onset (min)	Duration (h)	Comments
Methohexital[8,9] (Brevital®)	I.M.	5-10	5	1-1.5	Maximum concentration for I.M./I.V.: 50 mg/mL; maximum I.M./I.V. dose: 200 mg. Greater incidence of adverse effects with I.V. use.
	I.V.	0.75-2	1	7-10 min	
	P.R.	20-35	5-10	1-1.5	Shorter duration of action than thiopental; rectal given as a 10% solution in sterile water; maximum dose rectal: 500 mg
Pentobarbital	P.O./I.M./P.R.	2-6	10-25	1-4	Maximum I.M./I.V./P.O./P.R. dose: 100 mg
	I.V.	1-3	1	15 min	
Thiopental[10,4] (Pentothal)	I.V.	4-6	0.5-1	5-10 min	
	P.R.	25; immediately prior to procedure	10	1-5	Variable rectal absorption; may use additional 12.5 mg/kg if necessary; maximum rectal dose: 1-1.5 g

Note: See individual drug monographs for further information.

Sedatives Used to Produce Dissociative Anesthesia
(Monitor as if deep sedation)

Drug	Route	Dose (mg/kg)	Onset (min)	Duration	Comments
Ketamine	P.O.	6-10; 30 min prior	30-45	10-30	Use only under direct supervision of physicians experienced in administering general anesthetics; has analgesic effects; may use injectable product orally diluted in a beverage of the patient's choice
	I.M.	3-7	7	12-25	
	I.V.	0.5-2	1	5-10	

Note: See individual drug monographs for further information.

Footnotes

1. Committee on Drugs, Section of Anesthesiology, American Academy of Pediatrics, "Guidelines for Monitoring and Management of Pediatric Patient During and After Sedation for Diagnostic and Therapeutic Procedures," *Pediatrics*, 1992, 89:1110-5.
2. Yager JY and Seshia SS, "Sublingual Lorazepam in Childhood Serial Seizures," *Am J Dis Child*, 1988, 142(9):931-2.
3. Fell D, Gough MB, Northan AA, et al, "Diazepam Premedication in Children," *Anaesthesia*, 1985, 40:12-7.
4. Burckart GJ, White III TJ, Siegle RL, et al, "Rectal Thiopental Versus an Intramuscular Cocktail for Sedating Children Before Computer Tomography," *Am J Hosp Pharm*, 1980, 37:222-4.
5. Burtles R and Astley B, "Lorazepam in Children," *Br J Anaesth*, 1983, 55:275-9.
6. Roelofse JA, van der Bijl P, Stegmann DH, et al, "Preanesthetic Medication With Rectal Midazolam in Children Undergoing Dental Extractions," *J Oral Maxillofac Surg*, 1990, 48(8):791-7.
7. Wilton NC, Leigh J, Rosen DR, et al, "Preanesthetic Sedation of Preschool Children Using Intranasal Midazolam," *Anesthesiology*, 1988, 60(6):972-5.
8. Elman DS and Denson JS, "Preanesthetic Sedation of Children With Intramuscular Methohexital Sodium," *Anesth Analg*, 1965, 44(5):494-8.
9. Miller JR, Grayson M, and Stoelting VK, "Sedation With Intramuscular Methohexital Sodium," *Am J Ophthalmol*, 1966, 62(1):38-43.
10. "Drug Evaluations," *AMA*, 1980.

FEBRILE SEIZURES

A febrile seizure is defined as a seizure occurring for no reason other than an elevated temperature. It does not have an infectious or metabolic origin within the CNS (ie, it is not caused by meningitis or encephalitis). Fever is usually >102°F rectally, but the more rapid the rise in temperature, the more likely a febrile seizure may occur. About 4% of children develop febrile seizures at one time of their life, usually occurring between 3 months and 5 years of age with the majority occurring at 6 months to 3 years of age. There are three types of febrile seizures:

1. **Simple** febrile seizures are nonfocal febrile seizures of less than 15 minutes duration. They do not occur in multiples.

2. **Complex** febrile seizures are febrile seizures that are either focal, have a focal component, are longer than 15 minutes in duration, or are multiple febrile seizures that occur within 30 minutes.

3. **Febrile status epilepticus** is a febrile seizure that is a generalized tonic clonic seizure lasting longer than 30 minutes.

Note: Febrile seizures should not be confused with true epileptic seizures associated with fever or "seizure with fever." "Seizure with fever" includes seizures associated with acute neurologic illnesses (ie, meningitis, encephalitis).

Long-term prophylaxis with phenobarbital may reduce the risk of subsequent febrile seizures. The 1980 NIH Consensus paper stated that after the first febrile seizure, long-term prophylaxis should be considered under any of the following:

1. Presence of abnormal neurological development or abnormal neurological exam

2. Febrile seizure was complex in nature:

    duration >15 minutes

    focal febrile seizure

    followed by transient or persistent neurological abnormalities

3. Positive family history of afebrile seizures (epilepsy)

Also consider long-term prophylaxis in certain cases if:

1. the child has multiple febrile seizures

2. the child is <12 months of age

Anticonvulsant prophylaxis is usually continued for 2 years or 1 year after the last seizure, whichever is longer. With the identification of phenobarbital's adverse effects on learning and cognitive function, many physicians will not start long-term phenobarbital prophylaxis after the first febrile seizure unless the patient has more than one of the above risk factors. Most physicians would start long-term prophylaxis if the patient has a second febrile seizure.

Daily administration of phenobarbital and therapeutic phenobarbital serum concentrations ≥15 mcg/mL decrease recurrence rates of febrile seizures. Valproic acid is also effective in preventing recurrences of febrile seizures, but is usually reserved for patients who have significant adverse effects to phenobarbital. The administration of rectal diazepam (as a solution or suppository) at the time of the febrile illness has been shown to be as effective as daily phenobarbital in preventing recurrences of febrile seizures. These rectal dosage forms are just now available in the United States. Some centers in the USA are still using the injectable form of diazepam rectally. The solution for injection is filtered prior to use if drawn from an ampul. A recent study suggests that oral diazepam, 0.33 mg/kg/dose given every 8 hours only when the child has a fever, may reduce the risk of recurrent febrile seizures (see Rosman, et al). (**Note:** A more recent study by Uhari (1995) showed that lower doses of diazepam, 0.2 mg/kg/dose, were not effective.) Carbamazepine and phenytoin are **not** effective in preventing febrile seizures.

References

Berg AT, Shinnar S, Hauser WA, et al, "Predictors of Recurrent Febrile Seizures: A Meta-Analytic Review," *J Pediatr*, 1990, 116(3):329-37.

Camfield PR, Camfield CS, Gordon K, et al, "Prevention of Recurrent Febrile Seizures," *J Pediatr*, 1995, 126(6):929-30.

NIH Consensus Statement, "Febrile Seizures: A Consensus of Their Significance, Evaluation and Treatment," *Pediatrics*, 1980, 66(6):1009-12.

Rosman NP, Colton T, Labazzo J, et al, "A Controlled Trial of Diazepam Administration During Febrile Illnesses to Prevent Recurrence of Febrile Seizures," *N Engl J Med*, 1993, 329(2):79-84.

Uhari M, Rantala H, Vainionpää L, et al, "Effect of Acetaminophen and of Low Intermittent Doses of Diazepam on Prevention of Recurrences of Febrile Seizures," *J Pediatr*, 1995, 126(6):991-5.

CAUSES OF NEONATAL SEIZURES

1. Trauma
   a. subdural hematoma
   b. intracortical hemorrhage
   c. cortical vein thrombosis

2. Asphyxia — subependymal hemorrhage

3. Congenital abnormalities (cerebral dysgenesis)
   a. lissencephaly
   b. schizencephaly

4. Hypertension

5. Metabolic
   a. hypocalcemia
      • hypomagnesemia
      • high phosphate load
      • IDM (infants of diabetic mothers)
      • hypoparathyroidism
      • maternal hyperparathyroidism
      • idiopathic
      • DiGeorge's syndrome
   b. hypoglycemia
      • galactosemia
      • IUGR (intrauterine growth retardation)
      • IDM (infants of diabetic mothers)
      • glycogen storage disease
      • idiopathic
      • methylmalonic acidemia
      • propionic acidemia
      • maple syrup urine disease
      • asphyxia
   c. electrolyte imbalance
      • hypernatremia
      • hypomagnesemia
      • hyponatremia

6. Infections
   a. bacterial meningitis
   b. cerebral abscess
   c. herpes encephalitis
   d. Coxsackie meningoencephalitis
   e. cytomegalovirus
   f. toxoplasmosis
   g. syphilis

7. Drug withdrawal
   a. methadone
   b. heroin
   c. barbiturate (short-acting, such as secobarbital and butalbital)
   d. propoxyphene
   e. benzodiazepines (chlordiazepoxide, diazepam)
   f. cocaine
   g. ethanol
   h. codeine

8. Pyridoxine dependency

9. Amino acid disturbances
   a. maple syrup urine disease
   b. urea cycle abnormalities
   c. nonketotic hyperglycinemia
   d. ketotic hyperglycinemia
   e. Leigh disease
   f. isovaleric acidemia

10. Toxins
    a. local anesthetics
    b. isoniazid
    c. lead
    d. indomethacin (from breast feeding)
    e. fentanyl

11. Familial seizures
    a. neurocutaneous syndromes
       • tuberous sclerosis
       • incontinentia pigmenti
    b. genetic syndromes
       • Zellweger's
       • Smith Lemli Opitz
       • neonatal adrenoleukodystrophy
    c. benign familial epilepsy

12. Cerebral hemorrhage
    a. intraventricular
    b. subarachnoid
    c. subdural

Adapted from Painter MJ, Bergman I, and Crumrie P, "Neonatal Seizures," *Pediatr Clin North Am*, 1986, 33:91-107.

ANTIEPILEPTIC DRUGS

Antiepileptic Drugs for Children and Adolescents by Seizure Type and Epilepsy Syndrome

Seizure Type or Epilepsy Syndrome	First Line Therapy	Alternatives
Partial seizures (with or without secondary generalization)	Carbamazepine	Valproate, phenytoin, gabapentin, lamotrigine, vigabatrin, phenobarbital, primidone; consider clonazepam, clorazepate, acetazolamide
Generalized tonic-clonic seizures	Valproate or carbamazepine	Phenytoin, phenobarbital, primidone; consider clonazepam
Childhood absence epilepsy		
Before 10 years of age	Ethosuximide or valproate	Methsuximide, acetazolamide, clonazepam, lamotrigine
After 10 years of age	Valproate	Ethosuximide, methsuximide, acetazolamide, clonazepam, lamotrigine; consider adding carbamazepine, phenytoin, or phenobarbital for generalized tonic-clonic seizures if valproate not tolerated
Juvenile myoclonic epilepsy	Valproate	Phenobarbital, primidone, clonazepam; consider carbamazepine, phenytoin, methsuximide, acetazolamide
Progressive myoclonic epilepsy	Valproate	Valproate plus clonazepam, phenobarbital
Lennox-Gastaut and related syndromes	Valproate	Clonazepam, phenobarbital, lamotrigine, ethosuximide, felbamate; consider methsuximide, ACTH or steroids, pyridoxine, ketogenic diet
Infantile spasms	ACTH or steroids	Valproate; consider clonazepam, vigabatrin (especially with tuberous sclerosis), pyridoxine
Benign epilepsy of childhood with centrotemporal spikes	Carbamazepine or valproate	Phenytoin; consider phenobarbital, primidone
Neonatal seizures	Phenobarbital	Phenytoin; consider clonazepam, primidone, valproate, pyridoxine

Adapted from Bourgeois BFD, "Antiepileptic Drugs in Pediatric Practice," *Epilepsia*, 1995, 36(Suppl 2):S34-S45.

COMA SCALES

Glasgow Coma Scale

Activity	Best Response	Score
Eye opening	Spontaneous	4
	Responds to voice	3
	Responds to pain	2
	No response	1
Verbal Response	Oriented and appropriate	5
	Confused / disoriented conversation	4
	Inappropriate words	3
	Nonspecific sounds (incomprehensible)	2
	No response	1
Motor Response	Follows commands	6
	Localizes pain	5
	Withdraws to pain	4
	Abnormal flexion (decorticate posturing)	3
	Abnormal extension (decerebrate posturing)	2
	No response	1

Modified Coma Scale for Infants

Activity	Best Response	Score
Eye opening	Spontaneous	4
	Responds to voice	3
	Responds to pain	2
	No response	1
Verbal Response	Coos, babbles	5
	Irritable	4
	Cries to pain	3
	Moans to pain	2
	No response	1
Motor Response	Normal spontaneous movements	6
	Withdraws to touch	5
	Withdraws to pain	4
	Abnormal flexion (decorticate posturing)	3
	Abnormal extension (decerebrate posturing)	2
	No response	1

Interpretation of Coma Scale Scores
Maximum Score: 15; Minimum Score: 3
(low score indicates greater severity of coma)

Range of Score	Interpretation
3- 8	Coma. Severe brain injury. Immediate action needed. Notify ICU staff STAT. Will require intubation regardless of respiratory status.
9-12	Lethargic. Needs close observation in special care unit. Frequent neuro checks. Notify ICU staff.
13-14	Needs observation
15	Normal

References
James HE, "Neurologic Evaluation and Support in the Child With an Acute Brain Insult," *Pediatr Ann*, 1986, 15(1):16-22.
Jennett B and Teasdale G, "Aspects of Coma After Severe Head Injury," *Lancet*, 1977, 1(8017): 878-81.

ASTHMA

Expert Panel Report II: Guidelines for the Diagnosis and Management of Asthma

Stepwise Approach for Managing Asthma in Adults and Children >5 Years of Age: Classify Severity

Goals of Asthma Treatment

- Prevent chronic and troublesome symptoms (eg, coughing or breathlessness in the night, in the early morning, or after exertion)
- Maintain (near) "normal" pulmonary function
- Maintain normal activity levels (ie, exercise and other physical activity)
- Prevent recurrent exacerbations of asthma and minimize the need for emergency department visits or hospitalizations
- Provide optimal pharmacotherapy with minimal or no adverse effects
- Meet patients' and families' expectations of and satisfaction with asthma care

Clinical Features Before Treatment*

Symptoms**	Night-time Symptoms	Lung Function
STEP 4: Severe Persistent		
• Continual symptoms • Limited physical activity • Frequent exacerbations	Frequent	• FEV_1/PEF ≤60% predicted • PEF variability >30%
STEP 3: Moderate Persistent		
• Daily symptoms • Daily use of inhaled short-acting beta$_2$-agonist • Exacerbations affect activity • Exacerbations ≥2 times/week may last days	>1 time/week	• FEV_1/PEF >60% - <80% predicted • PEF variability >30%
STEP 2: Mild Persistent		
• Symptoms >2 times/week but <1 time/day • Exacerbations may affect activity	>2 times/month	• FEV_1/PEF ≥80% predicted • PEF variability 20% - 30%
STEP 1: Mild Intermittent		
• Symptoms ≤2 times/week • Asymptomatic and normal PEF between exacerbations • Exacerbations brief (from a few hours to a few days); intensity may vary	≤2 times/month	• FEV_1/PEF ≥80% predicted • PEF variability ≤20%

*The presence of one of the features of severity is sufficient to place a patient in that category. An individual should be assigned to the most severe grade in which any feature occurs. The characteristics noted in this figure are general and may overlap because asthma is highly variable. Furthermore, an individual's classification may change over time.

**Patients at any level of severity can have mild, moderate, or severe exacerbations. Some patients with intermittent asthma experience severe and life-threatening exacerbations separated by long periods of normal lung function and no symptoms.

Stepwise Approach for Managing Infants and Young Children (≤5 Years of Age) With Acute or Chronic Asthma Symptoms

Long-Term Control	Quick Relief
STEP 4: Severe Persistent	
Daily anti-inflammatory medicine • High-dose inhaled corticosteroid with spacer/holding chamber and face mask • If needed, add systemic corticosteroids 2 mg/kg/day and reduce to lowest daily or alternate-day dose that stabilizes symptoms	• Bronchodilator as needed for symptoms (see step 1) up to 3 times/day
STEP 3: Moderate Persistent	
Daily anti-inflammatory medication. Either: • Medium-dose inhaled corticosteroid with spacer/holding chamber and face mask **or** Once control is established: • Medium-dose inhaled corticosteroid and nedocromil **or** • Medium-dose inhaled corticosteroid and long-acting bronchodilator (theophylline)	• Bronchodilator as needed for symptoms (see step 1) up to 3 times/day
STEP 2: Mild Persistent	
Daily anti-inflammatory medication. Either: • Cromolyn (nebulizer is preferred; or MDI) or nedocromil (MDI only) tid-qid • Infants and young children usually begin with a trial of cromolyn or nedocromil **or** • Low-dose inhaled corticosteroid with spacer/holding chamber and face mask	• Bronchodilator as needed for symptoms (see step 1)
STEP 1: Mild Intermittent	
No daily medication needed	• Bronchodilator as needed for symptoms <2 times/week. Intensity of treatment will depend upon severity of exacerbation (see "Managing Exacerbations"). Either: – Inhaled short-acting beta$_2$-agonist by nebulizer or face mask and spacer/holding chamber **or** – Oral beta$_2$-agonist for symptoms • With viral respiratory infection: – Bronchodilator q4-6h up to 24 hours (longer with physician consult) but, in general, repeat no more than once every 6 weeks – Consider systemic corticosteroid if current exacerbation is severe **or** Patient has history of previous severe exacerbations

↓ **Step Down**
Review treatment every 1-6 months. If control is sustained for at least 3 months, a gradual stepwise reduction in treatment may be possible.

↑ **Step Up**
If control is not achieved, consider step up. First: review patient medication technique, adherence, and environmental control (avoidance of allergens or other precipitant factors)

ASTHMA *(Continued)*

Notes:

- **The stepwise approach presents guidelines to assist clinical decision making. Asthma is highly variable; clinicians should tailor specific medication plans to the needs and circumstances of individual patients.**

- Gain control as quickly as possible; then decrease treatment to the least medication necessary to maintain control. Gaining control may be accomplished by either starting treatment at the step most appropriate to the initial severity of their condition or by starting at a higher level of therapy (eg, a course of systemic corticosteroids or higher dose of inhaled corticosteroids).

- A rescue course of systemic corticosteroid (prednisolone) may be needed at any time and step.

- In general, use of short-acting beta$_2$-agonist on a daily basis indicates the need for additional long-term control therapy.

- It is important to remember that there are very few studies on asthma therapy for infants.

- Consultation with an asthma specialist is recommended for patients with moderate or severe persistent asthma in this age group. Consider consultation for all patients with mild persistent asthma.

Stepwise Approach for Managing Asthma in Adults and Children >5 Years of Age: Treatment

(Preferred treatments are in **bold** print)

Long-Term Control	Quick Relief	Education
STEP 4: Severe Persistent		
Daily medications: • **Anti-inflammatory: Inhaled corticosteroid (high dose) and** • Long-acting bronchodilator: Either **long-acting inhaled beta$_2$-agonist**, sustained-release theophylline, or long-acting beta$_2$-agonist tablets **and** • Corticosteroid tablets or syrup long term (2 mg/kg/day, generally do not exceed 60 mg per day).	• Short-acting bronchodilator: **Inhaled beta$_2$-agonists** as needed for symptoms. • Intensity of treatment will depend on severity of exacerbation; see "Managing Exacerbations" • Use of short-acting inhaled beta$_2$-agonists on a daily basis, or increasing use, indicates the need for additional long-term control therapy.	Steps 2 and 3 actions plus: • Refer to individual education/counseling
STEP 3: Moderate Persistent		
Daily medication: • Either – **Anti-inflammatory: Inhaled corticosteroid (medium dose)** or – **Inhaled corticosteroid (low-medium dose)** and add a long-acting bronchodilator, especially for night-time symptoms: Either **long-acting inhaled beta$_2$-agonist**, sustained-release theophylline, or long-acting beta$_2$-agonist tablets. • If needed – Anti-inflammatory: **Inhaled corticosteroids (medium-high dose) and** – **Long-acting bronchodilator**, especially for nighttime symptoms; either **long-acting inhaled beta$_2$-agonist**, sustained release theophylline, or long-acting beta$_2$-agonist tablets.	• Short-acting bronchodilator: **Inhaled beta$_2$-agonists** as needed for symptoms. • Intensity of treatment will depend on severity of exacerbation; see "Managing Exacerbations." • Use of short-acting inhaled beta$_2$-agonists on a daily basis, or increasing use, indicates the need for additional long-term control therapy.	Step 1 actions plus: • Teach self-monitoring • Refer to group education if available • Review and update self-management plan

Long-Term Control	Quick Relief	Education
STEP 2: Mild Persistent		
One daily medication: • **Anti-inflammatory:** Either **inhaled corticosteroid** (low doses) or **cromolyn or nedocromil** (children usually begin with a trial of cromolyn or nedocromil). • Sustained-release theophylline to serum concentration of 5-15 mcg/mL is an alternative, but not preferred, therapy. Zafirlukast or zileuton may also be considered for patients ≥12 years of age, although their position in therapy is not fully established.	• Short-acting bronchodilator: **Inhaled beta$_2$-agonists** as needed for symptoms. • Intensity of treatment will depend on severity of exacerbation; see "Managing Exacerbations." •Use of short-acting inhaled beta$_2$-agonists on a daily basis, or increasing use, indicates the need for additional long-term control therapy.	Step 1 actions plus: • Teach self-monitoring • Refer to group education if available • Review and update self-management plan
STEP 1: Mild Intermittent		
No daily medication needed.	• Short-acting bronchodilator: **Inhaled beta$_2$-agonists** as needed for symptoms. • Intensity of treatment will depend on severity of exacerbation; see "Managing Exacerbations" • Use of short-acting inhaled beta$_2$-agonists more than 2 times/week may indicate the need to initiate long-term control therapy	• Teach basic facts about asthma • Teach inhaler/spacer/holding chamber technique • Discuss roles of medications •Develop self-management plan • Develop action plan for when and how to take rescue actions, especially for patients with a history of severe exacerbations • Discuss appropriate environmental control measures to avoid exposure to known allergens and irritants

↓ **Step down**
Review treatment every 1-6 months; a gradual stepwise reduction in treatment may be possible.

↑**Step up**
If control is not maintained, consider step up. First, review patient medication technique, adherence, and environmental control (avoidance of allergens or other factors that contribute to asthma severity.)

Notes:

• **The stepwise approach presents general guidelines to assist clinical decision making; it is not intended to be a specific prescription. Asthma is highly variable; clinicians should tailor specific medication plans to the needs and circumstances of individual patients.**

• Gain control as quickly as possible; then decrease treatment to the least medication necessary to maintain control. Gaining control may be accomplished by either starting treatment at the step most appropriate to the initial severity of the condition or starting at a higher level of therapy (eg, a course of systemic corticosteroids or higher dose of inhaled corticosteroids).

• A rescue course of systemic corticosteroids may be needed at any time and at any step.

• Some patients with intermittent asthma experience severe and life-threatening exacerbations separated by long periods of normal lung function and no symptoms. This may be especially common with exacerbations provoked by respiratory infections. A short course of systemic corticosteroids is recommended.

• At each step, patients should control their environment to avoid or control factors that make their asthma worse (eg, allergens, irritants); this requires specific diagnosis and education.

ASTHMA *(Continued)*

Management of Asthma Exacerbations: Home Treatment*

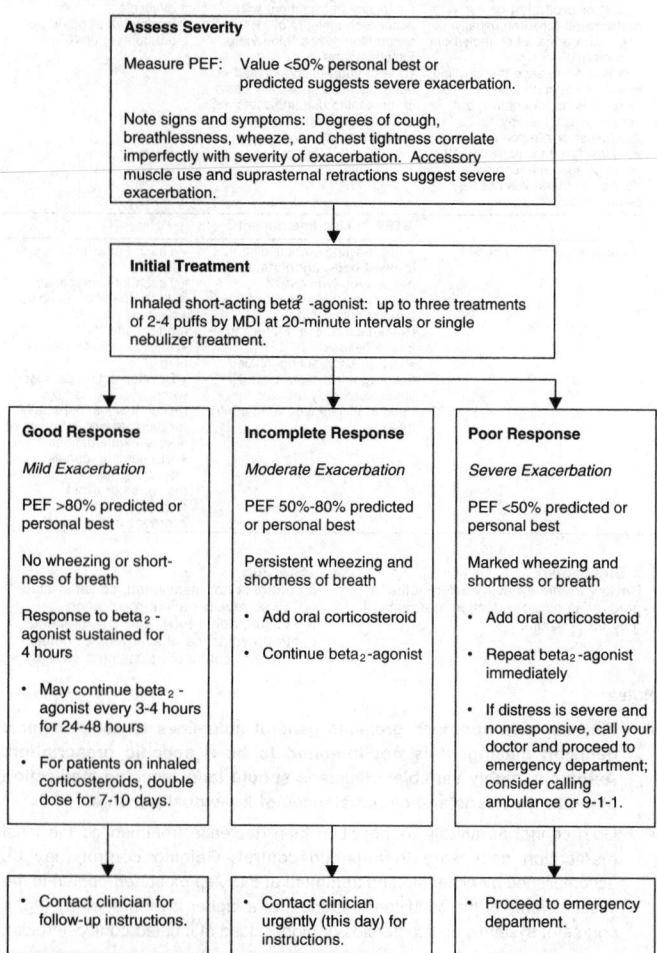

Assess Severity

Measure PEF: Value <50% personal best or predicted suggests severe exacerbation.

Note signs and symptoms: Degrees of cough, breathlessness, wheeze, and chest tightness correlate imperfectly with severity of exacerbation. Accessory muscle use and suprasternal retractions suggest severe exacerbation.

Initial Treatment

Inhaled short-acting beta$_2$-agonist: up to three treatments of 2-4 puffs by MDI at 20-minute intervals or single nebulizer treatment.

Good Response

Mild Exacerbation

PEF >80% predicted or personal best

No wheezing or shortness of breath

Response to beta$_2$-agonist sustained for 4 hours

- May continue beta$_2$-agonist every 3-4 hours for 24-48 hours

- For patients on inhaled corticosteroids, double dose for 7-10 days.

Incomplete Response

Moderate Exacerbation

PEF 50%-80% predicted or personal best

Persistent wheezing and shortness of breath

- Add oral corticosteroid

- Continue beta$_2$-agonist

Poor Response

Severe Exacerbation

PEF <50% predicted or personal best

Marked wheezing and shortness or breath

- Add oral corticosteroid

- Repeat beta$_2$-agonist immediately

- If distress is severe and nonresponsive, call your doctor and proceed to emergency department; consider calling ambulance or 9-1-1.

- Contact clinician for follow-up instructions.

- Contact clinician urgently (this day) for instructions.

- Proceed to emergency department.

*Patients at high risk of asthma-related death should receive immediate clinical attention after initial treatment. Additional therapy may be required.

Management of Asthma Exacerbations: Emergency Department and Hospital-Based Care

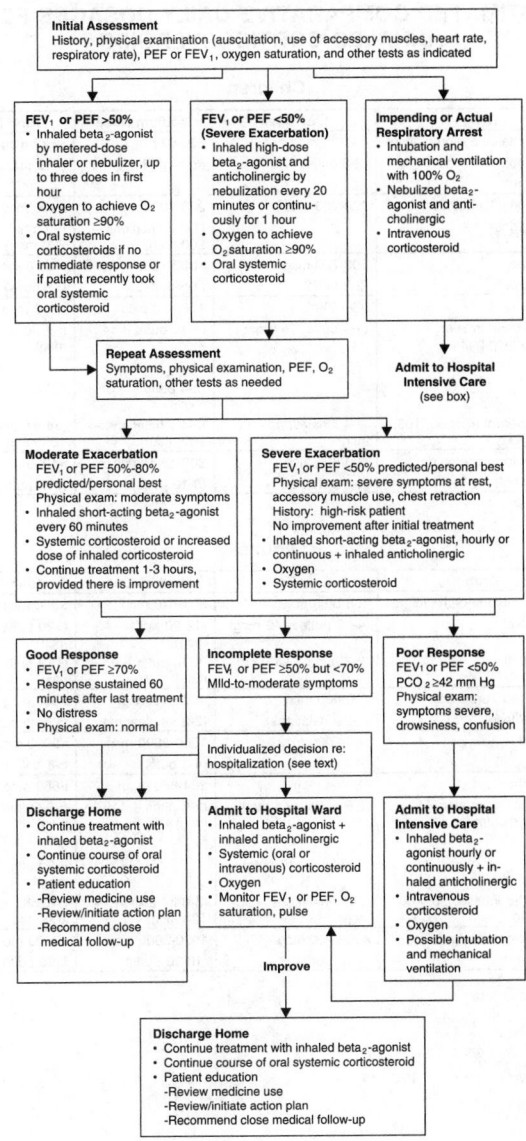

Initial Assessment
History, physical examination (auscultation, use of accessory muscles, heart rate, respiratory rate), PEF or FEV_1, oxygen saturation, and other tests as indicated

---

FEV_1 or PEF >50%
- Inhaled beta$_2$-agonist by metered-dose inhaler or nebulizer, up to three does in first hour
- Oxygen to achieve O_2 saturation ≥90%
- Oral systemic corticosteroids if no immediate response or if patient recently took oral systemic corticosteroid

FEV_1 or PEF <50% (Severe Exacerbation)
- Inhaled high-dose beta$_2$-agonist and anticholinergic by nebulization every 20 minutes or continuously for 1 hour
- Oxygen to achieve O_2 saturation ≥90%
- Oral systemic corticosteroid

Impending or Actual Respiratory Arrest
- Intubation and mechanical ventilation with 100% O_2
- Nebulized beta$_2$-agonist and anticholinergic
- Intravenous corticosteroid

Repeat Assessment
Symptoms, physical examination, PEF, O_2 saturation, other tests as needed

Admit to Hospital Intensive Care
(see box)

Moderate Exacerbation
FEV_1 or PEF 50%-80% predicted/personal best
Physical exam: moderate symptoms
- Inhaled short-acting beta$_2$-agonist every 60 minutes
- Systemic corticosteroid or increased dose of inhaled corticosteroid
- Continue treatment 1-3 hours, provided there is improvement

Severe Exacerbation
FEV_1 or PEF <50% predicted/personal best
Physical exam: severe symptoms at rest, accessory muscle use, chest retraction
History: high-risk patient
No improvement after initial treatment
- Inhaled short-acting beta$_2$-agonist, hourly or continuous + inhaled anticholinergic
- Oxygen
- Systemic corticosteroid

Good Response
- FEV_1 or PEF ≥70%
- Response sustained 60 minutes after last treatment
- No distress
- Physical exam: normal

Incomplete Response
FEV_1 or PEF ≥50% but <70%
Mild-to-moderate symptoms

Individualized decision re: hospitalization (see text)

Poor Response
FEV_1 or PEF <50%
PCO_2 ≥42 mm Hg
Physical exam: symptoms severe, drowsiness, confusion

Discharge Home
- Continue treatment with inhaled beta$_2$-agonist
- Continue course of oral systemic corticosteroid
- Patient education
  -Review medicine use
  -Review/initiate action plan
  -Recommend close medical follow-up

Admit to Hospital Ward
- Inhaled beta$_2$-agonist + inhaled anticholinergic
- Systemic (oral or intravenous) corticosteroid
- Oxygen
- Monitor FEV_1 or PEF, O_2 saturation, pulse

Admit to Hospital Intensive Care
- Inhaled beta$_2$-agonist hourly or continuously + inhaled anticholinergic
- Intravenous corticosteroid
- Oxygen
- Possible intubation and mechanical ventilation

Improve

Discharge Home
- Continue treatment with inhaled beta$_2$-agonist
- Continue course of oral systemic corticosteroid
- Patient education
  -Review medicine use
  -Review/initiate action plan
  -Recommend close medical follow-up

ASTHMA *(Continued)*

ESTIMATED COMPARATIVE DAILY DOSAGES FOR INHALED CORTICOSTEROIDS

Children

Drug	Low Dose	Medium Dose	High Dose
Beclomethasone dipropionate 42 mcg/puff 84 mcg/puff	84-336 mcg (2-8 puffs)	336-672 mcg (8-16 puffs)	>672 mcg (>16 puffs)
Budesonide Turbuhaler 200 mcg/dose	100-200 mcg	200-400 mcg (1-2 inhalations – 200 mcg)	>400 mcg (>2 inhalations – 200 mcg)
Flunisolide 250 mcg/puff	500-750 mcg (2-3 puffs)	1000-1250 mcg (4-5 puffs)	>1250 mcg (>5 puffs)
Fluticasone Metered dose inhaler: 44, 110, 220 mcg/puff	88-176 mcg (2-4 puffs – 44 mcg)	176-440 mcg (4-10 puffs – 44 mcg) or (2-4 puffs – 110 mcg)	>440 mcg (>4 puffs – 110 mcg)
Dry powder inhaler: 50, 100, 250 mcg/dose	(2-4 inhalations – 50 mcg)	(2-4 inhalations – 100 mcg)	(>4 inhalations – 100 mcg)
Triamcinolone acetonide 100 mcg/puff	400-800 mcg (4-8 puffs)	800-1200 mcg (8-12 puffs)	>1200 mcg (>12 puffs)

Adults

Drug	Low Dose	Medium Dose	High Dose
Beclomethasone dipropionate 42 mcg/puff 84 mcg/puff	168-504 mcg (4-12 puffs – 42 mcg) (2-6 puffs – 84 mcg)	504-840 mcg (12-20 puffs – 42 mcg) (6-10 puffs – 84 mcg)	>840 mcg (>20 puffs – 42 mcg) (>10 puffs – 84 mcg)
Budesonide Turbuhaler 200 mcg/dose	200-400 mcg (1-2 inhalations)	400-600 mcg (2-3 inhalations)	>600 mcg (>3 inhalations)
Flunisolide 250 mcg/puff	500-1000 mcg (2-4 puffs)	1000-2000 mcg (4-8 puffs)	>2000 mcg (>8 puffs)
Fluticasone Metered dose inhaler: 44, 110, 220 mcg/puff	88-264 mcg (2-6 puffs – 44 mcg) or (2 puffs – 110 mcg)	264-660 mcg (2-6 puffs – 110 mcg)	>660 mcg (>6 puffs – 110 mcg) or (>3 puffs – 220 mcg)
Dry powder inhaler: 50, 100, 250 mcg/dose	(2-6 inhalations – 50 mcg)	(3-6 inhalations – 100 mcg)	(>6 inhalations – 100 mcg)
Triamcinolone acetonide 100 mcg/puff	400-1000 mcg (4-10 puffs)	1000-2000 mcg (10-20 puffs)	>2000 mcg (>20 puffs)

Notes:

- **The most important determinant of appropriate dosing is the clinician's judgment of the patient's response to therapy.** The clinician must monitor the patient's response on several clinical parameters and adjust the dose accordingly. The stepwise approach to therapy emphasizes that once control of asthma is achieved, the dose of mediation should be carefully titrated to the minimum dose required to maintain control, thus reducing the potential for adverse effect.

- The reference point for the range in the dosages for children is data on the safety on inhaled corticosteroids in children, which, in general, suggest that the dose ranges are equivalent to beclomethasone dipropionate 200-400 mcg/day (low dose), 400-800 mcg/day (medium dose), and >800 mcg/day (high dose).

- Some dosages may be outside package labeling.

- Metered-dose inhaler (MDI) dosages are expressed as the actuator dose (the amount of drug leaving the actuator and delivered to the patient), which is the labeling required in the United States. This is different from the dosage expressed as the valve dose (the amount of drug leaving the valve, all of which is not available to the patient), which is used in many European countries and in some of the scientific literature. Dry powder inhaler (DPI) doses (eg, Turbuhaler) are expressed as the amount of drug in the inhaler following activation.

ESTIMATED CLINICAL COMPARABILITY OF DOSES FOR INHALED CORTICOSTEROIDS

Data from *in vitro* and in clinical trials suggest that the different inhaled corticosteroid preparations are not equivalent on a per puff or microgram basis. However, it is not entirely clear what implications these differences have for dosing recommendations in clinical practice because there are few data directly comparing the preparations. Relative dosing for clinical comparability is affected by differences in topical potency, clinical effects at different doses, delivery device, and bioavailability. The Expert Panel developed recommended dose ranges for different preparations based on available data and the following assumptions and cautions about estimating relative doses needed to achieve comparable clinical effect.

- **Relative topical potency using human skin blanching**

  - Standard test for determining relative topical anti-inflammatory potency is the topical vasoconstriction (MacKenzie skin blanching) test.

  - The MacKenzie topical skin blanching test correlates with binding affinities and binding half-lives for human lung corticosteroid receptors (see following table) (Dahlberg, et al, 1984; Hogger and Rohdewald 1994).

  - The relationship between relative topical anti-inflammatory effect and clinical comparability in asthma management is not certain. However, recent clinical trials suggest that different *in vitro* measures of anti-inflammatory effect is not certain. However, recent clinical trials suggest that different in vitro measures of anti-inflammatory effect correlate with clinical efficacy (Barnes and Pedersen 1993; Johnson 1996; Kamada, et al, 1996; Ebden, et al, 1986; Leblanc, et al, 1994; Gustaffson, et al, 1993; Lundback, et al, 1993; Barnes, et al, 1993; Fabbri, et al, 1993; Langdon and Capsey, 1994; Ayres, et al, 1995; Rafferty, et al, 1985; Bjorkander, et al, 1982, Stiksa, et al, 1982; Willey, et al, 1982.)

ASTHMA *(Continued)*

Medication	Topical Potency (Skin Blanching)*	Corticosteroid Receptor Binding Half-Life	Receptor Binding Affinity
Beclomethasone dipropionate (BDP)	600	7.5 hours	13.5
Budesonide (BUD)	980	5.1 hours	9.4
Flunisolide (FLU)	330	3.5 hours	1.8
Fluticasone propionate (FP)	1200	10.5 hours	18.0
Triamcinolone acetonide (TAA)	330	3.9 hours	3.6

*Numbers are assigned in reference to dexamethasone, which has a value of "1" in the MacKenzie test.

- **Relative doses to achieve similar clinical effects**
  - Clinical effects are evaluated by a number of outcome parameters (eg, changes in spirometry, peak flow rates, symptom scores, quick-relief beta$_2$-agonist use, frequency of exacerbations, airway responsiveness).
  - The daily dose and duration of treatment may affect these outcome parameters differently (eg, symptoms and peak flow may improve at lower doses and over a shorter treatment time than bronchial reactivity) (van Essen-Zandvliet, et al, 1992; Haahtela, et al, 1991)
  - Delivery systems influence comparability. For example, the delivery device for budesonide (Turbuhaler) delivers approximately twice the amount of drug to the airway as the MDI, thus enhancing the clinical effect (Thorsson, et al, 1994); Agertoft and Pedersen, 1993).
  - Individual patients may respond differently to different preparations, as noted by clinical experience.
  - Clinical trials comparing effects in reducing symptoms and improving peak expiratory flow demonstrate:
  - BDP amd BUD achieved comparable effects at similar microgram doses by MDI (Bjorkander, et al, 1982; Ebden, et al, 1986; Rafferty, et al, 1985).
  - BDP achieved effects similar to twice the dose of TAA on a microgram basis.

Reference
National Asthma Education and Prevention Program, February 1997

NORMAL RESPIRATORY RATES

Hour After Birth	Average Respiratory Rate	Range
1st hour	60 breaths/minute	20-100
2-6 hours	50 breaths/minute	20-80
>6 hours	30-40 breaths/minute	20-60

Age (years)	Mean RR (breaths/minute)
0-2	25-30
3-9	20-25
10-18	16-20

BLOOD LEVEL SAMPLING TIME GUIDELINES

Drug	Infusion Time	Therapeutic Range	When to Draw Levels
Amikacin sulfate			
I.V.	30 min	Peak: 20-30 µg/mL	Peak: 30 min after end of 30 min infusion
		Trough: <10 µg/mL	Trough: Within 30 min before next dose
I.M.			Peak: 1 h after I.M. injection
			Trough: Within 30 min before next dose
Carbamazepine		4-12 µg/mL	Just before next dose
Chloramphenicol			
I.V.	30 min	Peak: 15-25 µg/mL	Peak: 90 min after end of 30 min infusion
			Trough: Just before next dose
P.O.			Peak: 2 h post-P.O. dose
Cyclosporine			
I.V./P.O.		BMT 100-200 ng/mL	Just before next dose
		Liver transplant 200-300 ng/mL	
		Renal transplant 100-200 ng/mL	
Digoxin			
I.V./P.O.		Age and disease related: 0.8-2 ng/mL	6 h postdose to just before next dose
Ethosuximide			
P.O.		40-100 µg/mL	Just before next dose
Flucytosine			
P.O.		25-100 µg/mL	Peak: 2 h postdose after at least 4 d of therapy
Fosphenytoin (measure phenytoin levels)			
I.V.		Phenytoin: 10-20 µg/mL	Peak: 2 h after end of an infusion
I.M.			Peak: 4 h after I.M. injection
Gentamicin			
I.V.	30 min	Peak: 4-10 µg/mL	Peak: 30 min after end of 30 min infusion
		Trough: 0.5-2 µg/mL	Trough: Within 30 min before next dose
I.M.			Peak: 1 h after I.M. injection
			Trough: Within 30 min before next dose
Phenobarbital		15-40 µg/mL	Trough: Just before next dose
Phenytoin			
P.O., I.V.		10-20 µg/mL	Trough: Just before next dose
I.V.			Post-load/Peak: 1 h after end of infusion
Theophylline			
I.V. bolus	30 min	10-20 µg/mL	Peak: 30 min after end of 30 min infusion
Continuous infusion			16-24 h after the start or change in a constant I.V. infusion
P.O. liquid, fast-release tablet (Somophyllin®, Slo-Phyllin® liquid & tablet)			Peak: 1 h postdose Trough: Just before next dose

Drug	Infusion Time	Therapeutic Range	When to Draw Levels
P.O. slow-release (Theo-Dur®, Slo-Phyllin® GC, Slo-bid®)			Peak: 4 h postdose Trough: Just before next dose
Tobramycin			
I.V.	30 min	Peak: 4-10 µg/mL	Peak: 30 min after end of 30 min infusion
		Trough: 0.5-2 µg/mL	Trough: Within 30 min before next dose
I.M.			Peak: 1 h post-I.M. injection
			Trough: Within 30 min before next dose
Trimethoprim			
I.V., dose 20 mg/kg	60 min	Peak: 5-10 µg/mL	Peak: 30 min after end of 60 min infusion
I.V., dose 8-10 mg/kg		Peak 1-3 µg/mL	
P.O.			Peak: 1 h postdose
Valproic acid			
P.O.		50-100 µg/mL	Trough: Just before next dose
Vancomycin	60 min	Peak: 25-40 µg/mL	Peak: 20-30 min after end of 60 min infusion*
		Trough: 5-15 µg/mL	Trough: Within 30 min before next dose

*Some institutions may draw vancomycin peak 1 hour after 1-hour infusion and accept the lower range of therapeutic.

OVERDOSE AND TOXICOLOGY*

Drug or Drug Class	Signs/Symptoms	Treatment/Comments
Acetaminophen	Nausea, vomiting, diaphoresis, delirium, fever, coma, vascular collapse, hepatic necrosis, transient azotemia, renal tubular necrosis	Assess severity of ingestion; doses ≥150 mg/kg for children and 7.5 g for adults are thought to be toxic. Obtain serum concentration ≥4 hours postingestion and use acetaminophen nomogram to evaluate need for acetylcysteine. Empty stomach with ipecac (if <1 hour postingestion) or gastric lavage. May administer activated charcoal for one dose, this may decrease absorption of acetylcysteine if given within 1 hour of acetylcysteine. For unknown ingested quantities and for significant ingestion, give acetylcysteine orally (diluted 1:4 with juice or carbonated beverage); initial: 140 mg/kg then give 70 mg/kg every 4 hours for 17 doses.
Alpha-adrenergic blocking agents	Hypotension, drowsiness	Induce emesis, give activated charcoal, additional treatment is symptomatic; use I.V. fluids, dopamine, or ephedrine to treat hypotension. Epinephrine may worsen hypotension due to beta effects.
Aminoglycosides	Ototoxicity, nephrotoxicity, neuromuscular toxicity	Hemodialysis or peritoneal dialysis may be useful in patients with decreased renal function.
Anticholinergics, antihistamines	Coma, hallucinations, delirium, tachycardia, dry skin, urinary retention, dilated pupils	For life-threatening arrhythmias or seizures physostigmine may be used. See Physostigmine monograph *on page 9999* for dosage recommendation.
Anticholinesterase agents	Nausea, vomiting, diarrhea, miosis, CNS depression, excessive salivation, excessive sweating, muscle weakness	Suction oral secretions, decontaminate skin, atropinize patient; atropine dose must be individualized. Infants and children: Initial dose: 0.01-0.02 mg/kg/dose; may need to increase as high as 0.05 mg/kg. Adults: Initial atropine dose: 1 mg; may need to increase to 2-5 mg/dose; pralidoxime (2-PAM) may need to be added for severe intoxications.
Barbiturates	Respiratory depression, circulatory collapse, bradycardia, hypotension, hypothermia, slurred speech, confusion	Repeated oral doses of activated charcoal given every 3-6 hours will increase clearance: Children: 1-2 g/kg/dose; adults: 30-60 g. Assure GI motility, adequate hydration, and renal function. Urinary alkalinization with I.V. sodium bicarbonate will increase renal elimination of longer-acting barbiturates (eg, phenobarbital).
Benzodiazepines	Respiratory depression, apnea, hypoactive reflexes, hypotension, slurred speech, unsteady gait, coma	For comatose patient, use gastric lavage with endotracheal tube in place to prevent aspiration; flumazenil, a benzodiazepine antagonist, can be used to reverse the effects of benzodiazepines. See Flumazenil monograph *on page 9999* for dose. Action of flumazenil may be shorter than duration of benzodiazepine; repeat doses as needed. Norepinephrine, phenylephrine, or dopamine may be used to treat hypotension; dialysis is of limited value; support blood pressure and respiration.

Drug or Drug Class	Signs/Symptoms	Treatment/Comments
Beta-adrenergic blockers	Hypotension, bronchospasm, bradycardia, hyperglycemia, or hypoglycemia	Induce emesis, followed by activated charcoal; treat symptomatically; glucagon, atropine, isoproterenol, or cardiac pacing may be needed to treat bradycardia, conduction defects, or hypotension
Carbamazepine	Dizziness, drowsiness, ataxia, involuntary movements, opisthotonos, seizures, nausea, vomiting, agitation, nystagmus, coma, urinary retention, respiratory depression, tachycardia	Use supportive therapy, general poisoning management as needed; use repeated oral doses of activated charcoal given every 3-6 hours to decrease serum concentrations; children 1-2 g/kg/dose, adults: 30-60 g/dose; charcoal hemoperfusion may be needed; treat hypotension with I.V. fluids, dopamine, or norepinephrine; monitor EKG; diazepam may control convulsions but may exacerbate respiratory depression
Cardiac glycosides	Hyperkalemia may develop rapidly and result in life-threatening cardiac arrhythmias, progressive bradyarrhythmias, 2nd or 3rd degree heart block unresponsive to atropine, ventricular fibrillation, asystole	Obtain serum drug level, induce emesis or perform gastric lavage; give activated charcoal to reduce further absorption; atropine may reverse heart block, phenytoin will improve A-V conduction; digoxin immune Fab (digoxin specific antibody fragments) is used in life-threatening cases, each 38 mg of digoxin immune Fab binds with 0.5 mg of digoxin or digitoxin; see Digoxin Immune Fab monograph *on page 9999* for dosing recommendations
Heparin	Severe hemorrhage	1 mg of protamine sulfate will neutralize approximately 90 units of heparin sodium (bovine) or 115 units of heparin sodium (porcine) or 100 units of heparin calcium (porcine)
Hydantoin derivatives	Nausea, vomiting, nystagmus, slurred speech, ataxia, coma	Gastric lavage or emesis; repeated oral doses of activated charcoal may increase clearance of phenytoin. Children: 1-2 g/kg/dose, adults: 30-60 g/dose activated charcoal every 3-6 hours until nontoxic serum concentration is obtained; assure adequate GI motility, supportive therapy; dialysis may be helpful.
Iron	Lethargy, nausea, vomiting, green or tarry stools, hypotension, weak rapid pulse, metabolic acidosis, shock, coma, hepatic necrosis, renal failure, local GI erosions	Induce emesis if awake or lavage with saline solution; give deferoxamine mesylate I.V. at 15 mg/kg/hour in cases of severe poisoning (serum Fe >350 mcg/mL) and continue chelation therapy for 24 hours after child is excreting normal color urine; urine output should be maintained at >2 mL/kg/hour to avoid hypovolemic shock
Isoniazid	Nausea, vomiting, blurred vision, CNS depression, intractable seizures, coma, metabolic acidosis	Control seizures with diazepam; if suspected ingestion of >80 mg/kg, give pyridoxine I.V. equal dose to the suspected overdose of isoniazid; lavage after seizure control is reached; force diuresis with I.V. fluids; hemo- or peritoneal dialysis may be beneficial in severe cases
Nonsteroidal anti-inflammatory drugs	Dizziness, abdominal pain, sweating, apnea, nystagmus, cyanosis, hypotension, coma	Induce emesis; give activated charcoal via NG tube; provide symptomatic and supportive care.

OVERDOSE AND TOXICOLOGY* *(Continued)*

Drug or Drug Class	Signs/Symptoms	Treatment/Comments
Opiates and morphine analogs	Respiratory depression, miosis, hypothermia, bradycardia, circulatory collapse, pulmonary edema, apnea	Establish airway and adequate ventilation; give naloxone 0.1 mg/kg for children up to 5 years of age or 20 kg; for those >5 years or 20 kg give 2 mg naloxone; repeat doses every 2-3 minutes if needed; additional doses may be needed every 20-60 minutes. May need to institute continuous infusion, as duration of action of opiates can be longer than duration of action of naloxone.
Phenothiazines	Deep, unarousable sleep, anticholinergic symptoms, extrapyramidal signs, diaphoresis, rigidity, tachycardia, cardiac dysrhythmias, hypotension, or hypertension	Emesis or gastric lavage; do **not** dialyze; use I.V. benztropine mesylate 0.02-0.05 mg/kg/dose or for adults 1-2 mg/dose slowly over 3-6 minutes for extrapyramidal signs; use loading dose of phenytoin 10-15 mg/kg slow I.V. push for ventricular dysrhythmias; use I.V. fluids and norepinephrine or phenylephrine to treat hypotension; avoid epinephrine which may cause hypotension due to phenothiazine-induced alpha-adrenergic blockade and unopposed epinephrine B_2 action; dantrolene orally 0.5 mg/kg/dose every 12 hours may help with the rigidity
Salicylates	Nausea, vomiting, respiratory alkalosis, hyperthermia, dehydration, hyperapnea, tinnitus, headache, dizziness, metabolic acidosis, coma	Induce emesis or gastric lavage immediately; give charcoal with cathartic via NG tube; correct fluid imbalance by giving D_5LR at 10-20 mL/kg/hour for 1-2 hours, more rapid fluid resuscitation may be needed for patients in shock; use sodium bicarbonate to correct metabolic acidosis and enhance renal elimination by alkalinizing the urine; give supplemental potassium after renal function has been determined to be adequate. Monitor electrolytes; obtain serum salicylate level ≥6 hours postingestion; use poisoning nomogram to assess the significance of the ingestion and the need for more aggressive measures.
Tricyclic antidepressants	Agitation, confusion, hallucinations, urinary retention, hypothermia, hypotension, tachycardia, arrhythmias, widened QRS complex, prolonged PR intervals	Maintain normal temperature; correct acidosis with sodium bicarbonate to increase protein binding and decrease free fraction; correction of acidosis may decrease cardiovascular toxicities; avoid disopyramide, procainamide, and quinidine; lidocaine, phenytoin or propranolol may be necessary; reserve physostigmine for refractory life-treating anticholinergic toxicities. For life-threatening arrhythmias or seizures: Children: I.V., slow: Physostigmine 0.01-0.03 mg/kg/dose up to 0.5 mg/dose over 2-3 minutes, repeat in 5 minutes (maximum total dose is 2 mg). Adolescents and adults: 2 mg/dose physostigmine, may repeat 1-2 mg in 20 minutes and give 1-4 mg slow I.V. over 5-10 minutes if signs and symptoms recur.
Warfarin	Internal or external hemorrhage, hematuria	For moderate overdoses, give oral or I.V. phytonadione; for severe hemorrhage, give fresh frozen plasma or whole blood

Drug or Drug Class	Signs/Symptoms	Treatment/Comments
Xanthine derivatives	Vomiting, abdominal pain, bloody diarrhea, tachycardia, extrasystoles, tachypnea, tonic/clonic seizures	Induce emesis, except in a convulsive patient; give activated charcoal orally; repeated oral doses of activated charcoal may increase clearance; children: 1-2 g/kg/dose, adults: 30-60 g/dose of activated charcoal every 3-6 hours until nontoxic serum concentrations are obtained. Assure adequate GI motility, supportive therapy; charcoal hemoperfusion can also be effective in decreasing serum concentrations.

*As for all overdoses and toxic ingestions, provide airway, breathing, and cardiac support; use appropriate general poisoning management and give general supportive therapy when needed (eg, I.V. fluids, blood pressure support, control seizures, etc). Consult more specific toxicology references (eg, Leikin JB and Paloucek FP, *Poisoning & Toxicology Handbook*, Hudson, OH: Lexi-Comp Inc, 1998, and Poisondex®) for further information.

COMMONLY USED ANTIDOTES FOR ACUTE OVERDOSES

While certain drugs may modify symptoms produced by a toxin, only a relatively few toxins have specific antidotes. The purpose of this chart is to identify those drugs, non-medicinal chemicals, plants, snakes, and spiders to which specific antidotes exist. Please refer to the specific monograph for dosing information. This information does not preclude the use of "conventional" therapeutic modalities for the treatment of intoxication (eg, emesis, lavage, charcoal, etc).

Poisoning Agent	Antidote(s)	Indications	Comments
Chemicals, Nonmedicinal			
Arsenic	Dimercaprol (BAL in Oil®)	• Symptomatic arsenic exposure	• Monitor for hypertension, tachycardia, hyperpyrexia, and urticaria • Pretreatment with diphenhydramine may diminish side effects
Calcium oxide	Edetate calcium disodium (EDTA) (Calcium Disodium Versenate®)	• Eye exposure from calcium oxide	• Immediate irrigation with saline followed by an irrigation with 0.01-0.05 M EDTA solution for at least 15 minutes
Carbon monoxide	Oxygen	• Any suspected carbon monoxide intoxication • Hyperbaric oxygen for any patient with signs and symptoms of severe intoxication regardless of the carboxyhemoglobin concentration • Patients with ischemic heart disease, acute ECG changes, anemia, seizure history, or pregnancy should receive hyperbaric oxygen if the carboxy hemoglobin (COHB) >20% or if any acute symptoms are present	
Carbamate insecticides	Atropine	• Symptomatic bradycardia • Myoclonic seizures, severe hallucinations, weakness, arrhythmias, excessive salivation, involuntary urination and defecation	• Caution should be used in patients with narrow-angle glaucoma, cardiovascular disease, or pregnancy • Plasma and/or erythrocyte cholinesterase levels will be depressed from normal
Copper	Penicillamine (Cuprimine®, Depen®)	• Symptomatic copper intoxication	• Little experience with chelation therapy in the setting of acute ingestion
Cyanide	Amyl nitrite, sodium nitrite, sodium thiosulfate (cyanide antidote kit)	• Begin treatment at the first sign of toxicity if exposure is known or strongly expected	• Do not use methylene blue to reduce elevated methemoglobin levels • Oxygen therapy may be useful when combined with sodium thiosulfate therapy

Poisoning Agent	Antidote(s)	Indications	Comments
Ethylene glycol	Ethanol **OR** Fomepizole (Antizol®)	• Ingestion of >0.25 mL/ kg ethylene glycol • Ethylene glycol serum level >20 mg/dL • History or strong clinical suspicion of ingestion and at least two of the following criteria: Arterial pH <7.3 Serum bicarbonate <20 mEq/L Osmolality gap >10 mosm/L Urinary oxalate crystals present	• Goal: Blood ethanol concentration at least 100 mg/dL (22 mmol/L) • Indications for use of fomepizole over ethanol: Ingestion of multiple substances resulting in depressed level of consciousness, altered consciousness, lack of adequate intensive care staffing or laboratory support to monitor ethanol, critically-ill patient with anion gap metabolic acidosis of unknown origin and potential exposure to ethylene glycol, or patients with active hepatic disease • Continue therapy until ethylene glycol level <10 mg/dL • Monitor blood glucose especially in children as ethanol may cause hypoglycemia
Hydrazine	Pyridoxine (Vitamin B₆)	• Antidote for seizures and coma	
Hydrofluoric acid (HF)	Calcium gluconate	• Dermal burns (topical treatment with calcium gluconate gel for dermal exposures of HF <20% concentration) •S.C. injections of calcium gluconate for dermal exposures of HF >20% concentration or failure to respond to calcium gluconate gel	• Oral calcium also used as fluoride-binding agent following oral ingestion • Hypocalcemia occurs frequently following oral ingestion and dermal exposure • Topical calcium gels are not available commercially in U.S.; may be compounded; see Extemporaneous Preparations, Calcium Supplements *on page 9999* •Injections of calcium gluconate should not be used in digital area
Hydrogen sulfide	Amyl nitrite **AND** Sodium nitrite	• Severe anoxia, if therapy can be started early – within one hour of exposure	• Do **NOT** use sodium thiosulfate
Lead	Edetate calcium disodium (EDTA) (Calcium Disodium Versenate®) **with or without** Dimercaprol (BAL in Oil®)	Use both calcium EDTA and BAL: • Symptoms of lead encephalopathy and/or blood lead level >70 mcg/dL • Symptomatic without encephalopathy or asymptomatic with blood lead level >70 µg/dL Use only EDTA for: • Asymptomatic with blood lead level 45-69 µg/dL	• Do not confuse or interchange therapy of **calcium** disodium edetate with disodium edetate (Chealamide®, Disotate®, Endrate®) – tetany and possibly fatal hypocalcemia may occur • Calcium EDTA should only be administered after adequate urine flow is established • If urine flow is not established, hemodialysis must accompany calcium EDTA dosing
	Succimer (Chemet®)	• Lead level >45 µg/dL in patients without encephalopathy or protracted vomiting	• Do not use with calcium disodium edetate or BAL

COMMONLY USED ANTIDOTES FOR ACUTE OVERDOSES
(Continued)

Poisoning Agent	Antidote(s)	Indications	Comments
Manganese	Edetate calcium disodium (EDTA) (Calcium Disodium Versenate®)		• Do not confuse or interchange therapy of **calcium** disodium edetate with disodium edetate (Chealamide®, Disotate®, Endrate®) – tetany and possibly fatal hypocalcemia may occur • Calcium EDTA should only be administered after adequate urine flow is established
Methanol	Ethanol **OR** Fomepizole (Antizol®)	• Anion gap metabolic acidosis associated with a history of methanol ingestion • Methanol blood level >20 mg/dL (6.2 mmoles/L) • Any symptomatic patient with a history of methanol ingestion	• Goal: Ethanol blood level 100-130 mg/dL (22-28 mmoles/L) • Continue therapy until methanol blood level <10 mg/dL • Fomepizole therapy is considered investigational
Organophosphate insecticides	Atropine Pralidoxime (2-PAM, Protopam®)	• Symptomatic bradycardia • Myoclonic seizures, severe hallucinations, weakness, arrhythmias, excessive salivation, involuntary urination and defecation	• Caution should be used in patients with narrow-angle glaucoma, cardiovascular disease, or pregnancy •Most effective when used in initial 24-36 hours after exposure • Plasma and/or erythrocyte cholinesterase levels will be depressed from normal
Drug / Drug Class			
Acetaminophen	Acetylcysteine (Mucomyst®)	• Serum acetaminophen level >150 μg/mL at 4 hours postingestion (see Acetaminophen *on page 9999*) • Acute ingestion with dose ≥150 mg/kg (child) or 7.5 g (adolescent/adult) within 24 hours of presentation if results of plasma levels cannot be obtained within 8-10 hours of ingestion • Unknown quantity ingested and <24 hours have elapsed since the time of ingestion or unable to obtain serum acetaminophen levels within 12 hours of ingestion • Consider repeating an acetaminophen level 4-6 hours after an initial 4-hour level that is under the treatment range if extended release acetaminophen was ingested • Patients presenting >24 hours postacute ingestion who have measurable levels or biochemical evidence of hepatic injury	• Activated charcoal has been shown to adsorb acetylcysteine; therefore, administer activated charcoal before 4-hour acetaminophen level is drawn • If patient vomits within 1 hour of acetylcysteine dose, readminister the dose • I.V. N-acetylcysteine is available in the U.S. by investigational use only; contact a poison control center for further information

Poisoning Agent	Antidote(s)	Indications	Comments
Anticholinergics	Physostigmine (Antilirium®)	• Refractory seizures or arrhythmias unresponsive to conventional therapy • Symptoms should be life-threatening	• Due to potential for producing severe adverse effects, (eg, seizures, bradycardia) routine use of physostigmine is controversial • Atropine should be available to reverse life-threatening cholinergic effects of physostigmine
Baclofen	Physostigmine (Antilirium®)	• Distinguish anticholinergic delirium from other causes of altered mental status	• Long-lasting reversal of anticholinergic signs and symptoms is generally not achieved due to the relatively short duration of action of physostigmine • Atropine should be available to reverse life-threatening cholinergic effects of physostigmine
Benzodiazepines	Flumazenil (Romazicon®)	• Reverses sedative effects of benzodiazepines	• May precipitate benzodiazepine withdrawal in dependent patients • Not indicated for ethanol, barbiturate, general anesthetic, or narcotic overdose • Mixed drug overdose patients who have ingested drugs that increase the likelihood of seizures (eg, cocaine, lithium, cyclic antidepressants) are at extremely high risk for seizures when flumazenil is used • Action of flumazenil may be shorter than duration of benzodiazepines; repeat doses of flumazenil may be needed • Contraindicated in patients given benzodiazepines for potentially life-threatening conditions (eg, increased intracranial pressure, seizures) and patients with signs of serious cyclic-antidepressant overdosage
Beta-blockers	Isoproterenol (Isuprel®)	• Reversal of bradycardia and hypotension	
	Glucagon	• Reversal of bradycardia unresponsive to isoproterenol	• Glucagon activates adenyl cyclase system at a different site than isoproterenol • Requires liver glycogen stores for hyperglycemic response • I.V. glucose must also be given in treatment of hypoglycemia
Calcium channel blockers	Calcium chloride **OR** Calcium gluconate	• Reversal of cardiovascular effects of calcium channel blockers (calcium antagonists)	• Monitor serum calcium levels • Calcium is most effective in mild to moderate intoxications • May not be effective in correcting symptomatic bradyarrhythmias

COMMONLY USED ANTIDOTES FOR ACUTE OVERDOSES
(Continued)

Poisoning Agent	Antidote(s)	Indications	Comments
Digitalis glycosides	Digoxin immune Fab (Digibind®)	• Treatment of potentially life-threatening digoxin or digitoxin intoxication in carefully selected patients [serum digoxin level >10 ng/mL or ingestion of >4 mg (child) or >10 mg (adult)] • Life-threatening ventricular arrhythmias secondary to digoxin or digitoxin • Hyperkalemia (K⁺ >5 mEq/L) in the setting of digitalis toxicity • Life-threatening cardiac arrhythmias, progressive bradyarrhythmias, second or third degree heart block unresponsive to atropine	• Monitor potassium levels and continuous EKG • Digibind® interferes with the interpretation of serum digoxin/digitoxin levels
Heparin, Enoxaparin, Dalteparin	Protamine	• Severe hemorrhage	• Effect can be immediate and last for 2 hours • Protamine dosage related to anticoagulant dosage and time of anticoagulant administration • Monitor PTT • Monitor for hypotension
Insulin	Dextrose (25%-50%)	• Severe, symptomatic hypoglycemia	• Very hypertonic solutions; dilute with sterile water prior to I.V. administration
Iron	Deferoxamine (Desferal®)	• Serum iron level >350 μg/mL • Inability to obtain serum iron level within a reasonable time and patient is symptomatic	• Passing of vin rose colored urine indicates free iron was present • Discontinue therapy when urine returns to normal color • Monitor for hypotension during treatment
Isoniazid	Pyridoxine (Vitamin B₆)	• Ingestion of >80 mg/kg isoniazid	
Neuromuscular blocking agents, nondepolarizing (eg, pancuronium)	Edrophonium **OR** Neostigmine **OR** Pyridostigmine	• Reversal of neuromuscular blockade	• Atropine should be available to treat acute cholinergic crisis • Not effective for reversal of **depolarizing** neuromuscular blocking agents (eg, succinylcholine)

Poisoning Agent	Antidote(s)	Indications	Comments
Opiates	Naloxone (Narcan®)	• Reversal of symptoms associated with severe toxicity	• May precipitate withdrawal symptoms in patients with physical dependence to opiates • For prolonged intoxication, a continuous infusion may be used
Phenothiazines	Diphenhydramine (Benadryl®) **OR** Benztropine (Cogentin®)	• Reversal of phenothiazine-induced dystonic reactions	
	Sodium bicarbonate	• Reversal of "quinidine-like" cardiovascular effects (eg, prolonged QRS complex) – QRS duration >100 msec – Ventricular dysrhythmias and hypotension	• Goal is arterial pH of 7.45-7.55 and urine pH of 7.5-8 • Attempts at urine alkalinization may be dangerous in patients with renal dysfunction or where sodium and fluid overload may compromise respiratory or cardiac status
Tricyclic antidepressants	Sodium bicarbonate	• Reversal of "quinidine-like" cardiovascular effects (eg, prolonged QRS complex) – QRS duration >100 msec – Ventricular dysrhythmias and hypotension	• Goal is arterial pH of 7.45-7.55 and urine pH of 7.5-8 • Attempts at urine alkalinization may be dangerous in patients with renal dysfunction or where sodium and fluid overload may compromise respiratory or cardiac status
Warfarin	Phytonadione (Vitamin K_1)	• Large, acute ingestion • Prothrombin time greater than normal	• Vitamin K is relatively contraindicated in patients with prosthetic heart valves unless toxicity is life-threatening
Zinc	Edetate calcium disodium (EDTA) **and/or** Dimercaprol (BAL in Oil®)	• Symptomatic zinc ingestion	• Few case reports • Monitor zinc levels
Plants			
Foxglove Oleander	Digoxin immune Fab (Digibind®)	• Severely intoxicated patients who fail to respond to conventional therapy • Life-threatening ventricular arrhythmias, progressive bradyarrhythmias, or second- or third degree heart block not responsive to atropine • Hyperkalemia (K^+ >5 mEq/L) in the setting of digitalis toxicity	• Monitor potassium levels and continuous EKG
Mushroom (genus *Gyomitra*)	Pyridoxine (Vitamin B_6)		
Mushrooms containing muscarine (inocybe or clitocybe)	Atropine	•Myoclonic seizures, severe hallucinations, weakness, arrhythmias, excessive salivation, involuntary urination and defecation	•Atropine should only be used when indicated; otherwise use may result in anticholinergic poisoning

COMMONLY USED ANTIDOTES FOR ACUTE OVERDOSES
(Continued)

Poisoning Agent	Antidote(s)	Indications	Comments
Snake Bites			
Coral snakes (Eastern and Texas coral snakes only)	Antivenin *(Micrurus fulvius)*		• Not effective for Arizona or Sonoran coral snakes • Skin testing is recommended • Treatment for hypersensitivity reactions, including anaphylaxis, should be available
Pit vipers (Rattlesnakes, cottonmouths, copperheads)	Antivenin *(Crotalidae)* Polyvalent (equine origin)	• Administration within 4 hours of envenomation is ideal; however, administer within 30 hours in all severe cases of poisoning	• Skin testing is recommended • Treatment for hypersensitivity reactions, including anaphylaxis, should be available
Spiders, Scorpions			
Black widow spider	Antivenin *(Lactrodectus mactans)*	• Severe symptoms including respiratory failure, seizures, or pain and spasms not relieved by calcium, muscle relaxants, or analgesics • Symptomatic pregnant patients • Children <5 years or adults >60 years (at greatest risk for severe toxicity)	• Either dermal or conjunctival sensitivity testing should be done prior to administration of antivenin
Scorpion	Antivenin *(Centruroides)*		• No FDA-approved *Centruroides* antivenin in U.S.; only a *Centruroides exilicauda (sculpturatus)*-specific antivenin is available in Arizona (for intrastate use only)

Leikin JR and Paloucek FP, "Poisoning & Toxicology Compendium," Hudson, OH: Lexi-Comp, Inc, 1998.

Mowry JB, Furbee RB, and Chyka PA, "Poisoning," *Essentials of Critical Care Pharmacology,* 3rd ed, Baltimore, MD: Williams & Wilkens, 1994, 501-29.

Zed PJ and Krenzelok EP, "Treatment of Acetaminophen Overdose,"*Am J Health Syst Pharm,* 1999, 56(11):1081-91.

ANION GAP

Definition: The difference in concentration between unmeasured cation and anion equivalents in serum.

Anion gap = $Na^+ - Cl^- - HCO_3^-$
(The normal anion gap is 10-14 mEq/L.)

Differential diagnosis of increased anion gap

Organic anions
Lactate (sepsis, hypovolemia, large tumor burden)
Pyruvate
Uremia
Ketoacidosis (β-hydroxybutyrate and acetoacetate)
Amino acids and their metabolites
Other organic acids (eg, formate from methanol, glycolate from
ethylene glycol)

Inorganic anions
Hyperphosphatemia
Sulfates
Nitrates

Medications and toxins
Penicillins and cephalosporins
Salicylates (including aspirin)
Cyanide
Carbon monoxide

Differential diagnosis of decreased anion gap
Organic cations
Hypergammaglobulinemia

Inorganic cations
Hyperkalemia
Hypercalcemia
Hypermagnesemia

Medications and toxins
Lithium

Hypoalbuminemia

LABORATORY DETECTION OF DRUGS IN URINE

Agent	Time Detectable in Urine*
Alcohol	12-24 h
Amobarbital	2-4 d
Amphetamine	2-4 d
Butalbital	2-4 d
Cannabinoids	
Occasional use	2-7 d
Regular use	30 d
Cocaine (benzoylecgonine)	12-72 h
Codeine	2-4 d
Chlordiazepoxide	30 d
Diazepam	30 d
Ethanol	12-24 h
Heroin (morphine)	2-4 d
Hydromorphone	2-4 d
Marijuana	
Occasional use	2-7 d
Regular use	30 d
Methamphetamine	2-4 d
Methaqualone	2-4 d
Morphine	2-4 d
Pentobarbital	2-4 d
Phencyclidine (PCP)	
Occasional use	2-7 d
Regular use	30 d
Phenobarbital	30 d
Secobarbital	2-4 d

*The periods of detection for the various abused drugs listed above should be taken as estimates since the actual figures will vary due to metabolism, user, laboratory, and excretion.

Adapted from Chang JY, "Drug Testing and Interpretation of Results," *Pharmchem Newsletter*, 1989, 17:1.

OSMOLALITY

Definition: The summed concentrations of all osmotically active solute particles.

Predicted serum osmolality =

2 Na$^+$ (mEq/L) + glucose (mg/dL) / 18 + BUN (mg/dL) / 2.8

The normal range of serum osmolality is 285-295 mOsm/L.

Differential diagnosis of increased serum osmolal gap
(increased by >10 mOsm/L)

Medications and toxins
Alcohols (ethanol, methanol, isopropanol, glycerol, ethylene glycol)
Mannitol
Paraldehyde

SALICYLATE INTOXICATION

**Serum Salicylate Level and
Severity of Intoxication Single Dose
Acute Ingestion Nomogram**

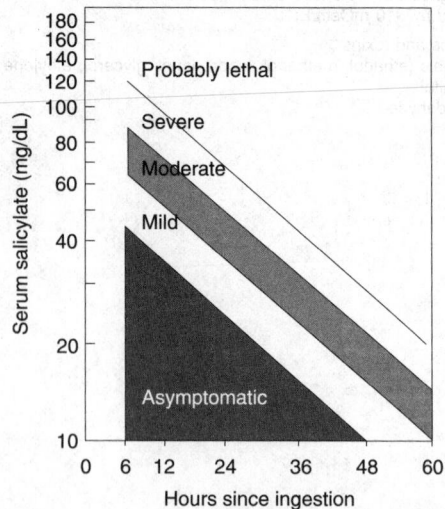

Nomogram relating serum salicylate concentration and expected severity of intoxication at varying intervals following the ingestion of a single dose of salicylate.
From Done AK, "Aspirin Overdosage: Incidence, Diagnosis, and Management," *Pediatrics*, 1978, 62:890-7 with permission.

ACETAMINOPHEN

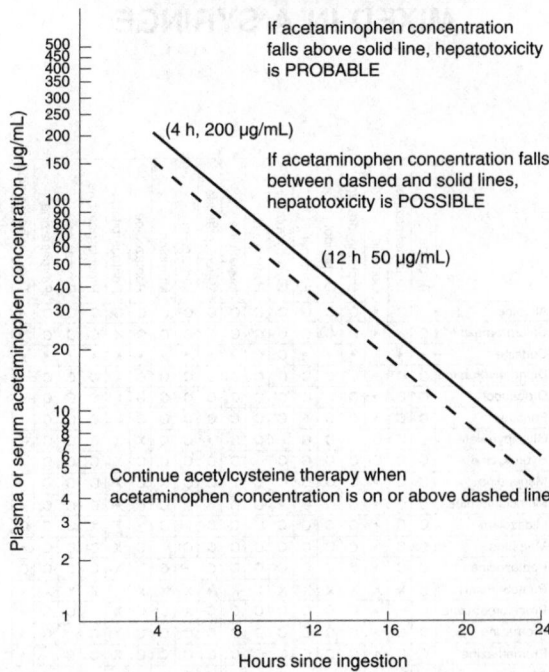

If acetaminophen concentration falls above solid line, hepatotoxicity is PROBABLE

(4 h, 200 µg/mL)

If acetaminophen concentration falls between dashed and solid lines, hepatotoxicity is POSSIBLE

(12 h 50 µg/mL)

Continue acetylcysteine therapy when acetaminophen concentration is on or above dashed line

Plasma or serum acetaminophen concentration (µg/mL)

Hours since ingestion

Nomogram relating plasma or serum acetaminophen concentration and probability of hepatotoxicity at varying intervals following ingestion of a single toxic dose of acetaminophen. Modified from Rumack BH, Matthew H, "Acetaminophen Poisoning and Toxicity", Pediatrics, 1975, 55:871-6,
© American Academy of Pediatrics, 1975, and from Rumack BH, et al, "Acetaminophen Overdose", Arch Intern Med, 1981, 141:380-5,
© American Medical Association.

COMPATIBILITY OF MEDICATIONS MIXED IN A SYRINGE

	Atropine	Chlorpromazine	Codeine	Diphenhydramine	Droperidol	Fentanyl	Glycopyrrolate	Hydroxyzine	Meperidine	Metoclopramide	Midazolam	Morphine	Pentazocine	Pentobarbital†	Prochlorperazine	Promazine	Promethazine	Trimethobenzamide
Atropine		C	•	C	C	C	C	C	C	C	C	C	C	C	C	C	C	•
Chlorpromazine	C		•	C	C	C	C	C	C	C	C	C	C	X	C	C	C	•
Codeine	•	•		•	•	•	C	C	•	•	•	•	•	X	•	•	•	•
Diphenhydramine	C	C	•		C	C	C	C	C	C	C	C	C	X	C	C	C	•
Droperidol	C	C	•	C		C	C	C	C	C	C	C	C	X	C	C	C	•
Fentanyl	C	C	•	C	C		C	C	C	C	C	C	C	C	C	C	C	•
Glycopyrrolate	C	C	C	C	C	C		C	C	•	C	X	X	C	C	C	C	C
Hydroxyzine	C	C	C	C	C	C	C		C	C	C	C	C	X	C	C	C	•
Meperidine	C	C	•	C	C	C	C	C		C	C	X	C	X	C	C	C	•
Metoclopramide	C	C	•	C	C	C	•	C	C		C	C	C	•	C	C	C	•
Midazolam	C	C	•	C	C	C	C	C	C	C		C	•	X	X	C	C	C
Morphine	C	C	•	C	C	C	X	C	X	C	C		C	X	C*	C	C	•
Pentazocine	C	C	•	C	C	C	X	C	C	C	•	C		X	C	C	C	C
Pentobarbital†	C	X	X	X	X	X	X	X	X	•	X	X	X		X	X	X	•
Prochlorperazine	C	C	•	C	C	C	C	C	C	C	X	C*	C	X		C	C	•
Promazine	C	C	•	C	C	C	C	C	C	C	C	C	C	X	C		C	•
Promethazine	C	C	•	C	C	C	C	C	C	C	C	C	C	X	C	C		•
Trimethobenzamide	•	•	•	•	•	•	C	•	•	•	C	•	C	•	•	•	•	

C = Physically compatible if used within 15 minutes after mixing in a syringe
X = Incompatible
• = No documented information
C* = Potential incompatibility produced by certain manufacturers
† = Compatibility profile is characteristic of most barbiturate salts, such as phenobarbital and secobarbital

The following combinations have been found to be compatible:
  atropine / meperidine / promethazine
  atropine / meperidine / hydroxyzine
  meperidine / promethazine / chlorpromazine

The following drugs should _not_ be mixed with any other drugs in the same syringe:
  diazepam, chlordiazepoxide

References
Forman JK and Sourney PF, "Visual Compatibility of Midazolam Hydrochloride With Common Preoperative Injectable Medications," Am J Hosp Pharm, 1987, 44(10):2298-9.
King JC, "Guide to Parenteral Admixtures," St Louis, MO: Cutter Laboratories, 1986.
Parker WA, Hosp Pharm, 1984, 19:475-8.
Trissel LA, "Handbook on Injectable Drugs," 5th ed, Bethesda, MD: American Society of Health-System Pharmacists, Inc, 1988.
Stevenson JG and Patriarca C, "Incompatibility of Morphine Sulfate and Prochlorperazine Edisylate in Syringes," Am J Hosp Pharm, 1985, 42:2651.

CONTROLLED SUBSTANCES

Note: These are federal classifications. Your individual state may place a substance into a more restricted category. When this occurs, the more restricted category applies. Consult your state law.

Schedule I = C-I

The drugs and other substances in this schedule have no legal medical uses except research. They have a **high** potential for abuse. They include opiates, opium derivatives, and hallucinogens.

Schedule II = C-II

The drugs and other substances in this schedule have legal medical uses and a **high** abuse potential which may lead to severe dependence. They include former "Class A" narcotics, amphetamines, barbiturates, and other drugs.

Schedule III = C-III

The drugs and other substances in this schedule have legal medical uses and a **lesser** degree of abuse potential which may lead to **moderate** dependence. They include former "Class B" narcotics and other drugs.

Schedule IV = C-IV

The drugs and other substances in this schedule have legal medical uses and **low** abuse potential which may lead to **moderate** dependence. They include barbiturates, benzodiazepines, propoxyphenes and other drugs.

Schedule V = C-V

The drugs and other substances in this schedule have legal medical uses and **low** abuse potential which may lead to **moderate** dependence. They include narcotic cough preparations, diarrhea, preparations, and other drugs.

FEVER DUE TO DRUGS

Aminosalicylic acid
Antihistamines
Asparaginase
Barbiturates
Bleomycin
Cephalosporins
Iodides
Methyldopa
Penicillins
Phenolphthalein
Phenytoin
Procainamide
Quinidine
Sulfonamides
Thiouracil

Abstracted from Harrison's *Principles of Internal Medicine*, 12th ed, Wilson JD, ed, New York, NY: McGraw-Hill Book Co, 1991 and Tabor PA, "Drug-Induced Fever," *Drug Intell Clin Pharm*, 1986, 20:413-20.

DISCOLORATION OF FECES
DUE TO DRUGS

Black
Acetazolamide
Alcohols
Alkalies
Aminophylline
Amphetamine
Amphotericin
Antacids
Anticoagulants
Aspirin
Betamethasone
Charcoal
Chloramphenicol
Chlorpropamide
Clindamycin
Corticosteroids
Cortisone
Cyclophosphamide
Cytarabine
Dicumarol
Digitalis
Ethacrynic acid
Ferrous salts
Floxuridine
Fluorouracil
Halothane
Heparin
Hydralazine
Hydrocortisone
Ibuprofen
Indomethacin
Iodine drugs
Iron salts
Levarterenol
Levodopa
Manganese
Melphalan
Methylprednisolone
Methotrexate
Methylene blue
Oxyphenbutazone

Paraldehyde
Phenacetin
Phenolphthalein
Phenylbutazone
Phenylephrine
Phosphorous
Potassium salts
Prednisolone
Procarbazine
Pyrvinium
Reserpine
Salicylates
Sulfonamides
Tetracycline
Theophylline
Thiotepa
Triamcinolone
Warfarin

Blue
Chloramphenicol
Methylene blue

Dark Brown
Dexamethasone

Gray
Colchicine

Green
Indomethacin
Iron
Medroxyprogesterone

Greenish Gray
Oral antibiotics
Oxyphenbutazone
Phenylbutazone

Light Brown
Anticoagulants

Orange-Red
Phenazopyridine
Rifampin

Pink
Anticoagulants
Aspirin
Heparin
Oxyphenbutazone
Phenylbutazone
Salicylates

Red
Anticoagulants
Aspirin
Heparin
Oxyphenbutazone
Phenolphthalein
Phenylbutazone
Pyrvinium
Salicylates
Tetracycline syrup

Red-Brown
Oxyphenbutazone
Phenylbutazone
Rifampin

Tarry
Ergot preparations
Ibuprofen
Salicylates
Warfarin

White/Speckling
Aluminum hydroxide
Antibiotics (oral)
Indocyanine green

Yellow
Senna

Yellow-Green
Senna

Adapted from Drugdex® — Drug Consults, Micromedex, vol 62, Rocky Mountain Drug
Consultation Center, Denver, CO: January, 1995.

DISCOLORATION OF URINE DUE TO DRUGS

Black
Cascara
Ferrous salts
Iron dextran
Levodopa
Methocarbamol
Methyldopa
Naphthalene
Phenacetin
Phenols
Quinine
Sulfonamides

Blue
Anthraquinone
Indigo blue
Indigo carmine
Methocarbamol
Methylene blue
Nitrofurans
Resorcinol
Triamterene

Blue-Green
Amitriptyline
Anthraquinone
DeWitt's pills
Doan's® pills
Indigo blue
Indigo carmine
Methylene blue

Brown
Anthraquinone dyes
Cascara
Levodopa
Methocarbamol
Methyldopa
Metronidazole
Nitrofurans
Nitrofurantoin
Phenacetin
Primaquine
Quinine
Rifampin
Senna
Sodium diatrizoate
Sulfonamides

Brown-Black
Quinine

Dark
Aminosalicylic acid
Cascara
Levodopa
Metronidazole
Nitrites
Phenacetin
Phenol
Primaquine
Quinine

Resorcinol
Riboflavin
Senna

Green
Anthraquinone
DeWitt's pills
Indigo blue
Indigo carmine
Indomethacin
Methocarbamol
Methylene blue
Nitrofurans
Phenols
Resorcinol
Suprofen

Green-Yellow
DeWitt's pills
Methylene blue

Milky
Phosphates

Orange
Chlorzoxazone
Dihydroergotamine mesylate
Heparin sodium
Phenazopyridine
Phenindione
Rifampin
Sulfasalazine
Warfarin

Orange-Red
Chlorzoxazone
Doxidan
Phenazopyridine
Rifampin

Orange-Yellow
Fluorescein sodium
Rifampin
Sulfasalazine

Pink
Aminopyrine
Anthraquinone dyes
Danthron
Deferoxamine
Merbromin
Phenolphthalein
Phenothiazines
Phenytoin
Salicylates

Red
Anthraquinone
Cascara
Daunorubicin
Dimethyl sulfoxide
DMSO
Doxorubicin

Heparin
Ibuprofen
Methyldopa
Oxyphenbutazone
Phenacetin
Phenazopyridine
Phenolphthalein
Phenothiazines
Phensuximide
Phenylbutazone
Phenytoin
Rifampin
Senna

Red-Brown
Cascara
Methyldopa
Oxyphenbutazone
Phenacetin
Phenolphthalein
Phenothiazines
Phenylbutazone
Phenytoin
Quinine

Red-Purple
Chlorzoxazone
Ibuprofen
Phenacetin
Senna

Rust
Cascara
Chloroquine
Metronidazole
Nitrofurantoin
Phenacetin
Riboflavin
Senna
Sulfonamides

Yellow
Nitrofurantoin
Phenacetin
Riboflavin
Sulfasalazine

Yellow-Brown
Cascara
Chloroquine
DeWitt's pills
Methylene blue
Metronidazole
Nitrofurantoin
Primaquine
Quinacrine
Senna
Sulfonamides

Yellow-Pink
Cascara
Senna

Adapted from Drugdex® — Drug Consults, Micromedex, vol 62, Rocky Mountain Drug Consultation Center, Denver, CO: January, 1995.

DRUGS AND BREAST-FEEDING

The following question and options should be considered when prescribing drug therapy to lactating women. 1) Is the drug therapy really necessary? Consultation between the pediatrician and the mother's physician can be most useful. 2) Use the safest drug, for example, acetaminophen rather than aspirin, for analgesia. 3) If there is a possibility that a drug may present a risk to the infant, consideration should be given to measurement of blood concentrations in the nursing infant. 4) Drug exposure to the nursing infant may be minimized by having the mother take the medication just after she has breast-fed the infant and/or just before the infant is due to have a lengthy sleep period.

In tables 1-6, the fact that a pharmacologic or chemical agent does not appear on the lists is not meant to imply that it is not transferred into human milk or that it does not have an effect on the infant; it only indicates that there were no reports found in the literature.

Table 1. Drugs That Are Contraindicated During Breast-Feeding

Bromocriptine	Ergotamine
Cocaine	Lithium
Cyclophosphamide	Methotrexate
Cyclosporine	Phencyclidine (PCP)
Doxorubicin*	Phenindione

*Drug is concentrated in human milk.

Table 2. Drugs of Abuse: Contraindicated During Breast-Feeding*

Amphetamine†	Marijuana
Cocaine	Nicotine (smoking)
Heroin	Phencyclidine

*The Committee on Drugs strongly believes that nursing mothers should not ingest any compounds listed in Table 2. Not only are they hazardous to the nursing infant, but they are also detrimental to the physical and emotional health of the mother. This list is obviously not complete; no drug of abuse should be ingested by nursing mothers even though adverse reports are not in the literature.

†Drug is concentrated in human milk.

Table 3. Radioactive Compounds That Require Temporary Cessation of Breast-Feeding*

Drug	Recommended Time for Cessation of Breast-Feeding
Copper-64 (^{64}Cu)	Radioactivity in milk present at 50 h
Gallium-67 (^{67}Ga)	Radioactivity in milk present for 2 wk
Indium-111 (^{111}In)	Very small amount present at 20 h
Iodine-123 (^{123}I)	Radioactivity in milk present up to 36 h
Iodine-125 (^{125}I)	Radioactivity in milk present for 12 d
Iodine-131 (^{131}I)	Radioactivity in milk present 2-14 d, depending on study
Radioactive sodium	Radioactivity in milk present 96 h
Technetium-99m (^{99m}Tc), ^{99m}Rc macroaggregates, ^{99m}Tc O4	Radioactivity in milk present 15 h to 3 d

*Consult nuclear medicine physician before performing diagnostic study so that radionuclide that has shortest excretion time in breast milk can be used. Before study, the mother should pump her breast and store enough milk in freezer for feeding the infant; after study, the mother should pump her breast to maintain milk production but discard all milk pumped for the required time that radioactivity is present in milk. Milk samples can be screened by radiology departments for radioactivity before resumption of nursing.

DRUGS AND BREAST-FEEDING *(Continued)*

Table 4. Drugs Whose Effect on Nursing Infants Is Unknown But May Be of Concern

Psychotropic drugs, the compounds listed under antianxiety, antidepressant, and antipsychotic categories, are of special concern when given to nursing mothers for long periods. Although there are no case reports of adverse effects in breast-feeding infants, these drugs do appear in human milk and thus could conceivably alter short-term and long-term central nervous system function.

Antianxiety
Diazepam
Lorazepam
Midazolam
Perphenazine
Prazepam*
Quazepam
Temazepam

Antidepressant
Amitriptyline
Amoxapine
Desipramine
Dothiepin
Doxepin
Fluoxetine
Fluvoxamine
Imipramine
Trazodone

Antipsychotic
Chlorpromazine
Chlorprothixene
Haloperidol
Mesoridazine

Miscellaneous
Chloramphenicol
Metoclopramide*
Metronidazole
Tinidazole

*Drug is concentrated in human milk.

Table 5. Drugs That Have Been Associated With Significant Effects on Some Nursing Infants and Should Be Given to Nursing Mothers With Caution*

Aspirin (salicylates)
Clemastine
Mesalamine
Phenobarbital

Primidone
Sulfasalazine
(salicylazosulfapyridine)

*Measure blood concentration in the infant when possible.

Table 6. Maternal Medications Usually Compatible With Breast-Feeding

Acebutolol	Dexbrompheniramine maleate with d-isoephedrine*	Morphine
Acetaminophen		Moxalactam
Acetazolamide		Nadolol†
Acitretin	Digoxin	Nalidixic acid*
Acyclovir†	Diltiazem	Naproxen
Alcohol (ethanol)*#	Dipyrone	Nefopam
Allopurinol	Disopyramide	Nefedipine
Amoxicillin	Domperidone	Nifedipine
Antimony	Dyphylline†	Nitrofurantoin*
Atenolol	Enalapril	Norethynodrel
Atropine	Erythromycin†	Norsteroids
Azapropazone (apazone)	Estradiol*	Noscapine
B₁ (thiamine)	Ethambutol	Oxprenolol
B₆ (pyridoxine)	Ethanol (cf. alcohol)	Phenylbutazone
B₁₂ (vitamin)	Ethosuximide	Phenytoin*
Baclofen	Fentanyl	Piroxicam
Barbiturate*	Flecainide	Prednisone
Bendroflumethiazide#	Flufenamic acid	Procainamide
Bishydroxycoumarin (dicumarol)	Fluorescein	Progesterone
	Folic acid	Propoxyphene
Bromide*	Gold salts	Propranolol
Butorphanol	Halothane	Propylthiouracil
Caffeine*	Hydralazine	Pseudoephedrine†
Captopril	Hydrochlorothiazide	Pyridostigmine
Carbamazepine	Hydroxychloroquine†	Pyrimethamine
Carbimazole*	Ibuprofen	Quinidine
Cascara	Indomethacin*	Quinine
Cefadroxil	Iodides*	Riboflavin
Cefazolin	Iodine (povidone-iodine/ vaginal douche)*	Rifampin
Cefotaxime		Scopolamine
Cefoxitin	Iodine*	Secobarbital
Cefprozil	Iopanoic acid	Senna
Ceftazidime	Isoniazid	Sotalol
Ceftriaxone	K₁ (vitamin)	Spironolactone
Chloral hydrate*	Kanamycin	Streptomycin
Chloroform	Ketorolac	Sulbactam
Chloroquine	Labetalol	Sulfapyridine*
Chlorothiazide	Levonorgestrel	Sulfisoxazole*
Chlorthalidone*	Lidocaine	Suprofen
Cimetidine†	Loperamide	Terbutaline
Cisapride	Magnesium sulfate	Tetracycline
Cisplatin	Medroxyprogesterone	Theophylline*
Clindamycin	Mefenamic acid	Thiopental
Clogestone	Methadone	Thiouracil
Clomipramine	Methimazole (active metabolite of carbi- mazole)	Ticarcillin
Codeine		Timolol
Colchicine		Tolbutamide*
Contraceptive pill with estrogen/proges- terone#	Methocarbamol	Tolmetin
	Methyldopa	Trimethoprim/sulfameth- oxazole
	Methyprylon*	
Cycloserine	Metoprolol†	Triprolidine
D (vitamin)	Metrizamide	Valproic acid
Danthron*	Mexiletine	Verapamil
Dapsone	Minoxidil	Warfarin
		Zolpidem

*Effects in infants have been reported in the literature.
†Drug is concentrated in human milk.
#Reported effect on lactation.
From "American Academy of Pediatrics Committee on Drugs: The Transfer of Drugs and Other Chemicals Into Human Milk," *Pediatrics*, 1994, 93(1):137-50, with permission.

MILLIEQUIVALENT FOR SELECTED IONS

Approximate Milliequivalents — Weights of Selected Ions

Salt	mEq/g Salt	mg Salt/mEq
Calcium carbonate ($CaCO_3$)	20	50
Calcium chloride ($CaCl_2 \cdot 2H_2O$)	14	73
Calcium gluconate (Ca gluconate$_2 \cdot 1H_2O$)	4	224
Calcium lactate (Ca lactate$_2 \cdot 5H_2O$)	6	154
Magnesium sulfate ($MgSO_4$)	16	60
Magnesium sulfate ($MgSO_4 \cdot 7H_2O$)	8	123
Potassium acetate (K acetate)	10	98
Potassium chloride (KCl)	13	75
Potassium citrate (K_3 citrate$\cdot 1H_2O$)	9	108
Potassium iodide (KI)	6	166
Sodium bicarbonate ($NaHCO_3$)	12	84
Sodium chloride (NaCl)	17	58
Sodium citrate (Na_3 citrate$\cdot 2H_2O$)	10	98
Sodium iodide (NaI)	7	150
Sodium lactate (Na lactate)	9	112
Zinc sulfate ($ZnSO_4 \cdot 7H_2O$)	7	144

Valences and Approximate Weights of Selected Ions

Substance	Electrolyte	Valence	Ionic Wt
Calcium	Ca^{++}	2	40
Chloride	Cl^-	1	35.5
Magnesium	Mg^{++}	2	24
Phosphate	PO_4^{3-}	3	95*
	HPO_4^{2-}	2	96
	$H_2PO_4^-$	1	97
Potassium	K^+	1	39
Sodium	Na^+	1	23
Sulfate	SO_4^{2-}	2	96*

*The atomic weight of phosphorus is 31, and of sulfur is 32.

SEROTONIN SYNDROME

Diagnostic Criteria for Serotonin Syndrome

- Recent addition or dosage increase of any agent increasing serotonin activity or availability (usually within 1 day).

- Absence of abused substances, metabolic infectious etiology, or withdrawal.

- No recent addition or dosage increase of a neuroleptic agent prior to onset of signs and symptoms.

- Presence of three or more of the following:

  Altered mental status (seen in 40% of patients, primarily confusion or hypomania)
  Agitation
  Tremor (50% incidence)
  Shivering
  Diarrhea
  Hyperreflexia (pronounced in lower extremities)
  Myoclonus (50% incidence)
  Ataxia or incoordination
  Fever (50% incidence; temperature >105°F associated with grave prognosis)
  Diaphoresis

Drugs (as Single Causative Agent) Which Can Induce Serotonin Syndrome

Specific serotonin reuptake inhibitors (SSRI)
MDMA (Ecstasy)
Clomipramine

Drug Combinations Which Can Induce Serotonin Syndrome*

Alprazolam – Clomipramine
Bromocriptine – Levodopa/carbidopa
Buspirone – Trazodone
Citalopram – Moclobemide
Clomipramine – Clorgiline
Clomipramine – Lithium
Dihydroergotamine – Sertraline
Dihydroergotamine – Amitriptyline
Fentanyl – Sertraline
Fluoxetine – Carbamazepine
Fluoxetine – Lithium
Fluoxetine – Remoxipide
Fluoxetine – Tryptophan
Lithium – Fluvoxamine
Lithium – Paroxetine
Lysergic acid diethylamide (LSD) – Fluoxetine
Moclobemide – Citalopram
Moclobemide – Clomipramine
Moclobemide – Fluoxetine
Moclobemide – Pethidine
Monoamine oxidase inhibitor – Fluoxetine
Monoamine oxidase inhibitor – Fluvoxamine
Monoamine oxidase inhibitor – Meperidine
Monoamine oxidase inhibitor – Sertraline
Monoamine oxidase inhibitor – Tricyclic antidepressants
Monoamine oxidase inhibitor – Tryptophan
Monoamine oxidase inhibitor – Venlafaxine
Nefazodone – Paroxetine

SEROTONIN SYNDROME *(Continued)*

Nortriptyline – Trazodone
Paroxetine – Dextromethorphan
Paroxetine – Dihydroergotamine
Paroxetine – Trazodone
Phenelzine, Trazodone – Dextropropoxyphene
S-adenosylmethionine – Clomipramine
Sertraline – Amitriptyline
Sumatriptan – Sertraline
Tranylcypromine – Clomipramine
Tramadol – Sertraline
Trazodone– Lithium – Amitriptyline
Trazodone – Fluoxetine
Valproic acid – Nefazodone
Venlafaxine – Tranylcypromine
Venlafaxine – Selegiline

*When administered within 2 weeks of each other.

TREATMENT OF SEROTONIN SYNDROME

Therapy is primarily supportive with intravenous crystalloid solutions utilized for hypotension and cooling blankets for mild hyperthermia. Norepinephrine is the preferred vasopressor. Chlorpromazine or dantrolene sodium may have a role in controlling fevers, although there is no proven benefit. Benzodiazepines are the first-line treatment in controlling rigors and thus, limiting fever and rhabdomyolysis, while clonazepam may be specifically useful in treating myoclonus. Endotracheal intubation and paralysis may be required to treat refractory muscular contractions. Tachycardia or tremor can be treated with beta-blocking agents; although due to its blockade of 5-HTIA receptors, the syndrome may worsen. Serotonin blockers such as diphenhydramine, cyproheptadine, or chlorpromazine have been used with variable efficacy. Methysergide and nitroglycerin (with lorazepam) also have been utilized with variable efficacy in case reports. It appears that cyproheptadine is most consistently beneficial.

Recovery seen within 1 day in 70% of cases; mortality rate is about 11%.

References

Gitlin MJ, "Venlafaxine, Monoamine Oxidase Inhibitors, and the Serotonin Syndrome," *J Clin Psychopharmacol*, 1997, 17:66-7.

Heisler MA, Guidery JR, and Arnecke B, "Serotonin Syndrome Induced by Administration of Venlafaxine and Phenelzine," *Ann Pharmacother*, 1996, 30:84.

Hodgman MJ, Martin TG, and Krenzelok EP, "Serotonin Syndrome Due to Venlafaxine and Maintenance Tranylcypromine Therapy," *Hum Exp Toxicol*, 1997, 16:14-7.

John L, Perreault MM, Tao T, et al, "Serotonin Syndrome Associated With Nefazodone and Paroxetine," *Ann Emerg Med*, 1997, 29:287-9.

LoCurto MJ, "The Serotonin Syndrome," *Emerg Clin North Am*, 1997, 15(3):665-75.

Martin TG, "Serotonin Syndrome," *Ann Emerg Med*, 1996, 28:520-6.

Mills K, "Serotonin Toxicity: A Comprehensive Review for Emergency Medicine," *Top Emerg Med*, 1993, 15:54-73.

Mills KC, "Serotonin Syndrome: A Clinical Update," *Crit Care Clin*, 1997, 13(4):763-83.

Nisijima K, Shimizu M, Abe T, et al, "A Case of Serotonin Syndrome Induced by Concomitant Treatment With Low-Dose Trazodone, and Amitriptyline and Lithium," *Int Clin Psychopharmacol*, 1996, 11:289-90.

Sobanski T, Bagli M, Laux G, et al, "Serotonin Syndrome After Lithium Add-On Medication to Paroxetine," *Pharmacopsychiatry*, 1997, 30:106-7.

Sporer, "The Serotonin Syndrome: Implicated Drugs, Pathophysiology and Management," *Drug Safety*, 1995, 13(2):94-104.

Sternbach H, "The Serotonin Syndrome," *Am J Psychiatry*, 1991, 146:705-7.

Van Berkum MM, Thiel J, Leikin JB, et al, "A Fatality Due to Serotonin Syndrome," *Medical Update for Psychiatrists*, 1997, 2:55-7.

SODIUM CONTENT OF SELECTED MEDICINALS

Name and Dosage Unit*	Sodium	
	mg	mEq
Antibiotics		
Amikacin sulfate, 1 g	29.9	1.3
Aminosalicylate sodium, 1 g	109	4.7
Ampicillin, suspension, 250 mg/5 mL, 5 mL	10	0.4
Ampicillin sodium, 1 g	66.7	3
Azlocillin sodium, 1 g	50	2.2
Carbenicillin disodium, 382 mg (tablet)	22	1
Cefazolin sodium, 1 g	47	2
Cefotaxime sodium, 1 g	30.5	2.2
Cefoxitin sodium, 1 g	53	2.3
Ceftriaxone sodium, 1 g	83	3.6
Cefuroxime, 1 g	54.2	2.4
Chloramphenicol sodium succinate, 1 g	51.8	2.3
Dicloxacillin, 250 mg (capsule)	13	0.6
Dicloxacillin, suspension 65 mg/5 mL	27	1.2
Erythromycin ethyl succinate, suspension 200 mg/5 mL	29	1.3
Erythromycin Base Filmtab®, 250 mg	70	3
Methicillin sodium, 1 g	66.7	2.9
Metronidazole, 500 mg I.V.	322	14
Mezlocillin sodium, 1 g	42.6	1.9
Moxalactam sodium, 1 g	88	3.8
Nafcillin sodium, 1 g	66.7	2.9
Nitrofurantoin, suspension, 25 mg/5 mL	7	0.3
Penicillin G potassium, 1,000,000 units I.V.	7.6	0.3
Penicillin G sodium, 1,000,000 units I.V.	46	2
Penicillin V potassium, suspension, 250 mg/5 mL	38	1.7
Piperacillin sodium, 1 g	42.6	1.8
Ticarcillin disodium, 1 g	119.6	5.2
Antacids, Liquid (content per 5 mL)		
Amphojel®	<2.3	<0.1
ALternaGEL®	2	0.1
Basaljel®	2.4	0.1
Extra Strength Maalox®-Plus	0.65	≅0.05
Gaviscon®	13	0.57
Maalox®	1.3	0.06
Tums E-X™	<4.8	<0.2
Sodium Content of Miscellaneous Medicinals		
Acetazolamide sodium, 500 mg	47.2	2.05
Chlorothiazide sodium, 500 mg	57.5	2
Cisplatin, 10 mg	35.4	1.54
Edetate calcium disodium, 1 g	122	5.3
Fleet® Enema, 4.5 oz	5000†	218
Fleet® Phospho®-Soda, 20 mL	2217	96.4
Hydrocortisone sodium succinate, 1 g	47.5	2.07
Hypaque® M 75%, injection, 20 mL	200	8.7

SODIUM CONTENT OF SELECTED MEDICINALS
(Continued)

Name and Dosage Unit*	Sodium	
	mg	mEq
Hypaque® M 90%, injection, 20 mL	220	9.6
Metamucil® Instant Mix (orange)	6	0.27
Methotrexate sodium, 100 mg vial	20	0.86
Methotrexate sodium, 100 mg vial (low sodium)	15	0.65
Naproxen sodium, 250 mg (tablet)	23	1
Neutra-Phos®, capsule and 75 mL reconstituted solution	164	7.13
Oragrafin® (capsule)	19	0.8
Pentobarbital sodium, 50 mg/mL, 1 mL vial	5	0.2
Phenobarbital sodium, 65 mg, 1 mL vial	6	0.3
Phenytoin sodium, 1 g	88	3.8
Promethazine expectorant, 5 mL	53	2.3
Shohl's solution modified, 1 mL	23	1
Sodium ascorbate, 500 mg acid equivalent	65.3	2.84
Sodium bicarbonate, 50 mL 8.4%	1150	50
Sodium nitroprusside, 50 mg	7.8	0.34
Sodium polystyrene sulfonate, 1 g	94.3‡	4.1
Thiopental sodium, 1 g	86.8	3.8
Valproate sodium, 250 mg/5 mL, 5 mL	23	1

*Product formulations and hence sodium content are subject to change by the manufacturer.

†Average systemic absorption 250-300 mg.

‡Total sodium content. Only about 33% is liberated in clinical use.

SUGAR-FREE LIQUID
PHARMACEUTICALS

The following sugar-free liquid preparations are listed by therapeutic category and alphabetically within each category. Please note that product formulations are subject to change by the manufacturer. Some of these products may contain sorbitol, xylitol, or other sweeteners which may be partially metabolized to provide calories.

Analgesics
Acetaminophen Elixir (various)
APAP/APAP Plus
Aspirin/Buffered Aspirin (Medique®)
Bufferin® A/F Nite Time
Children's Anacin-3® Infants Drops
Children's Myapap® Elixir
Children's Panadol® Drops, Liquid, and Chewable Tablets
Children's Tylenol® Chewable Tablets
Conex® Liquid
Cone® With Codeine Liquid
Dolanex® Elixir
Extra Strength Tylenol® PM
Febrol® and Febrol® EX
Methadone Hydrochloride Intensol
MS-Ai®
Myapap® Drops
No Drowsiness Tylenol®
Pain-Off®
Paregoric USP (Abbott)
Sep-A-Soothe® II
St Joseph® Aspirin-Free Liquid and Drops
Tempra® Chewable Tablets
Tylenol® Drops

Antacids/Antiflatulents
Alcalak®
Aldroxicon®
Almag® Suspension
Aludrox® Suspension
Aluminum Hydroxide Suspension
Calglycine® Tablets
Camalox® Suspension
Citrocarbonate® Granules
Creamalin® Suspension
Delcid®
Di-Gel® Liquid (mint, lemon & orange flavored)
Digestamic®
Dimacid®
Gaviscon® Liquid
Gelusil® II
Gelusil® Liquid
Gelusil® Liquid Flavor Pack
Gelusil-M® Liquid
Kolantyl® Gel
Maalox® Plus Suspension
Maalox® Suspension
Maalox® Therapeutic Concentrate
Magnatril® Suspension
Magnesia and Alumina Oral Suspension USP (Abbott, Phillips Roxane)
Mallamint® Chewable Tablets
Marblen® Suspension and Tablets
Medi-Seltzer®/Plus
Milk of Bismuth
Milk of Magnesia USP
Mylanta® Liquid

SUGAR-FREE LIQUID PHARMACEUTICALS *(Continued)*

Mylanta®-II Liquid
Mylicon® Drops
Nephrox® Suspension
Nutrajel®
Nutramag®
Pepto-Bismol® Liquid and Tablets
Phosphaljel® Suspension
Riopan Plus®
Riopan® Suspension
Silain-Gel® Liquid
Trisogel®
Titralac® Liquid
Titralac® Plus Liquid
WinGel® Liquid and Tablets

Antiasthmatics

Aerolate® Liquid
Alupent® Syrup
Choledyl® Pediatric Syrup
Droxine®
Elixophyllin® Elixir
Elixophyllin®-GG Liquid
Lanophyllin® Elixir
Lixolin® Liquid
Lufyllin® Elixir
Metaprel® Syrup
Mucomyst®-10
Mucomyst®-20
Mudrane® GG Elixir
Neothylline® Elixir
Neothylline® G
Organidin® NR
Slo-Phyllin® 80 Syrup
Somophyllin® Oral Liquid
Somophyllin®-DF Oral Liquid
Tedral® Elixir and Suspension
Theolair™ 80 Syrup
Theolixir®
Theon® Syrup
Theo-Organidin® Elixir
Theophylline Elixir (Phillips Roxane)

Antidepressants

Sinequan® Oral Concentrate

Antidiarrheals

Corrective Mixture With Paregoric
Diasorb® Liquid and Tablets
Di-Gon® II
Diotame®
Donnagel®
Infantol® Pink
Kalicon® Suspension
Kaolin Mixture With Pectin NF (Abbott)
Kaolin-Pectin Suspension (Phillips Roxane)
Konsyl® Powder
Lomanate®
Lomotil® Liquid
Paregoric USP (various)
Parepectolin® (various)
Pepto-Bismol®
St Joseph® Antidiarrheal

Antiepileptics
Mysoline® Suspension
Paradione® Solution

Antihistamine-Decongestants
Actifed® With Codeine
Actifed® Syrup
Actidil® Syrup
Bromphen® Elixir
Dimetane® Decongestant Elixir
Dimetapp® Elixir
Hay-Febrol® Liquid
Isoclor® Liquid and Capsules
Naldecon® Pediatric Drops and Syrup
Naldecon® Syrup
Novahistine® Elixir
Phenergan® Fortis Syrup
Phenergan® Syrup
Rondec® DM Drops
Ryna® Liquid
S-T® Forte® Liquid
Tavist® Syrup
Trind® Liquid
Veltap® Elixir
Vistaril® Oral Suspension

Anti-infectives
Augmentin® Suspension
Furadantin® Oral Suspension
Furoxone® Suspension
Humatin®
Mandelamine® Suspension/Forte®
Minocin® Suspension
Mycifradin® Sulfate Oral Solution
NegGram® Suspension
Proklar® Suspension
Sulfamethoxazole and Trimethoprim Suspension (Biocraft, Beecham,
    Burroughs Wellcome)
Vibramycin® Syrup

Antiparkinsonism Agents
Artane® Elixir

Antispasmodics
Antrocol® Elixir
Spasmophen® Elixir

Corticosteroids
Decadron® Elixir
Dexamethasone Solution (Roxane)
Dexamethasone Intensol Solution
Pediapred® Oral Liquid

Cough Medicines
Anatuss® With Codeine Syrup
Anatuss® Syrup
Brown Mixture NF (Lannett)
CCP® Caffeine Free
CCP® Cough/Cold Tablets
Cerose-DM®
Chlorgest-HD®
Codegest® Expectorant
Codiclear® DH Syrup
Codimal® DM
Colrex® Compound Elixir
Colrex® Expectorant
Conar® Syrup

SUGAR-FREE LIQUID PHARMACEUTICALS *(Continued)*

Conar® Expectorant Syrup
Conex® Liquid
Conex® With Codeine Syrup
Contac Jr® Liquid
Day-Night Comtrex®
Decoral® Forte®
Dexafed® Cough Syrup
Dimetane®-DC Cough Syrup
Dimetane®-DX Cough Syrup
Entuss® Expectorant Liquid
Fedahist® Expectorant Syrup and Pediatric Drops
Guaificon®-DMS
Histafed® Pediatric Liquid
Hycomine® Syrup and Pediatric Syrup
Lanatuss® Expectorant
Medicon® D
Medi-Synal®
Naldecon-DX® Pediatric Drops and Syrup
Naldecon-DX® Adult Liquid
Non-Drowsy Comtrex®
Noratuss®-II Expectorant and Liquid
Organidin® NR
Potassium Iodide Solution (various)
Prunicodeine®
Queltuss® Tablets
Robitussin-CF® Liquid
Robitussin® Night Relief Liquid
Rondec®-DM Drops
Rondec®-DM Syrup
Ryna® Liquid
Ryna-C® Liquid
Ryna-CX® Liquid
Scot-Tussin® DM Syrup
Scot-Tussin® Expectorant
Scot-Tussin® DM Cough Chasers
Silexin® Cough Syrup
Sorbutuss®
S-T® Expectorant, SF/D-F
S-T® Forte®, Sugar-Free
Sudodrin®/Sudodrin® Forte®
Terpin® Hydrate With Codeine Elixir (various)
Toclonol® Expectorant
Toclonol® Expectorant With Codeine
Tolu-Sed® Cough Syrup
Tolu-Sed® DM
Tricodene® Liquid
Trind-DM® Liquid
Tuss-Ornade®
Tussar® SF
Tuss-Organidin® DM NR
Tussirex® Sugar-Free

Dental Preparations and Fluoride Preparations
Cepacol® Mouthwash
Cepastat® Mouthwash and Gargle
Chloraseptic® Mouthwash and Gargle
Fluorigard® Mouthrinse
Fluorinse®
Flura-Drops®
Flura-Loz®
Flura® Tablets
Gel-Kam®
Karigel®
Karigel® N

Luride® Drops
Luride® SF Lozi-Tabs
Luride® 0.25 and 0.5 Lozi-Tabs
Luride® Lozi-Tabs
Pediaflor® Drops
Phos-Flur® Rinse/Supplement
Point-Two® Mouthrinse
Prevident® Disclosing Drops
Thera-Flur® Gel and Drops

Diagnostic Agents
Gastrografin®

Dietary Substitutes
Co-Salt®

Iron Preparations/Blood Modifiers
Amicar® Syrup
Beminal® Stress Plus With Iron
Chel-Iron® Drops
Chel-Iron® Liquid
Geritol® Complete Tablets
Geritonic™ Liquid
Hemo-Vite® Liquid
Iberet® Liquid
Iberet®-500 Liquid
Incremin® With Iron Syrup
Kovitonic® Liquid
Niferex®
Nu-Iron® Elixir
Vita-Plus H® Half Strength, Sugar-Free
Vita-Plus H®, Sugar-Free

Laxatives
Agoral® (plain, marshmallow, and raspberry)
Aromatic Cascara Fluidextract USP
Castor Oil
Castor Oil (flavored)
Castor Oil USP
Colace®, Liquid
Cologel®
Disonate™ Liquid
Doxinate® Solution
Emulsoil®
Fiberall® Powder
Haley's MO®
Hydrocil® Instant Powder
Hypaque® Oral Powder
Kondremul®
Kondremul® With Cascara
Kondremul® With Phenolphthalein
Konsyl® Powder
Liqui-Doss®
Magnesium Citrate Solution NF
Metamucil® Instant Mix (lemon-lime or orange)
Metamucil® SF Powder
Milk of Magnesia
Milk of Magnesia/Cascara Suspension
Milk of Magnesia/Mineral Oil Emulsion (various)
Milkinol® Liquid
Mineral Oil (various)
Neoloid® Liquid
NuLYTELY®
Phospho-Soda®
Sodium Phosphate & Biphosphate Oral Solution USP (Phillips Roxane)
Zymenol® Emulsion

SUGAR-FREE LIQUID PHARMACEUTICALS *(Continued)*

Potassium Products
Cena-K® Solution
EM-K®-10% Liquid
K-G® Elixir
Kaochlor-Eff® Tablets for Solution
Kaochlor® S-F Solution
Kaon® Elixir (grape and lemon-lime flavor)
Kaon-Cl® 20% Liquid
Kay Ciel® Elixir
Kay Ciel® Powder
Kaylixir®
Klor-Con®/25 Powder
Klor-Con® EF Tablets
Klor-Con® Liquid 20%
Klor-Con® Powder
Klorvess® Effervescent Tablets
Klorvess® Granules
Kolyum® Liquid and Powder
Potachlor® 10% and 20% Liquid
Potasalan® Elixir
Potassine® Liquid
Potassium Chloride Oral Solution USP 5%, 10%, and 20% (various)
Potassium Gluconate Elixir NF
Rum-K® Solution
Tri-K® Liquid
Trikates® Solution

Sedatives-Tranquilizers-Antipsychotics
Butabarbital Sodium Elixir
Butisol Sodium® Elixir
Haldol® Concentrate
Loxitane® C Drops
Mellaril® Concentrate
Serentil® Concentrate
Thorazine® Concentrate

Vitamin Preparations-Nutritionals
Aquasol A® Drops
BioCal® Tablets
Bugs Bunny™ Chewable Tablets
Bugs Bunny™ Plus Iron Chewable Tablets
Bugs Bunny™ With Extra C Chewable Tablets
Bugs Bunny™ Plus Minerals Chewable Tablets
Calciferol™ Drops
Caltrate® 600 Tablets
Ce-Vi-Sol® Drops
Cod Liver Oil (various)
Decagen® Tablets
DHT™ Intensol Solution (Roxane)
Drisdol® in Propylene Glycol
Flintstones™ Complete Chewable Tablets
Flintstones™ With Extra C Chewable Tablets
Flintstones™ Plus Iron Chewable Tablets
Incremin® With Iron Liquid
Kandium® Drops Tablets
Lanoplex® Elixir
Lycolan® Elixir
Oyst-Cal® 500 Tablets
Pediaflor®
PMS® Relief
Poly-Vi-Flor® Drops
Poly-Vi-Flor®/Iron Drops
Poly-Vi-Sol® Drops
Poly-Vi-Sol®/Iron Drops

Posture® Tablets
Spiderman™ Children's Chewable Vitamin Tablets
Spiderman™ Children's Plus Iron Tablets
Theragran® Jr Children's Chewable Tablets
Tri-Vi-Flor® Drops
Tri-Vi-Sol® Drops
Tri-Vi-Sol®/Iron Drops
Vi-Daylin® ADC Drops
Vi-Daylin® ADC/Fluoride Drops
Vi-Daylin® ADC Plus Iron Drops
Vi-Daylin® Drops
Vi-Daylin®/Fluoride Drops
Vi-Daylin® Plus Iron Drops
Vitalize®

Miscellaneous

Altace™ Capsules
Bicitra® Solution
Cibalith-S® Syrup
Colestid® Granules
Dayto® Himbin® Liquid
Digoxin® Elixir (Roxane)
Duvoid®
Glandosane®
Lipomul®
Lithium Citrate Syrup
Nicorette® Chewing Gum
Polycitra®-K Solution
Polycitra®-LC Solution
Tagamet® Liquid

References

Hill EM, Flaitz CM, and Frost GR, "Sweetener Content of Common Pediatric Oral Liquid Medications," *Am J Hosp Pharm*, 1988, 45:135-42.

Kumar A, Rawlings RD, and Beaman DC, "The Mystery Ingredients: Sweeteners, Flavorings, Dyes, and Preservatives in Analgesic/Antipyretic, Antihistamine/Decongestant, Cough and Cold, Antidiarrheal, and Liquid Theophylline Preparations," *Pediatrics*, 1993, 91:927-33.

"Sugar Free Products," *Drug Topics Red Book*, 1992, 17-8.

CARBOHYDRATE AND ALCOHOL CONTENT OF LIQUID MEDICATIONS FOR USE IN PATIENTS RECEIVING KETOGENIC DIETS

Generic Name	Carbohydrate g/5 mL				Ethyl Alcohol g/5 mL
	Sucrose	Sorbitol	Glycerin	Total	
Acetaminophen					
Tylenol® children's drops	0	0	0.43	0.43	0
Tylenol® children's elixir	1.6	1	0.43	3.03	0
Tylenol® children's suspension	3.7*	1	0.43	5.13	0
Tylenol® maximum strength liquid	5.49*	1	0	6.49	0
Acetaminophen/codeine					
Tylenol® elixir with codeine	3	0	0	3.0	0.35
Acyclovir					
Zovirax® suspension	0	0.3	0	0.3	0
Albuterol					
Ventolin® syrup	0	0	0	0	0
Proventil® syrup	0	0	0	0	0
AlOH/MgOH					
Maalox® Extra Strength Plus	0	0.5	0	0.5	0
Maalox® suspension	0	0.225	0	0.225	0
AlOH/MgOH/simethicone					
Mylanta® cherry cream liquid	0	0.6	0	0.6	0
Mylanta® double strength liquid	0	0.8	0	0.8	0
Mylanta® liquid	0	0.8	0	0.8	0
Mylanta® mint cream liquid	0	0.6	0	0.6	0
AlOH					
Alternagel®	0	0.6	0	0.6	0
Gaviscon® liquid	5.55§	0.36	0.51	6.42	0
AlOH gel (Roxane)					
Conc aluminum hydroxide gel	0	0.52	0	0.52	0
Alprazolam					
Alprazolam Intensol®	0	0	0	0	0
Aminocaproic acid					
Amicar® syrup	0	0.7	0	0.7	0
Amoxicillin					
Amoxicillin 125 suspension (Biocraft)	2	0	0	2	0
Amoxicillin 250 suspension (Biocraft)	3	0	0	3	0
Trimox® suspension	3.3	0	0	3.3	0
Amoxicillin 125 suspension (Lederle)	2.08	0	0	2.08	0
Amoxicillin 250 suspension (Lederle)	1.923	0	0	1.923	
Amoxicillin/clavulanate					
Augmentin® 125 suspension	0	0	0	0	0
Augmentin® 250 suspension	0	0	0	0	0
Ampicillin					
Ampicillin 125 suspension (Lederle)	4.021	0	0	4.021	0
Ampicillin 250 suspension (Lederle)	4.024	0	0	4.024	0
Ampicillin 125 suspension (Biocraft)	2.6	0	0	2.6	0
Ampicillin 250 suspension (Biocraft)	2.6	0	0	2.6	0
Azithromycin					
Zithromax® 100 suspension	3.86	0	0	3.86	0
Zithromax® 200 suspension	3.87	0	0	3.87	0
Calcium carbonate (Roxane)					
CaCO₃ oral suspension	0	1.4	0	1.4	0
Calcium glubionate					
Neo-Calglucon®	0	0.45	0	0.45	0
Carbamazepine					
Tegretol® suspension	2	0.6	0	2.6	0

Generic Name	Carbohydrate g/5 mL				Ethyl Alcohol g/5 mL
	Sucrose	Sorbitol	Glycerin	Total	
Cefaclor					
Ceclor® suspension	3	0	0	3	0
Cefadroxil					
Duricef® 125 suspension	2.55	0	0	2.55	0
Duricef® 250 suspension	2.43	0	0	2.43	0
Cefpodoxime					
Vantin® 50 suspension	2.94	0	0	2.94	0
Vantin® 100 suspension	2.94	0	0	2.94	0
Cefprozil					
Cefzil® suspension	2.03	0	0	2.03	0
Cefuroxime					
Ceftin® 125 suspension	3.214	0	0	3.214	0
Cephalexin					
Cephalexin 125 suspension (Lederle)	1.4	0	0	1.4	0
Cephalexin 250 suspension (Lederle)	1.2	0	0	1.2	0
Cephalexin 125 suspension (Biocraft)	2.6	0	0	2.6	0
Keflex® oral suspension	3	0	0	3	0
Cephradine					
Velosef® suspension	3.3	0	0	3.3	0
Chloral hydrate					
Chloral hydrate syrup (Geneva)	0	0	0.2	0.2	0
Chloral hydrate syrup (UDL Labs)	2.5	1.4	0	3.9	0
Chlorothiazide					
Diuril® oral suspension	2	0	0	2.0	0.025
Chlorpromazine					
Thorazine® concentrate	4.22	0	0	4.22	0
Cimetidine					
Tagamet® liquid	0	2.8	0	2.8	0.5
Cisapride					
Propulsid® suspension	0	3.85	0	3.85	0
Clarithromycin					
Biaxin® 125 suspension	3	0	0	3	0
Biaxin® 250 suspension	2.28	0	0	2.28	0
Clemastine					
Tavist® syrup	0	2.5	0	2.5	0
Clindamycin					
Cleocin® pediatric oral solution	1.825	0	0	1.825	0
Cloxacillin (Biocraft)					
Cloxacillin 250 suspension	2.4	0	0	2.4	0
Cyclosporine					
Sandimmune® oral solution	0	0	0	0	0.6
Dexamethasone (Roxane)					
Dexamethasone oral solution	0	1.2	0.5	1.7	0
Dexamethasone Intensol®	0	0	0	0	1.5
Diazepam					
Diazepam Intensol®	0	0	0	0	0.95
Diazepam solution	0	1	0	1	0
Dicyclomine					
Bentyl® liquid	0	0	0	4	0
Digoxin					
Lanoxin® elixir	1.5	0	0	1.5	0.5
Digoxin elixir (Roxane)	0	1	1	2.0	0.5
Diphenhydramine					
Benadryl® elixir cherry	0	0	0.3	0.3	0
Benadryl® elixir diet	0	2.25	0.6	2.85	0
EES					
EES	3.5	0	0	3.5	0
EES/Sulfisoxazole					
EES/Sulfisoxazole (Lederle)	2	0	0	2	0
Pediazole®	1.95	0	0	1.95	0

CARBOHYDRATE AND ALCOHOL CONTENT OF LIQUID MEDICATIONS FOR USE IN PATIENTS RECEIVING KETOGENIC DIETS *(Continued)*

Generic Name	Carbohydrate g/5 mL				Ethyl Alcohol g/5 mL
	Sucrose	Sorbitol	Glycerin	Total	
Ethosuximide					
Zarontin® syrup	3	0	0.625	3.625	0
Famotidine					
Pepcid® oral suspension	1.186	0	0	1.186	0
Felbamate					
Felbatol® suspension	0	1.5	0	1.5	0
Ferrous gluconate				*	
Fergon®	2	0	0	2.0	0.436
Ferrous sulfate					
Fer-in-Sol® drops	1.9	1.55	0	3.45	0
Fer-in-Sol® syrup	3	0.325	0	3.325	0
Fer-Gen-Sol®	2	0	0	2.0	0.436
Fluconazole					
Diflucan® 50 suspension	2.88	0	0	2.88	0
Diflucan® 200 suspension	2.73	0	0	2.73	0
Fluoxetine					
Furazolidone					
Furoxone® oral solution	0	0	0.1893	0.1893	0
Furosemide					
Lasix® oral solution	1.75	0	0	1.75	0.25
Furosemide solution (10 mg/5 mL)	0	2.4	0	2.4	0
Furosemide solution (40 mg/5 mL)	0	2.4	0	2.4	0
Griseofulvin					
Grifulvin V® oral suspension	3.5	0	0	3.5	0
Haloperidol					
Haldol® concentrate	3.9¶	0	0	3.9	0
Haldoperidol Intensol®	0	0	0	0	0
Hydrochlorothiazide					
Hydrochlorothiazide solution	0	0	2	2	0
Hydrocortisone cypionate					
Cortef® oral suspension	0.4	0	0	0.4	0
Hydroxyzine					
Vistaril® suspension	0	5	0	5	0
Ibuprofen					
Pedia-Profen® suspension	0	1.55	0	1.55	0
Kaolin/pectin (Roxane)					
Kaolin Pectin suspension	0	0	0.1	0.1	0
Kaopectin					
Kaopectate® concentrated antidiarrheal regular	0.6	0	0	0.6	0
L-carnitine					
Carnitor® oral solution	0.2385	0	0	0.2385	0
Lactulose					
Cephulac® syrup	4.67¶	0	0	4.67	0
Chronulac® syrup	4.67¶	0	0	4.67	0
Lithium citrate					
Lithium citrate USP	0	2.7	0	2.7	0
Loperamide					
Imodium A-D®	3.7¶	0	0.43	4.13	0.26
Loperamide oral solution	0	0	3	3	0
Loracarbef					
Lorabid®	3	0	0	3	0
Lorazepam					
Lorazepam Intensol®	0	0	0	0	0
Metaproterenol (Biocraft)					
Metaproterenol syrup	0	1.7	0	1.7	0

Generic Name	Carbohydrate g/5 mL				Ethyl Alcohol g/5 mL
	Sucrose	Sorbitol	Glycerin	Total	
Metaproterenol sulfate					
Alupent® syrup	0	1.4	0	1.4	0
Metaprel® syrup	0	1.4	0	1.4	0
Metoclopramide					
Metoclopramide syrup (Biocraft)	0	2.1	0	2.1	0
Metoclopramide Intensol®	0	1.4	0.5	1.9	0
Metoclopramide oral solution (Roxane)	0	1.4	0.5	1.9	0
Milk of Magnesia					
Concentrated Milk of Magnesia	0.4	1	0.2	1.6	0
Multivitamins					
Iberet® 250 liquid	0	3.61	0	3.61	0
Iberet® 500 liquid	0.62	2.1	0	2.72	0
Theragran® liquid	1.75	0	0	1.75	0
Poly-Vi-Sol® drops	0	0	4.25	4.25	0
Vi-Daylin® liquid	0.778	0	0.025	6.053	0
Vi-Daylin® multivitamin drops	0	0	4.8	4.8	0
Multivitamins with fluoride drops					
Poly-Vi-Flor® drops	0	0	4.25	4.25	0
Multivitamins with fluoride drops					
Tri-Vi-Flor® drops	0	0	4.25	4.25	0
Multivitamins with iron					
Poly-Vi-Flor® With Iron drops	0	0	3.9	3.9	0
Multivitamins with iron					
Tri-Vi-Flor® With Iron drops	0	0	3.9	3.9	0
Multivitamins with minerals					
Advanced Formula Centrum® liquid	1.67	0	0	1.67	0.335
Multivitamins/fluoride					
Vi-Daylin®/f	0	0	4.8	4.8	0
Naproxen					
Naprosyn® oral suspension	1.275	0.45	0	1.725	0
Nitrofurantoin					
Furadantin® suspension	0	0.7	0.7	1.4	0
Nystatin					
Nystatin oral suspension (Biocraft)	2.5	0	0.75	3.25	0.05
Nilstat® oral suspension	3	0	0	3	0
Oxybutynin					
Ditropan® syrup	4#	1.3	1.74	7.04	0
Paregoric					
Paregoric	0	0	0.25	0.25	2.25
PE/Triprolidine					
Children's Actifed® liquid	2.6	2.5	0	5.1	0
PE/PPA/chlorpheniramine/phenyltoloxamine					
Naldecon Ped® drops	0	1.14	0	1.14	0
Naldecon Ped® syrup	0	2	0	2	0
Naldecon syrup	0	2	0	2	0
Penicillin VK					
VeeTids®	3.5	0	0	3.5	0
Penicillin V Potassium (Biocraft)					
Penicillin VK 125® suspension	2.4	0	0	2.4	0
Phenobarbital (Lilly)					
Phenobarbital elixir	0.65	0	2.8	3.45	0.7125
Phenytoin					
Dilantin® suspension 125	1	0	0.385	1.385	0

CARBOHYDRATE AND ALCOHOL CONTENT OF LIQUID MEDICATIONS FOR USE IN PATIENTS RECEIVING KETOGENIC DIETS *(Continued)*

Generic Name	Carbohydrate g/5 mL				Ethyl Alcohol g/5 mL
	Sucrose	Sorbitol	Glycerin	Total	
Potassium chloride					
Rum-K®	0	0.54	1.72	2.26	0
Kay Ciel® liquid	0	0	0	0	0.14
Potassium chloride oral solution 10% (Roxane)	0	0	0.25	0.25	0.25
Potassium chloride oral solution 20%	0	0	0.25	0.25	0.25
Kaochlor S-F®	0	0	0	0	0.25
Kaon® elixir (potassium gluconate)	0	0	0	0	0.25
Kaon-Cl® 20%	0	0	0	0	0.25
Klor-Con® powder	0	0	0	0	0
Klor-Con/25® powder	0	0	0	0	0
Potassium citrate					
Polycitra-K®	0	0	0	0	0
Potassium citrate/sodium citrate					
Polycitra®	0	0	0	0	0
Potassium iodide					
SSKI®	0	0	0	0	0
Prednisolone					
Pediapred®	0	1.53	0	1.53	0
Prelone® syrup	1.84	0	0	1.84	0.18
Prednisone					
Prednisone Intensol®	0	0	0	1.5	1.5
Prednisone solution (Roxane)	1.8•	0	0	1.8	0.25
Primadone					
Mysoline® suspension	0	0	0	0	0
Prochlorperazine					
Compazine® syrup	3.15	0	0	3.15	0
Propranolol (Roxane)					
Propranolol oral solution (20 mg/5 mL)	0	3.2	0	3.2	0
Propranolol oral solution (40 mg/5 mL)	0	3.2	0	3.2	0
Ranitidine					
Zantac® syrup	0	0.5	0	0.5	0.375
Senokot					
Senokot® syrup	3.3	0	0	3.3	0.35
Simethicone					
Mylicon® drops	0	0	0	0	0
Phazyme® liquid	0	0	0	0	0
Sodium citrate/citric acid					
Bicitra®	0	0	0	0	0
Sodium polystyrene sulfonate (Roxane)					
Sodium polystyrene sulfonate suspension	0	1.2	0	1.2	0.1
Sucralfate					
Carafate® suspension	0	0.7	0.77	1.47	0
Sulfisoxazole					
Gantrisin® pediatric suspension	2.77	0	0	2.77	0.14
Tetracyline					
Sumycin®	2.2	1.5	0	3.7	0
Theophylline					
Theolair® liquid	2.5	0.48	0	2.98	0
Theoclear-80® syrup	0	4	3.5	7.5	0
Elixophylline® elixir	0	0	0.312	0.312	0.86
Elixophylline GG® elixir	0	2.3	1.625	3.925	0
Slo-Phyllin® 80 syrup	0	2.87	0	2.87	0
Slo-Phyllin GG® syrup	0.93	0.6	0.83	2.36	0
Aminophylline oral solution (105 mg/5 mL)	0	0.7	1	1.7	0
Theophylline oral solution (Roxane)	0	2.3	0.5	2.8	0.4

Generic Name	Carbohydrate g/5 mL				Ethyl Alcohol g/5 mL
	Sucrose	Sorbitol	Glycerin	Total	
Trimethoprim/Sulfamethoxazole					
Sulfamethoxazole/trimethoprim (Biocraft)	0	0.35	0.7	1.05	0
Septra® suspension	0	2.25	0	2.25	0
Bactrim® pediatric suspension	2.5	0.35	0.75	3.6	0
Valproic acid					
Depakene® syrup	3	0.75	0.75	4.5	0
Vancomycin					
Vancocin® oral solution	0	0	0	0	0
Vitamin A					
Aquasol A® drops	0	0	0	0	0
Vitamin D					
Drisdol®	0	0	0	0	0
Vitamin E					
Aquasol E® drops	0	1	0	1	0
Zidovudine					
Retrovir® syrup	3	0	0	3	0

Generic name abbreviations: DM: dextromethorphan; APAP: acetaminophen; PE: phenylephrine; Pyril: pyrilamine; PPA: phenylpropanolamine; EES: erythromycin ethylsuccinate

*Corn syrup

§Lactulose

•Fructose

¶Lactulose, galactose, lactose, and other sugars

#Glucose

Reference
Adapted from Feldstein TJ, "Carbohydrate and Alcohol Content of 200 Oral Liquid Medications for Use in Patients Receiving Ketogenic Diets," *Pediatrics*, 1996, 97:506-11.

TABLETS THAT CANNOT BE CRUSHED OR ALTERED

There are a variety of reasons for crushing tablets or capsule contents prior to administering to the patient. Patients may have nasogastric tubes which do not permit the administration of tablets or capsules; an oral solution for a particular medication may not be available from the manufacturer or readily prepared by pharmacy; patients may have difficulty swallowing capsules or tablets; or mixing of powdered medication with food or drink may make the drug more palatable.

Generally, medications which should not be crushed fall into one of the following categories.

- **Extended-Release Products**. The formulation of some tablets is specialized as to allow the medication within it to be slowly released into the body. This is sometimes accomplished by centering the drug within the core of the tablet, with a subsequent shedding of multiple layers around the core. Wax melts in the GI tract. Slow-K® is an example of this. Capsules may contain beads which have multiple layers which are slowly dissolved with time.

Common Abbreviations for Extended-Release Products

CR	Controlled release
CRT	Controlled-release tablet
LA	Long-acting
SR	Sustained release
TR	Timed release
TD	Time delay
SA	Sustained action
XL	Extended length
XR	Extended release

- **Medications Which Are Irritating to the Stomach**. Tablets which are irritating to the stomach may be enteric-coated which delays release of the drug until the time when it reaches the small intestine. Enteric-coated aspirin is an example of this.

- **Foul-Tasting Medication**. Some drugs are quite unpleasant to taste so the manufacturer coats the tablet in a sugar coating to increase its palatability. By crushing the tablet, this sugar coating is lost and the patient tastes the unpleasant tasting medication.

- **Sublingual Medication**. Medication intended for use under the tongue should not be crushed. While it appears to be obvious, it is not always easy to determine if a medication is to be used sublingually. Sublingual medications should indicate on the package that they are intended for sublingual use.

- **Effervescent Tablets**. These are tablets which, when dropped into a liquid, quickly dissolve to yield a solution. Many effervescent tablets, when crushed, lose their ability to quickly dissolve.

Recommendations

1. It is not advisable to crush certain medications.

2. Consult individual monographs prior to crushing capsule or tablet.

3. If crushing a tablet or capsule is contraindicated, consult with your pharmacist to determine whether an oral solution exists or can be compounded.

Drug Product	Dosage Forms	Reasons/Comments
Accutane®	Capsule	Mucous membrane irritant
Actifed 12® Hour	Capsule	Slow release†
Acutrim®	Tablet	Slow release
Adalat® CC	Tablet	Slow release
Aerolate® SR, JR, III	Capsule	Slow release*†
Afrinol® Repetabs®	Tablet	Slow release
Allerest® 12-Hour	Capsule	Slow release
Anaplex SR	Capsule	Slow release
Ansaid®	Tablet	Taste††
Artane® Sequels®	Capsule	Slow release*†
Arthritis Bayer® Time Release	Capsule	Slow release
Asacol®	Tablet	Slow release
A.S.A.® Enseals®	Tablet	Enteric-coated
Asbron G® Inlay	Tablet	Multiple compressed tablet†
Atrohist® LA	Tablet	Slow release
Atrohist® Plus	Tablet	Slow release
Atrohist® Sprinkle	Capsule	Slow release*
Azulfidine® EN-tabs®	Tablet	Enteric-coated
Baros	Tablet	Effervescent tablet¶
Bayer® Aspirin, low adult 81 mg strength	Tablet	Enteric-coated
Bayer® Aspirin, regular strength 325 mg caplet	Tablet	Enteric-coated
Bayer® Aspirin, regular strength EC caplet	Tablet	Enteric-coated
Betachron E-R®	Capsule	Slow release
Betapen®-VK	Tablet	Taste††
Biohist® LA	Tablet	Slow release♦
Bisacodyl	Tablet	Enteric-coated‡
Bisco-Lax®	Tablet	Enteric-coated‡
Bontril® Slow-Release	Capsule	Slow release
Breonesin®	Capsule	Liquid filled§
Brexin® L.A.	Capsule	Slow release†
Bromfed®	Capsule	Slow release†
Bromfed-PD®	Capsule	Slow release†
Calan® SR	Tablet	Slow release♦
Cama® Arthritis Pain Reliever	Tablet	Multiple compressed tablet
Carbiset-TR®	Tablet	Slow release
Cardizem®	Tablet	Slow release
Cardizem® CD	Capsule	Slow release*
Cardizem® SR	Capsule	Slow release*
Carter's Little Pills®	Tablet	Enteric-coated
Ceftin®	Tablet	Taste **Note:** Use suspension for children
Charcoal Plus®	Tablet	Enteric-coated
Chloral Hydrate	Capsule	**Note:** Product is in liquid form within a special capsule†
Chlorpheniramine Maleate Time Release	Capsule	Slow release
Chlor-Trimeton® Repetab®	Tablet	Slow release†
Choledyl® SA	Tablet	Slow release†
Cipro™	Tablet	Taste††
Claritin-D®	Tablet	Slow release
Cleocin®	Capsule	Taste††
Codimal-L.A.®	Capsule	Slow release
Codimal-L.A.® Half	Capsule	Slow release

TABLETS THAT CANNOT BE CRUSHED OR ALTERED
(Continued)

Drug Product	Dosage Forms	Reasons/Comments
Colace®	Capsule	Taste††
Comhist® LA	Capsule	Slow release*
Compazine® Spansule®	Capsule	Slow release†
Congess SR, JR	Capsule	Slow release
Contac®	Capsule	Slow release*
Cotazym-S®	Capsule	Enteric-coated*
Covera-HS™	Tablet	Slow release
Creon®	Capsule	Enteric-coated*
Creon® 10 Minimicrospheres™	Capsule	Enteric-coated*
Creon® 20	Capsule	Enteric-coated*
Cytospaz-M®	Capsule	Slow release
Cytoxan®	Tablet	**Note:** Drug may be crushed, but maker recommends using injection
Dallergy®	Capsule	Slow release†
Dallergy-D®	Capsule	Slow release
Dallergy-JR®	Capsule	Slow release
Deconamine® SR	Capsule	Slow release†
Deconsal® II	Tablet	Slow release
Deconsal® Sprinkle®	Capsule	Slow release*
Defen L.A.®	Tablet	Slow release
Demazin® Repetabs®	Tablet	Slow release†
Depakene®	Capsule	Slow-release-mucous membrane irritant††
Depakote®	Capsule	Enteric-coated
Desoxyn® Gradumets®	Tablet	Slow release
Desyrel®	Tablet	Taste††
Dexatrim® Max Strength	Tablet	Slow release
Dexedrine® Spansule®	Capsule	Slow release
Diamox® Sequels®	Capsule	Slow release
Dilatrate-SR®	Capsule	Slow release
Dimetane® Extentab®	Tablet	Slow release†
Disobrom®	Tablet	Slow release
Disophrol® Chronotab®	Tablet	Slow release
Dital®	Capsule	Slow release
Docusate	Capsule	Liquid filled§
Docusate with Casanthranol	Capsule	Liquid filled§
Donnatal® Extentab®	Tablet	Slow release†
Donnazyme®	Tablet	Enteric-coated
Doxidan® Liquigels	Capsule	Liquid filled§
Drisdol®	Capsule	Liquid filled§
Drixoral®	Tablet	Slow release†
Drixoral® Sinus	Tablet	Slow release
Dulcolax®	Tablet	Enteric-coated‡
Dynabac®	Tablet	Enteric-coated
Easprin®	Tablet	Enteric-coated
Ecotrin®	Tablet	Enteric-coated
E.E.S.® 400	Tablet	Enteric-coated†
Efidac/24®	Tablet	Slow release
Efidac® 24 Chlorpheniramine	Tablet	Slow release
Elixophyllin® SR	Capsule	Slow release*†
E-Mycin®	Tablet	Enteric-coated
Endafed®	Capsule	Slow release

Drug Product	Dosage Forms	Reasons/Comments
Entex® LA	Tablet	Slow release†
Entex® PSE	Tablet	Slow release†
Equanil®	Tablet	Taste††
Eryc®	Capsule	Enteric-coated*
Ergostat®	Tablet	Sublingual form•
Ery-Tab®	Tablet	Enteric-coated
Erythrocin Stearate	Tablet	Enteric-coated
Erythromycin Base	Tablet	Enteric-coated
Eskalith CR®	Tablet	Slow release
Exgest® LA	Tablet	Slow release
Fedahist® Timecaps®	Capsule	Slow release†
Feldene®	Capsule	Mucous membrane irritant
Feocyte	Tablet	Slow release
Feosol®	Tablet	Enteric-coated†
Feosol® Spansule®	Capsule	Slow release*†
Feratab®	Tablet	Enteric-coated†
Fergon®	Tablet	May cause excessive GI upset
Fero-Grad 500®	Tablet	Slow release
Fero-Gradumet®	Tablet	Slow release
Ferralet S.R.®	Tablet	Slow release
Ferrous Gluconate	Tablet	Film-coated
Feverall™ Sprinkle Caps	Capsule	Taste* **Note:** Capsule contents intended to be placed in a teaspoonful of water or soft food.
Fumatinic®	Capsule	Slow release
Gastrocrom®	Capsule	**Note:** Contents should be dissolved in water for administration.
Geocillin®	Tablet	Taste
Glucotrol® XL	Tablet	Slow release
Gris-PEG®	Tablet	**Note:** Crushing may result in precipitation of larger particles.
Guaifed®	Capsule	Slow release
Guaifed®-PD	Capsule	Slow release
Guaifenex® LA	Tablet	Slow release♦
Guaifenex® PSE	Tablet	Slow release♦
GuaiMAX-D®	Tablet	Slow release
Humibid® DM	Tablet	Slow release
Humibid® DM Sprinkle	Capsule	Slow release*
Humibid® LA	Tablet	Slow release
Humibid® Sprinkle	Capsule	Slow release*
Hydergine® LC	Capsule	**Note:** Product is in liquid form within a special capsule†
Hydergine® Sublingual	Tablet	Sublingual route†
Hytakerol®	Capsule	Liquid filled§†
Iberet®	Tablet	Slow release†
Iberet-500®	Tablet	Slow release†
ICAPS® Plus	Tablet	Slow release
ICAPS® Time Release	Tablet	Slow release
Ilotycin®	Tablet	Enteric-coated
Imdur™	Tablet	Slow release♦
Inderal® LA	Capsule	Slow release
Inderide® LA	Capsule	Slow release
Indocin® SR	Capsule	Slow release*†
Ionamin®	Capsule	Slow release
Isoptin® SR	Tablet	Slow release

TABLETS THAT CANNOT BE CRUSHED OR ALTERED
(Continued)

Drug Product	Dosage Forms	Reasons/Comments
Isordil® Sublingual	Tablet	Sublingual form•
Isordil® Tembid®	Tablet	Slow release
Isosorbide Dinitrate Sublingual	Tablet	Sublingual form•
Isosorbide Dinitrate SR	Tablet	Slow release
K+ 8®	Tablet	Slow release†
K+ 10®	Tablet	Slow release†
Kaon-Cl® 6.7	Tablet	Slow release†
Kaon-Cl® 10	Tablet	Slow release†
K+ Care® ET	Tablet	Effervescent tablet†¶
K-Dur®	Tablet	Slow release♦
K-Lease®	Capsule	Slow release*†
Klor-Con®	Tablet	Slow release†
Klor-Con/EF®	Tablet	Effervescent tablet†¶
Klorvess®	Tablet	Effervescent tablet†¶
Klotrix®	Tablet	Slow release†
K-Lyte®	Tablet	Effervescent tablet¶
K-Lyte®/Cl	Tablet	Effervescent tablet¶
K-Lyte DS®	Tablet	Effervescent tablet¶
K-Tab®	Tablet	Slow release†
Levsinex® Timecaps®	Capsule	Slow release
Lexxel®	Tablet	Slow release
Lodrane LD®	Capsule	Slow release*
Mag-Tab® SR	Tablet	Slow release
Meprospan®	Capsule	Slow release*
Mestinon® Timespan®	Tablet	Slow release†
Mi-Cebrin®	Tablet	Enteric-coated
Mi-Cebrin® T	Tablet	Enteric-coated
Micro-K®	Capsule	Slow release*†
Monafed®	Tablet	Slow release
Monafed® DM	Tablet	Slow release
Motrin®	Tablet	Taste†††
Motrin® IB	Tablet	Taste†††
Motrin® IB-Sinus	Tablet	Taste††
MS Contin®	Tablet	Slow release†
Muco-Fen-LA®	Tablet	Slow release
Naldecon®	Tablet	Slow release
Naprelan®	Tablet	Slow release
Nasatab LA®	Tablet	Slow release
Niaspan®	Tablet	Slow release
Nico-400®	Capsule	Slow release
Nicobid®	Capsule	Slow release
Nitro-Bid®	Capsule	Slow release*
Nitroglyn®	Capsule	Slow release*
Nitrong®	Tablet	Slow release
Nitrostat®	Tablet	Sublingual route•
Nitro-Time®	Capsule	Slow release
Noctec®	Capsule	**Note:** Product is in liquid form within a special capsule
Nolamine®	Tablet	Slow release
Nolex® LA	Tablet	Slow release
Norflex®	Tablet	Slow release
Norpace CR®	Capsule	Slow release form within a special capsule

Drug Product	Dosage Forms	Reasons/Comments
Novafed® A	Capsule	Slow release
Ondrox®	Tablet	Slow release
Optilets-500® Filmtab®	Tablet	Enteric-coated
Optilets-M-500® Filmtab®	Tablet	Enteric-coated
Oragrafin®	Capsule	**Note:** Product is in liquid form within a special capsule
Oramorph SR™	Tablet	Slow release†
Ornade® Spansule®	Capsule	Slow release
OxyContin®	Tablet	Slow release
Pabalate®	Tablet	Enteric-coated
Pabalate-SF®	Tablet	Enteric-coated
Pancrease®	Capsule	Enteric-coated*
Pancrease® MT	Capsule	Enteric-coated*
Panmycin®	Capsule	Taste
Papaverine Sustained Action	Capsule	Slow release
Pathilon® Sequels®	Capsule	Slow release*
Pavabid® Plateau®	Capsule	Slow release*
PBZ-SR®	Tablet	Slow release†
Pentasa®	Capsule	Slow release
Perdiem®	Granules	Wax coated
Peritrate® SA	Tablet	Slow release♦
Permitil® Chronotab®	Tablet	Slow release†
Phazyme®	Tablet	Slow release
Phazyme® 95	Tablet	Slow release
Phenergan®	Tablet	Taste†††
Phyllocontin®	Tablet	Slow release
Plendil®	Tablet	Slow release
Pneumomist®	Tablet	Slow release♦
Polaramine® Repetabs®	Tablet	Slow release†
Prelu-2®	Capsule	Slow release
Prevacid®	Capsule	Slow release
Prilosec™	Capsule	Slow release
Pro-Banthine®	Tablet	Taste
Procainamide HCl SR	Tablet	Slow release
Procan® SR	Tablet	Slow release
Procanbid®	Tablet	Slow release
Procardia®	Capsule	Delays absorption§#
Procardia XL®	Tablet	Slow release **Note:** AUC is unaffected.
Profen® II	Tablet	Slow release♦
Profen LA®	Tablet	Slow release♦
Pronestyl-SR®	Tablet	Slow release
Proscar®	Tablet	**Note:** Crushed tablets should not be handled by women who are pregnant or who may become pregnant
Proventil® Repetabs®	Tablet	Slow release†
Prozac®	Capsule	Slow release*
Quibron-T/ SR®	Tablet	Slow release†
Quinaglute® Dura-Tabs®	Tablet	Slow release
Quinidex® Extentabs®	Tablet	Slow release
Quin-Release®	Tablet	Slow release
Respa-1st®	Tablet	Slow release♦
Respa-DM®	Tablet	Slow release♦
Respa-GF®	Tablet	Slow release♦
Respahist®	Capsule	Slow release*
Respaire® SR	Capsule	Slow release

TABLETS THAT CANNOT BE CRUSHED OR ALTERED
(Continued)

Drug Product	Dosage Forms	Reasons/Comments
Respbid®	Tablet	Slow release
Ritalin-SR®	Tablet	Slow release
Robimycin®	Tablet	Enteric-coated
Rondec-TR®	Tablet	Slow release†
Roxanol SR™	Tablet	Slow release†
Ru-Tuss® DE	Tablet	Slow release
Sinemet CR®	Tablet	Slow release♦
Singlet for Adults®	Tablet	Slow release
Slo-bid™ Gyrocaps®	Capsule	Slow release*
Slo-Niacin®	Tablet	Slow release
Slo-Phyllin GG®	Capsule	Slow release†
Slo-Phyllin® Gyrocaps®	Capsule	Slow release*†
Slow FE®	Tablet	Slow release†
Slow FE® With Folic Acid	Tablet	Slow release
Slow-K®	Tablet	Slow release†
Slow-Mag®	Tablet	Slow release
Sorbitrate SA®	Tablet	Slow release
Sorbitrate® Sublingual	Tablet	Sublingual route
Sparine®	Tablet	Taste††
S-P-T	Capsule	**Note:** Liquid gelatin thyroid suspension.
Sudafed® 12-Hour	Caplet	Slow release†
Sudal® 60/500	Tablet	Slow release
Sudal® 120/600	Tablet	Slow release
Sudex®	Tablet	Slow release♦
Surfak® Liquigels	Capsule	Liquid filled§
Sustaire®	Tablet	Slow release†
Syn™-Rx	Tablet	Slow release
Syn™-Rx DM	Tablet	Slow release
Tavist-D®	Tablet	Multiple compressed tablet
Teczam®	Tablet	Slow release
Tedrol® SA	Tablet	Slow release
Tegretol XR®	Tablet	Slow release
Teldrin®	Capsule	Slow release*
Temaril® Spansule®	Capsule	Slow release†
Tepanil® Tentab®	Capsule	Slow release
Tessalon® Perles	Capsule	Slow release
Theo-24®	Tablet	Slow release†
Theoclear® L.A	Capsule	Slow release†
Theochron®	Tablet	Slow release
Theobid®	Capsule	Slow release*†
Theobid® Jr	Capsule	Slow release*†
Theo-Dur®	Tablet	Slow release†
Theo-Dur® Sprinkles	Capsule	Slow release*†
Theolair SR®	Tablet	Slow release†
Theo-Sav®	Tablet	Slow release♦
Theo-Time® SR	Tablet	Slow release
Theovent®	Capsule	Slow release†
Theo-X®	Tablet	Slow release
Thorazine® Spansule®	Capsule	Slow release
Toprol XL®	Tablet	Slow release♦
Touro A&H®	Capsule	Slow release
Touro DM®	Tablet	Slow release

Drug Product	Dosage Forms	Reasons/Comments
Touro EX®	Tablet	Slow release
Touro LA®	Tablet	Slow release
T-Phyl®	Tablet	Slow release
Trental®	Tablet	Slow release
Triaminic®	Tablet	Enteric-coated†
Triaminic®-12	Tablet	Slow release†
Triaminic® TR	Tablet	Multiple compressed tablet†
Trilafon® Repetabs®	Tablet	Slow release†
Tri-Phen-Chlor® Time Release	Tablet	Slow release
Tri-Phen-Mine® SR	Tablet	Slow release
Triptone® Caplets	Tablet	Slow release
Tuss-LA®	Tablet	Slow release
Tuss-Ornade® Spansule®	Capsule	Slow release
Tylenol® Extended Relief	Capsule	Slow release
ULR-LA®	Tablet	Slow release
Uni-Dur®	Tablet	Slow release
Uniphyl®	Tablet	Slow release
Valrelease®	Capsule	Slow release
Vanex® Forte	Caplet	Slow release
Vantin®	Tablet	Taste†††
Verelan®	Capsule	Slow release*
Volmax®	Tablet	Slow release†
Wellbutrin®	Tablet	Anesthetize mucous membrane
Wygesic®	Tablet	Taste
Zephrex LA®	Tablet	Slow release
ZORprin®	Tablet	Slow release
Zyban®	Tablet	Slow release
Zymase®	Capsule	Enteric-coated

*Capsule may be opened and the contents taken without crushing or chewing; soft food such as applesauce or pudding may facilitate administration; contents may generally be administered via nasogastric tube using an appropriate fluid, provided entire contents are washed down the tube.

†Liquid dosage forms of the product are available; however, dose, frequency of administration, and manufacturers may differ from that of the solid dosage form.

‡Antacids and/or milk may prematurely dissolve the coating of the tablet.

§Capsule may be opened and the liquid contents removed for administration.

††The taste of this product in a liquid form would likely be unacceptable to the patient; administration via nasogastric tube should be acceptable.

¶Effervescent tablets must be dissolved in the amount of diluent recommended by the manufacturer.

#If the liquid capsule is crushed or the contents expressed, the active ingredient will be, in part, absorbed sublingually.

•Tablets are made to disintegrate under the tongue.

♦Tablet is scored and may be broken in half without affecting release characteristics.

Adapted from Mitchell JF and Pawlicki KS, "Oral Solid Dosage Forms That Should Not Be Crushed: 1998 Update," *Hosp Pharm*, 1998, 33(4):399-415.

THERAPEUTIC CATEGORY & KEY WORD INDEX

PROGESTIN

PROSTAGLANDIN

PROTEASE INHIBITOR

PROTON PUMP INHIBITOR

RECOMBINANT HUMAN ERYTHROPOIETIN

RESPIRATORY STIMULANT

RETINOIC ACID DERIVATIVE

RICKETS, TREATMENT AGENT

SALICYLATE

SCABICIDAL AGENT

SEDATIVE

(Continued)

NOTES

NOTES

Other titles offered by

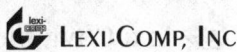 LEXI-COMP, INC

DRUG INFORMATION HANDBOOK (International edition available)
by Charles Lacy, RPh, PharmD, FCSHP; Lora L. Armstrong, RPh, PharmD, BCPS; Morton P. Goldman, PharmD, BCPS; and Leonard L. Lance, RPh, BSPharm

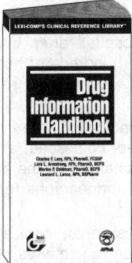

Specifically compiled and designed for the healthcare professional requiring quick access to concisely-stated comprehensive data concerning clinical use of medications.

The *Drug Information Handbook* is an ideal portable drug information resource, providing the reader with up to 29 key points of data concerning clinical use and dosing of the medication. Material provided in the Appendix section is recognized by many users to be, by itself, well worth the purchase of the handbook.

DRUG INFORMATION HANDBOOK P•O•C•K•E•T
by Charles Lacy, RPh, PharmD, FCSHP; Lora L. Armstrong, RPh, PharmD, BCPS; Morton P. Goldman, PharmD, BCPS; and Leonard L. Lance, RPh, BSPharm

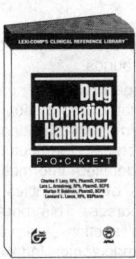

All medications found in the *Drug Information Handbook* are included in the abridged *Pocket* edition (select fields are extracted to maintain it's portability). It is specifically compiled and designed for the healthcare professional requiring quick access to concisely-stated comprehensive data concerning clinical use of medications.

The outstanding cross-referencing allows the user to quickly locate the brand name, generic name, synonym, and related information found in the Appendix making this a useful quick reference for medical professionals at any level of training or experience.

GERIATRIC DOSAGE HANDBOOK
by Todd P. Semla, PharmD, BCPS, FCCP; Judith L. Beizer, PharmD, FASCP; and Martin D. Higbee, PharmD, CGP

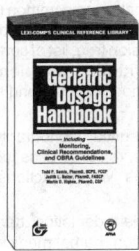

Many physiologic changes occur with aging, some of which affect the pharmacokinetics or pharmacodynamics of medications. Strong consideration should also be given to the effect of decreased renal or hepatic functions in the elderly, as well as the probability of the geriatric patient being on multiple drug regimens.

Healthcare professionals working with nursing homes and assisted living facilities will find the drug information contained in this handbook to be an invaluable source of helpful information.

An International Brand Name Index with names from 22 different countries is also included.

To order call toll free anywhere in the U.S.: 1-800-837-LEXI (5394)
Outside of the U.S. call: 330-650-6506 or online at www.lexi.com

Other titles offered by

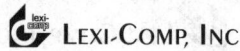
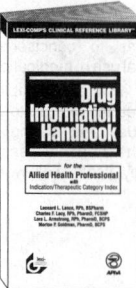
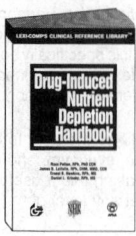
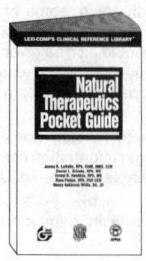

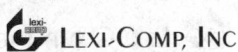
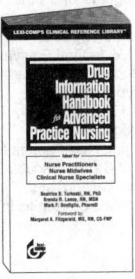
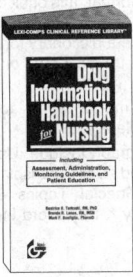
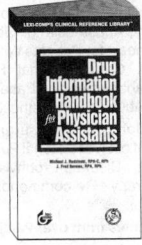

Other titles offered by

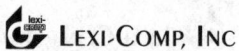
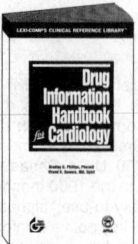
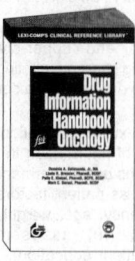
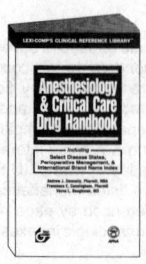

Other titles offered by

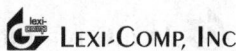

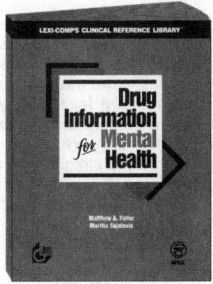
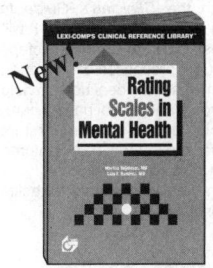
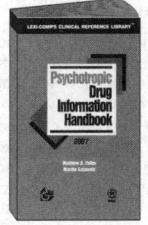

Other titles offered by

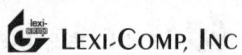

LEXI-COMP, INC

CLINICIAN'S GUIDE TO LABORATORY MEDICINE—A Practical Approach by Samir P. Desai, MD and Sana Isa-Pratt, MD

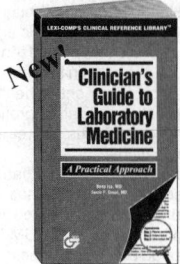

When faced with the patient presenting with abnormal laboratory tests, the clinician can now turn to the *Clinician's Guide to Laboratory Medicine: A Practical Approach*. This source is unique in its ability to lead the clinician from laboratory test abnormality to clinical diagnosis. Written for the busy clinician, this concise handbook will provide rapid answers to the questions that busy clinicians face in the care of their patients. No longer does the clinician have to struggle in an effort to find this information - *it's all here*.

CLINICIAN'S GUIDE TO DIAGNOSIS—A Practical Approach by Samir Desai, MD

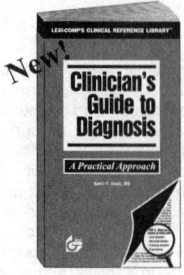

Symptoms are what prompt patients to seek medical care. In the evaluation of a patient's symptom, it is not unusual for healthcare professionals to ask "What do I do next?" This is precisely the question for which the *Clinician's Guide to Diagnosis: A Practical Approach* provides the answer. It will lead you from symptom to diagnosis through a series of steps designed to mimic the logical thought processes of seasoned clinicians. For the young clinician, this is an ideal book to help bridge the gap between the classroom and actual patient care. For the experienced clinician, this concise handbook offers rapid answers to the questions that are commonly encountered on a day-to-day basis. Let this guide become your companion, providing you with the tools necessary to tackle even the most challenging symptoms.

LABORATORY TEST HANDBOOK & CONCISE version by David S. Jacobs MD, FACP; Wayne R. DeMott, MD, FACP; and Dwight K. Oxley, MD, FACP

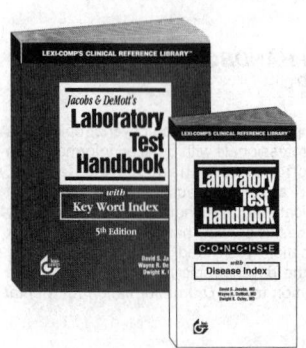

Contains over 900 clinical laboratory tests and is an excellent source of laboratory information for physicians of all specialties, nurses, laboratory professionals, students, medical personnel, or anyone who needs quick access to most routine and many of the more specialized testing procedures available in today's clinical laboratory.

Each monograph contains test name, synonyms, patient care, specimen requirements, reference ranges, and interpretive information with footnotes, references, and selected websites.

The *Laboratory Test Handbook Concise* is a portable, abridged (800 tests) version and is an ideal, quick reference for anyone requiring information concerning patient preparation, specimen collection and handling, and test result interpretation.

To order call toll free anywhere in the U.S.: 1-800-837-LEXI (5394)
Outside of the U.S. call: 330-650-6506 or online at www.lexi.com

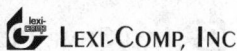
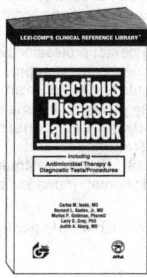
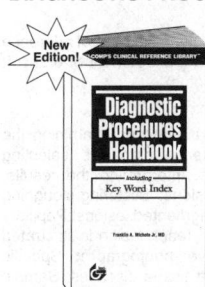
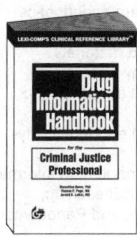

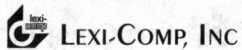
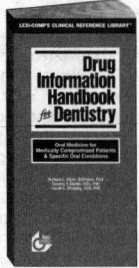
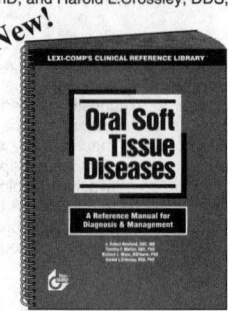
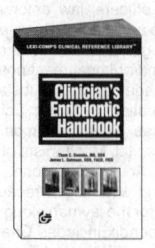

Other titles offered by
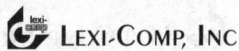
LEXI-COMP, INC

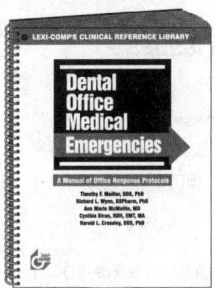
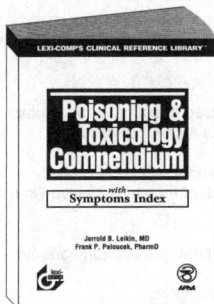
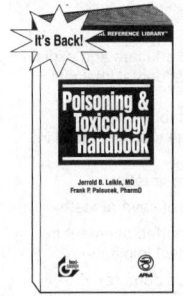

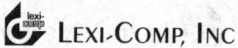
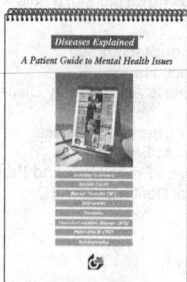
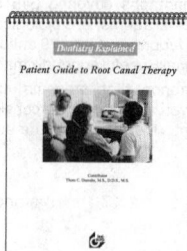
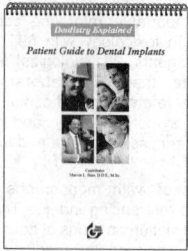

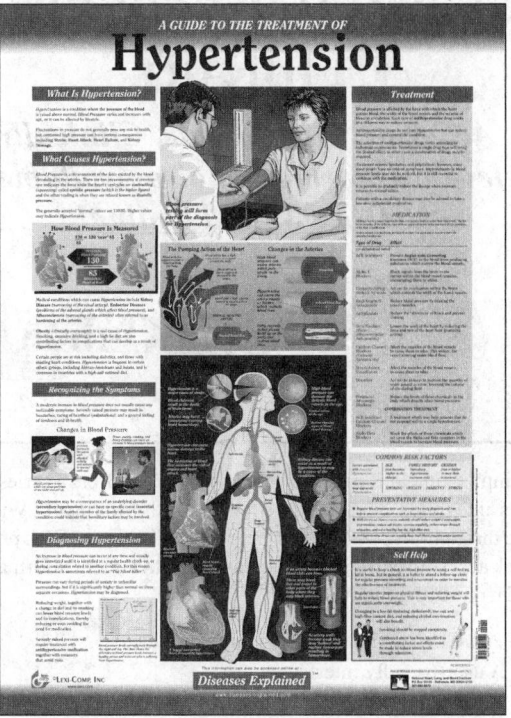

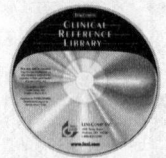 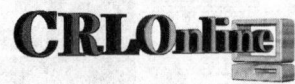